Willard and Spackman's
Occupational Therapy

FOURTEENTH EDITION

Willard and Spackman's
Occupational Therapy

FOURTEENTH EDITION

Glen Gillen, EdD, OTR/L, FAOTA

Professor
Programs in Occupational Therapy
Department of Rehabilitation and
    Regenerative Medicine
Vagelos College of Physicians and
    Surgeons
Columbia University
New York, New York

Catana Brown, PhD, OTR/L, FAOTA

Professor
Department of Occupational Therapy
Midwestern University—Glendale
Glendale, Arizona

Consulting Editor

Elelwani Ramugondo, BSc OT, MSc OT, PhD

Professor of Occupational Therapy
Department of Health and Rehabilitation Sciences
Deputy Vice Chancellor
Transformation, Student Affairs and Social Responsiveness
University of Cape Town
Cape Town, South Africa

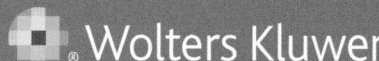 Wolters Kluwer

Philadelphia • Baltimore • New York • London
Buenos Aires • Hong Kong • Sydney • Tokyo

Acquisitions Editor: Lindsey Porambo
Development Editor: Amy Millholen
Project Manager: Laura S. Horowitz/York Content Development
Marketing Manager: Kirsten Watrud
Production Product Manager: Justin Wright
Design Coordinator: Stephen Druding
Manufacturing Coordinator: Margie Orzech
Prepress Vendor: S4Carlisle Publishing Services

Fourteenth Edition

9 8 7 6 5 4 3 2 1

Printed in Mexico

Library of Congress Cataloging-in-Publication Data

ISBN-13: 978-1-975174-88-0
ISBN-10: 1-975174-88-7

Library of Congress Control Number: 2023904004

shop.lww.com

When citing chapters from this book, please use the appropriate form. The APA format is as follows:

[Chapter author last name, I.] (2024). Chapter title. In G. Gillen & C. Brown (Eds.), *Willard and Spackman's occupational therapy* (14th ed., pp. x–x). Wolters Kluwer.

Johnson, K. R., & Anvarizadeh, A. (2024). What is occupation? In G. Gillen & C. Brown (Eds.), *Willard and Spackman's occupational therapy* (14th ed., pp. 2–10). Wolters Kluwer.

DEDICATION

Barbara A. Boyt Schell, PhD, OT/L, FAOTA
Professor Emerita
School of Occupational Therapy
Ivester College of Health Sciences
Brenau University
Gainesville, Georgia
Co-Owner
Schell Consulting
Athens, Georgia
Co-Editor, *Willard and Spackman's Occupational Therapy, 10th Edition, 11th Edition*
Lead Editor, *Willard and Spackman's Occupational Therapy, 12th Edition,*
    13th Edition

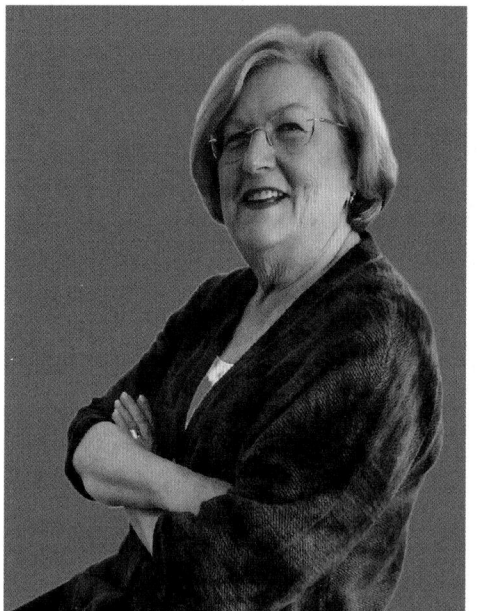

Dr. Barbara A. Boyt Schell—manager, academician, scholar, researcher, consultant, practitioner, thought leader, servant leader, and, of course, author. These are only a few of the professional roles that Dr. Schell has not only assumed but delivered above and beyond in her positions. One is hard pressed to find an occupational therapy (OT) practitioner who is not aware of Dr. Schell's influence on our profession. In fact, she has directly influenced literally thousands of individuals in their own work. By domino effect, Dr. Schell's influence has directly or indirectly impacted thousands of clients with outcomes skewing toward the positive.

Career highlights are too many to list. She is the founding director of Brenau University's School of Occupational Therapy. Her well-deserved current title is professor emerita at Brenau University. She was the lead editor of the last two editions of *Willard and Spackman's Occupational Therapy* and was coeditor of the preceding two editions. Most recently, she has completed updating several chapters for this edition. Dr. Schell and her husband are also in the process of writing and editing the next edition of *Clinical and Professional Reasoning in Occupational Therapy (3rd ed.)*. Beyond her textbooks, Dr. Schell has authored or coauthored multiple peer-reviewed papers, chapters, position papers, and official documents. Dr. Schell and her husband have owned Schell Consulting since 1990. In this capacity, they provide consultation to educational and healthcare organizations. Prior to her academic career, Dr. Schell spent the first 20 years of her career in clinical practice and management, first at the Tampa Veterans Administration Hospital, then the University of Missouri Hospital and Clinics, followed by Harmarville Rehabilitation Center. Throughout her career, she has held multiple leadership positions at both state and national levels. It was these experiences that fostered her lifelong commitment to helping others develop professionally and led to her research in professional reasoning.

On a personal note, she lives in Athens, GA, with her husband of 42 years, Dr. John Schell, a retired professor emeritus from the University of Georgia. Dr. Schell enjoys her many occupations beyond OT, including caring for their dog Brandy, painting watercolors (including several that have been publicly exhibited), being a grandmother, volunteering for her neighborhood association, singing in choirs, volunteering for leadership roles in her faith group, choral singing, and continuing periodic work with her state OT association. She swims, walks, or exercises each day in an effort to win the continuing battle with gravity. We are honored to have her husband John share the following:

> From a husband perspective, living with livewire and extravert Barbara is a treat … and challenge. In retirement, just some of her occupations include best wife ever, grandmother, artist, singer, exerciser, chef, and dog lover. And, oh, yeah, occupational therapist. Our marriage of 42-years is still fun and the product of a lifelong friendship.
>
> Then there are our immediate and extended families. Barbara's immediate family includes me and two grown stepchildren. In the extended family are 6 grandchildren, brothers, nieces and nephews. Barbara approaches grandparenthood as an active occupation. By the time you read this we will be welcoming our first great grandson.
>
> As husband and sometime colleague, I see Barbara's meaningful contributions as leader, administrator, mentor, cheerleader, and friend. Barbara has recruited and mentored many young therapists over the years first in clinical settings and later to join the Brenau faculty as novice OT faculty. Many young colleagues were encouraged to earn advanced degrees, were promoted within, have been honored for their teaching or have moved on to important positions elsewhere. Many are considered honorary "half-Schells". It is this sense of family and connection that best describes Barbara's lifetime of professional commitment, administrative skills, and personal leadership.

Glen Gillen and John W. Schell

We are pleased to dedicate this edition to Dr. Barbara A. Boyt Schell.

Glen Gillen
Lead Editor

Catana Brown
Coeditor

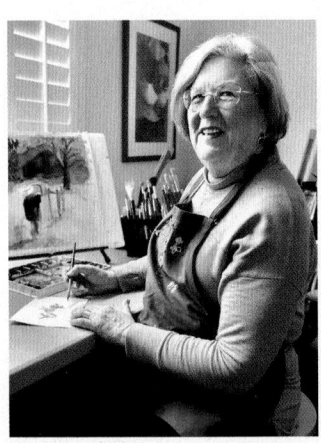 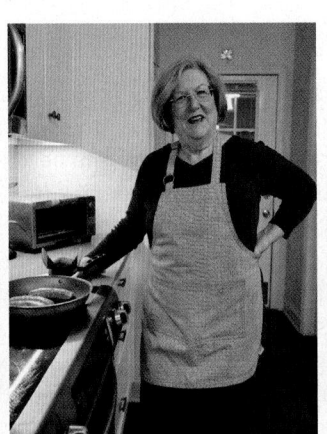 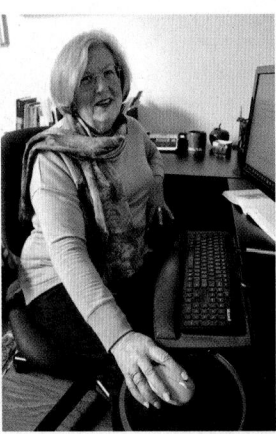 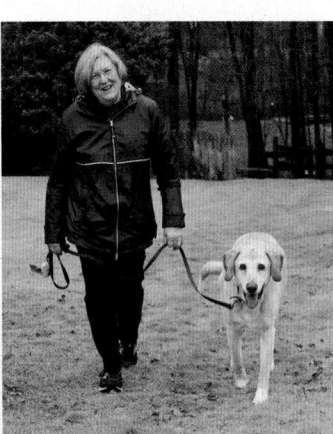

ON THE COVER

The cover shows a flat map of the world that has been altered to show a more accurate version of the relative size of each continent. We chose this image to enhance the theme of the 14th edition, which is to reflect the global and diverse practice of occupational therapy.

On the cover map shown here, we have added a push pin for each country represented by a contributor to the 14th edition. The countries include countries of origin and countries of current residence of those who contributed chapters, OT Stories, and "Expanding Our Perspectives" boxes.

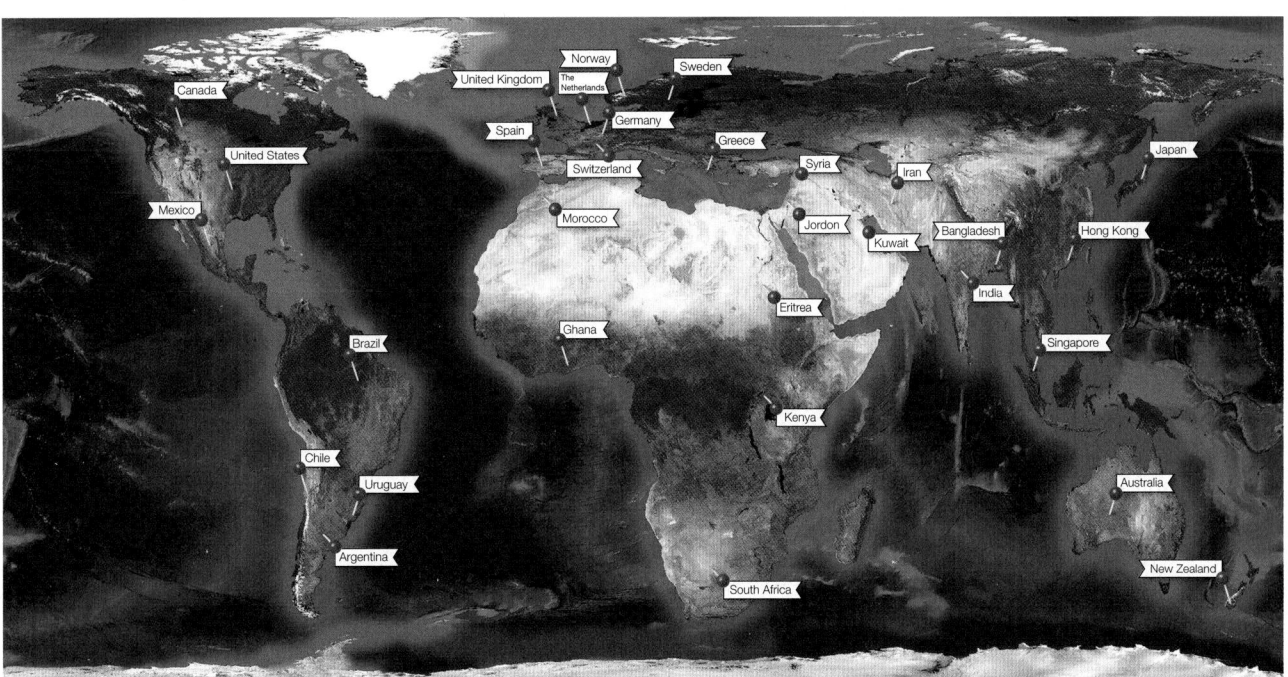

CONTRIBUTORS

The editors, in conjunction with our advisory group, specifically set out to recruit contributors from across the globe. Our team felt that it was time for the text to move beyond a U.S.-centric focus to a more realistic and inclusive focus of occupational therapy as a worldwide approach to enhancing occupational performance, participation, and quality of life.

Amanda Acord-Vira, EdD, OTR/L, CBIS (Chapter 62)
Associate Professor
Division of Occupational Therapy
West Virginia University School of Medicine
Morgantown, West Virginia

Diane E. Adamo, PhD, OTR (Chapter 15)
Associate Professor and Director of Research for the Health Sciences
Health Care Sciences
Wayne State University
Detroit, Michigan

Rawan AlHeresh, PhD, OTR/L (Chapter 66)
Associate Professor of Occupational Therapy
Occupational Therapy Department
MGH Institute of Health Professions
Boston, Massachusetts

Arameh Anvarizadeh, OTD, OTR/L, FAOTA (Chapter 1)
Director of Admissions
Associate Professor of Clinical Occupational Therapy
Chan Division of Occupational Science and Occupational Therapy
University of Southern California
Los Angeles, California

Md. Ariful Islam Arman, BSc, DU (Chapter 66)
Inclusion Officer
Centre for Disability in Development
Dhaka, Bangladesh

Nancy Bagatell, PhD (Chapter 7)
Associate Professor and Division Director
Division of Occupational Science and Occupational Therapy
University of North Carolina at Chapel Hill
Chapel Hill, North Carolina

Antoine Bailliard, PhD, OTR/L (Chapter 10)
Associate Professor
Division of Occupational Science and Occupational Therapy
University of North Carolina at Chapel Hill
Chapel Hill, North Carolina

Nancy A. Baker, ScD, MPH, OTR/L, FAOTA (Chapter 26)
Associate Professor and Chair
Department of Occupational Therapy
Tufts University
Medford, Massachusetts

Marci L. Baptista, OTD, OTR/L, CHT, CEAS (Chapter 64)
Assistant Professor
Occupational Therapy Department
Samuel Merritt University
Oakland, California

Skye Barbic, PhD, MSc, BScOT (Chapter 39)
Assistant Professor
Occupational Science and Occupational Therapy
The University of British Columbia
Vancouver, British Columbia, Canada

Kate Barrett, OTD, MPH, OTR/L (Chapter 13)
Program Director and Associate Professor
Occupational Therapy Department
DePaul University
Chicago, Illinois

Angela M. Benfield, PhD, OTR/L (Chapter 25)
Assistant Professor
Department of Occupational Therapy
UT Health San Antonio
San Antonio, Texas

Sue Berger, PhD, OTR/L, FAOTA (Chapter 23)
Clinical Associate Professor Emeritus
Department of Occupational Therapy
Boston University
Boston, Massachusetts

Christy Billock, PhD, OTR/L, DipACLM
(Chapter 59)
Former Professor and Founding OTD Program Director
Keck Graduate Institute
Claremont, California

Mary Black, MS, OTR/L (Chapter 66)
Occupational Therapist
Heartland Alliance Marjorie Kovler Center
Chicago, Illinois

Theo Bogeas, MSc (Chapter 66)
Occupational Therapist and Project Manager
HumanRights360
Athens, Greece

Angela K. Boisselle, PhD, OTR (Chapter 36)
Utilization Management Therapy Manager
Cook Children's Healthcare System
Fort Worth, Texas

Bette R. Bonder, PhD, OTR (Chapter 65)
Professor Emerita
Cleveland State University
Cleveland, Ohio

Cheryl Lynne Trautman Boop, MS, OTR/L,
BCP (Appendices I and II)
Clinical Lead of Homecare Clinical Therapies
Nationwide Children's Hospital
Columbus, Ohio

Helen Bourke-Taylor, PhD, MS, BAppSc OT
(Chapter 12)
Associate Professor
Department of Occupational Therapy
Monash University
Frankston, Victoria, Australia

Brent Braveman, PhD, OTR/L, FAOTA
(Chapter 73)
Director
Department of Rehabilitation Services
MD Anderson Cancer Center
Houston, Texas

Catana Brown, PhD, OTR/L, FAOTA
(Chapters 6, 34, 35, and 72)
Professor
Department of Occupational Therapy
Midwestern University—Glendale
Glendale, Arizona

Anita C. Bundy, ScD, OT/L, FAOTA, FOTARA
(Chapter 47)
Professor and Department Head
Occupational Therapy Department
Colorado State University
Fort Collins, Colorado

Susan M. Cahill, PhD, OTR/L, FAOTA
(Chapter 45)
Director of Evidence-based Practice
American Occupational Therapy Association
North Bethesda, Maryland

Jana Cason, DHSc, OTR/L, FAOTA
(Chapter 67)
Professor
Auerbach School of Occupational Therapy
Spalding University
Louisville, Kentucky

Dahlia Cavazos Castillo OTD, OTR
Assistant Professor
The University of Texas Rio Grande Valley
Edinberg, Texas

Karen Ching, BSc (Occupational Therapy),
PG Dip in Health Management, PG Dip in
Systems Thinking in Practice (Chapter 68)
Director of Strategy, Policy, and Planning
Western Cape Department of Health
Cape Town, South Africa

Denise Chisholm, PhD, OTR/L, FAOTA
(Chapter 18)
Professor and Vice Chair
Occupational Therapy Department
University of Pittsburgh
Pittsburgh, Pennsylvania

Charles H. Christiansen, EDD, OTR, FAOTA
(Chapter 2)
Professor Emeritus
Department of Occupational Therapy
School of Health Professions
University of Texas Medical Branch at Galveston
Galveston, Texas

Sherrilene Classen, PhD, MPH, OTR/L
(Chapter 20)
Professor and Chair
Occupational Therapy Department
University of Florida
Gainesville, Florida

Ellen R. Cohn, PhD, CCC-SLP, ASHA Fellow (Chapter 67)
Adjunct Professor
Department of Communication and Rhetoric
University of Pittsburgh
University of Maryland Global Campus
Pittsburgh, Pennsylvania

Ellen S. Cohn, ScD, OTR, FAOTA (Chapter 33)
Clinical Professor, Emeritus
Department of Occupational Therapy
Boston University
Boston, Massachusetts

Erin Connor, MA, OTR/L (Chapter 69)
Professor and Academic Fieldwork Coordinator
Quinsigamond Community College
Worcester, Massachusetts

Susan Coppola, OTD, OT/L, FAOTA (Chapters 4 and 5)
Clinical Professor
Division of Occupational Science and Occupational Therapy
University of North Carolina at Chapel Hill
Chapel Hill, North Carolina

Wendy J. Coster, PhD, OTR/L, FAOTA (Chapter 33)
Professor Emeritus
Department of Occupational Therapy
Boston University
Boston, Massachusetts

Diana Davis, PhD, OTR/L (Chapter 62)
Associate Professor
Division of Occupational Therapy
West Virginia University School of Medicine
Morgantown, West Virginia

Evan E. Dean, PhD, OTR, FAAIDD (Chapter 56)
Associate Director
Kansas University Center on Developmental Disabilities
University of Kansas
Lawrence, Kansas

Janet V. DeLany, DEd, OTR/L, FAOTA (Chapter 40)
Emerita Faculty and Graduate Dean, Retired
Department of Occupational Therapy & Occupational Science
Towson University
Towson, Maryland

Carmen Gloria de las Heras de Pablo, MS, OTR (Chapter 28)
International OT Professor and Consultant
Educational Authority of Model of Human Occupation in Latin America and Spain
Director of the Ibero-American Model of Human Occupation Community
Viña del Mar, Valparaíso, Chile

Regina F. Doherty, OTD, OTR/L, FAOTA, FNAP (Chapter 27)
Professor and Chair
Occupational Therapy Department
School of Health and Rehabilitation Sciences
MGH Institute of Health Professions
Boston, Massachusetts

Julie Dorsey, OTD, OTR/L, CEAS, FAOTA (Chapter 46)
Professor and Chair
Occupational Therapy Department
Ithaca College
Ithaca, New York

Winnie Dunn, PhD, OTR/L, FAOTA (Chapter 56)
Distinguished Professor
Occupational Therapy
School of Health Professions
University of Missouri
Columbia, Missouri

Sanetta Henrietta Johanna du Toit, MOT, MSc, PhD, Senior Fellow (HEA) (Chapter 47)
Master's Program Director
Faculty of Medicine and Health
Student Life Academic Director
Senior Research Fellow at the University of the Free State, South Africa
Occupational Therapy Department
The University of Sydney
Sydney, New South Wales, Australia

Emily Zeman Eddy, OTR/L, OTD, MS, OTR (Chapter 70)
Assistant Professor and Associate Director of Clinical Education
Occupational Therapy Department
MGH Institute of Health Professions
Boston, Massachusetts

Holly Ehrenfried, OTD, OTR/L, CHT (Chapter 46)
Occupational Therapist, Certified Hand Specialist, and Clinical Specialist
Lehigh Valley Health Network
Allentown, Pennsylvania

Mary E. Evenson, OTD, MPH, OTR/L, FAOTA (Chapters 60 and 70)
Professor and Director of Clinical Education
Occupational Therapy Department
MGH Institute of Health Professions
Boston, Massachusetts

Cynthia Lee Evetts, PhD, OTR (Chapter 17)
Professor and Director
School of Occupational Therapy
Texas Woman's University
Denton, Texas

Janet Falk-Kessler, EdD, OTR/L, FAOTA (Chapter 30)
Professor Emerita
Department of Rehabilitation and Regenerative Medicine / Occupational Therapy
Columbia University, College of Physicians and Surgeons
New York, New York

Maryam Farzad, PhD (Chapter 64)
Postdoctorate Associate
Hand and Upper Limb Centre
The University of Western Ontario
Landon, Ontario, Canada

Denise E. Finch, OTD, OTR/L, CHT (Chapter 46)
Assistant Professor
Occupational Therapy Department
Massachusetts College of Pharmacy and Health Sciences
Manchester, New Hampshire

Anne G. Fisher, ScD, OT, FAOTA (Chapter 52)
Professor Emeritus
Division of Occupational Therapy
Department of Community Medicine and Rehabilitation
Umeå University
Umeå, Sweden
University Distinguished Professor Emeritus
Department of Occupational Therapy
College of Health and Human Sciences
Colorado State University
Fort Collins, Colorado

Jami E. Flick, PhD, OTR/L (Chapter 57)
Assistant Professor and Academic Fieldwork Coordinator
Department of Occupational Therapy
College of Health Professions
University of Tennessee Health Science Center
Memphis, Tennessee

Kirsty Forsyth, PhD, OTR, FCOT (Chapter 34)
Department of Occupational Therapy
School of Health Sciences
Queen Margaret University
Scotland, United Kingdom

Roshan Galvaan, PhD (Occupational Therapy) (Chapters 15 and 66)
Professor
Division of Occupational Therapy
Department of Health and Rehabilitation Sciences
University of Cape Town
Cape Town, South Africa

Pablo A. Cantero Garlito, PhD, OTD (Chapter 14)
Professor
Department of Nursing, Physical Therapy and Occupational Therapy
Universidad de Castilla—La Mancha
Talavera de la Reina, Spain

Patricia A. Gentile, DPS, OTR/L (Chapter 74)
Clinical Assistant Professor and Professional Program Director
Department of Occupational Therapy
New York University Steinhardt School of Culture, Education, and Human Development
New York, New York

Glen Gillen, EdD, OTR/L, FAOTA (Chapters 4, 21, 42, 43, 53, 54, and 72)
Professor
Programs in Occupational Therapy
Department of Rehabilitation and Regenerative Medicine
Vagelos College of Physicians and Surgeons
Columbia University
New York, New York

Krista Glowacki, PhD, MSc (OT), BHKin (Chapter 39)
Postdoctoral Research Fellow
Occupational Science and Occupational Therapy
The University of British Columbia
Vancouver, British Columbia, Canada

Yael Goverover, PhD, OTR/L (Chapter 55)
Professor
Department of Occupational Therapy
New York University
New York, New York

Lenin C. Grajo, PhD, OTR/L (Chapter 36)
Director, Division of Professional Education
Associate Director, Program in Occupational Therapy
Associate Professor, Occupational Therapy and Psychiatry
Washington University School of Medicine in St. Louis
St. Louis, Missouri

Lou Ann Griswold, PhD, OTR/L, FAOTA
(Chapters 52 and 58)
Associate Professor and Department Chair
Department of Occupational Therapy
University of New Hampshire
Durham, New Hampshire

Mohammad Monjurul Habib, MPA (Chapter 66)
Project Delegate
International Federation of Red Cross and Red Crescent Societies (IFRC)
Damascus, Syria

Kristine L. Haertl, PhD, OTR/L, FAOTA
(Chapter 2)
Professor
Department of Occupational Therapy
St. Catherine University
St. Paul, Minnesota

Aster (né Elizabeth) Harrison, PhD, OTR/L
(Chapter 16)
Assistant Professor
Department of Occupational Therapy
Thomas Jefferson University
Philadelphia, Pennsylvania

Christine A. Helfrich, PhD, OTR/L, FAOTA
(Chapter 41)
Professor
Division of Occupational Therapy
American International College
Springfield, Massachusetts

Clare Hocking, PhD NZROT (Chapters 8 and 9)
Professor
Department of Occupational Science and Therapy
Auckland University of Technology
Auckland, Aotearoa New Zealand

Suzanne E. Holm, OTD, OTR/L, BCPR
(Chapter 32)
Associate Professor and OT Academic Program Coordinator
School of Physical Therapy
Regis University
Denver, Colorado

Barbara Hooper, PhD, OTR/L, FAOTA
(Chapter 3)
Division Chief and Program Director
Division of Occupational Therapy
Duke University
Durham, North Carolina

Spencer Hunley (Chapter 56)
LEND Trainee
Center for Child Health and Development
University of Kansas Medical Center
Kansas City, Kansas, United States

Moses N. Ikiugu, PhD, OTR/L, FAOTA
(Chapter 29)
Professor and Director of Research
Department of Occupational Therapy
University of South Dakota
Vermillion, South Dakota

Michael K. Iwama, PhD, BSc (OT)
(Chapter 37)
Professor
Occupational Therapy Doctorate Division
School of Medicine
Duke University
Durham, North Carolina

Lisa A. Jaegers, PhD, OTR/L, FAOTA
(Chapter 46)
Associate Professor
Occupational Science and Occupational Therapy
Doisy College of Health Sciences
College for Public Health and Social Justice, School of Social Work
Director, Transformative Justice Initiative
Associate Director, Health Criminology Research Consortium
Saint Louis University
St. Louis, Missouri
Owner
Work Interventions LLC
St. Louis, Missouri

Khalilah Robinson Johnson, PhD, OTR/L
(Chapter 1)
Assistant Professor
Division of Occupational Science and Occupational
Therapy
Department of Allied Health Sciences
University of North Carolina at Chapel Hill
Chapel Hill, North Carolina

Margaret Jones, PhD, NZROT (Chapter 9)
Senior Lecturer
Department of Occupational Science and Therapy
Auckland University of Technology
Auckland, New Zealand

Mary Alunkal Khetani, ScD, OTR/L
(Chapter 49)
Associate Professor
Department of Occupational Therapy
University of Illinois at Chicago
Chicago, Illinois

Laurie L. Knis-Matthews, PhD, OTR/L, FAOTA
(Chapter 50)
Professor
Occupational Therapy Department
Kean University
Hillside, New Jersey

Paula Kramer, PhD, OTR, FAOTA
(Chapter 75)
Professor Emerita
Department of Occupational Therapy
St. Joseph's University
Philadelphia, Pennsylvania

Angela M. Lampe, OTD, OTR/L (Chapter 76)
Associate Professor
Department of Occupational Therapy
Creighton University
Omaha, Nebraska

Leanne Leclair, PhD, MSc, BHSc (OT)
(Chapter 24)
Department Head and Associate Professor
Occupational Therapy Department
University of Manitoba
Winnipeg, Manitoba, Canada

Ritchard Ledgerd, MSc, BSc (OT), FWFOT
(Chapter 5)
Executive Director
World Federation of Occupational Therapists
Geneva, Switzerland

Lauren M. Little, PhD, OTR/L (Chapter 56)
Associate Professor
Occupational Therapy Department
Rush University
Chicago, Illinois

Helene Lohman, OTD, OTR/L, FAOTA
(Chapter 76)
Professor
Department of Occupational Therapy
Creighton University
Omaha, Nebraska

Catherine L. Lysack, PhD, OT (C) (Chapter 15)
Professor
Health Care Sciences
Wayne State University
Detroit, Michigan

Amanda Mack, OTD, MS, OTR/L (Chapter 70)
Instructor
Occupational Therapy Department
MGH Institute of Health Professions
Boston, Massachusetts

Inti Marazita, MS, OTR/L (Chapter 19)
Assistant Professor
University of St. Augustine for Health Sciences
St. Augustine, Florida

Elizabeth E. Marfeo, PhD, MPH, OTR/L
(Chapter 26)
Associate Professor
Departments of Occupational Therapy and Community Health
Tufts University
Medford, Massachusetts

John Lien Margetis, OTD, OTR/L (Chapter 32)
Associate Professor of Clinical Occupational Therapy
Chan Division of Occupational Science and Occupational
Therapy
University of Southern California
Los Angeles, California

Asako Matsubara, PhD, OT (Chapter 37)
Chief Occupational Therapist
Rehabilitation Department
Hiroshima City Rehabilitation Hospital
Hiroshima, Japan

Kathleen Matuska, PhD, OTR/L, FAOTA
(Chapter 13)
Professor and Chair of Occupational Therapy Programs
St. Catherine University
St. Paul, Minnesota

Daniel Emeric Meaulle, EdM (Rehabilitation)
(Chapter 14)
Occupational Therapist and Manager
Uzipen
Madrid, Spain

Mansha Mirza, PhD, OTR/L, MSHSOR
(Chapter 66)
Associate Professor
Department of Occupational Therapy
University of Illinois, Chicago
Chicago, Illinois

Jaime Phillip Muñoz, PhD, OTR/L, FAOTA
(Chapter 28)
Associate Professor
Pittsburgh, Pennsylvania

Bernard Austin Kigunda Muriithi, PhD, OTR/L
(Chapter 22)
Assistant Professor
Department of Occupational Therapy
University of Arkansas
Fayetteville, Arkansas

Dawn M. Nilsen, EdD, OTR/L, FAOTA
(Chapter 54)
Associate Professor and Associate Director
Programs in Occupational Therapy
Rehabilitation and Regenerative Medicine
Columbia University
New York, New York

Angela Patterson, OTD, OTR/L
(Chapter 76)
Assistant Professor
Department of Occupational Therapy
Creighton University
Omaha, Nebraska

Thais K. Petrocelli, OTD, MHA, OTR/L
(Chapter 19)
Assistant Professor and Doctoral Coordinator
Occupational Therapy Department
University of St. Augustine for Health Sciences
St. Augustine, Florida

Noralyn Davel Pickens, PhD, OTR/L, FAOTA
(Chapter 17)
Professor and Senior Associate Director
School of Occupational Therapy
Texas Woman's University
Denton, Texas

Doris Pierce, PhD, OT (Chapter 43)
Retired from Eastern Kentucky University
Richmond, Kentucky

Jennifer S. Pitonyak, PhD, OTR/L, SCFES
(Chapter 44)
Associate Professor and Associate Director
School of Occupational Therapy
University of Puget Sound
Tacoma, Washington

Elizabeth A. Pyatak, PhD, OTR/L, FAOTA
(Chapter 51)
Associate Professor
Chan Division of Occupational Science and Occupational
Therapy
University of Southern California
Los Angeles, California

Elelwani Ramugondo, PhD, MScOT, BScOT
(Chapter 11)
Professor of Occupational Therapy
Department of Health and Rehabilitation Sciences
Deputy Vice Chancellor
Transformation, Student Affairs and Social
Responsiveness
University of Cape Town
Cape Town, South Africa

Mehdi Rassafiani, PhD (Chapter 12)
Associate Professor
Occupational Therapy Department
Kuwait University
Kuwait City, Kuwait

S. Maggie Reitz, PhD, OTRL, FAOTA (Chapter 40)
Vice Provost
Office of the Provost
Towson University
Towson, Maryland

Panagiotis (Panos) A. Rekoutis, PhD, OTR/L
(Chapter 61)
Adjunct Faculty
Department of Occupational Therapy
New York University
Co-owner, ReDiscover Kids, OT PLLC
New York, New York

Jacquie Ripat, PhD, MSc, BMR (OT) (Chapter 24)
Associate Professor
Occupational Therapy Department
University of Manitoba
Winnipeg, Manitoba, Canada

Pamela S. Roberts, PhD, OTR/L, SCFES, FAOTA, CPHQ, FNAP, FACRM (Chapter 60)
Executive Director and Professor
Co-Director, Division of Informatics
Physical Medicine and Rehabilitation
Division of Informatics, Department of Biomedical Sciences
Office of the Chief Medical Officer
Cedars-Sinai
Los Angeles, California

Karen M. Sames, OTD, OTR/L, FAOTA (Chapter 31)
Professor
Occupational Therapy Department
St. Catherine University
St. Paul, Minnesota

Marjorie E. Scaffa, PhD, OTR/L, FAOTA (Chapter 57)
Professor Emeritus
Department of Occupational Therapy
University of South Alabama
Mobile, Alabama

Barbara A. Boyt Schell, PhD, OT/L, FAOTA (Chapters 4, 18, 25, 42, 43, and 53)
Professor Emerita
School of Occupational Therapy
Ivester College of Health Sciences
Brenau University
Gainesville, Georgia
Co-Owner
Schell Consulting
Athens, Georgia

Winifred Schultz-Krohn, PhD, OTR/L, BCP, SWC, FAOTA (Chapter 71)
Professor Emeritus
Occupational Therapy Department
San Jose State University
San Jose, California

Mary P. Shotwell, PhD, OT/L, FAOTA (Chapter 19)
Professor
Center for the Health Sciences
Rocky Mountain University of Health Professions
Provo, Utah

So Sin Sim, BSc OT (Hons), MSocSc (Professional Counselling), Grad Dip Child Psychotherapy, PhD OT (Chapter 12)
Lecturer
Department of Occupational Therapy
Monash University
Melbourne, Victoria, Australia

C. Douglas Simmons, PhD, OTR/L, FAOTA (Chapter 58)
Professor and Program Director
School of Occupational Therapy
Massachusetts College of Pharmacy and Health Sciences
Manchester, New Hampshire

Yda J. Smith, PhD, OTR/L (Chapter 66)
Associate Professor and Lecturer
Department of Occupational and Recreational Therapies
University of Utah
Salt Lake City, Utah

Helene Smith-Gabai, PhD, OTR/L, BCPR (Chapter 32)
Associate Professor
Department of Occupational Therapy
Brenau University
Gainesville, Georgia

Jo M. Solet, MS, PhD, OTR/L (Chapter 48)
Assistant Professor of Medicine
Division of Sleep Medicine
Harvard Medical School
Cambridge Health Alliance
Department of Medicine
Cambridge, Massachusetts

Daniel Sutton, PhD, PGDip (Mental Health), BHSc (OT) (Chapter 8)
Senior Lecturer
Occupational Science and Therapy
Auckland University of Technology
Auckland, New Zealand

Margaret Swarbrick, PhD, FAOTA (Chapters 50 and 63)
Professor and Associate Director
Center of Alcohol & Substance Use Studies
Rutgers Graduate School of Applied and Professional Psychology
Piscataway, New Jersey
Wellness Institute Director
Collaborative Support Programs of New Jersey
Freehold, New Jersey

Kimberly J. The, MS, PhD Candidate
(Chapter 16)
Department of Disability and Human Development
University of Illinois at Chicago
Chicago, Illinois

Linda Tickle-Degnen, PhD, OTR/L, FAOTA
(Chapter 26)
Professor Emerita
Department of Occupational Therapy
Tufts University
Medford, Massachusetts

Joan Pascale Toglia, PhD, OTR/L, FAOTA
(Chapter 55)
Adjunct Clinical Professor of Cognitive Science
Department of Rehabilitation Medicine
Cornell Weill Medical College
New York, New York
Professor Emerita
Mercy College
Dobbs Ferry, New York

Sivuyisiwe Khokela Toto, BSc (Occupational
Therapy) (Chapter 68)
Lecturer
School of Public Health and Family Medicine
University of Cape Town
Cape Town, South Africa

Concettina Trimboli, PhD Candidate,
MSc (Advanced Occupational Therapy),
BSc (Occupational Therapy) (Chapter 66)
Occupational Therapist
School of Allied Health
Curtin University
Perth, Western Australia, Australia

Tamara Turner, EdD, OTR/L (Chapter 72)
Associate Professor
Occupational Therapy Program
College of Health Sciences
Midwestern University—Glendale
Glendale, Arizona

Craig A. Velozo, PhD, FAOTA, OTR/L
(Chapter 20)
Professor
Division of Occupational Therapy
Department of Rehabilitation Sciences
Medical University of South Carolina
Charleston, South Carolina

Anna Wallisch, PhD, OTR/L (Chapter 56)
Postdoctoral Researcher
Juniper Gardens Children's Project
University of Kansas
Kansas City, Kansas

Steven D. Wheeler, PhD, OTR/L, FAOTA,
CBIS (Chapter 62)
Professor and Chairperson
Division of Occupational Therapy
West Virginia University School of Medicine
Morgantown, West Virginia

Kirsten L. Wilbur, EdD, OTR/L (Chapter 44)
Clinical Associate Professor
School of Occupational Therapy
University of Puget Sound
Tacoma, Washington

Jennifer L. Womack, PhD, OTR/L, FAOTA
(Chapter 7)
Professor
Division of Occupational Science and Occupational
Therapy
University of North Carolina at Chapel Hill
Chapel Hill, North Carolina

Wendy Wood, PhD, OTR/L, FAOTA
(Chapter 3)
Professor
Animal Sciences and Occupational Therapy
Colorado State University
Fort Collins, Colorado

Farzaneh Yazdani, PhD, MA, MSc
(Occupational Therapy), BSc (Occupational
Therapy) (Chapter 38)
Senior Lecturer
Sports, Life Sciences, and Social Care
Oxford Brookes University
Oxford, Oxfordshire, United Kingdom

Leanne Yinusa-Nyahkoon, ScD, OTR/L
(Chapters 23 and 49)
Clinical Assistant Professor
Department of Occupational Therapy
Boston University
Boston, Massachusetts

ADVISORY GROUP

The initial planning for the 14th edition of *Willard and Spackman* coincided with the murder of George Floyd and the ensuing Black Lives Matter protests. These events ignited a global movement of stopping hate focused on specific groups of individuals, diversity, equity, and inclusion. Glen Gillen and Catana Brown were challenged by members of the Justice-Based Occupational Therapy group to consider how we might respond in a tangible way to injustice and racism as it exists in our profession and in this text. Our response included the following:

- Dr. Elelwani Ramagundo was hired to serve as consulting editor and to oversee the advisory group process.
- An advisory group was formed made up of occupational therapist practitioners representing a variety of countries, ethnicities, sexual and gender identities, religions, and abilities.
- Each advisory group member was assigned a few chapters to review for (a) sensitivity to issues of diversity, justice, and inclusivity; (b) applicability to a broad audience; (c) addressing the pursuit of fair treatment, access, opportunity, and advancement for all while striving to identify and eliminate barriers that prevent full participation.
- A new feature was created for each chapter entitled "Expanding Our Perspectives." This feature was written most often by an advisory group member or someone selected by an advisory group member. The purpose of the "Expanding Our Perspectives" box is to present a different point of view on the content with an emphasis on presenting people and communities who are often missed or not seen in occupational therapy texts.

We recognize that this is an imperfect and partial response, but we do hope that these efforts have resulted in a more inclusive text that challenges the reader to pause and reconsider widely held assumptions and, most importantly, contemplate how they might work toward a more equitable and inclusive profession. We thank the following members of the advisory group for their contribution to the 14th edition:

Tara C. Alexander, OTR/L, CPC (Chapter 30)
Program Manager and Supervisor
Physical Medicine and Rehabilitation Service
VA North Texas Health Care System
Dallas, Texas

Arameh Anvarizadeh, OTD, OTR/L, FAOTA
(Chapters 15, 70, and 73)
Director of Admissions
Associate Professor of Clinical Occupational Therapy
Chan Division of Occupational Science and Occupational Therapy
University of Southern California
Los Angeles, California

Pamela Block, PhD (Chapters 24 and 50)
Professor
Anthropology Department
Western University
London, Ontario, Canada

Brent Braveman, PhD, OTR/L, FAOTA
(Chapter 34)
Director
Department of Rehabilitation Services
MD Anderson Cancer Center
Houston, Texas

Kaitlin Bristol, MSOT, OTR/L (Chapter 62)
Occupational Therapist
New York, New York

Dahlia Cavazos Castillo OTD, OTR
(Chapters 12, 13, 14, 18, 25, 28, and 31)
Assistant Professor
The University of Texas Rio Grande Valley
Edinberg, Texas

Chantal Juanita Christopher, BOT, Diploma in HIV Clinical Management, MPhil in Group Therapy (Chapter 37)
Lecturer
Discipline of Occupational Therapy
University of KwaZulu-Natal
Durban, KwaZulu Natal, South Africa

Erin Connor, MA, OTR/L (Chapters 22, 39, and 56)
Professor and Academic Fieldwork Coordinator
Quinsigamond Community College
Worcester, Massachusetts

Claudette Fette, PhD, OTR (Chapter 68)
Clinical Professor
School of Occupational Therapy
Texas Woman's University
Denton, Texas

Ellie Fossey, PhD, MSc, DipCOT (UK) (Chapter 35)
Professor and Head of Department
Department of Occupational Therapy
Monash University
Melbourne, Victoria, Australia

Karen Whalley Hammell, PhD, MSc, OT(C), Dip COT (UK) (Chapter 21)
Honorary Professor
Department of Occupational Science and Occupational Therapy
University of British Columbia
Vancouver, British Columbia, Canada

Aster Harrison, PhD, OTD, OTR/L (Chapters 17, 27, and 63)
Assistant Professor
Occupational Therapy Department
Thomas Jefferson University
Philadelphia, Pennsylvania

Sarah Selvaggi Hernandez, MOT, OTR/L (Chapter 61)
Autistic Advocate and Occupational Therapist
Advisory Board of NeuroClastic, Inc.
Enfield, Connecticut

Maggie Heyman Hotch, MOT, OTR/L (Chapter 55)
Owner and Lead Therapist
Four Ravens Occupational Therapy LLC
Haines, Alaska

Clover Hutchinson, OTD, MA, OTR/L (Chapters 23, 44, 46, 48, and 60)
Assistant Professor
Occupational Therapy Department
School of Health Sciences and Professional Programs
York College, City University of New York
Jamaica, New York

Moses N. Ikiugu, PhD, OTR/L, FAOTA (Chapters 8 and 36)
Professor and Director of Research
Department of Occupational Therapy
University of South Dakota
Vermillion, South Dakota

Frank Kronenberg, PhD, BSc OT, BA Ed (Chapters 3, 9, and 33)
International Lecturer and Consultant
Universities in North and South America, Europe, and Africa
Chair of Board of Directors, Grandmothers Against Poverty and AIDS (GAPA) NGO
Cape Town, South Africa

Lilian Magalhaes, PhD (Chapters 4, 6, and 66)
Adjunct Professor
Occupational Therapy
The Federal University of São Carlos (UFSCar)
São Carlos, Brazil
Professor Emeritus
Western University, Canada
London, Ontario, Canada

Lisa Mahaffey, PhD, OTR/L (Chapters 29, 32, and 57)
Professor
Occupational Therapy Department
Midwestern University
Downers Grove, Illinois

Asako Matsubara, PhD (Chapters 5, 42, 52, 53, and 54)
Chief Occupational Therapist
Rehabilitation Department
Hiroshima City Rehabilitation Hospital
Hiroshima, Japan

Jaime Phillip Muñoz, PhD, OTR/L, FAOTA (Chapter 58)
Associate Professor
Pittsburgh, Pennsylvania

Mohammed Sh. Nadar, PhD, OTR
(Chapters 1, 2, 43, 47, and 64)
Associate Professor
Faculty of Allied Health Sciences
Occupational Therapy Department
Kuwait University
Kuwait City, Kuwait

Said Nafai, OTD (Chapter 76)
Associate Professor
Occupational Therapy Department
American International College
Springfield, Massachusetts

Ingeborg Nilsson, PhD (Chapter 65)
Professor
Community Medicine and Rehabilitation
Umeå University
Umeå, Sweden

Raymond Nubla, MS, OTR/L (Chapter 14)
Occupational Therapist
Occupational Therapy Training Program
SSG, Inc.
San Francisco, California

Mariel Pellegrini, Mg, Lic. TO
(Chapters 41, 49, 59, and 67)
Director and Professor
Department of Occupational Therapy
Pontificia Universidad Católica Argentina
Professor
Department of Occupational Therapy
Universidad Nacional de Quilmes
Buenos Aires, Argentina

Elelwani Ramugondo, PhD, MScOT, BScOT
(Chapters 20 and 51)
Professor of Occupational Therapy
Department of Health and Rehabilitation Sciences
Deputy Vice Chancellor
Transformation, Student Affairs and Social Responsiveness
University of Cape Town
Cape Town, South Africa

Mehdi Rassafiani, PhD (Chapter 26)
Associate Professor
Occupational Therapy Department
Kuwait University
Kuwait City, Kuwait

Teresa Ricado, MOT, OTR/L (Chapter 14)
Clinical Supervisor and School Based Program Manager
Occupational Therapy Training Program
SSG, Inc.
San Francisco, California

Sabrina Salvant, EdD, MPH, OTR/L
(Chapters 38, 40, 52, 71, and 72)
Vice President
Education and Professional Development
Knowledge Division
American Occupational Therapy Association (AOTA)
North Bethesda, Maryland

Chi-Kwan Shea, PhD, OTR/L (Chapters 7, 11, and 19)
Professor
Department of Occupational Therapy
Samuel Merritt University
Oakland, California

So Sin Sim, PhD, Grad Dip (Psychotherapy), MSocSC (Professional Counselling0, BScOT (Hons) (Chapters 74 and 75)
Lecturer
Department of Occupational Therapy
Monash University
Melbourne, Victoria, Australia

Cristina Reyes Smith, OTD, OTR/L
(Chapter 45)
Associate Professor and Director of Admissions
Division of Occupational Therapy
Department of Rehabilitation Sciences
College of Health Professions
Medical University of South Carolina
Charleston, South Carolina

Selena Washington, PhD, MSPH, OTR
(Chapters 10 and 16)
Assistant Professor
Department of Occupational Science and Occupational Therapy
Saint Louis University
St. Louis, Missouri

This 14th edition of *Willard and Spackman's Occupational Therapy* maintains the rich history of the text as a comprehensive resource for the profession; however, the vision for this edition is to better reflect the global and diverse practice of occupational therapy (OT). Our goal is to help our students focus on the pursuit of fair treatment, access, opportunity, and advancement for all while striving to identify and eliminate barriers that prevent full participation. For example, we want our readers to learn to create environments in which any individual or group feels welcomed, respected, and valued enough to participate fully. Where appropriate, we want to provide students with examples of OT assessments and interventions that ignite the agency of the people we serve to fulfill their potential. While the editors focused on expanding this edition to represent a more global perspective, the American Occupational Therapy Association (AOTA)'s Practice Framework is used as anchor language in many instances as the text is still published in the United States. Therefore, the text still leans toward a U.S. perspective.

As always, chapters in this text summarize important and complex material in a way that is accessible and that challenges budding practitioners to think deeply about the many facets of occupation that emerge in the daily rounds of life. Furthermore, the process of OT is described across a wide array of practice arenas. This 14th edition continues these traditions, as Glen Gillen assumes the role of lead editor, with Catana Brown as a coeditor. Joining Gillen and Brown for the first time is Elelwani Ramugondo, who served as consulting editor and the coordinator of the advisory group described earlier. Dr. Ramugondo focused on our efforts to increase the diversity and inclusivity of the text by helping to identify contributors, reviewing chapters, writing the "Expanding Our Perspectives" features, and answering specific, pointed questions as they arose.

This revision of *Willard and Spackman's Occupational Therapy* builds on the successful revisions done in the last edition. Although users generally expressed strong satisfaction with the text, some organizational changes were implemented. This information, in addition to the perspectives of the editors and consulting editors, informed the reorganization of this edition as well as the addition of new chapters and materials. An overall summary of these changes is provided next, followed by an overview of each unit, highlighting the materials included in each.

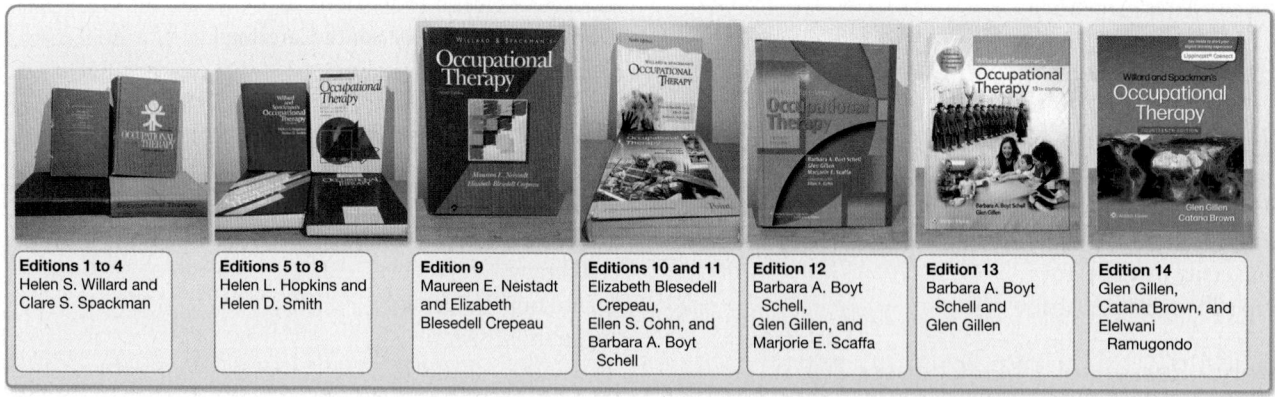

Willard and Spackman's Occupational Therapy, editions 1 to 14, with editors noted.

Editions 1 to 4	Editions 5 to 8	Edition 9	Editions 10 and 11	Edition 12	Edition 13	Edition 14
Helen S. Willard and Clare S. Spackman	Helen L. Hopkins and Helen D. Smith	Maureen E. Neistadt and Elizabeth Blesedell Crepeau	Elizabeth Blesedell Crepeau, Ellen S. Cohn, and Barbara A. Boyt Schell	Barbara A. Boyt Schell, Glen Gillen, and Marjorie E. Scaffa	Barbara A. Boyt Schell and Glen Gillen	Glen Gillen, Catana Brown, and Elelwani Ramugondo

Overall Changes in the Text and Web-Based Materials

Willard and Spackman's Occupational Therapy, 14th edition, retains materials focused on the centrality of occupation as the basis for practice, both as a means and an end of therapy. In this edition, we continue to acknowledge that evaluation and intervention processes are integrated with the theoretical perspectives of practitioners and the influences of the broader social and political environment on the day-to-day lives of practitioners and the clients they serve. This edition is much more reflective of the worldwide scholarship within OT, including the Global South, as indicated by the addition of numerous contributors, our consulting editor, advisory group members, and "Expanding Our Perspectives" authors coming from outside the United States. We have provided a more diverse range of examples across cultures, sexual and gender identities, life course, disability, and occupational performance concerns.

As in previous editions, we maintain that effective OT requires a collaborative process between or among OT practitioners and the clients they serve. For therapy to be optimally effective, a blending of current best evidence with therapist experience and client preferences must guide the process. Because this process is often complex, contributors were asked to provide many illustrations of the professional reasoning and underlying assumptions that guide practice. Furthermore, contributors were asked to acknowledge the challenges in implementing best practice and suggest approaches for overcoming these challenges.

As authors and editors, we acknowledge the power of language. Throughout this book, we have attempted to use language that is inclusive. That extends to appreciating the many different ways that humans are configured and the ways in which they engage in occupations. We have maintained the contributor's choice of language (e.g., client vs. patient vs. service-user) and have used the pronouns that were submitted within each chapter. For consistency, we have changed spelling and punctuation to American English. This text uses person-first language with the exception of communities that have vocalized other preferences. Unfortunately, we recognize that to maintain a reasonable textbook size, we cannot provide all perspectives on every topic. However, we have provided many more examples of OT as it is practiced throughout the world, while acknowledging when content is particularly reflective of U.S. perspectives.

In addition to the overall guiding principles just described, there were some noticeable changes in the book that include the following:

- The expansion of Web-based materials. Video resources inaugurated in the last edition were expanded to include children as well as adults and a greater variety of conditions/performance difficulties. These video cases of clients can be used in conjunction with the text to provide students with opportunities to observe and analyze applications of concepts and techniques. The appendices related to the OT assessments and interventions described in the text are available on Lippincott Connect. Finally, first-person narratives deleted from this edition will continue to be available to both students and faculty on Lippincott Connect. Web-based materials for instructors and students also include PowerPoint presentations, test questions, provocative questions, learning activities, etc.

- Overall the text is divided into fewer sections with some of the smaller units integrated into other units. The section on narrative perspectives was moved to the online platform as we have incorporated narrative within all of the chapters with our new feature, "Expanding Our Perspectives." Several units were reorganized and chapters were added. These changes are described in the Unit-by-Unit Summary section.

Unit-by-Unit Summary

The units in this edition were retained as the current general organization seemed to work well for users. We did add new chapters and, in some cases, renamed chapters to clarify the contents. In the description that follows, new chapters added to the text will be highlighted. Except where noted, all chapters returning from the 13th edition were either updated or completely rewritten; all chapters were reviewed by a member of the advisory group.

Unit openers contain a list of media (art, music, movies, videos, etc.) relevant to the content of the unit that can be used by faculty and students for inspiration or elucidation. These media can be assigned to enhance learning before, during, or after class time. They may be used to stimulate small group discussions, identify representation issues, apply to case studies, etc.

- **Unit I, Occupational Therapy: Profile of the Profession,** profiles the profession by opening with a chapter on occupation followed by the broad written history of the profession, which places OT history in the context of larger world events. This chapter now includes information on OT history from seven countries outside the United States. The remaining four chapters profile the philosophy, contemporary practice, organizations, and scholarship within the profession. By placing this material together in the opening unit, students are provided with important foundational material for the rest of the text.

- **Unit II, Occupational Nature of Humans,** describes the occupational nature of humans. The opening chapter explores how participation in occupation changes over the course of life. This is followed by a chapter on the relationships between occupation and health. The chapter on occupational science provides insight into the ongoing research about occupation, with updated examples of how such research informs OT practice. The Occupational Justice chapter was moved from the theories section to more accurately represent justice as an underlying principle of all OT practice. A new chapter on occupational consciousness was added to this section to reflect the impact of dominant practices and power on the things that people do every day.

- **Unit III, Occupations in Context,** contains a number of chapters designed to make a clearer connection with the broad array of contextual factors discussed in the *Occupational Therapy Practice Framework: Domain and Process*, 4th edition, and the World Health Organization's (WHO) International Classification of Functioning, Disability and Health (ICF). The chapters remain the same as the 13th edition, addressing family, patterns of occupation, culture, socioeconomic factors, disability, and physical and virtual spaces. However, in keeping with the vision of the 14th edition, these chapters have been heavily updated with several new authors to address contemporary perspectives on contextual factors such as family, culture, and disability rights.

- **Unit IV, Occupational Therapy Process,** contains chapters that explain the OT process. All the chapters from the previous edition return and are updated. The introductory chapter to this unit provides an overview of the OT process and outcomes of care. Then follows a chapter on determining client needs, which provides detailed examples of client evaluation in a variety of situations. Next, a chapter on critiquing assessments provides information on how to appraise traditional measurement procedures as well as current psychometric approaches in OT assessments. The process of intervention for individuals and for organizations, communities, and populations is fully explored in the next two chapters. The unit ends with a chapter about modifying performance contexts.

- **Unit V, Core Concepts and Skills,** addresses core concepts and skills such as professional reasoning; evidence-based practice; ethical practice; therapeutic relationships and client collaboration; group process and group intervention; professionalism, communication, and teamwork; and documentation in practice. A new chapter on safety, infection control, and personal protective equipment was added, as this content became particularly relevant during the COVID-19 pandemic.

- **Unit VI, Broad Conceptual Models for Occupational Therapy Practice,** discusses broad theories used by occupational therapists across practice areas. This unit starts with a chapter examining how theory guides practice. Following this are chapters focused on theories

for which there is a body of evidence to support their validity and utility, starting with the Model of Human Occupation. Next is a discussion of Ecological Models in Occupational Therapy, followed by a chapter on the Theory of Occupational Adaptation. Two new theories were added to this unit that offer new perspectives including a chapter on the Kawa River Model and a chapter on the Model of Occupational Wholeness. Included in this section are chapters of broad theories that inform practice but that are not specific to OT theories. These include the Recovery Model, Health Promotion Theories, and Principles of Learning and Behavior Change.

- **Unit VII, Evaluation, Intervention, and Outcomes for Occupations,** starts with an introductory chapter that provides an overview of evaluation, intervention, and outcomes for the major areas of occupation. Analyzing Occupations and Activity was moved from one of the small units that was deleted to this section where it fits well as an introductory chapter to the unit. This is followed by returning chapters on different areas of occupation, consisting of a chapter on basic and instrumental activities of daily living (BADLs and IADLs) followed by chapters on education, work, play and leisure, rest and sleep, and social participation. Two new chapters were added to the unit, one on Health Management and the other on Routines and Habits.

- **Unit VIII, Evaluation, Intervention, and Outcomes for Performance Skills and Client Factors,** addresses performance skills and client factors. The unit starts with an overview chapter on evaluating performance skills followed by another introductory chapter on body structures and functions. All specific topics from the last edition are retained, including motor control, cognition and perception, sensory processing in everyday life, emotional regulation, and a chapter on social interaction. A new chapter was added to this section on personal values, beliefs, and spirituality.

- **Unit IX, The Practice Context: Therapists in Action,** displays therapist decision-making as it is implemented in different therapy settings across various continuums of care. The first chapter explains the wide variety of practice settings in which occupational therapists practice. Subsequent chapters each provide a therapist explaining OT practice in a particular setting often including the thinking behind the evaluation and intervention strategies implemented for a particular client. Separate chapters address services for autistic individuals, older adults, and patients with traumatic brain injury, serious mental illness, and hand injuries. New chapters address the role of OT in forced migration, telehealth, the WHO model of primary care, and OT for persons who have experienced childhood trauma. The intent of this unit is to "bring alive" the various theories and intervention approaches by displaying real-world situations.

- **Unit X, Occupational Therapy Education,** contains updated chapters on fieldwork, practice education, professional entry, and competence and professional development. A new chapter discusses preparation for work in an academic setting.
- **Unit XI, Occupational Therapy Management,** addresses OT management, supervision, consultation, and payment for services.

End Matter

- The glossary contains definitions of key words from chapters and important terminology from other sources such as the WHO's ICF and the AOTA's *Occupational Therapy Practice Framework: Domain and Process*, 4th edition.
- There are three appendices related to the text, all of which can be found on Lippincott Connect. Appendix I is a table of interventions used in OT. Appendix II is an updated table of assessments used in OT. The third is a collection of narrative perspectives from previous editions of the book. Following an introductory chapter on the importance of narratives, these first-person narratives of people with various occupational challenges include first-person accounts by:
  - Laura and Craig Horowitz as they raised their son Will, a bright young man who is on the autism spectrum. Will describes his childhood and life from toddler days through high school, with an addendum about his recent years in community college.
  - Paul Cabell, a veteran who is an actor and comedian challenged by mental illness, substance abuse, and homelessness.
  - Gloria Dickerson and her successful narrative of her recovery process from the challenges of mental illness, which followed her abusive childhood. An addendum describes her recent activities in publishing.
  - Jean Westmacott, a sculptor and art director who brought her mother, Hildegard Viden Wilkins, home to live with Jean and her husband, in order to care for Hildegard in the final years of her life until her death at over 100 years old.
  - Beth Long, a Methodist minister who experienced a stroke while traveling to Ladakh, a northern province of India, who describes her personal and spiritual journey as she recovers, only to find that she has been "retired" from her ministerial position.

- A collection of narratives of people living with disability in Ecuador.
- Mary Feldhaus-Weber's experience of a head injury and an excerpt from *The Book of Sorrow, Book of Dreams: A First Person Narrative.*
- Alex McIntosh and his parents' Laurie S. and Lou McIntosh views on growing up with cerebral palsy.
- Donald Murray's poignant description of caring for his wife during her days with dementia.

Special Features

Special features are found both in the text and in the Web materials associated with this text. Special features include the following:

- **Expanding Our Perspectives**: This new feature is written by someone other than the author of the chapter to present a different point of view on the content. It is meant to increase the diversity of voices of occupational therapists and to provide students with thought-provoking examples of how to rethink practice.
- **OT Story**: The OT Stories present examples of OT evaluation and intervention modeling expert practice or in a few cases present the story of an occupational therapist. Each OT Story ends with questions to promote reflection and discussion.
- **Commentary on the Evidence**: This section succinctly discusses available evidence to support practice, including identification of where evidence is lacking or inconclusive and where further research is required.

With this edition, we are pleased to continue to offer specially selected video clips (described later) from International Clinical Educators, Inc. These may be found on Lippincott Connect. Also on Lippincott Connect are PowerPoint slides for each chapter, quiz and test banks, and additional learning materials.

Final Notes

Once again, we are grateful for the guidance provided by many experienced colleagues as we have created this 14th edition.

Glen Gillen
Catana Brown

ACKNOWLEDGMENTS

This edition of *Willard and Spackman's Occupational Therapy* was accomplished through the collective efforts of the contributors, editors, reviewers, photographers, students, colleagues, friends, and family. We are grateful for their many contributions to this effort and know that their commitment, scholarship, and generosity in sharing these traits have improved the quality of the work presented here.

Glen thanks the patients he has interacted with throughout his career. These interactions were oftentimes challenging, provocative, fun, thought-provoking, but always meaningful. I am a better person because of my career. Therefore, I also thank the profession of occupational therapy!

Tana thanks her mentors. I have been very fortunate to be taught, pushed, and inspired by these important people in my professional life: starting with Gail Fidler for encouraging me as a mental health practitioner, Carole Hays for recognizing skills I didn't see in myself, Winnie Dunn for furthering my research career, and Rue Cromwell who said at my dissertation defense, "you should write textbooks!"

Elelwani thanks various communities-in-struggle and her students from whom she continues to learn, her mentors, as well as Frank Kronenberg, a life partner whom she met through occupational therapy and with whom she shares a deep passion for the idea of occupational therapy. Lindsey Nichols saw me through occupational therapy undergraduate education alive and brought me back to my alma mater. Ruth Watson taught me the power of courage laced with grace. Seyi Ladele Amosun helped me own and assert my voice as a scholar. Diane Parham got me hooked on play scholarship and helped me see the political even in this otherwise mundane occupation. Thanks to each one of you for your commitment to each one of us.

Finally, each one of us is very proud of our universities and occupational therapy programs, which sustain us in our work and encourage us to greater accomplishments. Our students, faculty, and practitioners in our professional communities provide a background of inspiration for taking on a task such as this. We thank all those who helped us with their insights.

Professional Colleagues and Students

We thank our colleagues for their assistance, support, and insightful feedback.

Advisory Group

Special thanks go to the advisory group that helped us in so many ways. Beyond writing the amazing "Expanding Our Perspectives" boxes, they were all quick to respond to queries, help with other chapters as needed, and even help us to acquire permissions for photographs that we needed from countries where we didn't speak the language, but they did!

Wolters Kluwer/ Lippincott Williams & Wilkins

We are grateful to Matt Hauber for once again helping us to make this book a reality. Jennifer Clements, as always, did a wonderful job on the art program. And Stephen Druding's interior and cover designs incorporating the dynamic new map are perfect.

York Content Development

Our thanks to Wolters Kluwer for allowing us once again to have the special attention of this group. This is the fourth time that Laura and her staff have served to support us in this text, and their contributions are invaluable. Laura S. Horowitz provided overall guidance of the development of the manuscript through the production of the book. Her steady guidance, expertise, patience, emotional support, and good humor provided significant support to our efforts.

BRIEF CONTENTS

CONTENTS

Appendixes (available on Lippincott Connect)

APPENDIX I
Table of Interventions: Listed Alphabetically by Title

Cheryl Lynne Trautman Boop

APPENDIX II
Table of Assessments: Listed Alphabetically by Title

Cheryl Lynne Trautman Boop

APPENDIX III
First-Person Narratives

- A: Narrative as a Key to Understanding, *Ellen S. Cohn and Elizabeth Blesedell Crepeau*
- B: Who's Driving the Bus? *Laura S. Horowitz, Will S. Horowitz, and Craig W. Horowitz*
- C: Homelessness and Resilience: Paul Cabell's Story, *Paul Carrington Cabell III, Sharon A. Gutman, and Emily Raphael-Greenfield*
- D: While Focusing on Recovery, I Forgot to Get a Life, *Gloria F. Dickerson (updated for the 14th edition)*
- E: Mom's Come to Stay, *Jean Wilkins Westmacott*
- F: Journey to Ladakh, *Beth Long*
- G: Experiences With Disability: *Stories From Ecuador, Kate Barret*
- H: An Excerpt From *The Book of Sorrows, Book of Dreams, Mary Feldhaus-Weber and Sally A. Schreiber-Cohn*
- I: He's Not Broken—He's Alex, *Alexander McIntosh, Laurie McIntosh, and Lou McIntosh*
- J: The Privilege of Giving Care, *Donald M. Murray*

Expanding Our Perspectives

This feature is an important part of our effort to increase the diversity of occupational therapy (OT) voices in the text. The writers of this feature represent a variety of cultures, geographic locations, sexual and gender identities, life course, disability, and occupational performance interests. This feature presents a different point of view on the content of each chapter so that the reader may potentially rethink OT practice. We are grateful for the "Expanding Our Perspectives" writers for challenging us to be better!

OT Stories

OT Stories are descriptions of working with patients/clients/service users. Each OT Story ends with a few questions for readers to think about. Most OT Stories were written by the author(s) of the chapter. For those OT Stories contributed by others, their names are listed on the OT Story in the chapter and below. We thank them for their contribution.

Commentary on the Evidence

ONLINE VIDEO CLIPS

In addition to the features listed earlier, the 14th edition of *Willard and Spackman's Occupational Therapy* includes a video library on Lippincott Connect. The videos were selected from the International Clinical Educators, (ICE) Video Library (http://www.icelearningcenter.com/) to supplement various chapters. Although chapter suggestions are listed in the descriptions below, these suggestions are not exhaustive. The videos take place in various contexts (acute care hospitals, home-based services, outpatient services, school-based services, etc.) and across the life span and are not meant to represent all contexts and populations served by OT practitioners. Video clips are listed by their titles.

Dementia: Grooming and Hygiene
This video about the impact of dementia on activities of daily living (ADLs) is recommended as a supplement to Chapters 18, 19, 21, 44, 53–55, 60, and 65.

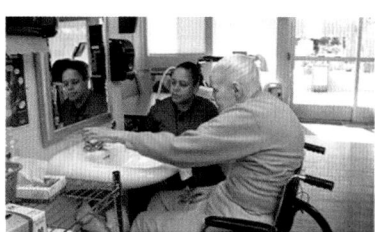

Dementia: Donning Socks
Dementia interferes with learning new tasks. This 75-year-old woman attempts to use a sock aid to don socks but has difficulty. The occupational therapist shares her thoughts on the patient's status and how to proceed.
May be used as a supplement to Chapters 18, 19, 21, 44, 53–55, 60, and 65.

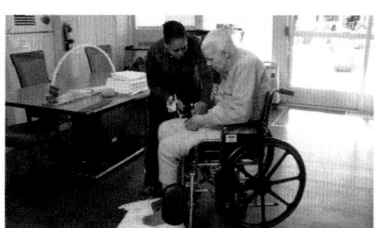

Dementia: Ambulation, Patient Refuses
It's not uncommon for patients in a skilled nursing facility (SNF) to refuse therapy. Observe how the physical therapist assistant attempts to help his patient ambulate, and how she responds.
May be used as a supplement to Chapters 18, 19, 21, 44, 53–55, 57, 60, and 65.

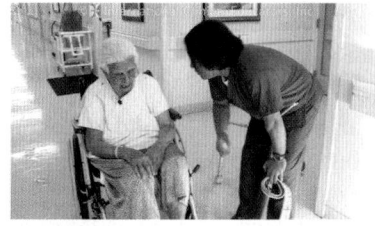

Pediatrics: Fine Motor: Letter Formation and Playdough
This video about improving coordination is recommended as a supplement to Chapters 18, 21, 47, and 52–54.

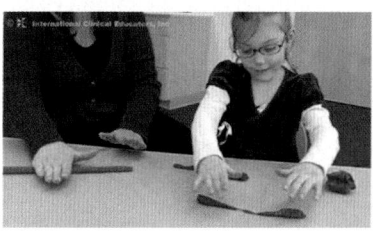

Pediatric Assessment: Administration of the Test of Visual Motor Skills
This video about assessing visual skills is recommended as a supplement to Chapters 18–20.

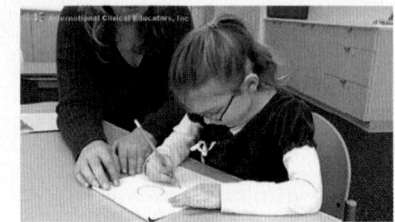

Pediatrics: Sensory Integration/Sensory Processing: Scooterboard and Letter Recognition Activity
This video about sensory interventions is recommended as a supplement to Chapters 47, 55, and 56.

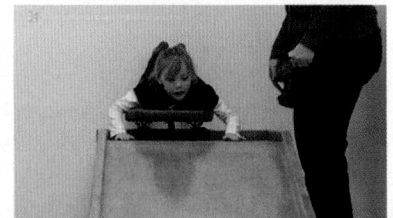

Pediatrics: Mat Activity: Sit to Stand
This video about functional mobility is recommended as a supplement to Chapters 18, 21, and 53.

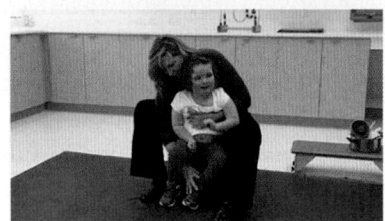

Early Childhood Development: Jack Feeding/Eating (9 Months)
Jack begins to feed himself finger foods. Observe how Jack grasps and eats small pieces of sweet potato and a teething biscuit while seated in his highchair.
May be used to supplement Chapters 18, 21, 24, 53, and 54.

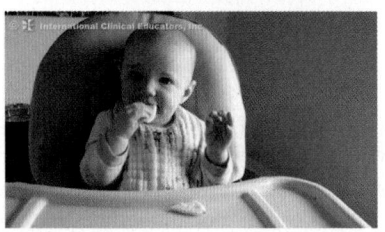

Pediatrics: Early Childhood Development: Jack Feeding/Eating (14 Months)
In this video, a utensil has been introduced. Observe Jack's attempts to use a fork to feed himself chicken and vegetables from the tray of his highchair.
May be used to supplement Chapters 18, 21, 24, 53, and 54.

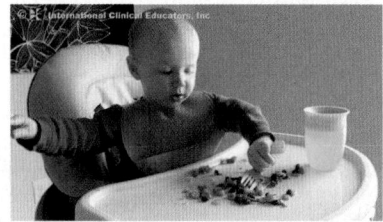

Pediatrics: Early Childhood Motor and Play Development: Standing/Walking (11 months)
In this video, Jack engages in a free play activity using a pop-up tent. He demonstrates several stages in the development of standing/walking. He also demonstrates various fine motor, visual motor, and cognitive skills while engaged in the activity.
May be used to supplement Chapters 18, 21, 24, 47, 53, and 54.

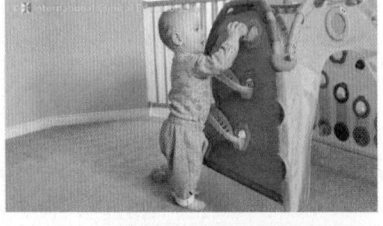

Multiple Sclerosis: Problems Observed in the Home: Part 1
This video about adaptations is recommended as a supplement to Chapters 18, 21, 23, 24, 44, and 46.

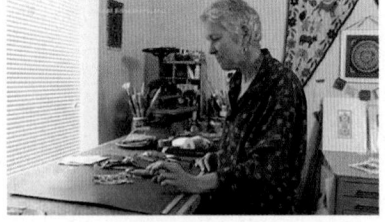

Self-Care: Dressing in Acute Care

The therapist demonstrates ADL training and upper extremity dressing techniques with a young stroke survivor exhibiting expressive aphasia, cognitive/perceptual deficits, and right hemiplegia in the acute care hospital. May be used to supplement Chapters 18, 21, 44, and 53–55.

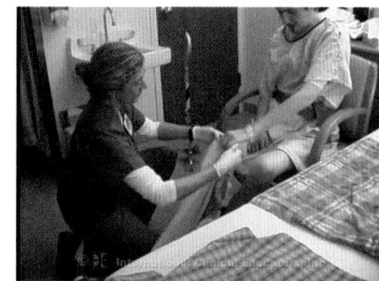

IADLs: Shining Shoes While Standing

This video about remediating motor function is recommended as a supplement to Chapters 18, 21, 44, 52–54, and 60.

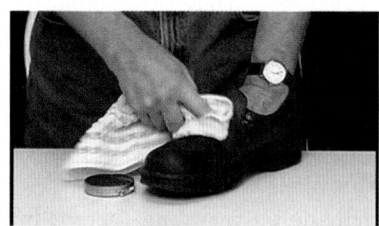

IADLs: Sweeping the Sidewalk

Functioning at a high level, this stroke survivor attempts to utilize his involved hand during an instrumental activity of daily living (IADL) task: sweeping the sidewalk. Recommended as a supplement to Chapters 18, 21, 44, 52–54, and 60.

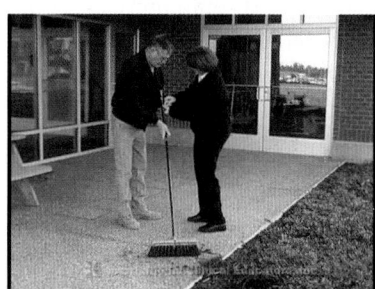

IADLs: Femur Fracture, 5 Weeks Post Surgery: Safety During Meal Preparation

This 71-year-old woman, 5 weeks post-surgery for a fractured femur, learns safety precautions in the kitchen. She uses a rolling walker to ambulate in the kitchen and learns to use appliances and equipment safely, in preparation for discharge to home. Recommended as a supplement to Chapters 18, 21, 23, 44, 52–54, and 60.

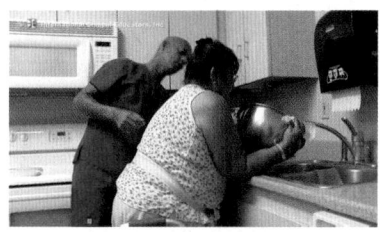

ICU: Treatment Begins: Sitting at the Edge of the Bed

This video about early mobilization is recommended as a supplement to Chapters 18, 21, 23, 32, 44, and 54.

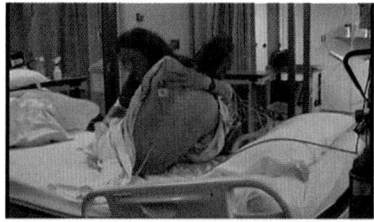

Rotator Cuff Repair: Measuring Range of Motion

This video about assessment is recommended as a supplement to Chapters 18, 19, 20, 21, and 52.

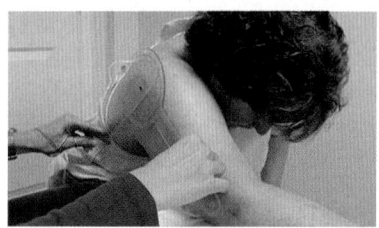

Radial Fracture, Ten Weeks Post Surgery: Paraffin Bath and Scar Mobilization

This video about preparatory interventions is recommended as a supplement to Chapters 18–21 and 52.

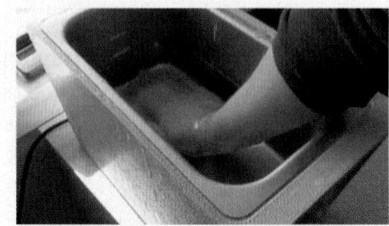

Ventilator: Self-Care at Edge of Bed

This video about acute ADL training is recommended as a supplement to Chapters 32, 44, and 60.

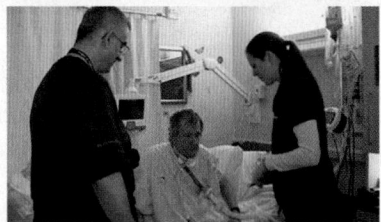

Participation: Expanding Therapy Into the Community

This video about community integration is recommended as a supplement to Chapters 44, 49, and 60.

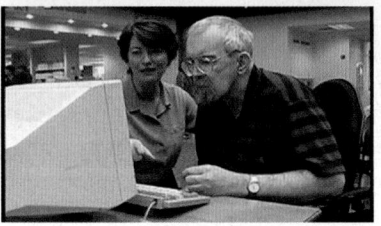

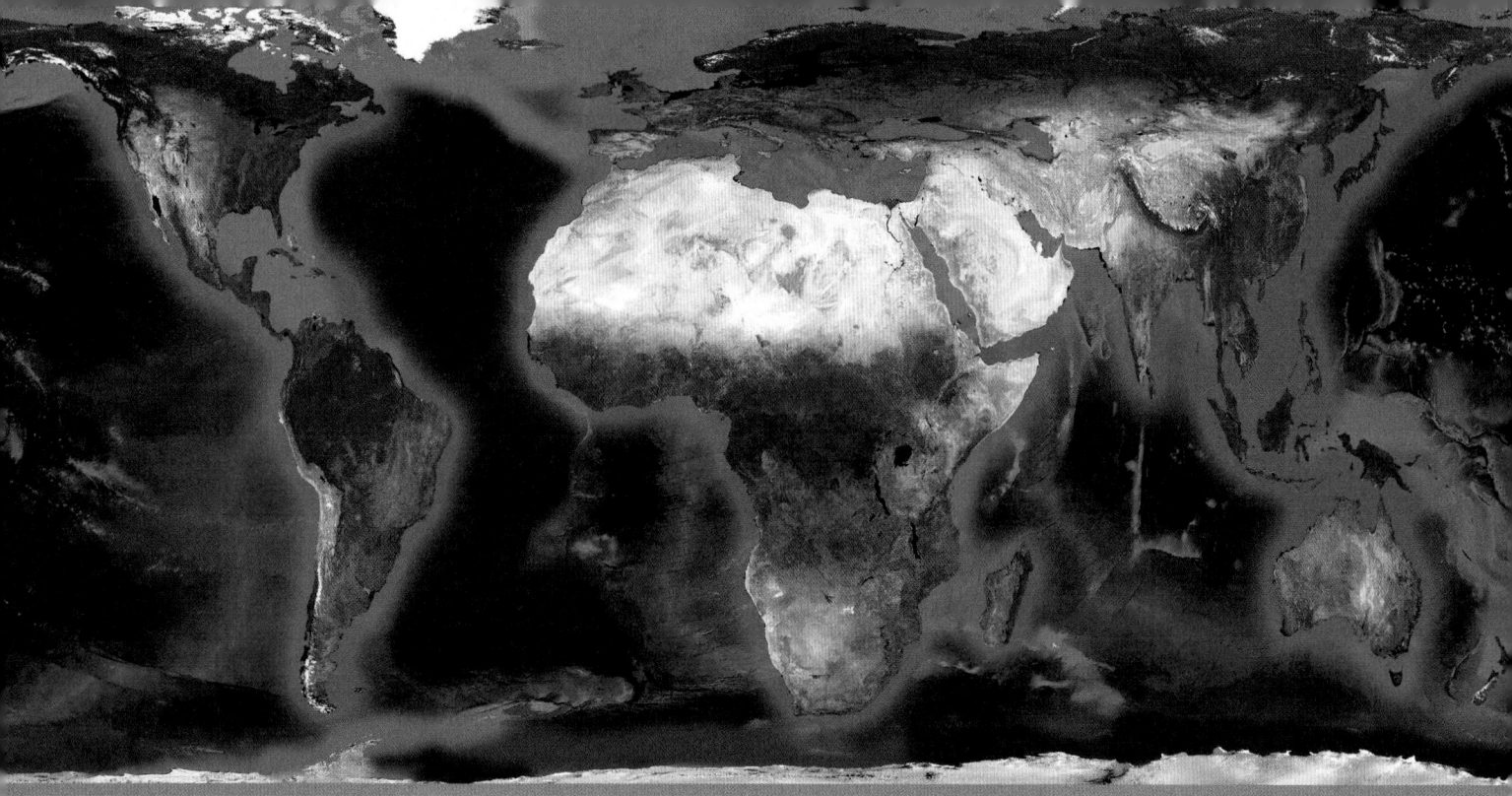

UNIT I

Occupational Therapy: Profile of the Profession

Media Related to Occupational Therapy: Profile of the Profession

Readings

- *Humans of New York:* This blog and two books by Hugh Garry started out as a photography project and later included interviews of people on the streets of New York. Eventually, he added 20 additional countries. The intimate stories depict the varied human experience. (www.humansofnewyork.com)

Movies

- *Murderball:* A documentary about the US wheelchair rugby team (mostly men with spinal cord injuries) who find purpose when they begin playing full-contact, and very competitive rugby. (2005)
- *Inside:* Bo Burnham created this comedy special that becomes more of a drama during COVID quarantine. It artistically depicts day-to-day life and Bo Burnham's deteriorating mental health. (2021)

Art

- *Walter Anderson:* An American artist known for his depictions of nature (1903–1965). He was diagnosed with schizophrenia and as a young adult, he spent time in psychiatric hospitals always managing to escape. Adolph Meyer was one of his psychiatrists. Although he was married and had four children, he led a reclusive life often alone creating artwork on a small island off the coast of Mississippi. (www.walterandersonmuseum.org)

Music

- *She Used to Be Mine:* Sara Bareilles's song about a woman who is disappointed in who she has become, but is still striving. (2015)

What Is Occupation?

Khalilah Robinson Johnson and Arameh Anvarizadeh

LEARNING OBJECTIVES

After reading this chapter, you will be able to:

1. Identify and evaluate ways of understanding occupation.
2. Articulate different ways of defining and classifying occupation.
3. Describe the relationship between occupation and context.

Knowing and Learning About Occupation

To be human is to be occupational. Occupation is a biological imperative, evident in the evolutionary history of humankind, the current behaviors of our primate relatives, and the survival needs that must be met through doing (Wilcock, 2006). Fromm (as cited by Reilly, 1962) asserted that people have a "physiologically conditioned need" to work as an act of self-preservation (p. 4). Humans also have occupational needs beyond survival. Addressing one type of occupation, Dissanayake (1992, 1995) argued that making art, or, as she describes it, "making special," is a biological necessity of human existence. According to Molineux (2004), occupational therapists now understand humans, their function, and their therapeutic needs in an occupational manner in which *occupation is life itself* (emphasis added). Townsend (1997) described occupation as the "active process of living: from the beginning to the end of life, our occupations are all the active processes of looking after ourselves and others, enjoying life, and being socially and economically productive over the lifespan and in various contexts" (p. 19).

In the myriad of activities people do every day, they engage in occupations all their lives, perhaps without ever knowing it. Many occupations are ordinary and become part of the context of daily living. Such occupations are generally taken for granted and most often are habitual (Gerlach et al., 2018; Hammell, 2009a; Wood et al., 2002). Listening to podcasts, laundering clothing, participating in religious activities, walking through a colorful market in a foreign country, and engaging with friends on social media platforms are occupations people do without ever thinking about them as being occupations.

Occupations are ordinary, but they can also be special when they represent a new achievement, such as getting a driver's license, or when they are part of celebrations and rites of passage. Preparing and hosting a holiday dinner for the first time and baking pies for the annual family reunion for the 20th time are examples of special occupations. Occupations tend to be special when they happen infrequently and carry symbolic meanings, such as representing achievement of adulthood or one's love for family. Occupations are also special when they form part of a treasured routine such as reading a bedtime story to one's child, singing "Twinkle, Twinkle, Little Star," and tucking the covers around the small, sleepy body. But even special occupations, although heavy with cultural nuances and tradition that transcend generations, change over time. Hocking et al. (2002) illustrated the complexity of traditional occupations in their study of holiday food preparation by older women in Thailand and New Zealand. The study identified many similarities between the groups (such as the activities the authors named "recipe work"), but the Thai women valued maintenance of an invariant tradition in what they prepared and how they did it, whereas the New Zealand women changed the foods they prepared over time and expected such changes to continue. Nevertheless, the doing of food-centered occupations around holidays was a tradition for both groups.

The Need to Understand Occupation

Occupational therapy (OT) practitioners need to base their work on a thorough understanding of occupation and its role in health and health behaviors, survival, and being in relation with others. That is, OT practitioners should understand what people need or are obligated to do individually and collectively to survive and achieve health and well-being. Wilcock (2007) affirmed that this level of understanding includes how people feel about occupation, how it affects their development, the societal mechanisms through which that development occurs, and how that process is understood. Achieving that understanding of occupation is more than having an easy definition (which is a daunting challenge in its own right). To know what occupation is, it is necessary to examine what humans do with their time, how they come to choose and coordinate such activities, what purposes they serve, and what they mean for individuals and society.

Personal experience of doing occupation, whether consciously attended to or not, provides a fundamental understanding of occupation—what it is, how it happens, what it means, what is good or harmful about it, and what is not. This way of knowing is both basic and extraordinarily rich.

Looking Inward to Know Occupation

To be useful to OT practitioners, knowledge of occupation based on personal experience demands examination and reflection. What do we do, how do we do it, when and where does it take place, and what does it mean? Who else is involved directly and indirectly? What capacities does it require in us? What does it cost? Is it challenging or uncomplicated? How has this occupation changed over time? What would it be like if we no longer had this occupation? To illustrate, Khalilah (first author) shares her experiences with cooking as she transitioned from home to college (OT Story 1.1).

Between college and the beginning of Khalilah's postgraduate career, cooking took on a different *form* (the need to prepare meals for herself as an independent adult), *function* (family-style meals were no longer reserved for times with family and friends but became a means to forge relationships with strangers), and *meaning* (a way to bridge and create new cultural experiences with her family and friends). These elements—the form, function, and meaning of occupation—are the basic areas of focus for the science of occupation (Larson et al., 2003).

Khalilah's cooking and communal mealtime example described in OT Story 1.1 illustrates how occupation is a *transaction* with the *environment* or *context* of other people and cultures, places, and tools. It includes the *temporal* nature of occupation—seasonal travel to particular destinations and the availability of specific ingredients based on the season of travel. That she calls herself a cook exemplifies how occupation has become part of her *identity* and suggests that it might be difficult for her to give up cooking.

Basic as it is, however, understanding derived from personal experience is insufficient as the basis for practice. Reliance solely on this source of knowledge has the risk of expecting everyone to experience occupation in the same manner as the therapist. So, although OT practitioners will profit in being attuned to their own occupations, they must also turn their view to the occupation around them and to understanding occupation through study and research.

Looking Outward to Know Occupation

As presented in this chapter and throughout this edition of *Willard and Spackman*, observation of the world through learning and observing others from differing backgrounds and experiences is another rich source of occupational knowledge. Connoisseurs of occupation can train themselves to new ways of seeing a world rich with occupations: the way a restaurant hostess manages a crowd when

OT STORY 1.1 COOKING "SOUTHERN" AT COLLEGE

My first real attempt at cooking a meal independently was my freshman year of college. My dorm had a full kitchen, and I, like many college students, loathed dining hall dinners. I had grown up in a home where my parents prepared dinner nightly and we ate together as a family. My grandparents cooked dinner for our extended family every Sunday, and as Southern culture would suggest, I learned the proper way to braise vegetables, season and smoke meat and fish, concoct gravies, and bake an array of casseroles prior to graduating high school. Meal preparation and meal execution generally adhere to rules and techniques according to the macro culture, local or home culture of the person(s) performing it. Going to college required that I translate that cultural knowledge and adapt those rules to my new environment, understanding that the same products and tools to which I was accustomed would not be available. To build community, I began to cook traditional Southern meals in several kitchens around campus, taking up new ideas and techniques as I "broke bread" with other students. It was not until I received recognition from my peers that I considered myself a true Southern cook. Since that time, I have taken my love of cooking to international spaces, where I learn to prepare traditional meals of the native culture in a local person's home (Figure 1.1).

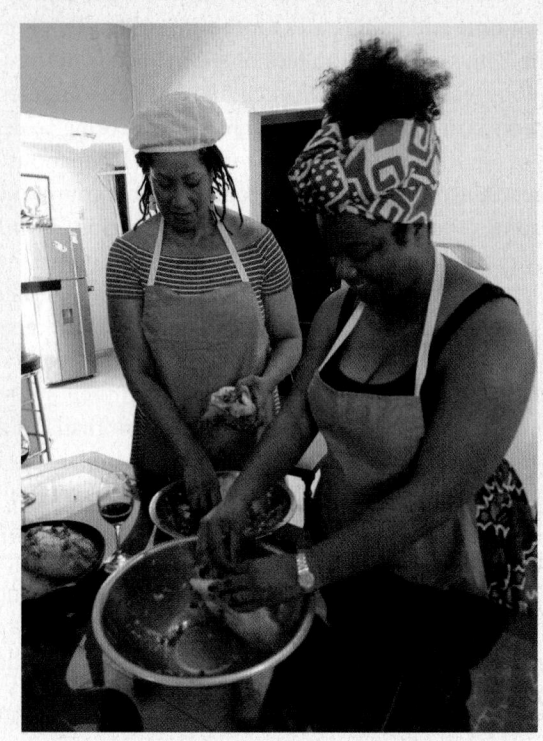

FIGURE 1.1 Khalilah (on the right) preparing fish.

the wait for seating is long, the economy of movement of a construction worker doing a repetitive task, the activities of musicians in the orchestra pit when they are not playing, the almost aimless social media scrolling on handheld devices as students take a break from class, and texting while engaging in social situations. Furthermore, people like to talk about what they do, and the scholar of occupation can learn a great deal by asking for information about people's work and play. By being observant and asking questions, people increase their repertoire of occupational knowledge far beyond the boundaries of personal interests, practices, and capabilities.

Observation of others' occupations enriches the OT practitioner's knowledge of the range of occupational possibilities (e.g., the types and ways of performing occupation that are deemed socially ideal) and of human responses to occupational opportunities (e.g., accessing and participating in occupation of one's choosing) (Laliberte-Rudman, 2010). But although this sort of knowledge goes far beyond the limits of personal experience, it is still bounded by the world any one person is able to access, and it lacks the depth of knowledge that is developed through research and scholarship.

Turning to Research and Scholarship to Understand Occupation

Knowledge of occupation that comes from personal experience and observation must be augmented with the understanding of occupation drawn from research in OT and occupational science as well as other disciplines. Hocking (2000) developed a framework of needed knowledge for research in occupation, organized into the categories of the "essential elements of occupation … occupational processes … [and the] relationship of occupation to other phenomena" (p. 59). This research is being done within OT and occupational science, but there is also a wealth of information to be found in the work of other disciplines. For example, in sociology, Duneier (1999) studied the economy of work for poor Black men in New York City neighborhoods; DeVault (1999) examined the dynamics of housework, in particular, family mealtimes; and Battle (2019) investigated the ways in which fathering is mediated through child support systems. Human geography researchers have studied the transactions between place, age, and care (Cutchin, 2005) and many other conceptualizations of home and community. Psychologists have studied habits (Aarts & Dijksterhuis, 2000; Wood et al., 2002) and a wealth of other topics that relate to how people engage in occupation. Understanding of occupation will benefit from more research within OT and occupational science and from accessing relevant works of scholars in other fields. Hocking (2009) has called for more occupational science research focused on occupations themselves rather than people's experiences of occupations. Refer to Chapters 6 and 11.

Defining Occupation

For many years, the word *occupation* was not part of the daily language of occupational therapists, nor was it prominent in the profession's literature (Hinojosa et al., 2003). According to Kielhofner and Burke (1977), the founding paradigm of OT was occupation, and the occupational perspective focused on people and their health "in the context of the culture of daily living and its activities" (p. 688). But beginning in the 1930s, the profession of OT entered into a paradigm of reductionism that lasted into the 1970s. One reason for the change was a desire to become more like the medical profession. During that time, occupation, both as a concept and as a means and/or outcome of intervention, was essentially absent from professional discourse. With time, a few professional leaders began to call for OT to return to its roots in occupation (Schwartz, 2003), and since the 1970s, acceptance of occupation as the foundation of OT has grown (Kielhofner, 2009). With that growth, professional debates about the definition and nature of occupation emerged and continue to this day.

Defining occupation in OT is challenging because the word is part of common language with meanings that the profession cannot control. The term *occupation* and related concepts such as *activity, task, employment, doing,* and *work* are used in many ways within OT. It seems quite logical to think of a job, cleaning house, or bike riding as an occupation, but the concept is fuzzier when we think about the smaller components of these larger categories. Is dusting an occupation, or is it part of the occupation of house cleaning? Is riding a bike a skill that is part of some larger occupation such as physical conditioning or getting from home to school, or is it an occupation in its own right? Does this change over time?

The founders of OT used the word *occupation* to describe a way of "properly" using time that included work and work-like activities and recreational activities (Meyer, 1922). Breines (1995) pointed out that the founders chose a term that was both ambiguous and comprehensive to name the profession, a choice, she argued, that was not accidental. The term was open to holistic interpretations that supported the diverse areas of practice of the time, encompassing the

elements of occupation defined by Breines (1995) as "mind, body, time, space, and others" (p. 459). The term *occupation* spawned ongoing examination, controversy, and redefinition as the profession has matured.

Nelson (1988, 1997) introduced the terms *occupational form,* "the preexisting structure that elicits, guides, or structures subsequent human performance," and *occupational performance,* "the human actions taken in response to an occupational form" (Nelson, 1988, p. 633). This distinction separates individuals and their actual doing of occupations from the general notion of an occupation and what it requires of anyone who does it.

Yerxa and colleagues (1989) defined occupation as "specific 'chunks' of activity within the ongoing stream of human behavior which are named in the lexicon of the culture.... These daily pursuits are self-initiated, goal-directed (purposeful), and socially sanctioned" (p. 5). Yerxa (1993) further elaborated this definition to incorporate an environmental perspective and a greater breadth of characteristics. She stated,

> Occupations are units of activity which are classified and named by the culture according to the purposes they serve in enabling people to meet environmental challenges successfully.... Some essential characteristics of occupation are that it is self-initiated, goal-directed (even if the goal is fun or pleasure), experiential as well as behavioral, socially valued or recognized, constituted of adaptive skills or repertoires, organized, essential to the quality of life experienced, and possesses the capacity to influence health. (Yerxa, 1993, p. 5)

According to the Canadian Association of Occupational Therapists (as cited in Law et al., 1998), occupation is "groups of activities and tasks of everyday life, named, organized and given value and meaning by individuals and a culture." In a somewhat circular definition, they went on to state that "occupation is everything people do to occupy themselves, including looking after themselves (self-care), enjoying life (leisure), and contributing to the social and economic fabric of their communities (productivity)" (p. 83). Occupational scientists Larson et al. (2003) provided a simple definition of occupation as "the activities that comprise our life experience and can be named in the culture" (p. 16). Similarly, after referencing a number of different definitions of occupation, the Occupational Therapy Practice Framework affirmed the statement from the World Federation of Occupational Therapists (WFOT) that occupation refers "to the everyday activities that people do as individuals, in families, and with communities to occupy time and bring meaning and purpose to life. Occupations include things people need to, want to and are expected to do" (WFOT, 2012a, para. 2 as cited by American Occupational Therapy Association [AOTA], 2020, p. S7). The previous definitions of occupation from OT literature help in explaining why occupation is the profession's focus (particularly in the context of therapy), yet they are open enough to allow continuing research on the nature of occupation. Despite, and perhaps because of, the ubiquity of occupation in human life, there is still much to learn about the nature of occupation through systematic research using an array of methodologies (e.g., Aldrich et al., 2017; Dickie, 2010; Johnson & Bagatell, 2017; Molke et al., 2004). Such research should include examination of the premises that are built into the accepted definitions of occupation.

At a more theoretical level, such an examination has begun. Several authors have challenged the unexamined assumptions and beliefs about occupation of Western occupational therapists (cf. Guajardo et al., 2015; Hammell, 2009a, 2009b; Iwama, 2006; Kantartzis & Molineux, 2011; Morrison et al., 2017; Ramugondo, 2015). These critiques center on the Western cultural bias in the definition and use of occupation across global contexts and the inadequacy of the conceptualization of occupation as it is used in OT in Western countries to describe the daily activities of most of the world's population. Attention to these arguments will strengthen our knowledge of occupation. In this text, the following chapters, among others, will expand on these issues: Chapters 10, 11, and 37.

Context and Occupation

The photograph of four children using a magnifying glass to examine leaves on the ground evokes a sense of a mildly temperate day during a season when leaves begin to shed from trees (Figure 1.2). Exploring in a forest and looking at leaves has a context with temporal elements (possibly autumn on the east coast of the United States, the play of children, and the viewer's memories of doing it in the past), a physical environment (wooded setting including pine

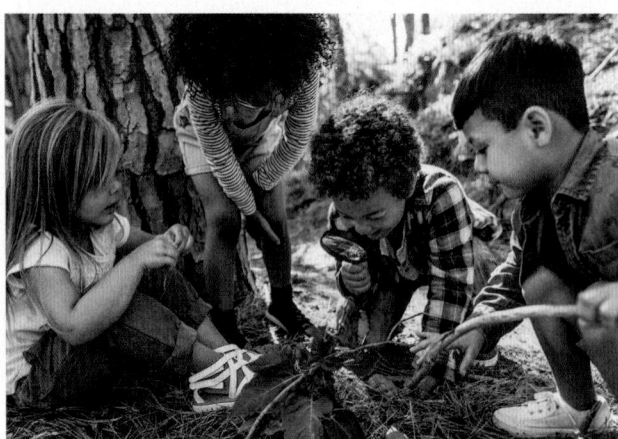

FIGURE 1.2 **Children in forest looking at leaves together with the magnifying glass.**

straw, sticks, and leaves), and a social environment (four children and the likelihood of an indulgent parent or educator). The children looking at leaves cannot be described or understood—or even happen—without its context. It is difficult to imagine that any of the children would enjoy the activity as much doing it alone as the social context is part of the experience. This form of exploration might also be set up in an indoor or outdoor garden, but not in a simulated environment with inanimate objects. Parents or educators would be unlikely to allow the children to wander in an outdoor wooded area alone. The contexts of the people viewing the picture are important, too; many will relate the picture to their own past experiences, but someone who lives in a place with less forestation might find the picture meaningless and/or confusing. In this example, occupation and context are enmeshed with one another.

It is generally accepted that the specific *meaning* of an occupation is fully known only to the individual engaged in the occupation (Larson et al., 2003; Pierce, 2001; Weinblatt et al., 2000). But it is also well accepted that occupations take place in *context* (sometimes referred to as the environment) (e.g., Baum & Christiansen, 2005; Kielhofner, 2002; Law et al., 1996; Schkade & Schultz, 2003; Yerxa et al., 1989) and thus have dimensions that consider other humans (in both social and cultural ways), temporality, the physical environment, and even virtual environments (AOTA, 2020).

Description of occupation as taking place *in* or *with* the environment or context implies a separation of person and context that is problematic. In reality, person, occupation, and context are inseparable. Context is changeable but always present. Cutchin (2004) offered a critique of OT theories of adaptation-to-environment that separate person from environment and proposed that John Dewey's view of human experience as "always situated and contextualized" (p. 305) was a more useful perspective. According to Cutchin, "situations are always inclusive of us, and us of them" (p. 305). Occupation occurs at the level of the situation and thus is inclusive of the individual and context (Cutchin & Dickie, 2013; Dickie et al., 2006). OT interventions cannot be context free. Even when an OT practitioner is working with an individual, contextual element of other people, the culture of therapist and client, the physical space, and past experiences are present.

Is Occupation Always Good?

In OT, occupation is associated with health and well-being, both as a means and as an end. But occupation can also be unhealthy, dangerous, oppressive, maladaptive, or destructive to self or others and can contribute to societal problems and environmental degradation (Blakeney & Marshall, 2009; Hammell, 2009a, 2009b; Kiepek et al., 2019; Lavalley & Johnson, 2022; Twinley, 2013). Among many examples, scholars have described how notions of acceptable and unacceptable sexual activity for particular gender groups are reinforced through social norms, the tensions between experiencing pleasure as good or bad by individuals who engage in illicit activities, sedentary employment environments and their negative impact on health outcomes, accessibility of various recreational sports have historically excluded racially minoritized groups, and more.

Further, the seemingly benign act of using a car to get to work, run errands, and pursue other occupations can limit one's physical activity and risk injury to self and others. Americans' reliance on the automobile contributes to urban sprawl, the deterioration of neighborhoods, air pollution, and overuse of nonrenewable natural resources. Likewise, industry and the work that provides monetary support to individuals and families may cause serious air pollution in expanding economies such as that of China and Nigeria (Egbetokun et al., 2020; U.S. Department of State, 2020).

Personal and societal occupational choices have consequences, good and bad. In coming to understand occupation, we need to acknowledge the breadth of occupational choices and their effects on individuals and society at large.

Categorizing Occupation

Categorization of occupations (e.g., into areas of activities of daily living [ADLs], work, and leisure) is often problematic. Attempts to define work and leisure demonstrate that distinctions between the two are not always clear (Snape et al., 2017). Work may be defined as something people *have* to do, an unpleasant necessity of life, but many people enjoy their work and describe it as "fun." Indeed, Hochschild (1997) discovered that employees in the work setting she studied often preferred the homelike qualities of work to being in their actual homes and consequently spent more time at work than was necessary. The concept of leisure is problematic as well. Leisure might involve activities that are experienced as hard work, such as helping a friend to build a deck on a weekend.

Take the two men plating salmon and vegetables (Figure 1.3) for example. Categorizing their activity presents a challenge. They are hovering over a kitchen counter, meticulously placing microgreens on top of the salmon using chef's tweezers. Their activity may be categorized as

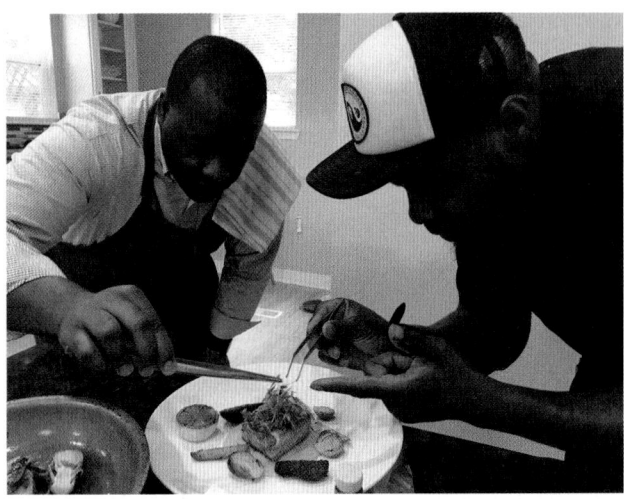

FIGURE 1.3 **Two men plating salmon and vegetables.**

engaging in work or other productive activity. However, what is not known is whether this is paid work, caregiving work (e.g., feeding others in the home), or leisure. Both men are dressed in a chef's coat and an apron and utilizing tools that are not commonly used in home kitchens. This may give the appearance that they are engaging in paid work—chefs preparing a meal for paying patrons. But only the gentleman on the left is a chef, which may lead you to interpret the situation as a leisure activity for the gentleman on the right. Categorizing the totality of this occupational situation is complicated. No simple designation of what is happening in the picture will suffice.

Another problem with categories is that an individual may experience an occupation as something entirely different from what it appears to be to others. Weinblatt and colleagues (2000) described how an older woman used the supermarket for purposes quite different from provisioning (that would likely be called instrumental activities of daily living [IADLs]). Instead, this woman used her time in the store as a source of new knowledge and interesting information about modern life. What should we call her occupation in this instance?

The construct of occupation might very well defy efforts to reduce it to a single definition or a set of categories. Many examples of occupations can be found that challenge other theoretical approaches and definitions. Nevertheless, the richness and complexity of occupation will continue to challenge occupational therapists to know and value it through personal experience, observations, and scholarly work. The practice of OT depends on this knowledge.

Lippincott® Connect *For additional resources on the subjects discussed in this chapter, visit* Lippincott Connect.

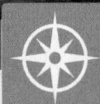

EXPANDING OUR PERSPECTIVE

The Value of Culture in Understanding Occupation

Arameh Anvarizadeh

Working in spaces that serve marginalized communities has been an enriching and humbling experience. One example of this is providing care to a child who recently immigrated to the United States from Iran to receive comprehensive rehabilitation services. He was a 7-year-old living with arthrogryposis and his parents were in dire need to have him engage in age-appropriate, meaningful occupations at home and in the school setting (e.g., playing with peers). Upon his arrival to the clinic, he was scheduled with occupational and physical therapists to complete his initial evaluation. However, there was one glaring issue—a language barrier. The therapists were having a difficult time identifying and understanding occupations that were important to the child and to his family. They were unable to define the context of the occupations his parents were describing to them.

As an occupational therapist who strives to demonstrate cultural fluidity and humility at all times, I lent myself to assist in the evaluation because I was able to speak their language, Farsi. Once that barrier was removed, the family and child instantly felt the ability to connect in identity, in context, and in understanding occupation. I was able to dive deep in gathering a thorough occupational profile, while also collecting information about what he wants to do, needs to do, but was unable to do because of physical limitations. We also were able to discuss his performance and satisfaction with the occupations that were important to him, such as dressing himself (donning socks and shoes specifically), playing with peers during recess (kicking a soccer ball), toileting, and feeding himself independently.

Questions such as "tell me about your favorite meal" were compelling because I, too, understood the common meals served in Iranian culture—not just what the dishes were, but how they smelled, how they were served, how individuals engaged in mealtime together as a family unit. Taking all of these factors into consideration were important and guided me in writing very client-centered, culturally responsive goals.

Attending Individualized Education Programs (IEPs) where I would observe educational staff and therapists speaking to the interpreter and not directly to the family, being in spaces where therapists would talk negatively about a client because they could not understand them, and watching clients experience frustration because of language barriers was difficult, yet a very valuable learning experience in advocating for all people, populations, and communities. More importantly, these experiences show why remaining grounded in cultural humility is critical in providing equitable care while maintaining client satisfaction.

This child and family were ultimately added to my caseload. We built rapport, addressed all of his goals, and were creative in ensuring that he had access to the occupations that were meaningful to him. This experience along with similar stories demonstrates that understanding occupation is one factor; however, knowing that occupation serves multiple meanings based on the cultural implications is a significant part of our role as practitioners, leading the way in holistic and justice-based care.

REFERENCES

Aarts, H., & Dijksterhuis, A. (2000). Habits as knowledge structures: Automaticity in goal-directed behavior. *Journal of Personality and Social Psychology, 78*(1), 53–63. https://doi.org/10.1037/0022-3514.78.1.53

Aldrich, R., Rudman, D., & Dickie, V. (2017). Resource seeking as occupation: A critical and empirical exploration. *American Journal of Occupational Therapy, 71*(3), 7103260010p1–7103260010p9. https://doi.org/10.5014/ajot.2017.021782

American Occupational Therapy Association. (2020). Occupational therapy practice framework: Domain and process—fourth edition. *American Journal of Occupational Therapy, 74*(Suppl 2), 7412410010p1–7412410010p87. https://doi.org/10.5014/ajot.2020.74S2001

Battle, B. P. (2019). "They look at you like you're nothing": Stigma and shame in the child support system. *Symbolic Interaction, 42*(4), 640–668. https://doi.org/10.1002/symb.427

Baum, C. M., & Christiansen, C. H. (2005). Person-environment-occupation-performance: An occupation-based framework for practice. In C. H. Christiansen, C. M. Baum, & J. Bass-Haugen (Eds.), *Occupational therapy: Performance, participation, and well-being* (3rd ed., pp. 243–266). SLACK.

Blakeney, A., & Marshall, A. (2009). Water quality, health, and human occupations. *American Journal of Occupational Therapy, 63*(1), 46–57. https://doi.org/10.5014/ajot.63.1.46

Breines, E. B. (1995). Understanding "occupation" as the founders did. *British Journal of Occupational Therapy, 58*(11), 458–460. https://doi.org/10.1177/030802269505801102

Cutchin, M. P. (2004). Using Deweyan philosophy to rename and reframe adaptation-to-environment. *American Journal of Occupational Therapy, 58*(3), 303–312. https://doi.org/10.5014/ajot.58.3.303

Cutchin, M. P. (2005). Spaces for inquiry into the role of place for older people's care. *Journal of Clinical Nursing, 14*(s2), 121–129. https://doi.org/10.1111/j.1365-2702.2005.01280.x

Cutchin, M. P., & Dickie, V. (2013). *Transactional perspectives on occupation*. Springer.

DeVault, M. L. (1999). Comfort and struggle: Emotion work in family life. *The ANNALS of the American Academy of Political and Social Science, 561*(1), 52–63. https://doi.org/10.1177/000271629956100104

Dickie, V. A. (2010). Are occupations "processes too complicated to explain"? What we can learn by trying. *Journal of Occupational Science, 17*(4), 195–203. https://doi.org/10.1080/14427591.2010.9686696

Dickie, V., Cutchin, M., & Humphry, R. (2006). Occupation as transactional experience: A critique of individualism in occupational science. *Journal of Occupational Science, 13*(1), 83–93. https://doi.org/10.1080/14427591.2006.9686573

Dissanayake, E. (1992). *Homo aestheticus: Where art comes from and why*. University of Washington Press.

Dissanayake, E. (1995). The pleasure and meaning of making. *American Craft, 55*(2), 40–45.

Duneier, M. (1999). *Sidewalk*. Farrar, Straus & Giroux.

Egbetokun, S., Osabuohien, E., Akinbobola, T., Onanuga, O. T., Gershon, O., & Okafor, V. (2020). Environmental pollution, economic growth and institutional quality: Exploring the nexus in Nigeria. *Management of Environmental Quality, 31*(1), 18–31. https://doi.org/10.1108/MEQ-02-2019-0050

Gerlach, A. J., Teachman, G., Laliberte-Rudman, D., Aldrich, R. M., & Huot, S. (2018). Expanding beyond individualism: Engaging critical perspectives on occupation. *Scandinavian Journal of Occupational Therapy, 25*(1), 35–43. https://doi.org/10.1080/11038128.2017.1327616

Guajardo, A., Kronenberg, F., & Ramugondo, E. L. (2015). Southern occupational therapies: Emerging identities, epistemologies and practices. *South African Journal of Occupational Therapy, 45*(1), 3–10. https://doi.org/10.17159/2310-3833/2015/v45no1a2

Hammell, K. (2009a). Sacred texts: A sceptical exploration of the assumptions underpinning theories of occupation. *Canadian Journal of Occupational Therapy, 76*(1), 6–13. https://doi.org/10.1177/000841740907600105

Hammell, K. (2009b). Self-care, productivity, and leisure, or dimensions of occupational experience? Rethinking occupational "categories." *Canadian Journal of Occupational Therapy, 76*(2), 107–114. https://doi.org/10.1177/000841740907600208

Hinojosa, J., Kramer, P., Royeen, C. B., & Luebben, A. J. (2003). Core concept of occupation. In P. Kramer, J. Hinojosa, & C. B. Royeen (Eds.), *Perspectives in human occupation: Participation in life* (pp. 1–17). Lippincott Williams & Wilkins.

Hochschild, A. R. (1997). *The time bind: When work becomes home and home becomes work*. Metropolitan Books.

Hocking, C. (2000). Occupational science: A stock take of accumulated insights. *Journal of Occupational Science, 7*(2), 58–67. https://doi.org/10.1080/14427591.2000.9686466

Hocking, C. (2009). The challenge of occupation: Describing the things people do. *Journal of Occupational Science, 16*(3), 140–150. https://doi.org/10.1080/14427591.2009.9686655

Hocking, C., Wright-St. Clair, V., & Bunrayong, W. (2002). The meaning of cooking and recipe work for older Thai and New Zealand women. *Journal of Occupational Science, 9*(3), 117–127. https://doi.org/10.1080/14427591.2002.9686499

Iwama, M. (2006). *The Kawa model: Culturally relevant occupational therapy*. Churchill Livingstone/Elsevier.

Johnson, K., & Bagatell, N. (2017). Beyond custodial care: Mediating choice and participation for adults with intellectual disabilities. *Journal of Occupational Science, 24*(4), 546–560. https://doi.org/10.1080/14427591.2017.1363078

Kantartzis, S., & Molineux, M. (2011). The influence of Western society's construction of a healthy daily life on the conceptualisation of occupation. *Journal of Occupational Science, 18*(1), 62–80. https://doi.org/10.1080/14427591.2011.566917

Kielhofner, G. (2002). *Model of human occupation: Theory and application* (3rd ed.). Lippincott Williams & Wilkins.

Kielhofner, G. (2009). *Conceptual foundations of occupational therapy practice* (4th ed.). F.A. Davis.

Kielhofner, G., & Burke, J. P. (1977). Occupational therapy after 60 years: An account of changing identity and knowledge. *American Journal of Occupational Therapy, 31*(10), 675–689.

Kiepek, N., Beagan, B., Laliberte-Rudman, D., & Phelan, S. (2019). Silences around occupations framed as unhealthy, illegal, and deviant. *Journal of Occupational Science, 26*(3), 341–353. https://doi.org/10.1080/14427591.2018.1499123

Laliberte-Rudman, D. (2010). Occupational terminology: Occupational possibilities. *Journal of Occupational Science, 17*(1), 55–59. https://doi.org/10.1080/14427591.2010.9686673

Larson, E., Wood, W., & Clark, F. (2003). Occupational science: Building the science and practice of occupation through an academic discipline. In E. B. Crepeau, E. Cohn, & B. Schell (Eds.), *Willard & Spackman's occupational therapy* (10th ed., pp. 15–26). Lippincott Williams & Wilkins.

Lavalley, R., & Johnson, K. R. (2022). Occupation, injustice, and anti-Black racism in the United States of America. *Journal of Occupational Science, 29*(4), 487–499. https://doi.org/10.1080/14427591.2020.1810111

Law, M., Cooper, B., Strong, S., Stewart, D., Rigby, P., & Letts, L. (1996). The person-environment-occupation model: A transactive approach to occupational performance. *Canadian Journal of Occupational Therapy, 63*(1), 9–23. https://doi.org/10.1177/000841749606300103

Law, M., Steinwender, S., & Leclair, L. (1998). Occupation, health and well-being. *Canadian Journal of Occupational Therapy, 65*(2), 81–91. https://doi.org/10.1177/000841749806500204

Meyer, A. (1922). The philosophy of occupational therapy. *Archives of Occupational Therapy, 1*(1), 1–10.

Molineux, M. (2004). Occupation in occupational therapy: A labour in vain? In M. Molineux (Ed.), *Occupation for occupational therapists* (pp. 1–14). Blackwell.

Molke, D., Laliberte-Rudman, D., & Polatajko, H. J. (2004). The promise of occupational science: A developmental assessment of an emerging academic discipline. *Canadian Journal of Occupational Therapy, 71*(5), 269–281. https://doi.org/10.1177/000841740407100505

Morrison, R., Gómez, S., Henny, E., Tapia, M. J., & Rueda, L. (2017). Principal approaches to understanding occupation and occupational science found in the Chilean Journal of Occupational Therapy (2001–2012). *Occupational Therapy International, 2017*, 5413628. https://doi.org/10.1155/2017/5413628

Nelson, D. L. (1988). Occupation: Form and performance. *American Journal of Occupational Therapy, 42*(10), 633–641. https://doi.org/10.5014/ajot.42.10.633

Nelson, D. L. (1997). Why the profession of occupational therapy will flourish in the 21st century. The 1996 Eleanor Clarke Slagle Lecture. *American Journal of Occupational Therapy, 51*(1), 11–24. https://doi.org/10.5014/ajot.51.1.11

Pierce, D. (2001). Untangling occupation and activity. *American Journal of Occupational Therapy, 55*(2), 138–146. https://doi.org/10.5014/ajot.55.2.138

Ramugondo, E. (2015). Occupational consciousness. *Journal of Occupational Science, 22*(4), 488–501. https://doi.org/10.1080/14427591.2015.1042516

Reilly, M. (1962). Occupational therapy can be one of the great ideas of 20th century medicine. *American Journal of Occupational Therapy, 16*(1), 1–9.

Schkade, J. K., & Schultz, S. (2003). Occupational adaptation. In P. Kramer, J. Hinojosa, & C. B. Royeen (Eds.), *Perspectives in human occupation: Participation in life* (pp. 181–221). Lippincott Williams & Wilkins.

Schwartz, K. B. (2003). History of occupation. In P. Kramer, J. Hinojosa, & C. B. Royeen (Eds.), *Perspectives in human occupation: Participation in life* (pp. 18–31). Lippincott Williams & Wilkins.

Snape, R., Haworth, J., McHugh, S., & Carson, J. (2017). Leisure in a post-work society. *World Leisure Journal, 59*(3), 184–194. https://doi.org/10.1080/16078055.2017.1345483

Townsend, E. (1997). Occupation: Potential for personal and social transformation. *Journal of Occupational Science: Australia, 4*(1), 18–26. https://doi.org/10.1080/14427591.1997.9686417

Twinley, R. (2013). The dark side of occupation: A concept for consideration. *Australian Occupational Therapy Journal, 60*(4), 301–303. https://doi.org/10.1111/1440-1630.12026

U.S. Department of State. (2020). China's air pollution harms its citizens and the world. https://ge.usembassy.gov/chinas-air-pollution-harms-its-citizens-and-the-world/

Weinblatt, N., Ziv, N., & Avrech-Bar, M. (2000). The old lady from the supermarket—Categorization of occupation according to performance areas: Is it relevant for the elderly? *Journal of Occupational Science, 7*(2), 73–79. https://doi.org/10.1080/14427591.2000.9686468

Wilcock, A. A. (2006). *An occupational perspective of health* (2nd ed.). SLACK.

Wilcock, A. A. (2007). Occupation and health: Are they one and the same? *Journal of Occupational Science, 14*(1), 3–8. https://doi.org/10.1080/14427591.2007.9686577

Wood, W., Quinn, J. M., & Kashy, D. A. (2002). Habits in everyday life: Thought, emotion, and action. *Journal of Personality and Social Psychology, 83*(6), 1281–1297. https://doi.org/10.1037/0022-3514.83.6.1281

Yerxa, E. J. (1993). Occupational science: A new source of power for participants in occupational therapy. *Journal of Occupational Science: Australia, 1*(1), 3–9. https://doi.org/10.1080/14427591.1993.9686373

Yerxa, E. J., Clark, F., Frank, G., Jackson, J., Parham, D., Pierce, D., Stein, C., & Zemke, R. (1989). An introduction to occupational science, a foundation for occupational therapy in the 21st century. In J. A. Johnson & E. J. Yerxa (Eds.), *Occupational science: The foundation for new models of practice* (pp. 1–17). Haworth Press.

A Contextual History of Occupational Therapy

Charles H. Christiansen and Kristine L. Haertl

LEARNING OBJECTIVES

After reading this chapter, you should be able to:

1. Understand how historical accounts are retrospective attempts to interpret the events of the past with the purpose of gaining improved insight into the present.
2. Identify key individuals and events that influenced the founding and development of occupational therapy.
3. Identify the milestones in occupational therapy's history.
4. Recognize how mind–body dualism and the competition between social and biomedical approaches to healthcare have been consistent points of tension since occupational therapy's founding.
5. Appreciate that occupational therapy has evolved into a globally recognized healthcare profession that is well established throughout the world.

Introduction

As a profession over a century old, occupational therapy (OT) has a rich and complex history. It has been influenced, as most professions have, by world events, key individuals, and social movements. In this chapter, we identify some of these factors as a way of understanding how OT came into being and evolved as a profession. Industrialization, romanticism, the civil rights struggles for women and children, world wars, economic shifts, healthcare legislation, globalization, and the digital age have been major influences on the evolution of the profession. The history of OT illustrates Faulkner's (1953, p. 73) observation that *"the past is never dead, it's not even past."* Moreover, although OT began in the United States, it is important to remember that many of the factors influencing its development originated in Europe and that the profession is now global in its reach and varied in its character.

In recognition that it is no longer appropriate to consider the evolution of OT from only a US-centric perspective, this chapter includes short summaries of past and current activities in various nations throughout the world. These expanded perspectives illustrate how developments in one country can have a global influence that expands rapidly in the digital world we now occupy. See Expanding Our Perspectives: The History of OT Around the World.

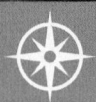

EXPANDING OUR PERSPECTIVES

The History of OT Around the World

Occupational Therapy in Australia

Lynne Adamson, PhD, Grad Cert UTL, MAppSc (OT), BAppSc (OT)

Beginnings: Building on the principles of humane treatment, OT emerged in the 20th-century Australia. Activities were part of treatment with injured World War I (WWI) soldiers and for people affected by poliomyelitis (Cusick & Bye, 2021). The first position in Australia using the title Occupational Therapist was in a psychiatric hospital in 1934. Early occupational therapists were educated in the United States and United Kingdom (Anderson & Bell, 1988).

Significant milestones: The first Australian OT education program, established during WWII, responded to increased demands for rehabilitation of injured soldiers. In 1945, the Australian Association of Occupational Therapists began, supporting establishment of the World Federation of Occupational Therapists (WFOT) in 1951 and hosting WFOT Congresses in 1999 and 2006.

The Australian Occupational Therapy Journal began as a bulletin for OTs during the 1940s, becoming a professional journal in 1952 (Cusick & Bye, 2021). During the 1980s and 1990s, development of research was promoted, along with postgraduate study and doctoral programs.

Since 2012, the Health Practitioner Regulation National Law requires all occupational therapists to be registered with the Occupational Therapy Board of Australia (OTBA).

Current status: More than 25,600 occupational therapists are registered to practice in Australia (OTBA, 2021). Areas of work are diverse, with pediatrics, aged care, rehabilitation, disability, and mental health as significant fields. Professional education programs are now offered by 19 universities, and opportunities for postgraduate qualifications and research are expanding. Inspired by Aboriginal and Torres Strait Islander occupational therapists, the profession identifies priorities as developing strengths-based approaches to practice, reconciliation, and cultural safety across the profession (Occupational Therapy in Australia, 2021; Ryall et al., 2021).

References

Anderson, B., & Bell, J. (1988). *Occupational therapy: Its place in Australia's history.* Association of Occupational Therapists.

Cusick, A., & Bye, R. (2021). History of Australian occupational therapy. In T. Brown, H. M. Bourke-Taylor, S. Isbel, R. Cordier, & L. Gustafsson (Eds.), *Occupational therapy in Australia: Professional and practice issues* (2nd ed., pp. 31–49). Routledge.

Occupational Therapy Board of Australia. (2021). *Registrant data reporting period: 01 April 2021 to 30 June 2021.* https://www.occupationaltherapyboard.gov.au/About/Statistics.aspx

Occupational Therapy in Australia. (2021). *Reconciliation.* https://otaus.com.au/about/reconciliation

Ryall, J., Ritchie, T., Butler, C., Ryan, A., & Gibson, C. (2021). Decolonising occupational therapy through a strengths-based approach. In T. Brown, H. M. Bourke-Taylor, S. Isbel, R. Cordier, & L. Gustafsson (Eds.), *Occupational therapy in Australia: Professional and practice issues* (2nd ed., pp. 130–142). Routledge.

Occupational Therapy in Chile

Erna Navarrete Salas, OT, MSc

Beginnings: OT began in Chile in 1963. This occurred through collaboration of a commission of Chilean academic and government authorities with the World Health Organization (WHO) to focus on the provision of rehabilitation services and the training of specialized professionals, including occupational and physical therapists (WHO & Candau, 1964). An American OT educator from Illinois, Beatriz Wade, provided guidance in the creation of an experimental training program for the region. Subsequently, an agreement between the University of Chile and the Pan American Health Office (PAHO) led to the creation of a cooperative educational program for occupational therapists, enabling students from Chile to train in Argentina.

Significant milestones: In its early years, OT theory and practice was focused on biomedical matters; later in 1990, emphasis was placed on human occupation.

In 1995, the creation of a 5-year bachelor's degree in the science of human occupation was officially introduced at the University of Chile. Since 2001, the School of Occupational Therapy has edited the *Chilean Journal of Occupational Therapy*, a scientific publication for the development of OT research in Chile and the world.

Current status: Today, OT practice in Chile has diversified beyond biomedicine to focus on community needs. As essential agents of change, over 7,400 occupational therapists apply person-centered practice that also advocates for human rights related to social inclusion and participation. Chilean therapists are preparing to meet the special needs of a growing population of older adults, as well as vulnerable populations created by poverty, migration, and natural disasters.

References

World Health Organization & Candau, M. G. (1964). *The work of WHO, 1963: Annual report of the Director-General to the World Health Assembly and to the United Nations.* World Health Organization. https://apps.who.int/iris/handle/10665/85765

Occupational Therapy in Germany

Sandra Schiller, PhD

Beginnings: Productive occupation was used in the treatment of German WWI veterans. In the 1920s, psychiatrist Hermann Simon propagated active engagement in occupation as a rehabilitative approach in mental institutions. The first training course for occupational

EXPANDING OUR PERSPECTIVES (*continued*)

therapists was offered in (West) Germany in 1947 with support of the British Red Cross (Junge et al., 2019).

Significant milestones: The German Association of Occupational Therapy was founded in 1954, joining WFOT as its 12th member in 1958, and the first professional journal for German occupational therapists (*Ergotherapie und Rehabilitation*) appearing in 1961. Working areas expanded in the 1970s and 1980s to include general and specialist hospitals; special needs education; geriatric institutions; medical, social, and vocational rehabilitation; and private practice (Marquardt, 2004). The 1977 legislation regulating the education and practice of OT enabled more autonomy from the medical profession. In the 1990s, engagement with English-language practice models and theories created an interest in the theoretical foundations of OT based on the profession's origins in social science. The first university-based education program was introduced in 2001. In the new millennium, practice areas like school-based OT, workplace health promotion, and social OT started to develop. The German Occupational Science group (dOS) was founded in 2017 and the German Society for Occupational Therapy Science (DGETW) in 2018.

Current status: There are over 60,000 practicing occupational therapists in Germany, almost half of them in private practice (Council of Occupational Therapists for the European Countries, 2019). Future developments include completion of the shift to university-based education, increased demand for OT owing to demographic changes, and a growing relevance for e-health and community-based services.

References

Council of Occupational Therapists for the European Countries. (2019). *Stat planet program with COTEC statistics: Practising OTs in your country.* https://www.coteceurope.eu/Statplanet/StatPlanet.html

Junge, I., Longrée, A., & Weber, B. (2019). Entwicklung des Berufes in Deutschland [Development of the profession in Germany]. In M. le Granse, M. van Hartingsveldt, & A. Kinébanian (Eds.), *Grundlagen der Ergotherapie* [*Foundations of occupational therapy*] (pp. 55–48). Thieme.

Marquardt, M. (2004). *Geschichte der Ergotherapie: 1954 bis 2004* [*History of occupational therapy: 1954 to 2004*]. Schulz-Kirchner.

Occupational Therapy in Ghana

Eric Nkansah Opoku, BSc (OT), MSc (OT)

Beginnings: The establishment of OT in Ghana dates back to the 1960s when selected psychiatric nurses were sponsored by the Ghana Ministry of Health (MOH) to study OT in the United Kingdom. They returned on completion to establish OT services in psychiatry until the 1980s when the OTs left the profession because of underfunding and low staff morale. OT services remained absent in the Ghana health system until 2010 when the MOH collaborated with the University of Ghana to start an OT undergraduate program. The 4-year program started in 2012, with a first cohort of 18 students graduating in 2016 (Opoku et al., 2021).

Significant milestones: The Ghana OT program received WFOT approval in 2016 and is currently the only WFOT-approved program in West Africa. Five cohorts have graduated, been licensed, and are practicing in settings, including hospitals, schools, nongovernmental organizations (NGOs), communities, and academia. The presence of OTs in the health system compelled the government to start a 3-year diploma in OT program in 2017 to train OT assistants (OTAs). In addition, the Occupational Therapy Association of Ghana (OTAG) was started in 2014 and became a full member of WFOT in 2016.

Current status: Currently, one university and one training college educate OT undergraduate students and OTA students, respectively. There are 52 OTs and 62 OTAs, with all being members of OTAG. Awareness creation and employment advocacy have been the Association's main focus over the years, alongside developing a research base to inform OT practice that is culturally relevant to the Ghanaian population.

Reference

Opoku, E. N., Van Niekerk L., & Khuabi, L.-A. J.-N. (2021). Exploring the transition from student to health professional by the first cohort of locally trained occupational therapists in Ghana. *Scandinavian Journal of Occupational Therapy*, 1–12. https://doi.org/10.1080/11038128.2020.1865448

Occupational Therapy in Iran

Mehdi Rassafiani, BOccThy, MSc, PhD

Beginnings: The WHO delegate Britta Pagh Jensen established OT in Tehran in 1971 at the Shafa rehabilitation hospital. Within 2 years, OT grew rapidly by attracting lecturers such as Fathiyeh Mezeo and establishing the School of Social Welfare and Rehabilitation Sciences in Tehran in 1973.

Significant milestones: At the time of formation, the primary focus of OT practice was on mental health, orthopedics, and vocational rehabilitation (Rassafiani et al., 2013). The Iranian Revolution in 1979 delayed OT in the early stages of its development. Following the revolution, many lecturers left the country and OT admission halted. Two years later, OT education resumed successfully. There were an additional Association of Occupational Therapy in 1994 and the approval of OT practitioners to

(*continued*)

EXPANDING OUR PERSPECTIVES (*continued*)

work independently in private sectors by the MOH in 2003. Iran became a full member of the WFOT in 2006 and established master's and PhD programs in 1991 and 2008, respectively (Rassafiani et al., 2018).

Current status: Currently, 14 universities across the country educate undergraduate and graduate (master's and PhD) students in OT. Occupational therapists work in settings such as hospitals, schools, communities, and NGOs. There are also several companies that produce therapeutic tools and equipment. Research and publication addressing the needs of local people with disabilities has grown alongside current practice.

References

Rassafiani, M., Sahaf, R., & Yazdani, F. (2018). Occupational therapy in Iran: Past, present, and future. *Annals of International Occupational Therapy, 1*(1), 49–56. https://doi.org/10.3928/24761222-20180212-04

Rassafiani, M., Zeinali, R., Sahaf, R., & Malekpour, M. (2013). Occupational therapy in Iran: Historical review. *Iranian Rehabilitation Journal, 11*(1), 81–84. http://irj.uswr.ac.ir/article-1-381-en.html

Occupational Therapy in Japan

Etsuko Odawara, PhD, OTR

Beginnings: After WWII, the government incorporated Western models to develop the Japanese national medical and welfare system. In the 1960s, an OT education and licensure system was started as a rehabilitation medicine profession.

Significant milestones: Originally based on knowledge and skills from the United States, the practice of OT increased rapidly, especially in medically based practice for physical disabilities. In 1970s, reimbursement was accepted, and the profession became protected as a medical-related profession working for social needs (Suzuki, 1986). OT moved from 3-year professional schools into universities in the 1990s. Higher-level OT education including master's and PhD programs began. The Japanese Association of Occupational Therapists' (JAOT) current definition of OT is occupation and community centered, which differs significantly from the legal, reductionistic definition dating to the 1960s.

Current status: According to Japanese Association of Occupational Therapy (JAOT) (2019), there were 94,255 registered occupational therapists in Japan, with 66% of them being the members of JAOT. The ratio of male-to-female occupational therapists is higher than any other nation. Although Japan's population has the world's largest percentage of older adults, the average age of Japanese occupational therapists is just over 30 years. Although JAOT emphasizes the importance of supporting people's participation in community daily life, more than 50% of therapists work in hospital-based physical disability practice and only 12% work in medical and community welfare

for the older adults, a critical need in Japan (Kondo, 2019). Developing an understanding of occupation-centered OT among the government, other professions, and people in our communities is vital for the future of OT in Japan.

References

Kondo, T. (2019). History and current practice of occupational therapy in Japan. *Annals of International Occupational Therapy, 2*(1), 43–52. https://doi.org/10.3928/24761222-20181116-01

Suzuki, A. (1986). *Nihon ni okeru sagyo ryoho no rekishi* [*History of occupational therapy education in Japan*]. Hokkaidou Daigaku Tosho Kanko Kai.

Occupational Therapy in the United Kingdom

Edward Duncan, PhD, BSc (Hons), Dip. CBT MRCOT

Beginnings: OT in the United Kingdom is rooted in the Enlightenment, which dominated European discourse during the 17th and 18th centuries. The Enlightenment stimulated the arts and crafts (1880s–1920s) and moral treatment (1900s) movements, which aimed to restore life balance and provide more humane care for people with mental illness. Both movements created a context in which meaningful occupation was valued as a means to influence health.

Significant milestones: OT's formal development was pioneered after WWI by Dr David Henderson, a Scottish psychiatrist. In 1924, Dr Elisabeth Casson heard Dr Henderson speak about OT, and by 1930, she had opened the first OT school in England. In 1932, an association of occupational therapists was formed in Scotland; with a similar association for the rest of the United Kingdom formed in 1938. The National Health Service was established in 1948, and in 1974, the two associations merged into the British Association of Occupational Therapists. In 1978, the College of Occupational Therapists was formed to address educational, professional, and research issues, becoming the Royal College of Occupational Therapists in 2017.

Current status: There are various routes to becoming an occupational therapist in the United Kingdom: an undergraduate honors degree, a postgraduate degree or diploma, or a degree-level apprenticeship. In 2020, there were approximately 52,400 occupational therapists in the United Kingdom (Statista, 2022). They work in physical and mental health hospital and community settings, social care, charitable organizations, public health, and universities (Perryman-Fox & Cox, 2020).

References

Perryman-Fox, M., & Cox, D. L. (2020). Occupational therapy in the United Kingdom: Past, present, and future. *Annals of International Occupational Therapy, 3*(3), 144–151. https://doi.org/10.3928/24761222-20200309-03

Statista. (2022). *Annual number of occupational therapists in the United Kingdom (UK) from 2010 to 2021*. Retrieved September 18, 2020, from https://www.statista.com/statistics/318909/numbers-of-occupational-therapists-in-the-uk/

Why Study History?

Students often ask about the relevance of history. After all, they reason that their studies should focus on the future because education should prepare them for what lies ahead. Yet, they also often wonder why seemingly illogical or inexplicable conditions exist.

The answer is that the study of history helps provide explanations for why important events occurred and how current situations evolved to their present state. History illustrates that conditions change, often quickly and dramatically, because of unexpected or calamitous events. It also shows that key people and ideas result in changes, especially when society supports them. Besides providing explanations for why change happened, an important reason to study history is that it frequently repeats itself and, therefore, provides important lessons that can help guide the decision-making for the future. Perhaps, this is the basis for the quote by author Robert Heinlein who wrote *"A generation which ignores history has no past and no future"* (Heinlein, 1987, p. 223).

What Is a Contextual History?

Of course, events happen in larger contexts. History shows that ideas that take hold may benefit from timing, the chance good fortune that is sometimes described "as being in the right place at the right time." The factors that have influenced OT during its history were not always related to healthcare, yet they helped shape attitudes and beliefs that made people and societies more or less amenable to ideas, innovations, and supportive actions. By providing a description of the contexts for events, historians offer *possible* explanations for why events occurred when and how they did. These explanations are of value if people are to derive lessons from the past. To present histories without contexts and without critical examination is to potentially oversimplify events and to miss opportunities to learn from them (Molke, 2009).

The Periods Covered by This Chapter

The periods identified for this chapter include 1700 to 1899 (a prehistory), 1900 to 1919, 1920 to 1939, 1940 to 1959, 1960 to 1979, 1980 to 1999, 2000 to 2019, and 2020 to present. Because the people, ideas, contexts, and events influencing OT during each time period varied significantly in their importance, no two eras can claim equivalent impact on the profession.

Bing (1981) identified the Age of Enlightenment as an especially fruitful time in the generation of ideas that influenced OT. Thus, we begin our chapter with a "prehistory" that explains the ideas from that age that ultimately led to the birth of the profession.

Occupational Therapy Prehistory: 1700 to 1899

Historical Context

During the first hundred years of this period in Western Civilization (roughly 1700–1799), significant social movements occurred that challenged authority and conventional thinking. This "age of enlightenment" marked the beginning of logical thinking as a trustworthy way of knowing (Paine, 1794). Great artists, composers, and thinkers in history flourished. The concepts of egalitarianism and idealism emerged, and the corruption, abuses, and intolerance of the church and state were challenged. Ideas broadened through intellectual discourse, conducted through regular social gatherings called salons and in academic societies (Sawhney, 2013). With the beginning of the Industrial Revolution, methods of mass production led to the printing and wide distribution of books, helping to spread ideas broadly (Hackett, 1992).

Industrialization brought new opportunities, yet it also brought resistance to mass production and a new respect for individual craftsmanship (Levine, 1987). Increased human migration during the era overwhelmed social infrastructures. Such migration, particularly in Great Britain and the United States, brought people from rural areas to the cities looking for work, often resulting in overcrowding and unsanitary living environments (Wilcock & Hocking, 2015). Many migrants, including children, took jobs in factories, and the exploitation that took place resulted in demands for reform, leading to many calls for reforms in labor practices, affecting women and children, workplace safety, and compensation for injuries (Hofstadter, 1955).

In the United States, this period also witnessed a collision of moral values and economic traditions that led to a civil war. Tensions between moral values and economics have recurred at several points in American history. These tensions continue to influence OT because its philosophy is strongly anchored in romanticism and transcendentalism, whose American proponents in the 19th century included abolitionists and advocates for women's rights (Christiansen, 2021).

Nowhere has this moral influence been more significant than in treatment for persons with mental illness. During the late 18th century, dramatic changes in how people with mental illness were viewed resulted in more humane treatment, first in Europe and later in the United States (Whiteley, 2004). An emerging belief influencing this change was that the "insane" were people reacting to difficult life situations and, therefore, must be treated with compassion (Gordon, 2009).

Although often associated with mental illness, moral treatment was also applied to physical illness because health and illness had been viewed as related to patient character and spiritual development (Luchins, 2001). This emergence of humanitarian treatment influenced the development of therapeutic communities and the emphasis on engagement of groups in productive activities (Whiteley, 2004).

The ideas of moral treatment also influenced social services, as exemplified by the settlement house movement. The settlement house movement originated in London at Toynbee Hall in 1884 (Harvard University Library, n.d.), a residence where middle-class men and women lived collectively with the goal to share knowledge, skills, and resources with the poor and those less educated living nearby (Wade, 2005). It quickly spread to the United States, first at Coit Hall in New York and later at Hull House established in Chicago by Jane Addams and Ellen Gates Starr in 1889 (Harvard University Library, n.d.). Funded through philanthropy, Hull House aimed to create opportunity, participation, and dignity for those served and also became a center for social activism (Carson, 1990). Volunteer workers often lived in the settlement house communities and taught crafts and other practical skills of living. A related and concurrent development, called the arts and crafts movement, also began in Britain and sought to counter the negative consequences of industrialization by encouraging a return to artistic design and the unique and genuine appeal of handmade articles (Levine, 1987). Both the settlement house and arts and crafts movements, originating in Europe, influenced the use of curative occupations in mental illness, and this ultimately led to the birth of OT.

People and Ideas Influencing Occupational Therapy

In his Eleanor Clarke Slagle lecture, Bing (1981) recounted many of the historical figures and ideas of the 18th and 19th centuries that he believed influenced the founding of OT. The figures he identified from the 18th century were John Locke, Philippe Pinel, and William Tuke. From the 19th century, Bing identified Adolf Meyer as a key figure.

John Locke, a physician and philosopher who lived in the late 17th century, is credited with advancing many ideas that later influenced the philosophy and practices of OT, including sensory learning and pragmatism (Faiella, 2006).

Philippe Pinel, a physician and superintendent of the Bicetre and Salpetriere asylums in Paris, is widely regarded as a pioneer for more humanitarian treatment. His work continues to have influence today as he advocated for occupation-based structured individualized treatment, which was a key emphasis of the moral treatment era (Fogan & Smith, 2019).

William Tuke, an English philanthropist who founded the York retreat, is credited with being the father of the

moral treatment movement. Tuke was appalled by the inhumane conditions he observed in asylums and sought a more compassionate approach to mental health treatment. He eliminated restraints and physical punishment and encouraged conditions where patients could learn self-control and improve self-esteem through participation in leisure and work activities (Digby, 1985; Stanley, 2010).

Adolf Meyer, a Swiss-educated physician who emigrated to the United States in 1892 and became head of an asylum in Kankakee, Illinois, introduced the concept of individualized treatment and began a long career of innovation and leadership in American psychiatry, emphasizing the importance of understanding the key events in the life history of each patient (Figure 2.1; Christiansen, 2007). While on a trip to the Chicago World's Fair in 1893, Meyer injured his leg and, during a brief convalescence in the city, visited Hull House. This experience was thought to influence Meyer's thinking about the connections between daily occupations and mental illness. These concepts appeared in an important paper ("the philosophy of occupation therapy") he would deliver three decades later at an early meeting of the newly created American Occupational Therapy Association (AOTA) (Lief, 1948; Meyer, 1922).

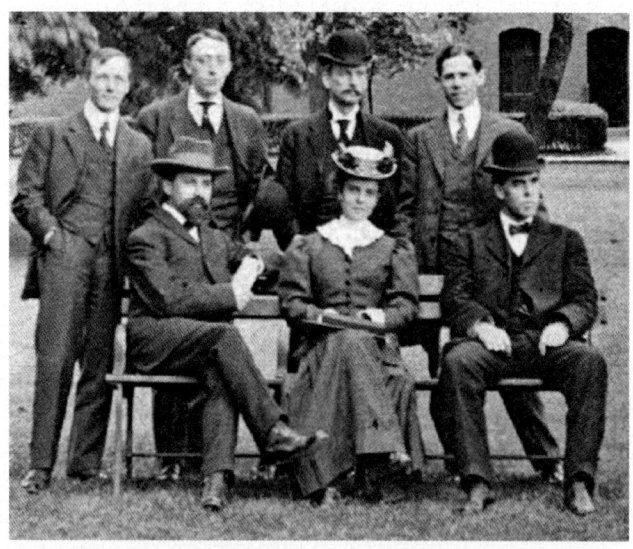

FIGURE 2.1 Dr Adolf Meyer (seated at far left), a Swiss immigrant known as the father of American Psychiatry, is shown with his staff at the Eastern Illinois Asylum at Kankakee, Illinois, around 1895. Dr Meyer later became the head of psychiatry at Johns Hopkins University and was a strong advocate for occupational therapy (OT) after its founding. His philosophy paper on OT, delivered at the Fifth Annual Meeting of the American Occupational Therapy Association, continues to be widely cited even today.

(Photo credit: Meyer Collection, Allen Chesney Memorial Library, Johns Hopkins University. Used with permission.)

Influences on the Evolution of Occupational Therapy

During OT's prehistory, the seeds had clearly been planted for the ideas that would lead to the founding of the profession. However, by 1899, its time had not yet come. In fact, the rise of large public asylums teeming with inmates, the shortage of well-trained physicians, and cost concerns led to a standard of care that fell far short of the individualized treatment and conditions idealized by the moral treatment movement. The ideas that eventually formed the beginning of the Society for the Promotion of Occupational Therapy would need to be nurtured and applied by several different people in diverse settings before the profession of OT would take root in the United States.

1900 to 1919

Historical Context

The first two decades of the 20th century in the United States and Europe marked a period of great optimism, driven by innovation and growing prosperity. The century began with the assassination of US President McKinley by an anarchist protesting corruption and social inequities tied to industrialization. McKinley was succeeded by his vice president, Theodore Roosevelt, an intelligent and audacious reformer. Although he was from a privileged background, Roosevelt was a populist who supported worker rights and consumer protection, fought cartels, started the Panama Canal project, created a powerful navy, lobbied for legislative rights of women, and established a national park system to preserve federal lands (Brinkley, 2009; Cordery, 2018).

This progressive era included leadership by Presidents William Taft and Woodrow Wilson, each of whom was a highly educated and task-oriented leader. Overall, significant social progress, including reforms in public health, education, and mental health, occurred during this period; thanks to the influence of John Dewey (an educator) and William James (a psychologist), both of whom were supporters of pragmatism (Schutz, 2011). Pragmatism advanced the belief that the value of an idea should be determined by the real-life consequences that resulted from it. The educational idea of learning through doing arose from this belief. This "thoughts into actions" practical perspective had a significant influence on how OT evolved (Ikiugu & Nissen, 2021).

The 19th Amendment of the US Constitution, ratified in 1920, afforded women the right to vote, providing a springboard for the advancement of women in American society (Pollitt, 2018). Owing to the preponderance of women in OT, the suffrage movement was significant for the profession.

Three years earlier, in 1917, after a period of neutrality and unsuccessful efforts to broker peace, the United States was drawn into WWI (the "The Great War"), a world conflict that began in 1914 and ended on November 11, 1918. Overall, WWI resulted in an estimated 40 million casualties, including around 20 million deaths and slightly more wounded (Mougel, 2011). As American soldiers prepared for battle, the War Department, at the request of General John J. Pershing, mobilized plans for the care of wounded soldiers whose disabilities would require rehabilitation and vocational reeducation (collectively called *reconstruction* at the time) to return them to civilian employment (Andersen & Reed, 2017). Importantly, the reconstruction aide "experiment" was deemed a success, thus assuring that reconstruction aides (and later a field called *rehabilitation*) would have a permanent place within American healthcare.

People and Ideas Influencing Occupational Therapy (1900–1919)

In 1910, educator Abraham Flexner completed a report on medical education for the Carnegie Foundation. His critical finding that most medical schools were substandard led to the closing of many "storefront" schools. His report recommended that only medical schools affiliated with large universities be recognized (Beck, 2004). The Flexner report ultimately led to increased emphasis on research and greater public awareness about the connection between science and its applications in healthcare. Although once considered the "father of modern medical education," in recent years, his work has received increased scrutiny by the Association of American Medical Colleges because of its racist and sexist content (Redford, 2020). Although Flexner's report led to many useful reforms, it also resulted in the closing of many medical schools and restricted opportunities for Black and women physicians (Redford, 2020; Steinecke & Terrell, 2010).

Flexner's standardization of American medical curricula emphasized science to the exclusion of social determinants of health, leading many to see it as dangerously myopic (Kielhofner & Burke, 1977; Matathia & Tello, 2020). Yet, even before Flexner, public sentiment supporting more holistic views of medicine and health was being expressed.

One such movement was Emmanuelism, started by an Episcopal minister named Elwood Worcester in Boston (Andersen & Reed, 2017; Quiroga, 1995). The Emmanuel movement was patient centered, holistic, community based, and comprehensive, involving social services and lay practitioners. In 1909, public awareness of the movement increased with a series of articles in the widely popular weekly magazine, *Ladies Home Journal* (Quiroga, 1995). This increased visibility brought criticism from conservative physicians, who questioned its church-based delivery and its use of lay practitioners (Williams, 1909).

During this period, Massachusetts-based physician **Herbert J. Hall** adopted a work-based approach for treating *neurasthenia*, a functional nervous disorder resulting in fatigue and listlessness thought to be caused by the stress of societal change and the new cultural emphasis on productivity and efficiency (Beard, 1880). Hall agreed that the "rest cure" (popular at the time) was the wrong treatment for neurasthenia. Instead, Hall's "work cure" at the Marblehead sanatorium in Massachusetts sought to actively engage patients in activities, such as weaving, basketry, and pottery, taught by skilled artisans, such as Jessie Luther, who had worked at Hull House in Chicago (S. H. Anthony, 2005). The new "work cure" approach became a suitable response to calls for improved mental healthcare. The "work cure" was also adopted at the Adams Nervine Asylum in Jamaica Plain, Massachusetts, where nurse **Susan E. Tracy** was hired to train nurses and develop an active approach for treating patients (Quiroga, 1995).

In 1910, Tracy wrote the first book on therapeutic use of occupations, sometimes referred to as the "work cure approach," called *Studies in Invalid Occupation* (Tracy, 1910). Although primarily a craft book, Tracy's work applied the ideas of William James's pragmatism and led to her involvement in the first course on occupations for patients in a general hospital setting at the Massachusetts General Hospital (Quiroga, 1995).

Tracy's book influenced **William Rush Dunton, Jr.,** a psychiatrist practicing at the Sheppard and Enoch Pratt Asylum in Baltimore, to teach his own course on occupations and recreations for nurses working there. In 1912, Dunton was placed in charge of programs in occupation and later wrote his own book on OT (Andersen & Reed, 2017). Dunton's enthusiasm was such that he later became a significant advocate and leader in developing the OT profession.

In 1908, **Clifford Beers,** a Yale-educated businessman wrote *A Mind That Found Itself,* a critical account of his treatment for mental illness in an asylum and his eventual recovery (Beers, 1908). His book spurred reforms in mental healthcare that led to the creation of the mental hygiene movement and emphasis on prevention and treatment outside asylums.

By 1910, many state mental hospitals were using occupations as a regular part of their treatment. Under the auspices of Hull House in Chicago and influenced by the mental hygiene movement, coursework in occupations and amusements for attendants at public hospitals and asylums began under the newly formed Chicago School of Civics and Philanthropy (Loomis, 1992; Quiroga, 1995).

Eleanor Clarke Slagle, a student at the school in a course called *curative occupations and recreations,* believed that the principles taught there could be applied usefully to idle patients in the state mental hospital at Kankakee,

Illinois (Christiansen, 2007; Quiroga, 1995). Slagle's interest in curative occupations led to an invitation by Adolf Meyer to develop a curative occupations therapy program at the prominent Phipps Clinic at Johns Hopkins University. There, she collaborated with Dr William Rush Dunton, Jr., at the nearby Sheppard and Enoch Pratt Asylum (Andersen & Reed, 2017).

Meanwhile, in 1912, Elwood Worcester of Boston, one of the founders of the Emmanuelism movement, was invited to the Clifton Springs Sanitarium in upstate New York to teach courses to the patients there. One of the patients was an architect, **George Edward Barton**, who was recovering from tuberculosis and hysterical paralysis. Barton was so influenced by his personal benefit from the work cure that he became an advocate for using occupations in the recovery of physical illness. Upon his discharge, from the sanitarium, he studied nursing at the facility's school and opened "Consolation House," a convalescence center through which he hoped to apply the ideas of the emerging curative occupation ("work cure") philosophy (Figure 2.2; Andersen & Reed, 2017; Quiroga, 1995).

Barton corresponded with prominent advocates for curative occupations, including Susan Tracy, **Susan Cox Johnson,** and William Rush Dunton, Jr. Johnson was an arts and crafts teacher who had gained recognition from a book on textile studies and later from her work with patients with tuberculosis and nervous disorder as director of occupations for public hospitals in New York City (Anderson & Reed, 2017). From 1914 to 1917, Barton wrote articles and developed plans for establishing a profession dedicated to

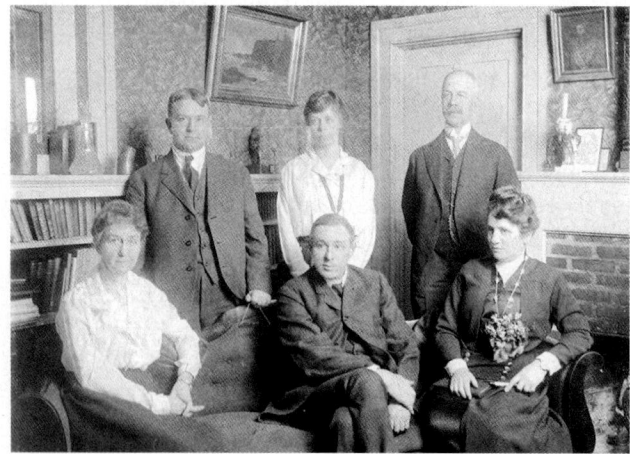

FIGURE 2.2 Society for the Promotion of Occupational Therapy Founders at Consolation House, Clifton Springs, New York, March 1917. Front row (left to right): Susan Cox Johnson, George Edward Barton, and Eleanor Clarke Slagle. Back row (left to right): William Rush Dunton, Jr., Isabel Newton, and Thomas Bessell Kidner.

(Photo credit: Archives of AOTA, Wilma L. West Library, AOTF, Bethesda, MD. Used with permission.)

the use of occupations in therapy. Dr Dunton assisted him, but Barton was initially hesitant to involve physicians, fearing that his own lack of medical credentials might diminish his role. In March 1917, the organizing meeting of the Society for the Promotion of Occupational Therapy was hosted by George Barton at Consolation House in Clifton Springs, New York (Andersen & Reed, 2017; Bing, 1961).

In attendance at that meeting were George Barton, Isabel Newton (his secretary and future wife), William Rush Dunton, Jr., Eleanor Clarke Slagle, Susan Cox Johnson, and Thomas Kidner, an expert from Canada assisting the US government to plan vocational rehabilitation programs for wounded soldiers (Friedland & Davids-Brumer, 2007; Friedland & Silva, 2008). Susan Tracy of Massachusetts had been invited but was not able to attend (Andersen & Reed, 2017). The participants at Consolation House drew up a charter of incorporation, drafted a constitution for the new society, named committees, planned for an annual conference, and elected officers, with Barton as the inaugural president and Slagle as the vice president (Andersen & Reed, 2017).

After the loss of American citizens with the sinking of the ocean liner *Lusitania* by German submarines, the United States entered WWI. The War Department, mindful of its terrible casualties, undertook careful planning to prepare for the wounded and disabled soldiers who would return from combat (Andersen & Reed, 2017; Quiroga, 1995).

Developments in Occupational Therapy (1900–1919)

During its mobilization planning for WWI, the United States anticipated the need for a significant number of facilities and rehabilitation workers. Although there were efforts to recruit men to these roles, the military soon realized that women could be recruited and be trained to support the effort (Crane, 1927, p. 57). Some existing programs for curative occupations added courses to meet the anticipated standards of the surgeon general, whereas others were established in large east coast cities explicitly for the war effort (Andersen & Reed, 2017; Quiroga, 1995).

Success in quickly establishing these important war training courses for reconstruction aides was made possible through the efforts of committed and prominent individuals who were able to organize the financial and political resources necessary to establish high-quality schools (Andersen & Reed, 2017; Quiroga, 1995). For various reasons, it was decided that a division of roles would be necessary with some reconstruction aides assigned to do orthopedic work, corrective exercise, and massage, whereas others, who became occupational therapists, provided handicrafts and support for "shell shock" that resulted from the stressful conditions of trench warfare, poisonous gas, and constant explosions from artillery (Low, 1992; see Figure 2.3).

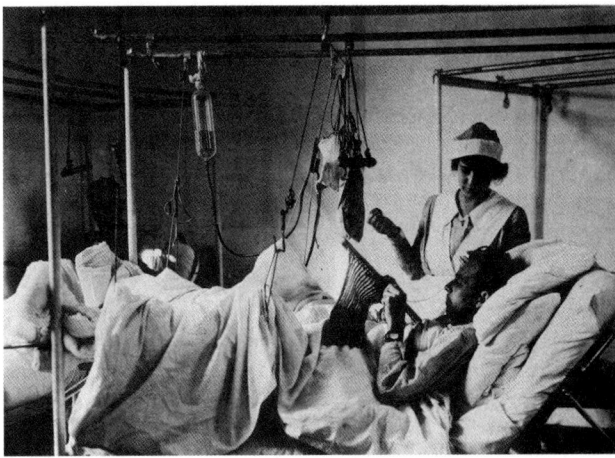

FIGURE 2.3 **Reconstruction aide providing bedside occupational therapy with a wounded soldier at Hospital 9, Chateauroux, France, during World War I.**

(Photo credit: Image Archive, History of Medicine Collection, National Library of Medicine.)

Despite the success in recruiting and training qualified reconstruction aides for the war effort, the initial placement of these trained aides proved to be difficult because some physicians continued to view OT as a fad, failing to appreciate that it could have a worthwhile role in the treatment of wounded soldiers. However, after OT reconstruction aides achieved success at base hospitals in France, attitudes began to change (Andersen & Reed, 2017; Low, 1992; Quiroga, 1995).

By November 1918, when Germany and its allies surrendered, at least 200 reconstruction aides were serving in 20 base hospitals in France (Quiroga, 1995). The war ended on November 11, 1918. Between 1917 and January 1, 1920, nearly 148,000 sick and wounded men were treated upon their return to the United States at 53 reconstruction hospitals (Office of the Surgeon General, 1918). The military specifications governing OT for returning soldiers declared that it should have a purely medical function and be prescribed for the early stages of convalescence to occupy the soldier's minds. Even at this early date, there was a lack of clarity and considerable ambiguity in the roles and functions of the reconstruction aides providing OT. However, leadership in the newly formed professional association for OT, which was now known as the American Occupational Therapy Association (AOTA), provided wise advocacy for the recruitment of high-quality trainees.

Dr William Rush Dunton, Jr. succeeded George Barton as the president of AOTA in 1917, and his friend Eleanor Clarke Slagle later succeeded him in the role. This provided a period of thoughtful and successful leadership that helped the new profession gain momentum and legitimacy after the war (Quiroga, 1995).

1920 to 1939

Historical Context

As the Treaty of Versailles following WWI was negotiated by the allies, President Woodrow Wilson proposed 14 principles for lasting peace including a standing body called the League of Nations where peaceful resolution of disputes could prevent such wars from recurring (Heckscher, 1991). Wilson was successful in getting these terms into the treaty, but he suffered a severe stroke and the US Congress never ratified them, reportedly because Wilson refused to compromise on minor details of the ratification (Eubank, 2004). The harsh conditions and reparations imposed on Germany at Versailles and the absence of US leadership to organize the League of Nations are viewed as contributing to political instabilities in Europe, economic shifts, and a rise in nationalism, which led to mistrust between various nations. Eventually, the rise of fascist leadership in Germany and Italy and additional tensions foreshadowed Hitler's decision to invade Poland in September 1939 and begin what was to become WWII (Zaloga, 2004).

Within the United States, the period from 1920 to 1939 framed the continuation of significant societal transformations as women asserted their right to vote. The first decade of this period is sometimes called the "roaring twenties" because the advancements of the era in manufacturing, transportation, and communication encouraged a sense of optimism and excess (Cooper, 1990). Profits in industry allowed increased earnings for workers, and the introduction of installment buying led to a very high level of consumerism that fueled a robust economy. Yet, new wealth encouraged widespread and irrational speculation in the stock market, which contributed to the stock market crash of 1929 and a long period of hardship that followed, known as the *Great Depression*.

In rural areas, the economic situation made more difficult by a persistent drought that was worsened in some areas by poor conservation (Egan, 2006). With unemployment at 25% and family incomes sliced in half, many people were desperate (McElvaine, 1993). President Herbert Hoover, an engineer, humanitarian, and respected administrator, was unable to contend with a crisis made worse by a financial disaster in Europe. In 1932, Franklin D. Roosevelt was elected to the first of four terms, and he quickly moved ahead with economic and social reform programs, collectively called the "New Deal" (Leuchtenburg, 1963). These included Social Security, higher taxes on the wealthy, new controls over banks and public utilities, and enormous work relief programs for the unemployed, including the Civilian Conservation Corps for rural conservation and environment projects and the Works Progress Administration focusing on constructing or repairing bridges, libraries, and public buildings (Kennedy, 1999). There were also efforts to support artists to create public murals, sculptures, and paintings and writers to produce books and plays. These government-sponsored programs contributed to the public's recognition that creative and productive activities were essential for both economic and social and psychological benefits.

People and Ideas Influencing Occupational Therapy (1920–1939)

The founders of the National Occupational Therapy Society had set events in motion for the rapid evolution of their new profession. After George Barton's abrupt resignation in 1917, **Dr William Rush Dunton, Jr.** helped to advance the new society, which was then focusing on standardizing educational programs. Dunton embraced Adolf Meyer's theory of psychobiology, which provided a commonsense approach to treating mental illness (Christiansen, 2007; Lief, 1948). Psychobiology was holistic and practical, emphasizing that mental disease was a reflective of habit disorganization in the lives of those affected. Meyer believed that humans organized time through doing things and that a balance of activities involving work and rest was essential for well-being. Both Meyer and Dunton shared the belief that occupational therapists had an important role in helping patients reorganize their daily habits and regain a sense of optimism through daily occupations. Meyer expressed these ideas in a paper given at the Fifth Annual Meeting of the AOTA held in Baltimore, Maryland, during October 1921 (Meyer, 1922).

Meyer's ideas were consistent with the emerging central beliefs of OT in that it recognized that forced idleness during convalescence was not only morally wrong but also disorienting and physically debilitating. Through engagement in occupations, Meyer asserted that patients could ward off depression and gain a sense of self-confidence that would help motivate them further (Christiansen, 2007). There were also socioeconomic reasons to normalize lives by enabling individuals to develop skills that would help them become self-sufficient.

Within psychiatry, other theoretical perspectives, including the work of Sigmund Freud, overshadowed Adolf Meyer's theory of psychobiology. Freud's emphasis on unconscious drives captured the interest of many psychiatrists as well as the general public (Burnham, 2006). Freudian psychoanalysis remained a contentious topic (Brunner, 2001), and many historians viewed the distraction it created as a scientific setback (Eysenck, 1985). Moreover, the progress made in general medicine in treating common diseases during that era led to biological explanations, such as infections, as a cause of mental illness. This led to unnecessary, unethical, and, sometimes, harmful experimental surgeries

(Scull, 2005). Electroconvulsive treatments and lobotomies began to be used with both positive and negative consequences, and these treatments remain controversial (Fink & Taylor 2007; Pressman, 1998).

The trend toward medicalization in OT that occurred in the 1920s and 1930s was purposely influenced by strategic decisions of the profession's leaders. In their quest for professional legitimacy, OT leaders perceived that there would be benefit in allying more closely with organized medicine (Andersen & Reed, 2017). The rise of physical medicine and rehabilitation as a medical speciality and leaders from that movement, especially *Frank H. Krusen, MD,* had a clear influence on the practice of occupational therapists in rehabilitation. Krusen believed that OT was simply a special application of physical therapy and that the two disciplines should merge (Krusen, 1934). This point of view had adherents in Canada, where training programs combined the theory and practices of both professions and produced graduates who, at one point, could be dually credentialed (Friedland, 2011).

During the 1920s and 1930s, the principles of OT were also viewed as beneficial in the care of persons with tuberculosis, a disease stigmatized through its association with immigrants and poverty. Thomas B. Kidner, the Canadian vocational education expert who had been a member of the AOTA founder's group, decided to remain in the United States after his temporary assignment to advise the surgeon general had concluded. Kidner, who served two separate terms as the president of AOTA, used his role as a vocational expert to plan facilities that included workspaces for OT and vocational training (Friedland & Silva, 2008).

Occupational Therapy (1920–1939)

In OT, the early part of this era was dominated by the continued "reconstruction" of wounded soldiers from WWI, which occurred at more than 50 hospitals established with reconstruction in mind (Quiroga, 1995). These facilities provided employment for occupational therapists in the early 1920s as did the curative occupation programs in place at mental hospitals (Hall, 1922).

The AOTA became an effective organization for promoting the profession through its network of members, annual meetings, and the publication of a journal under three different names (*Archives of Occupational Therapy*, *Occupational Therapy and Rehabilitation*, and *American Journal of Occupational Therapy* [now *AJOT*]) between 1917 and 1925, at which time the association had nearly 900 members listed in its registry (Dunton, 1925).

In order to continue the development and growth of the new profession during the 1920s, Eleanor Clarke Slagle, who served as president and later secretary-treasurer of the new society for 15 years, found creative ways to continue promoting the field through networking among women's clubs and the establishment of a national office in New York City (Figure 2.4; Andersen & Reed, 2017; Metaxas, 2000; Quiroga, 1995). Attendance in the association and in the society grew steadily during this time so that by 1929, there were 18 state and local OT associations and approximately 1,000 members of the AOTA (Slagle, 1934). The association leadership continued to foster stability and quality in the profession by emphasizing standards for educational programs and their graduates. The profession worked to gain legitimacy through aligning itself with other professionals, especially physicians (Andersen & Reed, 2017; Quiroga, 1995). In addition, a registry of qualified occupational therapists was published, with 318 members meeting standards to be listed in the inaugural 1932 edition (Anderson & Reed, 2017, p. 107) and eligible to use the designation OT. Reg. following their names.

In 1935, after several years of negotiation, the accreditation of OT educational programs was initiated in concert with the American Medical Association (Quiroga, 1995). The standards required that faculty be well qualified and that students complete a minimum of 100 weeks of full-time training, of which at least 36 weeks involved supervised practical training in hospitals. Curricula were required to include theoretical and lab instruction in anatomy,

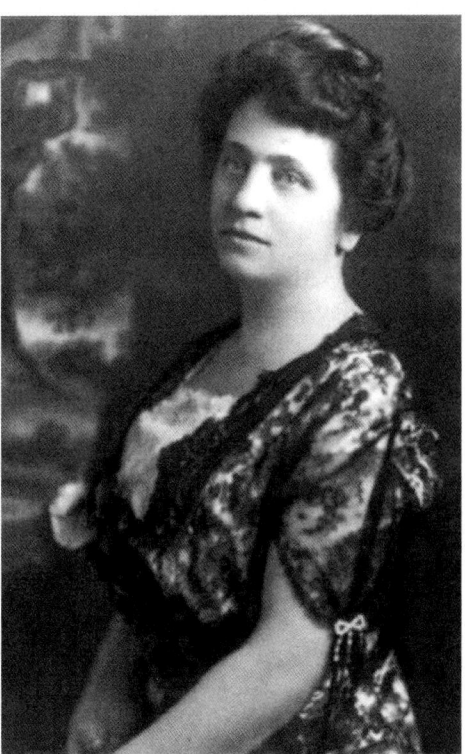

FIGURE 2.4 **Eleanor Clarke Slagle. Her work as founder and tireless leader is recognized through a prestigious lectureship named in her honor.**

(Photo credit: Archives of the AOTA, Wilma West Library, AOTF, Bethesda, MD. Used with permission.)

physiology, kinesiology, neurology, psychology, and psychiatry as well as theory in OT for treatment in a diverse range of conditions, including tuberculosis and contagious diseases, and instruction in practical occupations, including design skills and crafts involving textiles, wood, metal, leather, and plastic as well as recreational pursuits. Admitted students were required to be high school graduates and at least 21 years old at the time of course completion (Council on Medical Education and Hospitals, 1935).

During this period, male physicians dominated association leadership in OT; still, many more positions for occupational therapists were being created in specialized facilities for physical rehabilitation, mental health, and tuberculosis.

The emergence of physical medicine and rehabilitation in the mid-1930s, which had been influenced by physicians who used physical agents and practiced physical therapy, was reflected in many of the publications during this era (Slagle, 1934). Because occupational therapists assumed roles in rehabilitation units, they adopted goniometry and began adapting tools and equipment to enable patients to gain strength, endurance, and range of motion while doing crafts (Andersen & Reed, 2017).

During this period, polio epidemics and President Franklin Roosevelt's polio-related paralysis brought visibility and public awareness to the disease, leading to treatment facilities and research as well as specialized centers that employed occupational therapists and others for the care of patients. Polio epidemics peaked in 1952 and diminished after development of a vaccine by Jonas Salk a decade later (Oshinsky, 2005).

Aided by the advocacy of Thomas B. Kidner, tuberculosis hospitals had also become settings where many occupational therapists assumed roles providing recuperative, diversional, and vocational therapy for long periods of convalescence (Friedland & Silva, 2008; Kidner, 1922). The principle of activity graded to provide appropriate challenge and physical demand for patients was, by this time, a well-established part of the OT regimen in physical rehabilitation (Laird, 1923).

1940 to 1959

Historical Context

By 1940, Europe was well embroiled in turmoil; with Germany having already annexed Austria, it invaded Poland and Czechoslovakia. Those events were followed by declarations of war by Great Britain and France and German invasions of Denmark, Norway, Holland, Belgium, and France. The German Army was so dominant that it devastated French and British forces and caused their retreat at Dunkirk (Ward & Burns, 2007). Italy joined Germany,

and the war soon spread to North Africa. Meanwhile, Adolf Hitler exploited his occupation of the European continent to pursue massive genocide against the Jewish people (Bergen, 2016). In September 1940, Japan signed the Tripartite Pact, bringing together an alliance of Berlin, Rome, and Tokyo in the war (Yenne, 2020).

Despite the Neutrality Acts of the 1930s designed to prevent the United States from entering another war, the United States opposed Hitler, and when the Japanese attacked Pearl Harbor in December 1941, the United States entered WWII. With the numbers of men drafted to armed service, the severe unemployment of the late 1930s gave way to a workforce shortage that plagued all areas of industry. This led to an influx of women into the workforce. Many hospitals were understaffed and ill-equipped to meet healthcare needs of those at home as well as soldiers returning from combat. Health challenges of returning veterans included not only diseases such as tuberculosis, hepatitis, and rheumatic fever but also war injuries, including amputations and chemical wounds (Richards, 2011). Additional health challenges later discovered included exposure to environmental hazards, such as chemical hazards, extreme cold, radiation, and excessive noise (U.S. Department of Veterans Affairs, 2015).

According to the U.S. Department of Veterans Affairs (2015), WWII killed more people and was among the most devastating in history. Total estimates of global fatalities vary, but it is generally accepted that they exceeded 60 million. The economic and social effects of WWII brought changes in healthcare and the passage of a number of US legislative acts to fund research and services to returning veterans.

The Public Health Service Act gave the National Institutes of Health (NIH) permission to grant awards for nonfederal research, the GI Bill of 1944 funded efforts to aid veterans to transition back to civilian life, and in 1946, President Harry Truman signed the Mental Health Act, which was designed to provide funding for mental health services and research (Harlow, 2007). Rehabilitation expanded to assist veterans to return to work as the amendments in 1943 and 1954 of the Vocational Rehabilitation Act emphasized physical and mental restoration, leading to a rise in the development of curative workshops (Gainer, 2008).

The post-WWII era saw the start of the Cold War marked international tensions that were caused by the conflicting ideologies of Russia and Western democracies. Globally, as Japan started to rebuild post-WWII, the Korean War again brought armed forces from the United Nations (including the United States) to support the Republic of Korea (now South Korea). Postwar efforts to bring nations together included the formation of the United Nations in 1945 (United Nations, n.d.) designed to promote international peace and security and the development of the WHO in 1948 for the purposes of promoting global health and safety (WHO, n.d.).

Postwar in the 1950s, there was an increased emphasis on medical research and funding resulting in major healthcare advances, including triumph over polio, the discovery of the DNA double helix, the development of the pacemaker, and the formation of the Joint Commission on Accreditation of Healthcare Organizations (Gerber, 2007). Yet, despite these advances, there were still areas of healthcare in dire need of change. Mental health institutions were overcrowded, and the rate of alcoholism and juvenile delinquency skyrocketed (Dworkin, 2010). As the stigmatizing effects of mental illness persisted, patients and their families began organizing, and efforts were made to address concerns not only of the clients but also of their families (Brown et al., 2008). This, paired with the discovery of the antipsychotic effects of chlorpromazine (Thorazine), ushered in a new era of psychiatric treatments for those with mental illness. The reliance on pharmaceutical interventions and deinstitutionalization brought a new set of social and healthcare challenges.

Occupational Therapy (1940–1959)

Although occupational therapists did not serve overseas in WWII, US-based consultant positions were created along with emergency training programs to provide therapists for the treatment of veterans returning from war (Andersen & Reed, 2017). This was a time of immense growth and change in OT as the focus shifted from the use of arts and crafts toward rehabilitation techniques based on scientific methods, and OT was a woman-driven profession in a male-dominated scientific community of medicine (Peters, 2013). Emphasis was placed on reintegrating veterans into society; therefore, the use of activities of daily living (ADLs), ergonomics, and vocational rehabilitation gained favor in therapeutic communities (Gainer, 2008). With battlefield medicine focused on saving severely wounded soldiers, the development of prosthetics and orthotics gained momentum during this period and the US government sponsored research to improve the quality of assistive devices (Georgia Tech, 2021). Occupational therapists became involved in prosthetic training, which often entailed the use of adapted tools and involved strengthening and conditioning (Figure 2.5).

With the shift toward hospital-based therapy and the growth of rehabilitation, OT educational programs reorganized their curricula supported by the publication of the first OT textbook written in 1947 in the United States and edited by Helen Willard and Clare Spackman (Mahoney et al., 2017; Willard & Spackman, 1947). That same year, the first woman and registered occupational therapist, Winfred Kahmann, became the president of AOTA (Andersen & Reed, 2017). In 1949, guidelines for OT education were

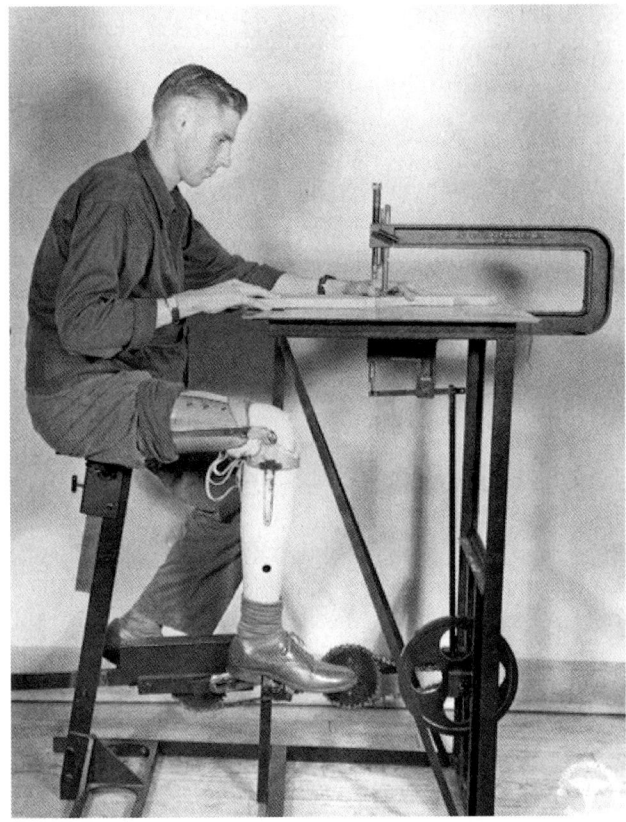

FIGURE 2.5 Bicycle jigsaw, common in physical rehabilitation occupational therapy clinics from the 1940s through the 1960s.

(Photo credit: Archives of the AOTA, Wilma L. West Library, AOTF, Bethesda, MD. Used with permission.)

expanded through the Council on Medical Education and Hospitals and the *Essentials of an Acceptable School of Occupational Therapy* were established (Council on Medical Education and Hospitals, 1950).

In 1956, OTA programs were started to help meet workforce needs, and in 1958, the AOTA took responsibility for accrediting assistant-level OT programs (AOTA, 2009). Since then, emphasis has been placed on collaborative work and education between occupational therapists and OTAs (AOTA, 2018). Although the term *certified occupational therapy assistant* did not take hold internationally, countries such as Canada, Australia, and the United Kingdom developed positions similar to the OTA in order to augment the workforce demands of the profession (Nancarrow & Mackey, 2005; Salvatori, 2001).

Globally, the number of occupational therapists continued to increase as educational programs expanded, and by 1950, there were seven OT educational courses in England and one in Scotland (Oxford Brookes University, 2011). In 1952, preliminary discussions took place for the eventual formation of the WFOT recognized in 1959 by the WHO, which was at that time just over a decade old (WFOT, 2022a).

People and Ideas Influencing Occupational Therapy (1940–1959)

Influences on the profession during this period came from OT leaders in the Army as well as from therapists working with individuals having motor paralysis. Here, we include the Bobaths (physiotherapists practicing in England), Ruth Robinson, and Margaret Rood.

Berta Bobath was a German physiotherapist, and her husband **Karel Bobath** was a Czech neuropsychiatrist. Together, they jointly developed a popular neurodevelopmental treatment (NDT), originally designed for persons with cerebral palsy but later applied to individuals with stroke or neurodevelopmental conditions. Their objective was to stimulate motor learning for efficient motor control (Conti, 2014). Although studies question the effectiveness of NDT for various populations, the Bobaths' techniques are still used by occupational and physical therapists throughout the world, and their work encouraged study of the sensory links to motor output (Levin & Panturin, 2011).

Col. Ruth A. Robinson of the US Army helped create OT educational programs for those preparing to serve in the military. Robinson proposed an accelerated training program to meet the needs for expansion during the Korean War (U.S. Army Medical Department, 2012). She continued in leadership positions, serving as the president of AOTA from 1955 to 1958 (Peters, 2011b). During her time in the Army, Col. Robinson became chief of the Army Medical Specialists Corps and served as a mentor to Wilma West and Ruth Brunyate (later Ruth Brunyate Wiemer), who later became colleagues and leaders in the AOTA.

Margaret Rood was an occupational and physical therapist credited as one of the earliest OT theorists on motor control. Rood stressed the importance of reflexes in early development and emphasized the use of facilitation and inhibition techniques, which were soon after used and expanded on by the Bobaths. In addition to clinical work, Margaret Rood took on leadership and educational positions including the development of the OT department of the University of Southern California (USC), where she served as its first chair (USC, n.d.).

1960 to 1979

Historical Context

During this period, Martin Luther King's famous speech "I had a dream" (M. L. King, 1963) symbolized decades of the civil rights movement seeking equality and justice for African Americans. This was also an era of unrest and change marked by the "cold war," a prolonged period of distrust between the Soviet Union (Union of Soviet Socialist Republics [USSR]) and the United States. This political tension led to continued division of Germany and the construction of the Berlin wall, advancements in space science as the two superpowers developed their defense technologies, the Cuban Missile Crisis, and, ultimately, a controversial war in the Vietnam War. Kennedy's decision to pursue civil rights legislation provided the foundation for President Johnson to sign the Civil Rights Act into law in 1964, protecting individual rights and freedom from discrimination in areas such as voting, education, and employment (Andrews & Gaby, 2015). Concerns were raised regarding poverty, access to healthcare, and quality education for all, leading President Johnson to institute a number of other domestic programs commonly known as the "Great Society" aimed at reducing poverty and providing increased funding in areas such as education, healthcare, and the establishment of the National Endowment for the Arts (Heath, 2017). Perhaps foremost among these was legislation in 1965, establishing Medicare and Medicaid, which provided healthcare access to millions of seniors and disabled and impoverished American citizens, many of whom previously did not have access to such care (Centers for Medicare & Medicaid Services, 2020). Similar efforts took place elsewhere during this period, with Canada instituting its federal–provincial universal coverage healthcare system in 1962 and many Western European countries instituting forms of social health insurance in the 1960s and 1970s (Saltman & Dubois, 2004).

By the 1960s, healthcare in industrialized nations modernized with updated equipment, electric beds, advanced communication systems, and innovative laboratories. The demographics of hospitalization shifted as new medicines were discovered and medical advances escalated. With the mass production of antibiotics and other pharmaceutical treatments for physical and mental health conditions, there was a move away from the treatment of acute epidemic illness (e.g., polio and smallpox) toward increased need for care of chronic conditions, such as rheumatism, arthritis, and heart conditions (U.S. Department of Health, Education, and Welfare, 1965). The rise of feminism also brought changes domestically and globally, bringing new emphasis to women's health and increased representation of women in medical schools (Rosser, 2002), yet women were still a small percentage of the medical workforce (Clancy, 2016). Health planning is increased in order to reduce duplication (Melhado, 2006), and private health insurance was widely provided by employers to compete for workers. Typically, these insurance plans had low deductibles and required little out-of-pocket cost by beneficiaries (Thomasson, 2002). This, alongside the legislation providing government payments under Medicare and Medicaid, contributed to an overuse of services and further stimulated the growth and cost of healthcare.

A move to close state institutions for the infirmed, particularly those with mental illness, caused additional challenges. The emergence of psychotropic medications paired with the overcrowding and deplorable conditions of many state hospital systems led to the deinstitutionalization movement and subsequent closure of state and psychiatric hospitals in both Canada and the United States, yet such deinstitutionalization has varied worldwide (Hudson, 2016; Koyangi, 2007). Although the aim was to contain costs and provide improved care in the community, the development of community mental health services was inadequate to address the demands (Koyangi, 2007). Many of those affected by deinstitutionalization wound up homeless or in the criminal justice systems and without adequate care (Yohanna, 2013). Efforts to shift the care for those with mental illness to the community have continued globally to the present day, yet challenges remain to provide adequate long-term care and housing.

Occupational Therapy (1960–1979)

The decades from 1960 to 1979 brought significant change to OT practice. During the reorganization of the AOTA in 1964 under the presidency of Wilma West, renewed emphasis was placed on supporting scientific endeavors in OT (Yerxa, 1967b). The board supported the idea of reorganization and expansion, and in 1965, the American Occupational Therapy Foundation (AOTF) was established to advance the science of the field and improve its public recognition (AOTA, 1969). Efforts to emphasize science and theory development led to increased graduate education in the field and later led to a proliferation of models, theories, and frames of references for practice. Continued emphasis on the legitimacy of the profession increased efforts to regulate practice through state licensure legislation as the US government, concerned about costs for outpatient therapy services, initiated the first caps on payments for services in 1972. In 1971, Puerto Rico became the first US state or territory to initiate licensure (AOTA, 2021a). Globally, WFOT received recognition as an NGO in 1963 by the United Nations (WFOT, 2022a).

The practice of OT during this period was heavily influenced by medical rehabilitation, which continued the post-WWII mechanistic paradigm, emphasizing neuromotor and musculoskeletal systems and their impact on function (Kielhofner, 2009). Advances in neuroscience motivated A. Jean Ayres to expand on the work of the Bobaths and Rood. Ayres used neuroscience to study perceptual motor issues in children and develop and apply a theory of sensory integration (Ayres, 1966, 1972). Influences on practice shifted from the holistic mind–body occupation-based philosophies to those with bottom-up approaches focusing on the underlying source of the problem, often with emphasis on reflex integration and motor function.

Various Great Society programs and the *Education for All Handicapped Children Act* (*1975*) expanded the scope and areas of practice for occupational therapists. Medicare and Medicaid laid the foundation for expanded services to the older adults, those with disabilities, and the poor, and the Education for All Handicapped Children Act mandated access to education for all children, including those with disabilities. These laws, governing provision for healthcare and educational services to expanded populations, led to an expansion of work for occupational therapists. In 1965, new guidelines were developed for accredited OT programs in the United States, and in 1967, AOTA celebrated the 50th year of OT (Andersen & Reed, 2017).

Internationally, OT was guided by theory-driven clinical models, but similar to the United States, it was also driven by the medical profession and the social and healthcare institutions because these were the main employers of occupational therapists (see Figure 2.6) (Clouston & Whitcombe, 2008). The ADL tools and adaptations were developed to accommodate for dysfunctions (Hocking, 2008), and the profession continued to emphasize scientific endeavors. There was also an increase in educational programs throughout the world, fostered in part by international efforts of representatives to the WFOT (Cockburn, 2001).

People and Ideas Influencing Occupational Therapy (1960–1979)

Mary Reilly was a clinician in the U.S. Army Medical Corps serving as a captain during the war and went on to earn her doctorate in education, serving as the chief of the

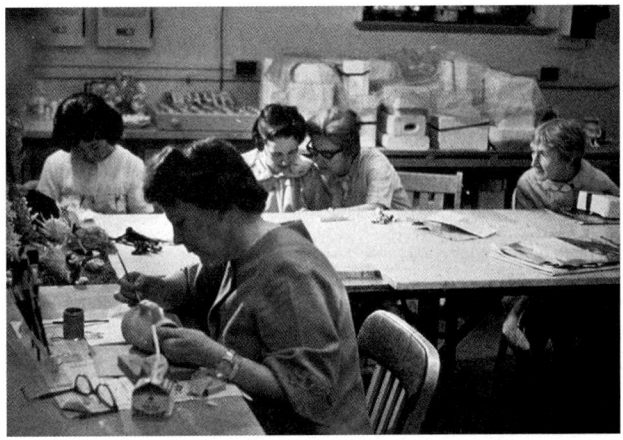

FIGURE 2.6 **Occupational therapist (with glasses, center top) with several patients doing slip cast ceramic pottery projects in an inpatient mental health facility (circa 1965).**

(Photo Credit: Image Archive. National Library of Medicine. In the public domain.)

rehabilitation department at the Neuropsychiatric Institute at the University of California, at Los Angeles. She later served as a professor and chair in OT at the USC, where she became an influential academician (USC Chan Division of Occupational Therapy, 2012). Through her graduate students, she is credited with evolving a theoretical framework known as the "occupational behavior" frame of reference, which emphasized the development of work skills and the societal importance of productive occupations. In her 1961 Eleanor Clarke Slagle lecture, Reilly challenged the profession to reclaim its roots in occupation and famously proclaimed, "Man [sic], through the use of his hands as they are energized by mind and will, can influence the state of his own health" (Reilly, 1962, p. 2).

A. Jean Ayres, an occupational therapist and licensed educational psychologist, applied neuroscience to practice. Dr Ayres was educated at the USC, where she served as a student, scientist, practitioner, and an educator. Within her research, Ayres developed tools for practice, including assessments of integrated sensory processing, later forming a battery known as the Sensory Integration and Praxis Tests (Ayres, 1989). In 1976, Ayres founded the Ayres Clinic, in which she combined teaching, research, and practice to develop her practice model of sensory integration (Kielhofner, 2009). Her theories and influence continue to present day.

Gail Fidler, graduated in 1942 from the Philadelphia School of Occupational Therapy, emphasized the use of occupation as a means for emotional expression. Fidler, a teacher and occupational therapist with a background in psychology, was influenced by her studies of interpersonal theory, self-esteem, and ego development (Miller & Walker, 1993). Gail Fidler became a leader in mental health OT, studied with her mentor Helen Willard, and worked in a settlement house while a student at the Philadelphia School of Occupational Therapy (Peters, 2011a). She and her husband wrote *Introduction to Psychiatric Occupational Therapy* (Fidler & Fidler, 1954), an early textbook that promoted the application of ego theory and therapeutic use of self in practice. Fidler's contributions include 13 books, numerous articles, and service on the executive board of AOTA (Gillette, 2005).

Ann Mosey advanced Fidler's ideas through development of the object relations/psychodynamic frame of reference, which offered concepts integral to understanding the use of activities and groups in therapy (Mosey, 1973). Other theorists also emerged at the time, increasing the theory base of OT. *Lorna Jean King* (1974) applied sensory integrative theories to persons with schizophrenia, *Claudia Allen* developed theories of cognition to guide therapy for persons with chronic mental illness (AOTA, 2019), and Kielhofner and Burke (1977) advocated an OT paradigm to refocus on human adaptation and occupation. The core concepts of this work later became the foundation of the widely recognized Model of Human Occupation (MOHO; Kielhofner & Burke, 1980).

Wilma L. West, a retired Army colonel who had served with Ruth Robinson during WWII, worked as executive director of the AOTA from 1947 to 1952 and became an influential advocate for the advancement of OT (Gillette, 1996; West, 1991). West served as the president of AOTF during its key formative years from 1972 to 1982, later becoming president emerita. She advocated strongly for the promotion of research and was instrumental in recruiting Charles Christiansen to become the founding editor of the profession's first research journal, *The Occupational Therapy Journal of Research* (*OTJR*), renamed *OTJR: Occupation, Participation and Health* in 2002. An extensive AOTF library, since discontinued, was named in her honor (Foto, 1997).

Elizabeth Yerxa, a successor to Mary Reilly, emphasized the importance of advancing theory to the benefit of practice. In her 1966 Eleanor Clarke Slagle lecture, she asserted the need for occupational therapists to take steps toward professionalism, produce research, and focus on the unique assets of the profession, including purposeful activity and the practice of authentic OT (Yerxa, 1967a). Yerxa later became involved in active promotion of research efforts and in promoting the development of occupational science as an academic discipline and foundation for practice. Yerxa retired in 1988 and was named a distinguished professor emerita at the USC.

Lela A. Llorens became the first person of color awarded the Eleanor Clarke Slagle lecture. Her 1970 lecture (Llorens, 1970) emphasized the role of occupation in human development and its influence on physical, psychosocial, neurophysiologic, and psychodynamic areas over the life span (AOTA, 2017a). Llorens later served as a member of the AOTA/AOTF Research Advisory Council.

1980 to 1999

Historical Context

The onset of the 1980s brought international change with the end of the Cold War, the collapse of the Soviet Union, and the removal of the Berlin Wall. Internationally, the Treaty of Maastricht was signed in the formation of the European Union, later paving the way for the development of the European Free Trade Association. Within the United States, Ronald Reagan took office, and the era of the space shuttle began along with an initiative to defend against missile attacks. With the advancement of the scientific age, perhaps one of the most pronounced shifts was the beginning of what was to become a dramatic new era of digital technology.

On January 3, 1983, *Time Magazine* featured a cover naming the home computer the "Machine of the Year" for 1982. This began an era where computer languages and new digital inventions proliferated (Bergin, 2007). As computer use extended to the World Wide Web, the Internet grew in popularity and use, affording unprecedented opportunities for cross-cultural communication and knowledge (Palfrey, 2010). By the late 1990s, computers were becoming integral to all areas of society, including business, education, and healthcare.

Driven by technological advances, the prevalence of chronic diseases, and Medicare funding, the healthcare industry expanded greatly. Health concerns shifted during the era as the WHO declared smallpox eradicated and the first case of HIV was identified (Hospitals and Health Networks, 2012). Advances in digital imaging technology brought increased diagnostic capabilities and costs. Between 1980 and 2000, annual age-adjusted costs per person for healthcare in the United States nearly tripled (Centers for Medicare & Medicaid Services, 2012).

Hospital stays grew shorter, telemedicine emerged, and increased emphasis was placed on patient choice and participation in healthcare decisions. Not only did telemedicine provide health professionals the opportunity to extend medical care, but also other digital advances evolved to maintain records and efficiently transfer information from one provider to another. These developments raised concerns about privacy and the protection of personal health information, leading to enactment of the Health Insurance Portability and Accountability Act of 1996 (HIPAA; Choi et al., 2006). Growing public use of the Internet for medical and health information added another influence of the digital age on healthcare (Hernandez, 2005).

Advances in psychiatric rehabilitation were influenced by a paradigm shift away from an expert model toward inclusion of the consumer in treatment decisions. The recovery model, influenced by W. A. Anthony (1993), highlighted the importance of skill training, consumer empowerment, self-determination, community involvement, and the development of cooperative alliances in psychiatric rehabilitation (Tilsen & Nylund, 2008). Goals of mental health recovery included reduced symptoms, enhanced quality of life, and emphasis on personal meaning, purpose, and values (Gagne et al., 2007).

The changing nature of the healthcare system, along with the renaming and reformulation of the Education for All Handicapped Children Act to the Individuals with Disabilities Education Act (IDEA) and President H. W. Bush's signing of the Americans with Disabilities Act (ADA) in 1990, focused attention on rehabilitation and independent living (see Figure 2.7). Overall, the legislation and trends affecting healthcare and education during this period influenced areas of OT practice, as increasing numbers of occupational therapists sought employment in school systems (AOTA, 2006b).

Occupational Therapy (1980–1999)

During this period, significant public attention was given to healthcare, especially following the election of William Jefferson Clinton as president. Clinton's healthcare reform

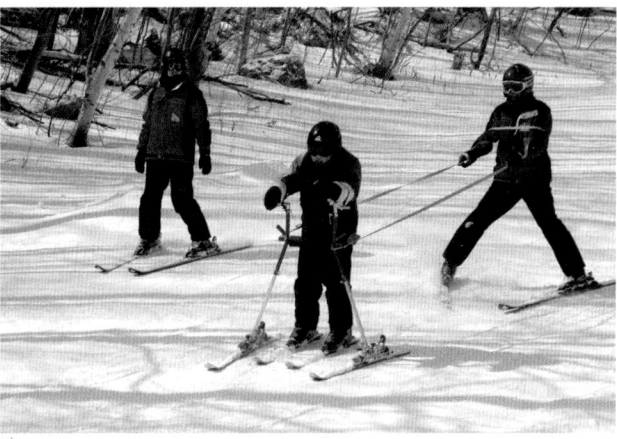

FIGURE 2.7 **Adolescent with cerebral palsy participating in an adaptive skiing program (circa 1999).**

(Photo courtesy of Maine Handicapped Skiing.)

agenda created much discussion but did not result in significant action, primarily due to heavy lobbying by the private health insurance industry, the complexity of the administration's plan, and lack of consensus among members of the majority party in Congress (Birn et al., 2003).

In OT, state professional associations continued their lobbying for legislative acts and licensure to regulate the practice of OT and increase the public safety, visibility, and legitimacy of the profession. During this period, emphasis was placed on research, efficacy, and defining the scope of practice for occupational therapists. As practice was defined, controversies emerged, such as whether physical agent modalities should be used by occupational therapists (West, 1991).

During this time, AOTF, under the leadership of President Wilma West and Executive Director Martha Kirkland, began a series of programs recommended by the Research Advisory Council to advance OT research. The most significant initiatives included the founding of a professional journal *The Occupational Therapy Journal of Research* in 1980 (Classen, 2017) and the creation of the Academy of Research in 1983, an honorary body to recognize outstanding scientists in OT (AOTF, 2012; Christiansen, 1991).

Within AOTA, discussions took place regarding the governance of certification activities. In 1986, the AOTA board of directors determined that certification activities and membership functions were not sufficiently independent to avoid potential liability under antitrust legislation. Accordingly, the board voted to create the American Occupational Therapy Certification Board, an independent body that later became known as the National Board for Certification in Occupational Therapy (Low, 1997). This action eventually led to a decline in the membership of the AOTA because membership was no longer required for certification purposes.

In 1997, the IDEA Amendments were signed into law providing strength and accountability for the education of children and adolescents with disabilities. OT was one of the specialized services provided for under this Act. The provisions for rehabilitation services in the law led to an increase in therapists practicing in the school system. By the mid-2000s, education and early intervention, as a practice area, accounted for the highest number of employed therapists (AOTA, 2006b).

The ADA enacted in 1990 became the most comprehensive piece of legislation in US history to provide protection against discrimination for persons with disabilities (Karger & Rose, 2010). The law defined disability and addressed issues of employment accommodation and ensured that persons with disabilities could access public services, transportation, and telecommunications (Hein & VanZante, 1993). The legislation was amended in 2008 to strengthen its provisions and clarify the scope of disabilities protected under the act.

Despite advances in opportunity enabled by legislation, OT employment growth slowed because of legislation to contain healthcare costs. The *Balanced Budget Act (1997)* was enacted largely to control Medicare's subacute care costs (Qaseem et al., 2007). However, it reduced rehabilitation positions and led to a decrease in applicants to OT programs, a few of which were eventually closed as a result of low enrollment.

During this era, occupational science was proposed as an academic discipline to provide an underlying foundation for OT (Yerxa, 1990). In 1989, Elizabeth Yerxa and colleagues started the first occupational science PhD program at the USC (Gordon, 2009). The intent was to establish an academic discipline focusing on occupation that would generate foundational knowledge to inform practice (Clark et al., 1998). Shortly thereafter, an "occupational science movement" expanded steadily and globally, with many academic units changing their names to "occupational science and OT." In Australia, Ann Wilcock and colleagues launched the *Journal of Occupational Science* in 1993. This was followed over the next decade by the creation of societies in several countries dedicated to the study of occupation. In the United States, this body is known as the Society for the Study of Occupation: USA (SSO: USA). There are also Canadian and international societies similarly organized.

Individuals who were influential during this period in advancing the study of occupation included Elizabeth Yerxa, Ruth Zemke, Ann Wilcock, and Gary Kielhofner. Yerxa asserted that systematic and foundational study into the occupational nature of humans was essential to the use of occupation as therapy (Yerxa et al., 1989). Earlier in the decade, Kielhofner and his colleagues had already published a series of articles on the MOHO (Kielhofner, 1980a, 1980b; Kielhofner & Burke, 1980). Influenced by Mary Reilly's work in occupational behavior and general systems theory,

MOHO emphasized motivation, performance, and patterns or routines. Wilcock's book, *An Occupational Perspective of Health*, emphasized the need for promoting health globally through a focus on the occupational nature of humans and the relationships between engagement in meaningful occupations, health, and well-being (Wilcock, 1988). Wilcock's work led to the concept of occupational justice, based on the assertion that if occupation is necessary for health, a truly just world must ensure human opportunities for such engagement (Stadnyk et al., 2010).

Additional occupation-based models such as the Person–Environment–Occupational Performance (PEOP) Model (Baum et al., 2015; Christiansen & Baum, 1997), the Ecology of Human Performance Model (Dunn et al., 1994), the Occupational Performance Process Model (Fearing et al., 1997), and the Canadian Model of Occupational Performance (Canadian Association of Occupational Therapists [CAOT], 1997; Townsend, 2002) laid a foundation for the growth of occupation-based practice.

In Canada, the government began programs to help older adults remain independent. In the early 1990s, a 30-month project began to emphasize health prevention and promotion in OT (CAOT, 1993). Soon after, a collaborative group from CAOT, the Client-Centered Practice Committee, met to develop guidelines on consulting, research, education, and practice. Initial representatives included Helene Polatajko, Tracey Thompson-Franson, Cary Brown, Christine Kramer, Liz Townsend, Mary Law, Sue Stanton, and Sue Baptiste. The eventual work resulted in publication of the monograph, *Enabling Occupation: An Occupational Therapy Perspective* (CAOT, 1997; Townsend, 2007).

People and Ideas Influencing Occupational Therapy (1980–1999)

Florence Clark completed her PhD in education at the USC and went on to serve as a faculty member, chair, and administrator. Clark was among a group of faculty who advocated the advancement of occupational science. Clark and colleagues demonstrated the benefit of lifestyle-oriented programs for maintaining health and preventing cognitive decline in well community-dwelling older adults (Clark et al., 1997, 2012). Clark served as the president of AOTA from 2012 to 2015.

Gary Kielhofner, a graduate student at the USC who studied the occupational behavior frame of reference under Mary Reilly, worked with colleagues to propose a comprehensive model for understanding the occupational nature of humans. This work evolved into a practice-oriented "Model of Human Occupation" (MOHO) described earlier. Kielhofner consulted globally and published extensively before his death in 2010 (Braveman et al., 2010; Christiansen & Taylor, 2011).

Mary Law, an OT scientist in Canada, co-founded the CanChild Centre for Childhood Disability Research at McMaster University in Hamilton, Ontario. Recognized by the AOTF Academy of Research, Law was instrumental in co-developing the Canadian occupational performance measure (COPM; Law et al., 1990), and the Person–Environment–Occupation Model (Law et al., 1996), a respected OT practice framework. Law was named an Officer of the Order of Canada in 2017 in recognition of her career accomplishments.

2000 to 2019

Historical Context

The dawn of the 21st century marked only the second recorded millennium change in documented history, and the transformations that were occurring in the world as the third millennium began were worthy of the occasion. As Thomas Friedman (2006) pointed out, global economic transformation, spawned by digital technology and the Internet, had created a new world that truly was connected economically, enabling China, India, and other emerging to participate more fully in world commerce, both for goods and for services. This increased global connectivity not only created rising middle classes in China and India but also enabled social transformations through the rapid sharing of ideas on social media platforms.

Ironically, in the United States, the 21st century began with remarkable events that were not related to the Internet. In 2000, the outcome of a historically close presidential election was decided by the Supreme Court, and George W. Bush became the 43rd president under contentious circumstances. Then, on September 11, 2001, during the first year of his presidency, the United States experienced a dramatic terrorist attack on the World Trade Center in New York City. This unprecedented event dominated the news for nearly a year and led to widespread efforts to increase security in ways that permanently changed the way people live their lives. These changes began with passage of the Patriot Act, which suspended some individual liberties in the service of national defense, and led to the creation of a Department of Homeland Security and the Transportation Safety Administration. These attacks also motivated the prosecution of controversial wars in Afghanistan and Iraq that were aimed at eradicating terrorist groups overseas.

In 2003, President George W. Bush signed legislation that expanded Medicare through provision of a prescription drug plan, known as Medicare Part D (117 Stat. 2066 Pub. L. 108-173). In his second term in 2008, speculative and unregulated real estate investments led to an economic collapse, which, because of the new global economics, resulted in a serious international market crisis that had profound economic consequences for the United States and most other countries in the world (U.S. Government Printing Office, 2011).

Barack H. Obama was elected president in 2008 just as the economic collapse was occurring. Obama worked with Congress to enact unprecedented legislation to restore market confidence (American Recovery and Reinvestment Act of 2009). In 2010, a significant healthcare reform bill called the Patient Protection and Affordable Care Act (popularly known as Obamacare) passed without bipartisan support. In addition to its provisions to subsidize premiums so that more people could afford health insurance (resulting in coverage of 30 million more people), the legislation also provided funding for research to promote patient-centered care through creation of the Patient-Centered Outcomes Research Institute (2017). Mr. Obama was elected to a second term, but a divided and partisan Congress continued a legislative stalemate that precluded significant progress on key national issues.

Donald W. Trump, a real estate businessman, was elected president in 2016. Mr. Trump proposed various measures, including immigration restrictions and a repeal of the Affordable Care Act, which was not successful. The Republican-controlled Congress was successful in passing significant tax reform legislation, but challenges to the Affordable Care Act failed.

The growth of digital communication accelerated through sales of digital devices, such as smartphones, tablets, and e-readers, which made use of cellular and wireless broadband networks. The growth of social networking websites and web-based commerce ushered in significant changes in communication and marketing.

Occupational Therapy (2000–2019)

In the millennium's first two decades, OT practice continued to be influenced in the United States by federal and state legislation and policy changes aimed at achieving cost containment and increasing quality, as determined by measurable outcomes and demonstrated effectiveness. In 2001, the WHO's *International Classification of Impairment, Disability, and Handicap* was revised to become the *International Classification of Functioning, Disability and Health* (*ICF*; WHO, 2001). This revision incorporated terminology and concepts that acknowledged the interrelationships between people, environments, and social influences on health and well-being, especially the importance of social participation as a desired outcome in rehabilitation. These changes implicitly gave credibility to OT's philosophy and practices, thus facilitating an improved understanding and appreciation for the profession.

In 2004, the NIH introduced a strategic plan to guide biomedical research called the NIH Roadmap (Zerhouni, 2003). Its purpose was to focus and coordinate biomedical research efforts toward areas deemed important to the health of the nation. This eventually led to the creation of an NIH strategic plan, specifically aimed at rehabilitation (Frontera et al., 2017). Research development in OT was bolstered in this period through NIH-funded training programs aimed at developing clinical scientists in physical therapy and OT.

Increasingly, the federal Centers for Medicare & Medicaid Services and the Agency for Healthcare Research and Quality (AHRQ) began to exert influence on healthcare practices and research by linking clinical studies of effectiveness to reimbursement through its Effective Health Care Program (Slutsky et al., 2010).

Increased emphasis of the federal government and private health insurers on cost containment and evidence-based practice led to greater emphasis on research within organized OT. Because hospitals experienced pressures to reduce patient length of stay in order to contain costs, the types of procedures offered to inpatients began to focus more on those needed for discharge. More therapy was offered on an outpatient basis or in the home as part of home health services.

Because OT developed globally, existing conceptual models were examined and challenged by the growing numbers of professionals outside North America, particularly in the Asia Pacific region, South America, and the European Union. A key development was the Kawa Model (Iwama, 2006; Iwama et al., 2009), which offered an alternative view of OT through the lens of Asian Pacific and other collectivist cultures. The influence of international perspectives was also fostered through the emergence of international societies for occupational science. The inaugural organizing meeting of the first SSO: USA was held in Galveston, Texas, in 2002; this was followed by the creation of similar organizations in the Asia Pacific region as well as in Canada and Europe.

In 2004, the AOTA board, under the leadership of Carolyn Baum, charged the vice president, Charles Christiansen, to lead a strategic planning initiative aimed at establishing a Centennial Vision. The aim was to identify goals necessary to position the profession for success beyond 2017 (the 100th anniversary of OT). The Centennial Vision, developed with significant AOTA member input, served as an ongoing goal-setting framework for the AOTA until 2017, emphasizing visibility, influence, research, evidence-based practice, diversity, global connectivity, and attention to the occupational needs of clients as key areas of focus (AOTA, 2006a).

In 2007, the AOTA and the AOTF published the Research Agenda for Occupational Therapy, recommended by a joint panel of OT scientists serving the two organizations (AOTA/AOTF Research Advisory Panel, 2011). This agenda emphasized the importance of providing a strong infrastructure for supporting research in OT that demonstrated the efficacy of services. In 2013, AOTF, in partnership with AOTA, launched a bold research grant program, providing significant funding for projects undertaken by promising emerging scientists with a focus on providing evidence for OT interventions (AOTF, 2014). This initiative was augmented with joint initiatives related to training OT scientists, including workshops and institutes (AOTF, 2015).

During this period, the US involvement in wars abroad resulted in significant and challenging injuries for many survivors of combat. These returning wounded warriors led to innovations in military OT and called attention to the need for services to reintegrate soldiers sustaining blast injuries that resulted in polytrauma, including brain injuries, severe burns, and amputations (see Figure 2.8; Howard & Doukas, 2006).

In OT education, the growth of clinical doctorate programs escalated during the period. Online and hybrid educational programs also increased, offering a significant portion of curricular content to be delivered over the Internet. This trend accelerated with the growth of online social networking and the development of new digital learning

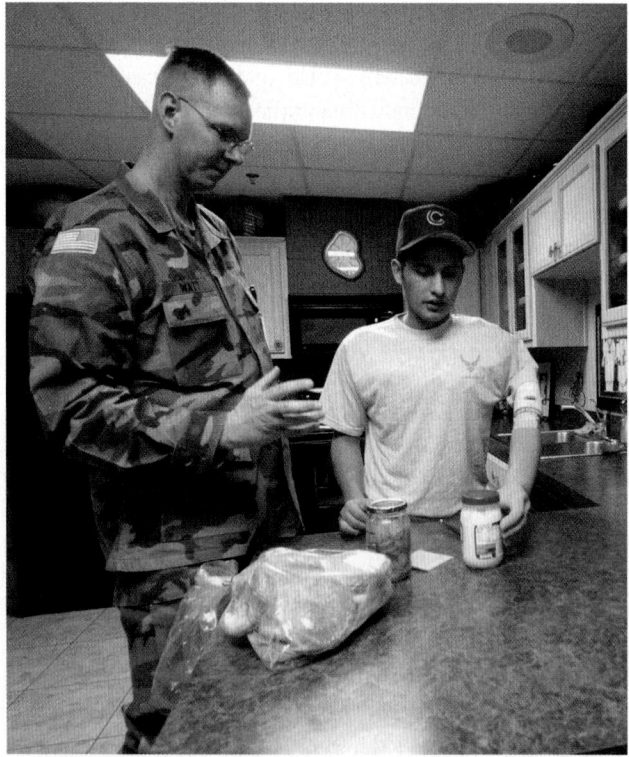

FIGURE 2.8 **Army Capt. James Watt, an occupational therapist, helps Senior Airman Dan Acosta make a sandwich in the life skills area of the amputee rehabilitation clinic at Brooke Army Medical Center in San Antonio. A mock apartment in the center helps patients get used to completing common tasks with their prosthetic limbs.**

(US Air Force photo/Steve White.)

technologies and the advent of mobile wireless smartphones and tablet computing devices.

People and Ideas Influencing Occupational Therapy (2000–2019)

Ann Wilcock of Australia proposed OT's role in population health. *Elizabeth Townsend*, a Canadian, worked with Wilcock to propose the concept of occupational justice (Townsend & Wilcock, 2004). These efforts ignited global advocacy by occupational therapists for conditions that enable access to and participation in meaningful occupation.

M. Carolyn Baum served as the president of AOTA from 2004 to 2007. She emphasized the links between practice, education, and research and the need for studies to support evidence-based practice. Baum worked with Charles Christiansen to develop the PEOP practice model in the 1980s. As professor and director of OT at Washington University in St. Louis, Baum organized an active program of research that focused on cognitive function.

In 2016, Hawaii became the 50th state to enact the licensure of OT practitioners. In the Spring of 2017, under the leadership of President Amy Lamb, the AOTA board undertook a strategic planning effort to determine goals beyond the centennial year (AOTA, 2017b, 2017c). These were focused on advocating for the importance of the association and promoting the distinct value of OT. These objectives were undertaken as part of the AOTA board's Vision 2025 initiative, which stated, "Occupational therapy maximizes health, well-being, and quality of life for all people, populations, and communities through effective solutions that facilitate participation in everyday living" (AOTA, 2017b).

In August 2017, the Accreditation Council for Occupational Therapy Education voted to mandate that the level of entry for occupational therapists and OTAs be at the clinical doctorate (OTD) and bachelor's degree (BS), respectively, by 2027 (AOTA, 2017d).

The international community came together in 2017 as the AOTA hosted the centennial celebration in Philadelphia. It was the largest gathering of occupational therapists in history. Events were hosted throughout the world commemorating the 100th anniversary of OT, and a dedicated website highlighted OT's history (www.otcentennial.org).

2020 to Present

Historical Context

This period has included a contentious US election won by President Joseph R. Biden, increased tensions in the Middle East, heightened activism related to social inequities, and the most serious pandemic in 100 years. The SARS-CoV-2 virus, responsible for the COVID-19 pandemic, spread quickly, given its transmission through close contact via respiratory droplets (see Figure 2.9; Centers for Disease Control and Prevention, 2021; WHO, 2020). The emergence of vaccinations in early 2021 significantly decreased infections, but 18 months into the pandemic, over 184 million had contracted the virus globally and nearly 4 million had died (World Meters, 2021). Public health concerns about resistance to vaccinations, often based on misinformation, and the emergence of resistant variants of the virus added global concern. In the United States, a number of incidents involving police killing persons of color in the line of duty, most notably George Floyd, led to worldwide protests and the growth of the Black Lives Matter (BLM) Movement. Social inequities and health disparities within and among nations were heightened, and renewed emphasis was placed on the importance of global health.

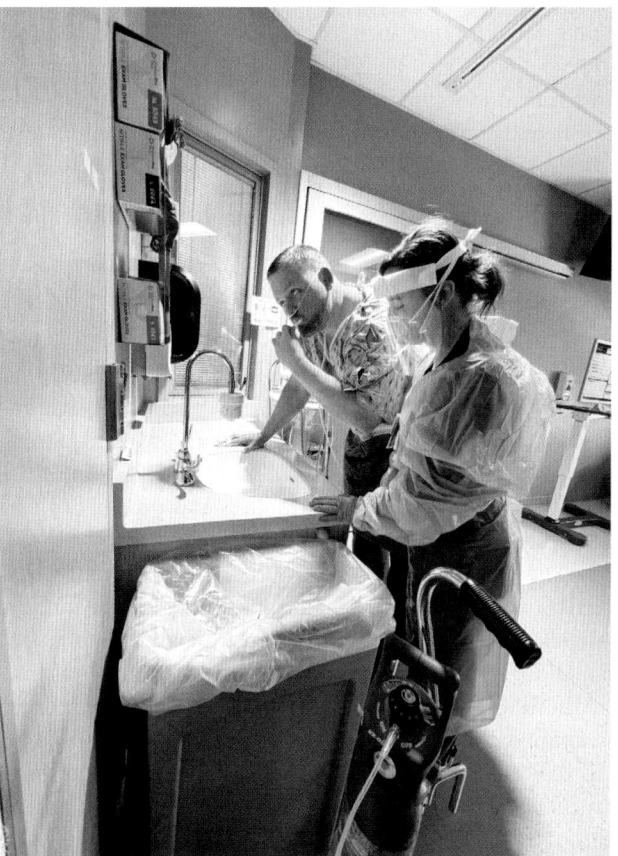

FIGURE 2.9 Susan Doolin, an occupational therapist at a level 1 trauma center, treating a COVID-positive patient who is working on activity tolerance while grooming at the sink.

(Photo courtesy of Susan Doolin.)

Occupational Therapy (2020 to Present)

The pandemic accelerated global changes to education and healthcare delivery. Healthcare workers were deemed essential in many countries, yet challenges existed with initial shortages of personal protective equipment and concerns about widespread transmission of COVID-19. Where possible, OT education used simulation, web-based, and hybrid instructional methods (Gustafsson, 2020). Some educational programs had established online educational platforms, yet others required rapid training of faculty, staff, and students. Concurrently, in developed regions with high-speed broadband, there was greater use of remote (virtual) delivery of services by practitioners (Garfinkel & Minard, 2021; Gitlow, 2021; Lunsford et al., 2016). The expanded insurance coverage for telehealth during the pandemic brought new opportunities and resources for online delivery of OT (AOTA, 2021b; Hoel et al., 2021), yet healthcare disparities were magnified as access to technology and other barriers limited services for some groups (Hoel et al., 2021). Societal movements in the United States to advocate for social justice prompted some professional groups, such as the Coalition of Occupational Therapy Advocates for Diversity (COTAD), to encourage widespread adoption of organizational commitments toward practices that promoted diversity, equity, and inclusion.

People and Ideas Influencing Occupational Therapy (2020 to Present)

In addition to telehealth and online education, advanced technologies, including the use of 3D printers, have enabled innovations in rehabilitation (Lunsford et al., 2016). A 3D printing has been applied to the fabrication of assistive technology devices, orthotics, and prosthetics and has fostered interdisciplinary collaboration in some OT educational curricula (Wagner et al., 2018). Although emphasis on interprofessional education increased in this era, Alotabi et al. (2019) found that while knowledge about occupational therapists by other health professionals was limited, attitudes were favorable. Interprofessional competence is emphasized in OT education and is incorporated into Accreditation Council for Occupational Therapy Education (ACOTE) standards as well as other educational standards throughout the world.

Frontline workers are among the groups most impacted during a pandemic. This includes service workers and those caring for the seriously ill. These groups often cannot work remotely and easily observe social distancing precautions, leading to disparities and inequities in how a pandemic is experienced—perhaps providing an example of occupational injustice, a concept advanced in occupational science. During the pandemic, WFOT conducted a survey of 100 country member organizations and found key priorities during the pandemic to be (a) collaborative efforts for the provision of information and education resources, (b) standards and supports for quality provision of services, and (c) advocacy to promote access to OT and address occupational justice (WFOT, 2022b). To augment local efforts and resources provided by individual countries, WFOT provided pandemic-related information to address the needs of OT globally.

OT continued to develop internationally, and this effort was enhanced by the evolution of the Internet, global virtual conferences, and international collaborations fostered by WFOT.

Conclusion

For much of its history, OT practitioners were doers, perhaps insufficiently interested in explaining or proving the theoretical ideas and practical benefits of their actions. This inattention placed the profession at a disadvantage to medicine and other disciplines, where science-based practice had received greater emphasis, until the Centennial Vision led to strategic research efforts to validate OT interventions (AOTF, 2014). Yet, the inherent flexibility of occupations as a therapeutic medium continued to offer creative opportunities for benefiting a wide range of patients and clients. As daunting health problems served by occupational therapists (e.g., tuberculosis, polio) faded into the history books of biomedical success, occupational therapists were able to mobilize in the service of emerging health problems and concerns deemed important by consumers (such as dementia and autism spectrum disorders). Moreover, the cooperative nature of the therapeutic relationship afforded a bridge to connect the body and mind, providing occupational therapists with a rare, important, and enduring place in the lives of their patients, serving as healers as well as technologists.

As OT moves ahead in an eventful 21st century, one must ask if these themes will continue to shape the story of the profession. Will an emphasis on science-based practice continue? Will therapists reinvent new approaches for addressing the emerging diseases of the 21st century, and will they preserve and capitalize on their unique position as both technologists and custodians of meaning (Engelhardt, 1983) to enable clients and populations to better manage their own health through occupation? Only the histories yet to be written will tell.

Lippincott® Connect *For additional resources on the subjects discussed in this chapter, visit* Lippincott Connect.

REFERENCES

Alotabi, N. M., Manee, F. S., Murphy, L. J., & Rassafini, M. (2019). Knowledge about and attitudes of interdisciplinary team members towards occupational therapy practice: Implications and future directions. *Medical Principles and Practice, 28*(2), 158–166. https://doi.org/10.1159/000495915

American Occupational Therapy Association. (1969). American occupational therapy organizations. *American Journal of Occupational Therapy, 23,* 519.

American Occupational Therapy Association. (2006a). *The road to the centennial vision.*

American Occupational Therapy Association. (2006b). *2006 AOTA workforce and compensation survey: Occupational therapy salaries and job opportunities continue to improve.* OT Practice Online.

American Occupational Therapy Association. (2009). *History of AOTA accreditation.*

American Occupational Therapy Association. (2017a). *100 Influential people: Lela Llorens.* http://www.otcentennial.org/the-100-people/llorens

American Occupational Therapy Association. (2017b). *Fiscal year 2018 board of directors strategic priorities.*

American Occupational Therapy Association. (2017c). Vision 2025. *American Journal of Occupational Therapy, 72,* 7103420010p1. https://doi.org/10.5014/ajot.2017.713002

American Occupational Therapy Association. (2017d). *AOTA board of directors statement on ACOTE decision (dated 8/21/2017).*

American Occupational Therapy Association. (2018). Importance of collaborative occupational therapist–occupational therapy assistant intraprofessional education in occupational therapy curricula. *American Journal of Occupational Therapy, 72*(Suppl. 2), 7212410030. https://doi.org/10.5014/ajot.2018.72S207

American Occupational Therapy Association. (2019). *In memoriam: Claudia Allen.*

American Occupational Therapy Association. (2021a). *Events from 1970-1979.* Author. http://www.otcentennial.org/events/1970

American Occupational Therapy Association. (2021b). *Telehealth.* https://www.aota.org/Practice/Manage/telehealth.aspx

American Occupational Therapy Association/American Occupational Therapy Foundation Research Advisory Panel. (2011). Occupational therapy research agenda. *OTJR: Occupation, Participation and Health, 31,* 52–54. https://www.aota.org/-/media/Corporate/Files/Practice/Researcher/AOTF-AOTA%20Occupational%20Therapy%20Research%20Agenda.ashx

American Occupational Therapy Foundation. (2012). *Academy of research in occupational therapy.* http://www.aotf.org/awardshonors/forresearch/academyofresearchinoccupationaltherapy.aspx American

American Occupational Therapy Foundation. (2014). *2013 report to donors.* Author.

American Occupational Therapy Foundation. (2015). *2014 report to donors.* Author.

American Recovery and Reinvestment Act. (2009). Pub. L. No. 111-5, 123 Stat. 115, H.R. 1.

Americans with Disabilities Act. (1990). 42 U.S.C.A. § 12101 *et seq.*

Andersen, L. T., & Reed, K. (2017). *The history of occupational therapy: The first century.* SLACK.

Andrews, K. T., & Gaby, S. (2015). Local protest and federal policy: The impact of the Civil Rights Movement on the 1964 Civil Rights Act. *Sociological Forum, 30*(Suppl. 1), 509–527. https://doi.org/10.1111/socf.12175

Anthony, S. H. (2005). Dr. Herbert J. Hall: Originator of honest work for occupational therapy 1904–1923 [part I]. *Occupational Therapy in Health Care, 19*(3), 3–19. https://doi.org/10.1080/J003v19n03_02

Anthony, W. A. (1993). Recovery from mental illness: The guiding vision of the mental health system in the 1990's. *Psychosocial Rehabilitation Journal, 16*(4), 11–23. https://doi.org/10.1037/h0095655

Ayres, A. J. (1966). Interrelationships among perceptual-motor functions in children. *American Journal of Occupational Therapy, 20*(2), 68–71.

Ayres, A. J. (1972). *Sensory integration and learning disorders.* Western Psychological Services.

Ayres, A. J. (1989). *Sensory integration and praxis tests.* Western Psychological Services.

Balanced Budget Act. (1997). Pub. L. No. 105-33, 111 Stat. 269.

Baum, C. M., Christiansen, C. H., & Bass, J. D. (2015). The person-environment-occupation-performance model. In C. H. Christiansen, C. M. Baum, & J. D. Bass (Eds.), *Occupational therapy: Performance, participation and well-being* (4th ed., pp. 49–56). SLACK.

Beard, G. M. (1880). *A practical treatise on nervous exhaustion (neurasthenia).* William Wood.

Beck, A. H. (2004). The Flexner report and the standardization of American medical education. *JAMA, 291*(17), 2139–2140. https://doi.org/10.1001/jama.291.17.2139

Beers, C. (1908). *A mind that found itself: An autobiography.* Longmans, Green and Company.

Bergen, D. L. (2016). *War & genocide: A concise history of the holocaust* (3rd ed.). Rowman & Littlefield.

Bergin, T. J. (2007). A history of the history of programming languages. *Communications of the ACM, 50*(5), 69–74. https://doi.org/10.1145/1230819.1230841

Bing, R. K. (1961). *William Rush Dunton, Jr.: American psychiatrist—A study in self* [Unpublished doctoral dissertation]. University of Maryland, College Park, MD.

Bing, R. K. (1981). Occupational therapy revisited: A paraphrastic journey. *American Journal of Occupational Therapy, 35*(8), 499–518. https://doi.org/10.5014/ajot.35.8.499

Birn, A., Brown, T. M., Fee, E., & Lear, W. J. (2003). Struggles for national health reform in the United States. *American Journal of Public Health, 93*(1), 86–91. https://doi.org/10.2105/ajph.93.1.86

Braveman, B., Fisher, G., & Suarez-Balcazar, Y. (2010). In memoriam: "Achieving the ordinary things": A tribute to Gary Kielhofner. *American Journal of Occupational Therapy, 64*(6), 828–831. https://doi.org/10.5014/ajot.2010.64605

Brinkley, D. (2009). *The wilderness warrior: Theodore Roosevelt and the crusade for America.* Harper Collins.

Brown, L. D., Shepherd, M. D., Wituk, S. A., & Meissen, G. (2008). Introduction to the special issue on mental health self-help. *American Journal of Community Psychology, 42,* 105–109. https://doi.org/10.1007/s 10464-008-9187-7

Brunner, J. (2001). *Freud and the politics of psychoanalysis.* Transaction.

Burnham, J. C. (2006). The "New Freud Studies": A historiographical shift. *Journal of the Historical Society, 6*(2), 213–233. https://doi.org/10.1111/j.1540-5923-2006.00176.x

Canadian Association of Occupational Therapists. (1993). *Seniors' health promotion project: Responding to the challenge of an aging population's final report.* Author.

Canadian Association of Occupational Therapists. (1997). *Enabling occupation: An occupational therapy perspective.* Author.

Carson, M. (1990). *Settlement folk: Social thought and the American Settlement Movement, 1885–1930.* University of Chicago Press.

Centers for Disease Control and Prevention. (2021). *Scientific brief: SARS-CoV-2 transmission.* https://www.cdc.gov/coronavirus/2019-ncov/science/science-briefs/sars-cov-2-transmission.html#:~:text=References-,SARS%2DCoV%2D2%20is%20transmitted%20by%20exposure%20to%20infectious%20respiratory,respiratory%20fluids%20carrying%20infectious%20virus

Centers for Medicare & Medicaid Services. (2012). *Office of the Actuary, National Health Statistics Group, National Health Care*

Expenditures Data. https://www.cms.gov/About-CMS/Agency-Information/History

Centers for Medicare & Medicaid Services. (2020). *History.* Author. https://www.cms.gov/About-CMS/Agency-Information/History

Choi, Y. B., Capitan, K. E., Krause, J. S., & Streeper, M. M. (2006). Challenges associated with privacy in health care industry: Implementation of HIPAA and the security rules. *Journal of Medical Systems, 30*(1), 57–64. https://doi.org/10.1007/s10916-006-7405-0

Christiansen, C. H. (1991). Nationally speaking: Research: Looking back and ahead after four decades of progress. *American Journal of Occupational Therapy, 45*(5), 391–392. https://doi.org/10.5014/ajot.45.5.391

Christiansen, C. H. (2007). Adolf Meyer revisited: Connections between lifestyles, resilience and illness. *Journal of Occupational Science, 14*(2), 63–76. https://doi.org/10.1080/14427591.2007.9686586

Christiansen, C. H. (2021). Romanticism and transcendentalism. In S. Taff (Ed.), *Philosophy and occupational therapy. Informing education, research and practice* (pp. 61–74). SLACK.

Christiansen, C. H., & Baum, C. (Eds.). (1997). Person-environment occupational performance: A conceptual model for practice. In C. H. Christiansen & C. Baum (Eds.), *Occupational therapy: Enabling function and well being* (2nd ed., pp. 47–70). SLACK.

Christiansen, C. H., & Taylor, R. (2011). In memoriam: Gary Wayne Kielhofner (February 15, 1949–September 2, 2010). *OTJR: Occupation, Participation and Health, 31*(1), 2–4. https://doi.org/10.3928/15394492-20101025-01X

Clancy, K. (2016). *Women in white: A retrospective look at medical education at one school before Title IX* [Theses and Dissertations]. Educational policy studies and evaluation. 42. https://uknowledge.uky.edu/epe_etds/42

Clark, F., Azen, S. P., Zemke, R., Jackson, J., Carlson, M., Mandel, D., Hay, J., Josephson, K., Cherry, B., Hessel, C., Palmer, J., & Lipson, L. (1997). Occupational therapy for independent-living older adults. A randomized controlled trial. *JAMA, 278*(16), 1321–1326. https://doi.org/10.1001/jama.1997.03550160041036

Clark, F., Jackson, J., Carlson, M., Chou, C. P., Cherry, B. J., Jordan-Marsh, M., Knight, B. G., Mandel, D., Blanchard, J., Granger, D. A., Wilcox, R. R., Lai, M. Y., White, B., Hay, J., Lam, C., Marterella, A., & Azen, S. P. (2012). Effectiveness of a lifestyle intervention in promoting the well-being of independently living older people: Results of the well elderly 2 randomised controlled trial. *Journal of Epidemiology and Community Health, 66*(9), 782–790. https://doi.org/10.1136/jech.2009.099754

Clark, F., Wood, W., & Larson, E. A. (1998). Occupational science: Occupational therapy's legacy for the 21st century. In M. Neistadt & E. Crepeau (Eds.), *Willard & Spackman's occupational therapy* (9th ed., pp. 13–21). Lippincott Williams & Wilkins.

Classen, S. (2017). OTJR's journey in becoming a world-class journal [editorial]. *OTJR: Occupation, Participation and Health, 37*(2), 59–61. https://doi.org/10.1177/1539449217699539

Clouston, T. J., & Whitcombe, S. W. (2008). The professionalization of occupational therapy: A continuing challenge. *British Journal of Occupational Therapy, 71*(8), 314–320. https://doi.org/10.1177/030802260807100802

Cockburn, L. (2001, May–June). The professional era: CAOT in the 1950's and 1960's. *Occupational Therapy Now,* 5–9.

Conti, A. A. (2014). Western medical rehabilitation through time: A historical and epistemological review. *The Scientific World Journal, 2014,* 1–5. Article 432506. https://doi.org/10.1155/2014/432506

Cooper, J. M. (1990). *Pivotal decades: The United States, 1900–1920.* Norton.

Cordery, S. A. (2018). Roosevelt, Theodore. In S. Bronner (Ed.), *Encyclopedia of American studies.* Johns Hopkins University Press.

Council on Medical Education and Hospitals. (1935, August 31). Essentials of an acceptable school of occupational therapy. *Journal of the American Medical Association, 105*(9), 690–691. https://doi.org/10.1001/jama.1935.02760350037011

Council on Medical Education and Hospitals. (1950). Essentials of an acceptable school of occupational therapy. *American Journal of Occupational Therapy, 4*(3), 125–128.

Crane, A. G. (1927). *The medical department of the United States Army in the world war: Volume XIII: Part one: Physical reconstruction and vocational education.* U.S. Government Printing Office.

Digby, A. (1985). *Madness, morality, and medicine: A study of the York retreat, 1796–1914.* Cambridge University Press.

Dunn, W., Brown, C., & McGuigan, A. (1994). The ecology of human performance: A framework for considering the effect of context. *American Journal of Occupational Therapy, 48*(7), 595–607. https://doi.org/10.5014/ajot.48.7.595

Dunton, W. R., Jr. (1925). Editorial. *Occupational Therapy and Rehabilitation, 4,* 73–75.

Dworkin, R. W. (2010). The rise of the caring industry. *Policy Review, 161,* 45–59. https://search.proquest.com/docveiw/609957271?accountid=45049

Education for All Handicapped Children Act of 1975. (1975). Pub. L. No. 94-142, 20 U.S.C. § 1401.

Egan, T. (2006). *The worst hard time: The untold story of those who survived the great American dust bowl.* Houghton Mifflin.

Engelhardt, H. T. (1983). Occupational therapists as technologists and custodians of meaning. In G. Kielhofner (Ed.), *Health through occupation* (pp. 130–144). F. A. Davis.

Eubank, K. (2004). *The origins of World War II* (3rd ed.). Wiley-Blackwell.

Eysenck, H. (1985). *Decline and fall of the Freudian empire.* Pelican.

Faiella, G. (2006). *John Locke: Champion of modern democracy.* Rosen.

Faulkner, W. (1953). *Requiem for a nun.* Random House.

Fearing, V. G., Law, M., & Clark, J. (1997). An occupational performance process model: Fostering client and therapist alliances. *Canadian Journal of Occupational Therapy, 64*(1), 7–15. https://doi.org/10.1177/000841749706400103

Fidler, G., & Fidler, J. (1954). *Introduction to psychiatric occupational therapy.* McMillan.

Fink, M., & Taylor, M. A. (2007). Electroconvulsive therapy: Evidence and challenges. *JAMA, 298*(3), 330–332. https://doi.org/10.1001/jama.298.3.330

Fogan, M., & Smith, M. (2019). State hospitals. In C. Brown, V. C. Stoffel, & J. P. Munoz (Eds.), *Occupational therapy in mental health: A vision for participation* (2nd ed., pp. 642–654). F. A. Davis.

Foto, M. (1997). Presidential address—Wilma West: A true visionary. *American Journal of Occupational Therapy, 51*(8), 638–639. https://doi.org/10.5014/ajot.51.8.638

Friedland, J. (2011). *Restoring the spirit: The beginnings of occupational therapy in Canada, 1890–1930.* McGill-Queens University Press.

Friedland, J., & Davids-Brumer, N. (2007). From education to occupation: The story of Thomas Bessell Kidner. *Canadian Journal of Occupational Therapy, 74*(1), 27–37. https://doi.org/10.2182/cjot.06.009

Friedland, J., & Silva, J. (2008). Evolving identities: Thomas Bessell Kidner and occupational therapy in the United States. *American Journal of Occupational Therapy, 62*(3), 349–360. https://doi.org/10.5014/ajot.62.3.349

Friedman, T. L. (2006). *The world is flat. A brief history of the 21st century.* Farar, Strauss, and Giroux.

Frontera, W. R., Bean, J. F., Damiano, D., Ehrlich-Jones, L., Fried-Oken, M., Jette, A., Jung, R., Lieber, R. L., Malec, J. F., Mueller, M. J., Ottenbacher, K. J., Tansey, K. E., & Thompson, A. (2017). Rehabilitation research at the National Institutes of Health: Moving the field forward (executive summary). *American Journal of Occupational Therapy, 71*(3), 7103320010. https://doi.org/10.5014/ajot.2017.713003

Gagne, C., White, W., & Anthony, W. A. (2007). Recovery: A common vision for the fields of mental health and addictions. *Psychiatric Rehabilitation Journal, 31*(1), 32–37. https://doi.org/10.2975/31.1.2007.32.37

Gainer, R. D. (2008). History of ergonomics and occupational therapy. *Work, 31*(1), 5–9.

Garfinkel, M., & Minard, C. (2021). Supporting occupational balance in children using everyday technologies: The distinct value of occupational therapy. *SIS Quarterly Practice Connections, 6*(1), 5–7. https://www.aota.org/publications/sis-quarterly/children-youth-sis/cysis-2-21

Georgia Tech. (2021). *History of prosthetics and orthotics.* https://mspo.gatech.edu/history/

Gerber, K. M. (2007). Eight decades of health care: The 1950's. *Hospitals & Health Networks, 81*(5), 10–13.

Gillette, N. P. (1996). Tribute to Wilma West. In R. Zemke & F. Clark (Eds.), *Occupational science: The evolving discipline* (pp. 403–412). F. A. Davis.

Gillette, N. P. (2005). A tribute to Gail S. Fidler: Our esteemed mentor. *American Journal of Occupational Therapy, 59*(6), 609–610. https://doi.org/10.5014/ajot.59.6.609

Gitlow, L. (2021). Assistive technology for college students with mental health conditions: Building on successful routines. *SIS Quarterly Practice Connections, 6*(1), 18–20. https://www.aota.org/publications/sis-quarterly/mental-health-sis/mhsis-2-21

Gordon, D. M. (2009). The history of occupational therapy. In E. B. Crepeau, E. S. Cohn, & B. A. Boyt Schell (Eds.), *Willard & Spackman's occupational therapy* (11th ed., pp. 202–215). Lippincott Williams & Wilkins.

Gustafsson, L. (2020). Occupational therapy has gone online: What will remain beyond Covid-19? *Australian Occupational Therapy Journal, 67*(3), 197–198. https://doi.org/10.1111/1440-1630.12672

Hackett, L. (1992). *The age of enlightenment: The European dream of progress and enlightenment.* Chicago Press.

Hall, H. J. (1922). *What is occupation therapy? Paper written for the General Federation of Women's Clubs.* American Occupational Therapy Foundation.

Harlow, J. (2007). Eight decades of health care: The 1940's. *Hospitals and Health Networks, 81*(5), 10–13.

Harvard University Library. (n.d.). *Aspiration, acculturation and impact: Immigration to the United States, 1789–1930.* http://ocp.hul.harvard.edu/immigration/settlement.html

Heath, K. P. (2017). Artistic scarcity in an age of material abundance: President Lyndon Johnson, the National Endowment for the Arts, and Great Society Liberalism. *European Journal of American Culture, 36*(1), 5–22. https://doi.org/10.1386/ejac.36.1.5_1

Hein, C. D., & VanZante, N. R. (1993). A manager's guide: Americans with Disabilities Act of 1990. *SAM: Advanced Management Journal, 58*(1), 40–45.

Heinlein, R. A. (1987). *Time enough for love.* Penguin Books.

Heckscher, A. (1991). *Woodrow Wilson.* Easton Press.

Hernandez, N. (2005). Telemedicine and the future of telemedicine. *AMT Events, 22*, 74–75; 116–117.

Hocking, C. (2008). The way we were: Thinking rationally. *British Journal of Occupational Therapy, 71*(5), 185–195. https://doi.org/10.1177/030802260807100504

Hoel, V., von Zweck, C., & Ledgerd, R. (2021). Was a global pandemic needed to adopt the use of telehealth in occupational therapy? *Work, 68*(1), 13–20. https://doi.org/10.3233/WOR-205268

Hofstadter, R. (1955). *The age of reform: From Bryan to F.D.R.* Alfred A. Knopf.

Hospitals and Health Networks. (2012). *Eight decades of health care.*

Howard, W. J., III, & Doukas, W. C. (2006). Process of care for battle casualties at Walter Reed Army Medical Center: Part IV. Occupational therapy service. *Military Medicine, 171*(3), 209–210. https://doi.org/10.7205/milmed.171.3.209

Hudson, C. G. (2016). A model of deinstitutionalization of psychiatric care across 161 nations: 2001-2014. *International Journal of Mental Health, 45*(2), 135–153. https://doi.org/10.1080/00207411.2016.116748

Ikiugu, M., & Nissen, R. M. (2021). Pragmatic foundations. Instrumentalism and transactionalism in occupational therapy. In S. D. Taff (Ed.), *Philosophy and occupational therapy. Informing education, research, and practice* (pp. 83–90). SLACK.

Individuals with Disabilities Education Act of 1997. (1997). Pub. L. No. 105-117, 20 U.S.C., §614, 672, 20 U.S.C.. http://www2.ed.gov/offices/OSERS/Policy/IDEA/index.html

Iwama, M. (2006). *The Kawa model: Culturally relevant occupational therapy.* Churchill Livingstone, Elsevier.

Iwama, M., Thomson, N. A., & Macdonald, R. M. (2009). The Kawa model: The power of culturally responsive occupational therapy. *Disability and Rehabilitation, 31*(14), 1125–1135. https://doi.org/10.1080/09638280902773711

Karger, H., & Rose, S. R. (2010). Revisiting the Americans with Disabilities Act after two decades. *Journal of Social Work in Disability & Rehabilitation, 9*(2), 73–86. https://doi.org/10.1080/1536710X.2010.493468

Kennedy, D. M. (1999). *Freedom from fear: The American people in depression and war 1929-1945.* Oxford University Press.

Kidner, T. B. (1922). Work for the tuberculous before and after the cure. *Archives of Occupational Therapy, 1*(5), 363–376.

Kielhofner, G. (1980a). A model of human occupation, part 2. Ontogenesis from the perspective of temporal adaptation. *American Journal of Occupational Therapy, 34*(10), 657–663. https://doi.org/10.5014/ajot.34.10.657

Kielhofner, G. (1980b). A model of human occupation, part 3, benign and vicious cycles. *American Journal of Occupational Therapy, 34*(11), 731–737. https://doi.org/10.5014/ajot.34.9.572

Kielhofner, G. (2008). *Model of human occupation: Theory and application* (4th ed.). Lippincott Williams & Wilkins.

Kielhofner, G. (2009). *Conceptual foundations of occupational therapy practice* (4th ed.). F. A. Davis.

Kielhofner, G., & Burke, J. P. (1977). Occupational therapy after 60 years: An account of changing identity and knowledge. *American Journal of Occupational Therapy, 31*(10), 675–689. https://doi.org/10.3233/WOR-131589

Kielhofner, G., & Burke, J. P. (1980). A model of human occupation, part 1. Conceptual framework and content. *American Journal of Occupational Therapy, 34*(9), 572–581. https://doi.org/10.5014/ajot.34.9.572

King, L. J. (1974). A sensory-integrative approach to schizophrenia. *American Journal of Occupational Therapy, 28*(9), 529–536.

King, M. L. (1963). I had a dream. Text of speech delivered August 28, 1963. Washington, DC.

Koyangi, C. (2007). *Learning from history: Deinstitutionalization of people with mental illness as precursor to long-term care reform.* Kaiser Foundation on Medicaid and Uninsured.

Krusen, F. H. (1934). The relationship of physical therapy and occupational therapy. *Occupational Therapy and Rehabilitation, 13*, 69–77.

Laird, A. R. (1923). Occupational therapy and vocational training in the tuberculosis sanitarium. *Archives of Occupational Therapy, 2*(5), 359–367.

Law, M., Baptiste, S., McColl, M., Opzoomer, A., Polatajko, H., & Pollock, N. (1990). The Canadian occupational performance measure: An outcome measure for occupational therapy. *Canadian Journal of Occupational Therapy, 57*(2), 82–87. https://doi.org/10.1177/000841749005700207

Law, M., Cooper, B., Strong, S., Stewart, D., Rigby, P., & Letts, L. (1996). The person-environment-occupation model: A transactive approach to occupational performance. *Canadian Journal of Occupational Therapy, 63*(1), 9–23. https://doi.org/10.1177/000841749606300103

Levin, M. F., & Panturin, E. (2011). Sensorimotor intervention for functional recovery and the Bobath approach. *Motor Control, 15*(2), 285–301. https://doi.org/10.1123/mcj.15.2.285

Levine, R. E. (1987). The influence of the arts-and-crafts movement on the professional status of occupational therapy. *American Journal of Occupational Therapy, 41*(4), 248–254. https://doi.org/10.5014/ajot.41.4.248

Leuchtenburg, W. E. (1963). *Franklin D. Roosevelt and the new deal, 1932-1940.* Harper & Row.

Lief, A. (1948). *The commonsense psychiatry of Adolf Meyer.* McGraw-Hill.

Llorens, L. (1970). Facilitating growth and development: The promise of occupational therapy. *American Journal of Occupational Therapy, 24*(2), 93–101.

Loomis, B. (1992). The Henry B. Favill School of Occupations and Eleanor Clarke Slagle. *American Journal of Occupational Therapy, 46*(1), 34–37. https://doi.org/10.5014/ajot.46.1.34

Low, J. F. (1992). The reconstruction aides. *American Journal of Occupational Therapy, 46*(1), 38–43. https://doi.org/10.5014/ajot.46.1.38

Low, J. F. (1997). The issue is: NBCOT and state regulatory agencies: Allies or adversaries? *American Journal of Occupational Therapy, 51*(1), 74–75. https://doi.org/10.5014/ajot.51.1.74

Luchins, A. S. (2001). Moral treatment in asylums and general hospitals in 19th-century America. *The Journal of Psychology, 123*(6), 585–607. https://doi.org/10.1080/00223980.1989.10543013

Lunsford, C., Grindle, G., Salatin, B., & Dicianno, B. E. (2016). Innovations with 3-dimensional printing in physical medicine and rehabilitation: A review of the literature. *PM&R, 8*(12), 1201–1212. https://doi.org/10.1016/j.pmrj.2016.07.003

Mahoney, M., Peters, C. O., & Martin, P. M. (2017). Willard and Spackman's enduring legacy for future occupational therapy pathways. *American Journal of Occupational Therapy, 71*(1), 7101100020p1–7101100020p7. https://doi.org/10.5014/ajot.2017.023994

Matathia, S., & Tello, M. (2020, August 27). Medical education needs retaining. *Scientific American.* https://www.scientificamerican.com/article/medical-education-needs-rethinking/

McElvaine, R. S. (1993). *The Great Depression: America 1929–1941.* Random House.

Melhado, E. M. (2006). Health planning in the United States and the decline of public-interest policymaking. *The Milbank Quarterly, 84*(2), 359–440. https://doi.org/10.1111/j.1468-0009.2006.00451.x

Metaxas, V. A. (2000). Eleanor Clarke Slagle and Susan E. Tracy: Personal and professional identity and the development of occupational therapy in progressive era America. *Nursing History Review, 8*, 39–70. DOI: 10.1891/1062-8061.8.1.39

Meyer, A. (1922). The philosophy of occupation therapy. *Archives of Occupational Therapy, 1*, 1–10.

Miller, R. J., & Walker, K. F. (1993). *Perspectives on theory for practice in occupational therapy.* Aspen.

Molke, D. (2009). Outlining a critical ethos for historical work in occupational science and occupational therapy. *Journal of Occupational Science, 16*(2), 75–84. https://doi.org/10.1080/14427591.2009.9686646

Mosey, A. (1973). *Activities therapy.* Raven Press.

Mougel, N. (2011). *World War I casualties.* Centre Européen Robert Schuman. http://www.centre-robert-schuman.org/userfiles/files/REPERES%20%E2%80%93%20module%201-1-1%20-%20explanatory%20notes%20%E2%80%93%20World%20War%20I%20casualties%20%E2%80%93%20EN.pdf

Nancarrow, S., & Mackey, H. (2005). The introduction and evaluation of an occupational therapy assistant practitioner. *Australian Journal of Occupational Therapy, 52*(4), 293–301. https://doi.org/10.1111/j.1440-1630.2005.00531.x

Office of the Surgeon General. (1918). *Carry on: A magazine on the reconstruction of disabled soldiers and sailors.* American Red Cross.

Oshinsky, D. M. (2005). *Polio: An American story.* Oxford University Press.

Oxford Brookes University. (2011). *The Churchill hospital years.* http://www.brookes.ac.uk/library/speccoll/dorset/dorsethist3.html

Paine, T. (1794). *The age of reason: Being an investigation of true and fabulous theology.* Barras.

Palfrey, J. (2010). Four phases of internet regulation. *Social Research, 77*(3), 981–996. https://ssrn.com/abstract=1658191

Patient-Centered Outcomes Research Institute. (2017). *About us.* Patient-Centered Outcomes Research. https://www.pcori.org/about-us

Peters, C. (2011a). History of mental health: Perspectives of consumers and practitioners. In C. Brown & V. C. Stoffel (Eds.), *Occupational therapy in mental health: A vision for participation* (pp. 17–30). F. A. Davis.

Peters, C. (2011b). Powerful occupational therapists: A community of professionals, 1950–1980. *Occupational Therapy in Mental Health, 27*(3), 199–410. https://doi.org/10.1080/0164212X.2011.597328

Peters, C. (2013). *Powerful occupational therapists: A community of professionals 1950-1980.* Routledge.

Pollitt, P. (2018). Nurses fight for the right to vote. *American Journal of Nursing, 118*(11), 46–54. https://doi.org/10.1097/01.NAJ.0000547639.70037.cd

Pressman, J. D. (1998). *Last resort: Psychosurgery and the limits of medicine.* Cambridge University Press.

Qaseem, A., Weech-Maldonado, R., & Mkanta, W. (2007). The Balanced Budget Act (1997) and the supply of nursing home subacute care. *Journal of Health Care Finance, 34*(2), 38–47.

Quiroga, V. A. (1995). *Occupational therapy: The first 30 years 1900–1930.* AOTA Press.

Redford, G. (2020). *AAMC renames its prestigious Abraham Flexner award in light of racist and sexist writings.* Association of American Medical Colleges. https://www.aamc.org/news-insights/aamc-renames-prestigious-abraham-flexner-award-light-racist-and-sexist-writings#:~:text=Who%20was%20Abraham%20Flexner%3F,part%20of%20the%2020th%20century

Reilly, M. (1962). Occupational therapy can be one of the great ideas of 20th century medicine. *American Journal of Occupational Therapy, 20*, 61–67.

Richards, E. E. (2011). Responses to occupational and environmental exposures in the U.S. military—World War II to the present. *Military Medicine, 176*(7), 22–28. https://doi.org/10.7205/milmed-d-11-00083

Rosser, S. V. (2002). An overview of women's health in the U.S. since the 1960's. *History and Technology, 18*(4), 355–369. https://doi.org/10.1080/0734151022000023802

Saltman, R. B., & Dubois, H. F. W. (2004). The historical and social base of social health insurance systems. In R. B. Saltman, R. Busse, & J. Figueras (Eds.), *Social health insurance systems in Western Europe* (pp. 21–32). Open University Press.

Salvatori, P. (2001). The history of occupational therapy assistants in Canada: A comparison with the United States. *Canadian Journal of Occupational Therapy, 68*(4), 217–227. https://doi.org/10.1177/000841740106800405

Sawhney, H. (2013). Analytics of organized spontaneity: Rethinking participant selection, interaction format, and milieu for academic forums. *The Information Society, 29*(2), 78–87. https://doi.org/10.1080/01972243.2013.758470

Schutz, A. (2011). Power and trust in the public realm: John Dewey, Saul Alinsky, and the limits of progressive democratic education. *Educational Theory, 61*(4), 491–512. https://doi.org/10.1111/j.1741-5446.2011.00416.x

Scull, A. (2005). *Madhouse: A tragic tale of megalomania and modern medicine.* Yale University Press.

Slagle, E. C. (1934). Occupational therapy: Recent methods and advances in the United States. *Occupational Therapy and Rehabilitation, 13*(5), 289–298.

Slutsky, J., Atkins, D., Chang, S., & Sharp, B. A. (2010). AHRQ series paper 1: Comparing medical interventions: AHRQ and the effective healthcare program. *Journal of Clinical Epidemiology, 63*(5), 471–473. https://doi.org/10.1016/j.jclinepi.2008.06.009

Stadnyk, R., Townsend, E. A., & Wilcock, A. (2010). Occupational justice. In C. H. Christiansen & E. A. Townsend (Eds.), *Introduction to occupation: The art and science of living* (2nd ed., pp. 329–358). Prentice Hall.

Stanley, J. (2010). Inner night and inner light: A Quaker model of pastoral care for the mentally ill. *Journal of Religion and Health, 49*(4), 547–559. https://doi.org/10.1007/s10943-009-9312-4

Steinecke, A., & Terrell, C. (2010). Progress for whose future? The impact of the Flexner report on medical education for racial and ethnic minority physicians in the United States. *Academic Medicine, 85*(2), 236–245. https://doi.org/10.1097/ACM.0b013e3181c885be

Thomasson, M. A. (2002). From sickness to health: The twentieth-century development of U.S. health insurance. *Explorations in Economic History, 39*(3), 233–253. https://doi.org/10.1006/exeh.2002.0788

Tilsen, J., & Nylund, D. (2008). Psychotherapy research, the recovery movement and practiced based evidence in psychiatric rehabilitation. *Journal of Social Work in Disability & Rehabilitation, 7*(3–4), 340–354. https://doi.org/10.1080/15367100802487663

Townsend, E. (Ed.). (2002). *Enabling occupation: An occupational therapy perspective*. Canadian Association of Occupational Therapists.

Townsend, E. (Ed.). (2007). *Enabling occupation II: Advancing an occupational therapy vision for health, well-being and justice through occupation*. Canadian Association of Occupational Therapists.

Townsend, E., & Wilcock, A. A. (2004). Occupational justice and client-centered practice. A dialogue in progress. *Canadian Journal of Occupational Therapy, 71*, 75–87. https://doi.org/10.1177/000841740407100203

Tracy, S. (1910). *Studies in invalid occupation*. Whitcomb and Barrows.

United Nations. (n.d.). *History of the United Nations*. https://www.un.org/en/about-us/history-of-the-un

University of Southern California. (n.d.). *USC occupational therapy: The 20th century*. http://ot.usc.edu/images/uploads/ot_timeline.pdf

U.S. Army Medical Department. (2012). *Occupational therapy educational programs April 1947–January 1961*. https://chan.usc.edu/about-us/history

USC Chan Division of Occupational Therapy. (2012). *Mary Reilly, 1916-2012*. https://chan.usc.edu/news/magazine/spring2012/mary-reilly-1916-2012

U.S. Department of Health, Education, and Welfare. (1965). *Part I: National trends in health education and welfare trends*. Author.

U.S. Department of Veterans Affairs. (2015). *Military health history pocket card for clinicians*. http://www.va.gov/oaa/pocketcard/worldwar.asp

U.S. Government Printing Office. (2011). *The financial crisis inquiry report: Final report of the national commission on the causes of the financial and economic crisis in the United States*. Author. https://www.gpo.gov/fdsys/pkg/GPO-FCIC/content-detail.html

Wade, L. C. (2005). *Encyclopedia of Chicago: Settlement houses*. http://www.encyclopedia.chicagohistory.org/pages/1135.html

Wagner, J. B., Scheinfeld, L., Leeman, B., Pardini, K., Saragossi, J., & Flood, K. (2018). Three professions come together for an interdisciplinary approach to 3D printing: Occupational therapy, biomedical engineering, and medical librarianship. *Journal of the Medical Library Association, 106*(3), 370–376. https://doi.org/10.5195/jmla.2018.321

Ward, J. C., & Burns, K. (2007). *The war: An intimate portrait*. Alfred K. Knopf.

West, W. L. (1991). The issue is: Should the representative assembly have voted as it did, when it did, on occupational therapists' use of physical agent modalities? *American Journal of Occupational Therapy, 45*(12), 1143–1147. https://doi.org/10.5014/ajot.45.12.1143

Whiteley, S. (2004). The evolution of the therapeutic community. *The Psychiatric Quarterly, 75*, 233–248. https://doi.org/0033-2720/040900/0233/0

Wilcock, A. A. (1998). *An occupational perspective on health*. SLACK.

Wilcock, A. A., & Hocking, C. (2015). *An occupational perspective of health* (3rd ed.). SLACK.

Willard, H. S., & Spackman, C. S. (1947). *Principles of occupational therapy*. J. B. Lippincott.

Williams, T. A. (1909). Requisite for the treatment of psycho-neuroses. The Kansas City medical index. *Lancet, 32*, 353–354.

World Federation of Occupational Therapists. (2022a). *History*. https://www.wfot.org/about/history

World Federation of Occupational Therapists. (2022b). *Covid-19 pandemic information and resources*. https://www.wfot.org/covid-19-information-and-resources-for-occupational-therapists

World Health Organization. (n.d.). *History*. https://www.who.int/about/history

World Health Organization. (2001). *International classification of functioning disability and health (ICF)*. Author.

World Health Organization. (2020). *Coronavirus disease (Covid-19): How is it transmitted?* https://www.who.int/news-room/q-a-detail/coronavirus-disease-covid-19-how-is-it-transmitted

World Meters. (2021). *Coronavirus cases*. Retrieved July 3, 2021 from https://www.worldometers.info/coronavirus/

Yenne, B. (2020). *The fourth axis power*. World War II, December 1, 2020, 63–69.

Yerxa, E. J. (1967a). The 1966 Eleanor Clarke Slagle lecture: Authentic occupational therapy. *American Journal of Occupational Therapy, 21*, 155–173.

Yerxa, E. J. (1967b). The American Occupational Therapy Foundation is born. *American Journal of Occupational Therapy, 21*(5), 299–300.

Yerxa, E. J. (1990). An introduction to occupational science, a foundation for occupational therapy in the 21st century. *Occupational Therapy in Health Care, 6*(4), 1–17. https://doi.org/10.1080/J003v06n04_04

Yerxa, E. J., Clark, F., Frank, G., Jackson, J., Parham, D., Stein, C., & Zemke, R. (1989) An introduction to occupational science: A foundation for occupational therapy in the 21st century. *Occupational Therapy in Health Care, 6*, 1-17. https://doi.org/10.1080/J003v06n04_04

Yohanna, D. (2013). Deinstitutionalization of people with mental illness: Causes and consequences. *AMA Journal of Ethics*. https://journalofethics.ama-assn.org/article/deinstitutionalization-people-mental-illness-causes-and-consequences/2013-10

Zaloga, S. (2004). *Poland 1939: The birth of Blitzkrieg*. Praeger.

Zerhouni, E. (2003). Medicine. The NIH roadmap. *Science, 302*(5642), 63–72. https://doi.org/10.1126/science.1091867

A Philosophy of Occupational Therapy

Barbara Hooper and Wendy Wood

LEARNING OBJECTIVES

After reading this chapter, you will be able to:

1. Describe elements of a philosophical framework and their transactions.
2. Explain how a philosophical framework guides practice.
3. Articulate occupational therapy's basic philosophical assumptions and their transactions, using a comprehensive philosophical framework.
4. Evaluate the fit of practice with occupational therapy's philosophy and create one or two strategies that could strengthen the congruence between practice and philosophy of occupational therapy, given an OT story.

Introduction

Occupational therapy (OT) has a philosophy, and it may be the most basic element of practice. A profession's philosophy is the foundation upholding all that practitioners, educators, and researchers do. A philosophy helps members of OT to (a) develop clear and coherent professional identities as *occupational* therapists, (b) hone a practice that is unique among healthcare providers, and (c) explain the hidden and often underestimated complexity of the profession to both themselves and others. Emphasizing how indispensable philosophy is, Wilcock (1999) stated that "the first essential for each individual in any profession is the acceptance of a philosophy that is the profession's keystone" (p. 192). A profession's *keystone* refers to a set of concepts that are shared at some level and provide boundaries for the profession's work, but which members continually debate, revise, and disrupt as needed. She proposed "occupation for health" as one such concept for OT's philosophy. Thus, Wilcock (2000), writing from an Australian context, proposed that professions need a "simple, usable philosophy that is sufficiently general" to distinguish the profession, yet allow for changes in ideas, context, research, and experience (p. 82).

It is noted in the previous paragraph how a philosophy is dynamic, being continuously refined by members of a profession. The refinement process is sometimes called *philosophizing*—an important skill if students and practitioners are to achieve what Wilcock called the "first essential" in joining a profession. In other words, a profession's philosophy is not static. It is the responsibility of all practitioners to critically appraise and evolve the intersections between particular contexts and the profession's concepts.

The philosophy presented in this chapter grew from a process of philosophizing. We compiled writings through a search of commonly cited sources describing aspects of OT history and which we deemed influential to the historical evolution of OT in a Western context. We also selected writings in which Western perspectives of OT theory and philosophy had been critiqued. In addition, we selected a framework that has traditionally been used in the field of philosophy in the United States and was used earlier in OT, and more recently in other fields, to represent elements of a philosophy. We used three elements of a philosophy to code the compiled readings and, ultimately, to narrate the philosophy presented here. The elements we used as the framework had been used independently of each other in other writings about OT philosophy, but not altogether and not as an analytic and narrative tool. Thus, we believed a broader approach to philosophizing was needed.

Moreover, because any philosophy is dynamic and emergent in response to its context, we refer readers to other content in this chapter that could help inform their own philosophizing for OT. For example, specific influences of many formal philosophies on the field have been detailed elsewhere (see Table 3.1). In particular, Taff and Babulal (2021) describe specific influences of formal philosophies and the movements they generated on the profession of OT. In Expanding Our Perspectives, Kronenberg critiques Western ways of philosophizing about OT.

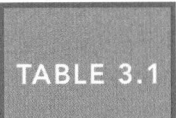

TABLE 3.1	Select Resources on the Influences of Formal Philosophies on Occupational Therapy
Formal Philosophy	**Select Resources**
Pragmatism	Breines (1986, 1987), Cutchin (2004), Hooper and Wood (2002), and Ikiugu and Schultz (2006)
Arts and crafts movement	Friedland (2003), Hocking (2008), Levine (1987), and Reed (1986, 2005)
European enlightenment	Ikiugu and Schultz (2006) and Wilcock (2006)
Structuralism	Hooper and Wood (2002)
Existentialism	Yerxa (1967)
Humanism	Bruce and Borg (2002), Devereaux (1984), and Nelson (1997)
Holism	Finlay (2001)
See also	Peloquin (2005), Punwar and Peloquin (2000), Reed and Sanderson (1999), West (1984), and Taff and Babulal (2021)

Our purpose in this chapter is to describe a philosophy of OT that was generated from the philosophizing process using three elements of a philosophical framework: ontology, epistemology, and axiology. We explore this profession-specific philosophy in relation to these elements, each of which suggests a question as captured in the chapter's headings:

- ***Ontology:*** What Is Most Real for Occupational Therapy?
- ***Epistemology:*** What Is Knowledge in Occupational Therapy?
- ***Axiology:*** What Is Right Action in Occupational Therapy?

We conclude the chapter with a comparison of philosophical and nonphilosophical thinking and case studies to apply the philosophical framework.

Philosophies, being constructions of people in particular places and times, will perpetually have gaps, including the OT philosophy proposed here. We have attempted to incorporate contemporary critiques of OT as well as new and renewed emphases in the profession worldwide. Some of the contemporary themes we reviewed for this revision include human rights and occupational justice; the indivisibility of individuals, communities, and populations; the indivisibility of individual's abilities and the social conditions of their lives; occupational issues related to violence against people in Black, indigenous, Asian, Pacific Island, Hispanic, LGBTQIA+, disability, and migrant communities; and social OT. In addition, our use of the term *clients* encompasses the continuum of individuals, families, organizations, communities, and populations. We also use the term *practice* to refer to OT across traditional and emerging settings and justice work with populations. These efforts at inclusivity noted, it is also the case that the philosophy represented herein remains predominantly a synthesis of the work of scholars and practitioners who have been informed primarily by Western cultural perspectives of OT, ourselves included.

The Meaning, Structure, and Use of Philosophy

At its root, the word *philosophy* refers to "The love, study, or pursuit of wisdom, truth, or knowledge" (Oxford University Press, 2021). Philosophy is built from a "network" of assumptions and beliefs (Paul, 1995). Assumptions are ideas or principles that are "taken for granted as the basis for argument and action" (Oxford University Press, 2021). **Assumptions** are sometimes referred to as "first principles" that form a bedrock for beliefs (Ikiugu & Schultz, 2006). **Beliefs** are convictions about what is true (Rogers, 1982b; Yerxa, 1979). Assumptions and beliefs function as a framework for thinking and action; in other words, they function as a philosophy.

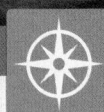

EXPANDING OUR PERSPECTIVES

Philosophizing Occupational Therapy Critically (POTC)

Frank Kronenberg

"It's not a measure of health to be well adjusted to a profoundly sick society."

– Jiddu Krishnamurti

Situating and Explaining POTC and Intention

Whereas the main text elaborates "the established philosophy of OT," this box, grounded in occupational consciousness (see Chapter 11), briefly addresses POTC, that is, to think, sense, imagine, and theorize our profession politically and in a historicized way. Here, *politically* refers to "being concerned with what is good or bad for mankind" (Aristotle, 1998), and *historicized* means employing a long-term approach to history that recognizes patterns of dehumanization. The intention of POTC is to contribute to positioning and preparing our profession to realize its ethical–political obligations to society through a process of acknowledging shortcomings, committing to resolve them, pursuing alternatives, and evidencing impact.

Exclusive to Inclusive Profession: Toward Serving Public Interests and Common Good

Like all professions, OT has both *private* and *public* duties, that is, we owe ethical–political obligations and responsibilities in service to private and individual clients *and* to the public or society as a whole (Jennings et al., 1987). However, an honest critical appraisal of our global and local practices and our institutional arrangements reveals two generatively disruptive truths: (a) our vision statements (American Occupational Therapy Association [AOTA], 2007, 2018) center not on societal needs but instead on our profession, which almost exclusively attends to private duties for individual clients, and (b) our global body of practitioners, educators, researchers, and governing structures grossly underrepresents the rich demographic, cultural, and socioeconomic diversity of the public we serve. The inclusion of this box acknowledges the need to start addressing the institutionalized exclusion (invisibilization) to date of the lived experiences and perspectives of peoples, populations, and communities whose full humanity may have been historically questioned, trivialized, or altogether negated, owing to systemic racism and other intersecting oppressions (AOTA, 2020; Kronenberg, 2020; World Federation of Occupational Therapists, 2020). This exclusion can also be seen in the virtual absence in our discourse of humanity terminologies (e.g., humanity–inhumanity, humanizing–dehumanizing, humanization–dehumanization) and in the still undertheorized core concept of society (Kronenberg, 2018; Kronenberg et al., 2015).

Phronesis and Set of Phronetic Questions

POTC employs a critical contemporary appreciation (Flyvbjerg, 2001) of Aristotle's three intellectual virtues: *phronesis*, *episteme*, and *tecne*, foregrounding the first virtue about "ends" to lead to the other two about "means" (see Figure A). Tellingly perhaps, OT training appears to be mostly occupied with obtaining the "means," much less so with our profession's ultimate "ends," particularly with regard to serving public interests and the common good.

Philosophizing Occupational Therapy Critically

A Critical Contemporary Appreciation of Aristotle's Three Intellectual Virtues

ENDS   VALUES & POWER RATIONALITIES   **PHRONESIS** Practical Knowledge 'Knowing WHY'   **OT**   INSTRUMENTAL RATIONALITIES   **EPISTEME** Theoretical Knowledge 'Knowing WHAT and HOW'   **TECNE** Technical Knowledge 'Knowing HOW to DO'   **MEANS**

Figure A Illustration by Frank Kronenberg.

POTC can be guided by the following set of phronetic questions, adapted from Flyvbjerg (2001):

1. Toward what private, public, and common-good ends is our OT profession occupied?
2. Who gains and who loses, and by what mechanisms of power?
3. How does what we are doing manifest on the continuum affirming or negating our humanity, generating health or harm, enabling liberation, or perpetuating oppression (see Figure B)?
4. What, if anything, should and can we do about it?

Politically–Historically Grounded OT Assumptions and Beliefs

Arguably, the established philosophy of OT is thought about and employed apolitically and ahistorically, particularly ignoring the racist tradition in Western humanism. It includes premises such as being human is a given, our interrelated core concepts of occupation and health can best be practically understood individualistically, and occupation is an object of study that can be separated from its subjects (humans) (Guajardo et al., 2015). These assumptions do not allow us to appreciate how historically unequal power relations have shaped OT and its practices, education, research, and governance.

A politically historicized appraisal of "reality, knowledge, and right action" may allow for a philosophy oriented more toward public interests and common good. Such a philosophy would be based on the following three assumptions (see Figure B):

1. Being human is not a given; instead, it is a political potentiality that manifests on a continuum of enacted harmful (pathogenic) negations and health-promoting (salutogenic) affirmations of our humanity, respectively, sustaining or disrupting oppressive forces and generating liberating practices (see Chapter 11).
2. Being human is radically relational, that is, we cannot be human by ourselves, we become human through how we relate to and interact with others.
3. Cultivation of being human as shared identity integrity can advance humanity health or Ubuntu, the African ethic of critical humanism (Kronenberg, 2018, 2020).

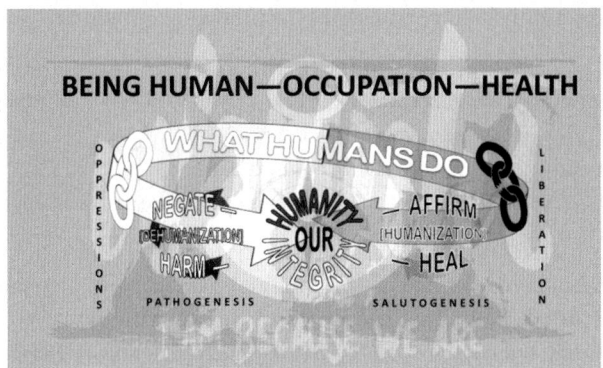

Figure B Illustration by Frank Kronenberg.

Toward a Public Philosophy of OT: How Are We Doing Together as Humanity?

A foregrounding of the ends of OT calls for a diversification and complexification of our profession's main concern and philosophy. Our private duties focus on *how some groupings of individual clients are doing ("functioning") within their everyday social contexts.* Mindful of Krishnamurti's (2020) opening quote in this box, serving public interests and the common good requires becoming occupied with "*how we [as humanity] are doing together as communities, organizations, societies,*" essentially adopting a collective occupations approach to our practices (Ramugondo & Kronenberg, 2013). Determining what may constitute "public interests" and the "common good" calls us to engage in ongoing civil deliberation and moral debates in everyday social contexts (e.g., school boards, community organizations, workplaces, social media platforms) about our societies' ultimate goals and public philosophies (Jennings et al., 1987),

to learn how we may indeed best contribute to serving societal needs.

Closing

In closing, POTC invokes the expression "the mother of all . . ." to ontologically position our profession to serve public duties and the common good: the mother of all traumas is dehumanization; the mother of all occupations and health is being human; and the mother of all OTs is humanizing and healing histories (Bockoven, 1972; Kronenberg, 2018; see Expanding Our Perspectives in Chapter 4).

References

American Occupational Therapy Association. (2007). AOTA's Centennial Vision and executive summary. *American Journal of Occupational Therapy, 61,* 613–614. https://doi.org/10.5014/ajot.61.6.613

American Occupational Therapy Association. (2018). *Vision 2025.* https://www.aota.org/aboutaota/vision-2025.aspx

American Occupational Therapy Association. (2021). *Position statement on justice and systemic racism.* https://www.aota.org/about/diversity-equity-and-inclusion/aota-statement-on-justice-and-systemic-racism

Aristotle. (1998). *Politics.* (C. D. C. Reeve, Trans.). Hackett.

Bockoven, J. S. (1972). Occupational therapy: A neglected source of community rehumanization. In J. S. Bockoven (Ed.), *Moral treatment in community mental health* (pp. 217–228). Springer.

Flyvbjerg, B. (2001). *Making social science matter: Why social inquiry fails and how it can succeed again.* Cambridge University Press.

Guajardo, A., Kronenberg, F., & Ramugondo, E. (2015). Southern occupational therapies: Emerging identities, epistemologies and practices. *South African Journal of Occupational Therapy, 45*(1), 3–10. https://doi.org/10.17159/2310-3833/2015/v45no1a2

Jennings, B., Callahan, D., & Wolf, S. M. (1987). The professions: Public interest and common good. *The Hastings Center Report, 17*(1), 3–10. https://doi.org/10.2307/3562447

Krishnamurti, J. (2020, July 30). *Chuck B philosophy blog post.* https://chuckbphilosophy.com/it-is-no-measure-of-success-to-be-well-adjusted-to-a-sick-society/

Kronenberg, F. (2018). *Everyday enactments of humanity affirmations in post 1994 apartheid South Africa: A phronetic case study of being human as occupation and health* [Doctoral thesis]. University of Cape Town. https://open.uct.ac.za/handle/11427/29441

Kronenberg, F. (2020, October 4). Commentary on JOS editorial board's anti-racism pledge. *Journal of Occupational Science, 28*(3), 398–403. https://doi.org/10.1080/14427591.2020.1827483

Kronenberg, F., Kathard, H., Laliberte Rudman, D., & Ramugondo, E. (2015). Can post-apartheid South Africa be enabled to humanise and heal itself? *South African Journal of Occupational Therapy, 45*(1), 20–26. https://doi.org/10.17159/2310-3833/2015/v45no1a4

Ramugondo, E. L., & Frank Kronenberg, F. (2013). Explaining collective occupations from a human relations perspective: Bridging the individual-collective dichotomy. *Journal of Occupational Science, 22*(1), 3–16. https://doi.org/10.1080/14427591.2013.781920

World Federation of Occupational Therapists. (2020). *Position statement on systemic racism.* https://wfot.org/wfot-statement-on-systemic-racism

Philosophies can be both unconscious and conscious. On the one hand, individuals and the groups, communities, and societies to which they belong can operate largely unaware of their active framework of assumptions and beliefs. When unaware, people and their various social groups are somewhat run by an inherited system of thinking and cannot easily evaluate the foundations that underlie their actions. Paul (1995) refers to this state as a personal and collective *nonphilosophical mind*. On the other hand, individuals and the groups, communities, and societies to which they belong can examine, choose, and organize their assumptions and beliefs. They form a conscious philosophy, which they intentionally use as a *framework for thinking* and a *mode of thinking*. Paul refers to this state as a personal and collective *philosophical mind*. Having adopted a philosophical mind, people and communities become keen to probe their thinking framework and how it drives their actions, methods, and policies; they do not confuse their thinking with reality and thus continuously seek to refine both the framework and actions for greater congruence over time.

We thus define *philosophy* as (a) a conscious framework of assumptions and beliefs that guides actions and (b) a mode of thinking that actively relies on the framework for processing and responding to experience, while remaining open to continuous refinement of the framework. In turn, *a philosophical mode of thinking* refers to "thinking with a clear sense of the ultimate foundations of one's thinking" (Paul, 1995, p. 436).

A Philosophical Framework: Ontology, Epistemology, and Axiology

A philosophical framework has at least three categories of assumptions and beliefs. One category, known as ontology, contains beliefs about reality. A second category, epistemology, contains beliefs about knowledge, and the third category, axiology, contains beliefs about appropriate actions (Lincoln et al., 2011; Ruona & Lynham, 2004; J. W. Schell, 2018a; Yerxa, 1979). In this section, we define and describe each category and how the three function as a dynamic framework for thinking.

Ontology is defined as the "science or study of being; that branch of metaphysics concerned with the nature or essence of being or existence" (Oxford University Press, 2021). Stated another way, ontology is concerned with the question *What is most real*? In other words, what aspects of reality are illuminated and foregrounded by one's perspective? The question itself implies that there are multiple realities and that there are dynamic processes by which communities form the realities receiving their foremost attention. Yerxa (1979), considering ontology in OT, phrased

the question as "What is 'really' real in the world?" (p. 26). Setting out an OT theory of humans, Wilcock and Hocking (2015) drew upon the question posed by Stevenson et al. (2004): "What is the nature of the universe and humans' relationship to it?" Therefore, the ontologic question is not new to OT and debate continues over the views of reality formed within OT.

The aspects of ontology in OT can be discerned by examining how the field's scholars and practitioners have addressed the following questions:

- What is an OT view of the human?
- What are the *most* real dimensions of life from an OT perspective?

Epistemology is defined as a theory of knowledge (Oxford University Press, 2021). Stated another way, epistemology asks the question *What is knowledge*? As noted about ontology, the question itself implies that there are multiple views of knowledge. The point in this chapter is not to answer this question definitively but to present a view that can be discerned by examining how the field's scholars and practitioners have addressed the following questions:

- What knowledge is most important to know and to demonstrate in OT?
- How is knowledge in OT organized?
- How is knowledge acquired and used?
- What is an OT view of the essence or nature of knowledge?

Axiology asks the question *What are right actions*? Axiology is defined as "the study of values including what is good, beautiful, and morally desirable" (Yerxa, 1979, p. 26). Values, in turn, help "make explicit how we ought to act" (Ruona & Lynham, 2004, p. 154). Similar to ontology and epistemology, the question about "right" actions implies there are many possible actions to take in a given situation and that some actions will align with the values of the situation and the profession better than other actions. Thus, axiology entails observable actions that manifest values; such actions are referred to as *methodologies and methods in service to one's values*. A **methodology** is a general approach to practice. **Methods** are the actual processes and procedures used when working within a given methodology. OT axiology can be discerned by examining how the field's scholars and practitioners have addressed the following questions:

- What are the enduring values of OT?
- What are the core methodologies and methods that practitioners use in practice that manifest its enduring values?

All three categories of belief—ontology, epistemology, axiology—are fluid, mutually influential, and continually interacting. These dynamic interactions form "a guiding framework for a congruent and coherent system of thought and action" (Ruona & Lynham, 2004, p. 154).

To illustrate, we borrow a visual representation from Palmer (2009). Figure 3.1 uses a Möbius strip to depict the dynamic nature and ongoing transactions among the ontologic, epistemologic, and axiologic premises of OT. Beliefs about reality and knowledge are commonly more internal to the profession and individual practitioners, sometimes held without full conscious awareness; they are, therefore, depicted on what seems to be the "inside" of the Möbius strip. Beliefs about what actions to take, which are expressed in observable methodologies and methods, are depicted on what seems to be the "outside" of the strip. On closer examination, however, there is no dichotomy between an inside and outside on a Möbius strip. Rather, according to Palmer, the two sides keep cocreating each other.

If Figure 3.1 were made into a three-dimensional object (we encourage readers to do so using instructions found on Lippincott Connect), one's finger could continuously move from ontology to epistemology to axiology and so on, indicating that these three elements can be considered one whole. That is, professional beliefs about reality flow into and shape beliefs about knowledge, which flow into and shape actions manifest in practice. In reverse, professional actions and values flow into, reflect, and shape one's beliefs about reality and continue around the Möbius strip.

The Relationship of Philosophy to Theory

As argued in Chapter 33, theories help people understand and address something in the world. Theories are, therefore, inextricably linked to ways of perceiving the world (ontology), constructing knowledge about the world (epistemology), and acting in the world (axiology) (Ruona & Lynham, 2004). A profession's philosophy consequently underpins its theories. Theory is like an intermediary that helps bind philosophy to practice and research.

The Philosophy of Occupational Therapy

Ontology: What Is Most Real for Occupational Therapy?

In her 1961 Eleanor Clarke Slagle lectureship, Reilly (1962) posed that the central belief of the profession could be stated in the form of this hypothesis: "That man, through the use of his hands, as they are energized through mind and will, can

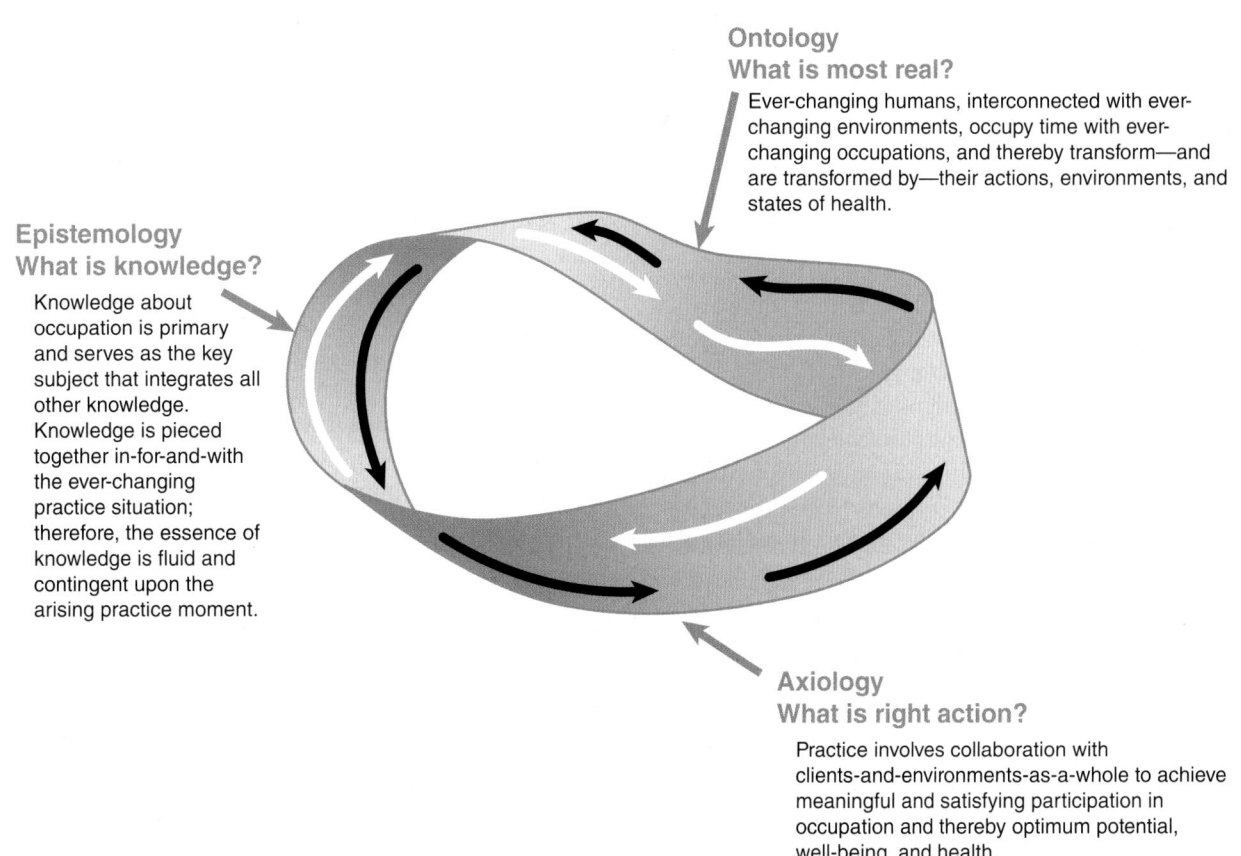

Ontology
What is most real?
Ever-changing humans, interconnected with ever-changing environments, occupy time with ever-changing occupations, and thereby transform—and are transformed by—their actions, environments, and states of health.

Epistemology
What is knowledge?
Knowledge about occupation is primary and serves as the key subject that integrates all other knowledge. Knowledge is pieced together in-for-and-with the ever-changing practice situation; therefore, the essence of knowledge is fluid and contingent upon the arising practice moment.

Axiology
What is right action?
Practice involves collaboration with clients-and-environments-as-a-whole to achieve meaningful and satisfying participation in occupation and thereby optimum potential, well-being, and health.

FIGURE 3.1 **An occupational therapy philosophical framework for practice.**

influence the state of his own health" (p. 6). Reilly's hypothesis has since been critiqued for privileging a view of humans as individuals who are decontextualized from, and exercise control over, their environments and circumstances (Dickie et al., 2006; Hammel & Iwama, 2012). Considering these critiques, we propose that the central ontologic premise for OT can be summarized today as follows (see Figure 3.1):

> Ever-changing humans, interconnected with ever-changing environments, engage with ever-changing occupations, and thereby transform—and are transformed by—their actions, environments and states of health.

We next elaborate on this statement, beginning with the ever-changing occupational human.

The Nature of Humans, Ever-Changing Occupational Beings

A profound view of human beings has served as a cornerstone of OT since its inception: human beings are infused with an innate, biological need for occupation; as humans engage in daily occupations, they meet needs for survival, growth, development, health, and well-being (Wilcock & Hocking, 2015; Wood, 1993, 1998a; Yerxa, 1998). Dunton (1919) described humans' biological need for occupation quite simply, "Occupation is as necessary to life as food and drink" (p. 17). Reilly (1962) described humans' biological requirement for occupation in neurologic terms. If the human organism is to grow and become productive, then there is a vital need for occupation; indeed, in her view, the central nervous system "demands the rich and varied stimuli that solving life problems provides" (Reilly, 1962, p. 5). Wilcock (2006) likewise argued that occupation activates the integrative functions of the central nervous system, making it possible not only for individuals to develop and experience health and well-being but also for the species to survive and evolve. Wilcock and Hocking (2015) further summarized that as humans engage in occupation, they simultaneously meet needs for doing, being, becoming, and belonging.

Embedded in these descriptions of humans' need for occupation is another long-standing belief: humans are an indivisible whole who possess an "inextricable union of the mind and body" (Bing, 1981, p. 515; Damasio, 1994). Mind, body, and spirit can be united in humans' pursuit of and engagement with occupation (Bing, 1981; Reed & Sanderson, 1999). A core philosophical assumption of the profession, therefore, is that by virtue of our biological endowment, people of all ages and abilities require occupation to survive, grow, thrive, and belong; in pursuing occupation, humans express the totality of their being, a mind–body–spirit union. Yet as noted by Wilcock (2000), saying that humans are occupational beings, or that occupation is indispensable to survival and health, or that mind, body, and spirit are inextricably linked, is much easier than grasping what these complex articles of faith mean. Stopping there, it would be easy to conclude

erroneously that these human qualities solely reside within the individual. As next discussed, one must also, therefore, consider how the environment calls forth, develops, and sustains the occupational essence of humans.

The Nature of Humans as Interconnected With Ever-Changing Environments

Being interconnected with the environment does not denote either being in harmony with the environment or being fully determined by the environment. The view of reality within OT includes simply the belief that human beings, as indivisible wholes, are part and parcel of their daily living environments (Reed & Sanderson, 1999). Kielhofner (1983) posited, for example, that "unity of the human system with the social environment is not a platitude but is an essential part of the human condition" (p. 76). Yerxa (1998) maintained that just like "water cannot be reduced to hydrogen and oxygen and still be wet and drinkable," neither can human beings be viewed as separate from their environments nor "be reduced to a single level, say that of the motor system, and retain their richness or identity" (p. 413).

Although an enduring belief of OT is that human beings are best understood in the context of their environments, beliefs about the person–environment relationship have evolved. Earlier conceptions of this relationship have been critiqued for separating the person and environment. According to Cutchin (2004), OT historically embraced a view of the environment "as a container" in which an individual carries out occupation. The individual was the focus; the environment was the background. This view allowed understandings of people to be too easily separated from understandings of environments as eliciting people's actions and influencing how they perform and experience occupation. According to Iwama (2006), some prominent models of OT that originated in Western cultural contexts similarly represented people and environments as distinct, even if mutually influential. As alternatives, these and other scholars have variously stressed the indivisibility of people and environments. For example, Dickie et al. (2006) advocated for a closer adherence to Dewey's transactionalism, in which the human is viewed as an "organism-in-environment-as-a-whole" (p. 83). Iwama (2006) and Wood (2017) developed practice models that are predicated on views of the indivisibility of people and environments. Thus, as expressed in this chapter, human beings and their environments constitute integrated and dynamic—that is, ever-changing—wholes.

The Nature of Transformation and Health

As ever-changing humans, interconnected with ever-changing environments, enact their biological needs for occupation, they and their environments continuously change as do the occupations in which they engage and how they so engage. Thus, people transform and are transformed by their actions as choreographed with the dynamics of their environments. Transformation refers to change on both small and grand scales, and change for both better and worse. On a small scale, for example, recall a time when participating in a favorite occupation transformed your outlook, emotional state, and body sense. For me (Barb), I can be in the throes of anxiety, feeling out of shape and out of time. Yet, in response to internal and external conditions, if I can go for a bike ride, I often experience change almost immediately. My anxiety falls away, contentment emerges, strength returns, and time opens. In such fashion, consider how often clients express that they feel much better after working with an occupational therapist to simply wash their face and brush their teeth for the first time after surgery. As Hasselkus (2011) persuasively illustrated, these taken-for-granted experiences and interactions reflect small-scale, yet still very important, transformations through occupation; they can even be epiphanous.

Especially prominent in OT is the more grand-scale belief that people's health changes as a function of their occupations over time (Blanche & Henny-Kohler, 2000; Friedland, 2011; Hasselkus, 2011; Kielhofner, 2004; Meyer, 1922; Peloquin, 2005; Quiroga, 1995; Reed & Sanderson, 1999; Reilly, 1962; West, 1984). In OT, health is not viewed as the absence of disease or pathology. Rather, relative states of good or ill health are viewed as inextricably related to people's access to a range of occupations and what they experience through, or what emanates from, their participation in those occupations. Consequently, health is highly dynamic. Health is also related to desirable effects, such as human thriving, well-being, and dignity; realization of potential and optimal functional capacities; and a good quality of life or satisfaction and meaning in life (Hasselkus, 2011; Peloquin, 2005; Rogers, 1982a; Wood et al., 2017; Yerxa, 1983, 1998). It is through occupation, therefore, that people and their environments exist in dynamic and mutually influential relationships, the optimal desired results of which are favorable states of health.

This is not to say that the occupations in which people engage are seen as inevitably positive. Because engagement in occupation is a biological necessity, when people are blocked from using—for whatever reasons—their powers to act, when they are deterred in developing their potentials, when they are thwarted in expressing their capacities for doing, or when they are marginalized, then the change is toward states of dysfunction, dissatisfaction, poor health, and ill-being. Occupationally limiting circumstances can lead to food insecurity, poverty, lack of shelter, boredom, anxiety, depression, alienation, dysfunction, and ill health. However, situations that block meaningful doing and thus give rise to unfavorable states of health are still viewed as malleable and subject to change through occupation, including the occupations of community organizing, advocacy, policy development, activism, education, and sustainability, among

others. Thus, people's persistent "doings" can change not only themselves for both better and worse, but their doings can also change communities, societies, and the health of the planet for better and worse (Wilcock & Hocking, 2015).

Within OT, the ontologic view of human beings and their situations remains ultimately a hopeful view. A hopeful view does not deny harsh realities of structural inequities worldwide or how the occupations of some groups suppress the occupations of others. Nor does a hopeful view imply that all situations invariably improve or progress in positive ways. Rather a hopeful view is one in which attention is given to the inherent potential of people to experience and cultivate, through occupation, a good life for members of their communities, their families, and themselves. As summarized by Peloquin (2005), a core belief of OT is that there is, in occupation, a capacity for people to "become hale and whole" (p. 614).

To be clear, we are not claiming a universal, theoretical consensus about occupation, which Iwama (2006) cautioned against and Hammel (2011) recognized as "theoretical imperialism" (p. 27). Rather, as Watson (2006) claimed, the profession "unifies around a belief in the power and positive potential of occupation to transform the life conditions of individuals and communities. This belief begins to capture the profession's 'essence'" (p. 151), even as that "essence" must be developed in and for specific societal conditions and cultural contexts.

Epistemology: What Is Knowledge in Occupational Therapy?

The OT's dominant perspective of reality and the nature of humans "sets priorities for knowledge" (Kielhofner & Burke, 1983, p. 43). As shown in Figure 3.1, we propose that the profession's most central epistemologic premises today can be summarized as follows:

> Knowledge about occupation is primary and serves as the key subject that integrates all other knowledge and clarifies the desired consequences of action. Toward that end, knowledge is pieced together in-for-and-with the present practice situation that is continuously changing; therefore, the essence of knowledge is both bound and fluid, contingent upon the arising practice moment.

We elaborate on this epistemologic premise by discussing each of its elements.

Knowledge of Occupation Is Primary for Occupational Therapists

Given the ontologic premises in OT, what is most important to know? Overwhelmingly, the answer is knowledge about occupation. As proclaimed by Weimer (1979), "Ours is, and must be, the basic knowledge of occupation" (p. 43). Reilly

(1962) advised that knowledge about anatomy, neurophysiology, personality theory, social processes, and medical conditions, although relevant, is not our distinctive content. Rather, in Reilly's (1962, 1974) view, the unique knowledge of OT is a deep understanding of the nature of work and productive activity, including the play–work continuum, a belief that she believed aligned with what the founders of OT saw as most central to the new field. That occupation continues to be held today as the foremost subject matter of OT has been corroborated extensively in the official documents of professional associations worldwide (AOTA, 2014, 2017; Craik et al., 2008; Hocking & Ness, 2004).

As the Primary Subject, Knowledge About Occupation Organizes and Integrates All Other Knowledge

In addition to what is most important to know, epistemology entails questions such as does knowledge have a structure? If so, then how is the structure to be conceptualized? Such questions are of particular interest because knowledge of occupation entails so many, and sometimes seemingly disparate, topics ranging from kinesiology to culture, to justice. Students can feel lost in the field's wide array of topics and, not perceiving any organization or coherence among them, may mistakenly think that they can pick and choose what is important to know based on their personal interests. It is reassuring, therefore, that scholars have promoted the view that knowledge in OT has an underlying structure. That structure has been portrayed differently over time; for instance, as hierarchical (Kielhofner, 1983; Trombly, 1995), heterarchical and transactional (Dickie et al., 2006; Kielhofner, 2004), and as subject centered (Hooper et al., 2020). Regardless of these different portrayals, however, some shared assumptions are evident concerning the structure of knowledge in OT.

Knowledge of occupation is commonly portrayed as having utmost importance and, accordingly, as regulating or constituting a vital lens through which other areas of knowledge (e.g., biological, psychological, or neuromusculoskeletal) are understood. Knowledge structured with a regulating concept shapes understandings of practice. For example, although two people may have the same injury, the injury will be understood as regulated by many factors, such as race, socioeconomic status, sociocultural context, access to healthcare, stigma, age, and the range of occupations in which someone must engage. Thus, as Kielhofner stated, "A hand injury to an accountant is not the same as a hand injury to a clock maker" (Kielhofner, 1983, p. 79). In the same way, a hip fracture for a retired, married man is not the same as a hip fracture for a woman who is the caregiver for an ailing spouse and two grandchildren. Each situation is unique because of the roles, values, goals, interests, meaning system, and culture into which the injury is introduced and

for which it has consequences. As a regulating influence, knowledge of occupation contextualizes each situation.

As the Primary Subject, Knowledge About Occupation Clarifies Desired Consequences of Action

What is most important to know and how that knowledge is organized are often linked to a group's vision for society or a set of desired consequences that a group would like to see realized (MacIntyre, 1990). Pragmatist philosophers described knowledge as continually being developed and evaluated in light of "a coveted future" (Hooper & Wood, 2002, p. 42). Thus, knowledge about occupation and how it is structured reflects a future, a set of desired consequences toward which the profession aims. That future is the optimal participation of individuals, groups, and populations in health-promoting occupations (Wilcock & Hocking, 2015). This desired future serves as the beacon toward which practitioners aim their knowledge. The exact path for moving toward this distant beacon is discovered through active experimentation that involves piecing OT knowledge together for a given injustice or practice situation and evaluating the results in light of how well it contributed to the desired consequence of participation in occupation.

Knowledge Is Pieced Together in-for-and-with the Ever-Changing Situations

Knowledge in OT is bound by subject, structure, and consequence. However, working within that boundary, practitioners continuously compose knowledge domains and modes of reasoning for each situation, whether traditional therapy situations or situations involving occupational injustices cut people off from occupation. For example, in Chapter 25, Schell and Benfield illustrate how practitioners assimilate and use knowledge in multiple domains, including knowledge of (a) their own beliefs, values, abilities, and experiences; (b) professional theories, evidence, and skills; (c) clients' beliefs, values, abilities, and experiences; (d) clients' goals and how health and life conditions impact their occupations; and (e) the practice culture and its influence on services. In addition, practitioners shift rapidly among and integrate multiple modes of reasoning, including scientific, narrative, pragmatic, ethical, and interactive reasoning (Mattingly & Fleming, 1994; B. A. Schell & Schell, 2018). Thibeault (2002) attested to how the OT reasoning process remains consistent when addressing political, cultural, and economic barriers with populations as well.

Practitioners not only integrate multiple knowledge domains through multiple reasoning processes but also do so again and again with each practice situation. Even if on the surface the situation seems routine, it is likely unique in subtle ways, such as the emotional state of the therapist or client, a change in schedule, or a change in the social or political environment, all of which can make the present practice situation one of a kind. Practitioners recognize that each practice situation is unique and changing even within a single therapy session or a single meeting with a grass-roots movement. Thus, practitioners continuously assemble knowledge with and in response to each practice situation as it presents itself in each moment. Another way of saying this is: practitioners use OT knowledge by configuring it for and with each practice situation.

The Essence of Knowledge Is Tentative, Fluid, and Contingent With the Arising Practice Moment

The earlier discussion culminates in the central consideration in epistemology: what is the nature of knowledge? In sum, knowledge in OT is bounded by its regulating subject, occupation, and its desired consequence, health, and well-being through occupational engagement of individuals, groups, and populations. In addition, there are structures for how knowledge about occupation relates to knowledge about its various elements. The subject, structure, and consequence of knowledge serve as boundaries for knowledge in the field. On the surface, these boundaries seem somewhat stable, yet they are always evolving in how we understand and talk about them. Thus, they are paradoxically enduring and tentative. On these seemingly stable foundations, OT knowledge is newly pieced together in-for-and-with each practice situation.

The essence of knowledge in OT is thus like a musical score. The practice of music is bounded by notes, music theory, and principles. These seemingly stable boundaries (understood and described in new ways over time) are continuously assembled into new pieces of music, and even the same pieces of music are experimented with and played with, given new interpretations in-for-and-with changing audiences and sociocultural situations.

That knowledge arises with the practice moment in a fluid and contingent manner is important for OT students to understand because it has everything to do with how students learn. That is, along with learning discrete content and skills, students need also to learn how to assemble knowledge, evaluate knowledge, and create knowledge in-for-and-with practice situations. To meet this epistemologic challenge, some students find they have to dramatically shift how they have viewed themselves for many years, from a learner who receives knowledge from experts to a learner who thoughtfully and reflectively acquires and integrates knowledge in order to apply it flexibly according to what is needed for a practice situation. This shift can be life-changing (Schell, 2018b).

Axiology: What Is Right Action in Occupational Therapy?

The profession's axiology answers the questions *Given the central beliefs in OT about reality and knowledge, how then shall we live day-to-day in practice? What do we value? What will we do?* As illustrated in Figure 3.1, views of reality and knowledge "shape and direct how we *act* in the world . . ." (Ruona & Lynham, 2004, p. 154). Coherence between how we act in practice and the other aspects of the field's philosophy is important to work out because as Wilcock (1999) cautioned:

> Skills without a philosophy can be a problem. It allows poaching outside a domain of concern, duplication of skills already available to those being served, the dropping of established skills for different ones when some other discipline changes its direction or sticking to familiar skills because of no mandate to inform the direction to be taken. (p. 193)

To illustrate links among skills and philosophy, we discuss three key practice methodologies. We do not believe that these methodologies are comprehensive; for example, they do not encompass important values and actions outlined in the Occupational Therapy Code of Ethics (AOTA, 2015). We do believe, however, that these methodologies help illustrate how actions flow from the field's ontologic and epistemologic premises as shown in Figure 3.1. In accordance with those premises, we propose that axiology within OT can be summarized as follows:

> Occupation practice involves contextually situated collaborations with clients to achieve meaningful and satisfying participation in occupation and thereby optimal potential, well-being and health.

Collaborative Practice

Because ever-changing humans, environments, and occupations are central to the beliefs in OT about reality, it follows that entering into a personal collaboration with clients is a fundamental methodology for practice (Taylor, 2008). That is, through collaborative relationships, practitioners explore the occupations and environments with which people seek to engage. Students will recognize this as client-centered practice but may not have considered how client-centered practice is an outward manifestation of a broader philosophical framework. Considering the philosophical framework in Figure 3.1, collaborative relationships express the profession's ontology. Similarly, if the central belief in OT about knowledge involves piecing knowledge together in-for-and-with each situation, it follows that collaboration is necessary for the practitioner to determine which elements of knowledge and experience to assemble for the current situation. Thus, collaborative, relationship-centered practice constitutes a methodology that manifests OT values and beliefs about reality and knowledge.

By using the term *methodology*, we do not mean to portray collaborative practice as a technical procedure; it is, rather, a long-standing, normative way of practicing OT and exhibiting the profession's values. As Peloquin (2005) stated, "occupational therapy *is* [emphasis added] personal engagement." Watson (2006) elaborated, stating that if we are true to the field's philosophy,

> We will make a personal connection with people in a personal way. The people we are, who we have become . . . and our earnest desire to be of service, will lead us to reach out to the "being" of the "other." (p. 156)

This textbook has much to say about the use of collaboration as a methodology in OT practice. Our purpose here is to highlight how collaborative practice as a methodology stems directly from and manifests the field's views of reality, knowledge, and right action. Collaborative practice can, therefore, serve as a stimulus for reflecting on the congruence between philosophy and practice by asking the following:

- Does this assessment or intervention or my way of being with this client reflect collaborative, relationship-centered care?
- Is collaboration at the center of my actions as an occupational therapist?

Each practitioner will have to work out specific methods for collaborative practice within the parameters of client populations served, cultural contexts for services, and practice setting, among others. But whatever challenges present, collaborative, relationship-centered care is one methodology that naturally expresses the field's core values, ontology, and epistemology.

Occupation-Centered, Occupation-Based, and Occupation-Focused Practice

Because occupation is at the very center of an OT view of reality and what practitioners most need to know, it follows that a core methodology for practice is to help clients participate in meaningful, satisfying, and health-promoting occupations. Since the field's origin, practitioners have provided opportunities for people to engage in occupation and, in so doing, to develop and transform their skills and potential (see, e.g., Christiansen et al., 2005; Kielhofner, 2004; West, 1984; Wood, 1998b). Students may associate these approaches with being occupation-centered and, therefore, with practicing in an occupation-based or occupation-focused manner. According to Fisher (2013), being occupation centered means having adopted a profession-specific perspective in OT, or "worldview of occupation and what it means to be an occupational being," as a guide to reasoning and action (p. 167). The methodology of occupation-based practice involves using occupation in

evaluation and intervention, but this is a complex process that emerges from within each practice situation through collaborated relationships with clients (Price & Miner, 2007). The methodology of occupation-focused practice involves keeping one's immediate, proximal focus on occupation. From the start of care, therefore, practitioners seek to understand clients' occupations and use those throughout the therapy process. At all times, practitioners make explicit how their therapeutic approaches relate to the occupations that clients want and need to do. Therefore, like collaborative practice, practice that is grounded in occupation manifests beliefs about the occupational nature of humans and about knowledge as continuously being put together in-and-with each situation.

This textbook has much to say about the use of occupation-centered practice as a methodology. Our purpose here is to highlight how occupation-centered practice is a natural right action directly stemming from and manifesting the field's views of reality and knowledge. Occupation-centered practice can thus serve as a stimulus for reflecting on the congruence between philosophy and practice by asking the following:

- Does this assessment or intervention or my way of being with this client reflect occupation-centered practice?
- Is occupation at the center of my actions as an occupational therapist?
- Am I making a credible and meaningful connection for clients between occupation, occupation, health, and well-being?

Once again, although each practitioner will have to work out specific methods for occupation-centered practice within the parameters of client populations served, cultural contexts for services, and practice settings, among others, occupation-centered practice is a methodology that naturally expresses the field's core values, ontology, and epistemology.

Context in Practice: Clients-and-Environments-as-Wholes

The emphasis in OT on a central belief about reality as an essential unity existing among people and environments leads to a third important methodology for practice, referred to as clients-and-environments-as-wholes. Occupations that are meaningful to clients—where they occur and with whom, the habits with which occupations are carried out, and the routines that help organize them, and even the musculoskeletal patterns used to perform them—occur in an interconnection between the environment and the client. This is equally true for the environments in which clients live and the environments in which they experience OT, for example, the hospital, rehabilitation center, outpatient clinic, skilled nursing facility, home, work, school, prison, refugee resettlement service, disaster relief center, homeless shelter, or other community organizations (Cutchin, 2004).

According to Hasselkus (2011), seeing clients as tightly knit together with their environments through memories of places, occupation, meanings, roles, routines, and intentions can positively influence therapy outcomes related to adoption and follow-through with environmental modifications. Conversely, when practitioners view clients as separate from environments, they may overly focus on clients' performance. For example, practitioners may make recommendations for environmental modifications from a template such as widen doorways, put in stair lifts, remove throw rugs, add medical equipment, rearrange furniture, and move items to within easy reach. But because these recommendations have been considered as separate from the clients-and-environments-as-a-whole, the family may refuse to implement them.

Like the other methodologies presented, this textbook has much to say about OT's use of the performance context as a methodology in practice. Our purpose here is to illustrate how clients-and-environments-as-a-whole constitutes a natural right action stemming directly from and manifesting the field's views of reality and knowledge. Clients-and-environments-as-a-whole can, therefore, serve as a stimulus for reflecting on the congruence between philosophy and practice by asking the following:

- Does this assessment or intervention or my way of being with this client reflect the unity reflected in clients-and-environments-as-a-whole?

Although each practitioner will, again, have to work out specific methods associated with this methodology within the multiple parameters previously mentioned, clients-and-environments-as-a-whole is a methodology that naturally expresses the field's core values, ontology, and epistemology.

Core Values in Occupational Therapy's Axiology

Lastly, although perhaps most importantly, the methodologies briefly presented earlier uphold and manifest core values of the profession that have been prominent throughout its history (e.g., Bing, 1981; Meyer, 1922; Peloquin, 1995, 2005, 2007; Yerxa, 1983). More specifically, inherent in these methodologies is a distinct valuing of and respect for:

- The essential humanity and dignity of all people
- The perspectives and subjective experiences of clients and their significant others
- Empathy, caring, and genuine engagement in the therapeutic encounter
- The use of imagination and integrity in creating occupational opportunities
- The inherent potential of people to experience well-being

Application to Practice: From a Philosophical Framework to a Philosophical Mode of Thinking

Application of the philosophy of OT to practice requires a philosophical mode of thinking. This mode of thinking requires that a practitioner of OT reflects on philosophical assumptions about reality, knowledge, values, and action and walk those assumptions forward into practices that intentionally manifest them. This mode of thinking also involves reflecting on one's practice and identifying the assumptions about reality, knowledge, values, and action that it seems to manifest. Practicing this mode of thinking will help a practitioner develop a philosophical mind, which may be the most indispensable element of practice.

The two scenarios in OT Story 3.1 and OT Story 3.2 (with additional learning activities on the Lippincott Connect) provide opportunities to build a philosophical mode of thinking. The two cases are real, and we have portrayed them as accurately as possible based on direct knowledge of

OT STORY 3.1 HIGH PRACTICE PHILOSOPHY CONGRUENCE

In Setting A, OT practitioners gather each morning to determine how the referrals and caseload will be distributed. As opportunities permit, the practitioners often consult with each other across the day on intervention ideas. Practitioners determine priorities for activities of daily living (ADLs) in collaboration with clients, and only the client's prioritized ADL tasks are addressed. In response to the many priorities of clients beyond basic and instrumental ADLs, practitioners created "occupational spaces" in the rehab gym, including an office area with computers and Internet access and a space in which clients can engage in various mechanical, leisure, and work-related activities. The OT kitchen is in constant use with clients whose priorities involve activities related to meal preparation, eating, and clean-up.

(continued)

OT STORY 3.1 HIGH PRACTICE PHILOSOPHY CONGRUENCE (*continued*)

After morning ADL sessions, the day is filled with individual client sessions, which range from 15 minutes to 1 hour, in addition to one group session. This scheduling approach meets productivity requirements. In individual sessions, therapists use familiar occupations to address clients' impairments, explore modifications to clients' desired occupations, educate significant others on how to assist clients, engage in mutual problem-solving of occupational challenges, revise goals, and so forth. The occupational therapists designed the group session to involve one realistic occupational project over 2 to 3 days, for instance, preparing a meal to share with family members, collecting clothing for a women's shelter, and shopping at a nearby store. Steps and tasks within these projects are assigned based on clients' interests, capacities, therapy goals, and the likelihood that they will be both challenged and successful. Although individual sessions may include exercises as a "warm-up," the focus is on both the client's occupational goals and the group's occupational project.

Clients are also often given "occupational homework" for weekends; that is, selecting an occupation they would like to engage in during weekend free time, reviewing related safety precautions, availability of needed materials, and relation to therapy goals. Examples include playing a game with visitors, sending e-mails, looking up information on the Internet, and visiting the gift shop. Significant others are encouraged to take part in both individual and group therapy sessions, as well as share in the weekend "homework." When possible, home visits are undertaken to help identify what occupations take place in what spaces and to collaborate with clients and their significant others about acceptable modifications. Discharge planning involves setting up environments and tasks as closely as possible to clients' usual contexts and performance patterns. As part of the OT department's continuous quality improvement plan, the OT manager conducts regular reviews, ensuring that therapists are centering their documentation on occupational performance. The manager tracks payment denials. Data indicate that there have been zero denials since increasing the focus on occupational performance.

Questions

1. Identify specific ways that practitioners in OT Story 3.1 take actions that are grounded in the philosophy of OT. Consider what features of their practice reflect
   a. An OT ontology.
   b. An OT epistemology.
   c. An OT axiology.
2. Summarize core values reflected in the practitioners' actions.
3. Are there points of incongruence between an OT philosophy and the approaches of the practitioners in this case? If so, what are they, and how might the practitioners modify to be more congruent with an OT philosophical framework?
4. Consider the practice context. What supports/shared commitments do you imagine would need to be in place in the practice environment to enable these practitioners to practice as they did in Setting A?

OT STORY 3.2 LOW PRACTICE PHILOSOPHY CONGRUENCE

In Setting B, OT practitioners meet each morning to determine how the referrals and caseload will be distributed. They go about their day largely independent of each other. All clients receive OT for basic ADLs in the morning; practitioners emphasize ADL independence and typically complete the same ADL tasks with all clients. The rest of the day consists of consecutive 15- to 45-minute individual sessions that incorporate documentation; this way of scheduling sessions is sufficient to meet the high productivity demand of the setting. Sessions emphasize physical components of function, such as range of motion, strength, and endurance. Prominently used activities include TheraBand or putty, items like the range of motion arc, weights, the upper extremity ergometer, pulleys, dowel exercises, various physical agent modalities, and ball or balloon toss.

Connections between impairment reduction and clients' occupational needs are seldom explained. Also addressed are visual–perceptual and cognitive components of function using activities such as paper-and-pencil activities, puzzles, pegboards, and computer-based exercises. Intervention is consistent client to client, and some clients question why they need to see the occupational therapist because they already had their "therapy," that is, physical therapy that day. There is a kitchen that is used for splinting and staff meetings. Significant others observe sessions with little direct involvement. When a client needs two people to complete a transfer or ambulate, an occupational therapist and a physical therapist may see the client together. Discharge planning may include bath transfers, dressing, and a kitchen activity such as making a cup of tea to determine safety for returning home. Clients' significant others receive training the last day of service before a client is discharged.

Questions

1. Identify specific ways that practitioners in OT Story 3.2 take actions that are not highly congruent with the philosophy of OT. Consider what features of their practice could be stronger in terms of
   a. An OT ontology.
   b. An OT epistemology.
   c. An OT axiology.

2. Even though the congruence with the philosophy of OT was lower in Setting B, can you identify some areas of congruence, even if weak, with ontology, epistemology, and axiology?
3. Summarize values reflected in the practitioners' actions.
4. What practices in Setting A were not identified in Setting B?
5. Consider the practice context. What features of the practice environment do you imagine contribute to how OT is enacted in Setting B?
6. Identify two changes that would seem possible in the context of Setting B to move toward higher congruence with the OT philosophy.

typical practices in each setting. We selected the cases because of their contrasts related to application of the philosophy of OT. Despite this divergence, both scenarios are from fast-paced, for-profit hospitals with subacute adult neurorehabilitation programs in which demands for productivity are equally high. Also in both settings, clients have various neurologic conditions and many have suffered from strokes or other brain injuries. OT is provided 2 or 3 times daily in both settings, and length of stay typically ranges from 3 to 10 days.

Conclusion

As is true of all professions, belonging to and working in OT requires ongoing philosophizing about what exactly makes OT distinct and what health and well-being needs in society the profession is best suited to address, and the value that meeting such needs holds for the overall good of societies.

In this chapter, we thus presented a philosophy that emerged from our own philosophizing about OT. As noted, this philosophy is largely, however not exclusively, influenced by our and others' Western perspectives on OT theory, philosophy, and practice. As is true of any profession-specific philosophy, moreover, this philosophy is not an exact replica of earlier philosophies of OT, nor is it set in stone as if a finished product. Far from it. Rather, the philosophy presented herein is properly understood as dynamic. By its very nature, therefore, this philosophy will evolve as new perspectives and needs emerge and become ascendant through the inclusion of increasingly diverse voices, cultural perspectives, and global experiences.

Ultimately, belonging to and working in OT requires that all members of the profession engage in the process of philosophizing. It requires that all members possess and

demonstrate fidelity to a sound philosophy of the profession. It requires that all members build congruence between their own personal philosophies and a sound philosophy of the profession. As Wilcock (1999) urged, if strong *incompatibilities* exist between a professional's (or student's) personal philosophy and the philosophy of OT, then that person's engagement with OT should likely cease not only for their own good but also for the good of their future clients and the profession itself. Conversely, if strong congruence exists between a professional's (or student's) personal philosophy and a sound philosophy of the profession, then that person will likely find their work in OT to be meaningful, satisfying, sustaining, and impactful. Thus, the stakes are high. They are high for adopting a philosophical mode of thinking, for philosophizing, and, most importantly, for ensuring deep fidelity to a sound philosophy of the profession.

Lippincott® Connect *For additional resources on the subjects discussed in this chapter, visit* Lippincott Connect.

REFERENCES

American Occupational Therapy Association. (2014). Occupational therapy practice framework: Domain and process, 3rd edition. *American Journal of Occupational Therapy, 68*(1), S1–S48. https://doi.org/10.5014/ajot.2014.682006

American Occupational Therapy Association. (2015). Occupational therapy code of ethics (2015). *American Journal of Occupational Therapy, 69*(3), 6913410030p1–6913410030p8. https://doi.org/10.5014/ajot.2015.696S03

American Occupational Therapy Association. (2017). Philosophical base of occupational therapy. *American Journal of Occupational Therapy, 71*, 7112410045. https://doi.org/10.5014/ajot.716S06

Bing, R. K. (1981). Eleanor Clarke Slagle lectureship—1981. Occupational therapy revisited: A paraphrastic journey. *American Journal of Occupational Therapy, 35*(8), 499–518. https://doi.org/10.5014/ajot.35.8.499

Blanche, E. I., & Henny-Kohler, E. (2000). Philosophy, science and ideology: A proposed relationship for occupational science and occupational therapy. *Occupational Therapy International, 7*(2), 99–110. https://doi.org/10.1002/oti.110

Breines, E. (1986). *Origins and adaptations: A philosophy of practice.* Geri-Rehab.

Breines, E. (1987). Pragmatism as a foundation for occupational therapy curricula. *American Journal of Occupational Therapy, 41*(8), 522–525. https://doi.org/10.5014/ajot.41.8.522

Bruce, M. A., & Borg, B. (2002). *Psychosocial occupational therapy: Frames of reference for intervention.* SLACK.

Christiansen, C. H., Baum, C. M., & Bass-Haugen, J. (Eds.). (2005). *Occupational therapy: Performance, participation, and well-being.* SLACK.

Craik, J., Townsend, E., & Polatajko, H. (2008). Introducing the new guidelines—Enabling occupation II: Advancing an occupational therapy vision for health, well-being, & justice through occupation. *Occupational Therapy Now, 10*(1), 3–5. Retrieved January 31, 2023, from https://www.proquest.com/trade-journals/introducing-new-guidelines-enabling-occupation-ii/docview/229522447/se-2

Cutchin, M. P. (2004). Using Deweyan philosophy to rename and reframe adaptation-to-environment. *American Journal of Occupational Therapy, 58*(3), 303–312. https://doi.org/10.5014/ajot.58.3.303

Damasio, A. (1994). *Descartes' error: Emotion, reason, and the human brain.* Putnam.

Devereaux, E. B. (1984). Occupational therapy's challenge: The caring relationship. *American Journal of Occupational Therapy, 38*(12), 791–798. https://doi.org/10.5014/ajot.38.12.791

Dickie, V., Cutchin, M. P., & Humphry, R. (2006). Occupation as transactional experience: A critique of individualism in occupational science. *Journal of Occupational Science, 13*(1), 83–93. https://doi.org/10.1080/14427591.2006.9686573

Dunton, W. R. (1919). *Reconstruction therapy.* W. B. Saunders.

Finlay, L. (2001). Holism in occupational therapy: Elusive fiction and ambivalent struggle. *American Journal of Occupational Therapy, 55*(3), 268–276. https://doi.org/10.5014/ajot.55.3.268

Fisher, A. G. (2013). Occupation-centred, occupation-based, occupation-focused: Same, same or different? *Scandinavian Journal of Occupational Therapy, 20*(3), 162–173. https://doi.org/10.3109/11038128.2012.754492

Friedland, J. (2011). *Restoring the spirit: The beginnings of occupational therapy in Canada, 1890–1930.* McGill-Queen's University Press.

Hammell, K. W. (2011). Resisting theoretical imperialism in the disciplines of occupational science and occupational therapy. *British Journal of Occupational Therapy, 74*(1), 27–33. https://doi.org/10.4276/030802211X12947686093

Hammell K. R. W., & Iwama, M. K. (2012). Well-being and occupational rights: An imperative for critical occupational therapy. *Scandinavian Journal of Occupational Therapy, 19*(5), 385–394. https://doi.org/10.3109/11038128.2011.611821

Hasselkus, B. R. (2011). *The meaning of everyday occupation* (2nd ed.). SLACK.

Hocking, C. (2008). The way we were: Romantic assumptions of pioneering occupational therapists in the United Kingdom. *British Journal of Occupational Therapy, 71*(4), 146–154. https://doi.org/10.1177/030802260807100405

Hocking, C., & Erik Ness, N. (2004). WFOT minimum standards for the education of occupational therapists: Shaping the profession. *World Federation of Occupational Therapists Bulletin, 50*(1), 9–17.

Hooper, B., Molineux, M., & Wood, W. (2020). The subject-centered integrative learning model: A new model for teaching occupational therapy's distinct value. *Journal of Occupational Therapy Education, 4*(2). https://doi.org/10.26681/jote.2020.040201

Hooper, B., & Wood, W. (2002). Pragmatism and structuralism in occupational therapy: The long conversation. *American Journal of Occupational Therapy, 56*(1), 40–50. https://doi.org/10.5014/ajot.56.1.40

Ikiugu, M., & Schultz, S. (2006). An argument for pragmatism as a foundational philosophy of occupational therapy. *Canadian Journal of Occupational Therapy, 73*(2), 86–97. https://doi.org/10.2182/cjot.05.0009

Iwama, M. (2006). *The Kawa model: Culturally relevant occupational therapy.* Churchill Livingstone, Elsevier.

Kielhofner, G. (1983). *Health through occupation: Theory and practice in occupational therapy.* F. A. Davis.

Kielhofner, G. (2004). *Conceptual foundations of occupational therapy* (3rd ed.). F. A. Davis.

Kielhofner, G., & Burke, J. (1983). The evolution of knowledge and practice in occupational therapy: Past, present, and future. In G. Kielhofner (Ed.), *Health through occupation: Theory and practice in occupational therapy* (pp. 3–54). F. A. Davis.

Levine, R. E. (1987). The influence of the arts-and-crafts movement on the professional status of occupational therapy. *American Journal of Occupational Therapy, 41*(4), 248–254. https://doi.org/10.5014/ajot.41.4.248

Lincoln, Y. S., Lynham, S. A., & Guba, E. G. (2011). Paradigmatic controversies, contradictions, and emerging confluences, revisited. In N. K. Denzin & Y. S. Lincoln (Eds.), *Handbook of qualitative research* (pp. 97–128). Sage.

MacIntyre, A. C. (1990). *First principles, final ends and contemporary philosophical issues.* Marquette University Press.

Mattingly, C., & Fleming, M. H. (1994). *Clinical reasoning: Forms of inquiry in a therapeutic practice.* F. A. Davis.

Meyer, A. (1922). The philosophy of occupation therapy. *American Journal of Physical Medicine & Rehabilitation, 1*(1), 1–10. https://journals.lww.com/ajpmr/Citation/1922/02000/The_Philosophy_of_Occupation_Therapy.1.aspx

Nelson, D. L. (1997). Why the profession of occupational therapy will flourish in the 21st century. The 1996 Eleanor Clarke Slagle lecture. *American Journal of Occupational Therapy, 51*(1), 11–24. https://doi.org/10.5014/ajot.51.1.11

Oxford University Press. (2021, September). *OED online.* Retrieved September 27, 2021, from https://www.oed.com/search?searchType=dictionary&q=philosophy&_searchBtn=Search

Palmer, P. J. (2009). *Hidden wholeness: The journey toward an undivided life.* Wiley & Sons.

Paul, R. (1995). *Critical thinking: How to prepare students for a rapidly changing world.* Foundation for Critical Thinking.

Peloquin, S. M. (1995). The fullness of empathy: Reflections and illustrations. *American Journal of Occupational Therapy, 49*(1), 24–31. https://doi.org/10.5014/ajot.49.1.24

Peloquin, S. M. (2005). The 2005 Eleanor Clark Slagle lecture—Embracing our ethos, reclaiming our heart. *American Journal of Occupational Therapy, 59*(6), 611–625. https://doi.org/10.5014/ajot.59.6.611

Peloquin, S. M. (2007). A reconsideration of occupational therapy's core values. *American Journal of Occupational Therapy, 61*(4), 474–478. https://doi.org/10.5014/ajot.61.4.474

Price, P., & Miner, S. (2007). Occupation emerges in the process of therapy. *American Journal of Occupational Therapy, 61*(4), 441–450. https://doi.org/10.5014/ajot.61.4.441

Punwar, A. J., & Peloquin, S. (2000). *Occupational therapy principles and practice* (3rd ed.). Lippincott Williams & Wilkins.

Quiroga, V. A. M. (1995). *Occupational therapy: The first 30 years 1900 to 1930.* American Occupational Therapy Association.

Reed, K. L. (1986). Tools of practice: Heritage or baggage? 1986 Eleanor Clarke Slagle lecture. *American Journal of Occupational Therapy, 40*(9), 597–605. https://doi.org/10.5014/ajot.40.9.597

Reed, K. L. (2005). Dr. Hall and the work cure. *Occupational Therapy in Health Care, 19*(3), 33–50. https://doi.org/10.1080/J003v19n03_04

Reed, K. L., & Sanderson, S. N. (1999). *Concepts of occupational therapy* (4th ed.). Lippincott, Williams & Wilkins.

Reilly, M. (1962). Occupational therapy can be one of the great ideas of 20th century medicine. *American Journal of Occupational Therapy, 16*, 1–9.

Reilly, M. (1974). *Play as exploratory learning*. Sage.

Rogers, J. C. (1982a). Order and disorder in medicine and occupational therapy. *American Journal of Occupational Therapy, 36*(1), 29–35. https://doi.org/10.5014/ajot.36.1.29

Rogers, J. C. (1982b). The spirit of independence: The evolution of a philosophy. *American Journal of Occupational Therapy, 36*(11), 709–715. https://doi.org/10.5014/ajot.36.11.709

Ruona, W. E. A., & Lynham, S. A. (2004). A philosophical framework for thought and practice in human resource development. *Human Resource Development International, 7*(2), 151–164. https://doi.org/10.1080/13678860310001630665

Schell, B. A., & Schell, J. W. (2018). Professional reasoning as the basis for practice. In B. A Schell & J. W. Schell (Eds.), *Clinical and professional reasoning in occupational therapy* (2nd ed., pp. 3–12). Wolters Kluwer.

Schell, J. W. (2018a). Epistemology: Knowing how you know. In B. A. Schell & J. W. Schell (Eds.), *Clinical and professional reasoning in occupational therapy* (2nd ed., pp. 229–257). Wolters Kluwer.

Schell, J. W. (2018b). Teaching for reasoning in higher education. In B. A. Schell & J. W. Schell (Eds.), *Clinical and professional reasoning in occupational therapy* (2nd ed., pp. 417–437). Wolters Kluwer.

Stevenson, L., Haberman, D. L., & Stevenson, L. F. (2004). Ten theories of human nature. In S.D. Taff (Ed.), *Philosophy and occupational therapy: Informing education, research, and practice*. SLACK.

Taff, S., & Babulal, G. M. (2021). Reframing the narrative on the philosophies influencing the development of occupational therapy. In S. Taff (Ed.), *Philosophy and occupational therapy: Informing education, research, and practice*. SLACK.

Taylor, R. R. (2008). *The intentional relationship: Occupational therapy and use of self*. F. A. Davis.

Thibeault, R. (2002). Occupation and the rebuilding of civil society: Notes from the war zone. *Journal of Occupational Science, 9*(1), 38–47. https://doi.org/10.1080/14427591.2002.9686492

Trombly, C. A. (1995). Occupation: Purposefulness and meaningfulness as therapeutic mechanisms. *American Journal of Occupational Therapy, 49*(10), 960–972. https://doi.org/10.5014/ajot.49.10.960

Watson, R. M. (2006). Being before doing: The cultural identity (essence) of occupational therapy. *Australian Occupational Therapy Journal, 53*(3), 151–158. https://doi.org/10.1111/j.1440-1630.2006.00598.x

Weimer, R. (1979). Traditional and nontraditional practice arenas. In AOTA's (Ed.), *Occupational therapy: 2001 AD* (pp. 42–53). American Occupational Therapy Association.

West, W. L. (1984). A reaffirmed philosophy and practice of occupational therapy for the 1980s. *American Journal of Occupational Therapy, 38*(1), 15–23. https://doi.org/10.5014/ajot.38.1.15

Wilcock, A. A. (1999). The Doris Sym memorial lecture: Developing a philosophy of occupation for health. *British Journal of Occupational Therapy, 62*(5), 192–198. https://doi.org/10.1177/030802269906200503

Wilcock, A. A. (2000). Development of a personal, professional and educational occupational philosophy: An Australian perspective. *Occupational Therapy International, 7*(2), 79–86. https://doi.org/10.1002/oti.108

Wilcock, A. A. (2006). *An occupational perspective on health* (*Vol. 2*). SLACK.

Wilcock, A. A., & Hocking, C. (2015). *An occupational perspective of health* (3rd ed.). SLACK.

Wood, W. (1993). Occupation and the relevance of primatology to occupational therapy. *American Journal of Occupational Therapy, 47*(6), 515–522. https://doi.org/10.5014/ajot.47.6.515

Wood, W. (1998a). Biological requirements for occupation in primates: An exploratory study and theoretical analysis. *Journal of Occupational Science, 5*(2), 66–81. https://doi.org/10.1080/14427591.1998.9686435

Wood, W. (Ed.). (1998b). Occupation centered practice [special issue]. *American Journal of Occupational Therapy, 52*(5).

Wood, W., Lampe, J. L., Logan, C. A., Metcalfe, A. R., & Hoesley, B. E. (2017). The lived environment life quality model for institutionalized people with dementia. *Canadian Journal of Occupational Therapy, 84*(1), 22–33. https://doi.org/10.1177/0008417416656207

Yerxa, E. J. (1967). 1966 Eleanor Clarke Slagle lecture. Authentic occupational therapy. *American Journal of Occupational Therapy, 21*(1), 1–9.

Yerxa, E. J. (1979). The philosophical base of occupational therapy. In AOTA's (Ed.), *Occupational therapy: 2001 AD* (pp. 26–30). American Occupational Therapy Association.

Yerxa, E. J. (1983). Audacious values: The energy source for occupational therapy practice. In G. Kielhofner (Ed.), *Health through occupation: Theory and practice in occupational therapy* (pp. 149–162). F. A. Davis.

Yerxa, E. J. (1998). Health and the human spirit for occupation. *American Journal of Occupational Therapy, 52*(6), 412–422. https://doi.org/10.5014/ajot.52.6.412

Contemporary Occupational Therapy Practice and Future Directions

Susan Coppola, Glen Gillen, and Barbara A. Boyt Schell

"People are most true to their humanity when engaged in occupation."
—YERXA ET AL. (1989)

LEARNING OBJECTIVES

After reading this chapter, you will be able to:

1. Define occupational therapy.
2. Discuss how context shapes practice, considering models of practice, culture, and systems influencing practice.
3. Explain the focus of the profession using professionally relevant terminology.
4. Discuss essential features of the occupational therapy process: client centered and relational, occupation centered, justice focused, evidence based, and culturally relevant.
5. Describe the current workforce and the societal needs that call for diversity and growth of the profession.
6. Describe the forces and possibilities that are likely to influence future practice.

Introduction

Contemporary and envisioned practices of occupational therapy (OT) are centered around the profession's core construct, occupation, a complex and essential aspect of human life. OT is grounded in a humanistic philosophy that people, regardless of their life situations, should have opportunities to participate in occupations that bring health and meaning. Occupation is the profession's core concern and means to bring about positive change in health, well-being, and life situations. Enacting these beliefs is why the profession exists and why OT must continually change to serve contemporary needs in society.

Throughout this chapter are linkages to other parts of the text that offer depth in key dimensions of this multifaceted profession. We address the profession globally, with emphasis on the United States, because of the origins of this text, and the challenge of representing the diversity of practice across cultures and continents. The profession has many roles, including educators, researchers, administrators, consultants, service providers, and others. The chapter addresses service provision. This is a challenging task because services are, and should be, wide ranging to reflect diversity of cultures, occupations, and places where people do occupations. The chapter offers tools to understand contemporary practice and consider how the profession can strive to enact values of human rights, equity, and inclusion.

Definition of Occupational Therapy

OT is a collaboration-focused health profession concerned with promoting health and well-being through occupation.* The profession's primary goal is to help people do the day-to-day activities that are important and meaningful in their lives. OT is a creative process that integrates art and science to care for people from newborns to those approaching the end of life. OT uses a variety of interventions designed to prevent occupational performance problems, enable health-promoting participation, reduce physical and social barriers to participation, and draw upon the strengths of clients to mitigate the impact of impairment and disability (American Occupational Therapy Association [AOTA], 2020a; World Federation of Occupational Therapists [WFOT], 2017). Occupation is something so ordinary and embedded in the everyday that we may fail to appreciate its complexity (Hasselkus, 2006). Occupations are instead extraordinary, as they form the complex network of day-to-day activities that enable people to sustain their health, meet their needs, contribute to the life of their families, and participate in the broader society (AOTA, 2020a). Occupations are constituents of our unique identities and meanings in life (Christiansen, 1999). Occupational engagement is well established as an integral to physical and mental health (AOTA, 2017a; Clark et al., 1997; Glass et al., 1999; Law et al., 1998).

OT practitioners provide individual and group interventions as well as consultative services to individuals, groups, and populations in a wide range of settings. The term *clients* is broad, to encompass persons, groups, and populations. Practice appears different from setting to setting. Yet, the desired outcome of OT intervention is that people will live their lives engaged in occupations

that sustain themselves, support their health and well-being, and foster involvement with others in their social world. OT practitioners and students comprise an international community that is centered on the significance of occupation in people's lives. OT is delivered in many languages by practitioners traveling by foot, plane, boat, wheelchair, car, and all other means of travel. OT practitioners can serve people of all ages in any place where people do occupations, and they can be found in health, education, social, community, and business arenas. Because people and their occupations are diverse, OT should look different at every encounter and context (Watson, 2006). Box 4.1 outlines definitions of OT from the AOTA and the WFOT.

BOX 4.1 DEFINITIONS OF OCCUPATIONAL THERAPY

American Occupational Therapy Association
Excerpt From the AOTA Philosophical Base of Occupational Therapy

The focus and outcome of occupational therapy are clients' engagement in meaningful occupations that support their participation in life situations. Occupational therapy practitioners conceptualize occupations as both a means and an end in therapy. That is, there is therapeutic value in occupational engagement as a change agent, and engagement in occupations is also the ultimate goal of therapy. Occupational therapy is based on the belief that occupations are fundamental to health promotion and wellness, remediation or restoration, health maintenance, disease and injury prevention, and compensation and adaptation. The use of occupation to promote individual, family, community, and population health is the core of occupational therapy practice, education, research, and advocacy. (AOTA, 2017b)

World Federation of Occupational Therapy
Excerpt From WFOT Statement on Occupational Therapy

Occupational therapy is a client-centered health profession concerned with promoting health and well-being through occupation. The primary goal of occupational therapy is to enable people to participate in the activities of everyday life. Occupational therapists achieve this outcome by working with people and communities to enhance their ability to engage in the occupations they want to, need to, or are expected to do, or by modifying the occupation or the environment to better support their occupational engagement. (WFOT, 2017, p. 1)

---

*According to the AOTA (2020a, p. S75), the term *client* refers to *persons* (including those involved in care of a client), *groups* (a collection of individuals having shared characteristics or common or shared purpose, e.g., family members, workers, students, and those with similar interests or occupational challenges), and *populations* (aggregates of people with common attributes, such as contexts, characteristics, or concerns, including health risks). However, in countries other than the United States, the term client often refers to persons who are paying for their care directly. In most countries, *patient* is used to describe persons who are in hospital or rehabilitation. *Service user* and *person* are terms in general use that describe those in need of OT services. For this chapter, we are using *client* without implying the source of payment for services.

Occupational Therapy in Action

Contemporary occupational therapists work with a vast array of clients in many settings. A selection of clients and settings are outlined in the vignettes in OT Story 4.1. See Unit VII for more details on the diversity of OT intervention.

OT STORY 4.1 EXAMPLES OF CLIENTS AND PRACTICE CONTEXTS

These scenarios convey the diversity of OT services around the world.

- Ya-Ning works in a retirement community composed of apartments, a skilled nursing facility, and a dementia care unit. In a typical week, Ya-Ning provides services for prevention of falls, developing routines for people with dementia, driving safety (including off-road and on-road assessments), strategies for low vision, home modifications, caregiver support, and rehabilitation for neurologic and orthopedic conditions. She works on an interdisciplinary team that meets twice per week to plan and coordinate care for residents. Ya-Ning's services are reimbursed by government health insurance policies. She regularly attends training for person-centered dementia care. Ya-Ning is active in her professional OT association in lobbying legislators to expand reimbursement for services to older adults.
- Raj works in an inner-city homeless shelter. He provides individual interventions as well as runs daily groups. His role at the shelter is to teach life skills so that residents can transition to supportive housing. Intervention topics include money management, home management, work preparation, anger management, and using public transportation.
- Kori works in a rural low-income school system. There are three OT practitioners who cover the schools. Kori divides her week between four schools, where she consults with teachers to provide inclusive services in the classrooms. The team meets with parents to develop a plan for students needing special services. Kori is leading a project at one of the schools, collaborating with physical therapists, speech-language pathologists (SLPs), school counselors, students with disabilities, and parents to build an accessible playground.
- Martin works with occupational therapists and occupational therapy assistants (OTAs) in a large psychiatric hospital with inpatient services and a day program. They conduct occupational profiles and assess functional cognition and psychosocial function of admitted clients. Client-driven goals are established in the evaluation, leading to a group activity program schedule for each client during their stay. These activities are led by interdisciplinary team members to build skills in leisure, work, parenting, money management, stress management, and other skills to prepare for life in the community. Upon discharge, many clients struggle to live in the community and thus return to the hospital programs. Martin is working with a social worker to develop home- and community-based programs that include supported employment for more successful transitions upon discharge.
- Atli works in an early intervention program for high-risk and developmentally delayed children, ages 0 to 3 years. It is a transdisciplinary team funded by the government to provide services in the home. Team members include nutritionists, social workers, nurses, and other disciplines. The program uses a coaching model to empower parents to problem-solve challenges and creatively uses natural objects within the home to promote occupational development. Many of the parents have mental health challenges and food insecurity. The team uses a primary provider model so that each family has a strong relationship with one team member who coordinates the many services to support the family. Increasingly, the family encounters are occurring over the phone or, where possible, via telehealth. Atli is collecting data on the outcomes of the remote encounters to compare with the in-person visits to inform decisions about service delivery context.
- Arjun owns a busy private practice serving children and youth. Because there are few OT practitioners in his country, he hires an occupational therapist from a nearby country as well as two trained rehabilitation technicians to provide services. His clients are self-pay, and for families without resources, there is a sliding fee scale. His team started a grant-funded, nonprofit organization to provide services in schools in nearby villages that have no occupational therapists. The nonprofit organization assesses children with special learning needs and collaborates with teachers to modify strategies and environments for inclusion.
- A team of OT practitioners is employed at a medical center for members of the military. Yet, each works in a different sector. Derron provides home-based primary care for people with disabilities, providing services through end-of-life care. Bjorn works in a program for housing insecure veterans, helping them to transition and remain in supportive housing. Aimee works in a community program for veterans with severe mental illness and

addictions. Carmen works with veterans experiencing a first psychotic episode. Other therapists work in the acute care, outpatient, assistive technology, and inpatient rehabilitation services throughout the medical center. The OT team meets regularly to share ideas and challenges of practices in these different programs and to discuss journal articles relevant to their work.

- Jaime works in a crowded prison facility. His work involves group activities for inmates to provide occupations that will offer structure to the day, skills for working in the community, and social relationships to support coping with the prison environment. He collaborates with a team including the warden, guards, and leaders of workshops for music and dance activities and LGBTQ+ programs. The team refers clients to Jaime for challenges in participation and coping and to prepare inmates for transition to community. Throughout the year, Jaime supervises many OT students who learn through providing evaluations, interventions, and teamwork. The students meet with Jaime to share the literature they are reading and collaborate to incorporate new ideas into practice.

- Mateo is a 26-year-old man who was hit by the shrapnel of a rocket-propelled grenade. He is missing his right upper limb, has burns across his chest wall, and has loss of vision in his right eye and loss of hearing in his right ear. He is working with Tacoya, an outpatient OT, to prepare for and learn to use an upper limb prosthesis. While waiting for his new artificial arm, Mateo's occupational therapist taught him how to care for his wounds from the burn and his surgical incisions. Mateo also worked on activities to strengthen his left arm and residual limb. Taylor, Mateo's OTA, taught him one-handed techniques to perform self-care and introduced assistive devices to help him be more independent in everyday tasks. See Figure 4.1 for an example of OT for a returning soldier.

- Isabella is an occupational therapist who has been hired by a museum to promote inclusion and diverse forms of engagement with art occupations. One aspect of her work is to help museum staff effectively support and communicate with visitors who have diversities, such as dementia, autism, and low vision. Her work extends to collaborations to make the museum more welcoming to older adults and minoritized individuals. She leads groups of people with varied abilities to learn about and enjoy participation in art. Isabella networks with OTs around the world to share stories, ideas, and evidence for their work.

As these scenarios demonstrate, OT practitioners provide services to a variety of clients in many settings, from

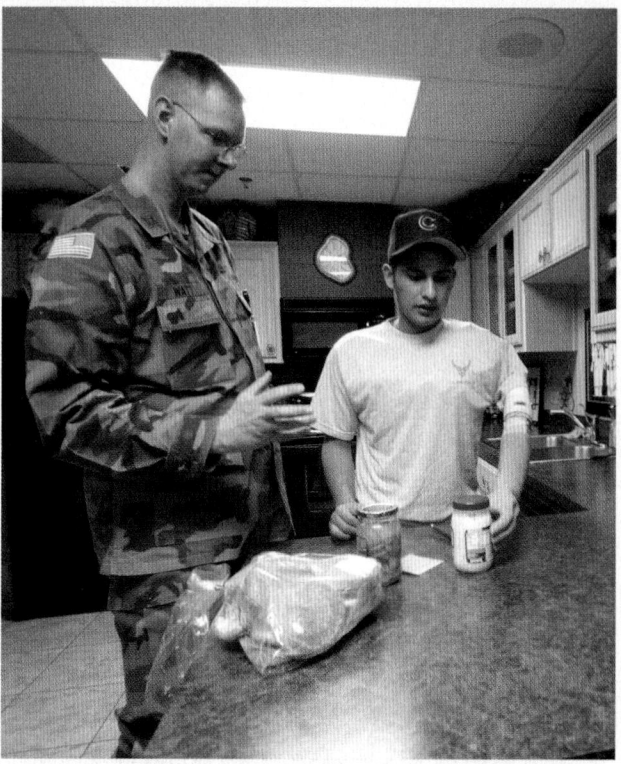

FIGURE 4.1 **Army Capt. James Watt, an occupational therapist, helps Senior Airman Dan Acosta make a sandwich in the life skills area of the amputee rehabilitation clinic at Brooke Army Medical Center in San Antonio. A mock apartment in the center helps patients get used to completing common tasks with their prosthetic limbs.**

(U.S. Air Force photo/Steve White.)

hospitals and schools to community programs and businesses. Some are examples of a medical model in which services are linked to health outcomes. The school-based practice example uses the education model, in which services are focused upon students' ability to participate in their education. Social and forensic models are also represented. Indeed, some settings have overlapping models. Knowing the model(s) of the setting or agency can explain the policies, practices, and purposes. Within these settings, OT practitioners may provide direct intervention with individuals and groups, consultation, and advocacy. Regardless of setting, the overarching goal of OT is to engage people in meaningful and important occupations to participate as fully as possible in life (Figure 4.2).

(*continued*)

OT STORY 4.1 EXAMPLES OF CLIENTS AND PRACTICE CONTEXTS (*continued*)

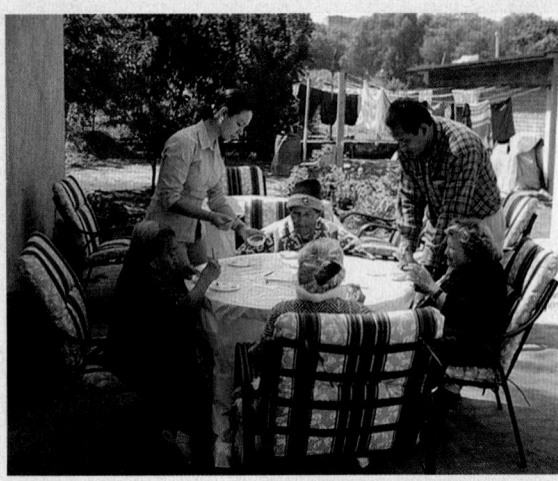

FIGURE 4.2 Occupational therapy students in Mexico City facilitate participation in a home for older adults.

Questions

As you read the sections that follow, think about:

1. What *OT processes* are described in OT Story 4.1?
2. What is the practice context, considering the *systems levels* in which these therapists work?
3. What fundamental *OT principles* are used by the therapists?

Occupational Therapy Process

What is the OT process that guides the provision of services across such a broad array of clients and situations? By understanding occupation and carefully analyzing many factors associated with occupation, practitioners can harness the therapeutic potential of *occupation* to improve function and quality of life. Occupational therapists must attend to the person or groups doing the occupation, the characteristics of the occupation itself, and the physical and social context in which the occupation occurs. Therapists also appreciate how various occupations are interwoven and have potential to evolve into new experiences, relationships, and meanings. Therefore, the evaluation process involves careful attention to what the person (or group) wants or needs to do and how both person and context are affecting actual performance and participation. Intervention then involves very carefully selecting those factors that most affect performance of occupations and figuring out ways to enable participation. Examples of common approaches in OT encounters include the following:

- Collaborating with clients to assess key abilities and problems affecting desired and necessary daily tasks
- Using occupations in a graded or modified form to promote the development or restoration of performance abilities

- Assessing and changing the physical space, objects, and assistive technologies to make performance and participation easier, safer, and more effective
- Changing the social context to support performance and participation
- Teaching alternate ways to perform tasks in order to improve performance and compensate for changes in the person's body functions
- Modifying routines and habits to promote health and participation in meaningful occupations
- Using preparatory activities that help the person be able to perform, such as activities and exercises to increase mobility, cognition, and emotional control (AOTA, 2020a)
- Incorporating prevention of disability, injury, or health decline (see Box 4.2)
- Advocating for clients or supporting self-advocacy in order to promote occupational participation
- Collaborating as part of a team, with other disciplines and people relevant to the lives of clients to plan, deliver, and modify services

In order to use these approaches, OT practitioners need a wide range of skills related to analyzing and modifying activities. They use interpersonal skills to encourage performance and they engage in education, consultation, and advocacy to help clients have desired performance opportunities (AOTA, 2014). Ultimately, improved performance in daily tasks and increased participation in life activities are the goals of OT. See Unit IV for chapters that explain the OT process in further detail.

Prevention is on the agenda of all global health strategies, targeting primary, secondary, and tertiary prevention. Most commonly, occupational therapists are associated with *tertiary prevention*, aimed at rehabilitation to prevent further decline or reducing secondary disability for people with disabilities. *Secondary prevention* by occupational therapists is directed toward identifying and intervening for populations at risk, for example, older drivers, childhood trauma survivors, premature infants, and people at risk for falls or other injuries. Occupational therapy increasingly contributes to *primary prevention* in public health measures include efforts to encourage vaccinations, workplace ergonomics, and backpack awareness (Jayaratne et al., 2012).

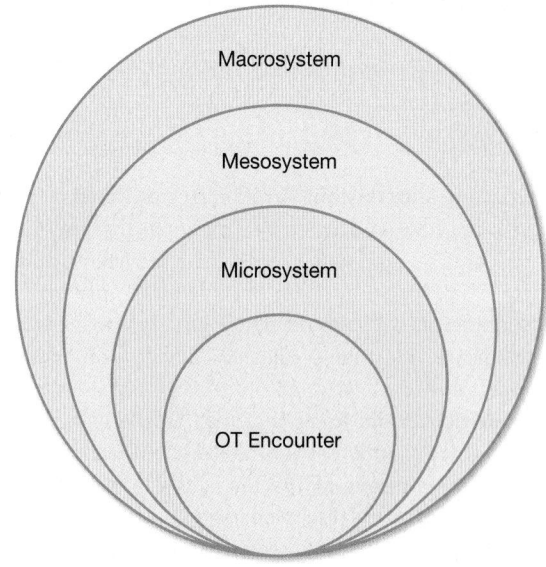

FIGURE 4.3 Diagram of systems based on Berwick (2002).

Systems Framework to Understand Practice

Practice is shaped by the context in which it occurs. The policies, norms, funding, equipment, team members, and many other contextual factors influence what therapists do in each setting. Pragmatics of practice situations enter into decisions therapists make every day (to learn about professional reasoning, see Chapter 25). It is, therefore, a challenge for OT students and practitioners entering new situations to understand "what is going on here."

A systems framework, as represented in Figure 4.3, can help practitioners analyze the layers of contexts that influence their day-to-day practice (Berwick, 2002). At first glance, we may see an OT *encounter* as composed of the client (including family) and OT practitioner. Encounters are typically situated in organizations, like a hospital, school, or home-based agency. Agencies are *microsystems* with cultures and practices relating to resources, teamwork, policies, documentation, and much more. The knowledge, habits, and skills of the occupational therapists may influence what and how services are delivered. The occupational therapist's role can be shaped by who else is on the team. For example, if there is not an SLP on the team, the occupational therapist may focus more on functional communication interventions. If there is a recreational therapist on the team, OT practitioners may focus less on leisure occupations. When OTAs are on the team, the occupational therapist may spend more time on evaluations than interventions. Teams can vary in how they operate as multidisciplinary, interdisciplinary, or transdisciplinary. The administrative culture of organizations influences how people communicate and work together to provide services. Key

to effectiveness and satisfaction in practice are the relationships fostered between team members in the microsystem through trust, communication, and shared responsibility.

At the next level is the *mesosystem*, the wider community culture, resources, and structures that may be at the local, village, county, district, or state level. Here are some examples of mesosystem influences. State or regional laws and regulations can define OT's legal scope of practice. Licensure laws may regulate whether services can be provided via telehealth (see Chapter 67). In the United States, a state Department of Education may determine processes by which occupational therapists obtain referrals to provide services to children and youth in schools. In the United States, Medicaid (a federal/state program) is administered at the state (mesosystem) level and includes rules for access, payment, and delivery of services for people who qualify with financial needs.

Broader yet are the *macrosystems* that exert broad influence, such as professional associations (see Chapter 5) and the sociopolitical context of the nation. There are formal influences such as national ministries of health, education, and social welfare. Some countries have national policies for school-based services for children and youth, or for injured workers. Countries with National Health Service provide care to people, regardless of their ability to pay. In countries in which healthcare is privatized, care is primarily through private businesses where access to care depends on a person's ability to pay or receive "charity" care. In the United States, where there is not a national health system, therapists find out what is covered by the myriad insurance policies and the processes to document, schedule, and justify services for clients based upon payer sources. Many countries have a hybrid of private and public services. See Chapter 76 for further information on reimbursement for services.

Analyzing a practice setting to interpret what levels of systems influence practice can be helpful for students, as can be seen in Box 4.3. Understanding "how things work" is part of successful adjustment to new practice settings. Van-Puymbrouck and Friedman (2022) found the system's perspective useful to interpret themes of students' experience of fieldwork during the first year of the COVID-19 pandemic. Understanding systems also guides targeted advocacy for OT services and client rights. Policy is often thought of as a problem, but it is actually helpful when it supports meeting client needs, such as payment policies that include OT. Advocacy for policy is an element of being a professional. Keep in mind that therapists can and do work at all systems levels, as administrators, policy makers, and government officials. Chapter 76 describes how payment for services is influenced by multiple levels of systems and varies by country.

Language for Occupational Therapy

As in any profession, OT uses terminology that has evolved to reflect the specific concerns of the profession. The OT process is not isolated: it is a collaborative endeavor with interprofessional and intraprofessional colleagues to plan and provide services. Through collaboration, it is possible to provide care experiences that honor and support the complex health and functional needs and preferences of the person and family as a whole (see Unit V). Essential to collaboration is common language that describes and explains client situations, interventions, and hoped-for outcomes.

Broad classifications or taxonomies are useful for understanding the scope of the field and for communicating core concerns and concepts to wider audiences. Because much of healthcare is provided in concert with other disciplines, resources described here play an important role in interprofessional communications. In this section, we explore classifications by the World Health Organization (WHO) and a sample of professional OT association models that offer language for practice (see Chapter 5).

World Health Organization International Classifications

The WHO provides several resources for scientists and healthcare professionals throughout the world to provide common language. One important document is the *International Classification of Diseases (ICD)*, which provides a standard classification of diseases and health problems (WHO, 2022). This resource is commonly seen when used in medical records and on billing sheets where the diagnosis is listed. In addition, it is an important resource for research as well as public health initiatives. In recent decades, the WHO recognized that the classification of diseases was not adequate to reflect the concerns of people with disabilities. After extensive development, the *International Classification of Functioning, Disability, and Health (ICF)* was developed (WHO, 2001). The WHO is in the process of constructing and testing yet another reference entitled the *International Classification of Health Interventions (ICHI)* (WHO, n.d.-a). It remains to be seen how the profession's contributions will be reflected in the new document. In summary, it is important to appreciate that OT has an important place in conceptual models and language that links occupations, activities, and participation to health.

International Classification of Functioning, Disability, and Health

The WHO developed the *ICF* as a framework and classification system that integrates social and medical models to represent how health conditions, performance, and performance contexts are interconnected (see Figure 4.4). At the same time, the *ICF* offers common language to communicate about the broad concept of *function* as it relates to health and ability. This language can be shared across disciplines and nations for collaboration to improve practice, research, and policy (Maritz et al., 2018). The *ICF* resonates with the OT conceptualization of the complexity

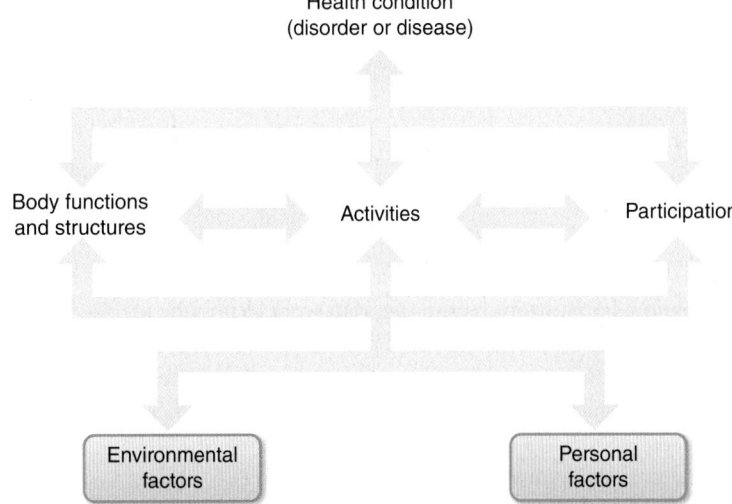

FIGURE 4.4 *International Classification of Functioning, Disability, and Health* (2001) illustrating the dynamic relationships of health with personal and environmental factors.

of function, which considers strengths, context, and health conditions. The *ICF* model was inspired by the disability rights movement to counter the myth that disabilities (formerly called *handicaps*) reside in a person. Stigma and inaccessible environments are instead central to disability. Ability is when the person *participates* in activities they wish to do and there is a good "match" between the person and the context in which the activities (or occupations) occur.

The *ICF* classifies functioning in three domains. At the human body level are the body structures (such as bones and nerves) and body functions (such as mental function or seeing). Problems of body function and structure are referred to as *impairments*. At the activity level, individuals have the capacity to do activities (e.g., ride a bike, dance, select clothing to wear), and problems at this level are *activity limitations*. *Participation* refers to actual engagement in life situations

(e.g., involvement in school, work, temple). Participation is an interaction of people in their physical and social life contexts, and problems at this level are called *barriers*. For example, social stigma about autism could be an obstacle to getting a particular job, when the autistic person is capable of the essential functions of the work. The domains of participation and activity have overlaps and are often combined. Similarly, in OT, we may think of nested occupations, such as eating and sharing a meal with family. Health conditions may influence function, yet they do not define or predict participation or disability for people with schizophrenia, cerebral palsy, arthritis, or other condition. Each person is unique and functions in a particular context. Importantly, the *ICF* supports the profession's strengths-based approach and complex understanding of occupation, as well as our focus on meaningful occupations in life situations. Table 4.1 contains

TABLE 4.1	International Classification of Functioning, Disability, and Health (ICF) Categories With Definitions (WHO, 2001)	
Aspect	**ICF Category**	**Problems, Difficulties**
Person	*Body structures:* Anatomic parts of the body, such as organs, limbs, and their components	Problems in body function or structure such as a significant deviation or loss are *impairments*.
	Body functions: Physiologic functions of body systems (including psychological functions)	
Actions (physical/mental)	*Activity:* The execution of a task or action by an individual (e.g., writing, planning a schedule, bathing)	Difficulties an individual may have in executing activities are called *activity limitations*.
	Participation: Involvement in a life situation (examples include participation in religious rituals, family dinner, school, work, leisure pursuits)	Problems an individual may experience in involvement in life situations are *participation restrictions*.
Context	*Environmental factors:* The physical, social, and attitudinal environment in which people live and conduct their lives and experience inclusion	*Barriers* is the term used to describe problems related to environmental factors.
	Personal factors: Includes things like age, race, coping styles, education, and behavior patterns	
Health	*Health:* Health is a state of complete physical, mental, and social well-being and not merely the absence of disease or infirmity.	Problems are *Health Conditions* listed in the *International Classification of Diseases, 10th revision (ICD-11)*.

definitions and examples of the components of *ICF*. The *ICF* Browser (https://apps.who.int/classifications/icfbrowser/) is a useful tool for applying the model to practice.

Broad Models and Frameworks for Occupational Therapy Practice

Professional organizations and theorists work to provide resources to define terms, scope, and processes of OT practice. OT models portray transactions of person–environment–occupation, based upon the cultural context of authors. The Canadian Model of Occupational Participation (CanMOP) emphasizes collaborative relationships in practice and the importance of engaging with factors of the micro, meso, and macro contexts to foster occupational possibilities and justice (Egan & Restall, 2022). The Kawa Model (see Chapter 37) uses a metaphor of a river to portray the OT process, derived from practice in Japan (Iwama, 2006). A Community-Centered Practice Model has emerged from an international collaboration (Hyett et al., 2019). In the United States, AOTA's Occupational Therapy Practice Framework (OTPF): Domain and process (4th ed.) offers terms, scope, process, and major outcomes of OT (AOTA, 2020a). See Unit VI for more information on various models that guide the OT process.

The AOTA's OTPF (AOTA, 2020a) presents interrelated constructs that describe OT practice. The current edition represents the evolution of a series of documents in which terminology is listed, definitions provided, and the general scope of practice is described. The authors, working on the behalf of the AOTA, attempt to gather commonly agreed-upon terms and concepts. Having this information in one resource promotes more effective communication between OT practitioners as well as among many others, such as those who pay for OT services and government groups who regulate services. Table 4.2 provides a listing

from the framework of the major domains that OT addresses. Note that there is overlap with the WHO's *ICF*, in that the AOTA adopted some of the same terminology for part of the OTPF (i.e., Body Functions and Structures in the Client Factors list and some of the same categories in Context and Environment). In contrast, careful comparison shows that the AOTA provided a much more nuanced look at the aspects of occupation by including not only major categories or areas of occupation (which are analogous to the WHO's use of the term *activities*) but also concepts related to various aspects of occupation and performance (i.e., skills, patterns). This detail is needed because occupation is the distinct focus of the profession's interests.

In addition to the major domain areas listed, the OTPF goes on to delineate the OT process and major outcomes of intervention. These are described in more detail in Chapter 18. The important point here is to recognize that there is professional language that helps occupational therapists communicate among themselves and with the larger worldwide audience.

Principles That Guide Occupational Therapy Practice

The diverse OT scenarios described previously characterize the historical roots of the profession based upon the focus and ethos of care. Meyer (1922/1977), in his address to the National Society for the Promotion of Occupational Therapy, stated, "Our role consists in giving opportunities rather than prescriptions. There must be opportunities to work, opportunities to do, to plan and create, and to use material" (p. 641). Engelhardt (1977) and Pörn (1993) asserted that health is measured by an individual's adaptive capacity and engagement in daily activities. In her Eleanor Clarke Slagle

---

| TABLE 4.2 | **Aspects of Occupational Therapy Domains** | | | |

Areas of Occupation	Client Factors	Performance Skills	Performance Patterns	Contexts
Activities of daily living (ADLs)[a] Instrumental activities of daily living (IADLs): • Rest and sleep • Education • Health management • Play • Leisure • Social participation	• Values, beliefs, and spirituality • Body functions • Body structures	• Motor skills • Process skills • Social interaction skills	• Habits • Routines • Rituals • Roles	• Environmental factors • Personal factors

The AOTA notes that all aspects of the domain have a dynamic interrelatedness. All aspects are of equal value and together interact to affect occupational identity, health, well-being, and participation in life (AOTA, 2020a, p. 6).
[a]Also referred to as basic activities of daily living (BADLs) or personal activities of daily living (PADLs).
Source: Based on American Occupational Therapy Association. (2020a). Occupational therapy practice framework: Domain and process (4th ed.). *American Journal of Occupational Therapy, 74*(Suppl 2), 7412410010.

lecture, Yerxa (1967) explained that authentic OT focuses on clients' humanity and their ability to choose and initiate occupations that provide the basis for the discovery of meaning. She further argued that authentic OT requires that the practitioner enter into a reciprocal relationship characterized by mutual care and that "to care means to be affected just as surely as it means to affect" (Yerxa, 1967, p. 8). OT practitioners intentionally form therapeutic relationships, and engage in therapeutic use of self, to create experiences that foster desired outcomes. Later in her address, Yerxa called for practitioner engagement in research to promote the development of the knowledge base of the profession. These themes translate into five interrelated principles that guide contemporary OT.

1. Client-centered and relational practice
2. Occupation-centered practice
3. Evidence-based practice and practice-based evidence
4. Culturally relevant practice
5. Occupational justice in practice

Client-Centered and Relational Practice

At the core of OT is a focus on the client as an active agent seeking to accomplish important day-to-day activities. As noted, the client can be an individual or a group such as a family whose occupations are interconnected or workers in a company. OT practitioners often work with people who are disempowered (Sakellariou & Pollard, 2017; Townsend & Polatajko, 2007). Clients seek care and professional help to "gain mastery over their affairs" (Rappaport, 1987, p. 122). To be client centered, practitioners must be willing to enter the client's world to create a relationship that encourages the client to enhance their life in ways that are most meaningful. Practitioners strive to understand the client as a person embedded in a particular context consisting of family and friends, socioeconomic status, culture, and other dimensions of their contexts.

Indeed, the focus of practice is the client. However, practice occurs through dynamic relationships between clients and therapists. The Canadian Occupational Therapy Inter-Relational Practice Process (COTIPP) framework (Egan & Restall, 2022) expands the notion of "client centered" beyond earlier conceptions of collaboration in a therapeutic process (Law et al., 1998). Mattingly (1991) asserted that this process is narrative in nature, which means that the practitioner and client create an understanding of the client's past, present, and future story. Mattingly further asserted that the future story is co-constructed and constantly revised in the midst of therapy. Practitioners strive to understand human feelings and intentions as well as the deeper meaning of people's lives through what Clark (1993) called *occupational storytelling*. In contrast, *occupational story-making* occurs during therapy. It is that

imaginative process through which clients create and then enact new occupational identities (Clark, 1993). For further exploration of intentional therapeutic relationships and client-centeredness in practice, see Chapter 28.

Occupation-Centered Practice

The profession originated from beliefs about the health and healing power of occupation. At times in the history of the profession, that focus was lost. Fortunately, in recent decades, the language, evidence, processes, and outcomes of practice are reclaiming our identity centered on occupational engagement. Clients seek OT because they need help engaging in their valued occupations—occupations they want to do, need to do, and/or have to do. Occupations are key to promote health and well-being (Reitz et al., 2020). The emphasis on occupational engagement stems from the profession's beliefs, substantiated by emerging research, that people's occupations are central to their identity and that they can reconstruct themselves through their occupations (Jackson, 1998). Occupations are not isolated activities; they are connected in a web of daily activities that help people fulfill their basic needs and contribute to their family, friends, and broader community (Hasselkus & Dickie, 2021). Occupation-centered practice focuses on meaningful occupations selected by clients and performed in their typical settings (AOTA, 2020a; Fisher, 2013). Systematic assessment of clients' occupations and priorities are vital to occupation-centered practice. This information—when coupled with careful analyses of the person's capacities, the task's demands, and the performance context—provides the basis for intervention. Intervention goals are directly connected to the person's occupational concerns, and intervention methods capitalize on the person's occupational interests. In this way, both the means (methods) and the ends (goals) of therapy involve intervention grounded in the occupations of the client (Cohn, 2019). Unit VII explores the evidence supporting the centrality of occupation in practice.

Evidence-Based Practice and Practice-Based Evidence

One of the important trends in healthcare is the increasing demand to base intervention decisions on "the conscientious, explicit, and judicious use of current best evidence" (Sackett et al., 1996, p. 71; Straus et al., 2011). This process, called *evidence-based practice*, entails being able to integrate research evidence and client preferences into the professional reasoning process to explain the rationale behind interventions and predict probable outcomes—or, as Gray (1998) asserted, "doing the right things right" (as cited in Holm, 2000, p. 576). Beyond "doing the right things right," evidence-based practice involves being able to explain the evidence and related OT recommendations in a language that the clients will understand (Tickle-Degnen, 2000). Furthermore, intervention based solely on how things have been done in the past no longer meets the ethical requirement that therapists provide therapeutic approaches that are evidence based and for which the client has been provided with understanding of benefits, risks, and potential outcomes of intervention (AOTA, 2020b).

The challenge for OT practitioners is 3-fold.

1. In order to practice evidence-based OT, practitioners must know how to access, evaluate, and interpret relevant research as well as to systematically attend to the data they are obtaining "in the moment" of intervention.
2. Practitioners must have the capacity to synthesize evidence from multiple sources to support their intervention recommendations.
3. Once practitioners understand the possible interventions and related outcomes, they need to communicate the probable outcomes to clients and/or their care providers so clients can make informed decisions about their participation in OT.

Evidence is often considered to be published literature; however, practice-based evidence is becoming an important source of data for practice in context. Practice-based evidence, using data collected and analyzed from practice about interventions and outcomes, is utilized to inform practice. Keeping data on interventions and outcomes provides rich information about what does and does not work, and for whom. At higher systems levels, collecting program evaluation data can inform broader programmatic and administrative decisions.

Evidence-based practice requires curiosity and flexibility. Not only must practitioners reflect upon their evaluation and intervention practices, but they must also be open to changes when the evidence suggests more effective approaches than the ones they typically use. Several sources available to OT practitioners for finding and critiquing current evidence are shown in Box 4.4. Chapter 26 provides extensive information on how to effectively use evidence for practice.

Culturally Relevant Practice

Every human activity of daily living is influenced by culture. Each person is influenced by their cultural experiences through intergenerational interactions and relationships with others and the structural conditions in which these occurred. Occupations as common as eating, bathing, and shopping can appear different, mean different things, and happen in different time and place, in part because of culture. It is not possible to think about OT without considering culture. According to Dickie (2004), culture is a tricky concept. Here we define *culture* as a set of shared attitudes, values, goals, and practices that shape occupations and

---

BOX 4.4 EXAMPLES OF RESOURCES FOR EVIDENCE-BASED OCCUPATIONAL THERAPY PRACTICE

- **OTseeker** (http://www.otseeker.com/) is a database that contains abstracts of systematic reviews and randomized controlled trials relevant to occupational therapy (OT). The included trials have been critically appraised and rated to assist the readers in evaluating their validity and interpretability. The ratings can be used by the readers to judge the quality and usefulness of the trials to informing clinical interventions.
- **OT Search** (http://www1.aota.org/otsearch/) is a bibliographic database covering the literature of OT and related subject areas, such as rehabilitation, education, psychiatry or psychology, and healthcare delivery or administration.
- **AOTA Evidence-Based Practice & Knowledge Translation** (https://www.aota.org/practice/practice-essentials/evidencebased-practiceknowledge-translation) contains links to relevant systematic reviews, critically appraised topics, and so on.
- **The Cochrane Library** (https://www.cochranelibrary.com/) is an online collection of databases that brings together, in one place, rigorous and up-to-date research on the effectiveness of healthcare treatments and interventions including, but not limited to, OT.

---

social expectations. Within cultural groups are further subtleties that enter into the process of client- and occupation-centered services. Taboo subjects, privacy, decision-making power, and more may vary within religions, families, and individuals.

An often-considered dimension of culture is the continuum of individualistic to collective orientation. In the United States, OT reflects a culture that emphasizes independence and capitalism. Clients are typically seen individually to optimize their independent function. In collectivist cultures, such as in South Africa, the concept of *ubuntu* or "I am because we are" (Ramugondo & Kronenberg, 2015) encourages services that center upon families, communities, or social networks.

In each encounter, OT practitioners and clients bring their own culture and understandings of others' cultures, which influence how and what occurs. The term "cultural fluency" refers to awareness, humility, learning mindset, empathy, respect, and adaptability (Inoue, 2007). These ingredients form the "ability to navigate the many dimensions of culture needed to build shared meaning and understanding with people from other cultures" (Inoue, 2007, p. 15).

OT practitioners who examine their own culture, assumptions, and biases and advocate to honor client cultural differences are positioned for culturally relevant practice. Ethical and culturally relevant OT practice involves humility to continuously learn the complex and dynamic cultural context of clients and groups (WFOT, 2010).

Practice increasingly involves cross-cultural encounters, as populations become more diverse and multiracial. Practice occurs in the contexts of systemic racism and stigmatization of groups (AOTA, 2021; WFOT, 2020). These disparities go beyond access to services to the imposition of dominant patterns and ways of doing occupations. The world population is shifting with mass human displacement. Throughout the world, people migrate to create better lives for themselves and their children and simply to survive from armed conflict, poverty, natural disasters, global warming effects, and oppression. There are few places where therapists are not engaged with clients of many cultures and lifestyles. Opportunities for practitioners to learn and grow personally abound in these cross-cultural encounters.

The diversity of cultures in which OT is practiced can be a source of strength for the profession (Hammell, 2019). This cultural richness of OT can be witnessed by visits to other countries. However, exporting of dominant Westernized ways of practice into other cultural situations is a widespread problem referred to as *colonialism* (Block et al., 2016; Hammell, 2019; Huff et al., 2020). Importing interventions and equipment used in Westernized practices does not honor the aesthetics and meanings of local cultures. Indeed, OT should be diverse because occupations are inseparable from culture (Watson, 2006).

Effective OT practice involves recognizing that occupations are inherently shaped by culture and that effective OT must attend to the culture of the client (see Figure 4.5). See Chapter 14 for more information on culturally relevant care.

Occupational Justice in Practice

When asked "what is occupational therapy?," a typical response is to explain what services we provide. Yet, a more powerful way to introduce the profession is to explain *why* the profession exists to serve individuals and society and, accordingly, why we chose to be part of this profession. OT is to enable people, regardless of their life situations, to participate in occupations that are meaningful. This deeply moral purpose is to enact occupational justice. The concept of occupational justice is integral to client- and occupation-centered practice. Townsend and Wilcock (2004) equate occupational justice with rights, equity, and fairness and argue that every individual has the right to have equal opportunities for and access to occupational participation. The concept of inclusion, not just accessibility, is a matter of justice. Rudman and colleagues (2014) note that institutional practices, such as those found in biomedical settings, can create forms

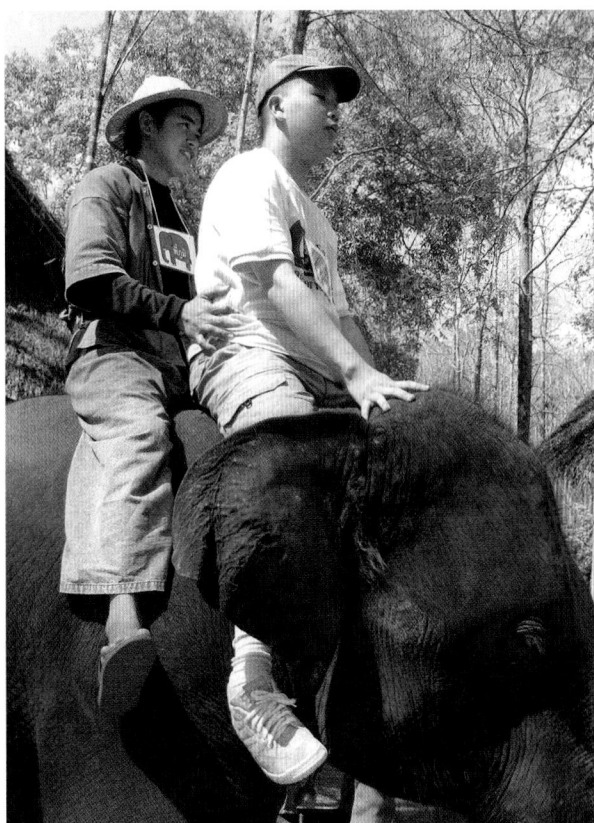

FIGURE 4.5 **A child with a developmental disability participates in an elephant camp implemented by occupational therapists in Thailand. Through carefully monitored interactions with the elephants, to improve higher level of adaptive responses and social/communication abilities in the children.**

of injustice through their focus on disease and inattention to important life activities of patients. In OT practice settings, there is evidence about disparities in access to and quality of healthcare based upon race, economics, gender identity, disability, and other minoritized identities is a call to speak out for change (Johnson & Lavalley, 2021; Lavalley & Johnson, 2020). Furthermore, a profession about justice must advocate for people who are disempowered in any way, including from laws, armed conflict, displacement, political upheavals, dictatorships, and natural disasters. OT initiatives to address instances of occupational injustice are being developed throughout the world, yet the profession is early in the journey to enact the ideals of an "occupationally just" world (Aldrich et al., 2017). See Chapter 10 for more information on occupational justice.

Neurodiversity and disability rights movements are shaping and improving our practice and our world. OT is delivered in the current context of rising awareness of diversity and disparities witnessed in the Black Lives Matter, Stop Asian Hate, and Muslim Lives Matter movements. At the same time, there are mass migrations of people displaced from untenable life situations. The COVID-19 pandemic has further revealed and created disparities at the intersections of race, age, socioeconomic status, and more. It is indeed a time of upheaval to the status quo and redefining and rebuilding communities. OT practitioners are navigating challenging contexts by doing justice, one by one for clients, and in advocacy at other systems levels. There is urgent need for the profession to "look like" the population served, for example, in North America and Europe where OT practitioners are predominantly White women. See Chapter 16 for more information.

Occupational Therapy Practitioners

Clients are, of course, the focus of OT intervention, but OT practitioners are also part of the equation. Just as clients have an occupational history, so do practitioners. Each practitioner brings a particular culture and educational background and repertoire of experiences to the therapeutic situation. OT education programs vary in level and curricular philosophy while also meeting standards for accreditation or approval. The WFOT Standards require a baccalaureate-level entry for occupational therapists (WFOT, 2016). In the United States, occupational therapists enter the profession with a graduate degree at the level of master's or clinical doctorate, OTAs are graduates of associate or baccalaureate-level programs. Practitioners are also obligated, ethically and in some places legally, to continue their education throughout their career so that clients receive up-to-date, competent practice.

Expert practitioners are aware of their own personal, social, and cultural contexts that shape their worldview and endeavor to see the world from the perspective of their clients (Higgs, 2003). Self-awareness, empathy, and professional reasoning abilities combine with preferred theories and interventions as practitioners actualize their knowledge, beliefs, and skills into therapy actions. OT practitioners enter therapeutic situations with the practical realities of their therapy environment and the team members with whom they work (Schell, 2018).

A Broad Profession Growing and Changing to Meet Society's Occupational Needs

In little more than a century, the OT profession has grown to more than 633,000 occupational therapists and 57,955 OTAs worldwide (WFOT, 2022). The WFOT, which began in 1952 with 10 member countries, is now composed of 105 member organizations. There are 120,000 students enrolled in WFOT-approved education programs (WFOT, 2022). In the United States, OT jobs are projected to grow by 17% and OTAs by 34% between 2020 and 2030 (Bureau of Labor Statistics, 2022). There is growing awareness of the need for OT because of advocacy efforts by the profession and people seeking our services. We will address the current unmet needs internationally in the subsequent section.

OT practice trends are reported by the AOTA Workforce Study (AOTA, 2019). In the United States, OT practitioners are concentrated in healthcare inpatient settings. However, trends are shifting toward outpatient and primary care services. Practice with children and youth in schools is a large sector (18%) of occupational therapists in the United States (AOTA, 2019). OTAs are more likely to work in long-term care, including skilled nursing facilities. Only than 3% of current practice is in mental health settings in the United States, yet this is likely to increase with the growing mental health crisis. In other countries, occupational therapists are more likely to work in mental health and less likely to work in school systems. In the United States, 80% of OT practitioners work in nongovernment positions, whereas in other countries, most work in jobs that are within government, such as in national health services (AOTA, 2019; WFOT, 2022).

Unmet Needs

Internationally, the number of people with identified disabilities is growing, and accordingly, there is an urgent need to scale up rehabilitation services (Cieza et al., 2020). The World Report on Disability (WRD) estimated that over 1 billion people (15% of the population) have some form of disability (WHO, 2011, 2020). These numbers may be underestimated because the data focus on body structures/functions and health conditions, whereas disability is associated with environmental conditions, including barriers of stigma, gender inequities, poverty, racism, unemployment, access to education, food insecurity, and other social determinants of health (Frier et al., 2018; Livingston, 2005). See Chapter 15, which addresses social, economic, and political factors that influence occupational performance. The historical notion of disability as fundamentally a medical problem has, in many parts of the world, concentrated practitioners in urban hospitals and medical settings.

The need for OT exceeds the number of professionals in most parts of the world (WFOT, 2020). Once in the workforce, practitioners' patterns of employment are driven by social, geographic, and economic factors. As noted, OT practitioners are concentrated in urban hospital-based services, with fewer serving people in their natural occupational environments. Where there is unmet need for OT practitioners, there are rehabilitation technicians and other personnel filling gaps, yet supervision is a challenge. In some underresourced contexts, there are more practitioners than jobs available, despite the unneed for services. Thus, job creation and distribution of practitioners to match needs is a global issue for the profession. The WFOT Human Resources Project collects data on the profession, including density of practitioners in nearly 100 countries in a report that is updated every 2 years (WFOT, 2022).

A factor that perpetuates inequity in services is when the profession does not reflect racial, ethnic, gender, and other diversities of the populations served. The profession is predominantly female, and in the United States, there is a disproportionate number of White women in the profession (AOTA, 2019; WFOT, 2020). Baseline data on the demographic makeup of the profession are needed to monitor and measure diversity, equity, and inclusion using a broad set of diversity indicators, such as race, ethnicity, and gender identity. As noted, OT practitioners tend to concentrate in urban areas, leaving a dearth of services in aging rural communities throughout the world (Laborda Soriano et al., 2021). Currently, access to and sharing information for OT education, research, and practice is limited by language barriers and the dominance of a few languages. Moreover, language is embedded in culture; thus, OT beliefs and concepts themselves cannot be translated word for word, even with the best intentions, in new contexts.

In the United States and other countries, a history of racism, oppression, and inequity is the context for documented disparities in health services, including OT (Freburger et al., 2011; Lavalley & Johnson, 2020; Nguyen et al., 2021). To varying degrees, societies are awakening to see privilege and disparities against marginalized people through justice movements and other critical discourses on disability, race, aging, gender, poverty, and human displacement. The profession is also taking steps to dismantle the structural racism and inequity that persists within the profession (AOTA, 2021; WFOT, 2020). Identifying intersections of disability and other minoritized groups is further increasing the profession's understandings of clients' experiences of daily life and occupations. We are in a potent time for awareness of bias, which can help advance the profession's capacity to better meet society's occupational needs. See Expanding Our Perspectives for an example.

Increasingly, population health data are revealing occupational needs (see, e.g., Malembaka et al., 2019). Advocacy is key to updating policies to grow services where they are needed. Practitioners are rising to the call to advocate and expand practice as the population ages, needs in mental health are revealed, and with increased survival from cancer, premature birth, chronic conditions, trauma, and infectious diseases like COVID-19 (Halle et al., 2018; Margetis et al., 2021; Novak & Honan, 2019; Pergolotti et al., 2019). Myriad specialized practices target issues such as low vision, hand rehabilitation, housing insecurity, dementia, transitions to adulthood, neurodiversity, falls risk, and driving. Our work is bolstered by human rights legislation in many places calling for accessibility and inclusion (see Chapter 16). Indeed, this profession evolves in tandem with a changing society at local, national, and international levels.

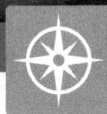

EXPANDING OUR PERSPECTIVES

Social Protest as a Legitimate Occupation

Michelle Lapierre

I am an occupational therapist from Chile, a country that has experienced deep social and political crises and social movements in recent years. I would like to speak to you from my experience as coordinator of the Report on Disability for the Human Rights Commission of the Constitutional Convention of my country.

On October 18, 2019, Chile began to experience the most important social movement in its contemporary history. That day, after the rise in public transport fares, the country literally exploded. The increase in transportation fares was the "straw that broke the camel's back" in a society that has suffered serious injustices and inequalities for many decades. Millions of people across the country took to the streets, for months, to protest in different ways, some of them peaceful and others considered violent. These protests were numerous and varied, and only diminished when society achieved a goal: starting a democratic, representative, participatory, and parity process to draft a new constitution.

The government tried to maintain order through extreme strategies of constitutional exceptions, which resulted in repeated violations of human rights by the state. Thus, street violence was combated with institutional violence, and citizen protest was criminalized.

With the appearance of the social protest on October 18, individuals with disabilities felt deeply called, they quickly joined the street protests and met with groups already organized, such as feminist, student, or indigenous groups. The first obstacle they faced was the lack of physical accessibility to participate in social activities. Once again, the participation of people with disabilities was seen as at risk. This allowed them to become aware of the importance of organizing, both in the streets and on social networks. From that moment on, numerous groups, assemblies, and councils of people with disabilities emerged throughout Chile.

People with disabilities, on behalf of themselves, decided to use their voice, to be recognized in their equality and difference, as part of a society, without being represented by others. They chose to resist to demand citizen recognition.

For a long time, people with disabilities were confined to the private space, institutionalization, and forced representation by family members, institutions, and professionals

(continued)

EXPANDING OUR PERSPECTIVES (continued)

(including ourselves). This has been one of the historical reasons for the low politicization of the movement of people with disabilities in Chile.

The slogan of the national social revolt focused on the concept of "Dignity." This was relevant for people with disabilities because the lack of dignity has been an historical reality for people with disabilities in Chile, and their demand, a struggle. The country has been characterized by the violation of the rights of people with disabilities and by generating precarious and undignified living conditions in multiple dimensions. Poverty, charity, forced institutionalization, homelessness, and social confinement have been the realities that have marked disability in Chile. Unfortunately, the profession of OT for a long time did not question this reality and, in many cases, even contributed to reproduce it.

Although the heat of the movement was still burning and the social pact for a new constitution had recently been signed, based on the social pressure imposed by the people, the commemoration of the International Day of Persons with Disabilities was approaching, on December 3, 2019. That day, the greatest national march for disability was organized, the most massive and politicized that can be remembered to date. From this event, the National Disability Collective (CONADIS), with more than 200 disability groups and organizations, was born.

People with disabilities became involved in social protest, through both peaceful and "violent" practices. Based on these facts, and the reflections on occupation from a critical perspective, I ask myself: When is protest a violent act? Is protest an occupation? Can violent social protest be a legitimate occupation? Is the concept of collective occupation sufficient to analyze the occupations associated with large social movements, or should we think of other notions to help us understand the occupation of a society on alert, in demand, and in nonpeaceful protest? What is the role of OT and occupational therapists in these social realities that flood the daily life of a country at any given time? These questions do not have a single answer, but here I want to raise them according to the experience that I have carried out with groups of people with disabilities during social protest period and later during their participation in the drafting of the new constitution.

Just as many of the people with disabilities committed violent acts, they also received violence from the state, were beaten, tortured, and were put in jail. Even new people with disabilities appeared as a result of the almost 500 victims of tear gas produced by the forces of public order. While this was happening, the same groups of people with disabilities supported the drafting of a new constitution, engaged in the institutional process, and fought for their democratic representation. During the process of drafting the new constitution, people with disabilities were heard in official public hearings and a historical truth report was made on their situation; they participated as advisers, theoretical references, references by experience, researchers, and communicators.

Considering the experience of people with disabilities in this Chilean social outbreak, we propose that social protest is a legitimate occupation, even if it takes forms that can be considered violent when analyzed out of context. Social protest is an occupation for agency, resistance, and reexistence. Social protest is an important occupation that contributes to massive social transformation, and it is shared by many civil society groups. Social protest is an occupation that can pave the way for other collective occupations that strive for dignity.

We believe that protest is not only a legitimate occupation but also a necessary occupation, especially in societies where people with disabilities have been historically oppressed and social protest emerges as a real possibility for representation. Today, the proposed new constitution includes articles that ensure the dignity and protection of people with disabilities. We believe that this is the concrete result of the experience of the occupation-based protest, and that without it, this civilizational advance would not be possible.

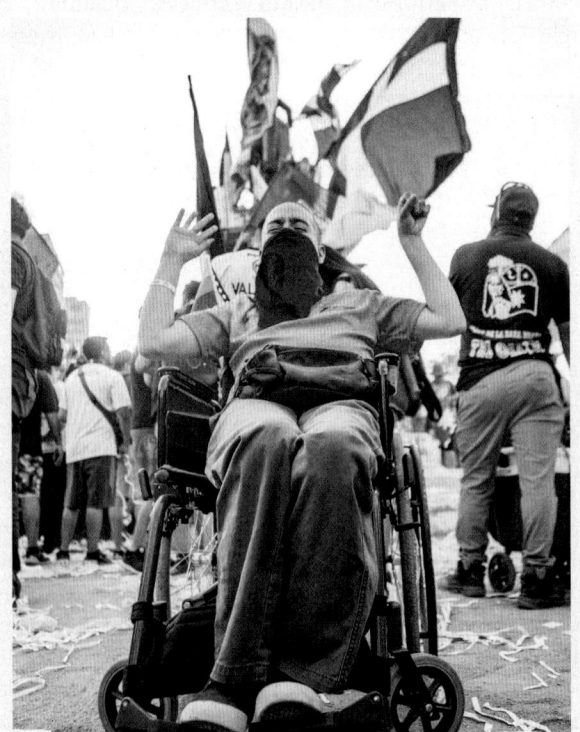

Jaime Ramírez (National Disability Collective), International Day of Persons with Disabilities on December 3, 2019, Santiago, Chile. By: @werkén_ fotografías (Mauricio Leiva Cullinao).

Vision for the Future

The arc of the moral universe is long, but it bends

toward justice.

—REVEREND MARTIN LUTHER KING, JR.

In countries and regions throughout the world, OT will continue to grow because of the profession's moral commitment to solve problems of daily living and contribute to prevention of disabilities. Professional organizations and individuals are compelled to change and expand where needs are unmet and as new problems arise. COVID-19 is a recent example, in which OT practitioners were innovators in developing services from intensive care units to communities for people with long-term COVID-19 (Mihevc et al., 2022). As always, the profession responded and modified services, by expanding telehealth delivery and addressing occupations in the context of quarantines and isolation. The profession grows because of continuous and connected innovations in research, theory, education, and service delivery. The profession's future will occur in tandem with scientific advances in other fields (e.g., neurosciences, technology, public health). Some of the broader forces include the following:

- Internet connectivity will support rapid development of worldwide technologies, including telehealth, virtual reality, driverless cars, robotics, artificial intelligence, and smartphone capabilities (Liu & Mihailidis, 2019).
- Climate change and resource depletion will impact occupations, particularly in low-income regions, drawing attention to environmental sustainability as part of future practice (Huss et al., 2020; Pollard et al., 2020).
- Decentralized care, primary care, and community-based care are contemporary shifts from urban medical centers toward local, accessible, and cost-effective services (Dahl-Popolizio et al., 2018; Jordan, 2019) (see Chapters 22 and 68).
- Systems for delivering and funding care will change along with shifts in policies about government versus private industry control of healthcare and other services.
- Evidence supporting evaluation and intervention strategies will increasingly drive practice (Lin et al., 2010).
- Evidence for the cost-effectiveness and cost savings will support growth, such as findings about OT reducing hospital readmissions (Edelstein et al., 2022).
- The human genome project will impact healthcare approaches and results (Reynolds & Lou, 2009).
- Investigation of social determinants of health will support occupational therapists' focus on occupational injustices that limit individuals and groups from their rights to engage in valued occupations (Braveman & Bass-Haugen, 2009; Kronenberg et al., 2011).
- Individual-, community-, and population-level disruptions and displacement that occur as a result of natural and man-made disasters and armed conflicts will influence where and how occupational therapists practice (AOTA, 2017a) (see Chapter 66).
- Attention to the value of assistive technology of all kinds, such as wheelchairs and hearing aids, will support participation for people with disabilities (WHO, 2022).
- With awareness of pervasive patterns of disparities, there is a rising movement to assess and create a more diverse workforce to guide appropriate and equitable services (Jesus et al., 2022).
- Human rights advocacy aims to expand policies for justice for people with disabilities and intersectionalities, in the forms of resources and participation in all aspects of society (De Beco, 2020; United Nations, 2018).
- Pharmaceutical and surgical advances will reduce impairments that interfere with occupations (e.g., drugs for multiple sclerosis and surgeries for arthritis). These treatments may also increase iatrogenic illnesses and disabilities.
- There is a proliferation of noncommunicable diseases (NCDs) that are lifestyle based, chronic, and disabling. Examples are heart disease, diabetes, obesity, and pulmonary conditions (WHO, n.d.-b).
- Societies are aging because of longevity and decreased birth rates. Premature infants and infants with disabilities are surviving at a higher rate. As the percentage of people with disabilities increases, caregiving needs will rise (United Nations, n.d.).
- Mental health and substance abuse are gaining increased attention. Recognition of these issues as health conditions, rather than personal failings, will support the society's sense of responsibility to provide care.
- United Nations Sustainable Development Goals call for a future of "Decent Work," including the right to work for all, regardless of gender, race, disability, religion, and other identities and distinctions, as well as fair income, hours, security, and conditions of work. The WFOT is engaging in a project to engage the profession in this broader economic and humanitarian effort (WFOT, 2018).

Occupational science research will increase our understanding of the nature, meanings, and power of occupation to better meet the needs of individuals and groups. These and many more unseen forces will shape future practice. With vision and strategic action to advance OT's effectiveness, leadership, collaboration, and accessibility, the profession is preparing to meet society's future needs.

Conclusion

Contemporary and envisioned practices of OT are centered around the profession's core construct, occupation, a complex and essential aspect of human life. OT is grounded in a humanistic philosophy that people, regardless of their life situations, should have opportunities to participate in occupations that bring health and meaning. OT practitioners offer unique knowledge and skills in the context of collaborative process with clients and team members to enable participation.

A systems approach can be useful to understand why practice does and should look different based upon practice context. Incorporating shared language and concepts within and outside the profession will advance the evidence and teamwork processes for care. OT is a broad profession that evolves with the needs and occupational challenges faced by society, with a vision for justice for groups that have been underserved or marginalized. Advocacy, innovation, and diversity of the profession itself will ensure the profession's continual relevance and contribution to society (Hammell, 2019).

OT services must be grounded in research and focused on clients' unique occupations and life situations. OT is a client-centered process that evolves as the practitioner and client work together to carefully analyze the client's occupations, performance limitations, and environment. Because OT involves doing *with* clients and not doing *to* them, there is an improvisational aspect of intervention that requires the OT practitioner and client to coordinate their actions to achieve the client's goal.

We end with a quote from Peloquin (2005) who concluded her Eleanor Clarke Slagle lecture with the following statement:

> The ethos of occupational therapy restores our clear-sightedness so that we see what is essential: We are pathfinders. We enable occupations that heal. We co-create daily lives. We reach for hearts as well as hands. We are artists and scientists at once. If we discern this in ourselves, if we act on this understanding every day, we will advance into the future embracing our ethos of engagement. And we will have reclaimed our magnificent heart. (p. 623)

Lippincott® Connect *For additional resources on the subjects discussed in this chapter, visit Lippincott Connect.*

REFERENCES

Aldrich, R. M., Boston, T. L., & Daaleman, C. E. (2017). Justice and US occupational therapy practice: A relationship 100 years in the making. *American Journal of Occupational Therapy, 71*(1), 7101100040p1–7101100040p5. https://doi.org/10.5014/ajot.2017.023085

American Occupational Therapy Association. (2017a). AOTA's societal statement on disaster response and risk reduction. *American Journal of Occupational Therapy, 71*(Suppl 2), 7112410060p1–7112410060p3. https://doi.org/10.5014/ajot.2017.716S11

American Occupational Therapy Association. (2017b). Philosophical base of occupational therapy. *American Journal of Occupational Therapy, 71*(Suppl 2), 7112410045p1. https://doi.org/10.5014/ajot.2017.716S06

American Occupational Therapy Association. (2019). *AOTA's workforce and salary survey.* AOTA Press.

American Occupational Therapy Association. (2020a). Occupational therapy practice framework: Domain and process (4th ed.). *American Journal of Occupational Therapy, 74*(Suppl 2). https://doi.org/10.5014/ajot.2020.74S2001

American Occupational Therapy Association. (2020b). Occupational therapy code of ethics AOTA 2020. *American Journal of Occupational Therapy, 74*(Suppl 3), 7413410005p1–7413410005p13. https://doi.org/10.5014/ajot.2020.74S3006

American Occupational Therapy Association. (2021). *AOTA statement on justice and systemic racism.* https://www.aota.org/about/diversity-equity-and-inclusion/aota-statement-on-justice-and-systemic-racism

Berwick, D. M. (2002). A user's manual for the IOM's "Quality Chasm" report. *Health Affairs, 21*(3), 80–90. https://doi.org/10.1377/hlthaff.21.3.80

Block, P., Kasnitz, D., Nishida, A., & Pollard, N. (Eds.). (2016). *Occupying disability: Critical approaches to community, justice, and decolonizing disability.* Springer.

Braveman, B., & Bass-Haugen, J. D. (2009). Social justice and health disparities: An evolving discourse in occupational therapy research and intervention. *American Journal of Occupational Therapy, 63*(1), 7–12. https://doi.org/10.5014/ajot.63.1.7

Bureau of Labor Statistics. (2022, April). *Occupational outlook handbook.* https://www.bls.gov/ooh/healthcare/occupational-therapists.htm

Christiansen, C. H. (1999). Defining lives: Occupation as identity—An essay on competence, coherence, and the creation of meaning. *American Journal of Occupational Therapy, 54*(6), 547–558. https://doi.org/10.5014/ajot.53.6.547

Cieza, A., Causey, K., Kamenov, K., Hanson, S. W., Chatterji, S., & Vos, T. (2020). Global estimates of the need for rehabilitation based on the Global Burden of Disease study 2019: A systematic analysis for the Global Burden of Disease Study 2019. *The Lancet, 396*(10267), 2006–2017. https://doi.org/10.1016/S0140-6736(20)32340-0

Clark, F. (1993). The 1993 Eleanor Clarke Slagle lecture—Occupation embedded in a real life: Interweaving occupational science and occupational therapy. *American Journal of Occupational Therapy, 47*(12), 1067–1078. https://doi.org/10.5014/ajot.47.12.1067

Clark, F., Azen, S. P., Zemke, R., Jackson, J., Carlson, M., Mandel, D., Hay, J., Josephson, K., Cherry, B., Hessel, C., Palmer, J., & Lipson, L. (1997). Occupational therapy for independent-living older adults: A randomized controlled trial. *JAMA, 278*(16), 1321–1326. doi:10.1001/jama.1997.03550160041036

Cohn, E. S. (2019). Asserting our competence and affirming the value of occupation with confidence. *American Journal of Occupational Therapy, 73*(6), 7306150010p1–7306150010p10. https://doi.org/10.5014/ajot.2019.736002

Dahl-Popolizio, S., Doyle, S., & Wade, S. (2018). The role of primary health care in achieving global healthcare goals: Highlighting the potential contribution of occupational therapy. *World Federation of Occupational Therapists Bulletin, 74*(1), 8–16. https://doi.org/10.1080/14473828.2018.1433770

De Beco, G. (2020). Intersectionality and disability in international human rights law. *International Journal of Human Rights, 24*(5), 593–614. https://doi.org/10.1080/13642987.2019.1661241

Dickie, V. A. (2004). Culture is tricky: A commentary on culture emergent in occupation. *American Journal of Occupational Therapy, 58*(2), 169–173. https://doi.org/10.5014/ajot.58.2.169

Edelstein, J., Walker, R., Middleton, A., Reistetter, T., Gary, K. W., & Reynolds, S. (2022). Higher frequency of acute occupational therapy services is associated with reduced hospital readmissions. *American Journal of Occupational Therapy, 76*(1), 7610510013p1. https://doi.org/10.5014/ajot.2022.76S1-RP13

Egan, M., & Restall, G. (2022). *Promoting occupational participation: Collaborative, relationship-focused occupational therapy.* Canadian Association of Occupational Therapists.

Engelhardt, H. T. (1977). Defining occupational therapy: The meaning of therapy and the virtues of occupation. *American Journal of Occupational Therapy, 31*(10), 666–672. https://pubmed.ncbi.nlm.nih.gov/341718

Fisher, A. G. (2013). Occupation-centred, occupation-based, occupation-focused: Same, same or different? *Scandinavian Journal of Occupational Therapy, 20*(3), 162–173. https://doi.org/10.3109/11038128.2012.754492

Freburger, J. K., Holmes, G. M., Ku, L. J. E., Cutchin, M. P., Heatwole-Shank, K., & Edwards, L. J. (2011). Disparities in post–acute rehabilitation care for joint replacement. *Arthritis Care & Research, 63*(7), 1020–1030. https://doi.org/10.1002/acr.20477

Frier, A., Barnett, F., Devine, S., & Barker, R. (2018). Understanding disability and the "social determinants of health": How does disability affect peoples' social determinants of health? *Disability and Rehabilitation, 40*(5), 538–547. https://doi.org/10.1080/09638288.2016.1258090

Glass, T. A., Mendes de Leon, C., Marottoli, R. A., & Berkman, L. F. (1999). Population based study of social and productive activities as predictors of survival among elderly Americans. *British Medical Journal, 319*(7208), 478–483. https://doi.org/10.1136/bmj.319.7208.478

Gray, J. M. (1998). Putting occupation into practice: Occupation as ends, occupation as means. *American Journal of Occupational Therapy, 52*(5), 354–364. https://doi.org/10.5014/ajot.52.5.354

Halle, A. D., Mroz, T. M., Fogelberg, D. J., & Leland, N. E. (2018). Occupational therapy and primary care: Updates and trends. *American Journal of Occupational Therapy, 72*(3), 7203090010p1–7203090010p6. https://doi.org/10.5014/ajot.2018.723001

Hammell, K. W. (2019). Building globally relevant occupational therapy from the strength of our diversity. *World Federation of Occupational Therapists Bulletin, 75*(1), 13–26. https://doi.org/10.1080/14473828.2018.1529480

Hasselkus, B. R., (2006). The world of everyday occupation: Real people, real lives. *The American Journal of Occupational Therapy, 60*(6), 627-640.

Hasselkus, B. R., & Dickie, V. A. (2021). *The meaning of everyday occupation* (3rd ed.). SLACK.

Higgs, J. (2003). Do you reason like a (health) professional? In G. Brown, S. A. Esdaile, & S. E. Ryan (Eds.), *Becoming an advanced healthcare practitioner* (pp. 145–160). Butterworth.

Holm, H. B. (2000). The 2000 Eleanor Clarke Slagle lecture—Our mandate for a new millennium: Evidence-based practice. *American Journal of Occupational Therapy, 54*(6), 575–585. https://doi.org/10.5014/ajot.54.6.575

Huff, S., Rudman, D. L., Magalhães, L., Lawson, E., & Kanyamala, M. (2020). Enacting a critical decolonizing ethnographic approach in occupation-based research. *Journal of Occupational Science, 29(1)*, 1–15. https://doi.org/10.1080/14427591.2020.1824803

Huss, N., Ikiugu, M. N., Hackett, F., Sheffield, P. E., Palipane, N., & Groome, J. (2020). Education for sustainable health care: From learning to professional practice. *Medical Teacher, 42*(10), 1097–1101. https://doi.org/10.1080/0142159X.2020.1797998

Hyett, N., Kenny, A., & Dickson-Swift, V. (2019). Re-imagining occupational therapy clients as communities: Presenting the community-centred practice. *Scandinavian Journal of Occupational Therapy, 26*(4), 246–260. https://doi.org/10.1080/11038128.2017.1423374

Inoue Y. (2007). Cultural fluency as a guide to effective intercultural communication: The case of Japan and the U.S. *Journal of Intercultural Communication, 15.* https://immi.se/oldwebsite/nr15/inoue.htm

Iwama, M. K. (2006). *The Kawa model: Culturally relevant occupational therapy.* Elsevier Health Sciences.

Jackson, J. (1998). The value of occupation as the core of treatment Sandy's experience. *American Journal of Occupational Therapy, 52*(6), 466–473. https://doi.org/10.5014/ajot.52.6.466

Jayaratne, K., Jacobs, K., & Fernando, D. (2012). Global healthy backpack initiatives. *Work, 41*(Suppl 1), 5553–5557. https://doi.org/10.3233/WOR-2012-0880-5553

Jesus, T. S., Mani, K., von Zweck, C., Kamalakannan, S., Bhattacharjya, S., Ledgerd, R., & World Federation of Occupational Therapists. (2022). Type of findings generated by the occupational therapy workforce research worldwide: Scoping review and content analysis. *International Journal of Environmental Research and Public Health, 19*(9), 5307. https://doi.org/10.3390/ijerph19095307

Johnson, K. R., & Lavalley, R. (2021). From racialized think-pieces toward anti-racist praxis in our science, education, and practice. *Journal of Occupational Science, 28*(3), 404–409. https://doi.org/10.1080/14427591.2020.1847598

Jordan, K. (2019). Occupational therapy in primary care: Positioned and prepared to be a vital part of the team. *American Journal of Occupational Therapy, 73*(5), 7305170010p1–7305170010p6. https://doi.org/10.5014/ajot.2019.735002

Kronenberg, F., Pollard, N., & Sakellariou, D. (2011). *Occupational therapies without borders: Vol. 2. Towards an ecology of occupationbased practices.* Churchill Livingstone, Elsevier.

Laborda Soriano, A. A., Aliaga, A. C., & Vidal-Sánchez, M. I. (2021). Depopulation in Spain and violation of occupational rights. *Journal of Occupational Science, 28*(1), 71–80. https://doi.org/10.1080/14427591.2021.1896331

Lavalley, R., & Johnson, K. R. (2020). Occupation, injustice, and anti-Black racism in the United States of America. *Journal of Occupational Science, 29*(2), 1–13. https://doi.org/10.1080/14427591.2020.1810111

Law, M. (1998). *Client-centered occupational therapy.* SLACK.

Law, M., Seinwender, S., & Leclair, L. (1998). Occupation, health, and well-being. *Canadian Journal of Occupational Therapy, 65*(2), 81–91. https://doi.org/10.1177/000841749806500204

Lin, S. H., Murphy, S. L., & Robinson, J. C. (2010). Facilitating evidence-based practice: Process, strategies and resources. *American Journal of Occupational Therapy, 64*(1), 164–171. https://doi.org/10.5014/ajot.64.1.164

Liu, L., & Mihailidis, A. (2019). The changing landscape of occupational therapy intervention and research in an age of ubiquitous technologies. *OTJR: Occupation, Participation and Health, 39*(2), 79–80. https://doi.org/10.1177/1539449219835370

Livingston, J. (2005). *Debility and the moral imagination in Botswana.* Indiana University Press.

Malembaka, E. B., Karemere, H., Balaluka, G. B., Lambert, A. S., Muneza, F., Deconinck, H., & Macq, J. (2019). A new look at population health through the lenses of cognitive, functional and social disability clustering in eastern DR Congo: A community-based cross-sectional study. *BMC Public Health, 19*, 1–13. https://doi.org/10.1186/s12889-019-6431-z

Margetis, J. L., Wilcox, J., Thompson, C., & Mannion, N. (2021). Occupational therapy: Essential to critical care rehabilitation. *American Journal of Occupational Therapy, 75*(2), 7502170010p1–7502170010p5. https://doi.org/10.5014/ajot.2021.048827

Maritz, R., Baptiste, S., Darzins, S. W., Magasi, S., Weleschuk, C., & Prodinger, B. (2018). Linking occupational therapy models and assessments to the ICF to enable standardized documentation of functioning. *Canadian Journal of Occupational Therapy, 85*(4), 330–341. https://doi.org/10.1177/0008417418797146

Mattingly, C. (1991). The narrative nature of clinical reasoning. *American Journal of Occupational Therapy, 45*(11), 979–986. https://doi.org/10.5014/ajot.45.11.998

Meyer, A. (1922/1977). The philosophy of occupational therapy. *American Journal of Occupational Therapy, 31*(10), 639–642. (Original work published 1922)

Mihevc, S., Sicherl, Z., & Galof, K. (2022). The consequences of COVID-19 pandemic on occupational therapy practice: A systematic review. *Journal of Family Medical and Primary Care Open Access, 6*, 182. https://doi.org/10.29011/2688-7460.100082

Nguyen, D. Q., Ifejika, N. L., Reistetter, T. A., & Makam, A. N. (2021). Factors associated with duration of rehabilitation among older adults with prolonged hospitalization. *Journal of the American Geriatrics Society, 69*(4), 1035–1044. https://doi.org/10.1111/jgs.16988

Novak, I., & Honan, I. (2019). Effectiveness of paediatric occupational therapy for children with disabilities: A systematic review. *Australian Occupational Therapy Journal, 66*(3), 258–273. https://doi.org/10.1111/1440-1630.12573

Peloquin, S. M. (2005). The 2005 Eleanor Clarke Slagle lecture— Embracing our ethos, reclaiming our heart. *American Journal of Occupational Therapy, 59*(6), 611–625. https://doi.org/10.5014/ajot.59.6.611

Pergolotti, M., Alfano, C. M., Cernich, A. N., Yabroff, K. R., Manning, P. R., de Moor, J. S., Hahn, E. E., Mohile, S. G., & Mohile, S. G. (2019). A health services research agenda to fully integrate cancer rehabilitation into oncology care. *Cancer, 125*(22), 3908–3916. https://doi.org/10.1002/cncr.32382

Pollard, N., Galvaan, R., Hudson, M., Kåhlin, I., Ikiugu, M., Roschnik, S., Shann, S., & Whittaker, B. (2020). Sustainability in occupational therapy practice, education and scholarship. *World Federation of Occupational Therapists Bulletin, 76*(1), 2–3. https://doi.org/10.1080/14473828.2020.1733756

Pörn, I. (1993). Health and adaptedness. *Theoretical Medicine, 14*(4), 295–303. https://doi.org/10.1007/BF00996337

Ramugondo, E. L., & Kronenberg, F. (2015). Explaining collective occupations from a human relations perspective: Bridging the individual-collective dichotomy. *Journal of Occupational Science, 22*(1), 3–16. https://doi.org/10.1080/14427591.2013.781920

Rappaport, J. (1987). Terms of empowerment/exemplars of prevention: Toward a theory for community psychology. *American Journal of Community Psychology, 15*(2), 121–145. https://doi.org/10.1007/BF00919275

Reitz, S. M., Scaffa, M. E., & Dorsey, J. (2020). Occupational therapy in the promotion of health and well-being. *American Journal of Occupational Therapy, 74*(3), 7403420010p1–7403420010p14. https://doi.org/10.5014/ajot.2020.743003

Reynolds, S., & Lou, J. Q. (2009). Occupational therapy in the age of the human genome: Occupational therapists' role in genetics research and its impact on clinical practice. *American Journal of Occupational Therapy, 63*(4), 511–515. https://doi.org/10.5014/ajot.63.4.511

Rudman, D. L., Stamm, T., Prodinger, B., & Shaw, L. (2014). Enacting occupation-based practice: Exploring the disjuncture between the daily lives of mothers with rheumatoid arthritis and institutional processes. *British Journal of Occupational Therapy, 77*(10), 491–498. https://doi.org/10.4276/030802214X14122630932359

Sackett, D. L., Rosenberg, W. M., Granny, J. A., Haynes, R. B., & Richardson, W. S. (1996). Evidence-based medicine. What it is and what it isn't. *British Medical Journal, 312*, 71–72. https://doi.org/10.1136/bmj.312.7023.71

Sakellariou, D., & Pollard, N. (Eds.). (2017). *Occupational therapies without borders: Integrating justice with practice* (2nd ed.). Elsevier.

Schell, B. A. B. (2018). Pragmatic reasoning. In B. A. B. Schell & J. W. Schell (Eds.), *Clinical and professional reasoning in occupational therapy* (2nd ed., pp. 203–223). Wolters Kluwer.

Straus, S. E., Glasziou, P., Richardson, W. S., & Haynes, R. B. (2011). *Evidence-based medicine: How to practice and teach it* (4th ed.). Churchill Livingstone, Elsevier.

Tickle-Degnen, L. (2000). Communicating with clients, family members, and colleagues about research evidence. *American Journal of Occupational Therapy, 54*(3), 341–343. https://doi.org/10.5014/ajot.54.3.341

Townsend, E., & Polatajko, H. (2007). *Enabling occupation II: Advancing an occupational therapy vision for health, well-being & justice through occupation.* Canadian Association of Occupational Therapists.

Townsend, E. A., & Wilcock, A. A. (2004). Occupational justice and client-centered practice: A dialogue in progress. *Canadian Journal of Occupational Therapy, 71*(2), 75–87. https://doi.org/10.1177/000841740407100203

United Nations. (2018). *Disability and development report: Realizing the sustainable development goals by, for and with persons with disabilities.* https://social.un.org/publications/UN-Flagship-Report-Disability-Final.pdf

United Nations. (n.d.). *Ageing.* https://www.un.org/en/global-issues/ageing

VanPuymbrouck, L. H., & Friedman, C. (2022). "We Weren't Taught How to Recover From a Pandemic": Recent occupational therapy graduates' reflections on COVID-19. *Journal of Occupational Therapy Education, 6*(2), 5. https://doi.org/10.26681/jote.2022.060205

Watson, R. M. (2006). Being before doing: The cultural identity (essence) of occupational therapy. *Australian Occupational Therapy Journal, 53*(3), 151–158. https://doi.org/10.1111/j.1440-1630.2006.00598.x

World Federation of Occupational Therapists. (2010). *Position statement on diversity and culture.* https://www.wfot.org

World Federation of Occupational Therapists. (2016). *Minimum standards for the education of occupational therapists revised 2016.* https://www.wfot.org

World Federation of Occupational Therapists. (2017). *Statement on occupational therapy.* Definitions of occupational therapy from member organizations. https://www.wfot.org

World Federation of Occupational Therapists. (2018). *Decent work project report.* Author. https://www.wfot.org

World Federation of Occupational Therapists. (2020). *WFOT statement on systemic racism.* https://wfot.org/wfot-statement-on-systemic-racism

World Federation of Occupational Therapists. (2022). *WFOT human resources project.* https://www.wfot.org

World Health Organization. (2001). *International classification of functioning, disability and health.* https://www.who.int/standards/classifications/international-classification-of-functioning-disability-and-health#:~:text=ICF%20is%20the%20WHO%20framework,and%20measure%20health%20and%20disability

World Health Organization. (2011). *World report on disability 2011.* Author. https://www.who.int/publications/i/item/9789241564182

World Health Organization. (2020). *Disability and health fact sheet.* https://www.who.int/news-room/fact-sheets/detail/disability-and-health

World Health Organization. (2022). *International classification of diseases* (11th ed.). https://www.who.int/standards/classifications/classification-of-diseases

World Health Organization. (2022). *Global Report on Assistive Technology.* https://www.who.int/publications/i/item/9789240049451

World Health Organization. (n.d.-a). *International classification of health interventions.* https://www.who.int/standards/classifications/international-classification-of-health-interventions

World Health Organization. (n.d.-b). *Non-communicable diseases.* https://www.who.int/health-topics/noncommunicable-diseases#tab=tab_1

Yerxa, E. J. (1967). The 1967 Eleanor Clarke Slagle lecture—Authentic occupational therapy. *American Journal of Occupational Therapy, 21*, 1–9.

Yerxa, E. J., Clark, F., Frank, G., Jackson, J., Parham, D., Pierce, D., Stein, C., & Zemke, R. (1989). An introduction to occupational science: A foundation for occupational therapy in the 21st century. *Occupational Therapy in Health Care, 6*(4), 1–17. https://doi.org/10.1080/J003v06n04_04

Occupational Therapy Professional Organizations

Susan Coppola and Ritchard Ledgerd

LEARNING OBJECTIVES

After reading this chapter, you will be able to:

1. Examine how member organizations, regulation, and educational standards are key elements that form the profession of occupational therapy.
2. Consider the importance of lifelong membership and participation in occupational therapy professional organizations for the individual and the profession.
3. Analyze the structure and function of state, national, and international occupational therapy professional organizations.
4. Determine the purpose and nature of regulatory bodies at state, national, and international levels.
5. Evaluate how professional and regulatory organizations serve the consumers of occupational therapy through standard setting and education.
6. Explain the roles that both volunteer and paid staff members in professional organizations play in developing and supporting all aspects of the occupational therapy profession and the clients served by its members.

Introduction

When students and practitioners from a profession come together to discuss mutual challenges and opportunities, the nucleus of a professional organization (association, society, or federation) is formed (Mata et al., 2010). These shared interests and relationships create the core of a profession. Professional organizations then work as a formal collective to *define and advance* the interests of practitioners to better serve the public needs. These are typically nonprofit organizations with evolving structures and functions that strengthen and unite the profession around a shared mission, vision, and strategic initiatives (Schneider & Somers, 2006). In occupational therapy (OT), these initiatives include setting standards for education and practice, defining and promoting a code of ethics, providing opportunities for professional education and networking, advocating in legislatures for practitioners and clients, and promoting the profession. Table 5.1 shows how associations are key elements of OT being a profession using Benveniste's

TABLE 5.1   What Makes Occupational Therapy a Profession?

What Makes a Profession a Profession?	What Makes OT a Profession?
1. Apply specialized knowledge and skills	OT knowledge, skills, and know-how applied to the art and science of practice
2. Have advanced education and training	Accreditation standards for OT education and opportunities for continuing education and professional development
3. Have demonstrated competency and have completed the requirements to be admitted to or maintained in the profession	Certification examination, field-based performance, continuing competence requirements
4. Have the support of a professional association	State, national, and international occupational therapy organizations
5. Are bound by a code of conduct or ethics	National associations and WFOT have Codes of Ethics
6. Feel a sense of responsibility for serving the public	Individual and collective ethos as well as regulation to protect the public

OT, occupational therapy; WFOT, World Federation of Occupational Therapists.

(1987) definition. These elements include applied knowledge, education, competency, associations, ethics, and social responsibility.

Another key element of a profession is *regulation* in order to protect the public from harm. Regulatory bodies provide a legal mechanism to ensure that persons who represent themselves as occupational therapists are educated, credentialed, ethical, and competent. Most countries with OT associations have a form of regulation. Box 5.1 identifies places where there is regulation of occupational therapists around the world (World Federation of Occupational Therapists [WFOT], 2022). Regulation of practice in the United States, for example, is through a national certification process for entry to practice, and each state requires a license to practice. Most countries have regulation only at the national/federal level.

This chapter explores how elements of the profession, professional organizations, and regulation work together at the local, national, and international levels to make OT a vibrant, valuable, and growing profession. Understanding these elements and the ability to engage with them is essential to being part of the advancement of the profession and to engage in legal and ethical practice in OT. Table 5.2 gives an overview of local, national, and international associations, regulatory bodies, and educational standards.

BOX 5.1 COUNTRIES WHERE OCCUPATIONAL THERAPY IS REGULATED AT THE NATIONAL/FEDERAL AND/OR STATE/REGIONAL LEVEL

Argentina	Germany	Macau	Singapore
Australia	Ghana	Madagascar	Slovenia
Austria	Greece	Malawi	South Africa
Bahamas	Guyana	Mexico	Spain
Belgium	Hong Kong	Mongolia	Sri Lanka
Bermuda	Iceland	Morocco	Sweden
Bosnia & Herzegovina	Indonesia	Namibia	Switzerland
Botswana	Iran	Netherlands	Taiwan
Brazil	Israel	New Zealand	Tanzania
Canada	Italy	Nigeria	Thailand
Chile	Jamaica	Norway	Trinidad & Tobago
China	Japan	Palestine	Uganda
Colombia	Jordan	Peru	United Kingdom
Costa Rica	Kenya	Philippines	United States of America
Croatia	Korea	Portugal	Venezuela
Cyprus	Kosovo	Romania	Zambia
Denmark	Latvia	Rwanda	Zimbabwe
Dominican Republic	Lebanon	Saudi Arabia	
Finland	Lithuania	Serbia	
France	Luxembourg	Seychelles	

TABLE 5.2	Relationship of Associations, Regulatory Bodies, and Education Standards		
	OT Professional Member Associations	**Regulatory Bodies for OT Practice**	**OT Education Standards**
Purpose	Build and promote the profession to serve societal needs	Protect the public from harm	Establish minimum standards for education in the profession
State/territory/ province	OT associations within states, territories, or provinces	State/regional licensure or certification board	
National	Over 90 countries have national associations. Some also include union representation.	77 countries have government regulation. This usually entails a fee and often registration with a government agency such as the Department or Ministry of Health. In the United States, passing the National Board for Certification in Occupational Therapy (NBCOT) exam is required to enter the profession. Ongoing NBCOT registration is elective for most states.	Some nations have curriculum standards. Others accept the standards from the World Federation. In the United States, AOTA's Accreditation Council for Occupational Therapy Education sets standards for OTA programs, and masters and doctorate entry-level programs for occupational therapists.
International	World Federation of Occupational Therapists (WFOT) member organizations have a national professional association with a constitution and a code of ethics. Full members of WFOT must also have an approved education program in their country. Of the 105 member organizations, 76 are full members.	No regulation at the international level	WFOT Minimum Standards for the Education of Occupational Therapists (2016). As of 2022, there were 1,141 WFOT education programs, and 367 nonapproved programs. As of 2016, WFOT recommended entry-level education is at the bachelor's level or equivalent. The WFOT does not approve OTA programs.

AOTA, American Occupational Therapy Association; OT, occupational therapy; OTA, occupational therapy assistant.

Professional Associations and the Importance of Lifelong Membership

Professional associations, sometimes referred to as societies or organizations, have made significant contributions as consultants to governments and academia. They have played a major role in establishing the profession and broadening the scope of practice and the scientific body of knowledge (Bickel, 2007). Associations are made up of members who elect individuals to fulfill leadership roles, such as president, vice president, directors, and so forth. If the association has sufficient funds, paid staff enact the administrative functions and strategic priorities. In most cases, volunteers perform many association activities. A strong association enables a profession to be self-defining in standards and scope rather than allowing other disciplines or policymakers delineate their role. Associations provide coherence and advancement of professions through official documents, publications, professional development activities, educational standards, conferences, linkage to core values, and the profession's code of ethics. Strong associations promote innovation in practice, monitor societal needs, and advance educational standards for entry to the profession and continuing competence.

Opportunities for guided interactions with mentors and professional peers are central to students' professional identity development (Greenwood et al., 2002). Association membership makes available socialization processes by enabling both the acquisition of specific knowledge and skills required for professional practice as well as the internalization of attitudes, dispositions, and self-identity that connect the individual to the larger profession. Members of a professional organization have access to various networks to pursue particular interests and professional goals. These networks are especially important for students and practitioners pursuing a new area of professional interest. Conferences, networking meetings, online practice communities, and professional journals offer guidance and expertise to enhance professional development, thus contributing to the advancement of the profession.

Each professional organization has its own unique benefits; many professional associations offer "members only" access to a variety of publications, resources, conferences, online communities, scholarships, grants, and professional development opportunities (Osborn & Hunt, 2007). Member dues are the major source of revenue and political strength of OT associations, although some also are supported by fees related to publications and continuing education. Lifelong membership can have the benefit of providing students and practitioners with access to knowledge, networks, and resources that can continually advance one's professional career.

The professional development that occurs through membership and active involvement in professional organizations is an important benefit of being a lifelong member of state, national, and international professional organizations (Ritzhaupt et al., 2008). Active participation in professional associations also has the benefit of building leadership in the profession, forming powerful collegial networks, and growing OT leaders in education, research, and practice settings. Leaders are important to the profession to interact with a diverse range of stakeholders from both inside and outside the profession while scanning the larger environment for emerging trends and opportunities that can benefit clients and the profession. Rather than seeing the future as a minor variation or logical extension of the present, professional organizations can strategize to invent a future using creativity and innovation to move the profession forward to meet societies' occupational needs.

World Federation of Occupational Therapists

The World Federation of Occupational Therapists (WFOT) was created in 1952 as the official international organization for the OT profession (Figure 5.1). It is registered as a nongovernmental organization (NGO) in Geneva, Switzerland. The WFOT has been in official relations with the World Health Organization (WHO) since 1959 and is recognized as a nonprofit NGO by the United Nations (UN). Since its inception, WFOT has worked to expand the profession to address the needs of an estimated 1 billion persons worldwide who have disabilities (WHO, 2018). As a worldwide body, WFOT sets the standard for OT education internationally, promotes excellence in research and practice, and represents the profession in its role of improving world health and well-being. At the time of writing, WFOT has 105 member organizations (national and regional), representing over 633,000 occupational therapists, 58,000 OT assistants (OTAs), and 120,000 students around the globe. Through its membership WFOT provides a platform for discussion and governance, bringing together a diverse range of cultures and perspectives of the profession globally. Each WFOT member organization is represented by an elected or appointed delegate who represents their organization at the biennial Council Meeting. The WFOT Council Meetings

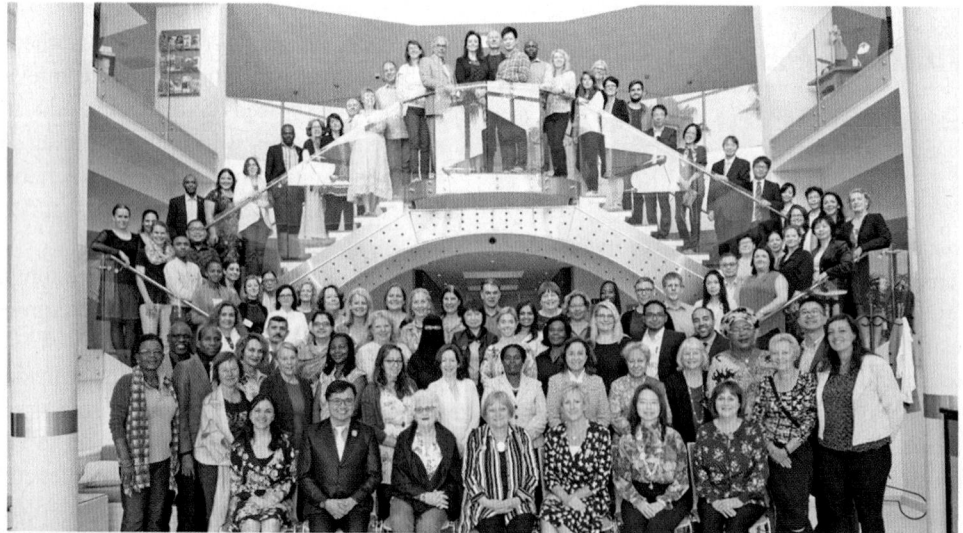

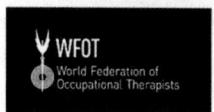

33rd Council Meeting
Cape Town, South Africa | May 2018

FIGURE 5.1 The World Federation of Occupational Therapists' 33rd Council Meeting in Cape Town, South Africa, May 2018. (Courtesy of World Federation of Occupational Therapists.)

enable meaningful interaction and debate to promote consensus and provide strategic direction for the profession. Throughout its history, WFOT has published, led, and advocated for human rights, diversity, and cultural safety (WFOT, 2020a), with the belief that it is a fundamental human right to participate in chosen meaningful occupations.

Examples of how the WFOT provides leadership and advocacy for the international OT profession include:

- *Strategy.* Provides a globally agreed strategic plan for the organization based on current and anticipated priorities for the profession. Provides OT expertise to inform and influence international policy and strategy development at a health systems level.
- *Standards and priorities.* Sets and maintains international standards for the education of occupational therapists, global research priorities, and resources to develop quality within practice.
- *Advocacy.* Ensures professional representation at key international stakeholder events and initiatives that progress the relevance of OT at a global level. Publishes Position Statements and Public Responses to critical issues to support advocacy and OT.
- *Engagement and representation.* Ensures that the WFOT's official status with the UN and WHO is maintained, enabling collaboration across a range of international and regional workplans including Disability and Rehabilitation, Mental Health, Human Resources, and humanitarian response. Interacts with national governments on policy and strategy to build the profession in countries where it is not yet established.
- *Education.* Enables the WFOT approval and reapproval process for OT education programs globally to ensure the Minimum Standards for the Education of Occupational Therapists are maintained across the world. Develops strategies to increase the number of entry-level education programs relevant to each country's cultural and resource context.
- *Human resources.* Works to identify and improve the supply of occupational therapists to meet health and social needs of local populations and communities.
- *Scholarship and publications.* Publishes the *WFOT Bulletin* twice per year as its official peer-reviewed journal and organizes the WFOT Congress, an international event that brings together occupational therapists from around the globe every 4 years. Provides an online learning environment with access to education modules on innovative and emerging areas of practice.
- *Policy development.* Influences policies at the international level with initiatives such as the WHO's Rehabilitation 2030: A Call for Action, the Global Strategy on Human Resources for Health: Workforce 2030, the World Report on Ageing and Mental Health, World Report on Disability, and Global Cooperation on Assistive Technology (GATE). Involvement in these initiatives by WFOT

helps to ensure that OT perspectives will influence the development of services globally.

- *Promotion and interaction.* Serves as a forum for global information sharing and monitoring of global trends affecting the OT profession through WFOT surveys, reports, and other communications. WFOT hosts World Occupational Therapy Day annually, an opportunity to celebrate and increase the visibility of the profession. It provides a dedicated interactive forum to engage with people around the world through the Occupational Therapy International Online Network (OTION) forum. The WFOT Occupational Narratives Database Project shares stories of doing and meaning from around the globe (https://occupational-narratives.wfot.org).

Information about WFOT's history, current initiatives, as well as information about OT in all member organizations can be found at www.wfot.org. Occupational therapists, students, and assistants can join WFOT as an individual member, which is administered through the national OT association in each country.

WFOT's collaborations often focus on occupational justice and the right for all people to engage in the occupations they need to survive, define as meaningful, and that contribute positively to their own well-being and the well-being of their communities. The WFOT has a detailed knowledge and understanding of the OT profession in most cultures of the world through its member organizations and can harness expertise and international perspectives on various subject areas whenever required.

National Member Organizations

Diversity of National Associations

National OT associations have an important role in providing leadership and advocacy for the profession. Each of the WFOT member organizations is shaped by the particular cultures, resources, and policies within the country. Most countries have a single national OT association. Some have several OT associations, one of which is identified as the WFOT member organization representing that country. Government policy may also determine how associations should be established, for example, requiring a minimum number of local nationals to form the basis of the organization. In some countries, OT associations provide union representation, which negotiate national pay structures and increases, terms of employment, and work conditions. Country geography, languages, and business practices influence how decisions are made, the nature of gatherings, and how organizations function. In countries with nationalized healthcare, OT is primarily delivered through government agencies with equal access to services. Advocacy approaches in those countries differ from countries like the United States where private businesses, including health insurance companies, dominate the healthcare landscape.

The growth of OT around the world can be characterized by data provided by national OT associations. The WFOT's Human Resources Project is a demographic scan of the OT profession globally. Between 2006 and 2022, the number of WFOT member organizations grew from 71 to 105 (48%). During the same period, there were similar percentage increases in the number of occupational therapists (137%) and between 2010 and 2022, a 58% increase in the number of students studying in WFOT-approved programs and a 37% increase in the number of OTAs. The demographic profile of the profession indicates the largest numbers of practicing occupational therapists are located in Germany, Japan, the United Kingdom, and the United States. However, when comparing the number of occupational therapists per 10,000 head of population, the countries with highest ratio of therapists are Denmark, Faroe Islands, Sweden, Belgium, Norway, and Iceland. It is from the work of national associations that the WFOT can amass data to analyze the profession's profile and needs globally.

American Occupational Therapy Association

The American Occupational Therapy Association (AOTA) is the national professional organization in the United States that is responsible for guiding and developing professional standards, professional development, and advocacy on behalf of OT practitioners and the clients served by OT (AOTA, 2022a). The AOTA was incorporated in New York in 1917 as the National Society for the Promotion of Occupational Therapy. The name was eventually changed in 1927 to AOTA. The AOTA's membership is composed of individual occupational therapists, OTAs, and students (Box 5.2).

BOX 5.2 ASSEMBLY OF STUDENT DELEGATES

Students are valued members of the American Occupational Therapy Association (AOTA) and belong to the Assembly of Student Delegates (ASD). Each educational program may select a student as its delegate to the ASD meeting that takes place during the AOTA annual conference and exposition. The ASD provides a platform for students to share their perspectives on student issues that affect the occupational therapy profession.

The AOTA members develop and refine AOTA's mission, vision, practice standards, professional development, and code of ethics, all of which shape the future success of the profession. Individual members work together as volunteers in the AOTA, serving in various leadership capacities. Members and volunteer leaders are supported by staff employed by AOTA. The staff is supervised by the AOTA executive director, who, in turn, is supervised by the AOTA Board of Directors (BOD). The BOD consists of elected directors, officers, and appointed consumer and public advisers. All board members have voice and vote during official meetings. The Representative Assembly (RA) is the policy-making body of the association that operates as a Congress (AOTA, 2022b). Each representative is elected nationally or by members of their state or jurisdiction. Representatives seek input from their members about policy decisions facing the profession. Policies, such as establishing the degree level required for entry to the profession, are deliberated and voted upon by the assembly. Practice standards and positions on the role of OT in various specialty areas, such as pain management and primary care, are ultimately approved by the RA.

The AOTA's federal and state policy departments are active with healthcare, social, and educational policy concerns. The national American Occupational Therapy Political Action Committee (AOTPAC), an entity distinct from AOTA, supports legislation, and many states have formed political action committees (PACs) as well. Evidence-based practice and practice-based evidence are essential to substantiate the efficacy of OT, and thus, member organizations actively develop these resources.

To illustrate the differences in organizations, Table 5.3 provides a profile of WFOT as the international OT organization and of the AOTA as an example of a national association. The selection of the AOTA for this is based in the origins of this text in the United States; however, the authors wish to acknowledge the diversity and importance of each national organization in representing and leading the profession.

Associations Within Countries at the State/Region/Territory Level

The municipalities within each country shape the nature of OT organizations, for example, some may be structured as states, provinces, regions, etc. In the United States, each state has a professional association that serves the needs of their OT practitioners (AOTA, 2022b). These state organizations are independent from AOTA, and thus, individuals join these state groups directly. State organizations are affiliated with AOTA to advance the profession and to advocate for clients who are served by OT. For example, AOTA

TABLE 5.3	Profiles of American Occupational Therapy Association and World Federation of Occupational Therapists	
	American Occupational Therapy Association (www.aota.org)	**Word Federation of Occupational Therapists (www.wfot.org)**
Volunteer leadership	President, vice president, secretary, treasurer (elected by membership) Board of Directors (elected by membership plus one consumer adviser and one public adviser)	President, vice president, VP-Finance, program co-ordinators (elected by Council)
Staff	Executive director that oversees a large staff that includes practitioners, attorneys, accountants, policy specialists, and administrative personnel	Executive director (ex officio) that oversees contracting staff to support the administration of the organization's work
Headquarters	Bethesda, Maryland	Geneva, Switzerland
Membership	Individual AOTA membership	105 member organizations. Individuals must join through their national association. Some national associations have automatic WFOT individual membership. Others, including the United States, have additional WFOT individual membership fees.
Estimated OT practitioners	142,007 practicing occupational therapists 55,628 OTAs	633,000 practicing occupational therapists 57,955 OTAs (approximately 95% are in the United States)
Policy-making structure	RA made up of one elected voting delegate from each state and one representing member living outside the United States meets 2 times per year. Responsible for professional practice policy for professional practice	WFOT Council composed of one voting delegate from each full member organization. All member organizations have alternate delegates but still one vote per country. Meets every 2 years. Executive management team meets annually.
Represents OT to key constituents that set or influence policy (examples)	• Members of Congress • Federal government agencies such as the Centers for Medicare & Medicaid, Office of Special Education, Rehabilitation Services Administration, and the Substance Abuse and Mental Services Administration	• National governments • WHO • UN • ILO
Publications	• *American Journal of Occupational Therapy* • *OT Practice* • *Special Interest Section Compendium* • AOTA Press publishes books, manuals, consumer guides, and other documents.	• *WFOT Bulletin* • *WFOT Newsletter* • Minimum Standards for the Education of Occupational Therapists • Position and public statements • Online modules and educational materials • Publications • World Occupational Therapy Day materials
Online forums	AOTA CommunOT (https://communot.aota.org/)	Occupational Therapy International Online Network (OTION) (http://otion.wfot.org/)
Conferences	Annual conference, education summit, and specialty conferences	World Congress of Occupational Therapists (held every 4 years)
States/regional groups	Affiliated state associations	Regional groups representing geopolitical regions of the UN
Interprofessional collaborations	Collegial professional organizations such as the American Speech and Hearing Association and the American Medical Association	International nongovernmental organizations, WHO, UN
Annual celebrations	April is OT Month.	October 27 is World Occupational Therapy Day.
Structures, organizations, groups	Commissions: • Commission on Practice • Commission on Education • Ethics Commission • Continuing Competence and Professional Development SIS ASD ACOTE	Programs: • Executive Program—Advocacy and Leadership • Research Program • Practice Development Program • Education Program IAGs International Review Teams

(continued)

	American Occupational Therapy Association (www.aota.org)	Word Federation of Occupational Therapists (www.wfot.org)
Examples of key current initiatives	• AOTA evidence-based practice resources • Continuing competence and professional development resources • Public policy and advocacy around healthcare reform • ACOTE educational standards for entry-level practitioners	• Human Resources Project is a demographic analysis of the profession including labor force statistics, regulation, education, and employment trends collected every 2 years. • OT and disaster management • Occupational Therapy and Displaced Persons • Quality Evaluation Strategy Tool • Development of the profession in countries where it does not exist • Minimum Standards for the Education of Occupational Therapists

TABLE 5.3 Profiles of American Occupational Therapy Association and World Federation of Occupational Therapists (*continued*)

ACOTE, Accreditation Council for Occupational Therapy Education; AOTA, American Occupational Therapy Association; ASD, Assembly of Student Delegates; IAGs, International Advisory Groups; ILO, International Labor Organization; OT, occupational therapy; OTA, occupational therapy assistant; RA, Representative Assembly; SIS, Special Interest Sections; UN, United Nations; WHO, World Health Organization; WFOT, World Federation of Occupational Therapists.

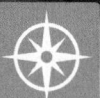

EXPANDING OUR PERSPECTIVES

Occupational Therapy Professional Organizations in Japan

Asako Matsubara

The number of occupational therapists and OT training programs in Japan has increased dramatically over the past two decades. As of February 2022, there were 104,286 licensed occupational therapists in Japan, qualifying it to be among the countries with the largest number of occupational therapists. This recent expansion of Japanese OT's capacity can be traced back to the Japanese government's response to the country's rapidly growing aging population and declining birthrate. The launch of "The Community Integrated Care System" was a comprehensive initiative that aimed to integrate Japan's living support, long-term care, medical care, and prevention programs. Until recently, rehabilitation care in Japan had been widely provisioned at hospitals and healthcare facilities. Now, rehabilitation care has shifted to the idea of supporting elderly and disabled citizens in the community. This major shift in the provision of healthcare services has resulted in an urgent need to prepare occupational therapists to play an active role in the community, as well as to reform OT pre- and postgraduate education.

The Japanese Association of Occupational Therapists (JAOT)—the country's national professional organization—was established on September 25, 1966, and became a regular member of WFOT in 1972. In addition to the national organization, there are OT associations in each prefecture, which work in cooperation with JAOT. The JAOT, like the AOTA, is also responsible for guiding and developing professional standards, professional development, governing policy, and administrative functions. The JAOT

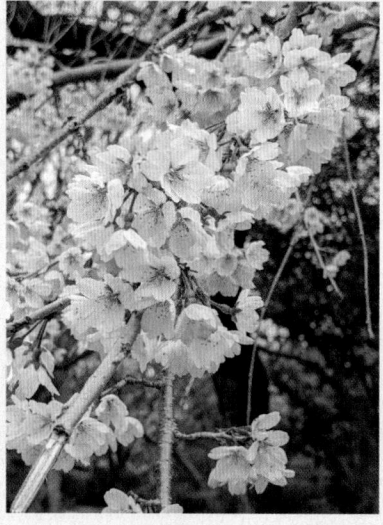

Photo courtesy of Asako Matsubara.

mainly consists of "the Corporate Administrative Affairs Section," which includes the Secretariat and Ethics Committee, among others. There is also "the Public Services Section," which includes the Education, Academics, Policy, and the International Affairs Department.

The Academic Department of the JAOT oversees the annual conference and exposition, publishes journals and manuals, makes OT guidelines and clinical practice guidelines, and awards research grants. Journals published by the JAOT include the *Asian Journal of Occupational Therapy* (AsJOT) and the *Japanese Occupational Therapy Research* (JOTR). The JOTR is published in Japanese. In addition, a peer-reviewed case study report registration system has been created for use on demand by JAOT members. The case study report system serves as

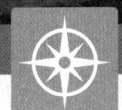

a repository to expand the evidence base for OT efficacy.

The Education Department of JAOT plays an important role in building and operating a postgraduate education system that supports continuing education. The Education Department oversees workshops and courses for the certifications of "Authorized Occupational Therapists" and "Specialized Occupational Therapists." The department also provides basic training for novice occupational therapists, which is conducted in collaboration with the prefectural OT associations. The Education Department also prepares and regularly revises the Minimum Standards for Japan's Occupational Therapy Education programs.

The health needs of OT clients are each unique, in the ever-changing contexts of medical institutions. The JAOT and prefectural OT associations play important roles in fostering the development and efficacy of occupational therapists who provide services suitable and relevant for their clients and the environments in which they live.

provides model language for state laws and regulations, but the state professional organization must work with the state government to include this language in state laws and policies. Membership in state organizations is critical for maintaining local networks and for mobilizing advocacy efforts related to state government–funded programs and state policies, including professional licensure.

Each state (or jurisdiction) regulates OT through a licensure board or regulatory agency (AOTA, 2022a). The definitions and guidelines are enacted by the legislature and are intended to protect the citizens of that state. The AOTA is a valued resource for these regulatory agencies, providing information about the profession and assisting with monitoring and advocating for OT in the state legislature. When students complete their academic programs and successfully pass the certification examination of the National Board for Certification in Occupational Therapy (NBCOT), they are eligible to apply for licenses and certificates to practice (NBCOT, 2018). These applications are handled through state government bodies.

How Professional Organizations Support Professional Development

OT students, OTAs, and occupational therapists can become members of their state, national, and international professional organizations (Mata et al., 2010). Such involvement builds professional identity beginning at the point at which an individual chooses OT as a career path and continues to develop throughout a career. Lifelong membership and participation in professional organizations is a key component to a successful OT career trajectory that begins as an OT student. Professional organizations provide the support needed for professional development, public awareness, advocacy, and standard setting. OT Story 5.1

Sumita is a recent graduate from an accredited OT program. Based on her academic and fieldwork experiences, she decided to pursue work with children with special needs.

Sumita as a Student

As an OT student, Sumita decided to join the AOTA, and on the AOTA membership application, she joined the WFOT. She also joined her state association. She attended her first AOTA conference to attend workshops and courses on innovative practice for autistic children and how to make a successful transition from student to practitioner. At the conference, she met OT students from around the country and found *many* shared her interests. She also found that the *American Journal of Occupational Therapy*, OT Practice, and the *Special Interest Section Compendium* contained interesting articles that she used in various course assignments (AOTA, 2022d). Using OT Connections, a social media site accessible on the home page of the AOTA website, she read posts from experienced practitioners about their intervention strategies. During her final Level II fieldwork placement, Sumita contacted the NBCOT and applied to take her certification examination near her home after completing her fieldwork.

Getting Ready to Work

Sumita interviewed at clinical sites in South Carolina and close to her home in Texas. Because she was not sure which position she would accept, she contacted the state

(*continued*)

OT STORY 5.1 SUMITA ENTERS THE OCCUPATIONAL THERAPY PROFESSION IN THE UNITED STATES (continued)

regulatory boards in both states to apply for licensure. She asked NBCOT to send her examination results to both of them. She anxiously awaited her certification examination results, and she was thrilled to learn that she had passed the examination and was now a registered occupational therapist. She accepted the offer from a private pediatric practice group in Texas and began her new job working with autistic children. When her practice obtained a contract to provide telehealth services to clients in Louisiana, Sumita used AOTA's Telehealth advisory resources to find out about licensure there. Later, when a client moved to Mexico and her parents wished to continue intervention, she consulted with the WFOT *Position Statement on Telehealth* (WFOT, 2021a).

When Sumita's student memberships expired, she renewed her memberships with the AOTA, WFOT, and her state association and joined both the Developmental Disabilities and the School System Special Interest sections so that she could communicate with other occupational therapists who worked with this population. In addition, Sumita learned from resources provided by these therapists and by her supervisor and coworkers. She also joined the Autism Society for interdisciplinary networking and conferences.

Practicing Abroad

Sumita was also interested in international practice opportunities, and through her membership with WFOT, she discovered the OTION, which facilitated her involvement in OT practice in Haiti. Sumita referred to the WFOT document *Occupational Therapy International Practice Guide* (WFOT, 2020b) to ensure she met regulatory standards for practice in Haiti. She learned of a new Haitian Association of Occupational Therapists, which she joined, and attended a meeting while in Haiti. While she was in Haiti, she was able to attend the regional group conference of the Association of Caribbean Occupational Therapists. There she learned from occupational therapists who provide community-based services on islands with shortages of OT personnel and the efforts to develop OT education programs in the Caribbean region.

Networking and Advocating Back Home

After returning from Haiti, Sumita learned that US federal and state funding for OT services for autistic children was at risk. She immediately went to the AOTA website to learn about the proposed cuts to services for children with autism and related conditions. Sumita used OT Connections to communicate with other practitioners regarding concerns for declining reimbursement rates and coverage for OT services. She decided to donate to the AOTPAC, which provides support to candidates for elected office who support OT services. Sumita also contacted the association to find out how she could get involved with advocating for fair reimbursement and coverage.

Becoming Part of the Solution

Sumita joined an ad hoc committee of practitioners to develop recommendations to the AOTA BOD on strategic priorities for advocating for OT and children with autism. Sumita also scheduled visits with her elected representatives to discuss her concerns regarding the proposed cuts to reimbursement and OT coverage for the children she served. She then invited her elected representatives and their legislative staff to tour her clinic to educate policymakers on the critical role of OT for autistic children. She followed up with each of the legislative representatives with a letter further advocating for reimbursement, and she included the AOTA document *Scope of Occupational Therapy Services for Individuals With Autism Spectrum Disorder Across the Life Course* and an AOTA evidence-based practice review article on autism. She then contacted her state association and joined a grassroots advocacy effort to contact state legislators to promote access to OT services for autistic children.

Summary

Through active participation in her state, federal, and international professional associations, Sumita witnessed the power of membership and participation in her professional organizations and committed to maintaining her lifelong state, national, and international professional organizational membership and to actively participate in shaping the future of the OT profession.

Questions

1. What professional OT organizations could you join at the international, national, and municipal (e.g., state, regional, province) level? Do they have conferences you could attend?
2. Does your country or region regulate OT practice? If so, what are the steps for you to acquire certification, licensure, or other credentials to practice?
3. In an area of your interest, what are professional organization resources or official documents to inform your practice from the WFOT, national association, or other sources?
4. Imagine practicing in another country. What information does the WFOT Occupational Therapy International Practice Guide (WFOT, 2020b) offer to plan your transition?
5. Think of people who are underserved or have unmet OT needs. What are professional association initiatives or resources for advocating to change practice or policy?
6. If a colleague in another profession says that OT cannot offer a particular service (e.g., interventions for cognitive, mobility, communication, or mental health issues), what professional organization documents serve as justification for your practice in these areas?

illustrates how OT professional organizations support professional development as an OT student enters the profession.

Benefits of Professional Associations

Continuing Education and Professional Development

Professional organizations may offer continuing education and professional development opportunities, including conferences and continuing education events in person and online often at reduced cost for members (AOTA, 2022a). OT state associations typically have an annual conference. The largest event in the United States is the AOTA annual conference and exposition, which includes continuing education, networking, and exhibit hall vendors and employers. The WFOT holds an international Congress that rotates among different regions of the world every 4 years. State, national, and WFOT conferences utilize volunteers to peer review abstracts for presentation. Volunteers also help provide the necessary human resources during conferences.

Occupational Therapy Foundations

Some countries have foundations to support education, scholarship, and research in the profession. The American Occupational Therapy Foundation (AOTF) is a nonprofit organization that was established in 1965 to advance the science and increase public awareness of OT. The AOTF is composed of OT practitioners, corporate partners, and sponsors who support OT education and research. The AOTF is financially supported by private contributions and through sponsors that value OT. Fundraisers are held at AOTA annual conference. The AOTF supports students and researchers through scholarships and grants (AOTF, 2022). AOTF publishes a scholarly journal, *Occupational Therapy Journal of Research: Occupation, Participation and Health (OTJR)* (AOTF, 2022).

Evidence for Practice

Professional associations can play a key role in creating a culture where use of evidence in OT is expected and fostered. They accomplish this "by promoting availability of research evidence and facilitating participation in professional development that is informed by best available evidence" (WFOT, 2021b, p. 1). Depending on resources, national associations may have initiatives that build and share evidence for practice. The AOTA and AOTF have an initiative to generate literature review articles and evidence-based practice briefs that therapists and students can use to inform their work

(AOTA, 2022c). The AOTA provides links to various publications and virtual resources providing additional information that supports practice.

Public Policy and Advocacy

Professional associations at all levels represent and advocate for the interests of OT practitioners and their clients in the areas of public policy. This involves communications with government agencies, such as the Ministry of Health and Education in some countries. In the United States, such work involves lobbying with legislators in Congress regarding initiatives that are important to the profession and to the people who are served by OT. At the federal level, this may also involve working with the policymakers from the Office of Special Education, the Rehabilitation Services Administration, and other governmental agencies regarding eligibility for service as well as guidelines for reimbursement. The AOTA staff members may provide information and testimony before congressional committees who make recommendations regarding the interpretation and implementation of legislation. State and national associations communicate with members about contacting their representatives to advocate for legislation affecting the profession and people with disabilities. Even students can get involved.

The AOTA State Affairs Department and the Federal Affairs Department also support the activities of state OT associations and licensure boards to ensure that language supportive of OT is included in state legislation. Further, these organizations work to prevent OT from being restricted or encroached upon by licensure rules of other professions (AOTA, 2022a). The AOTA also provides educational materials and individual support to members and state associations to prepare them to effectively advocate for the profession and those who are served in their area by OT.

American Occupational Therapy Political Action Committee

A PAC is a committee that provides financial support to candidates that support a profession and its initiatives through private donations from members. AOTA members can voluntarily donate to the AOTPAC to support candidates for elected office that support OT and the clients served by OT.

Publications

Many professional associations around the world have an official publication. These journals offer invaluable international and cross-cultural perspectives to inform best practice. Some examples of publications from national professional associations around the world include the following:

- *Asian Journal of Occupational Therapy*
- *Australian Occupational Therapy Journal*

- *British Journal of Occupational Therapy*
- *Hong Kong Journal of Occupational Therapy*
- *Scandinavian Journal of Occupational Therapy*
- *South African Occupational Therapy Journal*
- *Revista Ocupación Humana—(Colombian) Journal of Human Occupation*
- *American Journal of Occupational Therapy*—AOTA also publishes *OT Practice*, a bimonthly magazine, and a quarterly *Special Interest Section Compendium*.

Conclusion

OT professional organizations around the world offer the opportunity to collectively advance the profession in a way that cannot be achieved by an individual student or practitioner alone. Professional organizations are nonprofit organizations seeking to further the profession, the interests of individuals engaged in that profession, and the public interest. By building a strong community of students and practitioners that unite the profession around a shared mission and vision, strategies can be developed that advance practice and serve the public interest. These associations represent the interests of students and practitioners through legislative advocacy and public promotion of the profession. Occupational therapists, OTAs, and OT students are supported by state, national, and international OT professional organizations that provide the resources and information needed to practice effectively. Professionals have the opportunity and responsibility to support and participate in professional organizations to work toward continually developing, shaping, and promoting the OT profession through lifelong membership and active participation. Regulation of the OT profession is also critical for protecting the public from harm and ensuring that OT practitioners are ethical and competent to practice.

Acknowledgment

The authors would like to thank Shawn Phipps for his contribution to earlier editions of this chapter.

Lippincott® Connect *For additional resources on the subjects discussed in this chapter, visit Lippincott Connect.*

REFERENCES

American Occupational Therapy Association. (2022a). *Accreditation.* http://www.aota.org

American Occupational Therapy Association. (2022b). *Governance.* http://www.aota.org

American Occupational Therapy Association. (2022c). *Publications.* http://www.aota.org

American Occupational Therapy Association. (2022d). *Special interest sections.* http://www.aota.org

American Occupational Therapy Foundation. (2022). *Scholarships.* http://www.aotf.org

Benveniste, G. (1987). *Professionalizing the organization.* Josey-Bass.

Bickel, J. (2007). The role of professional societies in career development in academic medicine. *Academic Psychiatry, 31,* 91–94. https://doi.org/10.1176/appi.ap.31.2.91

Greenwood, R., Suddaby, R., & Hinings, C. R. (2002). Theorizing change: The role of professional associations in the transformation of institutionalized fields. *Academy of Management Journal, 45*(1), 58–80. https://doi.org/10.2307/3069285

Mata, H., Latham, T. P., & Ransome, Y. (2010). Benefits of professional organization membership and participation in national conferences: Considerations for students and new professionals. *Health Promotion Practice, 11*(4), 450–453. https://doi.org/10.1177/1524839910370427

National Board for Certification in Occupational Therapy. (2018). *NBCOT.* http://www.nbcot.org

Osborn, R. N., & Hunt, J. G. (2007). Leadership and the choice of order: Complexity and hierarchical perspectives near the edge of chaos. *Leadership Quarterly, 18*(4), 319–340. https://doi.org/10.1016/j.leaqua.2007.04.003

Ritzhaupt, A. D., Umapathy, K., & Jamba, L. (2008). Computing professional association membership: An exploration of membership needs and motivations. *Journal of Information Systems Applied Research, 1,* 1–22. http://jisar.org/1/4/

Schneider, M., & Somers, M. (2006). Organizations as complex adaptive systems: Implications of complexity theory for leadership research. *Leadership Quarterly, 17*(4), 351–365. https://doi.org/10.1016/j.leaqua.2006.04.006

World Federation of Occupational Therapists. (2016). *WFOT minimum standards for the education of occupational therapists.* www.wfot.org

World Federation of Occupational Therapists. (2020a). *WFOT statement on systemic racism.* http://www.wfot.org

World Federation of Occupational Therapists. (2020b). *Occupational therapy international practice guide.* http://www.wfot.org

World Federation of Occupational Therapists. (2021a). *Position statement on telehealth.* http://www.wfot.org

World Federation of Occupational Therapists. (2021b). *Guiding principles in the use of evidence in occupational therapy.* http://www.wfot.org

World Federation of Occupational Therapists. (2022). *WFOT human resources project.* http://www.wfot.org

World Health Organization. (2018). *World report on disability.* http://www.who.int/disabilities/world_report/2011/en/

CHAPTER 6

Scholarship in Occupational Therapy

Catana Brown

LEARNING OBJECTIVES

After reading this chapter you will be able to:

1. Recognize the difference between scholarship focused on knowledge acquisition and scholarship focused on knowledge development.
2. Describe why and how occupational therapists participate as lifelong learners to support their ability to practice competently.
3. Explain the processes to become and the activities of an occupational therapy researcher.
4. Discuss the benefits of clinicians and academics coming together to develop and apply new knowledge in the profession.

Introduction

Scholarship includes both knowledge acquisition and knowledge development. As an occupational therapy (OT) student, you are primarily engaged in knowledge acquisition. You are busy learning about the knowledge base of the profession. Much of what you are learning now is predicated on the research of others. Another component of scholarship is knowledge development. Knowledge development is crucial for the continued expansion of the theoretical and research base of OT. This chapter covers knowledge acquisition as it relates to scholarship in practice and also describes the development of new knowledge and possibly pique your interest in becoming a researcher. The chapter ends with a discussion about scholarship that can come from collaborations between practitioners and academics.

Acquiring Knowledge: Scholarship in Practice

Although you are currently a student, you have probably already heard that as an OT practitioner you are expected to be a lifelong learner. The knowledge base of our profession is complex and broad. The information you will acquire as an OT student is only a starting place. To develop expertise in your chosen area of practice requires learning more in-depth and specialized knowledge. Furthermore, OT is a rapidly expanding field, so throughout your career you will be required to keep up with new information as it accumulates so that you can continue to practice competently. There are many avenues for continuing your education and some of these are discussed below.

Continuing Education

Before deciding on a continuing education offering, it is important to do a self-evaluation of your learning needs. In your practice setting you will likely have identified many areas of knowledge that could be expanded. Perhaps there is an intervention technique you would like to learn more about, or you have found yourself asking a lot of questions about a population you are treating. After you've determined the content you are interested in, the next step is to determine the method for acquiring that information. For example, you can attend international, national, or local conferences. Offerings may be in person, virtual, or a hybrid option. In addition to acquiring new knowledge, conferences can be inspiring and reconnect you with your passion for the profession. Another benefit of attending conferences is the informal learning that happens when talking to colleagues. Especially when the conference is in person, you will have the opportunity to meet with peers, reflect on your practice, and find out what others are doing in their own practice settings. Besides professional organizations, there are many private businesses that offer continuing education courses. If the content is more extensive you could also consider taking a college class. OT Story 6.1 describes the importance of continuing education from the perspective of a provider of continuing education courses in Argentina, Mariel Pellegrini.

OT STORY 6.1 CONTINUING EDUCATION IN ARGENTINA

Mariel Pellegrini, Mgter. Lic. TO, Director of Alpha Occupational, www.alphaocupacional.com

Continuing education in Argentina is very important. Upon completion of the university degree, OT professionals have different options for further training that may include formal university graduate education or continuing education courses. Continuing education is important because there is a need for occupational therapists to learn new topics and deepen their understanding of previously studied topics. Continuing education courses may focus on theoretical models, evaluations, methodologies, or intervention strategies, among others.

For example, in Alpha Occupational Argentina, a national and Ibero-American benchmark institution for continuing education in OT, the offer of courses began in 2002. Originally, these courses were held in clinical spaces or rented rooms so that the training could take place in person. The courses were taught by occupational therapists with training experiences in other countries or Argentinian therapists with extensive clinical experience. Many therapists were interested in topics applicable to everyday clinical practice. The initial courses consisted of study group formats with assigned readings and discussion of theoretical material, clinical cases, evaluations, or intervention strategies. This format transformed into continuing education courses with occupational therapists from other countries (Canada, the United States, the United Kingdom, Spain, etc.) who were invited to come to Buenos Aires to give training for 2 to 5 days. This made many OT clinicians, who are not necessarily interested in formal postgraduate university training, able to update their knowledge and apply this knowledge to their daily work.

The modality of the courses during the first 10 years was face-to-face (Figure 6.1). Over the years, interest in continuing education continued to grow. The great distances and the cost of traveling for participants resulted in an expansion

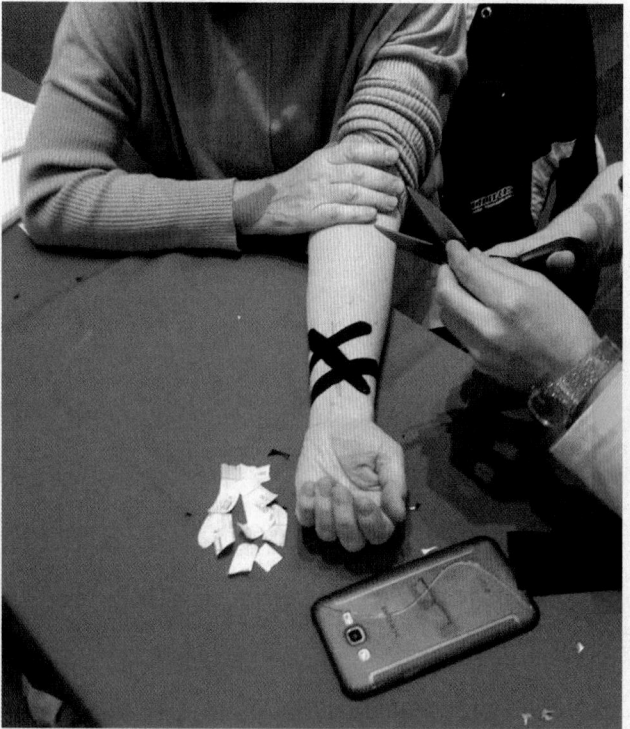

FIGURE 6.1 **Students receive practical skills while attending an in-person continuing education course on kinesiotaping.**

of the offerings to a hybrid synchronous training model in 2012. In this modality, the instructor gives their training in person in a room where some participants attend in person and others attend virtually from other cities in Argentina and from other Spanish-speaking countries. For virtual participants, there is a specialist technician in the room who plays the role of mediator between the face-to-face course and the online participants, reading their questions, facilitating the operation of group work, etc. If the instructor gives the course in a language other than Spanish, they are accompanied by a bilingual occupational therapist who performs the live translation.

When the pandemic arrived, the virtual format was the one that continued to be used (Figure 6.2). Currently, continuing education opportunities continue to grow, not only in the number of training topics but also in response to the needs and times of OT professionals. The hybrid format of courses with asynchronous and synchronous courses and with national and international instructors is well received.

We have continued to modify our formats to meet the needs of practicing therapists. Since 2020 we have implemented two new types of continuing education formats:

- Completely asynchronous recorded courses where participants enter with a link

- Hybrid courses that start with asynchronous training (recorded and reading material), followed by a hybrid live and virtual synchronous training

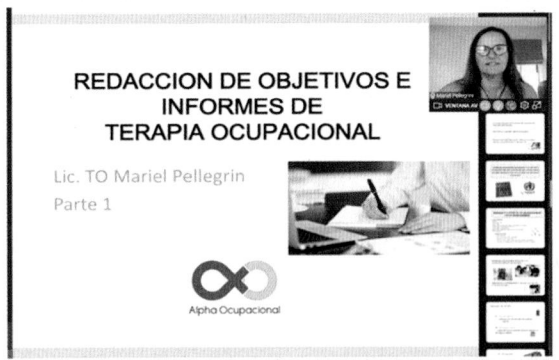

FIGURE 6.2 A virtual course on writing occupational therapy goals and reports.

To make the recorded asynchronous courses more dynamic, practical work is offered. Instructions are given and then questions are answered by the teacher in the same course. As a continuing education provider, it is important that I meet the needs and interests of the participants with a format this is accessible.

Question

1. The OT Story talks about the different formats for offering continuing education opportunities. Which format do you prefer the most when learning new material and why?

Certificate programs offer a more in-depth study in a specialty area of practice. For example, certified hand therapists (CHTs) in the United States have a minimum of 4,000 hours of direct practice in hand therapy but also pass a test of advanced clinical skills and theory (Hand Therapy Certification Commission, n.d.). To maintain the credential, CHTs must maintain an ongoing practice of continuing education. Recognition for qualified hand therapist occurs at the national level. The International Federation of Societies for Hand Therapy identifies 13 countries with certification for hand therapists including Argentina, Australia, Canada, Columbia, Denmark, Germany, Japan, the Netherlands, New Zealand, Portugal, Switzerland, the United Kingdom, and the United States. In addition, there is a European qualification process through the European Federation of Societies for Hand Therapy (International Federation of Societies for Hand Therapy, n.d.). In all cases, the pathways require an initial qualification in OT or physical therapy. Similarly, a certified psychiatric rehabilitation practitioner (CPRP) must pass a competency exam that demonstrates expertise for practitioners working within the adult mental

health system (Psychiatric Rehabilitation Association, n.d.). The CPRP certification is an international credential available to practitioners worldwide, and because the test is delivered via live virtual proctoring, it is accessible to anyone with an internet connection. In both cases, practitioners can use the designated credentials after their name. Chapter 71 provides more information about the topic of lifelong learning through the lens of continuing competency.

Evidence-Based Practice

A vital component of scholarship in practice is applying existing research to your work situation, otherwise known as **evidence-based practice** (EBP). OT students learn how to locate, understand, critique, and apply research to practice. The primary purpose of EBP is to improve the outcomes of our clients and to improve the quality of their care. As an evidence-based practitioner, you will be able to articulate what you are doing and why to your clients, team members, administrators, and payers. The evidence-based practitioner combines knowledge that comes from research, clinical experience, and the service recipient's situation and values to make informed decisions.

Although EBP is widely accepted as a quality standard in healthcare, and is integrated into OT accreditation standards, many practitioners do not regularly implement EBP. Self-reflection is highly associated with the adoption of EBP (Krueger et al., 2020). Therefore, as a student and beginning practitioner, it is useful to start working on reflection. This means that you approach practice experiences with cognitive intention and conduct a critical self-analysis to determine what knowledge you need to improve your practice. This self-analysis involves recognizing your knowledge gaps and coming up with a plan for acquiring new knowledge.

Sometimes accessing the literature and finding time to read and critique studies can be challenging; however, there are resources available to occupational therapists to facilitate the process. If you are a member of your professional association, you have access to a variety of resources including journals, practice guidelines, and summaries of research such as critically appraised papers or critically appraised topics. **Practice guidelines** are documents developed by organizations that synthesize and interpret the research and the expertise of clinicians to serve as a basis for making clinical recommendations for specific populations. For example, Occupational Therapy Australia (OTA) has a Guide to Good Practice for Working with Children (OTA, 2016), the Royal College of Occupational Therapists (RCOT) has a practice guideline on "Hand and wrist orthoses for adults with rheumatological conditions" (RCOT, 2020), and the American Occupational Therapy Association (Braveman & Hunter, 2017) has a practice guideline on Cancer Rehabilitation with Adults. At the same time, it is important to acknowledge that occupational therapists practicing in less-resource-rich areas may not have access to libraries and professional organizations with the type of literature mentioned here.

Another method for enabling EBP is to participate in a community of practice. This method of sharing resources and expertise may be more accessible for less-resource-rich areas. **Communities of practice** are informal or formal groups of people that have a common interest and come together for a process of sharing knowledge. The sharing may occur in face-to-face meetings, but many communities of practice meet virtually, making it possible to expand membership to people that are geographically distant. A review of communities of practice in OT found one benefit to be professional development through "boundary crossing" (Barry et al., 2017). Boundary crossing went beyond geography to include professional organizations, practice settings, and roles (e.g., practitioners and academics; clinicians and managers). These groups are not limited to sharing knowledge about research evidence, but this is a popular focus for healthcare communities. You can start your own community of practice by identifying an area of interest and then recruiting others to join your group. Perhaps you are working with persons with Parkinson disease, and you want to network with other occupational therapists with similar interests. After the community is formed, the group determines how they will work together to review the evidence on OT interventions for this population.

Galheigo et al. (2019) conducted a participatory action research project to explore a community of practice for occupational therapists in pediatric acute care in Brazil. Nine occupational therapists made up the community of practice, which met face-to-face but also had a virtual component that allowed for the exchange of materials and more informal chats. The study found that the community of practice was useful for providing opportunities to share stories and discuss challenges in the workplace. In addition, the community of practice affirmed professional identities, created a sense of belonging, and allowed participants to gain knowledge both through access to distributed resources and also through the sharing of practice-based expertise.

The American Occupational Therapy Association (n.d.) currently sponsors 19 communities of practice including topics such as Women's Health, Homelessness, Fitness to Drive, and Fieldwork Educators. The association provides training for groups interested in starting a community of practice.

An important component of EBP is shared decision-making. **Shared decision-making** is the process of information exchange that occurs between the practitioner and the service recipient to facilitate a collaborative agreement regarding the intervention plan. During the consensus-building process, the occupational therapist brings information about the research evidence and their clinical experience, whereas the service recipient shares their own values, preferences, and knowledge of the situation. At the end of the process, the two parties come to an agreement related to the intervention plan. Shared decision-making is also applicable to situations in which the occupational therapist is providing services to families, communities, or agencies. The therapist will want to include these groups in the decision-making process.

Lastly, the onus for translating and applying research to practice does not lie exclusively with the practitioner. It is important that researchers publish and present their findings in ways that support their implementation (Juckett et al., 2019). This includes developing implementation strategies such as training workshops for EBPs and reporting studies using language that is meaningful to practitioners (Proctor et al., 2011).

Developing New Knowledge: Scholarship of Discovery

As a science-driven profession, it is essential that OT has a cadre of researchers to generate new knowledge. Hopefully, some of you are considering the prospect of becoming an

OT researcher. Perhaps you are interested in developing a career as an independent researcher. This part of the chapter presents steps you can take that will lead to that career. Typically, a career in research means that you would work at a university in a position that supports and promotes research. Later in the chapter, clinical–academic partnerships will be presented as a means for clinicians to contribute to the development of new knowledge.

So, what is involved in becoming a researcher? There are a number of skills you will need to develop. Specific knowledge related to research design and data analysis is important for implementing a study. In addition, writing and communication skills are essential for obtaining grant funding and disseminating the findings. Research often involves teamwork, so researchers benefit from collaborative social skills. Developing the skills to become a researcher is facilitated by choosing the right academic path.

Doctoral Degrees in Research

The most common degree that is associated with independent research is the Doctorate of Philosophy (PhD). Other research degrees include a Doctor of Science or ScD, which is a research degree with a science emphasis such as engineering or health sciences. A Doctor of Education or EdD is a research degree with an emphasis on education. These research degrees are intense areas of study that typically take 4 to 6 years to complete.

In addition to content-oriented courses related to the specific area of study, a PhD, ScD, or EdD student takes courses that teach them how to design a study and how to conduct statistical analyses. These courses are taken in preparation for the dissertation. Although the student has a dissertation adviser and committee that guides the process, most of the work is done independently. The dissertation is intended to produce original research that is suitable for publication. The dissertation includes a written and an oral component. After the completion of the research, the student defends their study in front of a committee of experts. This deep

level of study and the production of a major work of original research can serve as the basis for a future career as a researcher. Some OT programs offer a PhD degree in a related field such as Occupational Science or Rehabilitation Science. However, many occupational therapists pursue PhDs in non-OT departments. The area of study can vary greatly but some examples include occupational therapists with PhDs in psychology, exercise science, and disability studies.

Some individuals go on to receive additional training beyond their PhD, ScD, or EdD in the form of **postdoctoral research**. A postdoctoral research position (postdoc) provides the individual with additional research experience and training in preparation for a career in academia/research. Postdocs work under a research mentor and contribute to the research mentor's body of work as well as developing their own research focus. In addition to conducting research, the postdoc gains experience in grant writing, publication, and presentation at professional meetings. In the United States, postdocs receive compensation for their work but at a level that is lower than a faculty position.

After receiving research training, occupational therapists should consider which academic environments are most likely to foster research. Research 1 universities is a designation used in the United States to indicate that the university is constructed to offer more support and infrastructure for research (Carnegie Classifications, n.d.); however, most OT education programs are not offered in Research 1 universities. Therefore, it is important that new faculty ask questions about the availability of financial support and time for conducting research. OT Stories 6.2, 6.3, and 6.4 present three occupational therapists at different stages of knowledge development, each of whom decided to pursue a career that involves research. Carly Cooper is pursuing a PhD with an emphasis in Research, Evaluation, Measurement, and Statistics (OT Story 6.2), So Sin Sim is just finishing up her PhD and is currently working on her dissertation (OT Story 6.3), while Ryan Bailey has completed his postdoctoral training and is a faculty member of the University of Utah where he has established a line of research (OT Story 6.4).

OT STORY 6.2 CARLY COOPER'S JOURNEY TO BECOME A RESEARCHER

Carly Cooper, OTR, MAJ, US Army Medical Specialist Corps*

From early on in my academic career, I was exposed to professors in the research realm that made an impact. I became interested in reading about and participating in research projects during my undergraduate athletic training program. This interest became a passion throughout my OT schooling where EBP initiatives fueled the importance of becoming a researcher in the profession. Just a few months out of OT school, I was recruited into the Army (Figure 6.3), where I

was immediately afforded the opportunity to pursue a post-professional doctorate degree through the Army-Baylor Doctor of Science (DSC) program. It was during this program that I was given opportunities to observe, participate in, and conduct various research projects being done within many professional disciplines, while expanding my own research knowledge and skills. I had always enjoyed statistics, so this program allowed me to delve deeper into statistical analysis procedures in a practical research context. I gained

(continued)

OT STORY 6.2 CARLY COOPER'S JOURNEY TO BECOME A RESEARCHER (continued)

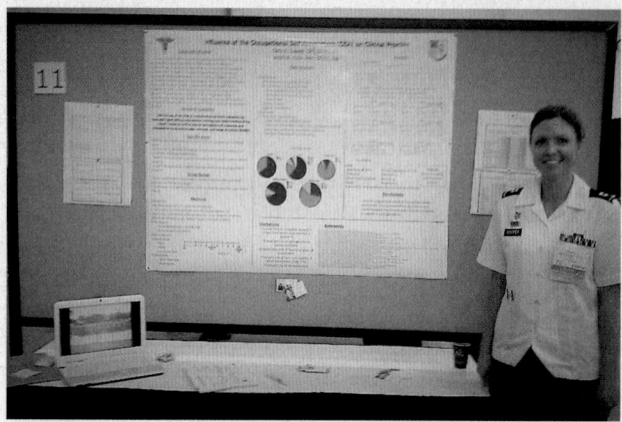

FIGURE 6.3 **Major Cooper.**

a deep understanding about the critical role research plays in continued progression of the profession while honing valuable knowledge translation skills.

My OT career so far has frequently involved demonstrating the necessity for OT services, and this wouldn't be possible without research production and dissemination within all areas and specialties of the profession. I've been afforded some amazing opportunities to develop research skills through projects in outpatient orthopedic rehabilitation, brain injury rehabilitation, and OT in behavioral health, but there is always a need for new and evolving evidence within the field. During my time in Afghanistan, I was even able to share knowledge about research in the rehabilitation field with local university representatives. Research projects

have proved a great way to collaborate with other disciplines, which provides unique opportunities to advocate for the OT profession and has often opened doors for further prospects by doing so.

After 10 years as an Army occupational therapist, I was again afforded an amazing opportunity to progress my passion as a researcher and attend a PhD program at the University of Kansas Educational Psychology program with emphasis in Research, Evaluation, Measurement, and Statistics. During this time, I've also been enjoying an appointment as volunteer faculty assisting with instructing EBP courses at the university OT program. OT researchers are critical to evolving EBP and ensuring the progression of the profession, so it's been great having the experience to develop those future leaders. It's an exciting time for the profession with all the emerging practice areas, which makes research in those areas that much more important. What fun it would be to be part of emerging research that has the potential to make huge impacts on everyday practice! It's a great feeling to know that I have contributed to professional progression and the continued evolution of OT practice. I look forward to doing so much more as I embark on my next adventure as an educator.

Question

1. Carly is getting her PhD in Educational Psychology with an emphasis in Research, Evaluation, Measurement, and Statistics. What other programs of study would benefit an occupational therapist that wants to get an advanced degree?

*The views and information presented are those of the authors and do not represent the official position of the U.S. Army Medical Center of Excellence, the U.S. Army Training and Doctrine Command, or the Department of Army, Department of Defense, or US government.

OT STORY 6.3 SO SIN SIM'S JOURNEY TO BECOME A RESEARCHER

So Sin Sim, PhD Candidate and Lecturer, Monash University, Australia

I worked as a mental health occupational therapist in Singapore for more than 15 years before deciding to become an academic. I am currently completing my PhD thesis in Australia (Figure 6.4).

Earlier in my career, I found it challenging to explain the science of what we do to other professionals I worked with. Even though they knew the OT sessions were benefiting their patients in unique ways, it was hard for them to understand what it was in the OT session that made changes in their patients.

Although we were often jokingly called the "art and craft teachers," the "basket weavers" the "job finder" or even

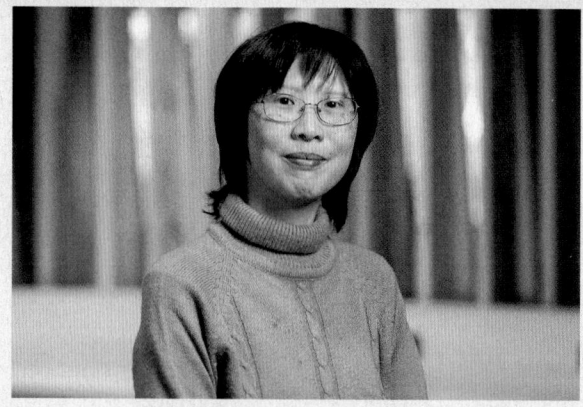

FIGURE 6.4 **Sin So Sim as a PhD candidate.**

OT STORY 6.3 SO SIN SIM'S JOURNEY TO BECOME A RESEARCHER (*continued*)

the "occupier" (frustrating for me), occupational therapists were valued and included in many consultations and projects. I was quietly confident in what I was doing, but not good at articulating the "science" of what we do. Our language of "occupations" seemed alien to everyone, and at times, in a multidisciplinary team, it could feel rather lonely. Sometimes I even felt a loss of professional identity.

With pressures from the healthcare system to include outcome measures, I knew that providing evidence of what we do and articulating the science of occupations in an understandable manner was unavoidable. I started to do little studies myself and worked on reporting on the daily interventions I was carrying out. I then started to apply for small grants to support my mini-projects.

One example was "The effectiveness of hydrotherapy on anxiety symptoms," where I carried out weekly OT sessions with a group of mental health clients using a particular intervention protocol. With the small grant, I was able to buy assessment tools and equipment, and pay for research assistant hours. In hindsight, it would have been good to be mentored and guided in this process. All I relied on then was my own readings and clinical experience, but I was inexperienced in the design of a rigorous study. Hence, along the way, I found that I had left out some important factors to consider, which potentially affected my results.

I was fortunate to work with professional colleagues who encouraged and guided me to publish my first papers together with them. They provided me with exposure and confidence in the research process. From there, I actively sought opportunities to provide evidence for our work in OT, in order to be moving the profession forward, as well as to be in sync with other mental health professionals who were much more advanced in their research work.

Finding time to do research in the midst of busyness was not easy. Together with like-minded occupational therapists, I continued to seek small projects and small grants, and each success was an encouragement that we were moving in the right direction. I also became more intentional in my participation in scientific meetings and conferences to showcase our findings.

Finally, when I moved into academia over the last 10 years, working with students on their research projects and community projects really ignited my interest in research. I found myself thinking more and more about the evaluation of practices, how to measure an outcome, and how to translate my observations into a hypothesis to be measured. Interacting with other international OT colleagues at conferences also further inspired me to grow my research skills. I hope to continue to contribute to the community and the profession through my current and future research work.

My advice to occupational therapists who are curious about the impact of the intervention they have provided to their clients and are passionate about contributing to the building of our professional identity is:

1. Start with small pilot studies.
2. Find a research mentor to guide you.
3. Work with like-minded people if you can.
4. Embark on a formal research training program at some stage.

Questions

1. So Sin talks about the importance of finding a mentor when she was doing small research projects as a clinician. How could you go about finding a mentor?
2. Who might you ask?

OT STORY 6.4 RYAN BAILEY'S JOURNEY TO BECOME A RESEARCHER

Ryan Bailey, PhD, OTR/L, Assistant Professor, University of Utah

I didn't plan on a career in academia and research when I entered OT school or when I started working as an occupational therapist. As a student, I completed a research elective where my mentor studied recovery of hand function following nerve injury. This experience piqued my interest in using neuroplasticity and motor control theories to maximize rehabilitation outcomes. Because of this interest, as a clinician I gravitated toward patients with neurologic conditions. After working as an occupational therapist for a few

years, I decided I wanted to contribute to research on stroke rehabilitation instead of just reading about it.

I decided to pursue a PhD instead of a Doctor of Occupational Therapy (OTD) because more time is devoted to research in PhD programs. Apart from research-centric coursework, time spent working under a mentor's supervision, conducting research, and writing scholarship papers was invaluable because doing research requires a skillset that can only be acquired through doing research—which requires a lot of time and energy. During my PhD studies, I was also fortunate to participate in a clinical research

(continued)

OT STORY 6.4 RYAN BAILEY'S JOURNEY TO BECOME A RESEARCHER (continued)

training program through my university that provided additional mentorship and training through journal clubs and research workshops that enhanced the training provided by my PhD curriculum. These "add-on" experiences covered information not usually taught in a class, and they were invaluable to learning about research culture and the unwritten "dos and don'ts" inherent to research.

While completing my PhD, I realized that I wanted to broaden my research interests beyond neurologic rehabilitation. Specifically, I wanted to learn about how to prevent stroke recurrence through lifestyle interventions, and I wanted to learn about different research methodologies. Accordingly, I participated in two postdoctoral training programs: the first to learn about gerontology and physical activity interventions, the second to learn about public health approaches to intervention and epidemiologic research methods. Throughout my postdoctoral training, I continued to work with mentors and conducted my own research studies under their guidance

As a result of the many years of post-OT school training I completed, I have a unique arsenal of content knowledge and skills in applying research and statistical methods. My training as an occupational therapist guides my thinking of humans as occupational beings, and my research aims to identify and investigate interventions to modify client factors, performance skills and patterns, and contexts and environments to enhance the health and well-being of people with stroke (see Figure 6.5).

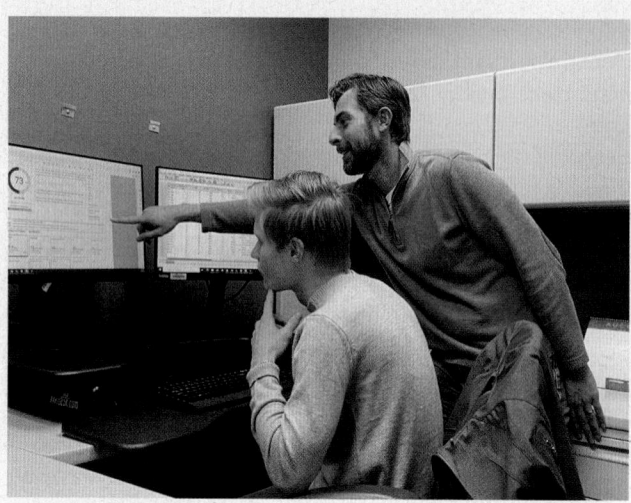

FIGURE 6.5 **Dr. Ryan Bailey (right) works with a research assistant to analyze data from a dietary behavior intervention for stroke survivors.**

Questions

1. Did you know that some researchers choose to continue their education beyond a PhD with postdoctoral training? What are the potential benefits for postdoctoral training for the postdoc?
2. Are there benefits for the mentor? For the profession of OT?

Grant Writing

Most significant research projects require funding to complete. To obtain funding, the researcher begins the process by writing a grant. There are different levels of grants. An RO1 grant from the National Institutes of Health (NIH) provides up to $250,000 per year for a 5-year period. However, before awarding such a large sum of money, the NIH requires that the investigator have strong preliminary data. Therefore, most researchers seek seed money from smaller grants to obtain that preliminary data. Universities often offer small grants so that researchers can get pilot data before applying for larger grant funding. In addition, professional organizations/foundations such as the American Occupational Therapy Foundation, the Canadian Occupational Therapy Foundation, and the RCOT Foundation provide grants to get occupational therapists started on a project.

Although the purpose of a grant application is to convince the funder that a project is worthy, the process of writing the grant application helps the researcher create a strong rationale for their study and a sound research plan. The grant application requires a process similar to a thesis or dissertation in that a background or rationale is presented along with hypotheses and research objectives, a detailed methods section is specified, and this is accompanied by timelines and a budget.

There are several strategies you can use to become a better grant writer. Taking a grant writing course is one of these. At a grant writing course, you will learn more about the process and writing style, and often have the opportunity to get feedback on your ideas. Another important strategy is to follow the grant's instructions. All grants have specific requirements regarding the application, and it is essential that these instructions are followed to the letter. It would be very disappointing to have a grant rejected just because of the font or line spacing used. Project directors that oversee a granting organization can be very helpful in facilitating a successful grant writing experience. Don't be hesitant to contact the project director and ask for guidance. In my own experience, a project director at NIH was willing to review my application before submission, and this made all the difference in getting funding! You might consider asking colleagues, especially others with a successful grant writing history, to review your grant application and provide you with feedback. Finally, the researcher should be prepared for rejection as the process of obtaining a grant can be highly competitive. However, many grants provide extensive feedback from reviewers to help the researcher prepare a stronger proposal for the next submission. A study of junior faculty found that many individuals were frustrated with the process of applying for grants and conducting research and had considered quitting (Stoykov et al., 2017). In addition, most had low confidence in their own research skills. The authors of this study recommended adequate training for a research career, the development of resilience strategies, and formal mentorship programs.

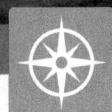

EXPANDING OUR PERSPECTIVES

International Opportunities for Research

Lilian Magalhaes

Opportunities to engage in research are not equally available to all practitioners and students. There are huge discrepancies among countries and even within the same country. Professionals who work in remote areas, for example, are less prone to join research projects than ones living in big cities. Language is another big hurdle for research collaboration that also disrupts the journey of novice researchers. Most labs and research groups carry material only in their own language, so people interested in joining the groups must find a way to translate and access material.

Currently the need for multilingual publications is an essential point to raise. Associations, research groups, and similar networks must acknowledge the importance of diversifying their audiences, to reach newer groups and engage wider perspectives. Everyone will benefit from that. Thankfully, online sources are one way to work around these hurdles to invite collaboration from different groups, if researchers understand the importance of working with frontline occupational therapists, as well as recognize the advantages of engaging students along the way. It goes without saying that research is a *collective endeavor* and, as such, we will need to engage in collective activities to succeed as researchers.

One strategy to find for partnership is to look for lab websites, such as the Laboratório de Estudos da Ocupação Humana e Tecnologias de Participação em Terapia Ocupacional (LEOH), which is headquartered in Rio de Janeiro, Brazil. In LEOH, the reader will find free videos and publications, although mostly available only in Portuguese. Also, by searching the internet under the keywords "research" and "occupational therapy" it is possible to find a myriad of sources that function as hubs for information, interaction, and networking among researchers and practitioners aspiring to be involved in and/or consume research. The same keywords translated into the language of interest may produce valuable information as well.

In the United States, OT Potential provides a network of professionals dedicated to evidence-based OT continuing education (https://otpotential.com/).

Worldwide, the Research | WFOT website (https://wfot .org/programmes/research) is part of the World Federation of Occupational Therapists (WFOT) communication venue. It describes the importance of research within OT and includes opportunities for research funds through the Thelma Cardwell Foundation Award for Research. There is also information about WFOT's current eight working projects, in which occupational therapists are welcome to engage.

In my home country of Brazil, the following sources provide information and opportunities for research and networking:

- Human Activities and Occupational Therapy Laboratory (Laboratório Atividades Humanas e Terapia Ocupacional, AHTO) dgp.cnpq.br/dgp/espelhogrupo/48834738 94010050
- Human Occupation and Technology Studies Laboratory LABOHETEC (Laboratório De Estudos Da Ocupação Humana E Tecnologia) https://institucional.ufpel.edu .br/projetos/id/u3107
- Laboratory of Memories, Territories and Occupations: Sensitive Traces (Laboratório de Memórias, Territórios e Ocupações: Rastros Sensíveis) http://dgp.cnpq.br/ dgp/espelhogrupo/210208#:~:text=dgp.cnpq.br/dgp/ espelhogrupo/9866519752585037
- LaFollia—Mental Health and Occupational Therapy (Laboratório de Terapia Occupacional e Saúde Mental) https:// www.dto.ufscar.br/pesquisa/laboratorios/laboratorio-de-pesquisa-em-saude-mental
- Metuia Lab, Social Occupational Therapy (Laboratório Metuia—Departamento do Terapia Ocupacional) https:// www.dto.ufscar.br/pesquisa/laboratorios/laboratorio-metuia

Conducting the Research

Researchers must take great care when carrying out their project so that they can maintain the reliability, validity, and trustworthiness of the findings. Rarely is a study conducted by only one person. The group of people involved in a study usually include coinvestigators and/or research assistants. Coinvestigators work together on the design, implementation, analysis, and dissemination of the research. Research assistants commonly assume a more specific role in a particular aspect of the study such as recruiting participants, administering assessments, providing the intervention, or entering data. To ensure that these tasks are carried out in a uniform way that is true to the purposes of the study, the research assistants will typically need to undergo some sort of training.

Another important step in the research process includes the recruitment and assignment of participants. Different methods may be used for this step depending on the design of the study, but again it is important that the researcher follow the procedures as first outlined in the research proposal. Data may be collected through various means such as surveys, interviews, observation, or standardized assessments. The process of data collection must be systematic and consistent especially when more than one data collector is involved. If the study is one that is determining the efficacy of an intervention, then the intervention ought to be administered in a manner that ensures its **fidelity**. This means that the intervention is implemented in a way that conforms to the basic principles of the treatment approach.

Once the data are collected, there is usually a great deal of anticipation surrounding the research analysis. The researcher will finally learn what they set out to accomplish. In other words, the researcher can answer their research question and, in the case of a hypothesis-driven study, determine whether their hypothesis was supported. Although this process sounds straightforward, data analysis often involves many steps, and then once the analysis is completed, the researcher must interpret the findings. From the researcher's perspective there is a great deal of gratification associated with completing a study and learning the results even when the results are not as expected! Sometimes it is the unexpected results that lead to the most important findings.

Sharing the Findings

When a study is completed, it is crucial that the results are shared so that others can be informed of the findings. Researchers share their findings through publications and presentations. The publication process can be time-consuming, so you may learn about a study first when attending a conference. Often, conferences will offer late-breaking poster sessions that provide researchers with the opportunity to share very recent findings.

Occupational therapists publish their findings in OT journals as well as in non-OT journals that address topics relevant to our areas of practice. For example, OT research can be found in the *Archives of Physical Medicine and Rehabilitation*, the *Psychiatric Rehabilitation Journal*, and *Infants and Young Children*. Similar to a grant application, when submitting research for publication it is essential that the specific guidelines are followed. For a peer-reviewed journal, the journal will send out your article for blind-review, meaning those who are reviewing the article will not know who submitted it. The reviewers will provide a recommendation to the editor of the journal. The recommendations typically include: (a) reject the article, (b) revise and resubmit, or (c) acceptance (with minor changes). Rarely is an article accepted outright. If not rejected, the author will be required to resubmit their article after a detailed revision that addresses the specific feedback of the reviewers. It is hurtful to be rejected, but the researcher should not lament. This is a common occurrence even among highly established researchers. Sometimes submission to a different journal is warranted and may result in an acceptance. Researchers may choose to first submit their manuscript to a journal with a high **impact factor** (a measure based on the number of citations of publications in that journal) with the plan to submit to a less prestigious journal if not successful.

As a practitioner it can be hard to understand why it takes so long for a study to be published. Now that you have read about the process of seeking seed money, obtaining preliminary data, writing a grant application, being awarded a grant, conducting the research, analyzing the data, writing the article, and then submitting for publication, perhaps you will have a greater awareness as to the time frame involved in the research process. An example of a research project that has been through the entire process but is still advancing is presented in OT Story 6.5. In this intervention study led by Stacey Schepens Niemiec, an OT wellness approach is examined for its efficacy with a Latino population in California.

Academic/Clinical Partnerships to Advance Scholarship in Occupational Therapy

Many OT practitioners want to contribute to new knowledge development, but they may not have the skills or resources to do so. Academic–clinical partnerships provide opportunities and benefits to both parties. University researchers may have knowledge in research methodology and statistical analysis, while the clinician has access to participants and knowledge about clinically meaningful

OT STORY 6.5 ¡VIVIR MI VIDA!: SCHOLARLY DEVELOPMENT OF AN OCCUPATION-BASED PREVENTIVE PROGRAM

When reading a published research study, it's easy to miss the full context of the project: both what led to the publication and also the work that continued afterward. The story associated with the development of the ¡Vivir Mi Vida! project illustrates the importance of many qualities of scholarly work: persistence, collaboration, and patience.

Stacey Schepens Niemiec, PhD, OTR/L, is the principal investigator for an intervention study named ¡Vivir Mi Vida! (¡VMV!). As a postdoctoral student at the University of Southern California (USC) in 2011, Dr. Schepens Niemiec's mentor was Florence Clark, PhD, OTR, FAOTA, the principal investigator of the landmark Well Elderly Studies and developer of OT Lifestyle Redesign® (Clark et al., 1997, 2001). Drs. Clark and Schepens Niemiec approached the Department of Health Services of Los Angeles County in an effort to apply OT Lifestyle Redesign® to a group of clients with more complicated needs. The health department suggested that the late middle age group of Latinos in the county had a high incidence of chronic health conditions and were not receiving the needed care. From there ¡VMV! was born.

Schepens Niemiec and colleagues conducted a needs assessment by interviewing 15 Latino adults between the ages of 50 and 60 who were at high risk for developing chronic conditions. A Spanish-speaking occupational therapist conducted the interviews, which included questions about health needs and what topics should be offered if a program like Well Elderly Lifestyle Redesign® were to be offered. It became clear that this group had unique needs not necessarily prominent in the Well Elderly study. Six areas of need were identified including weight management; disease management; mental health and well-being; personal finances; family, friends, and community (in relation to health-related activities); and stress management. The results of the needs assessment were published in the *American Journal of Occupational Therapy* (AJOT) (Schepens Niemiec et al., 2015).

Schepens Niemiec's team continued to expand, now including Jenny Martínez, OTD, OTR/L, BCG, as a coinvestigator and codeveloper of the program. The team then reached out to the Clinical and Translational Science Institute at USC, which links researchers with community partners. The institute connected Schepens Niemiec and Martínez with a local promotora, Laura Guzmán, who was then hired as staff on the research team. A promotora is a community health worker with deep ties to the Latino community who has shared lived experience with the clients and has specialized cultural knowledge. Schepens Niemiec, Martínez, and Guzmán coled the development and implementation of the intervention. OT Lifestyle Redesign® continued to serve as the primary theoretical foundation for the intervention, which along with results from the needs assessment served as the foundation for the development of intervention modules. The 16-week program included broad units focusing on planning, healthy eating and activity, healthcare navigation, chronic disease management, mental well-being, and wrap-up. Sessions included a combination of in-person home-based visits, video calls, and telephone check-ins. The team identified community health workers as the frontline interveners, with occupational therapists taking a supervisory role. The protocol for the intervention was described in an article published in the *Occupational Therapy Journal of Research* (Schepens Niemiec et al., 2019).

The first study of the efficacy of the intervention was funded through the USC Chan Division of Occupational Science and Occupational Therapy. There were 40 participants in the pilot study. Because of limited funds, the researchers were unable to include a control group and had to limit the intervention to 4 months when they originally wanted to provide a 6-month intervention. As planned, the intervention was provided primarily by community health workers trained by Guzmán. The occupational therapists on the team provided supervision in terms of grading and adapting activities and clinical intervention focused on the integration of healthful routines. The findings were very positive with improvements in symptom severity, perceived impact of symptoms on daily activity, general well-being, satisfaction with social roles, satisfaction with social activities, stress, and dietary intake. There was also an improvement in systolic blood pressure, although other physiologic parameters such as weight, cholesterol levels, and hemoglobin A_{1c} did not change. The project had a high retention rate, and the participants were very satisfied with the program (see Figure 6.6). These findings were published in *Primary Health Care Research and Development* (Schepens Niemiec et al., 2018).

All the while, Schepens Niemiec was completing grant applications so that she could obtain significant funding to implement the project with a larger group of people and with a controlled comparison. As of 2021, she has received encouraging responses from funding sources for R01-level proposals—major grants from the NIH. She will continue to pursue grants in the future.

In the meantime, the research team conducted a long-term follow-up study to determine whether participants in ¡VMV! maintained their improvements in health indicators. The findings indicated that the participants' outcomes continued to improve even after intervention conclusion in the areas of systolic blood pressure, stress, social role satisfaction, and activity satisfaction. These results were also published in AJOT (Schepens Niemiec et al., 2021).

(continued)

OT STORY 6.5 ¡VIVIR MI VIDA!: SCHOLARLY DEVELOPMENT OF AN OCCUPATION-BASED PREVENTIVE PROGRAM (*continued*)

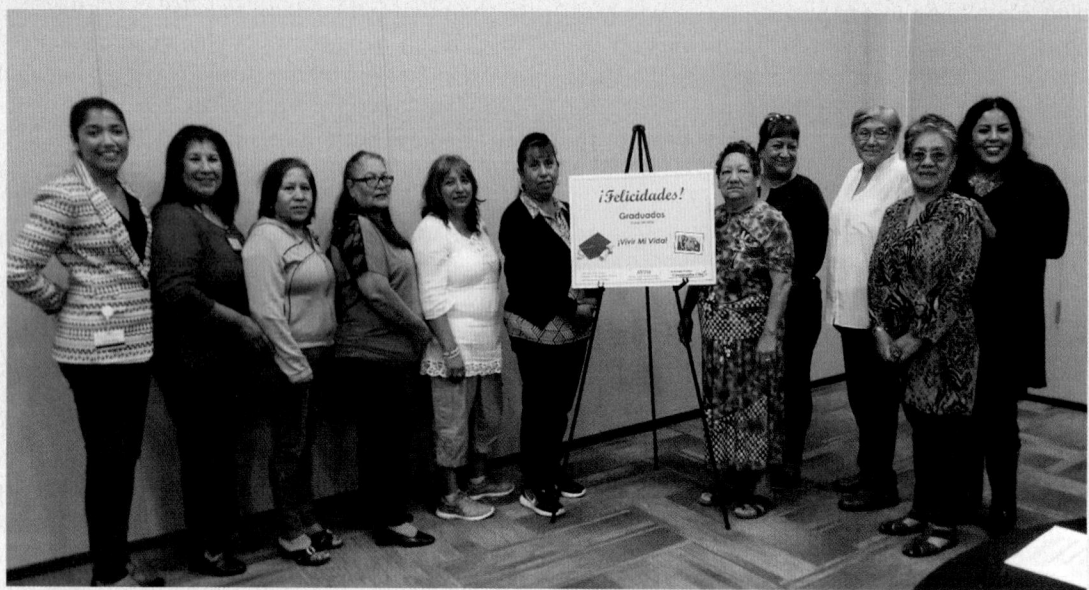

FIGURE 6.6 One graduating group of the ¡Vivir Mi Vida! program and the occupational therapist and promotoras de salud who supported them. Laura Guzmán (supervising promotora) is second from the left, Alyssa Concha (intervening OT) is on the far left, Joanna Ortego (intervening promotora) is on the far right. All others pictured were participants in the program.

Schepens Niemiec is hopeful that these findings will contribute to future funding, the opportunity to study the intervention with a randomized controlled trial, and the application of the intervention to a much larger group of people.

As can be seen, thus far, the project has involved multiple steps, many people, and several years of work. Through her work with a dedicated team, Schepens Niemiec has and will continue to contribute new knowledge to the practice of OT.

Question

1. What did you learn about the process of research by reading Stacey's story?

questions. For example, although there is a growing body of research that supports OT intervention, practitioners may not be able to implement these interventions under the same conditions that were used in the study (Juckett et al., 2021). Collaborations between practitioners and university settings can result in research that is more relevant and generalizable to everyday practice. As a practitioner you might consider contacting OT educational programs to explore opportunities for collaboration. You might be surprised by the interest among faculty. With greater opportunities using virtual interfaces, it is potentially easier to connect with faculty with specific interests that mirror your own.

Another role for academic–clinical partnerships relates to the adoption of EBPs. Clinicians can help researchers develop dissemination methods, such as continuing education opportunities or publications, that are relevant and meaningful to clinicians. This requires that the researchers be aware of and realistic about the pragmatics of certain practice settings. It is also useful if researchers can present information in a manner that is accessible to practitioners. Clinicians can help the researcher acquire knowledge about real-world practice.

Conclusion

Scholarship is necessary for the OT profession to advance. Occupational therapists may engage in scholarship either by acquiring and applying existing knowledge or by developing new knowledge. Research in OT provides the public and those receiving OT with a rationale for using our services. It also guides our practice so that we are more likely to make the best clinical decisions and improve outcomes for service recipients. It is important that clinicians and academics work together to generate evidence that is relevant for real-world practice. It is also crucial that clinicians and academics work together to design methods by which EBPs can be disseminated and applied.

Lippincott® Connect *For additional resources on the subjects discussed in this chapter, visit Lippincott Connect.*

REFERENCES

American Occupational Therapy Association. (n.d.). *Social learning through AOTA's Communities of Practice.* https://www.aota.org/community/communities-of-practice.

Barry, M., Kuijer-Siebelink, W., Nieuwenhuis, L., & Scherpbier-de Haan, N. (2017). Communities of practice: A means to support occupational therapists' continuing professional development. A literature review. *Australian Occupational Therapy Journal, 64*(2), 185–193. https://doi.org/10.1111/1440-1630.12334

Braveman, B., & Hunter, E. G. (2017). *Occupational therapy for cancer rehabilitation with adults.* AOTA Press.

Carnegie Classifications of Institutions of Higher Education. (n.d.). *Basic classification description.* https://carnegieclassifications.iu.edu/classification_descriptions/basic.php

Clark, F., Azen, S. P., Carlson, M., Mandel, D., LaBree, L., Hay, J., Zemke, R., Jackson, J., & Lipson, L. (2001). Embedding health-promoting changes into the daily lives of independent-living older adults: Long-term follow-up of occupational therapy intervention. *The Journals of Gerontology. Series B, Psychological Sciences and Social Sciences, 56*(1), P60–P63. https://doi.org/10.1093/geronb/56.1.p60

Clark, F., Azen, S. P., Zemke, R., Jackson, J., Carlson, M., Mandel, D., Hay, J., Josephson, K., Cherry, B., Hessel, C., Palmer, J., & Lipson, L. (1997). Occupational therapy for independent-living older adults. A randomized controlled trial. *JAMA, 278*(16), 1321–1326. https://doi.org/10.1001/jama.1997.03550160041036

Galheigo, S. M., Braga, C. P., Magalhães, L., & Kinsella, E. A. (2019). An occupational therapy community of practice within pediatric acute care: Fostering professional, social and cultural capital in resource challenged settings. *Brazilian Journal of Occupational Therapy, 27*(4). https://doi.org/10.4322/2526-8910.ctoAO1825

Hand Therapy Certification Commission. (n.d.). *Who is a certified hand therapist (CHT)?* https://www.htcc.org/about-htcc/CHT-Credential

International Federation of Societies for Hand Therapy. (n.d.). *How to become a hand therapist.* https://ifsht.org/how-to-become-a-hand-therapist/

Juckett, L. A., Robinson, M. L., Malloy, J., & Oliver, H. V. (2021). Translating knowledge to optimize value-based occupational therapy: Strategies for educators, practitioners, and researchers. *American Journal of Occupational Therapy, 75*, 7506090020. https://doi.org/10.5014/ajot.2021.756003

Juckett, L. A., Robinson, M. L., & Wengerd, L. R. (2019). Narrowing the gap: An implementation science research agenda for the occupational therapy profession. *American Journal of Occupational Therapy,* 73, 7305347010p1–7305347010p6. https://doi.org/10.5014/ajot.2019.033902

Krueger, R. B., Sweetman, M. M., Martin, M., & Cappaert, T. A. (2020). Self-reflection as a support to evidence-based practice: A grounded theory exploration. *Occupational Therapy in Health Care, 34*(4), 320–350. https://doi.org/10.1080/07380577.2020.1815929

Occupational Therapy Australia. (2016). *Guide to good practice for working with children.* https://www.otaus.com.au/practice-support/guides-to-good-practice

Proctor, E., Silmore, H., Raghavan, R., Hovmand, P., Aarons, G., Bunger, A., Griffey, R., & Hensley, M. (2011). Outcomes for implementation research: Conceptual distinctions, measurement challenges, and research agenda. *Administration and Policy in Mental Health and Mental Health Services Research, 38*, 65–76. https://doi.org/10.1007/s10488-010-0319-7

Psychiatric Rehabilitation Association. (n.d.). *Certified psychiatric rehabilitation practitioner.* https://www.psychrehabassociation.org/certification

Royal College of Occupational Therapists. (2020). *Hand and wrist orthoses for adults with rheumatological conditions: Practice guidelines for occupational therapists* (2nd ed.). Author.

Schepens Niemiec, S. L., Blanchard, J., Vigen, C. L. P., Martínez, J., Guzmán, L., Concha, A., Fluke, M., & Carlson, M. (2018). Evaluation of ¡Vivir Mi Vida! To improve health and wellness of rural-dwelling, late middle-aged Latino adults: Results of a feasibility and pilot study of a lifestyle intervention. *Primary Health Care Research & Development, 19*, 448–463. https://doi.org/10.1017/S1463423617000901

Schepens Niemiec, S. L., Blanchard, J., Vigen, C. L. P., Martínez, J., Guzmán, L., Fluke, M., & Carlson, M. (2019). A pilot study of the ¡Vivir Mi Vida! Lifestyle intervention for rural-dwelling, late-midlife Latinos: Study design and protocol. *OTJR: Occupation, Participation and Health, 39*(1), 5–13. https://doi.org/10.1177/1539449218762728

Schepens Niemiec, S. L., Carlson, M., Martínez, J., Guzmán, L., Mahajan, A., & Clark, F. (2015). Developing occupation-based preventive programs for late-middle-aged Latino patients in safety-net health systems. *American Journal of Occupational Therapy, 69*, 6906240010. https://doi.org/10.5014/ajot.2015.015958

Schepens Niemiec, S. L., Vigen, C. L. P., Martínez, J., Blanchard, J., & Carlson, M. (2021). Long-term follow-up of a lifestyle intervention for late-midlife, rural-dwelling Latinos in primary care. *American Journal of Occupational Therapy, 75*, 7502205010. https://doi.org/10.5014/ajot.2021.042861

Stoykov, M. E., Skarupski, K. A., Foucher, K., & Chubinskaya, S. (2017). Junior investigators thinking about quitting research: A survey. *American Journal of Occupational Therapy, 71*, 7102280010p1–7102280010p7. https://doi.org/10.5014/ajot.2017.019448

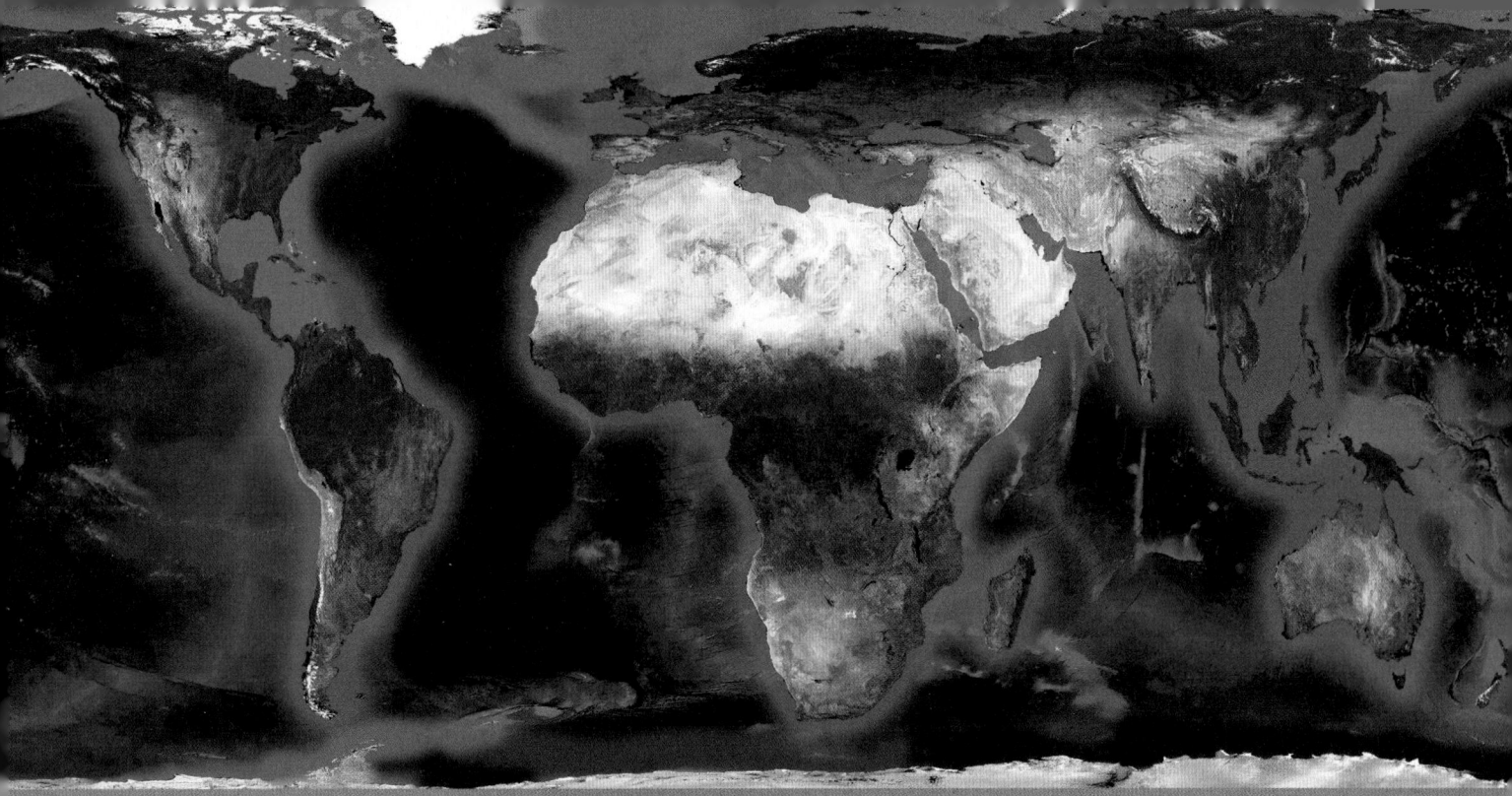

UNIT II
Occupational Nature of Humans

Media Related to the Occupational Nature of Humans

Readings
- *A River Runs Through It:* Norman Maclean's short story that includes fly fishing as a metaphor and occupation that connects a family. (1976)
- *Crying in H Mart:* Michelle Zauner's book recounts how cooking and eating traditional food nourishes memories of her Korean mother. (2021)

Movies
- *CODA:* Amelie grows up with deaf parents and she helps them with their business while pursuing her own passion of singing. (2021)

Art
- *Jean-Michel Basquiat:* Basquiat (1960–1988) was a Black American artist who was famous for depicting dichotomies such as wealth and poverty, integration and segregation, and inner and outer experiences. He combined painting, drawing, text, and poetry in his works.

Music
- *This Is Me:* Song from *The Greatest Showman,* which is about acceptance of unconventional people. (2017)

Emergence, Development, and Transformation of Occupations

Jennifer L. Womack and Nancy Bagatell

LEARNING OBJECTIVES

1. Differentiate between perspectives on human development based on biological and psychological maturation versus those grounded in occupational perspectives.
2. Synthesize current perspectives from occupational science and occupational therapy with concepts from other disciplines to enhance understanding of occupational development.
3. Analyze principles of the life course perspective to understand how individual agency is interwoven with sociohistorical time and place in shaping occupations over time.
4. Apply concepts of occupational emergence, development, and transformation in the context of clinical practice in order to enhance therapeutic interventions.

Introduction

Occupational therapy (OT) practitioners work with people across the life span to acquire, recover, and adapt life activities that are complex and contextually based. Within the OT profession, these life activities are labeled *occupations*. Throughout a life span, human beings take up, further develop, and at times change occupations. Within OT, these processes are often understood as intertwined with ways of thinking about the development of human bodies and minds as we age chronologically.

During the early decades of OT, the profession adopted prevailing theories from psychology and biology that emphasized predictable timing for human development through maturation. In other words, it was once believed that as soon as requisite skills developed at certain ages, an individual would be able to perform tasks that require those skills. As in most cases when long-held ideas break down, exceptions to those rules sparked transformations in thinking about development. Studies of twins adopted into different families first sparked debate about the relative impact of genetics versus environment, and their cumulative effect led to reexamining early developmental theories (Segal, 1997). Later developmental perspectives highlighted the interdependence of biological maturation along with the context in which humans develop, and even more recent conceptual contributions point out the relationships among sociocultural, historical, interpersonal, and individual factors as they influence the development and transformation of occupations across the span of human life. To illustrate the difference in these approaches, see the example of Felix in Table 7.1. This shift from foregrounding human maturation to emphasizing the development of occupations throughout a human lifetime calls for a deeper understanding as to how occupations emerge, develop, and transform over time, which is the focus of this chapter.

To address the complexity of these topics, we first present evolving knowledge about human development influenced by research in OT and occupational science (e.g., Humphry, 2002, 2005; Humphry & Wakeford, 2006, 2008; Leclair et al., 2018; Wiseman et al., 2005) and informed by a transactional perspective on occupation (Dickie et al., 2006). We will then introduce the life course perspective as first outlined by sociologist Glen H. Elder (1994) and furthered through the work of Elder and colleagues (Elder & Shanahan, 2006; Elder et al., 2003). The life course perspective has been influential for scholars in occupational science and therapy (e.g., Carroll et al., 2021; Pikkarainen et al., 2015; Rowles, 2008) and offers a beneficial framework for considering occupational development.

With this content, we challenge ourselves and readers of this chapter to consider how evolving views on human development and occupation influence clinical practice and research. What does it mean for an early interventionist to consider child development not only through the lens of developmental milestones but also from a sociocultural perspective? How might an understanding of teenage mental health informed by a lens of trauma exposure better prepare clinicians to design interventions? How do the cumulative effects of living through multiple large-scale sociohistorical events impact the health of a cohort of older adults differently than the cohort behind or before them? We invite you as the reader to engage with, critically examine, and challenge the ideas presented in this chapter as we all strive to better understand and serve the individuals, dyads, groups, communities, and populations with whom we partner.

Evolving Concepts of Occupational Development

OT practitioners, along with educators, psychologists, and other professionals concerned with human development, ascribed for many decades to a view of maturation based on developmental milestones. These milestones represented norm-based age thresholds at which children should, based on their biological maturation, acquire and use specific skills (Boyle, 2009; Rodger & Behr, 2017). Children who did not attain these milestones at the expected times were considered delayed or atypically developing. There was little to no consideration of occupation by developmental stage theorists (e.g., Erikson, Freud, Piaget), who were focused primarily on decontextualized components of motor, speech, and cognitive function. This was reflected for many decades in the assessments used by OT practitioners and others to test for developmental milestones (Coster, 1998).

TABLE 7.1   Evaluation of Felix

Felix is a 3-year-old boy recently adopted by a middle-class family living in the United States. He was evaluated because of concerns about challenges participating in everyday activities. Felix has cerebral palsy.

	Evaluation Based on Developmental Milestones	Evaluation Based on a Contextual Approach
Location	• Clinic	• Home
Assessment procedures	• Norm-referenced developmental assessment (performance and caregiver questionnaire)	• Caregiver interview to obtain information about family routines and occupations • Caregiver questionnaire to obtain information on Felix's performance with and without assistance and environmental/task modification • Observation in natural context • Assessment of engagement with contextual modifications (e.g., providing seating supports, adapted utensils)
Findings	• Felix's motor skills are equivalent to those of a 6-month-old as he has difficulty grasping objects and using toys/utensils functionally. He is able to sit independently but does not explore his environment as he is not able to crawl.	• Given caregiver and environmental supports, Felix demonstrates increased motivation to use toys, utensils, and explore his environment. • Parents have established routines that support Felix's participation in family occupations. • Trunk support, placement of objects, and physical prompts enable Felix to more actively participate.
Recommendations	• Work on fine and gross motor skills in developmental sequence.	• Provide environmental supports, including adapted toys, utensils, and mobility devices.

These dominant stage theories came to be viewed by many scholars and practitioners as too linear in nature, failing to account for the highly variable presence or absence of resources and opportunities that can alter developmental trajectories. They also effectively ignored developmental processes that extend throughout adulthood, later addressed by the emergence of life span theories of development (Peterson, 2003). Developmental theory was revolutionized during the latter part of the 20th century and into the early 2000s by emerging ideas that focused more heavily on the contextual nature of infant and child development (Gauvain, 2001; Ramey & Ramey, 1998; Stern, 1994), on changes across the entirety of the life span (Baltes, 1989), and on the importance of understanding the influence of relationships and social connectedness on individual development (Emde, 1989; Rogoff, 2003; Tronick, 1998). Scholars foregrounded the concept that there is more variability than uniformity as humans age (Crosnoe & Elder, 2002; Lachman, 2004; Westerhof et al., 2001), and that changes in performance are likely due not only to changing capacities of the individual human being but also to the sociocultural and historical contexts in which one lives.

Scholars in OT and occupational science embraced these emerging ideas, and pointed out the lack of attention in traditional developmental theories to contextual influences on developing occupations, such as interpersonal connections and sociocultural expectations (Humphry, 2002, 2005; Humphry & Wakeford, 2006, 2008; Lawlor, 2003; Rodger & Behr, 2017). The broadening of OT's views on human development shifted the field from an emphasis on the individual to a consideration of contextual influences at various levels. In addition, the term *occupational development* has entered international professional language, and is used in both official documents (e.g., Canadian Association of Occupational Therapists, 2016) as well as published scholarship (e.g., d'Entremont et al., 2017; Wiseman et al., 2005).

Scholars use the term *occupational development* to refer to the *repertoire* of what children can and choose to do at various times (Njelesani et al., 2020; Wiseman et al., 2005), as the establishment of occupational patterns that begin at birth (Townsend & Polatajko, 2007), and as opportunities offered through participation in everyday life (Leclair et al., 2018). The concept of occupational development is evolving as scholars grapple with the complexities of describing how humans take up and participate in occupation, and how occupations change over time. Humans are born into the world with varying potential for engagement in occupation based on their biological capacities, but the manifestation of that potential is heavily interdependent with contextual influences. Because individual capacities are covered in other chapters and texts, we focus here on contextual influences on occupational development. In particular, scholars in OT and occupational science have emphasized levels of influence on these processes that we will label, for the purposes

of this chapter, as *interpersonal*, *cultural*, and *societal*, acknowledging that these concepts are overlapping. We use them here to categorize the social realms in which humans are embedded.

Interpersonal Influences on Occupational Development

The interpersonal nature of occupational development is evident in research showing that even in utero, fetuses develop familiarity with the sound of the language of people around them (Choi et al., 2017) and that infants as young as 2 to 3 months mimic patterns enacted by their caregivers (Humphry, 2016). Price and Stephenson (2009) note that these interpersonal influences are not only critical to child development but also have a reciprocal impact on others in the situation. This is illustrated in their work describing a mother and preschool child who influence one another's occupational, social, and emotional development through co-occupation.

Humphry articulated these interpersonal influences in her Model of Processes Transforming Occupations (Humphry, 2005), integrating insights from previous research observing how children learn occupations (Humphry, 2002; McNamara & Humphry, 2008), as well as research about motor learning, child development, and communities of practice (e.g., Lave & Packer, 2008; Lave & Wenger, 1991; Siegler, 2000; Thelen, 2000). Humphry (2005) highlighted the combination of a human's self-organizing capabilities with interpersonal influences in suggesting mechanisms for change in occupational performance (Box 7.1). Throughout her work on the development and transformation of occupations, Humphry emphasizes the reciprocal nature of change for all persons involved in co-constructing occupation, the potential for change in the nature of the occupation being performed, and the possibility for transformation of occupational engagement across the life course (Humphry & Womack, 2019). In addition, Humphry (2005) maintained that although maturation of capacities cannot completely account for changes in occupational performance, individual capacities do change with use, pointing out the reciprocal nature of occupation within a human organism as well as in interactions between human beings.

Reciprocal influences on occupation are seen in the following example of intergenerational family members doing yoga together (OT Story 7.1).

Complementing Humphry's work, Lawlor (2003) described children as "socially occupied beings" (p. 426) engaged in the cocreation of occupation. She pointed out that developmental processes supporting occupation are more complex than was reflected in earlier thinking. Rather than the child representing an organism with the innate capacity to develop occupation, the latter emerges through

BOX 7.1 MECHANISMS BRINGING ABOUT CHANGE IN OCCUPATIONS

Interpersonal Influences on Occupational Engagement

- Novices learn about occupation through peripheral participation. As active onlookers, they learn how things are done, how objects are used, possible outcomes, and what is significant in the occupation.
- During co-constructed occupations between two or more people, the performance demands are distributed between participants; they learn from one another and alter their understanding of the outcomes and meanings.
- Explicit teaching and scaffolding brings a novice member's occupational performance to a higher level. The more experienced participant introduces culturally informed practices and ideas about outcome and meaning of the occupation to the novice participant.

Engagement in Occupation Is Transformational for That Occupation

- Challenges to familiar ways of doing, and/or altered experiences of the significance of an occupation, lead people to try new ways of using their capacities, which in turn leads to new strategies. Skilled action develops when people learn to select performance strategies to fit particular situations.
- Performance and capacities are interrelated with reciprocal influences. As a person uses current abilities in occupations, the repeated practice brings about further refinement of abilities and sustains skill. These changes in turn transform the occupation.

Source: Adapted from Humphry (2005).

OT STORY 7.1 INTERGENERATIONAL INFLUENCES ON LEARNING AN OCCUPATION

A grandmother, Harriet, her adult daughter, Lauren, and her granddaughter, Mariah, share a morning routine of yoga (see Figure 7.1). The photo was taken after Mariah's second birthday when she received her first yoga mat. Perhaps surprisingly, Harriet is the newest yoga learner in this scenario. Lauren first learned the practice of yoga in college from her partner and found it a great way to manage stress and be socially active. When their daughter Mariah was born, Lauren introduced her to yoga through a mother–baby class. Harriet became intrigued by their class and decided she wanted to try yoga as well. Lauren helped Harriet select poses and

practice moves until they became familiar with the poses. Unlike Mariah, who learned yoga by observing and being immersed in it from birth, Harriet learned more formally through being instructed and relating it to other forms of exercise in which she takes part. The family now gathers weekly for yoga as a way to socialize and exercise together.

All of the learners in this family scenario were influenced by interpersonal factors in their uptake of the occupation of yoga. The occupation reflects continuity with the history of a centuries-old wellness practice, as well as a shared interest in exercise for well-being. The ways in which each family member became involved and have developed their skills illustrate aspects of the mechanisms for change outlined in Box 7.1:

- As a novice to yoga, Harriet first observed others taking part in it, and began to understand the significance within her own family.
- Lauren, the more experienced partner, provided explicit teaching for Harriet, but also introduced Mariah to the practice and meaning of yoga through immersion.
- Both Harriet and Mariah's skill with the occupation changed as they practiced, and the occupation itself also changed as it developed into a new family routine.

Questions

1. How does Harriet's process of learning yoga reflect interpersonal influences on occupational development?
2. Think about intergenerational influences on one of your own occupations. How have people of different ages influenced your participation?

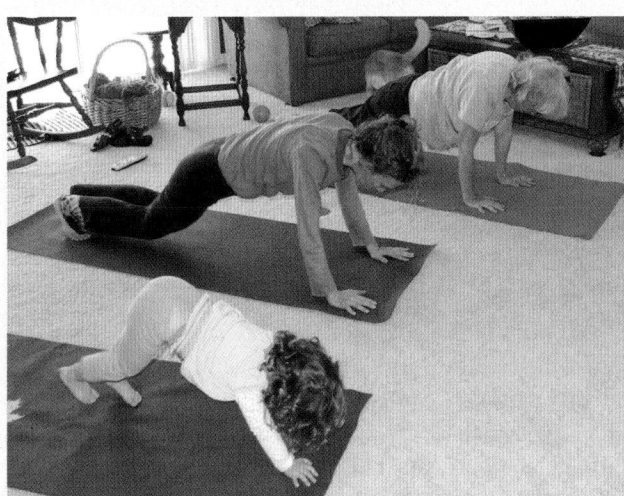

FIGURE 7.1 **Three generations in one family engaged in yoga.**

interrelationships between the human organism and its social and physical world. Lawlor proposed foregrounding experiences of children as a way to understand the interplay of actors within social and physical worlds, emphasizing that environment or context should be seen as integral to action rather than as a static site that can be regarded separately from the person. This change in thinking about the concept of *environment* is reflected in other seminal work in OT and occupational science.

Scholars Dickie, Cutchin, and Humphry (2006) drew from the work of philosopher and educational reformer John Dewey to propose a transactional perspective on occupation. Among the ideas that this perspective suggests is a move away from foregrounding the individual as a way to understand occupation and focusing instead on how people and context "co-constitute one another through their mutual relationship" (Aldrich, 2008, p. 151). The entirety of this theoretical perspective is beyond the scope of this chapter and is available in the OT and occupational science literature (e.g., Aldrich, 2008; Cutchin & Dickie, 2013; Dickie et al., 2006). For our purposes, the transactional perspective built on earlier concepts from chaos theory and systems theory to expand thinking about the relationship between human action and the environment or context, positioning the latter as a foundational element of a situation in which person, environment, and occupation cannot be separated, but are simultaneously and mutually active. These concepts informed developmental theorists in OT and occupational science as they began exploring the impact of broader cultural and societal contexts on the development of occupations.

Cultural Influences on Occupational Development

Culture is admittedly a complex construct, one that is used to describe domains of varying scale. Here we use the concept of culture to indicate customs and practices that extend beyond the immediate interpersonal realm but that are more intimate than a societal level that influences occupational development, such as the culture of a family or the culture of a group of people who share a specific identity representing this type of cultural sphere. OT scholars have introduced observations about cultural influence on development that again call into question an overemphasis on the individual. One interesting example of this is Bazyk et al.'s (2003) explication of Mayan cultural principles related to how children come to take up occupation:

> The first cultural principle, primacy of adult work, reflects the observation that children's daily activities are primarily structured around adult work activities. Children learn early that adult work must get done, that work should not be interrupted, and that they should help when needed and able. [...] The second cultural principle, importance of parental beliefs, considers the parents' view of the world and thoughts about the nature of children. All parents share a common goal of raising a child who will be able to [...] function as a competent member of the society. Cultures vary in how they believe children become competent adults. [...] For example, because the Maya believe that development is internally driven and automatic, parents are not concerned with [...] intentional teaching or encouragement to promote it. It is believed that children will naturally learn to work and be safe by participating in daily life within the family compound and community. (p. 274)

Bazyk's description is provocative in that even as she describes a belief of Mayan parents that "development is internally driven and automatic" (p. 274), she is simultaneously illuminating how culturally embedded their child-rearing practices are, and how shared concepts of work and independence influence how Mayan children engage with their world.

Although it may be argued that parental influences are more interpersonal than cultural in nature, here we are situating parents as actors within cultural contexts, acknowledging the influence of increasingly larger cultural spheres on parenting practices that in turn influence exposure to, and development of, occupations for children. d'Entremont et al. (2017), in their study reviewing the timing and types of engagement in productivity occupations among adolescents and teens, note the relatively stronger influence of parents and extended family over age-based factors. They concluded that environmental influences such as family structure, peer perceptions of work, and gendered societal expectations are more influential drivers of participation in work-related occupations than concrete age-based milestones.

Beyond the realm of family, the work of Ziviani et al. (2006) highlights community influences on physically active childhood occupations, citing the impact of culturally dominant sports, preferences of friends, and culturally prevalent gender expectations. Over a 2-year period, these influences were found to have varying impacts at different times, with gender expectations playing an increasing role relative to the waning participation of young girls as time progressed. These findings further problematize focusing solely on age as a developmental predictor, given the impact of gender stereotypes and other factors. These scholars emphasize that the ways in which children become engaged and know how to participate in physically active occupations are shaped by perceptions of safety, affordability, and accessibility shared between the children, their parents, their friendship circles, and their communities (Ziviani et al., 2006).

Communities influence the patterns of people's lives, shape their values, and provide structure in the form of opportunities and constraints (Diewald & Mayer, 2009; Elder & Shanahan, 2006; Engeström, 1999). People move through and participate in many communities over the life course (Hedegaard, 2009), occupying different roles, while also sharing with others in the community ways of doing things to achieve mutual goals. The timing of movement between communities, and participation within them, is often influenced by both informal and formal age-related normative expectations rather than capacities represented by age. Formal employment provides one example of these expectations: though child labor laws in the United States prevent children under the age of 14 from being employed in nonagricultural settings, within different communities the age-related expectations for this work vary widely. On the other hand, leaving paid employment to live on retirement income and savings cannot occur until a formally designated age in many cultures. There is a shared social understanding about engagement with work at both ends of the age spectrum. These concepts speak to an even broader societal realm of developmental influences explored by OT and occupational science scholars.

Societal Influences on Occupational Development

Wilcock (2006) suggested the occupational nature of people evolved simultaneously with the need to coordinate occupations for their immediate survival, and ultimately the sustained survival of the species. Hocking and Wright-St. Clair (2017) suggest the shared meaning of belonging to and doing with groups of people with common goals drives participation in occupations. From survival and basic subsistence to shared meaning, these scholars explore a wide range of societal influences on the development and continued participation in occupations. The give-and-take between human agency and broader societal presses demands or shapes certain actions. This tension is addressed by Rudman (2010) in her work on occupational possibilities.

Occupational possibilities are influenced by deeply ingrained social values and beliefs about what people can and should do in everyday life in relation to their life stage, gender, and social class. Rudman (2010) defines these possibilities as "the ways and types of doing that come to be viewed as ideal and possible with a specific sociohistorical context, and that come to be promoted and made available within that context" (p. 55). For example, Rudman (2010) explains how particular parenting occupations (e.g., feeding or disciplining) come

to be viewed as ideal and appropriate according to gender. Through policies, healthcare practices, and discourses on parenting, the "right" way to parent is idealized and becomes codified in the language and practices of a society.

Applying this same concept to an exploration of societal influences on later life transitions, Rudman (2015) demonstrated that ageism, enacted through governmental practices and social discourses, shapes the way in which adults enact retirement. Older adults in this study described ways in which employment practices and policies served to minimize their contributions and disempower their choices as they transitioned out of full-time work. Although retirement is often referred to as a "choice," these participants described how contextual factors such as social discourse around aging serve to constrain possibilities related to their leaving-work transition.

Other societal factors serve to promote, make available, or constrain occupational possibilities. Leadley and Hocking (2017) explored childhood poverty relative to its impact on the emergence and development of occupations in childhood as well as subsequent life prospects. Drawing on evidence that suggests social rather than biological determinants as predictive of lifelong health inequities (Attree, 2006), Leadley and Hocking (2017) noted poverty-driven disruptions to cognitive, motor, and emotional development that in turn negatively affect play, school, and social life and, ultimately, occupational choices and opportunities. These scholars also note, however, that negative outcomes may be mediated by personal and contextual factors such as caring and effective parenting, opportunities for educational attainment, positive social capital, and upward socioeconomic movement of the family (Leadley & Hocking, 2017).

In summary, there is an evolving interest not only in how human beings develop across the life course but also how occupations emerge, develop, and transform as they are influenced through human maturation and agency in transaction with social, historical, and cultural phenomena at particular times and in particular places. We next turn to a perspective external to our profession that foregrounds the influence of sociohistorical time and place on how human beings individually and collectively discover, learn, and adapt occupations.

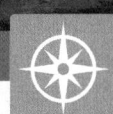

EXPANDING OUR PERSPECTIVES

Social History, Personal Contexts, and Occupations Transformed by COVID-19

Chi-Kwan Shea

The COVID-19 pandemic has significantly impacted our daily occupations. Reflecting on the past 2 years of on and off lockdowns and continuous insecurity in determining a safe social environment, I recognized several emergent

occupations that would likely persist beyond the pandemic. At the age of 65, a traditional retirement age in the United States, I am experiencing occupational transformation by adopting a new occupation of vegetable gardening, renewing a former occupation of pet caring, and expanding a current occupation of social activism.

The backyard of my suburban home is rather typical, with a few trees and a bunch of plants. Pre-COVID, my extent of gardening included pulling out a few weeds and

(continued)

trimming off a few dead branches every other month, usually no more than 15 minutes of yard work at a time. Teaching online afforded me more time to spend in my backyard, just to make connections with the outside world and get some fresh air. Growing vegetables became a peripheral idea that prompted my first attempt to plant a few herb seeds in a portable planter. Although the intended seeds did not germinate, an unintended tomato plant started to flourish. This serendipitous experience led me to plant vegetable seeds (cucumber, carrot, and lettuce) in a permanent planter. The only vegetable to emerge was the cucumber, which yielded bountiful. Having committed to eat organically since my breast cancer diagnosis 15 years ago, now I see the value of growing my own organic vegetables and tending my plants with thoughtfulness and care. This new occupation not only connects me to the mother earth but also brings me closer to my food source.

We had a family dog, Buster, for 15 years. Although the dog was intended for my children, I was the primary caregiver. After Buster died 13 years ago, I vowed not to care for another animal, feeling relieved from the burden of care and the sadness of loss. When my daughter decided to adopt a rescued dog during the pandemic, I first opposed vehemently but subsequently relented. Bucky became part of the family. As Bucky's grand-caregiver I spoil him as any grandparent would with their grandchildren. Once again, I take up the occupation of walking, feeding, playing, and cuddling with Bucky. Renewing this occupation brings me more joy than what I remembered when caring for Buster. I accept every opportunity to look after Bucky, who always lightens up my day.

From a young age, Catholicism taught me to care about social justice. Social activism is often in my mind and my heart but not much in my action. Certainly, I was marching with many others protesting a number of social justice issues over the years and had even spent a night in jail for blocking traffic. I often felt that these marches did not add up to anything. The murder of George Floyd by a police officer set off a worldwide storm of reaction

that I had never seen before. I took up serious reading, listened to lived experiences, attended trainings, and learned from experts about racism and self-reflection. As an Asian immigrant, I realized I was playing the role of a model minority, aligning myself with the dominant racial group, supporting policies that oppress others while not drawing attention to myself. This realization propelled me to commit to anti-racist activism, which started where I am employed. I assembled a Diversity, Equity, and Inclusion (DEI) task force to pursue holistic admission, DEI training for faculty, action-oriented support for the student chapter of the Coalition of Occupational Therapy Advocates for Diversity (COTAD), infusing DEI across academic curriculum, and better understanding the unique needs of our students of color. This expanded occupation of racial activism has been challenging but my commitment to DEI grows stronger by the day.

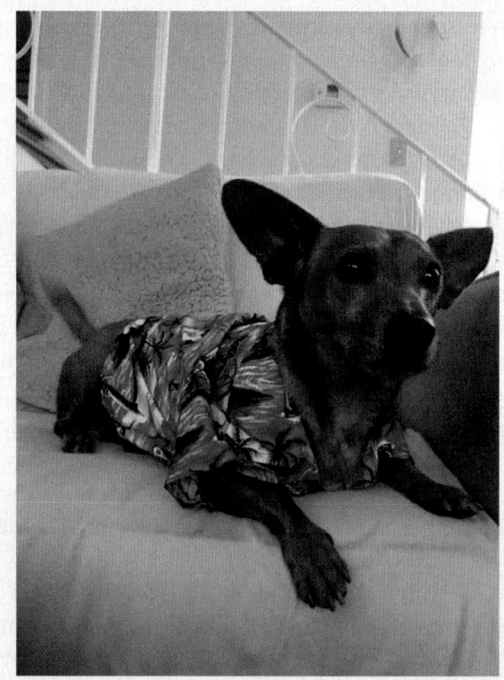

Bucky.

A Life Course Perspective on Occupational Possibilities

The ideas presented so far emphasize that the reasons people take up, change, or discontinue occupations extends beyond individual preferences and are contextually influenced. These changes represent dynamic transactions among people, places, and social and historical contexts, challenging us to think beyond conventional views of human development to understand how occupational changes occur. One theory external but complementary to OT that is useful in framing these processes is the life course perspective.

Originating with the work of sociologist Glen H. Elder, Jr. (1994, 1998) and evolving across multiple social sciences, the life course perspective, with its emphasis on sociohistorical influences on individual development and agency, serves as a guiding concept to understand how occupations emerge and transform over time. Life course theorists recognize that changes occur from birth to the end of life and are influenced across generations and within birth cohorts by sociohistorical events. Importantly, the life course perspective calls into question earlier developmental concepts emphasizing predictable age-based milestones, and instead argues for recognizing the impact of sociohistorical time and place on the physical, mental, social, and emotional changes occurring within the individual (Diewald & Mayer, 2009). For life course theorists, living is a highly situated, socially participatory process. They argue that we are born into birth cohorts or groups of people born at the same historical time, where the sum effect of the times and the people around us serves to create a trajectory or pathway for our lives (Elder & Shanahan, 2006). Within that pathway, we may have some individual agency, but that agency is more or less bounded depending on our life circumstances. Life transitions such as starting a family, emigration, or retirement are influenced by broader circumstances that shape these trajectories. Note the similarities between the life course perspective and Rudman's concept of occupational possibilities in the previous section.

Although life course theorists point us to consider the processes shaping people's lives, they do not explicitly use the term *occupation*. Nonetheless, the linkages made between individuals and context, viewed through the expanded temporality of a sociohistorical lens, are similar to the ways in which scholars and practitioners in occupational science and therapy are rethinking occupational development. Life course theorists consider *cohorts* as living through similar and particular social experiences. These experiences occur over the *trajectory* of a person's life and include typical *transitions*, or changes in roles and status,

as well as *turning points*, defined as changes that result in significant shifts in life trajectories. The types of experiences that shape a person's life, the things they do, and the things they are exposed to or have opportunities to do are reflected in the principles of life course theory outlined in Box 7.2.

The following story of a young girl named Coco shopping for food with her family (OT Story 7.2) is used to illustrate how a life course perspective expands our understanding of what people do that moves us beyond thinking about occupation in a given moment to embracing a more richly contextualized lens.

BOX 7.2 LIFE COURSE CONCEPTS AND PRINCIPLES

- *Sociohistorical time and place:* Historic times and societal events shape and alter what people do, how they do it, and give it meaning.
- *Linked lives:* People live interconnected lives, and these networks of relationships shape occupations.
- *Timing of lives:* Antecedents to an event or life transition and the consequences of such events for a person's occupations vary according to timing in the life course.
- *Human agency:* People make choices about their occupations, which reflect their circumstances and perceived occupational opportunities at that particular time.
- *Lifelong development:* Aging and transformations of occupations are lifelong processes; the accumulated experiences with past occupations impact current forms of engagement.

Sources: Adapted from Elder (1994) and Elder et al. (2003).

OT STORY 7.2 COCO SHOPPING FOR FOOD WITH HER FAMILY

Coco, a 6-year-old, is shopping with her uncle at an orchard and produce market in Durham, North Carolina, while visiting from out of town (Figure 7.2). She knows to carefully select just the right produce for the family's meal plans; this knowledge is linked not only to her immediate family's love of cooking but also to the choices they make about food that connects them to their community and their cultural heritage. This particular orchard where Coco and her uncle are shopping is a Black-owned independent produce market that has been in business for over 50 years, and is the largest and oldest business of its kind in the area (http://www.perkinsorchard.com). Currently managed by the grandson of its founder, who took it over at the age of 10 (!), it has grown into a thriving center for the community. For Coco and her family, supporting local fresh food growers

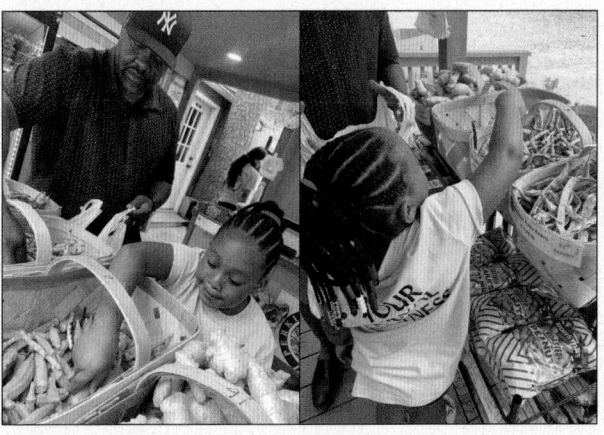

FIGURE 7.2 Coco shopping with her uncle.

(continued)

OT STORY 7.2 COCO SHOPPING FOR FOOD WITH HER FAMILY (*continued*)

and markets is an intentional commitment to honor African American traditions of gardening, sharing the fruit of the harvest, and continuing to use ancestral recipes.

From a life course perspective, Coco's occupation can be understood through several of the principles we have outlined in Box 7.2:

- *Sociohistorical time and place*: Coco is taught by her family the importance of honoring ancestral traditions at a time in US history when Black-owned businesses are experiencing increased support in response to racial unrest, despite challenges because of the COVID-19 pandemic (Keshner, 2021). At a more local level, the market where Coco and her family are shopping is situated in a city that has a history of Black entrepreneurism dating from the early 1900s. Today the city of Durham highlights Black-owned businesses via an online marketing arrangement in order to honor and further this legacy (Discover Durham, 2021).
- *Linked lives:* Coco is enacting a family occupation on an outing with her aunt and uncle, but her entire family and their wider social circles are involved in cooking and enjoying meals together. With the choice to shop at this particular orchard, Coco's life is also linked to that of the founders of the business, and to a Black community that chooses to intentionally support one another in business endeavors. She learns from these experiences the linkages to her ancestors as well as her immediate family through food-related occupations.
- *Timing of lives:* Had Coco been born earlier, she may have experienced a commitment to this business within her family and immediate community, but growing up in the current sociohistorical time and place also situates her

in a broader social conversation. Beyond the discourse related to racial equity, however, Coco is growing up in a time when the ways in which people obtain and consume food are being questioned from a standpoint of sustainability as well as ethics (Navin, 2014). Although we cannot know how Coco will regard her early exposure to food-related occupations later in her life, at present she is actively engaged in her family's commitment to locally grown food, which is a continuation of her heritage as well as a current social emphasis. Taking into account *lifelong development*, her experiences with food will continue to evolve but also remain anchored to the present time.

- *Human agency*: Coco is being actively taught to select food ingredients for cooking at a young age, and she enacts her role confidently in this context. Whereas societal norms in the United States suggest that children her age are not typically responsible for food shopping, her agency in this situation is supported by her uncle's presence and her previous experiences with food shopping as a co-occupation. She is also shopping in a context in which youth, as exemplified by the current manager of the orchard, is not a deterrent to knowledge about, or competence with, food-related occupations.

Questions

1. How is Coco's involvement in food shopping and preparation at a relatively young age supported by her context?
2. Consider an occupation that you have been involved in since childhood. Using the life course principles, explore the influences on how your occupation has developed over time.

Employing expanded concepts of human and occupational development to understand Coco's occupation of food shopping with her uncle allows us to grasp how this occupation is connected through time to others, to societal context, and to cultural traditions. Although we see a single young person enacting it, the occupational situation is simultaneously interpersonal, cultural, and societal in nature, reflecting both transactional (Dickie et al., 2006) and life course perspectives on human development (Elder, 1994; Elder & Shanahan, 2006; Elder et al., 2003) and pressing us to consider the actions of human beings within sociohistorical time and place.

For our final section, we turn to the implications of this expanded view of occupational development and its relationship to human development. Adopting terminology from the life course perspective, we situate recipients of OT as facing turning points in their life trajectories, and clinical practice as a mechanism that may shape those trajectories.

Turning Points: Implications for Clinical Practice

OT practitioners work with people who need or want to acquire new occupations, or to change existing occupations in anticipated or unanticipated ways. Turning points may be anticipated, such as a transition to college for a young adult, or a move to a new geographic location with a job change. Unanticipated turning points occur in situations such as traumatic accidents, or a medical diagnosis. For some, the turning points may alter their sense of self or relationship to others. For others, the turning points reinforce past life experiences, allowing them to draw from those experiences to further develop their occupations.

Returning to the example of Felix featured in Table 7.1, we see a child who is at a turning point. His life trajectory is altered by adoption into a family that is seeking services to evaluate and address his developmental delays. An OT practitioner who embraces a contextual view on human development will tap into factors beyond the structure and function of Felix's body, employing strategies to harness multilayered influences that will optimize his occupational development and participation.

Conclusion and Challenge

A colleague once observed that occupations are complex and messy. Embracing life course and transactional perspectives to understand occupational development helps to manage this messiness by recognizing a multitude of factors shaping how occupations emerge, develop, and transform over the span of life. In looking at the family engaged in yoga, we saw that age of the individual is not the primary factor in learning to do something new. Whereas the grandmother had reflected on the benefits of exercise and saw yoga offering a desired outcome, the granddaughter, without reflection, learned it as a natural family routine. In considering Coco and the co-occupation of food shopping, the influence of family and community, as well as sociohistorical influences on choices made about that occupation come into clearer focus. Coco's family members are passing on a cultural heritage and identity as well as food preparation skills through their intentional way of involving her in this occupation.

So, what does the content of this chapter challenge us as practitioners of OT to incorporate into our therapeutic processes in order to honor the myriad influences on occupational development? In closing, we offer four potential actions:

1. Choose assessment tools and procedures that reflect the complexity of occupation rather than focusing on discrete capacities of the human being.
2. Debunk the notions that optimal engagement in occupation can be predicted based on rigid notions of developmental milestones, age, or life stage.
3. Shift the view of the client from an individual perspective to a situational perspective in order to understand contextual factors influencing their occupational performance.
4. Become more familiar with policy and societal discourse that impacts practice as well as the lives of those who are service recipients.

Acknowledgment

The authors acknowledge Dr. Ruth Humphry, lead author of previous versions of this chapter, for her pioneering work in reconceptualizing human development through an occupational lens.

Lippincott® Connect *For additional resources on the subjects discussed in this chapter, visit* Lippincott Connect.

REFERENCES

Aldrich, R. M. (2008). From complexity theory to transactionalism: Moving occupational science forward in theorizing the complexities of behavior. *Journal of Occupational Science, 15*, 147–156. https://doi.org/10.1080/14427591.2008.9686624

Attree, P. (2006). The social costs of child poverty: A systematic review of the qualitative evidence. *Children & Society, 20*, 54–66. https://doi.org/10.1002/CHI.854

Baltes, P. B. (1989). The dynamics between growth and decline. *Contemporary Psychology, 34*, 983–984. https://doi.org/10.1037/030715

Bazyk, S., Stalnaker, D., Llerena, M. Ekelman, B., & Bazyk, J. (2003). Play in Mayan children. *American Journal of Occupational Therapy, 57*, 273–283. https://doi.org/10.5014/ajot.57.3.273

Boyle, M. (2009). Book Review of Occupational therapy with children: Understanding children's occupations and enabling participation (Eds: Rodger & Ziviani). *International Journal of Disability, Development & Education, 56*(1), 97–98. https://doi.org/10.1080/10349120802682125

Canadian Association of Occupational Therapists. (2016). *CAOT Lexicon. (Doc. No. 6647).* https://www.caot.ca/document/6647/CAOTLexicon.pdf

Carroll, A., Chan, D., Thorpe, D., Levin, I., & Bagatell, N. (2021). A life course perspective on growing older with cerebral palsy. *Qualitative Health Research, 31*(4), 654–664. https://doi.org/10.1177/1049732320971247

Choi, J., Cutler, A., & Broersma, M. (2017). Early development of abstract language knowledge: Evidence from perception–production transfer of birth-language memory. *Royal Society Open Science, 4*, 160660. https://doi.org/10.1098/rsos.160660

Coster, W. (1998). Occupation-centered assessment of children. *American Journal of Occupational Therapy, 52*, 337–344. https://doi.org/10.5014/ajot.52.5.337

Crosnoe, R., & Elder, G. (2002). Successful adaptation in the later years: A life course approach to aging. *Social Psychology Quarterly, 65*, 309–328. https://doi.org/10.2307/3090105

Cutchin, M. P., & Dickie, V. A. (Eds.). (2013). *Transactional perspectives on occupation.* Springer.

d'Entremont, L. Gregor, M. Kirou, E., Nelligan, L., & Dennis, D. (2017). Developmental milestones for productivity occupations in children and youth. *Work, 56*, 75–89. https://doi.org/10.3233/WOR-162466

Dickie, V., Cutchin, M., & Humphry, R. (2006). Occupation as transactional experience: A critique of individualism in occupational science. *Journal of Occupational Science, 13*, 83–93. https://doi.org/10.1080/14427591.2006.9686573

Diewald, M., & Mayer, K. U. (2009). The sociology of the life course and life span psychology: Integrated paradigm or complementing pathways? *Advances in Life Course Research, 14*, 5–14. https://doi.org/10.1016/j.alcr.2009.03.001

Discover Durham. (2021). *Durham's Black-owned businesses.* https://www.discoverdurham.com/community-culture/black-history/black-owned-businesses/

Elder, G. H. (1994). Time, human agency, and social change: Perspectives on the life course. *Social Psychology Quarterly, 57*(1), 4–15. https://doi.org/10.2307/2786971

Elder, G. H. (1998). The life course as developmental theory. *Child Development, 69*(1), 1–12. https://doi.org/10.1111/j.1467-8624.1998.tb06128.x

Elder, G. H., Johnson, M. K., & Crosnoe, R. (2003). The emergence and development of life course theory. In J. T. Mortimer & M. J. Shanahan (Eds.), *Handbook of the life course. Handbooks of sociology and social research.* Springer. https://doi.org/10.1007/978-0-306-48247-2_1

Elder, G. H., & Shanahan, M. J. (2006). The life course and human development. In R. M. Lerner & W. Damon (Eds.), *Handbook of child psychology: Theoretical models of human development* (pp. 665–715). John Wiley & Sons.

Emde, R. N. (1989). The infant's relationship experience: Developmental and affective aspects. In A. Sameroff & R. Emde (Eds.), *Relationship disturbances in early childhood: A developmental approach* (pp. 33–51). Basic Books.

Engeström, Y. (1999). Activity theory and individual and social transformation. In Y. Engeström, R. Miettinen, & R. L. Punamaki (Eds.), *Perspectives on activity theory* (pp. 19–38). Cambridge University Press.

Gauvain, M. (2001). Cultural tools, social interaction and the development of thinking. *Human Development, 44*, 126–143. https://doi.org/10.1159/000057052

Hedegaard, M. (2009). Children's development from a cultural-historical approach: Children's activity in everyday local setting as foundation for their development. *Mind, Culture, and Activity, 16*, 64–82. https://doi.org/10.1080/10749030802477374

Hocking, C., & Wright-St. Clair, V. (2017). Editorial: Special issue on inclusion and participation. *Journal of Occupational Science, 24*(1), 1–4. https://doi.org/10.1080/14427591.2017.1299560

Humphry, R. (2002). Young children's occupational behaviors: Explicating the dynamics of developmental processes. *American Journal of Occupational Therapy, 56*, 171–179. https://doi.org/10.5014/ajot.56.2.171

Humphry, R. (2005). Model of processes transforming occupations: Exploring societal and social influences. *Journal of Occupational Science, 12*, 36–41. https://doi.org/10.1080/14427591.2005.9686546

Humphry, R. (2016). Joining in, interpretative reproduction, and transformations of occupations: What is "know-how" anyway? *Journal of Occupational Science, 23*, 422–433. https://doi.org/10.1080/14427591.2016.1210000

Humphry, R., & Wakeford, L. (2006). An occupation-centered discussion of development and implications for practice. *American Journal of Occupational Therapy, 60*(3), 258–267. https://doi.org/10.5014/ajot.60.3.258

Humphry, R., & Wakeford, L. (2008). Development of everyday activities: A model for occupation-centered therapy. *Infants & Young Children: An Interdisciplinary Journal of Early Childhood Intervention, 21*(3), 230–240. https://doi.org/10.1097/01.iyc.0000324552.77564.98

Humphry, R., & Womack, J. (2019). Transformations of occupations: A life course perspective. In B. Schell & G. Gillen (Eds.), *Willard and Spackman's occupational therapy* (13th ed., pp. 100-112). Wolters Kluwer.

Keshner, A. (2021). *"If ever there's a time for progress, the time is now": Are more Americans supporting Black-owned businesses? MarketWatch.* https://www.marketwatch.com/story/more-consumers-have-been-looking-to-spend-money-at-black-owned-businesses-people-are-rallying-around-small-business-11619045035

Lachman, M. E. (2004). Development in midlife. *Annual Review of Psychology, 55*, 305–331. https://doi.org/10.1146/annurev.psych.55.090902.141521

Lave, J., & Packer, M. (2008). Towards a social ontology of learning. In K. Nielsen, S. Brinkmann, C. Elmholdt, & G. Kraft (Eds.), *A qualitative stance: In memory of Steinar Kvale, 1938–2008* (pp. 17–47). Aarhus University Press.

Lave, J., & Wenger, E. (1991). *Situated learning: Legitimate peripheral participation.* Cambridge University Press.

Lawlor, M. (2003). The significance of being occupied: The social construction of childhood occupations. *American Journal of Occupational Therapy, 57*, 424–434. https://doi.org/10.5014/ajot.57.4.424

Leadley, S., & Hocking, C. (2017). An occupational perspective on childhood poverty. *New Zealand Journal of Occupational Therapy, 64*, 23–31.

Leclair, L., Ali, S., & Finlayson, M. (2018). Creating opportunities for occupational development using the concerns report method. *Scandinavian Journal of Occupational Therapy, 25*(5), 313–324. https://doi.org/10.1080/11038128.2018.1502346

McNamara, P., & Humphry, R. (2008). Developing everyday routines. *Physical & Occupational Therapy in Pediatrics, 28*(2), 141–154. https://doi.org/10.1080/01942630802031826

Navin, M. C. (2014). Local food and international ethics. *Journal of Agricultural and Environmental Ethics, 27*, 349–368. https://doi.org/10.1007/s10806-014-9492-0

Njelesani, J., Davis, J. A., & Pontes, T. (2020). Occupational Repertoire Development Measure—Parent (ORDM-P): Face validity, comprehensiveness, and internal consistency. *British Journal of Occupational Therapy, 83*, 326–333. https://doi.org/10.1177/0308022619885247

Peterson, C. C. (2003) Lifespan human development. In J. P. Keeves et al. (Eds.), *International handbook of educational research in the Asia-Pacific region. Springer International Handbooks of Education* (Vol. 11). Springer. https://doi.org/10.1007/978-94-017-3368-7_27

Pikkarainen, A., Vähäsantanen, K., Paloniemi, S., & Eteläpelto, A. (2015). Older rehabilitees' life-course agency in Finnish gerontological rehabilitation. *Scandinavian Journal of Occupational Therapy, 22*(6), 424–434. https://doi.org/10.3109/11038128.2015.1057221

Price, P., & Stephenson, S. M. (2009). Learning to promote occupational development through co-occupation. *Journal of Occupational Science, 16*, 180–186. https://doi.org/10.1080/14427591.2009.9686660

Ramey, C. T., & Ramey, S. L. (1998). Early intervention and early experience. *American Psychologist, 53*(2), 109–120. https://doi.org/10.1037/0003-066X.53.2.109

Rodger, S., & Behr, A. K. (2017). *Occupation-centred practice with children: A practical guide for occupational therapists* (2nd ed.). Wiley Blackwell.

Rogoff, B. (2003). *The cultural nature of human development.* Oxford University Press.

Rowles, G. D. (2008). Place in occupational science: A life course perspective on the role of environmental context in the quest for meaning. *Journal of Occupational Science, 15*(3), 127–135. https://doi.org/10.1080/14427591.2008.9686622

Rudman, D. L. (2010). Occupational terminology: Occupational possibilities. *Journal of Occupational Science, 17*, 55–59. https://doi.org/10.1080/14427591.2010.9686673

Rudman, D. L. (2015). Situating occupation in social relations of power: Occupational possibilities, ageism and the retirement "choice." *South African Journal of Occupational Therapy, 45*(1), 27–33. https://doi.org/10.17159/2310-3833/2015/v45no1a5

Segal, N. L. (1997). Twin research perspective on human development. In N. L. Segal, G. E. Weisfeld, & C. C. Weisfeld (Eds.), *Uniting psychology and biology: Integrative perspectives on human development* (pp. 145–173). American Psychological Association. https://doi.org/10.1037/10242-003

Siegler, R. S. (2000). The rebirth of children's learning. *Child Development, 71*, 26–35. https://doi.org/10.1111/1467-8624.00115

Stern, D. N. (1994). One way to build a clinically relevant baby. *Infant Mental Health Journal, 15*(1), 9–25. https://doi.org/10.1002/1097-0355(199421)15:1<9::AID-IMHJ2280150103>3.0.CO;2-V

Thelen, E. (2000). Grounded in the world: Developmental origins of the embodied mind. *Infancy, 1*, 3–28. https://doi.org/10.1207/S15327078IN0101_02

Townsend, E., & Polatajko, H. (Eds.). (2007). *Enabling occupation II: Advancing an occupational therapy vision for health, well-being, and justice through occupation.* CAOT Publications ACE.

Tronick, E. (1998). Dyadically expanded states of consciousness and the process of therapeutic change. *Infant Mental Health Journal, 19*(3), 290–299. https://doi.org/10.1002/(SICI)1097-0355(199823)19:3<290::AID-IMHJ4>3.0.CO;2-Q

Westerhof, G. J., Dittmann-Kohli, F., & Thissen, T. (2001). Beyond life satisfaction: Lay conceptions of well-being among middle-aged and elderly adults. *Social Indicators Research, 56*, 179–203. https://doi.org/10.1023/A:1012455124295

Wilcock, A. A. (2006). *An occupational perspective of health* (2nd ed.). Slack.

Wiseman, J. O., Davis, J. A., & Polatajko, H. J. (2005). Occupational development: Toward an understanding of children's doing. *Journal of Occupational Science, 12*, 26–35. https://doi.org/10.1080/14427591.2005.9686545

Ziviani, J., Macdonald, D., Ward, H., Jenking, D., & Rodger, S. (2006). Physical activity and occupations of children: Perspectives of parents and children. *Journal of Occupational Science, 13*, 180–187. https://doi.org/10.1080/14427591.2006.9726514

Contribution of Occupation to Health and Well-Being

Clare Hocking and Daniel Sutton

LEARNING OBJECTIVES

After reading this chapter, you will be able to:

1. Describe, in occupational terms, what being healthy means and how that relates to the Ottawa Charter and Healthy People 2030.
2. Explore ways that being included in occupation contributes to the health and well-being of all people.
3. Drawing on the international literature, describe positive and negative health impacts of people's overall pattern of occupation.
4. Analyze how well-being and inclusion might be influenced by people's physical, social, and attitudinal environment.
5. Reflecting on your own community, identify a group whose "belonging through doing" is constrained and outline possible negative health impacts.
6. Analyze how having an impairment might affect well-being, taking environmental barriers into account.

Introduction

On a clear but cold Saturday morning, Amy joins hundreds of children playing team sports in her community. She locates her soccer team, the Blue Stars, for stretches and drills before their first game of the season. While they wait, their parents greet each other and share stories from the summer break, renewing the strong connections built up over the years the team has played together. Once the warm-up is completed, the coach gathers the team together to talk about the tactics and skills to work on: keeping their structure and accurate passing. Amy takes in his advice before joining in the team chant and taking her place on the pitch. The referee's whistle goes, and the game begins. From the sidelines, Amy's parents and grandparents cheer the team on. Her grandfather and both parents played soccer, so as she runs, tackles, and passes the ball, Amy is carrying on a family tradition.

Amy loves being part of a team. As a midfielder, she does a lot of running to link the backs and forwards. At times she runs out of breath and gets frustrated when she misses a tackle, but she thrives on the challenge and physicality of the game (Figure 8.1). There is a real sense of achievement when the team works together to score a goal. At half-time, the Blue Stars are winning, and they refresh with oranges and water while listening to their coach.

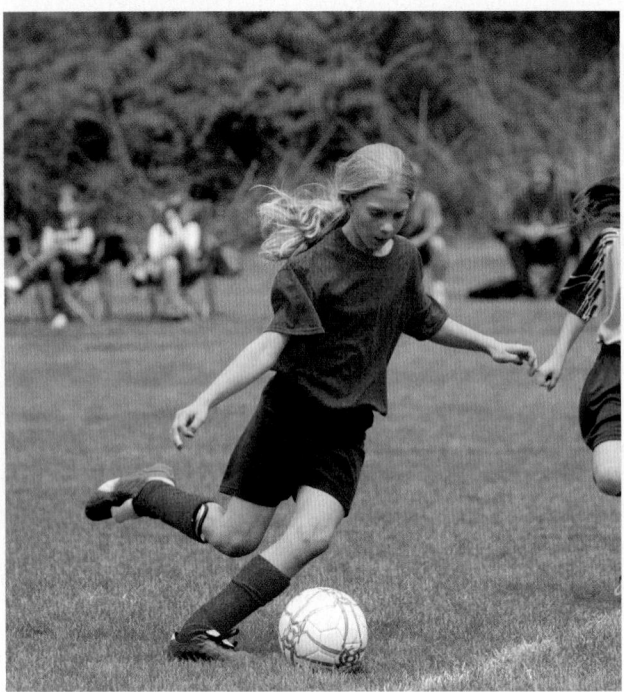

FIGURE 8.1 **Amy playing soccer.**

He is happy with their progress but encourages them to keep focusing on their roles in the team. When the final whistle blows the Blue Stars have won, and the teams exchange high fives before leaving the field physically exhausted. The coach calls them into a huddle to praise their performance and join the team chant. It is a great start to the season.

Although Amy doesn't think of it in these terms, her game of soccer epitomizes the interrelationship of occupation, health, well-being, and a sense of inclusion. We tease those relationships out in the first section of the chapter and, as a counterpoint, share Roshan Galvaan's confronting realization that social inequality can threaten those relationships. Mechanisms that help explain how occupation affects people's health, their sense of well-being, and social inclusion are addressed in the following section. To conclude the chapter, we turn to evidence that human development and our patterns of occupation impact health; that the amount of occupation we engage in is important for health; and finally, bring disability and ill-health into the picture. Overall, the chapter demonstrates that it is not just what we do as individuals, but also how well people get along and include each other that shape people's health and well-being.

Occupation, Health, Well-Being, and Inclusion

Playing soccer has many of the elements people in Western societies associate with being healthy, including physical, mental, emotional, and behavioral development, and functioning (Office of Disease Prevention and Health Promotion [ODPHP], 2021a). For this 13-year-old, there were physical benefits from exercising major muscle groups to maintain fitness, stamina, and balance. Amy was fully engaged, experienced a sense of accomplishment and pride in her team's efforts, and gained a sense of belonging from playing her part, supported by the coach, her parents, and grandparents. Playing soccer also stimulated the players' mental capacities through needing to understand and apply tactics, "read" the game, and follow the rules. The game afforded a challenge but was not beyond the players' capacity; rather, it was an exhilarating union of body, mind, and spirit. There were social rewards from inclusion in a culturally valued occupation and, for all involved, the renewal of friendships and team spirit reinforced the value of community and fair play. Other elements of the context were also beneficial to the soccer community's well-being: having safe open spaces to play, clean air and drinking water, and acceptance of girls' and women's right to participate in sports (United Nations, 2007). Consistent with the World Health Organization's (WHO) view that health is more than the absence of disease (WHO, 2018a), the soccer season will contribute to individual, team, and community well-being. Occupational therapists might also note the alignment of occupation and health, which people in Western societies often describe as being able "to do what and when you want to do it" and "take care of myself" (Tkatch et al., 2017), as well as how playing soccer fits Wilcock and Hocking's (2015) description of doing, being, belonging, and becoming.

Occupational therapy (OT) exists as a profession because, in some circumstances, people experience great difficulty engaging in occupations that support health and well-being. Unlike Amy, many people either cannot access or do not engage in opportunities for physical exercise. Only one in four adults in the United States, and only one in five adolescents, meet the physical activity guidelines in Healthy People 2030 (ODPHP, 2021d). For some sectors of the population, access to health-giving occupations can be hindered, or even barred, by "social problems, persistent poverty, economic restrictions, disease, social discrimination, displacement, natural and man-made disasters, armed conflict, [and] historic disadvantage" (World Federation of Occupational Therapists [WFOT], 2019). Paradoxically, taking up harmful occupations might be motivated by socially sanctioned goals, such as using substances to reduce anxiety or enhance "productivity especially in jobs that require stamina, long hours, and hard work" (Sy et al., 2020, p. 17). In addition, people can struggle to relinquish occupations with well-known detrimental health effects, such as cigarette smoking. Finally doing so may stimulate a cascade of health-promoting occupational changes, including restructuring eating habits, taking up exercise, and replacing smoking with more satisfying occupations that reinforce an identity of no longer being driven by addiction to nicotine

(Luck & Beagan, 2015). Societies play an important role in the reduction of harmful occupations, such as through legislation making provisions for smoke-free public places and taxes that make consuming tobacco, alcohol, and sugar increasingly unaffordable.

While occupational therapists working alone cannot ensure healthy lives and social inclusion for all, bringing an occupational perspective to these problems can generate powerful new insights. For example, findings across studies with people with mental illness indicate recovery is an ongoing occupational process that seems to involve experiences of gradual re-engagement, progressing from engaging within the stream of everyday occupational life to full community participation. Engaging in valued occupations appears to support recovery through fostering connectedness, hope, identity, meaning, and empowerment, and through establishing structured routines (Doroud et al., 2015). At a population level, opportunities for people in vulnerable circumstances to be, belong, and become through doing can be opened up through collaborative action guided by the Participatory Occupational Justice Framework (Whiteford et al., 2018).

An appreciation of the relationship between occupation and health—and how both of those hinge on inclusion—is also prominent in a WHO document, the Ottawa Charter (WHO, 1986). This influential public health policy document sought to promote broad understandings of the determinants of health. Its key concept is that health is a resource people create in their everyday lives, using their physical capacities and personal and social resources. More formally, that means having the capacity to function, meet one's needs, be productive, realize one's hopes and expectations, and participate in society. Conversely, ill-health is associated with having symptoms, such as low mood or pain that interrupt occupation, in contexts where not enough is done to enable people with a health condition to participate. While these perspectives on health are grounded in occupation, focusing on individual experiences and health conditions does not tell the full story. The "Black Lives Matter" movement is a powerful reminder that many groups in society are excluded from fair and just opportunities to experience health through doing, because of discrimination, poverty, colonization, and other circumstances (Farias & Simaan, 2020; McCartney et al., 2019). Thus, access to both occupation and health must be considered from the perspective of equity and human rights, because occupation can only confer health benefits on the people who are included, and experiences of being excluded can, in themselves, be detrimental to health.

One aspect of considering health and occupation from an equity perspective is whose definition of health and occupation is used as the reference point. The Indigenous perspectives beginning to be discussed in the OT literature are enriching the conversation. One important idea is the balance among physical, mental, emotional, and spiritual health, with no single aspect dominating (Fijal & Beagan, 2019), which fits well with understanding within OT that participation in occupation can be personally and culturally meaningful, as well as physically demanding, cognitively challenging, and elicit powerful emotional responses. Further, concepts of physical, mental, emotional, and spiritual health apply not only to the person. For example, Doyle et al. (2013) described how playing sports was a key facilitator in developing collective well-being, positive cultural identity, and spiritual strength for Aboriginal people of the Goulburn–Murray Rivers region in Australia. Others have described how the emotional health and well-being of Indigenous communities is nurtured through talking to Elders and regularly connecting with the land (Fijal & Beagan, 2019), and that fulfilling their responsibility to care for the land and other life forms can restore the health and well-being of the tribe (McNeill, 2017).

Another important message from the Ottawa Charter is that to attain complete well-being, "an individual or group must be able to identify and to realize aspirations, to satisfy needs, and to change or cope with the environment" (WHO, 1986, p. 1). In these days of escalating awareness of environmental degradation, we are reminded that human well-being is inextricably bound to the health of local and global ecosystems (Wilcock & Hocking, 2015). What we do affects the natural environment, while changes in the natural environment inevitably affect what we do. For instance, if Amy lived in a region with water shortages, access to sports might be restricted due to a lack of water for rehydration, inability to wash oneself and sports uniforms, lack of grass to play on, and limited time for training due the time spent fetching water from a distant source (Wrisdale et al., 2017). Therefore, changing global ecosystems may result in the need to reduce or adapt current occupations to ensure not only the well-being of humans but also the natural environment that sustains us.

As the discussion to this point reveals, the relationships between occupation, well-being, and inclusion are highly complex and multifaceted. In addressing that complexity, this chapter prioritizes understandings generated by occupational therapists and occupational scientists. Accordingly, the term *occupation* refers to the things people do that they find personally and culturally meaningful, whereas *participation* is used in the more restricted sense of whether a person actually engages in occupation. To give the discussion depth, evidence reported in literature from around the world is included. The discussion proceeds by considering some of the ways occupation contributes to health and well-being. That includes what can be learned by its absence, when people are deprived of sufficient occupation. There is also discussion of the ways occupation can be injurious to health. Contextual factors that act as barriers to achieving good health are also described before concluding with a brief summation of the evidence.

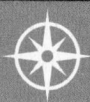

EXPANDING OUR PERSPECTIVES

Thinking, Doing, and Possibilities
in Everyday Life

Roshaan Galvan

Early in my study with young adolescents living in Lavender Hill, a low socioeconomic community in South Africa, I was driving with Monash and her friends, my research participants. Despite the differences in our age, educational achievement, and socioeconomic class, I felt that we were forming an open relationship in which, at times, she was comfortable to negotiate with me to drive her somewhere. As we approached her home, Monash and her friends started talking about the infant car seat in my car, and then, me. They were puzzled about my identity, discussing what differentiated us and tentatively concluded that I was a White person.

Since we shared a race identity, I was deeply perplexed by their conclusion. I had carefully and intentionally set out to form a collaborative relationship with them. Up to that point, I was confident that we had bridged the usual hierarchy of researcher and subject. Using colloquialisms, I inquired into what led them to think I was White. Their assumptions emerged: I was White because I was driving a car that I seemed to own, speaking English as my first language, had a car seat in the car, and worked at the university. Monash and her friends were alarmed as I explained myself to them, describing how, although constrained by socioeconomic factors, these markers could be accessible for people like us in South Africa. Learning more about the girls' assumptions revealed beliefs steeped in social inequality and White superiority.

I could see how our apartheid history and capitalistic ideals still showed up in their beliefs of inferiority. Listening to them opened up a space for us to reflect. Their imaginations and choices were tunnel visioned by what was available within their constraining context. Anything beyond were the assets, spaces, and occupations of White, or rich, people. Risk-taking behavior and poor mental health were part of their norm. While education may be one pathway out of such destiny, our education system conformed to Eurocentric norms and values. The curricula at local schools tended to alienate learners, leaving them with little confidence or pride in their cultural and linguistic heritages and wisdom. This meant that adolescents, like Monash, were often alienated and many learners ended up dropping out of high school.

As a therapist practicing in schools, I wanted to pursue fairer opportunities for adolescents. Catching opportunities for dialogue and talking about some of the gaps in their assumptions and beliefs gave space for something different to come about. Different thinking, different doing, possibilities for changing everyday life. Sometimes it was about doing something new, or, doing something in a new place. At other times it was about changing perspectives of what, how, or who could participate. We could recognize the past in the present. We strove to make changes that affirmed adolescents' power to not repeat age-old patterns. We saw possibilities and hope for a future that surpassed our restraining sociohistorical contexts. With this hope came power.

How Occupation Contributes to Health, Well-Being, and Inclusion

If we are to assert that occupation helps keep individuals and communities in good health, we need to understand how that comes about. Ann Wilcock, an eminent occupational scientist, considered that question from a biological perspective. She argued that occupation is essential to individual and species survival, because meeting basic biological needs requires people to act to secure sustenance, shelter, and safety and to keep themselves and their surroundings clean. Thus, societies across the globe have honed contextually relevant "skills, social structures and technology" (Wilcock, 1993, p. 20) to gather, grow, and cook nutritious food, construct clothing and dry homes, and negotiate ways of living peacefully with neighbors (see Figure 8.2).

Humans' capacity for occupation springs from our anatomical and cognitive characteristics: walking upright, opposable thumb and fingers to grasp objects, vocal cords

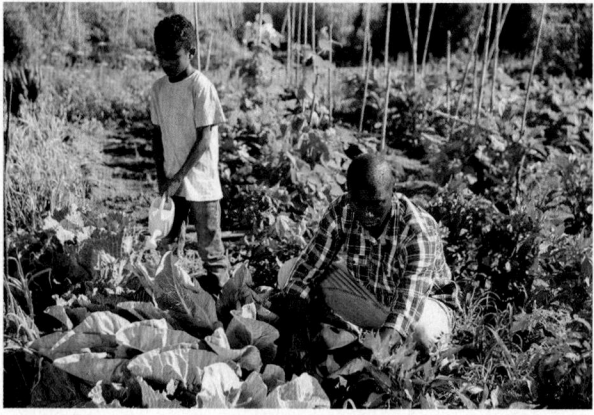

FIGURE 8.2 **Societies develop skills and technologies to grow nutritious food.**

and brain structures to produce and comprehend speech, and so on. In combination, those biological features allow us to, among other things, carry loads, design new tools and find novel uses for old ones, understand the workings of the universe, accumulate and pass on knowledge, predict what might happen and prepare for the future, play, form relationships, and express ourselves artistically and spiritually (Wilcock, 1993, 1995). Developing and exercising these capacities, Wilcock (1993) proposed, relates first to taking action to relieve the discomfort experienced from threats to our physiological state, such as seeking out shade when excessively hot or looking for food when hungry (Figure 8.3). Beyond ensuring a basic level of comfort, a surge of energy might propel us to acquire and practice skills that Wilcock termed protective and preventive, which enable us to solve problems and plan, interact with others, generate a livelihood, and so on. In so doing, at least before technology removed many of the physical demands of earlier lifestyles, people exercised their capacities for physical, mental, and social functioning. Feeling a sense of purpose, satisfaction, and fulfillment also prompts and rewards the use of our capacity to engage in occupation. According to Wilcock (1993), biological needs that stimulate occupation include:

1. Correcting threats to physiological state
2. Acquiring skills to protect and prevent
3. Engaging in occupations for prompts and rewards

Each person's capacities reflect their human potential via their genetic inheritance, brought into being through a developmental process and a unique life history of occupational engagement. The particular capacities a person develops reflect their natural aptitudes, as well as their preferences, choices, opportunities, and constraints. However, occupational opportunities and choices are not equally distributed. Youths growing up in an overcrowded and impoverished community established during the apartheid era in South Africa, for example, have few realistic options to choose from as they move into adulthood (Galvaan, 2015). From an occupational perspective, they are trapped in a vicious cycle. As members of a community living in vulnerable circumstances, they experience social exclusion, poor quality education, and limited access to resources. Their restricted opportunities diminish the capacities they can develop and their aspirations which, over time, see them turn to occupations they know will harm their health and longevity, and further impede their capacity for occupational pursuits that might lead to a better future.

At a societal level, failure to optimize citizens' occupational potential represents a tremendous waste. Everyone's health and well-being is optimized by living and working cooperatively, with each person benefiting from others' specialized skills, knowledge, resources, and labor. When diverse people are included, the whole community gains from the additional skills, knowledge, resources, and economic productivity they contribute (Wilcock & Hocking, 2015). Shared occupations are one means of enhancing cooperation and inclusion. Doing things together is a way to welcome and include people, helping them get to know and accept each other, while providing experiences of inclusion for all those who participate. Whichever way we view it, inclusive societies have health and well-being benefits for all.

Evidence That Occupation Affects Health and Well-Being

It is widely acknowledged that occupation benefits health. The Physical Activity Guidelines for Americans (U.S. Department of Health and Human Services, 2018) is one of many authoritative sources asserting that participation in occupations involving physical exertion improves "cardiovascular and muscle fitness, brain health, and ability to do tasks of daily life" (p. 81) (see Figure 8.4).

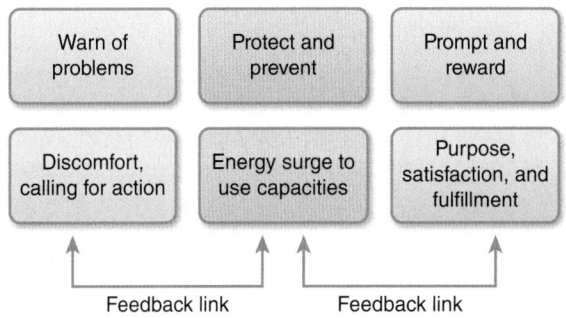

FIGURE 8.3 Biological hierarchy of need for occupation.

(Adapted from Wilcock, A. [1993]. A theory of the human need for occupation. *Journal of Occupational Science, 1*, 17–24. https://doi.org/10.1080/14427591.1993.9686375.)

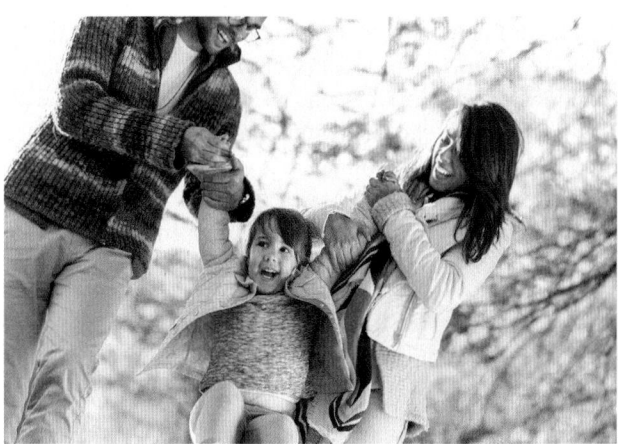

FIGURE 8.4 **Physical exertion through play.**

Healthy People 2030 promotes a broad range of occupations for health, including biking, playing ball games, community gardening, volunteering, and engaging in various sports (ODPHP, 2021b). It advances multiple strategies to encourage people to increase and sustain physical activity levels, such as setting up buddy systems or walking groups, or making a contract with someone to do a specific amount of exercise. All age and ability levels are targeted, including people with diagnosed health conditions and disabilities (ODPHP, 2021e). While emphasizing physical activity levels, Healthy People 2030 also addresses broader health and well-being outcomes (ODPHP, 2021a). These include promoting children's mental, emotional, and behavioral development by reading to them, helping them do well at school, and ensuring they get enough sleep. School curriculum changes are suggested to make it easier for children with obesity to eat healthy food and get sufficient exercise to reduce both their weight and the risk of being bullied. Increasing access to workplaces, homes, schools, and public venues is also recommended to decrease the stress experienced by people with disabilities as they struggle to get a job, go to school, and get around in their communities (ODPHP, 2021f).

The contribution of occupation to ill-health is also recognized, with smoking and alcohol abuse frequently singled out. Within occupational science, occupations that are harmful, illegal, or deviant have been labeled non-sanctioned (Kiepek et al., 2019) or "on the dark side"—meaning occupations that have been less studied (Twinley, 2021)—so that the practices themselves, their meanings, and how people are inducted into and desist from participation are less understood. The limited research undertaken to date points to complex identity, addiction, affiliation, thrill-seeking, experiential, and environmental factors that sustain participation despite the known risks. People's experience of occupations, and thus its contribution to health or ill-health, is affected by environmental and societal conditions. Discrimination based on ethnicity, gender, age, disability, or other individual characteristics is increasingly recognized to cause intentional or unintentional harm to physical and emotional health. Examples include everyday experiences of disrespectful and uncourteous behavior in shops and restaurants, unfair dismissal from work, and residential segregation, with flow-on effects to the quality of schooling and employment available. Routine discrimination is a chronic stressor, which increases vulnerability to physical illness, as well as being associated with risky occupations including smoking, alcohol abuse, and unprotected sex (ODPHP, 2021c).

Health, Development, and Patterns of Occupation

The overall pattern of people's occupations is also important. Breaking up active participation in occupation with rest contributes to health, whether that is a short break to stretch before returning to computer work, work/rest schedules to enhance the effects of training, or prolonged engagement in restorative leisure occupations. Having a rest confers many benefits, one of which is that it enhances memory, with evidence that preschoolers remember new words better if they have a nap rather than doing something active after learning them (Sandoval et al., 2017). Rather than resting, however, there is new evidence that going for a fast walk more effectively alleviates the fatigue associated with monotonous work (Aramaki & Hagiwara, 2018).

As well as these short-term effects, people's longer term patterns of occupation influence health. For children and youth, there is a cause-and-effect relationship between reducing screen time and reduced weight gain, which can be explained by the association between consuming calorie-rich food while viewing, the types of foods and beverages marketed to them while watching, and reduced hours of sleep (Robinson et al., 2017). Vocational opportunities and choices also shape patterns of occupation and the consequent risk of harm, with fishing, hunting, logging, roofing and working in construction having the highest rates of work-related fatalities in the United States (U.S. Bureau of Labor Statistics, 2021a, 2021b).

Where people live is another powerful influence on the pattern of occupation they set up for themselves and their families. Living in a neighborhood with unpredictable drug- and gang-related violence influences the decisions low-income Black mothers make for their daughters, with restrictions on outdoor play directly contributing to high levels of physical inactivity (Dias & Whitaker, 2013) (Figure 8.5). Moreover, environments can change. As the sociodemographic profile of their neighborhood deteriorated, older residents of Detroit experienced the loss of shared occupations, such as inviting a neighbor to sit and talk, doing things at different times of the day to avoid going outdoors after dark, and the need for heightened vigilance during daytime occupations (Fritz & Cutchin, 2017). Occupational

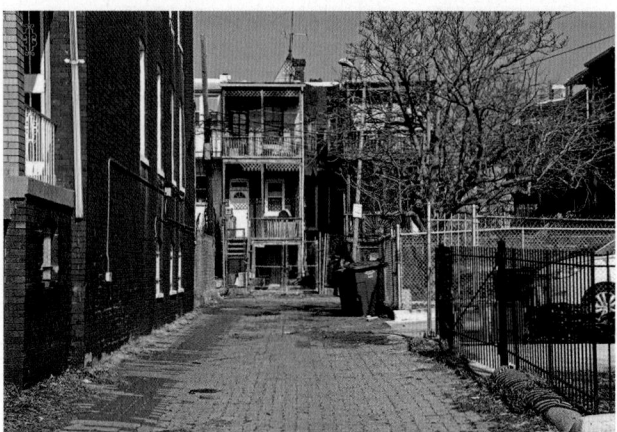

FIGURE 8.5 Mothers restrict girls' outdoor play if the neighborhood is perceived to be dangerous.

therapists are also increasingly aware that people's patterns of occupation can be restricted by discrimination, citizenship status, and other circumstances that deprive them of real opportunities to participate in productive, educational, and leisure occupations on an equal footing. Restricted opportunities amounting to occupational injustice are important determinants of health and development. Thus, young people who have experienced homelessness, foster care, or poverty, with its associated housing insecurity, are at risk of having poor working memory. In addition, compared to non-disadvantaged peers, those who are homeless or poor are more likely to have deficits in attention and executive functioning (Fry et al., 2017).

Ecological and sociopolitical factors also limit or disrupt access to health-giving occupations. Examples recently identified in the OT and occupational science literature include homelessness (Schultz-Krohn & Tyminski, 2018), unemployment (Huot et al., 2020), childhood poverty (Leadley et al., 2020), living in a supervised group home (Kåhlin et al., 2016), seeking asylum (Ingvarsson et al., 2016), and the COVID-19 pandemic (Lannigan & Tyminski, 2021). The interdisciplinary literature also recognizes the impact of natural disasters such as drought and tornados, lower educational attainment, and displacement (see OT Story 8.1). In recognition of the multiple impacts of disadvantageous social conditions that limit equitable access to occupation, the WFOT's (2016) standards for OT education now specify social inclusion as a focus for curricula content, student selection, and lecturers' professional development.

OT STORY 8.1 BEING, BELONGING, AND BECOMING THROUGH DOING

Having a positive sense of "*being*" someone in particular, "*belonging*" to valued social groups, and "*becoming*" the person you hope to be have been identified as being important for well-being and are inextricably linked to what we do. Wilcock and Hocking (2015) suggested that these elements of occupation are enacted by doing things that align with our "essential nature" (p. 135) with or for others, in contexts that we understand and feel accepted in. Whether learning new occupations in unfamiliar contexts or performing the traditional occupations of a particular location, family, or culture, we are constantly adapting and developing new ways of being and belonging in the world. The process of being, belonging, and becoming through doing is a dynamic transaction between an individual's unique identity, values, interests, and capacities and their sociocultural and physical context.

Accounts of migration illustrate how the development of new occupational patterns, while holding on to previous ways of doing things, can help shape being, belonging, and becoming in a new country. For example, older people who migrated from Finland to Sweden in their youth describe a dual sense of being and belonging through occupational patterns embedded in both the land of their birth and their host country (Arola et al., 2018). Over many years they had adapted to daily life in Sweden and felt at home there, where they had close family, friends, and established habits and ways of doing things. A sense of belonging was developed over time through occupational mastery in a new context and taking on elements of being Swedish, such as speaking the language. However, a sense of well-being was also associated with maintaining ties to their homeland by spending time with compatriots, speaking Finnish, keeping abreast of the news, exchanging phone calls, and visiting Finland when they could. Migration and the prospect of aging in a foreign nation seemed daunting, but maintaining well-being was possible for these older adults through the performance of meaningful occupations that reflected their essential nature and allowed them to belong in both Finland and Sweden simultaneously (Arola et al., 2018).

Similarly, young migrants and refugees in Auckland, New Zealand were able to successfully navigate a path between their old life and their new one, this time through engagement in creative occupations (Tischler, 2017). Spending Saturdays at a community arts project was a powerful means of feeling they belonged in their new surroundings. Mixing with people from diverse countries, languages, and religions, they sang, danced, played the drums, learned acrobatics, played board games, created graffiti art, and chatted together. As well as making friends, they learned that this was a safe place to be themselves and to develop new interests, capacities, and identities as artists and performers. In summer, they took to the stage to perform a routine they worked on, guided by a professional choreographer who also had an immigrant background.

Constraints on Doing, Being, Belonging, and Becoming

Not all migrants are welcome to participate in meaningful occupation in their host country. Lucia, Christina, and Ana worked in professional and service roles before they emigrated from Latin America to Spain. Since the economic crisis, the only work they were offered, when they are offered anything at all, was cleaning and caregiving in private homes (Rivas-Quarneti et al., 2018). There, employers told them they "have to be at my disposal" (p. 6). Even though they felt enslaved, these immigrant workers had no choice but to accept the low wages and exploitative work situations. Quitting would mean waiting for employment agencies to call

(continued)

them while "the days pass and your need gets sharper, and sharper" (p. 6). Despite restorative occupations like walking on the beach and the support they offered each other, the reality of having no resources beyond "my feet, my back and an attitude of overcoming the struggles to achieve" (p. 7) left them feeling frustrated, angry, and endlessly fatigued. The discriminatory attitudes they encountered as women, immigrants, and workers in precarious employment relegated them to the edges of society, with little hope of developing a secure and comfortable life in their new home country.

Even within countries, variations in occupational forms across groups are a means of identifying, othering, and marginalizing individuals. Examples linked to racism in the United States and United Kingdom include wearing baggy pants, playing hip-hop music, or particular styles of wearing one's hair, such as dreadlocks. The conflation of professionalism with "White" norms of comportment, clothing, ways of conducting business meetings is equally discriminatory and oppressive. Equally, the valuing of objective argument over narrative storytelling to impart information disadvantages children raised in Mexican homes in the United States (Bailliard et al., 2021). Internationally, asylum seekers are also

commonly subjected to legal constraints on engagement in educational opportunities and work, even in low paid jobs like the ones Lucia, Christina, and Ana had to accept. The imposed lack of valued and meaningful occupation might last for months or years while they wait to hear the outcome of their asylum application. Having nothing to do and nothing to mark one day from the next has been characterized as suffering. Not surprisingly, it gives rise to mental distress as well as self-harm and suicidal behavior (Crawford et al., 2016).

Questions

1. Research results cited in this story identify language, attitudinal, and legal barriers to occupation, which disrupt people's capacity to do well and derive a sense of belonging to the people and place where they live. In what ways might immigrants, asylum seekers, or other groups living in vulnerable circumstances also experience constraints on their capacity to be and become?
2. If you had an opportunity to work with youths living in a community that is new to them, how might you engage them in occupations that would create a sense of belonging?

Too Little and Too Much Occupation

Occupation's contribution to health is evident in accounts of the deleterious effects of not doing enough. Over the last 25 years, occupational scientists have reported the emotional, psychological, and societal harm caused when people experience externally imposed barriers to occupations that limit opportunities to engage in occupations that are meaningful and purposeful (Wilcock & Hocking, 2015). The populations studied include prisoners, people with disabling health conditions, those displaced by armed conflict, immigrants, refugees, and asylum seekers (Hocking, 2017b). More recently, the impact of reduced access to occupations during the COVID-19 pandemic has also been explored. A study of Belgian adults in "lockdown" found strong correlations between reduced mental health and the loss of meaningful occupations, such as work, school, social events, and community-based recreation (Cruyt et al., 2021). In the United States, the pandemic highlighted how access to employment directly shapes the distribution of both mental and physical health outcomes (Pratap et al., 2021). Being deprived of meaningful work has been linked to increased suicide rates, drug and alcohol abuse, increased depression, and greater rates of physical health conditions, such as cardiovascular disease and cancer (Antunes, 2016; Meneton et al.,

2015; Pratap et al., 2021). Unemployment is also associated with diminished access to health-promoting occupations, such as organized sports, social activities, and eating healthy food, and increased engagement in occupations with risk of poor health outcomes, such as smoking, eating unhealthy foods, and passive occupations (Nizalova & Norton, 2021).

It is not only people who are unemployed who experience health problems associated with too many passive occupations and not enough physically demanding ones. This is an issue across the populations of many Westernized societies as well as in countries in economic transition. Significant attention has been paid to the increased risk of cardiovascular disease, stroke, cancer, diabetes, osteoporosis, anxiety, depression, and dementia of people who do not regularly engage in physically active occupations such as gardening; household chores; swimming; riding a bicycle; planned exercise; and playing sport or games involving running, turning, or jumping. The scale of international concern and the strength of evidence from research is such that the WHO has published guidelines for the amount and types of physical activity required to achieve significant health benefits and mitigate health risks (WHO, 2018b). This includes guidance for children, adults, and older adults as well as people living with long-term health conditions and disabilities.

With the majority of people in affluent countries failing to meet activity guidelines, the health consequences of too much occupation tend to receive less attention. Nonetheless, one form of occupational imbalance, having too much to do, or doing things at too high intensity over a long time, are also associated with stress disorders, cardiac arrests, stress fractures, and other ill-health outcomes (Wilcock & Hocking, 2015).

Having a job with long hours or constant high demands can be equally detrimental to health as unemployment. Studies show that long working hours are associated with poor sleep, fatigue, increased injuries, and a range of other mental and physical health issues (Wong et al., 2019). Research has also explored "burnout" in workers, where a job exceeds an individual's personal and environmental resources, leading to exhaustion, negative attitudes, and reduced job performance (Bakker & de Vries, 2021). Here, rather than too much time spent in an occupation, it may be the intensity of the occupation that is too much. The health impacts of burnout include increased prevalence of depressive and anxiety disorders, alcohol dependence, and physical health issues, such as diabetes and heart attacks.

Issues with "too much" occupation may go beyond employment and be experienced as an imbalance across all of one's daily occupations. A study of African American working mothers (Parnell, 2020) found that participants experienced physical and cognitive overload due to too many competing occupational roles and tasks. With extended time focused on being a mother, other desired roles, such as being a partner, friend, or volunteer were neglected. Other important elements of their daily routines were missed as well, including rest, cooking nutritious meals, self-care occupations, and social events, leading to reduced well-being.

It is not always easy to judge what constitutes too much or too little occupation, as the experience of occupational balance is in many ways subjective and what is "too much" for one person may be manageable for another. Furthermore, specific occupations or routines can simultaneously have health-promoting elements and health risks. For example, occupations in the online or virtual world are becoming increasingly dominant in many people's lives and studies have explored the benefits and harms of social media and extended screen time. The findings of these studies are mixed and indicate the benefits of social connection and self-expression through online activity and social media, but also highlight disruption to occupational patterns through long hours online, social media or gaming addiction, and disrupted sleep (Keles et al., 2020). Interestingly, recent research into children and young people's screen time indicates that despite concerns, time spent in online occupations is not predictive of mental health issues and does not strongly influence engagement in other more physical recreational occupations (Lees et al., 2020; Vuorre et al., 2021). Rather, socioeconomic status was a far more significant factor in mental well-being and physical activity than screen time (Lees et al., 2020; Paulich et al., 2021).

As technologies develop, our occupational patterns also evolve. With virtual leisure pursuits becoming commonplace and work practices more time and cost efficient, people increasingly are at risk of becoming sedentary and disconnected from aspects of their being and belonging in other spaces, such as in nature and in face-to-face interactions. Even those with active leisure pursuits are at increased risk of obesity because of the many hours spent sitting rather than standing or walking. An occupational perspective of health and well-being offers unique insights into the factors that contribute to occupational imbalance and what might constitute "too much" or "too little" occupation. Risks inherent in the occupations people need, want, and are required to do can be identified, and effective ways of conveying that information to affected populations developed (Hocking, 2017a).

Disability, Health, and Occupation

Having an impairment associated with a health condition can impede participation in occupations that underpin well-being. Consistent with the *International Classification of Functioning, Disability and Health* (ICF; WHO, 2001), an impairment is defined as any problem with normal psychological or physiological function or with a body structure such as a joint or organ. The association between impairments and reduced capacity for participation is increasingly recognized. For example, in February 2021 the WHO estimated 568 million people were living with low back pain that, along with other musculoskeletal conditions, limited mobility, contributed to early withdrawal from work, and reduced the ability to participate in society (WHO, 2021b). Depression is another common cause of decreased functioning, affecting the capacity of approximately 280 million people worldwide to participate in occupations at work, school, and in the family (WHO, 2021a). Toxic social and environmental conditions such as discrimination, racism, and environmental degradation, along with poverty-related problems like malnutrition, also cause pervasive health problems, stunting human development and threatening capacity for occupation. Impairments can directly affect participation in occupation, for example not being sufficiently strong or flexible, having diminished cognitive capacity, or being too anxious to do things that in other circumstances people would choose to do. In addition, people tend to withdraw from occupation if health issues or social situations render participation too effortful, unpleasant, or harmful.

Occupational therapists are well aware of these risks to occupational performance. Accordingly, therapeutic processes to "enable people to engage in occupations that provide meaning and satisfaction and that support their physical and emotional well-being" are described (Taylor, 2017, p. 6). As people with disabilities readily identify, however, attitudinal barriers and lack of accommodations can disrupt inclusion much more than bodily and psychological impairments.

Legislative structures to implement universal design and mandate inclusion are helpful. For instance, Norway has a legislative requirement that organized sports be accessible to all children, regardless of disability (Asbjørnslett & Bekken, 2016), but the pace of environmental modifications and changes in people's attitudes about people's right to inclusion is frustratingly slow.

Just as impairments can affect occupational performance, the ICF makes clear that the opposite is also true; the things we do can threaten health and create impairments. Many commonplace occupations, such as driving a motor vehicle, have inherent health risks. Even leisure occupations can harm us. For instance, the National Safety Council (2021) reported 39,107 people died in motor-vehicle crashes in the United States in 2019 and an estimated 2,700,988 emergency department visits between 2013 and 2020 were due to sports and recreational activities, primarily riding bicycles and exercising. Over the long term, low-quality work, meaning jobs with low security, satisfaction, pay, and autonomy, is also associated with poor physical and mental health outcomes, which brings into question governmental efforts to get unemployed people into work without due consideration of the nature of the work (The Health Foundation, 2021).

Conclusion

Humans do many things to meet the biological need for sustenance and shelter. Occupation keeps us alive, and occupation in natural environments nourishes us. In the longer term, occupation can provide the physical activity, mental stimulation, and social interaction we need to keep our bodies, minds, and communities healthy. In addition, through participation in occupation, we express ourselves, develop skills, experience pleasure and involvement, and achieve the things we believe to be important. In short, we have opportunities for enhanced levels of well-being, to be, belong, and become what we have the potential to be. However, not all people have equal opportunity to engage in health-giving occupations. People with an impairment can experience limitations in their ability to engage in occupation and are known to have lower levels of engagement in physical exercise. People who live in poverty, are displaced by conflict or devastated by natural disasters, experience unemployment or homelessness, or have lower levels of educational attainment are also likely to experience barriers to participation in occupation, and thus lower levels of inclusion in society, that negatively affect health and well-being.

Equally, occupation can threaten or destroy health. Doing too much, doing too little, doing things that expose us to risk and harm, and exclusionary attitudes and practices that limit access to occupation can all have deleterious effects. It is also important to recognize that it is often through having trouble doing things that we become aware of health issues and the full impact of impairments. Furthermore, physical, social, or attitudinal barriers in the environment can exacerbate the impact of a health condition or impairment, sometimes to such an extent that participation in occupation is unsustainable.

Lippincott® Connect *For additional resources on the subjects discussed in this chapter, visit* Lippincott Connect.

REFERENCES

Antunes, J. L. (2016). The impact of unemployment on cancer mortality, and how to avoid it. *Annals of Translational Medicine, 4*(20), Article 404. https://doi.org/10.21037/atm.2016.08.46

Aramaki, K., & Hagiwara, H. (2018). Effect of walking upon fatigue due to monotonous work. *Advances in Intelligent Systems and Computing, 590,* 171–175. https://doi.org/10.1007/978-3-319-60483-1_18

Arola, A., Dellenborg, L., & Häggblom-Kronlöf, G. (2018). Occupational perspective of health among persons ageing in the context of migration. *Journal of Occupational Science, 25*(1), 65–75. https://doi.org/10.1080/14427591.2017.1368411

Asbjørnslett, M., & Bekken, W. (2016). Openness to difference: Inclusion in sports occupations for children with (dis)abilities. *Journal of Occupational Science, 23*(4), 434–445. https://doi.org/10.1080/14427591.2016.1199389

Bailliard, A., Carroll, A., & Peak, K. (2021). Laying low: Unmasking the contributions of science and education to racism. *Journal of Occupational Science, 28*(3), 441–448. https://doi.org/10.1080/14427591.2021.1893109

Bakker, A. B., & de Vries, J. D. (2021). Job demands–resources theory and self-regulation: New explanations and remedies for job burnout. *Anxiety, Stress & Coping, 34*(1), 1–21. https://doi.org/10.1080/10615806.2020.1797695

Crawford, E., Turpin, M., Nayar, S., Steel, E., & Durand, J.-L. (2016). The structural-personal interaction: Occupational deprivation and asylum seekers in Australia. *Journal of Occupational Science, 23*(3), 321–338. https://doi.org/10.1080/14427591.2016.1153510

Cruyt, E., De Vriendt, P., De Letter, M., Vlerick, P., Calders, P., De Pauw, R., Oostra, K., Rodriguez-Bailón, M., Szmalec, A., Merchán-Baeza, J. A., Fernández-Solano, A. J., Vidaña-Moya, L., & Van de Velde, D. (2021). Meaningful activities during COVID-19 lockdown and association with mental health in Belgian adults. *BMC Public Health, 21,* Article 1680. https://doi.org/10.1186/s12889-021-11699-4

Dias, J. J., & Whitaker, R. C. (2013). Black mothers' perceptions about urban neighborhood safety and outdoor play for their preadolescent daughters. *Journal of Health Care for the Poor and Underserved, 24*(1), 206–219. https://doi.org/10.1353/hpu.2013.0018

Doroud, N., Fossey, E., & Fortune, T. (2015). Recovery as an occupational journey: A scoping review exploring the links between occupational engagement and recovery for people with enduring mental health issues. *Australian Occupational Therapy Journal, 62*(6), 378–392. https://doi.org/10.1111/1440-1630.12238

Doyle, J., Firebrace, B., Reilly, R., Crumpen, T., & Rowley, K. (2013). What makes us different? The role of Rumbalara Football and Netball Club in promoting Indigenous wellbeing. *The Australian Community Psychologist, 25*(2), 7–21.

Farias, L., & Simaan, J. (2020). Introduction to the anti-racism virtual issue of the Journal of Occupational Science. *Journal of Occupational Science, 27*(4), 454–459. https://doi.org/10.1080/14427591.2020.1824567

Fijal, D., & Beagan, B. L. (2019). Indigenous perspectives on health: Integration with a Canadian model of practice. *Canadian Journal of Occupational Therapy, 86*(3), 220–231. https://doi.org/10.1177/0008417419832284

Fritz, H., & Cutchin, M. P. (2017). Changing neighborhoods and occupations: Experiences of older African-Americans in Detroit. *Journal of Occupational Science, 24*(2), 140–151. https://doi.org/10.1080/144 27591.2016.1269296

Fry, C. E., Langley, K., & Shelton, K. H. (2017). A systematic review of cognitive functioning among young people who have experienced homelessness, foster care, or poverty. *Child Neuropsychology, 23*(8), 907–934. https://doi.org/10.1080/09297049.2016.1207758

Galvaan, R. (2015). The contextually situated nature of occupational choice: Marginalised young adolescents' experiences in South Africa. *Journal of Occupational Science, 22*(1), 39–53. https://doi.org/10.108 0/14427591.2014.912124

Hocking, C. (2017a). Occupation and the risk message recipient. In R. Parrott (Ed.), *The Oxford encyclopedia of health and risk message design and processing* (pp. 1–16). Oxford University Press. https://doi .org/10.1093/acrefore/9780190228613.013.357

Hocking, C. (2017b). Occupational justice as social justice: The moral claim for inclusion. *Journal of Occupational Science, 24*(1), 29–42. https://doi.org/10.1080/14427591.2017.1294016

Huot, S., Aldrich, R. M., Laliberte Rudman, D., & Stone, M. (2020). Picturing precarity through occupational mapping: Making the (im)mobilities of long-term unemployment visible. *Journal of Occupational Science, 29*(4), 529–544. https://doi.org/10.1080/14427591.2020.1821244

Ingvarsson, L., Egilson, S. T., & Skaptadottir, U. D. (2016). "I want a normal life like everyone else": Daily life of asylum seekers in Iceland. *Scandinavian Journal of Occupational Therapy, 23*(6), 416–424. https://doi.org/10.3109/11038128.2016.1144787

Kåhlin, I., Kjellberg, A., & Hagberg, J.-E. (2016). Choice and control for people ageing with intellectual disability in group homes. *Scandinavian Journal of Occupational Therapy, 23*(2), 127–137. https://doi.org /10.3109/11038128.2015.1095235

Keles, B., McCrae, N., & Grealish, A. (2020). A systematic review: The influence of social media on depression, anxiety and psychological distress in adolescents. *International Journal of Adolescence and Youth, 25*(1), 79–93. https://doi.org/10.1080/02673843.2019.1590851

Kiepek, N. C., Beagan, B., Laliberte Rudman, D., & Phelan, S. (2019). Silences around occupations framed as unhealthy, illegal, and deviant. *Journal of Occupational Science, 26*(3), 341–353. https://doi.org/10.10 80/14427591.2018.1499123

Lannigan, E. G., & Tyminski, Q. (2021). Occupational therapy's role in addressing the psychological and social impact of COVID-19. *American Journal of Occupational Therapy, 75*(Supplement 1), 7511347030p1–7511347030p7. https://doi.org/10.5014/ajot.2021.049327

Leadley, S., Hocking, C., & Jones, M. (2020). The ways poverty influences a tamaiti/child's patterns of occupation. *Journal of Occupational Science, 27*(3), 297–310. https://doi.org/10.1080/14427591.2020.1738263

Lees, B., Squeglia, L. M., Breslin, F. J., Thompson, W. K., Tapert, S. F., & Paulus, M. P. (2020). Screen media activity does not displace other recreational activities among 9–10 year-old youth: A cross-sectional ABCD study*. *BMC Public Health, 20*, 1783. https://doi.org/10.1186/ s12889-020-09894-w

Luck, K., & Beagan, B. (2015). Occupational transition of smoking cessation in women: "You're restructuring your whole life." *Journal of Occupational Science, 22*(2), 183–196. https://doi.org/10.1080/14427 591.2014.887418

McCartney, G., Popham, F., McMaster, R., & Cumbers, A. (2019). Defining health and health inequalities. *Public Health, 172*, 22–30. https:// doi.org/10.1016/j.puhe.2019.03.023

McNeill, H. N. (2017). Maori and the natural environment from an occupational justice perspective. *Journal of Occupational Science, 24*(1), 19–28. https://doi.org/10.1080/14427591.2016.1245158

Meneton, P., Kesse-Guyot, E., Méjean, C., Fezeu, L., Galan, P., Hercberg, S., & Ménard, J. (2015). Unemployment is associated with high cardiovascular event rate and increased all-cause mortality in middle-aged socially privileged individuals. *International Archives of Occupational and Environmental Health, 88*(6), 707–716. https://doi .org/10.1007/s00420-014-0997-7

National Safety Council. (2021). *Injury facts.* https://injuryfacts.nsc.org/

Nizalova, O., & Norton, E. C. (2021). Long-term effects of job loss on male health: BMI and health behaviors. *Economics and Human Biology, 43*, Article 101038. https://doi.org/10.1016/j.ehb.2021.101038

Office of Disease Prevention and Health Promotion. (2021a). *Healthy people 2030: Child and adolescent development.* https:// health.gov/healthypeople/objectives-and-data/browse-objectives/ child-and-adolescent-development

Office of Disease Prevention and Health Promotion. (2021b). *Healthy people 2030: Objectives and data: Social determinants of health: Social determinants of health literature summaries: Civic participation.* https:// health.gov/healthypeople/objectives-and-data/social-determinants-health/literature-summaries/civic-participation

Office of Disease Prevention and Health Promotion. (2021c). *Healthy people 2030: Objectives and data: Social determinants of health: Social determinants of health literature summaries: Discrimination.* https:// health.gov/healthypeople/objectives-and-data/social-determinants-health/literature-summaries/discrimination

Office of Disease Prevention and Health Promotion. (2021d). *Healthy people 2030: Overview and objectives: Physical activity.* https:// health.gov/healthypeople/objectives-and-data/browse-objectives/ physical-activity

Office of Disease Prevention and Health Promotion. (2021e). *Healthy people 2030: Overview and objectives: Physical activity: Social support interventions in community settings.* https://health.gov/ healthypeople/tools-action/browse-evidence-based-resources/ physical-activity-social-support-interventions-community-settings

Office of Disease Prevention and Health Promotion. (2021f). *Healthy people 2030: People with disabilities.* https://health.gov/healthypeople/ objectives-and-data/browse-objectives/people-disabilities

Parnell, R. (2020). Occupational imbalance in hurried African American working mothers. *Journal of Occupational Science, 29*(1), 82–96. https://doi.org/10.1080/14427591.2020.1839785

Paulich, K. N., Ross, J. M., Lessem, J. M., & Hewitt, J. K. (2021). Screen time and early adolescent mental health, academic, and social outcomes in 9- and 10-year old children: Utilizing the Adolescent Brain Cognitive Development SM (ABCD) Study. *PLoS One, 16*(9), e0256591. https://doi.org/10.1371/journal.pone.0256591

Pratap, P., Dickson, A., Love, M., Zanoni, J., Donato, C., Flynn, M. A., & Schulte, P. A. (2021). Public health impacts of underemployment and unemployment in the United States: Exploring perceptions, gaps and opportunities. *International Journal of Environmental Research in Public Health, 18*(19), Article 10021. https://doi.org/10.3390/ijerph 181910021

Rivas-Quarneti, N., Movilla-Fernández, M.-J., & Magalhães, L. (2018). Immigrant women's occupational struggles during the socioeconomic crisis in Spain: Broadening occupational justice conceptualization. *Journal of Occupational Science, 25*(1), 6–18. https://doi.org/ 10.1080/14427591.2017.1366355

Robinson, T. N., Banda, J. A., Hale, L., Lu, A. S., Fleming-Milici, F., Calvert, S. L., & Wartella, E. (2017). Screen media exposure and obesity in children and adolescents. *Pediatrics, 140*(Suppl 2), S97–S101. https://doi.org/10.1542/peds.2016-1758K

Sandoval, M., Leclerc, J. A., & Gomez, R. L. (2017). Words to sleep on: Naps facilitate verb generalization in habitually and nonhabitually napping preschoolers. *Child Development, 88*(5), 1615–1628. https:// doi.org/10.1111/cdev.12723

Schultz-Krohn, W., & Tyminski, Q. (2018). *Community-built occupational therapy services for those who are homeless.* AOTA Continuing Education article. https://www.aota.org/~/media/Corporate/Files/ Publications/CE-Articles/CE-Article-June-2018.pdf

Sy, M. P., Bontje, P., Ohshima, N., & Kiepek, N. (2020). Articulating the form, function, and meaning of drug using in the Philippines from the lens of morality and work ethics. *Journal of Occupational Science, 27*(1), 12–21. https://doi.org/10.1080/14427591.2019.1644662

Taylor, R. R. (2017). *Kielhofner's model of human occupation* (5th ed.). Wolters Kluwer.

The Health Foundation. (2021). *Job quality: How does work affect our health?* https://www.health.org.uk/news-and-comment/charts-and-infographics/job-quality

Tischler, M. (2017). Wendy Preston, Mixit. *AA Directions*, 24–25.

Tkatch, R., Music, S., MacLeod, S., Kraemer, S., Hawkins, K., Wicker, E. R., & Armstrong, D. G. (2017). A qualitative study to examine older adults' perceptions of health: Keys to aging successfully. *Geriatric Nursing, 38*(6), 485–490. https://doi.org/10.1016/j.gerinurse.2017.02.009

Twinley, R. (Ed.). (2021). *The dark side of occupation*. Taylor and Francis.

United Nations. (2007). *Women, gender equality and sport.* https://www.un.org/womenwatch/daw/public/Women%20and%20Sport.pdf

U.S. Bureau of Labor Statistics. (2021a). *Injuries, illnesses, and fatalities.* U.S. Department of Labor. https://www.bls.gov/iif/oshwc/osh/case/cd_r9_2020.htm

U.S. Bureau of Labor Statistics. (2021b). *News release: National census of fatal occupational injuries in 2020.* U.S. Department of Labor. https://www.bls.gov/news.release/pdf/cfoi.pdf

U.S. Department of Health and Human Services. (2018). *Physical activity guidelines for Americans* (2nd ed.). https://health.gov/our-work/nutrition-physical-activity/physical-activity-guidelines/current guidelines

Vuorre, M., Orben, A., & Przybylski, A. K. (2021). There is no evidence that associations between adolescents' digital technology engagement and mental health problems have increased. *Clinical Psychological Science, 9*(5), 823–835. https://doi.org/10.1177/2167702621994549

Whiteford, G., Jones, K., Rahal, C., & Suleman, A. (2018). The Participatory Occupational Justice Framework as a tool for change: Three contrasting case narratives. *Journal of Occupational Science, 27*(1), 497–508. https://doi.org/10.1080/14427591.2018.1504607

Wilcock, A. (1993). A theory of the human need for occupation. *Journal of Occupational Science: Australia, 1*(1), 17–24. https://doi.org/10.1080/14427591.1993.9686375

Wilcock, A. (1995). The occupational brain: A theory of human nature. *Journal of Occupational Science: Australia, 2*(2), 68–72. https://doi.org/10.1080/14427591.1995.9686397

Wilcock, A. A., & Hocking, C. (2015). *An occupational perspective of health* (3rd ed.). SLACK.

Wong, K., Chan, A. H. S., & Ngan, S. C. (2019). The effect of long working hours and overtime on occupational health: A meta-analysis of evidence from 1998 to 2018. *International Journal of Environmental Research and Public Health, 16*(12), 2102. https://doi.org/10.3390/ijerph16122102

World Federation of Occupational Therapists. (2016). *Minimum standards for the education of occupational therapists.* Author.

World Federation of Occupational Therapists. (2019). *Position statement: Occupational therapy and human rights.* https://wfot.org/resources/occupational-therapy-and-human-rights

World Health Organization. (1986, November). *Ottawa charter for health promotion, 1986.* Paper presented at the First International Conference on Health Promotion. Ottawa, Ontario, Canada.

World Health Organization. (2001). *International classification of functioning, disability and health: A global model to guide clinical thinking and practice in childhood disability.* Author.

World Health Organization. (2018a). *Frequently asked questions.* Author. https://www.who.int/about/frequently-asked-questions

World Health Organization. (2018b). *Global action plan on physical activity 2018-2030: More active people for a healthier world.* Author.

World Health Organization. (2021a). *Depression.* https://www.who.int/news-room/fact-sheets/detail/depression

World Health Organization. (2021b). *Musculoskeletal conditions.* https://www.who.int/news-room/fact-sheets/detail/musculoskeletal-conditions

Wrisdale, L., Mokoena, M. M., Mudau, L. S., & Geere, J. (2017). Factors that impact on access to water and sanitation for older adults and people with disability in rural South Africa: An occupational justice perspective. *Journal of Occupational Science, 24*(3), 259–279. https://doi.org/10.1080/14427591.2017.1338190

Occupational Science
The Study of Occupation

Clare Hocking and Margaret Jones

LEARNING OBJECTIVES

After reading this chapter, you will be able to:

1. Apply an occupational science way of thinking and evidence-based practice to occupational therapy.
2. Distinguish between basic and applied occupational science knowledge underpinning practice.
3. Explain the importance of key aspects of the translational science research framework: theory development, testing, implementation, and collaboration.
4. Evaluate how well your own practice is guided by the existing and emergent basic and applied occupational science knowledge.

Introduction

This chapter explores how advances in knowledge, including the research undertaken by occupational scientists, inform developments in occupational therapy (OT) practice. Because occupational science exists, primarily, to inform OT, we begin by looking into occupational science as a basic science underpinning OT knowledge and then showcase recent developments in occupational science to illustrate its growth as an applied science. The process of turning knowledge from basic science into useful applications—that is, OT interventions and public health advice—is referred to as translational science. To explain and illustrate the process, a translational science research framework is presented, along with real-world translational science examples. Three OT Stories highlight how the "science" of occupational science is guiding *evidence-based occupational therapy practice*. Each story, in its own way, illustrates occupational science "in play" within the everyday practice worlds of occupational therapists.

Humans as Occupational Beings

Occupational science is founded on the idea that humans are occupational beings, which has two important implications. The first is the assumption that people "naturally" engage in occupation; it is part and parcel of being human (Wilcock & Hocking, 2015). When scholars like Wilcock refer to the occupational nature of being human, they are pointing to the way an array of human attributes come into play in the performance of occupation. Examples include:

- The anatomy of our hands, which enables us to handle something delicate without breaking it or grasp something firmly when needed
- The skeletal features that go along with being bipedal (standing on two feet), thus freeing our hands to manipulate tools
- Brain structures and functions to learn and remember how to do things, to use tools, and to work out what to do if it goes wrong
- Physiologic responses that keep our muscles supplied with oxygen and cause us to cool down by sweating if the occupation is effortful
- Binocular vision to perceive how far away things are and how fast they are approaching
- Speech and language skills to convey instructions, warnings, encouragement, and praise to others
- Self-consciousness to judge how others will perceive what we are doing

The second implication of viewing people as occupational beings is that human life can be interpreted from an occupational perspective, which encompasses not only what people do but also how the things we do occupy our minds, hearts, and relationships, including our relationship with other living things and the earth itself. In that sense, "what we do" extends well beyond individual doing—rather, occupation is a foundation stone in understanding how societies function, the possibilities for peace and war, our future as a species, and ultimately, the future of life on earth. Along with the occupational perspective we highlight in this chapter, we also acknowledge that humans can be viewed from Indigenous, biologic, psychological, sociologic, existential, economic, political, and evolutionary perspectives, to name a few.

Implicit in an occupational view of humans is the idea that, through the things we do, humans influence their state of health or ill-health of our relationships, communities, and the environment. To illustrate that, consider the COVID-19 pandemic that caused millions of deaths internationally (WHO, 2022). Living through the pandemic, we have observed impacts on national economies, poverty levels, school attendance, fertility rates, international shipping and air travel, mass gatherings such as sports events and religious observances, greenhouse gas emissions (because of decreased transport use), and so on. Interconnected with all those, taking an occupational perspective means attending to changes in occupation. Those changes were particularly pronounced during lockdowns, when citizens were directed to stay home, causing widespread disruption of people's daily routines, whether they could work, where and how school lessons were delivered, how groceries and other products could be acquired, cessation of occupations such as getting a haircut, and so on. Everyday actions were introduced or

intensified, such as frequent handwashing and putting on a mask before entering public places (Figure 9.1). The disruptions impacted people's sense of time, their sense of control over their lives, and generated a sense of social isolation for many (Donnelly et al., 2021).

Thinking about the COVID-19 pandemic from an occupational perspective illustrates what this chapter is about. It reveals how people's lives can change and suggests that communities, groups, and individuals will sometimes need support to engage in occupation and successfully adjust to changes in occupations. And it points toward understanding how an in-depth knowledge about *humans as occupational beings* can inform new ways for OT to contribute to healthy families and communities. But first, let us go back to the ideas behind this chapter.

Occupational science opens up new ways to explore the complexities of human engagement in occupations. As a basic science, Zemke and Clark (1996) proposed that the scope of this new science would encompass four focuses:

- The ***substrates*** of occupation are the physical and cognitive attributes of human anatomy, physiology, and consciousness that Wilcock identified as underpinning our capacity to engage in occupation. The substrates align with body structures and functions (AOTA, 2020) and are perhaps most apparent when something goes wrong; when you have cut your hand, hurt your back, lost the vision in one eye, or feel too fatigued or hot or depressed to do something.
- The ***form*** of an occupation is the knowledge people share about how something is usually done. The form might be explicitly stated, such as the rules for playing football, or just the "way things are done," such as making a hot drink in a coffee cup rather than a glass so that you do not burn your hand. Merely naming an occupation you intend to do will tell others a lot. Going for a run, for example, invokes an image of a leisure pursuit involving particular

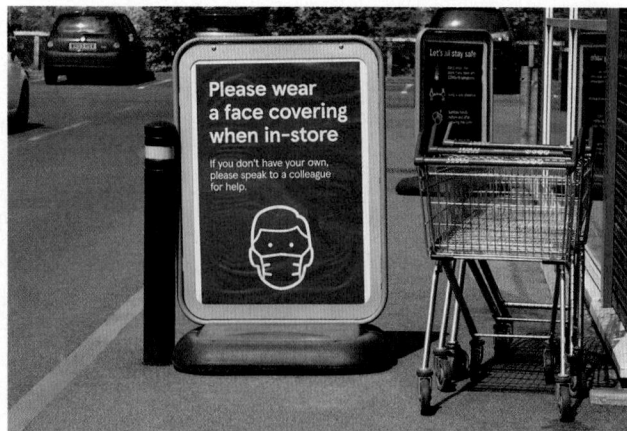

FIGURE 9.1 **Changes in everyday occupations: wearing a mask in public places.**

- clothing, footwear, level of exertion and pace, and perhaps running companions.
- The *function* of an occupation refers to its purpose or effect, such as writing a term paper to pass a class.
- The *meaning* of an occupation includes its significance at a personal level as well as how it is viewed by different groups in society.

As you can see, there are various ways of approaching and categorizing knowledge about occupation. In this chapter, we align the discussion with the two main research paradigms: quantitative (what can be directly observed and measured) and qualitative (what people experience). To explain the complex ideas behind studying both the visible and felt aspects of occupation, we draw on a study of mobile phone and tablet use by people with learning disabilities (Barlott et al., 2021). Some aspects could be observed and verified by others: the phone was charged, indicating the participant had remembered to plug it in. Messages were sent and received, demonstrating knowledge of the function of a phone and literacy skills. Podcasts and music were played, indicating access to the internet and content loaded onto the device. Understanding how these technologies were experienced relied on participant report. Dana murmured "Mmmm" and hugged her tablet when asked how it made her feel. Andrew explained he had to have his phone with him, that he depended on it. Doug's phone use was curtailed by his father saying "TOO MUCH PHONE!" (p. 9), conveying his preference to use it more than he was allowed. Sam laughed at the suggestion that texting "old man" to his support worker was calculated to be annoying, giving insight to his sense of humor.

Barlott and colleagues' (2021) study captures the two fundamentally different ways we as occupational therapists can study occupation as a basic science. One way is to examine its external, observable aspects. This way of coming to know things is underpinned by the assumption that the truth about occupations and the occupational nature of humans exists in the world. Therefore, we can come to know it by gathering data gained through our senses (de Poy & Gitlin, 2020). From this viewpoint, quantitative researchers can establish what is true or real, because it can be seen, touched, heard, or measured in some objective way. Additionally, if we accept there is not one but many truths—that there are multiple realities about occupations and the occupational nature of humans—then we can see the value of qualitative researchers exploring the internal, experienced aspects of occupation. This way of coming to know about occupation is underpinned by the assumption that, like Dana, Andrew, Doug, and Sam, people experience their own subjective, contextual reality. Across the two research traditions, the what, who, where, how, and why of occupations can all be studied as units of analysis within occupational science research.

Building a Basic Knowledge of Occupation

Attempting to give an overview of the knowledge occupational scientists are building is a complex task; there is no agreed way to go about it and the breadth of the field and diverse methodologies employed make it hard to convey its scope within a few paragraphs. Separating observable from experiential perspectives gives some structure. We have also chosen to focus on recent literature to give a sense of the whole of the science and its likely future directions.

Observable Aspects of Occupation

Comparatively little occupational science research has addressed the substrates involved in occupational performance: the anatomical structures to stabilize movement and apply force; the sensory and neurologic functions that direct movement; the physiologic functions that maintain homeostasis despite the rigors of performance; and the cognitive functions involved in initiating, monitoring, and communicating our actions, and judging the value of the outcome. That is perhaps because many of the client factors supporting the performance of an occupation are not directly observable, requiring neuroimaging and other technologies to "see" them. One example is an exploration of the sensory processing that occurs as people engage in occupation, which informs the "sense" people make of what they are doing and how they might adapt their actions to achieve a better result (Williams, 2017). Another is the proposal that lifestyle balance might best be interpreted as the balance of stressful occupations, such as exams and cognitively challenging work tasks, and restful occupations, such as gazing at a pleasant view, which decrease physiologic activation levels—observable as lowered heart rate and blood pressure, and activation of the hypothalamic-pituitary-adrenal (HPA) axis. The long-term aim of research of this nature would be to help people establish a lifestyle with reduced physiologic wear and tear, thus benefiting health and well-being (Hernandez et al., 2020).

The form our occupations take is readily observable, as we observe the steps involved, the duration from start to completion, how the tools required are handled, the number of people typically involved, and the pace of performance. Rules and norms guiding the performance can often be inferred, such as the kind of footwear suitable for outdoor play and whether running is acceptable. Research contributing to understanding of an occupation's form can be glimpsed in studies motivated by concern about participation in an occupation. For instance, an observational study of play occupations of autistic children was motivated by a general decline in outdoor play (Fahy et al., 2021). One occupation the children favored was running in a group, following a circular route around the playground. They were observed to follow the lead of the child in front of them and used pillars in the playground as obstacles to run around. Quantitative measures can also reveal aspects of an occupation's form, such as who does and does not participate in it and the equipment required to do so. For instance, disparities in older adults' access to mobile phones and computers have been noted and identified as contributing to systemic disadvantages for those living in poverty (Kottorp et al., 2016).

New understandings of the functions occupations serve are also coming into view. For example, interviews and observational methods revealed that children's sports can function as a means of including children with physical impairments (Asbjørnslett & Bekken, 2016), and shared occupations can function as a site for community members to learn how to help children with brain injuries participate (Jones et al., 2017). The increased use of critical methodologies also reveals aspects of the intersection of occupations and environments, such as how imposed restrictions on the occupations available to asylum seekers in Australia cause high levels of distress (Crawford et al., 2016).

Experienced Aspects of Occupation

We can study and come to understand experiential aspects of occupation through ideas (de Poy & Gitlin, 2020), which occupational scientists have typically accessed by asking individuals about their lived experiences of doing things. The substrates of occupation have not typically been the focus, even though the experience of doing things encompasses such understandings and is relevant to developing a science of occupation (Lala & Kinsella, 2011). Experiential accounts can generate insights, however, such as one evocative account of "turf cutting," that is, using a spade to cut a slice of wet turf from a peat bog that will be dried out to burn in the winter. McGrath and McGonagle (2016) described the skillful performance of this ancient occupation as "using your legs, you're using your arms, you're using your balance ... there's a bit of an art to it" (p. 316). Similarly, people's responses to occupational forms are less commonly reported, but are still present in the literature. For example, a study of the occupational rights of disabled people with direct funding to employ workers to assist them included Karen's account of going to bed at 8.15 in the evening, to fit in with the homecare agency's scheduling. Although the occupational form was observable from a quantitative perspective, in that others could see and affirm that this was her regular bedtime, it is Karen's account of its impact on her life as a university student that reveals how unwelcome

and restrictive it was to be in bed when it was still bright daylight in Ontario, Canada (Katzman et al., 2021).

The function of occupation has also been uncovered by studies asking people about their experiences. Taking on the role of peer educator in health promotion programs, for example, functioned to both maintain the physical fitness, psychological health, and social engagement of the volunteers and support participants in the program to stay in touch with their community (Turcotte et al., 2021). Finally, insights into the meanings occupations hold for particular people in specific contexts have been generated through studies using a wide range of methodologies. One recent study of older Sinhalese immigrants revealed how relocating to Canada involved surrendering long-held occupations, such as going to the temple, socializing with friends, and watching cricket, that had structured their days and contributed to a sense of identity, meaning, and purpose (Wijekoon et al., 2021).

Although we addressed them separately, what is important is not the study of occupation's observable *or* experienced aspects but the study of occupation's observable *and* experienced aspects. Both dimensions of knowledge are important to studying occupation as a basic science. One informs the other. One exists in accord with the other. It is a synergistic relationship. Beyond these aspects, moral philosophy offers an opportunity to think broadly about living a good life, such as the question of "what counts as an occupationally satisfying life" (Morgan, 2010, p. 217) or, guided by normative ethics, "How ought I practice to enable people to live occupationally satisfying lives?" Such understandings cannot be adequately addressed by observational or experiential approaches but may be addressed as the boundaries of occupational science scholarship extend to include more philosophical concerns.

The Occupational Nature of Being Human

Sitting alongside all the studies of observable and experienced aspects of occupation, there is an ongoing thread of discussion about the occupational nature of being human and the need to incorporate diverse cultural perspectives. One counterpoint to Western understandings of occupation as supporting individuals' identity and experienced in the present moment is the study by Núñez et al. (2021) of collective occupations of some Indigenous communities in Chile. Addressing their fishing practices and harvesting of medicinal plants, it is the collective and sustainable features of enacting these ancestral practices that come to the fore, along with their capacity to promote social cohesion. Further insights into an indigenous worldview frame occupation as deeply spiritual, demanding integrity, respect, and *aroha* (love, compassion) on the part of the performer (Smith, 2017). Critically informed understandings are also increasingly needed to expose the historical, political, and social forces that restrict people's occupational possibilities. This work unmasks misinformed assumptions about what people "choose" to do. For example, rather than racialized accusations of being noncompliant or disinterested in their children's well-being, the reluctance of Indigenous women in British Columbia to engage with the Aboriginal Infant Development Program can be more accurately understood to be informed responses to entrenched discrimination in the context of colonization, poverty, and a history of over-surveillance by the child welfare system (Gerlach et al., 2017). Over time, such perspectives will propel the development of knowledge of the occupational nature of humans that better represents the implicit relationship between occupation and well-being.

Occupational Science as an Applied Science

Thus far, we have considered occupational science as a basic science, yet it is more than that; it is emergent as an applied science. Applied sciences like biomechanics, ergonomics, and mental health rehabilitation provide a knowledge base informing what to do and how to go about practice for a given occupational disruption. Occupational therapists are already accustomed to using knowledge from those fields to guide their day-to-day decisions in practice. Although it may be a new addition to the applied sciences, over two decades on from its inception occupational science's latent potential exists in its capacity to be a "comprehensive translational science" (Clark & Lawlor, 2009, p. 7) that seeks insights into problems relating to engagement in occupation (basic science) to inform the development of health-promoting interventions (applied science). As will be explained, occupational science is already in the business of translating rigorous, basic science findings into evidence-based OT.

Systematizing Occupational Science Knowledge

Earlier in the development of occupational science, Clark and Lawlor (2009) asserted that it "is designed to systematize knowledge about occupation, especially in relation to health and well-being" (p. 4). So, let us look more closely at what is meant by systematizing knowledge. The origins, or etymology, of the word helps us to make sense of what it means to "systematize" knowledge. "Systema" in Greek was derived from the root words meaning "together" and to "cause to stand"; in other words, *systema* referred to something that stands as one in an "organized whole" (Harper, n.d.). Systematizing is about identifying, developing, analyzing, and optimizing knowledge for use. Thus, a process

that systematizes occupational science knowledge for OT is a methodical, rigorous way of developing a coherent set of rules or methods for application in practice.

Systematized occupational science knowledge is beginning to guide OT practice at all levels, from individual health to population health approaches. As we mentioned earlier, it is a translational process—translating findings from basic science into applied practice knowledge. As a translational science, occupational science generates theory-driven research aimed at resolving real-world concerns by informing occupation-based practice (Laliberte Rudman & Aldrich, 2017). Conversely, real-world, OT practice-based evidence (PBE) rigorously analyzed from systematized intervention outcomes has the potential to inform new ways of theorizing occupational science. Systematizing occupational science knowledge fits with the international call for health practitioners, including occupational therapists, to use best evidence to guide everyday practice.

A great number of frameworks to guide translational science research programs have been put forward internationally. Among the frameworks proposed within the health sciences, increasing emphasis is now given to engagement with communities, collaboration among researchers with diverse expertise, and involvement of practitioners implementing the recommendations or interventions being generated. There are good reasons for such collaborations. Engaging with communities experiencing the problem makes it more likely that research efforts address things that are important to the individuals affected, that theory development represents their perspective, and that the interventions developed make sense to them, are feasible in their context, and make enough difference to be worth investing effort, time, and resources. Research collaborations strengthen research designs and ensure research teams have access to the expertise they need. When researchers collaborate with occupational therapists in practice, there is increased likelihood that real-world considerations are taken into account, the interventions developed are workable within time and resource constraints, challenges with implementation are foreseen or resolved, and training materials and programs are trialed in preparation for implementation.

In addition to these collaborative practices, there is also explicit acknowledgment that knowledge generation is cyclical. For example, the testing and implementation phases might stimulate refinement or radical rethinking of interventions or recommendations, and theoretical insights that emerge as an outcome of the whole program of research can clarify the nature or occurrence of the initial problem. The contextual nature of all knowledge is also increasingly recognized, which means that there must be transparency and critique in relation to the worldview underpinning translational science research programs (e.g., an occupational perspective), the demographics of research participants (e.g., a representative sample of nursing home residents), and the context (e.g., high socioeconomic deprivation region).

The framework presented here is adapted from one developed at the Division of Occupational Science and Occupational Therapy, University of Southern California (USC), in the United States (Clark & Lawlor, 2009), which was designed as a rigorous way of developing OT practice knowledge to address issues about which little is known, but which may have an occupational foundation (see Figure 9.2). Community engagement and professional collaborations of communities, researchers, and practitioners are depicted as an encircling and indispensable part of the translational science research framework.

The process begins with identifying and articulating an observed or perceived problem with participation in occupation. Having defined the problem, research is conducted to gather a first layer of descriptive evidence to build a theoretical understanding of the nature of the problem, how it relates to people's occupations, and what might be possible to change. Equipped with that explanation, the research team proposes avenues for change: either things communities or individuals might do to produce a different outcome or development of an intervention. This might be something novel or a refinement of an existing intervention. Clearly, engaging with people experiencing the issue is imperative throughout this process of inquiry, given that occupation is always embedded in people's worldview. Possibilities for change that are not in accordance with their aspirations, priorities, resources, family and social structures, and culture will not be fully taken up—or if they are taken up, may disturb or disrupt the community researchers intend to assist. At an extreme, lack of engagement with the people researchers are trying to help can contribute to ongoing colonization by imposing "outside" perspectives and solutions that frame local knowledge as irrelevant, misguided, or erroneous. All such considerations require careful reporting, to aid communities and therapists in their judgment about the extent to which findings relate to their own context. Similar considerations hold true at all

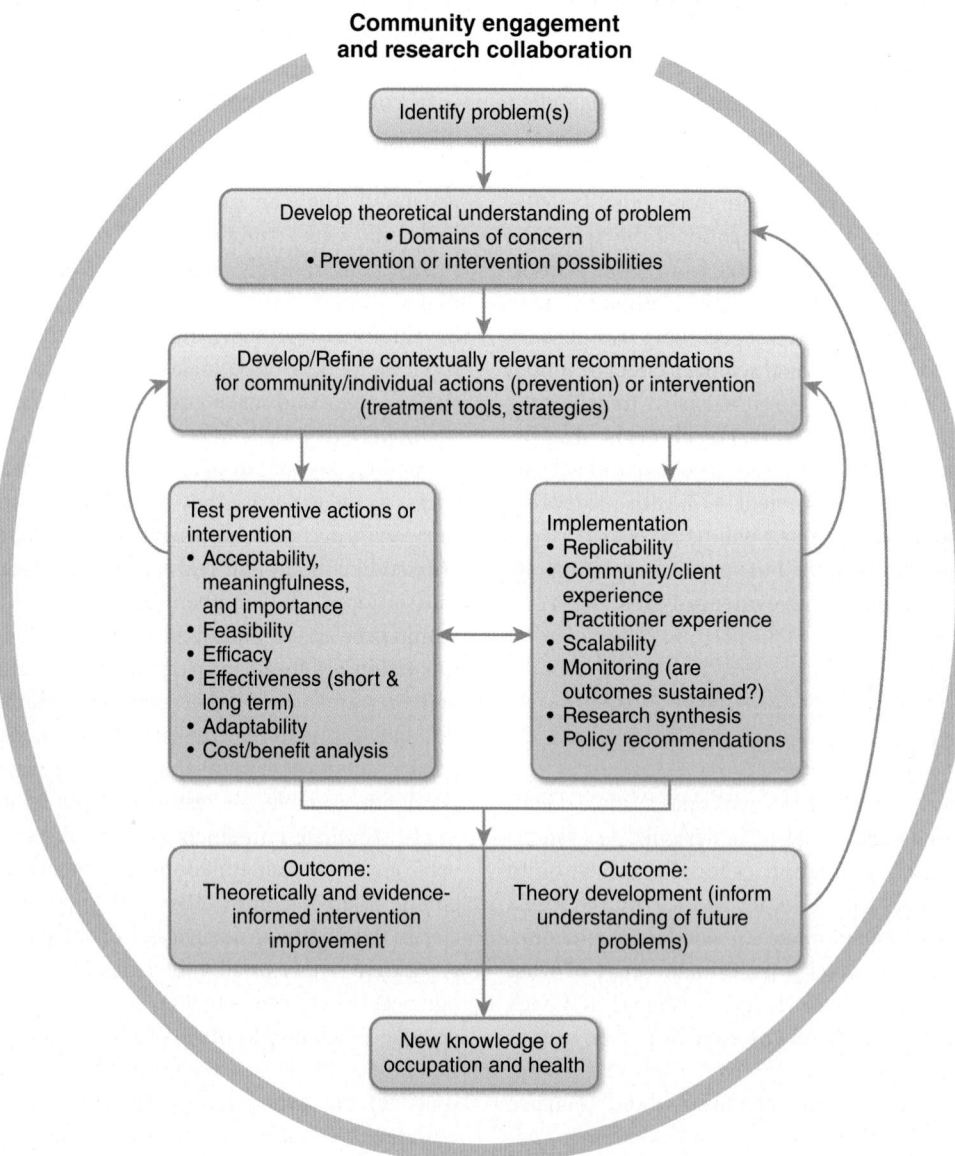

FIGURE 9.2 Framework for a translational science research program.

stages of translational science research programs. Having explored the nature of an issue and its physical and cultural context, preliminary testing of the recommendation or intervention can commence. Here, testing refers to establishing how reliable the intervention is in bringing about the desired outcome, then measuring its cost-effectiveness, and so on. Although initial testing is likely to occur under more controlled conditions, the implementation studies that follow are directed toward trials in real-world contexts; the recommendations are actioned, or interventions delivered, in diverse contexts with diverse people.

The testing and implementation phases we propose are elaborated in some detail in Figure 9.2, informed, initially, by occupational perspectives of the meaningfulness and importance of the issue in people's lives and the experience of delivering and participating in the intervention. The more "scientific" concerns such as efficacy, scalability, and monitoring are drawn from the translational science research framework proposed by the Sax Institute (2016). Considerations include any training required, funding and resource constraints, and any adaptations required to accommodate variations across populations involved or the form, function, and meaning of the target occupations. As the framework suggests, both testing and implementation require a whole program of research, most likely involving multiple studies with different purposes and outcomes. Both qualitative and quantitative studies are needed, for example, to capture people's experience of an intervention and their perception of what it achieved and to quantify that change.

The framework depicts the testing and implementation phases side by side to reflect the real-world practice of trialing implementation of preventive measures or targeted interventions while basic research into efficacy, effectiveness, acceptability, and so on continues. Again, knowledge of observable/measurable and experienced responses to the proposed and trialed recommendations and interventions is crucial, necessitating the inclusion of community members, people experiencing the occupational challenge, practitioners, health service planners, and so on in the research team.

The methodical steps involved in developing new recommendations and interventions might seem enough in themselves, but for this practice knowledge to "stand together" as an organized whole, understanding why interventions work is essential. A coherent body of causal evidence then opens the way to build an explanatory theory, bringing together the research observations with interpretive reasoning to explain outcomes of intervention and add to the body of occupation-based knowledge. That knowledge can then be called on as new problems are identified. Such a rigorous process shows the symbiotic relationship between the practice and research communities (Cogan et al., 2014). In the OT domain, questions for occupational science research might arise from practice-based issues, and the research findings, in return, provide knowledge for practice. Practice and research exist and thrive together. However, implementing the blueprint for generating new knowledge is not for the fainthearted; it takes years to undertake multiple studies and requires significant funding and researcher and community commitment. The following examples illustrate how occupational science research can underpin and come to life in the context of OT practice.

Occupational Science Informing Occupational Therapy

Occupational science informing OT is an idea whose time has come (Blanche & Henny-Kohler, 2000; Clark et al., 2004; Molineux, 2004; Pierce, 2011). The following three examples (OT Stories 9.1–9.3) show how scientific understandings about human occupation are informing practice across the international OT community. The systematic program of translational science research presented in Figure 9.2 is used explicitly as a way of illuminating the steps involved, and how they have played out differently in each example.

OT STORY 9.1 OCCUPATIONS AND PRESSURE INJURY RISK: THE USC/RANCHO LOS AMIGOS NATIONAL REHABILITATION CENTER PRESSURE ULCER PREVENTION RESEARCH PROGRAM

Identify the Problem

In the United States, pressure injuries are a frequent, multifaceted, and costly problem for people with spinal cord injury (SCI). Of particular interest to occupational scientists and therapists is the concern that pressure injuries are a recurrent barrier to participation in everyday occupations and could have an occupational causation (Clark et al., 2006).

As the researchers discovered, mundane occupations might hold hidden risks (Figure 9.3).

Develop Theoretical Understanding of the Problem

Occupational scientists at the USC and their research collaborators designed a holistic ethnographic, qualitative study,

(continued)

OT STORY 9.1 OCCUPATIONS AND PRESSURE INJURY RISK: THE USC/ RANCHO LOS AMIGOS NATIONAL REHABILITATION CENTER PRESSURE ULCER PREVENTION RESEARCH PROGRAM (*continued*)

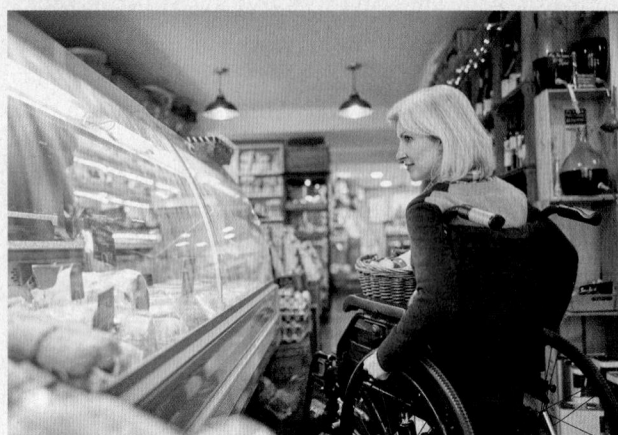

FIGURE 9.3 Mundane occupations might hold hidden risks of pressure injuries for wheelchair users.

now called the Pressure Ulcer Prevention Study I or PUPS I, to explore the everyday life contexts that contribute to the occurrence of pressure injuries in men and women from different socioeconomic backgrounds following SCI (Clark et al., 2007). Through a prolonged, in-depth process of observing and interviewing participants as they went about their usual days, the researchers sought to understand how their daily lives played out as risks for pressure injuries (Clark et al., 2006). For example, Robert's story illustrates the interplay between an individualized risk profile, the quest for occupation, and the development of pressure injuries. Robert spent much of his day riding around in his wheelchair and developed two pressure injuries as a consequence. After analyzing the narratives from diverse participants, the researchers developed a coherent series of pressure injury development models to account for the individualized and richly contextualized portfolio of occupations in relation to risk. These models incorporated the dynamic balance of liability and buffering factors, individualized risk profiles, a generalized pressure injury event sequence (Figure 9.4), and a long-term pressure injury event sequence. Although theoretical in nature, the models are grounded in qualitatively derived, occupational science data.

Among other results, the occupational scientists found that pressure injuries most commonly occurred, and recurred, for those who (a) had a moderately high-risk profile and (b) experienced a disruptive health or life event. What the findings highlight is the need for preventive interventions to take account of "the unique constellation of circumstances that comprise a person's everyday life" (Clark et al., 2006, p. 1516). The knowledge gained through this preliminary investigative work was ready to be further systematized and tested out in an applied study.

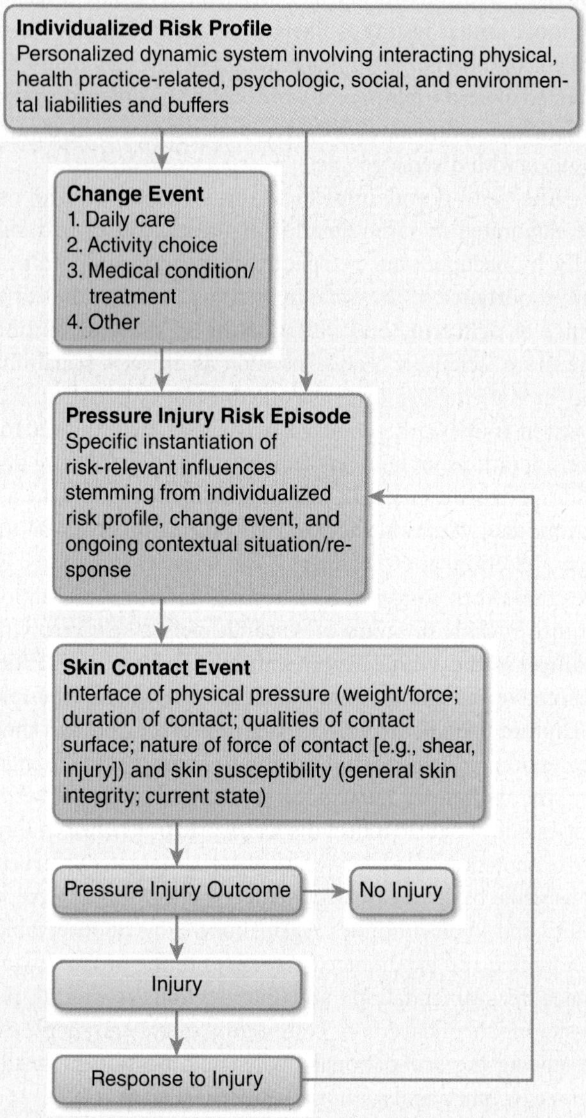

Individualized Risk Profile
Personalized dynamic system involving interacting physical, health practice-related, psychologic, social, and environmental liabilities and buffers

Change Event
1. Daily care
2. Activity choice
3. Medical condition/ treatment
4. Other

Pressure Injury Risk Episode
Specific instantiation of risk-relevant influences stemming from individualized risk profile, change event, and ongoing contextual situation/response

Skin Contact Event
Interface of physical pressure (weight/force; duration of contact; qualities of contact surface; nature of force of contact [e.g., shear, injury]) and skin susceptibility (general skin integrity; current state)

Pressure Injury Outcome → No Injury

Injury

Response to Injury

FIGURE 9.4 Overview of generalized pressure injury event sequence.

(Adapted from Clark, F. A., Jackson, J. M., Scott, M. D., Atkins, M. S., Uhles-Tanaka, D., & Rubayi, S. [2006]. Data-based models of how pressure ulcers developing daily-living contexts of adults with spinal cord injury. *Archives of Physical Medicine and Rehabilitation, 87,* 1516–1525. https://doi.org/10.1016/j.apmr.2006.08.329. Copyright [2006], with permission from Elsevier.)

Develop the Intervention

Armed with the ethnographic study findings, the occupational scientists now understood how pressure injury development was potentially modifiable. Their next step was to thoughtfully apply this basic knowledge they had gained to design an OT intervention based on lifestyle redesign.

OT STORY 9.1 OCCUPATIONS AND PRESSURE INJURY RISK: THE USC/ RANCHO LOS AMIGOS NATIONAL REHABILITATION CENTER PRESSURE ULCER PREVENTION RESEARCH PROGRAM (*continued*)

Test the Intervention

Putting the intervention to the test meant conducting an occupational science-driven randomized clinical trial (RCT) to determine the efficacy of the Pressure Ulcer Prevention Program (PUPP) in preventing medically serious pressure injuries. An early step was to manualize a rigorous therapeutic protocol to guide the therapist's focus on what matters, articulate the professional reasoning process, and map out the intervention procedures (Blanche et al., 2011). For the RCT, 144 men and 26 women who had sustained an SCI at least 6 months earlier, were nonambulatory, and had experienced at least one serious pressure injury were recruited. They were randomly assigned to either the 12-month occupation-based PUPP intervention group or standard care. The intervention included participants' self-selected goals, active problem-solving, and engagement in motivational interviewing. The incidence rate of new serious pressure injuries was the primary outcome measured before intervention, at 12 months, and at a 24-month follow-up (Clark et al., 2014). The unanticipated challenges of conducting an RCT in the real world, such as insufficient statistical power and the participants' chaotic life circumstances (Ghaisas et al., 2015), meant the researchers' ability to determine how much the lifestyle intervention *caused* positive change was compromised and the results of the intention-to-treat analysis were inconclusive (Carlson et al., 2019). A further study on the possibility of inadvertently altering the behaviors of the control group, by contacting them every 3 months to collect data about skin integrity, was also inconclusive (Carlson et al., 2019). Additional studies are needed to establish the efficacy of an occupation-focused intervention and its cost-effectiveness as an approach to reducing pressure ulcer incidence.

Implementation

Although the results of the RCT did not generate clear evidence of efficacy, it was still possible to examine the *relationship* between participants' lifestyle changes and pressure injury status. A secondary analysis of the treatment notes of the intervention group showed four patterns to the relationship between lifestyle changes and pressure injury development. The resulting case profiles can inform occupational therapists working in the field (Ghaisas et al., 2015) who use occupation-focused lifestyle interventions. In addition, the occupational scientists codesigned a comprehensive set of evidence-based, readily available online resources that can be employed by occupational therapists or consumers. For example, one provides guidance on pressure injury prevention techniques to families or carers. Perhaps most important, another provides information for people with SCI on the importance of everyday occupations as well as the risks associated with engagement in them (USC, 2013). More recently, the researchers published a PBE framework for methodically customizing the lifestyle intervention manual for therapy with a different group, US veterans (Cogan et al., 2014).

Outcomes

At a practice level, knowledge gained from this occupationally focused research on pressure injury prevention is now incorporated into an international guideline on prevention and treatment of pressure injuries (European Pressure Ulcer Advisory Panel, National Pressure Injury Advisory Panel, & Pan Pacific Pressure Injury Alliance, 2019). From a theoretical perspective, the PUPS research program has already generated considerable theory development. For example, its qualitative arms have produced overarching principles of pressure injury risk and data-based models therapists can employ to more comprehensively understand the elements that contribute to pressure injury risk (Clark et al., 2006; Jackson et al., 2010) and insights into the role habits play in sustaining recurrent pressure injuries (Fogelberg et al., 2016). Furthermore, a conceptual model was developed from the clinical trial. The model depicts how adherence to the lifestyle intervention and utilization of its components can have positive effects on recipients' self-efficacy, knowledge, and social support, which, in turn, can mediate pressure injury prevention (Clark et al., 2014). Systematizing occupational science knowledge means everyone wins: those with SCIs, their families and friends, the healthcare funders and providers, the greater community, and of course, the occupational therapists, who gain a theoretically guided, scientifically grounded, and evidence-based intervention approach for lessening pressure injury risk in people with SCI.

Questions

1. Propose one quantitative and one qualitative question you might ask Robert, to learn more about the pressure injury risks he faces from riding around in his wheelchair.
2. What are some of the advantages of codesigning resources for use by occupational therapists or consumers?
3. Why are replication studies important?

OT STORY 9.2 THE CO–OP™ APPROACH: PROMOTING PARTICIPATION IN OCCUPATION

Identify the Problem

It is well recognized that children with developmental coordination disorder (DCD) can struggle with everyday occupations, falling behind their siblings and peers. The occupational and social consequences can be profound, affecting their ability to master routine activities of daily living (ADLs), succeed at school, make friends, and establish positive self-esteem. Given the lifelong implications for these children and their families, occupational therapists at McMaster University in Canada have worked since the 1990s to find effective ways to improve children's performance and confidence in what they can do.

Develop Theoretical Understanding of the Problem

As a first step, the researchers consulted literature to understand that the difficulties associated with DCD should not be regarded as impaired maturation of the central nervous system substrates. Rather, as suggested by contemporary theories of motor learning and motor control, and consistent with OT theory, they reasoned that the children's performance resulted from interactions among the context, task demands, and children's unique physical, cognitive, and affective factors in the process of learning how to solve movement problems. They reasoned that the focus for intervention needed to be on occupational goals and enabling children to learn how to problem-solve ways to perform occupations in context (Missiuna et al., 2001). Determining that the difficulties experienced by children with DCD is best understood as a problem of skill acquisition and problem-solving opened up new avenues for supporting competent occupational performance (see Figure 9.5).

Develop the Intervention

The intervention initially developed was called Verbal Self-Guidance (Martini & Polatajko, 1998). As described in Missiuna et al. (2001), the intervention drew on relevant theories. (a) Children's use of self-talk as they work through difficult tasks came from Vygotsky's sociocultural theory. (b) Scaffolding learning with a global problem-solving process was grounded in Luria's and Meichenbaum's work. (c) Bringing adults in to mediate the learning and generalize meaning from it drew on theory proposed by Feuerstein and by Haywood. Care was also taken to ensure the intervention design was consistent with child- and family-centered care, using goals selected by children and their parents to ensure the intervention was both relevant in their context and empowering (Missiuna et al., 1998, 2001).

Test the Intervention

Testing and refining the intervention began with single-case experimental studies using the Goal-Plan-Do-Check process,

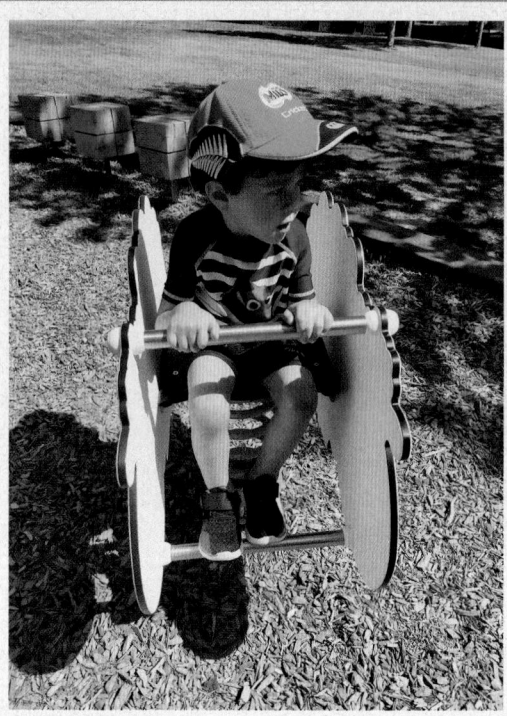

FIGURE 9.5 **Logan learning to use the playground equipment.**

(Courtesy of Kim Frenchman.)

where children verbalize instructions to guide themselves through a task. Initial evidence was that the intervention was effective in improving task performance, with outcomes sustained over 12 weeks. The studies also informed refinements in the intervention, such as including parents in its delivery so that they could support the children's continued use of the problem-solving strategy they had learned (Martini & Polatajko, 1998; Polatajko et al., 2001). Analysis of videos from those early studies revealed that the children additionally employed domain-specific cognitive strategies, which helped them acquire the skills necessary for competent performance (Mandich et al., 2001). This realization prompted the development of an intervention protocol, including domain-specific strategies, and the renaming of the intervention as the Cognitive Orientation to daily Occupational Performance (CO–OP) (Polatajko et al., 2001). The effectiveness of the CO–OP intervention was then tested in an RCT that showed it resulted in significantly greater improvements in performance than the current, eclectic treatments (Miller et al., 2001). Building on that early evidence base, collaborations with researchers, practitioners, and teachers internationally have been encouraged through the CANCHILD website (see https://canchild.ca), and more recently, by incorporating practitioners in different settings in the research process. Testing of the CO–OP approach is thus ongoing as its application is reported in the literature

OT STORY 9.2 THE CO–OP™ APPROACH: PROMOTING PARTICIPATION IN OCCUPATION (*continued*)

and through DCD conferences. Testing of the approach with other client groups, including children with acquired brain injuries and adults, is now underway.

Implementation

Once the effectiveness and efficacy of the CO–OP approach with children with DCD had been demonstrated in research settings, it was time to take it out into the real world. As indicated in Figure 9.2, these studies have been undertaken in parallel with ongoing testing and refinement of the intervention. Implementation studies began using data generated by occupational therapists at a university clinic who had been trained to deliver the CO–OP. Significant pre–post differences were found in children's general movement skills, their visual motor integration, and adaptive behavior. Together, these results suggested the skills learned had been generalized. Importantly, the children's rating of their performance and their satisfaction with the occupations they had worked on were also statistically significant (Polatajko et al., 2001). Subsequently, studies on the implementation of the CO–OP have been completed in Australia, Hong Kong, Brazil, and India. Qualitative studies of child and practitioner experiences of using the CO–OP have pointed to refinements that can support its implementation, including actively coaching parents (Gharebaghy et al., 2021) and ensuring adequate managerial support for the intervention within organizations (Hunt et al., 2021). Implementation is also supported through provision of continuing education courses on the CO–OP hosted by the Department of Occupational Science & Occupational Therapy at the University of Toronto, Canada.

Outcomes

Almost 30 years after work began on finding a more effective way to support children with DCD, the CO–OP is a well-known and well-regarded intervention. There is a comparatively strong body of evidence supporting its use although, as is true of many interventions that are tailored to clients' unique goals and contexts, both testing and implementation studies continue to be small scale. The underlying theory, of empowering people to set a performance goal and use cognitive processes to guide their performance of the steps required, informs understandings of the nature of DCD. It has also expanded knowledge of children's capacity to learn and apply strategies to enhance motor performance. That knowledge is being applied to other health conditions that impede cognitive functioning, furthering understandings of the part cognition plays in task performance and spawning new research directions.

Questions

1. As the CO–OP is increasingly implemented internationally, why might research evaluating its fidelity, or consistency of its delivery, be important?
2. What are some things an OT researcher might need to consider before replicating CO–OP research within an organization in your country?
3. How might you go about exploring the acceptability of the CO–OP intervention among Indigenous people in a community?

OT STORY 9.3 REDO PROGRAM: HELPING PEOPLE RETURN TO WORK AFTER LONG-TERM SICK LEAVE

Identify the Problem

Although occupational therapists have long assumed that a balance of occupations supports health, there is little evidence quantifying that relationship. Nonetheless, by the year 2000 it was clear that a problem existed. Increasing numbers of Swedish women were on long-term sick leave from their workplace because of work-related stress and anxiety. Faced with a worsening health situation that appeared to be implicitly occupational, occupational scientists recognized they had an important part to play in alleviating a growing social problem.

Develop Theoretical Understanding of the Problem

Reasoning that married women with children who work both inside and outside the home experience high levels of stress, Lena-Karin Erlandsson set out to develop a method of mapping the complexity of their daily occupational patterns. She asked 100 women to chart what they were doing over a 24-hour period, noting when they shifted from their main occupation to a hidden or unexpected occupation. Hidden occupations were defined as "performed with less notice, but considered as necessary elements of a daily

(*continued*)

routine, for example ironing a pair of trousers," whereas unexpected occupations are those "that interrupt the rhythm of main and hidden occupations and may be initiated by the performer's own thoughts or a stimulus from the environment" (Erlandsson & Eklund, 2006, p. 30). Analysis of the data revealed that women with more complex patterns of occupation characterized by frequent interruptions rate their health lower than women who can spend concentrated time on tasks they set out to complete.

Develop the Intervention

Increasing numbers of working mothers experience interruptions to their main occupation. Drawing on the results of the study outlined above, related studies, and the Value and Meaning in Occupations (ValMO) theory (Erlandsson et al., 2011), the Redesigning Daily Occupations (ReDO) program was developed to enable lifestyle changes that would support women with stress-related disorders to return to work. The development process was a collaboration between the main researcher and four occupational therapists who would go on to carry out the intervention. Together, they discussed the length of the program, the content of each session, the activities participants would engage in, and the practical arrangements to run the program. Over a 4-month period, a detailed written protocol was agreed on that would ensure consistency across different therapists, participants, and contexts. The protocol described a 16-week group rehabilitation program consisting of three phases: (a) complete an occupational self-analysis; (b) set goals and identify strategies for change; (c) begin a job placement program to implement the strategies identified in Stage 2 (Erlandsson, 2013).

Test the Intervention

The ReDO program has been described as taking a client-educating collaborative approach that provides "participants with knowledge and understanding of how their own unique patterns of daily occupations are developed and how they affect health" (Erlandsson, 2013, p. 97). In the initial trial of the effectiveness of the program, 42 women were enrolled. Twelve months after completing the program, data about their return to work, sick leave, perceived stress, and self-esteem were compared with a matched sample of women who had received usual care. Although the intervention succeeded in helping women resume work, decreased sick leave, and improved self-esteem, there was no difference in relation to stress reduction (Eklund & Erlandsson, 2011). Subsequent studies testing the efficacy, effectiveness, and adaptability of ReDo have expanded its application to diverse populations experiencing ill-health who would benefit from changing their everyday life patterns. Thus, testing the intervention has demonstrated its benefits well beyond the

original focus on "dual working" women. The acceptability of the ReDO program has also been tested, for example, by investigating quality of life and client satisfaction outcomes (Eklund & Erlandsson, 2013). Other studies have had a greater focus on how the working relationship between program participants and leaders affects outcomes (Eklund et al., 2015) and how women's perception of their workplace changes after participating in the program (Wästberg et al., 2016). Yet another study has investigated whether increases in perceived health and occupational balance predict participants' work ability (Olsson et al., 2020). Thus, knowledge of the program itself and the elements that make it successful are being strengthened over time.

Implementation

Alongside ongoing testing of the program, two other strands of work are underway. First, strategies to ensure the sustainability of the 1-week course to train occupational therapists to deliver the ReDO program are being put in place, including translation of the training package into English. Second, researchers are beginning to report the results of implementation studies. For example, a recent study in Ireland explored the feasibility of a 10-week version of the ReDO program, which had been developed for and tested in primary care settings, from the perspective of participants, the referring doctors, and occupational therapists (Fox et al., 2021).

Outcomes

The research described above is building a strong foundation of evidence supporting delivery of the ReDO program in its original format and the shorter 10-week version. Confidence in the program is also boosted by the level of engagement with OT practitioners in its initial design and with occupational therapists and referring doctors in later studies. Although participant perceptions of the program have been canvassed by researchers, they have not had direct input into its ongoing refinement. In addition to testing the program and its implementation, research is also generating new insights at a theoretical level, about the relationship between occupational imbalance and ill-health. For instance, one study found that occupational balance, rather than sociodemographic indicators such as age, gender, educational level, and number of children, was the main predictor of mental ill-health and, conversely, higher levels of occupational balance and having variety, recovery/sleep, and meaningful occupations are associated with higher levels of perceived health. This finding supports the approach taken in the ReDO program of intervening across people's entire pattern of daily occupations rather than focusing specifically on their paid work (Karlsson et al., 2021). As the diversity

OT STORY 9.3 REDO PROGRAM: HELPING PEOPLE RETURN TO WORK AFTER LONG-TERM SICK LEAVE (continued)

of research focuses makes evident, there is a great deal of information to gather about newly developed interventions before occupational therapists can be truly confident in recommending them, and even more to find out about the ways occupational balance and health interrelate.

Questions

1. Would refining the ReDO program based on participant perceptions of participating in it be an example of testing the intervention or an implementation study?

2. Can you pose an explanation why the results of one study testing the ReDO intervention found it helped women resume work and improved self-esteem, but did not reduce stress levels? How could researchers test your assumption?

3. Do you think the ReDo intervention would help people in your country improve their occupational balance and work ability? Why or why not?

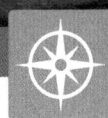

EXPANDING OUR PERSPECTIVES

Collaborations in Practice and Research

Arul Hamill and Lucy Charles

In our pediatric practice in Auckland, New Zealand, we're really committed to engaging with families, connecting with them and finding out what's important for them, and what actually would have the most impact for them. The main thing that drives us is the feedback from families such as "I can see my child in a different light" or "All of a sudden, we're having much more positive conversations about what our child can do, not what they can't do." Of course, we don't get it right every day, but we strive to be the best we can be … always questioning whether we're doing this, how we can do that differently …

The way we practice now has its origins, in a sense, in a community of practice set up some years ago with like-minded therapists. The discussions we had back then were like a broadening of our minds, based in relationships of trust and acceptance, and of being vulnerable to challenges to what we were thinking. Listening to each other and being open to the chaos that comes first help us when we are going through a period of change. We went on to learn different approaches that were being reported in the research literature, like Occupational Performance Coaching and CanChild's F-words,[1] which we added to our toolbox. The use of F-words enabled us to move on from a biomedical focus on impairments or "fixing" body

structures or functions. We moved to a biopsychosocial model of care, focusing on participation and what the child wanted and needed to do. When we applied our coaching knowledge, we really started handing over the control to children and families. We started to see people in a totally different light, because it was not about the tasks we were coming up with. Instead, families were bringing ordinary routines and tasks to us, saying, "Actually, this is what is happening to us. This is what we would love to see our child do more of."

After some time, we realized we needed to bring F-words and coaching together, to provide a voice for families and children. We created a resource and an approach, called the F-words Life Wheel, that enabled us to use coaching conversations with children and families in a way that really empowered them to express what was happening for them. It gave us a bird's-eye view of the whole of their life, including their *family, friends, fun, fitness, function* at school, home, and in the community and an insight into their vision for their *future* (the F-words). It enabled them to think about the next steps in their child's development, and what would enable them to have, for example, more fun or friends, or improve their function at school. As we went to share what we had developed with other people, we had to really unpack and question what we were doing. It was so exciting to have those discussions with both clinicians and researchers.

We happened to have a physical therapist working with us at that time, who had just been to the CanChild research and education center at McMaster University in Hamilton, Ontario, Canada. The research taking place there focuses on bettering the lives of children with developmental conditions and their families. The physical therapist said to us, "Look at what you've just done in terms of translating knowledge into practice, putting coaching and

---

[1] Occupational Performance Coaching is an evidence-based intervention that supports people with disabilities and their families to achieve their goals (Graham et al., 2021). The F-words for Child Development refer to six aspects essential to children's development: Functioning, Family, Fitness, Fun, Friends, and Future (Rosenbaum & Gorter, 2011). The application of the F-words in guiding effective practice with children with disabilities is the focus of ongoing research.

(continued)

EXPANDING OUR PERSPECTIVES (*continued*)

F-words together." So, she connected us with the research team at CanChild, and said to the team there, "You should see what these guys are doing!" So, we've been involved with CanChild for about 3 years, and now we are partnering with them in researching implementation of the F-words in practice with children and their families. We've had some really interesting conversations with researchers we've partnered with, not only in Canada, but in the United Kingdom, the United States, and Australia. It's been a sort of two-way reflective process. That's what it's like when we engage with CanChild: the researchers there, the communities, and their families. A two-way thing starts to happen, and everybody is enriched by those interactions. Like our work with families, partnering and collaboration are central to taking those next steps going forward. We don't know what that's going to look like yet but being research-engaged therapists means being open to new ideas and ways of doing things and having the flexibility to follow the evidence.

As we changed our practice, we needed to come to a place of acceptance of how we practiced before. We had the right heart and the vision for it, but that's all we knew. We had to come to that acceptance for ourselves, that it was okay. We often say, "Well, we only knew what was in our hands during that time." We did the best we could do with what we had. Now we are following the research, but also following our hearts, and listening to the stories of families and journeying alongside them.

Conclusion

As is already happening in numerous locations internationally, it is time for occupational science to take its place as a science informing OT practice. You might say that knowledge about the occupations people do, and their capacities and drive to do them, has always informed OT. At one level, this is true; at a far deeper and expansive level, the work done since the 1980s, beginning with researchers and colleagues at USC, is allowing a more profound philosophical, theoretical, and research knowledge base on humans as occupational beings to take root and flourish. There is a burgeoning of high-quality basic science available to practitioners to make sense of in the context of their own practice. Moreover, the quality and applicability of the knowledge generated is improving as researchers increasingly collaborate with the populations that experience occupational issues and practitioners who apply research evidence in practice. That is where occupational science's emergent capacity as a comprehensive applied science lies; in informing OT practice and society as a whole.

Lippincott® Connect *For additional resources on the subjects discussed in this chapter, visit Lippincott Connect.*

REFERENCES

American Occupational Therapy Association. (2020). Occupational therapy practice framework: Domain and process—Fourth edition. *American Journal of Occupational Therapy, 74*(Suppl 2), 7412410010p1–7412410010p87. https://doi.org/10.5014/ajot.2020 .74S2001

Asbjørnslett, M., & Bekken, W. (2016). Openness to difference: Inclusion in sports occupations for children with (dis)abilities. *Journal of Occupational Science, 23*(4), 434–445. https://doi.org/10.1080/14427 591.2016.1199389

Barlott, T., MacKenzie, P., Le Goullon, D., Campbell, L., & Setchell, J. (2021). A transactional perspective on the everyday use of technology by people with learning disabilities. *Journal of Occupational Science*, 1–17. Advance online publication. https://doi.org/10.1080/1442 7591.2021.1970616

Blanche, E. I., Fogelberg, D., Diaz, J., Carlson, M., & Clark, F. (2011). Manualization of occupational therapy interventions: Illustrations from the Pressure Ulcer Prevention Research Program. *American Journal of Occupational Therapy, 65*(6), 711–719. https://doi.org/10.5014/ ajot.2011.001172

Blanche, E. I., & Henny-Kohler, E. (2000). Philosophy, science and ideology: A proposed relationship for occupational science and occupational therapy. *Occupational Therapy International, 7*(2), 99–110. https://doi.org/10.1002/oti.110

Carlson, M., Vigen, C. L. P., Rubayi, S., Blanche, E. I., Blanchard, J., Atkins, M., Bates-Jensen, B., Garber, S. L., Pyatak, E. A., Diaz, J., Florindez, L. I., Hay, J. W., Mallinson, T., Unger, J. B., Azen, S. P., Scott, M., Cogan, A., & Clark, F. (2019). Lifestyle intervention for adults with spinal cord injury: Results of the USC–RLANRC Pressure Ulcer Prevention Study. *Journal of Spinal Cord Medicine, 42*(1), 2–19. https://doi.org/10.1080/10790268.2017.1313931

Clark, F. A., Jackson, J. M., & Carlson, M. (2004). Occupational science, occupational therapy and evidence-based practice: What the Well Elderly Study has taught us. In M. Molineux (Ed.), *Occupation for occupational therapists* (pp. 200–218). Blackwell.

Clark, F. A., Jackson, J. M., Scott, M. D., Atkins, M. S., Uhles-Tanaka, D., & Rubayi, S. (2006). Data-based models of how pressure ulcers develop in daily-living contexts of adults with spinal cord injury. *Archives of Physical Medicine and Rehabilitation, 87*(11), 1516–1525. https://doi .org/10.1016/j.apmr.2006.08.329

Clark, F. A., & Lawlor, M. C. (2009). The making and mattering of occupational science. In E. B. Crepeau, E. S. Cohn, & B. A. Schell (Eds.), *Willard & Spackman's occupational therapy* (11th ed., pp. 2–14). Lippincott Williams & Wilkins.

Clark, F. A., Pyatak, E. A., Carlson, M., Blanche, E. I., Vigen, C., Hay, J., Mallinson, T., Blanchard, J., Unger, J. B., Garber, S. L., Diaz, J., Florindez, L. I., Atkins, M., Rubayi, S., & Azen, S. P. (2014). Implementing trials of complex interventions in community settings: The USC–Rancho Los Amigos Pressure Ulcer Prevention Study (PUPS). *Clinical Trials, 11*(2), 218–229. https://doi.org/10.1177/1740774514521904

Clark, F. A., Sanders, K., Carlson, M., Blanche, E., & Jackson, J. (2007). Synthesis of habit theory. *OTJR: Occupation, Participation and Health, 27*(Suppl 1), 7S–23S. https://doi.org/10.1177/15394492070270S103

Cogan, A. M., Blanche, E. I., Diaz, J., Clark, F. A., & Chun, S. (2014). Building a framework for implementing new interventions. *OTJR: Occupation, Participation and Health, 34*(4), 209–220. https://doi.org/10.3928/15394492-20141009-01

Crawford, E., Turpin, M., Nayar, S., Steel, E., & Durand, J.-L. (2016). The structural-personal interaction: Occupational deprivation and asylum seekers in Australia. *Journal of Occupational Science, 23*(3), 321–338. https://doi.org/10.1080/14427591.2016.1153510

de Poy, E., & Gitlin, L. N. (2020). *Introduction to research: Understanding and applying multiple strategies* (6th ed.). Elsevier.

Donnelly, M. R., Fukumura, Y. E., & Richter, M. (2021). Untapped sources of contextualized knowledge: Exploring occupational disruption during COVID-19 as showcased through YouTube parodies. *Journal of Occupational Science, 29*(3), 417–429. Advance online publication. https://doi.org/10.1080/14427591.2021.1991841

Eklund, M., & Erlandsson, L.-K. (2011). Return to work outcomes of the Redesigning Daily Occupations (ReDO) program for women with stress-related disorders—A comparative study focusing on return to work. *Women & Health, 51*(7), 676–692. https://doi.org/10.1080/03630242.2011.618215

Eklund, M., & Erlandsson, L.-K. (2013). Quality of life and client satisfaction as outcomes of the Redesigning Daily Occupations (ReDO) programme for women with stress-related disorders: A comparative study. *Work, 46*(1), 51–58. https://doi.org/10.3233/WOR-121524

Eklund, M., Erlandsson, L.-K., & Wästberg, B. (2015). A longitudinal study of the working relationship and return to work: Perceptions by clients and occupational therapists in primary health care. *BMC Family Practice, 16*, 46. https://doi.org/10.1186/s12875-015-0258-1

Erlandsson, L.-K. (2013). The Redesigning Daily Occupations (ReDO)-program: Supporting women with stress-related disorders to return to work—Knowledge base, structure, and content. *Occupational Therapy in Mental Health, 29*(1), 85–101. https://doi.org/10.1080/0164212X.2013.761451

Erlandsson, L.-K., & Eklund, M. (2006). Levels of complexity in patterns of daily occupations: Relationship to women's well-being. *Journal of Occupational Science, 13*(1), 27–36. https://doi.org/10.1080/14427591.2006.9686568

Erlandsson, L.-K., Eklund, M., & Persson, D. (2011). Occupational value and relationships to meaning and health: Elaborations of the ValMO-model. *Scandinavian Journal of Occupational Therapy, 18*(1), 72–80. https://doi.org/10.3109/11038121003671619

European Pressure Ulcer Advisory Panel, National Pressure Injury Advisory Panel, & Pan Pacific Pressure Injury Alliance. (2019). Prevention and treatment of pressure ulcers/injuries: Clinical practice guideline. In E. Haesler (Ed.), *The international guideline*. Author. https://guidelinesales.com/page/About?&hhsearchterms=%22pressure+and+injury%22

Fahy, S., Delicâte, N., & Lynch, H. (2021). Now, being, occupational: Outdoor play and children with autism. *Journal of Occupational Science, 28*(1), 114–132. https://doi.org/10.1080/14427591.2020.1816207

Fogelberg, D. J., Powell, J. M., & Clark, F. A. (2016). The role of habit in recurrent pressure ulcers following spinal cord injury. *Scandinavian Journal of Occupational Therapy, 23*(6), 467–476. https://doi.org/10.3109/11038128.2015.1130170

Fox, J., Erlandsson, L.-K., & Shiel, A. (2021). A feasibility study of the Redesigning Daily Occupations (ReDO^TM-10) programme in an Irish context. *Scandinavian Journal of Occupational Therapy, 29*(5), 415–429. Online ahead of print. https://doi.org/10.1080/11038128.2021.1882561

Gerlach, A. J., Teachman, G., Laliberte Rudman, D., Aldrich, R. M., & Huot, S. (2017). Expanding beyond individualism: Engaging critical

perspectives on occupation. *Scandinavian Journal of Occupational Therapy, 25*(1), 35–43. https://doi.org/10.1080/11038128.2017.1327616

Ghaisas, S., Pyatak, E. A., Blanche, E., Blanchard, J., & Clark, F. (2015). Lifestyle changes and pressure ulcer prevention in adults with spinal cord injury in the Pressure Ulcer Prevention Study Lifestyle Intervention. *American Journal of Occupational Therapy, 69*(1), 6901290020p1–6901290020p10. https://doi.org/10.5014/ajot.2015.012021

Gharebaghy, S., Rassafiani, M., Vameghi, R., Akbarfahimi, M., Cameron, D., Polatajko, H. J., & Shafaroodi, N. (2021). Mothers' experience of being involved with the transfer of the CO-OP approach: A qualitative study. *British Journal of Occupational Therapy, 85*(5), 341–350. Advance online publication. https://doi.org/10.1177/03080226211026554

Graham, F., Kennedy-Behr, A., & Ziviani, J. (Eds.). (2021). *Occupational Performance Coaching (OPC): A manual for practitioners and researchers*. Routledge.

Harper, D. (n.d.). *Online etymology dictionary*. https://www.etymonline.com/search?q=systematize

Hernandez, R., Vidmar, A., & Pyatak, E. A. (2020). Lifestyle balance, restful and strenuous occupations, and physiological activation. *Journal of Occupational Science, 27*(4), 547–562. https://doi.org/10.1080/14427591.2020.1732229

Hunt, A. W., Allen, K. A., Dittmann, K., Linkewich, E., Donald, M., Hutter, J., Patel, A., & McEwen, S. (2021). Clinician perspectives on implementing a team-based metacognitive strategy training approach to stroke rehabilitation. *Journal of Evaluation in Clinical Practice, 28*(2), 201–207. Advance online publication. https://doi.org/10.1016/j.apmr.2013.05.021

Jackson, J., Carlson, M., Rubayi, S., Scott, M. D., Atkins, M. S., Blanche, E. I., Saunders-Newton, C., Mielke, S., Wolfe, M. K., & Clark, F. A. (2010). Qualitative study of principles pertaining to lifestyle and pressure ulcer risk in adults with spinal cord injury. *Disability and Rehabilitation, 32*(7), 567–578. https://doi.org/10.3109/09638280903183829

Jones, M., Hocking, C., & McPherson, K. (2017). Communities with participation-enabling skills: A study of children with traumatic brain injury and their shared occupations. *Journal of Occupational Science, 24*(1), 88–104. https://doi.org/10.1080/14427591.2016.1224444

Karlsson, L., Ivarsson, A., & Erlandsson, L.-K. (2021). Exploring risk factors for developing occupational ill health—Departing from an occupational perspective. *Scandinavian Journal of Occupational Therapy, 29*(5), 363–372. Ahead of Print. https://doi.org/10.1080/11038128.2021.1936160

Katzman, E., Mohler, E., Durocher, E., & Kinsella, E. A. (2021). Occupational justice in direct-funded attendant services: Possibilities and constraints. *Journal of Occupational Science, 29*(4), 586–601. Advance online publication. https://doi.org/10.1080/14427591.2021.1942173

Kottorp, A., Nygård, L., Hedman, A., Öhman, A., Malinowsky, C., Rosenberg, L., Lindqvist, E., & Ryd, C. (2016). Comment: Access to and use of everyday technology among older people: An occupational justice issue—but for whom? *Journal of Occupational Science, 23*(3), 382–388. https://doi.org/10.1080/14427591.2016.1151457

Lala, A. P., & Kinsella, E. A. (2011). Phenomenology and the study of human occupation. *Journal of Occupational Science, 18*(3), 195–209. https://doi.org/10.1080/14427591.2011.581629

Laliberte Rudman, D., & Aldrich, R. (2017). Occupational science. In M. Curtin, M. Egan, & J. Adams (Eds.), *Occupational therapy for people experiencing illness, injury or impairment* (pp. 17–27). Elsevier.

Mandich, A. D., Polatajko, H. J., Missiuna, C., & Miller, L. T. (2001). Cognitive strategies and motor performance in children with developmental coordination disorder. *Physical and Occupational Therapy in Pediatrics, 20*(2–3), 125–143. https://doi.org/10.1080/J006v20n02_08

Martini, R., & Polatajko, H. J. (1998). Verbal self-guidance as a treatment approach for children with developmental coordination disorder: A systematic replication study. *The Occupational Therapy Journal of Research, 18*(4), 157–181. https://doi.org/10.1177/153944929801800403

McGrath, M., & McGonagle, H. (2016). Exploring 'wicked problems' from an occupational perspective: The case of turf cutting in rural Ireland. *Journal of Occupational Science, 23*(3), 308–320. https://doi.org/10.1080/14427591.2016.1169437

Miller, L. T., Polatajko, H. J., Missiuna, C., Mandich, A. D., & Macnab, J. J. (2001). A pilot trial of a cognitive treatment for children with developmental coordination disorder. *Human Movement Science, 20*(1–2), 183–210. https://doi.org/10.1016/S0167-9457(01)00034-3

Missiuna, C., Malloy-Miller, T., & Mandich, A. (1998). Mediational techniques: Origins and application to occupational therapy in paediatrics. *Canadian Journal of Occupational Therapy, 65*(4), 202–209. https://doi.org/10.1177/000841749806500405

Missiuna, C., Mandich, A. D., Polatajko, H. J. & Malloy-Miller, T. (2001). Cognitive Orientation to Daily Occupational Performance (CO-OP): Part I – Theoretical foundations. *Physical and Occupational Therapy in Pediatrics, 20*(2–3), 69–81. https://doi.org/10.1080/J006v20n02_05

Molineux, M. (Ed.). (2004). *Occupation for occupational therapists.* Blackwell.

Morgan, W. J. (2010). What, exactly, is occupational satisfaction? *Journal of Occupational Science, 17*(4), 216–223. https://doi.org/10.1080/14427591.2010.9686698

Núñez, C. M. V., Hernández, S. S., & Alarcón, A. H. (2021). Collective occupations and nature: Impacts of the coloniality of nature on rural and fishing communities in Chile. *Journal of Occupational Science, 29*(2), 252–262. Advance online publication. https://doi.org/10.1080/14427591.2021.1880264

Olsson, A., Erlandsson, L-K., & Håkansson, C. (2020). The occupation-based intervention REDO™-10: Long-term impact on work ability for women at risk for or on sick leave. *Scandinavian Journal of Occupational Therapy, 27*(1), 47–55. https://doi.org/10.1080/11038128.2019.1614215

Pierce, D. (Ed.). (2011). *Occupational science for occupational therapy.* SLACK.

Polatajko, H. J., Mandich, A. D., Miller, L. T., & Macnab, J. J. (2001). Cognitive orientation to daily occupational performance (CO-OP):

Part II—the evidence. *Physical and Occupational Therapy in Pediatrics, 20*(2–3), 83–106. https://doi.org/10.1080/J006v20n02_06

Rosenbaum, P., & Gorter, J. W. (2011). The 'F-words' in childhood disability: I swear this is how we should think! *Child: Care, Health and Development, 38*(4), 457–463. https://doi.org/10.1111/j.1365-2214.2011.01338.x

Sax Institute. (2016). *Translational research framework: Testing innovation in policy, programs and service delivery.* https://www.saxinstitute.org.au/wp-content/uploads/Translational-Research-Framework.pdf

Smith, V. (2017). Energizing everyday practices through the indigenous spirituality of haka. *Journal of Occupational Science, 24*(1), 9–18. https://doi.org/10.1080/14427591.2017.1280838

Turcotte, S., DeBroux-Leduc, R., Aubry, C. V., Parisien, M., Levasseur, M., Daigle-Landry, D., Lorthios-Guilledroit, A., & Filiatrault, J. (2021). Older adults' experience as peer educators in health promotion programs. *Journal of Occupational Science,* 1–15. Advance online publication. https://doi.org/10.1080/14427591.2021.1944898

University of Southern California. (2013). *USC/Rancho Lifestyle Redesign* pressure ulcer prevention project. http://pups.usc.edu

Wästberg, B., Erlandsson, L.-K., & Eklund, M. (2016). Women's perceived work environment after stress-related rehabilitation: Experiences from the ReDO project. *Disability and Rehabilitation, 38*(6), 528–534. https://doi.org/10.3109/09638288.2015.1046567

Wijekoon, S., Laliberte Rudman, D., Hand, C., & Polgar, J. (2021). Late-life immigrants' place integration through occupation. *Journal of Occupational Science.* Advance online publication. https://doi.org/10.1080/14427591.2021.1960589

Wilcock, A. A., & Hocking, C. (2015). *An occupational perspective of health* (3rd ed.). SLACK.

Williams, K. (2017). Understanding the role of sensory processing in occupation: An updated discourse with cognitive neuroscience. *Journal of Occupational Science, 24*(3), 302–313. https://doi.org/10.1080/14427591.2016.1209425

World Health Organization. (2022). *WHO Coronavirus (COVID-19) dashboard.* https://covid19.who.int/

Zemke, R., & Clark, F. (1996). Preface. In R. Zemke & F. Clark (Eds.), *Occupational science: The evolving discipline* (pp. vii–xviii). F. A. Davis.

Occupational Justice

Antoine Bailliard

Quiet isn't always peace, and the norms and notions of what "just" is isn't always justice

AMANDA GORMAN (2021)

LEARNING OBJECTIVES

After reading this chapter, you will be able to:

1. Analyze the relationship between occupation, justice, health and inclusion for individuals, communities, and populations.
2. Describe the role of occupational justice within occupational therapy.
3. Describe the unique contribution of occupational justice in advancing justice for all.
4. Evaluate processes for advancing occupational justice and occupational rights.

Introduction

The purpose of this chapter is to introduce an occupational justice perspective and describe its relevance to occupational therapy (OT). The chapter will begin with an explanation of the relationship among occupation, health, justice, and the "good" to demonstrate that participation in occupation is a medical necessity and a right. The occupational justice perspective will be compared to other conceptualizations of justice to highlight its unique contribution to understandings of justice. Next, the relationship between OT and occupational justice will be discussed to demonstrate that incorporating an occupational justice perspective in OT practice is ethically necessary. The chapter will end with suggestions regarding how to undertake work to advance occupational rights and occupational justice.

An Occupational Justice Perspective—A Working Definition

The term **occupational justice** was originally mentioned by Wilcock (1998) in *An Occupational Perspective on Health*. Soon after, Wilcock and Townsend (2000) further developed the idea and proposed it in the *Journal* *of Occupational Science.* Since then, an occupational justice perspective has been embraced in many parts of the world and has been expanded upon by many other scholars and researchers. Similarly, but separately, social OT emerged in Brazil in the 1970s with the explicit goal to promote emancipation, inclusion, and social participation (Barros et al., 2011; Malfitano & Lopes, 2018; Malfitano et al., 2014). Both movements apply an occupational perspective to address social issues such as homelessness, mass migration, poverty, unemployment, marginalized groups, systemic racism, and systemic oppression of different sexualities (Malfitano et al., 2014; Townsend, 1997).

Prior to proposing a working definition of occupational justice, which generates and perpetuates knowledge, it is necessary to recognize that all knowledge is situated and emergent from a particular sociocultural perspective (Farias et al., 2016; Rudman, 2013). In doing so, it is possible to continue to refine the definition to improve its applicability and utility to different situations across the globe, including eliminating culturally biased assumptions regarding human nature.

Occupational justice came from a Western Anglo middle-class perspective, which is a unique and specific worldview that is not representative of all worldviews. Critiques have highlighted that occupational justice is poorly defined and not sufficiently distinguished from social justice (Durocher et al., 2014; Hammell, 2017). Others have critiqued it as another example of Western colonization that imposes a Western Anglo middle-class conceptualization of justice as universal (Córdoba, 2020; Emery-Whittington, 2021). Indeed, much research and scholarship on occupational justice continues to be marred by an individualistic and positivist frame that obscures systemic power relations (Benjamin-Thomas & Rudman, 2018; Farias et al., 2016; Galheigo, 2011a; Malfitano et al., 2014, 2019).

Despite these healthy critiques, this chapter will argue that an occupational justice perspective is beneficial and an essential aspect of OT. For OT practitioners, an occupational justice perspective can highlight the sociopolitical factors that affect engagement in occupation and encourage practitioners to reflect on how they and their clients[1] are situated in, and function through, sociopolitical power structures that affect their and their clients' relationships and participation. All forms of participation in occupation are

somehow affected by power structures (e.g., social, cultural, economic, and political) including writing this chapter.

An occupational justice perspective foregrounds the systemic inequities that simultaneously extinguish and privilege particular **occupational expressions**, which are the unique ways a person performs an occupation at a given moment including the form (i.e., step-by-step process) and style (e.g., cadence, intensity, rhythm, flair, and bodily comportment) of that occupation (see Box 10.1). It can serve as a protective force against reductionist perspectives that focus solely on "fixing" individual factors (e.g., performance skills, body structures, and body functions) and ignore the systemic factors that constrain participation. By encouraging OT practitioners to consider power structures and systemic factors that affect participation, an occupational justice perspective enhances a practitioner's understanding of their client's situation and expands the range of intervention targets that could be identified to support their participation. Considering the impact of systems and social structures on participation is ethically necessary for occupational therapists because those structures can suppress forms of occupational participation that promote health and impose forms of participation that are deleterious to health.

A *working definition* is proposed because understandings of occupation are emergent and evolving and, consequently, understandings of how occupation is intertwined with justice are also emergent and evolving as new occupational processes are explored. Prior to offering the working definition, the following sections will explore why an occupational justice perspective is needed.

BOX 10.1 OCCUPATIONAL EXPRESSIONS

- *Occupational expression* is the unique way a person performs an occupation at a given moment; it is
  - embodied through past experiences under the affordances and constraints of situational factors (e.g., sociocultural, geopolitical, temporal, and physical)
  - affected by social positioning
  - the basis for inclusion and exclusion in different environments
- *Form* refers to the step-by-step process
  - Varies across individuals, cultures, and time (e.g., steps for fashioning one's hair varies significantly across contexts and time)
- *Style* refers to the manner in which the form is carried out
  - Cadence, intensity, rhythm, flair, bodily comportments, etc.

[1]According to the American Occupational Therapy Association (AOTA, 2020, p. S75), the term *client* refers to *persons* (including those involved in care of a client), *groups* (a collection of individuals having shared characteristics or common or shared purpose, e.g., family members, workers, students, and those with similar interests or occupational challenges), and *populations* (aggregates of people with common attributes such as contexts, characteristics or concerns, including health risks). However, in countries other than the United States, the term *client* often refers to persons who are paying for their care directly. In most countries, *patient* is used to describe persons who are in hospital or rehabilitation. *Service user* and *person* are terms in general use that describe those in need of OT services. For this chapter, we are using *client* without implying the source of payment for services.

Occupation, Health, and the "Good"

The relationship between occupation and health is the cornerstone of medical OT practice and has been codified in professional associations across the world. Occupation is widely understood as a mechanism of health with the potential to generate both positive and negative effects on health and well-being. Because the occupational justice perspective emerged from a health-focused profession, historical accounts of occupational justice primarily focus on physical and mental health—the primary targeted outcome of healthcare.

However, occupation is more than a mechanism or expression of health, it is also a mechanism to and expression of "the good" (i.e., what a person, group, or community values). There are many potential "goods" (e.g., health, happiness, property, capital, joy, harmony with nature, and social integration) and what constitutes an important "good" varies considerably among individuals, groups, and populations. For example, in the West, self-determinism and independence are valued goods, whereas in Eastern cultures that value self-transcendence and interdependence, those are not considered "good" and are seen as paths to individual and collective unhappiness (Joshanloo, 2014). Therefore, it is risky to define an occupational justice perspective around one conceptualization of the "good." Despite the need to acknowledge the existence of, and unequal access to, many different "goods," it can be argued that it is logical to focus on "health" as a primary good because it affects the ability to achieve and express all other goods (Venkatapuram, 2011). However, health also has various conceptualizations depending on which theoretical perspective is adopted.

Occupation as a Medical Necessity: Social Participation, Inclusion, and Health

Health is more than the absence of illness or disease. In 2001, the World Health Organization (WHO) published the International Classification of Health, Functioning, and Disease (ICF), which proposed that health is the result of three personal factors: (a) body function and structure, (b) the ability to execute activities, and (c) participation or involvement in life situations. According to the WHO's model, health is not the absence of disease, rather it is the complete physical, mental, and social functioning of a person (WHO, 2001a, 2001b). The ICF model proposes that a person's meaningful participation is equally as important to their health as their body function and structure. Therefore, addressing a person's health should involve interventions that target a person's ability to perform activities and their participation in meaningful life situations. The movement clamoring for increased attention to meaningful participation is not new; indeed, scholars such as Salzer (2006) have long advocated for community participation as a medical necessity that should be prioritized in traditional healthcare systems.

Research that effectively captures the impact of meaningful participation on health is relatively rare because of difficulties with measurement and the scarcity of instruments that operationalize participation. This has complicated efforts to advocate for community participation as a medical necessity. However, existing evidence has demonstrated that the relationship between meaningful participation and health is significant. People who report having sufficient levels of participation report significantly higher quality of life than controls (Burns-Lynch et al., 2016). Participation in occupations with other people is also a significant contributor to mental and physical health.

Participation in social occupations is intimately related to feelings of inclusion and the absence of participation can lead to loneliness and isolation. Both loneliness and social isolation are associated with negative health outcomes (National Institute on Aging, 2021). Loneliness is the feeling of being alone and social isolation is having few social contacts. Loneliness is associated with higher use of healthcare (Gerst-Emerson & Jayawardhana, 2015), has a negative impact on physical and mental health (Cacioppo et al., 2015), and is a significant cause of mortality (Holt-Lunstad et al., 2015), whereas social isolation is associated with cognitive decline (Cacioppo & Hawkley, 2009).

Inclusion makes life more meaningful and people who participate in meaningful activities are able to build social connections that contribute to feelings of inclusion (Mezzina et al., 2006). Exclusion, even seemingly minor forms, makes life less meaningful. For example, in a controlled experimental game of catch, participants who did not have the ball tossed to them did not feel included in the activity and reported feeling the activity was less meaningful (Williams & Nida, 2011). Feeling excluded from a seemingly mundane occupation is sufficient to have a negative impact on a person's experiences with that occupation. In other words, the positive meanings experienced during an occupation can result from the occupation's social dimensions (i.e., feeling included) and not the objective nature of the occupation itself (i.e., playing catch). Unsurprisingly, a lack of social participation is at the core of experiences of loneliness (Morgan et al., 2007). Indeed, participation in social occupations is an important contributor to mental and physical health and, therefore, should be considered a medical necessity.

Cross-cultural research across the globe has revealed that family and social relationships are a key ingredient to happiness and well-being regardless of sociocultural origin (Delle Fave et al., 2011; Pflug, 2009). Yet social isolation and loneliness are on the rise across the globe (WHO, 2021a, 2001b). Because loneliness and social isolation are associated with negative health outcomes (Cacioppo et al., 2015; Gerst-Emerson & Jayawardhana, 2015; Holt-Lunstad et al., 2015), and a lack of social participation is at the core of loneliness and social isolation

(Morgan et al., 2007), interventions should prioritize targeting participation in social occupations that promote feelings of inclusion and social integration (Malfitano & Lopes, 2018; Malfitano et al., 2014; Young, 1990).

Unfortunately, many social structures, formal policies, and other power systems directly suppress people's ability to participate meaningfully in society and experience inclusion. People are often excluded because of their gender identity, racial ethnicity, socioeconomic origin, and many other social positionings that are arbitrarily assigned negative social values. These forms of exclusion lead to social isolation and loneliness with potentially devastating effects on mental and physical health. An occupational justice perspective highlights how individuals, communities, and populations can experience oppressions that exclude them from occupational participation or suppress forms of occupational expressions in a manner that prevents them from feeling included in society. Because participation in occupation is a medical necessity (i.e., sufficient participation in health-promoting occupations is necessary for health), and participation in occupation is at the mercy of power structures (e.g., sociocultural norms and political governance), then participation in occupation is a matter of justice.

Occupation and Justice

To standardize its approaches, Western medicine has historically championed an "objective" or "impartial" approach to conceptualizing health, science, and education (Bailliard

et al., 2021; Young, 1990). The body, disease, and illness are primarily understood in reductionist ways that take the body out of context and ignore environmental factors such as socioeconomic status and social positioning. As a result, Western medicine has long been considered "apolitical" and its interventions have focused on individuals instead of systems. Western OT came of age within these systems and has also historically focused on individual-level factors. Because its "dominant theories and models are deeply rooted in neoliberalism's White ableist norms and values, structural and social determinants of occupation and of health are overlooked" (Hammell, 2021, p. 7). However, in the past few decades, occupational therapists and scientists are increasingly attending to how sociopolitical and other power systems affect participation in occupation including social determinants of health. The link between occupation and justice is increasingly evident and impossible to ignore.

Social Determinants of Health—Access to Occupation Is Political

Social determinants of health are the structural conditions that affect the health of people (Artiga & Hinton, 2018). They include factors related to economic stability, neighborhood and physical environment, education, food, community and social context, and the healthcare system (Figure 10.1). They are not individual characteristics such as gender, race, or disability; rather, they are patriarchy, ableism, racism, sexism, colonialism, heteronormativity, or any other social and structural forces that establish inequity of privilege based

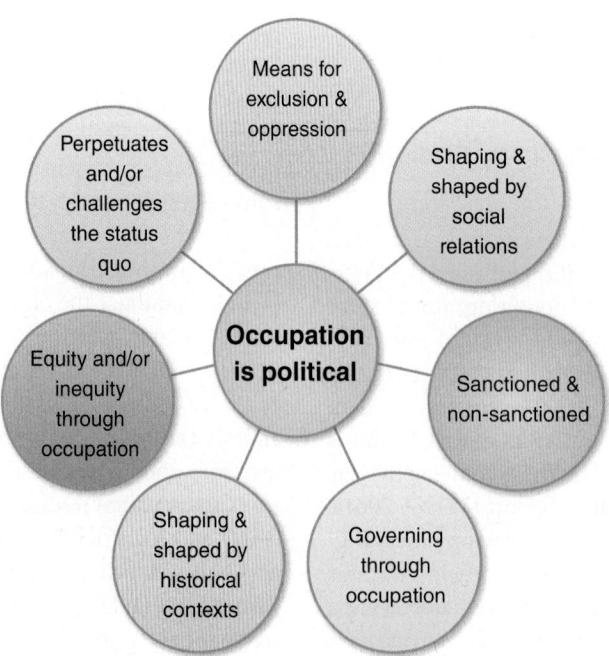

FIGURE 10.1 Occupation is political.

(Adapted from Rudman, D. L. [2021]. Mobilizing occupation for social transformation: Radical resistance, disruption, and re-configuration. *Canadian Journal of Occupational Therapy, 88*(2), 96–107. https://doi.org/10.1177/00084174211020836.)

on those characteristics (Hammell, 2021). Often, oppression of occupational expressions occurs formally through policies. For example, the occupations of transgender youth are consistently under attack by politicians and society at large as laws are proposed and passed that govern their access to bathrooms, changing rooms, athletics, and other typical youth occupations.

At the community level, an impoverished community with few resources will experience poorer health and fewer opportunities for health-promoting occupations than a wealthy community with numerous resources. For many individuals, groups, communities, and populations, the effective freedom to participate in health-promoting occupations is denied by political, economic, and social factors. Migrants, refugees, and people living under oppressive governments experience occupational injustice when their occupational habits and routines are suppressed and controlled. Simply put, there is inequitable access to health-promoting occupations and some people live in situations that are replete with occupations that are deleterious to health. For example, people experiencing homelessness and people living in poor socioeconomic conditions have fewer opportunities to access parks, playgrounds, or other venues for physical activity to promote physical health. They have less access to healthy foods in grocery stores to cook healthy meals. They have fewer opportunities to access forms of dignified employment or education. They are also more exposed to occupations that can be deleterious to health such as substance abuse, gang-related occupations, risky sexual activity, and sedentary lifestyles.

Inequitable access to health-promoting occupations is a matter of occupational justice. An occupational justice perspective entails consideration of how social, economic, political, and other power structures affect the ability of individuals, groups, and communities to participate in meaningful occupations that have a positive impact on health and well-being.

Participation in occupation is political (Figure 10.2) because it always involves power structures that directly impact the ability to participate (Pollard et al., 2008; Rudman, 2021). Political governance uses systems and laws to allocate vital resources and power across groups of constituents. Because of systemic racism, nepotism, greed, and the difficulty of matching resources to different needs, human history has been consistently plagued with inequitable distribution of resources and opportunities.

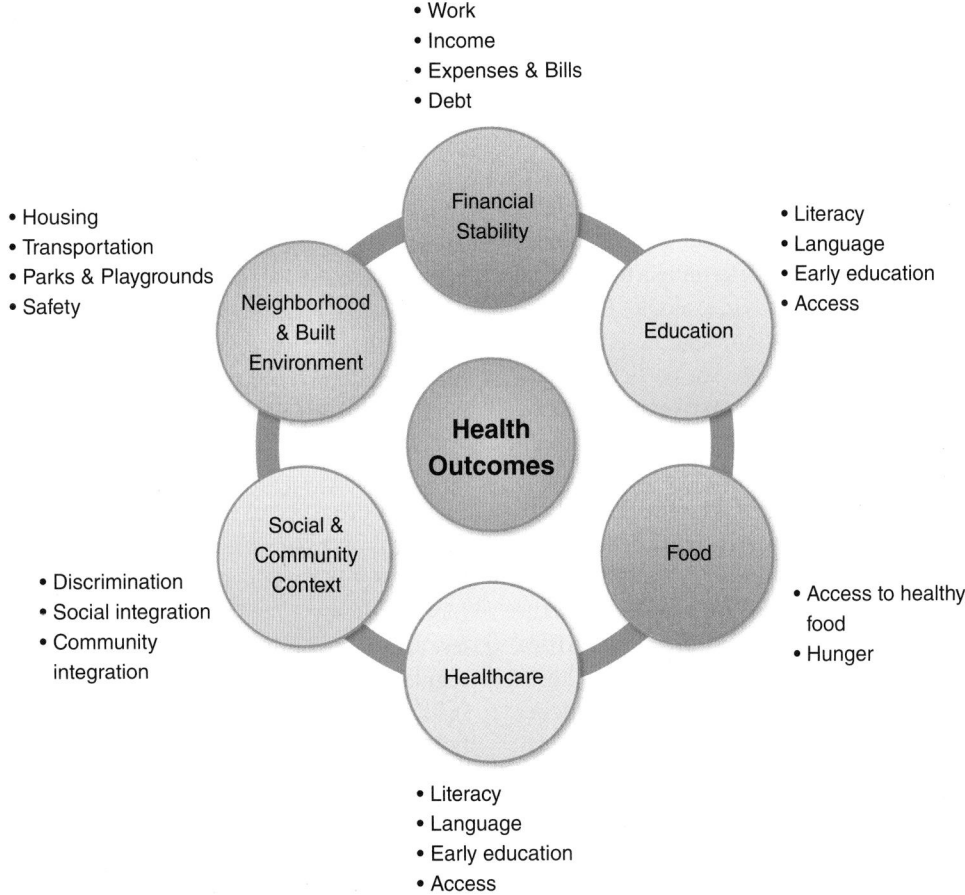

FIGURE 10.2 **Social determinants of health.**

(Adapted from Artiga, S., & Hinton, E. [2018]. *Beyond health care: The role of social determinants in promoting health and health equity.* K. F. Foundation.)

Occupations are also used to oppress and exclude people because they are shaped through historical social relations that determine whether or not they are sanctioned or disallowed by social norms (see Figure 10.2). History has shown that political and power inequities are self-sustaining and tend to reproduce the existing hierarchy of power such that the privileged experience and reproduce their privilege and the unprivileged are disempowered and unable to challenge power systems to increase their privilege (Bourdieu, 1998, 2004; Young, 1980, 1990). In other words, occupational injustices resulting from oppressive historical sociocultural forces are self-sustaining as a "natural" occurrence until they are explicitly challenged.

OT practitioners are well positioned in Western healthcare systems to enact changes that address occupational justice. Advances in medicine are increasingly attending to social determinants of health and studies have demonstrated their link to health outcomes such as mortality, morbidity, life expectancy, health status, and functional limitations (Artiga & Hinton, 2018). Indeed, many social determinants of health are also traditional intervention targets for OT practitioners. Stable employment, social integration, and community engagement are critical social determinants of health (Artiga & Hinton, 2018) that are frequently addressed in OT (albeit typically through individual-level factors). Access to transportation, parks, playgrounds, and education are also important social determinants of health addressed by OT.

Participation in leisure occupations is another important contributor to mental and physical health; however, the opportunity to participate in leisure occupations is also political because it is significantly affected by environmental factors and resources that are determined by political governance (Pollard et al., 2008). For example, Pressman et al. (2009) used the Pittsburgh Enjoyable Activities Test (PEAT) to measure associations between participation in leisure activities and physical health markers. The PEAT measures leisure participation across 10 different activities: spending quiet time alone; spending time unwinding; visiting others; eating with others; doing fun things with others; club, fellowship, and religious group participation; vacationing; communing with nature; sports; and hobbies. The study found that higher levels of participation on the PEAT were associated with lower blood pressure, cortisol, waist circumference, and body mass index as well as lower levels of depression and negative affect. Furthermore, higher levels of participation were associated with a higher perception of physical function and higher levels of positive psychosocial states (Pressman et al., 2009). They also found that higher socioeconomic class were also associated with higher scores on the PEAT. As demonstrated by the Pressman study, there is significant inequity in access to participation in health-supporting leisure occupations and that inequity is associated with socioeconomic class.

Health Justice

Because of such findings, scholars and philosophers of justice have argued that the close relationship between activity participation and health requires governments to create policies that support the equitable participation in meaningful activities of their constituents (Bailliard, 2016; Bailliard et al., 2021; Nilsson & Townsend, 2010; Nussbaum, 2011; Sen, 2009; Venkatapuram, 2011). Because access to health-promoting occupations is denied by socioeconomic and political circumstances which results in an unequal distribution of effective freedoms to participate in meaningful occupation, it is impossible to ignore that OT practitioners have a role in supporting the effective freedoms of others. It is a fundamental right for people to experience dignity and health through *being* and *doing* what they value (Bailliard, 2016; Bailliard et al., 2021; Nilsson & Townsend, 2010; Nussbaum, 2011; Sen, 2009; Venkatapuram, 2011).

Embodiment of Occupational Expressions and Justice

Beyond issues of access to health-promoting occupations, individuals and groups are often excluded from mainstream society because of differences in their occupational expressions (Box 10.1). Individuals, groups, communities, and populations can all experience occupational injustices because of sociocultural values and systems of understandings that position certain occupational expressions as being undesirable, deviant, and even morally "wrong." For example, local gender norms restrict what clothing is considered appropriate for different sexes such that transgressing normative expectations for dressing is often considered perverse and immoral. Other examples include policies that prohibit skateboarding in public spaces or public discourses that label graffiti as deviant. Social norms and expectations for occupational behavior are frequently the basis for excluding individuals from meaningful participation in society (Kiepek et al., 2019).

People learn to how to use their bodies to express their occupations in unique ways through repeated participation in their unique sociocultural contexts (Bailliard et al., 2018; Bourdieu, 2004; Cutchin et al., 2008; Hass, 2008; Merleau-Ponty, 1945/2012). From birth, people, their bodies, and their bodily expressions are subject to relentless regulation, control, and judgment (Young, 1980, 1990). Such instances occur as children learn and develop their occupations. For example, as a child learns to eat at the table, their caregivers may attempt to instill proper eating behaviors according to their sociocultural norms (e.g., how to hold oneself at the table, how to use utensils, and how to chew). Over time, children embody ways of doing that determine the extent to which they experience inclusion and exclusion when expressing their occupations in contexts that have different norms for doing those occupations (Bailliard et al.,

2022). For example, chewing food with an open mouth is considered "wrong" in some settings whereas it is considered insignificant in other settings. The "internalization of historico-racial schemas enables some bodies even and precisely as they disable other bodies" (Weiss, 2015, p. 88) such that bodily ways of being are the basis for social inclusion and exclusion (Bourdieu, 2004). The extent to which a person experiences inclusion and exclusion depends on how well a person's occupational expression (i.e., unique way of doing an occupation) fits with a context's dominant sociocultural norms (Bailliard et al., 2022).

Applying an embodied occupational justice perspective highlights how people's bodies can be sites of oppression when their unique occupational expression deviates from norms of bodily comportment. For example, White (Eurocentric) ways of being are the normative standard for professionalism in US workplaces (Bailliard et al., 2021; Frye et al., 2020) and these norms have been used to discriminate against people with non-White dress and appearance in those settings (Frye et al., 2020; Marom, 2019). An embodied occupational justice perspective highlights how OT practitioners must understand how their clients' bodies and bodily ways of being affect their capability to participate in occupations in society. It also highlights that practitioners must be mindful of how their interventions can transform their clients' bodily ways of doing in unjust ways that denigrate their natural expressions and supplant them with normative expressions. For example, an autistic child may express atypical bodily comportments (e.g., flapping, eye gaze, and sounds) while performing an occupation. Seeking to extinguish such behaviors through intervention is an act of oppression. An embodied occupational justice perspective encourages practitioners to critically assess their assumptions of how bodies *should* look, perform, and move.

An Occupational Justice Perspective—A Working Definition

There is no clear consensus regarding what occupational justice is or how to apply it in practice. The idea does not belong to any person or group and research from all over the world continues to develop understandings of occupational justice. Accordingly, this chapter proposes a working definition of an occupational justice perspective that will need to be tested and updated as more research and action apply it in real-world settings. ***An occupational justice perspective holds that people have the right to express their occupations to experience dignity, inclusion, health, and well-being in a context of associated living where their occupational expressions do not oppress the occupational expressions of others.*** According to the World Federation of Occupational Therapists (WFOT), occupational justice "is the fulfillment of the right for all people to engage in the occupations they need to survive, define as meaningful, and that contribute positively to their own well-being and the well-being of their

communities" (WFOT, 2019, p. 1). This right also entails "acknowledgement that with choice comes responsibility for other people, lifeforms and the planet" (p. 1).

Indeed, occupational justice does not entail unchecked formal freedoms to participate in whatever occupations one chooses regardless of the impact on others. Contrarily, the freedom to participate in occupation involves a responsibility to others and their freedom to participate in occupation. When one occupational expression directly oppresses the occupational expression of another, an injustice has occurred. This complicates analyses of occupational justice as humans are deeply entangled in complex webs of social relationships such that occupational expressions can have far-reaching consequences that cause injustice and oppression of occupation in other parts of the world (Bailliard, 2016). When participation in occupation entails consuming products or services that create the demand for denigrating and oppressive work conditions for others (e.g., purchasing clothes made with forced child labor), an occupational injustice has occurred. When a person shames another for an occupational expression that is causing no harm but is transgressive of social norms (e.g., eating or dressing in ways that do not adhere to local norms), an occupational injustice has occurred.

Occupational justice and injustice occur at micro, meso, and macro levels of human functioning. When applying an occupational justice perspective, expert practitioners can switch their analyses between micro, meso, and macro levels of functioning while understanding their interrelationship and being mindful of the whole.

Micro-level occupational injustices occur at the interpersonal level and involve mundane everyday actions. People commit, suffer, and witness micro-occupational injustices frequently throughout their everyday lives. Whenever someone experiences shame for not "doing" occupation in a way that does not match dominant social norms and expectations, they have experienced an occupational injustice. For example, if an adult tells a young boy with painted nails *Boys don't paint their nails, you don't want to be a sissy do you?*—this constitutes an explicit micro-occupational injustice that shames the boy for participating in an occupation that has historically not been socially sanctioned for boys (Bailliard et al., 2020, p. 148).

Children are persistently subject to micro-occupational injustices under the guise of their upbringing when their bodily expressions during occupations are disparaged and targeted through interventions by caregivers and teachers to modify their expressions to fit norms. Unless these interventions expand a child's capacities to be healthy and well, it is difficult to argue that transformations in bodily behaviors are not unjust. For example, children with sensory seeking needs may demonstrate difficulty sitting in one seat during long periods in a school classroom. Those students will frequently receive consequences for attempting to meet their sensory needs by moving or fidgeting with items regardless of the impact on their educational outcomes. The normative occupational expression for attending class requires students to stay seated, attentive, and quiet while the instructor teaches. However, some students need sensory input or fidgets to maintain their attention and focus so they can learn. The very behavior they need to learn is repressed under the assumed pretext that it negatively affects their learning. Their nonnormative occupational expression involves movement that is not socially sanctioned despite it enhancing their ability to learn.

Meso-level occupational injustices can occur through settings such as schools, workplaces, organizations, and neighborhoods and can occur through structures such as formal organizational policies, unspoken organizational sociocultural practices, or the built environment which prevent access to occupations or the occupational expressions of groups of people. Examples of meso-occupational injustices include school policies that prevent students with physical or behavioral diagnoses from being included in mainstream classes and occupations afforded to other students, work practices such as inviting a cohort of employees to a holiday party but excluding supportive staff, neighborhood policies that prohibit participation in occupations such as skateboarding or motorsports, institutional policies that restrict the occupations of residents, educational presentations that use pictures and stories solely representing the dominant culture, or safety policies on an inpatient psychiatric unit that severely restrict the availability of occupation for people on the unit.

Macro-occupational injustices result from population-level lifestyles, occupational patterns, geopolitical relationships, policies, standards, and formal regulatory texts that oppress occupation across wide geographic areas. Macro-occupational injustices can be caused by systemic racism (Bailliard et al., 2021; Lavalley & Johnson, 2020), climate change (Hocking & Kroksmark, 2013; Ung et al., 2020; WFOT, 2018; Wicks & Jamieson, 2014), forced migration (Khan et al., 2021; Trimboli et al., 2019), human trafficking (George & Stanley, 2019), and other oppressive forces and conditions that suppress occupational participation and expression.

Macro-occupational injustices also occur when broad sociocultural norms value certain occupational expressions over others. Mainstream sociocultural values and norms are based on the ways of being of the dominant group culture and are broadcasted as natural, healthy, and desirable (Bailliard, 2016; Kantartzis & Molineux, 2011; Young, 1990). These values and norms provide a hierarchy of desirable versus undesirable occupations that confer a hierarchy of power and prestige (Bourdieu, 1998). Certain occupations and forms of occupational expression are forms of capital that give members of the dominant culture privilege over others who have different ways of being (Bailliard, 2016; Bourdieu, 1998; Young, 1990). For example, the Common Core State Standards in the United States establish learning criteria that value and reward argumentative expressive styles over narrative styles. Accordingly, students enculturated in narrative styles of communication will be penalized in schools that celebrate debate and argument (Lin, 2014). Mexican cultural traditions embrace narrative communication styles and storytelling (Reese, 2012) and expressing oneself using narrative styles is a form of cultural capital in Mexican milieus and can help a person experience belonging and inclusion. However, in US school settings, such expressive styles are not similarly valued and negatively position Mexican students relative to other students who are enculturated with debating and argumentative communication styles (Lin, 2014).

Occupational Rights

The concept of occupational rights has also emerged to further the conceptualization of occupational justice where the "denial of occupational rights constitutes an occupational injustice" (Hammell, 2020, p. 388). Occupational rights are "the right of all people to engage in meaningful occupations that contribute positively to their own well-being and the well-being of their communities" (Hammell, 2008, p. 62). It has been argued that an occupational rights approach is conceptually clearer while providing a concrete mandate for OT practitioners (Hammell, 2017, 2020).

Rights-based theories have been critiqued for having a negative focus on freedom (i.e., absence of restrictions to secure goods) without sufficiently emphasizing the positive freedom of *being able* to secure basic goods (Guo et al., 2019). Indeed, when considering a person's real-world capability to participate in occupation, it is useful to consider the difference between *effective* and *formal* freedoms to participate (Boisvert, 1997). *Formal freedom* refers to the absence of legal or other formal restrictions to participate in an occupation, whereas *effective freedom* is the real-world capability or positive capacity to participate in that occupation. For example, a person may have the formal freedom to speak Spanish because there are no legal or social restrictions prohibiting it. But that person may not have the effective freedom to speak Spanish because they do not have both the personal ability and the contextual support to do so (Boisvert, 1997). These nuances are captured in the literature on occupational rights, which argues that the approach "requires a critical practice of occupational therapy: innovative practice that acts on the knowledge that human well-being cannot be achieved solely by enhancing individuals' abilities, and that consequently endeavors to address the inequitable conditions of people's lives" (Hammell & Iwama, 2012, p. 392). Accordingly, an occupational justice perspective is focused on the positive capability to express an occupation (i.e., effective freedom). ***Supporting occupational participation requires more than a context that is free from obstruction, it requires a supportive context that enables the conversion and expression of skills in the real world.*** Therefore, the pursuit of occupational justice involves the pursuit of effective freedoms to participate in occupation and not merely the formal freedom to participate.

The Unique Contribution of Occupational Justice

There are many theories of social justice and there is no consensus regarding how to define social justice. A person's understanding of justice is based on their moral values and upbringing, which reflect a specific social, cultural, political, and economic context. Through repeated exposure, these come to feel "natural" and difficult to imagine otherwise. As a result, there is no universal theory or understanding of justice that is accepted worldwide. Instead, there are many different theories of justice that offer very different conceptualizations that converge with local values and philosophies. For ages, scholars and philosophers from around the world have been theorizing and debating what constitutes "justice." Different theories have become dominant in different parts of the world at different times. Relationship-based, rights-based, goods-based, and virtue-based conceptualizations of justice have emerged from the East and West (Guo et al., 2019). This chapter will not attempt to provide a comprehensive overview of innumerable existing theories of justice; however, a few dominant theories from across the world are presented in order to situate an occupational justice perspective among them.

In the Global South, the relationship-based philosophy of *ubuntu* originated from south of the African Sahara in the precolonial era and has long dominated ethical theory in the area. Although there are many variations and interpretations of ubuntu, Ewuoso and Hall (2019) performed a systematic review of the literature and concluded that ubuntu

> prizes relationship[s] of interdependence, fellowship, reconciliation, relationality, community friendliness, harmonious relationships and other-regarding actions, and in which actions are morally right to the extent that they promote social integration and interconnectedness, honour communal relationships or the capacity for the same and reduce discord or promote friendly relationships with others, and in which the physical world (horizontal line) and the spiritual world (vertical line) are fundamentally united. (p. 100)

The integrated framework of ubuntu suggests it occurs at six levels: individual, family, community, society, environment, and spiritual wherein "an authentic individual human being is part of a larger and more significant relational, communal, societal, environmental and spiritual world" (Mugumbate & Chereni, 2020, p. 6). Merging an occupational justice perspective with ubuntu would highlight how social inclusion, social relationships, and interconnectedness are facilitated and hindered through occupational participation. The Brazilian approach to social OT (Barros et al., 2011), the South African Occupation-based Community Development Framework (ObCD; Galvaan, 2021), and the Social Transformation through Occupation Network (Laliberte Rudman et al., 2019) all adopt an occupational justice perspective to promote positive social transformation to enhance inclusion and community. Their respective approaches emphasize human interconnection and the need to nurture those connections.

In the Global East, Confucian and Mohist philosophies have influenced views of justice to be virtue-based wherein governments are obligated to care for their constituents through the provision of public goods and individuals demonstrate respect and virtue toward each other through their relationships (Guo et al., 2019). These models of justice emphasize the duty to care for others and to maintain the social order. Merging an occupational justice perspective with Confucian and Mohist philosophies highlights the duty and moral responsibility OT practitioners have toward others. It highlights the necessity of embracing an occupational justice perspective in practice to promote social cohesion.

In the Global West, John Rawls' social contract theory and theory of distributive justice as fairness has dominated the discourse on social justice (Sen, 1999, 2009). Rawls' theory proposes that resources, opportunities, income, and the social bases of self-respect should be distributed equally unless an unequal distribution is to everyone's advantage (Allingham, 2014). The latter part of his formulation has often been ignored in mainstream discourses, which often focus on how an equal distribution of resources will merely reproduce existing inequalities—a fact that Rawls had accounted for. Indeed, he defined injustice as inequalities that *do not benefit everyone* (Allingham, 2014). To achieve a just society, Rawls' theory emphasizes the need to create just rules and institutions that are impartial and applicable across diverse situations. Rawls argued that developing impartial institutions is possible if people set aside their biases and don a *veil of ignorance* wherein their decisions would not be influenced by what they will gain or lose. Yet, impartiality is based on assumptions of "a unified and universal moral point of view" (Young, 1990, p. 10) which "insists on only one subject position, that of the unified, disembodied reason identified with white bourgeois men" (p. 147). Impartiality is an impossibility because of the embodied nature of human cognition, ways of being, and sociocultural values. In other words, humans are unaware of their biases and perceptual orientations which operate subconsciously as habits of thinking which are embodied through repeated participation within specific sociocultural environments (Bailliard et al., 2018, 2022; Cutchin et al., 2008).

Transcendental-Focused Versus Realization-Focused Theories of Justice

Amartya Sen, an Indian economist and philosopher, has critiqued mainstream theories of distributive justice for relying on *transcendental institutionalism*, which depends on broad impartial rules that can be applied across all situations and complex contexts (Sen, 1999, 2009). Sen's critique highlighted the impossibility of impartiality including the problematic assumption that purportedly impartial rules can be applied fairly to the particularities and complexities of highly variable situations. Instead, Sen proposed that theories of justice should focus on what people can actually *be* and *do*. In other words, focusing on the distribution of resources or the creation of ideal social arrangements and rules is insufficient; it is necessary to adopt a *realization-focused* theory that focuses on what people have the real-world capacity to do (Bailliard et al., 2020; Sen, 2009). In response, Sen introduced the capabilities approach to justice which has been expanded upon by many scholars, most notably Martha Nussbaum and Sridhar Venkatapuram. For the purposes of this chapter, the following summary of the capabilities approach is very brief and does not address many nuances that have been identified as it has been developed.

Capabilities Approach

The capabilities approach to justice emphasizes the necessity of supporting people in their ability *to be* and *to do what they value* because of the close relationship between participation and health (Bailliard, 2016; Bailliard et al., 2021; Nilsson & Townsend, 2010; Nussbaum, 2011; Sen, 2009; Venkatapuram, 2011). Nussbaum (2000) introduced a list of 10 central capabilities that societies should support to be just (see Box 10.2). Sen, however, was opposed to creating such a list in light of the need for each society to self-determine which capabilities were most important for their particular situation. Despite these nuances, Sen, Nussbaum, Venkatapuram, and others have significantly developed this approach as an alternative to goods-based and distribution-based models of justice. Capabilities are incommensurable. In other words, people are uniquely and distinctly deprived of capabilities in a way that cannot be compared across capabilities—each is uniquely important (Venkatapuram, 2011).

In addition to being *realization-focused*, the capabilities approach provides additional nuance by distinguishing

between functionings (i.e., states of being and doings) and capabilities. Different combinations of actualized capabilities yield different functionings. Instead of imposing certain functionings on people, which would be an act of oppression, the capabilities approach focuses on supporting real-world capabilities to be and do. Applying these understandings to an occupational justice perspective highlights the importance of supporting people's capabilities to participate in occupation but cautions against imposing occupation or specific occupational expressions. Indeed, imposing certain occupations on people or specific styles of occupational expression is an act of injustice and cultural imperialism (Bailliard, 2016; Young, 1990). Accordingly, doing occupational justice "should promote the *capacity for occupational participation* [emphasis in original] and not a particular *form of occupational participation* [emphasis in original]" (Bailliard, 2013, p. 352).

One of the most important critiques levied against distributive conceptualizations of justice is that equitable distribution of goods and services is not enough for people to attain their capabilities. For any distribution to have a meaningful impact, people must be able to convert those goods and services into actual beings and doings (Sen, 2009; Venkatapuram, 2011). For example, to achieve the desired functioning of riding a bicycle, it is insufficient to merely provide someone with a bicycle. That person must have the appropriate conversion skill (knowledge of how to ride a bicycle) to convert the resource (bicycle) into a functioning (riding the bicycle) (Robeyns, 2005). According to Robeyns, there are *personal*, *social*, and *environmental conversion factors* that impact a person's conversion skills. Personal conversion factors include physical and psychological characteristics. Social conversion factors include policies, social norms, and power relations. Environmental conversion factors include characteristics of the physical environment. Societies must support the capabilities of their constituents beyond a minimal threshold "beneath which it is held that truly human functioning is not available to citizens; the social goal should be understood in terms of getting citizens above this capability threshold" (Nussbaum, 2000, p. 6). Therefore, doing occupational justice involves designing environments that support capabilities, by attending to social and environmental conversion factors, and ensuring people have the necessary conversion skills to actualize their capabilities into desired functionings or occupations (Bailliard, 2016).

Contribution of an Occupational Perspective

What distinguishes the occupational justice perspective from other theories of justice is its focus on everyday doings and happenings. Like the capabilities approach, an occupational justice perspective embraces a *realization-focused comparison* instead of *transcendental institutionalism*. This

BOX 10.2 CENTRAL HUMAN CAPABILITIES (NUSSBAUM, 2000)

1. Life
2. Bodily health
3. Bodily integrity
4. Senses, imagination, and thought
5. Emotions
6. Practical reason
7. Affiliation
8. Other species
9. Play
10. Control over one's environment

focus highlights the micro injustices that occur through everyday doing which can be overlooked because of the analytic lens of other theories of justice. For example, an occupational justice perspective magnifies the numerous daily injustices a transgender teenager would experience going throughout their daily occupations in society and at school (e.g., using gendered bathrooms, changing attire in gendered locker rooms, and gendered sports).

The occupational justice perspective is unique in that it focuses on how macro forces manifest in the microcosms of everyday experience. The occupational justice perspective does not stand in opposition to other theories of justice nor is the intent to supplant those theories; rather, it is complementary and useful because it foregrounds certain aspects of injustice that other theories of justice do not (i.e., those that occur through everyday doings). In other words, the occupational justice perspective provides an additional lens and framework of understanding of justice that supports the grander endeavor to make the world a better place for all.

Practitioners who embrace and understand an occupational justice perspective are able to see how occupations are a major conduit through which domination, oppression, and injustice occur and can harness occupation as a tool to promote justice. An occupational justice perspective is important to everyday OT practice and all OT practitioners should be aware of how issues of justice manifest in their everyday practices (Bailliard et al., 2020). In addition to sensitizing practitioners to the injustices in their everyday practices, an occupational justice perspective is also useful for alerting others outside the profession regarding the role of everyday occupations in fostering inclusive and exclusive practices. For example, an OT practitioner working on a community-based mental health outreach team can adopt an occupational justice perspective and demonstrate to their team how daily provider–client interactions that focus solely on symptom management at the expense of supporting meaningful and dignified participation in health-promoting occupations is an injustice that ignores that participation is a medical necessity. This approach also emphasizes the importance of attending to the social relations that generate health as health is "intrinsically bound up with social relations, it is both created as well as vulnerable to social relations" (Venkatapuram, 2011, p. 161).

Doing Occupational Justice

Occupational Justice and Occupational Therapy

An occupational justice perspective has been embraced by professional associations in OT and in educational standards by accrediting bodies for OT education. However, there remains ambiguity regarding how to implement an occupational justice perspective in practice to effect real-world change (Galvin et al., 2011). Despite these challenges, it is the responsibility of therapists to advance occupational justice.

Duty to Advance Occupational Rights and Occupational Justice

Integrating an occupational justice perspective is a central dimension of everyday practice and a duty for all occupational therapists (Bailliard et al., 2020). As described above, participation in occupation is a medical necessity and a right. Occupational injustices occur everywhere including in all traditional everyday OT practice settings. OT practitioners have the ethical responsibility to do no harm to their clients including not committing acts that oppress or denigrate unique occupational expressions. There is a moral imperative to support people and communities as dignified human beings to be and do what they value in the context of associated living (Bailliard, 2016; Bailliard et al., 2020; Boisvert, 1997; Hammell, 2020, 2021; Sen, 2009). Practitioners should view "justice as something that already intersects with practice, not something that practitioners must choose whether to take up" (Aldrich et al., 2017, p. 1). Because of the pervasive impact of structural factors on occupational participation, it is the duty of all occupational therapists to learn how to apply an occupational justice perspective to their everyday practices. Practitioners who fail to consider how structural factors affect the occupations of their clients are, in essence, upholding injustices, and they "collude in individualizing problems that are inherently social, in depoliticizing the systemic social and economic inequalities impacting people's lives, or in reinforcing the injustices inherent to the ableist neoliberal status quo" (Hammell, 2021, p. 6).

Applying an Occupational Justice Perspective to Advance Occupational Rights

The purpose of this chapter is to persuade readers to embrace an occupational justice perspective and to propose some strategies for applying the perspective. Doing occupational justice can involve a wide range of activities spanning from micro-level actions in inpatient settings to macro-level political activity and advocacy. The value of these activities is incommensurable, and each are noble and important endeavors. In the following section, a sample of existing approaches to occupational justice is provided followed by a discussion of how to apply an occupational justice perspective in micro, meso, and macro levels of OT practice.

Doing occupational justice is complicated because of the diversity of worldviews that conceptualize human nature differently. Most social systems adopt the worldview and ways of being of the dominant group and portray that group as the natural and desirable form of humanity (Bailliard et al., 2021; Young, 1990). Their ways of being are considered healthy, desirable, and the standard for living. Any deviations from dominant ways of being are labeled as deviant, immoral, and undesirable (Bailliard et al., 2021; Young, 1990). In response, societies create and reproduce ways of living that "members perceive to be the usual and 'healthy' way to live, the only possible way of doing things" (Kantartzis & Molineux, 2011, p. 62). Yet those possibilities are narrow and do not reflect the plurality in doings and ways of being among all communities. Failing to acknowledge the pluralism that exists among ways of being can lead OT practitioners to unintentionally impose their own ways of being on marginalized persons and groups when attempting to do occupational justice. In other words, naïve or uniformed attempts to promote occupational justice can unwittingly cause injustice and oppression (Bailliard, 2016).

Situational complexities challenge efforts to promote occupational justice. Social, cultural, and economic factors shape the repertoire of occupations that people think are available or appropriate for their particular situation and it may be difficult for them to imagine how things could be different (Galvaan, 2012; Laliberte Rudman, 2010). Therefore, it is necessary to understand how different societies construct their worlds, including what possibilities for doing and being are socially sanctioned and actually available to their constituents (Kiepek et al., 2019; Laliberte Rudman, 2014). Unmasking the sociocultural and political forces that privilege certain occupational expressions over others and deprive people of health-promoting occupations is an important step in supporting people to liberate themselves from oppression (Bourdieu, 1998; Freire, 1970). This requires adopting a critical perspective to question the status quo.

Occupational justice work is further complicated by the fact that humans and their doings are inextricably intertwined and interconnected through complex social, cultural, economic, and geopolitical relationships that are historical and continuously evolving. Interventions in one area, albeit well-intentioned and justice-focused, can ripple across those relationships in unpredictable ways that can cause injustice for others. For example, Thibeault (2013) described a situation when students representing a North American university distributed free wheelchairs to a community in Nicaragua. Despite their well-intentioned intervention, their provision of free wheelchairs caused a local wheelchair business to nearly collapse and the workers in that business to their lose jobs.

Accordingly, Hammell (2021) recommends that a core professional competency for OT should be *structural competence* or the "ability to discern the impact of institutional and social conditions—such as economic and policy decisions, colonialism, racism, heteronormativity, gender

binarism, ableism and disablism, ageism, sexism, patriarchy and misogyny, poverty and stigma—on health inequalities" (p. 5). Failure to develop structural competence when attempting to advance occupational justice can unintentionally result in unjust outcomes because of poor understandings of the complex intertwining of structural forces and human agencies (Bailliard, 2016; Thibeault, 2013).

Scholars have argued that OT educational programs should be more intentional in integrating an occupational justice perspective into their curricula and classroom activities (Aldrich et al., 2016; Hocking & Townsend, 2015; Sakellariou & Pollard, 2013). Habituating students to applying an occupational justice perspective will help in creating a more socially conscious and justice-oriented base of practitioners. It may also be helpful to teach students and practitioners to abandon SMART goals in favor of SMARTIE goals (Specific, Measurable, Achievable, Realistic, Timebound, *Inclusion, Equity*). The Centers for Disease Control and Prevention (CDC, 2021) suggests that using SMARTIE goals will habituate practitioners to stay focused on health equity and eliminating injustices. *Inclusion* refers to inviting and incorporating input from clients and community partners so their voices and priorities are included (CDC, 2021). *Equity* refers to considering whether the goal addresses the unique needs and circumstances of different clients to work toward equitable outcomes (CDC, 2021). Although SMARTIE goals began in the corporate world and the CDC recommends them in relation to cancer care, integrating them into typical OT practice promises to habituate practitioners to consider inclusion, equity, and justice in goal setting and intervention planning. In addition to these recommendations, different approaches to occupational justice have emerged across the world.

The following sections do not aim to provide a comprehensive overview of every approach that has been developed. The first section will outline some major developments in this area with the hope that practitioners will be able to select and develop approaches that are uniquely suited to their situation. The second section outlines interventions that target micro, meso, or macro levels of functioning or a combination of levels.

Approaches to Occupational Justice

Social Occupational Therapy. One of the earliest examples of an occupational justice approach can be found in the late 1970s in Brazil when Jussara de Mesquita Pinto presented about OT in the social field during the Fifth Scientific Meeting of Occupational Therapists in 1979 and when the Federal University of Sao Carlos and the Pontifical Catholic University of Campinas included Occupational Therapy Applied to Social Conditions in their curricula (Galheigo, 2021). Brazilian social occupational therapists were aware of the potential role of OT as a mechanism for social control and sought to harness

OT for positive social transformation (Galheigo, 2021). Social OT is presented as a specific subfield within OT that focuses on the emancipation of people whose social rights are violated through restriction of their actions and opportunities by socioeconomic factors (Malfitano, 2021; Malfitano et al., 2014). Social OT is distinguished from typical OT because of its explicit focus on the impact of socioeconomic conditions on the social position and life experiences of clients of OT. Accordingly, this subfield focuses on people experiencing homelessness, people who are incarcerated, individuals experiencing poverty, individuals in institutionalized care, immigrants, and other populations who are marginalized or alienated by socioeconomic and political forces (Malfitano, 2021).

To enact social OT, practitioners must constantly reflect on how macro-level forces manifest at the micro level and always understand the individual as part of a collective. Social occupational therapists foreground the following principles in their work: a "*collective perspective of understanding the reality of population groups* [italics in original] and the *articulation between the micro- and macro-social aspects*" (Malfitano, 2021, p. 52). These principles inform approaches that focus on the *cotidiano* (i.e., a commitment to everyday life and respect for the diverse ways it is expressed) and the *promotion of spaces of living together* (i.e., spaces that intentionally foster intermingling of beings and doings between diverse groups). In Brazil, social OT has been used with poor urban youth at a school and at a youth center using social technologies (i.e., workshops/activities, dynamics, and projects; individual territorial follow-ups, articulation of resources in the social field, and the dynamization of the support network) (Lopes et al., 2021). Youth participating in social OT are empowered to identify activities (e.g., making masks, making kites, cooking, participating in soccer tournaments, and displaying exhibits) that harness occupation to facilitate community building, challenge social inequity, and catalyze social transformation (Lopes et al., 2021). Activity workshops (e.g., developing individual profiles using memes, mapping spaces used by youth, planting and cleaning the neighborhood) facilitate exchanges between youth and communities that celebrate plural ways of being, challenge social inequity, foster discussion of identity issues, emphasize social inclusion, embrace collectivity, experiment with ideas, and challenge the status quo (Barreiro, 2021; da Silva & de Souza, 2021; de Silva, 2021).

The Capabilities, Opportunities, Resources and Environments Approach.
In Australia, the Capabilities, Opportunities, Resources and Environments (CORE) approach was developed to guide therapists in designing occupation-focused interventions that promote social inclusion (Pereira, 2017; Pereira & Whiteford, 2018). "The CORE approach provides a mechanism for occupational therapists to view practice through an inclusive lens, and *do* [emphasis in original] inclusive occupational therapy through applying reflexive questions" (Pereira et al., 2020, p. 163). Applying the CORE approach requires therapists to foreground its four key elements (capabilities, opportunities, resources, and environments) in their clinical reasoning. It also encourages therapists to address system-level and structural barriers to participation and inclusion. The CORE approach can inform efforts to advance occupational justice at all levels of functioning. It has been used in government-funded forensic mental health services in Sydney to illustrate how *resources* limited the occupational performance and recovery of those receiving services (Pereira et al., 2020). In this case, applying the CORE approach shifted practitioners' analytic foci to how the lack of *resources* directly stunted the *capabilities* of service recipients instead of focusing on their capabilities or symptoms. It demonstrated that institutional priorities of risk management had prevented service providers from promoting rehabilitation and recovery despite the institution's purported focus on recovery (Pereira et al., 2020). In clinical reasoning, applying the CORE approach foregrounds capabilities, opportunities, resources, and environments in a manner that shifts the focus away from symptom management. It "requires occupational therapists to critically engage with systems, structures, and policies that provide or delimit resources and (inter alia) opportunities and enable or constrain a capabilities approach" (Pereira et al., 2020, p. 168).

Practice-Based Enquiry.
Critical reflection is also a hallmark of practice-based enquiry (PBE), which has been used as a meso-level approach to advance occupational justice in the United Kingdom, Australia, and the United States. PBE can be used by OT practitioners in institutional settings to advance occupational justice through critical reflections that target their practices (Whiteford et al., 2020; Wilding et al., 2012). Critical reflexivity is necessary to understand how broad socioeconomic and political forces affect what therapists do and think is possible within their settings (Kinsella & Whiteford, 2009). The PBE process must be organic with no power differentials between members, although an experienced researcher is typically the facilitator. The PBE stages involve: (a) the formation of a group interested in addressing an aspect of their practice; (b) discussion of the aspect of practice informed by literature; (c) commitment to address the aspect of practice through PBE; (d) ethics approval; (e) data collection (i.e., repeated reflections on everyday practice changes in relation to the aspect of practice); (f) concurrent regularly occurring discussions of data and literature; (g) individual coding of narrative data; (h) group discussion and analyses of individual codes; and (i) refinement and finalization of themes. Whiteford et al. (2020) effectively used the PBE process with a group of occupational therapists in a forensic hospital in Sydney, Australia. Through

their participation, the therapists were guided in reflecting and interrogating their practices to implement iterative changes in their everyday practices. Participating therapists increasingly incorporated occupation into their practices and were able to confidently advance occupational justice to provide more opportunities for their clients. Gallagher et al. (2023) also used PBE in an acute mental health service in a large teaching hospital in the United States to transform their practices to be more justice-oriented and occupation-centered.

Participatory Occupational Justice Framework. Similar in philosophy to both CORE and PBE, the participatory occupational justice framework (POJF) was developed in Australia and Canada for use with populations who experience restrictions in their everyday participation (Townsend & Whiteford, 2005). The POJF adopts a nonlinear process (Figure 10.3) to raise awareness of occupational injustices and to address those injustices to promote social inclusion (Whiteford et al., 2018). Because of high variability in environmental contexts, population groups, and restrictions on participation, the POJF does not present a rigid step-by-step protocol and it is guided by critical epistemological foundations. Although there is no fixed starting point for the POJF process, Whiteford et al. acknowledge that *raising consciousness* would be a typical starting point. The POJF is founded on six Articles which focus on human rights, equalized power relations, social inclusion, social and cultural relevance, equitable opportunities and resources, and agency within adverse environments. The POJF process encourages practitioners to shed their professional stance in order to engage in *radical solidarity* with community partners using a critical perspective and reflexive practices to cocreate feasible real-world solutions that lead to social transformation (Whiteford et al., 2021).

Radical Sensibility. Similar to Whiteford et al.'s (2021) call for *radical solidarity*, Rudman (2021) argued that occupational therapists must adopt a *radical sensibility* to disrupt and transform social conditions that generate occupational possibilities. Rudman proposed the following six intersecting guideposts to foster the development and enactment of radical sensibility: resist fatalism and acquiescence (i.e., resist the idea that inequity is unavoidable and necessary), embrace critical optimism (i.e., resist the assumption that the existing social reality is natural and remain hopeful that it can be changed), engage a critical stance toward the "status quo" (i.e., adopt a critical worldview that is informed by diverse critical social theories), embrace a transformative model of participation (i.e., embrace cultural humility and authentic collaboration while

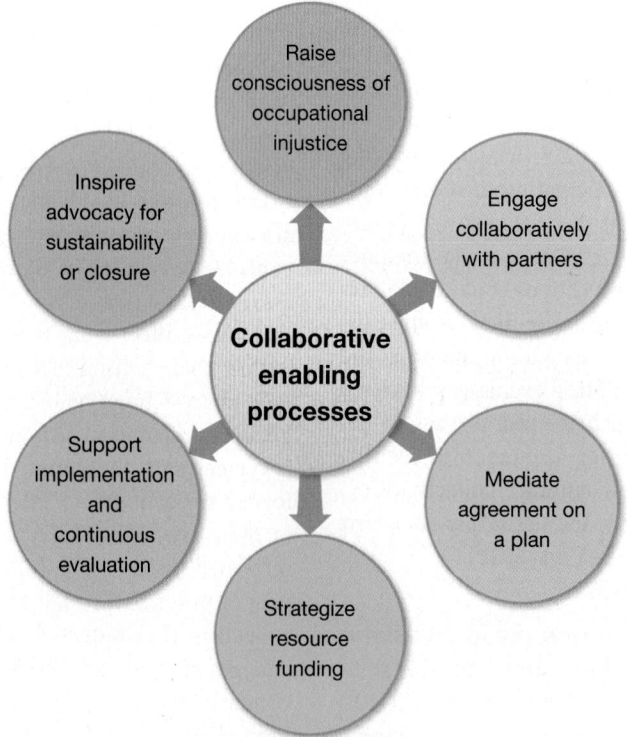

FIGURE 10.3 Participatory occupational justice framework (POJF) process.

(Adapted from Whiteford, G., Jones, K., Rahal, C., & Suleman, A. [2018]. The Participatory Occupational Justice Framework as a tool for change: Three contrasting case narratives. *Journal of Occupational Science, 25*(4), 497–508 (p. 498). https://doi.org/10.1080/14427591.2018.1504607)

resisting positioning oneself as the expert), enact Utopic imagination (i.e., imagine what society should be instead of limiting one's imagination to what one thinks is possible), and enact generative disruption through occupation (i.e., mobilize shared occupation to generate social transformation). Adopting a *radical sensibility* prepares practitioners to imagine what is possible without being constrained by the inertia of social habits.

Social Transformation Through Occupation. Rudman's call for a transformative agenda that leverages occupation to pursue a more just world has been echoed by many scholars over the years (Farias et al., 2016; Galheigo, 2011b). Engaging in social transformation through occupation is difficult (Farias & Rudman, 2019a) and requires communities of practice where practitioners can share examples of their work, including the challenges and successes they have encountered (Trimboli et al., 2019). The International Social Transformation through Occupation Network (ISTTON) emerged as an effort to form partnerships across the globe among individuals and organizations seeking to leverage occupation "as a means to enact social transformations that ameliorate social, health, and occupational inequalities" (Laliberte Rudman et al., 2019, p. 317). Occupations that are socially transformative must initiate personal and community-level growth to cause lasting societal change (Angell, 2014; Galheigo, 2011b). Farias et al. (2019) suggest that practitioners should engage in a critical dialogic approach with community partners to create spaces for challenging what is "taken for granted" such as how asymmetrical power relationships affect what people are able to do and how.

Despite the promise of these approaches, neoliberalism, healthism, and managerialism remain significant challenges in enacting social transformation through occupation-based practices (Farias & Rudman, 2019a). Neoliberalism individualizes occupation in a manner that hides sociopolitical influences and places personal responsibility as the primary factor influencing health choices and lifestyles. Healthism furthers the impact of neoliberalism by emphasizing the personal responsibility of individuals in making healthy choices that produce health. Managerialism involves the push to develop protocols and guidelines that control costs and ensure conformity in practices which encourage practitioners to think in oversimplified and reductionist ways that hide the complex influence of sociopolitical forces (Farias & Rudman, 2019b). Together, these challenges encourage placing "problems" and "intervention targets" within the individual while absolving political and sociocultural forces from responsibility. Responding to calls for social transformation through occupation, Benjamin-Thomas et al. (2021) collaborated with children with disabilities in rural South India as co-researchers in a participatory filmmaking project to critically analyze the occupational injustices they and their communities experienced. Together, the group made films and analyzed the visual data using a critical dialogue to uncover how systemic factors affected their participation in home, school, and community. Their work demonstrated how authentic collaboration and power sharing amplified the priorities for social transformation that were important to the children themselves (Benjamin-Thomas et al., 2021).

Occupation-Based Community Development Framework. Also embracing the importance of a critical perspective, the ObCD emerged from the University of Cape Town in South Africa through authentic collaborative work with the local community to represent the collective experience of marginalized groups (Galvaan, 2021). The ObCD framework applies a decolonial and critical perspective to do occupational justice and promote social inclusion. It recognizes that dominate geopolitical and social structures limit diverse occupational expressions by imposing specific ways of being. The ObCD framework encourages practitioners to carefully partner with their communities as equals and to get to know their communities through reading local newspapers, listening to the radio, and interacting with them (Richards & Galvaan, 2018). The ObCD framework process emphasizes generative disruption through collaborating with communities to engage in critical reflections regarding how power, privilege, and social norms are reproduced and challenged through their participation in occupation (Galvaan, 2021).

An Occupation-Based, Community-Building Process for Greater Occupational Justice. Another approach to community development in the occupational justice literature was offered by Rachel Thibeault. Thibeault (2013) argued that efforts to advance occupational justice at the community level are often naïve, rushed, and detrimental to the very community they portend to help. Over years collaborating with local partners, Thibeault developed a seven-step occupation-based, community-building process for greater occupational justice. Thibeault argued that this process cannot be rushed and usually takes 7 to 10 years because it is essential to tailor these steps to the unique sociocultural circumstances of the community. Step 1 involves befriending the community through participating in events, celebrations, and shared occupations that cultivate authentic collaborative relationships. Step 2 involves discovery and communication wherein bonds are continuously cultivated through shared occupations and a Communication Charter is established to acknowledge the possibility of communication breakdowns and potential solutions for managing those breakdowns. In Step 3, an occupation-focused approach is used to uncover core values. Step 4 involves performing an occupational analysis of the community with a focus on power, social status, and which groups experience unfair burden. During Step 5, the group identifies strong and positive community leaders who can lead the group in changing local mentalities. It is essential for leaders to have lived experience with the injustice(s) being addressed. In Step 6, community-building occupations are harnessed to build solidarity and identify social networks to enhance community cohesion and political influence. Step 7 is about sustaining the community's ability to discuss important issues and its cohesion through shared occupations. This process emphasizes humility and collaboration where "interventionists" shed the savior complex and "act as connectors, creating and strengthening networks that will embolden vulnerable communities" toward dignity and autonomy (Thibeault, 2013, p. 254).

Advancing Occupational Justice at Micro, Meso, and Macro Levels of Functioning

The abovementioned approaches are synergistic and share several conceptual similarities. They shift the focus away from individual factors to systemic factors, raise consciousness through critical reflection, establish authentic collaborative partnerships, minimize power differentials, embrace cultural humility, and harness occupation as a tool for social change. Practitioners can use these principles to advance occupational justice at micro, meso, and macro levels of functioning.

Micro-Level Approaches. Micro-level approaches occur at the interpersonal level and involve mundane everyday actions. Applying an occupational justice perspective to the micro level highlights the micro-occupational injustices that occur every day through interactions with a person's closest social circles. A micro-level approach to occupational justice would encourage practitioners to critically reflect on their social positioning in relation to their clients. Professional attire, name badges, clinical titles, and professional jargon are examples of cultural capital that give clinicians significant power over their clients. Enacting an occupational justice perspective at the micro level requires therapists to actively minimize power differentials with clients to engage in authentic client-centered collaborations (Bailliard et al., 2020). Most importantly, it requires therapists to avoid imposing their ways of beings and personal occupational expressions on their clients who may have very different values, priorities, and understandings of how to express their occupations. Indeed, a justice-oriented therapist avoids imposing specific meanings or forms of occupational expression and instead "invite their clients to co-create a therapeutic process that celebrates their clients' personal narratives, occupational meanings, and preferences regarding how to perform occupations" (Bailliard et al., 2020, p. 148). Other micro-level approaches to occupational justice involve equipping clients with

strategies to advocate for their rights and challenge stigma they may receive from society (Bailliard et al., 2020) and incorporating SMARTIE goals in practice to ensure interventions always consider inclusion and equity. Although such strategies do not address broader forces generating inequity and oppression of occupational expressions, they are necessary to help individuals experience dignity and humanity in the moment. Indeed, many meso- and macro-level approaches to advancing occupational justice effect changes to micro-level behaviors and practices.

Meso-Level Approaches. Meso-level approaches may occur at the organizational or institutional level. These may involve pushing for institutional or organizational policy change in places such as schools, workplaces, institutions, and neighborhoods. For example, to reduce violence and maltreatment, the WHO recommends programs that target life skills and social competence; however, programs typically favor targeting interpersonal and relationship factors rather than those that occur at the social and community level (Krug et al., 2002). Using an occupational justice perspective, practitioners can design and implement programs at the community or organizational level that harness occupation to habituate participants to engaging in inclusive practices that do not oppress or marginalize nonnormative occupational expressions in a manner that contributes to violence. Meso-level approaches also include creating safe spaces where people can participate in health-promoting and community-building occupations such as in social OT. Community-level OT interventions should always adopt an occupational justice perspective to promote community building, cohesion, and inclusion. Many of the abovementioned approaches to advancing occupational justice are meso-level interventions designed to change the behaviors of individuals.

A concrete example of a meso-level intervention is the Identity Development Evolution and Sharing (IDEAS) program (Wasmuth et al., 2020). IDEAS is an OT intervention that uses narratives of members from a marginalized group to produce a professional play and invites the audience to engage in a critical dialogue following the production. IDEAS focuses on systemic factors and intentionally eschews the medical model's focus on individual factors. Wasmuth et al. (2021) used IDEAS to advance occupational justice for transgender and gender-nonconforming people. The intervention involved writing a play based on the challenging stories of oppression and marginalization that participants had experienced throughout their lives. Findings suggest the intervention was effective in reducing social stigma in the community while providing an opportunity for transgender and gender-nonconforming people to experience positive social participation that enhanced their well-being.

Other meso-level interventions may include performing trainings, in-services, and workshops that enhance the capability of providers to advance occupational justice through intraorganizational change. For example, trainings might encourage practitioners to focus on systemic and environmental factors instead of symptom reduction. The trainings might also engage trainees in reflexive practices to "consider how their personal sociocultural backgrounds, biases, and occupational preferences can affect the selection of intervention targets and strategies" (Bailliard et al., 2020, p. 149). Meso-level interventions can also intentionally target and modify the culture of practice settings through systematic critical reflection such as those proposed by PBE, POJF, and CORE.

Macro-Level Approaches. Macro-level approaches involve practices such as mobilizing broad community partnerships, pushing for policy change with local or federal government, undertaking leadership roles at the regional or national level, developing regional and national intervention programs, or offering trainings at the regional or national level. These approaches involve targeting macro-level factors that generate the conditions of oppression and marginalization such as societal norms, cultural expectations,

and political relationships. For example, in 2002, the WHO released the World Report on Violence, which asserted that there is a need to examine social and cultural values and norms that have a significant role in perpetuating violence and injustice among vulnerable populations (Krug et al., 2002). An occupational justice perspective on this issue would encourage interventions that use meaningful community occupations to challenge and modify social and cultural values that denigrate and oppress others. Occupation is a medium through which social and cultural habits are formed, reproduced, and transmitted (Cutchin et al., 2008); therefore, occupation also has the potential to transform social norms (Townsend, 1997). Although macro-level transformations may seem daunting, it is important to imagine what could be possible and what an occupationally just society would look like instead of limiting possibilities to variations of a broken status quo (Rudman, 2021). Typically, macro-level changes advancing occupational justice will require establishing partnerships and collaborations with different stakeholders to ensure a plurality of views and expertise are represented and harnessed to effect meaningful and inclusive change.

OT STORY 10.1 SEEKING OCCUPATIONAL JUSTICE

Donna "Ara" Munier

Since childhood, I experienced multiple traumas but did not receive diagnoses until I was 28. I was often ridiculed for common signs of trauma, depression, and developmental disruption (i.e., interpersonal difficulties, difficulty expressing needs, social isolation, sensorimotor challenges, hypersensitivity to touch, decreased coordination, sleep disturbances, and poor impulse control).

School was a particularly challenging environment where I was frequently labeled a "problem." I spaced out in class, couldn't process homework, and felt empty. When I couldn't finish homework, I was forced to complete assignments in front of class. If I froze with a glazed expression, unable to speak, I was asked if I was an idiot. I became dysregulated and confused when attempting such tasks. Despite being an extroverted child who participated in sports and music, in high school I withdrew from social gatherings, extracurricular activities, and seeing friends. I couldn't bear encountering aggressive and authoritative individuals who left me in speechless terror—I was reliving trauma and had developed a pattern of avoidance for certain environmental triggers.

It wasn't enough to avoid people. Turning on the television showed depictions of mentally ill people as "psychopaths." As a Nurse Assistant, I was taught to distrust mentally ill patients as potential criminals, regardless of their

forensic history; yet experienced sexual harassment and intimidation from "sane" patients. I was frightened by how mental illness was stigmatized as a precursor to violence.

Health insurance never adequately covered treatment, and my physicians never inquired about mental health. When I first sought help for suicidal ideation, my physician responded: "You're cute. You'll find a boyfriend." People seldom understand that you can't simply "just stop thinking" about painful memories and that flashbacks are all-encompassing and resistant to cognitive control. I avoided the topic and lived with worsening symptoms for 15 years before learning that I had PTSD and MDD after being committed following a panic attack. Therapy helped, but I quickly realized that employers and educators weren't sensitized to mental illness as a valid medical condition. When I referenced the Americans with Disabilities Act to seek student accommodations, an instructor responded that it didn't apply to students. When experiencing severe symptoms after being reprimanded for sharing concerns with an instructor, I received a faith-based lecture, prayers, and advice to abandon my passions.

At 31, I finally began truly living. Life changed when I surrounded myself with growth-oriented people who were kind and respected my dignity and needs to regulate my nervous system with exercise, connection to supportive people,

(continued)

OT STORY 10.1 SEEKING OCCUPATIONAL JUSTICE (*continued*)

sunlight, consistent nutrition, meaningful activities, my service dog, and a system for self-monitoring my symptoms. Psychotherapy and medicine helped, but I believe kind words were what empowered me to overcome feelings of shame. How I identified with my thoughts and surroundings also changed. I no longer feel that something is disturbingly wrong with me. Now, I happily work multiple jobs as an occupational therapist, mentor students, attend speaking engagements, and enjoy several hobbies in the community.

Questions

1. What micro-, meso-, and macro-level occupational justice issues are present in this story?
2. Imagine you are an OT practitioner working with Ara as a client. How would applying an occupational justice perspective influence your work with her?
3. What micro-, meso-, and macro-level occupational justice interventions might address the injustices encountered by Ara?

EXPANDING OUR PERSPECTIVES

Occupational Justice Within Occupational Therapy Scholarship and Practice

Selena Washington

In recent years, I have continued to develop my practice as an occupational therapist, instructor, and researcher through the lens of occupational justice. I have utilized the concepts of occupational justice to challenge societal norms and examine power relations through an occupational perspective. As an assistant professor, I have incorporated the concepts of occupational justice to extend my students' knowledge of occupational function and engagement through an intersection of social identities (e.g., social class, gender, race/ethnicity, religion, disability, and sexual orientation) through an inclusive and reflexive approach. I have utilized the tenets of the participatory occupational justice framework (POJF) to promote the cultural sensitivity and humility necessary when forming relationships with patient, clients, community partners, and multifaceted communities. At this point you may ask "what does this all mean?" Let's explore further through an example of community-based OT research.

My research is centered within communities of color and with those aging with disability; the Social and Structural Determinants of Health (e.g., housing, discrimination, income, and race) as evidenced within this chapter, are associated with the safety and well-being of vulnerable aging adult populations. With the grounding of occupational justice, my research focuses on the understanding of my participants' lived experience and how to responsibly implement research protocols focused on client-driven directives, meaningful occupational engagement, and self-efficacy toward health-promoting activity. For example,

the decrease of engagement in social/community activity and wellness programs during the height of the COVID-19 pandemic placed older adults at greater risk of frailty, depression, and cognitive decline, which compromised their capacity for occupational engagement and daily functional activity. The threat of occupational injustice at the micro, meso, and macro levels of engagement as described within this chapter was imminent within this specific population. My research team utilized aspects of occupational justice to develop a social and occupation-based intervention at the height of the pandemic, specifically for those who were at risk of hospitalization and mortality based on race, underlying health conditions, and age (e.g., African American adults age 65 and older). Our intervention was group-based, participant-led (the content of the meetings was determined by the participants' interest/needs), and addressed areas of occupational interest and engagement, community resources, and environmental safety. As a result of this intervention, there were positive correlations between improved general health ratings, IADL functional activity, and self-reported depression symptoms, along with decreased environmental fall risk.

Finally, I acknowledge there is criticism of occupational justice, as this chapter identifies, specifying that occupational justice originated from a Western Anglo middle-class perspective that is not representative of all worldviews and is poorly defined. However, I hope that the examples I have provided demonstrate occupational justice as a foundational "start" to understand our own individual social positioning and how we must be conscious of our interactions with individuals whose historical, cultural, and current contextual factors differ from our own, and are unique and vital to the lived experience of those whom we serve.

Conclusion

This chapter proposes a working definition of an occupational justice perspective. It is important to continue developing and refining this definition to clarify what is meant by occupational justice, how it is situated among other theories of justice, and how to integrate an occupational justice perspective in practice.

OT practitioners have a moral duty and ethical responsibility to apply an occupational justice perspective to their practices. Doing occupational justice involves assessing occupational situations from micro, meso, and macro levels of functioning to identify micro-, meso-, and macro-level intervention targets that are oppressing occupational expressions. It involves rejecting reductionist individual-focused analyses and intervention in favor of holistic analyses and interventions which consider and target structural forces that oppress individuals and communities. It involves engaging in critical reflection to question the status quo and the various hierarchies of social positionings it attempts to impose. Most importantly, it emphasizes the need to protect the dignity and humanity of all persons, including their capabilities to be and do, in the context of oppressive political, cultural, and socioeconomic conditions.

Acknowledgments

I would like to extend a profound thanks to Dr. Barbara Hooper, Jody Bennett, Caroline Lass, and Kelsey McGregor for providing feedback on drafts of this chapter and to Noah Winstead and Laura Whiston for performing literature reviews.

Lippincott® Connect *For additional resources on the subjects discussed in this chapter, visit* Lippincott Connect.

REFERENCES

Aldrich, R. M., Boston, T. L., & Daaleman, C. E. (2017). Justice and U.S. occupational therapy practice: A relationship 100 years in the making. *American Journal of Occupational Therapy, 71*(1), 7101100040p1–7101100040p5. https://doi.org/10.5014/ajot.2017.023085

Aldrich, R. M., White, N. A., & Conners, B. L. (2016). Translating occupational justice education into action: Reflections from an exploratory single case study. *OTJR: Occupation, Participation and Health, 36*(4), 227–233. https://doi.org/10.1177/1539449216667278

Allingham, M. (2014). *Distributive justice.* Routledge.

American Occupational Therapy Association. (2020). Occupational therapy practice framework: Domain and process (4th ed.). *American Journal of Occupational Therapy,74*(Suppl. 2),7412410010. https://doi.org/10.5014/ajot.2020.74S2001.

Angell, A. M. (2014). Occupation-centered analysis of social difference: Contributions to a socially responsive occupational science. *Journal of Occupational Science, 21*(2), 104–116. https://doi.org/10.1080/14427591.2012.711230

Artiga, S., & Hinton, E. (2018). *Beyond health care: The role of social determinants in promoting health and health equity.* K. F. Foundation.

Bailliard, A. (2013). Laying low: Fear and injustice for Latino migrants to Smalltown, USA. *Journal of Occupational Science, 20*(4), 342–356. https://doi.org/10.1080/14427591.2013.799114

Bailliard, A. (2016). Justice, difference, and the capability to function. *Journal of Occupational Science, 23*(1), 3–16. https://doi.org/10.1080/14427591.2014.957886

Bailliard, A., Agostine, S., Bristol, S., & Syu, Y.-C. (2022). From embodiment to emplacement: Toward understanding occupation as body-mind-environment. *Journal of Occupational Science,* 1–16. https://doi.org/10.1080/14427591.2022.2031261

Bailliard, A., Carroll, A., & Peak, K. (2021). Laying low: Unmasking the contributions of science and education to racism. *Journal of Occupational Science, 28*(3), 441–448. https://doi.org/10.1080/14427591.2021.1893109

Bailliard, A. L., Carroll, A., & Dallman, A. R. (2018). The inescapable corporeality of occupation: Integrating Merleau-Ponty into the study of occupation. *Journal of Occupational Science, 25*(2), 222–233. https://doi.org/10.1080/14427591.2017.1397536

Bailliard, A. L., Dallman, A. R., Carroll, A., Lee, B. D., & Szendrey, S. (2020). Doing occupational justice: A central dimension of everyday occupational therapy practice. *Canadian Journal of Occupational Therapy, 87*(2), 144–152. https://doi.org/10.1177/0008417419898930

Barreiro, R. (2021). Activity workshops: Exploring the use of digital media by Brazilian youths. In R. Lopes & A. P. S. Malfitano (Eds.), *Social occupational therapy: Theoretical and practical designs* (pp. 212–216). Elsevier.

Barros, D., Ghiradi, M., Lopes, R., & Galheigo, S. (2011). Brazilian experiencs in social occupational therapy. In F. Kronenburg, N. Pollard, & D. Sakellariou (Eds.), *Occupational therapies without borders* (pp. 209–216). Elsevier.

Benjamin-Thomas, T. E., & Rudman, D. L. (2018). A critical interpretive synthesis: Use of the occupational justice framework in research. *Australian Occupational Therapy Journal, 65*(1), 3–14. https://doi.org/10.1111/1440-1630.12428

Benjamin-Thomas, T. E., Rudman, D. L., McGrath, C., Cameron, D., Abraham, V. J., Gunaseelan, J., & Vinothkumar, S. P. (2021). Situating occupational injustices experienced by children with disabilities in rural India within sociocultural, economic, and systemic conditions. *Journal of Occupational Science,* 1–18. https://doi.org/10.1080/14427591.2021.1899038

Boisvert, R. D. (1997). *John Dewey: Rethinking our time.* State University of New York Press. http://ebookcentral.proquest.com/lib/unc/detail.action?docID=3406907

Bourdieu, P. (1998). *Practical reason: On the theory of action.* Stanford University Press.

Bourdieu, P. (2004). The peasant and his body. *Ethnography, 5*(4), 579–599. https://doi.org/10.1177/1466138104048829

Burns-Lynch, B., Brusilovskiy, E., & Salzer, M. S. (2016). An empirical study of the relationship between community participation, recovery, and quality of life of individuals with serious mental illnesses. *Israel Journal of Psychiatry and Related Sciences, 53*(1), 46–54. https://cdn.doctorsonly.co.il/2016/08/09_Burns-Lynch_An-Empirical-Study.pdf

Caciopppo, J. T., & Hawkley, L. C. (2009). Perceived social isolation and cognition. *Trends in Cognitive Sciences, 13*(10), 447–454. https://doi.org/10.1016/j.tics.2009.06.005

Caciopppo, S., Grippo, A. J., London, S., Goossens, L., & Caciopppo, J. T. (2015). Loneliness: Clinical import and interventions. *Perspectives on Psychological Science, 10*(2), 238–249. https://doi.org/10.1177/1745691615570616

Centers for Disease Control and Prevention. (November 3, 2021). *From SMART to SMARTIE objectives.* https://www.cdc.gov/cancer/nbccedp/pdf/smartie-objectives-508.pdf

Córdoba, A. G. (2020). About new forms of colonization in occupational therapy. Reflections on the idea of occupational justice from a critical-political philosophy perspective. *Cadernos Brasileiros de*

Terapia Ocupacional, Ahead of Print. https://doi.org/10.4322/2526-8910.ctoARF2175

Cutchin, M. P., Aldrich, R. M., Bailliard, A. L., & Coppola, S. (2008). Action theories for occupational science: The contributions of Dewey and Bourdieu. *Journal of Occupational Science, 15*(3), 157–165. https://doi.org/10.1080/14427591.2008.9686625

da Silva, C., & de Souza, L. (2021). The planting has become a plantation: Germinating relationships to sow ties. In R. Lopes & A. P. S. Malfitano (Eds.), *Social occupational therapy: Theoretical and practical designs* (pp. 221–224). Elsevier.

de Silva, M. (2021). Under and between trees: Social occupational therapy in a public square. In R. Lopes & A. P. S. Malfitano (Eds.), *Social occupational therapy: Theoretical and practical designs* (pp. 217–220). Elsevier.

Delle Fave, A., Brdar, I., Freire, T., Vella-Brodrick, D., & Wissing, M. P. (2011). The eudaimonic and hedonic components of happiness: Qualitative and quantitative findings. *Social Indicators Research, 100*(2), 185–207. https://doi.org/10.1007/s11205-010-9632-5

Durocher, E., Gibson, B. E., & Rappolt, S. (2014). Occupational justice: A conceptual review. *Journal of Occupational Science, 21*(4), 418–430. https://doi.org/10.1080/14427591.2013.775692

Emery-Whittington, I. G. (2021). Occupational justice—Colonial business as usual? Indigenous observations from Aotearoa New Zealand. *Canadian Journal of Occupational Therapy, 88*(2), 153–162. https://doi.org/10.1177/00084174211005891

Ewuoso, C., & Hall, S. (2019). Core aspects of *ubuntu*: A systematic review. *South African Journal of Bioethics and Law, 12*(2), 93–103. https://doi.org/10.7196/SAJBL.2019.v12i2.679

Farias, L., Laliberte Rudman, D., & Magalhães, L. (2016). Illustrating the importance of critical epistemology to realize the promise of occupational justice. *OTJR, 36*(4), 234–243. https://doi.org/10.1177/1539449216665561

Farias, L., Laliberte Rudman, D., Pollard, N., Schiller, S., Serrata Malfitano, A. P., Thomas, K., & van Bruggen, H. (2019). Critical dialogical approach: A methodological direction for occupation-based social transformative work. *Scandinavian Journal of Occupational Therapy, 26*(4), 235–245. https://doi.org/10.1080/11038128.2018.1469666

Farias, L., & Rudman, D. L. (2019a). Challenges in enacting occupation-based social transformative practices: A critical dialogical study. *Canadian Journal of Occupational Therapy, 86*(3), 243–252. https://doi.org/10.1177/0008417419828798

Farias, L., & Rudman, D. L. (2019b). Practice analysis: Critical reflexivity on discourses constraining socially transformative occupational therapy practices. *British Journal of Occupational Therapy, 82*(11), 693–697. https://doi.org/10.1177/0308022619862111

Freire, P. (1970). *Pedagogy of the oppressed*. Bloomsbury Publishing.

Frye, V., Camacho-Rivera, M., Salas-Ramirez, K., Albritton, T., Deen, D., Sohler, N., Barrick, S., & Nunes, J. (2020). Professionalism: The wrong tool to solve the right problem? *Academic Medicine: Journal of the Association of American Medical Colleges, 95*(6), 860–863. https://doi.org/10.1097/acm.0000000000003266

Galheigo, S. (2021). Social occupational therapy in Brazil: A historical synthesis of the constitution of a field of knowledge and practice. In R. Lopes & A. P. S. Malfitano (Eds.), *Social occupational therapy: Theoretical and practical designs* (pp. 11–21). Elsevier.

Galheigo, S. M. (2011a). Occupational therapy in the social field: Concepts and critical considerations. In F. Kronenburg, N. Pollard, & D. Sakellariou (Eds.), *Occupational therapies without borders: Towards an ecology of occupation-based practices* (Vol. 2, pp. 47–56). Elsevier Science.

Galheigo, S. M. (2011b). What needs to be done? Occupational therapy responsibilities and challenges regarding human rights. *Australian Occupational Therapy Journal, 58*(2), 60–66. https://doi.org/10.1111/j.1440-1630.2011.00922.x

Gallagher, M., Bagatell, N., Godwin, K., & Peters, D. (2023). Using practice based enquiry to enact occupation-centered, justice-oriented practice in an acute mental health setting. *American Journal of Occupational Therapy.*

Galvaan, R. (2012). Occupational choice: The significance of socioeconomic and political factors. In G. Whiteford & C. Hocking (Eds.), *Occupational science: Society, inclusion, participation* (pp. 152–162). Blackwell Publishing.

Galvaan, R. (2021). Generative disruption through occupational science: Enacting possibilities for deep human connection. *Journal of Occupational Science, 28*(1), 6–18. https://doi.org/10.1080/14427591.2020.1818276

Galvin, D., Wilding, C., & Whiteford, G. (2011). Utopian visions/dystopian realities: Exploring practice and taking action to enable human rights and occupational justice in a hospital context. *Australian Occupational Therapy Journal, 58*(5), 378–385. https://doi.org/10.1111/j.1440-1630.2011.00967.x

George, E., & Stanley, M. (2019). Exploring the occupational injustices of human trafficking. *Journal of Occupational Science, 26*(3), 394–407. https://doi.org/10.1080/14427591.2018.1515104

Gerst-Emerson, K., & Jayawardhana, J. (2015). Loneliness as a public health issue: The impact of loneliness on health care utilization among older adults. *American Journal of Public Health, 105*(5), 1013–1019. https://doi.org/10.2105/ajph.2014.302427

Gorman, A. (2021). *The hill we climb: An inaugural poem for the country.* Viking.

Guo, S., Lin, X., Coicaud, J.-M., Gu, S., Gu, Y., Liu, Q., Qin, X., Sun, G., Wang, Z., & Zhang, C. (2019). Conceptualizing and measuring global justice: Theories, concepts, principles and indicators. *Fudan Journal of the Humanities and Social Sciences, 12*(4), 511–546. https://doi.org/10.1007/s40647-019-00267-1

Hammell, K. R., & Iwama, M. K. (2012). Well-being and occupational rights: An imperative for critical occupational therapy. *Scandinavian Journal of Occupational Therapy, 19*(5), 385–394. https://doi.org/10.3109/11038128.2011.611821

Hammell, K. R. W. (2017). Critical reflections on occupational justice: Toward a rights-based approach to occupational opportunities. *Canadian Journal of Occupational Therapy, 84*(1), 47–57. https://doi.org/10.1177/0008417416654501

Hammell, K. R. W. (2020). Action on the social determinants of health: Advancing occupational equity and occupational rights. *Cadernos Brasileiros de Terapia Ocupacional, 28*(1), 378–400. https://doi.org/10.4322/2526-8910.ctoARF2052

Hammell, K. W. (2008). Reflections on … well-being and occupational rights. *Canadian Journal of Occupational Therapy, 75*(1), 61–64. https://doi.org/10.2182/cjot.07.007

Hammell, K. W. (2021). Social and structural determinants of health: Exploring occupational therapy's structural (in)competence. *Canadian Journal of Occupational Therapy, 88*(4), 365–374. https://doi.org/10.1177/00084174211046797

Hass, L. (2008). *Merleau-Ponty's philosophy: Studies in continental thought.* Indiana University Press.

Hocking, C., & Kroksmark, U. (2013). Sustainable occupational responses to climate change through lifestyle choices. *Scandinavian Journal of Occupational Therapy, 20*(2), 111–117. https://doi.org/10.3109/11038128.2012.725183

Hocking, C., & Townsend, E. (2015). Driving social change: Occupational therapists' contributions to occupational justice. *World Federation of Occupational Therapists Bulletin, 71*(2), 68–71. https://doi.org/10.1179/2056607715Y.0000000002

Holt-Lunstad, J., Smith, T. B., Baker, M., Harris, T., & Stephenson, D. (2015). Loneliness and social isolation as risk factors for mortality: A meta-analytic review. *Perspectives on Psychological Science, 10*(2), 227–237. https://doi.org/10.1177/1745691614568352

Joshanloo, M. (2014). Eastern conceptualizations of happiness: Fundamental differences with western views. *Journal of Happiness Studies: An Interdisciplinary Forum on Subjective Well-Being, 15*(2), 475–493. https://doi.org/10.1007/s10902-013-9431-1

Kantartzis, S., & Molineux, M. (2011). The influence of western society's construction of a healthy daily life on the conceptualisation of occupation. *Journal of Occupational Science, 18*(1), 62–80. https://doi.org/10.1080/14427591.2011.566917

Khan, S. A., Kanji, Z., Davis, J. A., & Stewart, K. E. (2021). Exploring occupational transitions of Syrian refugee youth to Canada. *Journal of Occupational Science,* 1–18. https://doi.org/10.1080/14427591.2021.1975557

Kiepek, N. C., Beagan, B., Rudman, D. L., & Phelan, S. (2019). Silences around occupations framed as unhealthy, illegal, and deviant. *Journal of Occupational Science, 26*(3), 341–353. https://doi.org/10.1080/14427591.2018.1499123

Kinsella, E. A., & Whiteford, G. E. (2009). Knowledge generation and utilisation in occupational therapy: Towards epistemic reflexivity. *Australian Occupational Therapy Journal, 56*(4), 249–258. https://doi.org/10.1111/j.1440-1630.2007.00726.x

Krug, E. G., Mercy, J. A., Dahlberg, L. L., & Zwi, A. B. (2002). The world report on violence and health. *The Lancet, 360*(9339), 1083–1088. https://doi.org/10.1016/S0140-6736(02)11133-0

Laliberte Rudman, D. (2010). Occupational terminology. *Journal of Occupational Science, 17*(1), 55–59. https://doi.org/10.1080/14427591.2010.9686673

Laliberte Rudman, D. (2014). Embracing and enacting an 'occupational imagination': Occupational science as transformative. *Journal of Occupational Science, 21*(4), 373–388. https://doi.org/10.1080/14427591.2014.888970

Laliberte Rudman, D., Pollard, N., Craig, C., Kantartzis, S., Piškur, B., Algado Simó, S., van Bruggen, H., & Schiller, S. (2019). Contributing to social transformation through occupation: Experiences from a think tank. *Journal of Occupational Science, 26*(2), 316–322. https://doi.org/10.1080/14427591.2018.1538898

Lavalley, R., & Johnson, K. R. (2020). Occupation, injustice, and anti-Black racism in the United States of America. *Journal of Occupational Science,* 1–13. https://doi.org/10.1080/14427591.2020.1810111

Lin, C.-C. (2014). Storytelling as academic discourse: Bridging the cultural-linguistic divide in the era of the common core. *Journal of Basic Writing, 33*(1), 52–73. https://doi.org/10.37514/JBW-J.2014.33.1.04

Lopes, R., Malfitano, A. P. S., Silva, C., & de Oliveira Borba, P. (2021). Resources and technologies in social occupational therapy: Actions with poor urban youth. In R. Lopes & A. P. S. Malfitano (Eds.), *Social occupational therapy: Theoretical and practical designs* (pp. 169–176). Elsevier.

Malfitano, A. P. S. (2021). Social context and social action: Generalizations and specificities in occupational therapy. In R. Lopes & A. P. S. Malfitano (Eds.), *Social occupational therapy: Theoretical and practical designs* (pp. 48–56). Elsevier.

Malfitano, A. P. S., de Souza, R. G. d. M., Townsend, E. A., & Lopes, R. E. (2019). Do occupational justice concepts inform occupational therapists' practice? A scoping review. *Canadian Journal of Occupational Therapy, 86*(4), 299–312. https://doi.org/10.1177/0008417419833409

Malfitano, A. P. S., & Lopes, R. E. (2018). Social occupational therapy: Committing to social change. *New Zealand Journal of Occupational Therapy, 65*(1), 20–26. https://link.gale.com/apps/doc/A619090804/HRCA?u=anon~327d5aa&sid=googleScholar&xid=9c61bb8d

Malfitano, A. P. S., Lopes, R. E., Magalhães, L., & Townsend, E. A. (2014). Social occupational therapy: Conversations about a Brazilian experience. *Canadian Journal of Occupational Therapy, 81*(5), 298–307. https://doi.org/10.1177/0008417414536712

Marom, L. (2019). Under the cloak of professionalism: Covert racism in teacher education. *Race Ethnicity and Education, 22*(3), 319–337. https://doi.org/10.1080/13613324.2018.1468748

Merleau-Ponty, M. (1945/2012). *The phenomenology of perception.* Routledge.

Mezzina, R., Davidson, L., Borg, M., Marin, I., Topor, A., & Sells, D. (2006). The social nature of recovery: Discussion and implications for practice. *American Journal of Psychiatric Rehabilitation, 9*(1), 63–80. https://doi.org/10.1080/15487760500339436

Morgan, C., Burns, T., Fitzpatrick, R., Pinfold, V., & Priebe, S. (2007). Social exclusion and mental health: Conceptual and methodological review. *British Journal of Psychiatry, 191*(6), 477–483. https://doi.org/10.1192/bjp.bp.106.034942

Mugumbate, J. R., & Chereni, A. (2020). Now, the theory of Ubuntu has its space in social work. *African Journal of Social Work, 10*(1), 5–15. https://www.ajol.info/index.php/ajsw/article/view/195112

National Institute on Aging. (2021). *Understanding loneliness and social isolation.* Author.

Nilsson, I., & Townsend, E. (2010) Occupational justice—Bridging theory and practice. *Scandinavian Journal of Occupational Therapy, 17*(1), 57–63. https://doi.org/10.3109/11038120903287182

Nussbaum, M. (2000). *Women and human development.* Cambridge University Press.

Nussbaum, M. (2011). *Creating capabilities: The human development approach.* Harvard University Press.

Pereira, R. B. (2017). Towards inclusive occupational therapy: Introducing the CORE approach for inclusive and occupation-focused practice. *Australian Occupational Therapy Journal, 64*(6), 429–435. https://doi.org/10.1111/1440-1630.12394

Pereira, R. B., & Whiteford, G. (2018). Advancing understandings of inclusion and participation through situated research. In N. Pollard, H. van Bruggen, & S. Kantartzis (Eds.), *Occupation-based social inclusion* (pp. 129–145). Whiting & Birch.

Pereira, R. B., Whiteford, G., Hyett, N., Weekes, G., Di Tommaso, A., & Naismith, J. (2020). Capabilities, Opportunities, Resources and Environments (CORE): Using the CORE approach for inclusive, occupation-centred practice. *Australian Occupational Therapy Journal, 67*(2), 162–171. https://doi.org/10.1111/1440-1630.12642

Pflug, J. (2009). Folk theories of happiness: A cross-cultural comparison of conceptions of happiness in Germany and South Africa. *Social Indicators Research, 92*(3), 551–563. https://doi.org/10.1007/s11205-008-9306-8

Pollard, N., Sakellariou, D., & Kronenburg, F. (2008). *A political practice of occupational therapy.* Churchill Livingstone Elsevier.

Pressman, S. D., Matthews, K. A., Cohen, S., Martire, L. M., Scheier, M., Baum, A., & Schulz, R. (2009). Association of enjoyable leisure activities with psychological and physical well-being. *Psychosomatic Medicine, 71*(7), 725–732. https://doi.org/10.1097/PSY.0b013e3181ad7978

Reese, L. (2012). Storytelling in Mexican homes: Connections between oral and literacy practices. *Bilingual Research Journal, 35*(3), 277–293. https://doi.org/10.1080/15235882.2012.734006

Richards, L., & Galvaan, R. (2018). Developing a socially transformative focus in occupational therapy: Insights from South African practice. *South African Journal of Occupational Therapy, 48*(1), 3–8. http://www.scielo.org.za/scielo.php?script=sci_abstract&pid=S2310-38332018000100002&lng=en&nrm=iso&tlng=en

Robeyns, I. (2005). The capability approach: A theoretical survey. *Journal of Human Development, 6*(1), 93–117. https://doi.org/10.1080/146498805200034266

Rudman, D. L. (2013). Enacting the critical potential of occupational science: Problematizing the 'individualizing of occupation'. *Journal of Occupational Science, 20*(4), 298–313. https://doi.org/10.1080/14427591.2013.803434

Rudman, D. L. (2021). Mobilizing occupation for social transformation: Radical resistance, disruption, and re-configuration. *Canadian Journal of Occupational Therapy, 88*(2), 96–107. https://doi.org/10.1177/0008417421020836

Sakellariou, D., & Pollard, N. (2013). A commentary on the social responsibility of occupational therapy education. *Journal of Further and Higher Education, 37*(3), 416–430. https://doi.org/10.1080/0309877X.2011.645459

Salzer, M. (2006). *Psychiatric rehabilitation skills in practice: A CPRP preparation and skills workbook.* Psychiatric Rehabilitation Association.

Sen, A. (1999). *Development as freedom.* Oxford University Press. http://www.amazon.com/Development-as-Freedom-Amartya-Sen/dp/0385720270/ref=sr_1_1?s=books&ie=UTF8&qid=1310743622&sr=1-1

Sen, A. (2009). *The idea of justice.* Belknap Press of Harvard University Press.

Thibeault, R. (2013). Occupational justice's intents and impacts: From personal choices to community consequences. In M. P. Cutchin & V. Dickie (Eds.), *Transactional perspectives on occupation* (pp. 245–256). Wiley.

Townsend, E. (1997). Occupation: Potential for personal and social transformation. *Journal of Occupational Science, 4*(1), 18–26. https://doi.org/10.1080/14427591.1997.9686417

Townsend, E., & Whiteford, G. (2005). A participatory occupational justice framework: Population-based processes of practice. In F. Kronenburg, S. Algado Simó, & N. Pollard (Eds.), *Occupational therapy without borders: Learning from the spirit of survivors* (pp. 110–126). Elsevier.

Trimboli, C., Rivas-Quarneti, N., Blankvoort, N., Roosen, I., Simó Algado, S., & Whiteford, G. (2019). The current and future contribution of occupational therapy and occupational science to transforming the situation of forced migrants: Critical perspectives from a think tank. *Journal of Occupational Science, 26*(2), 323–328. https://doi.org/10.1080/14427591.2019.1604408

Ung, Y., Sarah, T. S., Drolet, M.-J., Simó Algado, S., & Soubeyran, M. (2020). Building occupational therapy practice ecological based occupations and ecosystem sustainability: Exploring the concept of eco-occupation to support intergenerational occupational justice. *World Federation of Occupational Therapists Bulletin, 76*(1), 15–21. https://doi.org/10.1080/14473828.2020.1727095

Venkatapuram, S. (2011). *Health justice: An argument from the capabilities approach.* Polity Press.

Wasmuth, S., Leonhardt, B., Pritchard, K., Li, C.-Y., DeRolf, A., & Mahaffey, L. (2021). Supporting occupational justice for transgender and gender-nonconforming people through narrative-informed theater: A mixed-methods feasibility study. *American Journal of Occupational Therapy, 75*(4), 7504180080. https://doi.org/10.5014/ajot.2021.045161

Wasmuth, S. L., Pritchard, K., Milton, C., & Smith, E. (2020). A mixed-method analysis of community-engaged theatre illuminates Black women's experiences of racism and addresses healthcare inequities by targeting provider bias. *Inquiry, 57*, 1–10. https://doi.org/10.1177/0046958020976255

Weiss, G. (2015). The normal, the natural, and the normative: A Merleau-Pontian legacy to feminist theory, critical race theory, and disability studies. *Continental Philosophy Review, 48*(1), 77–93. https://doi.org/10.1007/s11007-014-9316-y

Whiteford, G., Jones, K., Rahal, C., & Suleman, A. (2018). The Participatory Occupational Justice Framework as a tool for change: Three contrasting case narratives. *Journal of Occupational Science, 25*(4), 497–508. https://doi.org/10.1080/14427591.2018.1504607

Whiteford, G., Jones, K., Weekes, G., Ndlovu, N., Long, C., Perkes, D., & Brindle, S. (2020). Combatting occupational deprivation and advancing occupational justice in institutional settings: Using a practice-based enquiry approach for service transformation. *British Journal of Occupational Therapy, 83*(1), 52–61. https://doi.org/10.1177/0308022619865223

Whiteford, G., Parnell, T., Ramsden, L., Nott, M., & Vine-Daher, S. (2021). Understanding and advancing occupational justice and social inclusion. In P. Liamputtong (Ed.), *Handbook of social inclusion: Research and practices in health and social sciences* (pp. 1–30). Springer International Publishing. https://doi.org/10.1007/978-3-030-48277-0_10-1

Wicks, A., & Jamieson, M. (2014). New ways for occupational scientists to tackle "wicked problems" impacting population health. *Journal of Occupational Science, 21*(1), 81–85. https://doi.org/10.1080/14427591.2014.878208

Wilcock, A. A. (1998). *An occupational perspective of health.* SLACK.

Wilcock, A. A., & Townsend, E. (2000). Occupational terminology interactive dialogue. *Journal of Occupational Science, 7*(2), 84–86. https://doi.org/10.1080/14427591.2000.9686470

Wilding, C., Curtin, M., & Whiteford, G. (2012). Enhancing occupational therapists' confidence and professional development through a community of practice scholars. *Australian Occupational Therapy Journal, 59*(4), 312–318. https://doi.org/10.1111/j.1440-1630.2012.01031.x

Williams, K. D., & Nida, S. A. (2011). Ostracism: Consequences and coping. *Current Directions in Psychological Science, 20*(2), 71–75. https://doi.org/10.1177/0963721411402480

World Federation of Occupational Therapists. (2018). *Sustainability matters: Guiding principles for sustainability in occupational therapy practice, education and scholarship.* https://www.wfot.org/resources/wfot-sustainability-guiding-principles

World Federation of Occupational Therapists. (2019). *Position statement occupational therapy and human rights.* https://www.wfot.org/resources/occupational-therapy-and-human-rights

World Health Organization. (2001a). *International classification of functioning, disability, and health: ICF.* https://search.library.wisc.edu/catalog/999977181002121

World Health Organization. (2021b, July 29). *Social isolation and loneliness among older people: Advocacy brief.* https://www.who.int/publications/i/item/9789240030749

Young, I. M. (1980). Throwing like a girl: A phenomenology of feminine body comportment motility and spatiality. *Human Studies, 3*(1), 137–156. https://doi.org/10.1007/BF02331805

Young, I. M. (1990). *Justice and the politics of difference.* Princeton University Press.

Occupational Consciousness

Elelwani Ramugondo

LEARNING OBJECTIVES

After reading this chapter, you will be able to:

1. Describe the origin and key elements of the term *occupational consciousness*.
2. Describe and explain the philosophical foundations of occupational consciousness as a theoretical construct.
3. Analyze and explain how human occupation, health, and well-being have a political dimension.
4. Critique occupational therapy practice, scholarship, or research in terms of how these may perpetuate or disrupt dominant interests.

Introduction

The construct **occupational consciousness** has been defined as an ongoing awareness about the dynamics of hegemony, recognizing that dominant practices are sustained through what people do every day, with implications for both personal and collective health (Ramugondo, 2012, 2015). This chapter aims to provide background to the origin of the term, describing its key elements, offering its philosophical foundations, and reflecting on its implications for occupational therapy (OT) practice, scholarship, and research. The terms "concept" and "construct" are used interchangeably, recognizing that both are abstractions that form key building blocks to theorizing as a distinct scholarly practice, and theory as a product thereof (Neuman, 2011; Swedberg, 2012).

Construct Genesis

Occupational consciousness emerged as an occupational science construct out of a research project that I undertook toward my doctoral qualification. The project was aimed at describing and explaining the evolution of play across three generations within one Venda family. Bordering with Zimbabwe, Venda is an area located in the northern part of South Africa and is mostly rural. I was interested in exploring shifts and continuities in children's play in this region, investigating factors that explain why certain features persist, whereas others disappear. My interest in the evolution of play within African Black families grew after I detected a growing concern among older people in my community that children no longer played in ways that were familiar, and that at times, it seemed they did not play at all. These concerns were confirmed during my travels throughout each of the eight provinces of South Africa, in conversation with retired school teachers, traditional leaders, and community organizers, before I formally embarked on the research.

The research itself followed a case study approach, with embedded ethnography, and was located in rural Vhembe District, Limpopo Province, South Africa. The case study approach allowed for one Venda family to be bounded as a case, straddling early 20th to early 21st centuries South Africa, with each generation situated within its own historical, political, economic, and sociocultural contexts. Relying on oral storytelling from parents and the maternal grandmother, as well as accounts gleaned from early Christian missionary ethnographic texts, I was able to gain a reasonable picture of how children's play during the first and second generations looked. Ethnographic research tools were used to explore third generation's everyday culture in the here and now, allowing me to pay specific attention to how this generation played. Participant observation was the main data collection method, with me spending a month, including weekends, with the family, arriving early each morning and departing only after the last child had gone to bed.

What emerged as a key theme for the case study was the "complexification of the play rhetoric" (Ramugondo, 2012), signaling how, with the passing of time, this Venda family was rendered unable to sustain a coherent narrative about its children's play. On the one hand, the first and second generations could concur on play being one way of forming and asserting one's identity as part of family, community, and traditional society. On the other hand, the third generation, mainly through television, encountered a rapidly globalizing world and had to forge new meanings of play, often agreeing that theirs was hardly "real" play. Interestingly, although adults in the family were concerned about exogenous factors influencing their children's play, they omitted the role of the television in this, even as the television was the first thing to go on in the morning and the last device to be switched off at night.

Like in most families, the television was purchased by adults, prioritized over many other household items. Apart from being the first thing on and the last device off, the prominence of the television within the home was also evident in its location; a prime and central spot in the lounge, where family members spend most of their time together. The lounge was also where the family took their main meal of the day, supper. Supper often coincided with one of the family's favorite television shows: a local South African soapie "Generations." Family conversation often revolved around what was unfolding on the screen. On the days that mom arrived from work to find one of the other American soapies ("Days of Our Lives" or "The Bold and the Beautiful") already on, almost without fail, she would pose the question as she placed her bags down, "What did I miss?" On school days, one of the children, the youngest son at age 9, would first watch his favorite television show before getting ready for school. It is the omission of the television in adults' explanation of what influenced children's play, despite its prominence in the home, which inspired the coining of occupational consciousness as an occupational science and OT term.

Concept Elements

Reflected in the construct "occupational consciousness" are the key words "occupation" and "consciousness." The definition of the construct, however, invokes further terms "hegemony" and "health." Hegemony or "cultural hegemony" is a term often associated with Antonio Gramsci, an Italian Marxist intellectual and politician. It describes how the ruling capitalist elite and the state use institutions such as schools, universities, churches, the media, and popular culture to maintain power in society (Gramsci, 1975). It was Gramsci's observation that based on their ability to determine and organize society's economic activity, the ruling class effectively governed with the tacit consent of the subordinate masses. In other words, the ruling elite can exercise hegemonic influence over the rest of society because they have worked out how the latter will allow them to do so if some of their interests are protected. Hegemony thus implicates not only how society is politically organized but also how economic and social aspects of life find expression in what people do every day.

Health is a common term in OT and encapsulates the profession's ultimate concern. Yet, it is not always immediately clear whether health is understood to mean the same thing across different authors and contexts. Often, health and "well-being" are used interchangeably, or one is understood to be key aspect of the other. Both these terms are elaborated on in a later section.

Although not conspicuous, another term that is inferred in the construct is "human." Within OT and occupational science literature, the "human," otherwise always implicated in occupations, is often taken as a given. In this chapter, the human is made salient to make visible the political dimension of what people do every day: occupations, which otherwise often appear mundane and even benign. "Human occupation," therefore, is another term elaborated on further.

Construct Genealogy

Constructs that are associated with academic disciplines or professions come about in a variety of ways. Some emerge from classical theory, as part of what Swedberg (2012) describes, as theorizing in the context of justification. This refers to constructs that are part of already accepted theory that is applicable in practice. Others come about from everyday observations, which are then validated through systematic research that allows for deep contemplation and reflection, often accompanying the examination and distillation of research findings (Neuman, 2011). This is a process that can be described as theorizing in the context of discovery (Swedberg, 2012). The latter process matches how occupational consciousness as a construct came about. As a researcher, I did not have a theory "a priori," which I sought to confirm through data from the research field. What I pursued as a case study about the evolution of children's play across three generations spanning the early 20th through to 21st centuries in a rural South African Venda family, ended up being a case for occupational consciousness.

In retrospect, it should not be surprising that a study conducted in South Africa, a settler-colony with strong remnants of both colonialism and apartheid, should reveal the politics of human occupation, even as the phenomenon of interest in the research seemed rather benign: children's play. Almost intuitively, ontologically, epistemologically, and axiologically, the study was couched within the critical emancipatory paradigm. This, recognizing family not only as a social institution but also one that is located at the margins of a rapidly changing world, would be at the mercy of unequal power relations exerted upon it through globalized market forces. The emergence of the construct, occupational consciousness, in post-1994 South Africa, after apartheid had supposedly fallen, thus reflecting "the country's ongoing struggle with negotiating long-standing dynamics of power that were laid down during colonialism, and maintained under black majority rule" (Ramugondo, 2015, p. 488).

A key component to the construct, consciousness, is firmly rooted within liberation philosophy, with Stephen (Steve) Bantu Biko, Enrique Dussel, and Frantz Fanon as its key proponents.

The Proponents

Steve Biko is a prominent name in South Africa's liberation struggle, with his writings often associated with Black theology and the Black Consciousness Movement (BCM). Although Biko was not the only leader of BCM, he remains its most recognizable figure (Figure 11.1; South African History Online, 2021). Biko's prominence as a figure in South Africa's liberation struggle and within BCM is probably as a consequence of his brutal murder at the hands of the South African apartheid state security police, at the age of 30. He is also remembered for his sharp mind and ability to articulate his thoughts in writing, notably through his regular columns, under the pseudonym "Frank Talk," in the then-banned South African Student Organization's (SASO) newsletter (AZAPO, 1984). Following his incarceration in 1977, Biko was tortured by the police over a period of 22 hours. During this period, he was beaten, with several blows directed to the head, leading to a brain hemorrhage,

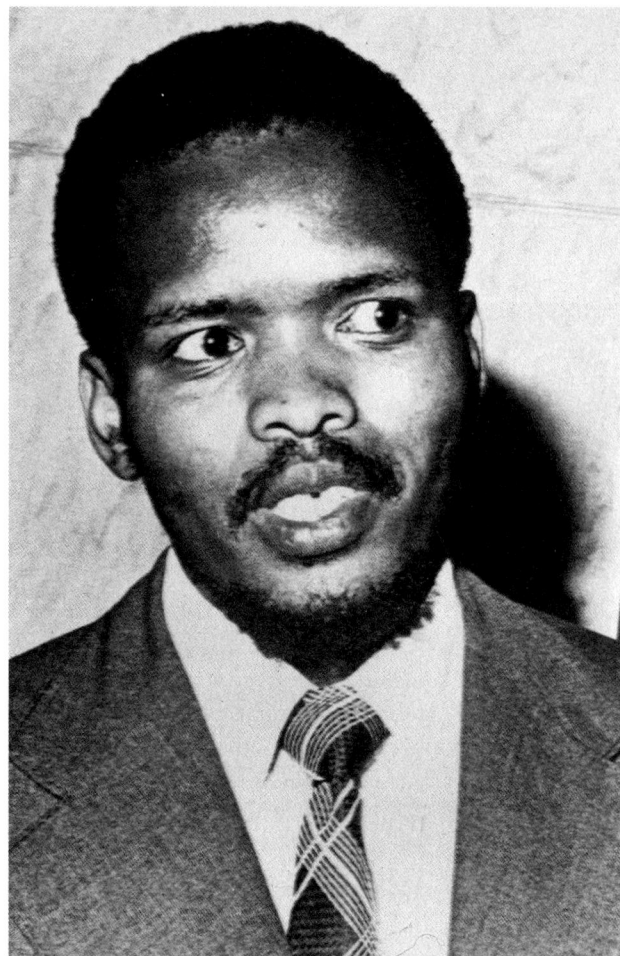

FIGURE 11.1 **Steve Bantu Biko.**

which, 8 years later, during an inquest, was found to be the leading cause of his death (South African History Online, 2019).

By the time they killed him, the apartheid government had pushed Biko to live in relative obscurity and enforced silence. He faced banning orders, restricting him to a small town, a long distance away from the metropolitan areas, and prohibiting him from making public utterances to be quoted and to function fully as a political person (Woods, 1978). His brutal murder served only to propel the global reach of his name and legacy.

Enrique Dussel is a historian, philosopher, and theologian who is regarded as one of the fathers of liberation philosophy (Burton & Osorio, 2011; Dussel, 2011; Mahvish, 2013). Born in Argentina, he was exiled to Mexico following targeted state violence, including death threats, dismissal from his university position, and the bombing of his home as part of events leading to the Argentinian military dictatorship of 1976 to 1983 (Burton & Osorio, 2011).

Frantz Fanon (Figure 11.2) was born in Martinique, during the time when the island was under the French

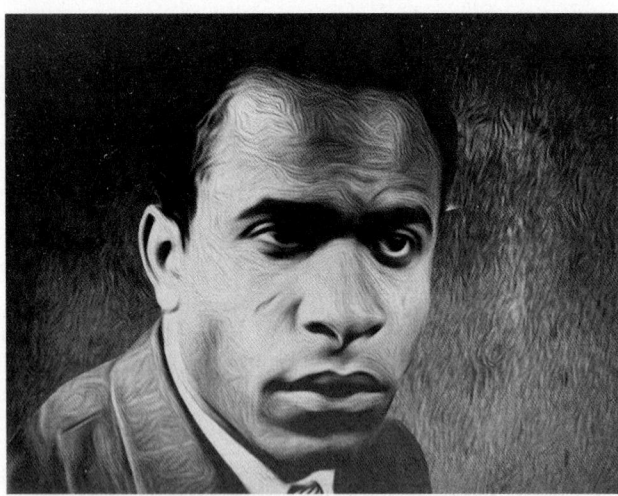

FIGURE 11.2 **Franz Fanon.**

colonial rule. Qualified as a psychiatrist, Fanon is well known for his two seminal works: *Black Skin, White Masks* (1967) and *The Wretched of the Earth* (1963). Fanon's participation in the Algerian revolutionary struggle makes him one of very few known theorist-philosophers to have translated his theorizations of blackness into pragmatic anticolonial struggle.

A Philosophy of Liberation

The philosophy of *liberation* refers to the articulation of what it means to be oppressed from the viewpoint of alterity, or the oppressed "other," and a critique of dominant explanations and accepted "truths" about the status quo (Dussel, 2011). In their writing, both Fanon and Biko also explain how oppressive systems are reinforced by both the oppressed and the oppressors. Fanon (1967), in describing internalized oppression and the "dependency complex" in *Black Skin, White Masks*, demonstrates how the successful colonization of Africa, the continent as a whole, was dependent not solely on the might of Empire but also on the implicit consent of oppressed Africans.

In the *Wretched of the Earth*, he writes:

> When we consider the efforts made to carry out the cultural estrangement so characteristic of the colonial epoch, we realize that nothing has been left to chance and that the total result looked for by colonial domination was indeed to convince the natives that colonialism came to lighten their darkness. The effect consciously sought by colonialism was to drive into the native's heads the idea that if the settlers were to leave, they would at once fall back into barbarism, degradation and bestiality. (Fanon, 1963, p. 169)

Liberation philosophy is thus not only about explaining the colonial situation as is but also about transcending it. Both Fanon and Biko centered their philosophy of liberation on the notion of consciousness as an awakening at both individual and collective levels. Those familiar with

Paulo Freire's writing will recognize in Fanon and Biko the same commitment to conscientization as a necessary tool toward liberation. Critical for Fanon and Biko, however, was a deep interrogation of how anti-Black racism comes to define both the social world and the subjectivities of Black and White people. Both Fanon and Biko were spurred on in their work by a deep anger toward not only anti-Black systemic racism and the perpetual domination of Western-led civilization, but they also shared a passion for justice and equity.

Initial reflections on the philosophical foundation of "consciousness" as a liberatory term first located it within postcolonial perspectives. Postcolonial theory or post-colonialism is a body of work in social science and the humanities, which is often associated with Edward Said, Homi Bhabha, and Gayatri Spivak. Said's seminal book, *Orientalism*, which was published in 1978, is credited with having inaugurated postcolonial theory (Azim, 2008). This perspective is primarily concerned with explaining the political, sociocultural, and economic impact the European colonial expansion has had globally, starting in the 15th century and continuing throughout the 20th century. Postcolonial theory helps us account for the impoverishment and bleak trajectories of the former colonies, on the one hand, and the wealth accumulation associated with Europe, Britain, and North America, on the other. It helps to clarify how the Euro American global domination not only in both material terms but also in the knowledge marketplace arises out of colonial entanglements in the rest of the world.

In recent years, the "post" in postcolonial theory has been placed under intense scrutiny, with many decolonial scholars suggesting that the prefix implies that colonialism ended. These scholars, particularly from Latin America, have argued instead for a theoretical framework that explicitly acknowledges the lingering forms of colonial authority even after imperial administrators have formally withdrawn from the territories (Cusicanqui, 2012; Dussel, 2011; Grosfoguel, 2011; Lugones, 2006; Maldonado-Torres, 2007; Mignolo, 2011; Quijano & Michael, 2000; Wynter, 2003). This critique has led to a reframing of global anticolonial struggles, shifting thinking away from decolonization being understood merely as a political and historical event, to decolonizing or decoloniality being adopted as a political movement and collective effort that is inspired by everyday struggles against anti-Black racism and the subjugation of indigenous populations toward new ways of being, doing, and knowing that are not dependent on domination and oppression.

Consciousness, as a liberatory term, borrows its genealogy from both postcolonial theory and decoloniality, with these two theoretical frameworks or philosophical foundations having emerged out of everyday struggle against oppression in general, and Western-led civilization as perpetual domination.

Elaborating on Key Elements

In this section, the three key components that constitute occupational consciousness as a theoretical construct are expanded on: human occupation, consciousness, and health and well-being. This elaboration is aimed at explaining how to apply occupational consciousness in OT practice, scholarship, and research.

Human Occupation

Human occupation is at the core of what OT is all about. A concern with what people do every day and how this impacts their health is what makes OT a distinct health profession. Given that occupational therapists often work with people in hospital settings, what is often forgotten is that human occupation occurs where people live, love, and do their work, and for that reason, it is best understood in context. Making explicit mention of the human in occupation helps us appreciate the extent to which occupation bears political relevance, an aspect that may otherwise remain obscure.

Human occupation as a concept has been defined in various ways in both OT and occupational science texts. The various definitions that exist not only signify the complexity of human occupation (Christiansen et al., 1995; Curtin et al., 2010; Hocking, 2000; Pollard & Sakellariou, 2012; Whiteford & Hocking, 2012; Wilcock, 2006) but also demonstrate that various authors may wish to emphasize some aspects and not others. Hammell (2009, 2011), Hocking (2009), Iwama (2005), and Kronenberg, Pollard, and Sakellariou (2011) have also cautioned that reflected in most of these definitions are perspectives of a minority of the global population. In recent times, however, there has been a concerted effort from OT and occupational science scholars to draw from a diversity of cultural perspectives, including ontologies and epistemologies of the South (Guajardo et al., 2015; Kronenberg, Pollard, & Ramugondo, 2011), to inform an expanded understanding of human occupation.

Reviewing the various definitions that exist, there are four themes that emerge that help deepen our understanding of human occupation as it relates to occupational consciousness.

Human Occupation as Both Ordinary and Extraordinary

The first theme highlights the fact that human occupation refers to both ordinary and extraordinary things that people do every day. Although it is important to point to the mundane aspects of human occupation, which Christiansen et al. (1995) refer to as the "the ordinary and familiar things that people do every day" (p. 1015), it is equally crucial to recognize that this presents an incomplete picture. Human occupations, as pointed out by Hocking (2003) and Watson (2004), can also be extraordinary. Here one can think about human occupations of motherhood, such as childbirth, or profound human inventions, such as finding a cure for a rare health condition.

Humans as Subjects Who Are Occupied

The second theme is around the ubiquitous nature of human occupation. Doing is an all-pervading aspect of human existence. It is as unavoidable as breathing, with some things done out of choice and many others executed through sheer necessity. Through human occupation, our resources of time, energy, and personal capacities are constantly engaged. In this way, it can be said that effectively, instead of us occupying the world as humans, we are occupied (Ramugondo & Kronenberg, 2015). This understanding of human occupation makes explicit the idea that as human beings who do in the world, we simultaneously become products of our actions in that world. This understanding is captured in Guajardo's summation that essentially, as human beings, "we are occupation" (Guajardo et al., 2015). In other words, instead of treating occupation as an object of study, it is ontologically repositioned as:

> People; relationships; subjects who think, act, decide; occupation is not separate from the subject; occupation is neither a mediating element to the environment, nor a method of intervention. To successfully separate occupation from people would mean that we have reified, naturalized and dehumanised subjects [and] our practices would as a result negatively affect the wellbeing of people. (Guajardo et al., 2015, p. 8)

Taking Guajardo's thinking further, Kronenberg has conceptualized human occupation as "*that (original emphasis) which occupies contextually embedded and embodied resources available to humans*" (Kronenberg et al., 2015, p. 25). Evident here is that we need to think of resources available to human beings as they engage in occupations as not only residing within them as individuals but also as embedded in context. This understanding of human occupation, inspired by thinking from the Global South, extends an understanding of humans as "subjects who occupy" to humans as "subjects who are occupied" and "objects of occupation" (dehumanized through oppressive forces) (Kronenberg, 2018, 2021).

Human Occupation and Meaning

The third theme revolves around meaning and meaninglessness. Meaning is widely associated with human occupation (Hagedorn, 2001; Hasselkuss, 2002; Nelson, 1988; Stein & Roose, 2000; Townsend & Polatajko, 2007). What is often foregrounded in OT literature is positive meaning, although there is growing appreciation that human occupation may also be associated with negative meaning (Galvaan, 2012; Russell, 2008). Kronenberg and Pollard (2006) have also pointed out that "the decision of when occupation is dignified and meaningful is not only culturally informed, but also likely to be politically negotiated" (p. 619).

Bridging the Individual-Collective Dichotomy

The fourth and last theme points to human occupation as both an individual and collective phenomenon. The dominant individualistic view of human occupation persists mainly because occupational therapists work predominantly with individuals as patients or clients in hospital settings. When situated and understood in context, it becomes immediately clear that human occupation, in fact, is hardly ever individual. Even solitary occupations such as brushing teeth or knitting always implicate others in how one gets to have access to resources that make such activities possible in the first place. Occupational therapists who interact with service users along the rehabilitation continuum, including access to where these individuals ordinarily live, often have an opportunity to appreciate the collective nature of human occupation. Beyond what occupational therapists do in their professional work, human occupation continues to be what it needs to be in the real world. The collective nature of human occupation has seen growing appreciation in occupational science literature in recent decades (Cutchin et al., 2008; Dickie et al., 2006; Fogelberg & Frauwirth, 2010; Hocking, 2000; Kuo, 2011; Ramugondo & Kronenberg, 2015). Critical in Ramugondo and Kronenberg's (2015) conceptualization of collective occupation was invoking the African notion of *ubuntu* in order to side-step the usual individual-collective dichotomy.

Ubuntu is an African philosophy centered on what it means to be human. It describes an ontic orientation within an interactive ethic to being human: a process through which one is dependent on others and yet responsible for them if both must realize their full humanity. In this way, *ubuntu* must be understood as a process of becoming more human (Cornell & Van Marle, 2005) or less so. Through *ubuntu* as an ethical and moral lens, society is judged according to how well those with means look after those with less, and individuals are afforded opportunities to reach their full potential. *Ubuntu* can be a useful lens through which groups, communities, and organizations can look at themselves and individuals within can ask themselves, "to what end am I, and are we occupied?"

Ramugondo and Kronenberg (2015) thus define collective occupations as those "that are engaged in by individuals, groups, communities and/or societies in everyday contexts" that "may reflect an intention towards social cohesion or dysfunction, and/or advancement of or aversion to a common good" (p. 10). They further assert that "these collective occupations may have consequences that benefit some populations and not others" (p. 10).

Consciousness

In the everyday English language, consciousness means to be aware of and responsiveness to one's surrounding environment. Consciousness, however, has also been adopted as a sociologic concept, and as has been indicated earlier, it is a term associated with liberation philosophy. In sociologic terms, consciousness has been understood in association with social inequity and systems of stratification; these two concepts themselves grounded on Marxian and Weberian thought and often invoked with reference to class and status. In this vein, Laumann and Senter (1976) define *class and status consciousness* as "the subjective awareness of class or status location and the implications of such awareness for social action" (p. 1307). Extending this understanding, Reay (2005) pointed to individuals' emotional and psychic response to social stratification, with Nash (2008) highlighting how social stratification creates unequal groups, with consequences to how these groups relate to each other in everyday life. Biko and Fanon's work gives us a glimpse of such consequences, from the perspective of the oppressed, with specific focus on racialized Black identities.

Biko on Consciousness

Although Biko is believed to have been heavily influenced by Fanon in his work (Ahluwalia & Zegeye, 2001; Gibson, 2008; Hook, 2004), it is fitting that his articulations on consciousness are presented as a distinct body of work. In writing about consciousness in his seminal work, *I write what I like*, Biko sought to clarify what Black consciousness means in ways that can be understood to be responding to three pertinent questions: What is consciousness? Who are the conscious? What does consciousness require? Answers to each of these questions follow in the subsequent sections.

What Is Consciousness?

First and foremost, Biko described consciousness as a mental attitude and a commitment to fight against all forces that seek to use racialized identity as a stamp that marks out subservience. This definition of consciousness is consistent with one of the most famous quotes Biko is known for: "The most potent weapon in the hands of the oppressor is the mind of the oppressed" (Biko, 1978, pp. 101–102). A liberation of the mind was thus central in how Biko understood consciousness. Biko's legacy is celebrated through a rich iconography that has become global. Figure 11.3 depicts fragments of this iconography.

Biko embodied the liberation of the mind by articulating his thoughts regarding political struggle with clarity and force, not only in writing but also in speech whenever he

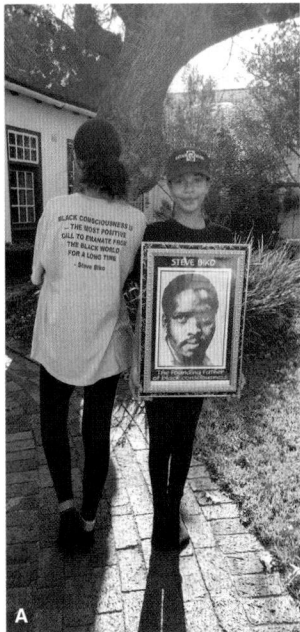 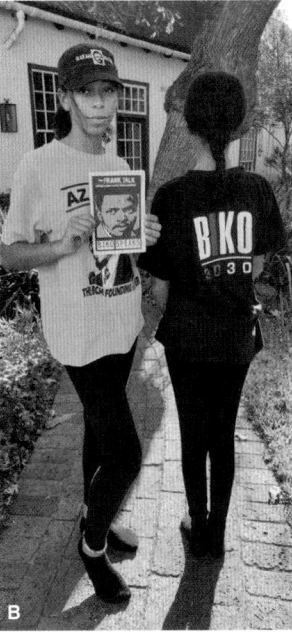

FIGURE 11.3 Present-day depictions of Biko's words: a T-shirt with Biko's image and one of many quotes, a framed portrait, and a cap with his image. The newsletter *Frank Talk* carries many of Biko's speeches.

was afforded an audience. This is also when confronting the apartheid regime through the courts. One example of this is when Biko acted as a defense witness at the 1975-1976 trial involving a charge of terrorism against his Black Power Convention (BPC) colleagues. In this example, it is evident that while choosing his words carefully so as not to incriminate his colleagues, Biko did not waste the opportunity to at once outwit his opponents but also communicate a powerful message, appealing for equity and justice toward a true humanity for all:

Attwell [senior prosecution lawyer for the apartheid state]: *Can you point to any document of SASO or BPC which specifically and unambiguously rejects violence?*

Biko: *You would have to give me a whole lot of documents to look through.*

Attwell: *It is not in the BPC constitution, is it, a rejection of violence?*

Biko: *No, it is not there. Nor is it anywhere in the constitution of the Nationalist Party* (The ruling governing party during apartheid South Africa).

(Woods, 1978, p. 231)

And,

Attwell: *Now, you know the accused are charged with causing or encouraging or furthering these feelings of hostility?*

Biko: *I understand that it is the charge.*

Attwell: *And you consider there is a difference between causing something, encouraging something, or furthering something?*

Biko: *Oh well, I am sure there is a difference because the actual words have different meanings. I think again that you have a wrong interpretation of Black solidarity. We are not envisaging getting a committed membership which constitutes almost what you might call a standing army. No, we are looking forward to getting a majority of Black people behind us, behind what we say, in the same way that the Nationalist Party has a majority of White people behind them at this moment. They do not constitute a homogeneous mass that can be called to action any day. There are wide differences even among them, but at least there is a central feeling. They constitute what you call die volk [the people] and the [Afrikaner] Nationalist Party, the Broederbond, these are their spokesmen. You cannot call them tomorrow to action because they are scattered throughout the country, but they have got an identity and they have got a vanguard in the form of the Nationalist Party, the Broederbond and all the other Afrikaner cultural organizations which speak for them. Now the same thing applies to Black people. We are trying to create a situation where BPC speaks for the people, gives them a home, gives them dignity, so that they can feel they are human once more, which is not what they are feeling now.*

Attwell: *You want to involve all the Blacks, do you not?*

Biko: *Not necessarily all. I am sure not all the Afrikaners are in the Nationalist Party.*

Attwell: *All right, how many Blacks are in South Africa?*

Biko: *More than twenty million.*

Attwell: *You see there are references in the documents to 30 million, about a third higher than you estimate?*

Biko: *Okay.*

Attwell: *Do you see any significance in this inflated figure?*

Biko: *No, I think the only significant thing about it is BPC's knowledge from experience that a lot of Black people are in fact not registered. For instance in Soweto, the current official figure is about 800,000. But there are about one and a half million in Soweto, because for every, say, six people who are registered, there are two who are not registered or something like that. Those figures come from that kind of thinking. There is no other significance beyond that.*

(Woods, 1978, pp. 233–234)

It needs to be mentioned that Biko, being a native Xhosa speaker, mounted this defense in a court of law in the English language that was not his home language. He was also not formally trained as a lawyer.

Given that the mind was so central in how Biko analyzed and understood oppression, it is devastating that it is the very same mind that the oppressive apartheid regime targeted in causing his death. Incarcerating Biko was clearly not enough. The system, instead, was deliberate in seeking to destroy the very part of Biko's body through which he was to liberate himself and others like him. What the South African apartheid state probably did not anticipate was that by brutally murdering him, they inadvertently elevated Biko into an important figure of the liberation struggle, not only in South Africa, but beyond. His famous quote continues to inspire everyday struggles globally, to this day. The student-led protests under the #RhodesMustFall banner, which were initially sparked off at the University of Cape Town and had global ramifications, including campaigns toward the removal of the Cecil John Rhodes statue at Oriel College at the University of Oxford, were partly inspired by Biko's articulation of what Black consciousness means.

Who Are the Conscious?

Crucial to Biko's conceptualization of Black, consciousness was that identifying as Black was not a matter of skin pigmentation, but "a reflection of a mental attitude" (AZAPO, 1984, p. 3; Biko, 1978, p. 52). To be Black was, however, associated with struggle, in that this identity was reserved for those who were by law or tradition discriminated against politically, economically, and socially as a group in South African society. To consider oneself Black was to claim solidarity with those who were disenfranchised and to reject any aspiration for whiteness. Biko made a distinction between those who were conscious and those who shared the same pigmentation but was somehow unable to identify with the liberation struggle:

> From the above observations therefore, we can see that the term black is not necessarily all inclusive; i.e. the fact we are all <u>not white</u> [original emphasis] does not necessarily mean that we are <u>black</u> [original emphasis]. Non-whites do exist and will continue to exist for quite a long time. If one's aspiration is whiteness but one's pigmentation makes attainment of this impossible, then one is a non-white. (AZAPO, 1984, p. 3; Biko, 1978, p. 52)

Importantly, those who are conscious necessarily admit that they are oppressed. This acknowledgment of oppression as part of becoming conscious has also been stressed by Freire (1998) and Dussel (2011). Freire (1998) saw it as the first crucial step to self-liberation, whereas Dussel (2011) noted that it is in being positioned as "the 'Other' and her Exteriority that the new truth-claims spring forth and demand explanation" (p. 21).

Paradoxically, consciousness is enhanced when those who recognize their oppression are also able "to hold their heads high in defiance rather than willingly surrender their souls" (AZAPO, 1984, p. 3; Biko, 1978, p. 52). In this statement, it becomes evident that Biko's ideologic views on

blackness were heavily influenced by the Negritude movement, which was developed mainly by francophone intellectuals of African descent, notably the Nardal sisters (Church, 2013), the eldest of whom is Paulette (see Figure 11.4).

Negritude became prominent during the 1930s in the African diaspora and laid the foundation for the African American "Black is Beautiful" cultural movement in the 1960s (Christian, 2008; Edwards, 2003). The term "negritude" is a derivative of the French term *Negre*, which, similar to its English equivalent, carries derogatory undertones. Adopting this term in order to affirm blackness and to affirm a pan-Africanist agenda was to invert its meaning and purpose. To be conscious, therefore, involves adopting a counterhegemonic stance toward the denigration that is often associated with blackness.

What Does Consciousness Require?

For both Biko (1978) and Fanon (1963, 1967), consciousness emerges as a mental attitude, always in continuous appraisal of the oppressive system. Those who are conscious need to be constantly aware about how the system operates. First, to be conscious requires that one is aware that people are oppressed by the same system. Although the process toward a conscious awakening begins with an individual, it does not end there. There is, instead, an "interrelationship between the consciousness of the self and the emancipatory programme" (AZAPO, 1984, p. 3; Biko, 1978, p. 53). This understanding begins to explore what sociology had long avoided—a theoretical analysis and interrogation of the complex patterns of relations that emerge in an unequal society, as well as the powerful dynamics that reinforce them. Biko's (1978) observations begin to unmask the deliberateness of the scheme, noting that the fact that people "are oppressed to varying degrees is a deliberate design to stratify [them] not only socially but also in terms of aspirations" (p. 56; AZAPO, 1984, p. 4).

Both Biko (1978) and Fanon (1963, 1967) sought to expose the instrumental mode of division as central to the colonial project, observing that regions within the colonies were often differently marked for privilege across history. This observation is certainly true even in the historical

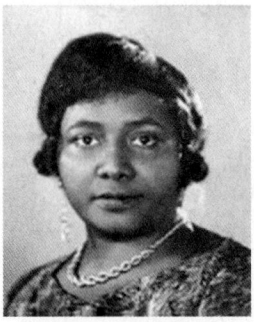

FIGURE 11.4 **Paulette Nardal (public domain, PD-US).**

events that ushered in the Rwandan genocide. Belgian colonial authorities, inspired by anthropometry, a branch of the Eugenics pseudoscience, introduced a hierarchized classification system that saw one side of the Rwandan people named *Tutsis* because of their facial traits that suggested Hamitic or Nilotic origin; were afforded privileges such as better schooling and wages, at the expense of those who were mostly descendants of the indigenous population (a pygmy people known as *Twa*); and were declared Hutus (Braeckman, 2021). This division and differential treatment cultivated resentment over time and resulted in one of the most horrific tragedies recorded on the African continent in recent years.

In apartheid South Africa, Biko (1978) observed how racialized identities were also used to stratify people in order to afford them different privileges and resources. People of lighter skin pigmentation, including those of Asian descent and others of mixed African and European ancestry, could ascend the social strata by successfully proving to the authorities that they were not Black. One of the methods to determine one's race is the infamous "pencil test," which involved a pencil being placed in one's hair (Thompsell, 2018). Failing the pencil test meant the pencil got stuck in the hair, proving that one was "Black African," or fell out with shaking, proving that one was "colored." Social stratification, however, did not begin and end at the point of racial classification but translated into people's aspirations. The education dark-skinned Black people received, dubbed Bantu education, was designed to limit their employment possibilities, mainly to cheap labor in the mines and White households as gardeners or cleaners, whereas those classified as "colored" or "Indian" could become professionals with relative ease (Shepherd, 1955). Stratified in this manner, the normative effect was that people in different social strata would view their positions as deserved. In Gramscian hegemonic terms, the governing apartheid regime had worked out how to gain relative consent from the subordinate masses. Those with greater possibilities to accumulate wealth were entrusted with the tools to preserve their relative privilege, whereas those with less resigned themselves to the limits prescribed for them. Profoundly, this scheme rendered differently oppressed people primed to participate in their own and each other's oppression. It was for this reason that Biko (1978) saw those who are conscious as carrying the responsibility not only to work out how the scheme works but also to seek to dismantle it.

Fanon on Consciousness

The most obvious similarity between Fanon and Biko's work is that both emphasize the role of the mind in achieving liberation. Critical in Fanon's writing is that informed by his psychoanalytic background, his analysis of consciousness seeps into the psyche, helping disentangle intersubjective relations between the Black and White world. Through racialized consciousness, Black subjectivity is dependent on White subjectivity, and vice versa. In *Black Skins, White Masks*, Fanon characterizes the colonized Blacks as having deeply ingrained within their souls an inferiority complex that arises out of the hyper-humanization of whiteness, partly cultivated through the elevation of European ways of being in the world (Fanon, 1967). For Fanon, the central task of conscientization toward liberation, therefore, is in exploring the possibilities of human existence that is no longer imprisoned, a product of a colonial psyche. Based on his observations as a Black person in Paris, as well as a Francophone-educated Black person on his return to Algeria, Fanon captures the profound alienation that results from colonialism.

In explaining the depth of psychic entanglement involving both the colonized and the colonizer, in *The Wretched of the Earth*, Fanon extends these intersubjective relations beyond the here and now, and invokes memory, and observes that:

> Colonialism is not satisfied merely with holding a people in its grip and emptying the native's brain of all form and content. By a kind of perverted logic, it turns to the past of the oppressed people, and distorts, disfigures and destroys it. This work of devaluing pre-colonial history takes on a dialectical significance today. (Fanon, 1963, p. 169)

Conscientization, therefore, by necessity in part, requires a reconstruction of history. Cognizant of how this attempt of going back in time to revive precolonial Africa, for instance, is certain to attract pity if not scorn, Fanon makes some comparison with how similar endeavors would be regarded if they concerned Europe and maintains:

> . . . but those who condemn this exaggerated passion are strangely apt to forget that their own psyche and their own selves are conveniently sheltered behind a French or German culture which has given full proof of its existence and which is uncontested. (Fanon, 1963, p. 168)

Political Education: A Necessity Toward Consciousness

Turning to African and Latin American states following the departure of colonial administrators, Fanon finds that the middle class and the political elite in these parts of the world, which he refers to as the "native bourgeoisie," often perpetuate colonialism. Failing to govern in ways that pay attention to new social relations that need to be understood and developed in the interest of the whole nation, he finds that instead they entrench social relations between unequal groups along the lines already laid down by colonialism. Nationalization, in this narrow sense, "has nothing to do with transforming the nation; it consists, prosaically, of being the transmission line between the nation and a capitalism, rampant though camouflaged, which today puts on the masque of neo-colonialism" (Fanon, 1963, p. 122).

For those who are keen to build anew in these former colonies, Fanon insists that the revolutionary struggle is paramount and emphasizes that it is through such a struggle that both a new consciousness and a new society are formed, based not only on "the disappearance of colonialism but also the disappearance of the colonised [person]" (1963, p. 197). Like Freire, Fanon also believed that political education was central to the forging of a new consciousness and that such political education should be focused on the entire population, as it is them that are integral to the process of transformation:

> Now, political education means opening their minds, awakening them, and allowing the birth of their intelligence; as Césaire said, it is 'to invent souls'. To educate the masses politically does not mean, cannot mean making a political speech. What it means is to try, relentlessly and passionately, to teach the masses that everything depends on them; that if we stagnate it is their responsibility, and that if we go forward it is due to them too, that there is no such thing as a *demiurge* [Original italic], that there is no famous [person] who will take the responsibility for everything, but that the *demiurge* [Original italic] is the people themselves and the magic hands are finally only the hands of the people. (1963, p. 159)

Consciousness, for Fanon, also meant doing away with gendered hierarchies, guarding "against the danger of perpetuating the feudal tradition which holds sacred the superiority of the masculine element over the feminine. Women will have exactly the same place as men, not in the clauses of the constitution but in the life of every day: in the factory, at school and in parliament" (1963, p. 163).

Ubuntu, Human Occupation, and Consciousness

Ultimately, Fanon's ideas regarding consciousness resonate strongly with *ubuntu* as a philosophy about how to sustain a true humanity: a process that takes collective effort at a national level:

> It is only when men and women are included on a vast scale in enlightened and fruitful work that form and body are given to that consciousness. Then the flag and the palace where sits the government cease to be the symbols of the nation. The nation deserts these brightly lit, empty shells and takes shelter in the country, where it is given life and dynamic power. The living expression of the nation is the moving consciousness of the whole of the people; it is the coherent, enlightened action of men and women. The collective building up of a destiny is the assumption of responsibility on the historical scale. Otherwise there is anarchy, repression and the resurgence of tribal parties and federalism. The national government, if it wants to be national, ought to govern by the people and for the people, for the outcasts and by the outcasts. (Fanon, 1963, p. 165)

Fanon, writing for his time, may be forgiven for taking a binary approach on gender, making reference only to women and men. Notwithstanding this gendered regard for personhood, Fanon does emphasize the need for society to work for all. The "people" in his view include those that are otherwise treated as "outcasts."

Tellingly, alongside *ubuntu*, human occupation is implicated in how Fanon explains political and social consciousness. "Fruitful" or productive work lies at the center of renewal efforts for the nation. Fanon's observations in this manner mirror the historical foundations of OT as a profession. The historical roots of OT can be traced back to the settlement house and the arts-and-crafts movements, both influenced by moral treatment and originated in England in the late 1800s (Harvard University Library, n.d.). These movements played a critical role in supporting poor people, particularly those presenting with mental health illness through social and cultural integration, as well as countering the effects of industrialization by encouraging a return to the aesthetics of design and handmade crafts (Levine, 1987). With the migration of various distressed refugees, largely from Europe, entering the United States between 1880 and 1910, the settlement house movement was translated to the United States, with Hull House being co-founded by Jane Addams and Ellen Gates Starr during 1889 in Chicago (Harvard University Library, n.d.). Hull House was, in 1917, to host the first training courses in OT, conducted by Eleanor Clarke Slagle, who, in 1922, became one of the founding members of an association for the promotion of OT, which later became the American Occupational Therapy Association (Pollock, 1942).

The Collective Unconscious, Mental Illness, and Consciousness

It should not come as a surprise that Fanon, a psychiatrist, would bring in psychopathology into his analysis of consciousness and blackness in an anti-Black racist world. In *Black Skin, White Masks*, he observes:

> Unless we make use of that frightening postulate – which so destroys our balance – offered by Jung, the collective unconscious [original emphasis], we can understand absolutely nothing. A drama is enacted every day in colonized countries. How is one to explain, for example, that a Negro who has passed his baccalaureate and has gone to the Sorbonne to study to become a teacher of philosophy is already on guard before any conflictual elements have coalesced round [them]? René Ménil accounted for this reaction in Hegelian terms. In his view it was "the consequence of the replacement of the repressed [African] spirit in the consciousness of the slave by an authority symbol implanted in the subsoil of the collective group and charged with maintaining order in it as a garrison controls a conquered city." (Fanon, 1967, p. 112)

Fanon goes further and observes:

> Very often the Negro who becomes abnormal has never had any relations with whites. Has some remote experience been repressed in his unconscious? Did the little black child see

[their] father beaten or lynched by a white man? Has there been a real traumatism? To all of this we have to answer <u>no</u> [original emphasis]. Well, then? If we want to answer correctly, we have to fall back on the idea of collective catharsis. In every society, in every collective, exists – must exist – a channel, an outlet through which the forces accumulated in the form of aggression can be released. This is the purpose of games in children's institutions, of psychodramas in group therapy, and, in a more general way, of illustrated magazines for children – each type of society, of course, requiring its own specific kind of catharsis. The Tarzan stories, the sagas of twelve-year-old explorers, the adventures of Mickey Mouse, and all those "comic books" serve actually as a release for collective aggression. The magazines are put together by white men for little white men. This is the heart of the problem. (Fanon, 1967, pp. 112–113)

Through this analysis, the first point that Fanon clarifies very poignantly is that mental illness arises from an encounter with an unjust world, whether this is in the form of real subjugation such as slavery or portrayed in popular culture. He makes similar observations in *The Wretched of the Earth*, where he describes three examples. The first example is around the etiology of puerperal psychosis, a severe form of prenatal and postnatal depression. Fanon notes that among Moroccan and Tunisian women refugees, this condition was as a result of the extreme poverty and precariousness of living conditions they were exposed to, following the decision of the colonial French government to execute their burnt-earth policy: frequent violent armed invasions and attacks over hundreds of kilometers covering Moroccan and Tunisian territories.

The second example is around the extensive instances of torture Algerian patriots suffered at the hands of the French colonizers, which manifested in a variety of mental illnesses such as depression, anxiety, and psychosomatic conditions. The third example is around how the general status of constant war in Algeria brought forth mental illnesses: "Quite apart from the pathology of torture there flourishes in Algeria a pathology of atmosphere, a state which leads medical practitioners to say when confronted with a case of which they cannot understand: 'This'll all be cleared up when this damned war is over'" (Fanon, 1963, p. 234). To make it patently clear that this atmosphere is not only a reserve of active wartime or direct armed resistance, but one that is generated by oppression, Fanon also states:

In this period of colonization when it is not contested by armed resistance, when the sum total of harmful nervous stimuli overstep a certain threshold, the defensive attitudes of the natives give way and they then find themselves crowding the mental hospitals. There is thus during this calm period of successful colonization a regular and important mental pathology which is the direct product of oppression. (Fanon, 1963, p. 201)

Yet, war in the usual sense played a critical role in influencing the development of OT (see Chapter 2). While planning for World War I, the United States anticipated the need for new facilities and a new cadre of worker, initially called "reconstruction aides" (Andersen & Reed, 2017; Quiroga, 1995). Some of these aides later became occupational therapists who were trained to provide treatment for "shell shock" resulting from the stress that comes with warfare; the treatment mostly entailed general support and participation in handicrafts (Low, 1992). Perhaps tellingly, it was during this period that Dr William Rush Dunton, Jr., a psychiatrist, became the president of the American Occupational Therapy Association, helping afford the necessary leadership alongside Eleanor Clarke Slagle and other founding members of the profession, to build on the impetus war provided for its legitimacy (Quiroga, 1995).

The second point of clarification from Fanon's observations with reference to Jung's collective unconscious is around the intersubjective entanglement between the Black and White world: the White construction of blackness, and vice versa. For Fanon, therefore, decolonization is not enough if it ends with the withdrawal of colonial administrators. What he strives for instead is a liberation that frees not only Black people but also White people, demonstrating to them that they are both perpetrators and victims of a delusion (Fanon, 1963). The work ahead, therefore, entails building an entirely new world:

Come, then, comrades, the European game has finally ended; we must find something different. We today can do everything, so long as we do not imitate Europe, so long as we are not obsessed by the desire to catch up with Europe. Europe now lives at such a mad, reckless pace that she has shaken off all guidance and all reason, and she is running headlong into the abyss; we would do well to avoid it with all possible speed . . . . Two centuries ago, a former European colony decided to catch up with Europe. It succeeded so well that the United States of America became a monster, in which the taints, the sickness and the inhumanity of Europe have grown to appalling dimensions. (Fanon, 1963, pp. 251–252)

Here Fanon brings back to our collective memory, the negative consequences brought upon all of humanity by Europe's colonization of much of the world, later emulated through slavery, by the United States. The historical period that is often celebrated as the "Age of Reason" or the "Age of Enlightenment" was birthed out of two centuries of pillage and human suffering that was part of the European colonial expansion, spear headed in part by Christopher Columbus in 1492. The colonization of "the Americas" ran in parallel with the Atlantic Captive Human Trade, bringing enslaved people, mostly from Africa, into the Americas. The dehumanization that is necessary for slavery to thrive, for instance, is what Fanon is warning us about. It is worth noting that Europe's colonization of much of the world and the U.S. dependence on enslaved human labor to achieve greatness happened at the hands of the ruling elite, with the tacit consent of the subordinate masses. This suggests that in a similar way that former colonies achieve a new consciousness by involving the entire population, former colonial states would require an awakening that involves ordinary citizens. This is necessary if humanity is to avoid repeating atrocities of the past.

Health and Well-being

Health and *well-being* are common terms in the nomenclature of the OT profession. Health, in particular, encapsulates the profession's ultimate concern. On close interrogation, both health and well-being are not terms whose meanings are to be taken for granted. A comprehensive understanding of these terms reveals their political dimensions as well.

Health

The World Health Organization's (WHO) definition of health remains instructive, having been accepted globally since its adoption in the late 1940s. It goes: "Health is a state of complete physical, mental, and social well-being and not merely the absence of disease or infirmity" (WHO, 1948). With such broad consensus on how health should be understood, it remains perplexing that health indicators remain so poor in much of the world's population and that global efforts to achieve and maintain population health remain so pathogenetic (disease focused) (Ramugondo, 2017).

A similar disjuncture between global aspirations for health and reality on the ground relates to health promotion. Also adopted by the WHO, this strategy was to enable world populations to exercise agency over their own health, shifting focus onto social determinants of health such as socioeconomic status, education level, access to sanitation, neighborhood environment, employment, and social support networks, addressing these as the root causes of ill health, not just treatment and cure (WHO, 2016). More than 40 years later, the promise ushered in by health promotion as a strategy toward better global health indicators has not borne much fruit (Ramugondo & Emory-Whittington, 2022). Instead, global health indicators have worsened over the years, especially in the Global South, with the burden of disease affecting indigenous populations the most (Raphael et al., 2008).

In trying to explain the poor translation of good intensions behind health promotion as a global strategy, to health practice on the ground, Dennis Raphael has focused on the discourses that inform such practices and policies that drive them (Raphael, 2011). In his analysis, Raphael found that health promotion fails as a strategy and at a policy level because social determinants of health and their distribution reflect ultimately "the power and influence of those who create and benefit from health and social inequalities" (Raphael, 2011, p. 225). Those with the means to accumulate wealth often lobby the political elite to advance their own financial interests, often with no regard for society's health outcomes in the long run. A pathogenetic approach to population health also fits well within this often-cannibalistic corporatized healthcare, as the illusion that every disease can be cured is a certain way to generate indefinite profit.

A more salutogenic approach to health, which was introduced by Aaron Antonovsky in the 1970s, focuses on factors that support human health (1979, 1987) and is consistent with the intention behind the development of health promotion as a population health strategy. Antonovsky's ideas about salutogenesis are also synergistic with perspectives of health from the first nations and indigenous populations (Ramugondo, 2017). These populations have always appreciated and recognized the complete and indivisible interdependence and interrelation of all things (Mji, 2019; Sasakamoose et al., 2016). Mji (2019), in particular, stresses how religion, education, and biomedicine introduced from the West and, without regard for traditional knowledge systems, can undermine the health indicators of indigenous populations.

Well-Being

Implicit in the WHO definition is that of the two embedded terms, health and well-being, the former is the bigger construct, encompassing the latter. Health is achieved, by implication, through the pursuit of physical, mental, and social well-being. All these three aspects of well-being have been comprehensively defined in OT literature and inform many of the profession's conceptual frameworks. Conspicuous, in its omission in the WHO definition, however, is spiritual well-being. Spiritual well-being and spirituality as concepts continue to be areas of marked contestation within OT discourse. This contestation is consistent with dominant Western approaches to health. Antonovsky's salutogenic approach to health, however, does recognize its spiritual dimension. Again, this is consistent with indigenous perspectives of health (Mji, 2019; Sasakamoose et al., 2016).

Implications for Practice, Scholarship, and Research

There are important implications to consider for occupational practice, scholarship, and research when occupational consciousness is a construct one tries to embody. Critically, occupational consciousness implicates the personal, professional, and political expression of human existence. Although this may be somewhat burdensome, it is also a human predisposition that is necessary if global injustices are to be confronted and addressed. Much of what props up coloniality and injustice are everyday actions, requiring a cultivation of consciousness and disobedient decolonial praxis (Ramugondo, 2020). Occupational consciousness highlights the need to adopt transgressive acts that disrupt the cycle of oppression for both individual and collective well-being.

Practice Implications

Given that occupational consciousness starts with an awakening at the personal level, it is not the case that one can simply point to others for their lack of consciousness. Consciousness starts with the self and then extends to those people one regards to be their own community. This is evident in how Biko and Fanon conceptualized the term, both doing so with constant reference to themselves and others facing the same predicament. The same can be seen in the manner that the term occupational consciousness emerged in the first place. The term emerges out of research informed by a growing concern among older people in my own community that children no longer played in ways that were familiar, reflecting a shared identity as part of family, community, and traditional society. Occupational consciousness thus implicates both the individual who sees the need for a reawakening and those whom they identify with. This was also observed in the second family from where I collected data, beyond what was required for my doctoral thesis. The father, a retired teacher, at one point during my month-long visit as part of participant observation says to me, "Elelwani, I see what you see," to which I respond, "What do you see?" His response was profound, and tears rolled down as he completed the sentence: "I no longer see myself in my own children. This, only one generation later. We are doomed!"

Given these reflections about occupational consciousness, it appears that the practice of OT as informed by the term cannot be limited to services that are necessarily prescribed and billed for. Further implications are that occupational therapists inspired by this term may need to embody and enact professional role transgression (Sonday et al., 2019). *Professional role transgression* refers to when individuals who find themselves within hegemonic and oppressive professional spaces or structures device strategies to enact their agency, in order to disrupt the status quo (Sonday et al., 2019).

For examples of occupational consciousness impacting practice, see OT Stories 11.1 and 11.2.

Implications for Scholarship and Research

Occupational consciousness again implicates both the individual and the collective with regard to scholarship and research. As a community of scholars and researchers, we are all implicated in how OT projects itself to the world in literature and in how further knowledge is generated. In what is written about OT, the reader may identify lapses in how the profession engages with both historical and ongoing injustice. Starting with historical injustice, it is a useful exercise to reflect on potential omissions in how the history

---

OT STORY 11.1 TACKLING CHILDHOOD OBESITY BEYOND THE INDIVIDUAL

Naledi is an occupational therapist employed in a district hospital that serves Soweto, a suburb just outside Johannesburg, South Africa. Soweto was established as a township (an underdeveloped racially segregated urban area) under the Group Areas Act during apartheid. It continues to be populated by Black people, with high levels of unemployment, financially destitute families, and crime. Naledi receives a referral letter for a 12-year-old female child, Zikho, who was diagnosed with morbid obesity, hypertension, and type 2 diabetes. The main reason Zikho was referred for OT is that she struggles to concentrate at school and has poor shoulder stability and fine-motor control.

Naledi, having grown up in a township herself, has also been noticing a growing number of children like Zikho in many other South African townships. After interviewing Zikho and her mother, and learning about the family's daily routine, Naledi realizes that it would not be sufficient to see Zikho for a few sessions and then discharge her with a home program. She then discusses her concerns with her supervisor, who confirms her fears that anything she does outside of the usual practice would have to be at her own cost and time. After a few discussions with her own family members and friends who share her concern about the rising number of children with noncommunicable diseases, Naledi decides to join a civic association in her community. After learning about how this association conducts its affairs, Naledi brings up the topic of rising noncommunicable diseases among children, and by then, she had developed a number of ideas around community-level engagements, including lobbying local government for safety in parks, street gardening, and regulation around fast-food chains in Black neighborhoods, nationwide.

Questions

1. Can you think of any neighborhood or community with rising morbid obesity, hypertension, and type 2 diabetes among children?
2. Are you able to identify civic organizations in your neighborhood or community, which are concerned with rising noncommunicable diseases among children and could work with occupational therapists to help address this concern?
3. What occupations may be affected by these diseases, and how would you address them in your community?

OT STORY 11.2 "I DO NOT DANCE!"

My name is Velaphi. In my final year as an OT student, I was placed for practice and service learning at Grandmothers Against Poverty and Aids (GAPA), a wide network of grannies-led self-help groups, in Khayelitsha, Cape Town, South Africa. Khayelitsha is a township made up of a majority of Black and isiXhosa-speaking population. While GAPA was founded based on challenges faced by grandmothers who lost their children to HIV/AIDS, and left to care for grandchildren, both the grannies and their grandchildren had become its protagonists and beneficiaries. GAPA continues to offer after-care services for school-going children who lost their parents to HIV/AIDS.

As part of my 8-week placement at GAPA, I was tasked with designing a contextually relevant OT intervention that responds to occupational needs for either the grannies or the after-care kids. In one of my supervision meetings, I was encouraged to think of an intergenerational approach that would engage both the children and the grannies meaningfully. At the time, GAPA had a White fitness instructor who led weekly sessions for the grannies focused on dance to maintain physical strength, endurance, and flexibility. Neither the music nor the dance moves were contextually relevant, bearing very strong North American influences.

After 3 weeks of struggling to identify an OT intervention that would appeal to both generations, my supervisor asked me to reflect on what I observed around me. She asked me to reflect specifically on what I observed the children participate in as part of unstructured play. With a little bit of reflection, I realized that the children used much of their free time dancing to the latest local musical hits and took pride in showcasing the latest dance moves. At that point, my supervisor asked me a pointed question: When last did you dance? My answer was simply, "I cannot remember . . . I do not dance." In giving that response, it suddenly dawned on me that even though these children were Black, like me,

until that moment, I struggled to see myself in them. The minute I took myself back in memory to when I was their age, with dance being a powerful way to express myself creatively in the world, it hit me!

Suddenly I recognized the absurdity of having the grannies dance to foreign music, following unfamiliar dance routines, when there was a readily available and untapped resource, their very own grandchildren. With that realization, I started working earnestly with the kids to create a repertoire of dance moves inspired by local South African music, targeting all the performance components that the grannies needed to keep strong and agile. The kids took great pride in putting together a video of the music and dance moves, as did the grannies in the kids' creativity. In writing my reflective piece on this intervention, the penny dropped when I realized that I stopped dancing after I came to study at the University of Cape Town, leaving a big part of myself behind in rural South Africa and conforming to the Western notion that it is unbecoming for a learned man to dance. This was an occupational consciousness moment for me. I had to ask myself: In what ways may I have perpetuated dominant expressions of doing, being, and becoming at GAPA through exercise and dance, had I not been challenged appropriately to disrupt this?

Questions

1. What may be the dominant factors at play that perpetuate North American influences on music and dance globally, and how may these be disrupted?
2. What are the potential consequences for local artistic forms of expression, including dance and music, not being actively promoted?
3. Who benefits or loses from dominant North American influences on music and dance, and in what ways?

of the profession's origins is recorded, for instance. While celebrating the profession's roots in moral treatment, as well as the settlement house and arts-and-crafts movements to help restore the humanity and dignity of displaced people in distress or casualties of war, it is important to pause and reflect on who were, at the same time, overlooked. That the United States was founded on colonial occupation and genocide affecting indigenous populations and that it was built on the back of slavery are historical facts. Yet, there is no record of service to native Americans or enslaved people, informed by the same ideals that lie at the foundations of the profession. Attending to this potential lapse in history is an important first step to acknowledging the colonial roots of the profession, allowing us to stay alert to possible ongoing patterns of exclusion.

Attending to similar concerns, Kronenberg (2018, 2021) proposed a framework toward understanding being human as occupation and health and suggests that rather than being a given, being human is radically relational and "a political potentiality which manifests on a continuum of enacted harmful negations and salutogenic affirmations of our humanity" (Kronenberg, 2018, pp. viii, 230). In reading about the profession's history and writing its ongoing story, it is important, therefore, to ask the questions: Whose humanity was/is being attended to and recognized, and whose humanity was/is questioned/diminished or all together being negated?

Occupational consciousness also helps elucidate that "performing the academy in Westernized universities follows a script that many are assimilated into, whether this is in front of the classroom, at conferences, in doing research or through citation practices. It is much easier to mimic behaviour and actions that are incentivized for upward mobility, than to disrupt and transgress these tendencies through one's own actions . . . . Withholding communicative reciprocity – through incomplete reading and listening, failed theoretic engagement, and flawed citation practices – typifies epicolonial knowledge relations" (Kessi et al., 2020, pp. 274–275). To disrupt this requires those within the academy "to attend on a daily basis to the active creation of equity, mutuality, and reciprocity that cuts against the grain of privilege and power" (p. 275). For OT, this requires that scholars and researchers do extra work to engage debates from the Global South "indigenous knowledge processes, and public discourses for the purposes of listening and dialogue, not commodification or co-optation. It requires both creating space for and ceding space to scholars from excluded and marginalized communities, whether they have been marginalized due to gendered, racialized, epistemic, religious, ethno-linguistic, or embodied hierarchies" (p. 275).

Clearly, all these take effort, but it is the necessary work to be done in embodying and enacting occupational consciousness.

Lippincott® Connect *For additional resources on the subjects discussed in this chapter, visit Lippincott Connect.*

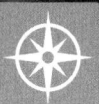

EXPANDING OUR PERSPECTIVES
Being Occupationally Conscious

Chi-Kwan Shea

Occupational therapy training program—San Francisco (OTTP-SF), a community-based program, serves children from 3 years old and young adults up to age 25, who experience psychosocial challenges. Their clients are predominantly self-identified people of color, including Black, Latinx, Asian Pacific Islander, and Indigenous. The life obstacles experienced by these persons often involve complex traumas, such as intersections of racism, gender and sexual prejudice, poverty, violence, interactions with the justice system, unstable homes, education deficiency, and mental health diagnoses. Staffed with occupational therapists and other licensed mental health practitioners, such as social workers and counselors, OTTP-SF's primary goal is to support their clients' occupational engagements during the critical developmental growth process. I have been a volunteer supporting this organization for over 22 years through primarily providing clinical consultations and conducting research studies.

Mostly funded by community and state grants, OTTP-SF steadily grew over the years, greatly due in part to the successful responses from this youth population to the interventions they received. The clients' complex needs demand the occupational therapists' utmost compassion, unconditional regard, and intentional flexibility in their daily practice. Therefore, my most recent study aimed to discover if the practitioners share similar practice concepts as they serve their clients. The grounded theory qualitative study of analyzing interview transcripts of one-on-one interviews with 25 occupational therapists illuminated three major shared practice concepts used to serve their clients. Conscious of the authentic everyday life their clients live, the occupational therapists deliberately exercise intellectual humility to recognize the youth as experts of their own lives, emphasizing their clients' strengths and taking leads from them in the intervention process. Conscious of the trauma that the clients experience, the occupational therapists consistently exemplify their shared humanity with the clients by cultivating emotional intelligence, emphasizing human interdependency, and employing flexibility that de-emphasize the clients' behaviors while addressing the underlying needs. Conscious of the clients' multilayered personal and environmental contexts, the occupational therapists mindfully and skillfully embed meaningful occupations within these contexts that enable successful co-participations.

Intentional intellectual humility, shared humanity between the client and the practitioner, and contextualized occupational engagement are basic concepts that every occupational therapist ought to embrace and so is the concept of occupational consciousness. Being occupationally conscious is a deliberate desire and act that requires continuous practice, self-reflection, and peer support to sustain. In OTTP-SF, occupational therapists are acclimated to these concepts with resources, administrative support, and autonomy and submerged in an explicitly caring, open, and yearning-to-learn culture. The weekly clinical meetings bring practitioners together to discuss complex cases and controversial subjects, giving and receiving peer support, collaborating on projects, and learning from each other. The very active racially conscious affinity groups provide a safe space for practitioners to work through aspects of racism. The ever-growing repository captures resources at the community, state, and national levels to support the practitioners serving their clients. Occupational therapists do their best work and thrive in this occupationally conscious environment.

REFERENCES

Ahluwalia, P., & Zegeye, A. (2001). Frantz Fanon and Steve Biko: Towards liberation. *Social Identities, 7*(3), 455–469. https://doi.org/10.1080/13504630120087262

Andersen, L. T., & Reed, K. (2017). *The history of occupational therapy: The first century.* SLACK.

Antonovsky, A. (1979). *Health, stress, and coping: New perspectives on mental and physical wellbeing.* Jossey-Bass.

Antonovsky, A. (1987). *Unravelling the mystery of health. How people manage stress and stay well.* Jossey-Bass.

AZAPO. (1984). Digital Innovation South Africa. *Frank Talk, 1*(1), 1–28. http://www.disa.ukzn.ac.za/ft16837118000000

Azim, F. (2008). Post-colonial theory. In C. Knellwolf & C. Norris (Eds.), *The Cambridge history of literary criticism* (pp. 235–248). Cambridge University Press.

Biko, S. B. (1978). *I write what I like.* Bowerdean Press.

Braeckman, C. (2021). Belgium's role in Rwandan genocide. *Le Monde Diplomatique.* https://mondediplo.com/2021/06/11rwanda

Burton, M., & Osorio, J. M. F. (2011). Introducing Dussel: The philosophy of liberation and a really social psychology. *Psychology in Society, 41*, 20–39. https://www.researchgate.net/publication/256474366_Introducing_Dussel_the_Philosophy_of_Liberation_and_a_really_social_psychology

Christian, F. (2008). *Negritude agonistes, assimilation against nationalism in the French speaking Caribbean and Guyane.* Africana Homestead.

Christiansen, C., Clark, F., Kielhofner, G., Rogers, J., & Nelson, D. (1995). Position paper: Occupation. *American Journal of Occupational Therapy, 49*(10), 1015–1018. https://doi.org/10.5014/ajot.49.10.1015

Church, M. E. (2013). In search of seven sisters: A biography of the Nardal sisters of Martinique. *Callaloo, 36*(2), 375–390. https://doi.org/10.1353/cal.2013.0100

Cornell, D. H., & Van Marle, K. (2005). Exploring ubuntu: Tentative reflections. *African Human Rights Law Journal, 5*(2), 195–220. https://hdl.handle.net/10520/EJC52032

Curtin, M., Molineux, M., & Supyk-Mellson, J. (2010). *Occupational therapy and physical dysfunction: Enabling occupation.* Elsevier/Churchill Livingstone.

Cusicanqui, S. R. (2012). Ch'ixinakax utxiwa: A reflection on the practices and discourses of decolonization. *The South Atlantic Quarterly, 111*(1), 95–109. https://doi.org/10.1215/00382876-1472612

Cutchin, M. P., Aldrich, R. M., Bailliard, A. L., & Coppola, S. (2008). Action theories for occupational science: The contributions of Dewey and Bourdieu. *Journal of Occupational Science, 15*(3),157–165. https://doi.org/10.1080/14427591.2008.9686625

Dickie, V., Cutchin, M. P., & Humphry, R. (2006). Occupation as transactional experience: A critique of individualism in occupational science. *Journal of Occupational Science, 13*(1), 83–93. https://doi.org/10.1080/14427591.2006.9686573

Dussel, E. (2011). From critical theory to the philosophy of liberation: Some themes for dialogue. *Transmodernity: Journal of Peripheral Cultural Production of the Luso-Hispanic World, 1*(2), 16–43. https://doi.org/10.5070/T412011806

Edwards, B. H. (2003). *The practice of diaspora: Literature, translation, and the rise of Black internationalism.* Harvard University Press.

Fanon, F. (1963). *The wretched of the earth* (R. Philcox Trans.). Grove Press. (Original work published 1961)

Fanon, F. (1967). *Black skin, white masks* (R. Philcox Trans.). Grove Press. (Original work published 1952)

Fogelberg, D., & Frauwirth, S. (2010). A complexity science approach to occupation: Moving beyond the individual. *Journal of Occupational Science, 17*(3), 131–139. https://doi.org/10.1080/14427591.2010.9686687

Freire, P. (1998). Cultural action and conscientization. *Harvard Educational Review, 68*(4), 499–521. https://www.proquest.com/scholarly-journals/cultural-action-conscientization/docview/212259583/se-2

Galvaan, R. (2012). Occupational choice: The significance of socio-economic and political factors. In G. E. Whiteford & C. Hocking (Eds.), *Occupational science: Society, inclusion, participation* (pp. 152–162). Blackwell Publishing.

Gibson, N. C. (2008). Upright and free: Fanon in South Africa, from Biko to the shackdwellers' movement (Abahlali baseMjondolo). *Social Identities, 14*(6), 683–715. https://doi.org/10.1080/13504630802462802

Gramsci, A. (1975). *Prison notebooks.* Columbia University Press.

Grosfoguel, R. (2011). Decolonizing post-colonial studies and paradigms of political economy: Transmodernity, decolonial thinking, and global coloniality. *Transmodernity: Journal of Peripheral Cultural Production of the Luso-Hispanic World, 1*(1), 1–34. https://escholarship.org/uc/item/21k6t3fq

Guajardo, A., Kronenberg, F., & Ramugondo, E. L. (2015). Southern occupational therapies: Emerging identities, epistemologies and practices. *South African Journal of Occupational Therapy, 45*(1), 3–10. http://www.scielo.org.za/pdf/sajot/v45n1/02.pdf

Hagedorn, R. (2001). *Foundations for practice in occupational therapy* (3rd ed.). Elsevier/Churchill Livingstone.

Hammell, K. W. (2009). Sacred texts: A skeptical exploration of the assumptions underpinning theories of occupation. *Canadian Journal of Occupational Therapy, 76*(1), 6–13. https://doi.org/10.1177/000841740907600105

Hammell, K. W. (2011). Resisting theoretical imperialism in the disciplines of occupational science and occupational therapy. *British Journal of Occupational Therapy, 74*(1), 27–33. https://doi.org/10.4276/030802211X12947686093

Harvard University Library. (n.d.). *Aspiration, acculturation and impact: Immigration to the United States, 1789–1930.* https://library.harvard.edu/collections/immigration-united-states-1789-1930

Hasselkuss, B. R. (2002). *The meaning of everyday occupation.* SLACK.

Hocking, C. (2000). Occupational science: A stock take of accumulated insights. *Journal of Occupational Science, 7*(2), 58–67. https://doi.org/10.1080/14427591.2000.9686466

Hocking, C. (2003). Creating occupational practice: A multidisciplinary health focus. In G. Brown, S. A. Esdaile, & S. E. Ryan (Eds.), *Becoming an advanced healthcare practitioner* (pp. 189–215). Butterworth-Heinemann.

Hocking, C. (2009). The challenge of occupation: Describing the things people do. *Journal of Occupational Science, 16*(3), 140–150. https://doi.org/10.1080/14427591.2009.9686655

Hook, D. (2004). *Critical psychology.* Juta Academic Publishing.

Iwama, M. K. (2005). Situated meaning: An issue of culture, inclusion, and occupational therapy. In F. Kronenberg, S. S. Algado, & N. Pollard (Eds.), *Occupational therapy without borders* (pp. 127–139). Elsevier/Churchill Livingstone.

Kessi, S., Marks, Z., & Ramugondo, E. (2020). Decolonizing African studies. *Critical African Studies, 12*(3), 271–282. https://doi.org/10.1080/21681392.2020.1813413

Kronenberg, F. (2018). *Everyday enactments of humanity affirmations in post 1994 apartheid South Africa: A phronetic case study of being human as occupation and health.* University of Cape Town. https://open.uct.ac.za/handle/11427/29441

Kronenberg, F. (2021). Commentary on JOS editorial board's anti-racism pledge. *Journal of Occupational Science, 28*(3), 398–403. https://doi.org/10.1080/14427591.2020.1827483

Kronenberg, F., Kathard, H., Laliberte-Rudman, D., & Ramugondo, E. (2015). Can post-apartheid South Africa be enabled to humanise and heal itself? *South African Journal of Occupational Therapy, 45*(1), 20–27. https://doi.org/10.17159/2310-3833/2015/v45no1a4

Kronenberg, F., & Pollard, N. (2006). Political dimensions of occupation and the roles of occupational therapy. *American Journal of Occupational Therapy, 60*(6), 617–625. https://doi.org/10.5014/ajot.60.6.617

Kronenberg, F., Pollard, N., & Ramugondo, E. L. (2011). Introduction: Courage to dance politics. In F. Kronenberg, N. Pollard, & D. Sakellariou (Eds.), *Occupational therapies without border. Volume 2: Towards an ecology of occupation-based practices* (pp. 1–16). Elsevier/Churchill Livingstone.

Kronenberg, F., Pollard, N., & Sakellariou, D. (2011). *Occupational therapies without borders. Volume 2: Towards an ecology of occupation based practices.* Elsevier/Churchill Livingstone.

Kuo, A. (2011):. A transactional view: Occupation as a means to create experiences that matter. *Journal of Occupational Science, 18*(2), 131–138. https://doi.org/10.1080/14427591.2011.575759

Laumann, E. O., & Senter, R. (1976). Subjective social distance, occupational stratification, and forms of status and class consciousness: A cross-national replication and extension. *American Journal of Sociology, 81*(6), 1304–1338. http://www.jstor.org/stable/2777006

Levine, R. E. (1987). The influence of the arts-and-crafts movement on the professional status of occupational therapy. *American Journal of Occupational Therapy, 41*(4), 248–254. https://doi.org/10.5014/ajot.41.4.248

Low, J. F. (1992). The reconstruction aides. *American Journal of Occupational Therapy, 46*(1), 38–43. https://doi.org/10.5014/ajot.46.1.38

Lugones, M. (2006). Heterosexualism and the colonial/modern gender system. *Hypatia, 22*(1), 186–209. https://doi.org/10.1353/hyp.2006.0067

Mahvish, A. (2013). The philosophy of liberation: An interview with Enrique Dussel (part I). *Naked Punch Review, 186.* http://nakedpunch.com/articles/

Maldonado-Torres, N. (2007). On the coloniality of being: Contributions to the development of a concept. *Cultural Studies, 21*(2), 240–270. https://doi.org/10.1080/09502380601162548

Mignolo, W. D. (2011). *The darker side of Western modernity: Global futures, decolonial options.* Duke University Press.

Mji, G. (2019). The heavy price paid by the Bomvana in questioning the Western modernity script of civilisation. In G. Mji (Ed.), *The walk without limbs: Searching for indigenous health knowledge in a rural context in South Africa* (pp. 187–217). AOSIS.

Nash, J. C. (2008). Re-thinking intersectionality. *Feminist Review, 89*(1), 1–15. https://doi.org/10.1057/fr.2008.4

Nelson, D. (1988). Occupation: Form and performance. *American Journal of Occupational Therapy, 42*(10), 633–641. https://doi.org/10.5014/ajot.42.10.633

Neuman, W. L. (2011). *Social research methods: Qualitative and quantitative approaches* (7th ed.). Pearson.

Pollard, N., & Sakellariou, D. (Eds.). (2012). *Politics of occupation-centred practice: Reflections on occupational engagement across cultures.* Wiley-Blackwell.

Pollock, H. M. (1942). Eleanor Clarke Slagle (1876–1942). *American Journal of Insanity, 99*(3), 473–474. https://ajp.psychiatryonline.org/doi/abs/10.1176/ajp.99.3.472-2?journalCode=ajp

Quijano, A., & Michael, E. (2000). Coloniality of power, eurocentrism, and Latin America. *Nepantla: Views from South, 1*(3), 533–580. https://www.muse.jhu.edu/article/23906.

Quiroga, V. A. (1995). *Occupational therapy: The first 30 years 1900–1930.* American Occupational Therapy Association.

Ramugondo, E. L. (2012). Intergenerational play within family: The case for occupational consciousness. *Journal of Occupational Science, 19*(4), 326–340. https://doi.org/10.1080/14427591.2012.710166

Ramugondo, E. L. (2015). Occupational consciousness. *Journal of Occupational Science, 22*(4), 488–501. https://doi.org/10.1080/14427591.2015.1042516

Ramugondo, E. L. (2017). Human occupation and health. In S. A. Dsouza, R. Galvaan, & E. L. Ramugondo (Eds.), *Concepts in occupational therapy: Understanding southern perspectives* (pp. 32–48). Manipal University Press.

Ramugondo, E. L. (2020). *Decoloniality of doing: A necessary disobedient praxis for health.* Paper presented at Decolonial Summer Schools at the University of Kwazulu Natal and the University of Cape Town.

Ramugondo, E. L., & Emory-Whittington, I. (2022). A decolonizing approach to health promotion. In S. Kessi, S. Suffla, & M. Seedat (Eds.), *Decolonial enactments in community psychology* (pp. 191–212). Springer Nature.

Ramugondo, E. L., & Kronenberg, F. (2015). Explaining collective occupations from a human relations perspective: Bridging the individual-collective dichotomy. *Journal of Occupational Science, 22*(1), 3–16. https://doi.org/10.1080/14427591.2013.781920

Raphael, D. (2011). A discourse analysis of the social determinants of health. *Critical Public Health, 21*(2), 221–236. https://doi.org/10.1080/09581596.2010.485606

Raphael, D., Curry-Steven, A., & Bryant, T. (2008). Barriers to addressing the social determinants of health: Insights from Canada. *Health Policy, 88*(2–3), 222–235. https://doi.org/10.1016/j.healthpol.2008.03.015

Reay, D. (2005). Beyond consciousness? The psychic landscape of social class. *Sociology, 39*(5), 911–928. https://doi.org/10.1177/0038038505058372

Russell, E. (2008). Writing on the wall: The form, function and meaning of tagging. *Journal of Occupational Science, 15*(2), 87–97. https://doi.org/10.1080/14427591.2008.9686614

Sasakamoose, J., Scerbe, A., Wenaus, I., & Scandrett, A. (2016). First nation and métis youth perspectives of health: An indigenous qualitative inquiry. *Qualitative Inquiry, 22*(8), 636–650. https://doi.org/10.1177/1077800416629695

Shepherd, R. H. W. (1955). The South African Bantu Education Act. *African Affairs, 54*(215), 138–142. https://doi.org/10.1093/oxfordjournals.afraf.a094285

Sonday, A., Ramugondo, E., & Kathard, H. (2019). Case study and narrative inquiry as merged methodologies: A critical narrative perspective. *International Journal of Qualitative Methods, 19*, 1–5. https://doi.org/10.1177/1609406920937880

South African History Online. (2019). *The inquest into Biko's death and his funeral.* Retrieved December 2021 from https://www.sahistory.org.za/article/inquest-bikos-death-and-his-funeral

South African History Online. (2021). *Stephen Bantu Biko.* Retrieved December 27, 2021, from https://www.sahistory.org.za/people/stephen-bantu-biko

Stein, F., & Roose, B. (2000). Pocket guide to treatment in occupational therapy. Singular Pub.

Swedberg, R. (2012). Theorizing in sociology and social science: Turning to the context of discovery. *Theory & Society, 41*(1), 1–40. https://doi.org/10.1007/s11186-011-9161-5

Thompsell, A. (2018). *Racial classification under apartheid.* https://www.thoughtco.com/racial-classification-under-apartheid-43430

Townsend, E. A., & Polatajko, H. J. (2007). *Enabling occupation II: Advancing an occupational therapy vision for health, well-being, & justice through occupation.* Canadian Association of Occupational Therapists.

Watson, R. M. (2004). New horizons in occupational therapy. In R. Watson & L. Swartz (Eds.), *Transformation through occupation* (pp. 3–18). Whurr.

Whiteford, G. E., & Hocking, C. (Eds.). (2012). *Occupational science: Society, inclusion, participation.* Wiley-Blackwell.

Wilcock, A. A. (2006). *An occupational perspective of health* (2nd ed.). SLACK.

Woods, D. (1978). *Biko.* Paddington Press.

World Health Organization. (1948). *Preamble to the constitution of the World Health Organization as adopted by the international health conference,* New York, 19–22 June 1946; signed on 22 July 1946 by the representatives of 61 states (official records of the World Health Organization, No. 2, p. 100) and entered into force on 7 April 1948.

World Health Organization. (2016). *What is health promotion?* https://www.who.int/news-room/questions-and-answers/item/health-promotion

Wynter, S. (2003). Unsettling the coloniality of being/power/truth/freedom: Towards the human, after man, its overrepresentation: An argument. *The New Centennial Review, 3*(3), 257–337. https://doi.org/10.1353/ncr.2004.0015

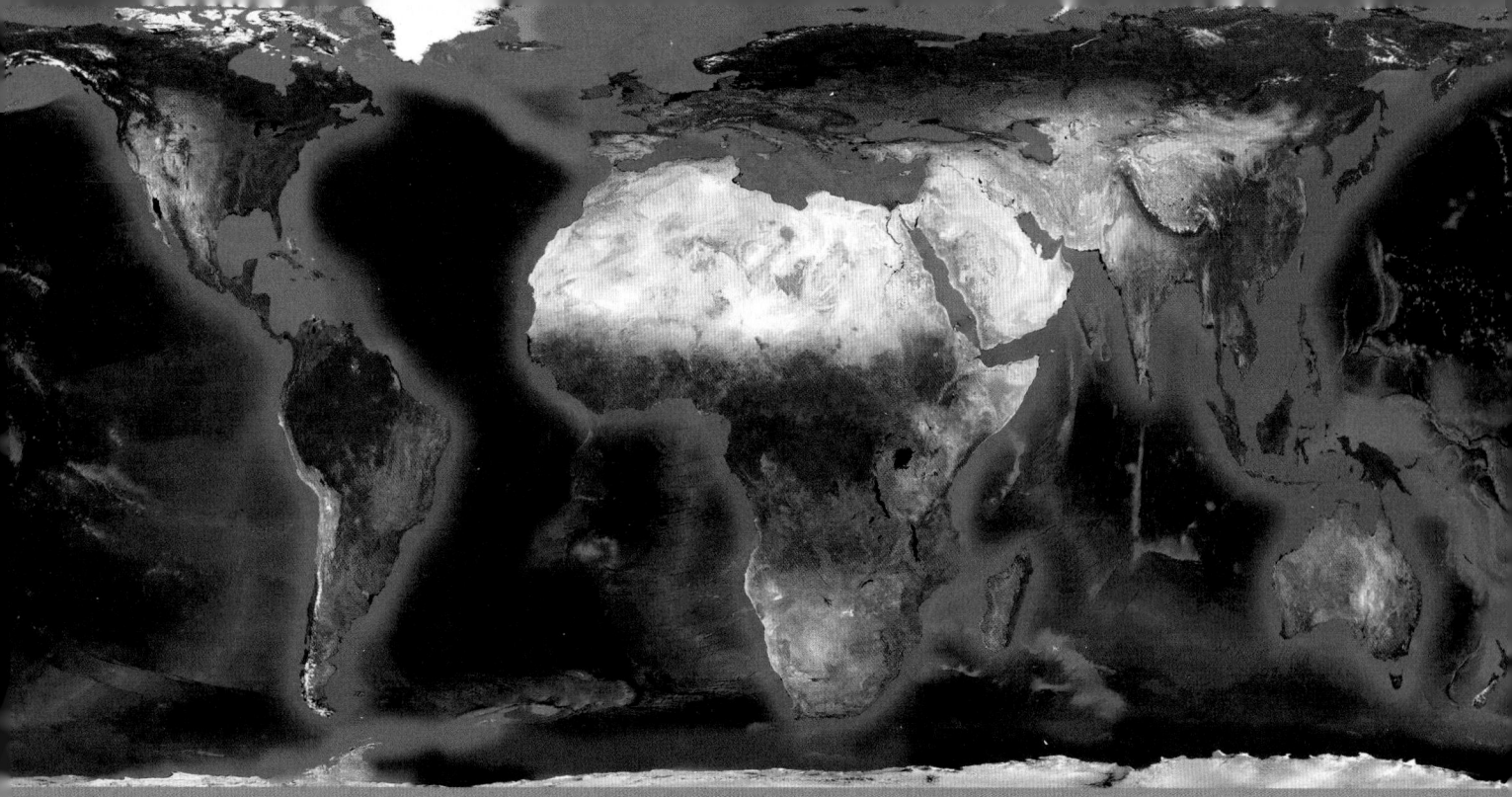

UNIT III

Occupations in Context

Media Related to Occupations in Context

Readings
- *The Lone Ranger and Tonto Fistfight in Heaven:* Sherman Alexie's short stories depict the struggles of Native Americans and efforts to reclaim their heritage. (1993)

Movies
- *My Flesh and Blood:* Documentary about a family with 11 adopted children, many of whom have disabilities. (2003)
- *Crip Camp:* Documentary about a camp for people with disabilities in the 1970s that led to the disability revolution. (2020)

Art
- *My Grandparents, My Parents, and I:* Painting by Frida Kahlo celebrating her mixed heritage. (1936)

Music
- *To Pimp a Butterfly:* Kendrick Lamar's influential album covering themes of Black America. (2015)

Social Media
- *Occupational Therapy & Disability Studies Network* (facebook.com/otdsnetwork/)

An Occupational Therapy Perspective on Families, Occupation, Health, and Disability

Helen Bourke-Taylor, So Sin Sim, and Mehdi Rassafiani

LEARNING OBJECTIVES

After reading this chapter, you will be able to:

1. Apply knowledge about the occupations, routines, and cultures of families to inform family-oriented occupational therapy assessment and interventions.
2. Analyze factors impacting families affected by disability to identify facilitators and barriers to the participation in family-related occupation and family occupations.
3. Synthesize research, family experiences, and individual needs to plan collaborative interactions with families to engage members' participation in the occupational therapy process.
4. Evaluate occupational therapy interventions that aim to promote family occupations, health, and well-being for individuals, families, and populations.

Introduction

This chapter presents foundational information and research on families in relation to occupational therapy (OT) practice. The Occupational Therapy Practice Framework recognizes clients as *individuals* who belong to families, *groups* including families, and whole *populations* made up of multiple and various family units and networks (American Occupational Therapy Association [AOTA], 2020b). This chapter discusses families, including family occupation, family-related occupation, family structure, family life cycles, family contexts, impact of disability on families, and communicating and collaborating with families.

Three sample scenarios of OT clients from diverse perspectives are included to demonstrate contrasting environmental and contextual influences on family-related occupation and family occupation. The chapter also includes examples of assessment tools and family-oriented interventions that occupational therapists might use in practice. Lastly, key professional behaviors that promote family-oriented practice are also described.

Defining Family

Families are the social units of society and have traditionally been viewed as the biologically related nuclear family, or the cohabiting groupings around the parent–child dyad (Dermott & Fowler, 2020). Defining families is difficult owing to the ramifications of the definition legally, economically, and in relation to health, education, and other services. Historically, definitions of family conveyed the majority of societal beliefs, which often excluded family units with less common makeup (Dermott & Fowler, 2020), for example, kinship carer families, single-parent families, and same-gender parent families.

In OT literature, a recent scoping review found that only 9 of 77 retrieved articles defined family (Ranger et al., 2021). Dermott and Fowler proposed a sociologic perspective of family groups that aligns strongly with an OT view. They state that ". . . the doing of family is central; families are sites of bundles of activities" (Dermott & Fowler, 2020, p. 4). In this chapter, we define **families** as groups of people who identify as family; who share emotional, biological, or cultural ties; and who participate in shared family occupations.

Families From an Occupational Therapy Perspective

OT considers clients within their social groupings and populations (AOTA, 2020b). Occupations are everyday activities that people perform to occupy their time meaningfully. Occupations are performed at various levels: individually, within families, and with communities (World Federation of Occupational Therapists, 2012).

What Are Family Occupations?

Family occupation refers to every meaningful activity and shared experience of family members during daily activities and special events that occur over time with input from family members who may participate in different ways (Bonsall, 2014; O'Brien & Kuhaneck, 2019; Segal, 1999). Family occupation is associated with the individual's health, identity, and sense of competence (AOTA, 2020b). Family occupations provide time and space for families to gather and may involve physical interactions, discussion, planning together, and shared emotions (DeVault, 1994; Sakellariou & Pollard, 2016). Family occupations include many activities such as eating together, morning routines around preparing to leave the family home for the day, or health management (e.g., routine dental or vaccination trips for family members). When engaging in family occupations, family members connect together, share meaning, communicate, and enjoy themselves (Smith et al., 2020). The occupational experiences of each family member when performing the same occupation might have different meaning and purposes depending on their role (Roberts & Bannigan, 2018). For example, a family occupation such as camping might be enjoyable to most family members; however, it might be considered as work for the parents who are responsible for orchestrating this leisure activity for the family.

Family occupation occurs when family members engage in occupation(s) together in-person or virtually (Sakellariou & Pollard, 2016; Zemke & Clark, 1996). Technological advances and the recent COVID-19 pandemic created more opportunities for families to perform family occupations in a "shared space," that is, the Internet or phones, with family use of the Internet and technology considered a "megatrend" by the United Nations (United Nations, 2021).

Family occupations are valued and meaningful, and every family balances their occupations within patterns and routines that influence the health, well-being, and participation of both the individuals of the family and the family as a unit in daily life opportunities (AOTA, 2020b; Ranger et al., 2021). Furthermore, family occupations can connect the family group to the broader community and populations with which the family identifies based on religion, culture, or other common beliefs and values.

What Are Family-Related Occupations?

Family-related occupations are central to an individual's role within their family, whereas family occupation relates to common occupation shared within the family group (AOTA, 2020b). An example of a family-related occupation is parenting occupations. A recent scoping review investigated parenting occupations, associating family occupations, and family-related occupations with the parenting role (Lim et al., 2022). The authors reviewed over 100 papers and proposed a conceptual framework of parenting occupation, identifying activities performed to address the child's basic, developmental, and social needs. Parenting occupations included teaching and facilitating the child's learning, playing and engaging in child-focused leisure, and creating a supportive environment for the child (Lim et al., 2022). Hence, parenting occupations and family occupations are related and have particular meaning and value. For example, managing family bills and finances is a significant productive family-related occupation for a parent, and it contributes to the performance of other related family occupations, such as financing and providing family meals, outings, and community activities.

Families, Occupations, and Scope of Practice

The occupations, routines, and the various environmental influences on both individuals and families are an essential consideration for occupational therapists during the intervention process. Multiple factors may be facilitators or barriers to the participation of clients in family-related occupation and family occupation.

Three OT Stories of clients and their family situations are presented next. Following the OT Stories, a comprehensive overview of families and perspectives on health and disability is provided with an emphasis on what occupational therapists need to know and do to practice competently with a family focus.

Families in Occupational Therapy Practice

OT practice is grounded in both a sophisticated and practical understanding of people, the families and groups to which they belong, and the homes and communities where they live and occupy their time. Most people identify with being a member of one or more families who may or may not be biologically related. Familial ties vary for every person, and the expert on a person's significant family ties is the person themselves. Hence, occupational therapists must keep an open-minded approach to gather information on meaningful and important familial relationships that may influence the client's social connections and participation in all occupations.

History of Family-Centered Practice

Historically, family-centered practice (FCP) has influenced OT practice when working in practice areas, such as with children, people with disabilities, and the aged. The family-centered paradigm stipulates that clients and their families need to be empowered to collaborate with professionals and that family forms a life context for the individual in receipt of OT (Bourke-Taylor, 2017; Rouse, 2012). Research suggests that health professionals need to better understand families and their needs to support more comprehensive care for families (Bellin et al., 2011; Jeglinsky et al., 2012). In fact, FCP has been criticized for being poorly defined and difficult to implement. A recent qualitative study found that occupational therapists experienced role confusion and believed that FCP can result in occupational therapists practicing outside their scope of practice (Pereira & Seruya, 2021).

Occupational therapists are inclusive practitioners when they accommodate different family structures, relationships, and the factors that influence family contexts. Being oriented to family issues and focused on family occupations means that occupational therapists focus on the family as a unit and the needs of individuals within the family (Skogøy et al., 2018). A recent scoping review proposed that health practitioners such as occupational therapists can engage in family-oriented practice by addressing client and family needs and promoting family capacity and wellness (King et al., 2017). The first step to becoming a family-oriented OT practitioner is to think about your own family (see Box 12.1). Consider who makes up your own family groupings (see also Figure 12.1).

Complexity of Family

Across the world, people live in different families, with different structures, cohabitation arrangements, beliefs, habits, and customs. In Western culture, families have traditionally been considered to be the "nuclear unit" with parents, offspring, and family pets, all dwelling in one place (Dermott & Fowler, 2020). In Eastern culture, extended families are common. More recently, families could sometimes be viewed as constellations of relations living together or apart; being biologically related or not; different roles and responsibilities within single or extended family groupings; and the different cultural influences that impact self-identity, occupations, values, beliefs, and customs. Family members relate differently on social, emotional, and physical levels and use various communication methods to maintain relationships. Similarly, families engage in various shared

---

BOX 12.1 REFLECT ON YOUR OWN FAMILY

Think about your own family. Your personal experiences of family will differ from others, including your clients. Consider the following questions and reflect on the case scenarios as you proceed with this chapter:

- Who are the members of your immediate family?
- Who are the members of your extended family network, and how do they relate to you and each other?
- How do you connect with biological/nonbiological relatives who are important to you?
- What role do you identify with within these different family groupings?
- What occupations, routines, and habits are associated with these relationships?
- What cultures, customs, and beliefs underpin these relationships and the associated occupations?

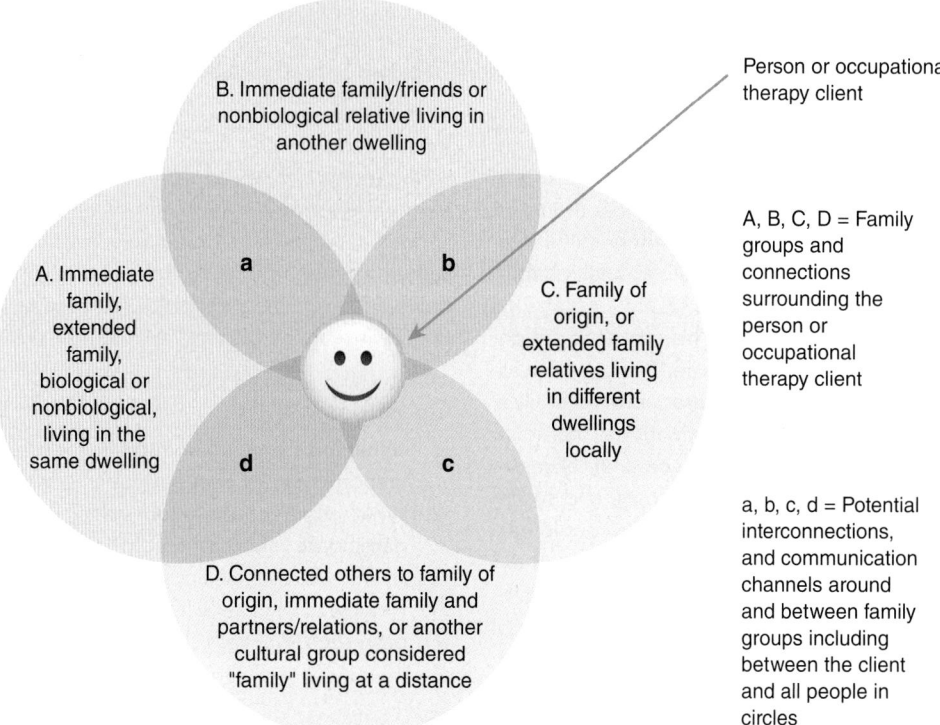

FIGURE 12.1 Family groupings that may surround clients.

occupations and routines to build, maintain, and develop relationships.

Families develop, link, separate, and change based on choice, external influences, the age and occupations of family members, and numerous other factors. Families are a complex phenomenon involving variation in interactions between members, interconnectedness, and interdependence.

Figure 12.1 provides a graphical representation of the circles of family groupings that may exist within a client's life.

Owing to the diversity of relationships within families, occupational therapists must remain open and curious about a client's family relationships: who plays a role in the client's life and how important are they to the client. Incorporating client family preferences is an important step in the provision of client-centered service. For example, if we consider OT Story 12.1, Michael has family members in several circles. In circle A, Michael was living with his wife Emily, although, currently, his daughter is living back within the family home to support Emily. In circle B, Michael has local adult children as well as their partners and children, as well as more distantly located adult children interstate and overseas. In circle C, Michael may have his own siblings or relatives living locally or distantly. In circle D, Michael may have lifelong friends who he considers brothers or a distant relative's partner who is an important family member.

Michael would be connected to all of his immediate family members, but independent from most of his adult-aged children. Since Emily's diagnosis of dementia, Michael's relationship with Emily may have changed to be one of interdependence as the couple managed their own self-care, domestic, and other occupations. This seems likely as Emily's daughter has moved in to provide the care that Michael is currently not able to provide. Considering the family groupings surrounding a client such as Michael is essential, if Michael's preferences and needs are to be included within his OT plan.

As shown in Figure 12.1, extensive family connections may exist around clients. When interacting with a client, it is important to gather information about family structure. The family-oriented OT practitioner is open minded and centers information gathering on the client's real-life situation. A client may be communicating with family members in the virtual space, and the relationship may be a major support to the client. Hence, when evaluating clients, occupational therapists must not assume that a lack of physical presence is associated with a lack of support for the client or an absence of family relationships. Other assumptions may include family structures or culture. Initial information gathering should involve identification of important family members, their roles and relationship to the client, communication modes and systems of support, and important occupations that the client prioritizes within family groupings. For example, in addition to his independent occupations such as self-care and leisure, Michael may value and prioritize many roles and relationships within his

OT STORY 12.1 MICHAEL IN A RURAL AUSTRALIAN TOWN

Michael is a 68-year-old man living in a single-story home with his 65-year-old wife in a close-knit regional town in Australia. Six weeks ago, Michael had a stroke that resulted in a mild left-sided hemiplegia and visual field loss (homonymous hemianopia). Michael spent 4 weeks in hospital in a nearby city and was transferred to the local regional rehabilitation unit as an inpatient 2 weeks ago.

Michael retired 12 months ago from his career as a high school teacher to provide care for his wife, Emily, who was recently diagnosed with dementia. Subsequent to Emily's diagnosis, Michael called on a local occupational therapist and had their home modified for ramp access, an accessible bathroom, and with shower chair, hand rails, and so on for disability access. Emily was a nurse, and the couple has seven children. Three adult children live locally with their own families, three adult children live in other Australian cities, and one son lives in the United States.

Michael and Emily were involved in picking up their grandchildren after school before Michael's stroke. When

Michael had the stroke, the couple's daughter, who lived locally, moved in to assist Emily who has some difficulties caring for herself. Michael has adequate health insurance for his inpatient rehabilitation and receives OT there.

Michael prioritizes being able to shower and dress himself independently, to be able to prepare a small lunch for Emily and himself, and to return home to live and care for Emily with family support.

Questions

1. What life stage influences Michael and his wife's participation in family occupations?
2. What interventions might assist Michael and Emily to participate successfully in family occupations after Michael is discharged from rehabilitation?
3. How will Michael's OT commence intervention that promotes Michael's success at home in the longer term?

family groups: the role of partner and carer, father, grandfather, and brother. Michael may prioritize occupations such as supporting his wife's self-care, sharing meal preparation with her, or driving Emily to medical appointments. Michael may value his grandparenting role and picking up his local grandchildren from school once per week. Without thorough and family-oriented information gathering,

the occupational therapist may miss identification of occupational problems that are a priority to Michael in his rehabilitation.

The client, or their carer, can describe the roles of family members, the values and habits of the family members, and the occupations and routines that relate to the client. Occupational therapists may facilitate participation for their

OT STORY 12.2 MENG IN URBAN SINGAPORE

Meng is a 22-year-old Singaporean Chinese man who has schizoaffective disorder with a history of early psychosis at 19, which was first diagnosed during his compulsory military service. Meng has been in remission until recently, when he entered his first year of university to pursue an engineering degree.

Meng lives with his parents, paternal grandmother, and a younger brother in a small three-room flat in high-rise public housing. Meng does not drive as his home has good accessibility for public transport. Meng's parents have always worked full time, and Meng and his brother were mainly cared for by their grandmother. Meng's parents were shocked that he had a "nervous breakdown" at military service and thought he was too stressed out by the army training. Upon his stabilization over the year, his parents felt that he should not be relying on medication anymore and that they did not want him to be labeled as "mentally ill," reducing his future prospects.

His grandmother, who had always been convinced that her grandson was possessed by evil spirits, insisted that Meng be brought to the temple for healing and also burned

incense for him to drink. Hence, Meng defaulted on his medication, became increasingly unable to complete his university work, was hearing voices, and getting paranoid of others. Meng is currently sharing a room with his brother and grandmother, living at home, and is cared for by his grandmother during the day while he receives OT in a community mental health program.

Meng prioritizes his family relationships, including meeting his obligations to respect his parents and grandmother's opinion about his condition, achieving a prestigious career to make his parents proud, and playing video games with his brother.

Questions

1. What environmental influences are impacting Meng's recovery and return to university?
2. What might an occupational therapist do to strengthen the supports Meng does have?
3. How will Meng's OT engage Meng's family to support his medication requirements?

OT STORY 12.3 ZAHRA IN URBAN TEHRAN, IRAN

Zahra is a 35-year-old single mother to four children living in Tehran, Iran. Zahra's son, Amin, is 9 years old and has diplegic cerebral palsy (CP). Amin is learning at his age level at school, and he has good verbal communication and bilateral hand skills. Zahra was a teacher, before full-time caring for Amin. The family lives in a second-story apartment that is not modified at all to accommodate Amin's mobility needs. Zahra and Amin share the same bedroom. Zahra's former husband's family pays the rent for Zahra, although there is no money available to make the apartment accessible for Amin.

Zahra's family assists with looking after Zahra's other three children. Amin receives monthly physiotherapy and OT that are provided by a government agency. Amin is currently transported in a pram and is due to receive his first wheelchair soon. There are no schools nearby that can accommodate a student with a physical disability. Consequently, Zahra has been Amin's full-time school aide for 3 years. Amin is dependent for toileting and moving around the school.

Zahra now experiences severe back and shoulder pain and reports feeling depressed all the time. Zahra's eldest daughter Azadeh is involved in Amin's care after school, such as carrying him up the two flights of stairs to their flat, assisting Amin with toileting, and preparing the family meal due to Zahra's current pain and depressed state. Consequently, Azadeh's grades and friendships have deteriorated at school. Zahra is concerned that she herself has lost contact with friends, is unable to participate in paid work, and is fearful that Azadeh is following suit. Zahra currently receives OT at a community rehabilitation program.

Zahra prioritizes managing her pain, improving her mood and well-being, supporting her children's education, and sharing enjoyable times together every day in their flat.

Questions

1. What family occupations are priorities for Zahra?
2. What family-oriented occupations are priorities for Azadeh?
3. How would the OT practitioner measure an increase in family occupations to support effective OT intervention?

client in their own daily family-related occupations or family occupations. For example, returning to OT Story 12.3, an occupational therapist may facilitate independent self-care skills at school (eating lunch, drinking, etc.) with Amin, as well as facilitate Amin's participation in family occupations such as the family meal or another occasion such as his sister's birthday event. The occupations of clients and the occupations of families change over time. Hence, the family life cycle requires understanding and consideration when planning OT intervention for a client's future participation.

The Family Life Cycle

The *family life cycle* is often referred to as the developmental stages that families go through across time. The concept of the family life cycle has been influenced by numerous theorists (Aldous, 1990; Allen & Henderson, 2016; Carter & McGoldrick, 1989; Duvall, 1988; Elder, 1998; White, 2002). Despite the many differences and arguments among family theorists, there are commonalities around the stages proposed. However, contemporary family life includes single adults, childless couples, adult friend groups who consider their group family, and so on. Hence, the next section acknowledges diversity in families and selects the most common family—child-rearing adult couples to expand the family life cycle. The reader is reminded that other families will have different life cycles.

A common trajectory of child-rearing adults would typically be singledom, adult transition into marriage, the couple with children at various developmental stages, growing children leaving their original family, and, finally, retired or aging (Carter & McGoldrick, 1989; Duvall, 1988). Such phases are major life transitions during which members take on new occupations and experience role changes with accompanying new occupational identities, which accompanies acquisition of new set of skills to perform their family roles. Each family would have different family role expectations and dynamics based on their values, which would be influenced by their family culture, upbringing, family history in the context of the larger society, generation, and culture in which they live in. The expectations for social conformity versus individual rights are different across different family groupings, further influencing differences in the family life cycle. For example, in many Asian families, multigenerational families are common and so clients may have families with members of different ages covering all of the proposed stages of family life cycle mentioned previously.

Despite the acknowledgment that each family and their family life cycle phases might differ, seven phases may be common to child-rearing couples (see Supplementary Online Table 12.S1):

Phase 1: Emerging young adults (singledom)
Phase 2: Couple formation

Phase 3: Families with young children

Phase 4: Families with adolescents

Phase 5: Moving on to midlife and launching children

Phase 6: Families in late middle age

Phase 7: Families entering later ages and new families forming

Family Life Cycle, Health Conditions, and Disability

Disability influences family occupations and family-related occupations (Laugesen, 2017; Werner, 2001). Changes in the family may be observed in all family-related and family occupations, including basic and instrumental activities of daily living (ADLs), rest and sleep, health management, leisure, and productive activities. Families adapt to disability by choosing particular occupations manageable by the family, restructuring occupations, modifying the family environment, and changing their family routines or patterns of family occupation to meet the needs of the family member with a health condition or disability (Bagby et al., 2012; Bedell et al., 2011; Bhopti et al., 2019). A recent scoping review investigated the patterns of family occupation when a family member had a disability or health condition (Ranger et al., 2021). The review identified evidence about the relationship between family occupation and health conditions or disability. First, research evidence indicates that health conditions and disability influence family occupations and routines. For example, research about the sensory or behavioral issues of children with autism spectrum disorder shows that they influence how, when, where, and what family occupation occurs. Second, emerging evidence suggests that family occupations and routines influence the management of the health condition or disability. For example, research about how changes in family routine and family or parenting occupations influenced changes in health conditions such as childhood obesity and asthma. The authors concluded that the OT profession needed to conduct more research to fully uncover the therapeutic potential of using family occupation and routines to impact health conditions (Ranger et al., 2021).

The OT Stories provide examples of OT clients at different life phases. Supplementary Online Table 12.S1 provides details about the family life cycle, occupations and roles, and impact of disability or health conditions. In OT Story 12.2, Meng lives with his grandmother and parents who are in the later phases of their individual life stages. Meng also has siblings, and as a family unit, they are approaching phase 5. Meng himself is at the first phase of the family life cycle—the emerging young adult phase. Meng was in the process of differentiating from his parents and engaging in independent occupations from his family, including his military service and university life. While recovering from his mental illness, Meng has experienced a disruption to his individual emerging roles and occupations, resulting in his increased dependence on his family. It is important to note that some disabilities may result in temporary dependence on other family members whereas some disabilities might result in permanent dependence.

Zahra's family in OT Story 12.3 is transitioning between phases 3 and 4 as she has children at different ages. Amin's needs influence Zahra's occupations and family occupations. Zahra's daughter is entering adolescence, and her assistance in helping her sibling with disability affects her participation in occupations necessary for adolescents. Depending on the severity of childhood disability and the levels of independence displayed across time, family members would typically adapt their individual life development to the family's needs. Some families may experience marital breakdown similar to Zahra's (Huang et al., 2011); however, research about the impact of having a child with disabilities on marital relationships is conflicting (Huang et al., 2011; Kwok et al., 2014; Lashewicz et al., 2018; Namkung et al., 2015).

Michael, from OT Story 12.1, is in phase 7, and his health issues and changing abilities may result in difficulties living independently without supports. In the cases of disability occurring at later phases of family life, many of these disabilities may reoccur or deteriorate, which might result in major changes in how families may organize themselves, or include new members into the family to assist in the caring of the older adults, particularly live-in helpers or distant relatives whose presence might have a great impact on family occupations.

Occupational therapists who work with Meng, Zahra, and Michael practiced in a family-oriented way and identified individual family-related occupations for intervention. Meng identified becoming more competent in video games to participate in a family leisure occupation with his brother. Zahra may eventually identify cooking the family meal every night so that the family can participate in the family occupation of eating together. Michael identified his ability to prepare a small, cooked lunch for himself and his wife. All of these prioritized goals were highly valuable to the clients as the occupations (family-related occupation) connected the client to their family and contribute to important family occupations of the family.

Family Health and Disability

OT is committed to health promotion among individuals, groups including families, and populations (AOTA, 2020a). The profession has asserted that the development and delivery of services that promote the health, well-being, and social participation of individuals, families, and communities occurs through engagement in occupation that brings meaning to life (AOTA, 2020a). Based on the US Healthy

People 2030, which commits to the health of people across the life span, five major goals of this initiative are summarized as follows:

1. Attain healthy, thriving lives and well-being, free of preventable disease, disability, injury, and premature death.
2. Eliminate health disparities, achieve health equity, and attain health literacy to improve the health and well-being.
3. Create social, physical, and economic environments that promote health and well-being for all.
4. Promote healthy development, healthy behaviors, and well-being across all life stages.
5. Engage leadership to address health and well-being (see https://health.gov/healthypeople).

Hence, the individual's participation in their own healthy occupation as well as family-oriented occupation and the family occupations of the group all promote health and well-being in families.

OT aligns with the World Health Organization (WHO) in this view of families and health. The WHO considered the family life cycle, demographic, and contextual factors as influential on the health of the family unit as early as 1978 (WHO, 1978). The WHO continues to identify and ameliorate risks to family health and healthy occupation currently through releasing news and research data and resources such as the Action for Healthier Families Toolkit that promotes health-related self-care, leisure, and productive occupation for family members (WHO, 2018). OT can contribute to health promotion in families through facilitating health-related occupation.

Impact of Disability on the Family

The family is impacted when a member becomes affected by a health issue or disability. Despite differences within families, when a chronic health condition or disability occurs within the family, it disrupts the family occupations in the present and in the future. Current family occupations and routines are interrupted and changed as families shift routines and occupations so that the new health or occupational status of their family member is accommodated. Future occupations are also disrupted as family members accommodate the needs of the member with disability.

Childhood Disability

When a child has a disability, it influences time use in daily activities and may create an imbalance in occupations for all members of the family (Boop et al., 2020; McKenna et al., 2009). Studies on time use in mothers of children with disabilities revealed that their time use is substantially different compared to mothers of children without disability. Mothers with higher care responsibilities spend more time taking

care of their children, and therefore, they spend less time with other family members, in paid work, in leisure activities, and in social interactions (Crowe & Florez, 2006; Johnson & Deitz, 1985; Rassafiani et al., 2012; Sawyer et al., 2011).

Family members typically go through a common pathway of shock and confusion, followed by a period of rapid knowledge acquisition as they learned about their child's condition and needs (Bourke-Taylor et al., 2010). The occupations of parents alter (Bhopti et al., 2019) and so does parental participation in health-maintaining occupation to the extent that mothers of children with a disability experience a sense of loss over their own health (Bourke-Taylor, Joyce, Morgan, et al., 2021; Dehghan et al., 2021). The occupations of family members are shaped around the child (Bhopti, 2017). Health disparity can be experienced by all family members, especially mothers (Bourke-Taylor, Joyce, Grzegorczyn, et al., 2021) and fathers (Bourke-Taylor, Cotter, et al., 2021; Marquis et al., 2020). These research findings are clearly occurring in Zahra's life situation (OT Story 12.3) as caregiving responsibilities are impacting her physical and mental health, a common experience for parents of children with high care needs (Chambers & Chambers, 2015).

Adult Disability

When a disability or health condition occurs in adulthood, where there are already established family routines and individual roles, there is a sudden interruption in all family members' routine, habits, and activities in response to the affected family members' temporal or permanent disability (Brott et al., 2007; Liang et al., 2017). Family members might also feel stressed, traumatized, or angry, and some families might benefit from support to manage and accept their disability (Brott et al., 2007). If the disability or health condition becomes longer term, the family may experience longer term financial, social, and occupational disruption accompanied by health consequences (Dionne-Odom et al., 2017; Lynch & Cahalan, 2017; Wubalem et al., 2019).

Family members all have to make adjustments according to the recovery trajectory of the individual with disabilities or health condition. For example, they have to quickly step up to take on roles and duties that were left vacant. They also have to take on the responsibility of caring and emotionally supporting the disabled individual. Sometimes, families might receive substantial support from one or more relatives who take on the role and occupations of unpaid family or primary carers (de Klerk et al., 2021). In the case of Meng (OT Story 12.2), his grandmother had always been a significant adult in his life and she would naturally be involved in his care. But the impact of caring for Meng would also affect her emotionally.

If disabilities occur in later family life-cycle phases, where adult children are assumed to be financially more independent, the family resources needed for caring for the older person might be different. Depending on whether the older person is working or in retirement, or caring for another family member, the impact on family-related occupations and family occupations would have to adjust. In Michael's case (OT Story 12.1) where he is a carer himself, his disability would impact his wife's care.

Regardless of when disability enters the life cycle for families, research indicates that family caregivers are impacted individually and as a unit (Chambers & Chambers, 2015; Lynch & Cahalan, 2017). It is one of the roles of OT to provide support to caregivers (Doll et al., 2020). Occupational therapists engage families in the recovery journey of our clients; hence, it is extremely important to understand the family life-cycle phases along with individual family members' life span development. Only then we can accurately assess and map out effective intervention to support not only family-related occupations for the primary client but also the family's valued occupations. Families are the immediate environment and source of support for individuals in recovery; hence, therapists need to take an interest in family occupations, family culture, values, history, interactions, and habits. When considering the impact of the family life cycle, occupational therapists must attend to the environmental context of families, that is, the family's living environment.

Impact of Family Environments

Families are influenced by a multitude of factors from the environment: cultural, geopolitical, education and service availability, and physical and social factors (see Figure 12.2). The United Nations keep constant surveillance on environment factors that influence families, such as the COVID-19 virus, megatrends in the use of technology in families, and affordances that the Internet offers to improve educational opportunities for families (United Nations, 2021).

Differences in family environments are evident in the contrasting OT Stories. For example, the health beliefs and attitudes of Michael and Zahra differ as they utilized services, compared to Meng's family who supported his noncompliance with medication. Hence, attitudes toward disability and recovery can be driven by the broader cultural or religious belief systems that surround families (Hu et al., 2022; Huang et al., 2020; Mohamed Madi et al., 2019).

Differences in the geopolitical environment are evident in the lack of equipment and technology available to Amin, compared to Michael's home that was already modified in anticipation of his wife's higher care needs. Differences in health and education are evident in Meng's access to OT to support return to university, whereas Amin's mother provided his access to education. Physical environmental differences are evident by comparing the modified home of Michael to Amin's inaccessible home.

From an OT perspective, a *family's living environment* refers to the specific social, physical, and attitudinal contexts, including the natural and human-made environment, products and technology, supports and relationships, attitudes, services, systems, and policies (see Figure 12.3) (AOTA, 2020b).

- ***Natural and human-made environment:*** The *natural and human-made environment* refers to the home and the contents, plants and animals, air, sound, light, and geographical areas that the family live in.

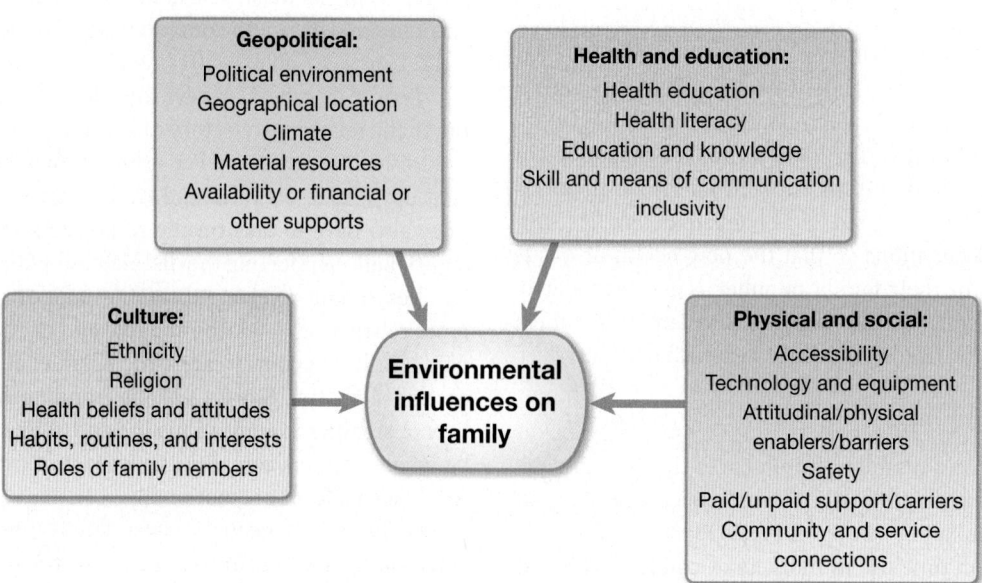

FIGURE 12.2 • Environmental factors impacting families.

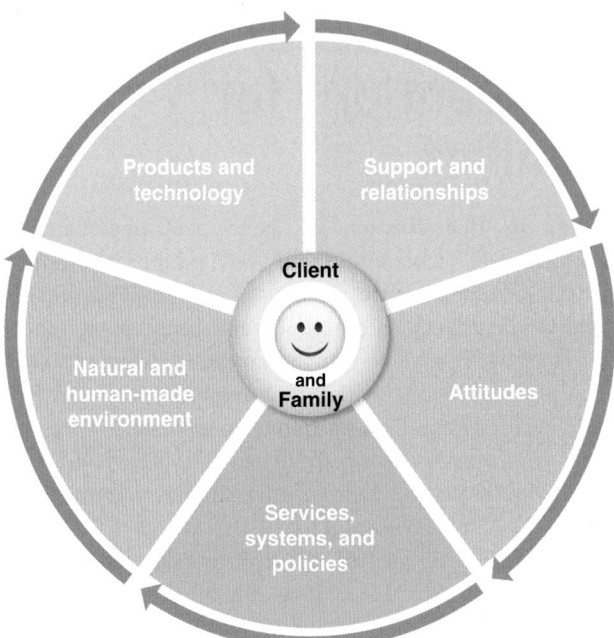

FIGURE 12.3 **An occupational therapy perspective of the environmental factors that influence clients and families.**

- *Supports and relationships:* Families have different supports and relationships if they live with an immediate or extended family, whether they are surrounded by friends, colleagues, neighbors, and being or not being a member of a community. Other supports may include paid carers inside the home or the availability of professional services inside or outside the home. Relationships may include family pets. All of these factors will influence both individual and family occupations. In the example of Meng, even though the family lived in a crowded physical environment, the access to Meng's grandmother is an enabler to his recovery as there is an additional significant support available. In the case of Michael, even though he does not live with his children, he has access to them. Amin's grandmother, although living about 10 minutes away from him, is a great asset to the whole family. She visits regularly and supports the family with cooking and cleaning activities.
- *Products and technology:* Another aspect of family environment are products and technology, such as natural and human-made tools, equipment, or even systems that family use for communication, education, employment, recreational activities, and practice of religion and spirituality and influence family occupation.
- *Attitudes:* Families are also living with other people inside and outside the family with their unique attitudes. Members of families and family groups have their own customs, religion, practice, values, norms, and beliefs that may be different from each other. Within families, different generations may hold different beliefs, values, and customs from each other. With Meng, even though

his grandmother and he were closely knitted, the family held attitudes that were not useful to support Meng's compliance to treatment. Numerous studies highlighted the stigma experienced by family members with mental illness or disabilities, such as Meng whose parents did not want him to be on medication (Hu et al., 2022; Huang et al., 2020; Mohamed Madi et al., 2019; Tsang, 2013).

- *Service, systems, and policies:* These are any developed structured programs and regulations designed to address the needs of persons, families, and society in various levels from local to international. Examples are economic services (e.g., retirement benefits, government support services for people with disabilities), health and medical services, transportation services, and housing policies. All these environmental dimensions are influencing the whole family members and their occupation. For example, in Amin's case, the limitation in school function and dependency on his mother was not caused by impaired client factors or performance skills, but instead was shaped by the context in which he functioned. This context included school policies covering only children without disabilities. There was not any policy that supported integration of children with disabilities in local schools, and school staff were not trained to include children with disability. The socioeconomic status of Zahra's family did not enable them to live in an area with access to a specialized school for Amin, and the community services provided by the government were not suitable to support the family's need. As a result, Zahra supported Amin during school, instead of going to work, and Azadeh took charge of family-related occupations such as shopping and meal preparation to maintain family occupation such as eating together.

Occupational therapists need to understand the influences of environmental factors on family life, the family-related occupations of members, and family occupation. Environmental factors influence OT evaluation, intervention plans, and practice. The environment impacts family members' motivation and their performance, and it can facilitate or hinder family occupation. Further, the health and occupations of family members can be influenced by the changes in family occupation that occur due to a member's disability or a health condition (AOTA, 2020b). Occupational therapists need to be able to skillfully assess all environmental enablers and barriers and work with them to maximize client's success in rehabilitation or recovery.

Family Communication and Dynamics

Occupational therapists communicate and collaborate with families to support individual clients and families as a whole. According to the family system perspective, the functioning of individuals is not limited to only intrapersonal factors but also in the push-and-pull factors existing in the system they find themselves in, and in the context of the family system (Watson, 2012). Families shape our role redefinition, expectations, personal boundaries, relationships with authority, and values (Watson, 2012). Hence, it is essential to have some understanding of family systems and dynamics in order to better facilitate the client outcomes. For example, Meng's occupational therapist needed to work with Meng's grandmother, parents, and sibling to supported Meng's medication compliance. In the case of Zahra, occupational therapists worked with Zahra to care for herself, ultimately maintaining her capacity to care for Amin.

Family cohesion is defined as emotional bonding between family members, and good family cohesion serves as a form of emotional support and well-being for individuals (Vandeleur et al., 2009). *Family dynamics* is the enduring pattern of interaction between family members. For occupational therapists, being aware of the level of family cohesion and dynamics is critical in understanding how support can be enabled around the individual with disabilities (Thomas et al., 2017). For example, when the occupational therapist understood the level of cohesion within Meng's family, she could activate them to support Meng. She worked on building rapport with Meng's brother, a trusted health professional, to deal with the family's disbelief about psychotropic medication. In contrast, if an occupational therapist identifies unhelpful patterns of interactions within the family that serve as barriers to the primary client's recovery, the occupational therapist must also manage these interactions. Examples of unhelpful patterns include abusive relationships, enmeshment, and co-dependency (Haines et al., 2020).

An assessment of family dynamics and perception of individuals and collaborative history from family members can help occupational therapists identify family function and family occupations. This helps generate an accurate picture of each individual's role in the family and their functioning within the social environment (Carr, 2014; Lachter & Ben-Sasson, 2020). The roles of partners differ from culture to culture, and family dynamics are different in hierarchical societies versus those that value equality. For example, Meng's grandmother's words hold a lot of weight in his family, and engaging his grandmother is an important part of his treatment success. In Michael's case, there is an understanding that his daughter would be a temporary support to the couple, while if a similar scenario occurred in an Asian society, there would be greater role expectations for longer term care involvement or even living together to care for the old couple. As occupational therapists, we need to be aware of the cultural influence on family systems so that we could activate resources appropriately for our clients (Smith & Melanson, 2020).

Assessments of and Interventions for Families

So far in this chapter, we have described families, family-related occupation, family occupations, the family life cycle, environmental influences on families, and the impact on the occupations, roles, and time use of family members when a person in the family is diagnosed with a medical condition or disability. We have proposed that the OT view of families as groups of people who relate and participate in activities that influence their health and well-being aligns with the view of international organizations, such as United Nations and the WHO. We have discussed the importance of identifying ways to relate and engage families because family systems surround and influence OT clients. Many client goals will include family-related occupation and family occupations. All of this knowledge is important for occupational therapists so that they practice in a family-oriented way. It is a core value of the profession to practice in a client-centered way (Hammell, 2013). Family-oriented practice supports and strengthens families when they are responsible for the care of a member with a health condition or disability (Bhopti et al., 2019; King et al., 2019). Nevertheless, research with families indicates that OT is still evolving as a family-oriented profession.

Occupational therapists do not always collaborate well with families. Family-oriented practice requires the establishment of meaningful therapist–family collaborations (Kruijsen-Terpstra et al., 2014). Consumer-oriented research informs occupational therapists about how to minimize barriers to understanding the family narrative (Hanna & Rodger, 2002). Families appreciate the use of measurement tools when collaborating to set goals with family members (Rodger et al., 2012). Family-oriented practice is synonymous with an outcome-oriented, strengths-based, collaborative practice model (King et al., 2017, 2019). Central tenets that facilitate therapists' mastery in applying family-oriented OT practice include shared knowledge and power, trustworthy relationships, respectful communication and partnerships with families, family involvement in goal setting, and shared informed decision-making with regard to the clients plan and intervention (King et al., 2019; Pereira & Seruya, 2021). A more recent example of family-oriented practice is health coaching for mothers of children with disabilities who were traditionally not considered the client in pediatric practice (Harris et al., 2022).

Family-Oriented Assessment

Occupational therapists are well placed to practice in a family-oriented way when conducting assessment and intervention planning with individuals and families.

Building a respectful and open communication with clients and their families takes effort and understanding on behalf of the occupational therapist. Occupational therapists can draw from a number of assessment tools during the evaluation process, although development of more tools should be a priority for the profession. Table 12.1 provides examples of assessments that may be used to measure family outcomes.

TABLE 12.1 Examples of Family-Oriented Assessment Tools

Assessment Tool	Journal Article/Source	Content/Purpose	Application to Family-Oriented Occupational Therapy
Family L.I.F.E. (Looking Into Family Experiences)	Honaker, D., Rosello, S. S., & Candler, C. (2012). Test–retest reliability of Family L.I.F.E. (Looking Into Family Experiences): An occupation-based assessment. *American Journal of Occupational Therapy, 66*, 617–620. https://doi.org/10.5014/ajot.2012.004002	Population: Families with a child with autism spectrum disorder Perspective: Self-report by family Assessment includes demographic section and a time diary of a typical weekday and a typical weekend day (helps to identify routines and rituals). Engages families and therapists in a collaborative partnership and promotes family-oriented practice.	Occupation-based assessment that engages families and therapists in a collaborative partnership to identify unique and relevant family occupations, evaluate these occupations, and measure perceived success in these occupations. Enables family occupation to be the focus for family intervention.
Life Participation for Parents (LPP)	Fingerhut, P. E. (2009). Measuring outcomes of family-centered intervention: Development of the Life Participation for Parents (LPP). *Physical & Occupational Therapy in Pediatrics, 29*(2), 113–128. https://doi.org/10.1080/01942630902784795	The LPP was developed to enhance family-centered practice by providing a self-report questionnaire to measure satisfaction with the efficiency and effectiveness of parental life participation while raising a child with special needs. The LPP correlated moderately with the Parenting Stress Index – Short Form ($n = 37$, $r = .54$).	Use of the tool recognizes that family-oriented practice goes beyond child-related goals to incorporate changing the quality of life for the whole family. Best practice involves therapists' identifying barriers to life participation for the child, parents, and other family members and setting goals to minimize impact and optimize other enablers.
Scale for Assessment of Family Enjoyment within Routines (SAFER)	Scott S., & McWilliam R. A. (2000). Scale for assessment of family enjoyment within routines (SAFER). Frank Porter Graham Child Development Center, University of North Carolina at Chapel Hill.	Routines-based interview for professionals working with families to develop functional intervention plans. By gathering information from the family about home and community routines, professionals can identify the independence, engagement, and social competence of the child and the concerns and priorities of the family.	Helps understand parental perspective of satisfaction with current family routines. Designed to assist with identifying intervention areas to improve family routine and occupation as well as child-related skill development.
Routines-Based Interview	Boavida, T., Akers, K., McWilliam, R. A., & Jung, L. A. (2015, July/September). Rasch analysis of the routines-based interview implementation checklist. *Infants & Young Children, 28*(3), 237–247. https://doi.org/10.1097/IYC.0000000000000041	This is a semi-structured clinical interview designed to help families decide on outcomes/goals for their individualized plans and provide a rich and thick description of child and family functioning.	Designed to help practitioners gather an understanding of current family routines and identify areas for intervention and parental perceptions of family routines.
Family Quality of Life Scale	Hoffman, L., Marquis, J., Poston, D., Summers, J. A., & Turnbull, A. (2006). Assessing family outcomes: Psychometric evaluation of the Beach Center Family quality of life scale. *Journal of Marriage and Family, 68*, 1069–1083. https://doi.org/10.1111/j.1741-3737.2006.00314.x	This 25-item inventory rates on a 5-point Likert-type scale to measure five domains of families' perceived satisfaction with family quality of life: Family Interaction, Parenting, Emotional Well-being, Physical/Material Well-being, and Disability-Related Support.	The practitioner might implement the use of this tool to better understand family satisfaction and identify areas for goal setting within the identified domains. The tool provides a starting point to identify family occupations and understand satisfaction and family functioning.

(continued)

| TABLE 12.1 | Examples of Family-Oriented Assessment Tools (*continued*) |

Assessment Tool	Journal Article/Source	Content/Purpose	Application to Family-Oriented Occupational Therapy
Family Goal Setting Tool	Rodger, S., O'Keefe, A., Cook, M., & Jones, J. (2012). Parents' and service providers' perceptions of the family goal setting tool: A pilot study. *Journal of Applied Research in Intellectual Disabilities: JARID, 25*(4), 360–371. https://doi.org/10.1111/j.1468-3148.2011.00674.x Jones, J., Rodger, S., Walpole, A., & Bobir, N. (2018). Holding the cards: Empowering families through an ASD family goal setting tool. *Topics in Early Childhood Special Education, 39*(2), 117–130. https://doi.org/10.1177/0271121418766240	Utilizes a pack of 80 picture cards with goal areas on them divided into nine categories such as communication, social participation, community access and participation, information, and support. Families sort cards into three categories to inform goal setting: (a) yes-now, (b) no-not now, and (c) maybe.	The practitioner is able to involve families in goal setting for interventions to ensure goal setting is driven by the family. Identifying and discussing the range of issues at the heart of family concerns provides the potential for facilitating problem-solving, prioritizing, and linking with services and service providers beyond the team. Strengths based and family oriented.
Parental Empowerment and Efficacy Measure (PEEM)	Freiberg, K., Homel, R., & Branch, S. (2014). The Parent Empowerment and Efficacy Measure (PEEM): A tool for strengthening the accountability and effectiveness of family support services. *Australian Social Work, 67*(3), 405–418. https://doi.org/10.1080/0312407X.2014.902980	This 20-item scale measures parental self-efficacy on a 1–10 scale. It targets needed areas around family support that would give parents time to participate and enable family occupation and family well-being. Correlates well with other scales of parental mental health.	Occupational therapists may use the scale to identify parents' capacity and competency to enact supports and services around their families. This enables identification of environmental enablers available to the family and acknowledges the capabilities within families that already exist.

Family-Oriented Interventions

Evidence-based practice uses the best available evidence to inform clinical reasoning when making decisions about effective interventions that may relate to a client's/family's goals. Several OT interventions have been deemed effective with individuals with family-focused goals. More research is required for the profession to advance evidence of effectiveness of family-focused interventions and the impact on clients. For example, a recent scoping review of OT interventions that influenced the sleep behaviors, toileting, and eating performance of young children aged 0 to 5 years concluded that effective interventions were characterized by changes in parenting behaviors, family routines around the target issue, and development of family goals (Gronski & Doherty, 2020). Table 12.2 provides an overview of a select number of research studies that describe OT interventions that promote health and well-being, along with individual occupations, family-related occupations, or family occupations.

Key Points to Family-Oriented Practice

Occupational therapists bring their own rich family history and understanding to daily practice with clients. Partnerships with families can only occur if therapists understand families diversity, environmental influences, culture, constellations, needs and resources, and understanding of family-focused occupation and family occupations. Several salient messages that may support occupational therapists to be competent family-oriented practitioners may be identified from this chapter. Key points for the reader to take away and apply to practice are summarized in Figure 12.4. A personal story about family of choice can be found in Expanding Our Perspectives.

TABLE 12.2	**Examples of Family-Oriented Interventions That Aim to Change Family-Related Occupations or Family Occupations and the Health and Participation of One or More Family Member**		
OT Intervention	**Research Evidence**	**Brief Description**	**Examples of Family-Related Occupation Changes and Family Occupation Changes**
Healthy Mothers Healthy Families (HMHF)	Bourke-Taylor, H. M., Joyce, K. S., Grzegorczyn, S., & Tirlea, L. (2022). Mental health and health behaviour changes for mothers of children with a disability: Effectiveness of a health and wellbeing workshop. *Journal of Autism Developmental Disorders, 52*(2), 508–521. Bourke-Taylor, H. M., Jane, F. J., & Peat, J. (2019). Healthy mothers healthy families workshop intervention: A preliminary investigation of healthy lifestyle changes for mothers of a child with a disability. *Journal of Autism and Developmental Disorders, 49*(3), 935–949.	This group-based health and well-being intervention aims to empower mothers of children with a disability to achieve occupational balance through increasing self-care and leisure in their own routines. Health-maintaining behaviors are important outcomes for mothers in the program with strategies to improve sleep, physical activity, connecting with others, bring support into the family, and engage with more family community activities and other individualized goals set by mothers. See https://healthymothers-healthyfamilies.com/	Mothers increase their participation in health-promoting behaviors and report statistically significant improvement in mental health and well-being. As mothers improve their health behaviors and community interactions, their child with a disability also experiences increased quality of life and family empowerment increases.
Occupational Performance Coaching (OPC)	Graham, F., Rodger, S., & Ziviani, J. (2014). Mothers' experiences of engaging in occupational performance coaching. *British Journal of Occupational Therapy, 77*(4), 189–197. https://doi.org/10.4276/0308022 14X13968769798791 Graham, F., Rodger, S., & Ziviani, J. (2013). The effectiveness of occupational performance coaching in improving children's and mothers' performance and mothers' self-competence. *American Journal of Occupational Therapy, 67*(1), 10–18. Foster, L., Dunn, W., & Lawson, L. M. (2013). Coaching mothers of children with autism: A qualitative study for occupational therapy practice. *Physical & Occupational Therapy in Pediatrics, 33*(2), 253–263. https://doi.org/10.3109/01942638.2012.747581	OPC targets goals in occupational performance for the mothers and their children. Coaching occurs between an occupational therapist and mother and consists of information sharing, action, and reflection. Mothers perceived OPC as a valuable means to support their children and themselves to attain occupational performance goals.	Mothers address their own family-related goals and identify family occupations that may be changed to enable their child's skill development or participation in line with mothers' goals for the family or child.
Training Special Care for Parents of Children with Cerebral Palsy (TSCP)	Nobakht, Z., Rassafiani, M., Hosseini, S. A., & Hosseinzadeh, S. (2020). A web-based daily care training to improve the quality of life of mothers of children with cerebral palsy: A randomized controlled trial. *Research in Developmental Disabilities, 105*, 103731. https://doi.org/10.1016/j.ridd.2020.103731 Johari, S., et al. (2016). Effects of maternal handling training at home, on development of fine motor skills in the children with cerebral palsy: A randomized clinical trial. *Journal of Occupational Therapy, Schools, & Early Intervention, 9*(4), 321–331.	TSCP was specifically developed to train mothers how to provide care to improve self-care activities for their child with cerebral palsy while caring for themselves. The program was delivered via a website and consisted of topics about caring, including feeding, bathing, toileting, and dressing children. Mothers were involved in all care activities with the child within the daily routine. A module was dedicated to self-care for mothers. The program aimed to assist mothers to manage the care provided to their child, improve their child's skills, and improve maternal mental and physical health.	Mothers receive advice and training about ways to facilitate their child's occupations and development. Mothers are also adjusting the way they provide care during family-related occupations (i.e., family eating together, morning dressing routine) to facilitate improvement in family occupations.

(continued)

TABLE 12.2	Examples of Family-Oriented Interventions That Aim to Change Family-Related Occupations or Family Occupations and the Health and Participation of One or More Family Member (*continued*)		
OT Intervention	**Research Evidence**	**Brief Description**	**Examples of Family-Related Occupation Changes and Family Occupation Changes**
Care of People in their Environments (COPE)	Clemson, L., Laver, K., Jeon, Y. H., Comans, T. A., Scanlan, J., Rahja, M., Culph, J., Low, L. F., Day, S., Cations, M., Crotty, M., Kurrle, S., Piersol, C., & Gitlin, L. N. (2018). Implementation of an evidence-based intervention to improve the well-being of people with dementia and their carers: Study protocol for 'Care of People with dementia in their Environments (COPE)' in the Australian context. *BMC Geriatrics*, *18*(1), 108. https://doi.org/10.1186/s12877-018-0790-7 Clemson, L., Laver, K., Rahja, M., Culph, J., Scanlan, J. N., Day, S., Comans, T., Jeon, Y.-H., Low, L.-F., Crotty, M., Kurrle, S., Cations, M., Piersol, C. V., & Gitlin, L. N. (2020). Implementing a reablement intervention, "Care of People With Dementia in Their Environments (COPE)": A hybrid implementation-effectiveness study. *The Gerontologist, 61*(6), 965–976. https://doi.org/10.1093/geront/gnaa105	COPE is an evidence-based dyadic intervention involving up to 10 consultations with an occupational therapist and up to 2 consultations with a nurse and offered over ~4 mo. The COPE program involves the occupational therapist assessing what the person living with dementia is able to do, their previous and current interests, and their physical environment and the carer, their level of stress, readiness of carer to engage with strategies, and identification of their primary care concerns. The program then incorporates collaborative problem-solving to address primary concerns, information and skills building in the carer, environmental assessment for safety and support of daily activities, stress management for the carer, and activity engagement of the person living with dementia. At the end of the program, the occupational therapist works with the carer to consolidate their learning and plan for future care.	Occupation-led intervention that addresses both the client with dementia and the carers occupational needs and health. The COPE program indicates that outcomes for carer well-being and coping and activity engagement of the person living with dementia were significantly increased. The COPE program addresses the individual occupational needs of the person with dementia, family-related occupations of the carer, and family-related goals of participants who are mostly older couples living alone together (families).

1. Understand families generally and your client's family specifically	• Acknowledge that families have different constellations. • Recognize the different roles within families in relation to the client. • Understand the family culture and narrative around health and disability, healthcare professionals, their family member, and their family's story. • Address the needs of family members that are involved the care of your client. If the person requires assistance from a family member to participate in daily occupations, that person is central in client-centered/family-oriented occupational therapy interventions.
2. Practice in a respectful collaborative way	• Interact with respect and form an authentic professional relationship. • Resource families with the information that they request and then step back to let the family make an informed choice. Accept that choice. • Collaborate to set family identified goals. • Celebrate, acknowledge, and harness the assets and resources within families in order to strengthened families. • Communicate with colleagues to improve coordination of care.
3. Facilitate family occupations and routines	• Make all reasonable and possible accommodations to suit the family when providing services. • Prescribe equipment that saves caregivers' backs, necks, knees, arms, hands, and mental health after collaborating with family members. • Advocate in all contexts (home, community, government, and policy) to ensure better resourcing for families and reduction of community barriers. • Direct families to community services with the capability to address all family members' participation in meaningful occupation.

FIGURE 12.4 **Three key professional behaviors to becoming a family-oriented occupational therapist.**

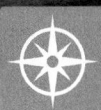

EXPANDING OUR PERSPECTIVES

The Family I Chose

Erin Connor

"Family," for some, can be an extremely emotionally charged word that has the power to bring forth even the most well-hidden insecurities and fears. As mentioned in the chapter, the vast differences in the way that people across the world define family, the cultural and societal expectations of what a family means, as well as the impact that family can have on a developing individual all combine to create a significant sense of loss or emptiness when your family does not meet the standards or "good enough" threshold. The Queer[a] community has a long history of redefining what the word "family" means. The term *families of choice* has been coined to honor the specialness of the relationships that the community has developed with each other to love, support, and care for each other in the absence of biological or cultural definitions of family. An article from SAGE publications outlines the origins of the term below:

> The idea of "families of choice" was framed as a form of political affirmation towards rights for homosexual ways of life, particularly in the USA (Weston, 1991). The context of the HIV/AIDS crisis was also significant, with the emergence of friends as providers of care for lesbian, gay and bisexual people, and the perceived failure of families of origin and the state to respond adequately to the situation. In this sense the term has its roots in a political project. (McCarthy & Edwards, 2011)

A unique and pervasive challenge that is faced by the LGBTQIA+ community is rejection from their family of origin. Whether this is due to religious or cultural beliefs, fear, or just outright ignorance, a significant percentage of the Queer community reports feeling alienated or not accepted by their biological families. At best, this can look like insensitive questions, such as asking a gay male "When are you going to settle down with a nice girl?" At worst,

this can be invasive rituals, such as conversion therapy or religious exorcisms, family abandonment and complete rejection from the home, and sadly even abuse, violence, or death. This creates a need within the community to develop support systems that meet those familial needs.

There is an unspoken bond that forms when people have been through the same type of oppression or rejection. A knowing that's visible to those who are wearing the same rainbow glasses so to speak. The importance of identifying a surrogate or chosen family is vital to an individual's health and well-being. In 2021, the Trevor Project surveyed 35,000 LGBTQ youth, and only one in three reported having affirming families. There is also significant research to suggest that familial rejection is a serious risk factor for mental health issues, including suicide.

I personally feel extremely lucky to have found and developed my own chosen family. My own biological family is wonderful, and they do their best to understand my life. It is just a different experience to be understood without words, accepted without questions, and loved without conditions. As OT practitioners, we hold our clients' views and needs as central to the OT process. Making space for how clients choose to define their family can go a long way toward honoring them.

References

McCarthy, J. R., & Edwards, R. (2011). Families of choice. In J. R. McCarthy & R. Edwards (Eds.), *Key concepts in family studies* (pp. 57–58). Sage. https://doi.org/10.4135/9781446250990.n13

The Trevor Project. (2021). *2021 national survey on LGBTQ youth mental health.* The Trevor Project. For additional information: Research@TheTrevorProject.org

---

[a]The term *Queer* is still controversial in many areas of the world, even within the community itself. It is used here to encompass all individuals who experience gender and sexuality outside of what is considered the majority culture. It includes, but is not limited to, Lesbian, Gay, Bisexual, Transgender, Questioning, Intersex, Asexual/Aromantic, Gender Fluid, Nonbinary, Two-Sprit, Polyamorous, or Pansexual. For more information on this topic, consider connecting with The Network for LGBTQIA+ concerns in OT at www.otnetworkmembers.org.

Conclusion

OT aligns with international recognition about the importance of family, the diverse nature of families, the impact of the environment on families, and the influence of a family members health or disability status on participation in not only their own occupations in the family but also the occupations of all family members. Further, the potential for occupational therapists to utilize family occupation and family routines as the primary intervention to impact the participation of all family members and family health and well-being remains a key focus for the profession going forward.

Lippincott® Connect *For additional resources on the subjects discussed in this chapter, visit Lippincott Connect.*

REFERENCES

Aldous, J. (1990). Family development and the life course: Two perspectives on family change. *Journal of Marriage and Family, 52*(3), 571–583. https://doi.org/10.2307/352924

Allen, K. R., & Henderson, A. C. (2016). *Family theories: Foundations and applications.* John Wiley & Sons, Incorporated.

American Occupational Therapy Association. (2020a). Occupational therapy in the promotion of health and well-being. *American Journal of Occupational Therapy, 74*(3), 7403420010p1–7403420010p14. https://doi.org/10.5014/ajot.2020.743003

American Occupational Therapy Association. (2020b). Occupational therapy practice framework: Domain and process—Fourth Edition. *American Journal of Occupational Therapy, 74*(suppl 2), 7412410010p1–7412410010p87. https://doi.org/10.5014/ajot.2020.74S2001

Bagby, M. S., Dickie, V. A., & Baranek, G. T. (2012). How sensory experiences of children with and without autism affect family occupations. *American Journal of Occupational Therapy, 66*(1), 78–86. https://doi.org/10.5014/ajot.2012.000604

Bedell, G. M., Khetani, M. A., Cousins, M. A., Coster, W. J., & Law, M. C. (2011). Parent perspectives to inform development of measures of children's participation and environment. *Archives of Physical Medicine and Rehabilitation, 92*(5), 765–773. https://doi.org/10.1016/j.apmr.2010.12.029

Bellin, M. H., Osteen, P., Heffernan, C., Levy, J. M., & Snyder-Vogel, M. E. (2011). Parent and health care professional perspectives on family-centered care for children with special health care needs: Are we on the same page? *Health & Social Work, 36*(4), 281–290. https://doi.org/10.1093/hsw/36.4.281

Bhopti, A. (2017, October). Promoting the occupations of parents of children with disability in early childhood intervention services: Building stronger families and communities. *Australian Occupational Therapy Journal, 64*(5), 419–422. https://doi.org/10.1111/1440-1630.12297

Bhopti, A., Brown, T., & Lentin, P. (2019). Opportunities for participation, inclusion and recreation in school-aged children with disability influences parent occupations and family quality of life: A mixed-methods study. *British Journal of Occupational Therapy, 83*(4), 204–214. https://doi.org/10.1177/0308022619883480

Bonsall, A. (2014). "This is what we do": Constructing postmodern families through occupations. *Journal of Occupational Science, 21*(3), 296–308. https://doi.org/10.1080/14427591.2014.914459

Boop, C., Cahill, S. M., Davis, C., Dorsey, J., Gibbs, V., Herr, B., Kearney, K., Metzger, L., Miller, J., & Owens, A. (2020). Occupational therapy practice framework: Domain and process—Fourth edition. *American Journal of Occupational Therapy, 74*(Suppl 2), 7412410010p1–7412410010p87. https://doi.org/10.5014/ajot.2020.74S2001

Bourke-Taylor, H. M. (2017). Occupational therapists working with children and families: Two decades of progress. *Australian Occupational Therapy Journal, 64*(Suppl 1), 11–13. https://doi.org/10.1111/1440-1630.12370

Bourke-Taylor, H. M., Cotter, C., Joyce, K. S., Reddihough, D. S., & Brown, T. (2021). Fathers of children with a disability: Health, work, and family life issues. *Disability and Rehabilitation, 44*(16), 4441–4451. https://doi.org/10.1080/09638288.2021.1910739

Bourke-Taylor, H. M., Howie, L., & Law, M. (2010). Impact of caring for a school-aged child with a disability: Understanding mothers' perspectives. *Australian Occupational Therapy Journal, 57*(2), 127–136. https://doi.org/10.1111/j.1440-1630.2009.00817.x

Bourke-Taylor, H. M., Joyce, K. S., Grzegorczyn, S., & Tirlea, L. (2021, September 9). Profile of mothers of children with a disability who seek support for mental health and wellbeing. *Journal of Autism and Developmental Disorders, 52*, 3800–3813. https://doi.org/10.1007/s10803-021-05260-w

Bourke-Taylor, H. M., Joyce, K. S., Morgan, P., Reddihough, D. S., & Tirlea, L. (2021). Maternal and child factors associated with the health-promoting behaviours of mothers of children with a developmental disability. *Research in Developmental Disabilities, 118*, 104069. https://doi.org/10.1016/j.ridd.2021.104069

Brott, T., Hocking, C., & Paddy, A. (2007). Occupational disruption: Living with motor neurone disease. *The British Journal of Occupational Therapy, 70*(1), 24–31. https://doi.org/10.1177/030802260707000107

Carr, A. (2014). *Positive practice: A step-by-step guide to family therapy*. Routledge.

Carter, E. A., & McGoldrick, M. (1989). *The changing family life cycle: A framework for family therapy* (2nd ed.). Allyn & Bacon.

Chambers, H. G., & Chambers, J. A. (2015). Effects of caregiving on the families of children and adults with disabilities. *Physical Medicine & Rehabilitation Clinics of North America, 26*(1), 1–19. https://doi.org/10.1016/j.pmr.2014.09.004

Crowe, T. K., & Florez, S. I. (2006). Time use of mothers with school-age children: A continuing impact of a child's disability. *American Journal of Occupational Therapy, 60*(2), 194–203. https://doi.org/10.5014/ajot.60.2.194

de Klerk, M., de Boer, A., & Plaisier, I. (2021). Determinants of informal care-giving in various social relationships in the Netherlands. *Health & Social Care in the Community, 29*(6), 1779–1788. https://doi.org/10.1111/hsc.13286

Dehghan, L., Dalvand, H., Hadian Rasanani, M. R., & Kelly, G. (2021). Exploring the process of health in mothers of children with cerebral palsy: Changing "clinical reasoning." *British Journal of Occupational Therapy, 85*(4), 283–291. https://doi.org/10.1177/03080226211020659

Dermott, E., & Fowler, T. (2020). What is a family and why does it matter? *Social Sciences, 9*(5), 83. https://doi.org/10.3390/socsci9050083

DeVault, M. L. (1994). *Feeding the family: The social organization of caring as gendered work*. University of Chicago Press.

Dionne-Odom, J. N., Demark-Wahnefried, W., Taylor, R. A., Rocque, G. B., Azuero, A., Acemgil, A., Martin, M. Y., Astin, M., Ejem, D., Kvale, E., Heaton, K., Pisu, M., Partridge, E. E., & Bakitas, M. A. (2017). The self-care practices of family caregivers of persons with poor prognosis cancer: Differences by varying levels of caregiver well-being and preparedness. *Support Care Cancer, 25*(8), 2437–2444. https://doi.org/10.1007/s00520-017-3650-7

Doll, J., Earland, T. V., & Dorsey, J. (2020). Role of occupational therapy in primary care. *American Journal of Occupational Therapy, 74*(Suppl_3), 7413410040p1–7413410040p16. https://doi.org/10.5014/ajot.2020.74S3001

Duvall, E. M. (1988). Family development's first forty years. *Family Relations, 37*(2), 127–134. https://doi.org/10.2307/584309

Elder, G. H. (1998). The life course as developmental theory. *Child Development, 69*(1), 1–12. https://doi.org/10.1111/j.1467-8624.1998.tb06128.x

Gronski, M., & Doherty, M. (2020). Interventions within the scope of occupational therapy practice to improve activities of daily living, rest, and sleep for children ages 0–5 years and their families: A systematic review. *American Journal of Occupational Therapy, 74*(2), 7402180010p1–7402180010p33. https://doi.org/10.5014/ajot.2020.039545

Haines, J., Matthewson, M., & Turnbull, M. (2020). Understanding and managing parental alienation: A Guide to Assessment and Intervention. Routledge. https://doi.org/https://doi.org/10.4324/9780429316111-14.

Hammell, K. R. W. (2013). Recentrer l'ergothérapie au Canada sur les valeurs fondamentales de la pratique centrée sur le client [Client-centred occupational therapy in Canada: Refocusing on core values]. *Canadian Journal of Occupational Therapy, 80*(3), 141–149. https://doi.org/10.1177/0008417413497906

Hanna, K., & Rodger, S. (2002). Towards family-centred practice in paediatric occupational therapy: A review of the literature on parent–therapist collaboration. *Australian Occupational Therapy Journal, 49*(1), 14–24. https://doi.org/10.1046/j.0045-0766.2001.00273.x

Harris, V., Bourke-Taylor, H. M., & Leo, M. (2022). Healthy Mothers Healthy Families, Health Promoting Activity Coaching for mothers of children with a disability: Exploring mothers' perspectives of programme feasibility. *Australian Occupational Therapy Journal*, 1–14. https://doi.org/10.1111/1440-1630.12814

Hu, R., Wang, X., Liu, Z., Hou, J., Liu, Y., Tu, J., Jia, M., Liu, Y., & Zhou, H. (2022). Stigma, depression, and post-traumatic growth among Chinese stroke survivors: A longitudinal study examining patterns and correlations. *Topics in Stroke Rehabilitation, 29*(1), 16–29. https://doi.org/10.1080/10749357.2020.1864965

Huang, Y.-P., Wang, S.-Y., Kellett, U., & Chen, C.-H. (2020). Shame, suffering, and believing in the family: The experiences of grandmothers of a grandchild with a developmental delay or disability in the context of Chinese culture. *Journal of Family Nursing, 26*(1), 52–64. https://doi.org/10.1177/1074840719895264

Huang, Y.-T., Ososkie, J., & Hsu, T.-H. (2011). Impact on marital and sibling relationships of Taiwanese families who have a child with a disability. *Journal of comparative Family Studies, 42*(2), 213–232. https://doi.org/10.3138/jcfs.42.2.213

Jeglinsky, I., Autti-Rämö, I., & Brogren Carlberg, E. (2012). Two sides of the mirror: Parents' and service providers' view on the family-centredness of care for children with cerebral palsy. *Child: Care, Health and Development, 38*(1), 79–86. https://doi.org/10.1111/j.1365-2214.2011.01305.x

Johnson, C. B., & Deitz, J. C. (1985). Time use of mothers with preschool children: A pilot study. *American Journal of Occupational Therapy, 39*(9), 578–583. https://doi.org/10.5014/ajot.39.9.578

King, G., Schwellnus, H., Servais, M., & Baldwin, P. (2019). Solution-focused coaching in pediatric rehabilitation: Investigating transformative experiences and outcomes for families. *Physical & Occupational Therapy in Pediatrics, 39*(1), 16–32. https://doi.org/10.1080/01942638.2017.1379457

King, G., Williams, L., & Hahn Goldberg, S. (2017). Family-oriented services in pediatric rehabilitation: A scoping review and framework to promote parent and family wellness. *Child: Care, Health and Development, 43*(3), 334–347. https://doi.org/10.1111/cch.12435

Kruijsen-Terpstra, A. J., Ketelaar, M., Boeije, H., Jongmans, M. J., Gorter, J. W., Verheijden, J., Lindeman, E., & Verschuren, O. (2014). Parents' experiences with physical and occupational therapy for their young child with cerebral palsy: A mixed studies review. *Child: Care, Health and Development, 40*(6), 787–796. https://doi.org/10.1111/cch.12097

Kwok, S. Y. C. L., Leung, C. L. K., & Wong, D. F. K. (2014). Marital satisfaction of Chinese mothers of children with autism and intellectual disabilities in Hong Kong. *Journal of Intellectual Disability Research, 58*(12), 1156–1171. https://doi.org/10.1111/jir.12116

Lachter, L. G., & Ben-Sasson, A. (2020). Evaluation of family-centered participation-based assessments: Content validity and clinical utility. *American Journal of Occupational Therapy, 74*(4), 7411500061p1. https://doi.org/10.5014/ajot.2020.74S1-PO8120

Lashewicz, B., Boettcher, N., Lo, A., Shipton, L., & Parrott, B. (2018). Fathers raising children with autism spectrum disorder: Stories of marital stability as key to parenting success. *Issues in Mental Health Nursing, 39*(9), 786–794. https://doi.org/10.1080/01612840.2018.1466943

Laugesen, B. (2017). *Children with ADHD: A mixed methods study on parental experiences, everyday life, and health care use.* Aalborg University.

Liang, P., Fleming, J., Gustafsson, L., & Liddle, J. (2017). Occupational experience of caregiving during driving disruption following an acquired brain injury. *The British Journal of Occupational Therapy, 80*(1), 30–38. https://doi.org/10.1177/0308022616668359

Lim, Y. Z. G., Honey, A., & McGrath, M. (2022). The parenting occupations and purposes conceptual framework: A scoping review of 'doing' parenting. *Australian Occupational Therapy Journal, 69*(1), 98–111. https://doi.org/10.1111/1440-1630.12778

Lynch, J., & Cahalan, R. (2017). The impact of spinal cord injury on the quality of life of primary family caregivers: A literature review. *Spinal Cord, 55*(11), 964–978. https://doi.org/10.1038/sc.2017.56

Marquis, S. M., McGrail, K., & Hayes, M. (2020). Mental health of parents of children with a developmental disability in British Columbia, Canada. *Journal of Epidemiology and Community Health, 74*(2), 173–178. https://doi.org/10.1136/jech-2018-211698

McKenna, K., Liddle, J., Brown, A., Lee, K., & Gustafsson, L. (2009). Comparison of time use, role participation and life satisfaction of older people after stroke with a sample without stroke. *Australian Occupational Therapy Journal, 56*(3), 177–188. https://doi.org/10.1111/j.1440-1630.2007.00728.x

Mohamed M. S., Mandy, A., & Aranda, K. (2019). The perception of disability among mothers living with a child with cerebral palsy in Saudi Arabia. *Global Qualitative Nursing Research, 6*, 2333393619844096. https://doi.org/10.1177/2333393619844096

Namkung, E. H., Song, J., Greenberg, J. S., Mailick, M. R., & Floyd, F. J. (2015). The relative risk of divorce in parents of children with developmental disabilities: Impacts of lifelong parenting. *AJMR: American Journal on Intellectual and Developmental Disabilities, 120*(6), 514–526, 569–572. https://doi.org/10.1352/1944-7558-120.6.514

O'Brien, J. C., & Kuhaneck, H. (2019). *Case-Smith's occupational therapy for children and adolescents—E-Book.* Elsevier Health Sciences. https://books.google.com.au/books?id=XNWxDwAAQBAJ

Pereira, I. J., & Seruya, F. M. (2021). Occupational therapists' perspectives on family-centered practices in early intervention. *The Open Journal of Occupational Therapy, 9*(3), 1–12. https://doi.org/10.15453/2168-6408.1848

Ranger, M. C., Bossé, S., & Martini, R. (2021, October). Occupational patterns of families living with a health condition: A scoping review. *Scandinavian Journal of Occupational Therapy, 28*(7), 498–519. https://doi.org/10.1080/11038128.2020.1766107

Rassafiani, M., Kahjoogh, M. A., Hosseini, A., & Sahaf, R. (2012). Time use in mothers of children with cerebral palsy: A comparison study. *Hong Kong Journal of Occupational Therapy, 22*(2), 70–74. https://doi.org/10.1016/j.hkjot.2012.11.001

Roberts, A. E., & Bannigan, K. (2018). Dimensions of personal meaning from engagement in occupations: A metasynthesis. *Canadian Journal of Occupational Therapy, 85*(5), 386–396. https://doi.org/10.1177/0008417418820358

Rodger, S., O'Keefe, A., Cook, M., & Jones, J. (2012). Parents' and service providers' perceptions of the family goal setting tool: A pilot study. *Journal of Applied Research in Intellectual Disabilities, 25*(4), 360–371. https://doi.org/10.1111/j.1468-3148.2011.00674.x

Rouse, L. (2012). Family-centred practice: Empowerment, self-efficacy, and challenges for practitioners in early childhood education and care. *Contemporary Issues in Early Childhood, 13*(1), 17–26. https://doi.org/10.2304/ciec.2012.13.1.17

Sakellariou, D., & Pollard, N. (2016). *Occupational therapies without borders E-Book: Integrating justice with practice.* Elsevier.

Sawyer, M. G., Bittman, M., La Greca, A. M., Crettenden, A. D., Borojevic, N., Raghavendra, P., & Russo, R. (2011). Time demands of caring for children with cerebral palsy: What are the implications for maternal mental health? *Developmental Medicine & Child Neurology, 53*(4), 338–343. https://doi.org/10.1111/j.1469-8749.2010.03848.x

Segal, R. (1999). Doing for others: Occupations within families with children who have special needs. *Journal of Occupational Science, 6*(2), 53–60. https://doi.org/10.1080/14427591.1999.9686451

Skogøy, B. E., Maybery, D., Ruud, T., Sørgaard, K., Peck, G. C., Kufås, E., Stavnes, K., Thorsen, E., & Ogden, T. (2018). Differences in implementation of family focused practice in hospitals: A cross-sectional study. *International Journal of Mental Health Systems, 12*(1), 1–11. https://doi.org/10.1186/s13033-018-0256-5

Smith, S., & Melanson, A. (2020). What families do together: An examination of family occupations affording family connection and identity cultivation. *American Journal of Occupational Therapy, 74*(4), 7411505235p1. https://doi.org/10.5014/ajot.2020.74S1-PO9116

Smith, S. L., Ramey, E., Sisson, S. B., Richardson, S., & DeGrace, B. W. (2020). The family meal model: Influences on family mealtime participation. *OTJR: Occupation, Participation and Health, 40*(2), 138–146. https://doi.org/10.1177/1539449219876878

Thomas, P. A., Liu, H., & Umberson, D. (2017). Family relationships and well-being. *Innovation in Aging, 1*(3), igx025. https://doi.org/10.1093/geroni/igx025

Tsang, H. W. H. (2013). Stages of change, self-stigma, and treatment compliance among Chinese adults with severe mental illness. *Hong Kong Medical Journal, 19*(6), 4–8. https://www.hkmj.org/system/files/hkm1306sp9p4_0.pdf

United Nations. (2021). Implementation of the objectives of the International Year of the Family and its follow-up processes (Report for the Secretary-General). United Nations, General Assembly Economic and Social Council.

Vandeleur, C. L., Jeanpretre, N., Perrez, M., & Schoebi, D. (2009). Cohesion, satisfaction with family bonds, and emotional well-being in families with adolescents. *Journal of Marriage and Family, 71*(5), 1205–1219. https://doi.org/10.1111/j.1741-3737.2009.00664.x

Watson, W. H. (2012). Family systems. In V. S. Ramachandran (Ed.), *Encyclopedia of human behavior* (2nd ed., pp. 184–193). Academic Press. https://doi.org/10.1016/B978-0-12-375000-6.00169-5

Werner, E. A. (2001). *Families, children with autism and everyday occupations.* Nova Southeastern University.

White, J. M. (2002). *Family theories* (2nd ed.). Sage.

World Federation of Occupational Therapists. (2012). *About occupational therapy: Definition "occupation."* https://www.wfot.org/about/about-occupational-therapy

World Health Organization. (1978). *Health and the family: Studies on demography of family life cycles and health implications.* Author.

World Health Organization. (2018). *Action for healthier families toolkit: A primer for policy-makers and health-care professionals.* https://www.who.int/publications/i/item/action-for-healthier-families-toolkit

Wubalem, F., Mihiretu, A., Craig, T. K. J., & Abebaw, F. (2019). Multidimensional impact of severe mental illness on family members: Systematic review. *BMJ Open, 9*(12). https://doi.org/10.1136/bmjopen-2019-032391

Zemke, R., & Clark, F. (1996). *Occupational science: The evolving discipline.* F.A. Davis.

CHAPTER 13

Patterns of Occupation

Kate Barrett and Kathleen Matuska

OUTLINE

LEARNING OBJECTIVES

After reading this chapter, you will be able to:

1. Examine roles, routines, rituals, and habits and their influence on health and well-being.
2. Compare/contrast measures of roles, routines, habits, and life balance and their usefulness for occupational therapy assessment.
3. Discuss intervention approaches that address problems in occupational patterns.
4. Analyze a theoretical model of life balance and its application to occupational therapy.
5. Describe how social determinants of health impact occupational patterns.

Introduction

Imagine the disruption to roles, routines, and habits that occurs when someone experiences housing insecurity. They often find themselves in overcrowded conditions, lacking regular access to clean water and sanitation, resulting in anxiety and frequent moves (Synovec & Aceituno, 2019). Their schedule and activities may be subject to the availability of a bed in a shelter, the availability of a friend to share a couch, or the hours of a food bank. It is important for occupational therapists to understand how systems and context shape habits and routines so that they can work with clients in meaningful ways within the systems. At the same time, occupational therapists can advocate for services and systematic change to remove barriers that prevent people from being able to fully participate in their communities.

This chapter discusses performance patterns and how they contribute to or detract from health and well-being. Other chapters in this book describe occupational therapy (OT) assessment and intervention for personal and environmental factors influencing occupational performance (the *what*, *why*, and *where*), and this chapter explores the patterns of occupations (the *how*) and how those patterns influence health and well-being. *The Occupational Therapy Practice Framework: Domain and Process*, 4th edition (American Occupational Therapy Association, 2020) identifies performance patterns as habits, routines, roles, and rituals used in the process of engaging in occupations or activities that can support or hinder occupational performance. This chapter also explores how social determinants of health influence life balance.

Roles

Occupational roles are normative models for behavior shaped by culture and society (Crepeau & Schell, 2009). Examples of roles in life are student, friend, worker, and parent. Roles are dynamic throughout the life course because new roles are learned and old roles are replaced. Individuals experience a sense of purpose, identity, and structure when carrying out roles (Kielhofner, 2009) and are learned through a process of socialization and acculturation.

Roles can be disrupted, altered, or ended by the presence of a disability. For example, a study by Davies Hallet et al. (1994) found that roles change significantly after traumatic brain injury (TBI). The study found that many persons with TBI experienced important role changes such as loss of a worker role, which resulted in feelings of anger, frustration, apprehension, confusion, boredom, and fear. Young adults who had a stroke also reported a disrupted sense of self because of altered worker and friendship roles (Lawrence, 2010). These effects of stroke are "invisible" but have significant impact on quality of life.

Caregiving can also disrupt valued roles. Caregivers of children or family members with disabilities influence how and which roles are performed (Crowe et al., 1996). The increased demands of caregiving can result in altered social roles, underemployment, and low levels of well-being (Bainbridge & Broady, 2017).

Occupational therapists help people to construct or reconstruct their roles when they have experienced a lack of engagement in desired roles or an unexpected/undesired loss or change in their roles.

While understanding a person's roles, we must be cautious to not overgeneralize their meaning. Roles do not easily translate from culture to culture and may limit us to singular or normative expectations of behavior and meaning (Jackson, 1998). Expectations of roles change from culture to culture; therefore, role assessments cannot always be used across cultures. When considering a person's roles, it is important for the OT practitioner to listen carefully to clients for their own interpretation of the meaning and responsibilities associated with their roles.

Assessment of Roles

There are several assessments commonly used in OT to learn about a client's roles. See Table 13.1 for a review of common role assessments.

TABLE 13.1   Common Role Assessments

Assessment Tools	Developers	Purpose	Method	Comment
Role Checklist	Oakley et al. (1986)	To assess a person's perception of participation in 10 major life roles (i.e., worker, caregiver, volunteer) and the value placed on these roles	The client identifies and rates the roles that he or she has done in the past and is currently engaged in as well as roles that he or she would like to have.	It is a relatively easy and quick way to assess how someone feels about the roles that he or she holds and to see changes in role patterns over time.
The Adolescent Role Assessment	Black (1976)	To assess four domains: developing aspirations, developing interpersonal competencies, developing self-efficacy, and developing autonomy	A semistructured interview that provides both narrative and quantitative information regarding worker role development.	It is based on the idea that during adolescence, one explores interests, assumes increased responsibility, and develops values and goals that influence occupational choice and work attitudes necessary for entering an occupation.
The Role Activity Performance Scale	Good-Ellis et al. (1987)	To assess a person's role performance in 12 major roles over a period of 18 months. The role activities assessed include work, education, home management, family of origin relationships, extended family relationships, partner/spouse relationship, social relationships, leisure, self-management, hygiene and appearance, and healthcare.	Interview process that allows for information to be collected from the client as well as other sources including family, medical record, and the healthcare team	It is used in mental health settings and is designed to guide intervention planning as well as be used as a research tool to measure intervention outcomes.

TABLE 13.1	Common Role Assessments (*continued*)			
Assessment Tools	**Developers**	**Purpose**	**Method**	**Comment**
The Role Change Assessment	Jackoway et al. (1987)	To assess the level of engagement and satisfaction experienced in these roles and how they have changed over time	A semistructured interview format to examine 48 roles in family and social, vocational, self-care, organizational, leisure, and healthcare categories for older adults	The interview format allows the OT practitioner to assess both role stability and change.
Worker Role Interview (WRI)	Braveman et al. (2005)	To assess psychosocial capacity in injured workers for readiness to return to work; to address both psychosocial and environmental factors that impact return to work	Semistructured interview formats for recently injured workers and persons who are chronically disabled	The information gathered complements other work/physical capacity assessments to ensure a well-rounded picture of the client and his or her needs that should be addressed to ensure return to work.

OT, occupational therapy.

Habits

Habits are specific, automatic behaviors that are performed repeatedly, relatively automatically, and with little variation. Because they can be performed in different contexts, they are not necessarily performed in exactly the same way each time (Clark, 2000). Habits can be useful, dominating, or impoverished and can be difficult to break.

An example of a useful habit is brushing teeth before bed every night. It is performed consistently without planning, and when barriers arise (such as when stranded overnight at an airport), the loss is noticed but is not incapacitating. Useful habits can help organize time and resources so that less cognitive energy is needed throughout the day. For example, with the habit of putting car keys on a hook by the door when entering the house, less time and energy are spent trying to find the keys when needed. Or when appointments are immediately recorded on a calendar, the cognitive load to remember the date is reduced. These useful habits reduce fatigue because they require less effort, free attention for other things, and allow novel actions without having to recall or attend to specific details (Clark as cited in Young, 1988). Simple, useful habits may be developed to manage time and reduce the stress that interferes with daily performance. For example, an occupational therapist may help a client with spinal cord injury (SCI) develop useful habits in the morning routine so time and energy are not wasted on locating and setting up supplies before going to work.

When people have difficulty learning new useful habits because of a dysfunctional internal state, they may have impoverished habits. People with Alzheimer disease, depression, or attention-deficit/hyperactivity disorder may not be able to develop new useful habits that help them adjust to their disability (Clark, 2000). Instead, the occupational therapist will consult with the caregivers for ways to modify the environment or the activity for optimal performance. For example, teaching the caregiver to have all lunch supplies available in one place every day can cue the individual with Alzheimer disease to make a sandwich.

Dominating habits are those that are consistently performed even if they interfere with optimal performance. Over time, some habits can become addicting and affect one's health, such as the need to smoke a cigarette when driving or consume snacks when watching TV. OT intervention may assist individuals to identify and practice alternative habits that are less harmful. Other dominating habits create stress or anxiety if they cannot be performed, such as needing to wash hands after touching anything. The anxiety from performing the handwashing and/or not being able to handwash makes it difficult to carry on with the other tasks in a day. Habit domination can occur with obsessive-compulsive disorder (OCD), autism, or other mental health disorders. These can be very difficult to change and are sometimes managed with medication or behavioral intervention.

Assessment of Habits

Structured interview with the client, family member, or caregiver is a useful assessment of habits. Questions should address how the individual performs activities of daily living (ADL) and instrumental activities of daily living (IADL) and the specific habits used during the performance of each activity. For example, "Describe the steps you take in the morning to get ready for the day." It is important to determine whether these habits are a help or hindrance to performance. See Table 13.2 for a summary of the LIFE-H 3.0 habit assessment.

TABLE 13.2 Assessments of Habits or Routines

Assessment Tools	Developers	Purpose	Method	Comment
The Assessment of Life Habits (LIFE-H 3.0)	Fougeyrollas et al. (2001)	To evaluate social participation of people with disabilities, regardless of the type of underlying impairment; to measure level of difficulty and type of assistance needed	Self- or therapist-administered; ratings for 12 life habit categories (nutrition, fitness, personal care, communication, housing, mobility, responsibility, interpersonal relationships, community, education, employment, and recreation)	Fits well in the International Classification of Functioning, Disability and Health (ICF) participation domains; measuring a person's involvement in a life situation
Daily activity log		Document a record of what occurs in people's lives. Could also include additional information such as location, other people involved, and how individual felt at the time	Record activities at regular intervals such as every 30 minutes in a 24-h day for 3 consecutive days.	While this is not a formalized tool, it is useful to capture how people spend their time and is easily adaptable.
The Model of Human Occupation Screening Tool (MOHOST) Version 2.0	Kielhofner et al. (2007); Parkinson et al. (2006)	To measure the Model of Human Occupation (MOHO) concepts of volition, habituation, communication/interaction skills, motor skills, process skills, and the environment	One of the six subscales measures performance patterns related to routines, adaptability, roles, and responsibility. Scoring reflects whether the individual's performance patterns facilitate, allow, inhibit, or restrict optimal performance.	The MOHOST has initial validity evidence for use as an overview of occupational performance and for use of the six subscales representing the MOHO concepts.
The Family Routines Inventory	Boyce et al. (1983); Jensen et al. (1983)	To measure the predictability of routine in the daily life of a family. It measures 28 positive, strength-promoting family routines and has demonstrated validity and reliability.	Scoring is based on the number of routines endorsed by the family (they do the routine), frequency of adherence to the routine (how often they do it), and how important the routine is to them.	Examples of items include "family eats at the same time each night," "each child has some time each day for playing alone," "family regularly visits with the relatives," and "parents and children play together some time each day."
The Scale of Older Adults' Routine (SOAR)	Zisberg et al. (2009)	To measure stability in activities on a daily and weekly basis for older adults. SOAR provides information about the stability or disruption of routine.	It is administered by in-person interview and includes 42 routine activities in five domains (basic, instrumental, leisure, social, and rest) measured on four dimensions (frequency, timing, duration, and sequence).	This assessment may be useful for occupational therapist in exploring altered routines during transitions such as from home to a retirement community, independent living to assisted living, or a nursing home.
The Social Rhythm Metric (SRM-5)	Monk et al. (1990); Monk et al. (2002)	To quantify daily lifestyle regularity (routines) with respect to event timing	Diary-like tool where participants record the timing of five daily events over the course of 1 week: when they get out of bed, have first contact with a person, start of work, school, volunteer or family care, have dinner, and go to bed	This measure was developed from the theory that social rhythms (i.e., eating and sleeping schedules) are important for structuring individuals' days and for maintaining circadian rhythms, and alterations in these rhythms lead to disengagement and poor health.

Routines

Routines are "a type of higher-order habit that involves sequencing and combining processes, procedures, steps, or occupations and provide a structure for daily life" (Clark, 2000, p. 128S). An example of a health-promoting routine is following a predictable series of stretches and exercises followed by a nutritious breakfast before going to work every day. For someone with a disability, a healthful routine may include taking care of medical equipment and setting up medications for the next day before going to bed. Older adults typically embed cues to take their medications into daily routines of mealtime and wake-up or sleep times (Sanders & Van Oss, 2013). People who have hired caregivers will be most efficient at managing their care if they have a predictable routine to teach their caregivers. Occupational therapists must help clients embed their newly learned strategies into everyday activities and routines to ensure greater compliance with recommendations (Radomski, 2011).

Because routines provide a useful daily structure, the loss of routines can also be disruptive. People who have chronic diseases may find it difficult to maintain a steady routine because managing their disease symptoms is challenging and often unpredictable. Dressing, for example, is typically done in a sequential way with similar steps and procedures used from day to day. However, research on women with rheumatoid arthritis (RA) and diabetes showed they altered their dressing routines because they had much more difficulty performing the steps (Poole & Cordova, 2004). Women with fibromyalgia who reported high levels of order and routine in their lives gained greatly from actively coping with their illness compared with women who did not have high levels of routine (Reich, 2000).

Routines can be a very important component of managing one's overall health but can also be damaging (Friese et al., 2002; Segal, 2004). Sometimes, people with chronic diseases avoid making future plans and limit social engagements to minimize potential discomfort. This pattern of avoidance leads to a vicious cycle of less positive social engagements (Zautre et al., 2000). Long-term patterns of sedentary or isolative behavior such as watching television every night for several hours can have a negative effect on health or well-being.

Performance patterns are disrupted with acute or chronic diseases or conditions. Several diseases have fatigue as one of the primary symptoms, and often, the additional requirement of managing disease symptoms taps into available energy reserves. Occupational therapists address performance patterns and help people create new habits or routines that maximize their available energy. For example, people who had an SCI recognized different levels of energy at different times of the day or week and learned to organize their time so that they were doing the most when they felt the best. This type of planning was viewed as a very useful strategy for participating in activities that were important to them (Chugg & Craik, 2002).

Chronic diseases such as multiple sclerosis, chronic fatigue syndrome, or fibromyalgia include symptoms of severe fatigue that interfere with routines and participation in everyday life.

Fatigue is often unpredictable and severe, making it difficult to follow desired routines or to make future plans. People who experience this type of fatigue are forced to make choices about how they are going to expend their limited energy and make reductions in the number and type of activities in which they participate (Matuska & Erickson, 2008).

Occupational therapists teach principles of energy conservation that address the importance of health-promoting routines in managing fatigue. Common energy conservation strategies include analyzing and modifying activities to reduce energy expenditures, balancing work and rest, delegating some activities, examining and modifying standards and priorities, using the body efficiently, organizing workspaces, and using assistive technologies to conserve energy (Matuska et al., 2007). All of these strategies create positive changes in daily routines, and when individuals integrate them into their lives, there has been an associated reduced fatigue impact and improved quality of life (Mathiowetz et al., 2001, 2005).

The experience of refugees provides another example. Transitioning into a new country and community requires learning new customs, roles, habits, and routines. In the United States, refugees are placed in "reception and placement" programs lasting approximately 3 months. These programs place refugees in housing, enroll them in employment services, register youth for school, and connect them with English learning programs (U.S. Department of State, n.d.). However, after 3 months, there is often a gap in resources and support as the refugees are still adjusting to a new culture and new ways of daily living. Daily activities that are typical in the United States such as riding a bus, cooking in an oven, or purchasing and managing refrigerated or frozen foods may be unfamiliar for people coming from rural settings and/or refugee camps where electricity was not readily available. As occupational therapists, it is important to work from a client-centered and culturally sensitive perspective to seek to understand the roles and routines that people want to learn more about and engage in (rather than assume they want to learn how to do everything the "American" way). Occupational therapists are uniquely positioned to work with refugees to identify ways in which they can participate in culturally relevant habits and routines in their new setting.

The COVID-19 pandemic has taught us how context shapes our habits and routines. Take a moment to reflect on how your own life changed with the pandemic. What habits and routines were disrupted by the pandemic? What new habits and routines did you create to help you cope and continue to function? How did the pandemic change your family life? Or your community? See OT Story 13.1 for an example of how one person's life became unbalanced due to the pandemic.

OT STORY 13.1 COVID IN A GROUP HOME

Rob is a 46-year-old man with Down syndrome. He lives in a group home with four other men. Before COVID-19, Rob worked in the mail room of a large law firm 25 hours a week. When he was not working, he enjoyed raking, sweeping, or shoveling outside his home, depending on the season. Rob also enjoyed getting together with other group homes for events such as picnics and field games. He is an avid fan of the local university basketball team and has season tickets.

When COVID-19 started, Rob's activities dramatically changed. The law firm decreased his hours to 5 hours a week to minimize the number of people in the building at one time. He no longer was able to attend basketball games. Gatherings with other homes were now prohibited. As a result, Rob started to show signs of depression—he did not want to get out of bed or eat.

The director of the group home had access to an occupational therapist and decided to call her into work with Rob and the house to come up with some ideas of how they could increase the activity level in the group home during COVID-19. The occupational therapist starts by asking the following questions.

Questions

1. In what ways have Rob's routines and habits been disrupted by COVID?
2. What habits and routines might Rob engage in to stay healthy during COVID?

Please refer to Chapter 51 to find out how the OT practitioner worked with Rob in his group home.

Family Routines

Family routines are important to address because they have been shown to be important in individual and family well-being (Denham, 2003; Friese, 2007; Friese et al., 2002). Family routines are observable and repetitive patterns involving family members that occur with predictable regularity in family life (Denham, 2002). Routines can help family members arrange everyday life in a way that helps them cope with illness or stress. When families are stressed, interventions are most effective when the new health routines are aligned with family values, meaningful, and applicable to family needs and when resources were available (Denham, 2002).

Assessment of Routines

Several assessment tools are available to assess routines. See Table 13.2 for a summary of common assessments for routines.

Rituals

Rituals are different from routines in that they include strong elements of symbolism (Crepeau, 1995). Rituals often are a reflection or enactment of one's culture. A strong sense of meaning and identity is experienced when a person feels engaged and included in a ritual. Many people associate the word *ritual* with religious activities such as a baptism, bar mitzvah, pilgrimage to Mecca, or other religious ceremonies. Rituals can also be secular such as a holiday parade, high school graduation, or initiation into a group of

people (gang, sorority, fraternity, etc.). Rituals often signify to a community of people a transition from one state of being to another, such as from child to adult, single to married, or student to graduate.

Rituals also exist in the context of families. Family rituals contain symbolic and affective components that serve to construct and affirm family identity (Segal, 2004). Examples of family rituals could include pizza nights, family reunions, or how families greet one another. Rituals occur at regular intervals or on special occasions. They may occur daily (kissing one another, hello), weekly (family dinner), annually (reunion), or only once in a lifetime (bar mitzvah). Figure 13.1 shows a group of friends having an iftar together during Ramadan.

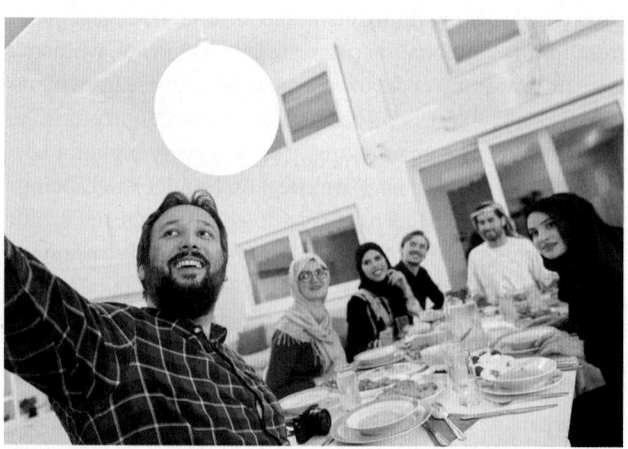

FIGURE 13.1 **A family and friends sharing dinner during Ramadan.**

Rituals offer individuals and groups of people an opportunity to carry out identified roles and to feel a sense of belonging and meaning. Although we do not have a formal way of assessing rituals in OT, it is important for occupational therapists to be aware that what may appear as "routine" may actually be experienced as a ritual by the person engaged. Rituals may also be thought of as a tool to be used in OT as we acknowledge the significant transitions one experiences in therapy: from nonacceptance to acceptance of a disability, meeting therapeutic goals, or transitioning off of a unit. See Expanding Our Perspectives.

Social Determinants of Health

The Centers for Disease Control and Prevention (2021) defines **social determinants of health (SDH)** as the conditions in the places where people grow, live, work, age, learn, and play that affect a wide range of health and quality of life outcomes. They are nonmedical factors that impact health. Healthy People 2030 groups SDH into five areas: economic stability, education, healthcare, neighborhood and built

EXPANDING OUR PERSPECTIVES

Collectivist Approach to Patterns of Occupation

Dahlia Castillo

Collectivism means giving priority to a group rather than an individual and has multiple contexts including political, social, religious, and economic life. Some terms regarding patterns of occupation associated with collectivism include community, cohesiveness, loyalty, interconnection, and group goals. Interconnectedness between and among people plays a large role in each member's individual identity.

I first became aware of a collectivist pattern of occupation while living in rural Mexico during an undergraduate study abroad experience. In the small town where I attended classes each morning, people took a daily siesta (nap). Before I traveled there, I decided I would not take a daily nap and instead get to know the community more. On the first day, I went to a local museum and arrived just before 2:00 PM. A man was closing the doors and told me to come back at 5:00 PM. I quickly discovered the whole town shut down every day between 1:00 PM and 2:00 PM for the siesta. Things began to reopen after 5:00 PM and stayed open until well past 8:00 PM and much later on the weekends.

Another example of collectivism was what I learned firsthand while visiting rural China. Each morning I saw large groups of people in front of office buildings doing movements in unison that I did not understand and had never seen before. I asked an interpreter to explain to me what was happening. She said, "It's a change of shift." I began to understand this pattern of occupation in the daily work of the people. Those employed at each building were coming together as one group was exiting and another group was entering the work environment. They completed twice daily Tai Chi exercises to prepare before entering their workday and again before leaving work.

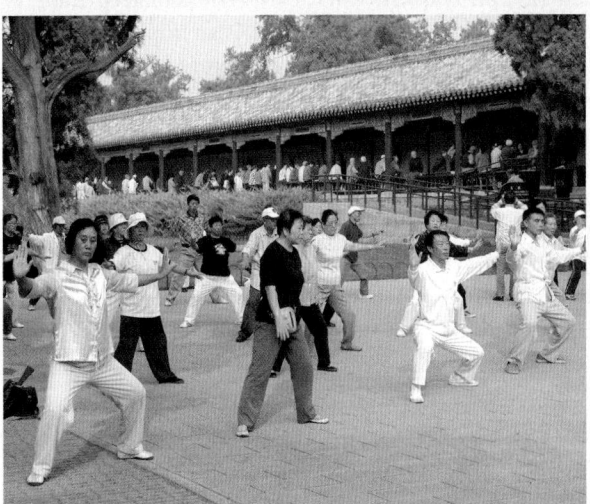

Tai Chi is practiced throughout China.

Before I understood this concept, I interpreted collectivism as individual disinterest in becoming independent. I did not understand that I was asking the person to disconnect from others. I was not coherent about how important it was to them, their community, and their well-being to follow the collectivist way to recovery from injury. I learned to appreciate that an individual who is part of a collectivist group requires a different approach to therapy services. When a person is injured or impaired, the group comes together to help the person, and roles are often assumed for a variety of supports the individual may need. It is important to include all members of the group that are potentially supporting the individual when determining patterns of occupation for the person at all phases of the therapy process. If the role of one person is to do all self-care for the other once they become injured, it is vital for them to be part of the therapy process that leads to independence with self-care for the individual.

environment, and social and community context. SDH impact health in positive and negative ways depending on the level of access to quality medical care, safe housing, education, employment, healthy food, transportation, and community participation. Access to these factors is shaped by the distribution of power and resources at local, national, and global levels. The unfair and avoidable differences in access to these factors result in health disparities among communities and countries (World Health Organization, 2021). SDH also have a significant influence on the roles, habits, routines, and rituals of individuals, groups, and populations.

Occupational Balance

OT was founded on the idea that practicing a kind of balanced rhythm between work, play, rest, and sleep leads to wholesome living (Meyer, 1977). OT is an important profession for addressing lifestyles in both preventive and restorative ways because of the expertise and understanding of occupational patterns. Lifestyles are unique patterns of everyday occupations including roles, habits, routines, and rituals and can lead to an overall life balance or imbalance with long-term consequences on health, well-being, and quality of life. **Occupational balance** refers to a perception that one's patterns of everyday occupations are satisfactory and include a range of meaningful occupations. **Life balance** is similar but uses words more commonly understood outside of the OT profession (Matuska, 2012; Matuska & Christiansen, 2009). *Life balance* is defined as "a satisfying pattern of daily activity that is healthful, meaningful, and sustainable to an individual within the context of his or her current life circumstances" (Matuska & Christiansen, 2008, p. 11).

The Life Balance Model (Matuska, 2012) depicts the relationships between occupational patterns, life outcomes, and the environment. Occupational patterns should enable people to meet important needs such as supporting biological health and physical safety (i.e., exercise, rest, medication management), contributing to positive relationships (i.e., friends and family), feeling engaged and challenged (i.e., hobbies, stimulating work), and creating a positive personal identity (i.e., caregiving, volunteering) (Matuska & Christiansen, 2008). When people are able to engage in

patterns of occupation that address all of these needs, they will perceive their lives as more satisfying, less stressful, and more meaningful, or *balanced*. People also need to have the skill to organize their time and energy in ways that enable them to meet their important personal goals and renewal (Matuska, 2012). In other words, life balance requires the skill to create a match between how much time one *desires* to engage in activities and how much time one *actually* engages in the activities that meet important needs.

Environmental factors may make it difficult to engage in a satisfactory pattern of occupations. Life balance positively correlates with having enough financial security to create a satisfactory life (Wagman et al., 2011). SDH such as safe housing and communities, access to clean water and healthy foods, and adequate sanitation, as well as access to education and employment, all contribute to one's sense of (or lack of) life balance. In addition to social determinants, a sense of belonging and acceptance of one's identity, free of racism, sexism, homophobia, and ageism impacts one's sense of well-being.

Finally, one's state of health impacts life balance. People who have disabilities experience life imbalance when they cannot participate in valued occupations because of physical or environmental barriers. An acute onset of shingles or a chronic condition such as diabetes may alter one's ability to experience life balance. For example, women with multiple sclerosis expressed how managing their health needs became a major factor in their lives and how they needed to make daily adaptations to continue doing things that were important to them (Matuska & Erickson, 2008). Their disease often dictated what their activity options were in a given day. People who do not have disabilities also experience life imbalance, and addressing this problem is an emerging role for OT practitioners. For example, people who are transitioning into retirement, caring for children and aging parents, single parents, and workaholics may benefit from coaching by an OT practitioner who could help them create more balanced patterns of occupation. To foster life balance for our clients, it is important for occupational therapists to understand how one's social, cultural, and economical contexts influence one's roles, habits, routines, and sense of life balance. See OT Story 13.2 for an example of a woman who has diabetes and hypertension.

OT STORY 13.2 KARINA

Karina is a 55-year-old woman who was referred to OT by her primary care physician for uncontrolled diabetes and hypertension. When the occupational therapist meets with Karina for the first time, they take a thorough occupational history, focusing particularly on Karina's habits and routines, and how they impact her ability to carry out health

management and other occupations relevant to managing her chronic conditions.

Karina lives in a townhouse with her husband, adult son and daughter, and 5-year-old grandson. She works the overnight shift stocking shelves at a grocery store where she has been employed for the past 8 years. She previously worked

OT STORY 13.2 KARINA (*continued*)

as a cashier, but 2 years ago changed her schedule to work overnight because it allows her to help care for her grandson, who has a developmental delay.

On a typical day, Karina leaves home at 11 PM for her 11:30 PM–7:30 AM shift at work. Before work, Karina has a "morning" routine during which she showers, takes her diabetes medication, and has a light meal such as eggs or toast with fruit. While at work, Karina is on her feet doing physically demanding work. She usually has a snack such as a yogurt or granola bar and a sports drink on her "lunch" break because she states "I need the energy to get through my shift" but does not like to eat a full meal because it gives her indigestion.

When Karina finishes her shift, she returns home to help her grandson get ready for school and then walks him to school. Upon returning home again, Karina has another light snack and gets ready for bed. She sleeps from around 9:00 AM to 2:30 PM, although her sleep is often disturbed by noise from people doing yardwork outside and traffic noise from the nearby expressway. She sometimes has difficulty sleeping because of neck and back pain caused by the repetitive lifting and reaching she does at work. After waking up, she walks to school to pick up her grandson at 3:00 PM and cares for him until his parents arrive home from work. Karina sometimes takes her grandson to the park or

to run errands before coming home to prepare dinner. Karina takes great pride in her cooking, and family dinners are a consistent routine in their household. Although she has tried to adjust her recipes to be mindful of nutrition recommendations to manage her diabetes and hypertension, her family loves her cooking and sometimes complains that her new versions of family favorites lack flavor.

After dinner, Karina usually watches television with her husband, reads magazines, or plays card games with her son and daughter. If she did not get enough sleep during the day, she sometimes naps before work, although she prefers not to because it makes her groggy. On the weekends, Karina does household chores, spends time with her family, and tries to catch up on sleep, but finds it difficult to fall asleep until late at night.

Questions

1. As Karina's occupational therapist, what routines and habits do you notice?
2. What is Karina doing to support her health?
3. Which habits and routines would you like to work on with Karina?

To find out how the occupational therapist worked with Karina, please refer to Chapter 51.

Lippincott® Connect *For additional resources on the subjects discussed in this chapter, visit Lippincott Connect.*

Conclusion

Roles, habits, routines, and rituals create the framework of people's lives and together make up lifestyles that are unique to each person. Well-being should be a consideration in any OT intervention. Are current lifestyle patterns contributing to a sense of overall well-being or taking away from a sense of well-being? When occupational patterns are dysfunctional, health and well-being are at risk. In turn, adapting or establishing satisfactory roles, habits, routines, and rituals may be used as tools in therapy to help a person improve life balance. OT practitioners can use the tools described in this chapter to work with clients to create new patterns that are satisfactory and contribute to their health. The desired outcome for any OT intervention is life satisfaction and improved quality of life.

For more specifics on interventions in these areas, see Chapter 51.

Acknowledgments

The authors of this chapter would like to acknowledge Beth Pyatak for writing the Karina OT Story. In addition, the authors would like to thank Dahlia Castillo for writing the Expanding Our Perspectives box.

REFERENCES

American Occupational Therapy Association. (2020). Occupational therapy practice framework: Domain and process—4th edition. *The American Journal of Occupational Therapy, 74*(Supplement_2), 741241 0010p1–7412410010p87. https://doi.org/10.5014/ajot.2020.74S2001

Bainbridge, H. T. J., & Broady, T. R. (2017). Caregiving responsibilities for a child, spouse or parent: The impact of care recipient independence on employee well-being. *Journal of Vocational Behavior, 101,* 57–66. https://doi.org/10.1016/j.jvb.2017.04.006

Black, M. M. (1976). Adolescent role assessment. *American Journal of Occupational Therapy, 30*(2), 73–79.

Boyce, W. T., Jensen, E. W., James, S. A., & Peacock, J. L. (1983). The family routines inventory: Theoretical origins. *Social Sciences Medicine, 17*(4), 193–200. https://doi.org/10.1016/0277-9536(83)90116-8

Braveman, B., Robson, M., Velozo, C., Kielhofner, G., Fisher, G., Forsyth, K., & Kerschbaum, J. (2005). *Model of occupational therapy clearinghouse.* https://moho-irm.uic.edu/default.aspx

Centers for Disease Control and Prevention. (2021). *Social determinants of health at CDC.* https://www.cdc.gov/socialdeterminants/about.html

Chugg, A., & Craik, C. (2002). Some factors influencing occupational engagement for people with schizophrenia living in the community. *British Journal of Occupational Therapy, 65*(2), 67–74. https://doi.org/10.1177/030802260206500204

Clark, F. (2000). The concepts of habit and routine: A preliminary synthesis. *OTJR: Occupation, Participation and Health, 20*(1), 123S–137S. https://doi.org/10.1177/15394492000200S114

Crepeau, E. B. (1995). Rituals. In C. B. Royeen (Ed.), *The practice of the future: Putting occupation back into therapy* (pp. 5–23). American Occupational Therapy Association.

Crepeau, E. B., & Schell, B. A. B. (2009). Analyzing occupations and activity. In E. B. Crepeau, E. S. Cohn, & B. A. B. Schell (Eds.), *Willard & Spackman's occupational therapy* (11th ed., pp. 359–374). Lippincott Williams & Wilkins.

Crowe, T. K., VanLeit, B., Berghmans, K. K., & Mann, P. (1996). Role perceptions of mothers with young children: The impact of a child's disability. *American Journal of Occupational Therapy, 51*(8), 651–661. https://doi.org/10.5014/ajot.51.8.651

Davies Hallet, J., Zasler, N. D., Maurer, P., & Cash, S. (1994). Role change after traumatic brain injury in adults. *American Journal of Occupational Therapy, 48*(3), 241–246. https://doi.org/10.5014/ajot.48.3.241

Denham, S. A. (2002). Family routines: A structural perspective for viewing family health. *ANS Advances in Nursing Science, 24*(4), 60–74. https://doi.org/10.1097/00012272-200206000-00010

Denham, S. A. (2003). Relationships between family rituals, family routines, and health. *Journal of Family Nursing, 9*(3), 305–330. https://doi.org/10.1177/1074840703255447

Fougeyrollas, P., Noreau, L., & St-Michel, G. (2001). *Life habits measure—Shortened version (LIFE-H 3.0)*. Canadian Society and Quebec Committee on the International Classification of Impairments, Disabilities, and Handicaps.

Friese, B. H. (2007). Routines and rituals: Opportunities for participation in family health. *OTJR: Occupation, Participation and Health, 27*(1), 41S–49S. https://doi.org/10.1177/15394492070270S106

Friese, B. H., Tomcho, T., Douglas, M., Josephs, K., Poltrock, S., & Baker, T. (2002). A review of 50 years of research on naturally occurring family routines and rituals: Cause for celebration. *Journal of Family Psychology, 16*(4), 381–390. https://doi.org/10.1037/0893-3200.16.4.381

Good-Ellis, M. A., Fine, S. B., Spencer, J. H., & DiVittis, A. (1987). Developing a role activity performance scale. *American Journal of Occupational Therapy, 41*(4), 232–241. https://doi.org/10.5014/ajot.41.4.232

Jackoway, I. S., Rogers, J. C., & Snow, T. L. (1987). The role change assessment: An interview tool for evaluating older adults. *Occupational Therapy in Mental Health, 7*(1), 17–37. https://doi.org/10.1300/J004v07n01_02

Jackson, J. (1998). Is there a place for role theory in occupational science? *Journal of Occupational Science, 5*(2), 48–55. https://doi.org/10.1080/14427591.1998.9686433

Jensen, E. W., James, S. A., Boyce, T., & Hartnett, S. A. (1983). The family routines inventory: Development and validation. *Social Science Medicine, 17*(4), 201–211. https://doi.org/10.1016/0277-9536(83)90117-X

Kielhofner, G. (2009). *Conceptual foundations of occupational therapy practice* (4th ed.). American Occupational Therapy Association.

Kielhofner, G., Fogg, L., Braveman, B., Forsyth, K., Kramer, J., & Duncan, E. (2007). A factor analytic study of the Model of Human Occupation Screening Tool of hypothesized variables. *Occupational Therapy in Mental Health, 25*(2), 127–137. https://doi.org/10.1080/01642120902856846

Lawrence, M. (2010). Young adults' experience of stroke: A qualitative review of the literature. *British Journal of Nursing, 19*(4), 241–248. https://doi.org/10.12968/bjon.2010.19.4.46787

Mathiowetz, V., Finlayson, M. L., Matuska, K., Chen, H. Y., & Luo, P. (2005). Randomized controlled trial of an energy conservation course for persons with multiple sclerosis. *Multiple Sclerosis, 11*(5), 592–601. https://doi.org/10.1191/1352458505ms1198oa

Mathiowetz, V., Matuska, K., & Murphy, M. (2001). Efficacy of an energy conservation course for persons with multiple sclerosis. *Archives of Physical Medicine and Rehabilitation, 82*(4), 449–456. https://doi.org/10.1053/apmr.2001.22192

Matuska, K. (2012). Validity evidence of a model and measure of life balance. *OTJR: Occupation, Participation and Health, 32*(1), 229–237. https://doi.org/10.3928/15394492-20110610-02

Matuska, K., & Christiansen, C. (2008). A proposed model of lifestyle balance. *Journal of Occupational Science, 15*(1), 9–19. https://doi.org/10.1080/14427591.2008.9686602

Matuska, K., & Christiansen, C. (Eds.). (2009). *Life balance: Multidisciplinary theories and research*. American Occupational Therapy Association.

Matuska, K., & Erickson, B. (2008). Lifestyle balance: How it is described and experienced by women with multiple sclerosis? *Journal of Occupational Science, 15*(1), 20–26. https://doi.org/10.1080/14427591.2008.9686603

Matuska, K., Mathiowetz, V., & Finlayson, M. (2007). Use and perceived effectiveness of energy conservation strategies for managing multiple sclerosis fatigue. *American Journal of Occupational Therapy, 61*(1), 62–69. https://doi.org/10.5014/ajot.61.1.62

Meyer, A. (1977). The philosophy of occupation therapy. Reprinted from the Archives of Occupational Therapy, Volume 1, pp. 1–10, 1922. *American Journal of Occupational Therapy, 31*(10), 639–642.

Monk, T. H., Flaherty, J. F., Frank, E., Hoskinson, K., & Kupfer, D. J. (1990). The Social Rhythm Metric: An instrument to quantify the daily rhythms of life. *Journal of Nervous and Mental Disease, 178*(2), 120–126. https://doi.org/10.1097/00005053-199002000-00007

Monk, T. H., Frank, E., Potts, J. M., & Kupfer, D. J. (2002). A simple way to measure daily lifestyle regularity. *Journal of Sleep Research, 11*(3), 183–190. https://doi.org/10.1046/j.1365-2869.2002.00300.x

Oakley, F., Kielhofner, G., Barris, R., & Reichler, R. (1986). The role checklist: Development and empirical assessment of reliability. *OTJR: Occupation, Participation and Health, 6*(3), l57–l70. https://doi.org/10.1177/153944928600600303

Parkinson, S., Forsyth, K., & Kielhofner, G. (2006). *The Model of Human Occupation Screening Tool (MOHOST) Version 2.0*. http://www.uic.edu/depts/moho/assess/mohost.htm

Poole, J., & Cordova, J. S. (2004). Dressing routines in women with chronic disease: A pilot study. *New Zealand Journal of Occupational Therapy, 51*(1), 30–35.

Radomski, M. V. (2011). More than good intentions: Advancing adherence to therapy recommendations. *American Journal of Occupational Therapy, 65*(4), 471–477. https://doi.org/10.5014/ajot.2011.000885

Reich, J. W. (2000). Routinization as a factor in the coping and the mental health of women with fibromyalgia. *OTJR: Occupation, Participation and Health, 20*(1), 41S–51S. https://doi.org/10.1177/15394492000200S104

Sanders, M. J., & Van Oss, T. (2013). Using daily routines to promote medication adherence in older adults. *American Journal of Occupational Therapy, 67*(1), 91–99. https://doi.org/10.5014/ajot.2013.005033

Segal, R. (2004). Family routines and rituals: A context for occupational therapy interventions. *American Journal of Occupational Therapy, 58*(5), 499–508. https://doi.org/10.5014/ajot.58.5.499

Synovec, C., & Aceituno, L. (2019). Social justice considerations for occupational therapy: The role of addressing social determinants of health in unstably housed populations. *Work, 65*(2), 235–246. https://doi.org/10.3233/WOR-203074

U.S. Department of State. (n.d.). *Reception and placement*. https://www.state.gov/refugee-admissions/reception-and-placement/

Wagman, P., Håkansson, C., Matuska, K., Björklund, A., & Falkmer, T. (2011). Validating the model of lifestyle balance on a working Swedish population. *Journal of Occupational Science*. Advance online publication. https://doi.org/10.1080/14427591.2011.575760

World Health Organization. (2021). *Social determinants of health*. https://www.who.int/teams/social-determinants-of-health

Young, M. (1988). *The metronomic society*. Harvard University Press.

Zautre, A. J., Hamilton, N., & Yocum, D. (2000). Patterns of positive social engagement among women with rheumatoid arthritis. *OTJR: Occupation, Participation and Health, 20*(1), 21S–40S. https://doi.org/10.1177/15394492000200S103

Zisberg, A., Young, H. M., & Schepp, K. (2009). Development and psychometric testing of the Scale of Older Adults' Routine. *Journal of Advanced Nursing, 65*(3), 672–683. https://doi.org/10.1111/j.1365-2648.2008.04901.x

Culture, Equality, Inclusion, Diversity, and Culturally Effective Care

Pablo A. Cantero Garlito, Daniel Emeric Meaulle, and Dahlia Castillo

"We are more alike, my friends, than unalike."

—MAYA ANGELOU

LEARNING OBJECTIVES

After reading this chapter, you will be able to:

1. Recognize the importance of cultural aspects in the practice of occupational therapy.
2. Explore how diversity is embedded in human occupations.
3. Understand the potential for safer, more inclusive, and more relevant interventions for service users.
4. Analyze the need for cultural awareness and culturally effective practice in occupational therapy.

Introduction

Over the past century, the world has changed significantly, and although occupational therapy (OT) has developed and grown, the emphasis on treatment and care for the individual has remained constant. A century ago, the language of culture including justice, equity, diversity, and inclusion was not found in OT literature, but early recognition of and sensitivity to client uniqueness found in the first set of standards for the profession (1920) set the foundation for today's focus on culturally effective care. At the third annual meeting of the National Society for the Promotion of Occupational Therapy, when developing the guidelines and standards for education, the committee stated that OT students "should know a little about the different racial groups, their habits, customs, beliefs, etc., in order to work with them more sympathetically and intelligently" (National Society for the Promotion of Occupational Therapy, 1919, p. 23). Although working with diverse clients and practitioners was not a focus in the early years of the profession, the creation of the World Federation of Occupational Therapists in 1951 pushed the profession to learn about and from a variety of countries and their people, expanding the worldview of US OT practitioners, educators/scholars, and scientists.

Understanding the strengths diversity brings to the profession has been of increasing interest, especially in the past two decades, for OT practitioners, researchers, and educators (Beagan & Chacala, 2012; Grenier et al.,

2020; Hammell, 2019). As a result, OT is widening its field of vision and adapting to the specific needs of individuals, groups, and communities. Likewise, the discipline has broadened the implementation of services and intervention programs to a variety of social, political, and cultural contexts (Balanta-Cobo et al., 2022; Fryer et al., 2019).

Although it may seem that this collective interest implies that the discipline of OT developed without sufficient sensitivity toward diversity, the profession has been working on these issues for many years (Iwama, 2004). However, the historical, political, and cultural aspects that undermine OT's capacity to meet the needs of people from nondominant communities are vast. As stated by Agner (2020), we need a paradigm shift to move from cultural competence to cultural humility. We must acknowledge that the road already traveled, especially regarding other sources and forms of knowledge generation and validation for the profession, remains insufficient (Agner, 2020; Sonn & Vermeulen, 2018).

In this chapter, we intend to contribute to a necessary critique and, above all, to generate a necessary debate that helps identify the problematic points that need attention. We attempt to point the way to a new, more open, and plural collective conscience that truly attends to the needs of those who have been traditionally left in the margins.

General Concepts

Culture

The concept of culture can have different meanings depending on the epistemologic or contextual point of view. Iwama (2004) states that culture is a "slippery concept, taking on a variety of definitions and meanings depending on how it has been socially situated and by whom" (p. 1). Yet, OT students and practitioners alike must have an understanding of what culture means. In the field of anthropology, *culture* is a common noun "indicating a particular way of life, of people, of a period, or of a human group" (Cardona & Agudelo, 2005, p. 86). In sociology, it is understood as "the abstract concept that describes processes of intellectual, spiritual and aesthetic development" of human affairs, including science and technology (Cardona & Agudelo, 2005, p.86). Fischer (1992, p.46) points out the sociologic perspective wherein *culture* is defined as "the intellectual and social progress of man in general, of collectivities, of humanity." However, more contemporary conceptualizations of culture point to understanding it as a set of meanings in an act of communication, both objective and subjective, between the mental processes that create the meanings and a significant environment or context. This is what Clifford Geertz stated when he said: "The concept of culture that I advocate . . . is essentially a semiotic concept. Believing with Max Weber that man is an animal embedded in webs of

meaning that he himself has woven, I consider that culture is that warp, and that the analysis of culture must therefore be, not an experimental science in search of laws, but an interpretative science in search of meanings" (Geertz, 2009, p. 5).

From an overall health perspective, Purnell and Fenkl (2019) define culture as "the totality of socially transmitted behavior patterns, beliefs, values, customs, lifeways, arts, and all other products of human work and thought characteristics of a population of people that guide their worldview and decision making" (p. 1). Furthermore, they state that the following attributes affect each person's worldview:

- Nationality
- Race
- Skin color
- Gender
- Age
- Religious affiliation
- Educational status
- Socioeconomic status
- Occupation
- Military experience
- Political beliefs
- Urban versus rural residence
- Enclave identity
- Marital status
- Parental status
- Physical characteristics
- Sexual orientation
- Gender issues
- Health literacy
- Length of time away from country of origin
- Reason for migration (sojourner, immigrant, or undocumented status)

Therefore, **culture** can be thought of as the interconnection of significant meanings we use to understand the phenomena or events of everyday life. It is not limited to ethnicity or race or simple expressions, such as dress or rituals. Castro and colleagues (2014), aiming to identify and describe how culture is expressed as a broad phenomenon, found that OT was at a crossroad between traditional taken-for-granted approaches based on Western and English-speaking perspectives and critical, more complex approaches that recognize multiple perspectives and the dynamic nature of culture. A complex view of culture allows the profession to address the political, ethical, and theoretical issues necessary to achieve the desired diversity that is essential to gain relevance in practice (Braveman & Gottlieg, 2014; Castro et al., 2014; Esquerdo et al., 2015; Iwama et al., 2009; Muñoz, 2014). For a glimpse at a few cultures from around the world, see Expanding Our Perspectives. See also the following Expanding Our Perspective features in other chapters:

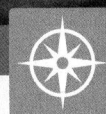

EXPANDING OUR PERSPECTIVES

Glimpses of Several Cultures

Recognizing that culture is multifaceted and dynamic, we present the perspectives of eight individuals and their respective cultures in their own words. A snapshot of their culture is presented along with considerations for OT practitioners.

isiXhosa Culture

Bongisa Shumane

My dominant culture is the isiXhosa—amaHlubi clan. The Xhosa people are recognized as part of the larger Nguni ethnic collective of the so-called Bantu people of sub-Saharan Africa, located predominantly in the Eastern Cape Province in South Africa. Within the Xhosa nation, there are various tribes that share traditional cultural practices, philosophies, and language dialects. These tribal variations are identifiable through the geographical location of the tribe within the Eastern Cape Province, and they present nuances in language dialects, traditional cultural practices, and philosophies. There is an idiom in isiXhosa that goes as "zikhala ngokhala ziphuma intabenye," which can then be directly translated into English as "they sound differently but come from the same mountain."

I identify with this culture because this is the culture I was born into, the culture that bred me to be the humble human that I am. Xhosa people are known to be fierce and upright. The Xhosa culture values respect for everyone, honesty toward self and others, and humility toward the community. I identify with these cultural values, and I espouse these philosophies in all my personal and professional interactions. These cultural values have enabled me as a therapist to form positive relationships with the healthcare users that I have worked with. These relationships are rooted in mutual respect and mutual appreciation of the therapeutic process that allows for shared growth and strengthens the potential of recovery.

Common traits/customs in my culture begin with gender-appropriate dress code, and when meeting others, one offers their hand for a handshake (customary greeting) and then facing the person that you are speaking to or addressing albeit in some cases when addressing an older adult, one might minimize eye contact.

An OT practitioner working with a member of my culture should remember:

1. *Respect:* The appropriate way of addressing individuals within their respective gender-related ages—mama, tata, bhuti, and sisi—is very important.
2. *Greet:* Greeting is very important to acknowledge that you see their presence (and the space they occupy and the space you are accessing). "Molo" for one person, or "Molweni" for a group, is the most common way of greeting people.
3. *Humility:* Humility and respect are very important. One should humble themselves and their opinion to show respect; this could mean that one must be quite conscious of their choice of words. The words that you utilize when addressing an older adult may be vastly different to when you are speaking to your peer group.

LGBTQ Culture

Cheranne Hunter Bennett

My dominant culture is the lesbian, gay, bisexual, transgender, questioning/queer community (LGBTQ). I am part of this community because I identify as a lesbian.

More recently, LGBTQ culture has embraced other communities, including persons who are asexual and intersex. In addition, the acronym often includes a + sign at the end to recognize individuals who identify as part of the LGBTQIA community but who do not necessarily identify with one of the defined labels. There is no monolithic LGBTQIA+ experience to point to, and there can be many other intersections of culture that impact individuals within this community. Within each layer of experience, an individual might have to endure oppression and struggles that are compounded. Each of these layers has its own implications for the health and well-being of your clients.

The overarching similarity between people who identify as part of the LGBTQIA+ culture is that we all have the experience of people assuming we are or *should be* part of the heteronormative society; therefore, we *and/or* our identities can be ignored. Our families, often "families of choice," are overlooked or undervalued when it comes to important life experiences and choices. In the instances when our sexuality or non-normative gender identity *is* recognized, people overlay heteronormative assumptions that limit the outsider's perspective.

(continued)

EXPANDING OUR PERSPECTIVES (continued)

An occupational therapist working with a member of my culture should remember the following:

1. Never assume the person before you is part of the heteronormative culture. Maintain an open mind and an open heart.
2. It is often not easy for the LGBTQIA+ individual to talk to you about their family relationships.
3. All persons within the LGBTQIA+ culture do not have the same experiences, and consideration should be given to identify intersectional experiences (e.g., socioeconomic status, gender, race, disability status, religious affiliation) that may compound oppression.

Native South Texas Mestizo (Hispanic) Culture

Dahlia Castillo

My dominant culture is Native South Texas Mestizo, also known as *Hispanic*. I identify with this culture because I was born in the southern part of Texas, USA, that was part of Mexico until a battle when the border moved south to the Rio Grande River. *Mestizo* is a term whereby Spanish conquerors mixed with natives.

Common customs in my culture are Catholicism, large extended family (that frequently attend appointments), and large family celebrations with attendance expectations. It is common for one or more family members to care for an ill family member, often taking turns.

An OT practitioner working with a member of my culture should remember the following:

1. Know their dominant language before initiating care. If it is not English, learn and practice the proper pronunciation for a greeting common in the region, followed by "No hablo espanol" (I don't speak Spanish).
2. Often, a family member will provide care and make decisions for the ill loved one. Always ask if there are one or more family members to include. Do not assume the client does not want to become independent; they might be adhering to long-held family roles and traditions. Cautiously proceed with educating the person and family on the benefits of improved independence.
3. When providing care in a home, you may be offered food and drink. They might take offense if you reject their hospitality and decline return visits.
4. Understand cultural nuances as they vary by region.

Culture of an African American Islamic Woman Who Has Experienced Homelessness

Richetta C as Told to Lee Westover

I am an African American woman. My dominant cultures are being an African American woman, homelessness, drug use, and Islam. I identify with this culture because I am an African American woman who has experienced homelessness and drug use. I identify with Islam because it gets me closer to God.

Common traits/customs in my culture include prayer, which is an important ritual in the day. I have learned to be more self-aware in order to not repeat my mistakes.

An OT practitioner working with a member of my culture should remember the following:

1. *Be flexible:* Meeting someone where they are in life is important because I feel that you never know what people are going through. Many people in my position have experienced physical abuse, sexual abuse, emotional abuse, or abandonment. You have to let them talk about themselves when they are ready. Bad experiences can make people distrustful, and building trust takes time.
2. *Respect:* Respect is important because you want your client to feel understood. They should never feel like you are looking down on them or know more than them. I spent 20 years sleeping on cardboard on the concrete. But I want the same things that you do—family, a safe place to live, education, and good relationships. Even though I have been through hardships, I have a whole life of experience and resources. Sometimes, I might have better resources than my provider.
3. *Compassion:* I may be in need of compassion. Sometimes, I just need to talk. Take your time to get to know me and learn what I am really like before you judge me. Sometimes, what you read in a book is not what real life looks like. Be open to listening about my experiences and believe me, not what you have heard about me.

Japanese Culture

Asako Matsubara

My dominant culture is Japanese. I identify with this culture because I value belonging and group harmony.

Common traits/customs in my culture are as follows:

- The "prime mover" may be located external to the self in the social frame, and the social situation strongly influences the interpretation, initiation, and shape of human agency.
- Belonging rather than doing may be the social ethos, and harmony between self and others is the cornerstone.
- People may be strongly reliant on the "here and now," rather than future oriented.

An occupational therapist working with a member of my culture should remember the following:

1. Family and the social situation may strongly influence decision-making when you decide something with clients because the prime mover of them may be located external to the self in the social frame.

EXPANDING OUR PERSPECTIVES (continued)

2. Clients may not like to do something different from other people because they may value group harmony.
3. It may be hard for clients to decide their goals because they may not be future oriented.
4. Some clients may be model patients and receive instructions from OT practitioners passively and obediently.

Mormon Culture

Tamara Turner

My dominant culture is Mormon. I identify with this culture because I belong to the Church of Jesus Christ of Latter-day Saints.

Common traits/customs in my culture are weekly church attendance, ministering to (checking in and helping out) those in our congregation. We often have a church calling (service assignment) that may involve teaching, running activities, or other service assignments. Commonly, children are baptized at the age of 8, can begin to attend the temple at the age of 11 or 12, and serve as full-time missionaries at 18 or 19. Christmas and Easter are important holidays, celebrating Christ's birth and death.

An OT practitioner working with a member of my culture should remember the following:

- Modesty is important, and the client may not want to undress or even wear sleeveless clothing in the gym. In addition, many people of my culture wear religious underclothes, called *temple garments*, that are to be kept sacred. If a client wants to wear their temple garments, the bottoms can go over incontinence briefs and the tops under a bra.
- Family responsibilities, weekly church attendance, church responsibilities, and community service are important roles and occupations.
- We have a health code that prohibits tobacco, coffee, tea, and alcohol, so dining and cooking may look a little different.
- Saying the name of God or Jesus Christ as an expletive, swear words, and other crass language may make the client uncomfortable.
- Keeping the sabbath day holy may mean they would prefer not to participate in therapy on Sundays.

Disability Culture

Dot Nary

I identify with disability culture for so many reasons. The main reason is that it supports a change in social culture that is making the United States and the world acknowledge disability as a common human condition and understand that disabled people deserve respect and accommodation as full participants in society. Disability culture embraces social justice and is reflected in the political, cultural, and personal spheres (Shakespeare, 1996). As disability activists demand change, as the arts reflect and interpret the lived experience of disability, and as people with disabilities acknowledge their shared experience of discrimination and resilience and their contributions to society, the world is a better place for all. My life is certainly enriched owing to disability culture.

Common traits/customs in my culture are the rejection of shame that has historically been associated with living with a disability, refusal to accept the second-class citizenship that has been assigned to this population, a demand for equity, and an acknowledgment of the need to educate and advocate to continue changing society. I would add that most disabled people who embrace disability culture acknowledge a responsibility to continue to improve opportunities for future generations of disabled people (e.g., by protecting and strengthening the Americans with Disabilities Act [ADA]) and to embrace intersectionality.

An OT practitioner working with a member of my culture should remember the following:

1. Not all disabled people would use the word "disabled" to describe themselves. Many are apolitical. They may not be familiar with the concept of disability culture, even though they benefit from it and would likely embrace it, if they understood the bigger picture. For example, some people deride the "militarism" of disability activists but certainly benefit from requirements of the ADA, such as accessible public accommodations.
2. Disabled people need allies who understand the importance of disability culture and support the social change that is needed (see Forber-Pratt et al., 2019). OT practitioners who understand the importance of disability culture and accessible communities should take any opportunity to educate their patients.

Mad and Neurodivergent Culture

Aster Harrison (They/Them pronouns)

I identify as Mad, neurodivergent, chronically ill, and disabled. I am also White, bisexual, nonbinary/genderqueer, and transgender. All of these identities are important to who I am as a person.

Here I focus on Mad and neurodivergent identities. I identify with Mad and neurodivergent identities because they give me a powerful way of understanding myself beyond the medical model. In medical terms, I am someone who has mental illness diagnoses. But my identity is so much more than diagnosis—the cultural, social, and political aspects of my Mad and neurodivergent identities are much more important to me.

Being part of Mad and neurodivergent communities has given me a way to understand my Madness and

(continued)

neurodivergence in a neutral or even positive light. Medical views of mental illness tend to be negative—portraying it as something to recover from or overcome. But many people see their mental differences as a natural and beautiful form of diversity. Many of us even see positive aspects to our Madness and/or neurodivergence and do not wish to eliminate our Mad or neurodivergent traits.

Within Mad and neurodivergent communities, we respect that there are many, many different ways of being and behaving in the world. We try to offer flexibility to each other to show up in different ways to meet our own access needs and personal preferences. We try to set up spaces where people can participate remotely or in-person, where stimming and sensory toys are welcome, and where different forms of communication (e.g., talking, typing, signing) are possible. We understand that some people might need more time or more support to get something done on a particular day.

We also acknowledge the role of oppression and trauma in creating mental distress. Many of us have distressing symptoms because of experiences of violence, oppression, and discrimination, which have left their traces on our bodies and/or minds. We work to take collective action against multiple forms oppression and support many forms of healing.

One of the most important things about our communities is the acknowledgment of diversity. Mad and neurodivergent people think about their Madness and neurodivergence in a million different ways. Some people want treatment, and others do not. Some people feel positively about their Madness or neurodivergence, and others do not. Our feelings about and experiences of our identities may shift over our lifetimes. We also have a wide variety of other intersecting identities—race, class, gender, religion, and sexuality—which affect our experiences of Madness and/or neurodivergence. No two people will have exactly the same experience of Madness or neurodivergence.

An occupational therapist working with a member of my culture should remember the following:

1. Mad and neurodivergent people are the experts of our own needs. When we tell you something about our brains or our access needs, listen.

2. Mad and neurodivergent people experience accessibility barriers. Environments are often not designed in inclusive ways for us. OT practitioners can help brainstorm and design disability accommodations and environmental modifications. OT practitioners can also advocate for disability rights, accommodations, and accessibility.

3. Mad and neurodivergent people experience discrimination and bias. Sanist bias is also built into the world around us in media, language, and policies. OT practitioners can work to question sanism within ourselves, our profession, and our world.

4. Not everyone wants to be cured or to minimize their Mad or neurodivergent traits. Many of us have pride in our Madness and neurodivergence. Everyone thinks about their identity differently and has the right to self-definition and self-determination.

5. Many Mad and neurodivergent people have experienced being medicalized or psychiatrized in a way that healthcare providers made decisions for us against our wishes. Being a trauma-informed OT practitioner requires returning power to Mad and neurodivergent people to make decisions about our own care—including respecting our right to refuse care we do not want.

Equality and Equity

The concepts of equality and equity are often used interchangeably to refer to the issue of social justice or injustice. But they are different.

The concept of **equality** arises from the recognition of others as equals, in that everyone is entitled to the same rights, resources, and opportunities as any other human being. On the other hand, **equity** recognizes that individuals and groups of people have different circumstances and needs. Therefore, to achieve the same outcome, different resources and opportunities are necessary (see Figure 14.1). The inclusion of ramps and elevators for public buildings is an example of the application of principles of equity for wheelchair users. In another example of equity, during the pandemic when children were receiving their education online, some communities provided free Wi-Fi hot spots and computers or tablets to children without access. These concepts help us understand the complex reality of public policies that create situations of inequality and inequity affecting the daily lives of many.

In this sense, it is worth mentioning the concept of *affirmative action*, which involves developing actions to improve the daily lives of certain populations who have experienced disadvantages. Such groups are "affected by a systematic and persistent state action that produces a specific result: placing the group in a position of disadvantage so deep that even if the barriers and discriminatory norms are eliminated and even if the same rights are guaranteed, that group will not be able to get out of its disadvantaged

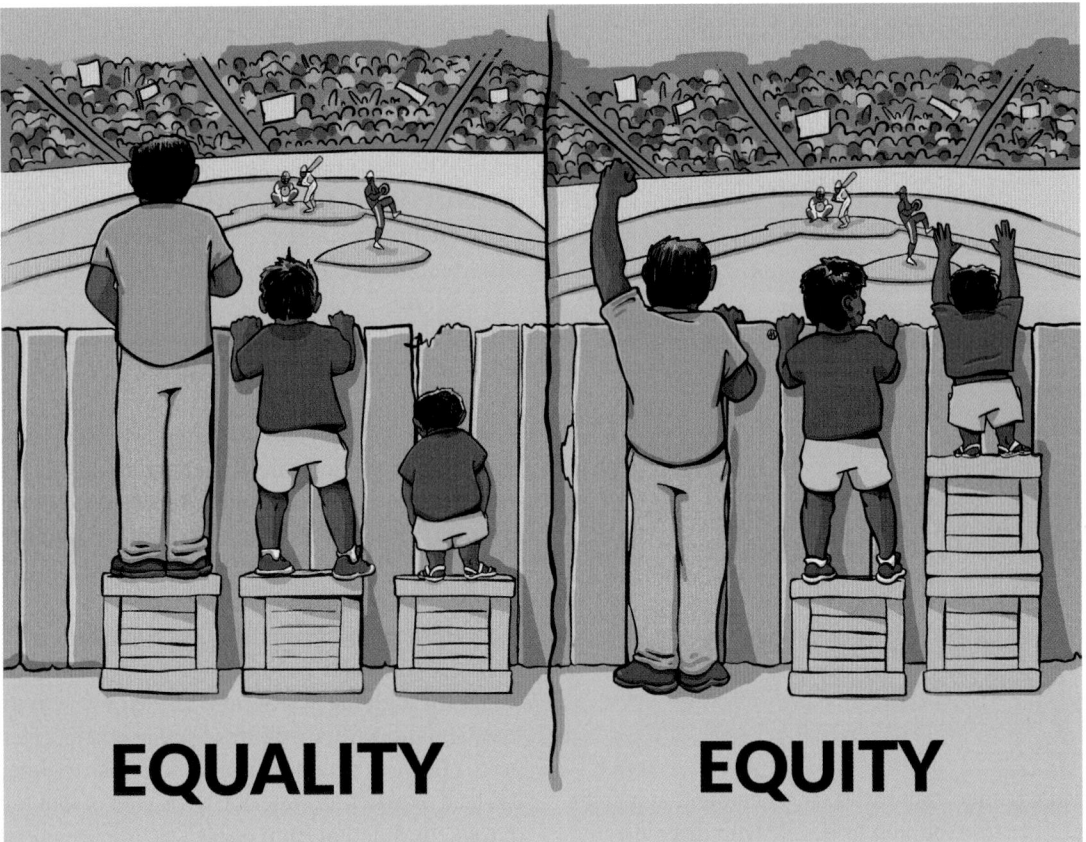

FIGURE 14.1 Illustration of equality versus equity.

(Courtesy of Interaction Institute for Social Change | Artist: Angus Maguire.)

situation or it could take a very long time" (Figueroa, 2015, pp. 195–196). Examples of affirmative action include setting aside slots for college admission for Black students in the United States at institutions where they were denied admissions in the past or targeting job advertisements to women for positions in which few women are working.

In relation to the practice of OT, Hammell (2015) raised how interesting it could be to incorporate the capabilities approach of the economist Amartya Sen and the philosopher Martha Nussbaum. Hammel states:

> It encourages us to consider, not just the abilities of disabled people and those with mental health issues, but their opportunities to envision, choose and accomplish what they wish to do and be. It incites us [OT practitioners] to refocus our endeavours, from solely endeavouring to change the abilities of individuals, to addressing the inequitable factors that determine the possibilities and the opportunities available to disadvantaged people to develop and exercise their abilities and attain their occupational rights. (Hammell, 2015, p. 83)

Inclusiveness

The concept of inclusive care in OT is multifaceted and requires that practitioners provide services that foster engagement in meaningful occupations. Inclusion includes aspects of full citizenship with access to resources in the community, connections with self-selected, reciprocal social networks, and opportunities to be a productive member of society. Therapists should repeatedly self-reflect to ensure they are providing services to everyone in an accepting manner that allows for a sense of belonging and inclusion.

The Commission of the European Communities (2003) defined *social inclusion* as "a process which ensures that those at risk of poverty and social exclusion gain the opportunities and resources necessary to participate fully in economic, social, political, and cultural life and to enjoy a standard of living that is considered normal in the society in which they live" (p. 9).

Gaining a better understanding of inclusiveness requires review of its origins from exclusion, a form of discrimination. Although the dynamic contexts of economic, political, and social dimensions are taken into consideration (Table 14.1), exclusion can be simply described ". . . as the process through which individuals or groups are wholly or partially excluded from full participation in the society within which they live" (Rawall, 2009, p. 164).

The set of potential qualities or individual differences that may be used as a justification or argument to limit, exclude, alienate, or segregate the occupational participation of individuals or communities is such that it should be

TABLE 14.1	Elements of Social Exclusion	

Axes	Dimensions	Aspects
Economic	Productive employment	• Lack of employment • Lack of income opportunities • Limited financial resources
	Consumerism	• Poverty • Deprivation of basic needs
Political	Citizenship	• Inequality • Inequitable access to resources • Voting restrictions • Political passivity
	Social citizenship	• Limited access to social protection systems: health, housing, and education
Social	Social ties	• Social isolation • Lack of social support
	Social relations	• Social conflict/violence • Family conflict (domestic violence) • Vulnerability to exploitation

reconsidered whether "minorities" are the potential beneficiaries of OT because the sum of people with diverse living conditions who experience some kind of occupational injustice or deprivation in the exercise of their occupational rights constitutes the vast majority of humanity.

The relationship between social exclusion and health is intertwined. Exclusion can lead to emotional distress, altered mood, decreased self-esteem, and a decreased sense of belonging (Mahar et al, 2013). Difficulties accessing certain goods intimately linked to independent selection of daily life choices (food, clothing, housing), the lack of paid work for long periods of time, or the performance of occupations in exploitative conditions negatively affect people's health. Similarly, frequently, limitations exist for people with disabilities or illness because of a lack of resources, resulting in inequality and social exclusion (Fundación FOESSA, 2019).

When providing inclusive services, having a connection is key to better outcomes. It is vital to incorporate both acceptance and a sense of belonging for each client served. Acceptance can best be described as a range on a continuum from simply tolerating another person to actively and intentionally including them (Leary, 2010). Mahar and colleagues (2013, p. 1026) define a "sense of belonging as a subjective feeling of value and respect derived from a reciprocal relationship to an external referent that is built on a foundation of shared experiences, beliefs, or personal characteristics. These feelings of external connectedness are grounded to the context or referent group, to whom one chooses, wants, and feels permission to belong. This dynamic phenomenon may be either hindered or promoted by complex interactions between environmental and personal factors."

Stereotyping and Ethnocentrism

Prejudice is often the result of *stereotyping* and *ethnocentrism*. **Stereotyping** occurs when one attributes certain characteristics to an entire group of people, or what Herbst (1997) defines as "an exaggerated image of their characteristics, without regard to individual attributes" (p. 212). These can be thoughts about people related to age, race, gender, sexuality, occupation, ethnicity, and physical and mental abilities.

Many of us have been raised in a society that teaches us stereotypical concepts. Although we often cannot control these thoughts, which are often unconscious, it is important to be aware of them and then choose not to listen to or act on them. This kind of thinking, which negates the importance of recognizing the uniqueness of each individual, may develop into prejudicial beliefs.

Ethnocentrism, on the other hand, is the "tendency of people to put their own group (*ethnos*) at the center; to see things through the narrow lens of their own culture and use the standards of that culture to judge others" (Herbst, 1997, p. 80). This is a common human response to difference and can lead to beliefs of superiority. Instead of looking at someone who is different from oneself as unique, interesting, and someone to learn about and from, a person with an ethnocentric viewpoint would judge the other person to be less than, not as good as, or inferior to oneself. It is apparent that this combination of stereotyping and ethnocentrism can promote prejudice that can lead to discrimination.

Diversity

Diversity, in modern usage, often refers to the inclusion of a wide variety of human differences with some sort of organization or institution (Hammell, 2019; Kinébanian & Stomph, 2010). From a traditional OT perspective, interest in diversity has always been present with a distinct focus on a concrete and specific interpretation of diversity: the existence of people whose different abilities derived from a particular disease and/or disability conditioned their performance in daily activities. Historically, however, the field was shaped by group leaders of nondiverse, predominantly White, Western backgrounds. Ethnocentric bias influenced OT practice, and until 2020, the profession neither explicitly placed value on diverse views nor intentionally sought to include varying perspectives (American Occupational Therapy Association [AOTA], 2020a; Kronenberg, 2021). Hammell (2019), in her keynote address at the Congress of the WFOT, addressed the development of OT concepts from the perspective of enculturation and English language supremacy and points out that our theories, models, assessments, and interventions have been formulated by people from areas considered high-income regions that comprise

20% of the population, a statistical minority. Theories on culture evolved from European colonialism and North American imperialism, without consideration for 80% of the world population residing in middle- and low-income regions. Nevertheless, we have an opportunity, as we embrace diversity, to grow as a profession and have a more relevant and significant impact globally.

The WFOT urges OT practitioners to increase their horizons of understanding about diversity individually and collectively in clinical, research, and teaching settings as well as in the institutional actions of occupational therapists worldwide. Kinébanian and Stomph (2010) identified four essential principles related to diversity and culture for OT professionals that include perspectives of both those we treat and those being educated in the OT profession:

1. *Diversity matters: the facts.* All societies have diverse populations requiring each OT practitioner to become familiar with people they encounter in their region. Therapists must consider disparities and differences with both those we serve and the professionals providing OT services that include, but are not limited to, gender, race, ethnicity, education level, income level, social class, able-bodied, non–able-bodied, sexual orientation, gender identify, and religious beliefs (AOTA, 2020b; Hammell, 2019; Kinébanian & Stomph, 2010; Wells et al., 2016). In addition, to reduce the disparity between professionals and those we serve, there is a need to advocate for a balance in workforce diversity of OT practitioners.

2. *Human rights and inclusiveness matter.* The right to meaningful participation in occupations of choice means inclusiveness is an ongoing process that warrants continual review. This means that OT practitioners need to have a sense of the individual and collective economic, political, and social dimensions that can interfere with inclusion and incorporate practices that ensure the individual dignity of everyone served. Moreover, academic institutions can contribute to the goal of becoming an inclusive profession by reviewing and reflecting on ways to intentionally admit and educate students from diverse backgrounds (AOTA, 2020b; Hammell, 2019; Kinébanian & Stomph, 2010; Kronenberg, 2021; United Nations, 1948).

3. *Language matters: the power of words.* It is important to be aware of personal biases and recognize past injustices and damages experienced by persons we serve and colleagues we work with. By avoiding professional jargon, and intentionally ascertaining if the messages sent are the same as messages received, OT practitioners can provide more culturally effective care. In both the professional and academic settings, mindfulness of the power language has on others is vital to ensure positive communication. Interactions can improve with individual awareness of potential stereotyping, judgmental,

and harmful discriminatory practices that can be associated with verbal and nonverbal communication (Iwama, 2004; Kinébanian & Stomph, 2010; Wells et al., 2016).

4. *Competence matters: attitudes, knowledge, and skills.* Ongoing competence includes a multidimensional process where individual practitioners, students, researchers, and educators pledge to the self-directed and lifelong practice of advancing their own attitude, knowledge, and skills toward being more inclusive. This action requires that OT practitioners are not only sensitive to diversity issues they encounter but also actively engage in meaningful ways to improve their own conscientious delivery of care to all in an equitable and competent manner. In addition, competence includes routine and systemic review of policies in clinical, research, and academic settings that involve individuals from diverse backgrounds, to ensure procedures guiding practice are objectively addressing diversity, equity, and inclusion in an impartial, nondiscriminatory, and unbiased manner (AOTA, 2020b; Iwama, 2004; Kinébanian & Stomph, 2010; Wells et al. 2016).

Practice of a Culturally Effective Occupational Therapy

Official Positions

OT organizations around the world are guided by statements related to the scope of practice of OT. Table 14.2 provides the most relevant official documents linked to cultural, equality, inclusion, diversity, and nondiscrimination aspects. The official documents from the AOTA, Canadian Association of Occupational Therapists (CAOT), and WFOT show an individual and collective commitment to addressing culturally effective practices in clinical, academic, and research contexts by addressing the complex, interconnected, and dynamic nature as well as the essential need for diverse perspectives to provide more inclusiveness to those served in OT.

- *From AOTA:* "Occupational therapy practitioners must commit to addressing challenges through evidence-based solutions to promote growth and development of the profession of occupational therapy. As such, occupational therapy is poised to lead in diversity, equity, and inclusion to maximize the health, well-being, and participation of all people, groups, and populations" (AOTA, 2020a, p. 5).
- *From CAOT:* "These systemic oppressions compromise occupational justice for under-represented equity-seeking and deserving groups, including but not limited

TABLE 14.2 — Relevant Documents Related to Culture From Occupational Therapy Organizations

Organization	Relevant Documents
American Occupational Therapy Association (AOTA)	*Position papers* • Occupational Therapy's Perspective on the Use of Environments and Contexts to Facilitate Health, Well-Being, and Participation in Occupations (2015) *Statements* • Occupational Therapy in the Promotion of Health and Well-Being (2019) • Occupational Therapy Services for Individuals Who Have Experienced Domestic Violence (2017) • Occupational Therapy's Commitment to Diversity, Equity, and Inclusion (2020)
Canadian Association of Occupational Therapy (CAOT)	• Occupational therapy and Indigenous peoples (2018 revised) • Joint Position Statement on Inclusive Occupational Therapy Education for Persons with Disabilities CAOT & ACOTUP (2018) • In development: A new position statement on equity and justice (2022)
World Federation of Occupational Therapists (WFOT)	• Inclusive Occupational Therapy Education (2008) • Diversity and Culture (2010) • Environmental Sustainability, Sustainable Practice within Occupational Therapy (2012) • Human Displacement (2014) • Occupational Therapy in Disaster Preparedness and Response (DP8:R) (2014) • Occupational Therapy in Disaster Risk Reduction (DRR) (2016) • Occupational Therapy and Community-Centered Practice (2019) • Occupational Therapy and Human Rights (revised) (2019)

to those who identify as Indigenous, Black, racialized, 2SLGBTQIA+, disabled and with mental health conditions, Mad, Deaf, and those living with invisible/episodic/fluctuating conditions among others. We recognize that intersections of ableism, ageism, classism, citizenship status, colonialism, the gender binary, heteronormativity, racism, saneism, sexism and/or structural poverty & structural violence produce differential experiences and outcomes" (CAOT, 2022).

• *From WFOT:* ". . . Justice through human rights for all to develop our occupational capabilities and social inclusion as individuals and in communities. We strongly encourage conversations on rights, inclusion, and justice with the key point being to start with an occupational

lens or perspective for seeing that occupation is a human right and human rights are exercised in real life through everyday occupations" (Hocking et al., 2021, p. 5).

Racism in Occupational Therapy Practice

Working with people who are in need of OT services requires first being aware of both the existing diversity in the spaces in which our professional work is developed and the situations of oppression linked to them. It is necessary to acquire a critical awareness that leads professionals to recognize the imbalances of power that can be produced by many different factors.

In this regard, it is pertinent to consider issues related to racism and systemic racism that may perpetuate social inequalities and occupational injustices. Kronenberg (2018) defines *occupational apartheid* as systemic discrimination that deprives individuals, groups, or communities from meaningful participation in daily life owing to oppressive social mechanisms (racism, classicism, sexism, homophobia, xenophobia, ableism, neoliberal individualism). Kronenberg argues that occupational therapists should become political and work toward eliminating these disparities, not just for people with disabilities but for all people. This includes confronting our own ignorance and prejudices that may contribute to unjust practices and calls on OT practitioners to assume leadership roles in promoting the value of occupation (Kronenberg & Pollard, 2006).

There is a risk of assuming that OT practitioners, by action or omission, could be contributing to the normative molding of people's ways of doing, belonging, and becoming potentially leading to another barrier to access to occupational rights, in other words, occupational oppression. Therefore, effective attention to diversity requires awareness, humility, respect, collaboration, commitment, and action. Ultimately, OT practitioners need to identify oppressive practices and ideas embedded in our identity and to discern what is fair in relation to the limits of desire and individual freedoms. It seems pertinent to wonder if the construction of the theoretical body, the instructions for practice, and the training received by all OT practitioners sufficiently contemplate this perspective and prepare us to adequately respond to the occupational needs of any person or community in the world.

Given the relationship between discrimination, occupations, and everyday life, it seems pertinent to integrate this vision and apply an ethical framework to public and private life, to the individual and the collective, and to the personal and the institutional. Schools that train future generations of occupational therapists have an essential role to make a firmer, more conscious, and constant commitment to eradicate all types of discrimination that may affect the occupational rights of all populations. See OT Story 14.1.

OT STORY 14.1 UNDERSTANDING SOCIAL INEQUALITIES AND OCCUPATIONAL INJUSTICES

Teresa Ricado and Raymond Nubla

The following case study and questions were adapted from the *Reflection on Occupation and Race (ROAR)*[a] tool.

Pediatric Outpatient

Tom is a 6-year-old Black male in the first grade at a local elementary school. Tom is diagnosed with attention deficit hyperactivity disorder (ADHD) and sensory processing disorder (SPD). He has been attending weekly sessions at the outpatient sensory clinic for 2 months.

Tom lives with his very supportive biological grandmother and a 5-year-old brother. They live in a studio apartment within a low-income housing complex. Tom and his brother were placed in their grandmother's care through the foster care system after their father was murdered by the police 5 years ago. Their mother had difficulty coping with her husband's death and began using substances. A Child Protective Services (CPS) call was made, resulting in Tom and his brother being temporarily placed in their grandmother's care.

While at home, Tom enjoys playing sports, especially soccer, with his brother. Tom likes to color but only maintains engagement for several minutes before getting bored. His grandma takes them out to play at a park 1 to 2 times per week and often takes them to her community meetings as well. She is a strong advocate for community involvement and tries to influence her grandsons to do the same.

While at the clinic, Tom habitually runs into the ball pit without being prompted to do so. He demonstrates poor activity tolerance for tabletop activities, though he is never opposed to engaging in them when prompted. When sitting on a chair, Tom is typically fidgety and easily distracted. He often runs into the ball pit without warning when engaging in nonpreferred activities for extended periods of time.

Tom's grandmother takes him to the clinic and waits in the lobby with Tom's brother. Tom has difficulty transitioning from the therapy sessions and tries to hide in the ball pit.

Questions

1. What strengths does Tom have that support his occupational engagement?
2. What are Tom's barriers to occupational engagement (consider context, environment, client factors, etc.)?
3. How does race impact the occupations of Tom and his family (consider access, type of occupation, implicit biases, etc.)?
4. How can racial and cultural inequalities affect Tom and his family's engagement throughout the clinical process?

[a]Nubla, R., Ricado, T., Borillo, R. M., Chilana, H., Mong, S., & Gagui, J. (n.d.). *Reflection on Occupation and Race (ROAR)*.

Cultural Humility

Many concepts and terms have been named to identify the skills, attitudes, and processes needed to further the goal of attaining occupational justice. Table 14.3 defines terminology relevant to the practice of OT.

Cultural humility is becoming increasingly important in both the provision of health services and other care programs delivered in social and health contexts. Recognition of power imbalances between people served and professionals is critical to improving interactions among different

TABLE 14.3 Terminology Related to Cultural Humility

Term	Definition
Cultural responsiveness	Cultural responsiveness "communicates a state of being open to the process of building mutuality with a client and to accepting that the cultural-specific knowledge one has about a group may or may not apply to the person you are treating" (Muñoz, 2007, p. 274).
Cultural humility	"An attitude and process in which providers strive to address issues of power differences between professionals and clients and to value and respect clients by continuous engagement in self-reflection and self-critique as life-long learners and reflective practitioners" (Tervalon & Murray-García, 1998, p. 118).
Cultural intelligence	"The ability to interact effectively with culturally different clients, and it relies on cultural metacognition—knowledge of one's own attitudes, values, and skills and those of clients—to ensure effective encounters" (Thomas et al., 2008, p.125).
Cultural dexterity	Refers to skills that facilitate effective collaboration and communication among people across multiple dimensions of diversity (Berger & Berger, 2011). In healthcare contexts, it is the "ability to comprehend and understand and adapt to the needs of patients, colleagues, and learners from diverse social and cultural backgrounds" (Erhunmwunsee et al., 2019, p. 1289).
Cultural safety	"A sociopolitical idea about the unconscious and unspoken assumptions of power held by health providers over groups that have been historically marginalized. It is about the trust and safety a client experiences when treated with respect and understanding and included in the decision-making process. Providers recognize their own culture, beliefs, and attitudes and know that building trust and empowering clients require power sharing" (Canadian Association of Occupational Therapists, 2011, p. 2).

cultures in the various contexts in which professionals carry out their work. Cultural humility is further defined as "a process of openness, self-awareness, absence of ego, and incorporation of self-reflection and critique after interacting willingly with diverse people" (Foronda et al., 2016). Cultural humility is a process-oriented approach used to enhance practitioners' ability to provide person-centered care, whereas cultural competence is a content-oriented approach aimed at increasing practitioners' knowledge, confidence, and self-efficacy in communicating with and dealing with diverse people (Singh et al., 2022). Occupational therapists work in diverse practice settings and with diverse subjects, making cultural humility central to ensuring ethical practice. The discipline emphasizes respect for the dignity and value of each person and the notion that subjects are diverse and unique.

Recognizing power dynamics is critical to understanding and improving the processes involved and making a strong commitment to better people-centered practice and, ultimately, to enabling the reduction of health inequalities. To this end, it is essential that the concept of cultural humility be incorporated into current training to better prepare future occupational therapists to address social and healthcare challenges with culturally appropriate care (Chang et al., 2012). For example, AOTA (2020b) has introduced the "Educator's Guide for Addressing Cultural Awareness, Humility, and Dexterity in Occupational Therapy Curricula" that provides information, strategies, and resources to enhance students' knowledge, skills, and attitudes through intentional and effective curriculum design practices.

For an example of OT with cultural humility, see OT Story 14.2.

OT STORY 14.2 CHANGES NEEDED FOR THE ADEQUACY OF SOCIAL AND HEALTHCARE SERVICES FOR A MAN FROM A ROMANY FAMILY

Part 1

A request for intermediary services was received from a clinic for people with addiction problems in Madrid for help with a 40-year-old male from a Romany family. He was having significant difficulties developing a therapeutic relationship with the clinic staff and adhering to the treatment plan. In addition, the clinic staff felt that the man's family was interfering with the treatment plan. The clinic wanted help convincing the service user to comply with the professional recommendations and to limit the family's interference in the process. The staff was concerned that systematic noncompliance with the commitments could lead to the man's expulsion from the clinic.

The intermediary service is available to service users and their relatives as a support aimed at improving the person's state of health, the satisfaction of all parties involved in the treatment process, and communication with the team of clinic staff. The service takes place in the community environment of the service user, accompanied also by an intercultural agent of reference for the service user's community.

A complete analysis of the situation was carried out by the intermediary, who interviewed the clinic's professionals, the management of the clinic, the participant himself, and the members of his family he identified as significant and/or relevant.

The interventions in which the most difficulties were observed were the psychological follow-ups, appointments with the social worker, and visits with OT services.

In the interview, the service user indicated a significant lack of regard for the assessment processes carried out by the professionals, as well as to the documentation linked to the treatment, because he did not understand their usefulness. Likewise, the family identified bad experiences in accessing the clinic and their family member because they were not considered relevant. They, therefore, had conflicts with admission and security personnel.

On the other hand, there is an evident interest on the part of the family to solve the service user's problems through medication and the physician's intervention, but the relevance of other professionals in the treatment was unclear to them. The treatment plan was interpreted as an intrusion in the family's life habits and an imposition from another culture. The opinion of a family member of the service user was playing an important role in the family's decisions.

The service user did show interest in some aspects of the OT program, where he felt that the professional respected his interests and motivations, especially in matters related to musical activities and handicrafts, where the user would like to be more involved. In this instance, he felt that his family did not understand the relationship between these activities and his medical treatment.

Questions

1. What interventions would you carry out with the user and his family?
2. How would you work with the institution and professionals?

Part 2

After this analysis, the following actions were carried out with the institution, the professionals, the service user, and his family:

- A meeting was held with the clinic's management to convey the need to incorporate a greater understanding of the influence of cultural factors in the service user's treatment process.

OT STORY 14.2 CHANGES NEEDED FOR THE ADEQUACY OF SOCIAL AND HEALTHCARE SERVICES FOR A MAN FROM A ROMANY FAMILY (*continued*)

- Training and awareness-raising activities were carried out for the professional team, and specific counseling activities were offered as a follow-up by the intermediary.
- Security, reception, and auxiliary services personnel were involved in the training and awareness-raising actions, as they were relevant in the access and maintenance of people in the clinic.
- The clinic's professionals and auxiliary personnel were trained in conflict resolution and intercultural mediation tools.
- Certain criteria limiting the participation of families (e.g., a limitation on the number of family members attending the clinic, or the exclusive reference to close relatives) were subject to review.
- The bureaucratic process of access to the clinic was simplified and the administration of complex evaluation tools was postponed to a later stage, when the service user was already linked to the resource.
- A common communication strategy was developed by all the professionals in order to try to adapt the message to the capacities of the service user and his family. This communication included more precise, clear, and adapted explanations as to the relevance of tests, the need to document the progress of the case, to have some agreements in writing, and the potential benefits of nonpharmacologic treatment programs offered by the center.
- Priority was given to medical and pharmacologic interventions, which were clearly identified by the service user and his family as elements that would mobilize their participation.
- The link with the OT service was used to address the culture of the Romany community, to invite relevant community members to hold meetings with other families of the community that have had successful experiences in the

clinic, and to contribute to improving the coexistence in the clinic as an anchoring element to the treatment. The service user played a leading role in the organization of these meetings, which served to make visible to his family the meaning and contribution of participation in other nonpharmacologic treatments.
- Group meetings were held with other families, where shared group needs were highlighted. In this process, the need to address issues related to the precariousness of the neighborhood expressed by the families was highlighted. The institution and the professionals of the clinic mobilized with the families to address this issue.
- Together with the clinic management, a joint procedure for monitoring culturally sensitive practices was established. Posters provided by the intermediary service with antidiscrimination messages were obtained and placed in the clinic.
- Through a family-centered practice, small assumable milestones were defined in the process of modifying habits and routines of the service user and his environment. Modifications related to daily life activities were progressively included, trying to respect the meanings, rhythms, and decisions of all the people involved.

Questions

1. It is not unusual for some people to be more amenable to medical and pharmacologic approaches and skeptical of nonmedical interventions. As an OT, how might you approach these concerns with service users and family members?
2. Why was it important to include the broader community and other families when addressing the concerns related to this family and service user?

Conclusion

Many occupational therapists practice culturally effective care within clinical, education, and scholarly arenas with varying amounts of attention to the global occupational needs of communities served. However, more is needed to address the ever-changing dynamics of those we serve. It was not until the emergence of relatively recent postulates that the conceptualization of "diversity" reached a broader dimension in OT and the profession started to be interested in other aspects of discrimination that influence, interfere, or limit peoples' participation and occupational rights.

Individual and collective characteristics that have to do with skin color, culture, purchasing power, ethnicity, ideology, gender identity, faith, and sexual orientation,

among others affect a multitude of people, conditioning their participation in daily life activities. This fact makes it necessary for OT practitioners to take a more conscious and active role in the recognition of these particularities that could lead to processes of inequality, inequity, exclusiveness, stereotyping, ethnocentrism, hatred, and/or occupational discrimination on which we are called upon to intervene.

As has been argued throughout this chapter, beyond a technical competence related to the procedures or practices to be implemented by occupational therapists, diversity should be understood as a value inexorably linked to occupational identity. Consequently, taking diversity into consideration is a guiding ethical principle of professional OT. Without such consideration, it is impossible to develop a practice that is truly centered on people and/or communities. Moreover, the lack of attention and commitment to diversity can also lead to explicit acts of discrimination and occupational injustice promoted by occupational therapists themselves.

In this regard, in addition to the individual commitment assumed by each professional in their daily practice, the existence of institutional antidiscrimination policies is essential. These should be created and promoted by organizations representing OT with input from diverse perspectives at the local and international levels, by training schools for future generations of professionals, and by institutions or societies in charge of research and/or scientific dissemination. It is pertinent that the promotion of active policies in favor of diversity and the development of best practices in this matter become an institutional priority on which concrete actions are anchored.

The principles of sensitivity, security, intelligence, responsibility, and cultural humility should be applied to the discipline of OT itself and will improve culturally effective practices. This improvement is an important component of OT practice to ensure that we do not contribute to processes in which people's occupational identity could be denied owing to a lack of recognition, attention, and/or validation of their diversity. To avoid the denial of individual and collective occupational identity, it is important to adhere to the commitments derived from the explicit recognition of human rights among all. Only from this starting point can human occupation be articulated within safeguards of the occupational rights of all people necessary to guarantee the survival of future generations.

Acknowledgments

The authors would like to thank Roxie Black for content used here from earlier editions of the chapter.

Lippincott® Connect *For additional resources on the subjects discussed in this chapter, visit* Lippincott Connect.

REFERENCES

Agner, J. (2020). Moving from cultural competence to cultural humility in occupational therapy: A paradigm shift. *American Journal of Occupational Therapy, 74*(4), 7404347010p1–7404347010p7. https://doi.org/10.5014/ajot.2020.038067

American Occupational Therapy Association. (2020a). Occupational therapy's commitment to diversity, equity, and inclusion. *American Journal of Occupational Therapy, 74*(Suppl 3), 7413410030p1–7413410030p6. https://doi.org/10.5014/ajot.2020.74S3002

American Occupational Therapy Association. (2020b). Educator's guide for addressing cultural awareness, humility, and dexterity in occupational therapy curricula. *American Journal of Occupational Therapy, 74*(Suppl 3), 7413420003p1–7413420003p19. https://doi.org/10.5014/ajot.2020.74S3005

Balanta-Cobo, P., Fransen-Jaïbi, H., Gonzalez, M., Henny, E., Malfitano, A. P. S., & Pollard, N. (2022). Human and social rights and occupational therapy: The need for an intersectional perspective. *Cadernos Brasileiros de Terapia Ocupacional, 30.* https://doi.org/10.1590/2526-8910.ctoED302022032

Beagan, B. L., & Chacala, A. (2012). Culture and diversity among occupational therapists in Ireland: When the therapist is the 'Diverse' one. *British Journal of Occupational Therapy, 75*(3), 144–151. https://doi.org/10.4276/030802212X13311219571828

Berger, L. A., & Berger, D. R. (2011). *The talent management handbook: Creating a sustainable competitive advantage by selecting, developing and promoting the best people.* McGraw-Hill Education.

Braveman, P., & Gottlieb, L. (2014). The social determinants of health: It's time to consider the causes of the causes. *Public Health Reports, 129*(1_suppl. 2), 19–31. https://doi.org/10.1177/00333549141291S206

Canadian Association of Occupational Therapists. (2011). *CAOT position statement: Occupational therapy and cultural safety.* Author.

Canadian Association of Occupational Therapists. (2022). *In development: A new position statement on equity and justice.* https://caot.in1touch.org/site/pt/caot_posn_stmt?nav=sidebar#gsc.tab=0

Cardona, A. D., & Agudelo, G. H. B. (2005). Construcción cultural del concepto calidad de vida. *Revista Facultad Nacional de Salud Pública, 23*(1), 79–90.

Castro, D., Dahlin-Ivanoff, S., & Mårtensson, L. (2014). Occupational therapy and culture: A literature review. *Scandinavian Journal of Occupational Therapy, 21*(6), 401–414. https://doi.org/10.3109/11038128.2014.898086

Chang, E., Simon, M., & Dong, X. (2012). Integrating cultural humility into health care professional education and training. *Advances in Health Sciences Education: Theory and Practice, 17*(2), 269–278. https://doi.org/10.1007/s10459-010-9264-1

Commission of the European Communities. (2003). *Equal opportunities for people with disabilities: A European Action Plan.* Commission of the European Communities.

Erhunmwunsee, L., Backhus, L. M., Godoy, L., Edwards, M. A., & Cooke, D. T. (2019). Report from the workforce on diversity and inclusion – The Society of Thoracic Surgeons members' bias experiences. *Annals of Thoracic Surgery, 108,* 1287–1292. https://doi.org/10.1016/j.athoracsur.2019.08.015

Esquerdo, R. R. E., Malfitano, A. P., Silva, C. R., & Borba, P. (2015). Historia, conceptos y propuestas en la terapia ocupacional social de Brasil. *Revista Chilena de Terapia Ocupacional, 15*(1), 73–84. https://doi.org/10.5354/0719-5346.2015.37132

Figueroa, R. G. (2015). Are gender quotas for congress constitutional? *Revista Chilena de Derecho, 42,* 189–214. DOI: 10.4067/S0718-34372015000100008

Fischer, G.-N. (1992). Campos de intervención en psicología social. *Narcea.* https://dialnet.unirioja.es/servlet/libro?codigo=235423

Forber-Pratt, A. J., Mueller, C. O., & Andrews, E. E. (2019). Disability identity and allyship in rehabilitation psychology: Sit, stand, sign, and show up. *Rehabilitation Psychology, 64*(2), 119–1129. https://doi.org/10.1037/rep0000256

Foronda, C., Baptiste, D.-L., Reinholdt, M. M., & Ousman, K. (2016). Cultural humility: A concept analysis. *Journal of Transcultural Nursing: Official Journal of the Transcultural Nursing Society, 27*(3), 210–217. https://doi.org/10.1177/1043659615592677

Fryer, V., Wright, St Clair, V. A., & Bright, F. (2019). Waiting for community occupational therapy services: A review. *New Zealand Journal of Occupational Therapy, 66*(3), 15–21. https://doi.org/10.3316/informit.776627946392701

Fundación FOESSA. (2019). *VIII Informe Sobre Exclusión Y Desarrollo Social En España 2019.* Fundación FOESSA.

Geertz, C. (2009). *La interpretación de las culturas*. GEDISA. https://www.casadellibro.com/libro-la-interpretacion-de-las-culturas/9788474323337/147019

Grenier, M.-L., Zafran, H., & Roy, L. (2020). Current landscape of teaching diversity in occupational therapy education: A scoping review. *American Journal of Occupational Therapy, 74*(6), 7406205100p1–7406205100p15. https://doi.org/10.5014/ajot.2020.044214

Hammell, K. W. (2015). Quality of life, participation and occupational rights: A capabilities perspective. *Australian Occupational Therapy Journal, 62*(2), 78–85. https://doi.org/10.1111/1440-1630.12183

Hammell, K. W. (2019). Building globally relevant occupational therapy from the strength of our diversity. *World Federation of Occupational Therapists Bulletin, 75*(1), 13–26. https://doi.org/10.1080/14473828.2018.1529480

Herbst, P. H. (1997). *The color of words: An encyclopaedic dictionary of ethnic bias in the United States*. Intercultural Press.

Hocking, C., Townsend, E., & Mace, J. (2021). World federation of occupational therapists position statement: Occupational therapy and human rights (revised 2019) – The backstory and future challenges. *World Federation of Occupational Therapists Bulletin*. https://doi.org/10.1080/14473828.2021.1915608

Iwama, M. K. (2004). Meaning and inclusion: Revisiting culture in occupational therapy. *Australian Occupational Therapy Journal, 51*(1), 1–2. https://doi.org/10.1111/j.1440-1630.2004.00429.x

Iwama, M. K., Thomson, N. A., Macdonald, R. M., Iwama, M. K., Thomson, N. A., & Macdonald, R. M. (2009). The Kawa model: The power of culturally responsive occupational therapy. *Disability and Rehabilitation, 31*(14), 1125–1135. https://doi.org/10.1080/09638280902773711

Kinébanian, A., & Stomph, M. (2010). Diversity matters: Guiding principles on diversity and culture. *World Federation of Occupational Therapists Bulletin, 61*(1), 5–13. https://doi.org/10.1179/otb.2010.61.1.002

Kronenberg, F. (2018). *Everyday enactments of humanity affirmations in post 1994 apartheid South Africa: A phronetic case study of being human as occupation and health* (Unpublished doctoral thesis). University of Cape Town. https://open.uct.ac.za/handle/11427/29441

Kronenberg, F. (2021). Commentary on JOS editorial board's anti-racism pledge. *Journal of Occupational Science, 28*(3), 398–403, https://doi.org/10.1080/14427591.2020.1827483

Kronenberg, F., & Pollard, N. (2006). Political dimensions of occupation and the roles of occupational therapy. *American Journal of Occupational Therapy, 60*(6), 617–626. https://doi.org/10.5014/ajot.60.6.617

Leary, M. R. (2010). *Affiliation, acceptance, and belonging: The pursuit of interpersonal connection*. In S. T. Fiske, D. T. Gilbert, & G. Lindzey (Eds.), *Handbook of social psychology* (pp. 864–897). John Wiley & Sons. https://doi.org/10.1002/9780470561119.socpsy002024

Mahar, A. L., Cobigo, V., & Stuart, H. (2013). Conceptualizing belonging. *Disability and Rehabilitation, 35*(12), 1026–1032. https://doi.org/10.3109/09638288.2012.717584

Muñoz, C. G. M. (2014). La labor de la terapia ocupacional en el marco de los determinantes sociales de la salud en Chile. *Revista Chilena de Terapia Ocupacional, 14*(1), 73–80. https://doi.org/10.5354/0719-5346.2014.32391

Muñoz, J. (2007). Culturally responsive caring in occupational therapy. *Occupational Therapy International, 14*(4), 256–280. https://doi.org/10.1002/oti.238

National Society for the Promotion of Occupational Therapy. (1919). *Minutes from the third annual meeting*. Author.

Purnell, L. D., & Fenkl, E. A. (2019). *Handbook for culturally competent care*. Springer.

Rawall, N. (2009). Social inclusión and exclusion: A review. *Dhaulagiri Journal of Sociology and Anthropology, 2*, 161–180. https://doi.org/10.3126/dsaj.v2i0.1362

Sen Amartya. (2010). *La Idea de la Justicia*. Taurus.

Shakespeare, T. (1996). Disability, identity and difference. In C. Barnes & G. Mercer (Eds.), *Exploring the divide* (pp. 94–113). The Disability Press.

Singh, H., Sangrar, R., Wijekoon, S., Nekolaichuk, E., Kokorelias, K. M., Nelson, M. L. A., Mirzazada, S., Nguyen, T., Assaf, H., & Colquhoun, H. (2022). Applying 'cultural humility' to occupational therapy practice: A scoping review protocol. *BMJ Open, 12*(7), e063655. https://doi.org/10.1136/bmjopen-2022-063655

Sonn, I., & Vermeulen, N. (2018). Occupational therapy students' experiences and perceptions of culture during fieldwork education. *South African Journal of Occupational Therapy, 48*(1), 34–39. https://doi.org/10.17159/2310-3833/2017/vol48n1a7

Tervalon, M., & Murray-García, J. (1998). Cultural humility versus cultural competence: A critical distinction in defining physician training outcomes in multicultural education. *Journal of Health Care for the Poor and Underserved, 9*(2), 117–125. DOI: 10.1353/hpu.2010.0233.

Thomas, D. C., Elron, E., Stahl, G., Ekelund, B. Z., Ravlin, E. C., Cerdin, J.-L., Poelmans, S., Brislin, R., Pekerti, A., Aycan, Z., Maznevski, M., Au, K., & Lazarova, M. B. (2008). Cultural intelligence: Domain and assessment. *International Journal of Cross Cultural Management, 8*(2), 123–143. https://doi.org/10.1177/1470595808091787

United Nations. (1948). *Universal declaration of human rights*. Author.

Wells, S. A., Black, R. M., & Gupta, J. (2016). *Culture and occupation: Effectiveness for occupational therapy practice, education, and research*. AOTA Press.

World Federation of Occupational Therapists. (2010). *Diversity and culture*. WFOT. https://www.wfot.org/resources/diversity-and-culture

World Federation of Occupational Therapists. (2022). *Diversity and culture*. WFOT. https://www.wfot.org/resources/diversity-and-culture

Social, Economic, and Political Factors That Influence Occupational Performance

Catherine L. Lysack, Diane E. Adamo, and Roshan Galvaan

LEARNING OBJECTIVES

After reading this chapter, you will be able to:

1. Distinguish between socioeconomic status, social class, and social inequalities.
2. Discuss how health is related to an individual's position in the social hierarchy.
3. List the five major social determinants of health categories, giving an example from each, and explain how socially (vs. biologically) determined factors shape people's health.
4. Explain how socioeconomic disadvantage experiences in childhood affect the health and occupational performance of those individuals as adults.
5. Describe three actions that occupational therapy practitioners can take to reduce the negative impact of social inequalities and health disparities in the lives of people they serve.

Introduction

The focus of this chapter is on the social, economic, and political factors that influence health and occupational performance across the life course. While most of us immediately recognize that a rare genetic disease or a sudden traumatic injury changes our health forever, it is less obvious that social, economic, and political causes shape our health as individuals and groups of people. What is noteworthy is that something that is often taken for granted, namely, socioeconomic status (SES), is one of the most reliable predictors of health, an even more powerful predictor of health than medical care. Individuals who have attained high levels of formal education and those who are economically well-off report better self-rated health and physical functioning and have lower levels of morbidity and mortality. In contrast, individuals with low formal educational attainment and economic hardship are associated with high rates of infectious and chronic illnesses, poor self-reported health, and lower life expectancy and expedited decline when sick (Centers for Disease Control and Prevention [CDC], 2021; Quiñones et al., 2019).

Decades of research have confirmed that SES, which is income, wealth, and social position in society, is linked to chronic stress, heart disease, ulcers, type 2 diabetes, rheumatoid arthritis, certain types of cancer, and premature aging (CDC, 2021; Ciciurkaite, 2021; Evans et al., 1994; Quiñones et al., 2019). Lower SES is also related to premature aging (Yegorov et al., 2020), reduced access to care, greater rates of hospitalization, and even death (Synovec & Aceituno, 2020).

The stratification of social class influences the choices and opportunities to participate that are available to different groups within contexts. For example, access to higher education and higher income are related to lower risk of ill health to the extent that it changes the range and quality of choices available and the way participation occurs (Galvaan, 2015). In general, adults with more formal education tend to get higher paying jobs with safer working conditions than those with little or no formal education. In the United States, those with paid work are also more likely to have health insurance, which helps to secure reliable access to quality healthcare as compared to those who are unemployed or those working for an hourly wage. Yet, there is more to the wealth–health story. In one analysis of this gradient in 16 countries, researchers showed that the positive association between wealth and health held in all countries *even after controlling for demographic attributes like education and household income* (Semyonov et al., 2013). Thus, there is something very fundamental about social stratification that has a real impact on health.

A term to describe these "fundamental social causes" of health is the **social determinants of health (SDOH)**. The World Health Organization (WHO, 2022) defines SDOH as "the conditions in which people are born, grow up, live, work and age" (p.1). These conditions influence a person's opportunity to be healthy, his/her risk of illness and life expectancy. There are many social determinants, but they can be grouped into five major categories: economic stability, educational access and quality, healthcare access and quality, neighborhood and built environment, and social and community context (Healthy People 2030 et al., 2022). It is beyond the scope of this chapter to fully review the literature on the SDOH, or the physiologic and sociopolitical mechanisms by which these factors affect our health and occupational participation in daily life. Nonetheless, the science is unequivocal—disadvantage in any of these five broad categories places your health at risk. One of the mechanisms is thought to be the physiologic toll that toxic stress and the deleterious effects of impoverished environments have on our body and mind. It is important to understand the complexity of experiences associated with these mechanisms and to appreciate the diverse situations that may be confronted. Social systems of oppression such as the classism of educational attainment together with heterosexism, racism, ageism, and ableism have intersubjective, organizational, and institutional influences on everyday experiences and health. As a starting point, all occupational therapists must recognize in basic terms what this means for the people they serve.

The SDOH contributes to health inequities, that is, the systematic differences in health status and health resources across different population groups. The literature is replete with studies that document how chronic stress, caused by a mix of social, economic, and cultural factors, harms human health. For example, early childhood stress and trauma negatively influence children's bodily systems and brain development (McEwen & McEwen, 2017). Research in human development has also clearly shown direct links between poverty and elevated rates of obesity, anxiety and depression, heart disease, and a range of other chronic conditions (Adler et al., 1999; Goyat et al., 2016; Loucks et al., 2011; Quiñones et al., 2019). Studies in South Africa with mothers who consume alcohol during pregnancy show how historical, socioeconomic, and cultural factors contribute to the prevalence of fetal alcohol syndrome (Cloete & Ramugondo, 2015). Systemic racism too, enacted through segregation policies as well as discrimination at the individual level, affects health by restricting equitable access to opportunities, such as higher socioeconomic attainment via educational and employment opportunities. Even perceived racial discrimination is, by itself, a psychosocial stressor, and laboratory studies have demonstrated an association between racism and physiologic reactivity, including increased cortisol and blood pressure, which may lead to accelerated degeneration of the body and premature illness (CDC, 2021; Ciciurkaite, 2021).

In this chapter, the focus is on those groups of people who are systematically disadvantaged—those rendered most vulnerable by underlying social structures and political and economic systems. Disadvantaged or marginalized groups in this sense include, for example, people who are older adults, poor, those belonging to ethnic and racial minorities, and persons with disabilities. These social identities may occur together, with each one bringing a distinct aspect to the experience of power and access to health resources in a specific place and time. For instance, the person who is an older adult may belong to an ethnic or racial minority and may have a disability. The composite dynamic of social stratification and intersecting identities is important as it contributes to the relationships between health and illness as described in this chapter.

Defining the Social Causes of Health and Illness

Social Inequalities and Health Disparities

Social inequality refers to uneven access to and distribution of resources across domains, such as education, employment, and health, which, in turn, lead to disparities across gender, race, and ethnicity. This results in a situation in which specific groups in a society do not have equal power to access opportunities that could maintain or promote their health. *Social inequalities put people at risk for poorer health overall.*

Stressful life experiences and impoverished environments contribute to poorer health in many ways. This means low-income families will live in neighborhoods that have fewer resources, such as playgrounds, libraries, parks, and good schools. In the United States, low-income families are more likely to live in substandard housing and have less access to nutritious food (Feeding America, 2021). Families with low income, often from racialized communities, do not have easy access to affordable and quick transportation either, which makes attending appointments more difficult and missing appointments more likely (Gower et al., 2013). These social causes lead to poorer health and less opportunity to achieve an optimal treatment outcome. Occupational therapists must guard against viewing these difficulties as the fault of the person in treatment. Attention to systemic, social, and economic factors and to each individual's real-life circumstances must be a central part of the therapists' problem-solving process if they expect to provide people with lower SES the best chance to benefit from their therapeutic interventions. Occupational therapists must be well informed and proactive in order to assist individuals to overcome obstacles with access to and quality of care. Increasing the diversity of the occupational therapy (OT) workforce so that it is more representative of Black and minority groupings would strengthen the quality of and access to OT services and education (Lucas & Washington, 2020). Referrals to pro-bono community clinics, particularly to those who live in geographic areas where reliable public transportation is scarce, is yet another way to connect low-income patients to the services they need (Gower et al., 2013). But of course, this means therapists need to do what they can, within the existing system, to find resources for the people in their care. This is a good step, but it does not change the underlying inequity; it merely compensates for it. Around the world, occupational therapists working within the realm of social inequalities are pushing for much more change—transformational social changes that would improve living conditions for marginalized and underserved groups more fundamentally (Hammel, 2020; Pooley & Beagan, 2021).

The US CDC defines *health disparities* as "preventable differences in the burden of disease, injury, violence, or opportunities to achieve optimal health that are experienced by socially disadvantaged populations" (Nambi & Artiga, 2021, p.2). Thus, it is inequity in the society itself that is ultimately responsible for the poorer health of some. Further, to change and improve that situation requires an orientation to social justice. One problem that arises from societal inequity in society is less powerful groups face considerable difficulty in *accessing quality, fair medical care, and treatment.* For example, studies have found that even after controlling for symptoms and insurance coverage, US doctors are more likely to offer White patients life-preserving treatments, including angioplasty and bypass surgery for cardiac disease, and are more likely to offer people of color various less desirable procedures such as amputations for diabetes (Institute of Medicine, 2002; Seabrook & Avison, 2012). And although every effort must be made to address problems in the clinical encounters between healthcare professionals and minority and/or marginalized groups, it must be recognized that this is only one small step to address health inequity. Even more critical than the challenges related to fair access to health services is the presence of stereotyping and institutional racism and other types of unfair treatment that are unacceptable and unjust, but continue to be encountered much too frequently in health systems everywhere. A recent study in India, for example, showed that reproductive and obstetrics care are strongly linked to SES and social discrimination, with those in lower income brackets and those from lower castes experiencing a greater risk of death and substandard care. In this case, like many others, the issue goes far beyond access and is much more deeply rooted in structural discriminatory practices that place some social groups at much greater disadvantage.

COVID-19 has also shown in dramatic manner how existing health inequities were worsened with the pandemic. Mackey and colleagues (2021) recently showed that the COVID-19 pandemic, in 2 short years, has increased hospitalizations and deaths for Black Americans dramatically as compared to Whites. Worldwide, even in high-income countries, poorer people have been more likely to be infected and die from COVID-19, due to existing health issues, worse living conditions, and work that could not be done from home (Ferreira, 2021; Mackey et al., 2021). In another example, researchers reported that nearly 77% of the world's COVID-related maternal deaths occurred in a single country, Brazil, with Black women and poor women dying at the highest rates of all (Pooler & Pulice, 2021). The global evidence is similar: those from low-income and racialized communities have died at higher rates than richer and White populations (WHO, 2022). And yet, although these facts are irrefutable, we must be conscious of all the complexities of gender, sexuality, and ability, and that rates of morbidity and mortality vary by the impacts brought by the intersectionality of race, gender, wealth, and ability. Continuing with the example of COVID-19 at a macro level, the distribution of the COVID-19 vaccine globally is another example of between-country health inequality: wealthier and more developed countries were able to buy the vaccine and effectively distribute it, whereas less developed countries could not. Research suggests that the mere fact of being born outside Europe and North American makes you 13 times less likely to receive even a single dose of COVID-19 vaccine (Inequality.org, 2022).

Even within a single country, workplace regulations for wages and health and safety and other types of protections differentially affect those most marginalized and powerless, whether due to economic disadvantage, racism, sexism, or ableism. Khazan (2022) has recently written passionately about the political choices of Americans when it comes to paying employees' living wages and paying for sick time. Investigating the facts about why some workers did not follow public health and self-isolate during the pandemic, she found about a fifth of all US workers do not have paid sick leave and that the lowest-paid workers—those who serve food, clean hotels, or stock groceries—are least likely to have it. A particularly hard-hit industry was the nursing home workforce, which has long been known for low wages and poor working conditions. Incidentally, the nursing home workforce is also disproportionally women and women of color. Work conditions were compounded by the high risk of COVID-19 exposure and a lack of resources to support childcare coverage and mental health. As a result, many workers left the industry forcing state and federal governments to modify licensing requirements to recruit new workers, to put in place policies for provision of basic needs such as personal protective equipment (PPE), and to create nonpunitive leave policies (Denny-Brown, 2021). Workers in higher paying jobs could transition to remote/virtual environments to conduct business, but this option was not possible in lower paying service-related jobs that were strictly hands-on. How can you be asked to choose between your health and that of your family when it will cost you your job? The social identities that these workers hold may have contributed to the difficulty in being able to navigate a different path. Perhaps learning from COVID-19 will bring a deeper examination of the foundational building blocks of meaningful work, a living wage, and the benefits to the individual and to society if a more equitable approach and better "occupational balance" can be found.

Social inequalities over the life course accumulate and adversely affect health and occupational performance in adults. Chronic stress affects every system in the human body, including the immune system, and puts people at increased risk for heart attacks, strokes, and cancer. Rates of anxiety, substance abuse, and depression are all higher in populations where chronic stress is high (Quiñones et al., 2019; Seabrook & Avison, 2012). External factors driving chronic stress include high unemployment and stressful work (USDHHS & Office of Minority Health, 2021). Research has shown that lack of personal autonomy and control in one's work (often characteristic of low-paying, low-skilled jobs) is significantly related to cardiovascular disease (CDC 2021; Ciciurkaite, 2021). Despite clear evidence that stress is bad for health, American workers work the most hours of any affluent country and earn the fewest vacation days (13 days, on average) compared to other countries. Spain, Denmark, France, Italy, Germany, and Portugal, for example, all give their workers more than 30 paid days off per year. A major problem is that the United States is the only industrialized nation in the world where paid vacation is not mandatory (Center on Economic and Policy Research, 2019). It is estimated that one in four workers in the United States accrue no vacation time whatsoever. The lasting pandemic has caused strained mental health, and "vacation deprivation" has never been higher.

Intersectionality, a theory developed from feminist critical race theory (Crenshaw, 1989) provides an analytical and conceptual tool with which to understand the dynamics of discrimination and oppression as it occurs in specific contexts. It focuses on how the interconnected relations between social categorizations such as race, gender, and social class apply to a group and create systems of disadvantage. This discussion highlighted how social practices in the labor market disadvantage persons who are of a lower SES, women, and persons of color, leading to prevalent precarious work with poor work conditions. Within a workplace, persons with different intersecting identities experience distinct discrimination that affects their daily experiences. These experiences are invisibly ingrained into everyday occupational performance and contribute to health risks. The barriers associated with the resulting poor work conditions and the accessible resources and opportunities available to persons in such positions contribute to marginalization. It limits people from substantively changing their occupational performance. An intersectional analysis thus reveals the distribution of power and resources within society (Yuval-Davis, 2015), showing the limitations of individual-oriented perspectives that do not consider how systemic factors influence health and participation in everyday life. Systemic and structural factors shape the economic benefits and contribute to creating poverty and wealth gaps, which reflects as social inequality.

Poverty and Health

The term *poverty* refers to the lack of material resources that are necessary for subsistence and experience of this deprivation relative to people's lives. Poverty increases exposure to factors that make people sick, and it effectively eliminates the chances of having high-quality medical insurance (and thus care) when the person needs it. Children, older adults, new immigrants, persons with disabilities, and members of ethnic minorities are at the greatest risk of poverty (U.S. Census Bureau, 2021). Historically, the official poverty rate in the United States had ranged from a high of 22.4% when it was first estimated for 1959 to a low of 11.1% in 1973. Since its initial rapid decline after 1964 with the launch of major War on Poverty programs, the poverty rate has fluctuated between around 11% and 15%. Back in 2019, the United States had seen 5 years of declining poverty rates and recorded the lowest average poverty rate ever at 10.5%.

Unfortunately, when the COVID-19 pandemic hit in 2020, this number rose by 8.5% to 11.4%, pushing an additional 3.3 million Americans into poverty (Self.Inc, 2022).

In the United States, economic and health policy experts are now both asking whether these pronounced levels of income and wealth inequality are taking a toll on the fabric of society (Wilkinson & Pickett, 2017). For example, "upward mobility," that is, doing better and having more than our parents, is not happening as much as in the past. Today, more than 40% of Americans born in the bottom wealth quintile remain there as adults (Braveman & Gottlieb, 2014; Surowiecki, 2014). Research on wealth inequality in the United States by Saez and Zucman (2019) shows that the gap between the richest and the poorest is growing. Astoundingly, today, America's wealthiest 5% of the population holds more than two-thirds of the nation's wealth. Furthermore, as America's richest have accumulated more wealth, they have paid a smaller share of total US taxes. In 2018, the tax share of the top 0.01% was close to what it was in 1953 (Inequality.org, 2022). With such pronounced inequality, how can we expect people with very limited economic resources to do well in health? Although the United States is not the only country that has seen wealth inequality rise over the past three decades, it is an extreme outlier (Piketty, 2022; Saez & Zucman, 2019).

The growing income and wealth gap has fueled the use of two terms in our popular lexicon: *the working poor* and *the new poor*. The working poor are people who work full time but whose wages do not raise them above the poverty line. In 2021, 78 million US workers aged 16 years and older were paid hourly rates, representing 59% of the total national workforce. Among those paid hourly wages, 1.8 million earned the federal minimum wage of $7.25 an hour (U.S. Department of Labor, 2011). President Joe Biden's proposed stimulus plan aims to increase the federal minimum to $15 an hour, more than doubling the current wage of $7.25, that package has not yet passed and it is unclear if it will. Unions that have long protected the wages of workers have fallen precipitously over the past number of decades. Federal and state regulations that permit part-time workers to be exempt from paid sick time is another example of political factors that shape our health. It is interesting to note how long these questions have been considered by American political leaders:

> Our nation, so richly endowed with natural resources and with a capable and industrious population, should be able to devise ways and means of insuring to all our able-bodied men and women, a fair day's pay for a fair day's work.
>
> —Franklin Delano Roosevelt, 1937

The new poor are those people who have fallen into poverty because of sudden or unexpected circumstances such as serious illness, divorce, or sudden job layoffs related to changes in the structure of our economy, including technology, which continues to replace human workers. Despite implementation of the Affordable Care Act, medical bankruptcy is still common. A study published in the *American Journal of Public Health* in 2019 found that 66.5% of bankruptcies in the United States were due to medical issues such as being unable to pay high bills or due to job loss (Himmelstein et al., 2019; Investopedia, 2021). Critics of the current American health system ask how the working poor and new poor can even survive (Econofact, 2021).

Socioeconomic Status, Class, and Social Mobility

Several terms are used to signal the influence of social and economic factors on health, and each has a different meaning. One of the most familiar terms is *socioeconomic status* or SES. Socioeconomic status refers to the occupational, educational, and income achievements of individuals or groups.

The term *class* is also used to indicate social differences between groups, as in *lower class, working class, middle class*, and *upper class*. The Online Dictionary of the Social Sciences (2022) defines class as a group of individuals sharing a common situation within a social structure, usually their place in the structure of ownership and control of the means of production. In capitalist societies, ownership of land or property brings wealth and power, which, in turn, provides the material resources to better quality medical care not only directly but also indirectly to provide a much less stressful and much more comfortable life that also improves chances for health. Although the more neutral term *social position* is quickly overtaking the term *social class* (Marmot, 2017), the impact of these social forces is powerful and evident in all societies around the world. The idea of social categories of people with more or less privilege was inspired by the theories of German sociologist Max Weber (1864–1920), who viewed the stratification of society as a result of the combined influences of economic class, social status (the level of a person's prestige or honor relative to others), and group power. Another sociologist, Pierre Bourdieu (1930–2002), viewed the symbolic power associated with different forms of capital as influencing social status. In addition to economic capital, he discussed the influence of social, cultural, and political forms of capital that influences power dynamics within society (Bourdieu, 1984). Around the world, it is easy to identify examples of people who have power and privilege and those who do not. The experience and consequences of social oppression and exclusion take a tremendous toll on health. There is evidence of this in every corner of the world (Bollyky et al., 2019).

Life expectancy is shorter, and most diseases are more common for people who have a lower social status. Research shows that the harms associated with social disadvantage and lower SES begin even before birth (e.g., a mother's prenatal nutrition, a safe family context), which can influence health even into the final years of life (Barker, 1998; Shonkoff, 2011). Lower SES occurs together with multiple interlocking social identities for each person and group that affect the opportunities and experiences of health and healthcare. Adults with lower SES are often disadvantaged by societal structures that discriminate against them, leaving them with little substantive support as they navigate lives filled with multiple stressors. In one of the earliest studies in the United States by an occupational therapist, Bass-Haugen (2009) showed how the activity profiles, home and work environments, experiences in health systems, and outcomes of healthcare services differed based on SES and social class. She concluded that occupational performance deficits are most notable for Indian American, Latino, mixed race, and low-income Americans through mechanisms related to restricted activity and participation. For example, when neighborhood quality was poor, children could not find safe places to play, and older adults were unable to walk in an environment that allowed them to exercise and socialize. In more recent research, Synovec and Aceituno (2020) showed how unstable housing in the United States negatively affects health and the many ways that occupational therapists can be better prepared to remove barriers to treatment for this population. Despite the potential for OT to contribute to reducing health inequalities, the literature in this field is very limited. Still, we urge further research. Occupational therapists are experts at occupational analysis in context.

There is great potential for OT, in collaboration with other dedicated to improving health, such as public health specialists, social workers, and even architects, sociologists, anthropologists, and others, to add to our knowledge about how to design healthy environments. To live healthily requires not only stable healthcare systems, but also neighborhoods and environments that are designed and built to be safer, more enriching and stimulating to ensure people of a wide array of ages and abilities can live well.

The Intersections of Gender, Race, Age, Disability, and Sexual Orientation

The range of factors that influence health and occupational performance are inextricably linked to the social categories to which individuals belong, including gender, ethnic heritage, age, sexual orientation, and whether or not they are disabled (America's Children, 2017; USDHHS & Office of Minority Health, 2021). This is true in higher income countries like those in North America and Europe, but it is especially true in the United States. Further, individuals often belong to more than one of these categories where inequalities operate. As occupational therapists, we must constantly ask ourselves if we are making assumptions about the people we serve based on the social categories they occupy, or are we truly seeing each individual and the force of their social position on their health. While the next section provides an overview of each of the categories of inequality, the intersecting and composite nature of these inequalities must be remembered.

Gender Inequalities

For some women, the experience of being a woman continues to be one of the inequalities. Research shows that in the United States, on average, women's pay is still only 82 cents for every 1 dollar a man earns (Payscale, 2022). The gender pay gap is partly explained by the number of women who perform jobs with lower salaries, but this does not explain the entire difference. Women also face more barriers to workplace advancement. The Pew Research Center (2021) reports that in the United States, 4 out of 10 women experience gender discrimination in the workplace, a rate twice that of men. There is also evidence that employers tend not to hire and promote women at the same rates as men because they anticipate women will step out of the workforce to have a family. The recent COVID-19 pandemic has also differentially affected women. Women have scaled back and quit their jobs in much higher rates in order to care for sick children at home and supervise children when school lockdowns were in place (Khazan, 2022). Even before COVID-19, many American women were at a relative social disadvantage. The United States is one of eight countries in the world and the only Organisation for Economic and Co-operation Development (OECD) country without a national paid parental leave policy; the United States is also one of the few high-income countries without a national family caregiver or medical leave policy (Bipartisan Policy Center, 2020). Although the US federal government passed the Family and Medical Leave Act (FMLA) in 1996, individual states vary in implementation of this law. In addition, employers are only required to offer FMLA benefits to their employees if they are a public agency, school, or private-sector business with more than 50 employees (U.S. Department of Labor, 2012). The lack of uniform and mandatory federal and state policies to support women takes a toll on women's health and their families. Yet, it does not have to be this way. In Sweden, for example, new parents are entitled to a total of 16 months of paid leave to split between them as they see fit (Bipartisan Policy Center, 2020). In America, the only rich country without legal entitlement to maternity leave, a quarter of women return to work within 10 days of giving birth. But many never return because they cannot bear the thought of leaving a newborn in child care or because paying for it would wipe out all or most of what they earn (Ceder, 2020).

Gender is also linked to health in more direct ways. Although, throughout the world, women live longer than men, women have higher rates of chronic illness at every age. For example, women account for two-thirds of all people diagnosed with arthritis in the United States (National Center for Health Statistics [NCHS], 2021), a phenomenon thought to be related to sex hormones, and women's stronger response to infections, vaccinations, and environmental triggers (Barnham, 2022). Similarly, depression is nearly twice as common in women as it is in men, and it is a worldwide phenomenon across the life span (Mayo Clinic, 2022). The higher rate of depression in women is not due to biology alone. Life circumstances and cultural stressors play a role, too. Although these stressors also occur in men, it is usually at a lower rate. Factors that may increase the risk of depression in women include unequal power and status, work overload, and sexual violence and abuse. Many women deal with the challenges of single parenthood, such as working multiple jobs to make ends meet. Also, women may be caring for their children while also caring for sick or older family members. Domestic violence is a common problem in the United States, affecting an estimated 10 million people every year; as many as one in four women and one in nine men are victims of domestic violence (Huecker et al., 2022). Intimate partner violence is a worldwide problem. The WHO indicates that globally, about one in three (30%) women worldwide have been subjected to either physical and/or sexual intimate partner violence or nonpartner sexual violence in their lifetime (WHO, 2021a). Virtually, all healthcare professionals will at some point evaluate or treat a patient who is a victim of sexual violence. Once again, COVID-19 has exposed who is most vulnerable in society and how their health is affected. Using data from 911 emergency calls and police data, researchers in the United States showed how a combination of sheltering in place, loss of wages, and lack of mental health support during the pandemic increased violence against women, many of whom are trapped in the home with their potential abuser (Hsu & Henke, 2020).

Racial Inequalities

Race affects life chances for health and a range of other societal opportunities like education and work. And a note about terms: "race" is not a biological reality; there are more genetic differences within "races" than between them. Yet racism, a social construct, is very real. It is based on notions of inferiority and superiority attached to social groups marked by physical attributes, and which groups become "racialized" is a result of social, political, and economic factors. Racism is oppression and a public health crisis. Discrimination and racism directly affect health through the mechanisms of chronic oxidative stress that are bad for every physiologic systems (Brosso et al., 2021; Yegorov et al., 2020). Structural inequality and oppression further worsen the situation for marginalized groups. Many health organizations recognize this and are actively advocating

for social justice. In June 2020, in part motivated by the events following police violence and the deaths of several Black Americans in the United States, the World Federation of Occupational Therapists (WFOT) released a powerful statement on racism:

> WFOT condemns systemic racism and stands in solidarity with the global Black Lives Matter movement . . . Systemic racism exists. Systemic racism is an abuse of human rights and actions need to be louder than words. Condemning racism is not enough, systemic racism needs to be addressed as a global priority. Occupational therapists, assistants, and students must be committed to freedom and justice in their own communities, and as professional global citizens . . . . Action is required to address the social determinants of health that currently impede justice and equity. Such determinants include racism, poverty, economic restrictions, discrimination, displacement, disasters, conflict, and historically oppressive systems. (WFOT, 2020)

Others have written we are in a moment of history where global health and human rights are being challenged more than ever before, and it is a moral imperative to respond (Marmot, 2017).

Individuals in racialized groups experience discrimination at much higher rates than those who are White, and their health status is much lower too (CDC, 2021; Ciciurkaite, 2021; Quiñones et al., 2019). The discrimination begins early. For example, there are studies to show that teachers give Black students less attention and assistance and that the teachers have lower expectations for their achievement (Brandmiller et al., 2020; Covay Minor, 2014; Econofact, 2022). Education is a critical factor in life because employment opportunities and, in turn, income provide the financial resources needed for healthcare; whether to buy healthcare insurance or to pay out-of-pocket costs is tied to educational success. Yet, educational quality is not equally distributed. The US government recognized this fact as early as the 1950s when it established the Head Start program, a national network of comprehensive child development programs that targeted low-income families and their communities. Low-income children are at the greatest risk because they grow up in poor-quality neighborhoods, which have poorer quality schools, staffed by teachers with fewer resources to enrich the learning environment. This example highlights the intersection of race, poverty, and health. Individuals with fewer opportunities in the early years seldom catch up (MacPhee et al., 2013). A sad fact is that in the United States in 2019, 14.4% of children (>10 million children) were living in poverty as measured by the official US poverty rate (Econofact, 2021). The official poverty thresholds are low: for one adult and two children, the federal poverty line is $20,598 per year; for two adults and two children, the federal poverty line is roughly $26,000 per year.

It can be challenging to see how powerful social forces like racism operate, perhaps especially so if you are young yourself and have grown up in a relatively privileged social position. Beagan (2021), a sociologist and occupational science scholar, writes:

> In capitalist cultures, there is a strong tendency to see everything through an individualist lens . . . Meritocracy is a cornerstone of capitalist belief systems, the notion that people rise and thrive (or not) based on our own merits—our skills, abilities, and efforts. It allows people to not-see White privilege, the system of unearned advantages that grants some of us extra resources and options at every turn. (p. 410).

She further argues that well-intentioned efforts initiated under the banners of "diversity, equity and inclusion" be carefully scrutinized to ensure that the solution to reducing the inequality is simply a "numbers game" where higher numbers of racial minorities are recruited to university, to certain jobs and professions, and so on. To Beagan and other allies, "it is time to change policies, to change structures and systems and institutions, trusting that change in ideas and minds will follow" (p. 412). Research in the United States has concluded that structural racism leads to poor access to quality healthcare, racial residential segregation, and discriminatory incarceration and that this leads to health inequity (Bailey et al., 2017).

Age Inequalities

Age is another factor that shapes health, but not only because of age-related health conditions. Social science research from around the world has shown that negative attitudes toward older people persist. For example, there are widespread views that older adults are unwilling to adapt to new technologies, lacking a desire to learn, and showing a resistance to change (WHO, 2021). *Ageism* can be defined as the systematic stereotyping of and discrimination against people on the basis of their age. Studies have verified that younger people often have negative attitudes toward older people, particularly if they have an aging-related condition or disability, such as slow walking speed (or driving speed), impaired hearing, or cognitive impairment (Warshaw et al., 2021). Ageism is not only pervasive; it can also lower self-esteem, reduce opportunities, and lead to isolation, loneliness, and depression (U.S. Administration on Aging, 2020; WHO, 2021).

Although many think of the United States as a country of equality and fairness, there remains a great deal of ageism in American society, and it may extend to hospitals and medical settings. For example, health professionals may assume that their older patients are incapable of accurately or effectively communicating their needs and as a result may be more likely to ignore or dismiss an older patient's complaints. Although decisions to withhold care based on age have been increasingly challenged in recent years, rates of application of lifesaving interventions, such as cardiovascular procedures and organ transplantation, continue to decline with increasing age; when resources are limited, youth is prioritized (Warshaw et al., 2021; WHO, 2021). Again, COVID-19 has exposed deep cracks in American systems of medical care. It has revealed, for example, the value our society puts on care for the older adults. Nursing home aids, critical to the care of older people in nursing homes, are low wage jobs, and these jobs are overwhelmingly done by women, especially women of color (Denny-Brown, 2021; Fekadu et al., 2021). As in other essential workers, this group has borne a disproportionate burden in terms of illness and death from exposures to this infectious disease (Khazan, 2022). Ageism and age discrimination are social problems found elsewhere in the world.

Are there countries that discriminate less on the basis of age and financial status, and do they have better health? The answer is a resounding yes (Nowatzki, 2012; Piketty, 2022). But the picture of aging societies, and individual views toward aging, is changing rapidly throughout the world too. Japan, the oldest country in the world, for example, is often held out to be a country where the treatment of older adults is more equitable. But Japan is also a country with considerable wealth, and they treat their children, not older adults, with great veneration. Although historically there is no doubt that Japanese culture may have been more equitable, and more equitable in regard to older adults, it appears the picture is changing as urbanization and modern values overtake tradition. Despite the appearance that SDOH and inequality are challenging societies more than ever, Thomas Piketty (2022) has written eloquently that the opposite is actually true. If we step back and consider the longer history of the planet, the picture is much more optimistic. Piketty shows that over time, human societies have moved fitfully toward a more just distribution of income and assets, a reduction of racial and gender inequalities, and greater access to healthcare, education, and the rights of citizenship. Our rough march forward is political and ideological, an endless fight against injustice. To keep moving, Piketty argues, we need to learn and commit to what works, to institutional, legal, social, fiscal, and educational systems that can make equality a lasting reality.

Irrespective of how the world's nations proceed with respect to social justice and health, it is undeniable that age and health status are tightly intertwined. Age-related health changes are real and cause poor health, particularly in the latest stages of life, wherever we live on this planet. Because age and illness are so closely tied, when the average age of the population increases, so does the prevalence of health problems. The US population aged 65 years and older, for example, will increase to approximately 71 million in 2030 and 98 million by 2060. People aged 65 years and older are expected to be 25% of the population by 2060 (Healthy People 2030 et al., 2022). The financial costs of meeting these needs are anticipated to be an enormous and challenge our nation's leaders. Is America prepared? We may need to look to other countries for guidance. For example, Japan, the oldest country in the world, currently has 26% of its population over age 65 years now; the comparable US figure is 15%. Other old countries such as Italy, Greece, and Germany have also had several more decades to adjust to population aging and may provide lessons for younger countries as they prepare for a society with fewer workers (and, in turn, fewer tax dollars) to offset the costs of illness that are associated with older age.

Inequalities Due to Disability

Disability is associated with disadvantage, regardless of individual skills or financial resources. According to the U.S. Census Bureau (2018), more than 55 million people or 17.6% of the population have a severe disability. This represents nearly 20% of the population aged 5 years and older living in the community. The WHO (2021) reports that 1 billion people or 15% of the world's population experience some form of disability, with disability prevalence higher for developing countries. Employment rates vary by type of disability. Employment rates are highest for people with hearing and vision disabilities and much lower for those with mobility and psychiatric disabilities (Fiorati & Elui, 2015; Goyat et al., 2016). The consequences for those who experience multiple inequalities are noteworthy. Women with disability are said to face the cumulative disadvantage or "double jeopardy" of being female and disabled (Chappell & Havens, 1980; Pentland et al., 1999). A marginalized social position and poverty only increase that disadvantage. Negative attitudes, discrimination, and social exclusion are all too familiar experiences for disabled people. The actions that led to the passage of the Americans with Disabilities Act, a policy to prevent such discrimination, reflect the long-standing efforts of the disability rights movement and its allies (including OT practitioners) to improve life conditions for people with disabilities (Colker, 2005; Hurst, 2003). Although it can be difficult to disentangle the physical from the social causes of ill health, the end result is the same. On virtually every metric of health, people with disabilities have worse health than those who are able bodied.

Inequalities Based on Sexual Orientation

Understanding the inequalities faced by individuals as a function of their sexual orientation is a significant challenge, given the tremendous lack of knowledge about the experiences and specific health needs of these populations. Individuals who identify as lesbian, gay, bisexual, asexual, transgender, nonbinary, queer, or intersex (LGBTQI+), as well as those who express same-sex or same-gender attractions or behaviors, will have experiences across their life course that differ from those of cisgender and heterosexual individuals (Healthy People 2030 et al., 2022).

It must be recognized that the experiences of LGBTQI+ individuals are not uniform and are shaped by factors such as race, SES, geographical location, and age, any of which can have an effect on health-related concerns and needs (National Academies of Sciences, Engineering, and Medicine, 2020). Individuals in same-sex relationships who are also older, or are visible minorities, may face a similar type of "double disadvantage" or even "triple disadvantage" mentioned earlier. Fredriksen-Goldsen and colleagues (2012), for example, found that lesbian and bisexual women experience higher rates of chronic diseases, such as lifetime asthma, arthritis, and obesity. Higher mental distress prevalence among all of these groups is also a challenging concern, related, in many instances, to prejudice, discrimination, and even physical violence (National Academies of Sciences, Engineering, and Medicine, 2020).

Research is also needed that goes beyond the individual level. LGBTQI+ individuals are in relationships, and many have children. When a child in an LGBTQI+ family encounters the medical system, how do occupational therapists respond? There can be unique challenges that more closely resemble those of new refugees, migrant workers, or even prison populations where a range of legal rights and statuses are relevant to the process of seeking care and gaining appropriate treatment. For example, children raised in same-sex households may not receive adequate healthcare if the parents' nontraditional partnership is not recognized as legal (Hacker et al., 2015). In a major step forward for gay rights, the US Supreme Court ruled same-sex legal in all 50 states in 2015. Still, there are new challenges. In schools, job sites, and public spaces in the United States, there have been strident social views, political clashes, and legal battles over the right to use a public washroom of one's choice National Academies of Sciences, Engineering, and Medicine, 2020). Inequalities and health disparities related to sexual orientation remind us that all laws and policies that govern education, the workplace, health insurance, and the health system are created by governments, with a power to shape their nation's health. In the realm of gay rights worldwide, progress has been much slower. The Human Rights Watch reports that there are 69 countries around the world where homosexuality is illegal, and in a few, long imprisonment, and even the death penalty, is the legally prescribed punishment for same-sex sexual acts (British Broadcasting Corporation, 2021). We are reminded that in so many aspects of human life, it is so much easier to be, and to care for, those who are "average," but as soon as an individual occupies a social position that is "different," the risk of unfair treatment grows.

In summary, regardless of beliefs in equal opportunity and a plethora of policies and legislation intended to prevent discrimination, life choices, opportunities, and access to health and meaningful occupations are not equal; they are mediated by an array of powerful social and economic and political forces that dictate the fate of individuals and, ultimately, their health. These factors are not easily changed or overcome through individual desire and effort, either our own as healthcare professionals or that of our patients. Much larger forces, including the structure of the health system in a given country, play an integral role. Previously, we have discussed how inequalities based on gender, age, race, poverty, and sexual orientation shape health. In addition, we have argued that the SDOH, that is, factors in the physical environment, such as healthy communities, safe schools and workplaces, and leisure spaces, also contribute to health and well-being. Next, we consider how the healthcare system itself influences the ways in which medical care and even OT interventions are delivered, and ultimately how it makes it easier (or harder) for people to achieve good health.

Mechanisms of Disadvantage Across the Life Course

There is an untested assumption that differences in health and health outcomes after treatment arise predominantly from basic biological and inherited genetic differences and less so from inadequacies in healthcare delivery systems and society. As a reader of this chapter, you already appreciate that a significant part of the problem is income and wealth inequality, as well as sexism, racism, and ableism, which leaves those most marginalized also the sickest. Figure 15.1 illustrates the many pathways by which SES at the individual level and the SDOH at the community level intersect to influence health.

Effects Over a Lifetime

It will be clear now to readers of this chapter that the foundations of adult health are generally laid in early childhood. Compared to women with high SES, women with low SES experience higher levels of stress, higher infection rates, and poorer nutrition during pregnancy that, in turn, lead to low birth weight and premature delivery, and the culprit is those range of deleterious effects that flow from impoverished environments (Quiñones et al., 2019). Wilkinson and Marmot (2003) have argued that the combination of a poor start and slow growth "become embedded in biology during the processes of development, and form the basis of the individual's biological and human capital, which affects health throughout life" (p. 14). Higher rates of depression, anxiety, attention problems, and conduct disorders plague children and adolescents from lower SES backgrounds (Merikangas et al., 2010). Slow physical growth in infancy is also associated with reduced cardiovascular, respiratory, pancreatic, and kidney function, which increases the risk of serious illness

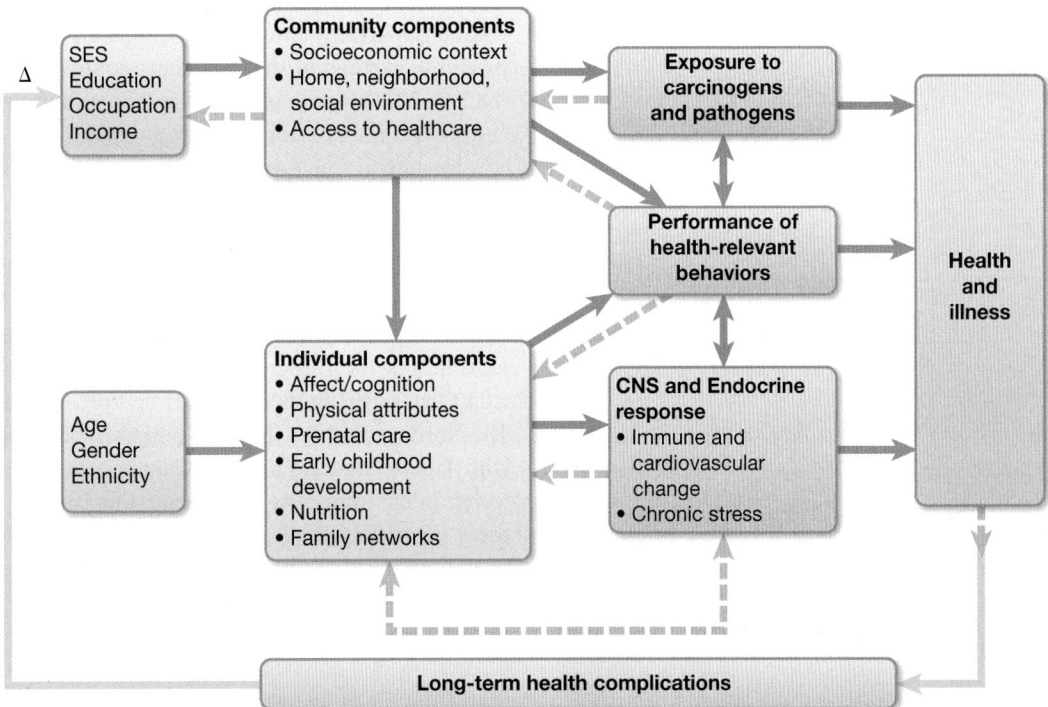

FIGURE 15.1 **A model of socioeconomic status (SES) influences and interactions on health. CNS, central nervous system.**

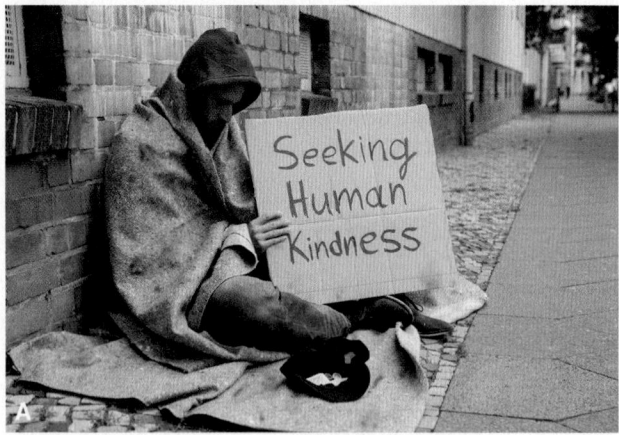

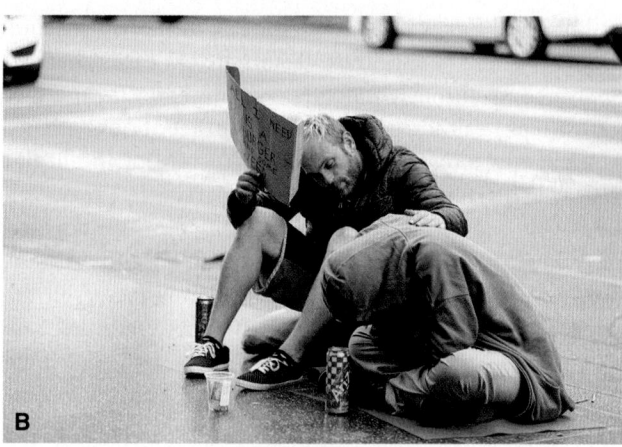

FIGURE 15.2 **Unsafe neighborhoods.**

in adulthood (Shonkoff & Phillips, 2000). The evidence is overwhelming. Disadvantage experienced in younger years stays with people over a lifetime and negatively affects cognition, emotion, and sensory systems until death.

Children learn and develop through play. Yet, the playing field is not equal. Seminal work by Kozol (1991, 1995) describes neighborhoods overrun by poverty, crime, and economic neglect. Such environments not only impede human development through a lack of stimulation and enrichment, they also put children at higher risk of injuries and diseases linked to environmental toxins and pollutants (Figures 15.2 and 15.3). Nearly a decade ago in the United Kingdom, Hutton et al. (2016) argued that significant inroads to improve the long-term health prospects of children living in chronic poverty could be achieved with only small changes to health legislation, suggesting OT be made universally accessible and free. Imagine the benefits to children and families if that occurred.

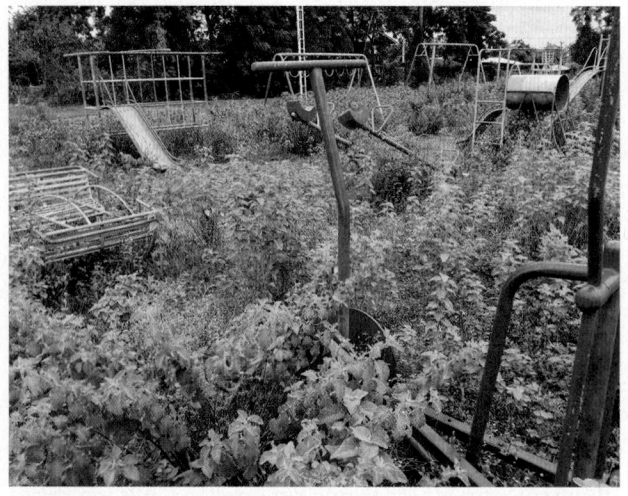

FIGURE 15.3 **No place to play.**

The Political Economy of the Healthcare System

To fully appreciate the influence of social and economic factors in the lives of individuals and families, these factors must be set against the backdrop of national healthcare systems. For instance, the US healthcare is the most expensive system in the world. Health expenditures in the United States in 2019 represented 16.9% of the country's gross domestic product, by far the highest share of any country in the OECD (2019). In 2019, the United States spent more than $10,500 per person on healthcare, an average of $3.3 trillion dollars, the most of any single OECD country and twice the average of the 30 richest countries in the world (NCHS, 2021). As the section that follows highlights, the investment is not providing a strong return.

Despite the huge amount spent, the United States ranks low on many health indicators (The Commonwealth Fund, 2021). Life expectancy in the United States in 2021 stands at 77.3 years, as compared to 81 years on average for the OECD countries (OECD, 2019). Japan, Italy, Spain, and Australia all have life expectancies above 81.5 years. Infant mortality in the United States is worse, too: 5.2 deaths per 1,000 live births in 2019, above the OECD average of 4.4. The Nordic countries (Iceland, Finland, and Sweden), along with Japan, Greece, Portugal, Canada, and Korea, all have lower infant mortality rates than the United States, and these countries spend a fraction of what the United States spends on healthcare. Is it reasonable to ask if the country is receiving the best value for that expenditure? Compared to peer nations, the United States also has the highest chronic disease burden and an obesity rate that is 2 times higher than the OECD average, and the highest number of hospitalizations from preventable causes and the highest rate of avoidable deaths (The Commonwealth Fund, 2020). In a system where financial resources are the means to access key screening tests as well as expensive medical interventions, those with low SES who are already residing in one of the countries with the greatest inequality between rich and poor (i.e., the United States) face even greater health disadvantage (Piketty, 2022).

The social and economic factors that impact health may be easier for occupational therapists to appreciate than political factors, and yet they are all important in shaping health. The type of health system we have is a direct result of the governments we have. In North America and most of Europe, elected democracies establish governmental priorities, and elected politicians are responsible for enacting the laws, regulations, and policies that organize every part of our life—including education, work, housing, and, of course, the type of health services we receive. While that is also true in nondemocratic countries like Russia, China, and many others, the government has much tighter control over the population. Evidence suggests that the less democratic the country, the poorer the health of the population. A recent study in the medical journal *The Lancet* analyzed the political leadership of more than 170 countries around the world and found overwhelming evidence that citizens in countries governed by autocratic leaders die much younger and have much poorer health than citizens who live in democracies (Bollyky et al., 2019).

The Role of Health Insurance in the United States

Health insurance (or, more accurately, medical insurance) is important because access to healthcare in the mostly private US system requires either a job with health benefits or the financial means to pay out of pocket. A substantial number of US citizens lack both. Currently, 44 million citizens are uninsured (U.S. Census Bureau, 2019) compared to 50.7 million in 2009, due largely to the implementation of the Affordable Care Act (Obama, 2016). Although these findings are encouraging, significant inequalities still exist. For example, research shows that out-of-pocket expense for pharmaceutical drugs is the fastest rising component of the healthcare system (Karim et al., 2021). For persons with low income, choices may be made between prioritizing between needed medications versus food and rent (Cohen & Villarroel, 2015; Feeding America, 2021) or other pressing needs. Within the health system itself, Americans should question why such a high proportion of expenditure is on hospital medical care versus other investments. It is noteworthy that the US healthcare system only spent 3% of all of its resources on community-based care (Healthy People 2030 et al., 2022). Can we envision a country where prevention and health promotion, delivered in the homes and neighborhoods where people live, receives a larger share of the healthcare spending pie?

There is no question that we need to care about the number of uninsured and underinsured Americans and the rising costs of healthcare whether based on social justice or simply as a matter of economic sense. Kawachi and Berkman (2003) warn that the least fortunate in society must be cared for, or spillover effects will adversely affect everyone. Wide income and wealth inequalities lead to stress, family breakdown, and also violence and crime (Mackey et al., 2021). Many countries outside the United States are also becoming more unequal. These facts challenge us to envision and work toward a more equal society. As citizens and healthcare professionals, we can make a difference.

The Role of Occupational Therapy in Addressing Health Disparities

Townsend and Wilcock (2003) asserted that it is an occupational injustice to ignore the social and economic determinants of health. We argue here that these factors affect opportunities for and engagement in occupation. Others have called on occupational therapists to address the segregation of groups of people based on a lack of meaningful participation in daily life occupations, something that Kronenberg and Pollard (2005) have provocatively called *occupational apartheid*.

There is little doubt that social and economic factors are real and exert a powerful influence on health and occupational performance, but what can occupational therapists do in the face of what appears to be intractable problems on a very large scale? After developing greater awareness of the influence of social inequalities on health and the extent of health disparities among the people OT practitioners serve, what are the next practical steps?

First, occupational therapists can apply the small but growing body of research evidence available that focused interventions early in a vulnerable child's life can produce lasting benefits throughout their life. For example, OT can effectively address sensory motor performance deficits, lack of peer–play relationships, and maladaptive family interaction (Pitonyak et al., 2015). Occupational therapists can also support parents to better understand their children's emotional and cognitive needs and modify school and home environments to facilitate occupational performance (Hammell, 2020; Synovec & Aceituno, 2020). All gains realized during childhood will positively affect the individual and their health throughout their life.

Second, occupational therapists are experts at person–environment fit and recognize the centrality of meaningful occupations to good health and can increasingly see how systemic factors contribute to this. Yet, there are serious gaps in knowledge. For example, little is known about meaningful occupational engagement for chronically unemployed people and what kinds of interventions might be effective. Recent research has shown how policies related to long-term unemployment should be expanded to offer better solutions for US citizens (Aldrich et al., 2020). Even less is known about occupational deprivation due to immigration, geographical isolation, and incarceration (Whiteford, 2000). Although these settings are not the major clinical settings where occupational therapists work, it is an important challenge to gain a deeper understanding of what meaningful occupation means in these settings and how to support marginalized individuals to achieve greater participation and inclusion and benefit from OT (Hammell, 2020; Pollard & Sakellariou, 2017; Pooley & Beagan, 2021).

Third, a unique strength of the profession is its appreciation for the person. This means therapists must learn about the people they serve in the terms of their world, their perceptions, their experiences, and their realities. This is easy to say but difficult to do. Purtilo et al. (2018) describe many difficulties that arise between practitioners and patients because of socioeconomic and cultural differences. These differences influence how individual therapists feel about the people they treat, and more education is needed to ensure that we truly understand their lives and daily routines and find ways to make our recommendations relevant to them.

Fourth, to act on issues of occupational deprivation and occupational injustice requires that therapists become more educated about economic and other institutional and structural barriers to treatment and fair allocation of medical and rehabilitation services (Pooley & Beagan, 2021). The WFOT has asked the profession to stand up for the injustice caused by systemic racism and inequity (WFOT, 2020). As healthcare professionals, we must all ask if we are doing enough to confront racism, poverty, economic restrictions, discrimination, displacement, disasters, conflict, and historically oppressive systems and do more to create a more equitable world.

The research in the United States and around the world confirms that medical services, including OT services, are not equally distributed (Fiorati & Elui, 2015; Hammell, 2020). Simply put, people who lack financial resources will not access needed services, or they will receive lower quality of services unless they are able to access alternative private pay or charity. Therapists regularly identify low SES as a risk to occupational performance but may be less attentive to factors in the physical and build environment that exert an influence, including the availability of affordable and accessible transportation, nutritious foods, and stable housing, for example (Figure 15.4). As stated earlier in this chapter, occupational therapists must go beyond addressing the clinical features and functional needs of their individual patients and focus more of their efforts and professional advocacy on effecting change at the level of social organizations

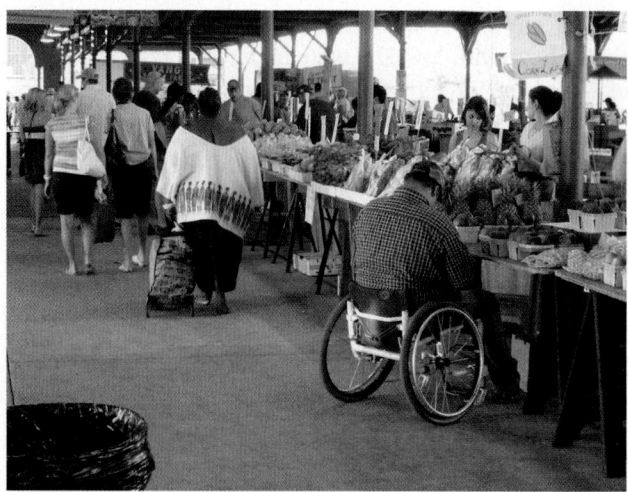

FIGURE 15.4 Farmer's market.

(e.g., schools, hospitals, housing administrators, transportation authorities) and social systems (e.g., health insurers, employers) and society.

This chapter explored the health consequences of powerful relationships between socioeconomic and political factors and their impact on occupational performance across the life course. To illustrate these issues, consider the story of Annie and Desmond and the role that social and economic forces have played in shaping their family's health (OT Story 15.1).

Many possible social causes of poor health are suggested in OT Story 5.1. Although Annie is recovering from a hip fracture, it is the context for her life that exerts a significant force on her chances at a positive outcome. First, the influence of race, gender, age, and class inequality in Annie's life limited her access to resources. The realities of these social categories must be considered as Annie's experience cannot be generalized to represent everyone. Second, Annie's deceased husband Desmond may have died because his work was dangerous and put him at higher risk of illness. Living in a lower income neighborhood near an industrial area, the entire family may have been exposed to unsafe levels of environmental pollutants. Although Annie is struggling to regain mobility and live safely and independently, her physical health is only one factor. A lifetime of limited financial means in a neoliberal, capitalist society and a neighborhood with possible higher exposure to pollutants puts Annie at risk for a poorer health outcome overall. These socioeconomic and political factors are out of her control. Annie and her family navigated these discriminatory and oppressive systems in how they participated and performed their occupations. Could we do more to change social and health systems and policies to improve health for all? See Expanding Our Perspectives for an example.

All OT practitioners in the United States as a group are overwhelmingly White and middle class (Perera & Douglas,

OT STORY 15.1 SEEING SOCIAL INEQUALITY IN THE INDIVIDUAL STORY

Annie is a 72-year-old, African American Black woman, and just spent 2 weeks in a hospital. As Annie described it, she "took a spell" and tumbled down her basement steps. She fractured her hip and two ribs. Annie uses a wheelchair and hopes it is temporary, but she is worried about managing at home alone. Annie lives in Detroit, Michigan. Her house has two bedrooms and a bathroom on the second floor, with laundry facilities in the basement. She is a widow, and her only surviving child, a son, lives a far way away, in Chicago. Her husband Desmond worked at an automotive supply company, and after 31 years of work, he became ill with lung cancer and died. Desmond was a nonsmoker. Desmond and Annie and other plant workers wondered if their jobs had made them sick, but this was not pursued. The plant that Desmond worked for declared bankruptcy during the COVID-19 pandemic, and this meant Annie lost the small pension she received as a surviving spouse. Now, she gets by on her Social Security check and Medicare. Her income is just over $24,000 per year.

Before discharge from the hospital, Annie was assessed by an occupational therapist who gave her recommendations for bathing and dressing and managing at home. Annie learned about Dial-a-Ride, a transportation service for older adults and people with disabilities, and the name of a senior center where she could take exercise classes and join social activities. Annie was appreciative of the advice, but she was disappointed that she would not get the needed assistive device, "a nice solid bath seat and grab bars" like her hospital roommate did. Annie's insurance covered none of this—not even the raised toilet seat her therapist told her would help prevent another fall. The advice from her occupational therapist focused on her medical condition and did little for systemic factors affecting her access to needed resources. Annie and her family were disadvantaged by their low SES, and this limited her past and current occupational performance.

After 3 weeks at home, Annie is worried about the slowness of her recovery and is discouraged and lonely. Occasionally, her church friends drop in with a meal and help with groceries, but Annie is anxious about the future. She feels unsteady and expressed that she does not trust her legs "not to buckle." She decided to not spend money on a class at a place where she feels she does not fit in. In a phone call to her son, she also expressed fear about the safety of walking in her neighborhood. Annie wonders whether the woman she met weeks ago in the hospital is faring better than she is, and how her life could be better if she could afford more help. Although she calls her friends her "lifeline," she is also praying "the good Lord will see [her] through" as she continues to navigate the systemic challenges of her everyday life.

Questions

1. Environmental and systemic factors contribute to health outcomes. Which environmental and systemic factors are a priority in this scenario, and what does intersectional analysis of Annie's story reveal?
2. Annie was disappointed that she would not get a "nice solid bath seat and grab bars" from her insurance company like others who have better insurance. How would an occupational therapist explain this inequity to Annie, and what else could an occupational therapist do in response to inequitable access to services? Are there any alternatives that might be suggested to her?
3. What evidence and types of arguments can an occupational therapist present to help obtain medical equipment, devices, and health services that their underserved patients need? Why would occupational therapists take on this advocacy?
4. What policy or systems change could an occupational therapist advocate for to reduce systemic discrimination (such as racism and sexism)?

 EXPANDING OUR PERSPECTIVES

Occupational Therapy's Impact on Addressing Social Determinants of Health

Arameh Anvarizadeh

Linda is a 58-year-old woman who immigrated to the United States when she was 15. She is a mother of three, a grandmother, a sister, and an aunt and is beloved in her community. She was a caregiver to her late father and grieved his passing heavily. Last year, she was diagnosed with stage 3 leukemia.

When Linda discovered she had cancer, she was in denial and refused to seek treatment. Linda continued to live a lifestyle that was counterproductive and unhealthy to possible recovery. A year later, Linda was hospitalized and placed in a medically induced coma. While in the hospital, she also received OT and physical therapy daily.

When Linda's children met with her physician, they expressed their desire to transfer her to a hospital specializing in oncology, which they felt was a better facility to care for their mother. Although her children felt a sense of urgency to do this, her physician continuously refused.

(continued)

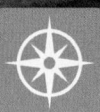

They pleaded with him to refer her to another physician. He refused that as well. This interaction immediately led to distrust and anger.

Based on society's standards of success, Linda is not college educated; she is unemployed, her living situation is unstable, and she has never been married. In addition, one of her main occupations is drug use, which she has engaged in for 30 years. Her three children are also not college educated and do not have the advocacy skills to address the systemic healthcare barriers they face with the physician's orders.

In addition, the medical team informed her children that Linda had stopped breathing and was placed in a medically induced coma because she had overdosed. The level of drugs combined with her opioid medication in her system compared to her extreme weight loss significantly impacted her heart function. Linda was embarrassed and did not want any visitors because of her shame. Her children felt that her physician was judging Linda's lifestyle choices, which they also felt contributed to his poor care for their mother.

Throughout his time managing Linda's care, her physician, a middle-aged male, not identifying from a minoritized group, demonstrated significant authoritative and paternalistic behaviors. As her occupational therapist, I felt deeply responsible for advocating for Linda's needs. I could not help but wonder if SES, class, economic disadvantage, stereotypes, and racism contributed to the lack of urgency from the physician's decision to transfer Linda. As mistrust grew, it became even more

evident why diversity and representation matter so much in healthcare. Was there judgment because of her social position in society? Was this a clear example of social inequities in health? By Linda being systemically disadvantaged, is her physician making assumptions and showing increased implicit bias? This mistreatment is not Linda's first; poor care occurred during her pregnancies, labor, and now during her cancer treatment. These stories are not new nor are isolated incidences; instead, they are far too commonly experienced by marginalized communities and populations.

As occupational therapists, it is critical to recognize when social inequities and health disparities occur. We have an opportunity to bridge health disparity gaps while focusing on achieving positive health outcomes. As significant members of the healthcare team, part of our advocacy and proactive leadership role is awareness of the social, economic, and political factors that influence health decisions and disparities. Acknowledging the disparities and having the skill set to navigate systemic barriers are essential to actualize Vision 2025, where all people, populations, and communities have quality of life and can participate in everyday living.

As I consulted with the medical team, we worked with Linda and her children to ensure her requests were heard, valued, and met. Linda was able to get the care she felt was best for her, and she continued to receive therapy services daily. Far too often, these experiences do not end in a positive outcome; however, our duty is always to fulfill our ethical responsibility to our clients and profession.

2020) and live more privileged lives than the populations that they serve (Pollard & Sakellariou, 2017). The profession has to invest in growing a more diverse demographic profile and also requires that all practitioners recognize their social position relative to the people they serve and actively reflect on how these differences create assumptions, unfounded judgments, and biases in the planning and delivery of care. Occupational therapists must work to reduce their implicit biases and take great care to ensure that they do not judge the people with whom they work and blame them for their relatively poorer health status that is often deeply rooted in social and economic structures, not individual traits of motivation and compliance. Occupational therapists are in a unique position to elicit change in the healthcare industry and speak as advocates for health equity in the care of the most vulnerable members of society.

Finally, if occupational therapists wish to see meaningful change in the health of the population, they must work more seriously to leverage their position within

the healthcare system to push for greater social change. Is there more OT can do? OT researchers have increasingly urged clinicians to go beyond their traditional assessments to measure the deleterious effects of the SDOH in their patients' lives, to provide objective evidence of their force in shaping treatment effectiveness and overall health outcomes (Hammell, 2020). Pooley and Beagan (2021) and Madsen et al. (2016) have asked more fundamental questions, including whether the profession is truly engaged in reflection on the deeper causes of social injustice and, once recognized, whether the profession is willing to confront its own history of colonialism, oppression, power, and privilege. Pollard and Sakellariou (2017) have critically analyzed OT's narrow demographic profile and dominance of a Northern discourse and challenged the profession to think more critically about working with marginalized groups. They urge greater attention to the lived experiences of our patients and examination of marginalized groups through the lens of social and political exclusion. Galvaan (2021) encouraged occupational therapists to embrace epistemic discomfort and to be more open to different ways of understanding the world as they pursued change. Through critically analyzing systemic issues that may present as individual situations and acknowledging the wisdom that marginalized bring, occupational therapists can partner with marginalized groups to advocate for and create equitable environments (Galvaan & Peters, 2017). There is significant potential for new investigations and new research to extend these lines of inquiry. And yet, we are individual therapists presented with new opportunities each day. Will occupational therapists step up and lend our expertise to the cause of positive social change? Each day in our work, we see the consequences of an unequal society and social and economic forces that marginalize and exclude social groups. We need to raise our collective hands and serve on school boards, boards of large health systems, prison parole boards, transit authority boards, and boards that lobby for every kind of health and social policy change. And we need more occupation-based research.

Conclusion

Person-centered OT emphasizes listening, asking the right questions, and truly understanding and empathizing with the person at the center of our interventions (Law, 1998; Lawlor, 2003; Wood, 1996). Although listening to and learning from individuals is paramount to effective OT interventions, this approach individualizes the underlying problems of health disparities that are fundamentally social in nature. Occupational therapists who work with socioeconomically disadvantaged people are well acquainted with this tension. More than a decade ago, in the OT literature, Dr Sandra Galheigo (2011) spoke boldly about the need to prepare the new generation of occupational therapists to engage in social transformation, not just individual change, and to address issues of social invisibility and lack of access to human rights. This reorientation could be a game changer. In a similar vein, Jennifer Creek, in her 2011 Hanneke van Bruggen lecture, challenges occupational therapists to ask themselves what they are really doing to help the people they serve. She states:

> We think that we want to hear what the client has to say but, in reality, we fear that we will not be able to understand or cope with a diversity of needs. It is safer to carry out a procedure or fill in a checklist than to confront our own inadequacy in the face of another's distress.

As stated earlier, some experts have argued that the path forward lies in large-scale professional coalitions aimed at major transformations of the healthcare system, including a universal single-payer system (Cutler, 2004), but this takes time to achieve, if ever. Very recently, even world renowned economists like Thomas Piketty are taking

an interest in the SDOH and how deeply health is linked to wealth inequality. In his latest book, Piketty (2022) argues that a simple solution would be to return to the societal equality that we used to have, where wealth taxes provided the economic stability needed for technological innovation, a robust economy and also a just and healthy society. In the meantime, occupational therapists must recognize they work in health systems that are imperfect, with many gaps and many pressing but unmet health needs. Recall once more Annie's illustrative story of struggle to recover from her hip fracture, against an array of social and economic inequalities, and also the story of Linda and her family's efforts to seek care for their mother. There are many "Annies" and "Lindas" who you will meet in clinical practice. To accomplish the true promise of OT undoubtedly requires better knowledge of the communities from which our patients come and the socioeconomic, historical, and political forces that have shaped their lives and their health. Identifying inequalities and disparities where they exist and working to ameliorate them are our ethical responsibilities as healthcare professionals. This is the only way to advance health for all.

Lippincott® Connect *For additional resources on the subjects discussed in this chapter, visit Lippincott Connect.*

REFERENCES

Adler, N. E., Marmot, M., McEwen, B., & Stewart, J. (Eds.). (1999). *Socioeconomic status and health in industrialized nations: Social, psychological, and biological pathways* (*Vol. 896*). Academy of Sciences.

Aldrich, R., Laliberte Rudman, D., Park, N. E., & Huot, S. (2020). Centering the complexity of long-term unemployment: Lessons learned from a critical occupational science inquiry. *Societies, 10*(3), 65. https://doi.org/10.3390/soc10030065

America's Children. (2017). *Child poverty and family income.* http://www.childstats.gov/americaschildren/eco1.asp

Bailey, Z. D., Krieger, N., Agénor, M., Graves, J., Linos, N., & Bassett, M. T. (2017). Structural racism and health inequities in the USA: Evidence and interventions. *Lancet, 389*(10077), 1453–1463. https://doi.org/10.1016/S0140-6736(17)30569-X

Barker, D. (1998). *Mothers, babies and disease in later life* (2nd ed.). Churchill Livingstone Elsevier.

Barnham, B. (2022). *Rheumatoid arthritis affects women differently than men.* https://www.verywellhealth.com/rheumatoid-arthritis-gender-differences-5070797

Bass-Haugen, J. D. (2009). Health disparities: Examination of evidence relevant for occupational therapy. *American Journal of Occupational Therapy, 63*(1), 24–34. https://doi.org/10.5014/ajot.63.1.24

Beagan, B. L. (2021). Commentary on racism in occupational science. *Journal of Occupational Science, 28*(3), 410–413. https://doi.org/10.1080/14427591.2020.1833682

Bipartisan Policy Center. (2020). *Paid family leave across OECD countries.* https://bipartisanpolicy.org/explainer/paid-family-leave-across-oecd-countries/

Bollyky, T. J., Templin, T., Cohen, M., Schoder, D., Dieleman, J. L., & Wigley, S. (2019). The relationships between democratic experience, adult health, and cause-specific mortality in 170 countries between 1980 and 2016: An observational analysis. *The Lancet, 393*(10181), 1628–1640. https://doi.org/10.1016/S0140-6736(19)30235-1

Bourdieu, P. (1984). *Distinction: A social critique of the judgement of taste*. Routledge.

Brandmiller, C., Dumont, H., & Becker, M. (2020). Teacher perceptions of learning motivation and classroom behavior: The role of student characteristics. *Contemporary Educational Psychology, 63,* 101893. https://doi.org/10.1016/j.cedpsych.2020.101893

Braveman, P., & Gottlieb, L. (2014). The social determinants of health: It's time to consider the causes of the causes. *Public Health Reports, 129*(Suppl 2), 19–31. https://doi.org/10.1177/00333549141291S206

British Broadcasting Corporation. (2021). *Homosexuality: The countries where it is illegal to be gay.* https://www.bbc.com/news/world-43822234

Brosso, S. N., Sheeran, P., Lazard, A. J., & Muscatell, K. A. (2021). Harnessing neuroimaging to reduce socioeconomic disparities in chronic disease: A conceptual framework for improving health messaging. *Frontiers in Human Neuroscience, 15,* 576749. https://doi.org/10.3389/fnhum.2021.576749

Ceder, J. (2020). *Childcare costs.* https://www.verywellfamily.com/affording-child-care-4157342#:~:text=The%20average%20cost%20of%20center-based%20daycare%20in%20the,Aware%20of%20America.%20Location%20matters%20when%20considering%20costs

Center on Economic and Policy Research. (2019). *No-vacation nation, revised.* https://www.cepr.net/report/no-vacation-nation-revised/

Centers for Disease Control and Prevention. (2021, April 19). *Health equity considerations and racial and ethnic minority groups.* https://www.cdc.gov/coronavirus/2019-ncov/community/health-equity/race-ethnicity.html

Chappell, N. L., & Havens, B. (1980). Old and female: Testing the double jeopardy hypothesis. *The Sociological Quarterly, 21*(2), 157–171. https://doi.org/10.1111/j.1533-8525.1980.tb00601.x

Ciciurkaite, G. (2021). Race/ethnicity, gender and the SES gradient in BMI: The diminishing returns of SES for racial/ethnic minorities. *Sociology of Health and Illness, 43*(8), 1754–1773. https://doi.org/10.1111/1467-9566.13267

Cloete, L. G., & Ramugondo, E. L. (2015). "I drink": Mothers' alcohol consumption as both individualised and imposed occupation. *South African Journal of Occupational Therapy, 45*(1), 34–40. https://doi.org/10.17159/2310-3833/2015/v45no1a6

Cohen, R. A., & Villarroel, M. A. (2015). Strategies used by adults to reduce their prescription drug costs: United States, 2013. *NCHS Data Brief,* (184), 1–8. https://pubmed.ncbi.nlm.nih.gov/25633356/

Colker, R. (2005). *The disability pendulum: The first decade of the Americans with Disabilities Act.* New York University Press.

Covay Minor, E. (2014). Racial differences in teacher perception of student ability. *Teachers College Record, 116*(10), 1–22. https://doi.org/10.1177/016146811411601004

Creek, J. (2011, November). *2011 ENOTHE inaugural Hanneke van Bruggen lecture "in praise of diversity."* Paper presented at the 2011 annual meeting of the European Network of Occupational Therapy in Higher Education (ENOTHE) in Ghent, Belgium. http://www.enothe.eu/activities/meet/ac11/Appendix3.4.pdf

Crenshaw, K. (1989). *Demarginalizing the intersection of race and sex: A black feminist critique of antidiscrimination doctrine, feminist theory and antiracist politics* (pp. 139–168). University of Chicago Legal Forum.

Cutler, D. (2004). *Your money or your life: Strong medicine for America's health care system.* Oxford University Press.

Denny-Brown, N. (2021). The impact of the COVID-19 pandemic on the long-term care workforce. *Health Services Research, 56*(Suppl 2), 15–16. https://doi.org/10.1111/1475-6773.13733

Econofact. (2021). *Child poverty in the U.S.* https://econofact.org/child-poverty-in-the-u-s

Evans, R. G., Barer, M. L., & Marmor, T. L. (Eds.). (1994). *Why are some people healthy and others not? The determinants of health of populations.* Aldine de Gruyter.

Feeding America. (2021). *Hunger in America, 2014.* https://www.feedingamerica.org/research/hunger-in-america

Fekadu, G., Bekele, F., Tolossa, T., Fetensa, G., Turi, E., Getachew, M., Abdisa, E., Assefa, L., Afeta, M., Demisew, W., Dugassa, D., Diriba, D. C., & Labata, B. G. (2021). Impact of COVID-19 pandemic on chronic diseases care follow-up and current perspectives in low resource settings: A narrative review. *International Journal of Physiology, Pathophysiology and Pharmacology, 13*(3), 86–93. https://pubmed.ncbi.nlm.nih.gov/34336132/

Ferreira, F. (2021). Inequality in the time of COVID-19. *Finance and Development,* 20–23. https://www.imf.org/external/pubs/ft/fandd/2021/06/pdf/inequality-and-covid-19-ferreira.pdf

Fiorati, R. C., & Elui, V. M. (2015). Social determinants of health, inequality and social inclusion among people with disabilities. *Revista Latino-Americana de Enfermagem, 23*(2), 329–336. https://doi.org/10.1590/0104-1169.0187.2559

Fredriksen-Goldsen, K. I., Kim, H. J., & Barkan, S. E. (2012). Disability among lesbian, gay, and bisexual adults: Disparities in prevalence and risk. *American Journal of Public Health, 102*(1), e16–e21. https://doi.org/10.2105/AJPH.2011.300379

Galheigo, S. M. (2011). What needs to be done? Occupational therapy responsibilities and challenges regarding human rights. *Australian Occupational Therapy Journal, 58*(2), 60–66. https://doi.org/10.1111/j.1440-1630.2011.00922.x

Galvaan, R. (2015). The contextually situated nature of occupational choice: Marginalised young adolescents' experiences in South Africa. *Journal of Occupational Science, 22*(1), 39–53. https://doi.org/10.1080/14427591.2014.912124

Galvaan, R. (2021). Generative disruption through occupational science: Enacting possibilities for deep human connection. *Journal of Occupational Science, 28*(1), 6–18. https://doi.org/10.1080/14427591.2020.1818276

Galvaan, R., & Peters, L. (2017). Occupation-based community development: A critical approach to occupational therapy. In S. Dsouza, R. Galvaan, & E. Ramugondo (Eds.), *Concepts in occupational therapy: Understanding southern perspectives* (pp. 172–187). Manipal University Press.

Gower, E., Silverman, E., Cassard, S., Williams, S., Baldonado, K., & Friedman, D. (2013). Barriers to attending an eye examination after vision screening referral within a vulnerable population. *Journal of Health Care for the Poor and Underserved, 24*(3), 1042–1052. https://doi.org/10.1353/hpu.2013.0134

Goyat, R., Vyas, A., & Sambamoorthi, U. (2016). Racial/ethnic disparities in disability prevalence. *Journal of Racial and Ethnic Health Disparities, 3*(4), 635–645. https://doi.org/10.1007/s40615-015-0182-z

Hacker, K., Anies, M., Folb, B. L., & Zallman, L. (2015). Barriers to health care for undocumented immigrants: A literature review. *Risk Management and Healthcare Policy, 8,* 175–183. https://doi.org/10.2147/RMHP.S70173

Hammell, K. W. (2020). Action on the social determinants of health: Advancing occupational equity and occupational rights. *Cadernos Brasileiros de Terapia Ocupacional, 28*(1), 378–400. https://doi.org/10.4322/2526-8910.ctoARF2052

Healthy People 2030, U.S. Department of Health and Human Services, & Office of Disease Prevention and Health Promotion. (2022). *Social determinants of health.* https://health.gov/healthypeople/objectives-and-data/social-determinants-health

Himmelstein, D. U., Lawless, R. M., Thorne, D., Foohey, P., & Woolhandler, S. (2019). Medical bankruptcy: Still common despite the Affordable Care Act. *American Journal of Public Health, 109*(3), 431–433. https://ajph.aphapublications.org/doi/abs/10.2105/AJPH.2018.304901?journalCode=ajph

Hsu, L. C., & Henke, A. (2020). COVID-19, staying at home, and domestic violence. *Review of Economics of the Household, 19*(1), 145–155. https://doi.org/10.1007/s11150-020-09526-7

Huecker, K., King, K., Jordan, G., & Smock, W. (2022, January). Domestic violence. In: *StatPearls* [Internet]. StatPearls Publishing.

Hurst, R. (2003). The international disability rights movement and the ICF. *Disability and Rehabilitation, 25*(11–12), 572–576. https://doi.org/10.1080/0963828031000137072

Hutton, E., Tuppeny, S., & Hasselbusch, A. (2016). Making a case for universal and targeted children's occupational therapy in the United Kingdom. *British Journal of Occupational Therapy, 79*(7), 450–453. https://doi.org/10.1177/0308022615618218

Inequality.org. (2022). *Wealth inequality in the United States.* https://inequality.org/facts/wealth-inequality/

Institute of Medicine. (2002). *Unequal treatment: Confronting racial and ethnic disparities in health care.* National Academies Press.

Investopedia. (2021). *Top 5 reasons why people go bankrupt.* https://www.investopedia.com/financial-edge/0310/top-5-reasons-people-go-bankrupt.aspx

Karim, M. A., Singal, A. G., Ohsfeldt, R. L., Morrisey, M. A., & Kum, H. C. (2021). Health services utilization, out-of-pocket expenditure, and underinsurance among insured non-elderly cancer survivors in the United States, 2011–2015. *Cancer Medicine, 10*(16), 5513–5523. https://doi.org/10.1002/cam4.4103

Kawachi, I., & Berkman, L. (2003). *Neighborhoods and health.* Oxford University Press.

Khazan, O. (2022). *The real reason Americans aren't self-isolating.* https://www.theatlantic.com/politics/archive/2022/01/lack-paid-sick-leave-undermines-covid-isolation/621233/

Kozol, J. (1991). *Savage inequalities: Children in America's schools.* HarperCollins.

Kozol, J. (1995). *Amazing grace: The lives of children and the conscience of a nation.* Crown.

Kronenberg, F., & Pollard, N. (2005). Overcoming occupational apartheid: A preliminary exploration of the political nature of occupational therapy. In F. Kronenberg, S. Algado, & N. Pollard (Eds.), *Occupational therapy without borders: Learning from the spirit of survivors* (pp. 58–86). Elsevier.

Law, M. (1998). *Client-centered occupational therapy.* SLACK.

Lawlor, M. C. (2003). Gazing anew: The shift from a clinical gaze to an ethnographic lens. *American Journal of Occupational Therapy, 57*(1), 29–39. https://doi.org/10.5014/ajot.57.1.29

Loucks, E. B., Almeida, N. D., Taylor, S. E., & Matthews, K. A. (2011). Childhood family psychosocial environment and coronary heart disease risk. *Psychosomatic Medicine, 73*(7), 563–571. https://doi.org/10.1097/PSY.0b013e318228c820

Lucas, C., & Washington, S. (2020). *Understanding systemic racism in the United States: Educating our students and ourselves.* AOTA.

Mackey, K., Ayers, C. K., Kondo, K. K., Saha, S., Advani, S. M., Young, S., Spencer, H., Rusek, M., Anderson, J., Veazie, S., Smith, M., & Kansagara, D. (2021). Racial and ethnic disparities in COVID-19–related infections, hospitalizations, and deaths: A systematic review. *Annals of Internal Medicine, 174*(3), 362–373. https://doi.org/10.7326/M20-6306

MacPhee, D., Farro, S., & Canetto, S. S. (2013). Academic self-efficacy and performance of underrepresented STEM Majors: Gender, ethnic, and social class patterns. *Analyses of Social Issues and Public Policy, 13*(1), 347–369. https://psycnet.apa.org/doi/10.1111/asap.12033

Madsen, J., Kanstrup, A. M., & Josephsson, S. (2016). The assumed relation between occupation and inequality in health. *Scandinavian Journal of Occupational Therapy, 23*(1), 1–12, https://doi.org/10.3109/11038128.2015.1075065

Marmot, M. (2017). Social justice, epidemiology and health inequalities. *European Journal of Epidemiology, 32*(7), 537–546. https://doi.org/10.1007/s10654-017-0286-3

Mayo Clinic. (2022). *Depression in women: Understanding the gender gap.* https://www.mayoclinic.org/diseases-conditions/depression/in-depth/depression/art-20047725

McEwen, C., & McEwen, B. S. (2017). Social structure, adversity, toxic stress, and intergenerational poverty: An early childhood model. *Annual Reviews of Sociology, 43*(1), 445–472. https://doi.org/10.1146/annurev-soc-060116-053252

Merikangas, K. R., He, J. P., Brody, D., Fisher, P. W., Bourdon, K., & Koretz, D. S. (2010). Prevalence and treatment of mental disorders among US children in the 2001–2004 NHANES. *Pediatrics, 125*(1), 75–81. https://doi.org/10.1542/peds.2008-2598

Nambi, N., & Artiga, S. (2021, May 11). *Disparities in health and health care: 5 key questions and answers.* https://www.kff.org/racial-equity-and-health-policy/issue-brief/disparities-in-health-and-health-care-5-key-question-and-answers

National Academies of Sciences, Engineering, and Medicine. (2020). *Understanding the well-being of LGBTQI+ populations.* The National Academies Press. https://doi.org/10.17226/25877

National Center for Health Statistics. (2021). *Health, United States, 2021.* https://www.cdc.gov/nchs/data/hus/hus18.pdf

Nowatzki, N. R. (2012). Wealth inequality and health: A political economy perspective. *International Journal of Health Services, 42*(3), 403–424. https://doi.org/10.2190/HS.42.3.c

Obama, B. (2016). United States health care reform progress to date and next steps. *JAMA, 316*(5), 525–532. https://doi.org/10.1001/jama.2016.9797

Online Dictionary of the Social Sciences. (2022). *Online resource.* http://bitbucket.icaap.org

Organisation for Economic Co-operation and Development. (2019). *Health at a glance.* http://www.oecd.org/els/health-systems/health-data.htm

Payscale. (2022). *2022 state of the gender pay gap report.* https://www.payscale.com/research-and-insights/gender-pay-gap/

Pentland, W., Tremblay, M., Spring, K., & Rosenthal, C. (1999). Women with physical disabilities: Occupational impacts of ageing. *Journal of Occupational Science, 6*(3), 111–123. https://doi.org/10.1080/14427591.1999.9686456

Perera, I., & Douglas, K. (2020, June 26). A here and now challenge for occupational therapists. *News Blog.* https://rehab.queensu.ca/blog/here-and-now-challenge-occupational-therapists

Pew Research Center. (2021). *Gender pay gap in U.S. held steady in 2020.* https://www.pewresearch.org/fact-tank/2021/05/25/gender-pay-gap-facts/

Piketty, T. (2022). *A brief history of equality.* Harvard University Press.

Pitonyak, J. S., Mroz, T. M., & Fogelberg, D. (2015). Expanding client-centered thinking to include social determinants: A practical scenario based on the occupation of breastfeeding. *Scandinavian Journal of Occupational Therapy, 22*(4), 277–282. https://doi.org/10.3109/11038128.2015.1020865

Pollard, N., & Sakellariou, D. (2017). Occupational therapy on the margins. *World Federation of Occupational Therapists Bulletin, 73*(2), 71–75. https://doi.org/10.1080/14473828.2017.1361698

Pooler, M., & Pulice, C. (2021, July 12). Brazil's COVID wave hits pregnant women especially hard. *Financial Times.* https://www.ft.com/content/a65810d5-5e14-4aac-8500-533115cc3e38

Pooley, E. A., & Beagan, B. L. (2021). The concept of oppression and occupational therapy: A critical interpretive synthesis. *Canadian Journal of Occupational Therapy, 88*(4), 407–417. https://doi.org/10.1177/00084174211051168

Purtilo, R., Haddad, A., & Doherty, R. (2018). *Health professional and patient interaction* (8th ed.). Saunders.

Quiñones, A. R., Botoseneanu, A., Markwardt, S., Nagel, C. L., Newsom, J. T., Dorr, D. A., & Allore, H. G. (2019). Racial/ethnic differences in multimorbidity development and chronic disease accumulation for middle-aged adults. *PLoS One, 14*(6), e0218462. https://doi.org/10.1371/journal.pone.0218462

Saez, E., & Zucman, G. (2019). *How would a progressive wealth tax work? Evidence from the economics literature.* https://eml.berkeley.edu/~saez/saez-zucman-wealthtaxobjections.pdf

Seabrook, J. A., & Avison, W. R. (2012). Socioeconomic status and cumulative disadvantage processes across the life course: Implications for health outcomes. *Canadian Review of Sociology, 49*(1), 50–68. https://doi.org/10.1111/j.1755-618x.2011.01280.x

Self.Inc. (2022). *Mapping poverty: The poverty rates in each U.S. state over time.* https://www.self.inc/info/poverty-rates-in-each-state/

Semyonov, M., Lewin-Epstein, N., & Maskileyson, D. (2013). Where wealth matters more for health: The wealth health gradient in 16 countries. *Social Science & Medicine, 81*, 10–17. https://doi.org/10.1016/j.socscimed.2013.01.010

Shonkoff, J., & Phillips, D. (Eds.). (2000). *From neurons to neighborhoods: The science of early childhood development.* National Academies Press.

Shonkoff, J. P. (2011). Protecting brains, not simply stimulating minds. *Sciences, 333*(6045), 982–983. https://doi.org/10.1126/science.1206014

Surowiecki, J. (2014, March 3). The mobility myth. *The New Yorker.* https://www.newyorker.com/magazine/2014/03/03/the-mobility-myth

Synovec, C., & Aceituno, L. (2020). Social justice considerations for occupational therapy: The role of addressing social determinants of health in unstably housed population. *Work, 65*(2), 235–246. https://doi.org/10.3233/WOR-203074

The Commonwealth Fund. (2020). *U.S. healthcare from a global perspective, 2020: Higher spending, worse outcomes?* https://www.commonwealthfund.org/publications/issue-briefs/2020/jan/us-health-care-global-perspective-2019

The Commonwealth Fund. (2021). *Mirror, mirror 2021: Reflecting poorly.* https://www.commonwealthfund.org/publications/fund-reports/2021/aug/mirror-mirror-2021-reflecting-poorly

Townsend, E., & Wilcock, A. (2003). Occupational justice. In C. Christiansen & E. Townsend (Eds.), *Introduction to occupation: The art and science of living* (pp. 243–273). Prentice Hall.

U.S. Administration on Aging. (2020). *Older Americans 2020: Key indicators of well-being.* https://agingstats.gov/docs/LatestReport/OA20_508_10142020.pdf

U.S. Census Bureau. (2018). *Americans with disabilities, 2014.* https://www.census.gov/content/dam/Census/library/publications/2018/demo/p70-152.pdf

U.S. Census Bureau. (2019). *Income, poverty, and health insurance coverage in the United States: 2019.* https://www.census.gov/newsroom/press-releases/2019/income-poverty.html

U.S. Department of Health and Human Services, & Office of Minority Health. (2021). *Infant mortality and African Americans.* https://www.minorityhealth.hhs.gov/omh/browse.aspx?lvl=4&lvlid=23

U.S. Department of Labor. (2011). *Employment standards administration wage and hour division.* http://www.dol.gov/dol/topic/wages/minimumwage.htm

U.S. Department of Labor. (2012). *Fact sheet#28: The Family and Medical Leave Act.* https://www.dol.gov/agencies/whd/fact-sheets/28-fmla

Warshaw, G., Potter, J., Flaherty, E., McNabney, M., Heflin, M., & Ham, R. (2021). Principles of care of older adults. In G. Warshaw, J. Potter, E. Flaherty, M. McNabney, M. Heflin, & R. Ham (Eds.), *Ham's primary care geriatrics* (pp. 3–15). Elsevier.

Whiteford, G. (2000). Occupational deprivation: Global challenge in the new millennium. *British Journal of Occupational Therapy, 63*(5), 200–204. https://doi.org/10.1177/030802260006300503

Wilkinson, R., & Marmot, M. (Eds.). (2003). *Social determinants of health: The solid facts* (2nd ed.). World Health Organization, Regional Office for Europe.

Wilkinson, R. G., & Pickett, K. E. (2017). The enemy between us: The psychological and social costs of inequality. *European Journal of Social Psychology, 47*(1), 11–24. https://doi.org/10.1002/ejsp.2275

Wood, W. (1996). Delivering occupational therapy's fullest promise: Clinical interpretations of "life domains and adaptive strategies of a group of low-income, well older adults." *American Journal of Occupational Therapy, 50*(2), 109–112. https://doi.org/10.5014/ajot.50.2.109

World Federation of Occupational Therapy. (2020). *Statement on systemic racism.* https://wfot.org/assets/resources/WFOT-Statement-on-Systemic-Racism.pdf

World Health Organization. (2021a). *Violence against women.* https://www.who.int/news-room/fact-sheets/detail/violence-against-women

World Health Organization. (2021b). *Disability and health.* https://www.who.int/news-room/fact-sheets/detail/disability-and-health

World Health Organization. (2021c). *Ageism is a global challenge.* https://www.who.int/news/item/18-03-2021-ageism-is-a-global-challenge-un

World Health Organization. (2022). *Social determinants of health.* https://www.who.int/health-topics/social-determinants-of-health#tab=tab_3

Yegorov, Y., Poznyak, A., Nikiforov, N., Sobenin, I., & Orekhov, A. (2020). The link between chronic stress and accelerated aging. *Biomedicines, 8*(7), 198. https://doi.org/10.3390/biomedicines8070198

Yuval-Davis, N. (2015). Situated intersectionality and social inequality. *Raisons Politiques, 58*(2), 91–100. https://doi.org/10.3917/rai.058.0091

Disability Rights in Action

Aster (né Elizabeth) Harrison (*Pronouns: They/Them*) and Kimberly J. The (*Pronouns: She/Her*)

OUTLINE

LEARNING OBJECTIVES

After reading this chapter, you will be able to:

1. Compare and contrast models of disability and relate these to occupational therapy practice.
2. Identify social, political, and environmental barriers to participation for people with disabilities and generate strategies for deconstructing those barriers.
3. Describe key disability movements, including the disability rights, Mad, self-advocacy, neurodiversity, and disability justice movements.
4. Critically reflect on the sociopolitical, economic, and cultural perspectives that influence your practice as an occupational therapist.
5. Identify key disability organizations and resources to consult to continue learning about disability movements.

Introduction

This chapter is just the beginning of your learning about disability rights. In order to make the most of it, review the tips for reading in Box 16.1.

BOX 16.1 THINKING ABOUT DISABILITY: TIPS FOR READING

1. Take out a piece of paper, start a note on your phone, or open up a document on your computer. As you read, make note of the disability resources and organizations mentioned. What do the authors mention that you would like to Google later? Which organizations interest you most?
2. Consider planning a break for halfway through your reading. You may want to pause for a few minutes when you reach Box 16.2: Thinking About Disability: A Moment to Reflect.

What Is Disability?

Disability has meant many different things throughout history and can mean different things depending on the context. For example, in the United States, disability means something different for Medicaid eligibility than it does when considering whether someone qualifies for reasonable accommodations under the Americans with Disabilities Act (ADA).

There is often a lot at stake when considering disability. Being considered disabled means that you could gain access to vibrant and proud disability communities with rich histories. It could mean that you become further subjected to oppression and stigma. It could mean anything in between. There are many different definitions of disability. Definitions of disability are debated, and which definition you choose informs how you think about disability and what to do about it.

The meaning of disability can vary based on the focus and function. The Centers for Disease Control and Prevention (n.d.) describes *disability* as "any condition of the body or mind (impairment) that makes it more difficult for the person with the condition to do certain activities (activity limitation) and interact with the world around them" (para. 1). This definition has a focus on disability as primarily located within the individual and how it impacts their ability to be a part of normative functions of society.

The ADA defines disability as "a physical or mental impairment that substantially limits one or more major life activities, a person who has a history or record of such an impairment, or a person who is perceived by others as having such an impairment" (ADA National Network, n.d.-a). The ADA definition of disability starts off similarly to the CDC definition of disability. However, it also introduces a broader scope with the reference to "records" and "perception of" being disabled. This definition comes with a recognition that some disabilities are visible and some are less visible. This definition also comes with an acknowledgment that physical and attitudinal environmental barriers create discrimination for people with different types of disabilities. Lydia X. Z. Brown (2014) describes that disability,

> arises when a person whose neurological, mental, emotional, and or physical differences are atypical and divergent enough from the neurologies and physicalities of the majority so that this person is forced to exist and live in a society and world not constructed to incorporate natural supports and full inclusion and access for people like this person. (pp. 39–40)

This definition of disability emphasizes that disability is created by the interaction between bodies and environments (Brown, 2014). Consider this question: Is someone whose vision can be corrected to 20/20 with glasses disabled? The answer depends on the environment. If you are a person with vision insurance or enough money to buy glasses, living in an area where vision care is readily available, you might not be disabled because your environment provides the necessary supports you need to participate in all of your desired occupations. If, on the other hand, you are unable to access glasses, you might be considered to have a disability; that is, your body will not be adequately supported by the available resources, and this may impact your participation.

Definitions of disability matter greatly to how we understand disability and what to do about it. Definitions of disability are also informed by the models of disability that we use.

Models of Disability

Models provide shortcuts for explaining phenomena, such as disability. As you read about these models, consider how they interact with your own understanding of disability. Also reflect on how you have seen people with disabilities treated in the media, in public, and in healthcare settings. How have various disability models shaped those interactions?

Two primary models of disability used today are the medical model of disability and the social model of disability. The *medical model of disability* (sometimes also referred to as the "individual model of disability") is the most commonly used model of disability in our society. This is the case not only in healthcare but also in media, policy, and everyday conversations. The *social model of disability* was developed by disabled[1] activists and disability studies scholars. The social model is preferred in the disability rights movement (DRM) and in disability communities. It is becoming more widely understood and used, but it still has not become as commonplace as the medical model. Figure 16.1 compares the medical, rehabilitative (functional), and social models of disability.

Medical Model of Disability

The medical model of disability views disability as an individual, bodily impairment that should be fixed by medical treatments (Oliver, 1990). The medical model of disability views disability as an objective fact about someone's body or mind, rather than as a social identity. The medical model of disability suggests that a person should cure or minimize their physical and/or mental impairments in order to return to full participation in occupations.

The rehabilitative model of disability (or "functional model of disability" in Figure 16.1) is closely related to the medical model of disability. A rehabilitative model shifts the focus slightly, considering the functional limitations that a

---

[1]Some people within disability communities prefer person first language (i.e., people with disabilities) while others prefer disability first or identity first language (i.e., disabled people). This chapter will utilize the two types of language interchangeably to reflect this complexity. It is important to ask people how they would like to be identified if you do not know. See the APA guide to bias-free disability language for more (APA Style, 2021).

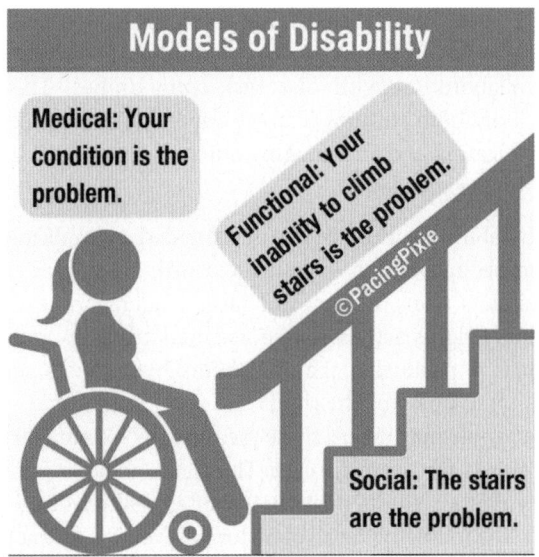

FIGURE 16.1 A graphical illustration created by Ankaret El Haj comparing the medical, functional (rehabilitative), and social models of disability. The person in the picture cannot get up the stairs. Who is to blame? The medical and rehabilitative models state that the person's bodily or functional impairment is the problem. The social model states that the stairs are the problem. (Reproduced with permission from Ankaret El Haj.)

person has because of their bodily impairments. However, the rehabilitative model still tends to put the responsibility on the disabled individual to overcome or minimize their functional limitations in order to participate fully. The rehabilitation model also emphasizes recovery and return to a normative state of being.

The medical and rehabilitative models are frequently used in occupational therapy (OT). These models are at work in OT interventions using the "establish, restore (remediation, restoration)" approach to maximize range of motion or strength, for example. Persons receiving OT services may sometimes desire a medical model or rehabilitative model approach to intervention. However, the Disability Rights Movement strongly criticizes the medical and rehabilitative models of disability because they fail to fully recognize the limiting barriers imposed by the social, political, cultural, and built environment. In order to address these critiques, disability activists propose we understand disability through a different lens—the social model of disability.

Social Model of Disability

The social model of disability highlights the role of the sociocultural and physical environment in creating many of the participation barriers faced by people with disabilities (Oliver, 1990). The social model of disability explains that bodily and mental impairments are not inherently negative. Moreover, impairments are not to blame for the participation restrictions disabled people experience. Rather, the inaccessible physical, social, and political environment is the problem. The social model explains that disability is not an individual issue, but rather a political and social issue. Rather than working to reduce impairments through medical treatments to bring disabled people closer to "normal" functioning, the social model argues that we should address disability by fighting for accessibility and disability rights. The social model argues that with proper accessibility and/or accommodations, impairments should not limit someone's participation in roles and occupations of their choosing. Proponents of the social model of disability often prefer the term "disabled person" to "person with a disability" because it indicates that a person with impairments is *disabled by* their environment (see Figure 16.1).

The minority group model is one variation of the social model of disability. The minority group model (Hahn, 1985) describes people with disabilities as a minority group that experiences systematic oppression, marginalization, alienation, and social and political isolation. The oppression that disabled people experience is called **ableism**. In addition to naming disabled people as a group who experience oppression, the minority group model also highlights strengths of the group. It opens up possibilities for pride in a common identity (otherwise known as *disability pride*). The minority group model was partially inspired by how other minority groups (e.g., based on race, gender, or sexual identity) in mid-century America had fought for their civil rights through political advocacy and activism. The minority group model pointed toward political solutions to breaking down barriers to social and political participation. This model incorporated terms and concepts from other rights campaigns that emerged as disability culture, disability pride, and disability identity.

Different models of disability offer contrasting views of what disability means and what society should do about it. From the classic medical model perspective, the individual with an illness or impairment is deficient and abnormal. A professional or team of professionals is required to heal, fix, or cure the deficiency in the individual's body through medication, surgery, and technology; and independence is the ultimate goal and measure of success. From a social model viewpoint, disability is simply another kind of human diversity (similar to skin color, gender, size, and ethnicity), and the real problem is inaccessibility and oppressive, ableist social structures. Like many differences, especially those attributed to minority groups, there are positive and negative aspects of the lived experience of disability, many of which are heavily influenced by social policies, practices, and attitudes. An OT practitioner working in alignment with the social model of disability would focus more on changing the world to accommodate disabled bodies rather than changing disabled bodies to better fit the existing world.

There are critiques of the social model that point out how some disabled people might want *both* social change *and* medical treatment to address their disabilities (Crow, 1996; Wendell, 1996); however, the social model is widely embraced as the best available way to understand disability. The social model is a foundation of disability rights work. If you are new to disability rights, developing a strong understanding of the social model is a powerful first step in your journey.

The social model of disability is compared with the medical model of disability in Table 16.1.

Disability Activism

Disabled people have engaged in activism to fight for civil rights and social justice in many different ways. These social change efforts can be categorized under the umbrellas of several different social movements, including the Disability Rights Movement (DRM), the Mad movement, the self-advocacy movement, the neurodiversity movement, and the disability justice movement. As you read about the movements, we encourage you to write down the organizations mentioned to further research them or follow them on social media to learn more.

The Disability Rights Movement

The history of the Disability Rights Movement is important for OT students and practitioners to understand for several reasons:

1. The DRM provides one way to understand people with disabilities outside the patient role they often occupy in interactions with occupational therapists.
2. Understanding the DRM is a way to understand sustained priorities of disability communities as a politicized and proud identity group.

3. OT has a role in sustaining the spirit of the laws that came out of the DRM. This should be done in strong collaboration with disability communities. This includes both within OT practitioners' daily practice and educating and encouraging others to uphold these disability rights laws.

Disability rights history is grounded in traditions of grassroots activism. It is connected with other civil rights movements along the lines of race, gender, and sexuality. Disability rights activists often use methods such as **direct action** (e.g., protesting, chaining themselves to buses, getting arrested) to push for the rights and services that they need. Some people may regard these measures as "extreme." However, this is far from the case. The rights and services disability rights activists push for are often matters of life and death. The following recall of historical events is meant to be brief and only highlights some key moments of the DRM. For a more comprehensive history of the US DRM, there are many great resources including University of California Berkeley's website on the disability rights and independent living movements (University of California, 2010) and the documentary *Crip Camp* on Netflix (LeBrecht & Newnham, 2020). A timeline of US disability rights events from 1780 to 2008 is also included in the online resources associated with this chapter on Lippincott Connect. Our overview of international disability rights events is even more brief than that of the US DRM. We recommend the database of international disability rights laws created by the Disability Rights Education and Defense Fund (DREDF) as a starting point to learn more about international movements (DREDF, 2021).

Although most scholars point to the 1960s or 1970s as the beginning of the international DRM (Charlton, 2000), roots of the movement stretch back to the 1940s and even earlier. Early disability rights organizations engaged in advocacy around employment for people with disabilities, including the poor working conditions at sheltered

| TABLE 16.1 | Comparing Models of Disability |

	Medical or Rehabilitative Model	Social or Minority Group Model
Impairment is...	Abnormal	A neutral difference
	Inferior	OK and natural
Participation restrictions are caused by...	Bodily or mental impairment, located within the person	Environmental and societal factors that oppress people with impairments
The solution is...	Cure or overcoming impairment through rehabilitation	Minimizing environmental and societal barriers, providing the person with support and resources, fighting for disability rights
The expert is...	The professional	The person with a disability

Adapted from Heffron, J. L., & VanPuymbrouck, L. (2015). *Introduction to disability studies theory* [Guest lecture]. OT 500: Theories of Occupational Therapy, University of Illinois at Chicago; and Hammel, J., Charlton, J., Jones, R. A., Kramer, J. M., & Wilson, T. (2014). Disability rights and advocacy. In B. A. Boyt Schell, G. Gillen, & M. E. Scaffa (Eds.), *Willard and Spackman's occupational therapy* (12th ed., pp. 1031–1050). Lippincott, Williams, & Wilkins.

workshops. Organizations such as the National Mental Health Foundation also advocated to improve conditions at state mental institutions (Pelka, 1997). The first Disabled Student's Program and the wheelchair basketball tournament began in Illinois toward the end of the 1940s. Additional disability organizations were founded in the United States and internationally throughout the 1950s (e.g., Aoi Shiba in Japan, see Hayashi & Okuhira, 2001).

Although early disability organizations lacked the broad political momentum of the later movement, they were important in bringing disabled people together. As disabled people gathered, they began to realize that the issues in their lives were not merely individual medical problems, but rather injustices that other disabled people also experienced (Charlton, 2000). Even when not formally engaged in advocacy, coming together with other disabled people in patient groups or sporting events allowed disabled people to build community. These community spaces provided the necessary conditions for a shared disability identity—and later a shared movement—to grow.

In the 1960s, the first state and national accessibility laws were passed in the United States. International disability rights laws also began to appear, such as the Handicapped Persons Act in Zambia and the Blind Persons Act in South Africa.

The 1970s were a time of explosive growth for the DRM around the world. In 1970, in Japan, patients of the Fuchu Ryoiku institution participated in a hunger strike to protest their cruel and inhumane treatment at the institution (Hayashi & Okuhira, 2001). In 1971, in the United States, the *Wyatt v. Stickney* decision was finally issued, which required that people held in institutions receive treatment—rather than simply being incarcerated. In 1972, a lawsuit was filed on behalf of the residents in the Willowbrook State School in New York in response to the horrific treatment of disabled children there (Pelka, 1997).

In 1972, the first Center for Independent Living (CIL) was founded in Berkeley, California. This center served as a hub for disability resources, socialization, and advocacy (O'Toole, 2015). The disabled people associated with the Berkeley CIL not only supported the local community but also educated and inspired disability leaders around the world. The foundation of this first CIL launched the Independent Living Movement, an important component of the international DRM (Charlton, 2000; University of California, 2010). CILs are cross-disability, community-oriented organizations that are "consumer controlled," meaning they are created by and for disabled people (National Council on Independent Living, n.d.). Most CILs in the United States were set up in the early 1980s. There are now more than 350 CILs in the United States. One requirement of CILs is that at least 51% of employees in each CIL need to be disabled (Independent Living Research Utilization, n.d.). CILs are good places for OTs to refer newly disabled clients to as it can

help them get connected to their local disability community as well as vital services to support their community living.

Thanks to the work of disabled activists, additional disability rights laws were created in the 1970s. Section 504 of the Rehabilitation Act of 1973 made it illegal to discriminate against disabled people in programs that receive federal funding and federal employment (DREDF, n.d.). When the Act was passed in 1973, disability activists were excited to see it enforced so that they could experience increased access to education, employment, and other services. However, Section 504 was not enforceable without further regulations. Activists pushed then-presidential-candidate Jimmy Carter to commit to issuing regulations, but after his election, Carter failed to do so in a timely manner. By 1976, disability activists were tired of waiting. They began sit-in protests in federal buildings in several states. The sit-in in the US Department of Health, Education, and Welfare (HEW) building in San Francisco lasted more than 25 days, making it the longest sit-in inside a federal building in US history (Shapiro, 1993). Organizations associated with the civil rights movement, the gay rights movement, the labor movement, and other rights struggles offered support and solidarity to disability activists during the sit-in (O'Toole, 2015; Schweik, 2011). The short film *The Power of 504* (DREDF, 2015) and the feature-length documentary *Crip Camp* (LeBrecht & Newnham, 2020) offer inside looks at this powerful protest.

The Education for All Handicapped Children Act (later known as the *Individuals with Disabilities Education Act* [IDEA]) was passed in 1975 and promised to guarantee a "free and appropriate public education" to disabled people aged 3 to 21 years. It also established funding for early intervention services for children under 3 years of age. It also requires public schools to provide Individualized Education Programs (IEPs) to meet the needs of children with disabilities. Transition services to support adolescents preparing for employment or college were also established by IDEA (U.S. Department of Education, 2017).

In the United Kingdom, the Union of the Physically Impaired Against Segregation (UPIAS) formed in 1972 (Charlton, 2000). In 1975, the UPIAS issued a document called "Fundamental Principles of Disability" with the Disability Alliance (1975). This document contained key ideas that would become the foundation of the social model of disability. More and more disability organizations popped up around the world, including the National Council of Disabled Persons of Zimbabwe (n.d.).

The movement continued to grow throughout the 1980s. At the 1980 Rehabilitation International (RI) conference, a group of attendees with disabilities protested the fact that RI was led almost entirely by nondisabled professionals. They demanded that at least half of the RI delegates should be people with disabilities. Their demands were not accepted; however, the event spurred the attendees with disabilities to form Disabled People's International (DPI)

(Charlton, 2000). Today, DPI groups exist in many different countries around the world (Charlton, 2000).

The United Nations declared 1981 the International Year of Disabled Persons, and many disability groups organized around this historic year. Important disability rights organizations were founded in the 1980s, including the Organization of the Revolutionary Disabled in Nicaragua, the Self-Help Association of Paraplegics (Soweto) (SHAP), the Program of Rehabilitation Organized by Disabled Youth of Western Mexico (PROJIMO), DPI-Thailand, and the Southern Africa Federation of the Disabled (SAFOD) (Charlton, 2000). Throughout the 1980s, the American Disabled for Accessible Public Transportation participated in acts of civil disobedience (such as sit-ins and blocking traffic) to protest the inaccessibility of the public transportation system (see Figure 16.2). They would go on to become a powerful national disability rights organization, now known as ADAPT (ADAPT, n.d.). The documentary *Piss on Pity: We Will Ride* (Grosz, 2019) offers a closer look at ADAPT's early work.

The 1990s started with a bang for the American DRM, with the passage of the ADA in 1990. The ADA is a comprehensive civil rights law that mandates equal opportunities for people with disabilities in American society in employment, public services, public accommodation, transportation, and telecommunication (ADA.gov, n.d.). The passage of the ADA was the result of decades of disability rights advocacy, civil disobedience, and protest that pressured lawmakers. This included a protest in which activists crawled up the steps of the Capitol building, called the *Capitol Crawl*, pictured in Figure 16.3.

The fight for disability rights did not stop with the ADA. The Olmstead decision is another key piece of disability rights history that was spurred by the efforts of two disabled women named Lois Curtis and Elaine Wilson. Curtis and Wilson were living at a state mental institution in Georgia. They wanted to live in the community, but the state denied

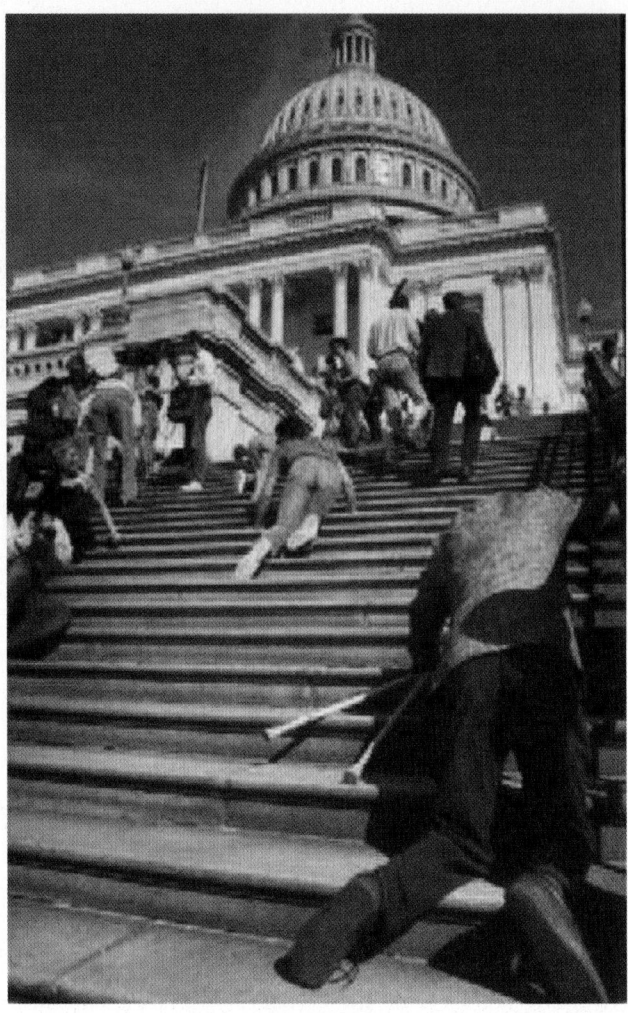

FIGURE 16.3 **The Capitol Crawl protest occurred on March 13, 1990. Disability activists crawled up the steps of the Capitol building to demand the passage of the Americans with Disabilities Act. (Photo by Tom Olin.)**

their request to be moved out of the institution. Curtis and Wilson filed a lawsuit, and in 1999, the Supreme Court ruled that their involuntary institutionalization was a violation of their rights under the ADA (Equip for Equality, 2019). This decision ignited activists and led to widespread systems change, particularly initiatives to rebalance long-term care financing toward community-based options and away from institutional care. These included changes to Medicaid rules and the formation of community-based waiver programs. The "Supporting Community Living" section in this chapter offers examples of OT practitioners working to support the rights of people with disabilities to live in the community, following the Olmstead decision.

The most comprehensive international disability rights agreement to date was introduced in 2006 by the United Nations: The Convention on the Rights of Persons with Disabilities (CRPD) (United Nations, n.d.). The CRPD offers

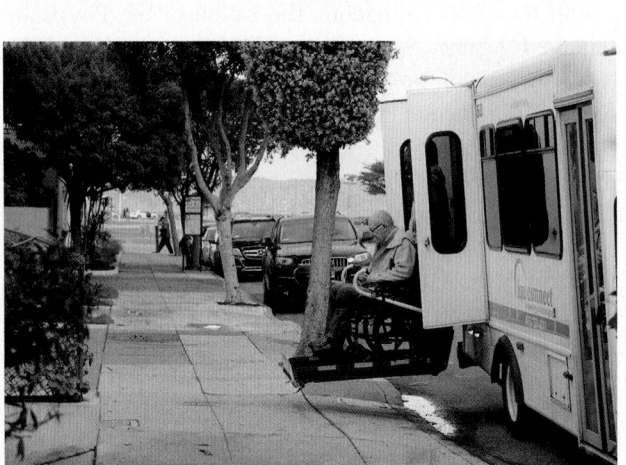

FIGURE 16.2 **Access to public transportation, such as this accessible bus, is a focus of the disability rights movement.**

comprehensive guidelines to reduce environmental barriers and improve the inclusion of people with disabilities across many spheres of public life. For another viewpoint on the CRPD, see Expanding Our Perspectives. As of this writing, 183 countries and the European Union have ratified the CRPD. The United States signed the CRPD (signaling initial agreement) but has failed to go through the necessary legal processes to ratify the convention. This means the United States is not currently bound by the CRPD. As we discuss later in this chapter, the DRM is ongoing.

The Americans With Disabilities Act

Now, let us take a closer look at the most comprehensive disability rights law in the United States: the ADA. Recall that the ADA defines disability as "(A) a physical or mental impairment that substantially limits one or more of the major life activities of an individual; (B) a record of such an impairment; or (C) being regarded as having such impairment" (ADA, 1990).

Each specific part of the ADA is useful for American OT practitioners to understand because there are practice implications associated with each title. The focus of the ADA definition on "major life activities" indicates the important role that OT should play in evaluating and recording these effects on major life activities. For example, an occupational therapist is well equipped to participate in the process that helps determine whether or not a person's disability qualifies for accommodations under the ADA or

---

EXPANDING OUR PERSPECTIVES
Disability Rights or Not?

Randa Abdelrahim

As of February 2022, 183 state members have signed the United Nations CRPD. Despite the high acceptance of the CRPD as a comprehensive human rights treaty, I often wonder if disability means the same thing across the nations. The CRPD was modeled after the "Western" social model, so ideas about disability migrated from the West to the East. I remember learning about the social model in OT school, but not about the movement that made it a language for disability rights.

I got my OT degree from Jordan. I do not recall thinking about the social model during my practice until one instance that changed my perspective. I was working in an outpatient clinic, and one day, I was in the elevator with a client—a child with cerebral palsy and a walker user—and another unrelated man. I was going to the therapy room for a session to work on fine motor skills with the child. A few seconds before the elevator door opened, the man said, "Praise be to Allah who saved me from what afflicted you and favored me over many of His creations." The man's voice was loud, and the child and I could hear him. We walked out of the elevator, and I could notice how distressed the child became even during the entire 1-hour session. I did not think about the social perspective of disability at that moment, but I asked myself if this is what Islam taught him, to be unmindful of the feelings of a 7-year-old child?

I have amblyopia in one eye. Even though I have 20/20 functional vision, some people who noticed or knew about my impairment made me feel like a victim, that I will not be able to live a fulfilling life like everyone else and that I need to be saved. During my PhD studies, meanings of the social model started to resonate. I know that I am socially disabled. My participation is sometimes limited because of social barriers related to how people perceive my

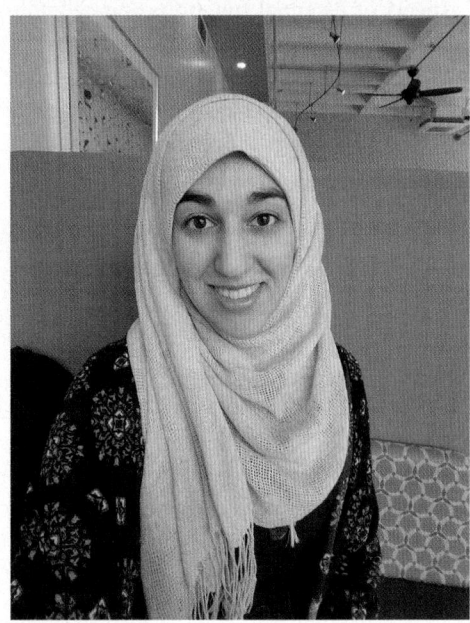

Randa Abdelrahim

impairment. But the social model may not be the best way to advocate for disability in my community. As Muslims, Islamic ideals dominate social relationships. The perception of a fulfilling life is related to Islam. I cannot go back to that elevator and talk about rights to a person who thought disability is a religious issue. So, I embarked on a journey to explore advocating for disability in Muslim communities. During my journey, I found that the prayer the man said in the elevator is socially constructed and falsely linked to the Prophet Muhammad peace be upon him. Disability is part of the human experience in Islam. It is not a hardship nor a bliss. As occupational therapists, we should recognize how disability forms in the life of our clients because they may not find a connection to disability rights if advocacy was placed outside the context they recognize.

the occupational therapist might serve as an expert witness (DeMaio-Feldman, 1987) in a disability discrimination case. OT practitioners are often called on to apply their skills in activity analysis to document the "essential functions" (Canelón, 1995) of a job to better determine whether or not people with disabilities can perform the job "with or without accommodation." The ADA has five "titles" or subsections that describe who and what is affected by the law.

Title I. Employers must offer "**reasonable accommodations**," an adaptation that helps the individual meet the "**essential functions**" of the job (a list of all the tasks and physical and cognitive demands of the work). The accommodations must be "readily achievable" and will not present an "undue hardship" on the employer (i.e., will not cost the employer a disproportionate amount relative to the value the typical worker produces and the size of the business).

- *OT implications:* OT practitioners can help identify ableist aspects of essential functions and redefine these functions to be more inclusive. Practitioners can also work with disabled people on reasonable accommodations and provide environmental modifications needed for disabled people to meet the essential functions of the work.

Title II. Title II affects publicly funded services and agencies, including public transportation.

- *OT implications:* OTs can support clients in self-advocating for their rights to transportation access. For an example of one way to advocate for transportation access, refer to OT Story 16.1.

Title III. Title III covers public accommodations and services that are operated by private entities, such as theaters, hotels, private schools, retailers, and restaurants. All construction after 1992 must comply with the ADA Accessibility Guidelines (ADAAG). The language and spirit of Title III is intended to provide a "vision of an inclusive public world" (Parmet, 1993, p. 128).

- *OT implications:* The ADAAG compliance regulations are worth knowing to support consultation with businesses that want to improve access and to identify noncompliant businesses. OT practitioners can educate people on the guidelines. In addition, OT practitioners can advocate on a local level by encouraging businesses to improve access and compliance, consulting with them on the standards, or reporting infractions.

OT STORY 16.1 OCCUPATIONAL THERAPIST WORKING IN DISABILITY RIGHTS SETTINGS

This story is based on a real-life event that took place in one of the author's (Kim The's) work as a community organizer for a disability rights activist group.

An OT student has been accepted into a semester-long service-learning placement in an activist group housed within a CIL. The organizer for the group explains that they need assistance with a direct action (referred to as an "action" for short) they have coming up. A direct action is an organizing tool used to pressure decision makers to create positive social change. Disability activists will be protesting the sub-par quality of services for paratransit. Paratransit provides door-to-door transportation for people with disabilities who are unable to take public transportation routes. Activists know that it is their right to have access to equal quality transportation as nondisabled people. However, paratransit services in the city are always late, the vehicles are unsanitary, and drivers will leave passengers behind if they are not immediately ready at the time of arrival. The direct action will take the form of a protest where disability activists will march around the building with signs while chanting. They will conclude with a press conference about their disappointing experiences with paratransit to push the paratransit agency to do better. Nearly all of the disability activists who will be involved love being front and center during protests. The action will take place in the suburbs,

where the agency is housed. However, the disability activists are in the city and will need to find a way to get there.

The organizer also needs help with figuring out how to get the disabled activists to use the signage that has been made for this action (see Figure 16.4). Protest signs are an effective way to gain public and media attention for social issues. Protest signs show the ineffectiveness of paratransit services that disability activists experienced. They also demonstrate how disability activists felt about the lack of quality of paratransit services. Many of the activists have physical disabilities, are wheelchair users, and cannot easily lift and wield signs. The organizer is wondering if there are other ways that they can use their voices to participate in the action too.

Lastly, the group has a large amount of props, food, and other necessary materials to carry with them to the action. The organizer asks for your advice on how to transport these materials around.

Questions

1. How does this story portray people with disabilities differently than what OTs typically see in patient or client roles?
2. What are two social model–oriented recommendations the OT student can make regarding accessibility of the action?

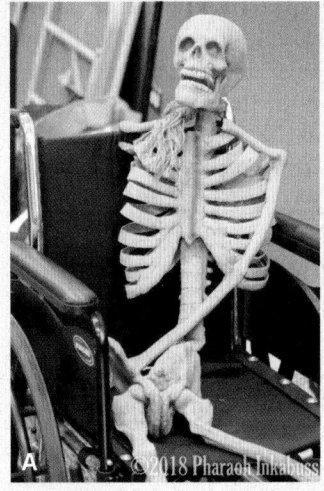 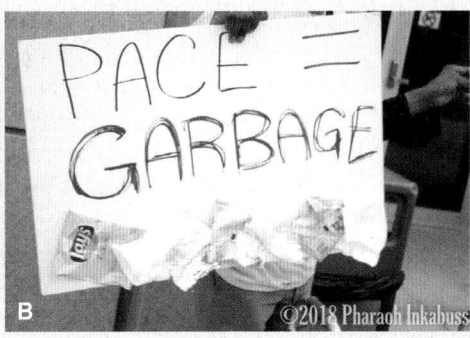 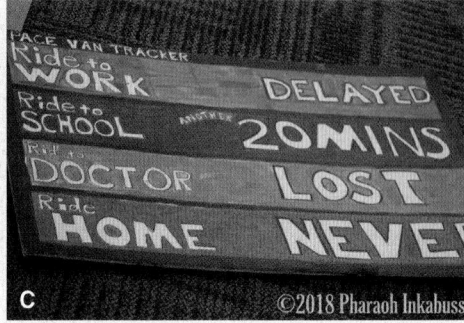

FIGURE 16.4 Protest signs used at the PACE paratransit protest described in OT Story 16.1. **A:** A skeleton in a wheelchair represents a person with a disability "dying waiting" for paratransit to show up. **B:** A sign titled "Pace van tracker" depicts a ride to work delayed, a ride to school delayed, getting lost on a ride to the doctor, and a ride home that never showed up. **C:** A sign with garbage glued to the bottom reads "PACE = GARBAGE." (Photos reproduced with permission from Timotheus Gordon, Jr. [Pharaoh Inkabuss].)

Title IV. Independent use of telecommunication services is the focus of Title IV, primarily in regard to people with hearing and speech impairments.

- ***OT implications:*** OT practitioners working with the Deaf or hard of hearing people will need to educate themselves on how to use teletypewriter (TTY) relay services. They can also have a role in educating non-Deaf or hard of hearing people on how to use TTY relay services.

Title V. Title V includes various "Miscellaneous Provisions" that describe the relationship of the ADA to other laws, such as the Rehabilitation Act of 1973. This title states that the ADA would not hold precedent over a law with stricter standards, for example, Sections 501 and 504 of the Rehabilitation Act of 1973. Title V further amended the Rehabilitation Act of 1973 to clarify that only drug and alcohol users whose job performance is not impaired by the use of such drugs can be considered disabled under this law (i.e., they must not be actively using substances).

- ***OT implications:*** A significant aspect of this section for OT practitioners is that workers who have drug or alcohol addictions can be protected as disabled under the ADA, so long as they are not actively using substances on the job. This information could be useful for those working

in addiction services, particularly in relation to teaching advocacy skills to combat discrimination.

Enforcement of the ADA is carried out by the Department of Justice (DOJ), but the DOJ does not actively seek out noncompliance. Therefore, it is left up to people with disabilities and their allies (like OT practitioners) to make this discrimination visible. OT practitioners can support the decision of the people experiencing the discrimination. They can also facilitate decision-making in regard to filing charges.

The ADA makes up the floor (is the minimum) of what should be provided in terms of accommodations. Refer to the DOJ (2020) *A Guide to Disability Rights Laws* for a comprehensive summary of what the ADA covers. For further support around the ADA, consult your regional ADA center (ADA National Network, n.d.-b).

Key Messages of the Disability Rights Movement

According to Charlton (2000), "Out of the different and often hard realities of everyday life, organizations of people with disabilities have appeared in virtually every country in the world. Most of these organizations embrace the principles of empowerment and human rights, independence and integration, and self-help and self-determination" (p. 130). Disability rights organizations all seek to address societal ableism that perpetuates the oppression of disabled people. Key goals of the DRM include the following (Charlton, 2000):

- Leadership of disabled people
- Self-determination
- Accessibility of public services and buildings
- Transportation access
- Affordable, accessible housing
- Community living
- Access to integrated, equitable education
- Reducing stigma and negative attitudes about disability

The Mad Movement

Another important activist movement for OT practitioners to understand is the Mad movement. The Mad movement has been referred to by several different names over the years and encompasses several related movements, such as the mental patient's liberation movement, the consumer/survivor/ex-patient (c/s/x) movement, and the Mad Pride movement. Each of these movements is worthy of study in its own right, but they are all referred to under the umbrella of "the Mad movement" for the sake of brevity in this chapter.

In the United States, beginning in the 1940s, mental patient groups brought together people living in mental institutions. (*Note:* Although we do not use language of "mental patient" today, this is how the groups were referred to at the time, so we use this historical language in places.) One example was "We Are Not Alone," a mental patients' group at Rockland State Hospital (Pelka, 1997). Patients in these groups organized for better treatment in psychiatric institutions, including an end to involuntary commitment and treatment.

In the 1960s, critique of mental healthcare systems in the United States, the United Kingdom, Europe, and Canada intensified. These critiques came from radical psychiatrists such as Thomas Szasz and R. D. Laing as well as from theorists such as Michel Foucault and Erving Goffman. Women's rights activists also critiqued the sexism in the mental healthcare system, drawing attention to instances wherein women were given psychiatric diagnoses or treatments for refusing to conform to gender norms (Menzies et al., 2013; Starkman, 2013). The growing lesbian, gay, bisexual, transgender, and queer (LGBTQ) rights movement also contributed to these critiques (Starkman, 2013). LGBTQ rights activists fought to have homosexuality removed from the *Diagnostic and Statistical Manual of Mental Disorders* (*DSM*). They argued that homosexuality was nothing to be ashamed about, and that it did not require psychiatric treatment or cures. In 1973, homosexuality was removed from the *DSM-II* as a result of this pressure from activists. Many of those critiquing the US mental healthcare system at this time argued that mental health providers assigned

psychiatric diagnoses to people who did not conform to societal norms. Then, once diagnosed, these people could be incarcerated in mental institutions or forcibly treated. In this way, mental healthcare served as a form of social control for minority populations. This critique of mental healthcare as a form of social control also applied to racial and ethnic minorities. For example, disability studies scholar Metzl pointed out that in the 1960s, psychiatrists sometimes applied the diagnosis of schizophrenia to Black civil rights organizers, saying that they had a "protest psychosis" rather than acknowledging their political views and arguments for civil rights (Metzl, 2011).

Both mental patients' groups and other minority movements spoke up against injustices they experienced in the mental healthcare system. Activists critiqued the cruel conditions inside mental institutions where people were stripped of their rights and held involuntarily. They critiqued inhumane "treatments," such as electroshock therapy, lobotomy, seclusion, and restraint. Throughout the 1970s, 1980s, and 1990s, Mad activists wrote about these issues in books like Judi Chamberlin's *On Our Own: Patient-Controlled Alternatives to the Mental Health System* (Chamberlin, 1979) and in magazines and newsletters such as "In a Nutshell" and "Phoenix Rising" (Menzies et al., 2013; Starkman, 2013). Activists engaged in protests such as bed pushes, where a group of protesters push hospital beds along city streets. Bed pushes symbolize the Mad movement's efforts to get people out of the beds of mental institutions and back into the community (Toronto Mad Pride, 2016). These efforts continue today. For example, the group MindFreedom International speaks out against electroshock therapy and helps people who are involuntarily committed to mental institutions get released (MindFreedom International, 2020).

OT is implicated in the history of injustices in mental institutions. The moral treatment movement is foundational to OT (see Chapter 2). One of the key arguments of the moral treatment movement was that people confined in mental hospitals should not be locked in chains, but rather should be engaged in activities. In the early 1900s, progressive era reformers in North American institutions began to advocate the "work cure." "Work cure" proponents argued that those in mental hospitals were better rehabilitated by work than by rest alone. Early OT practitioners engaged people confined in mental institutions in arts, crafts, and work-related activities (see Chapter 2). In some asylums, patients were involved in domestic labor and even in building the very walls that confined them (Reaume, 2011). Although it is arguably a positive development for patients to be engaged in labor as opposed to locked in chains, this labor was unpaid and, ultimately, of more benefit to the hospital owners than the patients themselves. Rehabilitation professionals contributed to the societal discourses that a normal citizen was a person who could work and that disabled people should be made normal through work training.

Today, historian and Mad studies[2] scholar Geoffrey Reaume offers tours of the wall of the former Asylum for the Insane (now called the *Centre for Addiction and Mental Health*) in Toronto, Ontario, Canada (Reaume, 2011). These tours serve to educate the public about the inhumane conditions that patients experienced and about the unpaid labor that they were made to complete to build the walls of the institution. OT practitioners should be educated about this critique of the moral treatment movement and of institutions. Much of OT began in institutions of confinement, and OT is still commonly practiced in places of confinement, such as segregated therapeutic schools for disabled children, nursing homes, mental hospitals, and medical hospitals. OT practitioners working in institutions can be mindful of this history as they consider how to return power and self-determination to the people they serve.

In addition to critiquing mental healthcare treatment, Mad activists also critique discrimination and bias against people who are labeled "mentally ill" in broader society. Discrimination against people who are thought to be mentally ill or "insane" is called **sanism**. Mad activists point out that sanism is widespread in our media, society, and personal beliefs. For example, many people hold sanist beliefs that people with mental illness are dangerous, feel they would not want to date or hire someone with a mental illness, or use sanist slurs such as "crazy" or "insane" to refer to things or people they do not like. OT practitioners have the power to combat sanism in our own profession and in broader society. For more about sanism, see Expanding Our Perspectives in Chapter 63.

Disability justice organizations such as Project LETS and Fireweed Collective make connections between sanism and other forms of discrimination, such as racism, sexism, ableism, cissexism, and heterosexism. For example, Project LETS educates people about how racism and sanism intersect during police encounters with Black people who have mental illnesses. More than 20% of people killed by police have a documented mental illness (*The Washington Post*, 2022), and police brutality disproportionately impacts Black people with mental illnesses. Mad and disability justice organizations make connections with movements such as Black Lives Matter that work against police brutality and racism.

Mad Pride is an important component of the Mad movement. Individuals in the Mad Pride contingency of the movement argue that their mental differences are a form of human diversity that should be celebrated (Diamond, 2013). They argue that not all mental illnesses need to be treated or cured. Although Mad activists agree that people should receive support for mental distress when and if they want it, they do not think that all symptoms need to be eliminated if they are not bothering the person. For example, the Hearing Voices Network hosts Unusual Belief groups for people who may believe, hear, or see things that other people do not. They do not necessarily pathologize these beliefs as hallucinations or delusions that need to be eliminated, but rather offer a space for people to share about their beliefs with peers (Hearing Voices Network, n.d.).

Like the DRM, the Mad movement is worldwide. Mad people organize against sanism in countries all around the world. For example, MindFreedom International has affiliate or sponsor groups in Australia, Canada, Germany, Ghana, Ireland, Japan, the Netherlands, South Korea, Taiwan, and the United States (MindFreedom International, 2020). Mad Pride events also occur in many different countries.

Although the Mad movement has many different contingencies (Diamond, 2013), there are some key beliefs that are important for OT practitioners to understand. The Mad movement argues that:

- People should never be forced to live in an institution against their will.
- People should never be forced to receive medication or other treatments against their will.
- Inhumane treatments such as electroshock, seclusion, and restraint should be ended.
- Peer support is extremely important.
- Mad people can and should be supported to live in the community, even when they have behaviors that are outside the norm.
- We should honor a wide variety of ways of thinking, being, and behaving in the world.

Self-Advocacy and Neurodiversity Movements

The self-advocacy and neurodiversity movements are also highly relevant to OT practitioners. The self-advocacy movement traces its beginnings to the 1960s and 1970s. Some self-advocates with intellectual and developmental disabilities were part of the DRM during this time, and some also began forming their own movement. The term "self-advocate" comes from the fact that people with intellectual and developmental disabilities were advocating for themselves. This stands in contrast to parents or practitioners advocating on their behalf. During this time, parent organizations were very common around the world. They gathered parents of people with disabilities who advocated for their children. However, the children or adults with disabilities had very little say in these organizations. One of the key origins of the self-advocacy movement was a meeting in Sweden in 1968, when people with intellectual and developmental disabilities began

---

[2]Mad studies is an academic discipline that critiques sanism and studies Mad people's history, community, culture. For more on Mad studies, we recommend the books *Mad Matters* (LeFrançois et al., 2013) and *Searching for a Rose Garden* (Russo & Sweeney, 2016).

speaking up about their own interests at a parents' meeting. This event is cited as a founding moment of the People First movement (People First, n.d.). The People First movement is now an international movement with actions and events taking place in at least 43 different countries, including the United States (People First, n.d.).

The self-advocacy movement is ongoing. For example, the annual Speak Up and Speak Out Summit provides training and opportunities for people with intellectual and developmental disabilities to engage in disability advocacy (Speak Up & Speak Out Summit, 2021). Self Advocates Becoming Empowered (SABE) is a key organization in the modern self-advocacy movement (SABE, n.d.).

The idea of person-first language can be traced back to the self-advocacy movement. Self-advocates with intellectual and developmental disabilities did not want to be seen as *only* their disabilities—they wanted to be seen as whole people with the power to direct their own lives. As discussed elsewhere in the chapter, many people in the DRM and later in the autistic and neurodiversity movements prefer identity-first language ("disabled person," "autistic person"). OT practitioners should always respect a person's preference for identity-first versus person-first language.

The self-advocacy movement also laid important groundwork for the Autistic Rights Movement, which traces its beginnings to the 1990s. A key moment in the beginning of this movement was a speech by Jim Sinclair (they/them) at the International Conference on Autism in Toronto in 1993. Sinclair, an autistic activist and co-founder of Autism Network International, spoke directly to the parents of autistic people in their speech. They offered a radically new perspective that autism was not a tragedy that parents should mourn, but rather that, "Autism is a way of being. It is not possible to separate the person from the autism" (Sinclair, 1993, para. 5). This argument is foundational to the autistic rights movement's call for identity-first language (e.g., calling themselves "autistic"), which acknowledges autism as a crucial part of someone's being (Brown, 2011). Sinclair's speech also aligned with the social model of disability.

> Yes, there is tragedy that comes with autism: not because of what we are, but because of the things that happen to us. Be sad about that if you want to be sad about something. Better than being sad about it, though, get mad about it—and then do something about it. The tragedy is not that we're here, but that your world has no place for us to be. (Sinclair, 1993, para. 20)

The neurodiversity movement arose from the autistic rights movement (and the self-advocacy movement before it). In 1998, Judy Singer coined the term **neurodiversity** (Singer, 2017). Singer was inspired by other minority rights movements, and she used the term to reflect an idea that autism and other neurodivergent ways of being should be considered forms of diversity, rather than pathologies that require elimination. This approach aligns with the minority model of disability.

Since the 1990s, the neurodiversity movement has continued to grow. Similar to the Mad Pride movement, many in the neurodiversity movement celebrate their mental differences as a beautiful form of diversity. Autistic rights and neurodiversity movement organizations also continue to fight for the rights of autistic people and other neurodivergent people. Two key autistic self-advocacy organizations in the United States are Autistic Self Advocacy Network (ASAN) and Autistic Women and Nonbinary Network (AWNN). These organizations continue work on a variety of important issues for autistic rights, including issues of employment, healthcare, education, and public attitudes. Readers are encouraged to look at their websites for updates on the latest issues.

Neurodiversity movement advocates envision a world that is accessible and accepting of many different ways of communicating, behaving, and being. Many autistic advocates criticize treatments like Applied Behavior Analysis (ABA), which emphasize that people with autism should "act normal." ABA is also criticized for its use of aversive conditioning, extreme repetition, and other interventions that autistic self-advocates have identified as traumatic (ASAN, 2021). OT practitioners should be aware of these critiques when clients and families ask about ABA. Advocates also critique Autism Speaks, an organization that engages in ableist advertising campaigns and emphasizes cures and treatments for autism as opposed to accessibility and support for autistic people (ASAN, 2020).

Similar to other disability movements, the self-advocacy and neurodiversity movements have a strong emphasis on self-determination. For example, autistic organizations such as ASAN and AWNN strongly critique the lack of autistic people in leadership at Autism Speaks (ASAN, 2020). The majority of board members at Autism Speaks are businesspeople, practitioners, or parents of people with autism.

Much of the work in the self-advocacy and neurodiversity movements are direct responses to organizations that represent the parents of people with disabilities. Self-advocates demanded the right to speak for themselves, and they critiqued the way that some parent organizations portrayed their disabilities as burdens to their families that were worthy of pity. Many disability rights organizations welcome parent allies, but they emphasize that people with disabilities themselves must always be in charge. OT practitioners can learn from this tension. Practitioners can work to promote the ability of children with disabilities to make choices about their own lives. Practitioners may also benefit from connecting children with disabilities and their parents to adult self-advocates and self-advocacy organizations. The OT stories of this chapter offer examples of how to do this.

The neurodiversity paradigm is becoming more commonly used in OT scholarship. For example, a 2021 special issue of the *American Journal of Occupational Therapy* (*AJOT*) examined OT with neurodivergent populations.

The editorial to this special issue was co-authored by two researchers: one is an OT professor who is a parent of adults with autism, and the other is an autistic researcher (Kornblau & Robertson, 2021). This approach to co-authorship demonstrates a commitment to ensuring that people with disabilities are represented in the research that concerns them and sets a powerful example for future OT scholarship.

The Disability Justice Movement

The DRM was—and remains—important in terms of disabled people gaining civil rights through legislation. However, there were some important critiques of the DRM that needed to be addressed. One issue was that the DRM tended to have a single-issue politic—meaning that they focused only on disability rights, rather than simultaneously considering other issues such as race, gender, or sexuality.

The disability justice movement aimed to address this problem by proposing a movement that was founded in intersectionality (Sins Invalid, 2019). **Intersectionality** is an idea that originated in Black feminism. Intersectionality explains that all systems of oppression (e.g., ableism, racism, sexism, heterosexism, cissexism, classism) are intertwined (Crenshaw, 1991; Sins Invalid, 2019). The disability justice movement explains that in order to achieve collective liberation, we need to address intersecting justice issues simultaneously and not leave anyone behind (Sins Invalid, 2019).

Disability justice was originally formed in 2005 by disabled queer people of color. There are 10 principles associated with disability justice: Intersectionality, Leadership of Those Most Impacted, Anti-Capitalist Politics, Cross-Movement Solidarity, Recognizing Wholeness, Sustainability, Cross-Disability Solidarity, Interdependence, Collective Access, and Collective Liberation (Sins Invalid, 2019).

Sins Invalid was the first disability justice organization. Another disability justice organization is the Disability Justice Culture Club. They describe themselves as a collective that centers disabled, queer, trans, Black, Indigenous people of color (disabled QTBIPOC) (Disability Justice Culture Club, n.d.). They made their own hand sanitizer during the start of the COVID-19 pandemic. They distributed this hand sanitizer, gloves, and N95 masks to people living in homeless encampments in Oakland. They carried this out as a form of mutual aid. This was during a time when there was little hand sanitizer available at stores because everyone wanted and needed it (Green, 2020).

Another example of disability justice organizing is the Power to Live campaign. This campaign pushed the PG&E power company in the Bay area to have better plans in place when they need to plan power shutdowns. Disability justice organizer Stacey Park Milbern explained that their disregard toward disabled people and the power they rely on for ventilators and keeping vital medications refrigerated demonstrated that they did not value disabled lives. This campaign demonstrates the importance of disabled people's wisdom about collective care and interdependence during times of crisis (Disability Visibility Project, 2019).

Disability justice work requires a radical approach that embodies all 10 principles, which may not be possible in most OT settings. For example, in a capitalist healthcare system, an OT practitioner may struggle to take an anti-capitalist approach. However, OT practitioners can learn from the principles and actions of the disability justice movement. For example, practitioners involved in advocacy can learn about the importance of taking an intersectional approach that acknowledges that different liberation struggles are interconnected. For more information on disability justice or the principles, the authors highly encourage readers to refer to the Sins Invalid website.

Disability Activism Today

The disability rights, Mad, self-advocacy, neurodiversity, and disability justice movements continue today. A few recent examples of such advocacy and activism are provided in the section that follows. For more, we encourage you to follow the organizations mentioned throughout this chapter for updates on current advocacy priorities and to pay attention to their calls for advocacy, including requests for support from healthcare providers.

ADAPT, a disability rights organization, is currently championing the Disability Integration Act (DIA). This legislation would support the right of people with disabilities to live in their homes, rather than institutions.

Organizations such as the National Disability Rights Network (n.d.) and the National Down Syndrome Society (n.d.) are working to end the subminimum wage for disabled people. In most states, it is legal for employers with a certificate under Section 14(c) of the Fair Labor Standards Act to pay people with disabilities less than the minimum wage (Association of People Supporting Employment First, n.d.). Disabled workers who are paid subminimum wage make $3.34 per hour on average, although there is no minimum requirement for pay and so some make just pennies per hour (U.S. Commission on Civil Rights, 2020). This undervaluation of disabled workers' time and labor represents a striking occupational injustice.

During the COVID-19 pandemic, particularly in the early months and years, disability justice organizations brought attention to the injustices occurring in COVID-19 care triage. In many states, legal documents assert the right of healthcare providers to deny lifesaving care (such as ventilators) to individuals based upon disability status. Such decisions about rationing care rely on myths about disability—including that disabled people do not have adequate quality of life and, therefore, are less worthy of lifesaving care. In Texas, Michael Hickson, a 49-year-old Black disabled man, was denied lifesaving treatment owing to a doctor's judgment that being disabled meant he did not have quality of life (Shapiro, 2020). Disability justice activists organized the #NoBodyIsDisposable campaign in response to such eugenics practices—"#ICUgenics"—which specifically targeted disabled, fat, queer, transgender, and older people, as well as Black and Indigenous people and other people of color (No Body is Disposable, 2020). Disability justice activists highlighted that COVID-19 eugenics practices represented an intersectional issue—one that affects people from many different marginalized groups, and especially people at the intersection of multiple marginalized groups (e.g., Black disabled people like Michael Hickson). OT practitioners work with disabled people every day on participation and assert that people can live quality lives with disability. Because of their firsthand knowledge of disability issues, OT practitioners can be strong advocates for issues of care rationing. Before reading further, take a moment to reflect by reading Box 16.2.

BOX 16.2 THINKING ABOUT DISABILITY: A MOMENT TO REFLECT

Take a moment to reflect on what you have read so far.

1. What surprised you about what you have read so far?
2. How is this different from what you have previously learned about disability?
3. What are the implications for practice?

After your reflection, keep reading to apply your new knowledge to OT practice.

Disability Critiques of Occupational Therapy

This chapter highlights many potential points of allyship between the DRM and the profession of OT. Despite these potentials, OT has sometimes been criticized as being unhelpful or actively harmful to disabled people and/or to disability movements (Kielhofner, 2005; Linton, 1998). This section highlights a few key critiques that we can learn from to improve the profession.

Need for More Person-Centered Approach

Disability scholars have pointed out that OT and other applied fields do not focus enough on the issues that disabled communities prioritize (Linton, 1998). There is a power differential in OT encounters, wherein the OT practitioner has more power to determine what happens to the patient. This includes the power to decide information that enters the patient's medical chart, resources that the patient has access to, and treatments they receive. Scholars within OT have also critiqued the profession for falling short of its stated goals of person-centeredness (Gupta & Taff, 2015; Whalley Hammell, 2013). Instead of letting disabled people set the priorities for OT research, practice, and education, these priorities are often set by nondisabled practitioners.

Our profession could also move to be more person centered in its national advocacy (Harrison et al., 2021). The American Occupational Therapy Association (AOTA) states that their advocacy works to "protect the profession and preserve access to occupational therapy services" and focuses on "billing and compensation" and "the scope and reach of occupational therapy" (AOTA, n.d.). Events such as Hill Day tend to focus on raising public awareness of OT as a profession and/or advocating for reimbursement of OT services. On the US national scale, OT advocacy for the recipients of OT services—disabled people—is barely visible in comparison to national advocacy for practitioners. While advocating for ourselves and our profession is certainly important, our profession is founded upon the ideas of person-centeredness. Our jobs depend upon disabled people, first and foremost. If our advocacy is to be centered on our patients, it must be disabled person centered. Allying with disability rights organizations in national advocacy would be a powerful step toward bringing OT into alignment with its values of person-centeredness.

Limitations of the Medical and Rehabilitative Models

Although the social model of disability aligns well with several aspects of OT, OT has been consistently criticized for overfocusing on the medical and individual aspects of disability. A recent study by Holler and colleagues found that although OT practitioners endorsed some social model ideas in theory, they were less likely to implement these ideas in practice (2021). Despite the theoretical emphasis of OT on the person–environment–occupation fit, in practice, interventions often focus on the person more than the environment and occupation. Part of this overfocus is due to reimbursement and billing structures that prioritize documentation of individual biomechanical outcomes, such as improvements in range of motion and muscle strength. OT practitioners who practice in ways that align with the social model sometimes find themselves doing it as "underground practice" that they cannot be fully documented in existing healthcare systems (Heffron et al., 2019).

Norman Kunc's foundational interview about the impact of OT and physical therapy (PT) services on his life provides an example of the possible negative impacts of rehabilitative model approaches on the identity and self-esteem of clients with disabilities,

> The implicit message that permeated all my therapy experiences was that if I wanted to live as a valued person, wanted a quality life, to have a good job . . . all I had to do was overcome my disability. No one comes up and says, "Look, in order to live a good life you have to be normal," but it's a powerful, implicit message. Receiving physical and occupational therapy were important contributors in terms of seeing myself as abnormal. (Giangreco, 1996, para. 10)

Kunc also described how therapists' emphasis on "function" and his experiences in a segregated school (a school exclusively for disabled children) negatively impacted his quality of life.

> Now there may be some therapists who say, "Wait a minute, I don't want to make people more normal. I want to help them function better so that they can do more things." Although that seems to be a far more enlightened perspective, I still have serious concerns about it because professionals mistakenly equate functioning level with quality of life and that may not be what's going on for some folks . . . Rather than functioning level, I think most people would agree that the quality of life has to do with important personal experiences, feelings, and events, like relationships, having fun, and making contributions to the lives of other people . . . Ironically, developing relationships, the opportunity to make contributions to your community, even fun itself is taken away from people with disabilities in the name of trying to get them to function better to presumably improve the quality of their lives. So I didn't get to go to regular school and then I missed the opportunity to make friends. Why? Because professionals were trying to improve my quality of life by putting me in a special school where I am supposed to learn to function better. So they take away the opportunity for me to have friends and subsequently they actually interfere with the quality of my life. (Giangreco, 1996, paras. 36–38)

A greater emphasis on the social model of disability would address many of Kunc's critiques. Examples of OT practice in alignment with the social model of disability are provided later in this chapter.

Experiences of Occupational Therapy Practitioners With Disabilities

The experiences of OT practitioners with disabilities also offer a critique of ableism within our profession. Research with OT practitioners with disabilities indicates that they experience inaccessibility in universities and workplaces, negative attitudes about disability, and outright discrimination (Bevan, 2014; The & Harrison, 2019). Despite working with individuals with disabilities every day, OT practitioners are not always welcoming to students and practitioners

with disabilities. Practitioners with disabilities have unique expertise in disability culture, advocacy, and accommodations, which are assets to the profession (Bevan, 2014; The & Harrison, 2019). Both authors of this chapter (Harrison and The) are occupational therapists with disabilities. We find that our experiences of disability identity, community, and activism inform our practice in powerful ways. Improving the treatment of OT practitioners with disabilities in our profession could also improve our profession's alignment with disability rights and help us better serve clients with disabilities. Support for OT practitioners with disabilities should be included in workforce diversity initiatives (The et al., 2017).

Disability Studies

Disability studies is an academic field associated with the disability community and the DRM. Disability studies is a minority studies discipline. Like other minority studies disciplines (such as women and gender studies, ethnic studies, queer studies, or African American studies), the field of disability studies is grounded in a view of disabled people as a minority group that experiences oppression—in this case, ableism. For many years, a small but growing group of OT scholars have worked to infuse disability studies perspectives into OT.

Disability scholars such as Linton (1998) critiqued OT and other rehabilitation fields, dating back at least to the 1990s. In response to some of these critiques and to the continuing DRM, a special issue on disability studies was compiled for the *American Journal of Occupational Therapy (AJOT)* in 2005. In the editorial for this issue, Kielhofner (2005) discussed disability studies critiques of OT. Such critiques included OT's tendency to take a medical model approach that overfocuses on impairment and neglects the potential for individuals to develop positive disability identities and participate in disability communities. The other studies in the issue brought attention to other disability studies topics, including methods for integrating disability studies into OT education (Block et al., 2005; Gitlow & Flecky, 2005), critiques of OT approaches to prevention (Neville-Jan, 2005), and calls for OT practitioners to engage in advocacy in support of the Olmstead decision and community living (Cottrell, 2005).

In 2021, scholars associated with the Occupational Therapy and Disability Studies (OTxDS) network guest edited a new special issue of *AJOT* on disability studies and OT. In the guest editorial, the authors called upon OT to better incorporate disability studies in practice, research, education, and advocacy (Harrison et al., 2021). Authors in the 2021 special issue referred back to the 2005 special issue and reflected that many of the problems raised in the original special issue continue more than 15 years later (Harrison et al., 2021, Sheth et al., 2021). These issues include moving from individual to more environmental interventions, using more disability theory in OT, and building partnerships with disability communities (Sheth et al., 2021).

Disability studies scholars also critiqued the lack of inclusion of disability perspectives in OT curricula (Harrison et al., 2021). Current OT programs tend to have a much stronger emphasis on the medical model than the social model (Sheth et al., 2021). Recent research on students at one OT program found that while students' explicit attitudes about people with disabilities improved over their years in the OT program, their implicit biases against people with disabilities did not improve. Most students graduated the program with an implicit bias favoring nondisabled people over disabled people (Friedman & VanPuymbrouck, 2021). Disability studies scholars argue that infusing more disability studies approaches into OT curricula could help bring the profession closer toward allyship with disabled people and disability movements (Harrison et al., 2021; Heffron et al., 2019; Sheth et al., 2021).

To see ongoing work of the OTxDS network, follow their Facebook page at https://www.facebook.com/otdsnetwork/.

Occupational Therapy Practice Informed by the Social Model of Disability and Disability Movements

Disability movements and disability studies have many concrete implications and direct applications for OT. In addition to those described throughout this chapter, this final section provides some key approaches to practice for the OT practitioner informed by the social model of disability and disability movements.

Becoming a Critical Occupational Therapist

Becoming a critical occupational therapist means being willing to examine, critique, and change your own practice and your profession. This chapter has provided many critiques of OT; however, there are practices that OT practitioners can adopt that could result in a closer alignment with the priorities of disability communities and movements. According to Whiteford and Townsend (2011), critical OT practice requires:

- Critical reflexivity
- Collaborative and participatory approaches
- Enabling social inclusion of marginalized groups
- Engaging people in meaningful occupations
- Transforming environments
- Collaborating in interdisciplinary teams

Each of these skills is highly relevant to the OT practitioner who wishes to support disability rights. Readers are highly encouraged to read more about the Participatory Occupational Justice Framework to support their development of skills for critical OT practice working toward occupational justice (Whiteford & Townsend, 2011; Whiteford et al., 2018). The section that follows gives the reader many examples of critical OT practice. We begin with OT Story 16.2 to see critical reflexivity in practice:

OT STORY 16.2 CRITICAL OCCUPATIONAL THERAPY IN ACTION

Francesca (she/her) is a first-year occupational therapist practicing in acute care. She is under a lot of pressure from her supervisor to maintain her productivity by treating patients for a certain number of units (billable minutes) per day. When a patient refuses treatment, her colleagues often circle back once or twice later in the day to ask the patient if they have changed their mind and are willing to do a session. Sometimes, the practitioners really try to talk the patient into it. Francesca understands why they do this is because of the pressure from her supervisor, but she also feels uncomfortable with the practice. She reflects on this and feels that pressuring clients to participate in therapy is not consistent with the OT values of *person-centeredness* and *autonomy*. Furthermore, it does not align with the disability rights value of *self-determination*. When a patient says no to Francesca, she asks them if they would like her to come back and ask again later that day. If they say no, she does not come back. When her supervisor asks her about this, she explains why she made this decision and advocates for a more person-centered approach on her team. She also brings up this issue at her state OT association conference, to spark a conversation about the possible conflicts between productivity demands and person-centeredness.

Questions

1. Describe an issue that you have encountered when a healthcare provider did not treat a patient with a person-centered approach.
2. Thinking of your example, what were the possible factors that led the provider to behave this way? Taking Francesca as an inspiration, how could you advocate to change those factors?

Working for Occupational Justice

Addressing occupational injustice is crucial for the critical occupational therapist. Occupational injustices occur when people, groups, or populations are not provided equitable access to fulfilling occupations (Whiteford & Townsend, 2011). The concept of occupational justice has taken a greater hold in the profession in recent years, especially with its prominent inclusion in the fourth edition of the Occupational Therapy Practice Framework (OTPF-4) (AOTA, 2020). The OTPF-4 names occupational justice a part of the OT domain (interwoven with contexts) and as a potential outcome of OT services (AOTA, 2020).

Disability movements brought (and continue to bring) attention to the many occupational injustices facing people with disabilities. In addition to those described previously, the restrictions associated with Social Security Disability Income (SSDI) provide another example of an occupational injustice facing disabled people. People who receive SSDI are severely limited in their ability to work for additional income (Astor, 2021). This prevents many disabled people from participating in a valued occupation of work and also means that disabled people on SSDI are forced to live in poverty. In addition, SSDI restrictions mean that many people with disabilities cannot get married, because if they got married, it would change their SSDI eligibility and they could lose access to needed services (Astor, 2021). The inability to freely select meaningful work and/or to get married represents significant occupational injustices for people who receive SSDI. OT Story 16.3 provides a window into the impacts of such restrictions.

See Chapter 10 for more on occupational justice.

Transforming Environments

The social model's focus on the interaction between a person and their environment in some ways parallels many OT models, particularly ecologic models such as the Person-Environment-Occupation (PEO), Person-Environment-Occupation-Performance (PEOP), and Ecology of Human Performance (EHP) models (see Chapter 35 for more on ecologic models). The fourth edition of the Occupational Therapy Practice Framework (OTPF-4) explains that occupational performance results from "the dynamic transaction among the client, their contexts, and the occupation" (AOTA, 2020, p. 8). Contexts are named in the OTPF-4 as a key aspect of the OT domain and encompass many different environmental factors. Although several approaches to intervention can align with the social model of disability, the "modify (compensation, adaptation)" (AOTA, 2020, p. 64) approach is particularly well suited to environmentally focused interventions in keeping with the social model. Interventions that focus on the environment are crucial to addressing the occupational injustices that

---

OT STORY 16.3 SCOTT: ADVOCACY, OCCUPATION, AND POLICY

Scott became disabled at age 19. Later in adulthood, he used work incentives like the Plan to Achieve Self-Support (PASS) and vocational rehabilitation to pay for tuition, books, and a computer in order to complete two bachelor of arts degrees and eventually his master of business administration (MBA). During college, Scott became very active in and eventually headed the campus for disabled student union, and he became a strong disability rights advocate and a consultant on navigating the complex disability benefit system. These roles helped him land a reasonably paid position with the state, supervising the office of disability affairs. After working there for 2 years, he was considered no longer disabled by Social Security Administration (SSA), because SSA defines disability solely based upon the ability to work. When Scott received a letter from the SSA that declared "you are no longer disabled," he replied with a wry smile, "So I guess I can sell my wheelchair now that I'm no longer disabled!"

During this time, Scott received health insurance through his employer and used Supplemental Security Income (SSI) support for his personal care assistant (PCA or PA). However, he was about to get a $300 per month raise. Unfortunately, this increase in income would have eliminated his eligibility for SSA funds, which he used to pay for his part-time PCA, so he felt compelled to quit work due to what are called "work disincentives." In having to pay for his healthcare, PCA, and other disability-related expenses (catheters, wheelchair maintenance, etc.) out of his salary, he would have less discretionary income than the approximately $100 per month he had on his SSDI check (that also made him eligible for Medicare and the PCA supplement). Thus, he chose to quit a job that he enjoyed and was successful in, not only because of the added income it provided but also because he had built a more active social life with coworkers. Through his frustrations, Scott was motivated to become more active in disability rights advocacy to decrease work disincentives.

Questions

1. What could you as an OT student or practitioner do to address the occupational injustice that Scott is experiencing?
2. Reflect on the intervention ideas you came up with to address this occupational injustice. Are they more aligned with the medical model of disability, or the social model of disability?

people with disabilities experience. According the Participatory Occupational Justice Framework,

> Occupational therapy is known to emphasize social change as well as individual change in transformation of the environment (context) to develop more equitable opportunities, resources, privilege and enablement for all to participate to their potential and to exert choice and control over what they do every day. (Whiteford & Townsend, 2011, p. 66)

Context-focused interventions are supported by a growing base of evidence. For example, Law and colleagues (2011) conducted a study examining OT and PT services for children with cerebral palsy. They assigned one group of practitioners to engage *only* in "child-focused" interventions that were intended to remediate client factors. They assigned a second group of practitioners to engage *only* in "context-focused" interventions for adapting tasks or modifying environments. A related article by the same team provided examples of this context-focused approach:

> For example, one child had difficulty independently stepping onto her school bus because of the height of the steps. Instead of working on improving the child's quadriceps muscle strength to climb the steps, the therapist phoned administrators in the school district, explained the problem, and requested a bus with steps that were less steep. The school complied and the next day the child achieved the identified goal of getting onto her school bus independently. In another situation, a parent's goal was for her child to finger-feed himself Cheerios independently. The therapist experimented with putting peanut butter on the tips of his fingers so that the Cheerios could stick to it. The child accomplished finger feeding in one intervention session, even though he did not have a pincer grasp. (Darrah et al., 2011, p. 618)

After 6 months of intervention, they found that child- and context-focused interventions were equally effective (Law et al., 2011). The researchers concluded that "a therapy approach focusing on changing the task and the environment rather than children's impairments can be a viable treatment strategy and merits further investigation" (Darrah et al., 2011, p. 615).

A greater focus on environmental interventions can also better align OT with the social model of disability and with the priorities of disability communities and movements. Adapting the environment and objects to serve a wide variety of people is a concept built into a universal design approach and is an essential tool of the occupational therapist (Figures 16.5 and 16.6). Universal design principles benefit a wide variety of people, not only disabled people. A worker delivering goods with a hand truck, parents with baby strollers, and travelers with roll-aboard luggage all benefit from ramps, sidewalk curb cuts, elevators, and automatic door openers (Figure 16.7). As you move about your environment, look for these accessibility features and consider the range of individuals that benefit from these adaptations. Readers are encouraged to learn about and use free accessibility checklists such as the ADA Checklist for

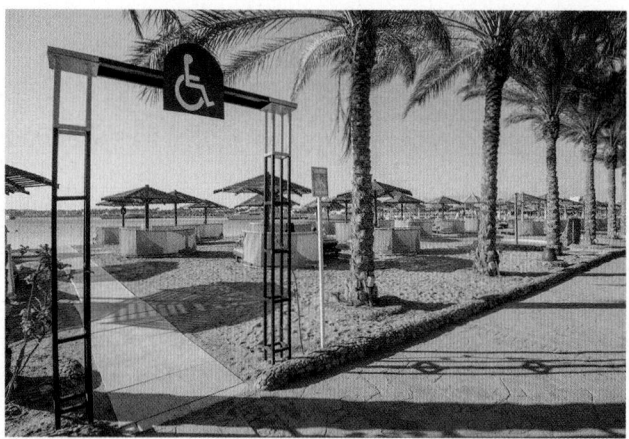

FIGURE 16.5 Universal design principles were employed at a beach to allow people with disabilities to access the ocean.

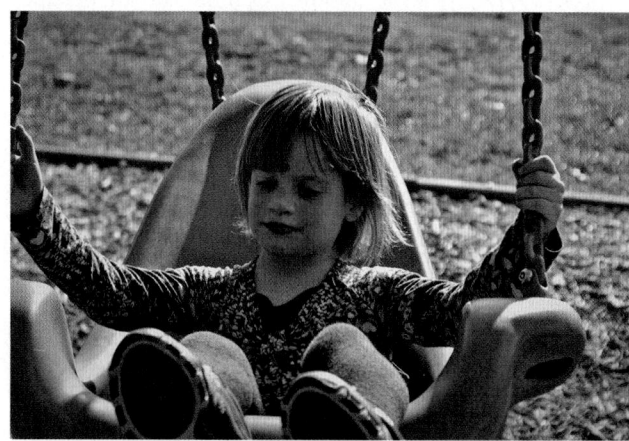

FIGURE 16.6 Universal design principles were employed at a playground to allow children with disabilities to play.

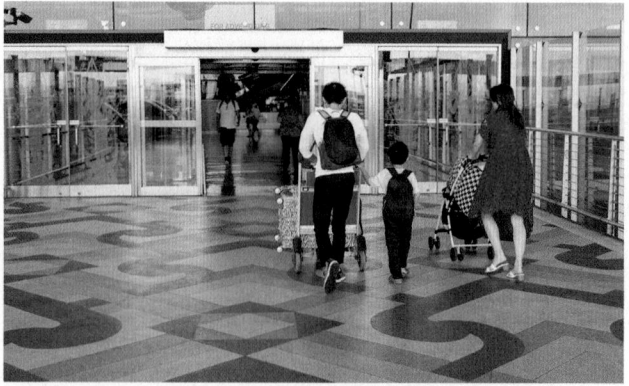

FIGURE 16.7 Universal design benefits a wide variety of people. Imagine this family trying to get through the doors of the airport if they did not open automatically.

Existing Facilities and the resources developed by occupational therapists under the brand *SafeScore* (Institute for Human Centered Design and ADA National Network, 2016; Pruett & Pruett, 2018). Some modern accessibility resources also address intersectional accessibility; that is, accessibility that promotes participation for members of multiple marginalized groups, and especially for those at the intersection of multiple marginalized groups like queer, disabled, people of color (e.g., Harrison & Kopit, 2020).

In addition to the physical environment, an OT practitioner inspired by the social model of disability and disability movements can also transform the other aspects of the environment. Table 16.2 offers examples of environmental interventions addressing each of the five categories of environmental factors included in the OTPF-4 (AOTA, 2020).

Chapters 15 and 17 further explore social, political, and environmental factors that impact occupational performance. See Chapter 24 for more about contexts and environmental factors.

Supporting Community Living

Although the Olmstead decision declared the right of people with disabilities to live in the community, unfortunately, many people with disabilities who would prefer to live in the community are stuck living in institutions because of the institutional bias in US healthcare. The institutional bias means that although the Centers for Medicare & Medicaid Services (CMS) requires states to fund long-term care in institutional settings like nursing homes, CMS does not mandate that states offer Medicaid services in homes and community-based settings. This means that access to home- and community-based services varies widely from state to state. Home- and community-based services include personal care assistants (PCAs) who can assist people with disabilities with activities of daily living (ADLs) to enable them to live in their own homes. These PCAs can be paid by Medicaid for people with home- and community-based services waivers. A disabled person with PCAs holds the responsibility for hiring, supervising, and—if necessary—firing their PCAs, giving them a great deal of control over their own care. OT practitioners can have a role in preparing a person for managing their team of PCAs. OT Story 16.4 offers an example.

In many states, class action lawsuits have been required to combat the state's noncompliance with the Olmstead decision. In Illinois, for example, three separate class action lawsuits were filed on behalf of people with disabilities who were unable to move into the community as they wished. Three consent decrees—the Colbert, Williams, and Ligas consent decrees—were issued as a result of these lawsuits to mandate Illinois to provide adequate funding for home- and community-based services. However, Illinois continues to fall out of compliance with these consent decrees (Equip for Equality, 2019).

An OT practitioner can support the right of their clients with disabilities to live in the community. This means advocating for their right to live at home and providing them with necessary supports. When working from a person-centered perspective, sometimes, this means supporting their self-determination even when our OT assessments suggest there may be safety concerns should the

TABLE 16.2 Environment-Focused Interventions

Environmental Factor	Example of OT Intervention Aligned With the Social Model of Disability and DRMs
Natural environment and human-made changes to the environment	An occupational therapist consults with the local parks and recreation department about the design of a new playground that will be accessible to a wide variety of kids with disabilities, using universal design principles.
Products and technology	An OT practitioner works in collaboration with a local CIL to create a lending library of adaptive equipment for people with disabilities in their city. They also create a website for the lending library that follows digital accessibility principles (e.g., NYU, n.d.).
Support and relationships	An occupational therapist speaks with a family who is distraught about their child's new autism diagnosis. The therapist not only expresses empathy with the difficulty of adjusting to big news but also provides the family with resources about self-advocacy organizations and the neurodiversity movement. They provide the family with links to organizations like ASAN and AWNN where they can hear the stories of adults with autism and learn about different ways of understanding the diagnosis.
Attitudes	An OT, Sal (they/them), overhears their colleague Martha (she/her) complaining about a patient whose chart she just reviewed. Martha has not met the patient yet, but upon seeing the client's diagnosis, she complains, "I hate working with people with Borderline Personality Disorder. They are so difficult and selfish." Sal speaks up and tells Martha they disagree with her applying a sanist stereotype to an individual before even meeting them.
Services, systems, and policies	An occupational therapist writes a letter to their state OT association asking the state association to sign on as a supporter of a new bill that would eliminate the subminimum wage for disabled people in their state.

ASAN, Autistic Self Advocacy Network; AWNN, Autistic Women and Nonbinary Network; CIL, Center for Independent Living; DRM, disability rights movement; OT, occupational therapy.

OT STORY 16.4 JAMAL: INTERDEPENDENCE AND COMMUNITY LIVING

Jamal (he/him) is a 70-year-old Black man who recently experienced a stroke and has been in inpatient rehabilitation for 3 weeks. Jamal's occupational therapist, Mohamed (he/him), is currently working with Jamal on discharge planning. Jamal's daughters are insistent that Jamal should go to a nursing home for at least a few months rather than returning home, and the physical therapist on Mohamed's team agrees because Jamal still requires moderate assistance with transfers. However, Jamal is insistent that he wants to return home. Mohamed works with Jamal to identify resources for home healthcare, including home- and community-based services waivers for PCAs. Mohamed works with Jamal's partner to conduct a home assessment via videoconference (telehealth) and provide recommendations for home modifications, durable medical equipment, and adaptive equipment for Jamal to use at home. Mohamed provides Jamal with a connection to the local CIL, which offers resources for peer support and funding for home modifications. Mohamed and Jamal work together to create a list of supportive neighbors and friends whom Jamal can ask

to help with errands and cooking in his first few weeks at home. They make a digital calendar where friends can sign up to help with tasks that Jamal requests. Through the CIL, Jamal attends a training about hiring and managing PCAs. In his last week in rehabilitation, Jamal hires his first PCA and invites the new PCA to come to the hospital for training. In preparation for the training session, Jamal and Mohamed practice how Jamal can self-direct the PCA through transfers and ADLs. During the training session, Mohamed lets Jamal lead but offers tips to the PCA as requested. Jamal is discharged home with a variety of social and community supports to help him keep living at home.

Questions

1. Do Mohamed's interventions align more with the medical model of disability or the social model of disability?
2. How could Mohamed advocate to or educate his coworkers to improve their ability to support clients' disability rights, self-determination, and interdependence?

person go home (Mahaffey et al., 2018). In these cases, the OT practitioner can work with the client to improve their safety at home by building up social supports, ensuring home accessibility, and connecting the client to resources. OT Story 16.4 provided examples of some of the supports that an occupational therapist can offer to someone who wants to live in the community. Some OT practitioners also work on teams that help people who are living in mental institutions and nursing homes transition to community living.

In Illinois, OT practitioners are part of community living, Assertive Community Treatment (ACT), and advocacy teams that support people with disabilities to transition out of institutional settings into less restrictive community housing, in alignment with the consent decrees mentioned earlier. Two examples are occupational therapists Nicole Barker and Kira Meskin.

- Nicole Barker is an occupational therapist who works on the community living team at Kenneth Young Center. Barker explains that her work can include working with clients on ADLs or environmental modifications in their new homes, or determining the need for daily equipment. She explains, "Sometimes it's as simple as teaching [clients] how to use grab bars in their showers, or as complex as crafting a new daily routine now that they are no longer institutionalized" (Kenneth Young Center, 2021, para. 10).

- Kira Meskin is a community reintegration advocate at the Progress CIL. She also works to help people who want to leave institutions move into the community. This includes making transition plans, connecting clients to resources, training in ADL skills, consulting on home modifications, and engaging in both individual- and systems-level advocacy (K. Meskin, personal communication, March 2, 2022).

Enabling Self-Determination

The right to determine one's own care and the direction of one's own life is a foundation of the DRM. This commitment underlies the famous disability rights slogan, "Nothing about us without us"—highlighting the demand of disability activists to be included in decisions that impact them (Charlton, 2000). Still, too often, OT practitioners and other healthcare providers have more weight in the decision-making about a patient's care than the patient themself (Gupta & Taff, 2015; Whalley Hammell, 2013). In order to align with the OT value of person-centeredness and the disability value of self-determination, we need to do more to return decision-making power to the clients and communities we serve. For example: Casey (he/him) is an occupational therapist working in a school-based setting. Inspired by the disability rights slogan, "Nothing about us without us," he advocates for all students to be included in their own IEP meetings.

Promoting Interdependence

Many OT assessments and approaches emphasize independence. This heavy focus on independence is not only reflective of nondisabled norms but also on cultural values that center white people, especially those from Europe and North America (Sins Invalid, 2019). However, *interdependence* is a reality of all human life. Our survival and flourishing is intertwined with the others in our social networks and communities. Members of the disability justice movement highlight the importance of interdependence, not only for disabled people but also for all people (Sins Invalid, 2019). A greater emphasis on interdependence could bring OT's values more in alignment with the priorities and realities of the populations we serve.

As you move into practice, consider how the typical focus on your clients becoming independent may be setting them up for failure with a goal that is unattainable even by nondisabled people. How might you use the language and concepts of interdependence to give them permission and affirmation in their reliance on adaptive equipment, PCAs, assistive technology, social support, and medical treatments? By stressing to your clients that we all need a supportive circle of social connections, you may help them flourish.

Engaging in Advocacy

OT practitioners partnering with disability communities to advocate for disability rights is important as it helps improve the range of interventions that OT practitioners can use to facilitate participation of their clients. Advocacy is described in the OTPF-4 as a type of OT intervention (AOTA, 2020). Advocacy means actively engaging in various political issues (Urrieta, 2005). Attention to power and oppression is needed. Advocacy is about putting the power that you have as an occupational therapist to work in ways that facilitate disability rights. OT practitioners can advocate on many different types of disability rights issues. For example, an occupational therapist could work with disability rights activist group ADAPT on pushing the DIA through Congress. An occupational therapist could also advocate by writing an appeal letter to an insurance company, arguing that the adaptive equipment that the client needs is medically necessary.

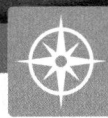 **EXPANDING OUR PERSPECTIVES**

It Takes a Village: Advocacy for Disability Rights

Selena Washington

"It takes a village" is a part of a well-known phrase derived from an African proverb. This proverb holds an entire *community* accountable to interact positively with *people* who are within vulnerable populations (e.g., based on disability, race, age, and social class) and provide meaningful life experiences for those individuals within a healthy and safe environment. For this specific context, we focus on *people* who live with disability and face discrimination at the structural/policy, organizational/community, and interpersonal/familial levels within society and need the support of the community or *village*; the *village* consists of the parents, caregivers, community organizations, disability leaders/stakeholders, medical community, and research community. The *village* contributes to quality-of-life aspects needed to address the discriminatory practices and the threat of societal marginalization. As an occupational therapist and community researcher working with adults aging with Down syndrome (DS), this African proverb is the center of my work and advocacy for the community

I support. Alcedo and colleagues (2017) summarized the challenges of people aging with disability well through this statement:

> We find ourselves facing a social phenomenon which poses significant, unexpected challenges, and key amongst those challenges will be the political and professional response to both the new needs these older people with intellectual disability present, and the exacerbation of already existing needs. (p. 39)

At this point, you might ask, How does an occupational therapist fit into a *village* to support people living with disability? Here are some examples (Washington et al., 2021):

- Listen to the intended community you are working with, go beyond work requirements, volunteer, and develop sustainable relationships with the community and its stakeholders. Engage in dialogue and advocacy to align with the needs and concerns of the intended community.
- Utilize current disability, disability studies, and evidence-based literature specific to your intended community to guide innovative practice and client-centered intervention (e.g., home modifications and universal design

(continued)

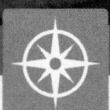

EXPANDING OUR PERSPECTIVES (*continued*)

recommendations for those living with cerebral palsy).

- Utilize trend data from government agencies or foundations to identify the most prevalent occupational, policy, and environmental issues within the intended community, including National Institute on Disability, Independent Living, and Rehabilitation Research (NIDILRR), Ford Foundation, and Aging and Disability Resource Centers.

References

Alcedo, M. Á., Fontanil, Y., Solís, P., Pedrosa, I., & Aguado, A. L. (2017). People with intellectual disability who are ageing: Perceived needs assessment. *International Journal of Clinical and Health Psychology, 17*(1), 38–45. doi: 10.1016/j.ijchp.2016.07.002

Washington, S. E., Johnson, K. R., & Hollenbeck, J. M. (2021). Environmental modifications and supports for participation among adults aging with intellectual and developmental disabilities: A scoping review. *American Journal of Occupational Therapy, 75*(4):7504180060. doi: 10.5014/ajot.2021.045336.

Conclusion

This chapter introduces different ways of thinking about disability and what to do about it. Disability movements and disability studies offer many opportunities for OT practitioners to ally ourselves with disability communities and their work for justice. The authors have presented ideas that you may have never heard before, that may seem more critical than what you are used to, and that may have surprised you. The authors encourage you to stay with these feelings and use them as a springboard for further reflection about the OT profession and practice. It is a process and journey to learn about disability rights and its associated movements. The authors encourage you to keep going. Let this chapter serve as your invitation to reflect, to learn more, and—we hope—to become a powerful advocate for disability rights. See Box 16.3 for the next steps you can take.

BOX 16.3 THINKING ABOUT DISABILITY: NEXT STEPS

1. Now that you've finished reading, refer back to the document where you recorded disability organizations mentioned in the chapter. Which of these organizations do you want to learn more about? Do they have social media accounts you can follow?
2. Which of the documentaries or readings mentioned in the chapter will you seek out to continue your learning?

Acknowledgments

The authors would like to acknowledge the authors of previous editions of this chapter, whose work provided a strong foundation for this latest edition. The previous authors are John White (13th Edition), and Joy Hammel, Jim Charlton, Robin A. Jones, Jessica M. Kramer, and Tom Wilson (12th Edition).

Lippincott® Connect *For additional resources on the subjects discussed in this chapter, visit* Lippincott Connect.

REFERENCES

ADA.gov. (n.d.). *Introduction to the ADA.* https://www.ada.gov/ada_intro.htm

ADA National Network. (n.d-a). *What is the definition of disability under the ADA?* https://adata.org/faq/what-definition-disability-under-ada

ADA National Network. (n.d.-b). *Map for contacting regional ADA center.* https://adata.org/find-your-region

ADAPT. (n.d.). *Welcome to American Disabled for Attendant Programs Today (ADAPT).* https://adapt.org/

American Occupational Therapy Association. (n.d.). *AOTA is advocating for you.* https://www.aota.org/advocacy

American Occupational Therapy Association. (2020). Occupational therapy practice framework: Domain and process—Fourth edition. *American Journal of Occupational Therapy, 74*(Suppl 2),7412410010p1–7412410010p87. https://doi.org/10.5014/ajot.2020.74S2001

Americans with Disabilities Act of 1990. (1990). 42 U. S. C. § 12101 et seq. (ADA). https://www.ada.gov/pubs/adastatute08.htm

APA Style. (2021). *Disability.* https://apastyle.apa.org/style-grammar-guidelines/bias-free-language/disability

Association of People Supporting Employment First. (n.d.). *Homepage.* https://apse.org/

Astor, M. (2021, July 30). How disabled Americans are pushing to overhaul a key benefits program. *The New York Times.* https://www.nytimes.com/2021/07/30/us/politics/disability-benefits-ssi-congress.html

Autistic Self Advocacy Network. (2020). *Before you donate to Autism Speaks, consider the facts.* https://autisticadvocacy.org/wp-content/uploads/2018/03/AutismSpeaksFlyer2020.pdf

Autistic Self Advocacy Network. (2021). *For whose benefit?:* Evidence, ethics, and effectiveness of autism interventions. https://autisticadvocacy.org/wp-content/uploads/2021/12/ACWP-Ethics-of-Intervention.pdf

Bevan, J. (2014). Disabled occupational therapists—Asset, liability … or "watering down" the profession? *Disability & Society, 29*(4), 583–596. https://doi.org/10.1080/09687599.2013.831747

Block, P., Ricafrente-Biazon, M., Russo, A., Chu, K. Y., Sud, S., Koerner, L., Vittoria, K., Landgrover, A., & Olowu, T. (2005). Introducing disability studies to occupational therapy students. *American Journal of Occupational Therapy, 59*(5), 554–560. https://doi.org/10.5014/ajot.59.5.554

Brown, L. (2011). *Identity-first language.* https://autisticadvocacy.org/about-asan/identity-first-language/

Brown, L. (2014). Disability in an ableist world. In C. Wood (Ed.), *Criptiques* (pp. 37–46). May Day. https://criptiques.files.wordpress.com/2014/05/crip-final-2.pdf

Canelón, M. F. (1995). Job site analysis facilitates work reintegration. *American Journal of Occupational Therapy, 49*(5), 461–467. https://doi.org/10.5014/ajot.49.5.461

Centers for Disease Control and Prevention. (n.d.). *Impairments, activity limitations, and participation restrictions.* https://www.cdc.gov/ncbddd/disabilityandhealth/disability.html

Chamberlin, J. (1979). *On our own: Patient-controlled alternatives to the mental health system.* McGraw-Hill.

Charlton, J. I. (2000). *Nothing about us without us: Disability oppression and empowerment* (1st ed.). University of California Press.

Cottrell, R. P. (2005). The Olmstead decision: Landmark opportunity or platform for rhetoric? Our collective responsibility for full community participation. *American Journal of Occupational Therapy, 59*(5), 561–568. https://doi.org/10.5014/ajot.59.5.561

Crenshaw, K. W. (1991). Mapping the margins: Intersectionality, identity politics, and violence against women of color. *Stanford Law Review, 43*(6), 1241–1299. https://doi.org/10.2307/1229039

Crow, L. (1996). Including all of our lives: Renewing the social model of disability. In J. Morris (Ed.), *Encounters with strangers: Feminism and disability* (pp. 206–226). The Women's Press.

Darrah, J., Law, M. C., Pollock, N., Wilson, B., Russell, D. J., Walter, S. D., Rosenbaum, P., & Galuppi, B. (2011). Context therapy: A new intervention approach for children with cerebral palsy. *Developmental Medicine & Child Neurology, 53*(7), 615–620. https://doi.org/10.1111/j.1469-8749.2011.03959.x

DeMaio-Feldman, D. (1987). The occupational therapist as an expert witness. *American Journal of Occupational Therapy, 41*(9), 590–594. https://doi.org/10.5014/ajot.41.9.590

Diamond, S. (2013). What makes us a community? Reflections on building solidarity in anti-sanist praxis. In B. A. LeFrançois, R. J. Menzies, & G. Reaume (Eds.), *Mad matters: A critical reader in Canadian mad studies* (pp. 64–77). Canadian Scholars' Press.

Disability Justice Culture Club. (n.d.). *Disability justice culture club.* https://www.facebook.com/disabilityjusticecultureclub/

Disability Rights Education & Defense Fund. (n.d.). *Section 504 of the Rehabilitation Act of 1973.* https://dredf.org/legal-advocacy/laws/section-504-of-the-rehabilitation-act-of-1973/

Disability Rights Education and Defense Fund. (2015). *The Power of 504.* https://dredf.org/web-log/2015/07/26/translating-the-power-of-504

Disability Rights Education & Defense Fund. (2021). *International disability rights laws.* https://dredf.org/legal-advocacy/international-disability-rights/international-laws/

Disability Visibility Project. (2019, October 19). *We need power to live.* https://disabilityvisibilityproject.com/2019/10/13/we-need-power-to-live/

Equip for Equality. (2019). *Olmstead—20 years of community integration.* https://www.equipforequality.org/olmstead-20-years-of-community-integration/

Friedman, C., & VanPuymbrouck, L. (2021). Impact of occupational therapy education on students' disability attitudes: A longitudinal study. *American Journal of Occupational Therapy, 75*(4), 7504180090. https://doi.org/10.5014/ajot.2021.047423

Giangreco, M. F. (1996). *"The stairs don't go anywhere!": A disabled person's reflections on specialized services and their impact on people with disabilities, an interview with Norman Kunc.* Physical disabilities: Education and related services. https://www.broadreachtraining.com/giangreco

Gitlow, L., & Flecky, K. (2005). Integrating disability studies concepts into occupational therapy education using service learning. *American Journal of Occupational Therapy, 59*(5), 546–553. https://doi.org/10.5014/ajot.59.5.546

Green, M. (2020, March 17). *Coronavirus: How these disabled activists are taking matters into their own (sanitized) hands.* https://www.kqed.org/news/11806414/coronavirus-how-these-disabled-activists-are-taking-matters-into-their-own-sanitized-hands

Grosz, P. (Director). (2019). *Piss on pity: We will ride* [Film]. Roustabout Media.

Gupta, J., & Taff, S. D. (2015). The illusion of client-centered practice. *Scandinavian Journal of Occupational Therapy, 22*(4), 244–251. https://doi.org/10.3109/11038128.2015.1020866

Hahn, H. (1985). Toward a politics of disability: Definitions, disciplines, and policies. *The Social Science Journal, 22*(4), 87–105. https://psycnet.apa.org/record/1987-07721-001

Harrison, E. A., & Kopit, A. G. (2020). Accessibility at the bisexual health summit: Reflections and lessons for improving event accessibility. *Journal of Bisexuality, 20*(4), 1–23. https://doi.org/10.1080/15299716.2020.1774834

Harrison, E. A., Sheth, A. J., Kish, J., VanPuymbrouck, L. H., Heffron, J. L., Lee, D., Mahaffey, L., & The Occupational Therapy and Disability Studies Network. (2021). Guest editorial—Disability studies and occupational therapy: Renewing the call for change. *American Journal of Occupational Therapy, 75*(4), 7504170010. https://doi.org/10.5014/ajot.2021.754002

Hayashi, R., & Okuhira, M. (2001). The disability rights movement in Japan: Past, present and future. *Disability & Society, 16*(6), 855–869. https://doi.org/10.1080/09687590120083994

Hearing Voices Network. (n.d.). *Hearing voices groups.* http://www.hearing-voices.org/groups/

Heffron, J. L., Lee, D., VanPuymbrouck, L., Sheth, A. J., & Kish, J. (2019). "The bigger picture": Occupational therapy practitioners' perspectives on disability studies. *American Journal of Occupational Therapy, 73*(2), 7302205100p1–7302205100p10. https://doi.org/10.5014/ajot.2019.030163

Holler, R., Chemla, I., & Maeir, A. (2021). Disability orientation of occupational therapy practitioners in physical rehabilitation settings: Tension between medical and social models in theory and practice. *American Journal of Occupational Therapy, 75*(4), 7504180010. https://doi.org/10.5014/ajot.2021.042986

Independent Living Research Utilization. (n.d.). *ILRU directory of Centers for Independent Living (CILs) and associations.* https://www.ilru.org/projects/cil-net/cil-center-and-association-directory

Institute for Human Centered Design & ADA National Network. (2016). *ADA checklist for existing facilities.* https://www.adachecklist.org/doc/fullchecklist/ada-checklist.pdf

Kenneth Young Center. (2021). *Staff spotlight: Meet Nicole, occupational therapist.* https://www.kennethyoung.org/blog/staff-spotlight-nicole

Kielhofner, G. (2005). Rethinking disability and what to do about it: Disability studies and its implications for occupational therapy. *American Journal of Occupational Therapy, 59*(5), 487–496. https://doi.org/10.5014/ajot.59.5.487

Kornblau, B. L., & Robertson, S. M. (2021). Special issue on occupational therapy with neurodivergent people. *American Journal of Occupational Therapy, 75*(3), 7503170010._https://doi.org/10.5014/ajot.2021.753001

Law, M. C., Darrah, J., Pollock, N., Wilson, B., Russell, D. J., Walter, S. D., Rosenbaum, P., & Galuppi, B. (2011). Focus on function: A cluster, randomized controlled trial comparing child- versus context-focused intervention for young children with cerebral palsy. *Developmental Medicine and Child Neurology, 53*(7), 621–629. https://doi.org/10.1111/j.1469-8749.2011.03962.x

LeBrecht, J., & Newnham, N. (Directors). (2020). Crip camp [Film]. Netflix Original Documentary.

LeFrançois, B. A., Menzies, R. J., & Reaume, G. (2013). *Mad matters: A critical reader in Canadian mad studies.* Canadian Scholars' Press.

Linton, S. (1998). Disability studies/not disability studies. *Disability & Society, 13*(4), 525–539. https://doi.org/10.1080/09687599826588

Mahaffey, L., VanPuymbrouck, L., & Harrison, E. A. (2018). *Ethical dilemma in practice: How to support a person's right to go home when our measures say they "shouldn't"* [Conference session]. Illinois Occupational Therapy Association conference, Lisle, IL.

Menzies, R., LeFrançois, B., & Reaume, G. (2013). Introducing mad studies. In B. A. LeFrançois, R. J. Menzies, & G. Reaume (Eds.), *Mad matters: A critical reader in Canadian mad studies* (pp. 1–22). Canadian Scholars' Press.

Metzl, J. (2011). *The protest psychosis: How schizophrenia became a black disease.* Beacon Press.

MindFreedom International. (2020). *MindFreedom International (MFI) sponsor and affiliate list.* https://mindfreedom.org/affiliates-sponsors/mfi-sponsor-affiliate-public-list/

National Council of Disabled Persons of Zimbabwe. (n.d.). *National Council of Disabled Persons of Zimbabwe.* https://www.ncdpz.org.zw/

National Council on Independent Living. (n.d.) *About independent living.* https://ncil.org/about/aboutil/

National Disability Rights Network. (n.d.). *Protection and advocacy for people with disabilities.* https://www.ndrn.org/

National Down Syndrome Society. (n.d.). *Homepage.* https://www.ndss.org

Neville-Jan, A. (2005). The problem with prevention: The case of spina bifida. *American Journal of Occupational Therapy, 59*(5), 527–539. https://doi.org/10.5014/ajot.59.5.527

New York University. (n.d.). *Digital accessibility how-to guides.* https://www.nyu.edu/life/information-technology/web-and-digital-publishing/digital-publishing/accessibility/how-to-guides.html

No Body is Disposable. (2020). *Fight discrimination in COVID-19 triage.* https://nobodyisdisposable.org/home/

Oliver, M. (1990). *Politics of disablement.* Macmillan International Higher Education.

O'Toole, C. J. (2015). *Fading scars: My queer disability history.* Autonomous Press.

Parmet, W. E. (1993). Title III: Public accommodations. In L. O. Gostin & H. A. Beyer (Eds.), *Implementing the Americans with Disabilities Act: Rights and responsibilities of all Americans* (pp. 123–136). Paul H. Brookes.

Pelka, F. (1997). *The ABC-CLIO companion to the disability rights movement.* ABC-CLIO.

People First. (n.d.). *History of people first.* http://peoplefirstwv.org/old-front/history-of-people-first/

Pruett, S., & Pruett, S. (2018). *Safescore: Universal design checklist.* https://safescore.org/checklists

Reaume, G. (2011). *Psychiatric built wall tours at the centre for addiction and mental health (CAMH), Toronto, 2000–2010.* http://activehistory.ca/papers/historypaper-10/

Russo, J., & Sweeney, A. (Eds.). (2016). *Searching for a rose garden: Challenging psychiatry, fostering mad studies.* PCCS Books.

Schweik, S. (2011). Lomax's matrix: Disability, solidarity, and the black power of 504. *Disability Studies Quarterly, 31*(1). https://dsq-sds.org/article/view/1371/1539

Self Advocates Becoming Empowered. (n.d.). *Self advocates becoming empowered.* https://www.sabeusa.org/

Shapiro, J. P. (1993). *No pity: People with disabilities forging a new civil rights movement.* Times Books.

Shapiro, J. P. (2020). *One man's covid-19 death raises the worst fears of many people with disabilities.* https://www.npr.org/2020/07/31/896882268/one-mans-covid-19-death-raises-the-worst-fears-of-many-people-with-disabilities

Sheth, A. J., Kish, J., VanPuymbrouck, L. H., Heffron, J. L., Lee, D., & Mahaffey, L. (2021). "A legitimate place in the profession": Author reflections on the 2005 disability studies special issue. *American Journal of Occupational Therapy, 75*(4), 7504180005. https://doi.org/10.5014/ajot.2021.045294

Sinclair, J. (1993). Don't mourn for us. *Our Voice, 1*(3). https://www.autreat.com/dont_mourn.html

Singer, J. (2017). *Neurodiversity: The birth of an idea.* Judy Singer.

Sins Invalid. (2019). *Skin, tooth, and bone: The basis of movement is our people* (2nd ed.). https://www.sinsinvalid.org/disability-justice-primer

Speak Up and Speak Out Summit. (2021). *Speak up and speak out summit (SUSO).* https://www.speakupspeakoutsummit.org/

Starkman, M. (2013). The movement. In B. A. LeFrançois, R. J. Menzies, & G. Reaume (Eds.), *Mad matters: A critical reader in Canadian mad studies* (pp. 27–37). Canadian Scholars' Press.

The, K. J., & Harrison, E. (2019, April 7–9). Cultures of OT and ableism [Conference session]. Society for Disability Studies Conference, Columbus, OH.

The, K. J., Heffron, J., & Harrison, E. A. (2017, April 2). Promoting a more diverse workforce through the inclusion of OT practitioners with disabilities [Conference session]. American Occupational Therapy Association Conference, Philadelphia, PA.

The Washington Post. (2022). *Fatal force database.* https://www.washingtonpost.com/graphics/investigations/police-shootings-database

Toronto Mad Pride. (2016). *Madness on parade—Mad bed push.* http://www.torontomadpride.com/2016/03/mad-pride-parade-bed-push/

Union of the Physically Impaired Against Segregation, & the Disability Alliance. (1975). *Fundamental principles of disability.* https://disability-studies.leeds.ac.uk/wp-content/uploads/sites/40/library/UPIAS-fundamental-principles.pdf

United Nations. (n.d.). *Convention on the rights of persons with disabilities (CRPD).* https://www.un.org/development/desa/disabilities/convention-on-the-rights-of-persons-with-disabilities.html

University of California. (2010). *The disability rights and independent living movement.* https://bancroft.berkeley.edu/collections/drilm/index.html

Urrieta, L. (2005). The social studies of domination: Cultural hegemony and ignorant activism. *The Social Studies, 96*(5), 189–192. https://doi.org/10.3200/TSSS.96.5.189-192

U.S. Commission on Civil Rights. (2020). *Subminimum wages: Impacts on the civil rights of people with disabilities.* https://www.usccr.gov/files/2020/2020-09-17-Subminimum-Wages-Report.pdf

U.S. Department of Education. (2017). *A transition guide: To postsecondary education and employment for students and youth with disabilities.* https://www2.ed.gov/about/offices/list/osers/transition/products/postsecondary-transition-guide-may-2017.pdf

U.S. Department of Justice. (2020). *A guide to disability rights laws.* https://www.ada.gov/cguide.htm

Wendell, S. (1996). *The rejected body: Feminist philosophical reflections on disability.* Routledge.

Whalley Hammell, K. R. (2013). Client-centred practice in occupational therapy: Critical reflections. *Scandinavian Journal of Occupational Therapy, 20*(3), 174–-181. https://doi.org/10.3109/11038128.2012.752032

Whiteford, G., Jones, K., Rahal, C., & Suleman, A. (2018). The participatory occupational justice framework as a tool for change: Three contrasting case narratives. *Journal of Occupational Science, 25*(4), 497–508. https://doi.org/10.1080/14427591.2018.1504607

Whiteford, G., & Townsend, E. (2011). Participatory occupational justice framework (POJF 2010): Enabling occupational participation and inclusion. In F. Kronenberg, N. Pollard, & D. Sakellariou (Eds.), *Occupational therapies without borders—Vol. 2: Towards an ecology of occupation-based practices* (pp. 65–84). Elsevier.

Physical and Virtual Environments

Meaning of Place and Space

Noralyn D. Pickens and Cynthia L. Evetts

LEARNING OBJECTIVES

After reading this chapter, you will be able to:

1. Explain why and how qualities of the physical environment and place are important dimensions of human life and experience.
2. Describe what a phenomenological approach to human experience entails and its usefulness in understanding human experience of environments and places.
3. Define place in terms of human experience using the concepts of insideness and outsideness.
4. Apply the concepts of home and at-homeness to people's lives and explain how home and at-homeness can be strengthened or undermined by physical features of dwellings and neighborhoods.
5. Explain the impact that displacement and temporary place may have on health and well-being.
6. Explain the relevance of virtual worlds and virtual places and apply them to occupational therapy conditions and contexts for engagement in occupation.
7. Explain the critical importance of physical and virtual environments in effective occupational therapy practice.

Environments, Places, and Occupational Therapy

Physical and virtual environments influence human health, well-being, and productive occupations (Eriksson & Dahlblom, 2020; Hasselkus & Dickie, 2021; Kylén et al., 2019; Mossabir et al., 2021; Wiederhold, 2020). How human beings *experience* environments, places, and spaces is central to understanding occupational therapy (OT). **Phenomenology** is the description and interpretation of human experience (Finlay, 2011; Hasselkus & Dickie, 2021). In this chapter, the phenomenological approach is briefly described, and four environmental themes important for occupational therapists and scientists are considered including (a) place, (b) environmental embodiment, (c) home and at-homeness, and (d) virtual technology and place.

Phenomenology and Occupational Therapy

To study human beings phenomenologically is to study human experiences, behaviors, situations, and meanings as they arise in the world of everyday life. For OT and occupational science, one significant phenomenological topic is the **lifeworld**—a person or group's everyday world of *taken-for-grantedness*, which is normally unnoticed and thus hidden as a phenomenon (Finlay, 2011; Seamon, 2018). One aim of phenomenological research is to see and describe the various lived structures and dynamics of the lifeworld more clearly—for example, the mostly unnoticed but crucial importance of places in people's daily lives (Seamon, 2018). An understanding of a client's lifeworld is central for occupational therapists because, typically, the taken-for-grantedness of their world has shifted or disappeared, including occupational dimensions (Marshall et al., 2018; Turpin et al., 2018).

Most of the time in everyday life, the lifeworld is *transparent* in the sense that day-to-day life *just happens* according to typical routine behavior and events (Seamon, 1979). An integral part of this lived transparency is good health, which is frequently taken for granted (Ahlzen, 2011; Stefanovic, 2008). In contrast, illness and disability can transform a usual lifeworld when feelings of awkwardness, unease, or discomfort arise. Daily life that simply unfolded before without the need for self-conscious awareness can become a continual event to be faced, whether because of pain, inconvenience, or inability to perform as usual. In this sense, one task of occupational therapists is to understand their clients' former mode of "being at home" and to locate pathways they can use to access and recover that mode (Ahlzen, 2011). As the next sections demonstrate, qualities of places and physical environments can help facilitate this return to "being at home."

Place and Occupational Therapy

The idea of place is an important aspect of the lifeworld. *Place* can be defined as any space that has meanings and intentions for an individual or group, and where related actions are carried out (Relph, 1976/2008). A place can be anything from a chair or room to a building, neighborhood, city, or region (Relph, 1976/2008; Seamon 2018). One of the most accessible publications about the phenomenology of place is geographer Edward Relph's *Place and Placelessness* (Relph, 1976/2008). Relph argued that the most important part of experiencing place is a feeling of *insideness*—in

other words, the more deeply a person or group feels themselves inside an environment, the more that environment becomes a place of meaning. The deepest experience of place attachment and identity is what Relph termed *existential insideness*—a situation where the person or group feels so much at home and at ease in place that they have no self-conscious recognition of its importance in their lives, unless the place or the people in it change in some way. Examples of such changes include when a home is destroyed by a flood or a client is no longer able to walk because of an injury. In one sense, a major aim of occupational therapists is working with a client to help them reestablish, as much as possible, a sense of existential insideness—feeling really at home.

In his phenomenology of place, Relph (1976/2008) described several other modes of place insideness and its lived opposite, *outsideness*. Outsideness is a situation where the person or group feels separate or alienated from place in some way. These modes of place experience are described in Table 17.1. The modes are useful for the occupational therapist because they provide accessible language for identifying particular place experiences in terms of the intensity of meaning and intention that a person and place hold for each other. Through illness or accident, for example, individuals' taken-for-granted sense of existential insideness can be ruptured, and they can fall into a particular mode of existential outsideness in which the lifeworld as it was before is now different, often in strange or uncomfortable ways. Relph's modes of insideness and outsideness offer a flexible means for distinguishing the lived experience of place from its material or assumed qualities. For example, when there is abuse or violence in someone's home, which is typically a place of existential insideness, their home becomes a place of existential outsideness.

The environmental themes discussed in this chapter are illustrated by the lifeworld of Alex, a person who experienced long COVID (see OT Story 17.1). For students learning to become occupational therapists, this story can be a powerful example of how occupation is transacted through environment and context.

Themes of place, insideness, and outsideness can offer occupational therapists valuable insights. Rowles and Bernard (2013) emphasized that their lifeworlds typically involve strong emotional attachments to place. Rowles identified three dimensions of place related to Relph's theme of existential insideness: first, *physical insideness*, a sense of being physically entwined with the environment; second, *social insideness*, whereby people feel an integral part of their community through social relationships and exchanges; and third, *autobiographical insideness*, the ways in which a place becomes an important part of one's personal and communal history (Seamon, 2018). Understanding place experience is important for occupational therapists in that

| TABLE 17.1 | Modes of Insideness and Outsideness |

Mode	Description
Existential insideness	Feeling completely at home and immersed in place, to such a degree the experience is not usually noticed unless the place dramatically changes in some way (e.g., one's home and community are destroyed by natural disaster). The mode of place experience most human beings strive for; typically, the mode of place experience that occupational therapists work toward recovering for their clients
Existential outsideness	Feeling alienated or separate from place, which may seem oppressive or unreal (e.g., the experience of homesickness or the deep sense of disjunction one feels, having suddenly become disabled because of an accident). The mode of experience that many people fall into after a disabling accident or after becoming ill or learning they are ill. A major task of the occupational therapist is to help clients shift, as much as possible, out of existential outsideness back toward existential insideness.
Objective outsideness	A dispassionate attitude of separation from place, which becomes an object of study or directed attention (e.g., designing a hospital using measurable criteria like the size of potential patient pool, square footage based on functional needs, building layout determined by staff efficiency)
Incidental outsideness	The experience in which place is a background or mere setting for activities (e.g., the short-term patient's limited relationship with the hospital environment in which she finds herself temporarily)
Behavioral insideness	A deliberate attending to the appearance of place (e.g., using environmental cues like landmarks and signage to find one's way around a place). The first stage in becoming an insider to a new place (e.g., mastering the layout of a hospital complex where one has just started working)
Empathetic insideness	Being open to place and attempting to understand it more deeply (e.g., the occupational therapist's effort to see and to understand the client's lifeworld as it really is and not as the occupational therapist supposes it to be)
Vicarious insideness	Deeply felt secondhand involvement with place (e.g., learning about worlds of illness or disablement through films, novels, or autobiographical accounts)

Reprinted with permission from Relph, E. (2008). *Place and placelessness.* Pion. (Original work published 1976.)

OT STORY 17.1 ALEX'S LIFEWORLD

Alex was experiencing the excitement of a total change in scenery. As a recent college graduate and newly admitted graduate student, Alex kissed their mom, high-fived their brother, and moved into a new apartment in a new town to attend a new school. Everything felt fresh and full of promise. Then the world came to a screeching halt in March 2020 when a global health crisis came to the United States and everything shut down, seemingly overnight. Alex's graduate program summer semester went online, and everybody learned how to Zoom, order groceries to be delivered, and make face masks for the rare occasion of venturing outside of their homes.

At first, all of the environmental change was novel and challenging—later it got boring. Alex felt their roommates were not always being safe, and with their mom's encouragement, they moved back home to their childhood room. Attending classes online felt lonely. It was hard meeting classmates over Zoom and doing DIY lab activities with whatever could be found at home. However, there was hope for a rapid end to the pandemic and a return to normal in the Fall semester. But, no, the pandemic raged on, and early in September, Alex got a sore throat and began to feel very tired. They remembered being in the car and realizing a really sick feeling: Alex had COVID.

While quarantined, Alex felt a lack of control. Their typical environments had switched from traditional college campus life to isolation in their childhood room and multiple clinical visits—often via telehealth (see Figure 17.1). Meals were delivered to their room to be eaten alone. The room they had grown up in did not feel comfortable and Alex experienced existential outsideness. Even worse, Alex was so sick they had to drop out of school. At one point, Alex remembers having eight doctor appointments within a single month. Their chief complaints were "no energy, head vibration, and feeling high, angry, and depressed." Anxiety built when Alex had difficulty breathing. Alex lost the sense of smell, and then everything smelled like "concrete, dog poop, and beer tacos—it's like that smell is stuck in my nose." Sixteen months later, they still have to keep regular appointments with a cardiologist because of pericarditis.

Drawing on their undergraduate degree, Alex went to work as an Early Childhood Intervention specialist. Employment has been a struggle primarily because of fatigue and "brain fog," making it difficult to pass tests that document required skills. Alex works with autistic children and has noticed that wearing a mask makes play and communication even more difficult. Even driving a new car between

(continued)

OT STORY 17.1 ALEX'S LIFEWORLD (continued)

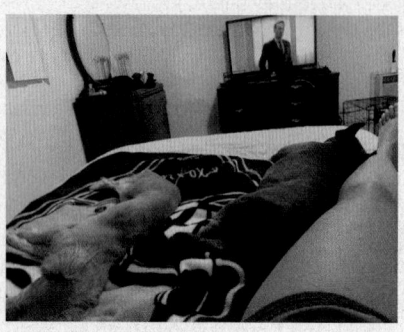
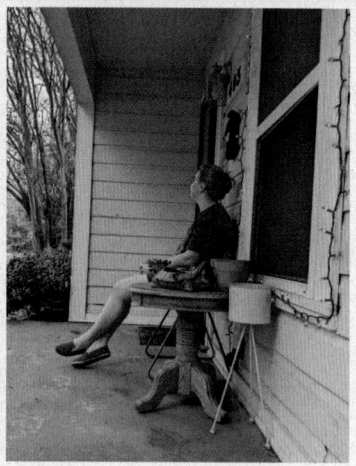

A   B

FIGURE 17.1 Alex's lifeworld (A) in their childhood bedroom with their dogs and (B) on their porch.

appointments, which used to be a favorite activity, is scary because the attacks of fatigue cause fears of having a crash.

Using a mode of empathic insideness, their occupational therapist explored Alex's experience of daily living and helped them learn to identify personal limits related to physical exertion during valued occupations. Alex monitors oxygen saturation levels and heart rate during activities with the help of wearable technology. Alex reported episodes of racing heart rate and difficulty breathing, even at rest. "My brain thinks I'm working out, even when I'm not."

Perhaps the most difficult thing about having the extended symptoms of "long COVID" has been "feeling like a burden." Alex feels like most of their friends are not able to comprehend what life is like now and feels like "I get on their nerves. . . . I have one friend who also has extended COVID symptoms so she gets it." Functional problems include needing extra time to accomplish tasks, being overstimulated by noise and bright lights, and difficulty focusing.

As a coping strategy, Alex develops "tunnel vision" to avoid getting overstimulated when, for example, going through a familiar grocery store.

To rest and restore energy, Alex enjoys petting or playing with their dogs, being in or near nature, and listening to music or watching TV. The back porch at home offers regeneration—both shelter and exposure to nature, with a comfortable and welcoming atmosphere where Alex can feel relaxed (see Figure 17.1).

Questions

1. How did Alex describe a sense of at-homeness?
2. What can be done to help Alex experience a greater sense of belonging?
3. How did interactions in virtual environments impact how Alex experienced different modes of insideness and outsideness?

its meaning shapes engagement in everyday occupation and conditioned responses to the environment.

Occupational therapists seek to understand the worldview of each client, but we are limited in some ways by our own experiences. In the absence of unlimited resources for study abroad and other global excursions, use of film and books in OT programs creates opportunities for students to develop *vicarious insideness*. That is, authors, filmmakers, and documentary producers offer us glimpses into worlds we might not have opportunity to experience otherwise. While being careful not to generalize and create stereotypes, these glimpses help us formulate questions rather than make assumptions based on our own limited lived experiences.

Experience of Home, At-Homeness, and Homelessness

The Lived Body and Environmental Embodiment

In exploring human experience, phenomenologists emphasize that humans are *bodily* beings, a lived fact important for OT's central focus on the well-being of the *whole person*.

Phenomenologists speak of the *lived body*—a body that simultaneously experiences, acts in, and is aware of a world that, normally, responds with immediate pattern, meaning, and contextual presence (Seamon, 2018). The lived body is the primary means of being in, experiencing, and encountering the world. The lived body falls ill, it experiences pain, it fails to heal, it heals badly, it becomes older, it remains impaired, it returns to good health, and it learns new ways to cope with illness and adapt to disabling conditions or contextual restrictions to participation.

An example is Curry's (2015) study of people experiencing homelessness in which she writes about the embodiment of body, home, and world and how the boundaries between these are permeable. Home, she writes, is often considered private, away from public sharing. Consider that not all people live in homes that are solid physical structures or that afford the privilege of privacy. For some, home is their tent, box, or sleeping bag (Figure 17.2). She tells the story of Jack, who one night in his bedding down habits and routines to prepare his sleeping bag in the park was nearly accosted by a weapon-wielding attacker. He was confused, as the near-attack (stopped by the oncoming headlights of a stranger) permeated his home. The space in the park was his temporary home, a private location without physical boundaries, yet of personal significance. Experiencing home is more about place than a structure; homelessness is a liminal state of not having permanent housing. We must consider how being houseless is one way of being in the world.

Sometimes, drawing on universal design (fabricating products and environments that work well for almost everyone), occupational therapists and other professionals have considered how architecture and environmental design can sustain and enhance patients' and clients' lifeworlds (Burns et al., 2017; Preiser & Smith, 2011; Söderback, 2009;

Ulrich et al., 2008). Brooks and colleagues (2011), for example, examined how patients in assisted living and rehabilitation settings made use of bedside table devices and then designed three improved "smart stand" prototypes that were more efficient in terms of object reach, placement, storage, and mobility. In a study that examined the walking behaviors of residents in assisted living, Lu (2010) developed recommendations to improve residential walkability, including looped indoor and outdoor walkways, alcoves in hallways with seating, and windowed interior walkways that offer residents a visual connection to the world outside, especially the natural environment (Ulrich et al., 2008). Pickens et al. (2019) demonstrated how addressing the accessibility needs of a father through design and modifications positively impacted the family's interactions and occupational engagement.

The onslaught of COVID-19 and the resulting global pandemic quite literally rocked our world off-balance. Phrases like "shut down," "stay at home," "social distancing," and the difference between "isolation" and "quarantine" became buzzwords and part of everyday conversation. But because of *virtual space* platforms such as Skype, GoTo Meeting, Google Meet, Zoom, and more, the threat of true isolation because of physical distancing was relieved for those who could maintain social connection through the internet, cellular connection, or both (Figure 17.3). Those who were fortunate to have access to video calling exchanged social distancing for physical distancing. People kept their distance but did not lose as much social connection. Some

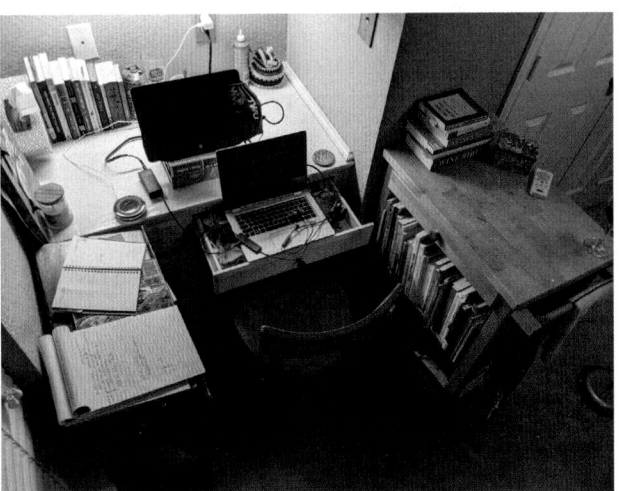

FIGURE 17.3 A built-in desk, a writing table, and a microwave cart were assembled to create a workspace in the corner of a bedroom. Technology to enhance the virtual space one enters from this seat includes an internet-connected laptop with webcam, extra monitor, earphones and microphone, phone charger, and remote control for the lights and ceiling fan.

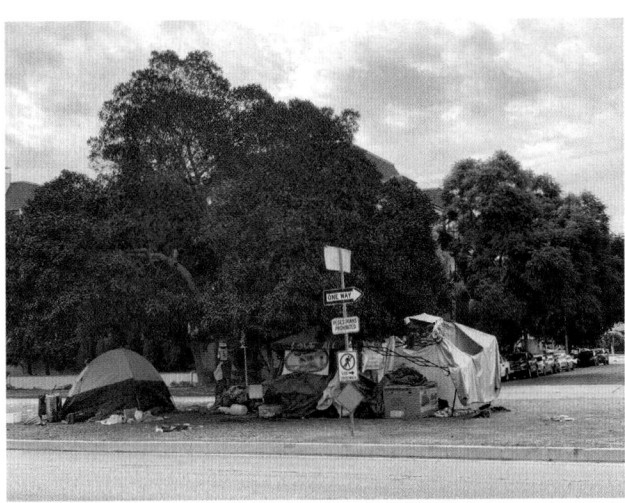

FIGURE 17.2 Homeless camp as a temporary place.

people missed the hugs and physical contact, the change of place and context—but they retained the ability to see faces, exchange smiles, and feel connected. Because of technology and virtual spaces, many people were able to retain a sense of belonging.

School went online, many people became remote workers with video meetings to stay in touch; clubs and groups of family and friends established meet-ups and game nights. Some people chose to attend cooking demonstrations, art classes, and virtual tours of museums and parks. They did this to avoid isolation, loneliness, and boredom—and they discovered a whole new way to take advantage of virtual spaces. However, this meant that now their homes also served as classrooms, workplaces, and leisure spaces. When possible, people set up boundaries in their homes to partition off work life from family life (Figure 17.4). Often separation was difficult, so some people created *virtual backdrops* that gave the illusion of a well-kept house, a place in nature or wherever they would rather have been, or a company logo as a reminder of their purpose.

Many of these virtual options were already available as the tech-savvy were well aware. But the pandemic pushed many more people to give it a try and, for a while, many expressed how they felt technology had saved them from the dreadful alternative of the shutdown. Additional buzzwords like "Zoom fatigue" would soon permeate the media, prompting many occupational therapists to pause and reevaluate the importance of occupational balance and meaningful activity.

Experience of Home

Another important aspect of the lifeworld is *home* and *at-homeness*. Studies by Ohlén et al. (2014) and Seamon (2018) indicate that all homes have specific physical,

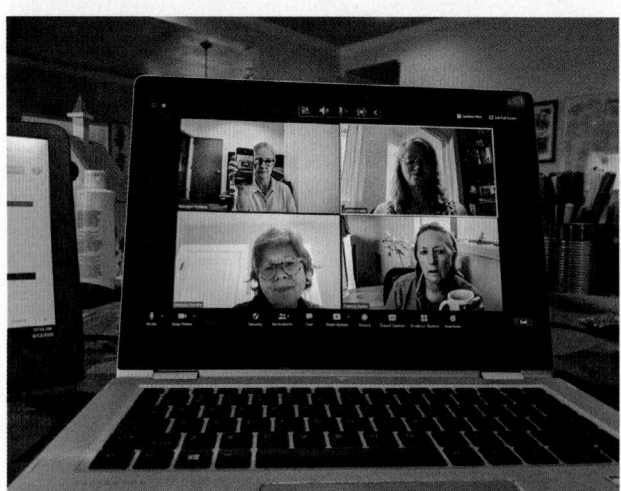

FIGURE 17.4 Coworkers in four different cities across the state sharing a moment of Zoom fatigue while simultaneously appreciating the virtual space.

personal, social, cultural, and political dimensions, but personal experience of how home comes together as a whole is unique to every individual. Home is not only a physical place but also a center of activities, an anchor of identity, a repository of memories bonding past and present, and a center of stability and continuity. At-homeness is conceptually related to wellness, regardless of illness or disability (Ohlén et al., 2014; Saarnio et al., 2019). This literature also emphasizes that some homes can involve a "shadow side" of discomfort, distress, and trauma—for example, in homes where there is violence or abuse (Mayock et al., 2021). At-home violence was especially problematic internationally during the pandemic lockdown (Fawole et al., 2021; Stockman et al., 2021; van Gelder et al., 2021).

There is also the question of how existing houses and dwelling units can be modified through design to match more closely the lifeworld needs of residents as they age or become ill or less abled (Kopec, 2006). Occupational therapists and other professionals have been actively involved in working out effective ways, through environmental interventions and assistive technology, to make home environments more accommodating—for example, widening doors, installing grab bars, adding entrance ramps, providing intercom systems, and so forth (Mendonca et al., 2017; Pickens & Burns, 2018; Söderback, 2009; Stark et al., 2017). Specific populations such as people who were formerly homeless and have premature aging may have special needs for home safety (Gutman et al., 2018). In some situations, however, environmental interventions and assistive technology in the home can disrupt residents' lives. This was demonstrated by Moore and colleagues (2010) in their study of the medical equipment and technology that many children with complex needs depend on in their homes: "The home space becomes an appropriated landscape—no longer a family landscape but a landscape of care, 'like a mini hospital,' with some parents feeling this particularly keenly" (Moore et al., 2010, p. 4).

Home as place offers a sense of well-being, safety, and comfort (Hasselkus & Dickie, 2021; Kylén et al., 2019). Healy-Ogden (2014) explored the meaning of place and dwelling in home care, finding that her participants dwelled in play space, creative space, nature's space, and spiritual space. When healthcare providers support well-being, they move beyond a simplistic view of a patient's house to understand the home as a meaning-filled dwelling. The experience of spaces may overlap. Pleasurable occupations such as gardening or table games with family and friends occur in play space. Play and creative spaces are nurturing and positive. Inside and outside spaces facilitate creative expression. Nature's space can be experienced inside or outside the home (Figure 17.5). Dwelling in spiritual space involves a connection through prayer or creative expression (Healy-Ogden, 2014). Being mindful of the home care client and their family member's sense of dwelling place opens possibilities of using the environment therapeutically to foster well-being.

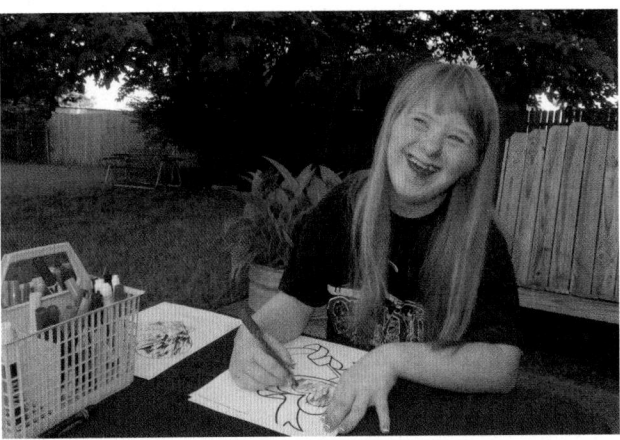

FIGURE 17.5 Addi Jo enjoys working at a backyard picnic table. Extending activity outside into the natural environment makes participation joyful, one way to create *warmth* in setting the stage for a just-right challenge.

Community as Place

If a dwelling is located in a car-dependent neighborhood, it cannot provide wider scale accessibility for residents who do not or cannot drive. Many health professionals, architects, and urban planners today favor compact, human-scaled communities providing easy access to a wide range of functions, services, and activities (Gunn et al., 2017; Hyde et al., 2019). Accessible neighborhoods might motivate residents to be more physically active and thus provide valuable health benefits (Christian et al., 2017). In addition, the higher densities and a more active street life might motivate residents to feel responsible for their neighborhood and be more willing to look out for each other (Gardner, 2011; Mehta & Bosson, 2010). Occupational therapists play a pivotal role in regard to housing needs because they have an intimate knowledge of clients' home requirements, restrictions, and possibilities. They can serve as an important go-between for helping clients articulate their environmental situation and needs to architects, interior designers, and contractors. Knowing clients' limitations firsthand, the occupational therapist can play a central role in "design teams" that plan aging in place or impairment-accommodating housing (Burns et al., 2017; Pickens & Burns, 2018) and community centers or environments (Figure 17.6).

At-Homeness and Occupational Therapy

Besides being a physical dwelling, home is also a constellation of experiences, meanings, and situations that relate to personal and communal senses of identity and belonging (Rowles, 2006; Rowles & Chaudhury, 2005; Stafford,

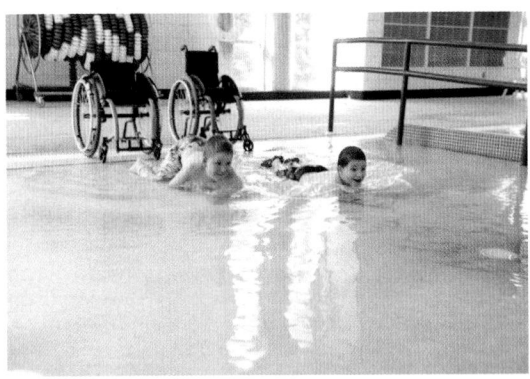

FIGURE 17.6 This recreation center, designed with an *objective outside* perspective, provides a space where all people can participate without segregation. An *empathic inside* understanding emerges among those who witness Simon and Manuel in an environment in which they are equally equipped to participate without restrictions or barriers. (Source: Reprinted with permission from http://committoinclusion.org/universal-design/)

2009). One phenomenological concept that helps integrate the lived dimensions of home is *at-homeness*, which is similar to the concept of existential insideness. At-homeness can be defined as the taken-for-granted situation of feeling completely comfortable and intimately familiar with the world in which one lives everyday life (Oldenburg, 1999; Seamon, 1979). For the clients of occupational therapists, at-homeness has often been disrupted or eroded. Understanding the lived dimensions of at-homeness helps occupational therapists to consider their clients' residential needs more precisely and think through routines that might be restored or better accommodated.

Table 17.2 describes aspects of at-homeness in terms of five lived qualities that can support or undermine a sense of familiarity and comfort (Seamon, 1979, 2010). First, *rootedness* refers to the idea that the home roots the person spatially, providing a place from which to come and go. When a client is impaired by illness, injury, or aging, rootedness may be displaced by *disconnectedness*, which can include spatial disorientation, bodily discomfort, or loss of mobility and accessibility. Second, *appropriation* refers to a resident feeling a sense of autonomy and control in regard to their home and immediate surroundings. But if a resident becomes disabled, appropriation devolves into *imposition*, a situation where the resident is less autonomous and more dependent or interdependent on external assistance.

A third quality of at-homeness is *at-easeness*, which refers to the "freedom to be." In a situation of at-homeness, residents can be who they most comfortably are and do what they most wish to do. At-easeness can shift into *uneasiness* when a lifeworld is upset in some way. Unlike appropriation,

TABLE 17.2	Aspects of At-Homeness: Sustaining and Undermining Dimensions			
Sustaining Aspect	Description	Spatial Expression	Undermining Aspect	Implications for Occupational Therapy
Rootedness	Organizes the habitual, bodily stratum of a person's life; intimately related to environmental embodiment and body-subject	Concentrated in places, paths, and points of use, especially favorite places within and around the home; undeveloped in unused portions	Disconnectedness: involves spatial disorientation, bodily discomfort, or loss of mobility and accessibility	Ensure meaningful daily occupations can be maintained through retraining and environmental supports. Focus on the client's bodily "doing" and "being" in and around the home, especially bodily routines and actions
Appropriation	Involves feeling a sense of autonomy and control in regard to home and immediate surroundings; typically includes a sense of privacy	Roughly concentric and generally strongest for most important "centers" in the home; intensity in proportion to use and attachment; relates to "centers," paths, places for things, and things themselves	Imposition: includes loss of autonomy; dependence on external assistance, whether human, environmental, or technological	Provide adequate human help and assistive technologies to support personal autonomy and self-worth (e.g., installing appropriate bathing equipment so client can maintain independence)
At-easeness	Involves "freedom to be" and contentment; relates to inner mood and sense of well-being; things and situations that give everyday satisfaction are readily available	Usually strongest in the home but possible in other places outside the home (i.e., third places) where person feels comfortable and relaxed	Uneaseness: involves a situation where comfortableness of lifeworld called into question by personal, social, or environmental changes	Enable satisfying occupations that can be engaged in alone or with others (e.g., working to maintain client's valued hobbies)
Regeneration	Relates to restorative powers of home and at-homeness; home not only as a site of relaxation and rest but also as a place of psychological recuperation and rejuvenation	Generally associated with the home but possible in other places with restorative powers (e.g., the route a person walks his or her dogs each day)	Degeneration: relates to disruption in rest and regeneration because of personal, social, or environmental changes.	Enable relaxing occupations through environmental modifications (e.g., incorporating more appropriate lighting or changing room use). Consider how such modifications may shift daily activities (e.g., if a living area is converted to a bedroom, where will the client go to relax and engage in leisure?)
Warmth	Relates to supportive ambience of sustenance and well-being; invokes positive emotions like kindness, cheerfulness, goodwill, and camaraderie	Most common in interior spaces and expressed by decoration, sense of order, and interpersonal harmony; also present in cared-for outside environments like gardens	Coldness: relates to an unpleasant or hostile environmental ambience; spirit of place devolves into raw material space	Work with client's values and find compromises (e.g., managing a level of cleanliness that is acceptable or decluttering a space but preserving what is most meaningful for client).

Adapted from Seamon, D. (1979). *A geography of the life world.* St. Martin's Press.

which relates more to physical and psychological control of the home, at-easeness relates to inner mood and sense of well-being. To be at ease is to have readily available the things and situations that give one everyday satisfaction and sustain the lifeworld's transparency and taken-for-grantedness. Fourth, *regeneration* refers to the restorative powers of home and at-homeness. Regeneration involves the home not only as a site of relaxation and rest but also as a place of psychological recuperation and rejuvenation. In a disrupted lifeworld, regeneration becomes *degeneration* because of stress, worry, or physical difficulties associated with sleeping and resting. Finally, *warmth* speaks to an intangible atmosphere of sustenance and well-being that often involves positive emotions like joy and happiness. Sometimes, the warmth of home life perseveres in times of illness or impairment, or it can disappear or devolve into *coldness*. When warmth is not sustained, a sense of place becomes spiritless space.

These five qualities of at-homeness are both personally experienced and broadly diagnostic in that they provide one way to think through a particular client's home situation in terms of daily occupations (Moore et al., 2010, pp. 4–5). Different clients' everyday worlds will involve different combinations and intensities of the five qualities of at-homeness. Their potential value is that each points toward a different set of possibilities and means for transforming negative aspects in a home toward more positive possibilities. For example, rootedness is grounded in the lived body, and one occupational aim is to find ways, through environmental intervention, assistive technology, and the client's rehabilitation efforts, to return their lifeworld to its former taken-for-grantedness in terms of bodily actions and routines. Or, in regard to at-easeness, the occupational therapist works to learn a client's daily pleasures and satisfactions and find ways whereby they might be reincorporated in their everyday life, although sometimes in revised or partial ways. The central aim in using at-homeness as a diagnostic focus is to envision the client's abled and impaired lifeworlds from a multidimensional perspective that might spur creative interventions not imagined otherwise (refer to OT Story 17.1).

There are other ways to create a sense of at-homeness for clients who are displaced temporarily (i.e., inpatients in hospital or rehabilitation centers) or for those who have experienced a permanent move yet have lost a feeling of being at home (i.e., those in assisted living facilities, refugees, and individuals and families experiencing houselessness). For people in these circumstances, simple tasks of daily living can feel foreign until they *adopt* a new location by *adapting* to change. Fischer and Hotchkiss (2008) proposed a Model of Occupational Empowerment that has been applied to mothers in recovery from addiction (Cardinale et al., 2014) and to men living in shelters (Hoffman, 2010). They identified that disempowering environments can lead to occupational deprivation, which reinforces learned helplessness. Further, they assert that OT programs can empower individuals through occupation to promote positive change (Fischer & Hotchkiss, 2008, p. 60).

Empowering occupations have positive outcomes. For example, a despondent new resident of a nursing home was not dressing or engaging in daily hygiene, nor leaving her room for any reason. After a conversation revealed that she did not at all feel at home and was not even aware of what personal possessions had been moved to this new place, the therapist and resident set about to explore her new space. Over the course of several sessions, they emptied her closet, assessed the contents, and rearranged it to suit her taste and ability to access what she wanted and needed. They did the same to the dresser, nightstand, and bathroom cabinets. Now familiar with this place through *behavioral insideness*, she could readily engage in familiar routines for self-care and as a result began to venture out to the dining area, chapel, and dayroom for activities. Although not yet an insider, she was beginning to feel more at home.

Impact of Temporary Places on Health and Well-Being

Individuals, families, groups, and populations are vulnerable to being displaced because of many factors, including homelessness (Alarcón & Khan, 2021; Bowpitt, 2020; Gunther, 2020), natural disasters (Gagné, 2020; Jinnouchi et al., 2020; Kawakami et al., 2020; Takahashi et al., 2020; Tsuchiya et al., 2019), seeking refuge from war and other forms of violence that threaten personal well-being (Turkoglu, 2022), and gentrification or urban renewal (Zeng et al., 2019). When people are displaced and given temporary housing, they can experience feelings of long-term disconnection, imposition, unease, degeneration, and coldness (lacking a warm sense of welcome and at-homeness). Poor health outcomes related to lack of a permanent place that provides a feeling of at-homeness include increased incidence of communicable diseases (Alarcón & Khan, 2021), decline in mental health (Gunther, 2020; Kawakami et al., 2020), musculoskeletal pain (Jinnouchi et al., 2020), exacerbation of chronic disease (Takahashi et al., 2020), and toothache (Tsuchiya et al., 2019). In fact, "symptoms such as feeling physically weaker or general pain, sleep disorders, and depression are commonly called 'temporary housing syndrome'" (Gagné, 2020, p. 712). See OT Story 17.2 for an example.

OT STORY 17.2 LESSONS FROM A TRIPLE DISASTER

On March 11, 2011, an earthquake shook Japan, which created a tsunami, which caused a nuclear meltdown that further decimated the island nation. This triple disaster created a rapid shift from being settled to homelessness, which was alleviated by temporary housing that extended beyond what was expected. Gagné (2020) interviewed people still in temporary housing from 2014 to 2018 to listen and tell the story of their ongoing recovery. The Pan Occupation Paradigm (POP; based on the seminal work of Wilcock, 1998) has been proposed as a bridge between occupational science and OT (Hitch, 2017; Hitch & Pepin, 2021). The POP can shed light on how displaced persons may be affected by their

(continued)

OT STORY 17.2 LESSONS FROM A TRIPLE DISASTER (*continued*)

environment, using the situation in Japan as an illustration. Used here, POP helps to bridge the research describing community recovery from a triple disaster to our understanding of the importance of place to the power of occupation.

- *Doing.* Although not an occupational therapist, Gagné (2020) saw that "after losing their job, their home, and loved ones simultaneously, many survivors felt alienated and isolated by not having anything to do with themselves day in and day out" (p. 171). Not having meaningful occupation—something to do—contributed to declining health and "temporary housing syndrome" among the survivors.
- *Being.* Waiting for a place to be, without meaningful occupation or access to jobs, schools, and community, the temporary residents exchanged their former identities for the solidarity of being victims of the triple disaster—something they all had in common. But this identity was also temporary because their individual differences related to opportunity and access began to emerge and dissolved the illusion of sameness (Gagné, 2020).
- *Belonging.* Many residents had been separated from their intergenerational family units and long-term neighbors when placed in temporary housing. "The disaster swept away not only their homes and neighborhoods, but the social nexus of community relations that had existed for a

long time in these areas" (Gagné, 2020, pp. 713–714). A sense of belonging was lost. Eventually, some residents of the temporary housing developments began to form relationships with their new temporary neighbors—but this caused further trauma when some were able to relocate, leaving the others behind and alone.
- *Becoming.* Gagné (2020) discovered that the residents' lives had been essentially put on hold when they were relocated to an area zoned for a temporary existence. The survivors' life experiences were disconnected because of the disruption in the flow of time before and after the disaster. Because the survivors experienced occupational disruption that lasted for years, it essentially put their lives on hold, halting the process of becoming or having a future orientation.

Questions

1. How would you go about determining what meaningful occupations could promote well-being for displaced persons?
2. How is your identity tied to being in place and in community with others?
3. If immediately and permanently displaced from your current housing, what steps could you take to facilitate belonging and becoming?

Physical Places, Virtual Places, and Occupational Therapy

There is considerable indication that virtual technologies are dramatically reshaping human life in the 21st century (Friesen, 2011; Relph, 2007). Currently, we can envision only glimpses of what robotics, virtual realities, and information and communication technologies (ICTs) might mean for occupations and OT (Fok et al., 2009; Rakoski, 2013). The desire of older people and people with disabilities to live independently has spurred the development of the smart house, which incorporates robotics, networked appliances, and other digital devices connecting residents with their home and the wider community (Sanchez et al., 2017). This integration of home services with technology is called domotics, which works to "improve safety, security, comfort, communication, and technical management in the home" (Rosenfeld & Chapman, 2008, p. 25). One example is digital lighting that automatically provides residents moving through their home with an illuminated pathway, helping

to reduce falls. Also significant are domestic robotic devices that include telerehabilitation, robotic pet therapy, and robotic assistants, the last of which can provide, among other home services, therapy and mental stimulation (Bedaf et al., 2015; Broekens et al., 2009; Cherry et al., 2017; Sicurella & Fitzsimmons, 2016). In addition, these robotic devices can monitor health and behaviors and connect residents to healthcare providers and to friends and relatives living elsewhere (Bedaf et al., 2015).

More transformative technological possibilities for occupational activities involve innovations in the brain–computer interface (BCI), which allows objects and images to be manipulated via sensory devices registering brain waves or facial movements (Graham-Rowe, 2011). By shifting the eyes or picturing an action or symbol cognitively, the user can direct a robotic assistant, activate networked appliances, or manipulate items on a computer screen (Corralejo et al., 2014; Miralles et al., 2015). For many older people and people with disabilities, this technology could well be life changing because they gain the mental and physical autonomy to control computers, wheelchairs, assistive technologies, and other aspects of their everyday environment. Perhaps even more compelling is the coupling of BCI with virtual reality technology, which allows users to generate and participate in online virtual worlds like "Second Life," where users (called "residents") meet other residents, socialize, create virtual homes and other virtual places, offer virtual goods and services, and so forth (Graham-Rowe, 2011).

Virtually connected homes are infusing place with technologies that link home dwellers to outside communities and supports for cognitive assistance, safety, and simple information. The concept of *at-homeness* will evolve as families and individuals weigh the functional and ethical balance of privacy and monitoring (Sanchez et al., 2017). The term *aging in place* suggests a continuous habitation of one's home in older years regardless of health impairment. Virtual monitoring of older adults comes at a cost of privacy and loss of connectedness to important others; that external monitoring would lessen the need for physically present social visits. Virtual monitoring reduces a sense of place by bringing "outsiders" into the home; the boundary created for the privacy of inhabitants is lost. To bring care closer is to bring the stranger in (Lopez & Sanchez-Criado, 2009).

Virtual worlds and virtual places may provide a radically innovative means for occupational therapists to assist clients in recovering and recreating what was called, at the start of this chapter, "being at home." In this sense, occupational therapists may help create virtual places that allow clients to become involved in virtual occupations that are unlikely or impossible in their physically present worlds. Clearly, virtual realities will create a new world of occupations in a dynamic context.

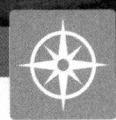

EXPANDING OUR PERSPECTIVES

Accessibility in Different Environments

Aster Harrison, PhD, OTD, OTR/L (pronouns: they/them)

"Access needs" refer to the supports and accommodations each of us needs to fully participate in a given space or event. Everyone has access needs, including nondisabled people. Some access needs can include comfortable seating, air-conditioning, wheelchair ramps, closed captioning, content warnings, language interpretation, or inclusive language—but the list is endless! Access needs can become more obvious in some environments than others. I often find that I don't fully realize all of my access needs until I change environments.

Recently, I experienced the important effects of environmental changes in my working life. During the first year of the COVID-19 pandemic, I worked from home. I purchased a small stand for my laptop to bring it to eye level and prevent neck pain. I also got an external keyboard and mouse. Otherwise, my workspace setup was not particularly adapted to my body. I sat in a regular kitchen chair at a small table. When I got a new job and started working in an office, I was shocked to find that I was able to sit and focus for hours longer than I previously could and that I was in much less pain at the end of the day. My new office had a comfortable, adjustable desk chair and an adjustable-height desk that could transform into a standing desk. It also had a large monitor that allowed me to split my screen or enlarge font to reduce visual strain. The difference was stark! I had come to think that my pain levels during my working days were unchangeable and just resulted from my chronic pain condition. My new work environment made me realize all of the access needs that my previous home office was not meeting.

Accessibility is not only about disability. People also have access needs associated with other marginalized identities. During the first year of the pandemic, I decided to publicly change my gender pronouns to they/them. I had been using different pronouns for a while with queer friends, but I hadn't felt ready to explain them at work. Working remotely made the shift feel a lot easier. I didn't feel like I needed to inform or correct coworkers face-to-face, but rather I could change how I referred to myself in my email signature, mention it in a quick message, and/or show new pronouns after my name on Zoom. Working from home also meant that I rarely heard anyone use the incorrect pronouns for me or interacted with people who were not transgender affirming. I was not very bothered by people using the wrong pronouns for me during that time, perhaps because it didn't happen very often.

When I started working in an office again, I was confronted with the daily experience of people using the wrong gender pronouns for me. Despite always introducing myself with my pronouns and educating coworkers, my coworkers really struggled to get it right. I was up close and personal with their difficulties honoring my gender expression, and I realized how tiring it is to be referred to incorrectly. Some days I found myself wanting to work from home just to avoid hearing people refer to me with the wrong pronouns. Using the correct gender pronouns for transgender and nonbinary people is an accessibility issue. When I am in a space where my gender expression is not respected, I feel less able to participate and more stressed.

As OT practitioners, we can play a role in helping people understand and meet their access needs. This can mean introducing people to adaptive equipment, making environmental modifications, or advocating for changes to workplace culture.

Conclusion

The physical environments that we inhabit have personal meanings and contribute to feelings of insideness and at-homeness. The experience of place is unique to every individual. However, when people encounter illness, disability, displacement, or other life disruptions, connections to place can be disturbed. Once familiar environments may no longer be supportive, or individuals may find themselves negotiating unknown spaces. Occupational therapists that are knowledgeable about the physical and virtual environment can use environmental interventions and assistive technology to ensure that places are sources of meaning, community, and well-being.

Acknowledgments

The authors would like to acknowledge David Seamon for his contribution to earlier editions of this chapter.

Lippincott® Connect *For additional resources on the subjects discussed in this chapter, visit Lippincott Connect.*

REFERENCES

Ahlzen, R. (2011). Illness as unhomelike being-in-the-world? Phenomenology and medical practice. *Medicine, Health Care and Philosophy, 14,* 323–331. https://doi.org/10.1007/s11019-011-9311-6

Alarcón, J., & Khan, T. V. (2021). Adapting backpack medicine in COVID-19 response for people experiencing homelessness in Southern California. *American Journal of Public Health, 111*(1), 58–61. https://doi.org/10.2105/AJPH.2020.305956

Bedaf, S., Gelderblom, G. J., & De Witte, L. (2015). Overview and categorization of robots supporting independent living of elderly people: What activities do they support and how far have they developed. *Assistive Technology, 27*(2), 88–100. https://doi.org/10.1080/10400435.2014.978916

Bowpitt, G. (2020). Choosing to be homeless? Persistent rough sleeping and the perverse incentives of social policy in England. *Housing, Care & Support, 23*(3/4), 135–147. https://doi.org/10.1108/HCS-07-2020-0010

Broekens, J., Heerink, M., & Rosendal., H. (2009). Assistive social robots in elderly care: A review. *Gerontechnology, 8*(2), 94–103. https://doi.org/10.4017/gt.2009.08.02.002.00

Brooks, J. O., Smolentzov, L., DeArment, A., Logan, W., Green, K., Walker, I., Honchar, J., Guirl, C., Beeco, R., Blakeney, C., Boggs, A., Carroll, C., Duckworth, K., Goller, L., Ham, S., Healy, S., Heaps, C., Hayden, C., Manganelli, J., … Yanik, P. (2011). Toward a "smart" nightstand prototype: An examination of nightstand table contents and preferences. *Health Environments Research & Design Journal, 4*(2), 91–108. https://doi.org/10.1177/193758671100400208

Burns, S. P., Pickens, N. D., & Smith, R. O. (2017). Interprofessional client-centered reasoning processes in home modification practice. *Journal of Housing for the Elderly, 31*(3), 213–228. https://doi.org/10.1080/02763893.2017.1280579

Cardinale, J., Malacari, L., Broggi, S., Savignano, J., & Fisher, G. (2014). Model of occupational empowerment and Gunnarsson's tree theme: Intervention for mothers in recovery. *Occupational Therapy in Mental Health, 30*(1), 43–68. https://doi.org/10.1080/0164212X.2014.878237

Cherry, C. O., Chumbler, N. R., Richards, K., Huff, A., Wu, D., Tilghman, L. M., & Butler, A. (2017). Expanding stroke telerehabilitation service to rural veterans: A qualitative study on patient experiences using the robotic stroke therapy delivery and monitoring system program. *Disability and Rehabilitation: Assistive Technology, 12*(1), 21–27. https://doi.org/10.3109/17483107.2015.1061613

Christian, H., Knuiman, M., Divitini, M., Foster, S., Hooper, P., Boruff, B., Bull, F., & Giles-Corti, B. (2017). A longitudinal analysis of the influence of the neighborhood environment on recreational walking within the neighborhood: Results from RESIDE. *Environmental Health Perspectives, 125*(7), 1–10. https://doi.org/10.1289/EHP823

Corralejo, R., Nicolas-Alonso, L. F., Alvarez, D., & Hornero, R. (2014). A P300-based brain computer interface aimed at operating electronic devices at home for severely disabled people. *Medical & Biological Engineering & Computing, 52,* 861–872. https://doi.org/10.1007/s11517-014-1191-5

Curry, H. R. (2015). *A semiotic phenomenology of homelessness and the precarious community: A matter of boundary* [Doctoral dissertation]. University of South Florida. http://scholarcommons.usf.edu/etd/5672

Eriksson, M., & Dahlblom, K. (2020). Children's perspectives on health-promoting living environments: The significance of social capital. *Social Science & Medicine, 258,* 113059. https://doi.org/10.1016/j.socscimed.2020.113059

Fawole, O. I., Okedare, O. O., & Reed, E. (2021). Home was not a safe haven: Women's experiences of intimate partner violence during the COVID-19 lockdown in Nigeria. *BMC Women's Health, 21*(1), 1–7. https://doi.org/10.1186/s12905-021-01177-9

Finlay, L. (2011). *Phenomenology for therapists: Researching the lived world.* Wiley-Blackwell.

Fischer, G. S., & Hotchkiss, A. (2008). A model of occupational empowerment for marginalized populations in community environments. *Occupational Therapy in Health Care, 22*(1), 55–71. https://doi.org/10.1300/J003v22n01_05

Fok, D., Miller Polgar, J., Shaw, L., Luke, R., & Mandich, A. (2009). Cyberspace, real place: Thoughts on doing in contemporary occupations. *Journal of Occupational Science, 16*(1), 38–43. https://doi.org/10.1080/14427591.2009.9686640

Friesen, N. (2011). *The place of the classroom and the space of the screen: Relational pedagogy and Internet technology.* Peter Lang.

Gagné, I. (2020). Dislocation, social isolation, and the politics of recovery in post-disaster Japan. *Transcultural Psychiatry, 57*(5), 710–723. https://doi.org/10.1177/1363461520920348

Gardner, P. J. (2011). Natural neighborhood networks—Important social networks in the lives of older adults aging in place. *Journal of Aging Studies, 25*(3), 263–271. https://doi.org/10.1016/j.jaging.2011.03.007

Graham-Rowe, D. (2011, July 2). *Control your home with thought alone: The latest brain-computer interfaces meet smart home technology and virtual gaming.* NewScientist, 2819. http://www.newscientist.com/issue/2819/

Gunn, L. D., Mavoa, S., Boulangé, C., Hooper, P., Kavanagh, A., & Giles-Corti, B. (2017). Designing healthy communities: Creating evidence on metrics for built environment features associated with walkable neighbourhood activity centres. *International Journal of Behavioral Nutrition & Physical Activity, 14*(1), 164. https://doi.org/10.1186/s12966-017-0621-9

Gunther, M. (2020). A place to call home: A bay area activist has persuaded tech giants like Cisco and government leaders to join forces to end homelessness by building homes rather than shelters. Now Covid might upend some of their gains. *Chronicle of Philanthropy, 32*(10), 16–20. https://www.philanthropy.com/article/bay-area-activist-enlists-tech-giants-to-help-end-homelessness

Gutman, S. A., Amarantos, K., Berg, J., Aponte, M., Gordillo, D., Rice, C., Smith, J., Perry, A., Wills, T., Chen, E., Peters, R., & Schluger, Z. (2018). Home safety fall and accident risk among prematurely aging, formerly homeless adults. *American Journal of Occupational Therapy, 72*(4), 1–9. https://doi.org/10.5014/ajot.2018.028050

Hasselkus, B. R., & Dickie, V. A. (2021). *The meaning of everyday occupation* (3rd ed.). Slack.

Healy-Ogden, M. J. (2014). Being "at home" in the context of home care. *Home Health Care Management Practice, 26*(2), 72–79. https://doi.org/10.1177/1084822313508646

Hitch, D. (2017.) Keeping occupation front and centre to address the challenges of transcending the individual. *Journal of Occupational Science, 24*(4), 494–509, https://doi.org/10.1080/14427591.2017.1374876

Hitch, D., & Pepin, G. (2021). Doing, being, becoming and belonging at the heart of occupational therapy: An analysis of theoretical ways of knowing. *Scandinavian Journal of Occupational Therapy, 28*(1), 13–25. https://doi.org/10.1080/11038128.2020.1726454

Hoffman, J. (2010). The model of occupational empowerment: Creating occupational change among men living in shelters. *Home & Community Health Special Interest Section Quarterly, 17*(4), 1–2.

Hyde, E. T., Omura, J. D., Watson, K. B., Fulton, J. E., & Carlson, S. A. (2019). Step it up! Prioritization of community supports for walking among US adults. *American Journal of Health Promotion, 33*(8), 1134–1143. https://doi.org/10.1177/0890117119856550

Jinnouchi, H., Ohira, T., Kakihana, H., Matsudaira, K., Maeda, M., Yabe, H., Suzuki, Y., Harigane, M., Iso, H., Kawada, T., Yasumura, S., Kamiya, K., & Mental Health Group of the Fukushima Health Management Survey. (2020). Lifestyle factors associated with prevalent and exacerbated musculoskeletal pain after the Great East Japan Earthquake: A cross-sectional study from the Fukushima Health Management Survey. *BMC Public Health, 20*(1), 1–10. https://doi.org/10.1186/s12889-020-08764-9

Kawakami, N., Fukasawa, M., Sakata, K., Suzuki, R., Tomita, H., Nemoto, H., Yasumura, S., Yabe, H., Horikoshi, N., Umeda, M., Suzuki, Y., Shimoda, H., Tachimori, H., Takeshima, T., & Bromet, E. J. (2020). Onset and remission of common mental disorders among adults living in temporary housing for three years after the triple disaster in Northeast Japan: Comparisons with the general population. *BMC Public Health, 20*(1), Article 1271. https://doi.org/10.1186/s12889-020-09378-x

Kopec, D. (2006). *Environmental psychology for design.* Fairchild.

Kylén, M., Löfqvist, C., Haak, M., & Iwarsson, S. (2019). Meaning of home and health dynamics among younger older people in Sweden. *European Journal of Ageing, 16*(3), 305–315. https://doi.org/10.1007/s10433-019-00501-5

Lopez, D., & Sanchez-Criado, T. (2009). Dwelling the telecare home: Place, location, and habitability. *Space and Culture, 12*(3), 343–358. https://doi.org/10.1177/1206331209337079

Lu, Z. (2010). Investigating walking environments in and around assisted living facilities: A facility visit study. *Health Environments Research & Design Journal, 3*(4), 58–74. https://doi.org/10.1177/193758671000300406

Marshall, C. A., Lysaght, R., & Krupa, T. (2018). Occupational transition in the process of becoming housed following chronic homelessness. *Canadian Journal of Occupational Therapy, 85*(1), 33–45. https://doi.org/10.1177/0008417417723351

Mayock, P., Parker, S., & Murphy, A. (2021). Family "turning point" experiences and the process of youth becoming homeless. *Child & Family Social Work, 26*(3), 415–424. https://doi.org/10.1111/cfs.12823

Mehta, V., & Bosson, J. K. (2010). Third places and the social life of streets. *Environment and Behavior, 42*(6), 779–805. https://doi.org/10.1177/0013916509344677

Mendonca, R., Pickens, N., & Smith, R. O. (2017). Environmental modifications: Ethics of assessment and intervention. In J. B. Scott & S. M. Reitz (Eds.), *Practical applications for the occupational therapy code of ethics (2015)* (pp. 283-294). AOTA Press.

Miralles, F., Vargiu, E., Dauwalder, S., Solà, M., Müller-Putz, G., Wriessnegger, S. C., Pinegger, A., Kübler, A., Halder, S., Käthner, I., Martin, S., Daly, J., Armstrong, E., Guger, C., Hintermüller, C., & Lowish, H. (2015). Brain computer interface on track to home. *The Scientific World Journal, 2015,* 623896. https://doi.org/10.1155/2015/623896

Moore, A. J., Anderson, C., Carter, B., & Coad, J. (2010). Appropriated landscapes: The intrusion of technology and equipment into the homes and lives of families with a child of complex needs. *Journal of Child Health Care, 14*(1), 3–5. https://doi.org/10.1177/1367493509360275

Mossabir, R., Milligan, C., & Froggatt, K. (2021). Therapeutic landscape experiences of everyday geographies within the wider community: A scoping review. *Social Science & Medicine, 279,* 113980. https://doi.org/10.1016/j.socscimed.2021.113980

Ohlén, J., Ekman, I., Zingmark, K., Bolmsjö, I., & Benzein, E. (2014). Conceptual development of "at-homeness" despite illness and disease: A review. *International Journal of Qualitative Studies on Health and Well-Being, 9*(1), 23677. https://doi.org/10.3402/qhw.v9.23677

Oldenburg, R. (1999). *The great good place: Cafés, coffee shops, bookstores, bars, hair salons, and other hangouts at the heart of a community* (3rd ed.). Marlowe & Company.

Pickens, N., & Burns, S. (2018). Home modifications. In B. A. Boyt Schell & J. Schell (Eds.), *Clinical and professional reasoning in occupational therapy* (2nd ed.). Lippincott Williams & Wilkins.

Pickens, N. D., Khimji, Z., & Lindgren, M. (2019). Effect of home modifications on the occupational participation of a family. *Annals of International Occupational Therapy, 3*(2). https://doi.org/10.3928/24761222-20191018-03

Preiser, W. F. E., & Smith, K. H. (Eds.). (2011). *Universal design handbook* (2nd ed.). McGraw-Hill.

Rakoski, D. R. (2013). The virtual context of occupation: Integrating everyday technology into everyday practice. *OT Practice, 18*(9), CE1–CE8. https://www.aota.org/publications/ot-practice/ot-practice-issues

Relph, E. (2007). Spirit of place and sense of place in virtual realities. *Techné: Research in Philosophy and Technology, 10*(3), 1–8. https://doi.org/10.5840/techne20071039

Relph, E. (2008). *Place and placelessness.* Pion. (Original work published 1976.)

Rosenfeld, J. P., & Chapman, W. (2008). *Home design in an aging world.* Fairchild.

Rowles, G. D. (2006). Commentary: A house is not a home: But can it become one? In H. W. Wahl, H. Brenner, H. Mollenkopf, D. Rothenbacher, & C. Rott (Eds.), *The many faces of health, competence and well-being in old age: Integrating epidemiological, psychological and social perspectives* (pp. 25–32). Springer.

Rowles, G. D., & Bernard, M., (2013). The meaning of and significance of place in old age. In G. D. Rorwles & M. Bernard (Eds.), *Environmental gerontology making meaningful places in old age* (pp. 129–152). Springer.

Rowles, G. D., & Chaudhury, H. (Eds.). (2005). *Home and identity in late life.* Springer.

Saarnio, L., Boström, A. M., Hedman, R., Gustavsson, P., & Öhlén, J. (2019). Enabling at-homeness for older people with life-limiting conditions: A participant observation study from nursing homes. *Global Qualitative Nursing Research, 6,* 2333393619881636. https://doi.org/10.1177/2333393619881636

Sanchez, V. G., Taylor, I., & Bing-Jonsson, P. C. (2017). Ethics of smart house welfare technology for older adults: A systematic literature review. *International Journal of Technology Assessment in Health Care, 33*(6), 691–699. https://doi.org/10.1017/S0266462317000964

Seamon, D. (1979). *A geography of the lifeworld.* St. Martin's Press.

Seamon, D. (2010). Gaston Bachelard's topoanalysis in the 21st century: The lived reciprocity between houses and inhabitants as portrayed by American writer Louis Bromfield. In L. Embree (Ed.), *Phenomenology 2010: Vol. 5. Selected essays from North America, Part I* (pp. 225–243). Zeta Books.

Seamon, D. (2018). *Life takes place: Phenomenology, lifeworlds, and place making.* Routledge.

Sicurella, T., & Fitzsimmons, V. (2016). Robotic pet therapy in long-term care. *Nursing, 46*(6), 55–57. https://doi.org/10.1097/01.NURSE.0000482265.32133.f6

Söderback, I. (2009). Adaptive interventions: Overview. In I. Söderback (Ed.), *International handbook of occupational therapy interventions* (pp. 39–51). Springer.

Stafford, P. B. (2009). *Elderburbia: Aging with a sense of place in America.* Praeger.

Stark, S., Keglovitis, M., Arbesman, M., & Lieberman, D. (2017). Effect of home modification interventions on the participation of community-dwelling adults with health conditions: A systematic review. *American Journal of Occupational Therapy, 71*(2), 7102290010p1–7102290010p11. https://doi.org/10.5014/ajot.2017.018887

Stefanovic, I. (2008). Holistic paradigms of health and place: How beneficial are they to environmental policy and practice? In J. Eyles & A. Williams (Eds.), *Sense of place, health and quality of life* (pp. 45–57). Ashgate.

Stockman, J. K., Wood, B. A., & Anderson, K. M. (2021). Racial and ethnic differences in COVID-19 outcomes, stressors, fear, and prevention behaviors among US women: Web-based cross-sectional study. *Journal of Medical Internet Research, 23*(7), e26296. https://doi.org/10.2196/26296

Takahashi, S., Tanno, K., Yonekura, Y., Shimoda, H., Sasaki, R., Sakata, K., Ogawa, A., & Kobayashi, S. (2020). Effect of temporary housing on incidence of diabetes mellitus in survivors of a tsunami-stricken area in 2011 Japan disaster: A serial cross-sectional RIAS study. *Scientific Reports, 10*(1), Article 15400. https://doi.org/10.1038/s41598-020-71759-4

Tsuchiya, M., Aida, J., Watanabe, T., Shinoda, M., Sugawara, Y., Tomata, Y., Yabe, Y., Sekiguchi, T., Watanabe, M., Osaka, K., Sasaki, K., Hagiwara, Y., & Tsuji, I. (2019). High prevalence of toothache among Great East Japan earthquake survivors living in temporary housing. *Community Dentistry & Oral Epidemiology, 47*(2), 119–126. https://doi.org/10.1111/cdoe.12433

Turkoglu, O. (2022). Look who perpetrates violence and where: Explaining variation in forced migration. *Political Geography, 94*, 102558. https://doi.org/10.1016/j.polgeo.2021.102558

Turpin, M., Kerr, G., Gullo, H., Bennett, S., Asano, M., & Finlayson, M. (2018). Understanding and living with multiple sclerosis fatigue. *British Journal of Occupational Therapy, 81*(2), 82–89. https://doi.org/10.1177/0308022617728679

Ulrich, R. S., Zimring, C., Zhu, X., DuBose, J., Seo, H., Choi, Y., Quan, X., & Joseph, A. (2008). A review of the research literature on evidence-based healthcare design. *HERD: Health Environments Research & Design Journal, 1*, 61–125. https://doi.org/10.1177/193758670800100306

van Gelder, N. E., van Haalen, D. L., Ekker, K., Ligthart, S. A., & Oertelt-Prigione, S. (2021). Professionals' views on working in the field of domestic violence and abuse during the first wave of COVID-19: A qualitative study in the Netherlands. *BMC Health Services Research, 21*(1), 1–14. https://doi.org/10.1186/s12913-021-06674-z

Wiederhold, B. K. (2020). Embodiment empowers empathy in virtual reality. *CyberPsychology, Behavior & Social Networking, 23*(11), 725–726. https://doi.org/10.1089/cyber.2020.29199.editorial

Wilcock, A. A. (1998). Reflections on doing, being and becoming. *Canadian Journal of Occupational Therapy, 65*, 248–256. https://doi.org/10.1177/000841749806500501

Zeng, H., Yu, X., & Zhang, J. (2019). Urban village demolition, migrant workers' rental costs and housing choices: Evidence from Hangzhou, China. *Cities, 94*, 70–79. https://doi.org/10.1016/j.cities.2019.05.029

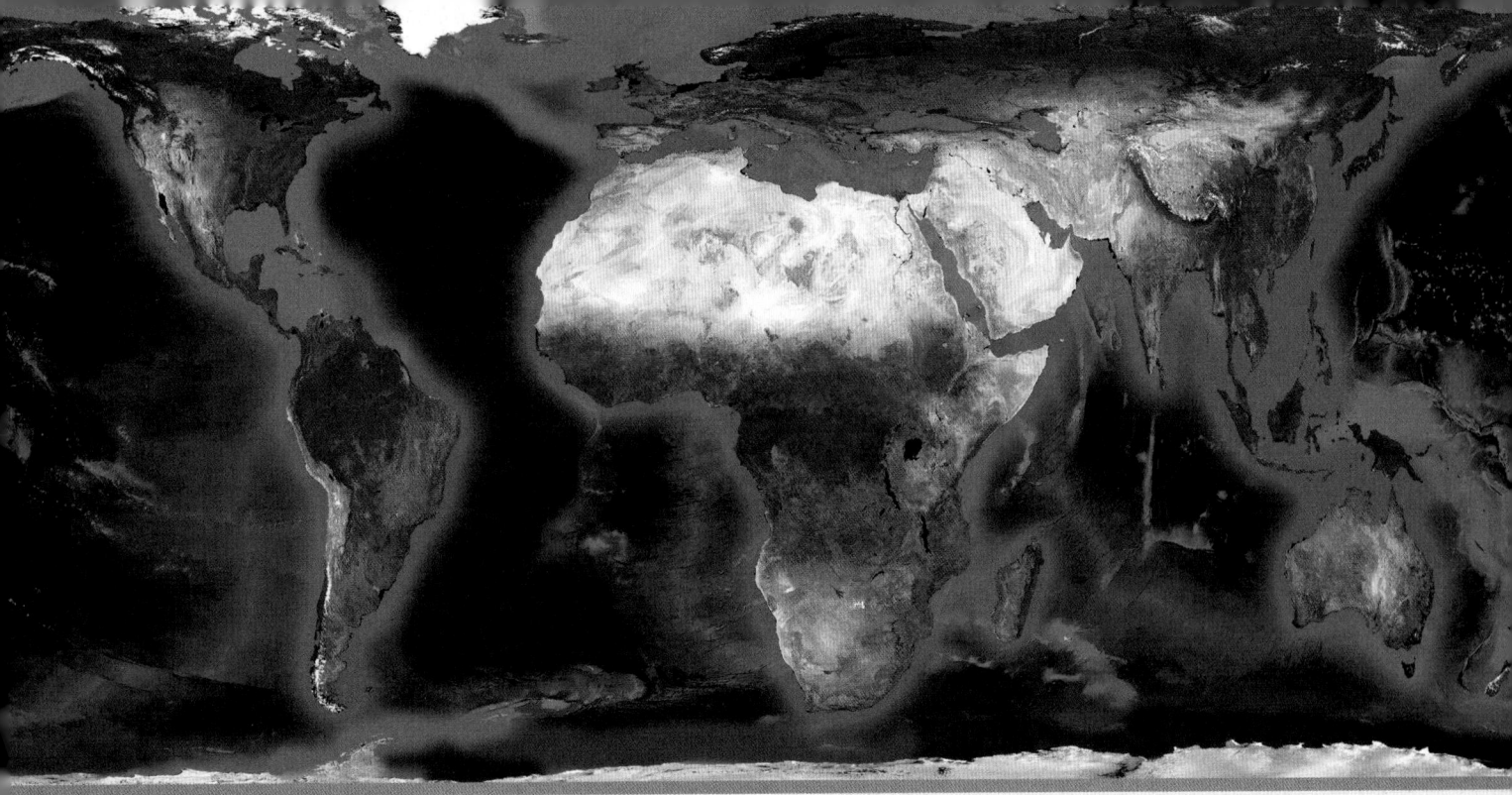

UNIT
IV
Occupational Therapy Process

Media Related to Occupational Therapy Process

Readings

- *Rules:* Twelve-year-old Catherine just wants a normal life, but she has a brother with autism and a family that revolves around his disability. But the summer Catherine meets Jason, a boy with paraplegia, and Kristi, the next-door friend she's always wished for, it's her own shocking behavior that turns everything upside down and forces her to ask: What is normal? (2006)
- *My Stroke of Insight: A Brain Scientist's Personal Journey:* Jill Bolte Taylor, a 37-year-old Harvard-trained brain scientist experienced a massive stroke in the left hemisphere of her brain. She observed her mind deteriorate to the point that she could not walk, talk, read, write, or recall any of her life—all within 4 hours. It would take her 8 years to fully recover. (2009)
- *The Autistic Brain: Helping Different Kinds of Minds Succeed:* Temple Grandin introduces the advances in neuroimaging and genetic research that link brain science to behavior, even sharing her own brain scan to show which anomalies might explain common symptoms. Dr Grandin argues that raising and educating kids on the autism spectrum should focus on their strengths to foster their unique contributions. (2014)
- *The Big Truck That Went By: How the World Came to Save Haiti and Left Behind a Disaster:* Jonathan M. Katz was the only full-time American news correspondent in Haiti on January 12, 2010, when the deadliest earthquake in the history of the Western Hemisphere struck the island nation. In this visceral firsthand account, Katz takes readers inside the terror of that day, the devastation visited on ordinary Haitians, and through the monumental—yet misbegotten—rescue effort that followed. (2014)

Art

- *Observing Everyday Life:* Food, friends and families, neighborhoods, work and leisure activities—these are the staples of everyday life. This chapter within the softcover book An Eye for Art: Focusing on Great Artists and Their Work features international artists who have taken notice of the people and objects that make up their world. (Observing Everyday Life [nga.gov])

Overview of the Occupational Therapy Process and Outcomes

Denise Chisholm and Barbara A. Boyt Schell

LEARNING OBJECTIVES

After reading this chapter, you will be able to:

1. Explain the components of the occupational therapy process.
2. Examine how evidence from research and practice is integrated into the occupational therapy process.
3. Analyze the professional reasoning typically associated with components of the occupational therapy process.
4. Apply the occupational therapy process to client cases.

Introduction

This chapter provides an overview of the occupational therapy (OT) process in preparation for understanding the more detailed information regarding assessing client needs as well as the provision of intervention services presented in the following chapters in this unit. First, we describe the general process of service delivery and its relationship with OT. In the second section of this chapter, an illustration or "road map" of the OT process is provided to assist you in visualizing the essential components and their dynamic and interactive relationships. Each component of the OT process—evaluation, intervention, reevaluation, and continuation/discontinuation of services based on client outcomes—will be expanded on in subsequent sections. Our hope is that the OT process road map will direct the services you provide as an OT practitioner. Evidence and professional reasoning have been embedded in the process road map as essential markers to assure accuracy in planning the most effective OT services. OT stories have been woven throughout this chapter to give you the opportunity to apply the OT process road map.

Occupational Therapy as a Process

Occupation is the central focus of OT services. The general process used in the delivery of OT services parallels the process used by other health-related professionals (e.g., nurses, physical therapists, physicians, and dietitians). It provides a structure for practitioners to employ therapeutic professional reasoning based on evidence to address the client's health-related problems.

The client is not only the person with the health-related problem but includes people important in the client's life, such as spouses, partners, family members, caregivers, employers, and teachers. The process is neither diagnosis-specific (i.e., disease, disorder, condition, and syndrome) nor age-specific, and it can be applied in any practice setting (i.e., hospital, outpatient clinic, school, workplace, community site, and client's home). OT practitioners customize the process with the end goal of "achieving health, well-being and participation in life through engagement in occupations" (American Occupational Therapy Association [AOTA], 2020a, p. 5). OT services incorporate the therapeutic use of occupation as a primary means for promoting the client's engagement in and performance of their preferred daily activities. The use of occupation as both an end goal and a means to achieve the goal is OT's unique application of the service delivery process. OT practitioners must deliver services that are occupation centered. In the words of Fisher (2009), if we are to practice as occupational therapists, we must use *occupation* as our primary form of therapy; that is, we must implement OT (p. 10).

The Occupational Therapy Process

Embarking on a trip without driving directions, a road map, or a public transportation guide and/or schedule—either virtual or paper—increases the risk of getting lost, which in turn results in confusion and frustration. This is analogous to what can occur when an OT practitioner provides therapy services without the guidance of a process "road map." Just as when taking a trip, OT practitioners need a clear diagram illustrating the road for traveling from the starting point—that is, evaluation—to the final destination or outcome of the therapy journey. We need to become competent in reading the markers that provide us with the evidence that supports taking the best route in both the evaluation and intervention portions of the trip. Our competency in "road map reading" is reliant on our professional reasoning, which is used to calculate and recalculate or problem-solve the best route options, assuring sound therapy decisions. With a thorough understanding of the process road map, you can effectively educate your clients about their OT services. When clients "know where they are going," they can actively and collaboratively participate in the process to support their health, well-being, and participation in life through engagement in occupation.

There are many different interpretations and illustrations of the OT process (AOTA, 2020a; Christiansen et al., 2014; Cole & Tufano, 2019; Fisher & Marterella, 2019; Law et al., 2016; Reed & Sanderson, 1999; Rogers & Holm, 1989, 2009; Taylor, 2017). Our OT process road map (Figure 18.1) is an adaptation of the process outlined in the "occupational therapy practice framework" (AOTA, 2020a).

Although the OT process is highly dynamic and cyclical, it does have a definitive starting point and important landmarks along the way. These are evaluation, intervention, reevaluation, and therapy outcomes.

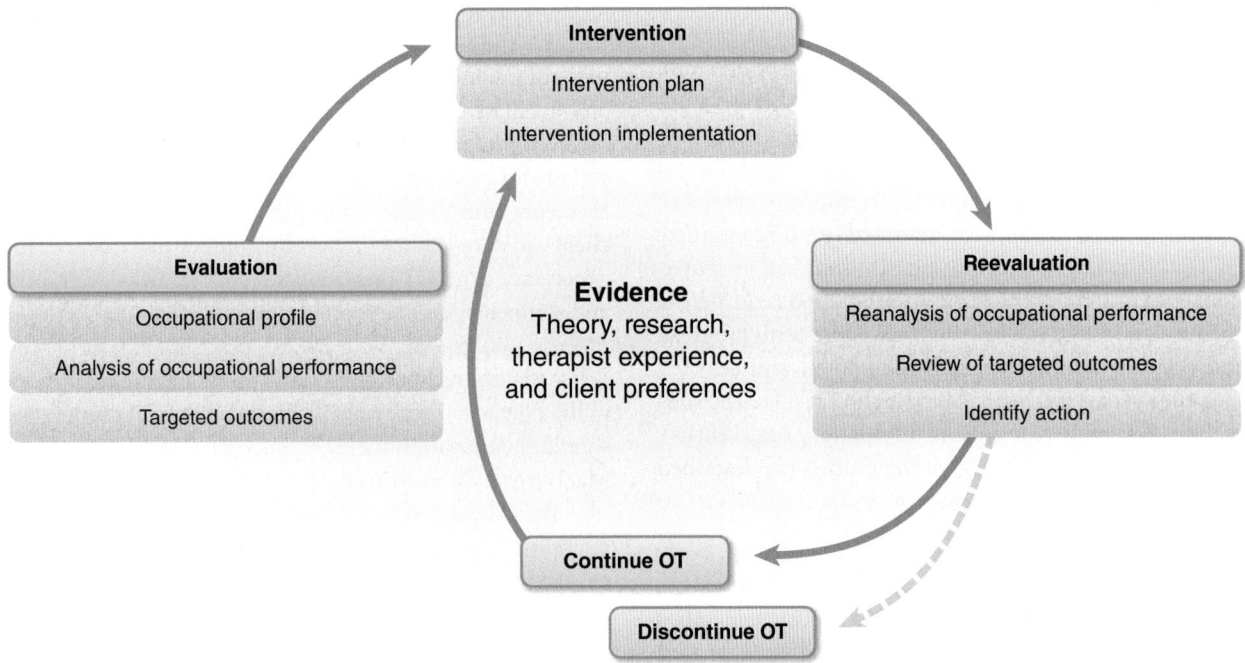

FIGURE 18.1 **The occupational therapy process.**

- **Evaluation** is the systematic collection and analysis of data needed to make decisions. OT practitioners use the evaluation results and conclusions to plan and implement interventions to assist clients in positively changing their occupational performance. Sometimes, the terms *evaluation* and *assessment* are used interchangeably; however, consistently using these terms based on distinct definitions can increase the efficacy of OT (Kramer & Grampurohit, 2020). We will delineate the terms as follows: evaluation is the comprehensive process of obtaining and interpreting data necessary to understand the person, system, or situation (AOTA, 2021, p. 2), and assessment refers to specific tools, instruments, or systematic interactions (e.g., observation of performance and context, interview with the client and significant others, record review, and measurement of specific aspects of performance) used during the evaluation process (AOTA, 2020a, p. 74, 2021, p. SX).
- **Intervention** is the implementation of skilled actions directed at facilitating the client's engagement in occupation related to health and participation (AOTA, 2020a, p. 78, 2021, p. SX). To determine the effectiveness of OT interventions, another evaluation or reevaluation must be conducted.
- **Reevaluation** can be conducted both *formally* and *informally*. *Formal reevaluation* compares the client's occupational performance data obtained during evaluation with the client's occupational performance after having received a period of intervention. Based on the formal reevaluation results, the occupational therapist makes one of two decisions—to continue or to discontinue OT services. If the decision is to discontinue services, intervention is ended, and the client is discharged from OT. If the decision is to continue services, intervention is resumed, although the original intervention plan may be modified based on the client's response to services and progress toward goals. The cycle continues with reevaluation being conducted at a designated time to again determine the effectiveness of OT interventions. Each formal reevaluation is a decision point to determine whether OT services will be continued, modified, or discontinued. *Informal reevaluation* also compares the client's occupational performance with goals but is focused more on the client's response to the intervention, short-term progress, and typically uses situational observation and selected measures versus full formal reevaluation results. The subsections for each component (evaluation, intervention, reevaluation, and outcomes) of the process are described in more detail later in this chapter.

The consideration of **outcomes** is inherent in every phase of the process. Outcomes are specifically identified results of OT interventions (AOTA, 2020a). In OT, outcomes include improved performance and participation in desired and meaningful occupations as well as increased abilities to adapt to occupational challenges. Additional outcomes include engaging in activities designed to prevent future limitation or to promote well-being, improve quality of life and role competence, and increase self-advocacy. As markers of achievement, outcomes guide the therapy process and help clients and therapists decide whether OT is effective. This in turn supports consideration about whether intervention is completed or needs to be modified. Modifications typically involve altering the goals, adding additional outcomes, or modifying approaches to improve progress.

Evidence provides the background that supports the OT process. The process is influenced and guided by a collection of evidence that includes theory, research, the therapist's experience, and the client's preferences (AOTA, 2020a). This facilitates evidence-informed practice, which combines the best current published evidence with practitioner expertise and client preferences (Brown, 2017; Cole & Creek, 2016; Law & MacDermid, 2013; Straus et al., 2019). Chapter 26 in Unit V specifically addresses evidence-based practice.

OT, like most health professions, is a multi-theory profession with occupational therapists applying one or more theories to examine and explain the occupational performance strengths and needs of each client. Theory reflects the operating assumptions that direct and guide the delivery of skilled services. Theories are a collection of concepts, definitions, and hypotheses that help occupational therapists make predictions about relationships between events (Kramer & Grampurohit, 2020). Theory is one piece of evidence that is important in the selection of assessment tools and interventions. In this chapter, the term *theory* is used synonymously with *frames of reference, conceptual models,* and *practice models,* which are other terms you may see. Unit VI addresses broad and specific models of practice.

The inclusion of research as an aspect of evidence reflects the data and science that verifies the OT evaluations and interventions used in service delivery. The best quantitative and qualitative research is information obtained from peer-reviewed journals. OT practitioners need research to establish validity for evaluation and intervention decisions. In addition to theory and research, the therapist's experience and the client's preferences are important sources of evidence. Your experience as an OT practitioner—your knowledge, training, and competencies—supports your implementation of the OT process. The experience of the OT practitioner provides evidence that the right professional is providing the right service in the right way, in the right place, and at the right time, which should then result in the right outcome (Holm, 2000; Law & MacDermid, 2013; Rice et al., 2019; Straus et al., 2019).

The OT process is accomplished through a collaborative relationship between clients and practitioners. Note that a *client* can be an individual, group, or population (AOTA, 2020a). For individuals, the term includes not only the person with the occupational performance problem but also their advocates (e.g., family members, significant others, caregivers, care managers, and community members). Clients that are groups are a collective of individuals (e.g., families, workers, and students), and populations are a collective of groups or individuals with the same or similar concerns (e.g., veterans and people with mental illness). Client preferences are based on life experiences, values, choices, needs, and priorities and are an integral piece of evidence supporting the OT process. Occupational therapists need to integrate the client's preferences consciously and systematically into all components of the OT process because they can significantly influence the outcomes. For clients to feel safe in expressing their preferences authentically, occupational therapists must create an inclusive, supportive environment throughout the OT process (AOTA, 2020a, 2020b). To do so, occupational therapists must use a lens of cultural humility throughout the OT process—be open to diversity within and across cultures; notice, recognize, and respond to each client's different viewpoints on health, wellness, family, and role expectations; and recognize the power dynamics in healthcare (Agner, 2020; Wells et al.,

2016). The best available evidence, including theory, research, therapist experience, *and* client preferences, must be used to achieve the best outcomes. Of significance is the choice of the word *and* in the previous sentence versus *or*. *All* available aspects of evidence must be used, including the client's preferences, for clients to gain maximum benefit from OT services (Cole & Creek, 2016; Holm, 2000; Law et al., 2016).

Just as each component of the OT process is supported by evidence, each component also requires professional reasoning. Professional reasoning, sometimes referred to as *clinical reasoning*, includes therapy decisions and problem-solving. Chapter 25 discusses the nature of professional reasoning. In this chapter, in addition to taking a closer look at the details of the OT process, we describe the professional reasoning and evidence focus for each component of the process. Subsequent chapters in this unit will provide further and more in-depth examination of evaluation and intervention and factors that connect with and shape the OT process.

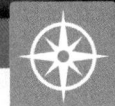

EXPANDING OUR PERSPECTIVE

The OT Process in a Nontraditional Setting

Dahlia Castillo

After reading the book *Occupational Therapy Without Borders* by Frank Kronenberg, I was inspired to treat individuals in areas with no OT services. I was unsure how I could do the OT process well without the usual resources at my fingertips in traditional settings. Each individual got a quick evaluation and interventions focused on home programming. It was a simple evaluation process, talk to the client and their family and observe the individual to ascertain their performance capacity, and finally hear their story to ascertain their goals and the meaningful occupations. Intervention happened briefly as I educated family members on what I was doing and instructed to do the same. I kept it extremely simple and focused on developmental milestones, as most were children with delayed development.

I met 7-year-old Armando and his family on the last day; he was diagnosed with cerebral palsy (CP) at birth. I quickly decide it was mild CP because he had normal tone in his extremities. I noticed occupational performance to be very limited although movement of all limbs was good, postural instability was evident, and he had slight flexor tone in the torso. His mother removed him from the too small umbrella stroller, hoisted him over one shoulder and then walked several paces before placing him on a therapy mat on the floor. His siblings played with him and took turns interacting and motivating him. A small plastic ball came toward him, and he kicked it. He then laughed uncontrollably as it hit one of the workers. I ask myself, just lucky, good aim, vision intact?

I ask mother about daily tummy time. She says she never places him on his tummy because that is a dangerous position for young children. I explain that may be true during sleeping, and asked if anyone ever told her that tummy time is good while awake. I place Armando on his belly, he immediately moved into prone on elbows and started to cry, wailing uncontrollably. Mother moved him on his back quickly. I asked the mother about goals for Armando. Father quickly answered that he wants Armando to go to school because they know he is smart. He is independent with toileting but cannot get to the toilet alone and the school requires him to do this before enrolling. I give my "development happens on the tummy" speech that I have said to most others I saw that day and encouraged them to start with 30 to 60 seconds at a time and increase to tolerance. I had done all components of the OT process: evaluation, intervention, and had a plan a reevaluation in 2 months. I was cautiously optimistic about his potential but skeptical about compliance from mother.

When I returned, I did not recognize Armando when he walked across the room independently. I was in a state of disbelief. Father explained that 13-year-old brother heard everything I said the last time I was there. When the parents were out of the house, brother began to play with Armando on his tummy. After a few days, Armando started to do it on his own. After 3 weeks, he was crawling and after 6 weeks, he started standing and creeping on the furniture. In the last 2 weeks, he started walking unsupported. He has been getting himself to the bathroom on his own since he began to crawl about a month ago. Armando's parents explain he will start school in 2 weeks. The reevaluation far exceeded my expectations and the decision to discharge him was clear.

Evaluation

Evaluation is the beginning of the OT process journey (Figure 18.2). The data occupational therapists collect and analyze are information about the client's occupational performance—strengths and problems. The occupational therapist is responsible for evaluating the client, administering, and interpreting the assessments, and integrating them to obtain the full picture of the client. The OT assistant may contribute to the evaluation using methods in which they have demonstrated competency and depending on licensure and payer regulations. For example, the OT assistant, under the supervision of the occupational therapist, may administer a standardized assessment such as a grip strength test, or perform an activities of daily living (ADLs) assessment. Occupational therapists are always responsible for the interpretation of assessment results and synthesis of those results into a full evaluation. There are professional guidelines to assist occupational therapists in determining when it is appropriate to delegate to OT assistants (see Chapters 73 and 74 for further discussion of these).

The primary question or therapy decision the occupational therapist must make during evaluation is "Who is my client and does my client need OT services?" To decide if the client needs OT services, we must first obtain information that will assist us in problem-solving answers to several secondary questions. These include but are not limited to the following:

- What is the client's occupational history and experience?
- What is the client's cultural context and personal identity?
- What is the client's pattern of activities during their daily routine?

- What are the occupations the client needs, wants, and is expected to perform?
- What is/are the client's problem(s)?
- Can OT assist in resolving the client's problem(s)?
- What are the client's priorities?
- What are the environment factors impacting the client's performance?
- Who are the significant people that will enhance and/or hinder the client's performance?
- What occupations are the client able to and unable to perform adequately?
- What skills, patterns, and aspects of context and environment affect the client's performance?
- What measurable and objective goals can address the client's targeted outcomes?

To effectively problem-solve the answers, we need to complete the occupational profile, perform an analysis of occupational performance, and identify targeted outcomes. It is essential that we use cultural humility when evaluating the client. Agner (2020) encourages practitioners to engage clients with open-ended questions about their goals and expectations while also considering questions that illustrate how systemic pressures and issues affect the client (p. 3). In addition to using a dialogue approach, we must engage in ongoing examination of our own assumptions and biases (both implicit and explicit) that may affect our relationships with our clients and recognize the role of power in the healthcare interaction.

Occupational Profile

A profile describes and summarizes information related to the client's history, resources, and performance. Because the focus of our skilled services is on occupation, we need to

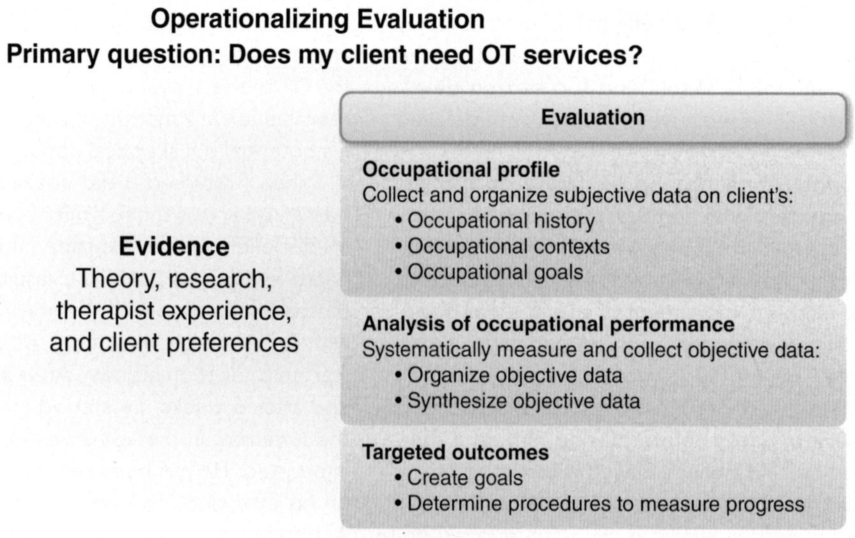

Operationalizing Evaluation
Primary question: Does my client need OT services?

FIGURE 18.2 Operationalizing evaluation. OT, occupational therapy.

create an occupational profile of our clients that describes their occupational performance. This involves collecting and organizing data on the client's occupational history, occupational contexts, and occupational goals (AOTA, 2020a). It is important to gather the client's perceptions about their occupations and related performance strengths and concerns as this information may or may not be consistent with what others might say who observe the client's performance. Remember that the client includes not only the person with an occupational performance concern but also other people important in the client's life, such as spouses, partners, family members, and caregivers, as well as those who are concerned about the client's performance, such as employers or teachers.

The historical information collected from and about clients needs to relate to the performance of their life activities, which include ADLs, instrumental ADLs, health management, rest and sleep, education, work, play, leisure, and social participation (AOTA, 2020a). The contextual information collected needs to describe the physical, social, attitudinal surroundings where the client lives and performs their preferred occupations and include features unique to the person (e.g., age, sexual orientation, gender identity, race and ethnicity, cultural identification, social background, education, professional identify, and lifestyle) (AOTA, 2020a). The occupational profile also needs to include information related to the client's occupational goals. OT practitioners need to know why their clients are seeking services; what their occupational performance concerns are; and what daily occupations they need, want, and are expected to perform. And finally, it is imperative that we know the outcomes the client wants and expects to attain through OT services. Refer to OT Story 18.1 to see how an occupational profile emerges during the evaluation process and how changes in contextual information unique to the client change the occupational profile, which then changes decisions related to analysis of occupational performance, targeted outcomes, and the planning and implementation of interventions.

OT STORY 18.1 OCCUPATIONAL PROFILE: WHO IS GEORGE?

Susan, an occupational therapist, receives a new client on her caseload. Based on the information she received with the referral for OT services, she knows his name is George, he is in the acute care unit, is 65 years old, and has multiple sclerosis. Susan knows she needs to find out more information about George as part of the evaluation process. She reviews George's medical record and learns that George is married, has three children, is a semiretired teacher, has had recent falls without injury, uses a cane, has type 2 diabetes and hypertension, and lives in a two-story house with a first floor bedroom and bathroom. Susan introduces herself to George and describes OT (refer to Box 18.1 to see approaches to describing OT). Through discussion with George, Susan finds out he is an engineer by profession, has been teaching college-level engineering courses for the past 15 years, and is currently an adjunct instructor, co-teaching two courses each year. George has four grandchildren (ages 4, 7, 8, and 11 years—all girls) and enjoys attending their school and sport events. He plays the violin and volunteers as an usher for symphony events. George enjoys cooking and playing cards. He has an office and music room on the second floor of his house, and there are 12 steps to enter the front door of his house and two steps to enter the back door. Through administration of the Canadian Occupational Performance Measure (COPM), Susan obtains data on George's priority daily activities—participating in volunteer activities at his church and the symphony, teaching, cooking, bathing, and ballroom dancing with his wife.

Questions

1. What is George's occupational history and experience?
2. What is George's cultural context and personal identity?
3. What is George's pattern of daily activities?
4. What are the occupations George needs, wants, and is expected to perform?
5. What are George's priorities?
6. What additional information would be beneficial for Susan to add to George's occupational profile?

What if George's contextual information was different? What if George's narrative was as follows: Susan, an occupational therapist, receives a new client on her caseload. Based on the information she received with the referral for OT services, she knows his name is George, he is in the acute care unit, is 65 years old, and has multiple sclerosis. Susan knows she needs to find out more information about George as part of the evaluation process. She reviews George's medical record and learns that George is married, has three children, is a semiretired teacher's aide, has had recent falls without injury, uses a cane, has type 2 diabetes and hypertension, and lives in a third-floor, two-bedroom apartment. Susan introduces herself to George and describes OT (refer to Box 18.1 to see approaches to describing OT). Through discussion with George, Susan finds out he retired 2 years ago with a state employee pension; however, he continues to work as a substitute teacher to supplement his income and reports he just has to make it to 67 when

(continued)

OT STORY 18.1 OCCUPATIONAL PROFILE: WHO IS GEORGE? (continued)

he can start collecting Social Security and stop working altogether. George has four grandchildren (ages 4, 7, 8, and 11 years—all girls) and enjoys attending their school and sport events. He plays the violin and volunteers as an usher for symphony events. George enjoys cooking and playing cards. He has two flights of stairs, each with 12 steps, to get to their third-floor apartment. The elevator is at the opposite side of the building and tightly fits one wheelchair and one other passenger. His two-bedroom apartment has large living and dining spaces, and a small bathroom with a combination bathtub/shower. George and his spouse each sleep in one bedroom. Through administration of the Canadian Occupational Performance Measure (COPM), Susan obtains data on George's priority daily activities—participating in

volunteer activities at his church and the symphony, teaching, cooking, bathing, and ballroom dancing with his wife.

Questions

Consider the same questions and how your responses are different based on the contextual differences.

1. What is George's occupational history and experience?
2. What is George's cultural context and personal identity?
3. What is George's pattern of daily activities?
4. What are the occupations George needs, wants, and is expected to perform?
5. What are George's priorities?
6. What additional information would be beneficial for Susan to add to George's occupational profile?

BOX 18.1 DESCRIBING OCCUPATIONAL THERAPY

Each OT practitioner has his or her own individual therapeutic style when describing the OT process to a client. Additionally, the description is tailored to make it relevant to the client. Although there is not a cookbook for what to say to your client, the following are some helpful hints when describing OT.

- Say occupational therapy, occupational therapist, and occupational therapy assistant versus "OT."

  Hello George. My name is Susan. I am your occupational therapist. My job as your occupational therapist is to help you do the things that you need and want to do throughout your day.

- Use examples of relevant daily occupations based on what you know about your client.

  Examples for George might include *safely getting dressed and showered, doing activities in your home such as making meals and yard work,* and *visiting with family and friends.*

  Examples for Nicholas might include *tying shoes, using a pencil, throwing a ball, organizing his desk and backpack,* and *playing board games.*

  Engage your client in a dialogue—ask questions and follow up on responses by asking additional questions to obtain more information.

  Have you ever heard of occupational therapy or known someone who had occupational therapy? If the person says, "Yes," ask them to tell you about the experience to determine whether it is similar to or different from the occupational therapy services they will have.

Ask the person about his or her daily routine:
Describe your daily routine to me.
Tell me about what you do at home.
Tell me about what you do at school.
Tell me about what you do at work.
Tell me about the daily activities you need or want to do.
Tell me about the people in your life that you would like to be involved in OT services.

Ask your client if they have questions.

- Don't use medical or healthcare buzzwords, acronyms, or abbreviations—they are likely meaningless to your client and can be confusing. Here are a few examples:
Instead of saying upper extremity, say arm
Instead of saying ADLs, say daily activities
Instead of saying orthosis, say splint or brace
Instead of saying don and doff, say put on and take off
Instead of saying fine motor skills, say hand coordination
If you need to use a medical or healthcare term, define it in user-friendly language.

- Emphasize that the OT process is collaborative.

  George, we are going to work together to help you get back to your volunteer activities at church and the symphony.

  Nicholas, you and I are a team; together we are going to make your school activities easier and more fun.

- Practice makes perfect. Practice describing occupational therapy . . . to your family, friends, colleagues, and to your clients. What did you say? Did you use person-centered communication? Did you address occupation? Did you customize your comments? How did you engage the person in the collaborative process?

As a reminder, the occupational profile is a "summary" of information, so although there is a wide range of data options, the occupational therapist collects what is most relevant to the specific client's occupational performance. Additionally, although much of the data are collected during the first session with the client, data can (and should) be added over sessions while working with the client.

Occupational Performance Analysis

Whereas the occupational profile addresses the collection and organization of primarily *subjective data* based on the client's perceptions, the analysis of occupational performance addresses the collection, organization, and synthesis of primarily *objective data* regarding the client's occupational performance (AOTA, 2020a). Objective data are descriptions that can be easily replicated by others observing the same phenomenon. To collect objective data, we have clients perform selected activities important to their occupations—that is, activities the client wants or needs to perform or that others expect the client to perform. Ideally, clients perform the priority occupations in their usual manner, with the objects and equipment they usually use, in the setting(s) they typically perform the occupation (Rogers & Holm, 2009). The ideal performance situation reflects the client's real-life situation. However, attainment of the real-life or ideal performance situation is dependent on the practice setting and may not always be feasible. Practitioners attempt to replicate real-life performance contexts and environments as closely as possible given the constraints of the practice setting. It is important for practitioners to understand that in the contrived setting of the OT clinic, the performance demands are different and thus may not fully reflect actual performance in the client's natural setting. Dr. Joan Rogers, well known for her research in task performance, highlights this issue well when she would challenge practitioners by saying "if you want to understand the importance of context, try going home and making dinner in your neighbor's kitchen . . . see how much longer it takes and whether you are able to do things as well."

To collect objective data, therapists need to rely on valid and reliable assessment tools specifically designed to measure factors that support and restrict occupational performance. Chapters 19 and 20 provide in-depth discussions about the importance of effective assessment tools. Performance may be supported or hindered by the person's body structures and functions, the environment, unique features of the person, and/or the transaction among them in the form of skills and patterns of performance. Therefore, depending on the client's needs, assessment tools may be used to measure client factors, contexts (environmental factors and personal factors), activity demands, performance skills, and performance patterns in one or more areas of occupation (AOTA, 2020a). As a reminder, although the occupational profile and analysis of occupational performance are presented sequentially, they are dynamic in nature and are typically integrated when evaluating a client. Data, both objective and subjective, should be collected about the client's strengths and limitations. See OT Story 18.2 to apply the concepts about evaluation discussed so far.

OT STORY 18.2 EVALUATION: DOES NICHOLAS NEED OCCUPATIONAL THERAPY SERVICES?

Mahmoud is 7 years old and was referred for school-based OT services because he has sloppy handwriting, difficulty sitting still in class, and easily becomes frustrated. Gina, the school occupational therapist, meets with Mahmoud's first grade teacher, his father, and Mahmoud to describe OT services (see Box 18.1) and to obtain information for Mahmoud's occupational profile. Gina finds out the following information: Mahmoud and his family are refugees; have lived in the United States with Mahmoud's aunt for approximately 2 years; Mahmoud's parents do not have health insurance; for emergent health needs they go to a local free clinic; Mahmoud's teacher has observed that he displays behaviors associated with attention deficit/hyperactivity disorder, however he has not been formally evaluated; his father and mother are reluctant to have him evaluated as they do not want to consider medications and wish to try behavior strategies; he has three older teenage siblings and a 5-month-old brother; Mahmoud has difficulty following rules at home and in the classroom; enjoys gym class and likes to swim; and he is slow to complete schoolwork, dress himself, and do his chores. Gina analyzed Mahmoud's occupational performance by observing him in the classroom, administering standardized assessment tools to Mahmoud, and requesting his parents and teacher complete standardized questionnaires, which his parents did with the assistance of Mahmoud's aunt. The data indicated that Mahmoud has problems with fine motor skills (difficulty holding and manipulating everyday objects—pencil, fork, toothbrush), dressing (difficulty fastening and adjusting clothes, unable to tie shoes), and cognitive skills (difficulty following directions and organizing himself and his environment and limited attention span). The data also indicated that Mahmoud has strengths in gross motor activities (swimming, running, and kicking and throwing balls), motivation (wants to do well in

(continued)

OT STORY 18.2 EVALUATION: DOES NICHOLAS NEED OCCUPATIONAL THERAPY SERVICES? (continued)

school and at home and please his parents and teacher), and social skills (gets along well with his siblings and peers).

Questions

1. What are Mahmoud's problems?
2. Does Mahmoud's problems relate to his occupational performance?
3. What are the contextual factors that may enhance and/or hinder Mahmoud's performance?
4. What outcomes would be appropriate for Gina to target in OT services in the school setting?
5. Can OT assist in resolving Mahmoud's problems?
6. What goals can address Mahmoud's targeted outcomes?

Targeted Outcomes

Once the data are collected and organized, the final task is to synthesize the data to define the performance problems that OT interventions can appropriately target. As part of the synthesis, the occupational therapist develops hypotheses about the client's occupational performance (Rogers & Holm, 1989, 2009). The hypotheses explain why the problem is occurring based on the subjective and objective data. Well-defined and highly specific problem statements and hypotheses are needed to develop relevant targeted outcomes. Creating short-term (i.e., goals achieved in a few days, week, or month) and long-term goals (i.e., ones achieved over a longer period—2 months to a year) and determining procedures to measure progress toward goal attainment are in the final aspect of evaluation—targeted outcomes (AOTA, 2020a).

Establishing goals is done in collaboration with the client and needs to reflect occupational performance problems relevant to the client's desired outcomes. Goals need to be written as objective, measurable statements with an identifiable time frame and predetermined objective methods to measure progress. Whether the problem limiting the client's performance is related to a client factor, performance skill or pattern, or context, the goal statement needs to address an occupation in addition to the performance problem.

In practice, short-term goals represent small steps along the way toward the long-term goals related to occupational engagement. Short-term goals may address aspects of body functions, sets of skills, or important contextual factors. For instance, a short-term goal may be to get food to the mouth effectively through therapeutic strategies such as engaging in graded eye–hand coordination activities as well as using adaptive feeding equipment. Long-term goals reflect performance of the client's meaningful and important daily occupations. Thus, a long-term goal in this example would be independence in all aspects of feeding and eating. The targeted outcomes, including long- and short-term goals, help predict what the client will achieve through OT intervention. See Chapter 31 for more information on documentation and writing goals.

Evidence Focus During Evaluation

The evidence focus for evaluation requires the therapist to use evidence-based information that supports the acquisition of information needed for the occupational profile, analysis of occupational performance, and targeted outcomes. For evaluation, we need to consider what theoretical principles or operating assumptions are most relevant for the client and practice setting. We need to identify and integrate the available *research* regarding the validity and reliability of appropriate assessment tools. Examples of relevant evidence for evaluation include studies addressing the use of a theoretical perspective with clients similar to your client and studies reporting the reliability of assessment tools appropriate to use with your client. The *therapist experience* is an essential consideration. The occupational therapist needs to reflect on the following questions: "What is my experience in evaluating this type of client?" and "What is my experience in administering the appropriate assessment tools?" Your responses to these questions are important in determining what your needs are to best evaluate your client. And finally, but essential in conducting the evaluation, is the evidence related to the *client's preferences*. Your client is central to the OT process and only clients can identify the occupations that give meaning to their lives, so the evidence indicating their preferred occupations must be systematically and meticulously collected because it provides the foundation for a client-centered, occupation-focused evaluation. The therapist must reason in a manner that considers the following:

- The client's preferred occupational outcomes
- The therapist's analysis of the factors affecting performance
- The agreed-on target outcomes

The results of the therapist's professional reasoning in turn affect the transition into the next component of the OT process—intervention. See OT Story 18.3 to problem-solve a professional dilemma related to providing an OT evaluation related to the client's preferences.

OT STORY 18.3 EVIDENCE-BASED EVALUATION: WHAT SHOULD RAUL DO?

Raul has just started his first job as an occupational therapist. He is working in a fast-paced outpatient clinic that specializes in rehabilitation for individuals with orthopedic conditions. Raul learns during orientation to his job responsibilities that the clinic has evidence-based protocols for evaluations and interventions based on diagnosis. The protocol lists the specific assessment tools that are to be administered and the problems that are to be addressed for clients with that diagnosis. Raul notices that the protocols do not include creating an occupational profile of the client. He also notices that the therapists do not seem to ask their clients questions about their occupational history, occupational contexts, or occupational goals. Based on his observation, Raul feels that the therapists follow the protocols and that all clients with the same or similar diagnosis receive the same evaluation process, have the same targeted outcomes, and engage in the same interventions. Raul learned (and believes) that the focus of OT services is on occupation and that to best understand a client's occupational performance, occupational therapists need to create an occupational profile, conduct an individualized evaluation, and provide customized interventions that support the client's goals. Raul asks some of the other therapists why they do not create an occupational profile for clients. The responses were "It's not on the protocol," "It takes too much time," and "Everyone has the same problems."

Questions

1. What is the problem/issue in Raul's situation?
2. What resources could Raul access to help address the problem/issue?
3. What are the potential courses of action that Raul can take? (Suggest as many as possible)
4. What are the potential consequences of each possible course of action?
5. Which course of action do you think is best for Raul to take?
6. Once Raul implements the best course of action, what are some ways Raul might evaluate the outcome of the course of action?
7. How can Raul follow up to determine if further action is necessary?

Intervention

Intervention follows evaluation in the OT process (Figure 18.3). The data collected and analyzed about the client's occupational performance during the evaluation provide navigational information for determining the best therapeutic route for the planning and implementation of OT interventions. The primary question or therapy decision the OT practitioner must make during intervention is "What OT interventions can best help my client?" To decide the appropriate intervention course, we must consider information obtained from answering secondary questions

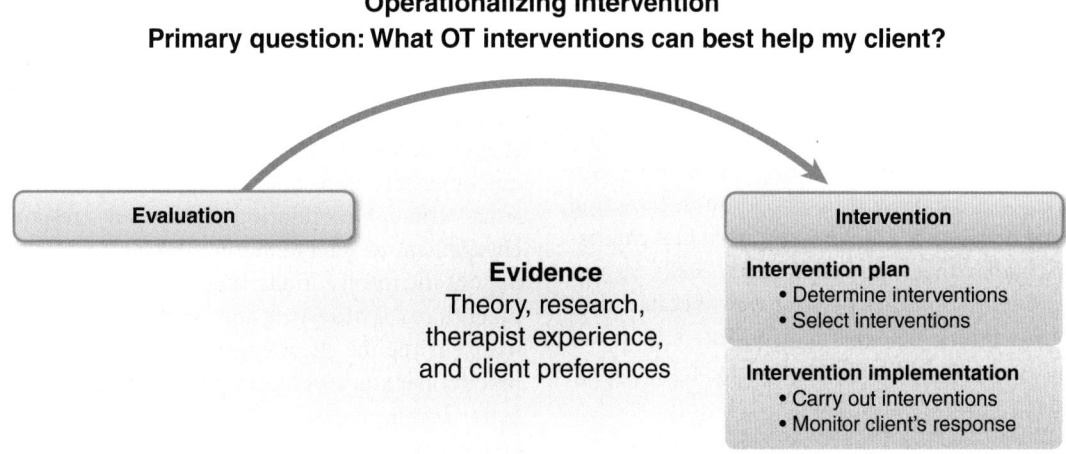

FIGURE 18.3 Operationalizing intervention. OT, occupational therapy.

relevant to intervention planning and implementation. These include but are not limited to the following:

- What is the range of appropriate interventions based on the evidence?
- Which interventions would the client prefer performing?
- Do the interventions align with the client's cultural context and identity?
- Who are the significant people that will enhance and/or hinder the client's performance?
- Which interventions are most effective?
- Which interventions can be implemented given the environment parameters of the therapeutic setting?
- How does the client respond to the interventions?
- Are the interventions addressing the client's occupational performance problems?
- Are the interventions promoting the client's engagement in and performance of their preferred daily activities?

OT practitioners need to continually ask themselves these questions throughout the intervention phase of the OT process. Discussing possible answers with colleagues can assist in increasing the breadth and depth of your professional reasoning. Think of these questions as road markers and billboard announcements directing you toward your objective of providing OT interventions that best help your client. Making therapy decisions based on answers to these questions will help focus your interventions on your clients' occupational performance needs.

The intervention component of the OT process includes the intervention plan and intervention implementation (AOTA, 2020a). To develop an intervention plan, we need to consider the client's current occupational performance and envision what the client will achieve through OT interventions. The results of the client's occupational profile and analysis of occupational performance provide subjective and objective information about the client's current occupational performance, and the targeted outcomes predict what the client will achieve through OT interventions. Therefore, although intervention is a separate component in the OT process, it is fully dependent on and explicitly interconnected with evaluation, and just as it is essential that we use cultural humility when evaluating the client, we also need to use cultural humility throughout the intervention phase. Cultural humility is a lifelong approach that emphasizes learning rather than knowing (Agner, 2020). So just as understanding each client's perspectives—because they are affected by multilayered cultural identities—requires an ongoing dialogue, cultural humility takes ongoing learning, practice, and reflection.

Intervention Plan

The intervention plan determines the selection of specific OT intervention approaches used to address the client's targeted outcomes (AOTA, 2020a). The intervention plan is developed in collaboration with the client. Although the occupational therapist is responsible for the development of the plan, it is the *client's* intervention plan, not the occupational therapist's intervention plan. The first step in developing the plan is to determine the range of intervention approaches appropriate to address the client's occupational performance problems. OT interventions can be categorized as occupations and activities, and interventions to support occupations (AOTA, 2020a). Occupations selected as interventions focus on the client engaging in client-directed daily life activities that match and support the client's targeted outcomes. Activities used as interventions are often components of occupations and engage clients in practicing activities related to occupations or help clients develop skills and patterns that enhance occupational performance. Interventions that support occupations are preparatory methods and tasks used as part of an intervention session in preparation for or concurrently with occupational and activities. Chapters 21 and 22 provide detailed information on OT interventions with individuals and for groups, communities, and populations.

Once the range of interventions appropriate to address the client's occupational performance problems are identified, the OT practitioner selects the interventions that have the greatest potential to improve performance and are the best match with the client's occupational profile. The final decision to include (or not include) a specific intervention is made in collaboration with the client and/or people important in the client's life. Doing so maximizes the client's understanding of the relationship between the selected interventions and their preferred daily occupations.

Intervention Implementation

Once the plan is established, the next step is to put the plan into action. Intervention implementation includes the process of carrying out the interventions and monitoring the client's response (AOTA, 2020a). The interventions clients engage in need to be appropriate to address the targeted outcomes related to their occupational performance problems. Although monitoring of the client's response to their engagement in interventions is listed separate from carrying out the interventions, they occur concurrently. The OT practitioner is observing and examining the client's performance while the client engages in the intervention(s). The practitioner adjusts aspects of the intervention as needed to better accommodate or challenge the client's occupational performance to achieve the client's targeted outcomes. Monitoring the client's response is part of the informal reevaluation described earlier in the chapter. See OT Story 18.4 for a clinical example of the intervention component of the OT process.

OT STORY 18.4 INTERVENTION: WHAT OCCUPATIONAL THERAPY INTERVENTIONS CAN BEST HELP ROSA?

Suraj, an OT assistant on an orthopedic rehabilitation unit, is assigned a new client, Rosa, on his caseload by the occupational therapist he works with. Rosa is 72 years old and was just transferred from the acute care unit where she had surgery to replace her hip. Rosa and her husband immigrated to the United States from Mexico when they were both in their 20s. She lives in an apartment building with elevator access; uses the public bus system; enjoys dancing, which she misses since her husband died; plays bingo at the local senior citizen center three nights a week; and does all of her own shopping, cooking, laundry, and cleaning of her apartment. The laundry facilities are in the basement of her apartment building; her bathroom has a tub with a shower—she prefers baths; she loves theater—she and her sister often attend the local community or school theater events; she is an avid reader of mystery novels, retired as a bank teller 7 years ago, and she and her sister have being saving for years to take a cruise to Alaska and the cruise is in a month. Rosa is currently using a walker; however, she anticipates

only needing a cane when she is discharged. Her upper extremity strength is limited, and she fatigues easily. Rosa has some pain in her hip and is fearful of falling. Rosa's priority is to be able to go on the cruise with her sister.

Questions

1. What is the range of appropriate interventions Suraj might include in Rosa's intervention plan? (Suggest as many as possible)
2. Do the interventions align with Rosa's cultural context and identity?
3. Who are the important people in Rosa's life to include in her care?
4. Which interventions do you think Rosa will prefer performing?
5. Which interventions would be most effective for Rosa?
6. How do the interventions promote Rosa's engagement in and performance of her preferred daily activities?
7. How do you think Rosa will respond to the interventions?

Evidence Focus During Intervention

Theory, research, the therapist's experience, and the client's preferences influence and guide intervention as much as they do evaluation but with a different focus. The focus for evidence to support intervention services is on the planning and implementation of interventions. Examples of information used to support intervention services are studies about the relative benefits of one intervention approach versus another, studies about common occupational challenges for clients with similar occupational performance problems, and medical and educational information about the client's condition. OT practitioners need to consider how each intervention identified within the range of potential interventions relates to the theoretical principles or operating assumptions most relevant for the client and the practice setting. In addition, practitioners need to reflect on personal competencies relative to the intervention, along with experiences administering them with clients. And last but certainly not least, we must identify the evidence related to the client's preferences. As during evaluation, the client's preferred daily occupations must be systematically and meticulously integrated into the plan and delivery of OT interventions. The combined evidence assists the OT practitioner in problem-solving and making therapeutic decisions that result in the selection and implementation of appropriate interventions. These therapeutic decisions reflect informal aspects of the next

component of the OT process—reevaluation. The occupational therapist informally reevaluates the client's response to each intervention and effectiveness in assisting the client in achieving their goals.

Reevaluation

The third component of the OT process is reevaluation (Figure 18.4). The formal reevaluation is a return to the evaluation component of the process. Data on the client's occupational performance are again collected and analyzed. As with evaluation, reevaluation provides navigational information for determining the best therapeutic route for the planning and implementation of intervention services. During reevaluation, the targeted outcomes established during evaluation are assessed using the same measures employed during the initial evaluation or last reevaluation. Ultimately, the occupational therapist is determining whether the best therapeutic intervention route was taken along with identifying the best therapeutic route to take from this point forward.

The primary question or therapy decision the occupational therapist must make during reevaluation is "How has OT services affected my client's occupational performance?" As with the other components of the OT process, to make the therapeutic decision about the continued need for services, we must first obtain information that will assist

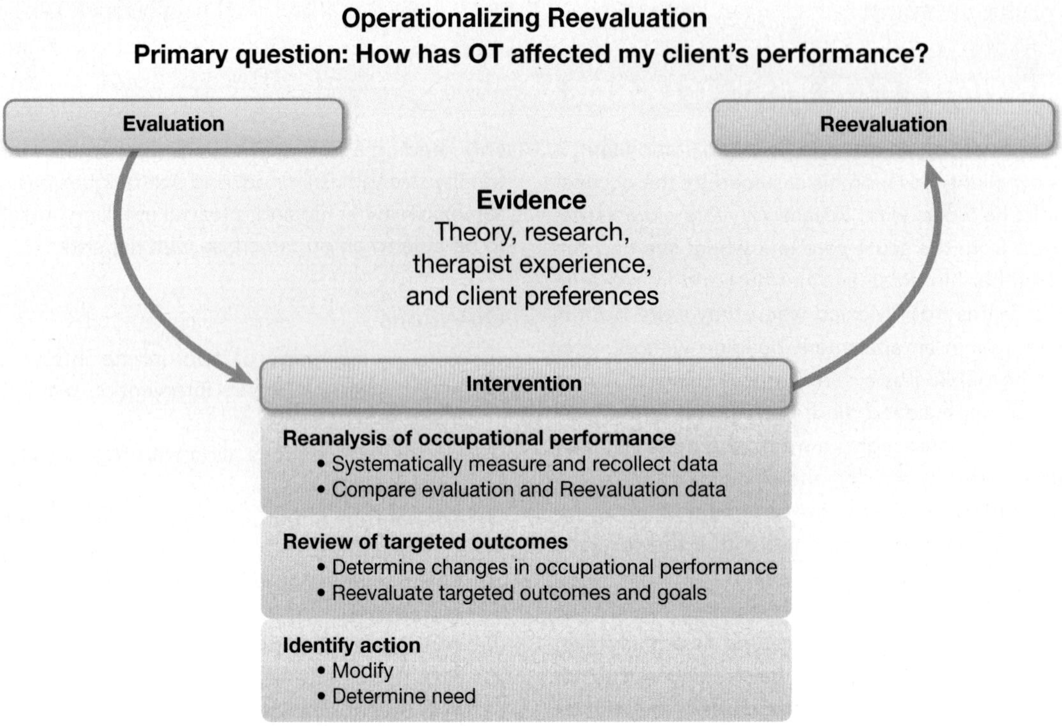

Operationalizing Reevaluation
Primary question: How has OT affected my client's performance?

FIGURE 18.4 Operationalizing reevaluation. OT, occupational therapy.

us in problem-solving answers to the secondary questions. These include but are not limited to the following:

- How has the client's occupational performance changed since the initial evaluation?
- What are the occupations the client is now able to perform?
- What are the occupations the client is still unable to perform or has problems performing?
- Can OT continue to assist in resolving the client's occupational performance problem(s)?
- How do the client's measurable and objective goals need to be modified to address the client's targeted outcomes?
- What are the environment factors impacting the client's performance and progress toward the targeted outcomes?
- Who are the significant people involved in the client's care and how are they enhancing and/or hindering the client's performance and progress toward targeted outcomes?

To effectively problem-solve the answers, we need to reanalyze the client's occupational performance, review the client's targeted outcomes, and identify the appropriate action to take regarding the continuation of OT services.

Reanalysis of Occupational Performance

Occupational therapists systematically measure and recollect data as the first step in the reanalysis of occupational performance. The next step in the reanalysis is to compare the data obtained during the initial evaluation with the data obtained during reevaluation. As with any comparison, occupational therapists need to ensure that they are comparing equivalent items. Therefore, it is essential that we use the same measures during reevaluation that were used during the initial evaluation phase. Doing so is the only dependable way the occupational therapist can measure change accurately. If we do not use the same measures, then we are not measuring comparable aspects of occupational performance. And if we are not measuring comparable aspects of occupational performance, we are not able to accurately and with valid evidence determine how OT has affected the client's performance. The comparison of data directly impacts the review of the targeted outcomes. The timing of the reevaluation is based on the occupational therapist's prediction of how long it will take for OT interventions to achieve the client's targeted outcomes. Additionally, some practice settings and payers have standard requirements for the timing of reevaluations.

Review of Targeted Outcomes

Changes in occupational performance are used to determine whether OT interventions achieved the intended targeted outcomes through goal attainment. Review of the targeted outcomes requires the occupational therapist to determine change in the client's occupational performance relevant to the client's goals established during the initial evaluation (AOTA, 2020a). The degree of goal attainment can be determined by comparing the client's performance measured at the initial evaluation with performance measured at reevaluation. The targeted outcomes and goals are then reviewed and reevaluated to identify the appropriate action (AOTA, 2020a).

Action Identification

After reevaluation, the therapist considers whether to continue OT, refer the client to another service or specialty, or discontinue services. Continuation of OT services is justified if the client is making progress toward targeted outcomes and goals or if there is reason to believe alternate approaches might work to improve progress. Additionally, new or altered targeted outcomes and goals may emerge because of the therapy process. In some situations, it may be apparent that the client could benefit from the services of other professionals, in addition to OT, or that a different specialty intervention within OT is warranted. In this situation, the occupational therapist refers the client to the appropriate resources. OT services are discontinued when the client has reached targeted outcomes or there is evidence to suggest that further intervention will not substantially improve occupational performance. When OT services are discontinued, the client is often provided with aftercare or follow-up recommendations to maintain and build on their therapy gains.

Reevaluation should be ideally scheduled at the end of the anticipated time for the OT intervention to have an effect on the client's occupational performance. Determining the "just right" time for reevaluation is a challenge (Rogers & Holm, 1989, 2009). If reevaluation occurs too early, a course of intervention may be prematurely considered unsuccessful because the client hasn't had enough time to show change in performance. In contrast, if reevaluation occurs too late, the client may have already achieved a targeted outcome and progression in occupational performance is not continuing because the targeted outcomes, measurable goals, and intervention plan have not been appropriately modified or advanced to accommodate the positive change.

There are other factors external to the occupational therapist's professional reasoning that determine the time for reevaluation. These factors include third-party payment sources, health organization policies and procedures, and practice guidelines. The evidence focus for reevaluation requires occupational therapists to consider the available research regarding reevaluation for the specific type of client and the assessment tools administered at evaluation. Evidence for reevaluation combines relevant information from studies supporting evaluation decisions with those addressing intervention options. Although we hope that the external factors impacting decisions regarding reevaluation are based on evidence, occupational therapists need to be aware that this is not always the case. We need to be advocates for the use of evidence-based decisions regarding all aspects of OT services, including reevaluation. See OT Story 18.5 for a clinical example of the reevaluation component of the OT process.

OT STORY 18.5 REEVALUATION: HOW HAS OCCUPATIONAL THERAPY AFFECTED TIM'S OCCUPATIONAL PERFORMANCE?

Tim is 29 years old and sustained a traumatic brain injury 2 months ago because of a car crash. One month ago, he was discharged from the hospital and referred for OT at the outpatient center. Prior to his accident, Tim was living with his father and grandmother. Since discharge, he has been living with his younger brother, the brother's husband, and their 4-year-old daughter. Mark, Tim's occupational therapist, collected data during the evaluation that indicated the following: Tim requires moderate physical assistance for putting on lower and upper body clothing because of decreased right arm strength and sequencing problems; Tim needs moderate physical and cognitive assistance to perform money management and meal preparation tasks; he requires constant supervision for safety when performing tasks because of impulsivity; and he easily becomes frustrated, exhibiting angry outbursts. Mark predicted that it would take 4 weeks to achieve the goals addressing the targeted outcomes he and Tim identified. Mark administered the same measures during the formal reevaluation that he had administered to Tim during the initial evaluation to accurately compare his initial and current occupational performance and determine progress. The following is Tim's current occupational performance: His right arm strength is now adequate for him to put on and take off his clothing; however, he is unable to fasten his clothing (buttons/zippers); Tim is able to independently sequence dressing tasks with the use of a written outline; he requires minimal assistance to physically perform money management and meal preparation tasks; however, he continues to require moderate cognitive assistance and supervision for safety in the kitchen environment; and Tim is now able to ask Mark for assistance when he becomes frustrated without display of anger.

Questions

1. How has Tim's occupational performance changed since initial evaluation?
2. What occupations are Tim now able to perform?

(continued)

OT STORY 18.5 REEVALUATION: HOW HAS OCCUPATIONAL THERAPY AFFECTED TIM'S OCCUPATIONAL PERFORMANCE? (*continued*)

3. What occupations are Tim still unable to perform?
4. Can OT continue to assist in resolving Tim's occupational performance problems?
5. How do Tim's goals need to be modified to address his targeted outcomes?

6. What are the possible environment factors that could be impacting Tim's performance and progress toward the targeted outcomes?
7. Who are the significant people involved in Tim's life and how could they be enhancing and/or hindering Tim's performance and progress toward targeted outcomes?

Outcomes: Continue or Discontinue

Outcomes are integrated throughout the OT process (Figure 18.5). As previously stated, "achieving health, well-being and participation in life through engagement in occupations" is the all-encompassing goal of the OT services (AOTA, 2020a). OT's unique focus on occupation is a primary factor in this inclusive outcome. As previously addressed in evaluation, targeted outcomes are identified that reflect the client's occupational performance problems. Measurable goals with an identifiable time frame and predetermined objective method to measure progress are essential in determining the attainment of targeted outcomes. The occupational therapist carefully considers the client's targeted outcomes when developing an intervention plan and implementing interventions. The targeted outcomes are revisited formally during reevaluation to address progress.

The primary question the occupational therapist must answer is "Does my client continue to need occupational therapy services?" As with all previous aspects of the process, the occupational therapist must obtain information to problem-solve secondary questions. These include the following:

- Has OT positively impacted the client's ability to perform daily occupations?
- Can OT continue to assist in resolving the client's occupational performance problems?
- Has the client achieved the maximum benefit from OT services?
- Does the client want to continue receiving OT services?
- Is there sufficient justification for continuing OT services?

The occupational therapist uses information from evaluation, intervention, and reevaluation to determine the

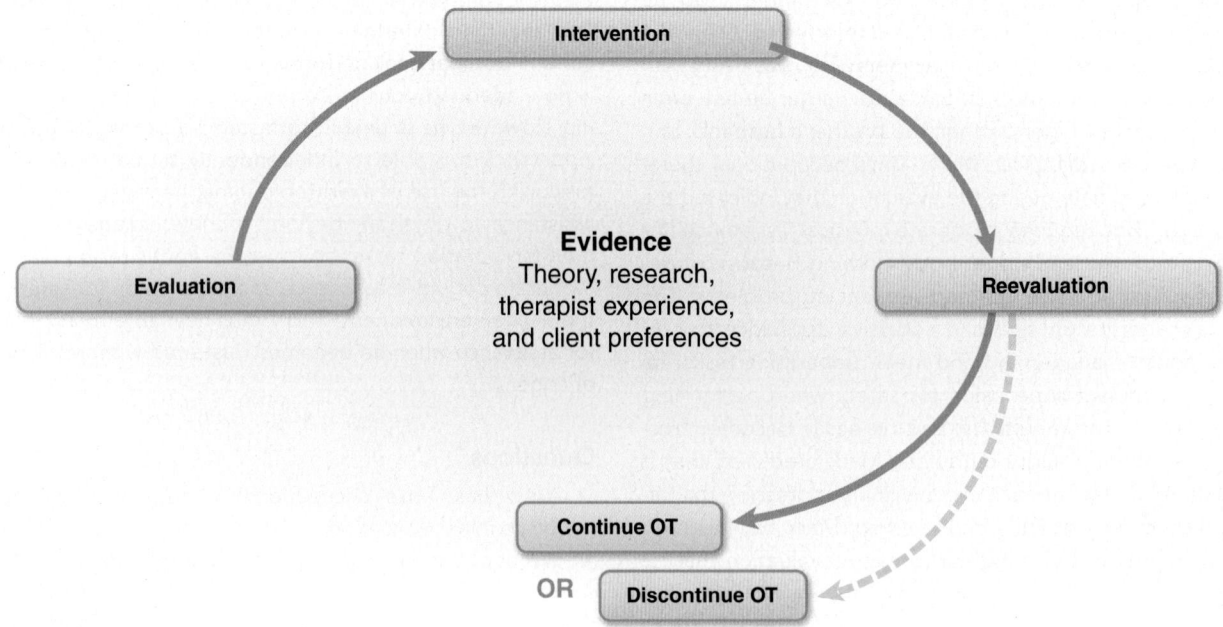

Operationalizing Outcome of Reevaluation
Primary question: Does my client continue to need OT services?

Intervention

Evaluation

Evidence
Theory, research, therapist experience, and client preferences

Reevaluation

Continue OT

OR   Discontinue OT

FIGURE 18.5 Operationalizing outcome of reevaluation. OT, occupational therapy.

answers to conclude whether OT services should be continued or discontinued. Just as with evaluation and intervention, cultural humility is essential when considering our client's outcomes and our client's decisions. It is important for us to examine our biases as they can significantly affect how services are delivered and the outcomes. For example, when a client doesn't want to receive (or continue receiving) OT services, we may not understand or find that client's decision reasonable and be uncomfortable with it based on our own cultural experiences and biases. We don't need to accept or agree with our client's decision, but if we are culturally humble, we recognize that both of our perspectives are culturally rooted and may or may not promote health (Agner, 2020).

As with all other aspects of the OT process, evidence provides the foundation for determining whether the client would benefit from continued OT services. The *evidence focus* requires the identification of the available research regarding the duration of services for the type of client based on evaluation and reevaluation results. Additionally, theoretical perspectives, the therapist's experience with the intervention route and attainment of targeted

outcomes for similar clients, and the specific client's preferences in addition to their evaluation and reevaluation data must be considered when making the therapy decision. If the evidence supports that the client would benefit from continued OT services, then the targeted outcomes, goals, and intervention plan are modified as needed and intervention is resumed. At a predetermined time, another reevaluation is completed to systematically measure and to collect new data using the previously administered assessment tools. Based on the new reevaluation results, a therapeutic decision is made based on the evidence—both prior and new evidence—that either supports the continuation or discontinuation of OT services, and intervention and reevaluation is repeated until the targeted outcomes are attained, and the evidence supports the discontinuation of OT services. The more frequently the OT process is navigated, the more observant we are of the markers directing us to the evidence that support our professional reasoning in all aspects of the process. See OT Stories 18.6 and 18.7 for clinical examples of the outcomes component of the OT process.

OT STORY 18.6 OUTCOMES: DOES MARGARET CONTINUE TO NEED OCCUPATIONAL THERAPY SERVICES?

Margaret is 57 years old and sustained a right wrist fracture. She has been receiving OT services at an outpatient center since her cast was removed 3 weeks ago. When Pam, her occupational therapist, completed her initial evaluation, she had limited range of motion in her left wrist; decreased strength; experienced increased pain with movement; and reported difficulty performing her work activities (using a cash register/computer, answering the phone; filing), opening doors, washing dishes, unloading/loading the washer/dryer, lifting objects (pots, bags of groceries), taking the bus, driving, watching her 4-year-old great niece, and vegetable gardening. Upon reevaluation, Margaret's range of motion is within functional limits; her strength has increased and she is able to lift medium-weight objects—prefers using two hands for heavy objects; Margaret is able to perform her work activities using the strategies that Pam taught her—taking breaks, performing stretching exercises, varying her activities, and so on; she is able to open doors, take the bus and drive; she has resumed watching her great niece and within the past few days was able to weed and begin

preparing her garden for planting for short periods of time. Margaret reports minimal pain and only when lifting heavy objects or when performing activities that require strength and resistance (e.g., gardening). Margaret can perform her home activity and exercise program independently and is able to use the strategies that Pam instructed her in to upgrade her activities and exercises. Margaret reports that she feels that her wrist has improved and that she is able to do almost all her daily activities.

Questions
1. Have OT services positively impacted Margaret's ability to perform her daily occupations?
2. Can continuation of OT assist in resolving Margaret's occupational performance problems?
3. Has Margaret achieved the maximum benefit from OT services?
4. Does Margaret want to continue receiving OT services?
5. Is there sufficient justification for continuing OT services with Margaret?

OT STORY 18.7 OUTCOMES: DOES CHENG CONTINUE TO NEED OCCUPATIONAL THERAPY SERVICES?

Cheng is 27 years old and has schizophrenia. He currently lives in a group home. Cheng's most recent hospitalization was 6 months ago, and since that time, he has been working

with Bonnie, his occupational therapist, one time a week. His OT sessions have primarily focused on his work-related goal to maintain a part-time job. Cheng's OT interventions

(continued)

OT STORY 18.7 OUTCOMES: DOES CHENG CONTINUE TO NEED OCCUPATIONAL THERAPY SERVICES? (continued)

have addressed appropriate grooming and hygiene for the work setting; interpersonal skills with coworkers and customers; time management; work skills and patterns; initiation, sustaining, and completing work tasks; and compliance with work norms and procedures. Cheng recently began working part-time at a local grocery store stocking shelves in the evening. Bonnie has continued seeing Cheng for OT sessions to assure continuation of his work performance; however, because he has achieved his goal, he may be appropriate for discharge in the next few weeks. During Cheng's last session, he said that because he is now working and has an income, he would like to pursue living in his own apartment.

Questions

1. Has OT services positively impacted Cheng's ability to perform his daily occupations?
2. Can OT continue to assist in resolving Cheng's occupational performance problems?
3. Has Cheng achieved the maximum benefit from OT services?
4. Does Cheng want to continue receiving OT services?
5. Is there sufficient justification for continuing Cheng's OT services?

Conclusion

Occupation is fundamental to the OT process and is embedded with both the best available and comprehensive evidence and the individual occupational therapist's professional reasoning. In this chapter, we have provided a road map of the primary components of the OT process—evaluation, intervention, reevaluation, and continuation/discontinuation of services—to assist you in successfully navigating the OT services you provide to your clients. As you gain experience in reading road maps and navigating the OT process, we are confident that your use of the evidence and professional reasoning will correspondingly develop, assuring sound therapy decisions and successful outcomes in the OT journey you take with your clients.

Lippincott® Connect *For additional resources on the subjects discussed in this chapter, visit Lippincott Connect.*

REFERENCES

Agner, J. (2020). Moving from cultural competence to cultural humility in occupational therapy: A paradigm shift. *American Journal of Occupational Therapy, 74*(4), 7404347010p1–7404347010p87. https://doi.org/10.5014/ajot.2020.038067

American Occupational Therapy Association. (2020a). Occupational therapy practice framework: Domain and process, 4th edition. *American Journal of Occupational Therapy, 74*(Suppl 2), 7412411010p1–7412411010p87. https://doi.org/10.5014/ajot.2020.74S2001

American Occupational Therapy Association. (2020b). Occupational therapy's commitment to diversity, equity, and inclusion. *American Journal of Occupational Therapy, 74*(Suppl 3), 7413410030p1–7413410030p6. https://doi.org/10.5014/ajot.2020.74S3002

American Occupational Therapy Association. (2021). Standards of practice for occupational therapy. *American Journal of Occupational Therapy, 75*(Suppl 3), 7513410030. https://doi.org/10.5014/ajot.2021.75S3004

Brown, C. (2017). *The evidence-based practitioner: Applying research to meet client needs.* FA Davis.

Christiansen, C. H., Bass, J. D., & Baum, C. M. (Eds.). (2014). *Occupational therapy: Performance, participation, and well-being.* SLACK.

Cole, M. B., & Creek, J. (2016). *Global perspectives in professional reasoning.* SLACK.

Cole, M. B., & Tufano, R. (2019). *Applied theories in occupational therapy: A practical approach* (2nd ed.). SLACK.

Fisher, A. G. (2009). *Occupational therapy intervention process model: A model for planning and implementing, top-down, client-centered, and occupation-based interventions.* Three Star Press.

Fisher, A. G., & Marterella, A. (2019). *Powerful practice: A model for authentic occupational therapy.* Center for Innovative OT Solutions.

Holm, M. B. (2000). The 2000 Eleanor Clarke Slagle lecture. Our mandate for the new millennium: Evidence-based practice. *American Journal of Occupational Therapy, 54*(6), 575–585. https://doi.org/10.5014/ajot.54.6.575

Kramer, P., & Grampurohit, N. (Eds.). (2020). Evaluation: Where do we begin? In P. Kramer & N. Grampurohit (Eds.), *Hinojosa and Kramer's evaluation in occupational therapy: Obtaining and interpreting data* (5th ed., pp. 1–12). AOTA Press.

Law, M., Baum, C. M., & Dunn, W. (2016). *Measuring occupational performance: Supporting best practice in occupational therapy* (3rd ed.). SLACK.

Law, M., & MacDermid, J. (2013). *Evidence-based rehabilitation: A guide to practice* (3rd ed.). SLACK.

Reed, K. L., & Sanderson, S. N. (1999). *Concepts of occupational therapy* (4th ed.). Lippincott Williams & Wilkins.

Rice, M. S., Stein, F., & Tomlin, G. (2019). *Clinical research in occupational therapy.* SLACK.

Rogers, J. C., & Holm, M. B. (1989). The therapist's thinking behind functional assessment. In C. Royeen (Ed.), *Assessment of function: An action guide* (pp. 1–29). American Occupational Therapy Association.

Rogers, J. C., & Holm, M. B. (2009). The occupational therapy process. In E. B. Crepeau, E. S. Cohn, & B. A. Schell (Eds.), *Willard & Spackman's occupational therapy* (11th ed., pp. 478–518). Lippincott Williams & Wilkins.

Straus, S. E., Glasziou, P., Richardson, W. S., & Haynes, R. B. (2019). *Evidence-based medicine: How to practice and teach EBM* (5th ed.). Elsevier.

Taylor, R. R. (Ed.). (2017). *Kielhofner's model of human occupation: Theory and application.* Wolters Kluwer Health.

Wells, S. A., Black, R. M., & Gupta, J. (2016). *Culture and occupation: Effectiveness for occupational therapy practice, education, and research* (3rd ed.). AOTA Press.

Evaluating Clients

Inti Marazita, Thais K. Petrocelli, and Mary P. Shotwell

LEARNING OBJECTIVES

After reading this chapter, you will be able to:

1. Differentiate screening, assessment, and evaluation.
2. Apply the Occupational Therapy Practice Framework (OTPF) to the evaluation process.
3. Identify strategies for interviewing about, observing, and assessing occupational performance.
4. Understand personal, logistical, and contextual factors that influence the evaluation process.

Introduction

Occupational therapy (OT) evaluation is a foundational process that facilitates OT practitioners collaborate with clients and families to develop goals and plans for intervention. Evaluation involves using professional reasoning to make decisions about what information is needed about a client, what assessment tools might help the occupational therapist learn about a client's strengths and challenges, and what the assessment/evaluation results mean in terms of collaborating with clients to generate goals and a plan for intervention. In this chapter, we will review the process of evaluation. We will begin by defining terminology and discussing components of evaluation including referral, interview and occupational profile, specific assessment measures, interpretation and findings, as well as making recommendations for intervention. To guide our discussion of the evaluation process, we will consider the Occupational Therapy Intervention Process Model (Fisher & Jones, 2017) and the Occupational Therapy Practice Framework (OTPF), 4th Edition (American Occupational Therapy Association [AOTA], 2020a). Lastly, we will explore factors associated with evaluation such as the practice setting, the therapist experience, assessment tools, documentation systems, and cultural and ethical factors associated with evaluation.

Terms Relevant to Evaluation

In terms of evaluation, there are distinctions made between the terms *screening*, *evaluation*, *assessment*, *reassessment*, and *outcome* (Kramer & Grampurohit, 2020).

Screening

Screening is often the first part of the OT process and consists of a quick review of the client's situation to determine whether an OT evaluation is warranted. It may occur when a referral is made or may be a routine activity that a therapist does any time a new client enters a given practice setting (Kramer & Grampurohit, 2020). For example, in long-term care settings, it is a routine practice for newly admitted residents to be screened for potential to benefit from OT services. Once the therapist determines that the client might be a candidate for OT and it is agreed that the client may benefit from OT services, the evaluation process begins.

Evaluation

Evaluation is the term used for the whole process of obtaining and interpreting information needed for intervention planning and effectiveness review. This includes planning for and documenting both the evaluation process and the results (AOTA, 2020a). Niestadt (2000) posited that "Occupational therapy evaluation is both a set of procedures and a thought process" (p. 1).

According to the OTPF (AOTA, 2020a), evaluation consists of an "Occupational Profile" as well as an "Analysis of Occupational Performance" (p. S16). The "Occupational Profile" typically uses an interview process to understand the history and life experience of the client along with patterns of engagement in meaningful occupation. An "Analysis of Occupational Performance" uses observations as well as formal and informal assessment strategies to identify the client's strengths and challenges related to engagement in occupation (AOTA, 2020a). The AOTA has a template available on their website for completing an Occupational Profile (AOTA, 2021a).

The procedural part of the OT evaluation can consist of performing interviews, observations, standardized and non-standardized assessments, and hands-on strategies to understand the client's strengths and challenges in occupational performance. In reality, it may not be possible to fully separate evaluation from intervention, because practitioners maintain an evaluative view of clients throughout the OT process (screening to discharge). The thought process of evaluation uses all types of professional and clinical reasoning as the therapist considers medical, social, and/or educational diagnoses; contextual factors in the client's world; and pragmatic factors that influence the client and the intervention process (Kramer & Grampurohit, 2020).

Reevaluation, which is closely related to evaluation, is defined in the OTPF as "Reappraisal of the client's performance and goals to determine the type and amount of change that has taken place" (AOTA, 2020a, p. S82). Reevaluation enables the therapist to assess the client's response to intervention and to collaborate with the client to determine changes to the intervention plan.

Assessment

As part of the evaluation, therapists may need to gather specific information via the use of assessment tools. Kramer and Grampurohit (2020) describe an **assessment** as ". . . a specific tool, instrument or systematic protocol used as part of an evaluation to gather data and describe a client's occupational profile, client factors, performance skills, performance patterns, environment, or activity demands" (p. 3). An assessment can be informal or non-standardized in that the therapist uses interview or clinical observations to obtain data about occupational performance. Standardized assessments typically involve a process in which the client performs specific actions that are graded or rated by the therapist according to a predetermined set of criteria. Assessments can be *criterion-referenced* where the client is graded in terms of some behavioral standard or *norm-referenced* where the client is compared to a group of other people who have taken the same measure. In today's practice environment, it is often not practical to perform numerous assessments; therefore, it is critical that therapists judiciously choose assessment tools that will best measure occupational performance. Chapter 20, Critiquing Assessments, provides guidance about factors to consider in choosing tools to assess client performance.

Professional Standards Related to Evaluation

The occupational therapist is responsible for all aspects of the evaluation process. The AOTA Standards of Practice (AOTA, 2021b) state that "An occupational therapist, in collaboration with the client (person, group, or population), completes both an occupational profile and an analysis of occupational performance to evaluate and identify the client's needs, supports, and barriers to occupational performance" (p. 3). Using appropriate and relevant assessment strategies or tools, the therapist gathers and synthesizes data from the occupational profile and the assessment of occupational performance during the evaluation process. The therapist interprets information and makes recommendations for OT intervention and/or referral to other services from which the client may benefit.

OT practitioners must respond to referrals and procedures in a manner that complies with regulatory, agency-specific, financial, and ethical requirements. Verbal and/or written communication of evaluation findings should be provided within time frames as specified by practice settings, legal/regulatory, accreditation, and payer requirements. All communication regarding clients should be conducted within boundaries of ethics related to client confidentiality (AOTA, 2021b).

Occupational therapists may ask occupational therapy assistants (OTAs) to contribute to the evaluation process. Under the supervision of an occupational therapist, OTAs may perform and report findings from selected assessments for which they have service competency (AOTA, 2020b,

2021b). Chapter 71, Competence and Professional Development, provides more information about the process of establishing competence, and Chapter 30 discusses the overall differences in practice roles between the OT and the OTA.

Factors Associated With Evaluation

The process of evaluation may be influenced by the practice setting and reimbursement system in which the client is receiving OT services. Over the last several years, payment for OT evaluations has shifted from a time-based model to a value-based model where the evaluation process is influenced by the complexity of the client's circumstance (AOTA, 2016). The Current Procedural Terminology (CPT®) OT evaluation codes (used to bill for services) recognize the importance of clinical decision-making in the evaluation process (American Medical Association [AMA], 2017). The structure for CPT® Codes for evaluations identify three components which must be attended to during the evaluation process:

1. Occupational profile and history (both medical and therapy)
2. Assessment of occupational performance (including identifying performance deficits and client factors that impact engagement in occupations)
3. Clinical decision-making

In funding systems that use CPT® codes, the three above-mentioned components are considered when determining the level of complexity (high, medium, and low) of the evaluation (which is ultimately associated with payment for evaluations). In addressing the three components, the process is not necessarily sequential or linear. For example, the occupational profile and history is typically the first step in the process, but the clinician is gathering occupational history data throughout the whole evaluation by interspersing interview and history questions with the client while performing assessment-related activities. For more information on reimbursement and documentation, see Chapter 76, Payment for Healthcare Services, and Chapter 31, Documentation in Practice.

Because the process of evaluation is complex, novice OT practitioners will likely need assistance from a supervisor or mentor to enhance clinical decision-making as well as improving skills in assessment of occupational performance. Fortunately, AOTA has a variety of resources available to assist in clinical decision-making regarding evaluation. In particular, the AOTA Occupational Profile Template (AOTA, 2021a) considers the client's concerns regarding engagement in occupations, occupational history, personal interests, and values, as well as the client's perceptions about barriers to engagement in occupations.

There is an ongoing debate within the OT profession regarding the use of a top-down (occupation-focused) versus a bottom-up (focus on client factors/performance deficits) approach when performing evaluations. Dirette (2013) argues against an exclusive focus on occupation:

> If we go back to the past, however, we must not forget what we have learned along the way. For example, if we only evaluate and treat a person's ability to perform occupations following an acquired brain injury, we dissociate from what we have learned about the underlying neurologic causes and process of recovery. We must instead build on our body of knowledge through a careful and constant critique of our ideas. (p. 4)

Dirette (2013) as well as Hinojosa (2017) contend that it is not an "either/or" proposition, but rather an approach where we consider both "client factors" and occupation in our evaluation and intervention.

At times, particularly with complex situations, practitioners struggle in knowing what areas should be focused on during the evaluation. AOTA provides practice guidelines for certain diagnostic groups/populations which help the practitioner know what areas should be focused on during evaluation and intervention. AOTA also has helped practitioners working in skilled nursing and in home health settings by creating the OT Skilled Nursing Facility Evaluation Checklist as well as a Home Health Evaluation Checklist & Quality Measures Document (AOTA, 2021c). Within the Quality Toolkit that AOTA (2021c) has developed, there are also recommendations about standardized assessments and screening tools to help the OT know what quality indicators are measured in each context. Many of these documents are updated periodically, therefore maintaining membership in national and state organizations is critical to being aware about updates to policies and practice documents related to evaluation and assessment.

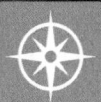

EXPANDING OUR PERSPECTIVES

Evaluating Holistically

Chi-Kwan Shea

I teach a course in OT evaluation of individuals who have neurologic deficits. My overarching goal is to instill in students a holistic approach to evaluating clients. Setting the tone of the course, I emphasize the importance of accurate evaluations and assessments to inform appropriate interventions. Furthermore, I repeatedly impress upon the students four major components in the evaluation process: (a) notice, (b) describe, (c) assess, and (d) interpret.

(continued)

Occupational therapists are uniquely trained in astute observation skills. When evaluating a client, the therapist ought to **notice** whatever matters to the client's participation and engagement in occupations. Whether reviewing documents, conducting interviews, or administering specific assessments, the therapist must heighten their awareness of all factors that could influence the client's occupations. As the therapist notices the influencing factors on occupations, the therapist must be able to **describe** them cogently in OT terms to clearly articulate the client's occupational profile, highlighting areas needing attention. These areas may be further **assessed** by collecting data to ascertain the client's current occupational performance status. Data collected from the assessments are then carefully **interpreted**, considering the complexity of the client, for the purpose of designing interventions to support occupational participation and engagement. This process repeats itself continuously throughout the therapeutic relationship. I gained these evaluation concepts from my volunteering at a community-based OT program for over 20 years.

As a volunteer occupational therapist for a grant-funded community-based program serving youth with psychosocial challenges, I occasionally evaluated youth clients such as Miguel. Sixteen-years-old, small in stature, articulate, and smiling often, Miguel was a student at a continuation high school, an alternative to traditional high schools for students who have experienced academic failure or behaviors identified by the school district as "problematic." During an interview to establish his occupational profile, Miguel shared with me his goal of going to college, although he had not been attending classes consistently and had only earned about 20% of academic units required for high school graduation. As the oldest of five siblings, he reported being very independent and hardworking. When not in school, Miguel assisted his uncle at construction sites, worked as a bouncer at a neighborhood night club, and often drank a six pack of beer with cousins on weekends. He was one of the 20% of students

in the continuation high school to have an Individualized Education Program, which addressed his reading and writing deficits as well as social-emotional regulation skill development. Miguel's school principal referred him to a life-skills training class provided by the OT program. The 60-minute weekly class throughout the semester comprised activities aimed at developing basic life skills such as leisure exploration, money management, vocational exploration, interpersonal communication, and health management.

Miguel's brief interview articulating his occupational goal to attend college is still memorable to me. I noticed and was able to describe his personal and environmental contexts as well as performance patterns, such as age, school factors and status, home factors and status, and work and social factors and status. Further assessments and interpretation were recommended, which included review of school records to identify alleged problem behaviors and school interventions, consultation with teachers and counselors to learn more about Miguel's academic strengths and challenges, assessments to discover his interests and strengths that may align with potential college majors, and investigation of home/family expectations, resources, potential barriers, etc. that might impact his education. Additionally, it was important to analyze his performance skills during the weekly OT life-skill training class. Throughout the semester-long OT intervention, the evaluation process was iterative. Miguel's therapists and I continued to notice and describe Miguel more deeply as a person and client as well as assess and interpret various aspects of his occupational performance, always with his college goal in mind.

I do not know about the eventual outcome of Miguel, as my volunteer assignments were not consistent, and I did not have the opportunity to follow through with most clients. However, as an occupational therapist, I marveled over what I learned about him through a holistic evaluation approach: Miguel was a whole person navigating a complex life and getting a little help from OT to pursue his goal of attending college.

Occupational Therapy Evaluation as Choreography

The practice of OT, like that of many service professions, is an art as well as a science. The science is evident in the methodical processes used by therapists as they explore client challenges and collaborate with the client to develop strategies for dealing with problems in daily living. The artistry in OT comes from the relationship or the connectedness with

the client's situation in order to generate individualized and creative solutions to help enhance quality of life (QOL). Part of the artistry in practicing OT is the ongoing dance that happens between evaluation and intervention throughout the OT process. Typically, throughout the evaluation phase, the therapist may be incorporating intervention strategies. Similarly, when implementing intervention, therapists gather data to evaluate the client's response and modify intervention accordingly. Evaluation does not only happen at the beginning and at the end of intervention; it should be happening throughout the OT process to explore effectiveness of intervention. The American Occupational Therapy

Association (AOTA) has published practice guidelines in many practice areas (e.g., Children and Youth; Productive Aging; Mental Health; Driving and Community Mobility. Available: www.aota.org) that give practice-specific strategies for evaluation and intervention for various diagnostic groups or populations.

The metaphor of dance provides a helpful way to examine the process, because in order to provide effective client-centered services, occupational therapists must "choreograph" the whole OT process (Figure 19.1). The process of choreography includes several components such as entering the studio, sources of inspiration, collaboration with others, elements of creation, making movement, composing the piece, and performing the piece (Canadian National Centre for the Arts, n.d.). Table 19.1 demonstrates parallels between choreographing a dance and the OT process.

Throughout the process of composing a dance, the choreographer must always keep in mind the "end product," which is the dance that will be performed before an audience. The choreographer considers all elements such as use of space, costume, set, and lighting, for example. Similarly, the occupational therapist must simultaneously consider evaluation, intervention, and discharge planning in light of

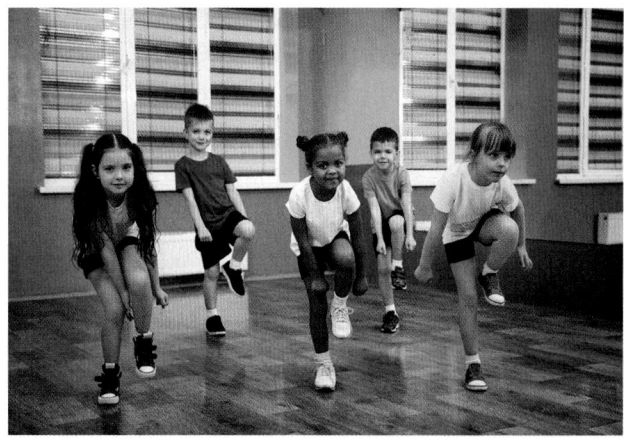

FIGURE 19.1 Just as these young dancers must attend carefully to each other in order to create an effective performance, occupational therapists must work with their clients to choreograph an evaluation that results in effective intervention.

client and contextual factors. Skilled practitioners carefully choose interview and assessment strategies that will most readily gather salient information to guide intervention.

TABLE 19.1	Metaphor of Dance Choreography of Dance to Occupational Therapy Process	
Element of Choreography in Dance	**Related Concept in the Occupational Therapy Process**	**Pragmatics With Clients in Occupational Therapy**
Collaboration Even the solo performer is dependent on stage people to adjust environmental factors including lighting, music, and costumes. The end product is a collaboration between the dancer and many other people.	Working "with" the client rather than "doing for" the client. Occupation therapists should also be aware of practitioners in other disciplines who might be working with the client and ensure collaboration in the best interest of the client.	Occupational therapist must ask the client what he or she wants to accomplish. Client must participate in goal setting rather than merely agree with goals you generate.
Studio The place where you do therapy (which may not be the place in which the skill is generalized)	The place where the dance is crafted, but the ultimate test is to perform the dance on a stage in front of an audience.	Occupational therapist must provide opportunities for skills to generalize to different settings, times, social situations, etc.
Elements The who, what, and where of the dance. What is the story the dance is trying to tell? Where will the dance be performed? What will the backdrop look like? What costumes will be worn?	Clients come with a multitude of factors that influence occupational performance. Similarly, therapists have their context that they bring to the OT process.	Occupational therapist's job is to figure out what needs to be emphasized during the OT process.
Making movement Deciding at what point in the music the dance will begin. Dancers must consider elements of timing, space, and props.	Typically, time must be spent on developing therapeutic rapport with the client, especially when dealing with sensitive or personal information. Therapists need to have some degree of logical flow through an assessment or an intervention session. In medicine, the physical assessment begins at the head and ends with private parts so as not to invade one's most intimate area at the beginning of the assessment.	Occupational therapist must consider time, tools, and therapist skills available for assessment.

(continued)

TABLE 19.1	Metaphor of Dance Choreography of Dance to Occupational Therapy Process (*continued*)	
Element of Choreography in Dance	**Related Concept in the Occupational Therapy Process**	**Pragmatics With Clients in Occupational Therapy**
Composition How does the piece flow from beginning to end? Are there "movements" in the piece that signify "chapters" in the story?	The more smoothly the assessment process flows, the more confidence the client has in the therapeutic relationship and in the potential outcomes of intervention. There needs to be some degree of transparency in the assessment process.	Occupational therapist must use time during an assessment wisely, often intertwining interviewing with other assessment measures.
Final step Any composition needs closure that signifies the conclusion and interpretation of the piece.	Clients typically expect some interpretation to be made at the end of the assessment session. Therapists are cautioned not to be too quick to make firm conclusions about the client's source of occupational performance problems; however, they should give some indication of possible sources and thus goals that might be used to address the occupational challenge.	Occupational therapist must know when to complete the evaluation process.

Novice therapists might not consider discharge planning until they are well into the intervention process, but more experienced practitioners know to treat each client visit as though it might be the last visit before discharge (or transfer to another setting). The OT evaluation typically follows a sequence that includes screening and referral, document review, interview and occupational profile, specific assessment measures, interpretation and findings, and recommendations for intervention.

Much like a beginning dancer, the novice OT practitioner is often somewhat clumsy and mechanical in interviewing, observing client performance, and in administering standardized assessments. Inexperienced therapists may be so concerned with their own performance (especially when being closely supervised) that they have limited ability to engage or enjoy the artistry of their practice. Focusing on the mechanics of performing an evaluation may result in limited mental reserves available for interpretation, synthesis, and documentation of findings. Expert occupational therapists seem to effortlessly flow through the "dance" of evaluation as they carefully choose interview questions and observe relevant performance factors. The seasoned therapist can demonstrate skilled reasoning to select appropriate assessment tools, seemingly knowing what questions to ask, what assessment tools to use, and when the evaluation is completed. Taking the metaphor of dance, a bit further, foundational texts on choreography will tell us that in order to compose a dance, there are factors that influence the outcome. Consideration of other factors that influence the process of evaluation will be our guide for the rest of this chapter.

Screening and Referral: Prelude to the Dance

In many practice settings, screening for services often occurs prior to referral for OT. In some settings, occupational therapists screen new clients as a matter of course, whereas in other settings, occupational therapists only screen clients as requested by other professionals such as nurses or teachers. In many long-term care settings, for example, all new residents are screened for their potential to benefit from therapy services as a way of potentially helping the client to transition to this new living environment. In school system practice, the therapist often engages with the teacher or a support team to screen students (often via observation or work samples) and makes recommendations (often in the form of adaptations) that the teacher might implement to see if problems can be abated. Should the child not respond to the support team recommendations, there is often a referral for an OT evaluation.

Screening involves gathering preliminary data about a client's challenges in occupational performance and determining whether the client may benefit from skilled OT services or perhaps referral(s) to other professionals. Screening is viewed as a "hands-off" approach where there is limited interaction between the client and the therapist, often taking the form of consulting with staff members or reviewing intake information on clients who are new to a facility or an agency. *The key things that the occupational therapist should look for in intake information are recent changes in living environment, health status, or occupational performance.* For example, in a long-term care environment, the client's records might be screened for recent history of falls or declines in performance of activities of daily living (ADL). In school system settings, screenings often take place after the student support team has recommended that the occupational therapist observe a student in a classroom and has given suggestions for the teacher to implement to enhance a child's classroom performance.

The mere presence of a diagnosis or clinical condition should not dictate whether a client is screened for or receives OT services; clients should be screened when they are experiencing challenges in occupational performance.

When dealing with caregivers, organizations, or populations, screening can be done by using results of surveys, needs assessments, incident reports, and population statistics that might influence occupational performance. Some examples of documents that might be used for determining whether OT screenings are needed for a group or population include the number of falls in a facility, the causes of back injuries to staff members, or national health statistics about secondary disability in a population of people with spinal cord injury.

Once it is determined that an OT evaluation is warranted, the practitioner receives the appropriate written referral as per agency policies and procedures. For example, in most medical settings, a physician order is necessary for an OT evaluation. In a school system setting, the referral for an OT evaluation usually comes from the student support team, the special education staff, or the school psychologist. Occupational therapists in the United States typically have the legal ability to provide OT services to a client without a referral from another professional, so clients can self-refer for OT services and they can self-pay; however, agency or payment requirements and mere pragmatics can be limiting factors in self-referral or self-payment.

Clients: The Source of Inspiration

In the arts, there are many sources of inspiration. In OT, an individual, group, or population could be the source that inspires the evaluation process. Fisher (2009) categorizes the client in three ways: (a) the "client" can be a "person" who seeks or is referred for OT services; (b) a "client constellation" that includes both the individual who seeks or was referred for services and others who are closely connected to that individual; and (c) a "client group" that includes people who share similar problems in occupational performance

(p. 3). Table 19.2 gives examples of terms and strategies for assessing different types of clients.

Regardless of the way in which we define the term *client*, a collaborative focus on occupation is critical in the OT process. This is true even when the therapist feels the client's goals are unrealistic.

Document Review: Understanding the Backdrop for the Dance

In many settings, there are client records that can provide useful information, such as demographic information, and often some type of history about the recent events or challenges experienced by the client. For example, in a medical or long-term care environment, the patient's record will discuss the reason for coming to the facility, procedures performed, and results of tests. In the educational setting, the student records may have reports from various professionals, results of educational testing, and an Individualized Education Plan (IEP) or a 504 Plan (student accommodations in educational settings) where appropriate. In the case of groups or populations, documents may include personnel files, incident reports, survey results, and statistics about a concern or health condition. For novice practitioners, as well as those new to a particular practice area, it can be difficult to identify which documents and what information should be the focus of the record review. Table 19.3 gives suggestions of potentially important documents to review by practice setting.

In medical settings, records will contain a history and physical, which reviews the systems in the body and the past medical history and provides consultation reports. The medical report, specialist consultation reports, progress notes, and results of testing can provide information vital

TABLE 19.2	Sample Terms and Assessment Strategies for Working With Different Types of Clients		
	Client	**Client Constellation**	**Client Group/Population**
Terms used to describe	• Patient • Student • Consumer • Resident • Member • Customer	• Family members • Caregiving staff • Teachers • Church groups • Support circle	• Class • Support group • Community • Staff • Organization or agency
Strategies for assessing needs	• Interview • Observation • Performance measures	• Interview • Self-efficacy surveys • Observation of performance	• Focus groups • Surveys • Reports • Performance measures
Considerations	• Client may self-advocate in a variety of ways to express their needs	• Being a caregiver does not necessitate OT involvement; caregivers must face challenges in their caregiving role to warrant intervention.	• Individual or group making the OT referral may have different opinions about the occupational performance challenges than do the individuals with whom you are directly working.

| TABLE 19.3 | Types of Documents Helpful in the Records Review Process | | |

Setting	Types of Documents Available	Important Notes	Tests and Lab Results
Medical	• Demographic sheet • Doctors' orders • Precautions • Consultation reports • Daily progress notes	• Nurses • Specialist notes • PT/SLP notes	• X-rays • Blood work • Cardiac/respiratory
Long-term care/ skilled nursing	• Demographic sheet • Doctors' orders • MDS/RUGs • Therapy plan of care • Daily notes	• Nurses • Specialist notes • PT/SLP notes	• X-rays • Blood work • Cardiac/respiratory
Educational	• Demographic sheet • Educational testing • Specialist reports • IEP/RtI (in public school systems)	• Teacher reports • Psychologist reports • Educational testing	• Hearing and vision screening • Psychological evaluation • Standardized testing
Outpatient/home health	• Demographic sheet • Discharge notes from medical setting • Initial evaluation from intake coordinator • OASIS • Therapy plan of care • IFSP (early intervention) • Progress notes	• Nurses • Specialist notes • PT/SLP notes	• X-rays
Mental health	• Demographic sheet • Doctors' orders • Consultation • Reports • Care plan	• Psychiatrist • Neuropsychology • Nursing • Mental health technician • Behavioral specialist	• Blood work (may be important to determine therapeutic levels of medications)
Group/ organization	• Reports of prior intervention • Incident reports • In-service logs • Meeting minutes • Survey or observation results	Must know who is requesting OT intervention. If the recipients are not the same people who requested the service, they may have a mistrust that the organization is employing OT services to find problems with individuals or groups.	Tests and lab results may be reported for groups and population, but these are typically reported by means and standard deviations and may not always be valuable in planning a group- or population-based intervention.
Population	• Request for proposal • Health statistics or community data		

IEP/RtI, Individualized Education Plan/response to intervention; IFSP, Individual Family Service Plan; MDS, minimum data set; OASIS, outcome and assessment information set; OT, occupational therapy; PT, physical therapy; RUGs, resource utilization groups; SLP, speech-language pathologists.

to the OT evaluation, such as reason for admission (e.g., diagnosis of a stroke or admission for a surgical procedure); and this "reason for admission" provides information about body systems/functions that might have an impact on occupational performance. During the review process, the practitioners must keep in mind the clients' occupational performance. A key understanding of the results of a history and physical can guide the therapist's choice of evaluation strategies as well as guide intervention. For example, a history and physical that lists sensory awareness as impaired would guide the therapist to interview and observe performance related to safety in the home environment. The history and physical, as well as sections regarding orders and test results, may guide the therapist to a particular action or precaution that may be indicated for a specific client. For example, when test results are indicative of a blood

clot, the client may be on bed rest; or when electrolytes are imbalanced, the therapist might notice that the client is mentally confused. When in doubt about anything in a client's records, the clinician should seek clarification from other staff members and/or the client/caregiver prior to initiating therapy.

The first thing that the OT practitioner should review is the reason for the OT referral. Often, the referral may read, "OT Eval and Treat," which is short for "perform an evaluation and provide interventions per OT guidelines." This open-ended language is good for our profession in that we can be client-centered; but for the novice practitioner, it provides little guidance about why the referral source believes this individual or group may need the services of an occupational therapist. The occupational therapist is cautioned against merely assuming that the diagnosis is the reason for the referral. For example, a client might be admitted to the hospital for a hip fracture and a walker is recommended for ambulation. However, the client has a former diagnosis of a left hemiplegia resulting from a stroke, which might impede use of a walker, which in turn may affect self-care. In this case, the occupational therapist may need to assist the client to compensate for inability to use their left upper extremity for holding onto the walker.

Once the clinician reviews the reason for the referral, the next step is to understand basic demographic information about the client. In many contexts in which individual services occur, there is a *face sheet* or some other introductory information sheet about the client that includes name, age, address, names of family members or guardians, diagnosis(es), education level or grade in school, and, in some settings, religious or spiritual preferences. This information can be used to get acquainted with the client more quickly by providing a starting point in the OT interview questions. For example, the client's *demographic sheet* in a medical setting might say that she is a retired teacher who lives with her sister in a large metropolitan area. These demographic characteristics might be used to ask the client about the sister's ability to help in the home or the availability of public transportation when the client returns home. In educational settings, there are often reports of the student's progress along with testing that also might be used to interview the student, teacher, or family member(s) about the student's strengths and challenges in the educational setting. In this way, the occupational therapist can begin to build an occupational profile of the client as well as anticipate possible occupational performance needs and challenges.

After reviewing the demographic information, the therapist then focuses on important data within a client's documentation that might be pertinent to the client, the setting, and the OT process. In a medical setting, particular attention might be paid to issues related to client safety that might include factors such as unstable medical status (vital signs, blood chemistry, seizures, presence of an infection, precautions, response to medication, etc.), history of falls or other injuries, unpredictable behavioral changes, and response to intervention thus far. Additionally, practitioners should consider social, emotional, contextual, and environmental impacts on the clients, such as traumatic events, marginalization experiences, homelessness, abuses, imprisonment, forced migration, etc. that would impact the client's readiness to communicate with or readily trust the practitioner. *In short, the therapist wants to know what to expect regarding potential adverse events that might influence evaluation and intervention.* The therapist might also use information about medical status to anticipate any potential communication difficulties in interviewing the client. For example, if the client is on a ventilator, it may be difficult or at least time consuming to obtain verbal responses. Similarly, if the record says that the client has unpredictable

behavioral changes, the therapist might want to modulate the initial interview so as not to agitate the client.

Understanding Client Precautions: Dancing Safely

In direct alignment with the concept of nonmaleficence from the OT Code of Ethics (AOTA, 2020c), a therapist must first "do no harm." Although implementation of this concept can take many forms within the OT process, in the evaluation phase practitioners must be aware of relevant precautions, as well as sociocultural and environmental factors that can impact physical and emotional safety. A therapist should review notes, doctors' orders, and other relevant documentation and note precautions that may impact the assessment process and client safety. In a best practice scenario, these precautions should also be reviewed with clients or caregivers at the start of the OT session if practical. Precautions may include those related to diet and swallowing, neurologic and orthopedic conditions (such as a lack of sensation or motion and weight-bearing restrictions), seizures, behavioral (particularly suicidal ideation) or cognitive impairments (particularly nighttime confusion in elderly clients), infection control (particularly important with clients who are immunosuppressed), open wounds or surgical sites, precautions related to medical devices, general cautions related to medications or blood chemistry (such as patients taking blood thinners need to take extra caution when shaving), and preparation for a procedure (such as restriction of water or food prior to testing). In addition, it is essential for an evaluating therapist to take note of facility-related precautions that may impact care. These might include disease-specific isolation protocols (such as COVID-19, MRSA, and *Clostridium difficile*), elopement precautions, specific patient handling techniques, behavior plans, color-coded fall precautions, and no-lift policies. See Chapter 32.

Critical Pathways: Script for the Dance

In many rehabilitation settings, therapists employ the use of interdisciplinary critical pathways as a guide for evaluation and intervention. Commonly used in settings with patient populations who have orthopedic impairments or strokes, rehabilitation teams generate typical pathways or "care maps" that guide clinicians about what evaluation and intervention activities should be done by each clinical discipline for each day or week of care. For example, a care plan for an older adult with a hip fracture in an acute care setting might include tasks to be accomplished on each day for the 3 days after an open reduction and internal fixation. Table 19.4 gives a sample of what might be included in the OT portion of a care plan.

TABLE 19.4	Sample of OT Aspects of a Care Plan for a Patient Who Has Received Surgical Procedure for a Hip Fracture	
	OT Assessment and Intervention	
Day 1	1. OT assessment completed within 24 hours after admission • Assessment of BADL • Interview regarding discharge plan and home environment • Assessment includes measurement of client factors such as ROM and strength in UE.	
Day 2	2. Client will sit up in chair. 3. Client will engage in and demonstrate use of long-handled equipment for dressing. 4. Client will be able to ambulate into bathroom with walker and transfer on and off commode with minimum assist.	
Day 3	5. Preparation for discharge home 6. Reassessment of neuromusculoskeletal factors, areas of occupation 7. Client will be able to perform transfers to and from toilet and tub bench with SBA. 8. Client will adhere to orthopedic precautions while performing mobility and ADL tasks.	

ADL, activities of daily living; BADL, basic activities of daily living; OT, occupational therapy; ROM, range of motion; SBA, stand by assist; UE, upper extremities.

Interview and Occupational Profile: Collaborating in the Dance

Once the "preparation" for the evaluation is completed, the therapist then meets the client and performs an interview to ascertain the client's perspective. Interviews can serve to uncover useful information regarding the client or proxy when standardized assessments are not appropriate. Interviews can span from highly structured to a free-flowing open-ended conversation depending on the needs of the client and the practice setting (Simon & Kramer, 2020). It can be structured in terms of using a standard agency-based form in which therapists ask questions and fill out a form. Conversely, there may be no guidance for the interview, and the therapist follows the client conversation to guide the interview questions. Just as we might learn about a dance partner while dancing with them, the interview is often interspersed with occupation-based assessment strategies. Regardless of the interview format, the therapist must ascertain some degree of information regarding the client's perceptions about occupational performance. As an occupational therapist, it is unique to our practice that invention should not proceed unless an appropriate occupational profile is conducted (AOTA, 2021d). The need for the completion of an appropriate occupational profile has been reflected in the recent changes in the American Medical Association CPT° evaluation codes for OT (AMA, 2017). As previously mentioned, AOTA has a template available for completing an occupational profile (AOTA, 2017c), although this task may take alternate formats depending on the practice setting and client.

Depending on the practice setting, therapists often find key questions that help them understand the occupational life of the client. Table 19.5 gives some typical questions asked in various practice settings along with typical spaces in which evaluations occur. A question such as "Tell me about a typical day?" often elicits information about what the client needs, wants, or is expected to do. The client response guides the therapist in knowing the occupations in which the client typically engages. To understand more about occupational challenges, therapists can ask the question: "What is the most stressful/least stressful time of day?" That may help the therapist know about activities that have different levels of demand for the client. Depending on the client's response to this question, the therapist may wish to probe further about why the client sees this time of day or a particular activity as challenging. For example, if you were to ask a client about the two times of day they find particularly challenging, the client might say (a) getting myself and my two adolescent children out of the house each morning and (b) coming home and deciding what to fix for dinner. The client's response might lead you to generate several hypotheses about their occupational challenges, which might include home or time management as well as caring for children, not to mention cooking.

A skilled therapist can quickly ascertain multiple patient factors while asking the patient simple, yet "high yield" interview questions. High yield questions are those few questions that will help us gather the most data. For example, knowing with whom a client lives or the type of housing that they anticipate returning to might be critical to discharge planning. The interview is an excellent opportunity to discover what patients need or want to do when they leave the hospital setting. The therapist gathers information about typical activities in which the client engages as well as the client's "home" environment and potential support the patient has, which may be critical factors in discharge planning. The interview is an excellent tool for gaining an overall picture of the patient's cognitive status (and is frequently the best and only method required, thus limiting embedding a cognitive evaluation). Finally, and most important, the interview helps establish rapport with clients. *A word*

TABLE 19.5	Sample Assessment Strategies in Various Practice Settings					
	Occupational Profile Questions	Focused Questions That May Elicit Rich Responses to Guide the OT Process	Observation Environments/Items Needed	Common Assessment Tools	Key Forms of Documentation	Important Considerations for this Setting
Acute care medical setting	• Before you came to the hospital, what was your typical day like? • What do you think a typical day will be like during the weeks after you are discharged from here?	What things might hinder you from going home?	Client's bed/chair and bathroom Wash basin, toothbrush, comb, etc.	• COPM • ROM • MMT • BADL • AMPAC 6-Clicks	• Standard evaluation form • Critical pathway • Daily progress notes	• Medical stability and necessary precautions. • Relationships with medical/nursing personnel.
Adult rehabilitation/long-term care setting	Tell me about a typical day for you. What do you need, want, or are required to do? In your home? In the community?	What things might hinder you from going home?	Client's bed/chair and bathroom, therapy area, ADL suite	• COPM • ROM/MMT • FIM • Cognitive-perceptual • BADL/IADL	• Standard evaluation form/plan of care • Daily/weekly progress notes	Medicare Part A requirements for clients' ability to tolerate therapy hours appropriate to the setting.
Home health	Tell me about a typical day for you. What do you need, want, or are required to do?	What do you need to be able to do to continue living at home?	Client's living, dining, and bedroom as well as kitchen BP cuff, gait belt, adaptive ADL equipment as needed	• COPM • BADL/IADL	• Standard evaluation form/plan of care • Daily/weekly progress notes	With Medicare funding, occupational therapists may not have permission to "open" a case; must be opened by nurse or physical therapist.
School system	To teacher: What is the student expected to do? To student: What kinds of things do you have to do at school? Like to do?	What subject is your (most/least) favorite? Who do you play with at recess? What games do you play at recess?	Classroom, playground, cafeteria, bathroom Pencil, paper, seating adaptations, visual and fine motor activities	• School function assessment • Quick neurologic screening test	• IEP; RtI • Daily or weekly progress notes • 6-month or annual reports • Handwriting assessment tools • Visual perceptual and visual-motor assessment tools	OT services are related and must be educationally relevant to educator-generated IEP goals.

(continued)

TABLE 19.5	Sample Assessment Strategies in Various Practice Settings (*continued*)					
	Occupational Profile Questions	Focused Questions That May Elicit Rich Responses to Guide the OT Process	Observation Environments/Items Needed	Common Assessment Tools	Key Forms of Documentation	Important Considerations for this Setting
Private pediatric setting	To parent: Tell me about your child and their role in your family. What things do you want them to be able to do?	For the parent: What is the worst/best time of day for you with your child? Tell me about your child's friends. Child: If you could do any play activity right now, what would it be?	Clinic, suspended equipment, tabletop activities, floor mobility activities, fine motor manipulatives	• Sensory Integration and Praxis Tests • Peabody Developmental Motor Scales • Bruininks-Oseretsky Test of Motor skills • Sensory Profile	• Initial evaluation report • Plan of care • Daily/weekly progress notes	Services often require prior authorization; therefore, therapists mustestimate number of visits requested.
Work-based setting	Tell me about your job. Tell me about your responsibilities at home. What do you do in your free time since you haven't been able to work?	What did you like best/least about your job? Your coworkers? Your boss? What do you see needing to happen for you to return to work or be retrained for another job? If you had a choice, would you return to your job or train for another job?	Actual or simulated work environment; work hardening setting/clinic	• Career interest inventories • Career aptitude measures • Focus on barriers to work performance, environment, body functions, performance skills	• Initial evaluation report • Plan of care • Daily/weekly progress notes	In order to delineate OT from other services, focus on the interaction of person-task-environment. Significant interaction with case managers.

ADL, activities of daily living; BADL, basic activities of daily living; COPM, Canadian Occupational Performance Measure; FIM, Functional Independence Measure; IADL, instrumental activities of daily living; IEP, Individualized Education Plan; MMT, manual muscle testing; OT, occupational therapy; ROM, range of motion; RtI, response to intervention.

of caution is advised about interviewing clients with cognitive impairment who may not have accurate insights about their performance or needs. In this case, the clinician may also interview family, friends, or staff who can offer insights about the client's occupational challenges. At the same time, one should still obtain the client's perspective, because the presence of cognitive impairment does not negate the need to understand and respond to the client's concerns.

The Canadian Occupational Performance Measure (COPM) (Law et al., 2014) is a standardized semi-structured client-centered interview to explore the client's perceptions about his or her current level of function in self-care, productivity, and leisure. The client is asked to identify the five most important problems in occupational performance. Using a visual analog scale ranging from 1 to 10, the patient is then asked to take each of these five problems and rate the importance and level of satisfaction with activity performance. The value in using the COPM is that a patient's perception can be used as an objective measure of progress,

which may be particularly valuable when progress is slower than expected or in cases where a client seems to be "higher functioning" but is having QOL concerns.

Therapists often intersperse observation of occupational performance or client factors with the interview. The most difficult part of this "dance" is knowing what questions to ask and when to ask them, because clients may not be able to focus on action and answering questions at the same time. It is also helpful to the client if the interview questions relate to the actions being performed. For example, the therapist may be asking the client to sit at the edge of the bed, and while the client is moving or resting after performing this action, the therapist may ask an interview question about anticipated difficulties getting in and out of bed when they go home. Brown (2009) notes that where possible, observation of a client in their natural environment can yield valuable information about the client's method of doing a particular occupation and can also help identify barriers to performing an occupation.

The Occupational Therapy Practice Framework: Backdrop for the Dance

The "Occupational Therapy Practice Framework" (OTPF) (AOTA, 2020a) notes the interview and occupational performance analysis to be effective tools to identify factors such as body functions that may be influencing occupational performance. During the interview, the therapist should ask clients about the following:

- **Occupations**
- **Contexts for occupational performance**—include cultural, personal, physical, social, temporal, or virtual
- **Performance patterns**—including habits, roles, and routines
- **Performance skills**—motor skills, process skills, and social interaction skills
- **Client factors**—body structure and function
- **Activity demands**—objects used, space demands, social demands, sequencing, required actions, and body functions or structures that the patient typically performs in his or her daily life activities

The online resources listed on the Willard & Spackman website provide a sample evaluation form, which is adapted from a sample evaluation by Shotwell et al. (2017) containing ideas similar to those of the OTPF.

Strategies for Assessment: Adding Elements to the Dance

Tables 19.6 to 19.13 provide examples of how a practitioner might incorporate concepts described in the OTPF (AOTA, 2020a). These tables are not necessarily in the order presented in the Practice Framework because the practice of OT is an art and a science in which the evaluation process may not follow a prescribed sequence. Nevertheless, the evaluation typically begins by understanding the client's perception of their own performance in areas of occupation. Clients should be asked about a typical day to understand the areas of occupation in which the client engages. In addition to interviewing and understanding client perceptions, the evaluation should also include if applicable the use of standardized assessment tools for areas in which the therapist seeks further information. The use of standardized assessment tools also contributes to the goal of our profession to provide evidence to support our practice.

In evaluating the areas of occupations, the therapist intends/aims to find out about basic or personal activities of daily living (BADL or PADL) as well as instrumental activities of daily living (IADL) that are necessary to "run our lives." Some of the IADL occupations include managing finances, cleaning the home, shopping for goods and services, and so forth. Therapists need to ascertain whether the client is having difficulties with sleep, rest, work, school, or participation in leisure activities. In acute medical situations, clients may not think about ADL or occupational performance and may assume that these skills will immediately return once the body functions or body structures are restored to health. Although this may be true in some cases, occupational therapists can often ease the process and reduce the time that it takes a client to engage in desired occupations. In many cases, this can alleviate the need to stay in a congregate care facility (e.g., hospital, nursing home, or assisted living facility) and help to enhance the individual's QOL. In institutional environments, it may be difficult to have the client engage in some of the IADL tasks during the evaluation process; so many times, information is gathered via interview rather than actual occupational performance. Table 19.6 gives some strategies for assessment of areas of occupation.

TABLE 19.6 Sample Strategies for Evaluation of Areas of Occupation

	Examples of Standardized Measures	Interview/Observational Strategies
Overall areas of occupation	• AOTA Occupational Profile • Canadian Occupational Performance Measure (COPM) • Occupational Performance History Interview II	• Ask the client about a typical day.
Basic activities of daily living (BADL)	• Barthel Index • Routine Task Inventory • Performance Assessment of Self-Care Skills	• Observe client dressing, bathing, feeding, etc.
Instrumental activities of daily living (IADL)	• Kohlman Evaluation of Living Skills • Executive Function Performance Test • Performance Assessment of Self-Care Skills	• Observe client doing a shopping, budgeting, or cooking task.
Health management	• Coping Inventory/Early Coping Inventory • Wellness Model Evaluation (Swarbrick & Yudof, 2015)	• When presented with a task that challenges a client's competence, does he or she become frustrated or defeated? • Is the client's response to his or her situation proportional to the magnitude of client's challenges?

(continued)

TABLE 19.6 Sample Strategies for Evaluation of Areas of Occupation (*continued*)

	Examples of Standardized Measures	Interview/Observational Strategies
Education/work	• School Function Assessment • School Assessment of Motor and Process Skills • Worker Role Interview	• Observe clients doing a work-related or school-related task.
Play/leisure	• Transdisciplinary Play-Based Assessment • Leisure Assessment Inventory	• Observe a child on the playground.
Social participation	• Evaluation of Social Interaction Skills • Social Interaction Scale of the Bay Area Functional Performance Evaluation (BaFPE)	• Note interaction during the interview. • Ask the client about his or her social life. • Observe in structured and nonstructured social environments.
Rest/sleep	• National Institutes of Health Activity Record • Pittsburgh Quality of Sleep Inventory	• Do you have difficulty with sleeping?

Assessing Overlapping Occupational Concerns: Composition of the Dance

To say that occupation is complex seems to be an understatement. Many times, it is not one occupation that is problematic, but, often, the interface among various occupational demands may be causing difficulty in occupational performance. This orchestration of various occupational demands can be challenging just as it can be challenging for dancers to combine different dance elements. For example, I am quite capable of cooking and cleaning, but my role as a worker and as a parent often supersede my engagement (or motivation) to engage in these tasks necessary for the "job of living." OT Story 19.1 provides an example of an individual who was working in a sheltered workshop setting. Although this client was successful in performing work-related tasks, the client had difficulty transitioning from sheltered to community-based employment because

of occupational performance concerns regarding hygiene and clothing management.

After understanding the client's areas of occupational engagement, the therapist begins to examine various factors that may facilitate or hinder occupational performance. Contexts should be first considered and then the performance pattern before looking at the performance skills and client factors. Client factors include values, beliefs, and spirituality; body functions; and body structures. In many settings, the focus of OT evaluation and intervention is on body functions, such as cognition, sensory, and neuromusculoskeletal functions; but therapists are cautioned to recognize the importance of values, beliefs, and spirituality on both the therapeutic relationship and the whole OT process.

A point worth mentioning in terms of client factors is that the term *spirituality* is meant in the broadest sense rather than religiosity. Although religion may provide a sense of spirituality, people may have many factors that influence their sense of inner peace and focus. When interviewing clients, the therapist may ask what activities give

OT STORY 19.1 TRAVIS: COMBINING WORK AND SELF-CARE FOR EFFECTIVE PARTICIPATION

Travis is a 47-year-old man who is participating in a vocational program that includes community placements and "sheltered workshop" employment. The goal of the agency is for all clients eventually to be employed in community-based settings; but the staff is concerned about Travis, not because of his work skills but because of his hygiene. Travis had been involved with this agency for the past 2 years, and the staff reports that he is capable of learning new jobs and could perform simple one- to two-step work tasks such as placing labels on boxes or repackaging materials for store display. The staff is concerned that they cannot move Travis into a community-based position because he needs constant cueing to brush his teeth and take a shower. When picking Travis up on the facility bus each morning, the bus

driver states that at least once or twice a month, she does not allow Travis to get on the bus because of his poor personal hygiene (which is a requirement for participating in the program). When Travis was told that he needed to go back into his home to shower, Travis would do so, but he seemed to have limited insight regarding why personal hygiene was necessary for successful work performance.

Questions

1. Why do you think that Travis has difficulty with his habits of self-care?
2. What contextual factors might be influencing Travis' difficulties in self-care?

them a sense of peace and calm. Client responses are often indicative of spirituality. Typical answers from clients might be "prayer," "meditation," "being out in nature," "petting my dog," and "being with family." Table 19.7 lists some possible measures and questions a therapist might attend to regarding values, beliefs, and spirituality. See Chapter 59.

In many practice settings, the focus of evaluation and intervention is on client factors such as the body functions of cognitive, sensory processing, or neuromusculoskeletal

factors that influence occupational performance. Body functions can be evaluated via the use of standardized assessment tools or through interview and observation. In medical or rehabilitation settings, typically, body functions such as sensory functions and neuromusculoskeletal functions are emphasized, but the therapist should always keep in mind that impairments in these functions do not necessitate dysfunction in occupation. Table 19.8 gives potential strategies for evaluating body functions.

TABLE 19.7 Sample Strategies for Evaluation of Client Factors—Values, Beliefs, and Spirituality

	Examples of Standardized Measures	Interview/Observational Strategies
Values, beliefs, spirituality	• Canadian Occupational Performance Measure (COPM) • Quality of Life Inventory • Health-Related Quality of Life • Multidimensional Measurement of Religiousness/Spirituality for use in Health Research.	• Tell me about your life . . . Family? Work? Social? • For some people, their religious or spiritual beliefs act as a source of comfort and strength in dealing with life's ups and downs; "is this true for you?" • Do you engage in any practices that enhance your spirituality? • What is the most important (occupation) for you to be able to do?

TABLE 19.8 Sample Strategies for Evaluation of Client Factors—Body Functions

Body Functions	Examples of Standardized Measures	Interview/Observational Strategies
Specific mental functions	• Allen Cognitive Level Screen • Executive Function Performance Test	• Have you noticed a change in your ability to remember, to pay attention, or to follow directions?
Global mental functions	• Montreal Cognitive Assessment • St. Louis University Mental Status Exam	• Have you noticed a change in your mental abilities?
Sensory functions and pain	• Sensory profile (all ages) • McGill pain questionnaire • Vision or hearing screening	• Do you have numbness or tingling anywhere in your body? • Do you have pain? Where? Type? Duration? What makes it better? • Do you have difficulty tuning out specific sensory things in the environment (noise, visual distractions, and things next to your body)? • Do you have difficulty getting aroused or calmed down?
Neuromusculoskeletal and movement-related functions	• Quick neurologic screening • Range of motion or manual muscle testing • Berg balance scale	• Notice coordination, strength (effort), or difficulty moving. • If you notice difficulty in the above, you might ask this: • Do you have a history of falls? • Do you have difficulty bending, reaching, or grasping?
Voice and speech functions	• Usually done by observation rather than formal assessment, which is typically done by a speech-language pathologist.	• During the interview, note particularly soft or loud voice, ability to articulate words, or difficulties in expressive or receptive language. • Ask client to talk after eating or drinking (a "wet" sounding voice may be indicative of swallowing problems).
Organ system function (cardiovascular, respiratory, hematologic, immunologic, digestive, metabolic, endocrine, genitourinary, and reproductive functions)	• Pulse oximetry, blood pressure; pulmonary function test. Occupational therapists may be involved in a modified barium swallow study, which is designed to view the swallowing functions, or they may administer the Swallowing Ability and Function Evaluation (SAFE)	• When working with clients who are on digital monitor, therapist can note changes in these numbers during the occupational therapy (OT) session. For example, a client may be comatose but have changes in heart rate or blood pressure when the therapist moves an extremity during fabrication of a splint. OT practitioners should be keenly aware by looking, feeling, and listening to changes in body functions as evidenced by changes in sweating, color of skin, respiration patterns, and so forth, because these may be signs of organ system changes.

In addition to understanding the client's body functions, therapists must have some appreciation for body structures that might have potential to influence occupational performance. Although these are not typically evaluated in a formal manner, therapists (particularly those working with clients with more acute medical concerns) must have awareness of these areas. Information about body structures can be gathered via test results such as the laboratory reports or x-rays. Many of the diagnostic procedures performed by medical specialists are designed to evaluate body structures. Table 19.9 lists potential strategies for evaluation of body structures.

Ultimately, it is the goal of OT to help a client enhance occupational performance. Our job as therapists is to identify which components of occupation, context, performance patterns, performance skills, and client factors are causing the greatest challenge and to remediate or compensate for these challenges to enable performance. Therapists must assess how clients use body functions and structures to perform given skills that comprise occupations. For example, the authors of this chapter could have the body "structures" necessary to see and to move their fingers to type this chapter, and they could have the body "functions" such as global and specific mental functions necessary to organize their thoughts for ideas to write this chapter, but they could have great difficulty in enacting the occupation of "professional writing." Their difficulties could be in performance skills (initiating, attending, or problem-solving to find good references) or with performance patterns (e.g., not making the time to write or conflicting roles between that of writer and parent). Tables 19.10 and 19.11 give potential strategies for how a therapist might evaluate occupational performance skills and performance patterns that may include both standardized assessment tools and interview.

TABLE 19.9 Sample Strategies for Evaluation of Client Factors—Body Structures

Body Structures	Evaluation Method	Interview/Observational Strategies
• Nervous system • Eyes, ear, and related structures • Structures involved in voice/speech • Structures related to movement • Skin and related structures • Organ system structures (cardiovascular, respiratory, immunologic, digestive, metabolic, endocrine, genitourinary, and reproductive systems)	Not typically evaluated by an occupational therapist because occupational therapists do not evaluate structures independent of a functional/purposeful activity. Many of the diagnostic procedures that physicians request would be used to assess body structures. An example might be an x-ray, an angiogram, or a magnetic resonance imaging, which are all designed to view structures and any potential abnormalities.	Much of this information can be found in clients' records. Look for history and physical that details prior injuries, procedures, and tests that the client may have undergone. Although the questions below are not necessarily indicative of a structural problem, positive client responses may be indicative of potential difficulties with body structures (and certainly warrant further evaluation and/or referral). • Do you have numbness, tingling, or difficulty moving? • Do you have any trouble with your eyes or hearing? • Do you have any wounds right now? Difficulty with skin healing? • Have you had any procedures for your heart, lungs, stomach, or reproductive system?

TABLE 19.10 Sample Strategies for Evaluation of Performance Skills

Performance Skills	Examples of Standardized Measures	Interview/Observational Strategies
Overall performance	• Assessment of Motor and Process Skills	Watch a client engage in an activity of daily living (ADL) that involves neuromusculoskeletal, cognitive, and social interaction, which may give some overall picture of performance.
Motor	• Jebsen Hand Function Test • Peabody Developmental Motor Scales	Observe the client as he or she engages in occupational tasks. Does he or she have a tremor? Slowness or problems with speed of movement? Is the accuracy of movement impaired? Does the client seem to have difficulty executing movements necessary for functional tasks?
Cognitive	• Executive Function Performance Test • Routine Task Inventory • Performance Assessment of Self-Care Skills	Does the client seem to have difficulty initiating, sequencing, terminating, problem-solving, and so forth, during occupational performance?
Social interaction skills	• Assessment of Communication and Social Interaction • Vineland Adaptive Behavior Scales	Is the client able to communicate his or her needs, wants, desires?

TABLE 19.11	Sample Strategies for Evaluation of Performance Patterns	
Performance Patterns	Examples of Standardized Measures	Interview/Observational Strategies
• Habits • Roles • Routines/rituals	• Role Checklist • Adolescent Role Assessment • Self-Discovery Tapestry • Worker Role Interview • National Institutes of Health Activity Record • OPHI; OCAIRS	• Tell me about a typical day for you. • May have to structure questions into categories for self-care, homemaking, work/school, social/leisure activities.

OCAIRS, Occupational Circumstances Assessment-Interview Rating Scale; OPHI, Occupational Performance History Interview.

Assessing the Environment and the Demands: The Setting for the Dance

The choreographer must know the setting for the dance and the type of dance to be performed. If the stage has a different type of flooring or lighting on which the dancers are not familiar, the rehearsal period may need to be extended. Additionally, if a dance requires a high degree of athleticism, the choreographer or director will choose dancers who excel in strength and endurance because of the demands of the piece to be performed. Similarly, the occupational therapist needs to understand the context in which occupations are performed and how those tasks are typically performed. When it is not possible to be in the real environment, the therapist asks questions about the environment and the ways in which the client typically performs tasks. This may include asking questions about location, surfaces, heights of various objects or surfaces, tools used, and social or cognitive aspects of task performance.

Table 19.12 gives strategies for evaluation of context and environment. Although many occupational therapists tend to focus on the physical environment, one must also consider other aspects of the environment that can influence occupational performance. Consider the case of Harlan in OT Story 19.2 who was gainfully employed but underproductive in his work environment. In this case, the OT practitioner's main interest was in a contextual evaluation of Harlan's work area(s), tools, tasks, and social and cultural aspects involved in productive employment.

In addition to looking at the client's context, we also need to understand the client's occupational performance; therefore, the therapist must have an appreciation of activity demands which are described in Table 19.13. In reviewing the "activity demands" of Harlan's position at this grocery store, the therapist reviewed the job description used for all people in his same position. Job descriptions can provide some guidance about the tools, space, and body functions required for a specific job. In the workplace, "essential functions" are often made explicit in job descriptions; however, for some roles, essential functions are not as clear (e.g., homemaker and hobbyist); therefore, the activity demands are evaluated by interviewing the client about how they perform the activity and the specific tasks associated with the activity. For example, one client may do laundry by going

TABLE 19.12	Sample Strategies for Evaluation of Context	
Area of Context in OTPF	Interview/Observational Strategies	Examples of Standardized Measures
Cultural	• Are there special rituals, foods, practices in which you engage?	• Alberta Context Tool
Personal factors	• Where do you live? Work? Engage in leisure? With whom? • Do you prefer to do things alone or with others? • With whom do you live? Other sources of social support?	• Work Environment Impact Scale • School Setting Interview • Classroom Environment Scale • Alberta Context Tool • World Health Organization (WHO) Quality of Life-BREF
Environmental factors	• Tell me about your home. • Try to identify potential barriers/strengths. • What is the best/worst time of day for you or your family? • Do you use the Internet, e-mail, cell phone, etc.? • For what purposes? Shopping, communicating?	• Safety Assessment of Function and the Environment for Rehabilitation (SAFER) • Person-Environment Fit • In-Home Occupational Performance Evaluation (I–HOPE) • National Institutes of Health (NIH) Activity Record • World Health Organization (WHO) Quality of Life-BREF

For further details, please see the OTPF. OTPF, Occupational Therapy Practice Framework.

OT STORY 19.2 HARLAN: CONTEXTUAL AND ACTIVITY DEMANDS

Harlan, who is cognitively impaired, is employed at a grocery store, and his manager noticed and questioned that Harlan's productivity and accuracy were not consistent with nondisabled employees in the same position. The occupational therapist observed Harlan in the grocery store and noticed that the store employers and employees had experienced and were currently working with clients with varying abilities. Additionally, there were posters around the break room that supported the company's efforts to promote diversity, which might be indicative that the cultural context of this organization was to support diversity practices including the hiring of people with disabilities. The therapist also noticed that all the associates took time to speak with each other, particularly the employees with disabilities to "make them feel special." Although this culture of social acceptance of people with disabilities was desirable, there seemed to be "lower" expectations of the employees with disabilities. The therapist observed that it took Harlan at least 15 minutes

to empty one trash can, and he took 30 minutes to sweep a small area near the pharmacy section. The therapist also noticed that most workers seemed to be hurried about their work and that the temporal context of the workplace was to enable customers to get out of the store as efficiently as possible. Harlan's slowness in work performance was not consistent with the temporal demands of the environment.

Questions

1. What aspects of this work environment/organization might be important to consider and evaluate?
2. When working within an organization, how do we balance the needs of the individual versus the group/organization in our evaluation?
3. In what ways might an OT address the group/population needs in the evaluation process to advocate for diversity, equity, and inclusion within an organization?

TABLE 19.13   Strategies for Evaluation of Activity Demands

Activity Demand	Interview/Observational Strategies
Relevance and importance	• How is this activity meaningful?
Objects used and their properties	• Do you have all the tools needed to do the activity? • Weight, size, amount of resistance of various objects/tools
Space demands	• Environmental considerations (social, cultural, physical, etc.) • Organization of space and materials
Social demands	• Do you "have" to do this task or "want" to do it? • Is this a task that you enjoy? If not, have you tried to get someone else to help you with the task?
Sequencing and timing	• Frequency; repetitions and duration of a task/subtask • Temporal components of the task (speed, sequencing, flow) • Is this a task that could be broken up into parts? Must all the steps of the task need to be done in one time period?
Required actions and performance skills	• What cognitive, motor, and social interaction skills are required to perform this activity?
Required body functions	• **Neuromusculoskeletal:** difficulty in bending, reaching, gripping, stiff or effortful movement; Does it involve climbing, stooping, and frequent bending or prolonged body position? • **Sensory functions:** missing one aspect of the visual field on a consistent basis; sensation related to position and balance; detection and discrimination of sound; feeling of touch from other and various textures; apparent lack of awareness of the body in space; what is the perception pain? • **Specific and global mental functions:** easily frustrated; tends to work alone; does not share materials; becomes easily discouraged; seeks constant reinforcement or never asks for help; passive; disinterested; hyper-focused; lack of ability to transition; forgetting the steps to a task; doing the task inaccurately or incorrect sequence; forget what you were doing during this or other tasks?
Required body structures	• Required strength, joint mobility, respiratory status, etc. • Do you need to sit or rest during this activity? Do you become short of breath or fatigued?

to a commercial laundry facility, whereas another client must go to the basement in her home to do laundry (see Figure 19.2). The fact that the demand for one person may require driving or walking a distance to access a laundry facility may be a barrier for the first client, whereas ascending and descending steps to do laundry may create a barrier for the second individual.

Typically, after the client has identified their valued activities, the therapist can probe further about the activity demands of these tasks because people vary greatly in task

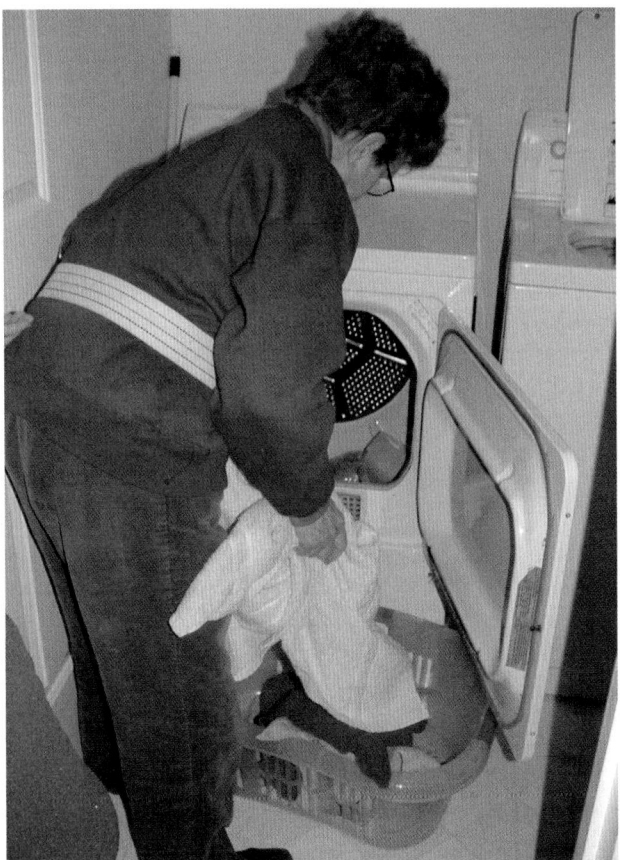

FIGURE 19.2 As part of the evaluation process, clients are observed performing tasks that are important to their daily routines. This requires attention to safety as well as the quality of performance. This client is wearing a gait belt because she has problems with balance when she bends over. In this way, the therapist can observe her routine performance but be ready to support her if needed. (Photo courtesy of Mary Shotwell.)

demands based on all the other factors involved in an analysis of occupation. Therapists are cautioned about making judgments about the "right or wrong" way to perform an occupation. If we are to facilitate occupational performance, we need to address strategies to learn or resume occupations that they are most comfortable, rather than using our preferred method of occupational engagement.

Another strategy for understanding the activity demands is to observe clients engaging in their valued occupation. The ability to see clients actually performing a task in their own environment using their own tools and space is most optimal, although this may not be possible in clinical settings. Therapists are encouraged to simulate occupational performance to best analyze the fit among the "person" (personal contexts, client factors, performance skills, performance patterns), the "environment" (cultural, physical, temporal, social, etc.), and the "task" (activity demands). In the case of Harlan, the therapist wanted Harlan to stay gainfully employed; however, the therapist questioned the match between the person, the task, and the environment. The therapist's report and recommendations for intervention would have to take person, task, and environment into account in order to help Harlan be successful in his employment. The chapters in Unit VII, as well as Chapter 35, Ecological Models in Occupational Therapy, provide more information about the unique interplay between person, environment, and occupation as we perform evaluations.

Factors Influencing the Evaluation Process

Just as the choreographer may be influenced by the potential audience, the space, the budget, and the artistic desires of various stakeholders, so, too, is the occupational therapist influenced by ethics, reimbursement, organizational factors, and requirements for documentation. First is the Occupational Therapy Code of Ethics (AOTA, 2020c), in which all principles seem to apply to evaluation and intervention. Beneficence and nonmaleficence apply to safety and doing what is in the best interest of the client. Autonomy and confidentiality relate to respecting the rights and privacy of clients throughout the OT process. The ethical principle of duty relates to maintaining professional competence and using the best evidence available to provide client care. Procedural justice relates to evaluation and intervention in that the occupational therapist must comply with laws and policies guiding the OT profession.

In terms of complying with laws and policies, occupational therapists speak to many audiences in their communication regarding evaluation and intervention. Not only do facilities have specific requirements for what should be included in evaluation and progress reports but accreditation agencies as well as funding organizations often require specific factors be attended to in OT practice. This being said, occupational therapists need to be mindful in preventing non-OT personnel dictating what should be included in OT evaluation and intervention planning as well as documentation. In order to advocate for OT, practitioners are advised to keep abreast of laws, policies, and the professional evidence regarding our practice.

Interpretation and Intervention Planning: Doing the Dance

Practitioners use their professional reasoning to interpret results of interview, observation, and assessment(s). Typically, the interpretation involves making some judgment about the client's strengths and challenges regarding occupational performance. The therapist makes a statement about the client's ability to benefit from therapy and predicts the duration, frequency, and type of intervention strategies that will likely be used. In some organizations, the use of a "critical pathway" may guide these decisions; however, one must keep in mind that critical pathways are based on statistical means and may not apply to all individuals.

Once the therapist determines that the client may benefit from OT services, long- and short-term goals are formulated in collaboration with the client. Long-term goals may be accomplished in days, weeks, or months depending on the intervention context. Therapists must estimate the number of visits that a client will require, so they must have some idea about typical lengths of stay or the number of visits that a client might need for their specific concerns. In the acute care setting, the length of stay can be as short as one day, so the evaluation, intervention, and discharge plan may all occur within the same day. For example, a client with an orthopedic condition may have an evaluation, receive adaptive equipment and education in its use, and be ready to go home. In this situation, the therapist may believe that the client will need follow-up OT services in his or her own home.

Client goals should be behaviorally oriented in terms of what the client will do. For example, the goal might read, "Client will participate in education regarding . . ." rather than "therapist will educate client about . . . ." Goals should be timed and measurable, which is often a challenge for the novice therapist who has little experience knowing how long it will take a client to achieve a goal, let alone being able to identify the benchmark for successful outcome(s) of services. When generating individualized goals and intervention plans, the therapist must consider person, task, and environment. Intervention plans typically consider a multitude of factors such as medical stability and contextual factors of the client, home environment, available social support, and task/activity demands.

Evaluation of Groups and Populations: A Group Dance

In recent years, there has been a shift toward maintaining one's health by engaging in meaningful health and wellness activities. OT's paradigm is shifting to include health and wellness at the group and the individual level to prevent illness. Pizzi and Richards (2017) note that a paradigm shift is necessary to direct focus onto well-being as well as QOL as a primary outcome of OT services delivered to individuals, communities, and populations. To that end, they advocate for evaluation strategies that focus on measurement of

QOL. As such, occupational therapists are becoming more involved within communities and providing services to groups and populations.

How would an occupational therapist screen and evaluate members of groups and populations? Just as a disc jockey or a dance instructor would scan the audience to determine the mood and the synchronicity of the group to decide the right song to dance to, the occupational therapist will screen (scan) the group or population by developing a community profile. Fazio (2017) defines a community profile as "a comprehensive description of the needs, resources, assets, and capacities of a population" (p. 99). An occupational therapist gathers information to establish a community profile by performing a needs assessment. The intent of a needs assessment is to uncover the current make-up of a community but most importantly to identify unaddressed needs within a group and/or population. Understanding the resources within a community can inform the occupational therapist of the types of supports, resources, and barriers that may enhance or impede occupational engagement. Having a thorough understanding of the landscape of a community will lead to developing effective occupation-based programming that will enhance the QOL of members within groups and populations.

When we think of populations, frequently we think about diagnostic populations. As mentioned previously, AOTA provides practice guidelines for various diagnostic groups and practice settings which mention evaluation. AOTA has also joined forces with the Emergency Care Research Institute Trust (ECRI, 2021) which has specific practice guidelines for certain populations with whom occupational therapists might work. The goal of ECRI is to be a clearinghouse for practice guidelines that are evidence based as well as promoting patient safety. Within many of these practice guidelines, there are specific suggestions for items which might be included in evaluations for certain diagnostic groups. Although the ECRI guidelines may be valued for certain groups, they are not inclusive of all populations including but not limited to homeless population, disaster victims, and imprisonment. The OTPF provides an overview of the evaluation process for groups and populations (AOTA, 2020a). See also Chapter 22, Occupational Therapy Interventions for Communities and Populations, for more specific guidance.

Conclusion

In this chapter, we have reviewed the OT process of determining needs for clients, groups, and populations. The therapist must be skilled/mindful at interspersing interviews with assessment and maximizing the time allotted to complete an evaluation in order to best reflect the client's concerns regarding occupational performance. Like well-planned choreography, effective evaluation requires attention to multiple factors. When done well, the "dance" of therapy flows from evaluation to intervention. In this process, the clinician is challenged to consider contextual factors of the client as well as the practice setting and to incorporate the use of interviews, observation, and standardized assessment tools where possible. Using guides for evaluation such as the AOTA Practice Framework (OTPF) (AOTA, 2020a) and the AOTA Standards of Practice (AOTA, 2021b) may aid the occupational therapists' reasoning by providing the range of factors affecting occupational performance.

Lippincott® Connect *For additional resources on the subjects discussed in this chapter, visit* Lippincott Connect.

REFERENCES

American Medical Association. (2017). New occupational therapy evaluation codes. *AMA CPT® Assistant, 27*(2). https://www.aota.org/advocacy/advocacy-news/coding/new-ot-cpt-evaluation-codes

American Occupational Therapy Association. (2016). *New occupational therapy evaluation coding overview.* https://www.aota.org/advocacy/advocacy-news/coding/new-ot-cpt-evaluation-codes

American Occupational Therapy Association. (2020a). Occupational therapy practice framework: Domain and process (4th ed.). *American Journal of Occupational Therapy, 74* (Suppl. 2), 7412410010p1–7412410010p87. https://doi.org/10.5014/ajot.2020.74S2001

American Occupational Therapy Association. (2020b). Guidelines for supervision, roles, and responsibilities during the delivery of occupational therapy services. *American Journal of Occupational Therapy, 74*, 7413410020p1–7413410020p6. https://doi.org/10.5014/ajot.2020.74S3004

American Occupational Therapy Association. (2020c). AOTA 2020 Occupational therapy code of ethics. *American Journal of Occupational Therapy, 74*, 7413410005p1–7413410005p13. https://doi.org/10.5014/ajot.2020.74S3006

American Occupational Therapy Association. (2021a). *Improve your documentation with AOTA's update occupational profile template.* https://doi.org/10.5014/ajot.2020.74S2001

American Occupational Therapy Association. (2021b). Standards of practice for occupational therapy. *American Journal of Occupational Therapy, 75*(Suppl. 3), 7513410050. https://doi.org/10.5014/ajot.2021.75S3004

American Occupational Therapy Association. (2021c). *12 ways to address the skilled nursing facilities patient driven payment model (PDPM).* https://www.aota.org/~/media/Corporate/Files/Practice/Manage/value/SNF-Evaluation-Checklist-Quality-Measures

American Occupational Therapy Association. (2021d). *Ten things patients and providers should question.* https://www.choosingwisely.org/societies/american-occupational-therapy-association-inc/

Brown, C. (2009). Functional assessment and intervention in occupational therapy. *Psychiatric Rehabilitation Journal, 32*, 162–170. https://doi.org/10.2975/32.3.2009.162-170

Canadian National Centre for the Arts. (n.d.). *The choreographic process.* http://artsalive.ca/en/dan/make/process/chprocess.asp

Dirette, D. (2013). Trading in our paradigm shifts for a staircase. *The Open Journal of Occupational Therapy, 1*(4), Article 1. https://doi.org/10.15453/2168-6408.1067

Emergency Care Research Institute. (2021). *About ECRI.* https://www.ecri.org/about/

Fazio, L. (2017). *Developing occupation-centered programs with the community* (3rd ed.). SLACK.

Fisher, A. G. (2009). *Occupational therapy intervention process model: A model for planning and implementing top-down, client-centered, and occupation-based interventions.* Three Star Press.

Fisher, A. G., & Jones, K. B. (2017). Occupational therapy intervention process model. In J. Hinojosa, P. Kramer, & C. B. Royeen (Eds.), *Perspectives on human occupation: Theories underlying practice* (2nd ed., pp. 237–286). F.A. Davis.

Hinojosa, J. (2017). How society's philosophy has shaped occupational therapy practice for the past 100 years. *The Open Journal of Occupational Therapy, 5*(2), Article 12. https://doi.org/10.15453/2168-6408.1325

Kramer, P., & Grampurohit, N. (2020). Evaluation: Where do we begin? In P. Kramer & N. Grampurohit (Eds.), *Hinojosa and Kramer's evaluation in occupational therapy: Obtaining and interpreting data* (5th ed., pp. 1–12). AOTA Press.

Law, M., Baptiste, S., Carswell, A., McColl, M. A., Polatajko, H., & Pollock, N. (2014). *The Canadian occupational performance measure* (5th ed.). CAOT.

Niestadt, M. E. (2000). *Occupational therapy evaluation for adults: A pocket guide.* Lippincott Williams & Wilkins.

Pizzi, M. A., & Richards, L. G. (2017). Guest editorial—promoting health, well-being, and quality of life in occupational therapy: A commitment to a paradigm shift for the next 100 years. *American Journal of Occupational Therapy, 71*(4), 7104170010p1–7104170010p5. https://doi.org/10.5014/ajot.2017.028456

Shotwell, M., Johnson, K. R., & Flecha, I. M. (2017). Evaluation of acute care patients. In H. Smith-Gabai & S. E. Holm (Eds.), *Occupational therapy in acute care* (pp. 37-62). AOTA Press.

Simon, P. L., & Kramer, P. (2020). Administration of evaluation and administration. In P. Kramer & N. Grampurohit (Eds.), *Hinojosa, and Kramer's evaluation in occupational therapy: Obtaining and interpreting data* (5th ed., pp. 63–75). AOTA Press.

Swarbrick, M., & Yudof, J. (2015). *Wellness in eight dimensions.* Collaborative Supportive Programs of New Jersey. https://www.center4healthandsdc.org/uploads/7/1/1/4/71142589/wellness_in_8_dimensions_booklet_with_daily_plan.pdf

Critiquing Assessments

Sherrilene Classen and Craig A. Velozo

LEARNING OBJECTIVES

After reading this chapter, you will be able to:

1. Discuss the application and importance of measurement theory relative to occupational therapy (OT) assessment.
2. Describe traditional versus modern testing approaches as they relate to OT practice.
3. Describe and apply a framework to evaluate assessments by type and structure.
4. Recognize the uses of standardized versus nonstandardized tests.
5. Define and apply the concepts of reliability to OT assessments.
6. Identify the components of validity and apply that knowledge to assessments.
7. Describe the basic components of item response theory (IRT).
8. Discuss factors important in critiquing IRT-based assessments.

Introduction

This chapter provides students and occupational therapy (OT) practitioners with the basic knowledge necessary for critiquing assessment tools used in practice. As noted in Chapter 28, the use of assessment tools is inherent in the OT evaluation process because they are important sources of evidence to inform effective decision-making for both therapists and clients.* Additionally, the prediction and measurement of occupational performance is a cornerstone for developing evidence to enhance therapy services. Therapists must critically evaluate which assessments are best to use in a given situation, and this in turn requires an understanding of the concepts of measurement and the process of using assessment tools. Key

---

*The term *client* refers to *persons* (including those involved in care of a client), *groups* (a collection of individuals having shared characteristics or common or shared purpose, e.g., family members, workers, students, and those with similar interests or occupational challenges), and *populations* (aggregates of people with common attributes such as contexts, characteristics or concerns, including health risks). However, in countries other than the United States, the term *client* often refers to persons who are paying for their care directly. In most countries, *patient* is used to describe persons who are in hospital or rehabilitation. *Service user* and *person* are terms in general use that describe those in need of OT services. For this chapter, we are using *client* without implying the source of payment for services.

information covered includes the concepts of measurement theory, how to evaluate potential assessment tools and their psychometric properties (including reliability, internal consistency, and validity), information on the implications of using standardized versus nonstandardized assessments, and the need to be aware if any cut points exist to understand the sensitivity and specificity of measures used. To help readers apply this information, an ongoing OT Story is provided featuring an occupational therapist, Dominique, as she seeks to evaluate a client who is at risk in terms of driving safety. See OT Stories 20.1 to 20.6.

Foundational to understanding measurement issues is an understanding of classical test theory (CTT) as well as generalizability theory approaches, which are part of traditional measurement. However, because measurement theory is advancing, Dominique may want to think about assessing and more specifically "measuring" her client's abilities. Traditional measurement approaches continue to have a prominent role in our understanding of assessment, but modern approaches are having a significant impact on how Dominique and others will assess clients, especially in the future. Therefore, this chapter includes information on both classical and modern approaches to critiquing assessments and provides recommendations for using open-access data collection resources and an open-access statistical program. The more modern approaches include presentations of a comparison of item response theory (IRT) to traditional test theory, advantages of IRT (efficiency and precision), linking assessments, computerized adaptive testing, and a modern approach to psychometric assessment. In this way,

the chapter provides foundational information for occupational therapists to critique assessments used in everyday practice and to be knowledgeable of resources efficient for data collection and analysis.

Traditional Approach to Critiquing Assessments

Measurement, in its simplest form, is defined as the rules for quantifying a classification of certain attributes or characteristics (Law, 1987). For example, occupational therapists use measures to reflect a child's performance in school tasks or an adult's ability to perform self-care or community living skills. The assignment of a number makes it possible to mathematically evaluate the attributes that are being measured in a standardized way. This allows comparisons of performance or capacity across individuals or groups of individuals. It also provides a way to document how an individual's performance has changed over time and across performance contexts. Because occupational therapists make judgments that affect the lives of our clients, it is an ethical responsibility to understand the strengths and limitations of any measure used as part of the evaluation process. The OT practitioner must understand aspects related to the types of assessments; their structural characteristics; and the basics of construction, standardization, reliability, and validity. Of importance, the practitioner is encouraged to reflect on the context in which assessments or measurements are conducted. Language, for example, is a significant barrier in contexts where English is not the dominant language used by patients/clients/service users, but assessments or measurements are presented in English. This barrier becomes even more pronounced when there is language discordance between the therapist and the service user/patient/client.

Nonstandardized Versus Standardized Assessments

As noted in Chapter 19, many OT evaluations include a blend of standardized and nonstandardized assessments. Although standardized assessments bring confidence in validity and reliability when used appropriately, nonstandardized assessments continue to be an important source of information gathering during the OT process. Luebben and Royeen argue that "every standardized assessment begins its life as a non-standardized test" and that "a new assessment moves along non-standardized continuum toward the standardize end as a result of rigorous development . . ." (as cited in Hinojosa et al. [2005, p. 125]).

Nonstandardized assessments, as the name implies, do not follow a standard approach or protocol. For instance,

---

OT STORY 20.1 DOMINIQUE EVALUATES A CLIENT FOR DRIVING

Dominique is an occupational therapist working in a regional medical center. She needs to evaluate Mr. Patel, a patient with Parkinson disease (PD). One concern is whether Mr. Patel should continue driving. For many individuals in the United States and other countries, the ability to drive has a far-reaching impact on community participation. Thus, Dominique has to carefully select and administer the best possible assessments for her to make an informed recommendation to Mr. Patel, his family, and the appropriate medical and legal authorities.

Questions

1. Why are the fitness-to-drive abilities of a client within the scope of OT practice?
2. Are you aware of any fitness-to-drive screening tools that may assist Dominique in screening her client before an in-depth evaluation is necessary?

they may not involve a consistent set of questions, directions, or conditions for administration, testing, or scoring. Such assessments may contain data collected from observations or interviews (e.g., with the referring physician, the client, or the family member) as well as during the OT evaluation via questionnaires (e.g., demographic, health, or medication) and observation of performance. Data obtained from this method are most effective when they reflect attention to the issues raised in Box 20.1 (Hinojosa et al., 2005). Additionally, these data are most useful when combined with the following approaches. See an example of a nonstandardized assessment in the Expanding Our Perspectives box.

BOX 20.1 QUESTIONS TO ASK IN CRITIQUING NONSTANDARDIZED ASSESSMENTS

- Is it guided by theoretical frameworks and/or models of practice?
- Does it inform further clinical reasoning and decision-making?
- Is it client centered?
- Is it a means to an end and not an end in itself?
- Is it based on having a good rapport with the client?
- Does it acknowledge the diversity of clients?

EXPANDING OUR PERSPECTIVES

Assessing School Readiness Using Dance and Humor

Elelwani Ramugondo

My first assignment as a newly graduated young occupational therapist was to establish the first Occupational Therapy Department at a school for children with barriers to learning in rural Limpopo, South Africa. A key responsibility that emerged for me in this role was assessing whether applicants were school ready. This example shows how, seeing the human first, in context, and within their community, immediately brings collective occupations to the surface, even if one were to think of OT in the traditional sense. It was also, however, possible to miss this opportunity to do OT differently.

On advice from educationalists and psychologists, the school had purchased an aptitude test and had one of the teachers in the past administer this as part of selecting those who would be admitted to the school. The aptitude test was developed in the United Kingdom. Given that this aptitude test was in English and used puzzles, which I knew rural kids would never have seen before, I indicated to the school authorities that the test was not a suitable measure of aptitude for these kids. Although my reservations about the test were understood, the school authorities felt that an alternative test should still be deemed objective. After consulting with other occupational therapists nationally, I was pointed to a newly developed test, developed in South Africa, specifically for environmentally disadvantaged preschool children. I was still skeptical, given the diversity of South Africa in terms of language, and was unconvinced about whether at the time, in the 1990s, "disadvantage" was a clearly defined construct that applies across contexts. The school authorities, however, felt this test would be a suitable substitute for the previous one.

As an inexperienced occupational therapist, I was not about to challenge authority and place myself at risk for insubordination. Given that I was the only OT at the school and was left to work independently most of the time, I decided to use the test only on paper, while in practice, I used other means to determine whether the child was school ready or not. Usually these kids, with various disabilities (postpolio, osteogenesis imperfecta, cerebral palsy, etc.), would present at the school between ages six to nine. I used interviews with these children and their caregivers as the most reliable means to assess their school readiness. Two questions proved particularly useful: What is your favorite song that you dance to at home? Can you share a joke with me that you think is the funniest you have ever heard, or something you saw that you thought was the funniest ever? As a backup, I always had a recorded cassette with the latest music trending locally. I would play a song closest to the genre the child had said was their favorite song and begin to dance. Often, I did not even have to invite the child and their caregiver to join in the dance. If the child had rhythm and could sing or hum along, it meant they were fairly school ready.

The answer to the second question was particularly telling and gave me a good sense of whether the child would benefit from being in the school or not. Once the child was admitted, and I still had a niggly worry that perhaps I had made a mistake, I would watch the child engage in unstructured play with others. If they were able to negotiate their place in a game, and know when to lead or follow, I was sold on the child being school ready.

There are profound implications when we insist on practice that derives from seeing the human in people we work with, humans in context, engaged in collective occupations embedded in context. A child who is deemed not school ready goes back to a community, where this diagnosis should make sense. When this is not the case, the community may be left with less faith in itself to identify problems and find workable solutions.

A standardized assessment is developed using prescribed procedures. It is administered and scored consistently under the same conditions and test directions. The standardization of test questions, directions related to performance, conditions of testing, and scoring is needed to make test scores comparable and to assure, as much as possible, that clients have equal, unbiased opportunities to demonstrate what they know and can do (Association of American Publishers, n.d.). Standardized assessments have typically undergone extensive development. Usually, the developers of such assessments provide a user manual detailing the process of development, a protocol for administration, a procedure for scoring, rules for interpretation, criteria or norms for performance, and the psychometric properties of the assessment. Research on the development of the assessment should be available in peer-reviewed journals to demonstrate that the quality of the assessment has been critically appraised. Box 20.2 provides a list of the different aspects of a standardized test that need to be considered in choosing an assessment, each of which is defined in the sections that follow, along with issues to consider regarding each of these factors.

Types of Assessments

Generally, assessments can be classified as descriptive, evaluative, or predictive. In addition, assessments can be classified as norm referenced and criterion referenced. An assessment can have multiple classifications, but for illustrative purposes, we provide examples of each type.

Descriptive Assessments

Descriptive assessments use items to describe individuals within groups and to characterize the differences between individuals on the attribute being measured. This information can be used by the therapist to assess the specific characteristics of an individual to determine whether and what type of intervention is needed. An example of a descriptive assessment is the Clinical Dementia Rating, a clinical staging assessment for dementia (Morris, 1993). Broadly, it characterizes six domains of cognitive and functional performance: memory, orientation, judgment and problem-solving, community affairs, home and hobbies, and personal care. The information for each rating is obtained through a semistructured interview with a client and a reliable collateral source, such as a caregiver or family member. The Clinical Dementia Rating table provides descriptors that guide the clinician in making appropriate ratings based on interview data and clinical judgment. In addition to ratings on a 5-point scale for each domain (except personal care, which is rated on a 4-point scale), an overall Clinical Dementia Rating score is derived. This score is useful for globally staging the level of impairment: 0 = no impairment, 0.5 = very mild dementia, 1 = mild dementia, 2 = moderate dementia, and 3 = severe dementia (Morris, 1993).

BOX 20.2 COMPONENTS TO CONSIDER WHEN CRITIQUING STANDARDIZED ASSESSMENTS

1. Type
   a. Descriptive
   b. Evaluative
   c. Predictive
2. Structural
   a. Format
   b. Cost
   c. Orientation
   d. Clinical utility
3. Construction
   a. Levels of measurement
      i. Nominal
      ii. Ordinal
      iii. Interval
      iv. Ratio
4. Psychometric evaluation
   a. Reliability (classical test theory vs. generalizability theory)
      i. Measurement error
         1. Random
         2. Systematic
         3. Sources
      ii. Type
         1. Test–retest
         2. Rater (interrater and intrarater)
         3. Internal consistency (split-half, Cronbach α, Kuder–Richardson formulas)
   b. Validity (evidence to support the construct)
      i. What the instrument looks like
         1. Face
         2. Content
      ii. How the instrument acts
         1. Construct (convergent, discriminant)
         2. Criterion (concurrent, predictive)
   c. Screening
      i. Sensitivity
      ii. Specificity
      iii. Positive predictive value
      iv. Negative predictive value
   d. Item response theory
      i. Unidimensionality (fit statistics/factor analysis)
      ii. Local independence
      iii. Precision
      iv. Person–item match
5. Summary of strengths and weaknesses of the assessment

OT STORY 20.2 ASSESSING MR. PATEL'S DRIVING PERFORMANCE— NONSTANDARDIZED ASSESSMENT

Before selecting assessments to measure Mr. Patel's driving ability, Dominique first wants to know a little more about him. Dominique reviews the personal and medical history available from his chart and decides that her first step is to interview Mr. Patel to get his self-report on potential problems that may impact his driving ability. Dominique also interviews his spouse, asking her about his driving performance to form a more comprehensive approach of his driving abilities. As a result of her nonstandardized assessments (chart review and interviews), she finds that Mr. Patel is a 72-year-old man who is retired from business and lives in the community with his wife. He has some college after high school graduation. Mr. Patel has had PD for 17 years and is on antiparkinsonian drugs. He also has arthritis in his knees and neck and wears trifocals to see well. He was referred by

a neurologist from a movement disorders center with a concern about his continued safe driving. Mr. Patel tells Dominique that he feels sleepy during the day, and she notes that he demonstrates a flat affect during the interview. He has a driver's license and drives about 3 to 4 days per week, mainly with his spouse. His spouse adds that he has had two citations and a fender bender in the last 3 years. Dominique is now ready to think through which standardized evaluations she wishes to use to complete her initial evaluation.

Questions

1. What are the client factors that Mr. Patel exhibit that will be of concern considering his abilities to drive? Why?
2. What environmental factors may be considered barriers or facilitators for his continued driving?

Evaluative Assessments

Evaluative assessments use criteria or items to measure an individual's trait or attribute over time. The most appropriate characteristics included in an evaluative assessment are those that can be sensitive to change within an individual. The Simulator Sickness Questionnaire (SSQ; Kennedy et al., 1993), used to quantify simulator sickness symptoms as a result of being exposed to a driving simulator, is an example of an evaluative measure. The SSQ can be administered at various time points during the simulator drive so that comparisons can be made to assess whether simulator sickness symptoms are increasing. This is important clinically to determine whether the client will be able to tolerate the use of the simulator without becoming ill. Essentially, the SSQ

rates 16 symptoms across three domains, which include the oculomotor, disorientation, and nausea domains. Clients report the degree to which they experience each symptom on a scale from 0 to 3, with 0 = none, 1 = slight, 2 = moderate, and 3 = severe. The total SSQ score is derived by using a weighted scale and a standard algorithm (a step-by-step procedure for calculations). By comparing the scores after the first 5 minutes of driving with the scores obtained after 15 minutes of driving, the OT practitioner may be able to intervene with clients who show an increase in simulator sickness symptoms. For a description of the use of the SSQ and clinical application with returning combat veterans with mild traumatic brain injury (TBI), please see Classen and Owens (2010).

OT STORY 20.3 ASSESSING MR. PATEL'S DRIVING PERFORMANCE—SELECTING STANDARDIZED ASSESSMENTS

Knowing that advanced stages of PD can also affect cognition, especially executive functions, Dominique decides that she will have to assess Mr. Patel's general cognition. Recently, she has also read in one of her journals that divided attention, a critical important function for driving, may be affected in people with neurological disorders. Thus, Dominique decides to use the Mini-Mental State Examination (MMSE; Folstein et al., 1975) to assess Mr. Patel's general cognition and the Trail Making Test Part B (Trails B; Reitan, 1958) to assess Mr. Patel's divided attention, which is also known as set shifting. She is also concerned about visual changes that may have occurred because of the chronic neurological progression of PD as well as his impaired range of motion (ROM) due to arthritis in his neck and trunk. Dominique decides to also include a comprehensive visual battery using the Optec 2500 visual analyzer (registered trademark of Stereo Optical Co.,

Inc.) that measures visual acuity, peripheral vision, contrast sensitivity, depth perception, lateral and vertical phorias, and color discrimination. Finally, she used her knowledge of ROM and Manual Muscle Testing (MMT) to assess the corresponding functions in Mr. Patel's neck and trunk. All of these assessments are considered standardized, but Dominique is aware that she must delve a bit deeper into the published literature as well as the assessment manuals to be sure that she has identified good measures that she is justified in using to make a reasonable fitness-to-drive recommendation for Mr. Patel.

Questions

1. What alternative assessment may be considered instead of the MMSE?
2. If the Optec 2500 is not available in the clinic, what reasonable substitutes can be considered?

OT STORY 20.4 DESCRIPTIVE, PREDICTIVE, AND EVALUATIVE ASSESSMENTS

After reviewing the nature of the assessments she has selected, Dominique is convinced that Trails B is a *predictive assessment*, especially after reading in a journal article that Trails B was highly correlated with passing/failing an on-road test in people with PD (Classen et al., 2009). In the same study, Dominique also read that the MMSE was moderately correlated to on-road outcomes. She is not sure whether the MMSE is sufficiently predictive or not. Knowing that using the Optec 2500 visual analyzer to determine Mr. Patel's visual function can characterize his visual acuity, peripheral visual fields, contrast sensitivity, ocular movements, and depth perception, Dominique decides that these assessments fit the *descriptive* criteria well. Certainly,

the ROM tests as well as the MMT tests can be considered *evaluative tools*, especially because Dominique can expect changes (improvements) in Mr. Patel's measures based on interventions to improve his neck and trunk mobility and strength.

Questions

1. Based on the information obtained from these assessments, will Dominique have adequate information about Mr. Patel's performance skills for driving?
2. Should Dominique also assess Mr. Patel's view and his goals pertaining to the occupation of driving? What relevant questions might she ask?

Predictive Assessments

Predictive assessments use criteria to classify individuals to predict a certain trait in comparison to set criteria. For example, a predictive tool can measure skills underlying driving performance to predict whether an older adult will be able to successfully return to driving. The Useful Field of View™ (UFOV), a computer-based assessment of visual attention (subtest 1), divided attention (subtest 2), and selective attention (subtest 3), is an example of a predictive assessment (Edwards et al., 2006). The first UFOV subtest involves identifying a single object (either a car or a truck) presented centrally on the touch screen. Subtest 2 (divided attention) required the client to identify a peripheral target while still attempting to correctly identify the central target (car or truck). Subtest 3 (selective attention) involves the same procedure as subtest 2, except for distracter triangles being present surrounding the peripheral target. After completion, threshold scores are provided as well as a risk index (low, moderate, and high) for all tasks. Higher scores indicate longer times to process the information and thus poorer performance. The UFOV is one of the best predictors of crash involvement and poor on-road performance for drivers with Alzheimer disease (Owsley & McGwin, 1999). The divided attention component (subtest 2) is rated as the best predictor of (at-fault) crash involvement among older adults (Owsley, McGwin, & Ball, 1998).

Norm-Referenced Assessments

Norm-referenced assessments compare a person's score to the scores of a norm group. This comparison is often in the form of standard scores, standard deviations, and percentile ranks. A common example of norm-referenced measures is the Centers for Disease Control and Prevention (CDC) clinical growth charts. These charts allow physicians and

families to evaluate a child's height and weight relative to a large sample of children within the same age group. For example, for a child who is in the 40th percentile of height, 40% of children in their age group are shorter than the child, and 60% of children are taller than the child. Norm-referenced assessments are commonly used in pediatric and school settings. For example, the Peabody Developmental Motor Scale, widely used in early intervention settings, provides norm-reference scores for fine and gross motor skills in children from birth to 5 years old.

Criterion-Referenced Assessments

Criterion-referenced assessments compare a person's score against a predetermined standard rather than the scores of a norm group. The written driving test at the Division of Motor Vehicles is criterion referenced. The examinee has to get a certain percentage of the exam questions correct to pass the test. Occupational therapists do not typically set an overall standard for an individual receiving treatment. Criterion-referenced assessments are not as common as norm-referenced assessments in OT.

Structure of Assessments

The previous section introduced the reader to the types of assessments. We next discuss the structure of the assessments as it pertains to their characteristics, clinical utility, and basic information on constructing items. Characteristics of the assessments may include the format, cost, and orientation of the test.

Format

Assessments may appear in a paper-and-pencil format, for example, the Mini-Mental State Examination (MMSE), or as a computerized test, for example, the UFOV. The paper-and-pencil tests are very common in the state, national, and international organizations, but computer-based testing (CBT) is becoming increasingly popular. Some advantages of CBT include reduced administration time, fewer data entry errors, worldwide testing via the Web, and rapid results (Kraut et al., 2004; Streiner & Norman, 2008a). However, limitations of CBT include questionable reliability and validity, apprehension for individuals not skilled with computers, and concerns about the security of test materials.

Cost

Cost of the assessment is an important consideration because some assessment tools may be available free of charge, for example, the Craig Handicap Assessment and Reporting Technique (CHART; Whiteneck et al., 2009). Others, such as a driving simulator, may be very expensive in terms of equipment, training, updating, and maintenance costs.

Orientation

Knowledge about the *orientation*, whether the assessment is invasive or not and insight into how much cooperation from the client and/or other stakeholders is needed, must be considered. Therefore, the OT practitioner must also consider the *clinical utility* of the test. It is fitting to refer to the importance of explaining assessments to clients and/or their family members. Here, the issue of language as a possible barrier becomes relevant. When needed, the OT practitioner should involve a language translator to explain an assessment presented in English and should also consider the value of translating available OT assessments into relevant languages.

Clinical Utility

Clinical utility refers to how *acceptable* the assessment will be among OT practitioners when used in the clinic. As such, acceptability may be influenced by the clinical applicability of the assessment (usefulness of the assessment for making interpretations to facilitate interventions), time demands (time to complete the assessment, time allocated to the scoring of the test, and time required to be trained to administer the assessment), and acceptability of the assessment to the clients (Rudman & Hannah, 1998).

In general, OT practitioners need to make decisions regarding which test to use (descriptive, evaluative, or predictive) based on the specific purpose of the assessment, characteristics of the assessment, and clinical utility of the tool, including the practical steps in administering the tool.

Construction

Construction of a test pertains to devising or writing the items in such a way that they will match the purpose of the assessment. For a more detailed discussion on aspects of construction, please see the document entitled "Constructing Assessments" on Lippincott Connect. Items can be constructed to include different levels of measurement and is discussed next in detail. Refer to Box 20.3 for a summary of measurement levels and scales. These are important because they dictate the kinds of statistical analyses that can be done using the assessment results across clients. It is helpful to realize that measurement exists on different levels and that the scale itself limits or determines the analysis of the data.

OT STORY 20.5 DOMINIQUE CONSIDERS ASSESSMENT CHARACTERISTICS

Dominique knows that the assessment tools she has selected use the paper-and-pencil method for scoring (MMSE, Trails B), except for the Optec 2500 visual analyzer, which is computer based. The cost of all the assessments, apart from the Optec 2500 visual analyzer machine, is reasonably low. Luckily, Dominique's facility has invested in Optec to measure the visual function of the low-vision clients; thus, no further financial expenses are necessary for her to use this assessment. She also realizes that the ROM and MMT may be a little invasive because they require hands-on testing. However, since these functions are important for neck and trunk movement during driving, and Mr. Patel shows observable signs of such related impairment, Dominique decides to evaluate those—especially for backup functions during driving. She doesn't think that it will pose a problem and thus is satisfied that she has identified tools that are feasible to use in her setting.

Dominique is confident that all the assessments that she has chosen will help her clinical reasoning to assess Mr. Patel's abilities important for driving performance. She has calculated that it will take her about 28 minutes to assess Mr. Patel's visual (15 minutes with the Optec), cognitive (5 minutes for the MMSE and 3 minutes for Trails B), and physical abilities (gross MMT and ROM for 5 minutes). True to following a person-centered approach, she discusses the type of assessments with Mr. Patel, and he concurs to participate as she conducts this part of her evaluation.

Questions

1. Will Dominique be able to make clinical judgments related to Mr. Patel's visual-cognitive functions? Why or why not?
2. Will Dominique be able to discern Mr. Patel's driving performance patterns based on this evaluation? Why or why not?

BOX 20.3 SCALES OF MEASUREMENT

Assigning numbers to traits results in measurement scales. The four scales of measurement are nominal, ordinal, interval, and ratio (Portney & Watkins, 2009).

- **Nominal.** The nominal scale represents the first level of measurement. This involves mutually exclusive categories (e.g., female vs. male, driving vs. nondriving). Assigned numbers are simply used as labels or means of identification with no attempt to quantify or order the differences.
- **Ordinal.** The second level is the ordinal scale. In this scale, the numbers represent the relative rank order of the trait under investigation. For example, driving evaluators often use a Global Rating Scale, indicating whether a client who has taken an on-road test should fail = 1, fail with options for remediation = 2, pass with recommendations = 3, or pass = 4 (Justiss et al., 2006). The assigned numbers merely indicate the rank order; they do not represent absolute quantities, and the intervals between the ranks cannot be presumed equal. In this example, someone who is passing the on-road test is not twice as competent as someone who is passing with recommendations. Thus, no inference can be made about the magnitude of the difference between scores.
- **Interval.** The interval scales represent the third level. The intervals between scores are equal so that comparisons can be made between individuals. Also, a characteristic of an interval scale is that there is no true zero value. An example of an interval scale that is commonly used in OT surveys is the bipolar (goes in both directions) Likert scale (e.g., 0 = strongly disagree, 1 = disagree, 2 = agree, 3 = strongly agree) and the unipolar (goes in one direction)

adjectival scale, (e.g., 0 = cannot do, 1 = very difficult, 2 = somewhat difficult, 3 = a little difficult, 4 = not difficult).[a] Although a client can get the lowest value (a zero) on a driving assessment that uses the adjectival scale, there is no true "absence of driving safety." Although not having an absolute zero limits some mathematical operations, most psychometric operations such as calculations of means and standard deviations are commonly performed on interval scales.
- **Ratio.** The ratio scales reflect the fourth and highest level scale in measurement. It has equal distances but, in addition, has a meaningful zero point. The zero point indicates a total absence of whatever trait is being measured. To use these scales, the absence of the attribute being measured must be meaningful. Range of motion (ROM) measurements assessed by a trained clinician with standardized equipment, such as a goniometer, will yield ratio data. All mathematical operations can be accomplished with ratio scale data (addition, subtraction, multiplication, division) and statistical (means, standard deviations, and standard errors) calculations. In this case, it is correct to indicate that a person has gained twice as much movement between measurements of 20° elbow flexion and 40° elbow flexion.

---

[a]Some measurement experts believe that Likert scales are not interval scales. Although Likert scales look like they are interval in nature, for example, the distance between a value of 1 to 2 and 2 to 3 are equal, we cannot be assured that there are equal distances between the qualifiers that these numbers represent (e.g., maximum assistance, moderate assistance, and minimum assistance) (Bond & Fox, 2007).

For example, if ordinal data are to be analyzed, then the scale from which these data are derived must contain defined ranks and intervals to approximate rank order. Moreover, critiquing measures must be pursued with knowledge of their rules, the nature of the trait being measured, and a consideration of the purpose of measuring.

In addition to how a test is constructed, a psychometric evaluation or an empirical way to evaluate the quality of the assessment tool must include testing related to reliability (Does the test yield the same or similar scores consistently?), external validity (Can generalizations be made to the general population?), internal validity (Does the assessment measure what it is supposed to measure [i.e., a specific trait, behavior, construct, or performance]?), sensitivity (predictor test's ability to obtain a positive test when the condition exists), and specificity (predictor test's ability to obtain a negative test when the condition does not exist). Each of these components of the psychometric evaluation is discussed next.

Reliability—Traditional Approaches

Reliability pertains to the reproducibility of test results and the amount of variation measured that is real and not due to error. Reliability, generally, is based on a correlation coefficient or a measure of agreement and referred to as a reliability coefficient, which can range from 0 to ± 1 (0 = no reliability and 1 = perfect reliability). Two theoretical concepts related to reliability are CTT and generalizability theory.

CTT, also called classical reliability theory, centers around the notion that each observation or test score has a single true score and yields a single reliability coefficient (Nunnally & Bernstein, 1994). CTT postulates that a test score has two components: the true score and the measurement error score. Although many sources of error exist, only one source (e.g., either the rater or the assessment itself) is estimated, meaning that the difference therefore between the observed score and the true score is due to random error (Portney & Watkins, 2009). This model is overly restrictive and often unrealistic in situations where there may be multiple sources of error. Examples of multiple error sources include differences among raters (see interrater reliability) and differences in testing context (e.g., driving assessed in one's car or driving assessed in an evaluator's car). Additionally, measures themselves are heterogeneous (e.g., driving can be operationalized, and therefore measured, in various ways such as driving awareness, driving behaviors, driving confidence, driving habits, driving fitness, driving performance, and/or driving safety).

Generalizability theory provides a framework for conceptualizing, investigating, and designing reliable observations. It was originally introduced by Cronbach and colleagues (1963, 1972) in response to the limitations of CTT. Generalizability theory recognizes different sources of error and attempts to quantify the sources of those various errors. So, not all variations in the administration of an assessment are attributed to random error. Relevant testing conditions that may influence test scores are identified (e.g., time of day such as driving in the midmorning vs. driving in peak traffic where there are many more demands from the driving environment). In identifying the different sources of error, one may be better able to identify why an assessment score changes and thus provide additional explanations beyond the assumption of random error (Portney & Watkins, 2009).

Measurement Error

Measurement error arises when there is a difference between the true value, such as one's absolute weight measured with a precise scale (e.g., an electronic scale in a doctor's office), and the observed value (e.g., weight as measured by a spring-based bathroom scale). The observed value (X) is therefore a function of two components: a true score (T) and an error component (E), expressed as:

$$\text{Observed Score} = \text{True Score} \pm \text{Error}$$

$$X = T \pm E$$

An error can appear as a random error or systematic error. *Random error* is represented by inconsistencies that cannot be predicted, for example, fatigue or mechanical inaccuracy of the measurement assessment, causing the error. *Systematic error* refers to predictable fluctuations occurring during measurement. Systematic error may occur in design flaws such as accessing convenient pools for subject selection, for example, recruiting from a pool of clients lacking diversity. Usually, systematic errors occur in one direction and consistently overestimate or underestimate the true score. When the error is identified, it may be easier to manage or correct the systematic error compared to when the random error occurs as outlined in Box 20.4.

BOX 20.4 SOURCES OF SYSTEMATIC MEASUREMENT ERROR

- The individual taking the measurements (e.g., raters or evaluators that are biased in expecting the client to have improved due to driving training)
- The measurement assessment (e.g., poorly calibrated mechanical parts of a driving simulator)
- The variability of the characteristics being measured (e.g., ROM, when measured early in the morning, may be different than when measured late in the day)

Types of Reliability

Several types of reliability relate to assessments. See Table 20.1 for a synopsis of reliability testing.

Test–Retest Reliability

The test–retest method estimates the reliability or stability of measurements when the same test is given to the same people after a period of time. One obtains a correlation between scores on the two administrations of the same test. It is presumed that responses to the test will correlate because they reflect the same true score; however, the correlation of measurements across time will be less than perfect. This may occur because of the *instability* of measurements taken over various time points. For example, a client may be distracted, have a bad (or good) day, or be influenced by the test administrator (Carmines & Zeller, 1979; Portney & Watkins, 2009). Other factors that can influence (increase or decrease) test–retest reliability are the following:

- *A construct may change,* such as the influence of environmental changes, for example, the use of in-vehicle technology, on the driving task and thus the fitness-to-drive construct (please see detailed discussion under "Construct Validity" section).
- *Reactivity,* or change in the measured trait or behavior occurring because of the testing. For example, drivers may alter their performance due to their awareness of being observed. Therefore, drivers may perform more optimally when driving with a driving evaluator than when they drive by themselves under natural conditions.
- *Overestimation or underestimation.* In the driving literature, older drivers (and most other drivers) overestimate their driving ability as they report that they are better drivers than what they really are when compared to their performance on a road test. Similarly, older drivers may underestimate the number of citations received when their self-report data are compared to official citation records.

TABLE 20.1 Reliability by Type, Use, Source or Error, and Method of Testing

Type	Use	Sources of Error	Method to Test
Test–retest reliability	The test is given to the same people after a period of time	How time, changes in the construct, reactivity, over or underestimation, and changes in the environment effect the reliability of a measure	Intraclass correlation coefficient (ICC)[a]
Rater reliability	To illustrate the stability of data collected		ICC or κ
• *Intrarater reliability*	To illustrate the stability of data collected by one rater on two or more trials over time	Tool administration procedures, calibration of the instrument, untrained rater, recall, or other forms of bias	ICC or κ
• *Interrater reliability*	To determine rater variability between two or more raters who measure the same clients	The effect of time, rater interaction with the client, or variables that may influence the observation skills of the raters	ICC or κ
Internal consistency	To determine the degree of agreement between the items in a test that measure an underlying trait or construct		Cronbach coefficient α
• *Alternate form*	Tests the same group of people on two separate occasions using two distinct but parallel forms of the test	Length of the test	ICC
• *Split-halves*	The same group of people partakes in the test where the total set of items in the test is divided in half	Method of splitting	Spearman–Brown Prophecy statistic
• *Cronbach α or Kuder–Richardson formulas*	To estimate the reliability of scales or commonality of one item in a test with other items in a test	Consistency of content of the test	Cronbach coefficient α

[a]A perfect correlation is indicated by a correlation coefficient expressed as $r = 1.0$, $P \leq .05$. A strong correlation is indicated if $r \geq 0.75$, a moderate correlation if $r = 0.50$ but <0.75, and a weaker correlation if $r < 0.50$ when $P \leq .05$. Also note that acceptability of correlation strength may vary according to the purpose for reliability testing. For example, one may tolerate lower reliability estimates to indicate differences/similarities of groups, but values required for making accurate predictions in terms of diagnoses will need to have a high correlation coefficient. Correlations can be conducted with various methods, such as κ and ICC through Cronbach coefficient α (Portney & Watkins, 2009).

Rater Reliability

Intrarater reliability refers to the stability of data collected by one rater on two or more trials over time. The objective nature of scientific inquiry demands that even when experts are used, intrarater reliability should be tested. Error in this type of reliability can be reduced by training the rater in the use of the tool(s), using the tool administration procedures, calibrating measurement assessments, training rater skills to avoid deterioration over time, and assessing the rater for bias based on memory, training, views, and/or assumptions. Developing objective grading criteria may be conducive to limiting measurement error occurring as a result of intrarater reliability (Hinojosa et al., 2005; Portney & Watkins, 2009).

Interrater reliability concerns detecting rater variability between two or more raters who measure the same clients (Portney & Watkins, 2009). To establish interrater reliability, the raters should view the same clients at the same point in time. In driving research, for example, the use of a driving simulator, which allows for video playback versus on-road testing, is particularly helpful for raters to rate a subject and useful for researchers to establish interrater reliability. Not only can one include a wide variety of raters with this testing method but also disagreements among the raters may be resolved through consensus and rewatching the video.

Should the raters test the client during an on-road driving test, their scores may be influenced by their seating position in the vehicle as well as the interaction of the evaluator with the tester. For example, the optimal seating position for the driving evaluator is the right front seat and the worst seating position is the back left seat because observation of many driver responses, such as eye movements or positioning of the vehicle, may be restricted as a result of the seating position. Likewise, the evaluator that is providing travel directions to the driver may rate the driver differently than the raters without any interaction with the driver.

Internal Consistency

Internal consistency determines the degree of agreement between the items in a test that measure an underlying trait or construct. It is essentially an estimation of the *homogeneity* of the test. Ways to test for internal consistency are alternate form, split-halves, Cronbach α, or Kuder–Richardson formulas.

• **Alternate form** tests the same group of people on two separate occasions using two distinct but parallel forms of the test. Although more expensive and time-consuming, because two forms of the test need to be developed, this method is obviously superior to test–retest method. Specifically, it reduces the effect to which the individual's memory can bias the results (i.e., result in improved score due to recall of the test questions) and therefore also the strength of the correlation.

- **Split-halves method** (in contrast to the alternate form method) can be conducted in one time period. Specifically, the same group of people partakes in the test wherein the total set of items in the test is divided in half. The scores on the halves are then correlated to obtain an estimate of reliability. One limitation is that how the items are subdivided will affect the reliability coefficient (Carmines & Zeller, 1979; Portney & Watkins, 2009; Streiner & Norman, 2008b). The Spearman–Brown prophecy formula, a statistical method, can be used to correct such incongruent results (Carmines & Zeller, 1979).

- **Cronbach** α (also referred to as *coefficient* α) and *Kuder–Richardson formulas* are used to estimate the reliability of scales or the commonality of one item in a test with other items in a test. The difference is that Cronbach α is used when the test scale is composed of *nondichotomous* responses (i.e., rating scale), whereas the Kuder–Richardson formulas are used for *dichotomously* scored items (e.g., correct/incorrect). Essentially, the purpose of applying these formulas is to identify the items that do not contribute to the overall construct that is being measured and therefore, such items may be lowering a test's reliability. The reader is referred to select references (Carmines & Zeller, 1979; Portney & Watkins, 2009; Streiner & Norman, 2008a) for more information on these methods.

Validity—Traditional Approaches

Validity is defined as the extent to which any assessment measures what it is intended to measure. The definition of validity is straightforward, but it is imperative to realize that although an assessment may yield valid data when being used to measure certain population traits under certain conditions, the same assessment may not be replicated if traits of a different population are being measured. Likewise, the same assessment may not be replicated if the same population is being measured under different conditions. For example, the Driving Habits Questionnaire has been developed and tested psychometrically for use among older adults in a research setting (Owsley et al., 1999). As such, if this tool is being used in a group of novice drivers (different populations) or used to record the history of night driving in older drivers (different conditions), the validity may be impacted. The question then becomes *if the assessment is still valid when measuring attributes of different populations or the same population but under different conditions.* The

practitioner needs to cautiously consider these aforementioned points before using an assessment.

To determine the accuracy of a measurement tool, one may ask what the assessment *looks* like and also how it *acts*. The "look" pertains to whether the assessment has *face validity* (e.g., Does it overall look like the assessment is measuring what it is supposed to measure?) and/or *content validity* (e.g., Do expert raters rate the items in that they comprehensively represent the content area?). The "act" pertains to a more rigorous process in assessment development that includes *construct validity* or how the assessment compares to other assessments measuring the same construct (*convergent*) or different (*divergent*) constructs, as well as *criterion validity*, which may be *concurrent* (measured at the same point in time) or *predictive* (measured at some point in future). See Table 20.2 for a synopsis of validity.

Face Validity

Face validity indicates that a measure is testing what it is supposed to and that the items are viewed as plausible. No statistical manipulation of the data is involved in this process, and the measure is peer reviewed (i.e., reviewed by experts in the field) to determine the plausibility of the items. For example, in the development of the items of the Safe Driving Behavioral Measure (SDBM), face validity was tested by asking a group of doctoral students and researchers to evaluate the chosen items based on ease of reading, content, clarity, appropriateness, and time that it took to answer the items. Recommendations from the peer review were followed in refining the items before content validity testing (Classen et al., 2010).

Content Validity

Fundamentally, content validity depends on the extent to which an empirical measurement reflects a specific domain of content. Following the guidelines of Lynn (1986), Classen and colleagues (2010) invited four expert raters to complete a *content validity index* (CVI)—an index of consensus related to the relevance of the items—on each of the items in the SDBM. Apart from rating each SDBM item on a 4-point Likert scale (1 = not relevant, 2 = relevant with major revisions, 3 = relevant with minor revisions, and 4 = very relevant), the experts also gave feedback on item accuracy, purpose, organization, clarity, appearance, understandability, and adequacy (Grant & Davis, 1997). Usually, content validity can be claimed if the rater agreement on the item relevance is 80% or higher (House et al., 1981).

Construct Validity

Construct validity establishes whether the assessment measures a construct and the theoretical components underlying the construct. A construct is an abstract idea that

TABLE 20.2 Validity by Type, Use, and Method to Test and Strength of Estimate			
Type	**Use**	**Method to Test**	**Strength of Estimate**
Face validity	Is the measure testing what it is supposed to measure? Are the items plausible?	Peer review	No statistical inference testing
Content validity	Does the measurement instrument reflect a specific domain of content?	Content validity index (CVI)	CVI ≥ 80%
Construct validity	Does the assessment measure a construct and the theoretical components underlying the construct?	Tests of correlation	Higher correlation coefficients are better, thus $r \geq 0.80$, $P \geq .05$.
• Convergent validity	Is the level of agreement between two tests that are being used to measure the same construct acceptable?	Tests of correlation	Higher correlation coefficients are better, thus $r \geq 0.80$, $P \leq .05$.
• Discriminant validity	Is the level of disagreement (poor or zero correlation) when two tests measure a trait, behavior, or characteristic acceptable?	Tests of correlation	Higher correlation coefficients are better, thus $r \geq 0.80$, $P \leq .05$.
Criterion validity	Can the outcome of one assessment be used as a substitute test to the established *gold standard criterion* test?	Prediction methods	See later
• Concurrent validity	Do the results of a criterion measure and a target test, given at the same relative time point, concur with one another?	Receiver operating characteristics (ROC) curves	Area under the curve (AUC) ≥ 0.70, with $P \leq .05$
• Predictive validity	Does the outcome of a target test predict a future criterion score or outcome?	Prediction methods, for example, regression analyses	The higher the R^2 in the prediction model, the better the validity.

Note: The above statistical tests are examples to illustrate the points raised. To evaluate the validity, other methods may be explored with biostatistician or psychometrician colleagues because the reader gets more accomplished in applying principles of validity testing.

we cannot observe directly. Many, if not all, occupational assessments measure abstract ideas that we can only indirectly observe through behaviors. For example, we cannot directly observe job satisfaction but can indirectly assess it by direct observation (e.g., watching an individual in a job situation) or through questionnaires (e.g., asking the client about satisfaction with different aspects of the job). Two different types of construct validity can be established, *convergent* and *discriminant*.

• **Convergent validity** is the level of agreement between two tests that are being used to measure the same construct. For example, if one wants to determine whether *lane maintenance* is challenging for a novice driver, one may test the driver on a driving simulator and on the road. Should there be a high correlation between lane maintenance under these two testing conditions (simulator and on road), one may infer construct validity pertaining to the lane maintenance aspect of driving.
• **Discriminant validity** is the level of disagreement (poor or zero correlation) when two tests measure a trait, behavior, or characteristic. Let's assume that community-dwelling older drivers are screened before taking an on-road test. The driving rehabilitation specialist will administer an MMSE to assess cognitive functioning and a visual acuity test to assess distant vision before participating in an on-road test (Folstein et al., 1975, 2010). A successful evaluation of discriminant validity will show that the test

of cognition (MMSE) is poorly correlated with a test of visual acuity because these tests are designed to measure different concepts.

The process of establishing construct validity involves at least three steps (Carmines & Zeller, 1979):

1. Determine the theoretical relationship between the concepts themselves.
2. Determine the empirical relationship between the measures of the concepts.
3. Interpret the empirical evidence to clarify the construct validity of a measure.

Because safe driving is an *abstract* idea and a *multidimensional* construct (e.g., includes aspects of the driver, the vehicle, and the environment), it may be challenging to determine the construct validity. Testing the construct, therefore, must be an ongoing process, and statistical methods used may include factor analysis or hypothesis testing, next described.

• **Factor analysis** is based on the idea that a construct contains one or more dimensions or theoretical components. As such, thinking about safe driving, one may assume that at least three dimensions are involved to execute a driving maneuver such as exiting a ramp and merging with traffic. Those are the person dimension (e.g., vision, cognition, and motor functions), the environment dimension (e.g., highway ramp, lanes on a highway, traffic, weather, light), and the vehicle dimension (e.g., roadworthiness of vehicle and working status of all vehicle controls). Factor analysis helps to tease out the underlying dimensions of an assessment by grouping variables or items that correlate highly with one another.

- *Hypothesis testing* can be used to determine whether an assessment can distinguish between people at different levels of safe driving. For example, one may postulate that older women who resume driving after the death of a spouse may have a greater number of errors related to driving skills when compared to older men who are the primary drivers in a family. If the assessment can detect such differences and affirm the hypothesis, one may infer construct validity pertaining to the population for the given test conditions.

Challenges to construct validity may include *changes in the environment or society over time* which influences the construct of the measurement tool. For example, the Fitness-to-Drive Screening Measure (FTDS), developed from 2008 to 2015 (Classen et al., 2015), included items reflective of fitness to drive before the onset of the semiautonomous or autonomous revolution currently evolving in the automobile industry (Denaro et al., 2014). Nowadays, many vehicles are equipped with in-vehicle technologies such as advance driver assistance systems (ADAS) or in-vehicle information systems (IVIS) (Alvarez & Classen, 2017). *ADAS*, for example, a collision avoidance system, are integrated systems that can directly help drivers with vehicle control, especially in high-risk situations (Wilschut, 2009). *IVIS, such as* a lane departure warning system with haptic (vibration) feedback, are technologies that provide information or warnings to drivers but do not assume functions related to driving tasks such as steering, accelerating, or braking. The use of such technologies may impact fitness-to-drive abilities. The absence of including items that accurately reflect the presence of ADAS or IVIS may compromise the construct validity and the stability of the FTDS. This (not having items reflective of ADAS or IVIS) is no small matter as this screening tool is making *predictions* on the risk probability of older adults' fitness-to-drive abilities. The construct validity of an instrument (in this case using items reflective of the fitness-to-drive construct) contributes to the ability to predict the risk associated with fitness to drive. Because construct validity is a key factor in the prediction of an outcome, systematic measurement error may be introduced if the FTDS does not reflect the inclusion of ADAS and IVIS items.

Criterion Validity

Criterion validity implies that the outcome of one assessment can be used as a substitute test for the established gold standard criterion test. Criterion validity can be tested as concurrent validity or predictive validity.

- *Concurrent validity* is inferred when two measures, the criterion measure and a target test, are given at relatively the same point in time and the results of the two tests concur with one another. Most often, when proven more efficient and/or cost-effective than the criterion test, the target test may be used as a substitute for the gold standard test. Currently, a comprehensive driving evaluation (CDE) conducted by a driving rehabilitation specialist is considered the industry or gold standard to determine driving ability (Di Stefano & Macdonald, 2005). However, the CDE is expensive, time-consuming, offers limited access (i.e., presently, there is a shortage of driving rehabilitation specialists), and invites an element of risk because it is conducted in the real world. To overcome many of these challenges, researchers are investigating the concurrent validity between the driving simulator and the CDE (Bédard et al., 2010).
- *Predictive validity* establishes that the outcome of a target test can be used to predict a future criterion score or outcome. For example, in a review of vision impairment and driving, the UFOV was shown to be one of the best predictors of crash involvement as tested in a simulator and on road (gold standard criterion) in drivers with Alzheimer disease (Owsley, Ball, et al., 1998). Thus, one may infer that the UFOV has predictive validity with the criterion (on-road testing) for the population under study.

Ecological Validity

Ecological validity implies that the outcome of an assessment can "hold up" in real-world circumstances. For example, if Mr. Patel, our OT Story participant, is deemed to be able to drive based on the findings of an assessment, one must ask whether that assessment outcome will also hold true in the real world. If so, one can infer ecological validity.

Screening Tools

Many assessments are specifically developed to be used as a *screening* tool. A screening is a brief measure that tests the presence or absence of a disease, condition, or outcome. Because screening tools are often used by clinicians to determine whether a client will require further treatment, it is very important to verify their validity (see Box 20.5 and Figure 20.1 for an example).

Sensitivity and Specificity

Sensitivity is defined as the predictor test's ability to obtain a positive test when the condition exists (a true-positive).

OT STORY 20.6 DOMINIQUE CRITIQUES HER ASSESSMENTS AND COMPLETES HER EVALUATION

Dominique is ready to critique her assessments. She has developed a matrix displayed in Table 20.3 and included information from the published studies that she has read to assess whether she is on the right track.

Dominique has chosen assessments with a structure that is conducive to Mr. Patel's needs. Two of the assessments (Trials B, ROM) provide interval-level data, two more (MMSE, Vision) ratio data, and the other (MMT) ordinal data. Even though not all the components of reliability and validity are known (through the publications that she has read), the overall psychometrics of the tools are acceptable and suggest that Dominique's decision to use these tools is evidence based.

Dominique proceeds to assess Mr. Patel using the MMSE and Trails B. She also assesses his vision with the Optec 2500 along with selected ROM and MMT pertinent to driving. From these results, she finds that he is demonstrating some mild difficulty with divided attention, impaired contrast sensitivity, and limitations in his neck and trunk mobility. All these impairments may affect Mr. Patel's ability to continue to drive. Based on these results, she recommends an on-road driving evaluation to be conducted by a certified driving rehabilitation specialist, both to determine a baseline for his fitness-to-drive abilities and to make recommendations for any modifications, adaptations, compensatory strategies, or referrals (e.g., to an ophthalmologist) needed to assure appropriate fitness-to-drive abilities.

Questions

1. Where might Dominique obtain a listing of all certified driving rehabilitation specialists?
2. What other alternatives exist to further assess Mr. Patel's fitness-to-drive abilities if he has no access to a certified driving rehabilitation specialist?

TABLE 20.3 Matrix to Critique Assessments

Assess-ment	Structure				Level of Measurement				Reliability			Validity			
	Format	Cost	Orien-tation	Clinical Utility	Nom-inal	Ordi-nal	Ratio	Inter-val	Test–Retest	Rater Reliability	Internal Consistency	Face	Con-tent	Con-struct	Crite-rion
MMSE	x	x	x	x			R		x	x	?	x	x	x	x
Trails B	x	x	x	x				I	x	x	x	x	x	x	x
Vision	x	x	x	x			R		x	?	?	x	x	x	x
ROM	x	x	x	x				I	x	x	?	x	x	x	?
MMT	x	x	x	x		O			x	x	?	x	x	x	?

Note: The "x" indicates a positive response to reflect that the component of the assessment that is being rated is acceptable. The "?" indicates that the component of the assessment being rated is not known.

I, interval; MMSE, Mini-Mental State Examination; MMT, Manual Muscle Testing; O, ordinal; R, ratio; ROM, range of motion.

For example, when a predictor test suggests that the client will fail an on-road test, and this prediction is then verified by the actual outcome of the on-road test, sensitivity is evident. Specificity is defined as the predictor test's ability to obtain a negative result when the condition is absent (a true-negative). An example here is whether the predictor test suggests that the client should pass, and this result is then verified by the client passing the on-road test (Portney & Watkins, 2009).

Positive and Negative Predictive Value

Positive predictive value is the probability of the client, given a certain cut point on the predictor test failing in the actual situation (e.g., the on-road test). Negative predictive value is the probability of the client, given a cut point on the predictor test, to pass (in this case to pass the on-road test).

It is important to note that the number of false-positives (those who receive a failing score but pass the road test) and false-negatives (those who receive a passing score but fail the road test) and thus the sensitivity and specificity values, change with the cutoff value. Ultimately, one wants the false-positives and false-negatives to be as close to zero as possible. The formulas for calculating these values are well described in many of the texts cited in this chapter.

Modern Approaches to Critiquing Assessments

Although most OT clinicians and researchers have been trained on traditional psychometric methods (CTT and

BOX 20.5 USING EVIDENCE TO EVALUATE SCREENING TOOLS: AN EXAMPLE FROM THE LITERATURE

Occupational therapists are encouraged to make decisions regarding screening tools by examining the evidence that the tool is effective to predict the relevant criterion outcome. For example, in a pilot study with 19 drivers with Parkinson disease (PD) who underwent a clinical battery of tests and an on-road driving test, the researchers wanted to determine which of the screening tests were most predictive of those clients who failed the on-road test. Figure 20.1 demonstrates how to calculate sensitivity, specificity, positive predictive value, and negative predictive value for the Useful Field of View (UFOV) Risk Index in a 3-point cutoff value (N = 19 drivers with PD). The researchers determined that the sensitivity (true-positives or those drivers with PD who failed the road test and who were predicted to fail by the UFOV) was 87%. The specificity (true-negative or those drivers with PD who passed the road test and who were predicted to pass by the UFOV) was 82%. The positive predictive value (probability of the driver with PD, given a cut point of 3 on the UFOV Risk Index to fail the on-road test) was 78%. The negative predictive value (probability of the PD drivers, given a cut point of 3 on the UFOV Risk Index to pass the on-road test) was 90%. In this study, the authors concluded that among this sample of drivers with PD tested and compared to other clinical measures of disease, cognition, and vision, the

		Global rating scale (fail/pass)	
		+ (FAIL)	− (PASS)
UFOV risk index	+ (UFOV ≥3)	a true-positives (hits) [n = 7]	b false-positives (misses) [n = 2]
	− (UFOV ≤3)	c false-negatives (false alarms) [n = 1]	d true-negatives (correct rejections) [n = 9]

FIGURE 20.1 Calculating sensitivity, specificity, positive predictive value, negative predictive value, and error for the Useful Field of View (UFOV) Risk Index value of 3 (N = 19 drivers with Parkinson disease). Sensitivity = $a/(a + c)$ [7/(7 + 1) = 0.87]; specificity = $d/(b + d)$ [9/(2 + 9) = 0.82]; positive predictive value = $a/(a + b)$ [7/(7 + 2) = 0.78]; negative predictive value = $d/(c + d)$ [9/(1 + 10) = 0.90]; total error = 1 − sensitivity + 1 − specificity [0.13 + 0.18 = 0.31].

UFOV was a superior screening measure for predicting on-road outcomes (Classen et al., 2009).

---

generalizability theory), unfortunately, these approaches have several shortcomings. First, traditional assessments generate *scores* versus *measures*. Scores are simply the sum of the frequency of answers marked as "correct" or if using a Likert or adjectival scale, the sum of the ratings of each item. Although our scores on our assessments may look more sophisticated when converted into a percentage of the total score, in essence, they still simply reflect a frequency count. Second, the traditional analyses are specific to the sample from which they were derived. That is, although most researchers report on the reliability and validity of an assessment as if it is a stable characteristic, it is not. Reliability and validity are *sample dependent*. That is, reliability and validity values are unique to the particular sample from which they were derived. Although such actions require a research-intensive process, we must reevaluate the reliability of any assessment being used for diverse populations that did not include diverse populations in the original research samples.

Third, scores are *test dependent*. That is, a score on one assessment cannot be readily translated to a score on a second assessment. For example, a score of 50 on one road test does not carry the same meaning as a score of 50 on any other road test. Test scores are dependent on the difficulty of the items (tasks or questions) of the assessment.

An individual with a particular level of ability (e.g., someone who can drive well only in their hometown) will get a low score on a challenging driving assessment (e.g., one that only involves complex driving situations such as negotiating traffic in peak traffic hours) and a high score on an easy driving assessment (e.g., one that only involves simple driving situations such as putting the car in gear and pulling out of the driveway). Finally, in most cases, traditional assessments require clients to take all items of the assessment. Obviously, if clients take fewer of the items and the items are summed for a total score, they will get a lower score on the assessment even though their ability has not changed.

In recent years, there have been dramatic advances in measurement theory in healthcare. Modern test theory (MTT), more commonly referred to as IRT and Rasch measurement theory, which emerged from the field of education, has had a dramatic impact on clinical assessments in OT and healthcare (Cella & Chang, 2000). For purposes of this chapter, we use the term *item response theory*. Several OT assessments have been developed using IRT methods, as shown in Box 20.6. The purpose of this part of the chapter is to introduce IRT or Rasch measurement theory and its applications in critiquing OT assessments.

- Assessment of Motor and Process Skills (AMPS) (A. G. Fisher, 1993)
- School AMPS (Munkholm et al., 2012)
- Fitness-to-Drive Screening Measure (Classen et al., 2015)
- Occupational Performance History Interview (Kielhofner et al., 2005)
- Pediatric Evaluation of Disability Inventory (Haley et al., 1993)
- School Function Assessment (Coster et al., 1998)
- DriveSafe and DriveAware (Kay et al., 2009)
- Automated Vehicle User Perception Survey (Mason et al., 2021)
- Worker Role Interview (Velozo et al., 1999)

Item Response Theory

In contrast to traditional psychometrics that focuses on the entire "test," IRT, as the name implies, focuses on the items of the test. As a measurement theory, IRT addresses many limitations of traditional test theory. First, IRT is *sample free*. That is, one should expect that the results from an IRT analysis should be the same no matter what sample is chosen from a population. Second, IRT is *test free*. The basis of an assessment being test free is that in IRT, the items of an assessment measure a latent trait. A *latent trait* is a hypothesized construct or attribute that is not directly observed but is inferred from responses on an assessment (R. M. Smith, 2000). For example, driving, as assessed by a specific driving assessment, is represented by the particular items from that assessment. Tasks such as stopping at stoplights, turning at an intersection, and passing another vehicle on a highway only represent a small sample of the almost infinite number of driving tasks that can represent the latent trait of driving. Finally, in contrast to scores (frequency counts) generated from traditional assessments that are only ordinal in nature, the measures generated for some IRT models are interval in nature. Note that we are using the term *scores* to refer to the numbers obtained from traditional assessments and the term *measures* for values derived from IRT-based assessments. That is, measures have equal intervals between their values (i.e., there are equal "distances" between a one and two, two and three, etc.). Interval-level data are necessary for any level of mathematics, from the simplest addition of two numbers to complicated statistical analyses.

The aforementioned unique characteristics of IRT offer advantages of measurement that have not been achievable with traditional psychometric approaches. First, because IRT is sample free, norms are not *necessary* for measurement. That does not mean that norms are unimportant in OT. On the contrary, for example, developmental norms are extremely important in determining whether a client is within the range of what is "normal" or "typical," for instance, for a developing child. But norms are not necessary for measurement (i.e., norms are not necessary to determine whether you have more or less of something). Because IRT is sample free, an assessment should perform the same way for every sample from a particular population. That is, the relative challenge of the items on an instrument should have the same difficulty for every sample taken from a population. For example, for the population of elder drivers, pre-driving skills (e.g., opening a car door, inserting a key into the ignition) will always be easier than on-the-road driving skills (e.g., taking left-hand turns against traffic, merging onto a highway), independent of whether they have low or high driving ability. When using IRT, one should be confident that measures are replicable across different samples.

Advantages of Item Response Theory

Because IRT is test free, two important advantages arise. First, it is unnecessary to use all the items from an assessment to measure a client. Although typically, when using traditional assessments, one sums the responses on all the items of the assessment to determine the "ability" of the client, with IRT, instead of using all the items or an assessment, one can use only the most relevant items to measure a particular client. Figure 20.2 shows items of different challenges for driving. Items to the far left (obey traffic lights and stay in proper lane) represent easy driving items, and items to the far right (drive at night and drive in heavy wind and rain) represent hard items. For example, if individuals are capable of driving in heavy wind and rain, they are very likely to be capable of obeying traffic lights and staying in the proper lane. If a client is successful at a more challenging task, it is unnecessary to test them on a very easy task. This feature of IRT provides considerable efficiency for both the client and the therapist. Clients do not have to be burdened by taking all the items of an assessment, and therapists can save time by only assessing items that are most relevant to a client.

The second advantage of the test-free nature of IRT is communication between assessments. With traditional assessments, the scores generated from one assessment are not readily comparable to the scores generated from another assessment. For example, even though most activities of daily living (ADL) assessments have similar items (e.g., eating, grooming, dressing, bathing), the scores generated from each assessment carry different meanings (i.e., a score of 50 on the Functional Independence Measure [FIM™] has a different meaning than a 50 on the Barthel ADL Index). When using an IRT-based assessment, the concept of the

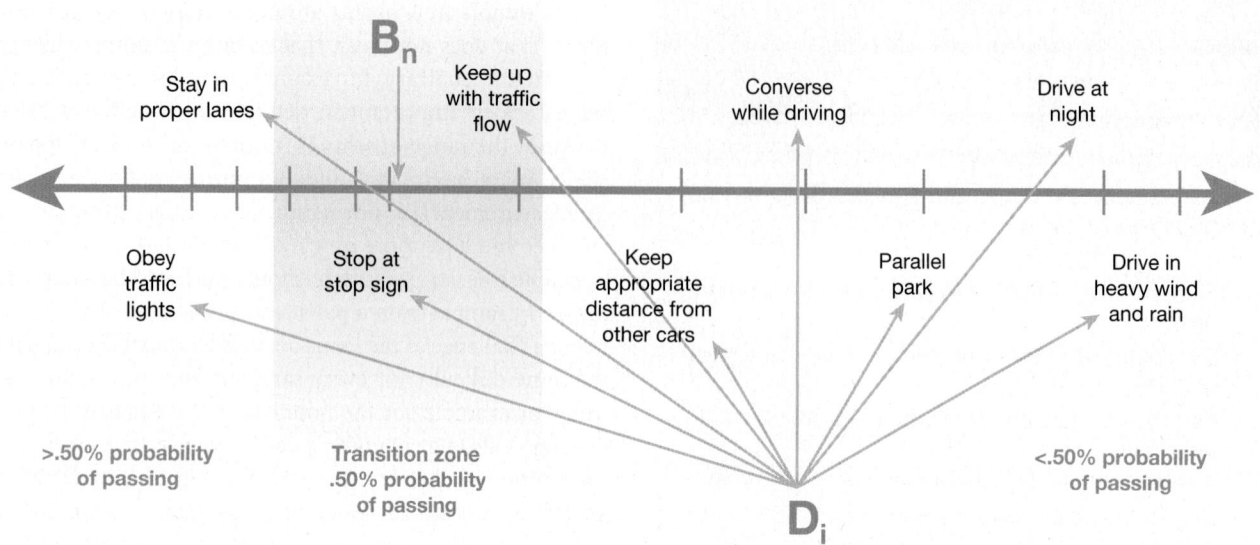

FIGURE 20.2 **Comparison of person ability (B_n) to item difficulty (D_i) for a driving assessment.**

individual assessment fades. Instead, all assessments measuring a particular latent trait represent subsets of the "infinite" number of items that can represent that latent trait. If specific assessments represent subsets of items from the same latent trait (e.g., ADL), then measures from one assessment should be readily translatable to another assessment. W. P. Fisher and colleagues (1995) used this principle to translate measures between two ADL scales, the FIM and the Patient Evaluation Conference System (PECS). Velozo et al. (2007), have also used this principle to translate measures between the FIM and the ADL items of the Minimum Data Set (MDS). Because different assessments are often used in different facilities (e.g., FIM in inpatient rehabilitation facilities and MDS in skilled nursing facilities), linking assessments provides the capability of monitoring a client's progress as they move from facility to facility even when those facilities use different assessments.

Basic Formula Underlying Item Response Theory

As noted previously, there are several IRT models with the most basic IRT models being the one-parameter Rasch model. Despite their complexity, all IRT models compare *person ability* to *item difficulty*. If it is a math test, it is whether or not the student (person ability) can pass the question (item), "8 + 8 = ?" If the person is more able than the question, they get it correct, but if the person is less able than the question, they get it wrong. This basic principle works for all assessment situations, even the assessment of clients in OT. If someone is assessed on driving, the critical question is whether the client (person) can pass the driving task (item). For example, is the client successful in taking a

left-hand turn against traffic? If the client is more able than the task, they pass the task, but if the client is less able than the task, they fail the task.

A basic statistical formula that expresses this comparison of person ability and item difficulty is the one-parameter IRT or Rasch formula (Figure 20.3). The left side of the formula represents the probability of the person passing a specific item (P_{ni}) divided by the person failing an item ($1 - P_{ni}$). The right side of the equation represents the comparison of person ability versus item difficulty ($B_n - D_i$).

Figure 20.2 presents how this formula "works" when assessing someone on a driving assessment. B_n from the formula is represented by B_1, a person with a "low" driving ability level. D_i from the formula is represented by nine driving items of different difficulty levels. To the far left are easy items, represented by predriving activities such as opening a car door and adjusting mirrors. To the far right are difficult items, such as driving at night, driving in complex situations, and driving in heavy rain and wind. Client B_1 will have a higher than .50 probability of passing the easy items such as opening a car door and a much lower than .50

$$\log [P_{ni}/1-P_{ni}] = B_n - D_i$$

P_{ni} = probability of person n passing item i
$1 - P_{ni}$ = probability of person n failing item i
B_n = ability of person n
D_i = difficulty of item in i

FIGURE 20.3 **Rasch one-parameter item response theory formula.**

probability of passing the difficult items such as driving in heavy rain and wind. But for the items that are close to their ability level (e.g., staying in the proper lane when turning), they will have a .50 probability of passing. These items are at "just the right" challenge for the individual.

This IRT model of relating a person's ability to item difficulty can be applied to assessing any client on any assessment. If we can think of our assessments as a series of items or tasks that have different challenges, we would expect that our client would have a high probability of being successful with items that were "below" their ability (the easiest items). These items could be "easy" ADL tasks such as eating and grooming, easy motor development items such as being able to roll from prone to supine, or easy upper extremity movement tasks such as moving one's arm in a gravity-eliminated position. We would expect that our client would have a low probability of being successful on items that were above their ability level. Challenging ADL tasks could be bathing or walking up the stairs, challenging motor development items could be running and jumping, and challenging upper extremity movement tasks can be lifting one's arm while extended holding a 10-lb object. As an occupational therapist, a major interest is determining the ability of a client. From a clinical perspective, IRT can be described as finding the "just right" challenge for a client. That is, not what is too easy or too hard, but the tasks that are appropriately challenging for a client.

One of the advantages of an IRT perspective for critiquing an assessment is that it provides solutions to increasing assessment efficiency (reducing respondent burden) and maximizing assessment precision. Because one acquires the most information from an assessment by using items that match a client's ability, it is logical that all of the items of an assessment are not necessary. Items that are too easy or too hard provide fairly little information about a client. This leads to the concept of "efficiency," assessing clients on only the most relevant items. This has the advantage of reducing respondent (client) burden and therapist assessment time. The IRT perspective also allows for maximizing measurement precision. For example, a low-functioning client may be assessed only by testing them on only predriving activities (e.g., opening a car door and adjusting mirrors), but a client with more ability may be assessed on only higher-level activities, such as basic driving skills (e.g., maintain lane when turning, stop at stop sign) tasks. This logic can also be used to eliminate floor effects (the inability of the assessment to discriminate among clients of low ability) and ceiling effects (the inability of the assessment to discriminate among clients of high ability). To remove a floor effect, easy items can be administered (e.g., more predriving tasks), and to remove a ceiling effect, hard items can be administered (e.g., challenging driving tasks). Although this approach is logical, the obvious question is "How do I find the most relevant assessment items for an individual?" If an assessment has a logical hierarchy in terms of the difficulty of items, such as a motor development test, this can be quite easy to find the most appropriate items. This can be accomplished by starting with easy items and progressively administering more difficult items until the client fails several items (e.g., DENVER II, previously known as the Denver Developmental Screening Test [Frankenburg et al., 1992]).

IRT-based assessments are also effectively designed for goal setting and treatment planning. As indicated in Figure 20.2, the client ability measure (B_n) is associated with the client having a .50 probability of being successful with items at their ability level (e.g., maintaining a lane when turning) and has a lower probability of being successful for items above their ability level (e.g., stopping at a stop sign, merging on the highway, driving in a complex situation). Logical short-term goals would be to increase the client's success on items at their ability level, and logical longer-term goals would be to increase the client's success on items above their ability level.

A useful way to demonstrate a client's performance on an IRT-based measure is through a keyform that presents the responses on individual items of the instrument. Figure 20.4 presents part of the keyform of the FTDS. The top of the keyform presents the scale of the instrument from 0 to 100 with the dashed vertical line representing the measure of a client (about 51). The right side of the keyform presents the items of the keyform with the easier items at the bottom (e.g., altering driving after health changes, stay focused) and the harder items at the top (e.g., drive icy road, use paper map). The numbers 1 to 4 which stair-step to the right are the ratings of the instrument (i.e., 1 = very difficult, 2 = somewhat difficult, 3 = a little difficult, and 4 = not difficult). The typical pattern shows higher ratings on easier items and lower ratings on more difficult items. Keyforms can be used to set treatment goals. For example, short-term goals could be for the client to improve on items that are rated 2 to 3 to ratings of 3 to 4, and long-term goals could be for the client to improve on items that are rated with 1's to ratings of 2 to 3. Coster et al. (1998) show how keyforms that include the item ratings on the School Function Assessment can be used to set realistic goals (e.g., moving from a rating of a 3, inconsistent performance, to 4, consistent performance, on more challenging items). Velozo and Woodbury (2011) have used similar keyforms of the Fugl–Meyer Assessment of upper extremity to suggest short- and long-term goals for clients recovering from upper extremity movement impairments following stroke. Keyforms for a variety of rehabilitation instruments are available at https://patientprogress.org, a noncommercial website affiliated with the Medical University of South Carolina that has been designed to distribute keyform recovery maps to OT and other rehabilitation professionals.

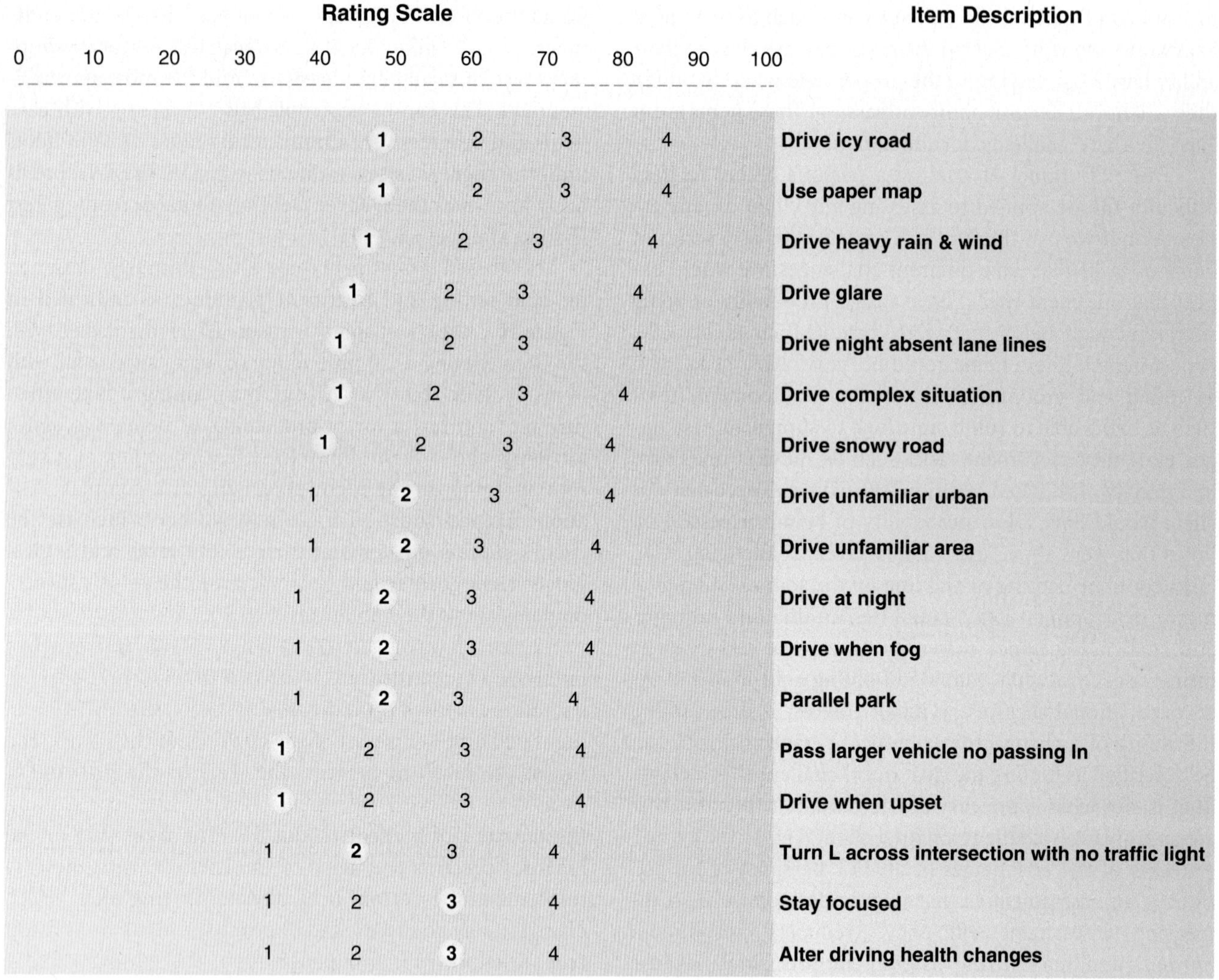

Rating Scale   **Item Description**

	0	10	20	30	40	50	60	70	80	90	100	Item
						1	2	3	4			Drive icy road
						1	2	3	4			Use paper map
						1	2	3	4			Drive heavy rain & wind
					1	2	3	4				Drive glare
					1	2	3	4				Drive night absent lane lines
					1	2	3	4				Drive complex situation
					1	2	3	4				Drive snowy road
				1	2	3	4					Drive unfamiliar urban
				1	2	3	4					Drive unfamiliar area
				1	2	3	4					Drive at night
				1	2	3	4					Drive when fog
				1	2	3	4					Parallel park
			1		2	3	4					Pass larger vehicle no passing In
			1		2	3	4					Drive when upset
			1		2	3	4					Turn L across intersection with no traffic light
			1		2	3	4					Stay focused
			1		2	3	4					Alter driving health changes

FIGURE 20.4 Part of the fitness-to-drive screening measure keyform.

Computerized Adaptive Testing

For assessments in which we do not have a clear item difficulty order, paper-and-pencil administration techniques may be ineffective. We would have to search through our assessment for the most appropriate items for our client. For example, if we find our client failing items, we would have to locate easier items. Similarly, if we found our client passing items, we would have to locate harder items. Unfortunately, for many of our assessments, the item difficulty order is not clear, thus making the selection of the most relevant items for a client even more challenging. In those cases, computer technology provides the solution. Computer software programs can be programmed to select items, even from hundreds of items (often referred to as an item bank), to administer the most relevant items to a client.

IRT, in combination with computer application of assessment items, can be used to automate both efficiency and precision in measurement. Computers can be programmed with algorithms (i.e., sets of rules) to direct only the most appropriate items to the client to maximize efficiency (use the fewest number of items) and maximize precision (use those items that differentiate one client from another or differentiate a client from one stage of progress to another) (Figure 20.5). In general, computerized adaptive testing involves presenting questions to a client until a desired level of precision (reduced error) is reached. At the beginning of the assessment, before we present any items, we have little idea of the client's ability (e.g., they could be a poor driver or could be an excellent driver), our error is large, and we have a large confidence interval. But every time we assess the client on an item or task, we get more information on the client, reduce our error of measurement, and get a smaller confidence interval. A simple computerized adaptive testing algorithm can be described in six steps (see Figure 20.5). At the beginning of an assessment, we have little idea of the client's ability (ADL, driving, depression, etc.); therefore, we typically estimate the client's ability to be at the "middle

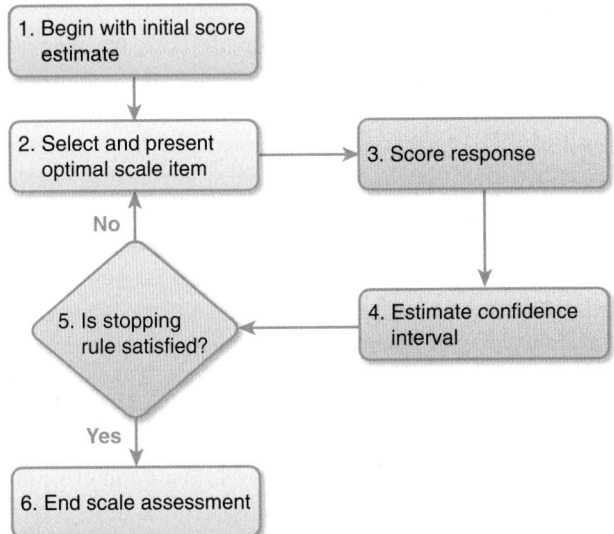

FIGURE 20.5 **Computer adaptive test algorithm.** (Adapted from Wainer, H., Dorans, N. J., Eignor, D., Flaugher, R., Green, B., Mislevy, R. J., Steinberg, L., & Thissen, D. [2000]. *Computerized adaptive testing: A primer* [2nd ed.]. Lawrence Erlbaum Associates.)

difficulty" of the items. Steps 2 through 5 represent the item administration process. The computer presents the item that most closely matches the client's initial ability estimate and/or the item that provides the most information about a client (e.g., "Do you stop at stop signs?") (step 2), and the client is scored on the item (step 3). That is, they either pass or fail (successfully stop or fail to stop) or get a particular rating (1 = failed to stop, 2 = partially stopped, 3 = stopped completely). After answering each question, the computer algorithm estimates a confidence interval or amount of precision we have in our measurement of a client (step 4). Upon answering each question, we get a smaller confidence interval and more precision. The computer continues to administer questions until we have reduced the confidence interval to a designated level (step 5); we then end the assessment and provide the client with a final assessment measure (step 6).

Presently, there are few specific OT computerized adaptive tests available for clinical use. This is probably because most assessments in OT are performance-based and computerized adaptive tests are typically self-report (often referred to as patient-reported) or proxy-report assessments. For general rehabilitation assessment, basic mobility, daily activity, and applied cognition are available in the AMPAC™ CAT (http://am-pac.com/cat/). For pediatrics, the Pediatric Evaluation of Disability Computer Adaptive Test (PEDI-CAT) is a caregiver report that measures daily activities, mobility, and social/cognitive and responsibility (pearsonassessment.com). For general healthcare, the National

Institutes of Health invested in the development of a large number of patient and proxy reported computerized adaptive measures of global, physical, mental, and social health for adults and children with chronic conditions (Patient Reported Outcomes System—PROMIS) and similar computerized adaptive measures for adults and children with neurological conditions (Neuro-QoL) (healthmeasures. net). As these assessments become readily available via the Web and via electronic health record (EHR) systems, occupational therapists and other rehabilitation professionals are likely to incorporate these assessments in clinical practice.

Critiquing Item Response Theory–Based Assessments

IRT, being a different psychometric theory than CTT and generalizability theory, demands a different set of evaluation methods. IRT is based on a set of strong psychometric assumptions or requirements. Although most of these methods are beyond the scope of the typical occupational therapist practice, we generally describe them here. There are four general areas in which IRT is typically critiqued: unidimensionality, local independence, precision, and person–item match.

Unidimensionality

Unidimensionality is the determination of whether an assessment measures a single trait. Although it is often argued that human beings are multidimensional, assessing multiple dimensions at the same time often leads to confusion. For example, ADL assessments often involve both physical function and cognitive items when evaluating a total score on the assessment; it is difficult to know what combination of attributes makes up that total score. Does the score reflect equal amounts of physical function and cognition items? Does the score represent a person with a lot of physical function ability and little cognitive ability or a lot of cognitive ability and little physical function ability? This becomes a more complex interpretation following the treatment of the client. Let's say that a client improves in their overall ADL score from admission to discharge. Has the individual improved in both physical and cognitive functioning? Improved just in physical functioning or improved just in cognitive functioning? Measuring a single or unidimensional trait is less confusing.

There are several psychometric methods to determine unidimensionality. One method is "item fit." This statistic determines how well items fit the IRT model. Items that do not fit the IRT model may be erratic or may be measuring a second trait (Bond & Fox, 2007). A second, more preferred method of determining unidimensionality is factor analysis. In general, factor analysis groups items that correlate with each other. An indication of unidimensionality is when all assessment items show a high correlation or "load" on a single factor (e.g., all load on physical functioning). An indication of multidimensionality is when items load on separate factors (e.g., physical functioning and cognitive functioning).

Local Independence

Local independence is an indication of whether the items of an assessment independently contribute to the measurement of a particular trait. That is, are some items redundant or not adding anything new to the measuring of a particular trait? This can be a particularly confusing concept and may seem in conflict to assess a client. For example, from a *qualitative* perspective, one would want to know every aspect of a client's driving ability (e.g., can the individual insert a key into the ignition, open the window, and press the gas pedal?). But some of these items may be redundant in terms of measuring driving ability. For example, pressing the gas pedal may be essentially equivalent to pressing the break or doing some other lower extremity activity. Turning a key may be essentially equivalent to adjusting a car mirror. If this is the case, then one can remove redundant items. Fairly sophisticated analyses, such as polychoric correlations or the correlation of item residuals, identify that selected items are redundant and can be removed from an assessment (Reeve et al., 2007).

Precision

Precision of an assessment is a critical feature of measurement in IRT. Obviously, we would like to have assessments that are as precise as possible because we would expect that the more precise assessment will be more effective in differentiating our patients from one another and, more importantly, effective in detecting the change in our clients following OT intervention. There are several indices of precision used in IRT. Two important indicators of precision are error and information. Although in traditional testing, one gets only one value of error for an assessment in IRT, the error can be plotted across the range of an assessment (across easy to hard items). Typically, we find that the error of an assessment is lower at the middle of the assessment and increases at the extremes of the assessment. That is, there is usually more error at the easy and hard items of an assessment. Information is the reciprocal or inverse of error; therefore, the more information provided by an assessment, the more precise it is.

Person–Item Match

Person–item match, as noted earlier, characteristic of all IRT models is the comparison of person ability to item difficulty. This relationship can tell us how well the items of our assessment match the abilities of the clients under study. This can be exemplified by ceiling and floor effects in our assessments. Ceilings effects are when an assessment cannot differentiate

the most able clients (i.e., clients are more able than what our assessment can assess), and floor effects are when an assessment cannot differentiate the least able clients that (i.e., clients are less able than what our assessment can assess). Based on IRT models, this is related to whether or not we have items that match a client's ability. For ceiling effects, we do not have items that differentiate the most able clients. For example, if we have good drivers in our sample and our hardest item is driving in our hometown, it is likely that all of these clients will get "perfect" measures on our assessment. The reality may be that if we tested these clients on more challenging items, for example, merging onto a highway, we would then be able to differentiate these clients of high ability. Similarly, a floor effect suggests that we do not have items that differentiate the lowest ability-level clients and likely indicate that we do not have easy enough items to differentiate these clients. For example, if we do not have predriving tasks on our assessment, we may not be able to differentiate those individuals who cannot do on-the-road driving. If one has a good conceptual model for an assessment, that is, an understanding of the relative challenge of the items of our assessment, resolving these problems can be easy. Ceiling effects can be eliminated by creating more challenging items, and floor effects can be eliminated by creating easy items.

Conclusion

The purpose of this chapter is to provide an overview of the many methods used to critique assessments. As evident by the number of areas covered in this chapter, critiquing assessments is not an easy task. It requires both clinical knowledge of one's specialty area and statistical knowledge of reliability and validity. Critiquing assessments becomes more daunting with the addition of new measurement theories such as IRT and new test administration methods such as computerized adaptive testing. Obviously, the practicing therapist cannot be up to date on all OT assessments. But as a practicing occupational therapist, one must be able to critique the assessments that one uses in daily practice.

Lippincott® Connect *For additional resources on the subjects discussed in this chapter, visit Lippincott Connect.*

REFERENCES

Alvarez, L., & Classen, S. (2017). In-vehicle technology and driving simulation. In S. Classen (Ed.), *Driving simulation for assessment, intervention, and training: A guide for occupational therapy and health care professionals* (pp. 265–278). AOTA Press.

Association of American Publishers. (n.d.). *Standardized assessment: A primer* (Rev. ed.). Author.

Bédard, M. B., Parkkari, M., Weaver, B., Riendeau, J., & Dahlquist, M. (2010). Assessment of driving performance using a simulator protocol: Validity and reproducibility. *American Journal of Occupational Therapy, 64*(2), 336–340. https://doi.org/10.5014/ajot.64.2.336

Bond, T. G., & Fox, C. M. (2007). *Applying the Rasch model: Fundamental measurement in the human sciences*. Lawrence Erlbaum Associates.

Carmines, E. G., & Zeller, R. (Eds.). (1979). *Reliability and validity assessment*. Sage.

Cella, D., & Chang, C. H. (2000). A discussion of item response theory and its applications in health status assessment. *Medical Care, 38*(9 Suppl), II66–II72. https://doi.org/10.1097/00005650-200009002-00010

Classen, S., McCarthy, D. P., Shechtman, O., Awadzi, K. D., Lanford, D. N., Okun, M. S., Rodriguez, R. L., Romrell, J., Bridges, S., Kluger, B., & Fernandez, H. H. (2009). Useful field of view as a reliable screening measure of driving performance in people with Parkinson's disease: Results of a pilot study. *Traffic Injury Prevention, 10*(6), 593–598. https://doi.org/10.1080/15389580903179901

Classen, S., & Owens, A. B. (2010). Simulator sickness among returning combat veterans with mild traumatic brain injury and/or post-traumatic stress disorder [Special issue]. *Advances in Transportation Studies, 2010*, 45–52. https://trid.trb.org/view/1118219

Classen, S., Velozo, C. A., Winter, S. M., Bédard, M., & Wang, Y. (2015). Psychometrics of the fitness-to-drive screening measure. *OTJR: Occupation, Participation and Health, 35*(1), 42–52. https://doi.org/10.1177/1539449214561761

Classen, S., Winter, S. M., Velozo, C. A., Bédard, M., Lanford, D., Brumback, B. A., & Lutz, B. J. (2010). Item development and validity testing for a safe driving behavior measure. *American Journal of Occupational Therapy, 64*(2), 296–305. https://doi.org/10.5014/ajot.64.2.296

Coster, W., Deeney, T., Haltiwanger, J., & Haley, S. (1998). *School function assessment user manual*. The Psychological Corporation.

Cronbach, L. J., Gleser, G. C., Nanda, H., & Rajaratnam, N. (1972). *The dependability of behavioral measurements: Theory of generalizability for scores and profiles*. Wiley.

Cronbach, L. J., Nageswari, R., & Gleser, G. C. (1963). Theory of generalizability: A liberation of reliability theory. *The British Journal of Statistical Psychology, 16*(2), 137–163. https://doi.org/10.1111/j.2044-8317.1963.tb00206.x

Denaro, R. P., Zmud, J., Shladover, S., Walker Smith, B., & Lappin, J. (2014, May). Automated vehicle technology: Ten research areas to follow. *TR News, 292*, 19–24.

Di Stefano, M., & Macdonald, W. (2005). On-the-road evaluation of driving performance. In J. M. Pellerito (Ed.), *Driver rehabilitation and community principles and practice* (pp. 255–274). Mosby.

Edwards, J. D., Ross, L. A., Wadley, V. G., Clay, O. J., Crowe, M., Roenker, D. L., & Ball, K. K. (2006). The useful field of view test: Normative data for older adults. *Archives of Clinical Neuropsychology, 21*(4), 275–286. https://doi.org/10.1016/j.acn.2006.03.001

Fisher, A. G. (1993). The assessment of IADL motor skills: An application of many-faceted Rasch analysis. *American Journal of Occupational Therapy, 47*(4), 319–329. https://doi.org/10.5014/ajot.47.4.319

Fisher, W. P., Jr., Harvey, R. F., Taylor, P., Kilgore, K. M., & Kelly, C. K. (1995). Rehabits: A common language of functional assessment. *Archives of Physical Medicine & Rehabilitation, 76*(2), 113–122. https://doi.org/10.1016/S0003-9993(95)80020-4

Folstein, M. F., Folstein, S. E., & McHugh, P. R. (1975). "Mini-mental state." A practical method for grading the cognitive state of patients for the clinician. *Journal of Psychiatric Research, 12*(3), 189–198. https://doi.org/10.1016/0022-3956(75)90026-6

Folstein, M. F., Folstein, S. E., White, T., & Messer, M. A. (2010). *Mini-mental state exam: User's guide* (2nd ed.). PAR.

Frankenburg, W. K., Doods, J., Archer, P., Bresnick, B., Maschka, P., Edelman, N., & Shapiro, H. (1992). *DENVER II training manual*. Denver Developmental Materials.

Grant, J. S., & Davis, L. L. (1997). Selection and use of content experts for instrument development. *Research in Nursing & Health, 20*(3), 269–274. https://doi.org/10.1002/(SICI)1098-240X(199706)20:3<269::AID-NUR9>3.0.CO;2-G

Haley, S. M., Ludlow, L. H., & Coster, W. J. (1993). Pediatric Evaluation of Disability Inventory: Clinical interpretation of summary scores using Rasch rating scale methodology. *Physical Medicine and Rehabilitation Clinics of North America, 4*(3), 529–540. https://doi.org/10.1016/S1047-9651(18)30568-0

Hinojosa, J., Kramer, P., & Crist, P. (Eds.). (2005). *Evaluation: Obtaining and interpreting data* (2nd ed.). AOTA Press.

House, A. E., House, B. J., & Campbell, M. B. (1981). Measures of interobserver agreement: Calculation formulas and distribution effects. *Journal of Behavioral Assessment, 3*, 37–57. https://doi.org/10.1007/BF01321350

Justiss, M. D., Mann, W. C., Stav, W., & Velozo, C. (2006). Development of a behind-the-wheel driving performance assessment for older adults. *Topics in Geriatric Rehabilitation, 22*(2), 121–128. https://doi.org/10.1097/00013614-200604000-00004

Kay, L. G., Bundy, A. C., & Clemson, L. M. (2009). Predicting fitness to drive in people with cognitive impairments by using DriveSafe and DriveAware. *Archives of Physical Medicine & Rehabilitation, 90*(9), 1514–1522. https://doi.org/10.1016/j.apmr.2009.03.011

Kennedy, R. S., Lane, N. E., Berbaum, K. S., & Lilienthal, M. G. (1993). Simulator Sickness Questionnaire: An enhanced method for quantifying simulator sickness. *The International Journal of Aviation Psychology, 3*(3), 203–220. https://doi.org/10.1207/s15327108ijap0303_3

Kielhofner, G., Dobria, L., Forsyth, K., & Basu, S. (2005). The construction of keyforms for obtaining instantaneous measures from the Occupational Performance History Interview rating scales: Empirical quantitative study. *OTJR: Occupation, Participation and Health, 25*(1), 23–32. https://doi.org/10.1177/153944920502500104

Kraut, R., Olson, J., Banaji, M., Bruckman, A., Cohen, J., & Couper, M. (2004). Psychological research online: Report of Board of Scientific Affairs' Advisory Group on the Conduct of Research on the Internet. *The American Psychologist, 59*(2), 105–117. https://doi.org/10.1037/0003-066X.59.2.105

Law, M. (1987). Measurement in occupational therapy: Scientific criteria for evaluation. *Canadian Journal of Occupational Therapy, 54*(3), 133–138. https://doi.org/10.1177/000841748705400308

Lynn, M. R. (1986). Determination and quantification of content validity. *Nursing Research, 35*(6), 382–385. https://doi.org/10.1097/00006199-198611000-00017

Mason, J., Classen, S., Wersal, J., & Sisiopiku, V. (2021). Construct validity and test–retest reliability of the automated vehicle user perception survey. *Frontiers in Psychology: Quantitative Psychology and Measurement, 12*, Article 626791. https://doi.org/10.3389/fpsyg.2021.626791

Morris, J. C. (1993). The clinical dementia rating (CDR): Current version and scoring rules. *Neurology, 43*(11), 2412–2414. https://doi.org/10.1212/WNL.43.11.2412-a

Munkholm, M., Löfgren, B., & Fisher, A. G. (2012). Reliability of the school AMPS measures. *Scandinavian Journal of Occupational Therapy, 19*(1), 2–8. https://doi.org/10.3109/11038128.2010.525721

Nunnally, J. C., & Bernstein, I. H. (1994). *Psychometric theory* (3rd ed.). McGraw-Hill.

Owsley, C., Ball, K. K., McGwin, G., Jr., Sloane, M. E., Roenker, D. L., White, M. F., & Overley, E. T. (1998). Visual processing impairment and risk of motor vehicle crash among older adults. *JAMA, 279*(14), 1083–1088. https://doi.org/10.1001/jama.279.14.1083

Owsley, C., & McGwin, G., Jr. (1999). Vision impairment and driving. *Survey of Ophthalmology, 43*(6), 535–550. https://doi.org/10.1016/S0039-6257(99)00035-1

Owsley, C., McGwin, G., Jr., & Ball, K. K. (1998). Vision impairment, eye disease, and injurious motor vehicle crashes in the elderly. *Ophthalmic Epidemiology, 5*(2), 101–113. https://doi.org/10.1076/opep.5.2.101.1574

Owsley, C., Stalvey, B. T., Wells, J., & Sloane, M. E. (1999). Older drivers and cataract: Driving habits and crash risk. *Journal of Gerontology: Series A: Biological Sciences & Medical Sciences, 54*(4), M203–M211. https://doi.org/10.1093/gerona/54.4.M203

Portney, L., & Watkins, M. P. (2009). *Foundations of clinical research: Applications to practice* (3rd ed.). Prentice Hall.

Reeve, B. B., Hays, R. D., Bjorner, J. B., Cook, K. F., Crane, P. K., Teresi, J. A., Thissen, D., Revicki, D. A., Weiss, D. J., Hambleton, R. K., Liu, H., Gershon, R., Reise, S. P., Lai, J. S., Cella, D., & PROMIS Cooperative Group. (2007). Psychometric evaluation and calibration of health-related quality of life item banks: Plans for the Patient-Reported Outcomes Measurement Information System (PROMIS). *Medical Care, 45*(5 Suppl 1), S22–S31. https://doi.org/10.1097/01.mlr.0000250483.85507.04

Reitan, R. M. (1958). Validity of the trail making test as an indicator of organic brain damage. *Perceptual and Motor Skills, 8,* 271–276. https://doi.org/10.2466/pms.1958.8.3.271

Rudman, D., & Hannah, S. (1998). An instrument evaluation framework: Description and application to assessments of hand function. *Journal of Hand Therapy, 11*(4), 266–277. https://doi.org/10.1016/S0894-1130(98)80023-9

Smith, R. M. (2000). Fit analysis in latent trait measurement models. *Journal of Applied Measurement, 1*(2), 199–218.

Streiner, D. L., & Norman, G. R. (Eds.). (2008a). Devising the items. In *Health measurement scales: A practical guide to their development and use* (4th ed., pp. 17–36). Oxford University Press.

Streiner, D. L., & Norman, G. R. (Eds.). (2008b). *Health measurement scales: A practical guide to their development and use* (4th ed.). Oxford University Press.

Velozo, C. A., Byers, K. L, Wang, Y. C., & Joseph, B. R. (2007). Translating measures across the continuum of care: Using Rasch analysis to create a crosswalk between the functional independence measure and the minimum data set. *Journal of Rehabilitation Research and Development, 44*(3), 467–478. https://doi.org/10.1682/JRRD.2006.06.0068

Velozo, C. A., Kielhofner, G., Gern, A., Lin, F. L., Azhar, F., Lai, J. S., & Fisher, G. (1999). Worker role interview: Toward validation of a psychosocial work-related measure. *Journal of Occupational Rehabilitation, 9*(3), 153–168. https://doi.org/10.1023/A:1021397600383

Velozo, C. A., & Woodbury, M. L. (2011). Translating measurement findings into rehabilitation practice: An example using Fugl–Meyer assessment-upper extremity with patients following stroke. *Journal of Rehabilitation Research and Development, 48*(10), 1211–1222. https://doi.org/10.1682/JRRD.2010.10.0203

Wainer, H., Dorans, N. J., Eignor, D., Flaugher, R., Green, B. F., Mislevy, R. J., Steinberg, L., & Thissen, D. (2000). *Computerized adaptive testing: A primer* (2nd ed.). Lawrence Erlbaum Associates.

Whiteneck, G., Brooks, C. A., Charlifue, S., Gerhart, K. A., Mellick, D., Overholser, D., et al. (2009). *Guide for use of the CHART: Craig handicap assessment and reporting technique.* www.craighospital.org/Research/CHART

Wilschut, E. S. (2009). The impact of in-vehicle information systems on simulated driving performance: Effects of age, timing and display characteristics [Unpublished doctoral dissertation]. University of Groningen, The Netherlands.

CHAPTER 21

Occupational Therapy Interventions for Individuals

Glen Gillen

LEARNING OBJECTIVES

After reading this chapter, you will be able to:

1. Understand the overarching themes that occupational therapists embrace when choosing interventions for their clients.
2. Differentiate between interventions that are categorized as "occupation as ends" and "occupation as means."
3. Develop and choose interventions that combine the principles of occupation as ends and occupation as means.
4. Compare and contrast a variety of specific intervention approaches that are used for individuals receiving occupational therapy services.
5. Begin to understand when to choose one type of intervention over another, combine interventions, and/or switch the intervention plan.
6. Understand the concept of grading interventions.

Introduction

When developing intervention plans for clients,[1] occupational therapy (OT) practitioners work under the guidance of three overarching and interrelated themes. Interventions must be client centered, evidence based, and chosen based on sound professional reasoning. The term *client-centered practice* has been defined as

> an approach to providing occupational therapy, which embraces a philosophy of respect for and partnership with people receiving services. It recognizes the autonomy of individuals, the need for client choice in making decisions about occupational needs, the strengths clients bring to an occupational therapy

---

[1] According to the American Occupational Therapy Association (AOTA, 2020, p. S75), the term *client* refers to *persons* (including those involved in care of a client), *groups* (a collection of individuals having shared characteristics or common or shared purpose, e.g., family members, workers, students, and those with similar interests or occupational challenges), and *populations* (aggregates of people with common attributes such as contexts, characteristics or concerns, including health risks). However, in countries other than the US, the term *client* often refers to persons who are paying for their care directly. In most countries, *patient* is used to describe persons who are in hospital or rehabilitation. *Service user* and *person* are terms in general use that describe those in need of OT services. For this chapter, we are using *client* without implying the source of payment for services.

encounter and the benefits of client-therapist partnership and the need to ensure that services are accessible and fit the context in which a client lives. (Law et al., 1995, p. 253)

Sumsion and Law (2006) have reviewed and analyzed subsequent definitions of client-centered practice and concluded that the various definitions share many similar components including " . . . a strong emphasis on a collaborative approach or partnership, respect for the client, facilitating choice and involving the client in determining the occupational goals that emerge from his or her choices" (p. 154). The reader is referred to Chapter 28 for further discussion on this topic.

Sumsion and Law (2006) further point out that the development of the literature regarding client-centered practice parallels the development of our understanding of the evidence-based practice. Sackett and colleagues (2000) define evidence-based practice as "the integration of best research evidence with clinical expertise and patient values" (p. 1). Client values include "the unique preferences, concerns, and expectations each patient brings to a clinical encounter" (Sackett et al., 2000, p. 1). A major component of evidence-based practice is the clear message that we, as OT practitioners, must use evidence to inform our intervention choices (Bennett et al., 2003). Bennett and Bennett (2000) summarize that the research literature can provide guidance concerning the effectiveness and choices of OT interventions, how interventions are best implemented, and whether there are any associated difficulties related to the intervention. They conclude that "occupational therapists can use this sort of research evidence to help clients understand, plan and cope with their situation" (Bennett &

Bennett, 2000, p. 173). See Chapter 26 for more detail regarding evidence-based practice.

The literature regarding evidence-based decision-making has consistently emphasized that research evidence alone is not adequate to guide the choice of interventions. Rather, clinicians must apply their clinical expertise and professional reasoning to assess the patient's deficits while at the same time incorporating the research evidence (Haynes et al., 2002). Bennett and Bennett (2000) also stress that evidence needs to be integrated with clinical expertise and reasoning so that practitioners can decide if valid and potentially useful results from a research study can apply to the individuals that they are working with. They proposed the following questions to guide the application of evidence:

1. "Do these results apply to my client? (i.e., is my client so different from those in the study that its results cannot help me?)
2. Does the treatment fit in with my client's values and preferences?
3. Are there resources available to implement the treatment?" (Bennett & Bennett, 2000, p. 177)

In addition to these questions, the OT practitioner must consider how or whether the evidence relates to our profession's underlying assumptions and philosophy (AOTA, 2020). It is important to remember that just because an intervention is deemed effective does not automatically mean that it is an appropriate OT intervention. The reader is further referred to Chapter 25 for detailed information regarding the professional reasoning process and Expanding Our Perspectives for another viewpoint.

EXPANDING OUR PERSPECTIVES

Challenging Occupational Therapy's Assumptions about Its "Client-Centered" Practices

Karen Whalley Hammell

The OT profession claims to be both "client centered" and "evidence based." This has caused me to ponder two questions: Has evidence derived from clients' perspectives informed the profession's conception of "client-centered" practice? And: Does evidence support the premise that clients perceive their OT interventions to be "client centered"? The dearth of research addressing these basic questions challenges OT's claims to be either "evidence based" or client centered. I suggest that this embarrassing shortcoming reflects both the ongoing absence of scholarly debate about what constitutes "best evidence" in the context of OT and the inadequacy of attempts to generate relevant, actionable knowledge through recourse to just one

research approach. Critical scholars contend that purportedly "context neutral," quantitative research methods are of little use for understanding complex, context-dependent human experiences—such as occupation—or subjective perspectives—such as of being a client. Striving to adhere to borrowed "hierarchies" of evidence, while simultaneously ignoring the robust critiques of evidence-based practice articulated within medicine has led to the priorities, perceptions, and judgments of potential former and current recipients of OT being excluded from our research. Thus, we do not know whether our plethora of "standardized" assessments are measuring what matters most to clients or whether the interventions informed by these assessments are either valuable or relevant.

It is rarely acknowledged that a significant body of evidence generated by critical disability researchers contests the assumption that clients consistently perceive OT to be a client-centered profession. Indeed, therapists have

EXPANDING OUR PERSPECTIVES (*continued*)

been described as being hierarchical and disempowering, intent on dictating clients' lifestyles, slavish adherents to procedural "red tape," and accountable to employers rather than to clients. OT's research reinforces these findings, reporting that some therapists "prescribe" activities; some act as gatekeepers to the equipment, resources, and services clients need; and some abuse their professional power through tactics of coercion and intimidation. This contradicts our profession's claim to be client centered.

It has therefore been encouraging to discover—in rigorous research reports published in international OT journals—that practices worthy of the descriptor "client centered" do exist! Moreover, these studies inform us that from clients' perspectives, client-centered practices are undertaken by OT practitioners who listen to clients, who strive to reduce power inequalities, who are neither authoritarian nor judgmental, who do not tell clients what to do but who work on behalf of, for, and with clients toward those goals that are of importance to them, such

that interventions are responsive to clients' lives rather than their deficits, diagnoses or "conditions." These studies indicate that "client-centered" practices are enacted by OT practitioners who demonstrate clearly that clients are respected, valued, and cared about; who treat clients as equals; who choose closeness over distance and detachment; who seek and respect clients' experience and knowledge; who create supportive and accepting relationships with clients; who are trustworthy and reliable; and who are kind.

If OT's reality is going to match its rhetoric, we must employ diverse research methods amenable to exploring clients' priorities and perspectives; we must seek out and learn from innovative and inspirational work undertaken by our international colleagues; and we must commit to practicing in ways that are ethically consistent with our public proclamations. (For references to the research sketched in this box, see Hammell, K. W. [2020]. *Engagement in living: Critical perspectives on occupation, rights and wellbeing.* CAOT.)

OT Story 21.1 was developed to provide the reader with insight into the OT intervention process that is described in detail in this chapter. As you read, note that the various interventions were developed based on the clients' needs and desire to maintain access to their community. The interventions were planned based on the findings of a variety

of evaluation techniques. Finally, note that the combinations of interventions were used to meet client-centered goals. This story is focusing the critical occupation of community mobility and driving (Dun et al., 2020; Krasniuk et al., 2022; Samuelsson et al., 2019). More stories are provided at the end of this chapter to further illustrate intervention processes.

OT STORY 21.1 BENJAMIN AND BESS: A MARRIED OLDER COUPLE WHOSE FAMILY IS CONCERNED ABOUT THEIR DRIVING ABILITIES

Occupational Profile

Benjamin is a 79-year-old male who lives with his wife Bess in a retirement community. Benjamin and Bess have always enjoyed visiting their children and grandchildren who live in neighboring towns. Benjamin had a myocardial infarction about 7 years ago and underwent bypass surgery. Although Benjamin remains independent in his basic activities of daily living (ADL), plays cards with his longtime buddies, and enjoys walks about the community's gardens, he can get short of breath with exertion. One year ago, Bess experienced a mild/moderate stroke with residual left-sided weakness and a visual field cut. She has not driven since the stroke, needs assistance with transfers, and uses a scooter except for short distances, thus making road trips more stressful due to mobility and vision issues. Up until a year ago, Benjamin and Bess shared driving responsibilities, functioning as a team for navigation. Since Benjamin assumed full

responsibility for driving and navigation, Bess has reported several "near misses" while driving, but Benjamin is quick to report that these incidents were the fault of other drivers. Recently, they both were upset after a "fender bender" that Benjamin insisted was the fault of a driver who "came out of nowhere." Bess tearfully admits that she struggles to assist in navigation and there have been some tense moments as they struggled to find their way home when returning from a trip to see their grandchildren. She relies on her husband for transportation, so she waffles back and forth with her concerns. The adult children are now worried for both of their parents' safety and discussed the issue with Benjamin and Bess's physician. The physician referred Bess to a general practice OT practitioner to address her mobility issues, and Benjamin was referred to an OT practitioner who is a driver rehabilitation specialist for a comprehensive driving evaluation.

(continued)

OT STORY 21.1 BENJAMIN AND BESS: A MARRIED OLDER COUPLE WHOSE FAMILY IS CONCERNED ABOUT THEIR DRIVING ABILITIES (continued)

Assessment Findings

Benjamin, Bess, and their adult children were interviewed by the driver rehabilitation specialist to review Benjamin's medical and driving history as well as to understand the environmental context for community mobility resources. The OT practitioner reviewed Benjamin's medications and cardiac history and administered an array of clinical assessments to cover his cognitive, motor, and visual abilities. Specifically, assessments include (a) functional range of motion and strength of the neck, arms, and legs; (b) visual acuity; (c) contrast sensitivity; (d) visual fields and tracking; (e) Short Blessed cognitive exam; (f) Trail-Making Test A and B; (g) the Useful Field of View (UFOV) (computer-based screen for selective attention); (h) clock drawing; and (i) brake reaction timer; and the OT practitioner observed Benjamin making a meat and cheese sandwich and coffee. Benjamin wore his glasses for the vision testing and demonstrated very poor contrast sensitivity and vision that was 20/70. When asked, Benjamin had not had a vision evaluation for more than 10 years. There were no field cuts or difficulty tracking visually. Benjamin's cognitive abilities did not show any sign of significant dementia, but his processing speeds were slow with the Trail-Making Test, UFOV, and brake reaction timer. He also had some range of motion restrictions with his neck. The behind-the-wheel (BTW) evaluation was delayed until Benjamin was able to see an optometrist. After the optometrist evaluated Benjamin's vision and prescribed new glasses, his visual acuity increased to 20/30. However, the contrast sensitivity remained poor, not unusual for his age. The BTW assessment demonstrated that Benjamin follows the rules of the road and did not make any significant errors but was slow in making decisions at unprotected turns and drove significantly slower than other traffic on the highway component of the evaluation.

Goal

Several goals were established: (a) Their automobile would be modified with a swing front seat for improved transfer for Bess; (b) Benjamin would remain independent in driving with a recommended restricted license; and (c) Benjamin, Bess, and their children would make plans for alternative transportation when needed and eventual driving retirement.

Intervention

Bess was seen by an OT practitioner generalist who recommended that their motor vehicle be modified with a scooter lift as well as a swing-out seat for ease of transfers from the scooter to the front passenger seat to decrease the physical toll when using their automobile (adaptation). Both Benjamin and Bess would be educated on the proper use. The therapist also evaluated Bess's instrumental ADL (IADL) in the home and assisted her in modifying the kitchen and bathroom to improve her independence (environmental modifications).

Using a prevention approach, the driver rehabilitation specialist made the recommendation to restrict Benjamin's license to daytime driving only due to the poor contrast sensitivity because evidence demonstrates the relationship between contrast sensitivity and crashes (Owsley & McGwin, 1999; Owsley et al., 1983, 1999). The therapist also recommended that highway driving be eliminated and that planning be done for local routes to avoid unprotected turns or yield signs because evidence shows that the risk of crashes at these types of intersections increases significantly with slowed processing (Stutts et al., 2009). The driving rehabilitation specialist reviewed Benjamin and Bess's community mobility needs and planned routes that posed less risk for crashes, including right-hand turns and intersections with signals. Meeting with the adult children, Benjamin, and Bess, the OT practitioner devise alternative transportation plans that included the children picking up their parents when an activity might involve nighttime driving, and the grandchildren alternating picking up their grandparents for visits. Benjamin and Bess began to use the retirement community's transportation for some events. Three months later, Bess and Benjamin indicated that traveling had become much easier with the scooter lift and transfer seat. No further "close calls" were reported, and Benjamin and Bess reported it was sometimes delightful to be chauffeured by their grandchildren.

Questions

1. Describe the roles of the OT generalist compared to the driver rehabilitation specialist for this case.
2. Why was it important to include Benjamin's whole family as team members?

Occupation as Therapy

As OT practitioners, our outcomes are focused on improving occupational performance. We achieve this goal by using occupation as a therapeutic change agent. Therefore, we believe in the therapeutic value of occupational engagement and that engagement in occupations is also the ultimate goal of therapy (AOTA, 2017). The therapeutic occupations we use are ideally both *meaningful* and *purposeful*. Meaningful suggests that the task at hand is motivating and has some level of significance (Trombly, 1995). The task may be something the person wants to do, has to do, or needs to do throughout the day. The purposeful component may serve to organize and enhance performance as it pertains to the client's aim, the reason for doing it, or personal goal (Fisher, 1998; Trombly, 1995). Interventions may involve changing occupations in ways that either foster development or improvement in desired performance or allow for participation in spite of limitations. Based on the intervention choices that are outlined in the following discussion, occupations can be graded to create "just the right challenge." The term *grading* refers to systematically increasing the demands of an occupation to stimulate improved function or reducing the demands to respond to client difficulties in performance.

When grading, the OT practitioner increases the demands of the task at hand to potentially reduce an underlying impairment or performance skill deficit. In other cases, the OT practitioner may downgrade the demands so that the task can be achieved despite a client's limitations. A person who is recovering from cardiac transplant surgery that was preceded by a long period of bed rest may be engaged in occupations that are systematically graded to improve strength and endurance to foster participation in meaningful occupations. The therapist may grade therapeutic occupations based on the posture assumed while performing

tasks (standing as opposed to sitting), duration of the task, number of rest breaks, use of adaptive equipment, and vanishing cognitive and physical assistance by the therapist to complete the task. OT practitioners may also downgrade demands and modify the task or the environment so that a client can still participate despite persistent impairments. A therapist may work with an adult who is living with schizophrenia to circumvent daily life problems by teaching the use of a daily planner to help organize and complete home and work tasks. The therapist may grade the number of verbal cues required for organization and sequencing when teaching the client to use the planner to create a grocery list.

Fisher (1998) describes occupation as a "noun of action" that has the power to enable people "to perform the actions they need and want to perform so that they can engage in and 'do' the familiar, ordinary, goal directed activities of every day in a manner that brings meaning and personal satisfaction" (p. 511). She further outlines groups of activities and their attributes that can be implemented as OT (Table 21.1).

TABLE 21.1 Intervention Methods Potentially Used by Occupational Therapy Practitioners

Activity Type	Examples	Focus of Therapy	Source of Meaning and Purpose	How Real or Natural	OT Practice Framework Classification
Exercise: rote exercise or practice	Elastic bands, weight lifting, practice line drawing for eye–hand coordination	Remediation of impairments	Practitioner-chosen for therapy benefits Client expected to "comply"	Contrived—typically only done in therapy situation	Interventions to support occupation
Contrived occupation: exercise with added purpose and occupation with a contrived component	Practice picking up balls from the floor and placing them in a bucket, placing cones on a shelf pretending they are dishes, hammering nails into wood, throwing bean bags at a target	Remediation of impairments or skill development	Practitioner-chosen for therapy benefits Client expected to "comply"	Contrived, therapy using culturally common objects	Purposeful activity
Therapeutic occupation[a]: graded occupations to treat impairments, direct intervention of impairments in the context of occupation	Challenging balance skills via organizing library book shelves for a client who loves to read, working on social skills during a group focused on adolescents making a cake for one of their mothers, using a favorite card game to improve attention	Remediation of impairments or skill development	Chosen collaboratively for meaning to client and therapy potential	More naturalistic, uses authentic aspects of occupation (tools, context)	Occupation-based intervention
Adaptive/compensatory occupation[a]: assistive devices, teach compensatory strategies, modify physical or social environments	Adapting a shopping task to compensate for poor endurance Learning to drive again after an orthopedic injury Working in a job for a person with developmental disabilities	Improved occupational performance	Chosen collaboratively based on occupations, with therapy processes selected to support performance	Naturalistic activity in natural contexts	Occupation-based intervention

Note that current trends in the field suggest that occupation-based approaches (indicated by [a]) are often the most effective and provide a clearer external reflection of the occupational therapy (OT) profession's contribution to healthcare. Additionally, interventions may involve a mix of methods to both minimize the effects of impairment and promote occupational functioning.

Data from Fisher, A. G. (1998). Uniting practice and theory in an occupational therapy framework, 1998 Eleanor Clarke Slagle lecture. *American Journal of Occupational Therapy, 52*(7), 509–522. https://doi.org/10.5014/ajot.52.7.509

Occupation as Ends as Intervention

In her Eleanor Clarke Slagle Lecture, Catherine Trombly (1995) described the **occupation as ends** as being "not only purposeful but also meaningful because it is the performance of activities or tasks that a person sees as important" (p. 963). Occupation as ends refers to engaging your client in occupations that constitute the end product of therapy (i.e., the occupations to be learned or relearned). Occupation as ends has been described by Trombly as the following:

- Directly teaching the activity or task
- Using whatever abilities clients have at their disposal to learn a task
- Providing adaptations to learn a task or activity
- A rehabilitative approach
- A skills training approach
- An approach in which the therapist serves as a teacher or adapter of a task
- Influenced by learning and cognitive information–processing theories regarding the therapeutic principle behind this approach
- *Not* being used to make a therapeutic change of underlying capabilities such as strength or memory

Using occupation as ends as an intervention serves as the goal to be learned or achieved. It refers to the ultimate goal of OT intervention, which is to restore, improve, and enable clients to engage in purposeful occupations (Che Daud et al., 2016).

For example, Rashad, who is undergoing inpatient rehabilitation after a spinal cord injury (SCI) left him paraplegic, may have a goal to independently transfer from his wheelchair to his car or his bathtub. If you were to watch the therapist and Rashad in action, they would be engaged in specifically chosen areas of occupation, and you may observe the actual practice of these mobility skills: the therapist teaching Rashad how to use a sliding board to move from surface to surface; the therapist suggesting environmental modifications such as a tub bench and nonslip bath mats; and/or the therapist gradually decreasing the amount of physical, cognitive, and emotional support required to perform the task as the client becomes more independent. The occupations chosen are based on the occupations that the client wants to, needs to, or has to resume or continue various life roles. Using occupation as ends as an intervention approach makes the focus of OT quite clear, particularly when a collaborative approach to intervention planning is used (Box 21.1).

Occupation as Means as Intervention

Occupation as means refers to "the occupation acting as the therapeutic change agent to remediate impaired abilities or capacities" (Trombly, 1995, p. 964). Occupation as means as an intervention can be described as follows:

- Including a variety of interventions, such as arts and crafts, games, sports, and specifically chosen daily activities
- Requiring more constrained responses as compared to occupation as ends
- Chosen based on both client interest and potential to remediate an underlying impairment
- Providing a challenge that is slightly beyond what the client can easily achieve. This concept has also been described as finding "just the right challenge."

An assumption inherent in this intervention approach is "that acquisition or reacquisition of motor, cognitive, and

---

BOX 21.1 EXAMPLES OF USING OCCUPATION AS ENDS

- Teaching a person who has just had a hip replacement to adapt positions so that sexual activities can be engaged in safely
- Practicing one-handed shoe tying after stroke or upper limb amputation
- Repetitive practice of components of meal preparation
- Teaching a child living with developmental delays to use an augmentative communication device
- Recommending magnifying devices so that a person living with macular degeneration can read the newspaper
- Recommending and training with vehicular hand controls so that a person who does not have use of their lower extremities after a spinal cord injury can drive again

- Teaching an adult living with schizophrenia a new leisure activity, such as photography
- Task-specific practice of handwriting, such as writing out a weekly grocery list
- Teaching a person who has survived a stroke how to propel a wheelchair using one arm and leg for functional mobility within the home
- Demonstrating and teaching the use of bilateral upper limb prostheses to eat a meal after upper limb amputations
- Demonstrating and teaching an adaptive swallowing technique to promote independent and safe self-feeding

psychological skills will ultimately result in successful performance of activities of daily living" (Weinstock-Zlotnick & Hinojosa, 2004, p. 594). It is used as a remediation agent and a way to improve a client's function (Che Daud et al., 2016). Box 21.2 provides examples of using occupation as means as an intervention. Unlike occupation as ends, simply observing a client engaged in an occupation as means may not provide the observer with a clear understanding of why the intervention was chosen. In many cases, this understanding emerges after a discussion with the OT practitioner as to the rationale for the choice of the intervention. Teaching someone a new board game may be considered occupation as ends if the client's goals include expanding their repertoire of leisure-based occupations. A board game may also be chosen as a therapeutic mechanism for a variety of reasons that may classify the intervention choice as occupation as means. Examples include using manipulation of game pieces to acquire or reacquire dexterity, placing game pieces out of reach to promote postural control, using the game to develop social skills such as turn-taking, grading how long the client plays the game to improve sustained attention skills, and using the game to enhance self-efficacy or lessen anxiety. When this approach is used, the therapist

---

BOX 21.2 EXAMPLES OF USING OCCUPATION AS MEANS

- Rolling out dough to strengthen an older adult's upper limbs so that they can regain independence in homemaking tasks such as washing dishes
- Engaging a child in a playground climbing activity to promote body awareness and motor planning so that they can engage in age-appropriate play such as bike riding
- Playing a game of Connect Four with game pieces placed on the left side to promote spatial awareness so that a person may be able to locate grooming items placed on the left side of the sink
- Using arts and crafts activities to improve self-esteem and/or lessen anxiety so that a person feels more confident when socializing with others
- Leading a group of adults in a session of water aerobics to promote joint flexibility so that they can maintain independence in home activities such as putting away groceries
- Engaging in a gardening task to develop reach and coordination skills that may then be used during self-care activities
- Engaging a client in a challenging occupation such as money management to promote awareness of cognitive deficits. This improved awareness may then result in the client understanding the need for adaptive cognitive strategies to manage at home

---

must link the potential change in underlying skills and client factors to improved occupational performance. Improved dexterity would not be considered the end product of OT. However, regaining the ability to manipulate fasteners to independently dress, independently finger feed, or be able to manipulate scissors while making holiday cards in school would all be considered examples of desired outcomes depending on client preference and the context of therapy.

When using occupation as means as the intervention, it is particularly important that the OT practitioner choose occupations that have meaning and that the rationale for the intervention is made explicit. Otherwise, clients may find it difficult to understand the focus of OT. It is important that clients do not leave a session simply thinking "we played cards in OT today."

Combining Occupation as Means and as Ends

It is possible to combine aspects of occupation as ends and occupation as means (Figure 21.1). Using this method, a collaborative approach is used to determine goals and to understand a client's interests. The OT practitioner then uses their skills of occupational analysis to determine which underlying performance skills and/or client factors may need to be challenged. In her discussion of combining occupation as ends and means, Gray (1998) states,

> Rather than completing an assessment and using problem areas (components) to decide which activities to use for treatment (e.g., macramé is great for coordination, parquetry puzzles are assumed to help visual perceptual deficits), the occupational therapist has the added challenge of looking into the client's occupational history and selecting activities related to the client's occupations and interests that can be modified and structured to improve coordination and visual perception. Perhaps that particular client enjoyed waxing the car, making fried chicken, or playing with his or her nieces. The occupational therapist could, with a little creativity and ingenuity, tailor those occupations to treat the very same coordination or visual perceptual deficits. (p. 358)

Che Daud et al. (2016) examined the OT experience of hand therapy in Malaysia. The researchers concluded that although occupation as a means and as an end have different purposes, the ultimate goal is to enhance the clients' maximum level of functioning both can be used for the successful rehabilitation of hand injuries. Although occupation as a means and an end has different purposes, the ultimate goal is the same: to promote independence and enhance the quality of life of the clients.

To be successful, this approach requires that the OT practitioner has mastered the skill of occupational analysis. See Chapter 43 for detailed information on occupational analysis. In summary, occupation is always the ends and is

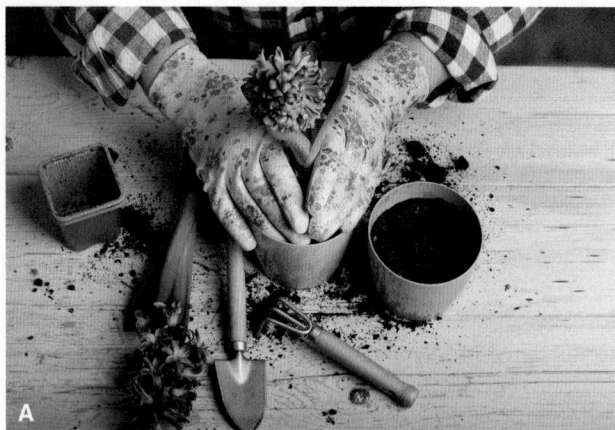
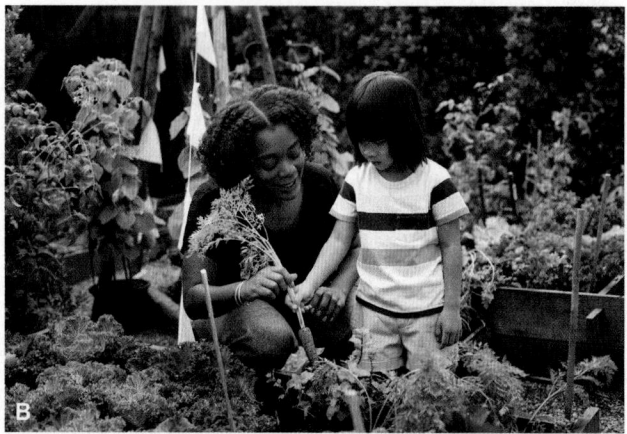

FIGURE 21.1 **A:** Gardening may be considered occupation as ends or means or both. If the client's goal is to resume leisure activities in their garden or work in a nursery, this would be considered occupation as ends. If the therapist chooses an enjoyable activity such as gardening as a way to improve endurance, balance, coordination, or organization skills, it would be considered occupation as means. Just by observing one cannot tell. The therapist's rationale and client's goals must be investigated. **B:** For a child, gardening is most likely an occupation as means.

the most frequent means with the addition of purposeful and preparatory methods as needed. See Table 21.2 for examples of combining occupation as ends and means. See Box 21.3 for further discussion regarding classifying interventions.

Specific Intervention Approaches

OT practitioners address the interaction among client factors, performance skills, performance patterns, contexts and environments, and activity demands that influence occupational performance within those occupations the person needs and wants to do. The intervention focus is on the following (AOTA, 2020) (Table 21.3):

- Therapeutic use of occupations and activities
- Preparatory methods/Interventions to support occupations
- Education and training
- Virtual interventions
- Advocacy (e.g., advocacy, self-advocacy)
- Group interventions

TABLE 21.2   Combining Occupation as Means and Occupation as Ends

Goal: Independently Manage/Navigate a Subway System to Attend Alcoholics Anonymous Meetings	Goal: Independent in Toileting
Occupation as ends: Task-specific training of the occupation using graded physical and verbal cues for difficult aspects of the task such as interpreting a subway map. Helping the client perform parts of the task that are difficult (e.g., money management) so that the task can be completed. Adapting the task so that it can be completed (e.g., providing a prepaid fare card so that the client does not need to manage money).	**Occupation as ends:** Task-specific training of the occupation using graded physical and verbal cues for difficult aspects of the task such as maneuvering from a wheelchair to the commode. Helping the client perform parts of the task that are difficult (e.g., clothing management) so that the task can be completed. Adapting the task so that it can be completed (e.g., providing grab bars or a raised toilet seat).
Occupation as means: Managing and navigating the subway is used to challenge a variety of underlying skills and factors such as the following: • Manipulation of money • Way finding in new environments • Social skills development such as appropriately waiting in line for the attendant • Problem-solving if there is a schedule or service change • Calculation of change after money exchange • Maintaining balance when the train is in motion • Endurance for ambulation, stair climbing, and standing tolerance	**Occupation as means:** Using aspects of toileting to challenge a variety of underlying skills and factors such as the following: • Postural control when transitioning from sitting to standing • Motor planning during manipulation of toilet paper • Sequencing the steps of the toileting task • Promoting safety awareness in reference to locking brakes and manipulating footplates out of the way • Challenging sitting balance • Manipulation skills when fastening pants • Awareness of body position in space when transitioning from chair to commode • Lower extremity strength and control to transition from sit to stand and stand to sit

BOX 21.3 INTERVENTIONS ARE NOT ALWAYS EASY TO CLASSIFY

It would be nice if we could neatly classify our occupational therapy (OT) interventions as occupation as means or occupation as ends. In reality, OT interventions are complex and often involve elements that address impairments, relate to caregivers, and involve both the client and the client's environment. This makes them difficult to name or fit into neat categories. For example, consider interventions focused on clinical challenges such as the following:

- Decreasing self-injurious behavior for people living with traumatic brain injury, dementia, autism, etc.
- Protecting caregivers from harm (e.g., biting) during activities of daily living assist
- Preventing wandering behaviors
- Preventing interaction with potentially dangerous substances such as household chemicals

These interventions may be categorized in a variety of ways beyond means and ends. Categories may include preparatory, education-based, behavioral-based, sensory-based, or as a combination of categories. These interventions are clearly under our domain of concern as occupational therapists as they promote safe participation in occupation in the least restrictive environment.

TABLE 21.3 Types of Interventions Outlined in the American Occupational Therapy Association Practice Framework

Type of Intervention	Non-Inclusive Examples
Occupations and activities Occupations (client-directed life activities that match participation goals)	Bathing a child Completing morning self-care Applying for job Building a Lego castle Participating in a bowling team Paying monthly bills Participating in a peaceful protest or rally Visiting parent in the hospital Attending and participating in religious services
Activities (selected to improve or develop performance skills and patterns to improve occupational performance; components of occupation that hold meaning and relevance)	Practicing car transfers Shuffling cards Climbing a playground ladder Engaging in handwriting or keyboarding activities to type the alphabet Manipulating tools, locks, fasteners Writing out a medication schedule
Preparatory methods/Interventions to support occupations and tasks (prepares the client for occupational performance; used as *part* of a session; these methods are used in preparation for our concurrently with occupation and activities) (see Box 21.4)	Thermal modalities Electrical modalities Edema massage Relaxation activities Splinting Experiencing a sensory room Strengthening via elastic bands or therapeutic putty Assistive technology Self-Regulation
Education and training Education (imparting knowledge and information) (see Chapter 23)	Teaching energy conservations skills to a group undergoing cancer treatments Educating a parent as to the best sleep position for their child with torticollis Educating a company that is planning expansion on universal design Developing a cumulative trauma prevention training course for a local factory
Training (training for the acquisition of everyday skills)	Instructing how to utilize a sip-and-puff wheelchair control Training a child to use a new prosthesis to self-feed Teaching a shelter dweller how to apply for housing or fill out a job application Teaching deep breathing to address anxiety before engaging in social situations Teaching a person who has lost communication skills to access an augmentative communication device with an adapted switch

(continued)

TABLE 21.3	Types of Interventions Outlined in the American Occupational Therapy Association Practice Framework (*continued*)

Type of Intervention	Non-Inclusive Examples
Advocacy and self-advocacy (efforts toward promoting occupational justice and empowering clients to obtain resources to participate in everyday life)	Collaborating with an employer to enact the Americans with Disability Act to make reasonable accommodations for your client with mental illness Becoming a board member of the local parks department to assure playgrounds are inclusive Connecting with local museums and arts initiatives to promote sensory-friendly experiences A graduate student requests an accommodation for his attention-deficit disorder via the university office of students with disabilities. A group of intensive care unit (ICU) nurses reach out to the administration concerned over the recent increase in experienced back pain.
Group interventions (facilitate learning and skill acquisition through the dynamics of a group and social interaction) (see Chapter 29)	Running a group for recent widows and widowers to learn skills that were previously performed by their deceased spouses Engaging in a support/education group for those who have experienced a recent amputation Developing a group for children/adolescents with poor social skills to engage in social skills role-playing

Adapted from American Occupational Therapy Association. (2020). Occupational therapy practice framework: Domain and process—Fourth edition. *American Journal of Occupational Therapy, 74*(Suppl. 2), 7412410010p1–7412410010p87. https://doi.org/10.5014/ajot.2020.74S2001

A variety of intervention approaches are available. In some cases, only one category of intervention is used to meet client goals. Other clinical situations require the use of several categories of intervention or a change in intervention choice based on a poor response, reimbursement issues, or a change in client status. Practitioners base their choice of interventions on a variety of factors including client choice (see Chapter 28), interpretation of assessment findings (see Chapter 19), evidence (see Chapter 26), clinical experience and professional reasoning (see Chapter 25), knowledge of disease and disability, setting (see Chapter 60), and length of stay and reimbursement (see Chapter 76). The following paragraphs describe the specific approaches, give examples of evidence that support the approaches, and provide further examples in Table 21.4.

TABLE 21.4	Examples of Specific Intervention Approaches

Intervention Approach	Examples
Remediation or restoration of personal factors, performance skills, and/or performance patterns to improve occupational performance	• Therapeutic exercise to strengthen a muscle • Use of a video game to improve sustained attention • Goal-oriented reaching to improve upper limb function • Constraint-induced movement therapy to improve upper limb control • Mall walking program to improve endurance • Using homemaking tasks to challenge cognitive functions such as safety and judgment • Sensory integration techniques
Occupational skill acquisition	• Teaching meal preparation skills • Task-specific practice of handwriting • Mental practice of IADL • Teaching adaptive coping skills • Using motor learning principles such as random practice schedules to learn or relearn self-care skills • Teaching a recently widowed woman how to manage monthly bills (which her husband had previously taken care of) • Developing crawling ability in a nonambulatory child with developmental delays
Adaptation/compensation approach to improve occupational performance	• Using a wrist extension orthosis to allow keyboarding • Using a checklist system to perform assigned tasks in a supported employment program • Using a tub seat, handheld shower, and long-handled sponge to enable bathing • Using lightweight cookware during meal preparation • Using built-up handles on school supplies • Using a power scooter during grocery shopping • Using an augmentative communication device to interact with other students

TABLE 21.4	Examples of Specific Intervention Approaches (*continued*)
Intervention Approach	**Examples**
Environmental modifications to improve occupational performance (see Chapter 24)	• Performing a home visit and suggesting removing throw rugs, sliding shower doors, and unnecessary furniture to promote wheelchair access • Recommending appropriate playground equipment for children with varying skills • Recommending minimizing environmental stimuli (e.g., television on in the background, many people talking at once) for those who are easily distracted • Providing specific information regarding the gradient for a wheelchair ramp • Removing trip hazards in a home or work setting to decrease fall risks • Setting up a bathroom so that needed grooming and hygiene items are placed on the right for those who do not attend to the left • Assisting a family in developing a caretaker schedule for a loved one with a disability • Assisting parents in understanding the type and timing of verbal cues required for their child to focus on homework • Demonstrating how the ground floor of a two-story dwelling can be set up so that a nonambulatory person can live independently on one floor • Providing sensory input such as music to improve alertness during a therapy session
Educational approach to improve occupational performance (see Chapter 23)	• Instructing caretakers on proper transfer techniques • Informing a person as to the signs and symptoms of emerging depression • Leading a stroke education group focused on community resources and leisure opportunities • Providing information about alternative community access after a driver's license is lost due to visual impairment • Instructing a client or caregiver on skin inspection techniques and the signs of skin breakdown
Prevention approach to maintain occupational performance	• Instructing a stock person in a retail store on proper lifting techniques • Instructing nursing staff on an appropriate in-bed turning schedule to prevent the development of decubitus ulcers • Educating a person who types most of the day on proper posture, rest breaks, and so forth to prevent carpal tunnel syndrome • Preventing social isolation by suggesting appropriate leisure-based after-work activities such as a bowling league, participation in a chorus, etc.
Palliative approaches	• Prescribing positioning equipment that allows more time out of bed • Engaging in reminiscence activities • Engage in activities related to leaving a legacy such as finally writing down and sharing a secret recipe, engagement in creative arts, scrapbooking, etc. • Physical agent modalities, positioning, edema management, and fabricating an orthosis to reduce pain • Teaching caregivers handling techniques for bed mobility assist as the client's physical status declines
Therapeutic use of self (see Chapter 28)	• Developing rapport • Appropriate use of humor • Maintaining open communication • Being empathetic • Establishing trust • Being motivational • Maintaining a caring attitudeActive listening

IADL, instrumental activities of daily living.

Preparatory Interventions/ Interventions to Support Occupations

Preparatory interventions or Interventions to support occupations have been defined as "methods and tasks that prepare the client for occupational performance, used as *part of a treatment session* in preparation for or concurrently with occupations and activities or provided to a client as a home-based engagement to support daily occupational performance"

(AOTA, 2020, p. 59). Indeed, a systematic review (Amini, 2011) of OT for individuals with work-related injuries and illnesses as summarized by Arbesman et al. (2011) documented

> the effectiveness of several preparatory activities such as exercise, the use of the thermal modality of heat, and early mobilization after fractures and acute trauma. Other preparatory methods have been found to be effective for specific clinical conditions, including splinting for osteoarthritis and carpal tunnel syndrome; scar massage to prevent hypertrophic scarring and promote extensibility; the use of sensory focusing, a cognitive pain control technique during burn dressing changes; and the use of pressure garment work gloves after burns. (p. 14)

More recently, Wheeler et al. (2022) examined the evidence for the effectiveness of interventions that address psychosocial, behavioral, and/or emotional skills to improve social participation and other everyday activities and occupations for persons with traumatic brain injury (TBI). They concluded that OT practitioners use interventions to support occupations, including self-regulation tasks which may be used as preparatory or concurrently with occupations and activities to improve social participation and other everyday activities and occupations for persons with TBI. Their review included preparatory activities such as yoga, music, and mindfulness.

Indeed, the preparatory activity of mindfulness is receiving increased attention in the OT literature. Goodman et al. (2019) examined mindfulness and occupation in their review of articles from Canada, the United States, England, and Israel. The researchers identified an overarching theme of mindful occupation, with five sub-themes including occupational presence; occupational awareness; occupational engagement; occupational well-being; and occupational fulfillment. They recommended that future directions focus on more depth and breadth of empirical research about mindful engagement in a human occupation that can be used to implement and evaluate mindfulness in occupation-based theory and practice.

These interventions are only used in preparation for or concurrently with occupation-based interventions (Box 21.4).

Remediation or Restoration of Client Factors, Performance Skills, and/or Performance Patterns to Improve Occupational Performance

The **remediation** or restoration approach is used to enhance client factors (body functions and body structures) such as range of motion, strength, endurance, thoughts, feelings, cognitive processing, and so on, to improve occupational performance. The approach is also used to enhance performance skills and patterns to support occupational performance. Clinicians must link potential changes in underlying abilities to changes in occupational performance. For example, an objective improvement in strength on a manual muscle test or improved cognitive testing without a resultant change in performance may reveal that this is the incorrect intervention approach for a client or that the underlying impairment being treated was incorrectly chosen. Although some impairments are not amenable to remediation (e.g., severe memory loss, denervated muscles, endurance impairments that emerge during the end stages of disease), others are amenable but require substantial time, motivation, and commitment to achieve a positive outcome. These factors must be considered carefully when choosing

> **BOX 21.4 EXAMPLES OF PREPARATORY METHODS AND INTERVENTIONS USED IN CONJUNCTION WITH OR PREPARATION FOR ENGAGEMENT IN OCCUPATION**
>
> - Applying a therapeutic hot pack to and stretching both shoulders before a remediation session that uses reaching into kitchen cabinets as a means to improve shoulder range of motion
> - Teaching a person with an anxiety disorder to use deep breathing and guided imagery to promote relaxation before interviewing for a new job
> - Teaching a morning flexibility program to be completed after a warm morning shower to prepare for a variety of morning activities such as making breakfast
> - Having a hospitalized child who survived a burn interact with a therapy dog to decrease anxiety before a potentially painful therapy session
> - Suggesting morning yoga as a method of promoting mental focus before facing the day
> - Using biofeedback to manage increased muscle tone and maximize the use of an involved limb after traumatic brain injury
> - Massaging edema out of a swollen hand to improve finger range of motion to enable coin manipulation

this approach. See Figure 21.2 for an example of using pet therapy as part of an intervention designed to remediate coordination problems.

Therapists working with a variety of shoulder conditions such as adhesive capsulitis, tears of the rotator cuff, and humeral fractures tend to adopt a remediation approach as part of an overall intervention plan. Marik and Roll (2017) evaluated the evidence for interventions within the OT scope of practice that address pain reduction and increase participation in functional activities. Seventy-six studies were reviewed. Strong evidence was found that range of motion, strengthening exercises, and joint mobilizations can improve function and decrease pain.

Nielsen et al. (2022) aimed to assess the effectiveness and describe the contents of OT interventions aimed at improving older adults' occupational performance by strengthening their problem-solving skills. The author's systematic review included five studies comprising a total of 685 participants. In four studies, OT with a problem-solving approach outperformed control conditions postintervention. The interventions involved problem identification, analysis, strategy development, and implementation. However, the quality of evidence was deemed low due to inconsistent and imprecise results.

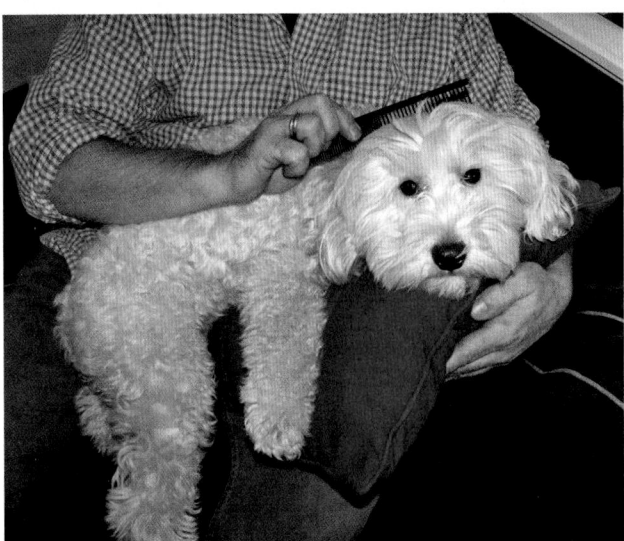

FIGURE 21.2 Occupation as means. Pet therapy can be used to increase the range of motion, develop motor planning skills, improve coordination, or lessen anxiety. If the client was a pet owner with the goal of resuming care for his pet, this intervention may be considered occupation as ends.

A remediation approach called sensory integration may also be adopted when working with children who have varying abilities related to processing incoming sensory information (see Chapter 56). A recent systematic review addressed the question "What is the efficacy of occupational therapy using Ayres Sensory Integration® (ASI) to support functioning and participation?" The authors found that ASI intervention demonstrated positive outcomes for improving individually generated goals of functioning and participation as measured by Goal Attainment Scaling for autistic children. Moderate evidence supported improvements in impairment-level outcomes of improvement in autistic behaviors and skills-based outcomes of reduction in caregiver assistance with self-care activities. Child outcomes in play, sensory-motor, and language skills and reduced caregiver assistance with social skills had emerging but insufficient evidence (Schaaf et al., 2018).

Occupational Skill Acquisition (Development and Restoration of Occupational Performance)

Interventions that focus specifically on skill development (**occupational skill acquisition**) are frequently used in OT and often described as "skills for the job of living." Skills may include those that were previously developed and are now limited or lost. This situation may occur, for example, with an adolescent or adult who sustains a head trauma. It is also an appropriate approach to develop skills for those

with developmental delays such as a young adult with an intellectual delay or a child with a developmental coordination disorder. Finally, it is appropriate for those who are required to learn new skills based on a change in their role. An example is that of a young adult who has sustained an SCI and needs to learn car transfers (Figure 21.3).

Social skills training is an example of this intervention, and evidence supports the use of this intervention for particular populations (see Chapter 58). Gol and Jarus (2005) compared the daily living skills of children with and without attention-deficit/hyperactivity disorder (ADHD) and the influence of a social skills training group on these skills. Children in the group with ADHD were randomly selected to attend group treatment that focused on social skills training through meaningful occupations such as art, games, and cooking. The children were evaluated at the beginning of group treatment and after 10 sessions using the Assessment of Motor and Process Skills (AMPS). Ten children without ADHD were evaluated at similar intervals. Children with ADHD initially achieved significantly lower scores on the AMPS in all process skills and the coordination motor subtest than children without ADHD. Children with ADHD significantly improved from the first to the second evaluation and no longer differed from the children without ADHD after treatment. The authors concluded that the results emphasize the need for a focus on occupation in the assessment and treatment of children with ADHD (Gol & Jarus, 2005).

Charlton et al. (2021) examined the manual wheelchair skills training program. It is used to structure teaching manual wheelchair use for people following injury or disability. Their pilot study aimed to explore the outcomes of introducing a group wheelchair skills training program The study found that The Wheelchair Skills Training Program can improve wheelchair performance, confidence, and frequency to

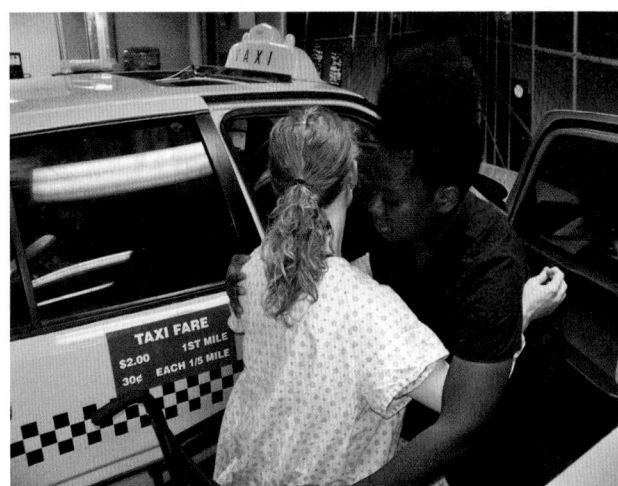

FIGURE 21.3 Occupation as ends. The therapist is using physical assistance during a session focused on functional retraining of mobility using an adaptive transfer technique.

support enhanced safety, independence, and quality of life for people with lower limb amputation on skill performance, confidence, and frequency of wheelchair use for people with lower limb amputation in a rehabilitation setting from the perspective of participants and group facilitators.

Community reintegration training also serves as an example of this intervention. Gillen and colleagues (2007) carried out an experiment to examine the effect of an OT intervention focused on improving community skills after a lower extremity major joint replacement. One hundred and seven subjects who had a total hip or total knee replacement were examined pre- and postcommunity reintegration intervention involving the practice of community skills in a natural environment. Skills included safely transferring out of the vehicle, managing outdoor obstacles such as uneven surfaces, ambulating throughout the destination, and appropriately transferring back into the car. Participants reported significantly higher scores postintervention on measures of satisfaction, performance, and confidence related to community living skills. Self-reported scores were significantly higher for individual community skills as well as the overall score (Gillen et al., 2007).

Adaptation/Compensation Approach to Improve Occupational Performance

The **adaptation** or compensation approach is used in a variety of situations. These include when a disability is considered permanent (e.g., after the amputation of a limb), underlying client factors or performance skills are not expected to improve (e.g., prolonged and severe short-term memory loss or severe and persistent lower limb weakness after an SCI), limited access to therapy prevents engagement in a remediation program, and/or clients and their families prefer this approach. This intervention is frequently combined with environmental modifications that are described next. Many times, this approach is also used in conjunction with a remediation approach. A person who is recovering from the resection of a brain tumor may use adaptive ADL methods while they are undergoing motor control remediation interventions. Specific areas of occupation are the focus of this approach, with an emphasis on modifying the demands of the task and using adaptive equipment/assistive devices (Figure 21.4).

Gentry (2008) evaluated the effects of an OT training protocol using personal digital assistants (PDAs) as assistive technology for people with cognitive impairment related to multiple sclerosis. Following the training period, participants demonstrated the ability to learn how to use basic PDA functions and retain learning for at least 8 weeks. Functional performance increased significantly with PDA use, and this gain was maintained at an 8-week follow-up.

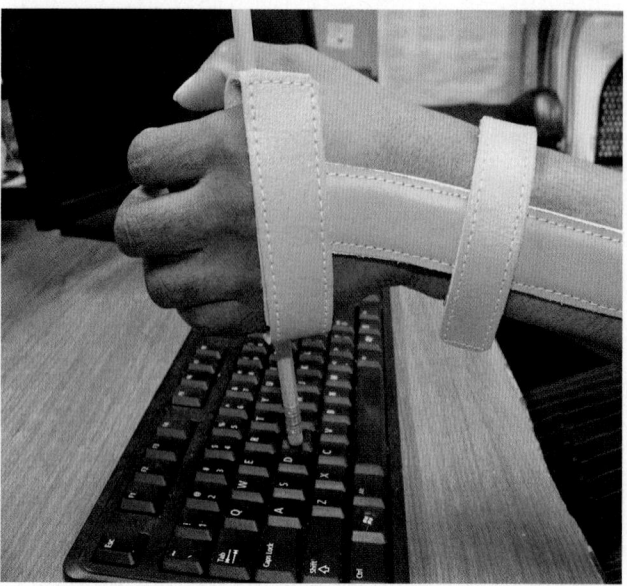

FIGURE 21.4 **An adaptive device used to promote independence in typing, writing, feeding, and so forth for those with wrist and hand weakness.**

This approach can also be useful within the cognitive rehabilitation domain. Another example of evidence to support the use of this approach is a study that examined the effect of cognitive adaptation training (CAT) on a sample of people living with schizophrenia who had been in the community for at least 3 months. CAT is a series of adaptive supports and environmental modifications (see later) designed to compensate for deficits in cognitive functioning. Examples of supports include signs, alarms, labels, and organization of belongings to cue and sequence adaptive behavior in the client's home and work environments. Forty-five participants were randomly assigned to one of three conditions: (a) CAT, (b) a condition that controlled for therapist time and provided environmental changes unrelated to cognitive deficits, or (c) follow-up only. Results of repeated measures indicated that those participating in CAT had better adaptive function and quality of life and fewer positive symptoms than those in the two non-CAT conditions. The authors concluded that compensatory strategies may improve various outcomes in those living with schizophrenia (Velligan et al., 2002).

Environmental Modifications to Improve Occupational Performance

Modifying the environment (**environmental modification**) is also considered an adaptive approach as described earlier. It includes modifying both the physical environment that includes the natural (geographic terrain, sensory qualities of the environment, plants, and animals) and built nonhuman environment (buildings, furniture, etc.) as well as the social environment (relationships and expectations of persons, organizations, populations) (AOTA, 2020). Physical environment modifications may include incorporating aspects of barrier-free and universal design into intervention plans. An example of social environment modifications would be teaching caregivers the most efficient curing method to assure that the person living with dementia can continue to participate in family meals.

A variety of sources of evidence for the efficacy of environment-based interventions on the affect, behavior, and performance of people with Alzheimer disease and related dementias exist. Jensen and Padilla (2017) evaluated the effectiveness of environment-based interventions that address behavior, perception, and falls in the home and other settings for people with Alzheimer disease and related major neurocognitive disorders. The authors documented that strong evidence indicates that person-centered approaches can improve behavior. Moderate evidence supports noise regulation, environmental design, unobtrusive visual barriers, and environmental relocation strategies to reduce problematic behaviors. On the other hand, they found that evidence is insufficient for the effectiveness of mealtime ambient music, bright light, proprioceptive input, wander gardens, optical strategies, and sensory devices in improving behavior or reducing wandering and falls.

Meuser et al. (2022) examined school environments related to the participation of children with special needs. The authors concluded that a shift from individual child-focused to environment-focused approaches that target all children's participation could impact classroom setup and teachers' roles. OT practitioners' expertise in matching school environments and task requirements with individual children's needs could be valuable in their collaboration with schools to support this transition.

Another study examined the short-term effects of a home environmental intervention on self-efficacy and upset in caregivers and the daily function of dementia patients. One hundred and seventy-one families were examined and were randomized to intervention or usual care control group. The intervention involved five 90-minute home visits by OT practitioners who provided education and physical and social environmental modifications. The intervention involved the following:

- Educating caregivers about the impact of the environment on dementia-related behaviors
- Helping caregivers simplify objects in the home (e.g., remove clutter), break down tasks (e.g., one- or two-step commands, lay out clothing in the order in which it is to be donned)
- Involving other members of the family network or formal support in daily caregiving tasks

The authors demonstrated that, as compared with controls, intervention caregivers reported fewer declines in patients' IADL, less decline in self-care, and fewer behavior problems in patients. The intervention spouses reported reduced upset, women reported enhanced self-efficacy in managing behaviors, and women and minorities reported enhanced self-efficacy in managing functional dependency. The authors concluded that the environmental program appeared to have a modest effect on those with dementia IADL dependence as well as improve self-efficacy and reduce upset in specific areas of caregiving (Gitlin et al., 2001).

Educational Approach to Improve Occupational Performance

OT practitioners frequently take on the role of teacher and use an education-based approach when working with clients. Education approaches may be used in both individual and group settings. This approach may be aimed directly at the clients, their caregivers, significant others, employers, and so on.

Teaching joint protection techniques would serve as an example of this approach. Researchers have assessed the effects on pain, disability, and health status of an educational joint protection program in a group of people with moderate-to-severe rheumatoid arthritis (RA). Eighty-five subjects were enrolled in the study and randomized into either an experimental group or a control group. The intervention consisted of four educational meetings. These included information on the pathophysiology and evolution of RA, joint protection during ADL, suggestions on how to adapt to the surrounding environment, and self-learning exercises to perform at home. The study showed that 8 months after attending an educational joint protection program, subjects with moderate-to-severe RA presented with less pain and disability and thus an enhanced health status (Masiero et al., 2007).

Teaching those with fatigue issues how to manage and conserve their energy throughout the day would also fall under this category of intervention. A study assessed the impact of a one-to-one fatigue management course on participants' fatigue, self-efficacy, quality of life, and energy conservation behaviors. Participants showed significant reductions in fatigue and significant increases in self-efficacy and quality of life at the posttest. These beneficial effects were maintained at follow-up. The authors concluded that the one-to-one fatigue management course is a beneficial intervention for people with chronic conditions and fatigue (Van Heest et al., 2017).

Prevention Approach to Maintain Occupational Performance

The prevention intervention approach can be used for those living with or without a disability but who are at risk for developing limitations in occupational performance

(AOTA, 2020). It can also be used to prevent secondary impairments that may limit occupational performance such as pain, contracture, skin breakdown, depression, and so on.

The Lifestyle Redesign* for pressure injury prevention in SCI falls under this approach. The specific aim of this program is to develop a lifestyle intervention that promises to significantly reduce pressure injuries in the population of adults with SCI. The intervention was developed based on the results of a qualitative investigation of lifestyle and pressure injury risk among adults with SCI (Clark et al., 2006; University of Southern California, 2013).

Another example of a prevention approach is discussed in a systematic review that explored the impact of fall prevention programs and home modifications on falls and the performance of community-dwelling older adults. The authors concluded that the strongest results were found for multifactorial programs that included home evaluations and home modifications, physical activity or exercise, education, vision and medication checks, or assistive technology to prevent falls. Positive outcomes included a decreased rate of functional decline, a decrease in fear of falling, and an increase in physical factors such as balance and strength. The strength of the evidence for physical activity and home modification programs provided individually was moderate (Chase et al., 2012).

More recently, Keglovits et al. (2020) examined fall hazards in the homes of older adults. This scoping review validated a previous list of home fall hazards that were most frequently attributed to the cause of falls among older adults identifying several new areas for priority focus when observing for fall hazards. From the 14 articles reviewed in this scoping study, 17 home fall hazards were identified. These included icy surfaces, pets, flooring, footwear, uneven surfaces, poor illumination, obstacles/clutter, and so on.

Palliative Approaches

The **palliative** approach focuses on providing clients with relief from the symptoms, pain, and stress of a serious illness regardless of the diagnosis. The goal is to improve the quality of life for both the client and their family. Unlike hospice care (end-of-life care), it can be carried out throughout the disease course and not just during the last months of life. Curative care interventions also may be considered under the umbrella of the palliative approach; however, curative services are not provided when a client is receiving hospice care (AOTA, 2016). Palliative care is often part of end-of-life care.

The AOTA (2016) defines the roles and focus of the OT practitioner related to end-of-life care as the following:

- OT practitioners' distinct value in end-of-life care is to facilitate quality of life for clients and their caregivers through engagement in occupations during the client's remaining days.

- The chosen occupations of a dying person or their caregiver may be familiar and routine, such as a goal of sharing a final family meal, or they may be dynamic and tied specifically to say goodbye in a good way, such as resolving unfinished business or crafting a final gift for family members.

- OT practitioners recognize the purpose of these occupations as twofold: (a) providing a means of self-expression and engagement while (b) serving as a vehicle by which the client finds peace with the dying process and prepares for death.

- OT practitioners facilitate a good death experience for all involved in the dying process by enabling occupation.

- Practitioners consider environmental and contextual factors (e.g., accessibility of objects or places in the environment, caregiver training, social contacts available to prevent isolation) as well as personal factors (e.g., decreased endurance, increased anxiety) that may be limiting a client's abilities and satisfaction when performing desired occupations.

- Practitioners collaborate with the client and family members throughout the OT process to identify occupations that are especially meaningful and to incorporate strategies that support participation and quality of life rather than rehabilitation.

The AOTA (2016) further defines the roles and focus of the OT practitioner related to end-of-life care as it relates to caregivers as the following:

- OT practitioners recognize the interdependent nature of relationships at end of life and caregivers' potential need for support in their caring role. At times, the needs of the caregiver may exceed the needs of the person who is dying yet be overshadowed by the immediate needs of the loved one.

- OT practitioners extend services to caregivers in their own right.

- Practitioners are uniquely qualified to boost caregiver recognition and support by identifying people in caregiving roles and assessing their needs and preferences about potential interventions.

Home-based OT is a typical context in which palliative care is delivered. A study examined OT for patients in the palliative stage of cancer care from the perspective of the patients and carers. This study defined the palliative stage of cancer care as the point from which the patient is no longer responsive to curative treatment until death. The study examined 30 clients and their primary informal carers via a structured interview. The results suggested that both patients and their carers valued the service provided and report high levels of satisfaction, although there were gaps identified in service provision. The authors concluded that there is a need to build on the good work being done by home-based OT practitioners in the area of palliative cancer care and increase education and resources to ensure that a client-centered, holistic approach to care is used, addressing both the needs of the patient and their carers (Kealey & McIntyre, 2005).

Further education needs of practitioners working in this area persist (Talbot-Coulombe et al., 2022). The author's survey found that the 67 survey participants mainly optimized comfort and safety in meaningful occupations such as mobility, transfers, and hygiene. Barriers to their practice included organizational obstacles and unfamiliarity with their role. The authors concluded that the findings highlight the need to improve education and awareness among OT practitioners and other healthcare professionals about the scope of what OT practitioners can do in palliative and end-of-life care.

Therapeutic Use of Self

Therapeutic use of self, a component of the therapeutic relationship, should not be considered a separate intervention but should instead influence and inform all of the aforementioned intervention approaches. Although there is no consensus on a definition, therapeutic use of self has been defined as the "planned use of his or her personality, insights, perceptions, and judgments as part of the therapeutic process" (Punwar & Peloquin, 2000, p. 285). This term is also used to refer to therapists' conscious efforts to optimize their interactions with clients (Punwar & Peloquin, 2000).

Although this area of clinical practice can benefit from further research emphasis and attention in education programs (Taylor et al., 2009), it is a foundation of practice. A survey of 129 OT practitioners practicing in various areas found that therapists strongly emphasized empathy, rapport, and open communication as being important in the therapeutic relationship. Participants also perceived the therapeutic relationship as critical to therapy outcomes (Cole & McLean, 2003).

The therapeutic use of self is not always clearly defined (Solman & Clouston, 2016). However, Eklund and Hallberg (2001) reported the results from a survey investigating psychiatric OT practitioners' ($n = 292$) use of verbal interaction regularly with their clients. Among predefined areas, verbal interaction, routine occupations, self-image, and ego-strengthening interventions were among the most frequently given alternatives. The content analysis indicated that the OT practitioners used verbal interaction to:

- Enhance the therapeutic relationship. This was expressed as efforts to make contact, stimulate motivation in the patient, or enhance mutuality and make the patient participate actively.
- Give the patients opportunities to reflect on and articulate feelings and experiences (e.g., formulate feelings and opinions; make their thoughts, feelings, and actions clear; have the patient reflect on their behavior in the OT sessions).
- Make assessments (i.e., to assess capacities, resources, functions, liabilities, problems, and motivation).
- Make treatment plans to arrive at an appropriate treatment plan together with the patient and set goals.
- Provide interventions in order to reach certain goals—the intention of acting to remedy problems and give support in order to reach certain goals.
- Evaluate and follow up on their practice.

See Table 21.4 for specific examples of interventions. See Chapter 28 for more detail on therapeutic relations.

Client Stories

One may note that the aforementioned approaches are not mutually exclusive. As described earlier, you may use an *education*-based approach to *prevent* joint destruction and a further decline in occupational performance for those living with arthritis. A therapist involved in *palliative* care with a client with a nonoperable brain tumor may use *adaptive* seating in a wheelchair to decrease back pain. In many cases, therapists use a variety of approaches with the same client, whereas in other cases may focus on one approach. The following client stories highlight this point. Each case includes an occupational profile, relevant assessment findings, goals, and intervention choices (OT Stories 21.2–21.4).

OT STORY 21.2 SAHAR: AN 8-YEAR-OLD GIRL LIVING WITH CEREBRAL PALSY

Occupational Profile

Sahar is an 8-year-old girl who attends a mainstream school. Sahar receives occupational, physical, and speech therapy in school to manage her spastic cerebral palsy. She has an attendant with her at all times. Sahar enjoys art, pop music, playing with her dog, and, until recently, school. Until the recent past, she particularly enjoyed spelling and English classes. She recently started to make comments to her parents that she "does not fit in," is "tired of being teased," "does not want to feel different," and that she "is a bad friend." Her parents are concerned about her self-esteem and her new disinterest in school. They are getting reports from her teacher that she is "falling behind" and seems "disinterested."

(continued)

OT STORY 21.2 SAHAR: AN 8-YEAR-OLD GIRL LIVING WITH CEREBRAL PALSY (continued)

Sahar recently started working with a new OT practitioner. Her assessment findings included the following:

- **Environmental:** Sahar's power wheelchair was ill-fitting. Her seating system was not providing enough support, and she tended to lean to the left and sit with a flexed spine and neck. This position limited her eye contact, which resulted in difficulty seeing the teacher and the information written on the blackboard. In addition, she has recently started to drool occasionally because of her neck position. The wheelchair was too high to pull up to the desks and tables in the classroom so she was always positioned behind the class with her aide, which also added to her difficulty interacting with peers and seeing her teacher. Finally, due to her poor seated position, she was having trouble controlling the wheelchair, and her aide was now assisting her in navigating the school.
- **Children's Assessment of Participation and Enjoyment (CAPE):** The CAPE was used to measure Sahar's participation in activities outside of school. Sahar presented with overall low participation in activities. Specifically, she reported low participation in recreational, physical, and social activities. Many activities were engaged in alone and many were confined to her bedroom.
- **School Function Assessment (SFA):** Sahar scored 2 (participation in a few activities) for most items on the participation scale, 1 or 2 (moderate-to-extensive assistance and adaptations) for most items on the task supports scale, and 1 or 2 (does not perform or partial performance) for most items on the activity performance scale.
- **Evaluation of Social Interaction (ESI):** Sahar's score on the ESI was indicative of problematic social interactions severe enough to limit interactions with others (moderately to markedly ineffective and/or immature social interaction skills). Particular items that were difficult for Sahar included not approaching/starting interactions, physical difficulties not supporting interaction (looks, turns toward), not replying, and at times not taking turns.
- **Vision:** Sahar has worn glasses since she was 3 years old. The therapist found that Sahar's acuity was decreased (20/60) for far vision using a Snellen chart.

Goals

(a) Sahar will navigate her school in a power wheelchair with distant supervision. (b) Sahar will answer two questions per day during teaching lessons. (c) Sahar will improve her overall academic performance as indicated by her quarterly report card. (d) Sahar will initiate two conversations per day with peers during recess or other group activities.

Interventions

Sahar's new therapist took the lead in terms of managing this change in Sahar's function. He focused on maximizing her social and academic participation in school, making Sahar feel more comfortable about fitting in with peers and improving her self-esteem. He used a variety of approaches including *environmental modifications* and *adaptive* and *acquisition* approaches. In addition, he referred Sahar to an eye care specialist to change the prescription for her glasses. Sahar's OT practitioner first collaborated with a wheelchair vendor to update the chair that she has outgrown and update her seating system. An *adapted* wheelchair frame that has the ability to tilt in space was ordered. A tilt system changed Sahar's orientation in space while maintaining fixed hip, knee, and ankle angles. This tilt helped to promote proper alignment including an extended spine. A headrest was provided to maintain Sahar's head in extension, expand her field of vision, and decrease the tendency to drool. Lateral supports were added to the system to further help maintain Sahar's posture. A removable lap tray was provided so that Sahar could use it as a work/play space when not at a table or desk. The OT practitioner ordered an *adapted* joystick with a "t-bar" to compensate for Sahar's poor hand function and promote independent mobility. The OT practitioner spent time with Sahar teaching her to *acquire* the skill of controlling the wheelchair both indoors and outdoors. Time was spent learning how to navigate doorways, ramps, and curb cuts. Particular attention was spent teaching Sahar how to safely navigate the playground and recess areas.

The OT practitioner collaborated with Sahar's teacher to *modify the environment*. Desks/tables were rearranged to assure that Sahar's chair could easily navigate the classroom. The therapist placed table risers on one table so that Sahar's wheelchair could fit underneath it. With these modifications, Sahar was able to navigate the classroom and sit with other students. This also served to facilitate her interactions with peers and her teacher during lesson plans.

Although these changes resulted in Sahar making statements that reflect improved esteem, the OT practitioner and Sahar's parents were concerned about her feeling socially isolated. The therapist then shifted back to an *acquisition* approach focused on social skills training. The therapist tapped into Sahar's love of art and collaborated with Sahar's teacher to integrate an arts and crafts lesson once a week. The focus of the lesson was for the students to make seasonal decorations for a bulletin board. The therapist provided *adaptive* art supplies such as a loop scissor mounted on the table and a paintbrush that was built up with foam. As Sahar's physical participation began to improve, the

OT STORY 21.2 SAHAR: AN 8-YEAR-OLD GIRL LIVING WITH CEREBRAL PALSY
(continued)

therapist used the arts and crafts sessions to encourage Sahar to initiate conversations, maintain eye contact, and answer appropriately when spoken to. Because Sahar had limited manipulation abilities, as her confidence grew, she took on the primary role of deciding the overall theme and design of the bulletin board while her peers took main responsibility for the implementation of the design. The interventions in total helped Sahar reach her goals.

Questions

1. Several assessments were used in this case. Please prioritize the two that are most important. Justify your answers.
2. Going forward, how could the therapist include Sahar's teacher and parents in developing the intervention priorities?

OT STORY 21.3 ANGEL: AN A 22-YEAR-OLD ADULT IMMIGRANT LIVING IN A SHELTER IN A LARGE URBAN AREA

Occupational Profile

Angel (who uses the pronouns they/them) arrived in New York City from Venezuela with the plan of living with a distant cousin. This plan did not work out and Angel had no choice but to enter the complicated homeless shelter system. Angel's given name is Lauro but Angel decided to change it recently as they struggle with gender identity. Angel was disowned by their biological family as they began experimenting with makeup and a more feminine style of dress. Angel's family is quite religious and these beliefs were the impetus to disinvite them from the family. Angel is unemployed with little to no social support in their new community.

Assessment Findings

An informal interview was conducted with Angel by Sam who works part time as an OT with those living in the shelter. Angel appeared fatigued, somewhat disheveled, and was overall suspicious of any questions they perceived as personal.

Angel reports being fearful as the shelter is designated as a men's shelter by the city and Angel can't present as their authentic self. Angel expressed being lonely and yearning for support from people that understood their situation. Angel is new to the city and does not understand transportation systems. Angel is anxious to work but does not know where to start.

Three standardized measures were administered:

- On the Beck Depression Inventory (range 0–63), Angel scored a 25 indicating moderate depression. Angel reports that suicidal ideation is not a concern.
- On the Kohlman Evaluation of Living Skills (range 0–17), Angel scored an 8 indicating that they require assistance

to live in the community. Specific areas of concern were: self-care (Angel is struggling with achieving the physical appearance he is striving for), community mobility, and employment.

- On the Community Integration Questionnaire (range 0–29), Angel's scores indicate difficulty in all three subscales including home integration, social integration, and productivity.

Assessment results and observations were discussed between Sam and Angel. As many occupational performance issues were identified, Angel and Sam worked together to prioritize areas for intervention.

Goals

Based on the assessments and follow-up discussion, two initial goals were set for Angel: (a) Angel will navigate two routes on the subway system with supervision and two to three specific verbal cues; (b) Angel will participate in one to two weekly events at the Lesbian, Gay, Bisexual & Transgender Center.

Interventions

Acquisition, education:

Sam took on an *educator's* role to help Angel *acquire* the skills required to master the New York City subway system. Specific skills that were taught included:

- Accessing the subway system
- Preplanning start and end points to the journey
- Resources for navigation assistance (transit police, transit authority workers)
- Troubleshooting if preplanning failed (e.g., train lines out of service)
- Subway social skills and etiquette

(continued)

OT STORY 21.3 ANGEL: AN A 22-YEAR-OLD ADULT IMMIGRANT LIVING IN A SHELTER IN A LARGE URBAN AREA (*continued*)

Sam and Angel made several trips to the LGBT Center to identify offerings and events that were appropriate for Angel. They identified several offerings possibly participating in:

- *Center Works* helps LGBTQ young adults ages 18+ to enter the job market, advance their careers, and become financially stable, while building community with their peers.
- The Center's gender identity programming fosters the healthy development of transgender and gender nonconforming people, partners, family, and communities.

- A variety of social and leisure offerings such as art classes, trauma-informed yoga, and music events.

Questions

1. What strategies can be used to continue to assist Angel in his goal of seeking employment as an immigrant?
2. What data can you use to continue to monitor Angel's symptoms of depression?

OT STORY 21.4 MICHELLE: RECEIVING HOME HOSPICE WITH END-STAGE AMYOTROPHIC LATERAL SCLEROSIS

Occupational Profile

Michelle is a 60-year-old woman who was diagnosed with amyotrophic lateral sclerosis (ALS) 1 year ago. The OT practitioner in this case, Yin, first met Michelle when she was diagnosed and monitored her functional status during monthly clinic visits. Michelle is now homebound and receiving end-of-life care via home hospice. Michelle was a homemaker; and her pride and joy are her two children and, more recently, her three grandchildren, all younger than 3 years old. OT was ordered for three to four home visits to implement *palliative* and *prevention* interventions and maximize the family's ability to care for her using both *adaptive* and *education* approaches, with an overarching theme of the *therapeutic use of self* during this difficult time.

Assessment Findings

Before the home visit, Yin reviewed Michelle's medical record. Her last documented ALS Functional Rating Scale-Revised was 15. This tool estimates the degree of functional impairment. The scores range from 0 to 48 (best). An informal interview indicated that the family was most concerned about keeping Michelle pain free as she recently started to wince when they were assisting her to move in bed, transfer, and dress. Michelle's husband, Tom, reported that he wanted to be very hands-on with her care despite having the hospice team. He reported that his low back has been hurting him ever since Michelle developed a substantial loss of strength in her legs and trunk. Before this latest decline in status, Michelle had been typing letters to her three young grandchildren. Her plan was to give these letters to her children in a sealed envelope to be given to the grandchildren when they turned 16. Tom reported that Michelle was devastated that she would not see them grow up and she wanted to be remembered by them. Michelle

was not able to talk despite being grossly cognitively intact. Yin established a yes/no system of responses using eye movements (one blink indicated "yes," two "no," and wide eyes indicated "pain"). Through this blinking system, Michelle was able to indicate that she was highly motivated to finish the letters and that it was painful in her low back, shoulders, and hips when she was being assisted with ADL/mobility. The Caregiver Burden Scale was administered to Tom. Findings suggested that Tom felt quite burdened in all five domains (general strain, isolation, disappointment, emotional involvement, and environment). In addition, Yin observed Tom assisting Michelle in and out of bed and from her bed to her wheelchair. Tom was noted to hold Michelle tightly under her arms during transfers and demonstrated poor body mechanics (twisting his back) during the transfer.

Goals

Based on Michelle and her family's concerns, the following goals were established: (a) Tom will demonstrate proper body mechanics and safe technique when transferring Michelle to her wheelchair with supervision; (b) Michelle will, with supervision, complete writing three letters with assistive devices; and (c) Tom will independently and safely position Michelle in bed.

Interventions

The first intervention was *education based* to *prevent* injury to Tom's back as well as to *prevent* Michelle from becoming injured during transfers and mobility. Yin demonstrated and discussed proper body mechanics and demonstrated proper transfer techniques. As Tom was still having difficulty, Yin further *adapted* the transfer method and showed Tom how to use a sliding board to assist Michelle from her bed to the wheelchair. Tom reported that he felt more secure with this technique. Continuing with an *education* approach, Yin demonstrated proper positioning in bed to keep Michelle's joints in neutral as to *prevent* contractures and pain. While Michelle was in bed, Yin additionally taught Tom to perform a gentle passive range of motion following the application of heating pads on Michelle's shoulders and hips to help control pain (*palliative* approach). Yin told Tom that the heat could be used two to three times per day for 20 minutes to help control Michelle's pain.

At the next home-based session, Yin observed that Michelle was in a much better position in her bed. Yin asked to observe Tom transfer Michelle to her wheelchair. He transferred her safely and effectively. Yin borrowed three pieces of equipment from the ALS clinic to allow Michelle to complete her letters using an *adaptive* approach. Yin applied a static wrist orthosis to Michelle's right wrist for stability and applied a universal cuff to her right hand (refer back to Figure 21.4). The cuff is designed to give persons with limited grip or dexterity-controlled use of items such as eating utensils and writing tools. A pencil was inserted into the universal cuff with the eraser side facing down. Next, Yin attached an overhead suspension sling to Michelle's wheelchair. Using this device, Michelle's arm was supported by a sling and suspended by an overhead rod. This device is used for people presenting with proximal weakness, with muscle grades in the 1/5 to 3/5 range. The sling acts to unweight Michelle's weak arm to allow her to use her remaining muscle strength to guide her hand to the proper letters on the keyboard. Using these adaptations, Michelle was able to complete her letters, albeit slowly.

Questions

1. How would you evaluate Michelle's wheelchair for proper fit and cushioning?
2. Develop goals for Tom based on his evaluation findings.

Conclusion

OT practitioners have a variety of intervention approaches available to choose from and combine. The correct choices of interventions are based on a variety of data including client choice, knowledge of disease/disability, assessment findings, clinical experience, and professional reasoning. No matter which approach is chosen, occupation is always the end and is the most frequent means with the addition of purposeful and preparatory methods as needed.

Acknowledgments

The author would like to acknowledge the contributions of Anne E. Dickerson, PhD, OTR/L, FAOTA, and Elin Schold Davis, OTR/L, CDRS, for contributing to the driving vignette. The author would also like to acknowledge Emily Raphael-Greenfield, EdD, OTR/L, and Debra Tupé, PhD, OTR, for useful feedback. Thank you to Cathy Peirce, PhD, OTR/L, for thoughtful discussions on occupation.

Lippincott® Connect *For additional resources on the subjects discussed in this chapter, visit* Lippincott Connect.

REFERENCES

American Occupational Therapy Association. (2016). The role of occupational therapy in end-of-life care. *American Journal of Occupational Therapy, 70*(Suppl. 2), 7012410075p1–7012410075p16. https://doi.org/10.5014/ajot.2016.706S17

American Occupational Therapy Association. (2017). Philosophical base of occupational therapy. *American Journal of Occupational Therapy, 71*(Suppl. 2), 7112410045p1. https://doi.org/10.5014/ajot.2017.716S06

American Occupational Therapy Association. (2020). Occupational therapy practice framework: Domain and process—Fourth edition. *American Journal of Occupational Therapy, 74*(Suppl. 2), 7412411010p1–7412411010p87. https://doi.org/10.5014/ajot.2020.74S2001

Amini, D. (2011). Occupational therapy interventions for work-related injuries and conditions of the forearm, wrist, and hand: A systematic review. *American Journal of Occupational Therapy, 65*(1), 29–36. https://doi.org/10.5014/ajot.2011.09186

Arbesman, M., Lieberman, D., & Thomas, V. J. (2011). Methodology for the systematic reviews on occupational therapy for individuals with work-related injuries and illnesses. *American Journal of Occupational Therapy, 65*(1), 10–15. https://doi.org/10.5014/ajot.2011.09183

Bennett, S., & Bennett, J. W. (2000). The process of evidence-based practice in occupational therapy: Informing clinical decisions. *Australian Occupational Therapy Journal, 47*(4), 171–180. https://doi.org/10.1046/j.1440-1630.2000.00237.x

Bennett, S., Hoffmann, T., McCluskey, A., McKenna, K., Strong, J., & Tooth, L. (2003). Evidence-based practice forum. Introducing OTseeker (Occupational Therapy Systematic Evaluation of Evidence): A new evidence database for occupational therapists. *American Journal of Occupational Therapy, 57*(6), 635–638. https://doi.org/10.5014/ajot.57.6.635

Charlton, K., Murray, C., Boucaut, R., & Berndt, A. (2021). Facilitating manual wheelchair skills following lower limb amputation using a group process: A nested mixed methods pilot study. *Australian Occupational Therapy Journal, 68*(6), 490–503. https://doi.org/10.1111/1440-1630.12759

Chase, C. A., Mann, K., Wasek, S., & Arbesman, M. (2012). Systematic review of the effect of home modification and fall prevention programs on falls and the performance of community-dwelling older adults. *American Journal of Occupational Therapy, 66*(3), 284–291. https://doi.org/10.5014/ajot.2012.005017

Che Daud, A. Z., Yau, M. K., Barnett, F., & Judd J. (2016). Occupation-based intervention in hand injury rehabilitation: Experiences of occupational therapists in Malaysia. *Scandinavian Journal of Occupational Therapy, 23*(1), 57–66. https://doi.org/10.3109/11038128.2015.1062047

Clark, F. A., Jackson, J. M., Scott, M. D., Carlson, M. E., Atkins, M. S., Uhles-Tanaka, D., & Rubayi, S. (2006). Data-based models of how pressure ulcers develop in daily-living contexts of adults with spinal cord injury. *Archives of Physical Medicine and Rehabilitation, 87*(11), 1516–1525. https://doi.org/10.1016/j.apmr.2006.08.329

Cole, B., & McLean, V. (2003). Therapeutic relationships re-defined. *Occupational Therapy in Mental Health, 19*(2), 33–56. https://doi.org/10.1300/J004v19n02_03

Dun, C, Swan, J, Hitch, D, & Vlachou, V. (2020). Occupational therapy driver assessments with mental health consumers: A mixed-methods study. *Australian Occupational Therapy Journal, 67*(4), 330–340. https://doi.org/10.1111/1440-1630.12652

Eklund, M., & Hallberg, I. R. (2001). Psychiatric occupational therapists' verbal interaction with their clients. *Occupational Therapy International, 8*(1), 1–16. https://doi.org/10.1002/oti.128

Fisher, A. G. (1998). Uniting practice and theory in an occupational therapy framework, 1998 Eleanor Clarke Slagle lecture. *American Journal of Occupational Therapy, 52*(7), 509–522. https://doi.org/10.5014/ajot.52.7.509

Gentry, T. (2008). PDAs as cognitive aids for people with multiple sclerosis. *American Journal of Occupational Therapy, 62*(1), 18–27. https://doi.org/10.5014/ajot.62.1.18

Gillen, G., Berger, S., Lotia, S., Morreale, J., Siber, M., & Trudo, W. (2007). Improving community skills after lower extremity joint replacement. *Physical and Occupational Therapy in Geriatrics, 25*(4), 41–54. https://doi.org/10.1080/J148v25n04_03

Gitlin, L. N., Corcoran, M., Winter, L., Boyce, A., & Hauck, W. W. (2001). A randomized, controlled trial of a home environmental intervention: Effect on efficacy and upset in caregivers and on daily function of persons with dementia. *The Gerontologist, 41*(1), 4–14. https://doi.org/10.1093/geront/41.1.4

Gol, D., & Jarus, T. (2005). Effect of a social skills training group on everyday activities of children with attention-deficit-hyperactivity disorder. *Developmental Medicine and Child Neurology, 47*(8), 539–545. https://doi.org/10.1017/s0012162205001052

Goodman, V., Wardrope, B., Myers, S., Cohen, S., McCorquodale, L., & Kinsella, E. A. (2019). Mindfulness and human occupation: A scoping review. *Scandinavian Journal of Occupational Therapy, 26*(3), 157–170. https://doi.org/10.1080/11038128.2018.1483422

Gray, J. M. (1998). Putting occupation into practice: Occupation as ends, occupation as means. *American Journal of Occupational Therapy, 52*(5), 354–364. https://doi.org/10.5014/ajot.52.5.354

Haynes, R. B., Devereaux, P. J., & Guyatt, G. H. (2002). Clinical expertise in the era of evidence-based medicine and patient choice. *ACP Journal Club, 136*(2), A11–A14. https://doi.org/10.1136/ebm.7.2.36

Jensen, L., & Padilla, R. (2017). Effectiveness of environment-based interventions that address behavior, perception, and falls in people with Alzheimer's disease and related major neurocognitive disorders: A systematic review. *American Journal of Occupational Therapy, 71*(5), 7105180030p1–7105180030p10. https://doi.org/10.5014/ajot.2017.027409

Kealey, P., & McIntyre, I. (2005). An evaluation of the domiciliary occupational therapy service in palliative cancer care in a community trust: A patient and carers perspective. *European Journal of Cancer Care, 14*(3), 232–243. https://doi.org/10.1111/j.1365-2354.2005.00559.x

Keglovits, M., Clemson, L., Hu, Y.-L., Nguyen, A., Neff, A. J., Mandelbaum, C., Hudson, M., Williams, R., Silianoff, T., & Stark, S. (2020). A scoping review of fall hazards in the homes of older adults and development of a framework for assessment and intervention.

Australian Occupational Therapy Journal, 67(5), 470–478. https://doi.org/10.1111/1440-1630.12682

Krasniuk, S., Crizzle, A. M., Toxopeus, R., Mychael, D., & Prince, N. (2022). Clinical tests predicting on-road performance in older drivers with cognitive impairment. *Canadian Journal of Occupational Therapy*. Advance online publication. https://doi.org/10.1177/00084174221117708

Law, M., Baptiste, S., & Mills, J. (1995). Client-centred practice: What does it mean and does it make a difference? *Canadian Journal of Occupational Therapy, 62*(5), 250–257. https://doi.org/10.1177/000841749506200504

Marik, T. L., & Roll, S. C. (2017). Effectiveness of occupational therapy interventions for musculoskeletal shoulder conditions: A systematic review. *American Journal of Occupational Therapy, 71*(1), 7101180020p1–7101180020p11. https://doi.org/10.5014/ajot.2017.023127

Masiero, S., Boniolo, A., Wassermann, L., Machiedo, H., Volante, D., & Punzi, L. (2007). Effects of an educational-behavioral joint protection program on people with moderate to severe rheumatoid arthritis: A randomized controlled trial. *Clinical Rheumatology, 26*(12), 2043–2050. https://doi.org/10.1007/s10067-007-0615-0

Meuser, S., Piskur, B., Hennissen, P., & Dolmans, D. (2022). Targeting the school environment to enable participation: A scoping review. *Scandinavian Journal of Occupational Therapy*. Advance online publication. https://doi.org/10.1080/11038128.2022.2124190

Nielsen, T. L., Winstrup Holst-Stensborg, H., & Nielsen, L. M. (2022). Strengthening problem-solving skills through occupational therapy to improve older adults' occupational performance: A systematic review. *Scandinavian Journal of Occupational Therapy, 30*(1), 1–13. https://doi.org/10.1080/11038128.2022.2112281

Owsley, C., & McGwin, G., Jr. (1999). Vision impairment and driving. *Survey Ophthalmology, 43*(6), 535–550. https://doi.org/10.1016/s0039-6257(99)00035-1

Owsley, C., Sekuler, R., & Siemsen, D. (1983). Contrast sensitivity throughout adulthood. *Vision Research, 23*(7), 689–699. https://doi.org/10.1016/0042-6989(83)90210-9

Owsley, C., Stalvey, B. T., Wells, J., & Sloane, M. E. (1999). Older drivers and cataract: Driving habits and crash risk. *The Journals of Gerontology, 54*(4), M203–M211. https://doi.org/10.1093/gerona/54.4.m203

Punwar, J., & Peloquin, M. (2000). *Occupational therapy: Principles and practice* (3rd ed.). Lippincott Williams & Wilkins.

Sackett, D. L., Strauss, S. E., Richardson, W. S., Rosenberg, W., & Haynes, R. B. (2000). *Evidenced-based medicine: How to practice and teach.* Churchill Livingstone.

Samuelsson, K., Tropp, M., Lundqvist, A., & Wressle, E. (2019). Development, concurrent validity and internal consistency of a simulator tool for assessing continued car driving after a brain injury/disease. *British Journal of Occupational Therapy, 8*(9), 544–552. https://doi.org/10.1177/0308022619836935

Schaaf, R. C., Dumont, R. L., Arbesman, M., & May-Benson, T. A. (2018). Efficacy of occupational therapy using Ayres Sensory Integration®: A systematic review. *American Journal of Occupational Therapy, 72*(1), 7201190010p1–7201190010p10. https://doi.org/10.5014/ajot.2018.028431

Solman, B., & Clouston, T. (2016). Occupational therapy and the therapeutic use of self. *British Journal of Occupational Therapy, 79*(8), 514–516. https://doi.org/10.1177/0308022616638675

Stutts, J., Martell, C., & Staplin, L. (2009). *Identifying behaviors and situations associated with increased crash risk for older drivers* (Report No. DOT HS 811 09). National Highway Traffic Safety Administration.

Sumsion, T., & Law, M. (2006). A review of evidence on the conceptual elements informing client-centred practice. *Canadian Journal of Occupational Therapy, 73*(3), 153–162. https://doi.org/10.1177/000841740607300303

Talbot-Coulombe, C., Bravo, G., & Carrier, A. (2022). Occupational therapy practice in palliative and end-of-life care in Québec. *Canadian Journal of Occupational Therapy, 89*(2), 201–211. https://doi.org/10.1177/00084174221084466

Taylor, R. R., Lee, S. W., Kielhofner, G., & Ketkar, M. (2009). Therapeutic use of self: A nationwide survey of practitioners' attitudes and experiences. *American Journal of Occupational Therapy, 63*(2), 198–207. https://doi.org/10.5014/ajot.63.2.198

Trombly, C. A. (1995). Occupation: Purposefulness and meaningfulness as therapeutic mechanisms. 1995 Eleanor Clarke Slagle lecture. *American Journal of Occupational Therapy, 49*(10), 960–972. https://doi.org/10.5014/ajot.49.10.960

University of Southern California. (2013). *USC/Rancho Lifestyle Redesign® pressure ulcer prevention project.* http://www.usc.edu/programs/pups/

Van Heest, K. N. L., Mogush, A. R., & Mathiowetz, V. G. (2017). Effects of a one-to-one fatigue management course for people with chronic conditions and fatigue. *American Journal of Occupational Therapy, 71*(4), 7104100020p1–7104100020p9. https://doi.org/10.5014/ajot.2017.023440

Velligan, D. I., Prihoda, T. J., Ritch, J. L., Maples, N., Bow-Thomas, C. C., & Dassori, A. (2002). A randomized single-blind pilot study of compensatory strategies in schizophrenia outpatients. *Schizophrenia Bulletin, 28*(2), 283–292. https://doi.org/10.1093/oxfordjournals.schbul.a006938

Weinstock-Zlotnick, G., & Hinojosa, J. (2004). Bottom-up or top-down evaluation: Is one better than the other? *American Journal of Occupational Therapy, 58*(5), 594–598. https://doi.org/10.5014/ajot.58.5.594

Wheeler, S., Davis, D., Basch, J., James, G., Lehman, B., & Acord-Vira, A. (2022). Self-regulation and relaxation-based interventions for adults with traumatic brain injury (2013–2020). *American Journal of Occupational Therapy, 76*(Suppl. 2), 7613393150. https://doi.org/10.5014/ajot.2022/76S2015

Occupational Therapy Evaluation and Intervention for Communities and Populations

Bernard Austin Kigunda Muriithi

LEARNING OBJECTIVES

After reading this chapter, you will be able to:

1. Define client factors, performance skills, performance patterns, and context when considering communities or populations as a client.
2. Discuss the importance of considering diverse intervention approaches to meet unique community and population health needs.
3. Demonstrate an understanding of the process and considerations made when developing community programs.
4. Discuss the benefits of considering different theories to inform interventions for communities and populations.
5. Describe how practitioners may promote evidence-based practices while serving programs in different roles.

Introduction

Occupational therapists work with individuals, groups, organizations, communities, and populations. The American Occupational Therapy Association (AOTA, 2020) considers a *client* to be either a person group or a population, whereas the World Federation of Occupational Therapists (WFOT, 2019) includes *organization* and *community* in addition to the other three. Groups, organizations, communities, and populations are seen as clients if interventions impact aggregates of people rather than single individuals. *Group* refers to a "collection of individuals having shared characteristics or a common or shared purpose" (AOTA, 2020, p. 2). Examples of groups include family members, students, workers, or a sports team. Interventions for groups address the challenges that face a group of people rather than single individuals. As interventions designed for organizations, communities, and populations involve groups of people with shared needs, this chapter uses the term *group* to refer to a collection of individuals receiving an intervention due to similarities in needs and goals.

Organization refers to an "entity composed of individuals with a common purpose or enterprise, such as a business, industry, or agency" (AOTA, 2020, p. 80). Organizations can provide an institutional venue and support in which groups of people can receive intervention programs that may improve health or performance within the organization. The term *population* refers to "an aggregate of people who may or may not know each other but share at least one characteristic such as age, race, ethnicity, gender, health habit or condition, geographical location, cultural identity, socioeconomic status or education" (Scaffa & Reitz, 2020, p. 8). Population as client describes a group of people who, due to *shared attributes,* have similarities impacting health, well-being, or inclusion in comparable ways. Examples of populations are older adult survivors of stroke, refugees resettled in new countries, adults who are addicted to substances, students, and school-aged children with autism, among others.

Groups, organizations, and populations exist within communities. Thus, the term *community program* has been used to refer to interventions that address the needs of groups of people (Fazio, 2017). The goal of such programs is to "promote health, prevent injury and illness, improve well-being and inclusion, and reduce burden of disease" (WFOT, 2019, p. 2). A *community* is defined as "a collection of populations that is changeable and diverse and includes various people, groups, networks, and organizations" (AOTA, 2020, p. 2). This definition parallels the World Health Organization (WHO) definition of community as a "specific group of people, often living in a defined geographical area, who share a common culture, values, and norms, are arranged in a social structure according to relationships which the community has developed over a period of time" (1998, p. 5). Community thus entails the sharing of identity and collective regard for certain values, beliefs, and norms, along with proximity and/or ability to gather as a group for collective action.

Current understandings of the community can exclude the necessity for geographical proximity between members due to possibilities for *virtual groups and communities.* This possibility means that occupational therapy (OT) services can be delivered to groups of people via *telehealth,* which is the "use of information and communication technologies to deliver health-related services when the provider and client are in different physical locations" (WFOT, 2021, p. 1). Telehealth is a service delivery model that relies on technology and possibilities for virtual communities that can improve access to underserved communities in which in-person service delivery is impractical (WFOT, 2021). As the efficacy of telehealth has been documented, it is an alternative that yields comparable results to services delivered in person (WHO & World Bank, 2011). Virtual communities provide an alternative to community service programs where unexpected benefits could be witnessed (see Expanding Our Perspectives). This also provides possibilities for sharing of information between providers who may be in different geographical locations, with the possible benefit of promoting evidence-based practices by sharing knowledge across the globe (see Chapter 67 for more information on telehealth).

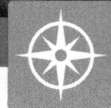

EXPANDING OUR PERSPECTIVES

Developing a Cancer Survivorship Program for Latina Women

Yanet Ybarra, OTD, OTR/L

The Latino population is a marginalized group in the United States. The group faces barriers in accessing health services due to a variety of reasons, including limited familiarity with the healthcare system, limited financial resources making health insurance unaffordable, and language and cultural barriers that negatively affect communication with providers.

As an occupational therapist with Latino background, whose own mother had ovarian cancer and whose first language was Spanish, I decided to explore the possibility of creating a program to service this population at Wesley Community Center (WCC) in Phoenix, Arizona. I reviewed the available information regarding the mission, vision, goals, and objectives of the community center and consulted widely with individuals and leadership at WCC. I completed a needs assessment by interviewing individual women and holding group discussions to identify their priorities. Major priorities emerging from this process included a need to address physical and mental health problems affecting women's quality of life (QOL). I collaborated with WCC and a group of women to create the *Cancer Survivorship Program* (CSP), aiming to support women recovering from various forms of cancer.

The CSP was designed to educate and equip women with knowledge and skills to empower women to better manage their own health. As the women's goal was to improve QOL, the World Health Organization Quality of Life (WHO-QOL) scale was selected for outcome measures. While the original plan was to implement the program at WCC, the COVID-19 pandemic emerged before program implementation, and the WCC facility was closed to prevent coronavirus infections.

I was able to test the efficacy of the program, however, by implementing it via telehealth. Qualifying women who received services at WCC were invited to sign up if they had access to a computer and internet and were

(continued)

able to meet via Zoom. Program implementation occurred 3 times per week for 8 weeks. A different intervention type was implemented each week, alternating interventions for physical problems with those of mental health. Interventions for physical needs included education for lymphedema management and strategies to maintain or improve strength, range of motion, and endurance. Interventions for mental health included education on sleep hygiene, stress management techniques, coping and resiliency, emotional regulation, and self-advocacy.

The effectiveness of the CSP in improving QOL was tested by administering the Spanish version of the WHO-QOL scale before and after CSP implementation. The overall results demonstrated that QOL for all participants improved in all four domains (physical, psychological, social relationships, and environment). Telehealth proved to be an effective delivery model in providing women with the help they needed. Additionally, the intervention process resulted in a virtual community in which the women would continue to support one another at a time when physical gatherings were restricted.

Interventions for groups, communities, organizations, and populations are known as *programs*, and the process of developing them is *community program development*. Programs are designed to "achieve preplanned objectives such as changes in knowledge, attitudes, skills, and behaviors to maintain or improve function and/or health" (Flecky et al., 2020, p. 75). OT practitioners play an important role in developing programs, but they may also take other roles given that community programming often involves teams that include other professionals, agencies, and organizations within communities.

Community and Population Characteristics and Context

Community programs are developed to modify specific aspects of the target population (i.e., context, performance patterns, performance skills, or client factors), any one of which can promote or interfere with occupational performance and influence health in positive or negative ways. *Performance patterns* are the "acquired habits, routines, roles, and rituals used in the process of engaging consistently in occupations and can support or hinder occupational performance" (AOTA, 2020, p. 12). Routines are observable, regular, and repetitive patterns of behavior, which may satisfy, promote, or damage the well-being of a population (AOTA, 2020). For example, parents with young children have routines for daily care for their children, but a community may support parents and children by creating supportive after-school programs. Activities such as the one shown in Figure 22.1 are common in many communities, and they can involve whole communities or certain groups within them.

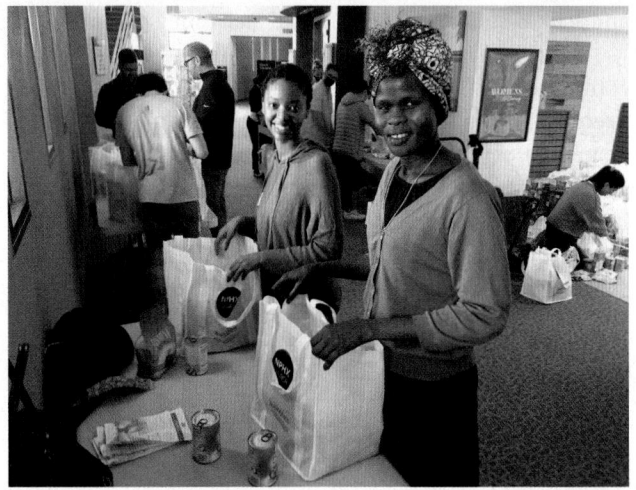

FIGURE 22.1 Left to right, Jahrae Andrews (United States) and Ageta Bui (Ethiopia) volunteering to pack Thanksgiving dinners for the needy people in the city of Phoenix, Arizona. Jahrae is a volunteer with a nonprofit agency Abounding Service, which offers refugees (like Ageta) English learning programs supported by volunteer "Encouragers" like Jahrae. Location: North Phoenix Church, Phoenix, AZ. (Photo courtesy of Derek DeVelder.)

Performance skills are goal-directed actions that include motor skills, process skills, and social interaction skills (AOTA, 2020). Impairment in these skills has a significant impact on occupational performance and may affect certain populations more than others. For example, autistic young adults may struggle with social interaction skills as they transition from high school to community living. An independent-living community program can play a supportive role for this population. Similarly, programs can be developed to support populations that struggle specifically with motor or processing skills within a community.

Client factors are the "specific capacities, characteristics, or beliefs that reside within a person, group, or population and influence performance of occupations" (AOTA, 2020, p. 15). They include (a) body structures and body functions and (b) values, beliefs, and spirituality (AOTA, 2020). Values, beliefs, and spirituality may be shared by a group as may be reflected when freedom of religion, conviction that group action can transform society, and shared search for meaning by a church congregation, are seen within a community. Programs may be designed to influence client factors, for instance, when they are developed to promote values like social justice and equity within diverse communities.

Context includes both *environmental* and *personal* factors. Environmental factors "are aspects of the physical, social and attitudinal surroundings in which people live and conduct their lives" (AOTA, 2020, pp. 9–10). Environmental factors can limit individual participation necessitating community programs to help specific populations. For example, ramps may be created to facilitate access to public facilities and buildings for individuals using wheelchairs. Personal factors are stable and unique features of a person such as age, sexual orientation, gender identity, race and ethnicity, and education (AOTA, 2020), which can affect how an individual functions within a community. Table 22.1 shows examples of contexts associated with groups, communities, and populations. These factors have historically influenced how different groups of people interact in communities. Programs may target specific populations based on these factors.

The Evaluation and Program Development Process

All OT services, including programs, involve *evaluation*, *intervention*, and *outcome* measures. **Community programs** require extensive planning, collaboration, and partnership with stakeholders within communities for several reasons. First, community programs often do not receive reimbursement in the same way as individual interventions. Therefore, a plan to acquire funding may be a necessary step. Second, the client is a community that includes individuals who may not agree on important aspects of the process, which can delay or prevent program development. An important way to deal with possible disagreements is exercising democratic principles that allow participants to make suggestions and vote so they can take ownership of the process. Third, communities may have individuals and entities willing to provide support in skilled manpower, volunteer hours, space, funding, and equipment. Harnessing community resources and persuading a community to act requires skillful collaboration, networking, and organizational skills.

Community programming is a relatively new intervention type among OT practitioners. It has been suggested that instead of developing programs *for a community*, OT

TABLE 22.1	Examples of Environments and Contexts Associated With Groups, Communities, and Populations
Environment or Context	**Examples**
Natural Environment and Human-made Changes to the Environment	
Group (family, workers, students)	Home, neighborhood, office, factory, school, hospital complex
Community/population	Public transportation system, city parks, natural resources
Support and Relationships	
Group (family, workers, students)	Interaction with extended family, communication and social support among workers, appreciation from supervisors, positive feedback from teachers and peers
Community/population	Influence of city government, nonprofit agencies, and other community organizations on occupational performance and/or participation
Attitudes	
Group (family, workers, students)	Interaction patterns and behavioral expectations within the group; for example, family prayer, dress-down Fridays, professional behavior
Community/population	Cultural activities such as siestas, afternoon tea, Mardi Gras, etc.
Services, Systems, and Policies	
Group (family, workers, students)	Family-centered programs, peer support for members with mental illness, wellness groups or clubs
Community/population	Public utilities (e.g., water and electricity), political systems, transportation systems
Products and Technology	
Group (family, workers, students)	Hearing aids for family members in need, wheelchairs for non-ambulatory group members, bathroom with grab bars and raised toilet, gaming consoles
Community/population	Churches, temples, mosques, fitness facilities, bicycle trails, elevators for multistory buildings, internet access

practitioners should develop programs *with the community* (Fazio, 2017). This is acknowledging that the more a community is involved in the process, the greater the chances of creating a successful program. How OT practitioners have worked with communities and populations has been changing as more is learned about best practices. Scaffa and Reitz (2020) propose a new *Community and Population Health Practice* (CPHP) paradigm, in which they incorporate elements that are seen as important in OT programs. Their proposed paradigm is client centered, occupation based, supported by evidence, based on dynamic systems theory, ecologically sound, and strengths based (Scaffa & Reitz, 2020). The CPHP offers a set of principles that practitioners can use as guidelines for creating programs that are evidence based and occupation centered.

Regardless of the approach taken, developing community programs is a complex process that differs from that of interventions for individuals (see Figure 22.2). The phases of program development include *preplanning, needs assessment* (evaluation), *program design and implementation* (intervention), and *evaluation* (outcome measures). This, however, is not to be viewed linearly because certain forms of outcome measures contribute to program design and implementation in a continuing process.

In the *preplanning* phase, research is conducted to identify the health needs of a group (AOTA, 2020). Research should include not only the occupational priorities of the present group but also a careful environmental scan and analysis of trends or future forecasts (AOTA, 2020; Fazio, 2017). Some important tasks at this stage include a review of public health information, a review of secondary data regarding the prevalence of health problems, an analysis of demographic data, and an analysis of social and economic data. After the preplanning phase, a *needs assessment* is performed to establish the interests and needs of a community by directly engaging community members through interviews, surveys, or group discussions to determine their priorities. Such primary sources of information also enable one to create a *community profile,* which reveals not just priorities but also opportunities for collaboration

with specific individuals, agencies, or organizations (AOTA, 2020). A community profile indicates both resources that may support and barriers that may impede program development and implementation. The evaluation process is completed after analysis and interpretation of data to inform the course of action, which is done collaboratively with the community partners (Fazio, 2017).

Program design and implementation involves creating and implementing an occupation-based plan to meet program goals. This plan includes goals, objectives, activities, and desired outcomes (Doll & Domina, 2020). It is important to evaluate a community in collaboration with partners and carefully select outcomes that are consistent with the needs and desires of the community; therefore, the needs assessment always precedes program design. According to AOTA (2020), outcomes for groups or populations are like those of individuals and include:

1. Enabling *occupational performance*—developed ability to do and accomplish an occupation or activity
2. Improved occupational performance—reducing the effects of barriers
3. Enhancement of performance—augmented skills and patterns, where no performance limitations are present
4. *Prevention*—improved knowledge and health promotion skills that reduce the incidence and minimize the risk of disease, or injury
5. *Health and wellness*—improved physical, mental and social well-being, the capacity of individuals and groups to make healthy choices for a balanced life
6. *Quality of life*—improved satisfaction with one's overall life
7. *Occupational participation*—making engagement personally satisfying
8. Developed *role competence*—effectively meeting demands of specified roles
9. *Well-being*—contentment with one's health and having a "good life"
10. *Occupational justice*—access to the full range of occupations afforded to others, or inclusion.

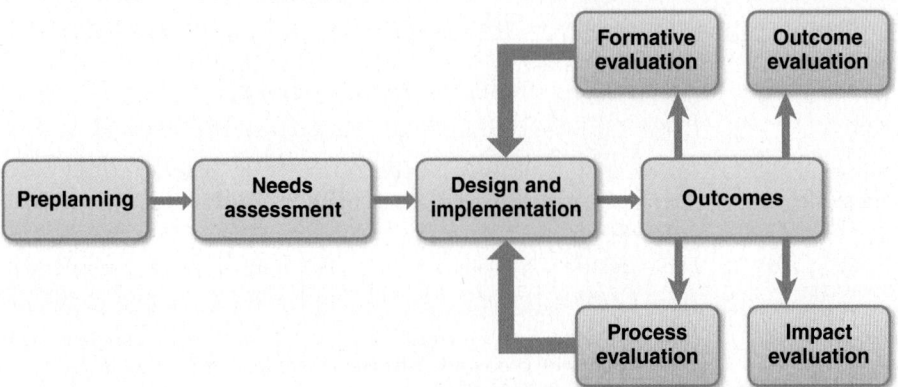

FIGURE 22.2 **The process of community program development.**

Any one of the above outcomes may be what a community or population wants or needs, but a single program may address one or more of these outcomes.

After the outcomes are collaboratively selected by the community members and program developer, the implementation plan is created. This plan must include a timeline for the major tasks such as obtaining space, acquiring materials and/or supplies, hiring staff and personnel, recruiting participants, and administrating outcome measures. The implementation plan also describes the roles and responsibilities of entities such as community groups or agencies, hired personnel and staff, and volunteers (Doll & Domina, 2020; Fazio, 2017). It may be important for the OT practitioners developing programs to seek support from an advisory board, which helps establish stronger links with community partners, organizations, government agencies, and networks, and provides the program with valuable feedback (Doll & Domina, 2020). Selection of advisory board members should be done purposefully to ensure diversity and representation of all members of a community, and representatives of marginalized groups should be particularly encouraged to articulate the concerns of those who are not viewed as mainstream in a particular community. Finally, the implementation plan may show how the program is presently funded and how it may be funded or sustained in the future.

Program evaluation is the last phase in community program development. Evaluation may gather information regarding program implementation or improvement (formative evaluation), evaluate efficiency in implementation (process evaluation), measure the impact of a program after implementation (impact evaluation), and evaluate achievement of program goals (outcome evaluation). Program evaluation results should be shared with community partners to provide a basis for further program development, generate support for expanding programs and for public relations, and demonstrate good use of sponsor funds (Ensminger et al., 2020).

Intervention Approaches for Communities and Populations

An evaluation of the client's performance patterns, performance skills, client factors, and context help to identify the unique needs of a community or population. When the needs are identified and goals and objectives are known, the program developer selects a suitable approach collaboratively with community partners. Intervention approaches are "specific strategies selected to direct the evaluation and intervention processes on the basis of the client's desired

outcomes, evaluation data and research evidence" (AOTA, 2020, p. 63). They include remediation, restoration, prevention, maintenance, health promotion, and compensation.

Remediation is an approach that aims to develop a skill that has not yet been developed in the client. For example, a program might be designed for developing social and interaction skills for children in a community. *Restoration*, on the other hand, aims to recover skills or resources that were lost. Communities in which the needs of all people are addressed fairly can decline due to policy changes or diminished resources, but community programs can respond to restore skills or resources that were previously present to serve the needs of the specified population. For example, government policy changes may result in the loss of highly valued after-school programs for children with special needs, but specific communities can develop alternative programs to address the same needs using comparable or same approaches. Remediation and restoration approaches are often supported by established reimbursement programs in cases of individual intervention, whereas the intervention programs at the community or population level often require a different source of funding, such as grants, state funding, or individual sponsorships.

Compensation is the approach that aims to find "ways to revise the current context or activity demands to support performance in the natural setting" (Dunn et al., 1998, p. 533). That is, rather than develop skills in a person or group, the context (including the environment) or task is altered to facilitate occupational performance. A community center can be designed, for instance, in a way to provide access and recreational options to people with physical and mental health conditions, so that it supports and encourages participation for all members of a community.

Prevention is "an anticipatory action taken to reduce the possibility of an event or condition from occurring or developing or to minimize the damage that may result from the event or condition if it does occur" (Pickett & Hanlon, 1990, p. 81). This approach is used in programs that address the needs of groups or populations who are at risk of developing occupational performance problems. For instance, weight reduction programs may prevent serious health complications such as heart disease for young adults with obesity. OT Story 22.1 demonstrates that preventive measures can prevent serious injuries or even death.

Maintenance enables clients to "preserve the performance capabilities that they have regained and that continue to meet their occupational needs" (AOTA, 2020, p. 63). The maintenance approach regards it likely that without intervention occupational performance would decrease and health would be affected negatively. For instance, exercise programs may help maintain strength and endurance for seniors in a community, while without such a program this population is likely to experience a faster decline because of aging.

OT STORY 22.1 FALL REDUCTION PROGRAMMING FOR OLDER ADULTS IN ASSISTED LIVING

A group of occupational and physical therapists noted that a large percentage of deaths among older adults living in multiple assisted living facilities of a large metropolitan city, where they worked, were due to falls. These falls also increased fear of falling among residents, restricting participation in everyday activities for some of the adults. The therapists saw a need to provide an intervention but did not have availability in their very busy schedules to provide programming for fall prevention (intervention approach: prevention). The occupational and physical therapists were expected to focus on treating residents with more serious difficulties in mobility or self-care activities like walking, bathing, or dressing (approaches: remediation or restoration).

An occupational therapist from this group contacted a local university to inquire about possibly collaborating with the Department of Occupational Therapy and Department of Physical Therapy to meet this need (role of advocate). He partnered with the university in seeking possible interventions by researching available evidence and looking at publicly available data regarding older adults in the city (preplanning). The collaborating team decided to consult residents and other team members at the assisted living facilities to hear their thoughts. They presented basic evidence to stakeholders and residents in group discussions where they assessed the needs, interests, and resources available (needs assessment). The research findings they shared included a definition of fall as "the unintentional coming to rest on the ground, floor, or lower surface" (Hauer et al., 2006; WHO, 2007); that falls occur in everyday occupations that all people need and want to do (Johansson et al., 2018); that prevalence for falls among older adults is 22% to 33% (Peel, 2011); and that the WHO (2004) urged that individuals should be encouraged to participate in all aspects of life, and they should be assured safety in daily tasks.

Similar evidence and discussions were held with residents (collaboration), while the therapists assessed the level of interest and gathered their feedback on what they wanted in the falls prevention program (needs assessment). This collaborative process led to a development of a program for fall prevention focusing on home safety, exercises for strength and endurance, balance, and fear of falling (program design). The program was later implemented in all six assisted living facilities. The university had agreed with the facilities that the occupational and physical therapy students would implement the program under supervision (collaboration and partnership). The program was manualized with clear instructions to students. The older adults were asked to sign up if they wanted to participate in the program. Enrolled participants received 2 hours of training weekly for 8 weeks in all facilities.

Residents who completed the falls prevention program performed better (outcomes) on the Timed Up and Go (TUG), Performance-Oriented Mobility Assessment (POMA), and the Functional Reach Test, in comparison to a control group. The program was repeated annually for several years, while data regarding falls and deaths were collected and shared with the stakeholders. Both the number of falls and the number of deaths decreased during the years of program implementation compared to previously (outcomes). This community program later became a sought-after learning experience for students at the university, making the program sustainable. The partnership between a local university and six assisted living facilities in the city proved beneficial to both the university and community residents.

Questions

1. How would such a program be sustained had this university not been in the area?
2. What other kinds of interventions could you develop to promote health among community-dwelling seniors?
3. What type of interventions could be done using compensatory strategies to minimize fall risk?

Health promotion is the approach that involves creating or promoting "any planned combination of educational, political, regulatory, environmental, and organizational supports for actions and conditions of living conducive to the health of individuals, families, communities and populations" (Scaffa, 2020, p. 22). This approach does not assume that a disability is present or likely in the future but seeks to enrich occupational performance for all people in their natural contexts (Dunn et al., 1998). For example, a meditation program may promote emotional, mental, and social well-being for high school students who struggle with anxiety.

Value of Diverse Theories in Program Development

An important element of evidence-based practice is the application of theories that are supported by evidence. Theory selection is made based on the nature of the problem and the approach being taken, but it is recognized that theories that consider interrelations between various levels of society have high relevance in community programs (Scaffa, 2019).

These theories, collectively called ecological theories, are supported by evidence from health education, health promotion, and public health (Scaffa, 2019). They can and have informed OT interventions, and they have influenced well-known conceptual models.

One of the most widely known ecological theories is Bronfenbrenner's Ecological Systems Theory. Bronfenbrenner (1977) identified four levels of the environment that influence a developing child and postulated that these levels influence each other in a reciprocal fashion. Beginning with the most intimate to the furthest from a person, the levels are *microsystem*, *mesosystem*, *exosystem*, and *macrosystem*. The microsystem is the smallest and most immediate environment (family, daycare, peers), whereas the mesosystem encompasses interactions between microsystems, for example, interactions between a family and school environment, where the child is directly involved in both. Exosystems are linkages between two or more settings but include one setting in which a child is not directly involved. For example, a parent's interactions at the workplace can affect the child, although the child does not directly interact at the parent's workplace. Macrosystem refers to the broadest elements of an environment which include cultural, political, and economical systems. These levels can be used to inform interventions at various levels, as indicated in Table 22.2, which shows an example of addressing childhood obesity from the individual to the microsystem level of society.

Popular OT *conceptual models* integrate the environment in theory and can inform program development in important ways as well. These models usually present the view that the environment is modifiable and could be the root cause of health problems. The focus of intervention is therefore not entirely on an individual, but on a range of environmental factors that may be involved. Some examples of these models are the Ecology of Human Performance model (Dunn et al., 1994), the Person–Environment–Occupation model (Law et al., 1996), the Canadian Model of Occupation Performance and Engagement (Townsend & Polatajko, 2013), the Model of Human Occupation (Kielhofner & Burke, 1980), the Occupational Adaptation model (Schkade & Schultz, 1992), and the Person–Environment–Occupation–Performance model (Christiansen & Baum, 1997) (see the chapters in Unit VI for overviews of these models). Given their broad understanding of the environment and its interaction with person and occupation/task, these theories have high applicability in community programs. Better participation of OT practitioners in program development would build the evidence needed to support the wider application of such occupation-centered theories in intervention programs.

The *Participatory Occupational Justice Framework (POJF)* was first developed by Townsend and Whiteford (2005) as a framework specifically focused on the occupational injustices of everyday living. The framework is grounded in *critical occupational therapy*, a philosophical view that looks at power relations and their application in the everyday life of people within communities (Whiteford & Townsend, 2011; Whiteford et al., 2017). POJF is an appropriate framework for community programs targeting occupational justice, which is now recognized as an outcome of intervention (AOTA, 2020). OT literature has considerably expounded on occupational injustices. Authors from across the world are included in the book series *Occupational Therapy(ies) Without Borders* (Kronenberg et al., 2005, 2011; Sakellariou & Pollard, 2017), where themes related to this topic are discussed. There is growing consensus regarding specific forms of occupational injustice. These are occupational deprivation, occupational imbalance, occupational alienation, occupational marginalization, and occupational apartheid (Hocking, 2017; Durocher et al., 2014; Townsend & Wilcock, 2004). The various types of restricted participation in occupation may call for different intervention approaches. However, the POJF generally calls for the inclusion of politically oriented methods such as raising the consciousness of injustice, collaboration, sharing plans with community partners, strategizing on funding, active involvement of participants in the implementation and evaluation of programs, and advocacy for sustainable action (Whiteford & Townsend, 2011; Whiteford et al., 2017). The POJF invites occupational therapists to consider interventions that involve politically oriented occupations, which often are necessary to meet the needs of marginalized populations.

TABLE 22.2	Addressing Childhood Obesity at Multiple Levels of Intervention
Level of Intervention	**Potential Occupational Therapy Role**
Individual	Facilitate regular physical activity through engagement in meaningful and enjoyable occupations (leisure participation, health management and maintenance)
Microsystem	Teach children and their parents how to develop and implement healthy meal plans for the family (meal preparation)
Mesosystem	Consult with local agencies to provide developmentally appropriate after-school active play or leisure activities for children (play exploration and play participation)
Exosystem	Advocate for accessible and safe walking and biking paths for persons of diverse abilities (safety and emergency maintenance, community mobility)
Macrosystem	Lobby for improvements in the nutritional value of school lunches and vending machine snacks (health management and maintenance)

One other theory that is concerned with the problems of injustice, inequality, and disempowerment is the *theory of occupational reconstruction (OR)*, which is philosophically grounded in American pragmatism (Frank & Muriithi, 2015). The theory of OR suggests seven principles that can guide collective action, drawn from analyzing the actions and outcomes of the civil rights protests in the United States as well as the struggle against apartheid in South Africa. The action begins when people *realize* they have no choice but to do something (first principle) to address a shared social problem. Communities should act to *ameliorate a situation* (second principle) if not fully resolve it. *Embodied practice*, the real action taken by the group, is a critical component of OR (third principle). OR has a *narrative structure*, which allows for anticipation of positive change when action is undertaken (fourth principle). As indicated by the outcomes of the civil rights movement, OR opens spaces for the *creative transformation* of society (fifth principle), and outcomes may go beyond meeting the goals originally targeted, because OR embraces new ways of thinking and acting in society. At all times OR involves *voluntary* participation and democratic values, not authoritarianism (sixth principle). Finally, OR assumes *hopeful experiments* in that actors are not assured of specific outcomes (seventh principle). As the theory of OR encourages collective action rather than despair in certain highly problematic situations, it suggests community programs should be considered even if the chances of meeting narrowly defined outcomes are not high, and the evaluation of outcomes should include analyzing more broadly how a program impacts a community because OR has potential to transform communities in ways that are difficult to predict.

Given that social problems take different forms, and contexts vary significantly across the globe, different theories should be considered to inform community programs depending on the type of problem they aim to address and the unique attributes of individual communities. The paucity of evidence to support the application of various theories in occupation-based community programs should not deter OT practitioners because community programs are a relatively new type of intervention in OT, and using theories sheds light on the practice guidelines used.

The benefits of considering diverse and/or multiple theories in program development, as indicated by the unique strengths of the theories described above, include but are not limited to increased:

1. Chance of selecting a theory that has *strong evidence*
2. Chance of selecting a theory that promotes *occupation-centered* interventions
3. Chance of addressing *occupational injustice*, an underlying cause of many health problems
4. Chance of promoting collective actions that may lead to unexpected *societal transformation* in healthy ways

Promoting Evidence-Based Programs in Diverse Roles

There is limited, but increasing, evidence of the effectiveness of community programs (see Commentary on the Evidence and Table 22.3), and there is a need to increase the search for evidence in various roles that occupational therapists may take (see Figure 22.3). OT practitioners are equipped with skills for a variety of roles in community programs. In each of these roles, the practitioners can bring their expertise in evidence-based practice. OT practitioners can be *program developers*. They are equipped with skills for evaluation, development of evidence-based programs, implementation, and analysis of outcomes to inform further action. In this role, their effectiveness relies on how well they collaborate and partner with other community stakeholders. Unlike most of the current forms of practice, which are based on established reimbursement programs, community program development may require skills for grant application and financial management to develop sustainable programs. Good skills in this role can enable OT practitioners to bring evidence into community programs in addition to acquiring justice for populations that may be marginalized in society.

OT practitioners can also enable programs to optimize the use of available evidence in the role of *supervisor*. Supervisors are responsible for leading and managing teams. As supervisors, they are responsible for the day-to-day running of the program and must determine how to delegate tasks based on the skill sets of team members. Team members may include fellow OT practitioners, related professionals like speech-language pathologists and physical therapists, physicians, nurses, social workers, certified OTAs, rehabilitation aides, and volunteers, among others (Fazio, 2017). Supervisor roles require the ability to recruit, train, and evaluate the performance of employees (Scaffa & Reitz,

> ## COMMENTARY ON THE EVIDENCE
>
> Evidence to support OT interventions at the group, community, and population levels is limited at present. However, evidence from health education, health promotion, and public health can guide the design and evaluation of OT interventions. Evidence-based techniques vary depending on the desired outcomes and level of intervention. A few studies from OT and other disciplines providing evidence for the efficacy of interventions for groups, communities, and populations are briefly described in Table 22.3.

TABLE 22.3	Selected Studies Providing Evidence of the Efficacy of Interventions for Organizations, Communities, and Populations
Authors	**Findings**
Lai et al. (2021)	Demonstrated the effectiveness and acceptability of telemedicine in breast perioperative rehabilitation via videoconference which included functional assessment, exercises, and education
Pan et al. (2018)	Demonstrates through neuroimaging techniques that Tai Chi intervention cortical thickness, functional connectivity, homogeneity of the brain, and executive network neurological functioning among healthy older adults
Coker-Bolt et al. (2017)	Demonstrates the effectiveness of a community-based program on women's hygiene through the use of health education and the distribution of sustainable personal hygiene supplies
Umeda et al. (2017)	Describes the provision of organization-level consultation to maximize community social participation of individuals with intellectual and developmental disabilities
Wenborn et al. (2016)	Discusses the importance of adapting complex community-based OT interventions to specific national contexts using an example of a program for persons with dementia and their family caregivers
Webb et al. (2010)	Investigates the characteristics of effective Internet-based health promotion interventions. The use of theory, multiple behavior change techniques, and various methods for interacting with participants were deemed to be significant factors
Classen et al. (2007)	Identified 11 factors in three categories (behavioral, health, and environmental) related to safe driving for older adults that can be used as elements of a population-based health promotion intervention
Lamontagne et al. (2007)	A systematic review indicated the efficacy of organizational-level primary prevention strategies addressing the causes and consequences of workplace stress in improving work productivity and decreasing job stress
Maller et al. (2006)	Presents empirical and theoretical evidence of the important contact with nature plays in human health and well-being and describes public health strategies to optimize the health-promoting effects of nature-based interventions
McClure et al. (2005)	An evidence-based review of the characteristics of effective population-based approaches to the prevention of falls among older people

2020). A skilled OT practitioner in this role can identify and recruit professionals who have expertise and certification to provide interventions that are supported by evidence.

The role of a *consultant* allows an OT practitioner to "suggest the best strategies and methods without becoming enmeshed with the day-to-day operations of an organization" (Fazio, 2017, p. 178). This role enables the OT

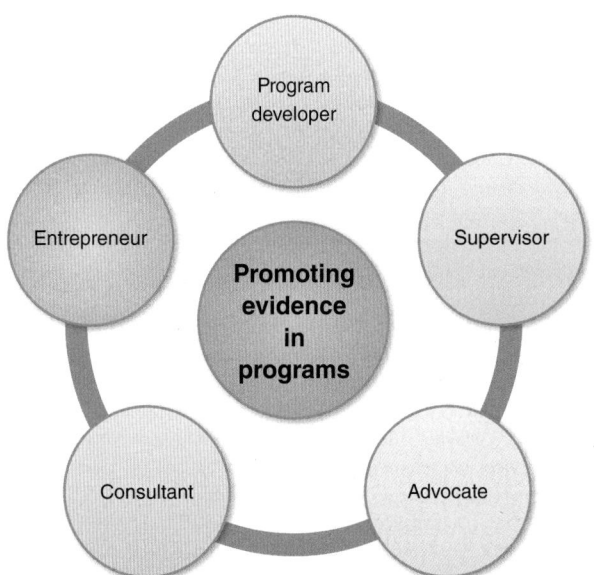

FIGURE 22.3 **The various roles in which OT practitioners can promote evidence-based practices.**

practitioner to recommend the most evidence-based approaches because their vision is not clouded by internal organizational factors (Fazio, 2017). The practitioner can be consulted at any stage in the program development process, including the evaluation and goal setting phase, program development and implementation, and outcome measures. This role can make community programs strongly grounded in the available evidence.

In the role of *entrepreneurs*, OT practitioners utilize evidence to develop new innovative programs for communities. An entrepreneur is a risk taker, optimist, and visionary who sees opportunities that emerge in communities and seeks to meet the needs through for-profit or nonprofit practices (Fazio, 2017; Scaffa & Reitz, 2020). *Social entrepreneurs* are individuals who seek "righting the unrightable wrong and finding your mission" (Scofield, 2011, p. 1). Because the focus for social entrepreneurs is the public good (Fazio, 2017), this role can facilitate the development of community programs that benefit many who would otherwise experience occupational injustice. Closely related to the role of social entrepreneurs is the role of community *advocates*. The advocate responds to problems of occupational injustice using methods such as lobbying with legislators or government agencies to provide community resources and pass just laws. Entrepreneurs and community advocates can utilize evidence, including data regarding *social determinants of health*, to promote practices that address the needs of marginalized populations within communities.

Conclusion

There is growing recognition that OT practitioners should be involved in developing interventions for communities and populations. This is, however, met with barriers in most parts of the world. New approaches that embrace greater collaboration with community stakeholders are needed, new ways of thinking and acting are required, new sources of funding are often needed, and new theories are needed to frame social problems in ways that inspire rather than constrain group action. OT practices should always rely on evidence to make informed decisions. With communities and populations, it can be seen as *colonial* to develop programs based on evidence without carefully getting the community to accept the evidence-based approaches which can be applied differently between contexts. Program developers must recognize that communities have values that differ significantly across the globe, so an approach that works for one community may not be effective in another part of the world. Although evidence is essential perhaps the best principle should be collaborative efforts between program developers and community partners that would directly be involved in the action, for interventions need to be created and implemented *by the community*, not *for the community*. Evidence can be used to educate communities about what has worked in other places so that the community can make informed decisions.

Acknowledgments

The author would like to acknowledge the following two contributors: Marjorie Scaffa authored part of this chapter, including Tables 22.1 to 22.3 and the Commentary on the Evidence, which was part of the 13th edition of Willard and Spackman's Occupational Therapy. OT Story 22.1 is based on a true story provided by a colleague, Jennifer Radziak, OTD, CHT.

Lippincott® Connect *For additional resources on the subjects discussed in this chapter, visit Lippincott Connect.*

REFERENCES

American Occupational Therapy Association. (2020). Occupational therapy practice framework: Domain and process (4th ed.). *American Journal of Occupational Therapy, 74*(Suppl. 2), 7412411010p1–7412411010p87. https://doi.org/10.5014/ajot.2020.74S2001

Bronfenbrenner, U. (1977). Toward an experimental ecology of human development. *American Psychologist, 32*(7), 513. https://doi.org/10.1037/0003-066X.32.7.513

Christiansen, C., & Baum, C. (1997). *Occupational therapy: Enabling function and wellbeing.* Slack.

Classen, S., Lopez, E., Winter, S., Awadzi, K. D., Ferree, N., & Garvan, C. W. (2007). Population-based health promotion perspective for older driver safety: Conceptual framework to intervention plan. *Clinical Interventions in Aging, 2,* 677–693. https://www.ncbi.nlm.nih.gov/pmc/articles/PMC2686324/

Coker-Bolt, P., Jansson, A., Bigg, S., Hammon, E., Hudson, H., Hunkler, S., Kitch J., Richardson, H., Tiedemann, E., O'Flynn, J., & Laurent, M. D. (2017). Menstrual education and personal hygiene supplies to empower young women in Haiti. *OTJR: Occupation, Participation, and Health, 37,* 210–217. https://doi.org/10.1177/1539449217719866

Doll, J. D., & Domina, A. (2020). Program design and implementation. In M. E. Scaffa & S. M. Reitz (Eds.), *Occupational therapy in community and population health practice* (pp. 94–111). F. A. Davis.

Dunn, W., Brown, C., & McGuigan, A. (1994). The ecology of human performance: A framework for considering the effect of context. *American Journal of Occupational Therapy, 48*(7), 595–607. https://doi.org/10.5014/ajot.48.7.595

Dunn, W., McClain, L. H., Brown, C., & Youngstrom, M. J. (1998). The ecology of human performance. In M. E. Neistadt & E. B. Crepeau (Eds.), *Willard and Spackman's occupational therapy* (9th ed., pp. 525–535). Lippincott Williams & Wilkins.

Durocher, E., Gibson, B. E., & Rappolt, S. (2014). Occupational justice: A conceptual review. *Journal of Occupational Science, 21*(4), 418–430. https://doi.org/10.1080/14427591.2013.775692

Ensminger, D., Scaffa, M. E., Doll, J. D., & Messer, M. (2020). Program evaluation. In M. E. Scaffa & S. M. Reitz (Eds.), *Occupational therapy in community and population health practice* (pp. 114–133). F. A. Davis.

Fazio, L. S. (2017). *Developing occupation-centered programs with the community.* Slack.

Flecky, K., Doll, J., & Scaffa, M. E. (2020). Community-based and population health program development. In M. E. Scaffa & S. M. Reitz (Eds.), *Occupational therapy in community and population health practice* (pp. 73–152). F. A. Davis.

Frank, G., & Muriithi, B. A. K. (2015). Theorising social transformation in occupational science: The American civil rights movement and South African struggle against apartheid as "occupational reconstructions." *South African Journal of Occupational Therapy, 45*(1), 11–19. http://www.scielo.org.za/scielo.php?script=sci_arttext&pid=S2310-38332015000100003

Hauer, K., Lamb, S. E., Jorstad, E. C., Todd, C., & Becker, C. (2006). Systematic review of definitions and methods of measuring falls in randomised controlled fall prevention trials. *Age and Ageing, 35*(1), 5–10. https://doi.org/10.1093/ageing/afi218

Hocking, C. (2017). Occupational justice as social justice: The moral claim for inclusion. *Journal of Occupational Science, 24*(1), 29–42. https://doi.org/10.1080/14427591.2017.1294016

Johansson, E., Jonsson, H., Dahlberg, R., & Patomella, A. (2018). The efficacy of a multifactorial falls-prevention program, implemented in primary health care. *British Journal of Occupational Therapy, 18*(8), 474–481. https://doi.org/10.1177/0308022618756303

Kielhofner, G., & Burke, J. P. (1980). A model of human occupation, part 1. Conceptual framework and content. *American Journal of Occupational Therapy, 34*(9), 572–581. https://doi.org/10.5014/ajot.34.9.572

Kronenberg, F., Algado, S. S., & Pollard, N. (2005). *Occupational therapy without borders: Learning from the spirit of survivors.* Elsevier/Churchill Livingstone.

Kronenberg, F., Pollard, N., & Sakellariou, D. (Eds.). (2011). *Occupational therapies without borders: Towards an ecology of occupation-based practices* (Vol. 2). Elsevier Health Sciences.

Lai, L. L., Player, H., Hite, S., Satyananda, V., Stacey, J., Sun, V., Jones, V., & Hayter, J. (2021). Feasibility of remote occupational therapy services via telemedicine in a breast cancer recovery program. *The American Journal of Occupational Therapy, 75*(2), 7502205030p1–7502205030p9. https://doi.org/10.5014/ajot.2021.042119

Lamontagne, A. D., Keegel, T., Louie, A. M., Ostry, A., & Landsbergis, P. A. (2007). A systematic review of the job-stress intervention evaluation literature, 1990–2005. *International Journal of Occupational and Environmental Health, 13,* 268–280. https://doi.org/10.1179/oeh.2007.13.3.268

Law, M., Cooper, B., Strong, S., Stewart, D., Rigby, P., & Letts, L. (1996). The person-environment-occupation model: A transactive approach to occupational performance. *Canadian Journal of Occupational Therapy, 63*(1), 9–23. https://doi.org/10.1177/000841749606300103

Maller, C., Townsend, M., Pryor, A., Brown, P., & St. Leger, L. (2006). Healthy nature healthy people: "Contact with nature" as an upstream health promotion intervention for populations. *Health Promotion International, 21(1)*, 45–54. https://doi.org/10.1093/heapro/dai032

McClure, R. J., Turner, C., Peel, N., Spinks, A., Eakin, E., & Hughes, K. (2005). Population-based interventions for the prevention of fall-related injuries in older people. *The Cochrane Database of Systematic Reviews, 25*(1), CD004441. https://doi.org/10.1002/14651858.CD004441.pub2

Pan, Z., Su, X., Fang, Q., Hou, L., Lee, Y., Chen, C. C., Lamberth, J., & Kim, M. L. (2018). The effects of Tai Chi intervention on healthy elderly by means of neuroimaging and EEG: A systematic review. *Frontiers in Aging Neuroscience, 10*, 110. https://doi.org/10.3389/fnagi.2018.00110

Peel, N. M. (2011). Epidemiology of falls in older age. *Canadian Journal on Aging, 30*(1), 7–19. https://doi.org/10.1017/S071498081000070X

Pickett, G., & Hanlon, J. J. (1990). *Public health: Administration and practice.* Times Mirror/Mosby.

Sakellariou, D., & Pollard, N. (2017). *Occupational therapies without borders: Integrating justice with practice* (2nd ed.). Elsevier.

Scaffa, M. E. (2019). Occupational therapy interventions for groups, communities, and populations. In B. A. B. Schell & G. Gillen (Eds.), *Willard and Spackman's occupational therapy* (13th ed., pp. 436–447). Wolters Kluwer.

Scaffa, M. E. (2020). Community and population health concepts. In M. E. Scaffa & S. M. Reitz (Eds.), *Occupational therapy in community and population health practice* (pp. 22–35). F. A. Davis.

Scaffa, M. E., & Reitz, S. M. (2020). Historical and philosophical perspectives of community and population health practice. In M. E. Scaffa & S. M. Reitz (Eds.), *Occupational therapy in community and population health practice* (3rd ed., pp. 1–19). F. A. Davis.

Schkade, J. K., & Schultz, S. (1992). Occupational adaptation: Toward a holistic approach for contemporary practice, part 1. *American Journal of Occupational Therapy, 46*(9), 829–837. https://doi.org/10.5014/ajot.46.9.829

Scofield, R. (2011). *The social entrepreneur's handbook: How to start, build, and run a business that improves the world.* McGraw-Hill.

Townsend, E., & Polatajko, H. J. (2013). *Enabling occupation II: Advancing an occupational therapy vision for health, well-being, & justice through occupation.* Canadian Association of Occupational Therapists.

Townsend, E., & Whiteford, G. (2005). A participatory occupational justice framework: Population-based processes of practice. In F. Kronenberg, S. S. Algado, & N. Pollard (Eds.), *Occupational therapists without borders* (pp. 110–126). Elsevier/Churchill Livingstone.

Townsend, E., & Wilcock, A. (2004). Occupational justice and client-centred practice: A dialogue in progress. *Canadian Journal of Occupational Therapy, 71*(2), 75–87. https://doi.org/10.1177/000841740407100203

Umeda, C. J., Fogelberg, D. J., Jirikowic, T., Pitonyak, J. S., Mroz, T. M., & Ideishi, R. I. (2017). Expanding the implementation of the Americans with Disabilities Act for populations with intellectual and developmental disabilities: The role of organization-level occupational therapy consultation. *American Journal of Occupational Therapy, 71(4)*, 7104090010p1–7104090010p6. https://doi.org/10.5014/ajot.2017.714001

Webb, T. L., Joseph, J., Yardley, L., & Michie, S. (2010). Using the internet to promote health behavior change: A systematic review and meta-analysis on the impact of theoretical basis, use of behavior change techniques, and mode of delivery on efficacy. *Journal of Medical Internet Research, 12(1)*, e4. https://doi.org/10.2196/jmir.1376

Wenborn, J., Hynes, S., Moniz-Cook, E., Mountain, G., Poland, F., King, M., Omar, R., Morris, S., Vernooij-Dassen, M., Challis, D., Michie, S., Russell, I., Sackely, C., Graff, M., O'Keeffe, A., Crellin, N., & Orrell, M. (2016). Community occupational therapy for people with dementia and family carers (COTiD-UK) versus treatment as usual (Valuing Active Life in Dementia [VALID] programme): Study protocol for a randomised controlled trial. *Trials, 17*, 65. https://doi.org/10.1186/s13063-015-1150-y

Whiteford, G. E., & Townsend, E. (2011). Participatory occupational justice framework (POJF 2010): Enabling occupational participation and inclusion. In F. Kronenberg, N. Pollard, & D. Sakellariou (Eds.), *Occupational therapies without borders: Towards an ecology of occupation-based practice* (Vol. 2, pp. 65–84). Elsevier/Churchill Livingstone.

Whiteford, G. E., Townsend, E., Branton, O., Wicks, A., & Pereira, R. (2017). The participatory occupational justice framework: Salience across contexts. In D. Sakellariou & N. Pollard (Eds.), *Occupational therapies without borders* (2nd ed., pp. 163–174). Elsevier.

World Federation of Occupational Therapists. (2019). *Occupational therapy and community-centred practice* [Position statement]. https://www.wfot.org/resources/occupational-therapy-and-community-centred-practice

World Federation of Occupational Therapists. (2021). *Occupational therapy and telehealth* [Position statement]. https://wfot.org/resources/occupational-therapy-and-telehealth

World Health Organization. (2004). *Towards age-friendly primary health care.* https://apps.who.int/iris/handle/10665/43030

World Health Organization. (2007). *WHO global report on falls prevention in older age.* https://www.who.int/ageing/publications/Falls_prevention7March.pdf

World Health Organization, Division of Health Promotion, Education, and Communication. (1998). *Health promotion glossary.* https://apps.who.int/iris/handle/10665/64546

World Health Organization & World Bank. (2011). *World report on disability.* https://www.who.int/teams/noncommunicable-diseases/sensory-functions-disability-and-rehabilitation/world-report-on-disability

CHAPTER 23

Best Practices for Health Education

Leanne Yinusa-Nyahkoon and Sue Berger

"You can't transform something you don't understand."

—ANNETTE FRANZ

LEARNING OBJECTIVES

After reading this chapter, you will be able to:

1. Understand and synthesize key factors that contribute to effective client education.
2. Analyze how personal and organizational health literacy influence client education.
3. Implement strategies to support comprehension and use of educational content for clients of varying abilities.
4. Choose and/or develop appropriate written, digital, or web-based client education materials based on client needs.

Introduction

Education and Training is one of the six core categories of occupational therapy (OT) interventions as stated in our Practice Framework (American Occupational Therapy Association [AOTA], 2020). Educating clients decreases anxiety, increases knowledge, improves satisfaction with services, and leads to better clinical outcomes (Agency for Healthcare Research and Quality [AHRQ], 2020; Berkman et al., 2011; Fredericks & Yau, 2017). Client education may shorten hospital stays and decrease costs of healthcare (Hosseini et al., 2019). Client education maximizes an individual's ability to participate in daily activities.

To be effective clinicians, we must know what specific strategies to teach our clients and we need to know *how* to teach our clients. For this to occur, OT practitioners need to communicate information clearly, and more importantly, they need to understand their client and ensure the client understands the material conveyed. This chapter begins by discussing health literacy and the role it plays for clients and practitioners in client education. We then continue by discussing the who, what, where, and when of client education. Finally, we focus on strategies to use when providing client education, including strategies for educating in person, in writing, and virtually (OT Story 23.1).

OT STORY 23.1 EDUCATING THE CHUNG FAMILY

The Chung family came to the United States from Hong Kong 1 year ago. Their primary language is Cantonese, and they live in a multigenerational household. Their son, Wei Xiang (威翔/Wēi Xiáng) Chung, is 4 years old and has been diagnosed with autism spectrum disorder (ASD). At his preschool, he is able to participate in most learning activities with teacher support, but he often plays alone and at times appears overstimulated. At home, Wei Xiang enjoys playing with his toy cars and running outside, but he cries for extended periods of time when these activities end. He is able to eat independently with a utensil, but only eats a few preferred foods. Wei Xiang primarily uses gestures to communicate with family members. The Chung family attend temple weekly and receive healthcare at their neighborhood community center where they also attend cultural and social events. Many healthcare professionals at the center speak Cantonese, including community connectors who refer families to specialty services and help families navigate unfamiliar systems including healthcare and public education.

Wei Xiang's pediatrician referred him to OT services. Mr. Chung has limited English proficiency but is able to communicate some ideas in English. Mr. Chung reports that he and his wife have limited information about ASD and would like to "meet with an expert" to learn more about the diagnosis and plan next steps for Wei Xiang who will soon be "old enough to attend his sister's elementary school."

The parents and grandparents' goals are for Wei Xiang to play with his 6-year-old sister as well as peers at preschool and the community center, eat more foods that the family prepares, and cry less when his preferred activities end. As you read the remaining sections of this chapter, think about the following questions.

Questions

1. What are the five most important guidelines to consider to ensure educational materials and recommended resources are accessible to the Chung family?
2. What are ways to facilitate effective communication while utilizing interpretation and translation services?
3. The Chung family has shared that they plan to use complementary and alternative medicine (CAM), specifically traditional Chinese medicine (TCM), alongside OT services. How might the Chung family's desire to use TCM influence your client education plan and strategies?

Health Literacy

Health literacy is essential to health and illness management, effective healthcare delivery, and improved health outcomes. Increasing healthy literacy of the US population is an objective for Healthy People 2030 (US Department of Health and Human Services [USDHHS], 2021b). Initial definitions were developed from a deficit model and approached health literacy as a clinical risk factor, implying that the inability to access health information was solely due to personal factors such as age, gender identity, race, ethnicity, native language, income, educational attainment, and employment status (Institute of Medicine, 2004; Rikard et al., 2016). Standardized health literacy assessments have been rarely validated with specific racial and linguistic groups, and consequently Black, Indigenous, and other people of color (BIPOC) as well as **multilingual learners (MLLs)** were often identified to have limited health literacy levels (Health Literacy Tool Shed, 2021; Nguyen et al., 2015; Rikard et al., 2016).

Health literacy is related to health equity and recent national initiatives remind the healthcare community to reflect on historical circumstances and life experiences as contributing factors to clients' capabilities and challenges (USDHHS, 2018b, 2021a). Emerging public health perspectives and health promotion initiatives have reframed health literacy from an individual asset and now recognize the social and environmental factors contributing to inequities in assets such as health literacy (Rikard et al., 2016; USDHHS, 2018b).

Therefore, current definitions of health literacy are separated into (i) personal and (ii) organizational health literacy. **Personal health literacy** is defined as "the degree to which individuals have the ability to find, understand, and use information and services to inform health-related decisions and actions for themselves and others" (Centers for Disease Control and Prevention [CDC], 2021a). **Organizational health literacy** is described as "the degree to which organizations equitably enable individuals to find, understand, and use information and services to inform health-related decisions and actions for themselves and others" (CDC, 2021a). Approaching health literacy from both a personal and organization lens has the potential to positively impact client outcomes and long-standing health disparities. It is the responsibility of health professionals to meet the needs of the clients they serve and provide equitable, accessible, and comprehensible health information (Santana et al., 2021; USDHHS, 2021a, 2021b).

Who Needs to Know the Information?

It is important to note who the client[1] is when providing education, as the values, priorities, preferences, and learning needs of one client may differ from another client or those of their caregiver. For example, when addressing meal preparation, embrace food options, cooking practices, and eating habits that are familiar to the client (e.g., culturally appropriate vegetables and fruits, specific sauces or spices, food storage containers, use of cooking and eating utensils, adaptive equipment, or hands). Anti-racism practices are integrated throughout the chapter as a reminder that anti-racism is an ongoing process and key to effective client education (Kendi, 2019).

What Information Needs to Be Conveyed?

One of the most challenging aspects of client education is determining what the client needs and wants to know (Marcus, 2014). Several studies have found large discrepancies between what clients want to know and what health professionals believe is most important. For example, Kang-Yi et al. (2018) found that clients within the Korean-American community have different beliefs about autism than some healthcare professionals, and recommend that initial discussions focus on general topics like developmental milestones rather than diagnosis and a plan of care. When clients don't receive the information from healthcare professionals that they want to know or are ready to receive, they seek out desired information on their own, often through the Internet. However, with so much material available of varying quality and accuracy, clients, especially those with limited literacy, struggle to know which information to trust (Diviani et al., 2015; Sbaffi & Rowley, 2017). Collaborative goal setting can support OT practitioners in understanding what information is important to the client.

---

[1]According to the American Occupational Therapy Association (AOTA, 2020, p. S75), the term *client* refers to *persons* (including those involved in care of a client), *groups* (a collection of individuals having shared characteristics or common or shared purpose, e.g, family members, workers, students, and those with similar interests or occupational challenges), and *populations* (aggregates of people with common attributes such as contexts, characteristics or concerns, including health risks). However, in countries other than the United States, the term *client* often refers to persons who are paying for their care directly. In most countries, *patient* is used to describe persons who are in hospital or rehabilitation. *Service user* and *person* are terms in general use that describe those in need of OT services. For this chapter, we are using *client* without implying the source of payment for services.

Where Is the Best Place to Communicate the Information?

Information should be shared in a safe and judgement-free environment (Osborne, 2018), with minimal distractions where the client feels free to ask questions, admit needing clarification, or ask for repetition. For example, before providing services ask for permission to turn off the television, turn down background music, or find a time when the client is not engaged in preferred activities. If communicating with the client virtually, let the client know you are in a private space and ask if they are alone or okay to speak with others present. If the client is reading educational material, be sure there is adequate lighting with little or no glare. A gooseneck task light is ideal to illuminate the material. Aiming the light on the paper and not toward the person, along with directing the individual to face away from a window, are key factors to reduce glare (Warren, 2013).

When Is the Best Time to Communicate the Information?

Internal distractions such as pain, anxiety, hunger, or need to use the restroom affect clients' ability to absorb and understand information. When possible, resolve these distractions prior to client education. Consider the timing of all client education. When working with clients and their caregivers, consider offering various time options and in-person and virtual options to provide caregiver education. Caregivers with limited weekday availability or who need to take time off from work to attend a meeting may participate while feeling frustrated or angry, and therefore are less able to receive and process new information. A rushed or time-pressured environment can increase anxiety for the client and the practitioner and limit client comprehension (Marcus, 2014). It is also important to consider timing of information over the course of care. For example, educational needs in the acute phase of healthcare differ from those during rehabilitation.

Communicating Health Information

Best practices for the delivery of health information align with many of the recommended approaches to client and person-centered care and ensure that communication methods are equitable across client communities and practice contexts (Adebayo et al., 2020; Constand et al., 2014). Initial considerations include using active listening and establishing rapport with the client and any caregivers so that information shared will be individually tailored and perceived as trusted and relevant. Next, eliciting the client's educational agenda and negotiating educational priorities that may differ between the client and the practitioner will help create an optimal environment for information to be exchanged. Lastly, creating a plan to disseminate health information either over time or all at once in small chunks maximizes client learning and informational uptake (Constand et al., 2014).

Communication is most efficient when consistent words and plain language are used. **Plain language** is described as terms an audience perceives as familiar, understands the first time, and feels comfortable with (CDC, 2021b). During a session on feeding skills, for example, the words *fork* and *spoon* represent plain language, whereas the terms such as *silverware* and *utensil* do not. The use of clear and consistent plain language with clients improves the clarity of communication, saves time and money by minimizing misunderstandings, improves a client's response to the healthcare professional's message, and connects the speaker with those they are communicating with (CDC, 2021b; National Institutes of Health [NIH], 2021b). The CDC offers plain-language alternatives and replaces healthcare jargon and technical terms with words public audiences and clients use most frequently (CDC, 2021c).

Unusual or challenging words used in conversation should be defined, and acronyms should be explained (CDC, 2021b). Most people understand the phrase *thinking skills* better than they do *cognition*. If it is important to use the term *cognition*, define it and use it consistently. Acronyms such as *ROM* and *ADL* should be used only after they have been fully explained; even then, be sure to verify comprehension. If you are unsure of word choice, ask the client what word they use to describe an item, and use that word consistently. For example, you might ask your client if they refer to rubber soled shoes with laces as *shoes, sneakers, tennis shoes, running shoes*, kicks, footwear, tenis, or some other term.

Organized and clear presentation of content helps clients understand and apply information, especially those who are in a new environment, are learning new information, are in pain, or are anxious. Therefore, plan the information to be conveyed before talking and remember to sequence the information logically (Centers for Medicare & Medicaid Services [CMS], 2020). For example, if you are working with a group of children to help them lighten their backpacks, begin by stating, "First, decide what needs to go inside the backpack; second, put heavy books at the back of the pack; and third, put lighter objects such as pencils in the front of the backpack." When using numbers to represent quality, the higher number should always convey better quality (Berkman et al., 2011). Information that is given as a concrete suggestion is recalled more often than a general suggestion (NIH, 2021a). For example, "Walk briskly for 30 minutes three times a week" would be recalled more often than "Exercise several times a week."

Using demonstrations, models, and pictures along with oral communication also helps people to understand information (Berkman et al., 2011; NIH, 2021a). When teaching clients about the importance of eliminating clutter for safety, show before and after pictures of a kitchen and point out safety hazards and ways they were resolved. When teaching use of adaptive equipment, explain and demonstrate. Use multiple teaching methods, especially when working with groups of individuals, because different people learn differently. Even when working with one client, multiple teaching methods help to emphasize key information and facilitate comprehension and memory.

Finally, it is important to verify understanding. The OT practitioner might believe that the information was clear, organized, and consistent, but if the client did not understand the message, the practitioner was not successful. The client who is passive or constantly nodding in agreement might not fully understand or adhere to the recommendations. Therefore, whenever possible, employ the **teach-back technique**, having clients return demonstration, repeat in their own words, or explain a concept using a different example (Caplin & Saunders, 2015; Osborne, 2018). This technique is effective in making sure that clients understand the information and, more importantly, in improving health outcomes. If appropriate, the practitioner can ask one client to demonstrate to or teach other clients. Clients are more likely to ask questions and admit lack of understanding with a peer than with a therapist.

In general, there are three ways to educate clients: in person, in writing, and virtually. We present information in these categories for clarity but acknowledge that there is overlap in strategies among each of the communication methods.

In-Person Education

Communicating with clients in person allows participants to use familiar conversational style, facilitates rapport building and trust between clients and healthcare professionals, and provides nonverbal cues that healthcare professionals can interpret when determining client comfort, confidence, and comprehension (van Servellen, 2020). Speaking with someone in person provides an opportunity for clients to demonstrate understanding through action and for the OT practitioner to observe task performance.

When communicating with clients who are hard of hearing, choose an environment that minimizes noise and distractions, get the client's attention before speaking, and position oneself directly in front of the client (Osborne, 2018). If the person wears hearing aids or uses other assistive hearing devices, make sure they are in place and working. If hearing is severely impaired, use other methods of communication along with, or instead of, speaking.

Knowing the individual characteristics of a client is critical to providing effective education (see Expanding Our Perspectives). It is important to include educational topics that are relevant to the intended audience, perceived as appropriate rather than invasive or overly sensitive, and use generally acceptable terminology recognizing that term preferences may differ among clients who identify similarly (Refugee Health Technical Assistance Center, 2011a). Communication should be in a person's primary language, and when the healthcare professional and client's primary language differ, a trained **healthcare interpreter** should support the communication exchange (Certification Commission for Healthcare Interpreters, 2021). Partnering with a trained healthcare interpreter and following interpreter guidelines can reduce medical liability, increase healthcare utilization, improve client satisfaction with service delivery, and increase follow-through with healthcare recommendations (Refugee Health Technical Assistance Center, 2011a). Use of plain language when speaking supports the ease and accuracy of interpretation (USDHHS, 2021a). Interpreting by family members or friends of a MLL in their native or heritage language should be avoided as it compromises client confidentiality and provides an opportunity for the interpreter's own perspectives and reactions to be conveyed in addition to or instead of the client's (Brega et al., 2015; USDHHS, 2021c).

Some individuals wear a face covering when communicating in person, which can make facial expressions hard to interpret (Isautier et al., 2020; Marler & Ditton, 2021). The American Speech-Language-Hearing Association (n.d.) recommends using a barrier with a clear panel or transparent shield, instead of a solid colored mask, if using the covering to prevent the spread of infectious respiratory droplets. When wearing a cloth covering as part of your daily routine or dress, consider accentuating key phrases, speaking clearly, adjusting voice volume as needed, and using emotion and intonation in your voice. Similarly, if appropriate and feasible, use gestures and body language and incorporate visuals (York, 2020).

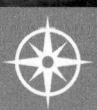

EXPANDING OUR PERSPECTIVES

Tips on Client Education

Donald Cunnigen, Ph.D.[1]

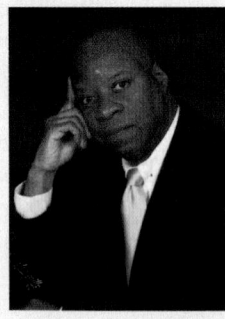

As a stroke survivor, I had to quickly learn to make the best out of any situation. Through necessity and misfortune, my new poststroke life has required me to become more flexible and adaptable. As a result, I politely accept any and all assistance proffered by student clinicians. Like all therapists, caregivers, and care partners, students must realize that progress is best made when working in tandem with the client. It is a reciprocal process that demands the characteristics of patience, respect, understanding, encouragement, and cheerful dispositions on everyone's part. The last characteristic is hardest to acquire and maintain. For the stroke survivor who faces the daily reality of a terribly altered life, it is very difficult to get and keep a cheerful and hopeful countenance. Student clinicians must realize that goals are best achieved with a happy client or at least a client who thinks you care. With those general comments in mind, here are some tips to facilitate happiness and demonstrate care.

Intake and Initial Engagement

My initial encounters with student clinicians featured "in-taking" information, or an opportunity for student clinicians to get to know me and vice versa. During initial intake interviews, they allowed me to speak freely. Given my vocal challenges with dysarthria, this was fantastic! It is very common among therapists and others to ignore stroke survivors while valuing their own points more and our perspectives less. Moreover, we are often made to feel "invisible" by being frequently interrupted or talked over. It is a horrible feeling but you learn to live with it, especially when you have made an enormous effort just to get a word out.

Codesigning the Intervention Agenda

I recommend that student clinicians design an intervention agenda in conjunction with the client. It makes the client feel more part of therapy activities. This was done by all of my student clinicians. For example, they selected the African Mancala game as a treatment activity as it deeply aligned with my personal and professional identity. Similarly, the student clinicians devoted intervention time to improving my computer proficiency so that I could use my laptop to write and publish my personal memoir about my stroke and subsequent therapy. I believe in the therapy world this is called client-centered care.

Implementing Client Education

You can only successfully teach what a client wants to or is able to learn, therefore it is best to engage in cooperative teaching activities with the client. Very often, student clinicians have a goal they want the client to achieve but their expectations are too high or too low. Set realistic expectations. Client education should teach clients how to accomplish their goals based on individual abilities and beliefs. For example, I hold on to a deep faith and believe that I can only go so far and then God does the rest. I "use what I got to get what I need" and understand that this may differ from what a student clinician wants me to accomplish.

[1]B.A., Tougaloo College; M.A., University of New Hampshire; A.M., Harvard University; Ph.D., Harvard University; Professor Emeritus of Sociology, University of Rhode Island.

Written Education

Most people forget much of what they are told during a patient–physician interaction, and what they believe they remember, they remember incorrectly (Sandberg et al., 2012). Written forms of communication reinforce, record, and remind participants of the information conveyed. Written material can be provided on paper or accessed virtually in many forms. For example, the AOTA develops fact sheets about specific conditions and related OT services. OT practitioners develop written home exercise programs or share images of suggested home modifications as reminders to clients of information shared.

Educational materials should be provided in the client's primary language, and trained **healthcare translators** can adapt health education materials (Refugee Health Technical Assistance Center, 2011b). Healthcare organizations are encouraged to post educational materials with visible signage translated into the languages commonly used by the clients they serve (Brega et al., 2015; USDHHS, 2021c). For example, a "Client information" or "Take one!" sign in English and translated into other primary languages used by clients should be posted above infographics and fact sheets displayed in waiting areas. When providing written material, note whether the client states something similar to "I'll read this later" or if they appear to read the material but are unable to follow the instructions. These behaviors might indicate challenges with reading or understanding written material and therefore, using other modes of communication might be best.

Although some rules apply to all written material (i.e., paper and web-based), there are important distinctions to consider. Therefore, after summarizing the readability of general written material, we highlight best practices for communicating in writing for web-based and other digital formats.

Readability of Written Material

Presentation of educational material includes the reading level of the content, type and color of paper, font type, size, and style, organization, and visuals. All of these factors affect clients' ability and motivation to see, read, and understand the material.

Word Choice, Style, and Reading Level. Individuals often refer to reading level when they consider readability of material, but engagement with content, word choice, and style of writing also influence readability. Consider using an engaging opening statement, conversational writing style, relatable stories, positive messaging, and active voice to capture the client's attention and encourage continued reading (USDHHS, 2018a). See Table 23.1 for examples of word choice and style.

The Simplified Measure of Gobbledygook (SMOG) formula (McLaughlin, 1969) and online programs are used to assess the reading level of some health materials (Microsoft Support, 2021; Wang et al., 2013). Readability formulas, however, do not predict comprehension or consider reading fluency (AHRQ, 2015). For example, most readability formulas would score, "I wave my hand" and "I waive my rights" similarly, whereas more individuals would understand the first phrase than the second phrase. Generally, use short and medium length sentences, one- or two-syllable words, and plain language, and trial the material with the intended audience, whenever possible (Parnell, 2015).

Font, Paper, and Color. To ensure that most people can see the written material, the font should be at least 12 points and easy-to-read (NIH, 2021a). Serif font (font with small lines at the end of characters, such as the text you are reading now) is recommended for information in the body of a text. Sans serif is suggested for headings (such as the headings used in this book) as it contrasts the font in the

TABLE 23.1	Strategies and Examples of Best Practices for Written Material		
Strategy	**Correct Example**	**Incorrect Example**
Use active wording.	When providing instructions, state, *Put your right arm in first when getting dressed.*	Avoid passive voice such as, *Your right arm should be put in first when getting dressed.*
Use positive terminology.	When providing instructions, state, *Raise your arm slowly.*	Avoid phrasing things negatively such as, *Don't raise your arm quickly.*
Use common words, when possible.	Use words like *doctor and blood pressure.*	Avoid words like *physician and hypertension,* but if needed, define these words.
Use language that is simple to visualize.	*No bigger than a shoe box*	*No bigger than 2 ft × 1 ft × 1 ft*
Use large font size.	Font size should be at least 12 points; 14 points or larger for people with low vision.	Small font, such as a 9 point, makes items difficult to read.
Use simple fonts and a combination of serif and san serif.	San serif fonts are suggested for headings. Use serif fonts for the body of the text.	*Fancy fonts like this make reading more challenging.*
Use a combination of uppercase and lowercase letters.	It is easier to read a combination of uppercase and lowercase letters.	IT IS HARDER TO READ MATERIAL IN ALL CAPITALS.

primary text and enables readers to skim material by reading headings easily (USDHHS, 2018a).

ALL CAPITAL LETTERS are more challenging to read than a combination of uppercase and lowercase letters as readers use the shapes of words to help read. When typed in all capitals, AND looks like a rectangle and is visually similar to other three-letter words such as FOR and THE (CMS, 2020; Osborne, 2018). If typed with lowercase letters, *and*, *for*, and *the*, all have different shapes, making it easier to quickly determine each word. Table 23.1 provides examples of easy and difficult to use layouts and fonts.

Matte paper is recommended because glossy paper can cause glare, making reading difficult. Black print on white paper is most effective for contrast (CMS, 2020; Osborne, 2018). Multiple colors can be distracting and make material hard to read. However, if using color, do so in a way that supports comprehension (e.g., green for positive actions and red for negative actions).

Organization. Highlighting, bolding, underlining, and listing key information captures clients' attention and helps them remember the information (USDHHS, 2018a). Headings help group information and including white space supports the reader's willingness to read the text (NIH, 2021a; Parnell, 2015). Looking at a brochure that is crammed with information can be discouraging for clients, regardless of the content.

Visual cues such as more spacing above headings and subheadings than below ties information together at a quick visual glance (NIH, 2021a; USDHHs, 2018a). Chunking information into five or fewer categories and using simple questions as headers, such as "What is energy conservation?" and "What are the key principles of energy conservation?" facilitates recall. When possible, personalize educational material by writing the client's name at the top or by leaving space for adding individualized suggestions (AHRQ, 2020).

Visuals. The old saying "A picture is worth a thousand words" is true only if the picture is clear and relevant. Health literacy literature emphasizes the importance of visuals that are familiar and identifiable to the client, easy to understand, positive, and includes simple captions (NIH, 2021a; Parnell, 2015). For example, when teaching bed mobility, be sure to use photos and images relevant to the client's sleeping environment (e.g., hammock, couch, floor, bed, crib, and car). In educational materials about mealtime routines, include pictures of familiar healthy foods rather than sugary snacks with a line through them. The purpose of using visuals is to facilitate comprehension and enhance the message in the text (Parnell, 2015).

Web-Based Material

Web-based written material may include a webpage, fact sheet, infographic, or an e-book. Fact sheets provide brief, easy-to-read information about a specific topic and include action steps. Infographics provide visual representations of data to make statistics and complex information easy to understand (USDHHS, 2018a). E-books are digital full-length books or long-form text documents that can be accessed via e-book readers and apps, cell phones, and desktop devices (USDHHS, 2018a). For example, a social story to support a child managing medical treatments or a flipbook that offers adaptive clothing ideas for wheelchair users might be presented as an e-book (see Figure 23.1).

Using web-based materials requires both reading and computer literacy. If using computer technology for client education, be sure to consider the client's information technology knowledge, the client's motivation and interest, the usability and functionality of the application, the costs of implementation and use, and the infrastructure and support. Health Literacy Online (Office of Disease Prevention and Health Promotion [ODPHP], 2016) and the Health Communication Playbook (USDHHS, 2018a) provide helpful guides to support the development of accessible websites.

Printed material and material on the web may be similar in content but differ in presentation. For example, printed material is static, whereas material on the web may include video, audio, and interactive activities along with written words (CMS, 2020). Access to the web varies and may include scrolling, clicking, or downloading and may be displayed differently across devices. Users with limited income, less education, and younger adults tend to rely on smartphones for online access more than others (Pew Research Center, 2021). Social media and mHealth technology has successfully engaged BIPOC individuals, underserved communities, and young adult populations in health education and health behavior change (Alvidrez et al., 2019; Anderson-Lewis et al., 2018). Providing resources regarding health, appointments, or "homework" reminders through a mobile device is an important mechanism to use to reach clients who may experience difficulty accessing and interpreting other types of health information. Below are some key strategies to consider when writing for the web to make it accessible.

- ● *Write actionable content:* Users of the web are usually looking for specific information on the center of the screen and rarely stay on a page for more than 15 seconds (Haile, 2014). Therefore, the most important information should appear first, and content should include an action step.
- ● *Display content clearly on the page:* Although most of the guidelines are similar to general written text regarding headings, font, and white space, there are a few specific strategies for web-based content.
  - ■ The term "above the fold" means you can see information without scrolling. Above the fold content is different depending on the device. Review content on multiple devices and if content continues "below the fold," the best way to cue someone to continue reading is to have the paragraph continue below the fold (ODPHP, 2016).
  - ■ Users may become distracted by links and icons, choose the first clickable option, and struggle to navigate some material (ODPHP, 2016). Therefore, limit the number of links and ensure they are clickable

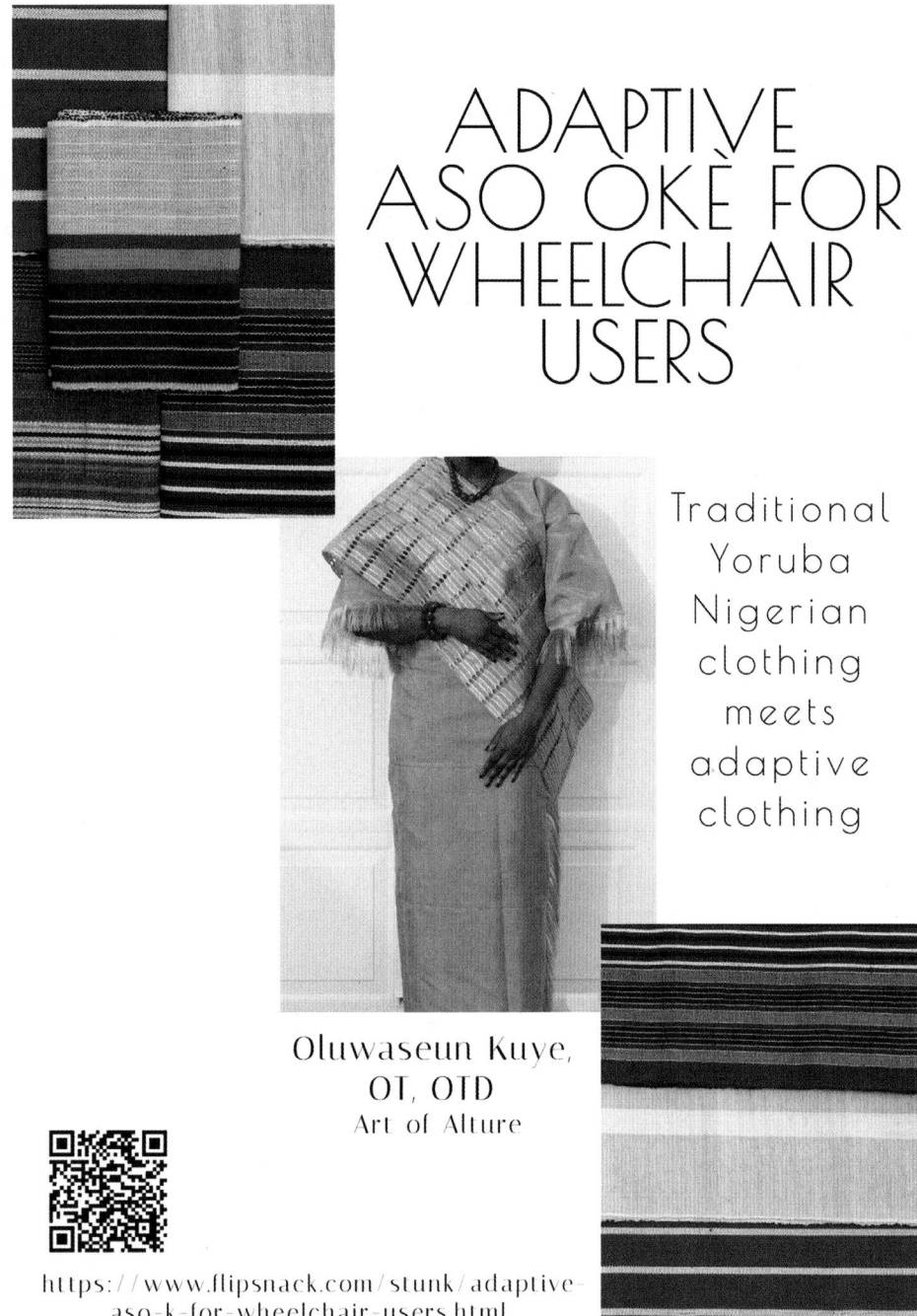

FIGURE 23.1 E-book featuring adaptive clothing strategies for Aso Òkè.

(ODPHP, 2016). Use descriptive links so the user knows what they are linking to and ideally, begin the link with an action word such as, "Read about…"

■ Assure that recommended web pages are accessible to clients using assistive technology (e.g., screen reader).

● *Simplify navigation:* It is usually easier for people to scroll versus click on links, but ideally, provide multiple ways to browse information. For example, you could have a page that someone could scroll along with direct links to the section of interest. Including a search button along with an "A-Z" search provides options for those who might struggle spelling a search term (ODPHP, 2016).

● *Engage users:* One of the benefits of electronic information is that it can easily be presented in multiple formats, including written, video, and audio. Video testimonials and interactive activities can make written material engaging (CMMS, 2023; Osborne, 2018).

There is evidence regarding the effectiveness of asynchronous, web-based professional development on clinical practice, yet few studies provide objective data regarding patient outcomes (Sinclair et al., 2016). Clearly, there is still much information we do not know regarding the benefits and challenges of electronic forms of education.

Assessing Written Material

The best way to develop effective written material is to engage members of the intended audience in the development of the material, ask potential users for feedback on a draft, and revise accordingly (NIH, 2021a). The Suitability Assessment of Materials (SAM) (Doak et al., 1996) and the Patient Education Materials Assessment Tool (PEMAT) (AHRQ, 2013) are two of several published assessments that can be used to ensure that written materials are developed well. In addition, A Plain Language Checklist for Reviewing Your Document (see Figure 23.2) provides guidelines

---

A Plain-Language Checklist for Reviewing Your Document

Do I know my audience?

☐ **Consider your potential readers.**
Who is your audience, exactly? Are there multiple audiences? Remember, there is no "general public."

☐ **Evaluate the needs of your readers.**
What do they want to know? How much detail do they need? What is the right tone for this audience? What action do you want readers to take?

☐ **Engage your audience.**
Use style, word choice, voice, organization, and visuals to draw your readers into your message.

Did I organize my document or product for my reader?

☐ **Provide a clear take-away message.**
Your document should convey a clear, specific message, such as *Consider participating in a clinical trial at NIH.*

☐ **Put your main message first.**
In most cases, readers appreciate documents that begin with the main point.

☐ **Answer their questions.**
Before writing your document, write down the questions your readers have about your topic. Make sure each section or paragraph of your document answers a reader's question.

Have I used an easy-to-read style?

☐ **Use first-person and second-person pronouns when appropriate.**
Using the pronouns *I, you,* and *we* make your document more converstational and help your reader focus on your message.

☐ **Use familiar, concrete, non-technical words.**
Unless you are writing for a group of experts such as *bombesin peptide receptor* scientists, limit the use of jargon and technical terms.

☐ **Consider whether each adjective and adverb adds meaning.**
Avoid padding your writing with words like *very, really, actually,* or *carefully.*

Have I written this as concisely as possible and kept the message?

☐ **Keep sentences and paragraphs short.**
Try to write paragraphs of no more than 5 to 7 sentences and sentences of 10 to 20 words.

☐ **Write sentences focused on one idea.**
Write paragraphs that have a single theme. Sentences and paragraphs that focus on developing an idea are easier for readers.

Have I used the right visuals?

☐ **Use illustrations or visuals.**
Visuals, such as lists, tables, and infographics, can help the reader understand your message.

☐ **Use typography and white space appropriately.**
Fonts and other typographical elements should make your document more readable, not fancier. Having enough blank space in the margins and between sections also increases readability.

Have I written in the active voice?

☐ **Use the active voice whenever possible.**
The active voice makes it clear who or what (the subject) is doing the action (the verb). Passive sentences often do not clearly identify who is performing the action.

Did I make my document "skimmable"?

☐ **Use headings.**
Headings enable your reader to skim your document. Write headings in the form of questions, sentences, or phrases.

☐ **Use vertical lists (numbers or bullets).**
Lists, which group similar items, are easy for readers to skim. Choose numbers when presenting a list with items in a specific sequence or rank order. Use bullets when the items listed are equivalent in importance.

For more information, visit Plain Language: Getting Started or Brushing Up at www.nih.gov/plainlanguage/gettingstarted

A PLAIN-LANGUAGE CHECKLIST FOR REVIEWING YOUR DOCUMENT | 2013 ■

FIGURE 23.2 A plain-language checklist for reviewing your document (with permission): Complete checklist accessed at https://www.nih.gov/sites/default/files/institutes/plain-language/nih-plain-language-checklist.pdf.

to use during document development (CDC, 2013). The Plain Language Checklist adheres to fact sheet guidelines, chunking information into bold headings with indented subheadings. Language throughout is simple, positive, active, and succinct and examples are included. The document includes white space and is personalized with boxes to check off as needed.

Virtual Education

The explosion of technology has expanded the ways we educate individual clients and inform large audiences. Previously, print material, television, and radio were the primary multimedia approaches to reinforce important knowledge and skills. Currently, many US adults use computers, tablets, and smartphones to access, share, and consume health-related videos, podcasts, images, posts, blogs, embodied conversational agents, and other innovative tools (Brega et al., 2015; Jack et al, 2020; Neiger et al., 2012).

Social Media

Social media has become a common and effective approach to disseminating health information. Social media is defined as "the use of online and electronic tools to create, share, and exchange content and ideas in communities and networks" (USDHHS, 2018a). Social media allows for the timely dissemination of evidence-based messaging, can be intentionally repeated, is accessible from various geographic locations at any time, can be tailored to diverse audiences, and benefits clients across literacy levels. Social media uses a multisensory approach to engage individuals with different learning preferences, and allows clients to consume health information in a method they individually trust and find credible (CDC, 2011).

Social media has multiple formats or tools that are interactive and facilitate active participation and conversations about health. Increasingly, clients with chronic health conditions use social media networking platforms to learn from and with one another. Healthcare professionals' use of social media tools to educate clients and engage virtual communities is emerging, and is used to introduce client education, review and reinforce learned skills, and support generalizability of therapeutic recommendations into the client's natural contexts.

Social media tools including image sharing, video sharing, and social networking have the potential to positively influence clients' health decisions, approach to health management, and health behavior change (CDC, 2011; USDHHS, 2018a). A clear plan, or social media strategy, will help sustain social media use within the identified timeline and ensure that key messages are relevant, accessible, coordinated, and engaging for clients, caregivers, and other consumers of health information. The social media strategy should also identify key performance indicators and other metrics (e.g., number of followers, likes, retweeted posts,

and comments) that are monitored and periodically evaluated to determine whether the social media strategy meets communication expectations and goals (CDC, 2011; Neiger et al., 2012; Yinusa-Nyahkoon et al., 2020).

In choosing or developing social media materials, similar considerations should be used as for written materials, keeping accessibility principles in mind. For example, use plain language and present key information first. Use voice tones and vocabulary familiar to the intended audience, and for video, ensure that viewers can identify with the images featured.

Telehealth

Telehealth is defined as the "application of evaluative, consultative, preventive, and therapeutic services delivered through information and communication technology" (AOTA, 2018). Similar terms used include tele-OT, telerehabilitation, teletherapy, telecare, telemedicine, and telepractice (World Federation of Occupational Therapists [WFOT], 2014).

It is expected that telehealth services meet the same standards of care as in-person service delivery (WFOT, 2014). For example, interpreter services are recommended for telehealth sessions where the client and the OT practitioner do not have the same language proficiency (see Figure 23.3) (Refugee Health Technical Assistance Center, 2011a). Using plain language, active voice, and accommodating clients' preferred meeting times are examples of best practices for client education via telehealth. The benefits of telehealth include increased ability to assess and understand occupational performance within the client's home environment and natural contexts, decreased travel time, easier involvement of caregivers and family members, and increased client access to therapy sessions and specialty services, especially for clients in rural areas, using public transit, or with competing time demands (AOTA, 2018; Serwe et al., 2017). There are challenges to telehealth, as well,

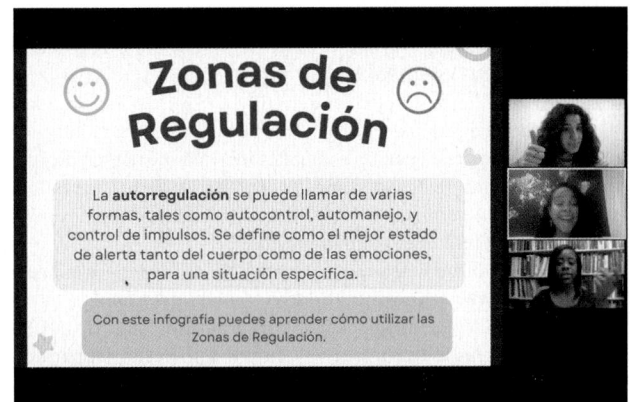

FIGURE 23.3 **Caregiver, OT practitioner, and healthcare interpreter reviewing a translated, plain language fact sheet during a telehealth session.**

including reimbursement in some states, limited technology and broadband infrastructure in under-resourced communities, privacy concerns during synchronous sessions, and licensure regulations, especially when practicing remotely across state lines (AOTA, 2018; Doerr, 2021; WFOT, 2014).

Conclusion

No single approach to client education is effective for all individuals (van Servellen, 2020). Some material is best suited for certain methods of teaching, and some individuals learn best via particular teaching strategies. It is our responsibility, as OT practitioners, to use best practices to assure that our clients understand the information they need to know. Although more research is needed to determine the best ways to provide client education, specifically when using virtual platforms, considering multiple modes of communication and the specific needs of the client will help convey valuable information.

> Without clear communication, we cannot expect people to adopt the healthy behaviors and recommendations that we champion. (USDHHS, 2010)

Lippincott® Connect *For additional resources on the subjects discussed in this chapter, visit Lippincott Connect.*

Acknowledgments

The authors would like to thank Lilian Wang, OT/s for the insight, research evidence, and cultural humility she contributed to the OT story and the spirit of belongingness woven throughout the chapter.

REFERENCES

Adebayo, C. T., Walker, K., Hawkins, M., Olukotun, O., Shaw, L., Sahlstein Parcell, E., Dressel, A., Luft, H., & Mkandawire-Valhmu, L. (2020). Race and blackness: A thematic review of communication challenges confronting the Black community within the US healthcare system. *Journal of Transcultural Nursing: Journal of the Transcultural Nursing Society, 31*(4), 397–405. https://doi.org/10.1177/1043659619889111

Agency for Healthcare Research and Quality. (2013). *The Patient Education Materials Assessment Tool (PEMAT) and user's guide.* https://www.ahrq.gov/sites/default/files/publications/files/pemat_guide.pdf

Agency for Healthcare Research and Quality. (2015). *Tip 6. Use caution with readability formulas for quality reports.* https://www.ahrq.gov/talkingquality/resources/writing/tip6.html

Agency for Healthcare Research and Quality. (2020). *About health literacy.* https://www.ahrq.gov/health-literacy/about/index.html

Alvidrez, J., Castille, D., Laude-Sharp, M., Rosario, A., & Tabor, D. (2019). The National Institute on Minority Health and Health Disparities research framework. *American Journal of Public Health, 109*(S1), S16–S20. https://doi.org/10.2105/ajph.2018.304883

American Occupational Therapy Association. (2018). Telehealth in occupational therapy. *American Journal of Occupational Therapy,* *72*(Suppl. 2), 7212410059p1–7212410059p18. https://doi.org/10.5014/ajot.2018.72S219

American Occupational Therapy Association. (2020). Occupational therapy practice framework: Domain and process (4th ed.). *American Journal of Occupational Therapy, 74*(Suppl. 2), 7412410010p1–7412410010p87. https://doi. org/10.5014/ajot.2020.74S2001

American Speech-Language-Hearing Association. (n.d.). *Communicating effectively while wearing masks and physical distancing.* https://www.asha.org/public/communicating-effectively-while-wearing-masks-and-physical-distancing/

Anderson-Lewis, C., Darville, G., Mercado, R. E., Howell, S., & Di Maggio, S. (2018). mHealth technology use and implications in historically underserved and minority populations in the United States: Systematic literature review. *JMIR mHealth and uHealth, 6*(6), e128. https://doi.org/10.2196/mhealth.8383

Berkman, N. D., Sheridan, S. L., Donahue, K. E., Halpern, D. J., Viera, A., Crotty, K., Holland, A., Brasure, M., Lohr, K. N., Harden, E., Tant, E., Wallace, I., & Viswanathan, M. (2011). *Health literacy interventions and outcomes: An updated systematic review (Evidence Report/Technology Assessment, 199. AHRQ Pub. No. 11-E006).* Agency for Healthcare Research and Quality.

Brega, A. G., Barnard, J., Mabachi, N. M., Weiss, B. D., DeWalt, D. A., Brach, C., Cifuentes, M., Albright, K., & West, D. R. (2015). *AHRQ health literacy universal precautions toolkit* (2nd ed.). Agency for Healthcare Research and Quality.

Caplin, M., & Saunders, T. (2015). Utilizing teach-back to reinforce patient education: A step-by-step approach. *Orthopedic Nursing, 34,* 365–368. https://doi.org/10.1097/NOR.0000000000000197

Centers for Disease Control and Prevention. (2011). *The health communicator's social media toolkit.* Author. https://www.cdc.gov/healthcommunication/toolstemplates/socialmediatoolkit_bm.pdf

Centers for Disease Control and Prevention. (2013). *A plan language checklist for reviewing your document.* https://www.nih.gov/sites/default/files/institutes/plain-language/nih-plain-language-checklist.pdf

Centers for Disease Control and Prevention. (2021a, August 1). *What is health literacy?* https://www.cdc.gov/healthliteracy/learn/index.html

Centers for Disease Control and Prevention. (2021b, August 1). *Health literacy: Plain language materials and resources.* https://www.cdc.gov/healthliteracy/developmaterials/plainlanguage.html

Centers for Disease Control and Prevention. (2021c, August 1). *Everyday words for public health communication.* https://www.cdc.gov/healthcommunication/everydaywords/

Centers for Medicare & Medicaid Services. (2023). Writing for the web: Tips to help you improve online communications. https://www.cms.gov/files/document/writing-web.pdf

Certification Commission for Healthcare Interpreters. (2021). *Certification Commission for Healthcare Interpreters: National, accredited, inclusive.* https://cchicertification.org/

Constand, M. K., MacDermid, J. C., Dal Bello-Haas, V., & Law, M. (2014). Scoping review of patient centered-care approaches in healthcare. *BMC Health Services Research, 14,* 271. https://doi.org/10.1186/1472-6963-14-271

Diviani, N., van den Putte, B., Giani, S., & van Weert, J. C. M. (2015). Low health literacy and evaluation of online health information: A systematic review of the literature. *Journal of Medical Internet Research, 17*(5), e112. https://doi.org/10.2196/jmir.4018

Doak, C. C., Doak, L. G., & Root, J. H. (1996). *Teaching patients with low literacy skills* (2nd ed.). J. B. Lippincott.

Doerr, B. (2021). *Board support crucial to telehealth success.* https://trustees.aha.org/advancing-rural-telehealth-and-addressing-its-challenges

Fredericks, S., & Yau, T. (2017). Clinical effectiveness of individual patient education in heart surgery patients: A systematic review and meta-analysis. *International Journal of Nursing Studies, 65,* 44–53. https://doi.org/10.1016/j.ijnurstu.2016.11.001

Haile, T. (2014, March 9). What you think you know about the web is wrong. *Time.* http://time.com/12933/what-you-think-you-know-about-the-web-is-wrong/

Health Literacy Tool Shed. (2021). *Health literacy tool shed: A database of health literacy measures.* http://healthliteracy.bu.edu/

Hosseini, H. M., Pai, D. R., & Ofak, D. R. (2019). COPD: Does inpatient education impact hospital costs and length of stay? *Hospital Topics, 97*(4), 165–175. https://doi.org/10.1080/00185868.2019.1677540

Institute of Medicine, Committee on Health Literacy, Nielsen-Bohlman, L., Panzer, A. M., & Kindig, D. A. (Eds.). (2004). Health literacy: A prescription to end confusion. National Academies Press. https://www.ncbi.nlm.nih.gov/books/NBK216032/pdf/Bookshelf_NBK216032.pdf

Isautier, J. M., Copp, T., Ayre, J., Cvejic, E., Meyerowitz-Katz, G., Batcup, C., Bonner, C., Dodd, R., Nickel, B., Pickles, K., Cornell, S., Dakin, T., & McCaffery, K. J. (2020). People's experiences and satisfaction with telehealth during the COVID-19 pandemic in Australia: Cross-sectional survey study. *Journal of Medical Internet Research, 22*(12), e24531. https://doi.org/10.2196/24531

Jack, B. W., Bickmore, T., Yinusa-Nyahkoon, L. S., Reichert, M., Julce, C., Sidduri, N., Martin-Howard, J., Zhang, Z., Woodhams, E., Fernandez, J., Loafman, M., & Cabral, H. J. (2020). Improving the health of young African American women in the preconception period using health information technology: A randomized controlled trial. *Lancet Digital Health, 2,* e475–e485. https://doi.org/10.1016/S2589-7500(20)30189-8

Kang-Yi, C. D., Grinker, R. R., Beidas, R., Agha, A., Russell, R., Shah, S. B., Shea, K., & Mandell, D. S. (2018). Influence of community-level cultural beliefs about autism on families' and professionals' care for children. *Transcultural Psychiatry, 55*(5), 623–647. https://doi.org/10.1177/1363461518779831

Kendi, I. X. (2019). *How to be an antiracist.* Bodley Head.

Marcus, C. (2014). Strategies for improving the quality of verbal patient and family education: A review of the literature and creation of the EDUCATE model. *Health Psychology and Behavioral Medicine, 2*(1), 482–495. https://doi.org/10.1080/21642850.2014.900450

Marler, H., & Ditton, A. (2021). "I'm smiling back at you": Exploring the impact of mask wearing on communication in healthcare. *International Journal of Language & Communication Disorders, 56*(1), 205–214. https://doi.org/10.1111/1460-6984.12578

McLaughlin, G. H. (1969). SMOG grading—A new readability formula. *Journal of Reading, 12,* 639–646. http://www.jstor.org/stable/40011226

Microsoft Support. (2021). *Get your document's readability and level statistics.* Get your document's readability and level statistics (microsoft.com)

National Institutes of Health. (2021a). *Clear and simple.* https://www.nih.gov/institutes-nih/nih-office-director/office-communications-public-liaison/clear-communication/clear-simple

National Institutes of Health. (2021b). *Plain language at NIH.* https://www.nih.gov/institutes-nih/nih-office-director/office-communications-public-liaison/clear-communication/plain-language/

Neiger, B., Thackeray, R., Van Wagenen, S., Hanson, C., West, J., Barnes, M., & Fagen, M. (2012). Use of social media in health promotion: Purposes, key performance indicators, and evaluation metrics. *Health Promotion Practice, 13,* 159–164. https://doi.org/10.1177/1524839911433467

Nguyen, T. H., Park, H., Han, H. R., Chan, K. S., Paasche-Orlow, M. K., Haun, J., & Kim, M. T. (2015). State of the science of health literacy measures: Validity implications for minority populations. *Patient Education and Counseling, 98*(12), 1492–1512. https://doi.org/10.1016/j.pec.2015.07.013

Office of Disease Prevention and Health Promotion. (2016). *Health literacy online: A guide for simplifying the user experience.* https://health.gov/healthliteracyonline/

Osborne, H. (2018). *Health literacy from A to Z: Practical ways to communicate your health message* (2nd ed.). Aviva Publishing.

Parnell, T. A. (2015). *Health literacy in nursing: Providing person-centered care.* Springer Publishing Company.

Pew Research Center. (2021). *Mobile fact sheet.* https://www.pewresearch.org/internet/fact-sheet/mobile/

Refugee Health Technical Assistance Center. (2011a). *Best practices for communicating through an interpreter.* https://refugeehealthta.org/access-to-care/language-access/best-practices-communicating-through-an-interpreter/

Refugee Health Technical Assistance Center. (2011b). *Translated health education materials.* https://refugeehealthta.org/access-to-care/language-access/translated-health-education-materials/

Rikard, R. V., Thompson, M. S., McKinney, J., & Beauchamp, A. (2016). Examining health literacy disparities in the United States: A third look at the National Assessment of Adult Literacy (NAAL). *BMC Public Health, 16,* 975. https://doi.org/10.1186/s12889-016-3621-9

Sandberg, E. H., Sharma, R., & Sandberg, W. S. (2012). Deficits in retention for verbally presented medical information. *Anesthesiology, 117,* 772–779. https://doi.org/10.1097/ALN.0b013e31826a4b02

Santana, S., Brach, C., Harris, L., Ochiai, E., Blakey, C., Bevington, F., Kleinman, D., & Pronk, N. (2021). Updating health literacy for Healthy People 2030: Defining its importance for a new decade in public health. *Journal of Public Health Management and Practice, 27,* S258–S264. https://doi.org/10.1097/PHH.0000000000001324

Sbaffi, L., & Rowley, J. (2017). Trust and credibility in web-based health information: A review and agenda for future research. *Journal of Medical Internet Research, 19*(6), e218. https://doi.org/10.2196/jmir.7579

Serwe, K. M., Hersch, G. I., Pickens, N. D., & Pancheri, K. (2017). Caregiver perceptions of a telehealth wellness program. *American Journal of Occupational Therapy, 71,* 7104350010p1–7104350010p5. https://doi.org/10.5014/ajot.2017.025619

Sinclair, P. M., Kable, A., Levett-Jones, T., & Booth, D. (2016). The effectiveness of internet-based e-learning on clinician behavior and patient outcomes: A systematic review. *International Journal of Nursing Studies, 57,* 70–81. https://doi.org/10.1016/j.ijnurstu.2016.01.011

US Department of Health and Human Services. (2018a). *Health communication playbook: Resources to help you create effective materials.* https://www.cdc.gov/nceh/clearwriting/docs/health-comm-playbook-508.pdf

US Department of Health and Human Services, Office of Disease Prevention and Health Promotion. (2010). *National action plan to improve health literacy.* Author.

US Department of Health and Human Services, Office of Disease Prevention and Health Promotion. (2021a, October 26). *Health literacy and health equity: Connecting the dots.* https://health.gov/news/202110/health-literacy-and-health-e

US Department of Health and Human Services, Office of Disease Prevention and Health Promotion. (2021b, August 1). *Healthy People 2030: Health communication.* https://health.gov/healthypeople/objectives-and-data/browse-objectives/heal

US Department of Health and Human Services, Office of Minority Health. (2021c, August 1). *National culturally and linguistically appropriate services standards.* https://thinkculturalhealth.hhs.gov/clas/standards

US Department of Health and Human Services, Secretary's Advisory Committee for Healthy People 2030. (2018b). *Issue briefs to inform development and implementation of Healthy People 2030.* https://www.healthypeople.gov/sites/default/files/HP2030_Committee-Combined-Issue%20Briefs_2019-508c.pdf

van Servellen, G. (2020). *Communication skills for the health care professional: Context, concepts, practice, and evidence* (3rd ed.). Jones & Bartlett Learning.

Wang, L. W., Miller, M. J., Schmitt, M. R., & Wen, F. K. (2013). Assessing readability formula differences with written health information materials: Application, results, and recommendations. *Research in Social and Administrative Pharmacy, 9*(5), 503–516. https://doi.org/10.1016/j.sapharm.2012.05.009

Warren, M. (2013). Promoting health literacy in older adults with low vision. *Topics in Geriatric Rehabilitation, 29*(2), 107–115. https://doi.org/10.1097/TGR.0b013e31827e4840

World Federation of Occupational Therapists. (2014). *Position statement: Telehealth*. Author.

Yinusa-Nyahkoon, L., Woodall, K., Pluviose-Philip, J., Williams, A., Sidduri, N., Julce, C., Wangari Walter, A., & Jack, B. W. (2020). A little bird tweeted me: Using social media to provide equitable access to evidence-based health initiatives. *Occupational Therapy Practice Magazine, 25*(12), 21–23. https://www.aota.org/publications/ot-practice/ot-practice-issues/2020/social-media-equitable-access

York, D. (2020). How to build rapport while wearing a mask. *Harvard Business Review*. https://hbr.org/2020/09/how-to-build-rapport-while-wearing-a-mask

Modifying Performance Contexts

Leanne Leclair and Jacquie Ripat

LEARNING OBJECTIVES

After reading this chapter, you will be able to:

1. Define context and explore its importance to occupational participation.
2. Examine context at the micro, meso, and macro levels.
3. Analyze the interrelationship between positionality, intersectionality, and context.
4. Examine approaches and interventions used to modify and adapt contexts across the life course and settings.
5. Critically reflect on how context influences your practice as an occupational therapist.

Introduction: Context in Occupational Therapy Practice

The focus of this chapter is on modifying performance contexts. To enable occupational participation, occupational therapists need to understand the importance of context. Throughout this chapter, the term *client* may refer to individuals, families, groups, organizations, or communities who experience barriers to occupational participation. We recognize there is tension in using the term client as it can imply an imbalanced power relationship between the person and the occupational therapist. We suggest throughout this chapter that occupational therapists need to be critically reflexive about this power dynamic and use a collaborative relationship focused approach. Occupations occur within a context that is unique to a client's circumstances (Dunn et al., 1994). Consequently, the context will influence a client's engagement in occupation, and this may vary across time.

Although there is no single definition of context, Dunn et al. (1994) in their depiction of the Ecology of Human Performance Model described context as the physical, social, cultural, and temporal factors external to the person that together influence occupational performance. Shogren and colleagues (2014) examined "context as a concept that integrates the totality of circumstances that comprise the milieu of human life and human functioning" (p. 100). They highlighted that context includes the interaction between personal characteristics and the environmental factors that hinder or enhance functioning. Similar to the definition proposed by Shogren et al. (2014), the International Classification of Functioning, Disability and Health (ICF) (World Health Organization [WHO], 2001) defines context as the interconnection of personal factors such as gender, race, age, lifestyle, social background, education, occupation, and psychological characteristics with environmental factors (WHO, 2001). Environmental factors, as described in the ICF, can include physical elements (products and technology and natural environment and human-made changes to the environment); social elements (social support and relationships); attitudes (arising from customs, practices, ideologies, values, norms, and beliefs); and services, systems, and policies (Schneidert et al., 2003).

Occupational therapists recognize that personal and environmental factors have an important influence on a clients' engagement in and performance of occupations (American Occupational Therapy Association [AOTA], 2014; Townsend & Polatajko, 2013). The person and environment feature prominently in numerous models of occupational behavior, performance, and engagement (e.g., Dunn et al., 1994; Kielhofner, 2008; Law et al., 1996; Townsend & Polatajko, 2013). Occupational therapy (OT) models emphasize the transactional person-environment-occupation (PEO) relationship. Conceptually, the outcome of a congruent PEO relationship or good PEO fit is optimal occupational performance (Law et al., 1996). When there is less congruence or a poor PEO fit, modifying the environment becomes an important strategy to improve fit and occupational performance. Environmental modifications result in modifications to the context, as they change the totality of the circumstances surrounding the client.

Occupational therapists understand that clients' occupational experiences cannot be separated from contextual influences (AOTA, 2014). The context plays an important role in shaping human experience and behavior over time. At the same time, people actively shape and influence the contexts in which they live, work, and play. Contexts can afford people with or impede possibilities for actions, which, depending on an individual's previous and current experiences, can be viewed as opportunities and resources or demands and barriers. In Chapter 17, the meaning of place and space was explored and explained. Those concepts and recommendations for OT practice are critically important when considering interventions to modify the performance context.

Understanding Context at the Micro, Meso, and Macro Levels

Context is multidimensional with mediating factors at the micro, meso, and macro levels that continuously interact to influence performance outcomes (Shogren et al., 2021). When considering modifying performance contexts, occupational therapists first need to understand the concepts

and relevance of the micro, meso, and macro levels that hinder or support occupational participation. For this chapter, we define each level as follows (Egan & Restall, 2022; Shogren et al., 2021):

- **Micro:** The micro level includes the immediate social settings such as physical spaces, technology, and social supports including family, friends, teachers, caregivers, and others.
- **Meso:** The meso level includes the structures, services, policies and processes embedded in the health, employment, education, justice, and social systems.
- **Macro:** The macro level is made up of the larger socioeconomic, historical, cultural and political systems and structures—including societal values and beliefs, laws, and public policies.

This understanding of micro, meso, and macro levels stems from earlier work by Bronfenbrenner (1979) which has long influenced thinking in OT (Dunn et al., 1994; Law, 1991). In Bronfenbrenner's model, people are believed to engage within contexts in different ways throughout their lives. Although Bronfenbrenner's model is primarily concerned with human development over time, the dynamic interplay of the various levels is particularly relevant for OT's focus on occupational participation.

Furthermore, occupational therapists agree that modifying performance contexts can be easier to achieve and have more immediate enabling effects than using interventions that try to change the person (Anaby et al., 2014; Law et al., 2010). Framing success or failure in occupational participation as an individual choice, attribute, or effort is problematic and flawed (Galvaan, 2012, 2021; Hammell, 2020; Rudman, 2021). Hammell (2020) contends that not all people have the same occupational choices because of varying contexts. Systemically excluded groups experience greater inequality because of contexts that favor privileged groups (Gerlach et al., 2018; Hammell, 2020). Chapters 14 and 15 address social, economic, political, and cultural contexts that influence occupational performance. Occupational therapists must also move beyond the micro level and address contextual factors at the meso and macro levels that limit occupational opportunities and participation. To effect change at these levels requires a critically reflexive stance.

The Interconnectedness of Positionality, Intersectionality, and Context

Being critically reflexive about positionality relates to modifying performance contexts. Positionality has long been discussed as part of reflexivity in qualitative research (Jacobson & Mustafa, 2019) but is also relevant for practice.

Positionality suggests that our perspectives are based on our position in society and relates to the many factors that comprise our social identities: class, citizenship, ability, age, race, sexual orientation, cis/trans status, and gender, to name a few (Collins, 2015; Dhamoon & Hankivsky, 2011). Critical reflexivity draws attention to taken-for-granted assumptions and the broader social structures that shape one's knowledge and positionality within issues of power and privilege (Farias & Rudman, 2019; Galvaan, 2021; Kinsella & Whiteford, 2009). Clarifying our social positions and how they influence our beliefs, values, and taken-for-granted assumptions is an essential part of our practice as it impacts one's approaches, interactions, and interpretations (Jacobson & Mustafa, 2019). Intersectionality focuses on the intersection of multiple social identities (e.g., race, gender, and ability) and how together they shape structural, political, and representational aspects of an individual's context (Crenshaw, 1991).

Understanding one's social positions, particularly how they relate to a client's social positions, helps to understand the power relations that exist in practice. Ongoing critical reflexivity related to one's positionality and intersectionality is imperative as they shape how one views and addresses all aspects of our practice and life (Rudman, 2021). They are inherently part of who we are and how we view the world.

Being critically reflexive includes acknowledging implicit bias and problematizing the context within which occupational therapists practice and clients engage in occupation. Occupational therapists must recognize the dominance of white Western Eurocentric worldviews that shape OT and oppress and disadvantage diverse worldviews. They must seek to dismantle the colonial structures that perpetuate health inequities (Emery-Whittington & Maro, 2018; Gibson, 2020; Hammell, 2021). Critical reflexivity that questions what is taken for granted can lead to generative disruption and "naming and enacting possibilities for promoting social change and social inclusion" (Galvaan, 2021, p. 8). Although reflexivity is an important aspect of praxis, putting theory into practice, it is also susceptible to solipsism or becoming self-absorbed and thus fraught with challenges for dismantling structural privilege and oppression (D'Arcangelis, 2018). Critical self-reflexivity alone will not eradicate oppressive systems and structures. For that, other skills and practices are also needed (D'Arcangelis, 2018).

The Pursuit of Systems and Social Transformation

Pursuing systems and social transformation should be at the forefront of modifying performance contexts. Systems change has long been identified as key to lasting social change (Kania et al., 2018). Noticing what is invisible and taken for granted are at the core of systems change. The *Water of Systems Change* (Kania et al., 2018) highlights the six conditions that hold a problem in place, and the need to shift these six conditions to effect systems change. The six interconnected conditions are at three different levels of change shaped in an inverted pyramid with explicit conditions at the top, semi-explicit conditions in the middle, and implicit conditions at the bottom (Figure 24.1). The three explicit conditions at the top focus on structural change: (i) policies, (ii) practices, and (iii) resource flows. The two semi-explicit conditions in the middle center on relational

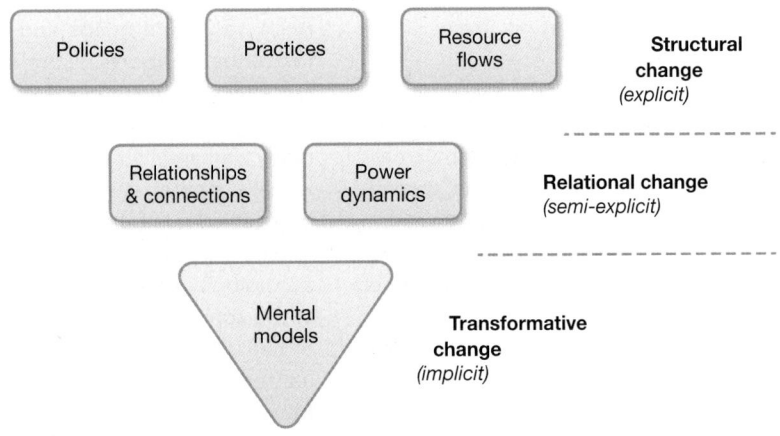

FIGURE 24.1 **The six conditions of systems change.** (Reprinted from Kania, J., Kramer, M., & Senge, P. [2018]. *The waters of systems change.* https://www.fsg.org/publications/water_of_systems_change)

change: (iv) relationships and connections, and (v) power dynamics. One implicit condition at the bottom emphasizes transformative change: (vi) mental models. Mental models are deeply held beliefs and assumptions that influence ways of thinking and acting. Kania et al. (2018) further defined each of these six conditions. Each level of change poses its own challenges, but all must be addressed for sustainable systems change. The six conditions for systems change can inform work at the macro, meso, and micro levels.

Nixon (2019) introduced the Coin Model as a framework for transformative change (Figure 24.2). The Coin

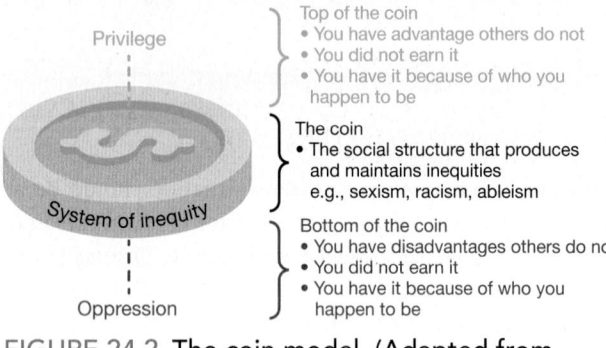

FIGURE 24.2 **The coin model. (Adapted from Nixon, S. A. [2019]. The coin model of privilege and critical allyship: Implications for health.** *BMC Public Health, 19,* 1637. https://doi.org/10.1186/s12889-019-7884-9)

Model uses an intersectional approach to highlight how social structures produce both unearned advantage and disadvantage. It illustrates how social identities produced by systems of inequality interact with one another to create power, privilege, and oppression. Nixon frames health inequities around the social structures that create oppression and unearned disadvantage for some, and unearned privilege and advantage for others. Occupational therapists need to reflect on how systems of inequality are played out in existing policies and practices that influence their client's context. Like the Coin Model, the capabilities approach (Sen, 2003) highlights advantages and disadvantages afforded to people. The capabilities approach asserts that not all individuals or collectives have the same advantages and opportunities (capabilities) to access and convert available resources into the things that they value doing (functionings). For example, social norms and cultural expectations that are unjust and inequitable disadvantage and constrain people and result in socioeconomic disadvantage that limits people's opportunities to make choices (Hammell, 2022). Nixon (2019) identifies that all healthcare providers need to recognize their positions of unearned privilege and advantage and use this understanding to reorient their approach with a focus on redressing systems and structures of inequality rather than on saving "unfortunate people." Practicing critical allyship can support systems change and address health inequities. As an example, see OT Story 24.1.

OT STORY 24.1 INTRODUCING JAMAL

Jamal is a 10-year-old boy born with spastic quadriplegia cerebral palsy. Jamal experiences sensory processing differences and speech delays. He recently received a power wheelchair from a local non-profit agency to mobilize as he has limited movement and control of his upper limbs, lower limbs, and trunk.

Jamal lives with his Mom and Dad and 13-year-old sister Aya. The family recently immigrated from Afghanistan and have no extended family in Canada. Although Jamal's mom was trained as an engineer and dad as an accountant in Afghanistan, their credentials are not recognized in Canada. Consequently, mom is employed as a housekeeper and dad as a bookkeeper for a small business. Jamal's older sister Aya was diagnosed with attention-deficit/hyperactivity disorder (ADHD) with significant hyperactivity. She is very active, loud, and talkative. Her hyperactivity often causes Jamal to become dysregulated.

Currently, Jamal and his family live in a subsidized housing complex for refugees. This housing is temporary; it is intended to support the family as they adjust to living in Canada and the family will have to find other housing in 1 year. Their two-bedroom suite is wheelchair accessible using a manual wheelchair; Jamal transfers from his manual wheelchair to his power wheelchair whenever leaving the suite. Jamal currently has no formal supports such as home care or respite. Mom is providing support for Jamal's basic care needs and does not know how to apply for formal supports. Mom is exhausted, has injured herself multiple times while caring for Jamal, and struggles to fulfill her work duties and provide care for Jamal. The many demands limit the family's community participation. Jamal's mother is extremely grateful for the support the other residents of the housing complex have offered their family, but she often states that "they have no life." Many accessibility barriers limit the family's ability to participate in the community.

Jamal is currently in fifth grade. He receives individualized support from an educational assistant, including full support with activities of daily living (ADLs) during the school day. Jamal recently received a tablet to support communication. The occupational therapist completed several lengthy funding applications and advocacy letters seeking support for equipment and technology. The school playground has limited accessibility, which prevents Jamal from engaging with other classmates during recess. Despite the school's efforts in encouraging Jamal's participation in gym (e.g., as goalie during soccer or hockey), Jamal has expressed he would prefer to participate in other forms of play and physical activity in gym class. He has limited adapted equipment for sport. Jamal loves watching soccer with his dad and streaming videogames. He enjoys going for walks with his family in the community. Jamal wishes there was an accessible playground nearby that would allow him to play with other kids in the neighborhood. He spends a lot of time with his sister who sometimes takes care of him after school when his parents are still at work.

Questions

1. Consider your social identities (e.g., race, gender, class, sex, education, religion, citizenship, and ability). How might your positionality influence your work with Jamal and his family?
2. What are the macro, meso, and micro level contextual factors impacting Jamal's occupational participation at home, school, and in the community?
3. How can you influence systems change for Jamal and his family?
4. How can you practice critical allyship with Jamal and his family to support systems change that addresses health and occupational inequities?

When working with Jamal, the occupational therapist must first examine their positionality and intersectionality. Critical reflexivity on issues of power, privilege, and advantage should be part of the therapist's ongoing process for social and systems transformation. Identifying the impact of policies and practices on the occupational participation of Jamal and his family should foreground the occupational therapist's work with Jamal. However, reflexivity alone will not result in social and systems transformation. Praxis, or the act of moving theory to action, to address inequities and promote justice are paramount at the meso and macro levels. The next section of this chapter describes approaches to modifying and adapting performance contexts.

Approaches for Modifying and Adapting Performance Contexts

Contextual factors at the micro, meso, and macro levels support or hinder occupational participation. Although all levels should be considered when modifying or adapting performance contexts, occupational therapists need to understand and develop strategies that will extend beyond the micro level to effect change at the broader meso and macro levels. OT publications have pressed occupational therapists to support changes at the macro level to promote equity and justice for all clients (Gibson, 2020; Hammell, 2022; Rudman, 2021). As outlined earlier, the macro level is made up of the larger socioeconomic and political environments around the client—societal values and beliefs, laws, and public policies. There is a small but growing body of OT literature to guide work at the macro level (Fleming-Castaldy, 2015). This section will explore some of these approaches and how occupational therapists can apply them to their practice.

Taking an Occupational Justice and Rights-Based Approach

When modifying performance contexts, justice and equity should be a primary concern for occupational therapists. Bailliard et al. (2020) demonstrated how occupational justice is part of all OT practice and how it is enacted at the micro, meso, and macro levels. In growing discourse, OT writers have highlighted the need for practitioners to become aware of the impacts of occupational injustice (Galvaan, 2021; Leclair et al., 2016; Stadnyk et al., 2010; Townsend & Polatajko, 2013). Chapter 10 is devoted to exploring occupational justice. Wolf et al. (2010) applied the occupational justice framework to reframe dilemmas in everyday practice as occupational injustices related to environmental and systems barriers. This approach provides a thinking frame to assist occupational therapists to consider occupational justice issues at the micro, meso, and macro levels. Bailliard and colleagues (2020) contended that when promoting occupational justice the capabilities approach that "melds human rights and people's opportunities to do" (Sen, 2003, p. 48) should also be considered. The World Federation of Occupational Therapist's (WFOT, 2019) and Hammell (2017, 2022) highlighted the importance of the capabilities approach to achieve occupational rights for all people. However, Hammell (2017) and others (Durocher et al., 2014) have been critical of the lack of conceptual clarity related to occupational justice. Emery-Whittington (2021) critiques the lack of examination of colonialism in occupational justice approaches and promotion. Ongoing work to clarify this concept and its application to practice continues.

The WFOT (2019) position statement on Occupational Therapy and Human Rights outlines occupational therapists' obligations to promote occupational rights in the realization of human rights. To promote and support a rights-based approach, occupational therapists must be aware of and understand the Universal Declaration of Human Rights (United Nations, 1948) that outlines the rights and freedoms to which all humans are entitled regardless of their status, including race, color, sex, social origins, or other status. In addition, the United Nations Convention on the Rights of Persons with Disabilities (UNCRPD; United Nations, 2016) adopted in 2006 is a binding international treaty reaffirming that all persons with disabilities must enjoy all human rights and fundamental freedoms. Other important declarations and conventions from the United Nations relating to human rights that occupational therapists should be familiar with include, but are not limited to, the Declaration on the Rights of Indigenous Peoples (United Nations, 2007), the Convention on the Rights of the Child (United Nations, 1990), the Convention on the Elimination of Forms of Racial Discrimination (United Nations, 1969), and the Convention on the Elimination of all Forms of Discrimination Against Women (United Nations, 1979).

From these declarations and treaties, legislation has been developed across the world, bridging the gap from international treaties to state-level, municipal, or organizational policies. They all shape how social groups or individuals are included or not in the public domain and are important in guiding occupational therapists' thinking and advocacy efforts when working with clients. For example, Gibson and colleagues (2015) highlighted the importance of partnering with Indigenous peoples in the development and delivery of OT programs and services to facilitate human rights-based practice that recognizes self-determination of Indigenous peoples. Although legislation may exist, implementation and enforcement vary across contexts. Therefore, occupational therapists need to be aware of the various legislations that impact on client's occupational participation to support its implementation.

Antidiscrimination laws have been developed in many jurisdictions to ensure inclusion of historically and currently excluded groups, including peoples of minority ethnic, religious, or sexual identities. Many of these policies were hard-won achievements and, like the American Civil Rights Act of 1964, came at the expense of tremendous effort and even the lives of people dedicated to making the world a more socially inclusive place for all people. Efforts that continue today. At an organizational level, companies and public institutions have developed employment equity policies that ideally prevent discrimination. These laws and policies seek to ensure that all people have access to housing, work, education, and other publicly and privately funded opportunities. In essence, they enable or disable occupational engagement. Though oppressive systems and structures continue to perpetuate health and social inequities.

The rights of people with disabilities are also typically protected in many countries through human or civil rights laws. For example, the Americans with Disabilities Act (ADA, 1990) was designed to create equal opportunity and equal access to public environments, services, employment, accommodations, telecommunications, and transportation across the United States. The ADA Amendments Act of 2008 (ADA, 2016) provides a revised definition of "disability" to more broadly encompass impairments that substantially limit a major life activity, such as going to work. The ADA Standards for Accessible Design outline how both public and private sector services, programs, and facilities must comply with and implement accessibility requirements (U.S. Department of Justice, 2010). The focus of the ADA, and of similar legislation in many countries, is to enable people with disabilities to achieve social inclusion and participation. Chapter 16 provides additional insight about these issues. Occupational therapists should become familiar with the policies and laws that influence historically and currently excluded populations, including persons with disabilities, as this knowledge will affect their practice.

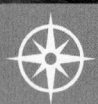

EXPANDING OUR PERSPECTIVES

Collective Access

Pamela Block

Collective Access is one of the 10 Principles of Disability Justice outlined by Sins Invalid: "As brown, black and queer-bodied disabled people we bring flexibility and creative nuance that go beyond able-bodied/minded normativity, to be in community with each other" (Sins Invalid, n.d., https://www.sinsinvalid.org/blog/10-principles-of-disability-justice). The concept of collective access is further outlined by Aimi Hamraie in their book Building Access: Universal Design and the Politics of Disability (2017) and in Berne et al. (2018). Rather than a static set of regulations or guidelines, collective access is an improvisational process where people work together to create the most accessible setting possible for the largest number of people. Successful articulation of collective access can lead to what Mia Mingus calls access intimacy (Mingus, 2011). Access intimacy happens in spaces and relationships where people feel safe in the knowledge that their access needs are important, and that people are working together to ensure they are being met.

Collective access is a process not a product. It is something that people dynamically strive to produce together knowing that it is impossible to fully achieve because of access conflicts and the reality that access needs change over time. An access conflict is when something that improves access for one person creates an access barrier to another. For example, someone needs a service animal, causes harmful allergies for another person, or someone needs bright florescent lighting, which gives someone else a headache. Unfortunately, the reality for many disabled people is closer to the experience of what Annika Konrad (2021) refers to as access fatigue. Access fatigue takes place when the role of ensuring access is left as the sole responsibility of the disabled person. The labor of constantly fighting for access creates access fatigue where people might give up even trying to ensure access for themselves (Konrad, 2021). Occupational therapists can play a crucial role in striving for collective access for disabled people across many social contexts. However, it is important to always ensure that efforts are led by disabled people themselves, and that their own perceptions of their needs (vs. what other people think they might need) are prioritized.

References

Berne, P., Morales, A. L., Langstaff, D., & Invalid, S. (2018). Ten principles of disability justice. *WSQ: Women's Studies Quarterly, 46*(1&2), 227–230. https://doi.org/10.1353/wsq.2018.0003

Hamraie, A. (2017). *Building access: Universal design and the politics of disability*. University of Minnesota Press.

Konrad, A. (2021). Access fatigue: The rhetorical work of disability in everyday life. *Urbana, 83*(3), 179–199.

Mingus, M. (2011). *Access intimacy: The missing link.* https://leavingevidence.wordpress.com/2011/05/05/access-intimacy-the-missing-link/

Sins Invalid. (n.d.). *10 Principles of disability justice.* https://www.sinsinvalid.org/blog/10-principles-of-disability-justice

Engaging in Social and Political Advocacy

Policy shapes society and guides actions to influence every aspect of life (Torjman, 2005). Policies are socially constructed and are a reflection of the values held by a society, institution, and/or organization. Policy links individuals with their community (Urbanowski et al., 2013). Understanding how policies impact client's occupational participation is critical for modifying performance contexts. Ultimately, policy affects occupational therapists, but occupational therapists can also affect policy. Occupational therapists practice in political systems and structures and can be seen as political actors (Aldrich & Rudman, 2020; Pollard & Sakellariou, 2014). Kronenberg and Pollard (2006) stressed that occupational therapists need to develop a political consciousness and capacity to fulfill their roles.

Regardless of the practice setting, occupational therapists can be seen as "street-level bureaucrats [who] respond to inter-related policies and systems in ways that can perpetuate, resist, or transform opportunities for doing and being" (Aldrich & Rudman, 2020, p. 137). Occupational therapists can exercise discretion when implementing policies in everyday practice to privilege client's needs. With Jamal (from OT Story 24.1) this may mean the occupational therapist provides support to the family in accessing health and social services they are currently not receiving through assisting with navigating complex bureaucracies. Their role may shift from consultative to more direct care providing intervention because of gaps and limitations in support services until the other services are in place. Whenever there is discretion in implementing policies, occupational therapists should consider how they can use this opportunity to support client needs.

Advocacy is an important strategy for policy and structural change (National Collaborating Centre for Determinants of Health, 2015). Occupational therapists predominantly focus on addressing health equity for individuals and groups, but advocacy is most effective when it combines bottom-up and top-down approaches along the upstream-downstream continuum (Carlisle, 2000). Moving further upstream toward policy and structural change will have the most significant impact on health equity (National Collaborating Centre for Determinants of Health, 2014). Political advocacy requires public engagement. Advocating with clients for systems change requires a particular set of knowledge, skills, and attitudes. Lewis (2020) outlined seven competencies health professionals need for political advocacy. They include collaboration, communication, critical thinking, research and analysis, relationship building, resource management, and understanding the policy process. Occupational therapists need to develop competencies to be effective advocates for systems change. Picotin et al. (2021) examined factors that influence occupational therapists' actions as social agents of change. They identified nine personal factors (adaptability/flexibility, confidence in their expertise, effective communication, directed collaboration, discovery, observation/analysis, planning, positivism, and reactivity) and 11 environmental factors organized under six themes that included development of the profession, micro, meso, and macrosystems, organizational culture, and resources. By recognizing the influence of personal and environmental factors on their ability as social agents of change, occupational therapists could adapt their actions to support equity and justice while working in collaboration with clients.

The 4 P's model (Power, Perception, Potency, and Proximity) outlines the factors that can influence public policy agenda setting (Zahariadis, 2016).

- **Power** is the most important of the four factors. The power to persuade others to focus on or to dismiss certain issues is crucial. Occupational therapists must develop political literacy or the "capacity to understand power relations and one's position within power relations—that may currently constrain occupational therapists' abilities to leverage their positioning and actions relative to broader policies and systems" (Aldrich & Rudman, 2020, p. 140). Occupational therapists need to be critically reflexive about how their practices can maintain or alter power relations (Gerlach et al., 2018). Occupational therapists as political actors can gain strength by strategically allying with organizations that have a wide audience and a network of support within society and supporting clients in doing the same. By joining coalitions or committees, participating in mobilization campaigns, taking part in actions that are intended to disrupt, and engaging in power dynamics (National Collaborating Centre for Healthy Public Policy, 2020), occupational therapists in collaboration with clients can exercise influence on public policy.

- **Perception** of the public about the issue also matters. Issues that can evoke public empathy or an emotional response while also humanizing those most affected will provoke decision makers to act. Persuasion and storytelling are essential elements of this strategy rather than just simply providing evidence. When it comes to policymaking, evidence alone is not sufficient (Cairney & Oliver, 2017). Telling compelling stories that require evidence can influence agendas (Cairney & Kwiatkowski, 2017). Led by the client's knowledge and understanding of their context and constraining or inequitable policies

and systems, occupational therapists are well-positioned to work with clients and coalitions to support efforts and influence public perception.

- **Potency** is about the severity of the consequences if an issue is not addressed. The greater the severity, the greater the attention from decision makers to act. Conveying the severity of inaction can provoke reaction.

- **Proximity** to the issue geographically and temporally incites greater response from decision makers. An issue that presents an imminent threat to the public will get a much greater response from government. The global response to COVID-19 highlights how the 4 P's can influence policy agendas. Occupational therapists cannot sit on the sidelines of political processes if they genuinely want to modify performance contexts to support occupational participation.

In the OT Story, the occupational therapist working with Jamal and his family takes steps to influence context at the macro and meso levels by following the 4 P's. An inaccessible playground limited Jamal's occupational participation and social engagement. This barrier existed because of macro level issues related to gaps between policy and implementation. Therefore, the occupational therapist not only made recommendations to Jamal's school to make adaptations, but also made efforts to address the larger macro level barriers by supporting the community of parents of children with disabilities to bring concerns to the school division. The occupational therapist and parents strategically allied with other school division representatives to bring the issue to government levels. They shared stories about the importance of accessibility and inclusion for all children and the number of children impacted in their community. They highlighted changes in policy to ensure all playgrounds were accessible for children and caregivers with different abilities. For another example of advocacy, see Expanding Our Perspectives.

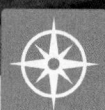

EXPANDING **OUR** PERSPECTIVES

Wrong Answers

Dot Nary

My husband and I attended the wedding of a colleague, north of Sacramento. After growing up on the ocean, it always feels like coming home when I can view the expanse of a bay from the air.

After landing in San Francisco, renting a car, driving north, and arriving at the motel where we'd reserved a room, we entered it only to discover that I could get inside the door but no further. We'd requested and reserved a wheelchair accessible room but this one was so small and the furniture so big that I could not get around the bed to reach the bathroom. The paths within the room were

much less than the 36 inches wide required by the Americans with Disabilities Act.

I called to speak to the manager.

"Well, an ADA room means that you can get into it but nothing else," he replied when I explained that we must have been given the room in error.

Wrong answer.

I called another nearby hotel and reserved an accessible room. We checked out of the Day's Inn, got a refund on our credit card, and relocated to a comfortable room where I could use the toilet and take a shower.

The wedding was simple and lovely. At the ceremony, I remembered the bride's brother playing Bachianas Brasileiras No. 5 beautifully on the guitar, accompanied by

EXPANDING OUR PERSPECTIVES (*continued*)

a soprano. The reception was held at a recreation center in Folsom, in a room charmingly decorated with flowers where a delicious buffet was served—I remember the grilled vegetables. The bride was gorgeous in her full-skirted gown, the couple joyous, and it was an honor to celebrate with them.

Before driving south to San Francisco for some site seeing, I called to reserve tickets for half-day bus trip to Muir Woods to see the redwoods. I'd checked the bus company website for options.

"Hello, I'd like to reserve two tickets for the Muir Woods trip on Tuesday afternoon."

"Okay, that will be $62.00 dollars plus tax. What card will you be using?"

"I want to let you know that I use a wheelchair. Your website notes that you will provide an accessible bus if given 48 hours' notice."

"Oh, I am sorry that we cannot accommodate you on Tuesday."

"OK, how about Wednesday?"

"I'm sorry we cannot accommodate you that day,"

"Well, what day can you accommodate us?"

"I'm sorry, we cannot accommodate you this week."

Wrong answer.

"Well, what you're telling me is a clear violation of a federal law, the Americans with Disabilities Act, so I am going to give you the opportunity to check with your supervisor and come back and give me a different answer."

Within 5 minutes, I had purchased two tickets for the Tuesday trip and gained assurance that we would be picked up at our hotel by a wheelchair accessible bus.

We stopped in Sacramento to check out the state capitol building, reached San Francisco, dropped another wedding guest off at the airport, and then pulled up to the hotel. I had driven that leg of the trip, so my husband went in to register and get the key to the room. He gave our names and the reservation confirmation number that we had obtained several weeks earlier.

"I'm sorry, that room is not available and there are no other accessible rooms available."

"What do you mean, we made a reservation weeks ago?"

"I'm sorry, we have no accessible rooms available."

Wrong answer.

"We need an accessible room, we reserved an accessible room, and now you just need to give us the key to an accessible room." My husband, who is short-statured and has a very deep voice, assured me that he spoke loud enough for everyone in the crowded lobby to hear him.

Within 10 minutes, after many whispered conversations among the staff, he emerged with the key to a room. It was a large room that smelled of chlorine from the pool and lacked a deadbolt. As our stay progressed, we learned that the hotel employed many young people from Ireland. We guessed that the room, with multiple beds and a fold-out sofa, was typically used by staff. But it was comfortable, had an accessible bathroom, and was conveniently close to Union Square.

For several days, we were immersed in the wonders of San Francisco. Muir Woods was breathtaking. Wandering among those huge, ancient trees in a light mist was soul-sustaining and we wouldn't have missed it for the world. The bus tour stopped in Sausalito on the way back and we enjoyed lunch with a view of the bay. We got off the bus at the Palace of Fine Arts, after crossing the Golden Gate, and then spent the afternoon meandering through the Marina District on the way back to the hotel. We visited the Cannery, Chinatown, took a boat tour of the harbor around Alcatraz, and met friends for dinner at a restaurant on Pier 39, where we stuffed ourselves with seafood and sourdough bread.

Overall, our trip was made possible by our refusal to be unable to move about the country like nondisabled people, or to miss out on a good friend's wedding. In terms of social isolation, I think about what it would be like if we had been unable to attend that wedding, tour the state capitol with another guest, or have a great dinner with friends on the pier. Life would be so less rich and rewarding without these social connections. This is precisely why I worked to pass the ADA. It's also why disabled people need to be aware of their rights—had we not known them, we probably would have missed out on Muir Woods and had to search for another hotel in San Francisco on a busy summer weekend.

By the way, upon returning home, I filed a federal complaint against that first motel with the inaccessible room. That franchise owned a dozen other chain motels across the northern California coast. When the complaint was addressed, I learned that, under the Americans with Disabilities Act passed 10 years earlier, the owners of the franchise were forced to renovate all of their facilities to implement accessibility standards and comply with the law.

Maybe, we helped other travelers to avoid getting wrong answers.

Promoting and Facilitating Community Engagement and Participation

Political and social advocacy at the macro and meso levels is closely aligned with strategies of community mobilization, development, and empowerment. These strategies promote and facilitate community participation and engagement. *Community participation* refers to active participation of individuals who both benefit and contribute to the community through their actions, ideas, knowledge, or skills. Community participation is about relating to others and developing relationships with community. Communities or, at the very least, a sense of community can be fostered by the social spaces that occupational therapists work within, such as congregate living environments or neighborhoods. Communities engage in collective occupations that provide a shared sense of purpose and meaning (Leclair, 2010). Communities can be fostered, developed, built, enhanced, created, or organized with the aim to enhance the health and wellness of their members. As illustrated in Jamal's case study, socially exclusive environments with poor accessibility can negatively affect the community participation of people with disabilities and other marginalized groups.

The ethical space of engagement is an important framework for building respectful community relationships (Ermine, 2006). It is the space in between two worldviews that supports the development of a framework for dialogue between "human communities" (p. 193). Ermine proposed this framework as a process for reconciliation to allow for exploring the diversity of worldviews and positionality of Indigenous peoples and Western society by understanding that the difference and diversity of each human community is "moulded from a distinct history, knowledge tradition, philosophy, and social and political reality" (p. 194). This framework has relevance for discussion related to addressing oppression of systemically excluded communities. The ethical space is a neutral zone between human communities and cultures that requires stepping out of allegiances, where dialogue can occur, and hierarchical structures are abandoned. It requires the creation of a level and ethical playing field where universality is not the goal, but rather equality of worldviews, allowing diverse groups to assert and define their rights to create a partnership model between human communities that overrun old ways of thinking. Embracing the ethical space of engagement can support greater health equity for OT clients. In the Global South, de Sousa Santos (2013) identified the value of knowledge from worldviews that challenge only legitimizing knowledge that the Global North deems scientific allowing historically excluded people's ways of knowing and being to shape what is known and how individuals practice. Santos (2013) termed this approach cognitive justice. Occupational therapists

can practice in an ethical space of engagement and enact cognitive justice through listening and giving voice to systemically excluded groups so that their knowledge and experiences are at the center in a community development process (Galvaan, 2021).

Community development strategies aim to create supportive environments and strengthen the capacity of communities to respond to health problems (WHO, 1986). Hoffman and Duponte (1992) state, "community development is about . . . helping people to develop the skills they need and removing the structural barriers that prevent them from achieving their full potential as members of the community" (p. 21). Rothman and Tropman's (1987) classic taxonomy of three community development approaches can be helpful for occupational therapists considering this type of work.

1. A *locality development* approach views the change process as involving many people, most often within one geographic community, in determining goals and action. Emphasis is placed on process components and on strengthening the connections among community members. An example is the community coming together to create a garden that would address food insecurity for members of the local community.
2. *Social planning* uses a top-down process where a governing body typically defines issues and solutions. This approach is not considered community-centered (Hyett et al., 2015; Reitz et al., 2014) but when community is included in the process and their interests and issues align with governing bodies, this approach can lead to important social change that will benefit the community. An example is the government providing food subsidies to address food insecurity among low-income earners.
3. Finally, *social action* demands a critical social analysis based on class, gender, ability, and race to create change and views problems as rooted within inequitable power structures (Alinsky, 1971); thus, efforts are directed at changing power structures. Community coalitions and advocacy groups often engage in these efforts. An example is a community coalition advocating for social housing that is affordable and accessible to low income earners.

Social action approaches share many assumptions with the concept of social OT. Social OT in Brazil is practice outside of the health system that focuses on addressing social inequities and injustices in a "territory" or geographically delimited place (Malfitano et al., 2014). It draws attention to the inseparability of micro and macro contexts when addressing individual needs and issues to enable the rights of individuals disadvantaged by social conditions (Malfitano & Lopes, 2018). Social OT is committed to social action and change.

Occupational therapists can move beyond individualist assumptions within OT theory to consider the notion of shared or collective occupations as a helpful construct in their work aimed at community change (Leclair, 2010). Occupational therapists can engage in multilayered work with individuals, groups, communities, and society as a continuum of OT services by bridging individual work with broader community issues and practice (Lauckner et al., 2019). Lauckner et al. (2011) emphasized the role of the occupational therapist to enable "power sharing between sectors to create opportunities for meaningful engagement with(in) communities" (p. 267). They can promote and support community actions aimed at producing shifts in power structures.

There is a growing body of literature that highlights occupational therapists' work with communities.

- Galvaan and Peters (2013) introduced the Occupation-based Community Development (ObCD) Process based on practice in Cape Town, South Africa (Galvaan & Peters, 2013, 2017a, 2017b). This framework is about long-term relationships with community (i.e., "groups of people who share binding social bonds based on their histories, interests, locality, values or occupations": Galvaan & Peters, 2013) that challenge power, privilege, structural inequalities, and entrenched thinking. The ObCD is composed of the iterative processes of Initiating Intervention, Designing, Implementation and Monitoring Reflection and Evaluation.
- Leclair et al. (2019) developed an OT community development practice process based on work with Canadian occupational therapists engaged in community development practice. The process consists of five key elements: (i) getting to know the community, (ii) getting the ball rolling/planning together, (iii) building (upon) occupational opportunities, (iv) revisiting the approach, and (v) striving for sustainability. Leclair et al. (2019) shared examples of occupational therapists' work with communities in Canada.
- The European Network of Occupational Therapy in Higher Education (ENOTHE) published case studies on social transformation through occupation that highlight the work of occupational therapists with communities in several countries (Van Bruggen et al., 2020).

These examples provide evidence of the contributions that occupational therapists are making to community development practice and the transformation of performance contexts at the micro, meso, and macro levels. Considering Jamal's story, where he and his family have limited formal supports, the occupational therapist could partner with families, community leaders, and other stakeholders in the community to highlight the lack of supports provided to families of children with disabilities. The occupational therapist could use one of the OT community development frameworks described to address this issue with the community.

Using Design Strategies and Technologies

Occupational therapists use principles of universal design (UD) and accessible design (AD) to create and modify performance contexts that are more usable for everyone. These principles can be used at the micro, meso, and macro levels. Similarly, the implementation of assistive technologies and smart technologies supports occupational participation in a variety of contexts.

Universal Design

Universal design is an approach to design to create products and environments that are more usable by everyone, regardless of age or ability (Steinfeld & Maisel, 2012). UD involves thinking about a range of human abilities before the environment is built. The seven principles of UD developed by the Centre for Excellence in Universal Design (2020) integrate accessibility and usability features in design. Today, UD is considered across most settings, including housing, office buildings, airports, restaurants, and parks. It recognizes human differences in shapes, sizes, ages, abilities, and cultures and promotes inclusion and ergonomic design for all people. For example, the level entrance and power sliding doors at the entrance to a grocery store make the store accessible to everyone. In this case, the entrance design accommodates people who are pushing the grocery carts, those moving large objects on a cart, caregivers pushing strollers, as well as those using wheelchairs or mobility devices.

As indicated by the dwelling design illustrated in Figure 24.3, this universal housing includes such features as stepless entrances with flush thresholds; kitchen and laundry appliances at convenient heights; bathing fixtures allowing multiple bathing options; and clear sight lines and adequate space for wheelchair use, including wide hallways, pocket doors, roll-under sinks, and wheelchair-height fixtures. See Box 24.1 for principles of universal design.

Accessible Design

Accessible design, also referred to as *barrier-free design*, adds accessibility to otherwise inaccessible buildings, products, and services to enable persons with disabilities to function independently (Iwarsson & Ståhl, 2003). For example, braille can be added to elevator keypads to enable persons with visual impairments to select the floor number they want. Often, AD responds to specific requirements and standards as laid out in legislation, such as the ADA and in building codes. It can be applied to make buildings, products,

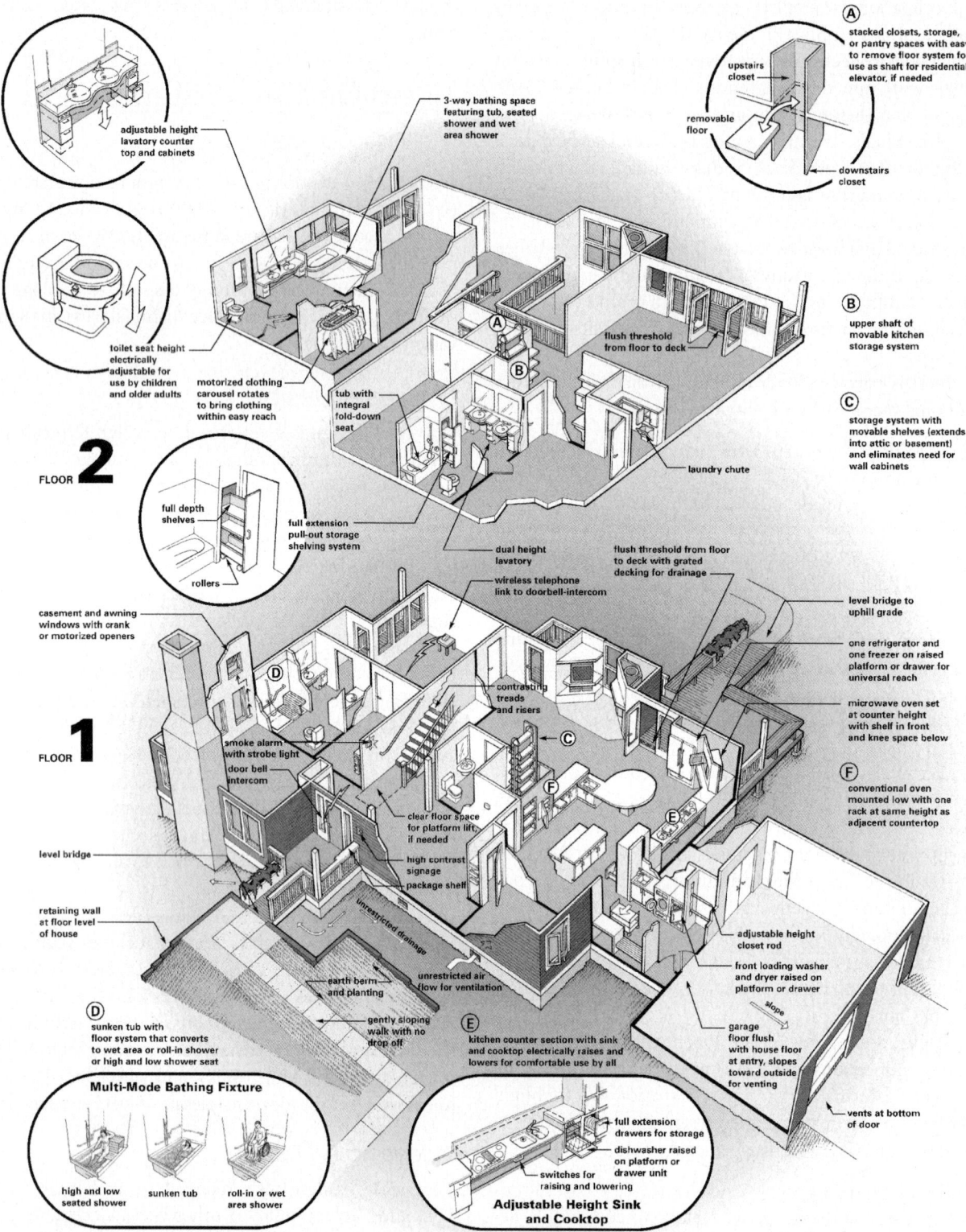

FIGURE 24.3 Two-story universal house. (Adapted from Preiser, W. F. E., & Smith, K. H. [Eds.]. [2011]. *Universal design handbook* [2nd ed., p. 24.6]. McGraw-Hill. Illustration by Ron Mace and Rex Pace, Center for Universal Design, North Carolina State University, Raleigh; used with permission of the Center for Universal Design.)

and services more accessible. AD can also be applied at the micro level with changes made to specific aspects of the environment in the home, school, or workplace to achieve PEO fit for individual clients. Occupational therapists routinely apply their knowledge about AD in their daily practice. For example, the home modifications such as the ramp added to Jamal's home in the OT Story exemplify AD.

Assistive Technologies

Assistive technologies (ATs) are devices, adaptive equipment, or products that are designed to enable persons with disabilities to engage in daily occupations within their homes, schools, workplaces, and communities (Cook & Polgar, 2015). They fall into the products and technology category within the environmental factors domain of the ICF (Schneidert et al., 2003). As will be shown when discussing modifying settings, ATs are routinely prescribed by occupational therapists to address specific occupational performance goals of their clients, including those for ADL, mobility, and communication and typically modify context at the micro level. These technologies range from simple devices such as grab bars and raised toilet seats to more complex devices such as powered wheelchairs and speech-generating devices (Figure 24.4).

ATs are widely used by persons with disabilities. There is growing evidence that ATs can improve occupational

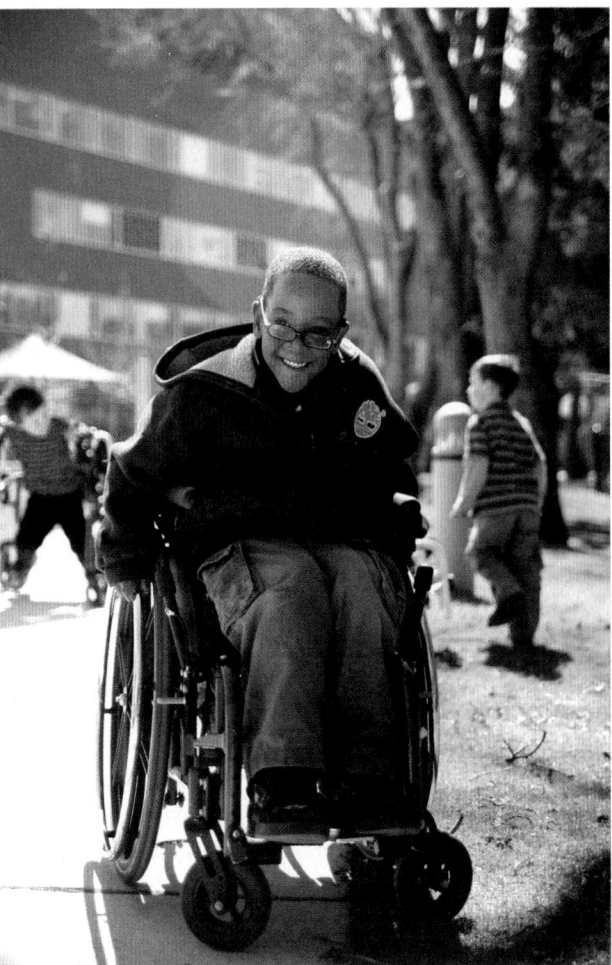

FIGURE 24.4 **Wheelchairs are a commonly used assistive technology for mobility and enable participation in daily life.**

performance and participation (e.g., McNicholl et al., 2021; Ripat et al., 2018, 2019), enhance quality of life (e.g., Baldassin et al., 2018; Rigby et al., 2011), and reduce caregiver burden (e.g., Marasinghe, 2016; Mortenson et al., 2012). In many jurisdictions, funding for ATs is provided by the state and/or charitable organizations. Occupational therapists assist their clients to obtain this funding.

Smart Technologies

Computers and smart technologies are transforming how people live and perform their daily occupations. Smartphones and mobile computers are rapidly developing, and many have been developed using UD principles, making them very user-friendly and accessible. For example, many have easy-to-use and see LCD touch screens, enlarged keyboards, and menu-driven software. It is common to see many people, from children through older adults, using smartphones, computer tablets, and laptop computers in public spaces. Occupational therapists find many features and new applications made for these technologies helpful for enabling their clients' occupational performance

(Verdonck & Maye, 2016). For example, persons with memory impairments can use the schedule reminder on their smartphone to organize their day (Andreassen et al., 2020) and persons with motor impairments can use voice commands to operate their phone.

Modifying Community Spaces

Public spaces are typically designed to meet the needs of average individuals and are based on general guidelines such as the ADA-Architectural Barriers Act (ABA) Accessibility Guidelines (U.S. Access Board, 2004). Greater accessibility can be achieved by working directly with clients, by working with community property owners or consultants, and by working as advocates in the community. For example, people with activity or participation restrictions may face barriers navigating public transportation systems, an important component of occupational performance. Iwarsson et al. (2003) described collaborative work between OT, traffic planning, and engineering in an initiative to understand the accessibility of transportation systems. Physical barrier removal might not always be possible. In some cases, without regulatory incentives in place (e.g., mandatory accessibility guidelines), it might not be possible to make changes. It is the occupational therapist's role, however, to understand current legislation and minimum standards and to help clients advocate for change. It is also possible to identify barriers through the assessment process to help clients make decisions about how they could access and use spaces.

For example, walkability of a community is an important aspect for promoting occupational participation. One way to document walkability is to use the Walkability Checklist (available at https://www.nhtsa.gov/sites/nhtsa.dot.gov/files/walkingchecklist.pdf). The United States National Highway Traffic Safety Administration created the checklist to guide a survey of safety for pedestrians in a particular area. For each problem identified, specific potential short-term and long-term solutions are suggested. Short-term actions are aimed at immediate safety; actions that may require more time include ways to advocate for safe neighborhoods and communities. Walkability assessments look at neighborhoods as places in which goods and services should be walkable. After safety is evaluated, the rater determines what common destinations, such as grocery stores, dry cleaners, salons, banks, medical clinics, and parks, are within a 10-minute walk (AARP has a range of assessment tools available at https://www.aarp.org/livable-communities/archives/info-2014/walkability.html). Understanding the physical environment is the goal, even though modification might not always be possible.

Playgrounds

Playgrounds are an important community space for children's social, emotional, and physical development (Ripat & Becker, 2012), and are often a constructed area within a schoolyard or park where play is usually unstructured. With an interest in promoting inclusive play experiences for children with disabilities, occupational therapists may be involved in developing plans for new construction, modifying existing playgrounds, and advocating for funding. Accessibility standards may be applicable to the construction of new playgrounds in some jurisdictions and consulting these documents is one step. However, playground design should go beyond accessible toward becoming a place of inclusivity (Ripat & Becker, 2012). In a scoping review of the literature, Brown et al. (2021) identified best-practice recommendations for the development of inclusive playgrounds in the areas of entrance, surfacing, features, supervision, and design process. The development of playgrounds and spaces must also be guided by cultural meanings of play (Brown et al., 2019). Figure 24.5 illustrates two different accessible playgrounds that meet the needs of different cultural communities.

In Jamal's early years, his playground was not accessible and did not promote his participation and inclusion in play

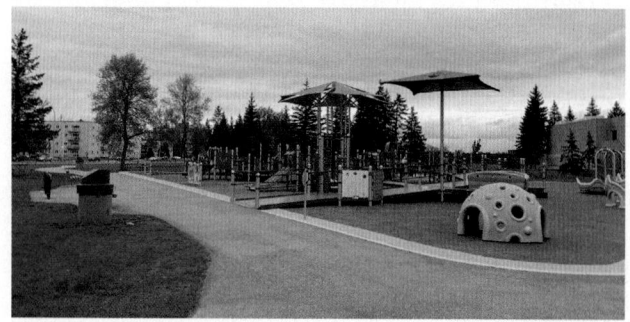
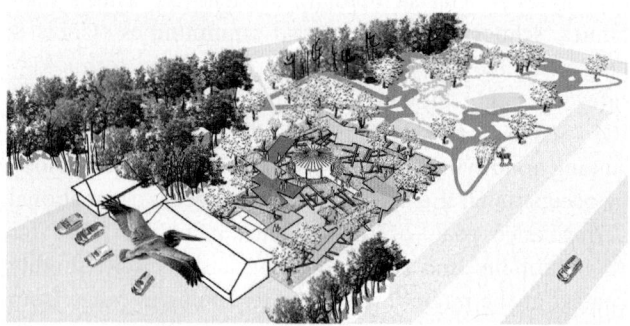

A   **B**

FIGURE 24.5 Accessible playgrounds that meet the needs of different cultural communities. **A:** An urban playground in Winnipeg, Canada. **B:** Design for a First Nations playground. (Source: Part B: Zaagaate Garden & Zaagaate Trail and Pollinator Meadow, Pelican's Eye View, Design and Drawing by Straub Thurmayr Landscape Architects.)

with peers. The occupational therapist took steps to make recommendations that the school could implement in their playground and brought the issue to school division administrators to provide education on the gap in accessibility standards that perpetuate barriers for children with disabilities.

Modifying Educational Settings

Occupational therapists play a critical role in enabling students with various conditions and disabilities to succeed and participate in school (AOTA, 2016). Various contextual factors, for example social and physical environments, can help or hinder students' participation in school-based occupations (Bonnard & Anaby, 2016). Occupational therapists use strategies to modify the physical, social, cultural, and organizational school environments. Modifying the performance context in schools can take many forms and should consider the macro, meso, and micro levels. Although there are many ways to support a student through accommodation, there are also many ways to go beyond accommodation to support broader inclusion within the school setting. In the case example of Jamal, the occupational therapist saw it as her role to influence both the *social structures* and physical access concerns of Jamal's school and playground (see OT Story 24.2). Further information about school-based practice is provided in Chapter 49.

The UNCRPD provides some important statements regarding education. Children with disabilities should have access to inclusive quality and free primary and secondary education on an equal basis with other children in their community. Reasonable accommodation and individualized supports are provided to maximize development with a goal of full inclusion. It is important that occupational therapists working in a school setting familiarize themselves with relevant legislation and policies that support the inclusion of students with disabilities where they exist, such as the Individuals with Disabilities Education Act in the United States. Relevant state or federal laws and policies will govern services and supports available to the student with a disability, such as availability and access to educational assistants and assistive technology. Furthermore, there may be local school policies designed to support students with disabilities. Understanding school, school division, and/or school board governance structures is imperative for knowing where and with whom to communicate, consult and advocate.

At the meso level, the focus may be on making schools accessible for persons with disabilities, including students, staff, and family members. School culture and attitudes of teachers and classmates have an important influence on inclusion, and occupational therapists can work with school administrators and staff to promote inclusive environments (Bourke-Taylor et al., 2018). Examples include sensitivity

education for school staff and students, capacity building in school staff, and advocating for social supports in the classroom (e.g., teaching assistants or peer mentors). Critical reflexivity is required so that assumptions are not made about how children want to participate in their school context. Respecting the views of the student and assisting them to express how they uniquely define and experience inclusion and participation in their school is an important role for the occupational therapist. This notion of perceived participation and inclusion was illustrated in the Jamal case example where Jamal was often assigned to be the goalie in gym class. Jamal expressed that this was not how he wished to participate in sport or gym class. Exploring Jamal's wishes to participate in gym class would support greater inclusion.

Although physical environment barriers, such as heavy doors, raised thresholds at doors, and absence of elevators in multilevel schools, are still common, examples of specific modifications can include installing electronic door openers, lever-style taps at sinks, and grab bars in the toilet stall. Therapists can consult about and advocate for architectural accessibility and the use of UD principles within schools. They can also consult with individual schools or school boards to prepare annual accessibility plans or to assist in the design and planning of new schools and planning for major renovations to make schools more accessible. The occupational therapist should also become familiar with the conditions and terms for funding environmental modifications and special or adapted furniture and ATs for schools. Some environmental modifications can be made at little expense, whereas others will be costly and involve applying to the school board or a government agency for special funding (Table 24.1).

Therapists may collaborate with teachers to modify and adapt curricula and educational materials to support students' learning, and coach teachers to use specific teaching strategies tailored for individual students but that may also support the whole class. At a meso level, the concept of UD for Learning refers to the ways that all students are given an equal opportunity to learn and succeed. Key concepts include providing multiple options for engagement, for representing information or materials, and for action and expression (CAST, 2022). Occupational therapists can bring an understanding of the importance and multifaceted nature of occupation to work with teachers to support implementation of UD for Learning in classrooms that can promote the success of all students (Collins, 2014).

Classroom environments can have high levels of sensory stimuli in terms of noise, visual clutter, and the physical activity of a classroom full of students, which can have a disorganizing effect on children with sensory processing disorders. Occupational therapists assess the classroom environment to identify the sensory features that either facilitate or hinder students' ability to complete schoolwork and recommend modifying the space to better fit students' sensory processing needs (Benson et al., 2019; Mowell et al., 2022). For example, sound-absorbing partitions and low lighting

TABLE 24.1	Context-Based Interventions at the Micro, Meso, and Macro Levels to Support Jamal's Occupational Participation
Occupational Participation Barriers and Factors	**Context-Based Interventions**
Client-Identified Goal: Increase social inclusion and participation in school	
Micro • Negative attitude of peers at school related to disability and use of AT/adapted equipment • Delay of adaptive equipment access	**Micro** • Classroom and staff education on disabilities and use of adaptive equipment • Assessment and recommendations for adaptations to the playground environment to increase accessibility (e.g., play equipment that is accessible to all children—raised sand boxes or sand tables, firm and stable surface at base of playground, staff to promote playground inclusion)
Meso • Limitations to accessibility of playground at the school • Limited organizational programming for social-emotional development and disability awareness • Attitudinal barriers, negative perceptions related to disability and use of AT	**Meso** • Help the school develop social opportunities/structured social opportunities between classmates and children with disabilities (increased contact experiences) • Provide school with evidence about elements required for meaningful participation for Jamal and his family in the school community (choice, control, acceptance, safety, accessibility, accommodation, making connection with other families)
Macro • Limitations in policies supporting accessible playgrounds, limited education and reference guides—difference between technically accessible and functionally accessible • Barriers to AT and adapted equipment access in schools because of policies not including them in their list of approved assistive devices	**Meso/Macro** • Collect evidence to support advocacy efforts to expand list of approved assistive devices covered to eliminate barriers and share at a school board meeting • Coordinate a project that allows children and youth with disabilities and who use technology to raise awareness of negative attitudes and promote inclusion • Work with school district to provide education materials on inclusion and disabilities to use system wide and implement in early years • Discuss accessibility issues in the school playground with school administrators. Partner with school community (e.g., students, parents, and teachers) to raise the issue at the district level. Work with school community to highlight the issue of lack of guidance and gaps in policy for accessible playgrounds to government levels.

can enable some students to focus their attention while working on individual assignments. The therapist might recommend setting up a quiet space in the classroom where a student with autism can use a rocking chair to seek calming sensory input and put on a headset to listen to music or an audiobook story. To support inclusion at a classroom level, Wener and colleagues (2009) described the use of a sensory processing workshop designed to address exclusionary attitudes toward peers with sensory processing differences.

Students with disabilities may use assistive technologies to participate in their curricular and extracurricular activities, and occupational therapists may work with students, families, teachers, and educational assistants to identify, train, and support the student to use appropriate options (Karlsson et al., 2018). Software options such as speech-to-text for input into computers, and text-to-speech or screen readers for students with low vision or learning disabilities may be options for some students. An increasing number of applications are available to support students in writing, reading, math skills, and organizational skills. Alternate input methods such as specialized switches to access laptops

and tablets, or recommendations for positioning devices may also be recommended.

In Jamal's early years of school, he experienced barriers to his social participation and inclusion because of social attitudes and limited programming and education related to disabilities and use of adapted aids, limitations in the accessibility and inclusivity of the playground environment, and limitations and delay in access to assistive technologies and adaptive equipment that could promote participation. The occupational therapist was able to provide some assessment findings and recommendations to the school to mitigate the immediate impact of these barriers, such as an education session for staff and peers related to disability and advocacy letters for funding for expedited assistive technology (tablet), adaptive equipment (adapted bicycle), and modifications to the existing playground. However, the occupational therapist also targeted the overarching cause of these barriers by facilitating the development of education, training and programming for the future, and escalating concerns regarding gaps in supports and policies to school division and government levels through partnership.

Jamal is now 18 years of age and is coming up on his high school graduation. Throughout high school the educational system provided Jamal with access to AT devices to support his communication and his ability to do other activities independently, such as his banking, schoolwork, and playing videogames. The occupational therapists initiated the process to get funding and assessment for AT in the adult system. Despite beginning the process early, Jamal may still experience a gap in his access to AT, affecting his hobbies and postsecondary education.

As an adult, Jamal will no longer receive the all-day ADL support provided while he was at school, or regular rehabilitation services such as physiotherapy and OT. Jamal does not qualify for many adult community support services such as respite to support him in the community. Rehabilitation services will be more intermittent, which will not meet Jamal's need for continued therapy to manage his chronic condition. Jamal's parents continue to be unable to practice in their respective professions, which has limited their income for many years.

As a young adult, Jamal is experiencing decreased occupational participation. Jamal is finding the decreased control he has over his personal care very frustrating. He would like to establish his independence from his family who are his main support for his care needs. It has been difficult for Jamal to navigate his family's desire to care for him while asserting his independence. Jamal has begun considering other living arrangements to assist with this process for him and his family.

In exploring housing options with Jamal, funding and eligibility is a question. Jamal wants to continue living close to his community and social networks. Jamal does not qualify for publicly funded group homes because of not having a mental health diagnosis or intellectual disability. Nearby, there is a personal care home option; however, Jamal is reluctant to live in a facility that has mainly older adults as residents. Independent living with home care will not provide enough support for Jamal, as home care policy does not provide sufficient time in the home.

In his spare time, Jamal enjoys watching and streaming videogames. He has developed strong skills in programming using his AT setup during high school and has an interest in sports statistics. Jamal is aware he has difficulties with aspects of learning; however, he has been motivated to pursue continued education and possibly career opportunities in these fields. But there are many barriers to him pursuing this, including: (i) barriers to accessing AT for learning, (ii) the need for accommodations/adaptations to university courses to be successful, (iii) home care supports not being allowed to go out into the community with Jamal, and (iv) financial costs of attending university.

Questions

1. How might an occupational therapist use the 4 P's approach to address Jamal's housing issue?
2. How could a community development process be used to modify the meso and macro level contexts that limit Jamal's participation in postsecondary education?

Postsecondary Institutions

As young adults, clients will have graduated or transitioned out of child and youth health, rehabilitation, educational, and social services that may have been an integral part of their childhood experience with service providers. In comparison with children's services that may have been centered around the child and family, adult services are often more individually oriented. For students attending postsecondary education settings, there may be additional needs related to capacity building, systems navigation, and teaching self-advocacy skills. Postsecondary institutions may have a student accessibility services center that can support accommodations, provide notetakers, assist with assistive technology needs, and address overall campus access and accessibility. Occupational therapists may be part of this team. Linking students with existing services will be crucial to their academic success. With increasing options for virtual and online learning, some students may elect to study remotely. The role of the occupational therapist may be to identify assistive technology or other strategies to support notetaking, studying, and learning.

Recognizing the importance of lifelong learning, postsecondary universities worldwide have formed a network of institutions that have adopted Age-Friendly University Principles as they apply to programs, spaces, and policies (Dublin City University, 2021; The Gerontological Society of America, 2021). Occupational therapists are well-positioned to become allies in initiatives such as this, providing their unique understanding of occupation and ways to adapt and modify context to meet the diverse learning needs of students across the life span. As Jamal approaches adulthood, his ability to go to university and live independently is limited by contextual factors at the micro, meso, and macro levels. Although the occupational therapist can assess Jamal's occupational issues and make recommendations for equipment and environmental modifications specific to his situation, Jamal and his peers will continue to experience meso and macro level systemic barriers such as barriers in eligibility criteria for funding and adult services and limited housing options.

Modifying Work Settings

For many people, the ability to work is an occupational goal that holds importance and contributes to self-efficacy. However, the workplace can contribute to illness and injury and can pose barriers to those with various chronic conditions and disabilities who wish to enter the workforce, return to work, or volunteer in a work environment. The scope for OT in the workplace is broad; the focus can be on health promotion and wellness, injury prevention, or return to work. All these areas involve making modifications to the work environment and can range from micro to macro levels and address physical, social, and attitudinal factors. The role of the occupational therapist in the workplace is explored in detail in Chapter 46. This chapter focuses on modifications to the workplace to enable individuals with occupational participation challenges to enter or return to work and successfully perform their jobs.

The ADA and similar human rights legislation in many countries support the individual's right to work by prohibiting discrimination against people with disabilities. In the United States, when people with disabilities can perform the essential functions of a job with accommodations, they can apply for and maintain a job. The concept of reasonable accommodation is an important consideration when modifying workplace contexts; it is outlined in Article 27 of the CRPD (United Nations, 2006) and enacted in legislation in many countries. Reasonable accommodation refers to an equity-based approach that outlines an employer's legal responsibility to adapt or modify the physical work environment, working conditions or schedules, policies and/or duties to meet the needs of the worker with a disability, as long as it does not constitute "undue hardship" or "undue burden" for the employer. For instance, a small company that has a very small profit margin might not be required to pay for an elevator if it would cause the company bankruptcy, but the employer might be required to move the office of an employee with a mobility impairment to the first floor if space was available. The outcome of the job accommodation should be evaluated, and the continued success of the accommodations should be monitored over time to ensure the best worker-job-environment fit.

When workplace accommodations are necessary, the occupational therapist can lead a team to identify the environmental resources and barriers that influence an employee's ability to work and help to access resources and/or remove these barriers. In addition to the occupational therapist, the team members typically include the employer, key employees, and the group that is responsible for implementing the environmental modifications. There is a growing body of evidence for the efficacy of workplace accommodations and modifications, but more research is needed to develop best practices (Padkapayeva et al., 2017; Wong et al., 2021; Zafar et al., 2019). The Job Accommodation Network (n.d., https://askjan.org/) provides an excellent resource for therapists, employers, and employees with disabilities to identify possible workplace modifications in relation to specific work performance challenges. Many useful modifications are not expensive or complex (Denny-Brown et al., 2015). Assistive technologies are commonly prescribed, such as a one-handed keyboard with a reduced number of keys to depress when typing or use of voice recognition software that enters data to the computer via voice. Equipment and tools used in the workplace may require modification. Therapists may recommend ergonomic modifications for workstations to improve function, safety, and work efficiency. Architectural changes to the environment, such as installing electronic door openers and modifying a bathroom, can make the workplace accessible for employees and others who use mobility aids such as a wheelchair.

In the OT Story of Jamal, accommodations are imperative for his success in employment. Jamal's regular care needs are provided on a limited schedule. The occupational therapist provides assessment and recommendations regarding Jamal's need for alternative access for computer use and the need for physical modifications to increase accessibility. The employer may support working from home to support Jamal's care needs, but Jamal may not wish to work from home. The occupational therapist can take this opportunity to address inclusivity and accessibility at a meso level by working with the employer to develop education and workplace sensitivity training, as well as support the employer in feeling more comfortable making changes in the workplace to increase accessibility for all in the workplace.

The occupational therapist can recommend how social, cultural, and organizational aspects of the workplace can be modified to be more supportive and inclusive (Padkapayeva et al., 2017). For instance, employers could assign a peer mentor to assist the worker to break down daily tasks into achievable steps, create daily to-do lists, or hire job coaches to provide daily guidance. Employers might offer job-sharing options, flexible work hours, or work-from-home options. In some instances, workplace cultures and attitudes have been described as exclusionary when a worker uses assistive technology or other accommodations to support their work duties (Ripat & Woodgate, 2017). Disclosure of disability status to employers may be a difficult decision for some individuals, and the occupational therapist may assist in supporting the individual to disclose, and to work with the employer and employee to identify appropriate accommodations (Lindsay et al., 2018). Employees with disabilities could be encouraged to be engaged in discussions and decisions regarding workplace policy. Greater emphasis on shifting societal attitudes toward individuals with disabilities continues to be essential.

Modifying Home Settings

Home is a setting for engaging in a broad range of occupations, from basic ADLs like bathing to social events and celebrations with family. Home is a multidimensional concept, which includes a physical space within a geographic location along with emotional, cultural, and personal elements (Mitty & Flores, 2009). Home is frequently one of the most cherished settings in people's lives, and people make meaning out of their life events through their homes (Cristoforetti et al., 2011). Another important aspect of the lifeworld is *home* and *at-homeness* (Ohlén et al., 2014; Rioux & Werner, 2011; Seamon, 2018). These studies indicate that home has specific physical, personal, social, cultural, and political dimensions but, experientially, is lived as a human and environmental whole that incorporates and facilitates a wide range of existential significances. Home is not only a physical place but also a locus of activities, an anchor of identity, a repository of memories bonding past and present, and a center of stability and continuity. Home as place offers a sense of well-being, safety, and comfort (Hasselkus & Dickie, 2021; Kylén et al., 2019). At-homeness is conceptually related to wellness, regardless of illness or disability (Ohlén et al., 2014; Saarnio et al., 2019). This literature also emphasizes that some homes can involve a "shadow side" of discomfort, distress, and trauma—for example, homes where there is domestic violence or abuse (Mayock et al., 2021), especially problematic internationally during pandemic lockdown (Fawole et al., 2021; Stockman et al., 2021; van Gelder et al., 2021).

When dealing with clients' homes, several intervention strategies can be considered in the environment to maximize people's ability to engage in their occupations (Siebert et al., 2014). These can range from building a new home following a catastrophic injury to making minor changes to the living space like rearranging furniture or installing a grab bar. The home has been described as having three elements: physical, social, and personal (Tanner et al., 2008). The implications of modifications to a physical aspect of a home should be considered in light of these other elements. In some situations, however, environmental interventions and assistive technology in the home can disrupt residents' lives. For example, what may be viewed as clutter to a therapist concerned about falls prevention could be seen as a threat to personal self-expression by an older adult with many important possessions. Moore and colleagues (2010) also demonstrated this in their study of medical equipment and technology for children with complex needs: "The home space becomes an appropriated landscape—no longer a family landscape but a landscape of care, 'like a mini hospital,' with some parents feeling this particularly keenly" (Moore et al., 2010, p. 4).

Beyond considering the home as a physical space and the need for modifications of the physical environment within clients' homes, therapists need to be attentive to the nature of home as a social sphere, which might also be modified to support clients' return to or remaining home. Social supports at home can sometimes be implemented as an environmental intervention that can overcome physical barriers associated with the home environment. The elements of the social and personal meanings of home may help therapists and others understand the importance of home beyond its physical layout and features. Home modifications can incorporate formal or informal supports, ranging from personal care workers to help with bathing to family assistance with meal preparations. Supports from others are often also important to consider. Sometimes, help from others can make it possible for someone to remain in his or her home environment. For example, having a neighbor collect mail from a community mailbox can not only overcome challenges with outdoor mobility but can also provide a social connection for an older adult living alone. Having a personal support worker assist with ADLs can be an alternative or addition to installing assistive devices. When the occupational therapist originally met Jamal and his family, the family was not accessing social supports. By modifying Jamal and the family's social context such as adding home care and respite supports, it greatly influenced Jamal and the family's occupational performance. In Jamal's context, his family was eligible for home care assistance for daily dressing and twice weekly bathing assistance. In addition, specific assessment and recommendations for ADL adaptive equipment and specific caregiver training and education bolstered Jamal's micro level context to better support his needs.

At the macro level, it is important to be aware of relevant federal or local laws and regulations that impact access to housing. For instance, the Fair Housing Act in the United States protects people from housing discrimination based on race, color, nationality, religion, sex, family status, or disability when renting or buying a home. Within this law, housing providers are required to provide reasonable accommodations and modifications to allow persons with disabilities to function in their housing. Jamal's family required a ground-floor suite for ease of access using his wheelchair and several grab bars to be installed in the bathroom to facilitate bath and toilet transfers.

Occupational therapists should also keep in mind that any modifications to different types of homes, whether they are situated in suburban neighborhoods, urban apartments or condominiums, or within congregate living arrangements such as group homes or retirement homes, are contingent on different regulations and processes. Personal environments, such as a private dwelling, are generally not subject to the same accessibility laws and requirements. However, these laws may be applicable to public housing or other residential multiunit buildings. Prior to making recommendations, therapists should inform themselves of the various policy and legal considerations and guidelines that apply to the various housing types. In addition, therapists must be aware of how home modifications will impact other residents. This is particularly an issue when working in congregate living settings.

Funding of home modifications can sometimes present a barrier to implementation of the optimal solution. Renovations can be expensive, and, depending on the client's circumstances, insurance companies may not provide financial supports. Occupational therapists assist in locating funding sources and providing input into applications. Occupational therapists have an important duty to help justify the need for home modifications to payers (whether insurers, social service agencies, or other funding bodies). Local or federal grants may be available to support changes needed to function in the home that could be used to add ramps for entrance and egress, modify kitchens and bathrooms, or widen doorways. Some countries may have tax credits that can be used to offset expenses related to modifications required. People often rely on personal resources or social service agencies to fund the modifications. Occupational therapists should be familiar with their local social service agencies that provide such modifications and may need to work collaboratively with the client to apply for funding supports. Although home renovations are costly, paid support workers are also expensive. Justification for modifications to the physical environment may in part be that the increased independence of the client will decrease costs associated with paid support workers.

Occupational therapists may provide consultation to clients if accessible housing is being sought or built. As discussed in this chapter, universally designed housing is housing design that serves to meet the widest range of needs for people of all sizes and abilities without the need for adaptations. Based on design principles rather than regulations, the concepts are useful in considering a wide range of occupants' abilities. Accessible homes are homes that allow full access to all levels and uses by the occupants and have been designed or modified to meet functional abilities. For people requiring accessible housing, ideal features vary depending on their needs. Most frequently, accessible housing is sought when people have issues related to mobility, requiring use of a mobility device such as a walker or manual or power wheelchair.

Considerations to Implementing Home Modifications

Occupational therapists may conduct home visits to identify home adaptations or modifications that can be implemented to promote accessibility, safety and autonomy within the home. By focusing on the goals of the client, the therapist can generate several possible environmental strategies that can be implemented. There is often more than one environmental solution available to address an occupational performance issue.

In newer areas of research, virtual reality (VR) and augmented reality (AR) technology have been used to co-create design ideas and discuss recommended home modifications with clients. As an immersive technology, VR can be used to evaluate a home setting without the need to conduct an in-home visit, and to engage the client in decision-making about modifications (Hwang & Shim, 2021). AR functions by superimposing 3D images on pictures of real environments and can be used to engage clients in envisioning placement of assistive technologies or adaptations within their homes (Aoyama & Aflatoony, 2020).

A final consideration related to home modifications is the relationship between the various parties involved in any renovations. Although occupational therapists may recommend major or minor modifications to the physical environment, the implementation of any modifications is completed by others and should be overseen by the client or family. The AT vendor or a skilled family member can sometimes do minor modifications, such as installing grab bars. Major modifications or home renovations involve a complex team that might include an architect, contractor, trades people, AT vendors, or even builders in the case of a new home. However, occupational therapists can advise clients on strategies to consult and collaborate with all parties to oversee modifications to the home environment.

Major Home Modifications

Not all clients are able to find accessible housing. Other clients are reluctant to move away from their family home. Both of these situations may result in a need to consider modifying the physical environment of the home in which the client is currently residing. The Canada Mortgage and Housing Corporation (CMHC, 2018) has created a series of consumer-friendly fact sheets that highlight accessibility and safety considerations when adapting a home, addressing changing needs, or purchasing or installing new products in homes.

Entrances are most frequently modified with the installation of either ramps or porch lifts. A major consideration in recommending these relates to the height from the ground level to the entrance. Ramps are most useful when the distance from ground to entrance is 30″ or less (CMHC, 2018) and a front or side door can be designated for access. It is important to be aware of local building codes that stipulate maximum slope on ramps. A common permissible slope is a minimum of 12″ in length for each inch of rise (1:12) but individuals with reduced strength or stamina may find this slope too difficult to manage and may opt for a 1:15, 1:18, or 1:20 slope. However, these reduced slope ramps will be longer and may require landings to be built between sections of the ramp. Portable ramps may be an option for temporary access or lower changes in level. However, there may be occasions when a ramp is simply not feasible.

Some individuals may be interested in installing a lift at the entrance. Some considerations in the selection of lifts include backup electrical or manual systems in case of power failures and a need to consider the climate in which the home is located. Ideally, there will be more than one entrance/exit accessible to the client so that in case of an emergency such as a fire, at least one exit is available. If there is only one accessible entrance, escape plans in case of emergencies are advised.

Bathrooms often require major modifications because they are typically small, making mobility within the space challenging. In addition, transferring to and from a toilet and bath/shower can present challenges. Although minor modifications such as grab bars and handheld showers might be adequate in some circumstances, other clients require major modifications in the bathroom. These modifications can range from moving or removing fixtures to installation of new fixtures such as roll-in shower stalls, higher toilets, and sink and tap fixtures that can be readily managed.

Kitchens often serve the needs to many household members as a place for food preparation and consumption, and as a social space. Modifications may require consideration of the needs of many different users and application of UD principles in kitchen design might be considered, such as installation of lever-style faucets, lowered working areas for those in a seated position, and consideration of layout and maneuverability between preparation, cooking, and cleanup zones (CMHC, 2018). Because major modifications are costly, it is important for the therapist to work closely with the client and family to consider current as well as possible future needs.

Minor Home Modifications

Major modifications to the physical environment of a client's home are not always required. There are many times when minor modifications provide solutions to challenges experienced in the home. Assistive technologies such as a bath bench and handheld shower for someone who is unable to enter and stand for a shower is a common minor modification that occupational therapists provide. Wall-mounted or adjustable height grab bars mounted to fixtures such as the toilet may be added to improve safety when transferring. Therapists also recommend off-the-shelf products that support performance such as adding a handrail to the wall or stairs to the basement or an automatic shutoff kettle for someone with early cognitive decline.

Occupational therapists can also suggest that clients modify the way they use the physical environment. For example, they can teach individuals to make use of features of their existing environment in ways that make it safer or easier to perform daily activities. This may mean rearranging furniture, placing chairs with arms for extra support in commonly used areas, organizing items in a basket to be carried up and down stairs, or programming the telephone to make use of autodial functions to make it easy for someone with memory issues to contact family.

Aging in Place

Drawing on the principles of UD, architects, interior designers, and technology specialists have made major efforts to envision housing and other environments that accommodate the needs of users, regardless of their age or degree of impairment. A newer concept is the understanding of the social experiences, challenges, and needs of diverse populations called "empathic design" (Altay, 2017; Dalton & Kahute, 2016; O'Shea et al., 2016). This work is grounded partly in understanding how people function at different stages of life and in regard to different degrees of ableness and social needs. One aim is homes that support aging in place—in other words, dwelling units that residents, if they so choose, can occupy from childhood to old age unless illness or impairment come into play (Steinfeld & White, 2010; Young, 2011). Many older adults want to continue living in their own homes for as long as possible (AARP, 2014). Aging in place is a concept that has been defined as, "having the health and social supports and services you need to live safely and independently in your home and community for as long as you wish and are able" (Canada Ministers Responsible for Seniors, 2016, p. 2). Older adults may feel safe and connected to the familiarity of their house or community and aging in place provides older adults with a sense of autonomy and independence over their lives (Wiles et al., 2012). To support aging in place, home modifications and strategies are implemented to support older adults to remain in their home as long as possible. Enabling older adults to age in place typically requires home modifications such as the addition of ramps for home entry/egress or grab bars in the bathroom. These types of modifications have been shown to positively impact the older adult's ability to stay longer in current housing (Hwang et al., 2011).

If a universal dwelling is located in a car-dependent neighborhood, it cannot provide wider scale accessibility for residents who do not or cannot drive—an increasingly important group as the populations of countries age. Many health professionals, architects, and urban planners today favor compact, human-scaled communities providing easy access to a wide range of functions, services, and activities (Gunn et al., 2017; Hyde et al., 2019). Such walkable, neighborhoods might motivate residents to be more physically active and thus provide valuable health benefits (Christian et al., 2017). In addition, the higher densities and a more active street life might motivate residents to feel responsible for their neighborhood and be more willing to look out for each other (Gardner, 2011; Mehta & Bosson, 2010). Occupational therapists play a pivotal role in regard to housing needs because they have an intimate knowledge of clients' home requirements, restrictions, and possibilities. They can serve as an important go-between for helping clients articulate their environmental situation and needs to architects, interior designers, and contractors. Knowing clients' functional abilities firsthand, the occupational therapist can play a central role in "design teams" that plan aging in place or impairment-accommodating housing (Burns et al., 2017; Pickens & Burns, 2018) and community centers or environments (Figure 24.6).

Home Safety

Home safety is often an overriding concern for clients and families when physical or cognitive abilities change because of injury, illness, or aging. Home safety assessment tools such as the SAFER-HOME tool (Chiu, 2011) are available to occupational therapists to use to evaluate the ability of clients with cognitive and/or physical disabilities to safely manage within their homes. It addresses physical environmental features of the home along with occupational performance tasks conducted by the client. Consumer-friendly checklists and guides are available for community dwelling adults and their social supports to self-identify fall risk hazards in and around areas of their home, and to provide

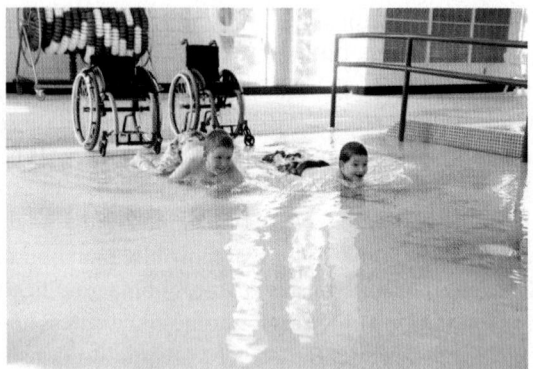

FIGURE 24.6 This recreation center, designed with an *objective outside* perspective, provides a space where all people can participate without exclusion. An *empathic inside* understanding emerges among those who witness Simon and Manuel in an environment in which they are equally equipped to participate without restrictions or barriers. (Source: Reprinted with permission from http://committoinclusion.org/universal-design/)

suggested solutions. For instance, the Home Safety Self-Assessment Tool (HSSAT) and a checklist created by the Centers for Disease Control and Prevention (2015) ask occupants to consider safety hazards with in the home, along with suggestions to improve safety and reduce falls.

Because contexts may need to change in the case of natural disasters or emergencies, occupational therapists may work with clients to develop emergency preparedness plans. The plans may include development of an emergency support network and contacts, evacuation plan, emergency kit that includes medications and medical and/or assistive devices, and items for service animals if applicable. Checklists and suggestions are available to support these conversations (https://www.getprepared.gc.ca/cnt/rsrcs/pblctns/pplwthdsblts/index-eng.aspx)

Smart Home Technologies

The development of smart home technology is rapidly evolving and there is growing evidence of its efficacy (Liu et al., 2016). Smart home technologies, or home automation systems, support persons with physical, sensory, and/or cognitive disabilities to live in their own home, and older adults to age in place. They consist of electronic sensors and actuators used in the home to allow individuals to achieve greater independence and safety within their home and reduce the need for caregiver assistance. They can be used to monitor health wellness, emergency detection and response, and to prompt behaviors, such as steps to completing ADL. Although dedicated AT devices to control a home environment are available (e.g., for locking and unlocking entrances, opening and closing blinds, and manipulating home electronics such as the television), the range and function of commercially available smart home devices to automate home access is rapidly expanding. Control of heating and cooling systems, speakers, light bulbs, lamps, doorbells, door locks, security cameras, smoke detectors are just a few of the smart home products that might be considered by clients to support functioning in their homes. Jamwal et al. (2020) conducted a scoping review of the impact of smart home technologies when used by people with disabilities and concluded that studies reported the use of this technology increased the sense of safety, security, and independence. However, downsides to the use of technology were also identified, particularly regarding the use of monitoring technologies and the potential for loss of privacy.

Visitable Housing

An important social aspect of place incorporates participation in community life through visiting others at home. Building and remodeling homes with *visitability* creates home as a place to gather others. Issues of convenience, mobility, accessibility, and visitability are not limited to the dwelling alone but extend to the realm of the dwelling's immediate surroundings and larger neighborhood (Steinfeld & White, 2010). The concept of visitability supports the social value of the home. Visitable housing is a concept of housing design and construction that includes basic accessibility features. Three requirements need to be met for a home to be "visitable": (i) one zero-step entrance, (ii) doors with 32″ of clear passage space, and (iii) one bathroom on the main floor accessible by wheelchair (Scovel & Lichter, 2016). (See http://www.visitability.org for more information.) Although not considered fully accessible or universally designed, visitable homes can improve access for everyone, including movers, and those pushing strollers.

Institutional/Residential Care Settings

Occupational therapists may work with individuals whose home is an institutional context such as a skilled nursing facility or long-term care home. Although older adults may be more frequently encountered in these settings, working-age individuals may also require institutional or residential care for financial, care, or safety reasons, or because of lack of accessible housing. Levack and Thornton (2017) highlighted that a lack of opportunity for social participation and personal growth in institutional settings were overriding concerns for working-age adults. As with other settings, adapting or modifying institutions require consideration of the social, physical, and cultural structures and relationships (Shin, 2015).

In these contexts, macro considerations (such as policy and regulations) and meso considerations (such as philosophy of care of an institution, routines, communication processes, and roles of formal caregivers) need to be understood as a first step toward implementing changes in a context. Framing institutional or residential facilities as "micro-communities" that can mutually benefit and support the well-being and participation of residents, families, and staff is a useful way to consider these settings (Morgan-Brown & Chard, 2014).

Helping clients to personalizing their rooms, including displaying personal belongings and furnishings, can support self-identity, promote familiarity and attachment, and encourage social interactions and engagement (Falk et al., 2013; Shin, 2015). Occupational therapists can recommend assistive technologies for bed mobility and toilet transfers, or technologies to support individuals' engagement in social activities, such as magnifiers, task lighting or large-print materials. Clinicians can suggest cueing strategies such as reminders and signage. For instance, when privacy and personal space are desired, environmental cues can be communicated by shutting a door or through signage directing nonresidents to knock. Occupational therapists can facilitate autonomy and choice by assisting individuals to advocate and negotiate for their desired routines, for instance for timing of baths or meals, or choosing where to sit in the dining room (Wada et al., 2020).

Common spaces in residential facilities can be considered occupational spaces that promote occupational participation and engagement (Du Toit et al., 2019). At a meso level, clinicians can recommend space layouts of shared spaces that promote social interaction and engagement of residents (Wada et al., 2020). Advocating for residents to engage in familiar home-based occupations such as meal preparation, baking, cleaning and tidying, laundry, gardening and yard work alongside paid staff may provide meaning and social engagement otherwise lacking in this context.

Conclusions and Future Considerations

Contexts can create barriers or provide resources and supports toward enabling optimal occupational participation. Occupational therapists have considerable experience and have demonstrated leadership and success with modifying home, school, work, and community settings to support the participation of their clients in their daily pursuits. Today, more people who have previously been marginalized, excluded, or discriminated against are able to live with greater autonomy, go to school, return to work, and actively participate in their communities through efforts made by occupational therapists to reduce barriers and harness resources at the micro, meso, and macro levels. To provide this leadership, it is critical that occupational therapists maintain a strong working knowledge about applicable policies, legislation, and guidelines that can improve the overall occupational participation of individuals and collectives. Beyond this awareness, however, as enablers of occupation, therapists can serve their clients by boldly participating in efforts to shape more inclusive social and public policies and to join the efforts of others, including their clients, in creating the spaces and opportunities that foster meaningful participation in life for all.

Acknowledgments

We would like to acknowledge the contributions of Patty Rigby, Lori Letts, and Barry Trentham—the authors of an earlier edition of this chapter. We would also like to acknowledge support from Janelle Swiderek for assisting with development of the case study and gathering resources for inclusion in the chapter.

Lippincott® Connect *For additional resources on the subjects discussed in this chapter, visit Lippincott Connect.*

REFERENCES

AARP. (2014). *Home and community preference of the 45+ population.* https://www.aarp.org/content/dam/aarp/research/surveys_statistics/il/2015/home-community-preferences.doi.10.26419%252Fres.00105.001.pdf

ADA Amendments Act. (2016). *ADA Amendments Act of 2008, U.S. Equal Employment Opportunity Commission.* https://www.eeoc.gov/statutes/ada-amendments-act-2008

Aldrich, R. M., & Rudman, D. L. (2020). Occupational therapists as street-level bureaucrats: Leveraging the political nature of everyday practice. *Canadian Journal of Occupational Therapy, 87*(2), 137–143. https://doi.org/10.1177/0008417419892712

Alinsky, S. D. (1971). *Rules for radicals: A practical primer for realistic radicals.* Random House.

American Occupational Therapy Association. (2014). Occupational therapy practice framework: Domain and process (3rd ed.). *American Journal of Occupational Therapy, 68*(S1), S1–S48. https://doi.org/10.5014/ajot.2014.682006

American Occupational Therapy Association. (2016). *Occupational therapy's role with school settings.* https://www.aota.org/~/media/Corporate/Files/AboutOT/Professionals/WhatIsOT/CY/Fact-Sheets/School%20Settings%20fact%20sheet.pdf

Americans with Disabilities Act. (1990). *Americans with disabilities act of 1990, U.S. equal employment opportunity commission.* https://www.eeoc.gov/americans-disabilities-act-1990-original-text

Anaby, D., Law, M., Coster, W., Bedell, G., Khetani, M., Avery, L., & Teplicky, R. (2014). The mediating role of the environment in explaining participation of children and youth with and without disabilities across home, school, and community. *Archives of Physical Medicine and Rehabilitation, 95,* 908–917. https://doi.org/10.1016/j.apmr.2014.01.005

Andreassen, M., Hemmingsson, H., Boman, I.-L., Danielsson, H., & Jaarsma, T. (2020). Feasibility of an intervention for patients with cognitive impairment using an interactive digital calendar with mobile phone reminders (RemindMe) to improve the performance of activities in everyday life. *International Journal of Environmental Research and Public Health, 17*(7), 2222. https://doi.org/10.3390/ijerph17072222

Aoyama, H., & Aflatoony, L. (2020). *HomeModAR: A home intervention augmented reality tool for occupational therapists.* Extended abstracts of the 2020 CHI conference on human factors in computing systems. ACM. 1–7. Web.

Altay, B. (2017). Developing empathy towards older adults in design. *Educational Gerontology, 43*(4), 198-208. DOI: 10.1080/03601277.2016.1273733

Bailliard, A., Dallman, A., Carroll, A., Lee, B., & Szendrey, S. (2020). Doing occupational justice: A central dimension of everyday occupational therapy. *Canadian Journal of Occupational Therapy, 87*(1), 144–152. https://doi.org/10.1177/0008417419898930

Baldassin, V., Shimizu, H. E., & Fachin-Martins, E. (2018). Computer assistive technology and associations with quality of life for individuals with spinal cord injury: A systematic review. *Quality of Life Research, 27*(3), 597–607.

Benson, J. D., Breisinger, E., & Roach, M. (2019). Sensory-based intervention in the schools: A survey of occupational therapy practitioners. *Journal of Occupational Therapy, Schools, & Early Intervention, 12*(1), 115–128. https://doi.org/10.1080/19411243.2018.1496872

Bonnard, M., & Anaby, D. (2016). Enabling participation of students through school-based occupational therapy services: Towards a broader scope of practice. *British Journal of Occupational Therapy, 79*(3), 188–192. https://doi.org/10.1177/0308022615612807

Bourke-Taylor, H. M., Cotter, C., Lalor, A., & Johnson, L. (2018). School success and participation for students with cerebral palsy: A qualitative study exploring multiple perspectives. *Disability and Rehabilitation, 40*(18), 2163–2171. https://doi.org/10.1080/09638288.2017.1327988

Bronfenbrenner, U. (1979). *The ecology of human development.* Harvard University Press.

Brown, C., Campbell-Rempel, M. A., Diamond-Burchuk, L., Johnson, L., Leclair, L., Mendez, L., Restall, G., & Ripat, J. (2019). Together we are stronger: Collective reconciliation action. *Occupational Therapy Now, 21*(4), 20–21. https://caot.ca/document/6761/July_OTNow_2019_test.pdf

Brown, D. M., Ross, T., Leo, J., Buliung, R. N., Shirazipour, C. H., Latimer-Cheung, A. E., & Arbour-Nicitopoulos, K. P. (2021). A scoping review of evidence-informed recommendations for designing inclusive playgrounds. *Frontiers in Rehabilitation Sciences, 2,* 3. https://doi.org/10.3389/fresc.2021.664595

Burns, S. P., Pickens, N. D., & Smith, R. O. (2017). Interprofessional Client-Centered Reasoning Processes in Home Modification Practice. *Journal of Housing for the Elderly, 31*(3), 213–228, DOI: 10.1080/02763893.2017.1280579

Cairney, P., & Kwiatkowski, R. (2017). How to communicate effectively with policymakers. *Palgrave Communications, 3,* Article 37. https://doi.org/10.1057/s41599-017-0046-8

Cairney, P., & Oliver, K. (2017). Evidence-based policymaking is not like evidence-based medicine, so how far should you go to bridge the divide between evidence and policy? *Health Research Policy and Systems, 15,* Article 35. https://doi.org/10.1186/s12961-017-0192-x

Canada Ministers Responsible for Seniors. (2016). *Thinking about aging in place.* https://www.canada.ca/en/employment-social-development/corporate/seniors/forum/aging.html

Canada Mortgage and Housing Corporation. (2018). *Accessible housing by design.* CMHC-SCHL. https://www.cmhc-schl.gc.ca/en/professionals/industry-innovation-and-leadership/industry-expertise/accessible-adaptable-housing/accessible-housing-by-design

Carlisle, S. (2000). Health promotion, advocacy and health inequalities: A conceptual framework. *Health Promotion International, 15*(4), 369–376. https://doi.org/10.1093/heapro/15.4.369

CAST. (2022). *The UDL guidelines.* https://udlguidelines.cast.org/

Centre for Excellence in Universal Design. (2020). *The 7 principles.* https://universaldesign.ie/what-is-universal-design/the-7-principles/

Centers for Disease Control and Prevention. (2015). *Check for safety: A home fall prevention checklist for older adults.* https://www.cdc.gov/steadi/pdf/check_for_safety_brochure-a.pdf

Christian, H., Knuiman, M., Divitini, M., Foster, S., Hooper, P., Boruff, B., Bull, F., & Giles-Corti, B. (2017). A Longitudinal Analysis of the Influence of the Neighborhood Environment on Recreational Walking within the Neighborhood: Results from RESIDE. *Environmental Health Perspectives, 125*(7), 1–10. DOI: 10.1289/EHP823

Chiu, T. (2011). *Safety assessment of function and the environment for rehabilitation-health outcome measurement and evaluation: SAFER-HOME version 4 manual.* VHA Home HealthCare.

Collins, B. (2014). Universal design for learning: What occupational therapy can contribute. *Occupational Therapy Now, 16*(5), 22–23.

Collins, P. H. (2015). Intersectionality's definitional dilemmas. *Annual Review of Sociology, 41,* 1–20.

Cook, A. M., & Polgar, J. M. (2015). *Cook and Hussey's assistive technologies: Principles and practice* (4th ed.). Elsevier/Mosby.

Crenshaw, K. (1991). Mapping the margins: Intersectionality, identity politics, and violence against women of color. *Stanford Law Review, 43*(6), 1241–1299. https://doi.org/10.2307/1229039

Cristoforetti, A., Gennai, F., & Rodeschini, G. (2011). Home sweet home: The emotional construction of places. *Journal of Aging Studies, 25,* 225–232. https://doi.org/10.1016/j.jaging.2011.03.006

Dalton, J., & Kahute, T. (2016). Why Empathy and Customer Closeness is Crucial for Design Thinking. *Design Management Review. 27.* 20–27. DOI: 10.1111/drev.12004

D'Arcangelis, C. L. (2018). Revelations of a white settler woman scholar-activist: The fraught promise of self-reflexivity. *Cultural Studies ↔ Critical Methodologies, 18*(5), 339–353. https://doi.org/10.1177/1532708617750675

de Sousa Santos, B. S. (2013). *Epistemologies of the south: Justice against epistemicide.* Paradigm Publishers.

Denny-Brown, N., O'Day, B., & McLeod, S. (2015). Staying employed services and supports for workers with disabilities. *Journal of Disability Policy Studies, 26*(2), 124–131. https://doi.org/10.1177/1044207315583899

Dhamoon, R., & Hankivsky, O. (2011). Why the theory and practice of intersectionality matter to health research and policy. In O. Hankivsky (Ed.), *Health inequities in Canada: Intersectional frameworks and practices* (pp. 16–50). UBC Press.

Du Toit, S. H., Casteleijn, D., Adams, F., & Morgan-Brown, M. (2019). Occupational justice within residential aged care settings–time to focus on a collective approach. *British Journal of Occupational Therapy, 82*(9), 578–581. https://doi.org/10.1177/0308022619840180

Dublin City University. (2021). *Principles – Age-friendly university.* https://www.dcu.ie/agefriendly/principles-age-friendly-university

Dunn, W., Brown, C., & McGuigan, A. (1994). The ecology of human performance: A framework for considering the effect of context. *American Journal of Occupational Therapy, 48*(7), 595–607. https://doi.org/10.5014/ajot.48.7.595

Durocher, E., Gibson, B. E., & Rappolt, S. (2014). Occupational justice: A conceptual review. *Journal of Occupational Science, 21,* 418–430. https://doi.org/10.1080/14427591.2013.775692

Egan, M., & Restall, G. (2022). The Canadian model of occupational participation. In M. Egan & G. Restall (Eds.), *Promoting occupational participation: Collaborative relationship-focused occupational therapy* (pp. 75–95). CAOT.

Emery-Whittington, I. G. (2021). Occupational justice—Colonial business as usual? Indigenous observations from Aotearoa New Zealand. *Canadian Journal of Occupational Therapy, 88*(2), 153–162. https://doi.org/10.1177/00084174211005891

Emery-Whittington, I., & Maro, B. T. (2018). Decolonising occupation: Causing social change to help our ancestors rest and our descendants thrive. *New Zealand Journal of Occupational Therapy, 65*(1), 12–19.

Ermine, W. (2006). The ethical space of engagement. *Indigenous Law Journal, 6.* https://jps.library.utoronto.ca/index.php/ilj/article/view/27669/20400

Falk, H., Wijk, H., Persson, L. O., & Falk, K. (2013). A sense of home in residential care. *Scandinavian Journal of Caring Sciences, 27*(4), 999–1009. https://doi.org/10.1111/scs.12011

Farias, L., & Rudman, D. L. (2019). Challenges in enacting occupation-based social transformative practices: A critical dialogical study. *Canadian Journal of Occupational Therapy, 86*(3), 243–252. https://doi.org/10.1177/0008417419828798

Fawole, O. I., Okedare, O. O., & Reed, E. (2021). Home was not a safe haven: women's experiences of intimate partner violence during the COVID-19 lockdown in Nigeria. *BMC Women's Health, 21*(1), 1–7. https://doi.org/10.1186/s12905-021-01177-9

Fleming-Castaldy, R. P. (2015). A macro perspective for client-centred practice in curricula: Critique and teaching methods. *Scandinavian Journal of Occupational Therapy, 22*(4), 267–276. https://doi.org/10.3109/11038128.2015.1013984

Galvaan, R. (2012). Occupational choice: The significance of socio-economic and political factors. In G. Whiteford & C. Hocking (Eds.), *Occupational science: Society, inclusion, participation* (1st ed., pp. 152–162). Blackwell Publishing.

Galvaan, R. (2021). Generative disruption through occupational science: Enacting possibilities for deep human connection. *Journal of Occupational Science, 28*(1), 6–18. https://doi.org/10.1080/14427591.2020.1818276

Galvaan, R., & Peters, L. (2013). *Occupation-based community development framework.* https://vula.uct.ac.za/access/content/group/9c29ba04-b1ee-49b9-8c85-9a468b556ce2/OBCDF/pages/intro.html

Galvaan, R., & Peters, L. (2017a). Occupation-based community development: A critical approach to occupational therapy. In S. Dsouza, R. Galvaan, & E. Ramugondo (Eds.), *Concepts in occupational therapy: Understanding southern perspectives* (pp. 172–187). Manipal University Press.

Galvaan, R., & Peters, L. (2017b). Occupation-based community development: Confronting the politics of occupation. In D. Sakellariou & N. Pollard (Eds.), *Occupational therapies without borders: Integrating justice with practice* (pp. 283–291). Elsevier.

Gardner, P. J. (2011). Natural neighborhood networks—Important social networks in the lives of older adults aging in place. *Journal of Aging Studies, 25,* 263–271.

Gerlach, A. J., Teachman, G., Laliberte-Rudman, D., Aldrich, R. M., & Huot, S. (2018). Expanding beyond individualism: Engaging critical perspectives on occupation. *Scandinavian Journal of Occupational Therapy, 25*(1), 35–43. https://doi.org/10.1080/11038128.2017.1327616

Gibson, C. (2020). When the river runs dry: Leadership, decolonization and healing in occupational therapy. *New Zealand Journal of Occupational Therapy, 67*(1), 11–20.

Gibson, C., Butler, C., Henaway, C., Dudgeon, P., & Curtin, M. (2015). Indigenous peoples and human rights: Some considerations for the occupational therapy profession in Australia. *Australian Occupational Therapy Journal, 62*(3), 214–218. https://doi.org/10.1111/1440-1630.12185

Gunn, L. D., Mavoa, S., Boulangé, C., Hooper, P., Kavanagh, A., & Giles-Corti, B. (2017). Designing healthy communities: creating evidence on metrics for built environment features associated with walkable neighbourhood activity centres. *International Journal of Behavioral Nutrition & Physical Activity, 14,* 1–12. DOI 10.1186/s12966-017-0621-9

Hammell, K. R. W. (2017). Critical reflections on occupational justice: Toward a rights-based approach to occupational opportunities. *Canadian Journal of Occupational Therapy, 84*(1), 47–57. https://doi.org/10.1177/0008417416654501

Hammell, K. W. (2020). Making choices from the choices we have: The contextual-embeddedness of occupational choice. *Canadian Journal of Occupational Therapy, 87*(5), 400–411. https://doi.org/10.1177/0008417420965741

Hammell, K. W. (2021). Social and structural determinants of health: Exploring occupational therapy's structural (in)competence. *Canadian Journal of Occupational Therapy, 88*(4), 365–374. https://doi.org/10.1177/00084174211046797

Hammell, K. W. (2022). Securing occupational rights by addressing capabilities: A professional obligation. *Scandinavian Journal of Occupational Therapy, 29*(1), 1–12. https://doi.org/10.1080/11038128.2021.1895308

Hasselkus, B. R., & Dickie, V. A. (2021). *The meaning of everyday occupation* (3rd ed.). Slack Incorporated.

Hoffman, K., & Dupont, J. (1992). *Community health centres and community development.* Health and Welfare Canada.

Hwang, E., Cummings, L., Sixsmith, A., & Sixsmith, J. (2011). Impacts of home modifications on aging-in-place. *Journal of Housing for the Elderly, 25*(3), 246–257. https://doi.org/10.1080/02763893.2011.595611

Hwang, N.-K., & Shim, S.-H. (2021). Use of virtual reality technology to support the home modification process: A scoping review. *International Journal of Environmental Research and Public Health, 18*(21), 11096. https://doi.org/10.3390/ijerph182111096

Hyde, E. T., Omura, J. D., Watson, K. B., Fulton, J. E., & Carlson, S. A. (2019). Step It Up! Prioritization of Community Supports for Walking Among US Adults. *American Journal of Health Promotion, 33*(8), 1134–1143. DOI 10.1177/0890117119856550

Hyett, N., McKinstry, C. E., Kenny, A., & Dickson-Swift, V. (2015). Community-centred practice: Occupational therapists improving the health and wellbeing of populations. *Australian Occupational Therapy Journal, 63*, 5–8. https://doi.org/10.1111/1440-1630.12222

Iwarsson, S., & Ståhl, A. (2003). Accessibility, usability and universal design—Positioning and definition of concepts describing person-environment relationships. *Disability and Rehabilitation, 25*, 57–66. https://doi.org/10.1080/dre.25.2.57.66

Iwarsson, S., Ståhl, A., & Carlsson, G. (2003). Accessible transportation: Novel occupational therapy perspectives. In L. Letts, P. Rigby, & D. Stewart (Eds.), *Using environments to enable occupational performance* (pp. 235–251). SLACK.

Jacobson, D., & Mustafa, N. (2019). Social identity map: A reflexivity tool for practicing explicit positionality in critical qualitative research. *International Journal of Qualitative Methods, 18*, 1–12. https://doi.org/10.1177/1609406919870075

Jamwal, R., Jarman, H. K., Roseingrave, E., Douglas, J., & Winkler, D. (2020). Smart home and communication technology for people with disability: A scoping review. *Disability and Rehabilitation Assistive Technology, 12*(9), 1–21. https://doi.org/10.1080/17483107.2020.1818138

Job Accommodation Network. (n.d.). *A to Z of disabilities and accommodations.* https://askjan.org/

Kania, J., Kramer, M., & Senge, P. (2018). *The waters of systems change.* https://www.fsg.org/publications/water_of_systems_change

Karlsson, P., Johnston, C., & Barker, K. (2018). Influences on students' assistive technology use at school: The views of classroom teachers, allied health professionals, students with cerebral palsy and their parents. *Disability and Rehabilitation: Assistive Technology, 13*(8), 763–771. https://doi.org/10.1080/17483107.2017.1373307

Kielhofner, G. (2008). *Model of human occupation: Theory and application* (4th ed.). Lippincott Wilkins & Williams.

Kinsella, E. A., & Whiteford, G. E. (2009). Knowledge generation and utilisation in occupational therapy: Towards epistemic reflexivity. *Australian Occupational Therapy Journal, 56*, 249–258. https://doi.org/10.1111/j.1440-1630.2007.00726.x

Kronenberg, F., & Pollard, N. (2006). Political dimensions of occupation and the roles of occupational therapy. *AJOT: American Journal of Occupational Therapy, 60*(6), 617–625. https://link.gale.com/apps/doc/A208275868/HRCA?u=univmanitoba&sid=bookmark-HRCA&xid=964f7a4e

Kylén, M., Löfqvist, C., Haak, M., & Iwarsson, S. (2019). Meaning of home and health dynamics among younger older people in Sweden. *European Journal of Ageing, 16*(3), 305–315. https://doi-org.ezp.twu.edu/10.1007/s10433-019-00501-5

Lauckner, H., Krupa, T., & Paterson, M. (2011). Conceptualizing community development: Occupational therapy practice at the intersection of health services and community. *Canadian Journal of Occupational Therapy, 78*, 260–268. https://doi.org/10.2182/cjot.2011.78.4.8

Lauckner, H., Leclair, L., & Yamamoto, C. (2019). Moving beyond the individual: Occupational therapists' multi-layered work with communities. *British Journal of Occupational Therapy, 82*(2), 101–111. https://doi.org/10.1177/0308022618797249

Law, M. (1991). The environment: A focus for occupational therapy. *The Canadian Journal of Occupational Therapy, 58*(4), 171. https://doi.org/10.1177/000841749105800404

Law, M., Cooper, B., Strong, S., Stewart, D., Rigby, P., & Letts, L. (1996). The person-environment-occupation model: A transactive approach to occupational performance. *Canadian Journal of Occupational Therapy, 63*, 9–23. https://doi.org/10.1177/000841749606300103

Law, M., Di Rezze, B., & Bradley, L. (2010). Environmental change to improve outcomes. In M. Law & M. A. McColl (Eds.), *Interventions, effects, and outcomes in occupational therapy: Adults and older adults* (pp. 155–182). SLACK.

Leclair, L. (2010). Re-examining concepts of occupation and occupation-based models: Occupational therapy and community development. *Canadian Journal of Occupational Therapy, 77*, 15–21. https://doi.org/10.2182/cjot.2010.77.1.3

Leclair, L., Ashcroft, M., Canning, T., & Lisowski, M. (2016). Preparing for community development practice: A Delphi study of Canadian occupational therapists. *Canadian Journal of Occupational Therapy, 83*(4), 226–236. https://doi.org/10.1177/0008417416631773

Leclair, L. L., Lauckner, H., & Yamamoto, C. (2019). An occupational therapy community development practice process. *Canadian Journal of Occupational Therapy, 86*(5), 345–356. https://doi.org/10.1177/0008417419832457

Levack, W., & Thornton, K. (2017). Opportunities for a meaningful life for working-aged adults with neurological conditions living in residential aged care facilities: A review of qualitative research. *British Journal of Occupational Therapy, 80*(10), 608–619. https://doi.org/10.1177/0308022617722736

Lewis, A. L. (2020). *Developing competencies for public policy advocacy: A comparative case analysis* [Electronic thesis and dissertation repository]. 7500. https://ir.lib.uwo.ca/etd/7500

Lindsay, S., Cagliostro, E., & Carafa, G. (2018). A systematic review of workplace disclosure and accommodation requests among youth and young adults with disabilities. *Disability and Rehabilitation, 40*(25), 2971–2986. https://doi.org/10.1080/09638288.2017.1363824

Liu, L., Stroulia, E., Nikolaidis, I., Miguel-Cruz, A., & Rios Rincon, A. (2016). Smart homes and home health monitoring technologies for older adults: A systematic review. *International Journal of Medical Informatics, 91*, 44–59. https://doi.org/10.1016/j.ijmedinf.2016.04.007

Malfitano, A., & Lopes, R. (2018). Social occupational therapy: Committing to social change. *New Zealand Journal of Occupational Therapy, 65*(1), 20–26.

Malfitano, A. P. S., Lopes, R. E., Magalhães, L., & Townsend, E. A. (2014). Social occupational therapy: Conversations about a Brazilian experience. *Canadian Journal of Occupational Therapy, 81*(5), 298–307. https://doi.org/10.1177/0008417414536712

Marasinghe, K. M. (2016). Assistive technologies in reducing caregiver burden among informal caregivers of older adults: A systematic review. *Disability and Rehabilitation, 11*, 353–360. https://doi.org/10.3109/17483107.2015.1087061

Mayock, P., Parker, S., & Murphy, A. (2021). Family "turning point" experiences and the process of youth becoming homeless. *Child & Family Social Work, 26*(3), 415–424. DOI 10.1111/cfs.12823

Mehta, V., & Bosson, J. K. (2010). Third places and the social life of streets. *Environment and Behavior, 42*, 779–805.

McNicholl, A., Casey, H., Desmond, D., & Gallagher, P. (2021). The impact of assistive technology use for students with disabilities in higher education: a systematic review. *Disability and Rehabilitation: Assistive Technology, 16*(2), 130–143. https://doi.org/10.1080/17483107.2019.1642395

Mitty, E., & Flores, S. (2009). There's no place like home. *Geriatric Nursing, 30*, 126–129. https://doi.org/10.1016/j.gerinurse.2009.01.004

Moore, A. J., Anderson, C., Carter, B., & Coad, J. (2010). Appropriated landscapes: The intrusion of technology and equipment into the homes and lives of families with a child of complex needs. *Journal of Child Health Care, 14*, 3–5.

Morgan-Brown, M., & Chard, G. (2014). Comparing communal environments using the Assessment Tool for Occupation and Social Engagement: Using interactive occupation and social engagement as outcome measures. *British Journal of Occupational Therapy, 77*(2), 50–58. https://doi.org/10.4276/030802214X13916969446994

Mortenson, W. B., Demers, L., Fuhrer, M., Jutai, J., Lenker, J., & DeRuyter, F. (2012). How assistive technology use by individuals with disabilities impacts their caregivers: A systematic review of the research evidence. *American Journal of Physical Medicine & Rehabilitation, 91,* 984–998. https://doi.org/10.1097/PHM .0b013e318269eceb

Mowell, M., Richter, L., & Jewell, V. (2022). Exploration of common sensory interventions utilized in school-based occupational therapy. *Journal of Occupational Therapy, Schools, & Early Intervention.* https://doi.org/10.1080/19411243.2022.2027839

National Collaborating Centre for Determinants of Health. (2014). *Let's talk: Moving upstream.* http://nccdh.ca/images/uploads/ Moving_Upstream_Final_En.pdf

National Collaborating Centre for Determinants of Health. (2015). *Let's talk: Advocacy and health equity.* National Collaborating Centre for Determinants of Health, St. Francis Xavier University. https://nccdh .ca/resources/entry/lets-talk-advocacy-and-health-equity

National Collaborating Centre for Health Public Policy. (2020). *Understanding public policy agenda setting using the 4P's model: Power, perception, potency and proximity.* https://ccnpps-ncchpp.ca/ understanding-public-policy-agenda-setting-using-the-4-ps-model- power-perception-potency-and-proximity/

Nixon, S. A. (2019). The coin model of privilege and critical allyship: Implications for health. *BMC Public Health, 19,* Article 1637. https:// doi.org/10.1186/s12889-019-7884-9

Ohlén, J., Ekman, I., Zingmark, K., Bolmsjö, I., & Benzein, E. (2014). Conceptual development of "at-homeness" despite illness and disease: a review. *International journal of qualitative studies on health and well-being, 9,* 23677. doi.org/10.3402/qhw.v9.23677

O Shea, E. C., Pavia, S., Dyer, M., Craddock, G. & Murphy, N. (2016) Measuring the design of empathetic buildings: a review of universal design evaluation methods. *Disability and Rehabilitation: Assistive Technology, 11*(1), 13–21. DOI: 10.3109/17483107.2014.921842

Padkapayeva, K., Posen, A., Yazdani, A., Buettgen, A., Mahood, Q., & Tompa, E. (2017). Workplace accommodations for persons with physical disabilities: Evidence synthesis of the peer-reviewed literature. *Disability and Rehabilitation, 39*(21), 2134–2147. https://doi.org/ 10.1080/09638288.2016.1224276

Pickens, N., & Burns, S. (2018). Home Modifications. In B. A. Boyt Schell & J. Schell (Eds.), *Clinical and professional reasoning in occupational therapy* (2nd ed.). Lippincott Williams & Wilkins.

Picotin, J., Beaudoin, M., Hélie, S., Martin, A. É., & Carrier, A. (2021). Occupational therapists as social change agents: Exploring factors that influence their actions. *Canadian Journal of Occupational Therapy, 88*(3), 231–243. https://doi.org/10.1177/ 00084174211022891

Pollard, N., & Sakellariou, D. (2014). The occupational therapist as a political being. *Cadernos de Terapia Ocupacional da UFSCar, 22*(3), 643–652. https://doi.org/10.4322/cto.2014.087

Reitz, S. M., Scaffa, M. E., & Merryman, M. B. (2014). *Theoretical frameworks for community-based practice. Occupational therapy in community-based practice settings* (2nd ed., pp. 31–50). F. A. Davis.

Rigby, P., Ryan, S. E., & Campbell, K. A. (2011). Electronic aids to daily living and quality of life for persons with tetraplegia. *Disability and Rehabilitation: Assistive Technology, 6,* 260–267. https://doi.org/10.31 09/17483107.2010.522678

Rioux, L., & Werner, C. (2011). Residential satisfaction among aging people living in place. *Journal of Environmental Psychology, 31,* 158–169.

Ripat, J., & Becker, P. (2012). Playground usability: What do playground users say? *Occupational Therapy International, 19*(3), 144–153. https://doi.org/10.1002/oti.1331

Ripat, J., Verdonck, M., & Carter, R. J. (2018). The meaning ascribed to wheeled mobility devices by individuals who use wheelchairs and scooters: A metasynthesis. *Disability and Rehabilitation: Assistive Technology, 13*(3), 253–262. https://doi.org/10.1080/17483107.2017.1306594

Ripat, J., Verdonck, M., Gacek, C., & McNicol, S. (2019). A qualitative metasynthesis of the meaning of speech-generating devices for people with complex communication needs. *Augmentative and Alternative Communication, 35*(2), 69–79. https://doi.org/10.1080/07434618 .2018.1513071

Ripat, J., & Woodgate, R. (2017). The importance of assistive technology in the productivity pursuits of young adults with disabilities. *WORK: A Journal of Prevention, Assessment, and Rehabilitation, 57,* 455–468. https://doi.org/10.3233/WOR-172580

Rothman, J., & Tropman, J. E. (1987). Models of community organization and macro practice perspectives: Their mixing and phasing. In F. M. Cox, J. L. Erlich, J. Rothman, & J. E. Tropman (Eds.), *Strategies of community organization: Macro practice* (4th ed., pp. 26–63). Peacock.

Rudman, D. L. (2021). Mobilizing occupation for social transformation: Radical resistance, disruption, and re-configuration. *Canadian Journal of Occupational Therapy, 88*(2), 96–107. https://doi .org/10.1177/00084174211020836

Saarnio, L., Boström, A.-M., Hedman, R., Gustavsson, P., & Öhlén, J. (2019). Enabling At-Homeness for Older People With Life- Limiting Conditions: A Participant Observation Study From Nursing Homes. *Global Qualitative Nursing Research.* DOI 10.1177/2333 393619881636

Schneidert, M., Hurst, R., Miller, J., & Ustün, B. (2003). The role of environment in the International Classification of Functioning, Disability and Health (ICF). *Disability and Rehabilitation, 25*(11–12), 588–595. https://doi.org/10.1080/0963828031000137090

Scovel, G., & Lichter, M. (2016). Come on in. *Paraplegic News, 70*(1), 29–33.

Seamon, D. (2018). *Life takes place: Phenomenology, lifeworlds, and place making.* Routledge.

Sen, A. (2003). Development as capability expansion. In S. Fukuda-Parr & A. K. S. Kumar (Eds.), *Readings in human development* (pp. 41–58). Oxford University Press.

Shin, J. H. (2015). Declining body, institutional life, and making home—Are they at odds? *HEC Forum, 27*(2), 107–125. https://doi .org/10.1007/s10730-015-9269-5

Shogren, K. A., Luckasson, R., & Schalock, R. L. (2014). The definition of "context" and its application in the field of intellectual disability. *Journal of Policy and Practice in Intellectual Disabilities, 11*(2), 109–116. https://doi.org/10.1111/jppi.12077

Shogren, K. A., Luckasson, R., & Schalock, R. L. (2021). Leveraging the power of context in disability policy development, implementation, and evaluation: Multiple applications to enhance personal outcomes. *Journal of Disability Policy Studies, 31*(4), 230–243. https://doi .org/10.1177/1044207320923656

Siebert, C., Smallfield, S., & Stark, S. (2014). *Occupational therapy practice guidelines for home modifications.* AOTA Press.

Stadnyk, R., Townsend, E., & Wilcock, A. (2010). Occupational justice. In C. H. Christiansen & E. A. Townsend (Eds.), *Introduction to occupation: The art and science of living* (2nd ed., pp. 329–353). Pearson.

Steinfeld, E., & Maisel, J. (2012). *Universal design: Creating inclusive environments.* Wiley.

Steinfeld, E., & White, J. (2010). *Inclusive housing: Design for diversity and equality.* Norton.

Stockman, J. K., Wood, B. A., & Anderson, K. M. (2021). Racial and Ethnic Differences in COVID-19 Outcomes, Stressors, Fear, and Prevention Behaviors Among US Women: Web-Based Cross-sectional Study. *Journal of Medical Internet Research, 23*(7), e26296. https://doi .org/10.2196/26296

Tanner, B., Tilse, C., & de Jonge, D. (2008). Restoring and sustaining home: The impact of home modifications on the meaning of home for older people. *Journal of Housing for the Elderly, 22,* 195–215. https://doi.org/10.1080/02763890802232048

The Gerontological Society of America. (2021). *Age-friendly university global network.* https://www.geron.org/programs-services/education-center/age-friendly-university-afu-global-network

Torjman, S. (2005). *What is policy?* https://maytree.com/wp-content/uploads/544ENG.pdf

Townsend, E. A., & Polatajko, H. J. (2013). *Enabling occupation II: Advancing an occupational therapy vision for health, well-being, & justice through occupation* (2nd ed.). Canadian Association of Occupational Therapists.

United Nations. (1948). *Universal declaration of human rights.* https://www.un.org/en/about-us/universal-declaration-of-human-rights

United Nations. (1969). *International convention on the elimination of all forms of racial discrimination, United Nations Human Rights Office of the High Commissioner.* https://ohchr.org/EN/ProfessionalInterest/Pages/CERD.aspx

United Nations. (1979). *Convention on the elimination of all forms of discrimination against women.* https://www.ohchr.org/sites/default/files/cedaw.pdf

United Nations. (1990). *Convention on the rights of the child, UNICEF.* https://www.unicef.org/child-rights-convention/convention-text

United Nations. (2006). *Article 27. Convention on the rights of persons with disabilities.* https://www.ohchr.org/EN/HRBodies/CRPD/Pages/ConventionRightsPersonsWithDisabilities.aspx#27

United Nations. (2007). *Declaration on the rights of indigenous peoples.* https://undocs.org/A/RES/61/295

United Nations. (2016). *Convention on the Rights of Persons with Disabilities (CRPD).* https://www.un.org/development/desa/disabilities/convention-on-the-rights-of-persons-with-disabilities.html\

Urbanowski, R., Shaw, L., & Chemmuttut, L. C. (2013). Occupational science value propositions in the field of public policy. *Journal of Occupational Science, 20*(4), 314–325. https://doi.org/10.1080/14427591.2013.806208

U.S. Access Board. (2004). *A federal agency committed to accessible design.* https://www.access-board.gov/

U.S. Department of Justice. (2010). *ADA standards for accessible design.* http://www.ada.gov/2010ADAstandards_index.htm

Van Bruggen, H., Craig, C., Kantartzis, S., Laliberte Rudman, D., Piskur, B., Pollard, N., Schiller, S., & Simó, S. (2020). Case studies for social transformation through occupation. *European Network of Occupational Therapy in Higher Education.* https://enothe.eu/wp-content/uploads/2020/06/ISTTON-booklet-final.pdf

van Gelder, N. E., van Haalen, D. L., Ekker, K., Ligthart, S. A., & Oertelt-Prigione, S. (2021). Professionals' views on working in the field of domestic violence and abuse during the first wave of COVID-19:

a qualitative study in the Netherlands. *BMC Health Services Research, 21*(1), 1–14. DOI: 10.1186/s12913-021-06674-z

Verdonck, M., & Maye, F. (2016). Enhancing occupational performance in the virtual context using smart technology. *British Journal of Occupational Therapy, 79*(6), 385–390. https://doi.org/10.1177/0308022615591172

Wada, M., Canham, S. L., Battersby, L., Sixsmith, J., Woolrych, R., Fang, M. L., & Sixsmith, A. (2020). Perceptions of home in long-term care settings: Before and after institutional relocation. *Ageing & Society, 40*(6), 1267–1290. https://doi.org/10.1017/S0144686X18001721

Wener, P., Diamond-Burchuk, L., Ripat, J., Belton, L., & Schwab, D. (2009). Promoting inclusive social environments using a sensory processing simulation. *Occupational Therapy Now, 11*(5), 20–22.

Wiles, J. L., Leibing, A., Guberman, N., Reeve, J., & Allen, R. E. S. (2012). The meaning of "aging in place" to older people. *Gerontologist, 52*(3), 357–366. https://doi.org/10.1093/geront/gnr098

Wolf, L., Ripat, J., Davis, E., Becker, P., & MacSwiggan, J. (2010). Applying an occupational justice framework. *Occupational Therapy Now, 12,* 15–18. https://doi.org/10.1111/j.1440-1630.1968.tb00253.x

Wong, J., Kallish, N., Crown, D., Capraro, P., Trierweiler, R., Wafford, Q. E., Tiema-Benson, L., Hassan, S., Engel, E., Tamayo, C., & Heinemann, A. W. (2021). Job accommodations, return to work and job retention of people with physical disabilities: A systematic review. *Journal of Occupational Rehabilitation, 31*(3), 474–490. https://doi.org/10.1007/s10926-020-09954-3

World Federation of Occupational Therapy. (2019). *Occupational therapy and human rights.* https://wfot.org/resources/occupational-therapy-and-human-rights

World Health Organization. (1986). Ottawa charter for health promotion. *Health Promotions, 1,* iii–v. https://doi.org/10.1093/heapro/1.4.405

World Health Organization. (2001). *International classification of functioning, disability and health.* Author. https://www.who.int/standards/classifications/international-classification-of-functioning-disability-and-health

Young, L. C. (2011). Universal housing: A critical component of a sustainable community. In W. Preiser & K. H. Smith (Eds.), *Universal design handbook* (2nd ed., pp. 24.3–25.13). McGraw-Hill.

Zafar, N., Rotenberg, M., & Rudnick, A. (2019). A systematic review of work accommodations for people with mental disorders. *Work, 64*(3), 461–475. https://doi.org/10.3233/WOR-193008

Zahariadis, N. (Ed.). (2016). *Handbook of public policy agenda setting.* Edward Elgar.

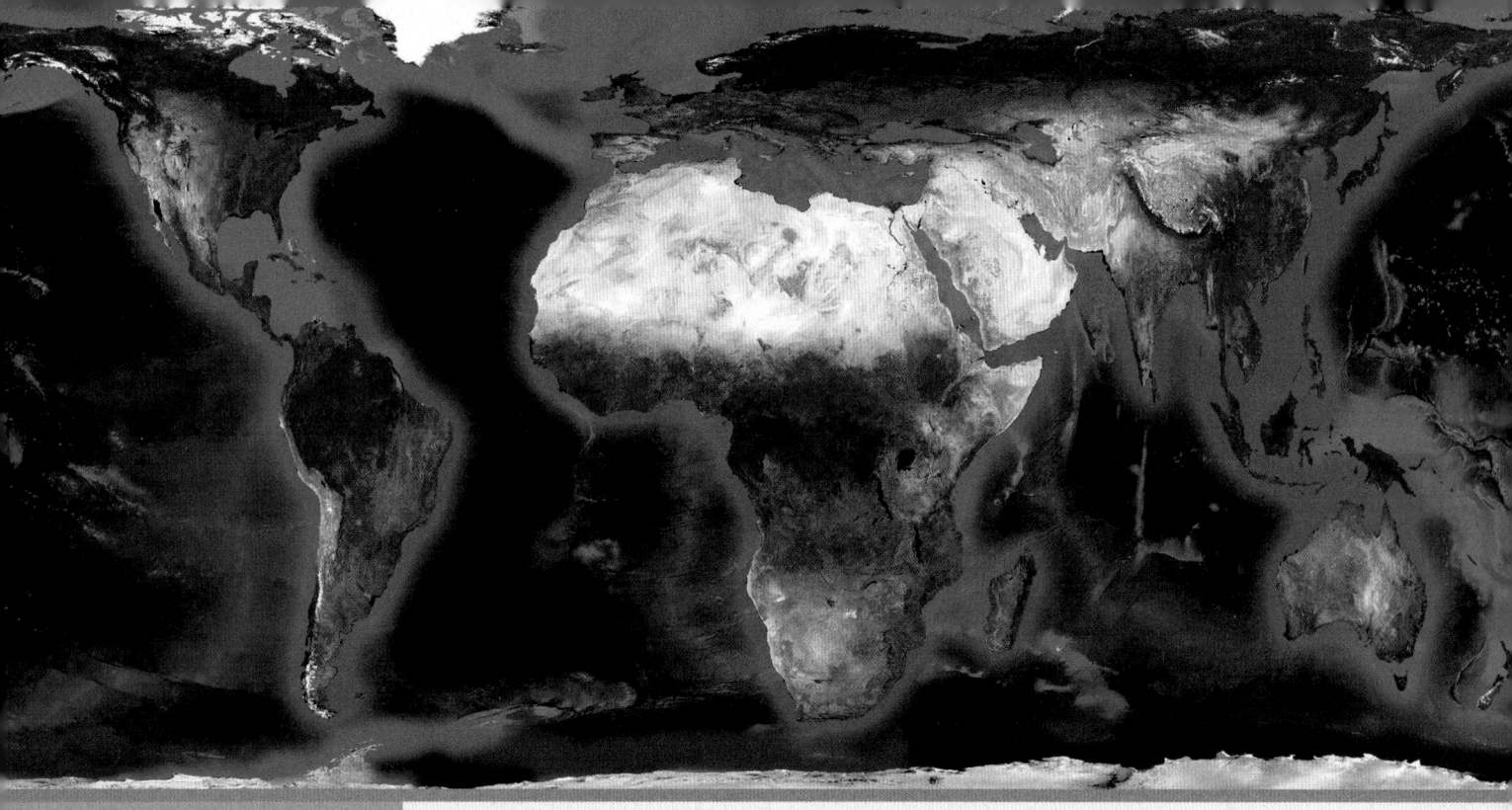

UNIT V

Core Concepts and Skills

Media Related to Core Concepts and Skills

Readings

● *Pandemic:* This poem by Lynn Ungar addresses how to deal with the anxiety of the coronavirus outbreak and the imposition of stay-at-home orders. It addresses spirituality more broadly. (2020) (Pandemic [lynnungar.com])

Movies

● *Twelve Angry Men:* An American courtroom drama written by Reginald Rose concerns the jury of a homicide trial. The play explores the deliberations and process of a jury on a homicide trial, in which a dozen "men with ties and a coat" decide the fate of a teenager accused of murdering his abusive father. At the beginning, they are nearly unanimous in concluding the youth is guilty. One man dissents, declaring him "not guilty," and he sows a seed of reasonable doubt. (1957)

● *The Biomedical Ethics in Film Program:* Launched in 1998 under the leadership of Dr Maren Monsen, this program specializes in producing innovative films on biomedical ethics. The films are created to inspire both medical students and the general public to experience and question the magnitude of the ethical dilemmas in healthcare facing our society today. (https://www.med.stanford.edu/medethicsfilms/films.html)

● *28 Days:* Gwen Cummings knows that she drinks a lot, but she doesn't believe it's a problem, and she decides that if it becomes an issue that she could stop drinking on her own. For Gwen to make progress, she has to acknowledge that she has a problem that requires support during 28 days in a facility. She needs the support not only of the staff, but also of the other patients who are going through their own issues with addiction. If she does eventually acknowledge the problem, she will also have to reconcile the events of her life. (2000)

● *Dopesick: Dealers, Doctors, and the Drug Company That Addicted America:* Account of America's opioid epidemic from the boardroom to the courtroom and into the living rooms of Americans. (2019)

Professional Reasoning in Practice

Barbara A. Boyt Schell and Angela M. Benfield

LEARNING OBJECTIVES

After reading this chapter, you will be able to:

1. Analyze important aspects of reasoning in occupational therapy (OT) practice.
2. Discuss how the reasoning process is embedded in the transactions that occur among the practitioner, client and practice context.
3. Identify the different facets of professional reasoning based on personal reflection, practitioners' descriptions, and OT stories.
4. Describe the process of developing competency and expertise in professional reasoning.
5. Explore the use of critical reflection and decision supports for effective professional reasoning.
6. Appreciate the challenges and benefits of interprofessional reasoning within teams for better client outcomes.

Introduction

Professional reasoning is the process that practitioners use to develop and provide occupational therapy (OT) services with individuals, groups, or populations. Providing ethical OT services requires the therapist to use professional knowledge and skills to plan, direct, perform, and reflect on client care. It is a complex and dynamic process that is connected directly to therapy action. Practitioners must reason in a given session. The process is called different names by different authors and professions, with the most common term being **clinical reasoning** (Young et al., 2020). In this chapter, and across the profession, the term *professional reasoning* is used because it reflects OT's range of practice settings, many of which are outside medical contexts, and because it more accurately reflects the thinking at various levels of care, such as planning care routines and practice standards (American Occupational Therapy Association [AOTA], 2020; Schell & Schell, 2018; Unsworth & Baker, 2016). When using these labels, the authors are talking about how therapists *actually think* when they are engaged in practice. This requires metacognitive analysis or, in simple terms, *thinking about thinking*. This is important because newcomers to the field might incorrectly understand professional reasoning as something that practitioners "choose to do" or confuse it with the many OT intervention theories. It is neither of those things. Whenever you are thinking about or doing OT for an identified individual or group, you are engaged in professional reasoning. It is not a question of *whether* you are doing it, but a question of *how well* you are doing it.

This chapter examines professional reasoning from several perspectives. To help you see real examples of the material discussed, OT Story 25.1 describes an encounter between an occupational therapist Terry and her client Mrs. Munro. This case is adapted from a real situation that was observed as part of a research study, although the names have been changed. Read this OT Story before continuing with the text, paying special attention to the different kinds of issues and problems that the OT practitioner must address. Then, keep referring to it as you read about the nature of professional reasoning.

OT STORY 25.1 TERRY AND MRS. MUNRO: DETERMINING APPROPRIATE RECOMMENDATIONS

Terry, an occupational therapist, goes up to a client's room in the neurology unit of a regional medical center. The client, Mrs. Munro, is a widow who lives alone in a house in town. She had a stroke—a right cerebrovascular accident (CVA)—and was brought by a neighbor to the hospital. Mrs. Munro has made a rapid recovery and demonstrates good return of her motor skills. She still has some left-sided weakness and incoordination, along with some cognitive problems. She is a delightful, pleasant older woman and is anxious to return home.

Terry is seeing this client for the third time, and her primary concern is to assess whether Mrs. Munro has any residual cognitive effects from her stroke that would put her at serious risk if she returned home alone. Terry plans to do some more in-depth activities of daily living with Mrs. Munro to see how well she demonstrates safety awareness. Terry thinks that she will probably have Mrs. Munro get out of bed, obtain her clothing and hygiene supplies, perform her morning hygiene routines at the sink, and then get dressed. Terry wants to see the degree to which Mrs. Munro is spontaneously able to manage these tasks as well as how good her judgment appears to be. Terry's thought is that if she can engage Mrs. Munro in several multistep activities that also require her to perform in different positions, Terry should be able to detect any cognitive and motor problems that pose a serious safety threat.

When Terry arrives at the room, she greets Mrs. Munro who says, "I am so excited. The doctor says I can go home today."

Terry thinks to herself, "I thought so." On the way to the room, Terry was worried that Mrs. Munro's physician tended to think that as soon as clients could physically get up, they should go home. Terry mentally defends the physician as she knows that in today's cost-conscious environment, doctors are under a lot of pressure not to keep patients in the hospital.

As Terry converses with Mrs. Munro about generalities, she notices that Mrs. Munro is already dressed in her housecoat. When she talks to Mrs. Munro about doing some self-care activities, it becomes apparent that Mrs. Munro has already completed her bathing and dressing routines, with help from a nurse. When Terry suggests that she perhaps brush her teeth and comb her hair, Mrs. Munro is happy to get up out of bed but notes that her neighbor never did bring in her dentures. Mrs. Munro sits on the edge of the bed and, after a reminder from Terry, puts on her slippers. She then stands and walks to the nearby sink, finds her comb, and combs her hair. While she is doing this, Terry looks around for some other ideas about what to do because Mrs. Munro has already completed the self-care tasks Terry had planned to do with her.

Terry's eyes light on some wilted flowers by the bed. She suggests to Mrs. Munro that she might want to dispose of the flowers and clean the vase so that it will be ready to pack when it is time to go home. Mrs. Munro agrees and proceeds to walk somewhat unsteadily over to the vase, picks it up and carries it to the sink, pulling out the dead flowers. Terry follows her, staying slightly behind and within reach of Mrs. Munro. When Mrs. Munro stops after removing the flowers, Terry suggests that she rinse out the vase, which she does. She then dries it and returns the vase to the bedside table. Terry reminds her to throw out the dead flowers. While Mrs. Munro does this, they talk some more about her plans to return home. She then sits with Mrs. Munro and has her complete a weekly planning activity.

Mrs. Munro tells Terry that she has lived in her home for 40 years, and even though her husband died more than 10 years ago, she still feels his presence there. He used to love her cooking, and she still cooks three meals a day for herself. Mrs. Munro starts to cry when they talk about cooking but then cheers up. Terry tells her that it might be safer if she had someone around the house for a few weeks until she recovers a bit more from her stroke. Mrs. Munro thinks that she can get some help from her neighbor. Terry says she is also going to suggest some home care therapy, just to make sure Mrs. Munro is safe in the kitchen, bathroom, and so on, noting, "We sure don't want to see you have a bad fall just when you are doing so well after your stroke."

After reviewing some coordination activities for Mrs. Munro's left hand, Terry says goodbye and leaves the room. Terry stops at the nurses' station to note in the chart that Mrs. Munro demonstrated good safety awareness in familiar tasks at her

(continued)

OT STORY 25.1 TERRY AND MRS. MUNRO: DETERMINING APPROPRIATE RECOMMENDATIONS (*continued*)

bedside but did require cueing to complete multistep tasks. She demonstrated mild difficulty with executive function, which could lead to unsuccessful discharge and subsequent readmission. Terry also notes some motor instability in task performance during ambulation. Terry recommends a referral to a home health OT practitioner "to assess safety and equipment needs during bathroom activities, meal preparation, and routine homemaking tasks." As she walks off the unit, Terry thinks to herself that Mrs. Munro did fairly well, but Terry remains concerned about the risks once Mrs. Munro goes home, particularly when she is tired. Terry wants someone to monitor Mrs. Munro in a familiar setting to see whether she handles her daily routines adequately. Terry would really like to see Mrs. Munro start to consider a more supported living environment, but the client does not have

either long-term care insurance or the personal finances to support that. Terry believes that she might at least be able to get one home care visit to evaluate home safety, particularly fall prevention. Staying in her own home seems to be Mrs. Munro's major goal, and Terry is going to do what she can to try to help her attain that goal. Terry will catch up with the social worker later to discuss the need for Mrs. Munro to have good support from any neighbors, friends, or relatives.

Questions

1. How did Terry develop her concerns about Mrs. Munro?
2. How did Terry know what to do when her initial plans did not work out?
3. What factors seem to guide Terry's recommendations at the end?

Reasoning in Practice: Using the Whole Self

With the OT Story in mind, let us explore the nature of reasoning during practice. First, all the reasoning in practice revolves around problem-solving: defining occupational performance concerns, determining the client's fit with their occupational requirements, and developing interventions that improve participation and function with the targeted occupations. Reasoning in practice relies heavily on heuristic reasoning because of the speed of interactions (Facione & Facione, 2008). Heuristic reasoning is thinking based on experience, and that sort of thinking relies on the mental model used by the individual therapist (Evans, 2003). These mental models represent a therapist's synthesis of formal professional theories, personal theories, and lived experiences that are used to define the problem and goal, identify the relationship between the factors (e.g., person, occupation, environment), and select intervention(s) that are likely to affect the outcome. Importantly, these mental models are dynamic and evolve with every interaction and reflection (Waldmann & Hagmayer, 2013).

Professional reasoning is also an **embodied process** involving the therapist's whole self as well as the context in which therapy occurs, which can be highly intuitive and beyond one's attention and grasp (Arntzen, 2018). That is one reason why reading an OT Story and being the practitioner in the situation are different experiences. Some professional reasoning involves straightforward thinking processes that the practitioner can easily describe. Examples include assessing occupational performance, such as daily living skills

and work behaviors. OT practitioners use their mental models to select assessment activities, attribute meaning to the observations, and identify relevant client factors that they believe contribute to occupational performance problems. Practitioners also attend to the contextual factors that affect performance. For instance, Terry was concerned about Mrs. Munro safety during self-care and home management activities in her home setting. Terry analyzed relevant contextual factors about the home setting and Mrs. Munro's social and financial situation. Terry had identified some impairments in cognition and motor control that were affecting her client's occupational performance skills. This was all information that Terry could readily share.

Part of Terry's professional reasoning involved knowledge that she gained from her senses. For instance, Terry used her sense of touch to feel the muscle tension (or lack of tension) in Mrs. Munro's affected arm when she was doing an activity. During her evaluation, Terry did some quick stretches to Mrs. Munro's elbow and wrist to determine whether she could feel evidence of spasticity, an abnormal reflex response that is commonly found in individuals who are recovering from a stroke. When Mrs. Munro stood up, Terry gauged the distance she stood from Mrs. Munro because Mrs. Munro was at some risk of falling. Terry was careful to stand not so close that she crowded or overprotected Mrs. Munro but close enough to protect her should she lose her balance. While close to Mrs. Munro, Terry could smell her, gaining a quick sense of possible hygiene or continence problems. Terry used her voice quality to display encouragement and support. Terry watched and listened carefully for clues about the nature of Mrs. Munro's emotional state. In particular, she watched facial expressions and listened for evidence of fear or insecurity during Mrs. Munro's performance of activities. All these sensations contributed to an image of Mrs. Munro that influenced Terry's practice.

There are other aspects of reasoning during therapy that are even harder to describe. Fleming (1994a) described this as "knowing more than we can tell" (p. 24). She explained that much of the profession's knowledge is practical knowledge, which is "seldom discussed and rarely described" (Fleming, 1994a, p. 25). This tacit knowledge, combined with the rich sensory aspects of actual practice, helps to explain why reading about therapy and doing therapy are such different experiences. Kinsella summarizes this deeper understanding of reasoning when she notes "the mind can be revealed in the embodied *doings* of a person, mind is revealed in *practices*" (Kinsella, 2018, p. 111). Hooper (2018) has also noted the importance of each practitioner's values, beliefs, and assumptions underpin their grasp of the therapy process. So, keep in mind that therapy always happens in the real world with real people, and you will see variations because each therapist is different. Therefore, it is critically important for thinking therapists to be conscious of their own beliefs, values, and assumptions and how they affect the decision-making process.

Theory and Practice

The outcome of the decision-making process by a therapist using their mental model is an action or a lack of action. Theories help practitioners to make decisions, although Cohn (1989) noted that the problems of practice rarely present themselves in the straightforward manner described in textbooks. Professional reasoning involves the naming and framing of problems based on a personal understanding of the client's situation (Schön, 1983). This mental model represents the individual's integration of professional knowledge; personal theories, values, beliefs, and experiences; and their interpretation of the client's mental model. Evidence suggests that even members of the same profession will have different conceptualizations of the same client and that these models may not be consistent with formal evidence/theory nor their professional paradigm (Fava & Morton, 2009; Pilecki et al., 2011). In other words, practitioners blend theories with their own personal and practice experiences to guide their actions. Importantly, evidence suggests that an individual's mental models may not represent what is known about the causal relationships between the factors affecting person–occupation–environment fit (Friston et al., 2014). An evidence-informed mental model (including local outcomes data) helps the practitioner to avoid unjustified assumptions or the use of ineffective therapy techniques (Benfield & Krueger, 2021) and supports ethical practice. Therefore, effective professional reasoning explicitly requires OT practitioners to reflect on the effect of

their actions on clients and the accuracy of their mental model used in the decision-making process. This reflection is used to compare how their experience and intervention activities were similar to or different from actions expected from theoretical understandings (Gambrill, 2012; Motycka et al., 2010). Self-assessment and reflection are improved by using outside sources of information against which to assess oneself. In Chapter 33, you will find more information about how theories inform practice as well as how our underlying assumptions shape our therapy actions. The point here is that although practice can (and should) be informed by professional and empirical theories, it is ultimately a result of how each therapist interprets each therapy situation and then acts on that understanding.

Cognitive Processes Underlying Professional Reasoning

In the OT Story, Terry had to remember, obtain, and manage a great deal of information quickly to provide effective and efficient intervention. How did she do it? Research findings from the field of cognitive psychology and medical clinical reasoning help to explain how practitioners process information and how experience combined with reflection fosters increasing routine expertise. *Routine expertise* is defined as the mastery of procedures that are highly efficient and accurate for addressing common problems (Bohle Carbonell & Dailey-Hebert, 2021). Individuals receive, store, and organize information in *frames* or *scripts*, which are complex representations or simulations representing typical problems and client situations gained from their experiences (Bruning et al., 1999; Carr & Shotwell, 2018; Norman, 2005). Through experience and critical reflection, they develop mental models that have rich relational connections between the factors causing or influencing the problem and those that are not important. This allows for faster decision-making (Durning et al., 2015; Klein, 2015).

The cognitive process underlying professional reasoning involves both working memory and long-term memory. Working memory is where the thinking occurs, and it can hold very few thoughts at a time. For example, the limitations on short-term memory are why you must look at the directions 2 or 3 times to correctly assemble something unfamiliar, such as a new toy or piece of furniture. Similarly, students and new practitioners find it challenging to try to keep all the important considerations in mind when dealing with a client or attempting a new assessment or intervention procedure. Practitioners with extensive experience have this information organized and stored in their long-term memories and thus do not have to actively juggle all the details. Norman's research with physicians suggests that practitioners create exemplars in their minds that serve to guide analysis of new cases (Norman, 2005).

In the OT Story, Terry probably learned many of the common problems associated with someone who has had a stroke when she was a student. Since graduation, she also has seen perhaps 100 people with strokes over the past several years. She has built up a general representation in her mind of what to expect when she receives a referral for someone who has had a stroke. She anticipates that many of these individuals will have extensive medical charts because they almost always have prior medical problems, such as diabetes and high blood pressure. She will not be surprised if the person is overweight. She expects to see impairments in cognition that often affect the person's ability to do everyday tasks, such as dressing, cooking, and driving. As part of her frame, Terry has built-in mental rules that help her to categorize and detect differences. For instance, although she knows that many people who have strokes have movement impairments, she knows that not all do. Furthermore, when movement is impaired, she expects individuals with a left CVA to have right-sided weakness and those with a right CVA to have left-sided weakness. In addition, she knows that a person's social support system is critical for promoting an adaptive response to disability. She may use certain cues, such as the presence or absence of frequent family visits, to prompt her to categorize a family as supportive or nonsupportive.

In addition to framing or "chunking" information, Terry also creates and uses scripts or procedural rules that guide her thinking (Bruning et al., 1999; Carr & Shotwell, 2018). Just as her mental frames help her to organize and retrieve her knowledge about common aspects of stroke, scripts help her to organize common occurrences or events. For instance, she understands that her role involves responding to the referral by seeing the client, writing her findings on the correct form, providing interventions, communicating verbally with the other team members, and developing discharge plans. Terry likely has scripts about the implications for clients with supportive families and those without. In her experience, a supportive family cares for its family member at home, regardless of the family's financial resources. Alternatively, clients with little family support are more likely to face institutional care. Terry knows the procedures for obtaining care for those who need support, and she works to balance the clients' preferences and abilities against her understanding of the environmental, financial, and social constraints. Again, these scripts are formed by Terry's observations and experiences over time and serve the purpose of helping her to anticipate likely events.

The mind appears to use frames, scripts, and exemplars to support effective processing of information by providing efficient mental frameworks for handling complex information (Carr & Shotwell, 2018; Norman, 2005). Each person individually constructs them. Critically, evidence suggests that these mental scaffolds can be highly influenced by cognitive biases and prone to errors (Saunders et al., 2019). Later in this chapter, we discuss strategies to avoid bias and improve professional reasoning.

Given all this complexity, it is no surprise that students and new practitioners often struggle to retain and effectively use their therapy knowledge. It takes time, repetition of experiences, and critical reflection on experience to develop effective reasoning. This reasoning is based on efficient storage in long-term memory, allowing for targeted use of short-term memory as therapy happens. Important aspects of the process are as follows (Roberts, 1996):

- **Cue acquisition:** Searching for helpful and targeted information through observation and questioning
- **Pattern recognition:** Noticing similarities and differences among situations
- **Limiting the problem space:** Using patterns to help focus cue acquisition and knowledge application on the most fruitful areas
- **Problem formulation:** Developing an explanation of what is going on, why it is going on, and what a better situation or outcome might be
- **Problem solution:** Identifying courses of action based on the problem formulation

These cognitive processes are interactive and rarely occur in a linear manner. Rather, the mind jumps around between the information at hand and that which has been stored up from prior learning while attempting to make sense of the situation.

Now that we have a better understanding of the basic systems our mind uses to support our professional reasoning, we turn our attention to research on the different aspects of professional reasoning that have surfaced from research on occupational therapists.

Aspects of Professional Reasoning

The purpose of professional reasoning is to effectively identify client problems addressed by OT. Although common processes underlie reasoning in practice, the focus of that mental activity appears to vary with the demands of the problems to be addressed (Fleming, 1991). Professional reasoning includes the systematic and routine integration of the information gathered from each of the perspectives. To effectively apply the OT process, the following reasoning about different aspects are likely to be needed over the course of intervention—scientific, narrative, pragmatic, ethical, and interactive—each of which is described in the following sections. The most agreed-upon elements of professional reasoning are listed in Table 25.1, along with the

TABLE 25.1	Aspects of Reasoning in Occupational Therapy	
Reasoning Aspect	Clues for Recognizing in Therapist Discussions	Examples of the Therapy Problems or Questions That Draw Out This Reasoning
Scientific		
Reasoning involving the use of applied logical and scientific methods, such as hypothesis testing, pattern recognition, theory-based decision-making, and statistical evidence	Impersonal, focused on the diagnosis, condition, guiding theory, evidence from research, or what "typically" happens with clients like the one being considered	What is the nature of the illness, injury, or development problem? What are the common impairments or disabilities resulting from this condition? What are the typical contextual factors that affect performance? What theories and research are available to guide assessment and intervention?
Diagnostic		
Investigative reasoning and analysis of cause or nature of conditions requiring OT intervention can be considered one component of scientific reasoning	Uses both personal and impersonal information. Therapists attempt to explain why client is experiencing problems using a blend of science- and client-based information.	What are the occupational performance problems this client has or may have in the future? What are the factors contributing to this problem (impairments, performance context)? How are these problems manifest (skills, habits, routines, occupational roles)?
Procedural		
Reasoning in which therapist considers and uses intervention routines for identified conditions; may be science based or may reflect the habits and culture of the intervention setting	Characterized by therapist using therapy regimes or routines thought to be effective with problems identified and that are typically used with clients in that setting	What evaluation and intervention protocols are applicable to this person's situation? How are clients like this usually handled in my setting?
Narrative		
Reasoning process used to make sense of people's particular circumstances; prospectively imagine the effect of illness, disability, or occupational performance problems on their daily lives; and create a collaborative story that is enacted with clients and families through intervention	Personal, focused on the client, including past, present, and anticipated future. Involves an appreciation of client culture as the basis for understanding client narrative; relates to the "so what" of the condition for the person's life	What is this person's life story? What is the nature of this person as an occupational being? How has the health condition affected the person's life story or ability to continue their life story? What occupational activities are most important to this person? What occupational activities are both meaningful to this person and useful for meeting therapy goals?
Pragmatic		
Practical reasoning that is used to fit therapy possibilities into the current realities of service delivery, such as scheduling options, payment for services, equipment availability, therapists' skills, management directives, and the personal situation of the therapist	Generally not focused on client or client's condition but rather on all the physical and social "stuff" that surrounds the therapy encounter as well as the therapist's internal sense of what they are capable of and have the time and energy to complete	Who referred this person, and why? Who is paying for services, and what are their rules? What family or caregiver resources are there to support intervention? What are the expectations of my supervisor and workplace? How much time do I have to see this person? What therapy space and equipment are available? What are my practice competencies?
Ethical		
Reasoning directed toward analyzing an ethical dilemma, generating alternative solutions, and determining actions to be taken; systematic approach to moral conflict	Tension is often evident as therapist attempts to determine what is the "right" thing to do particularly when faced with dilemmas in therapy, as in competing principles, risks, and benefits.	Are the benefits of therapy worth the cost? Are the risks of therapy worth the benefits? How should I prioritize my caseload? What are the limits of how I change my documentation to maximize payment? What should I do when other members of the treatment team are operating in ways that I feel conflict with the goals of the person receiving services?

(continued)

TABLE 25.1	Aspects of Reasoning in Occupational Therapy (*continued*)	
Reasoning Aspect	**Clues for Recognizing in Therapist Discussions**	**Examples of the Therapy Problems or Questions That Draw Out This Reasoning**
Interactive		
Thinking directed toward building positive interpersonal relationships with clients, permitting collaborative problem identification and problem-solving	Therapist is concerned with what client likes or does not like; use of praise, empathetic comments, and nonverbal behaviors to encourage and support client's cooperation.	How can I best relate to this person? How can I put this person at ease? What is the best way for me to encourage this person? What nonverbal strategies should I use in this situation? Where should I place myself relative to this person so that I support them but do not "invade" the person? What cultural factors do I need to consider as I engage with the person?
Conditional		
A blending of all forms of reasoning for the purposes of flexibly responding to changing conditions or predicting possible client futures	Typically found with more experienced therapists who can "see" multiple futures based on the therapist's past experiences and current information	Where is this person going? How will the various therapy options play out, given this person's health condition, social situation, economic status, and culture? Given these future possible trajectories, what is the best action I can take now?

For more additional summaries of these aspects, refer to Carrier, A., Levasseur, M., Bédard, D., & Desrosiers, J. (2010). Community occupational therapists' clinical reasoning: Identifying tacit knowledge. *Australian Occupational Therapy Journal, 57*, 356–365. https://doi.org/10.1111/j.1440-1630.2010.00875.x; Schell, B. A. B., & Schell, J. W. (2018). *Clinical and professional reasoning in occupational therapy* (2nd ed.). Wolters Kluwer; Unsworth, C. A. (2012). The evolving theory of clinical reasoning. In E. A. S. Duncan (Ed.), *Foundations for practice in occupational therapy* (5th ed., pp. 209–231). Elsevier/Churchill Livingstone; and Unsworth, C.A. (2011). Gaining insights to the clinical reasoning that supports an on-road driver assessment. *Canadian Journal of Occupational Therapy, 78*, 97–102. Doi: 10.2182/cjot.2011.78.2.4

typical focus clues for recognizing when that sort of reasoning is occurring. Most of the studies involved occupational therapists, with few studies on OT assistants (Doumanov & Rugg, 2003; Humbert, 2004; Lyons & Crepeau, 2001). Note that other authors may name and characterize these somewhat differently, but all agree that there are multiple aspects that surface in research about professional reasoning within OT (Unsworth, 2021) as well as across many healthcare professions (Higgs & Jones, 2019).

Fleming (1991) was the first within OT to describe how occupational therapists seemed to use different thinking approaches depending on the nature of the clinical problem they were addressing. She referred to this process as the "therapist with the three-track mind" (p. 1007).

Scientific Reasoning

Therapists use scientific reasoning to understand the condition affecting an individual and to decide on interventions that are in the client's best interest. It is a logical process that parallels scientific inquiry. Forms of scientific reasoning that are described in OT are diagnostic reasoning (Rogers & Holm, 1991) and procedural reasoning (Fleming, 1994b), in addition to the general use of hypothetical-deductive reasoning (Tomlin, 2018).

Diagnostic reasoning is concerned with clinical problem sensing and problem definition. The process starts in advance of seeing a client. OT practitioners, because of their domains of concern, look primarily for occupational performance problems. Furthermore, the nature of the problems they expect to find is influenced by the information in the requests for services. Some of Terry's diagnostic reasoning, described earlier, included information about the typical symptoms associated with having a stroke.

Procedural reasoning occurs when practitioners are "thinking about the disease or disability and deciding which intervention activities (procedures) they might employ to remediate the person's functional performance problems" (Fleming, 1991, p. 1008). This may involve an interview, an observation of the person engaged in a task, or formal evaluations using standardized measures. Although one hopes that procedural reasoning is science based, Tomlin makes the important observation that procedural reasoning can become an unquestioned implementation of therapy protocols, in which case it becomes less scientific in nature (Tomlin, 2008). That is why there is such an emphasis on evidence-based practice (EBP), which challenges the practitioner to routinely evaluate customary therapy approaches in light of the best information currently available (Holm, 2000; Law & MacDermid, 2008). Some researchers suggest that scientific reasoning is part of an evidence-informed process versus EBP (Dougherty et al., 2016; Tomlin, 2018). Chapter 26 speaks on the importance of evidence-informed practice. All the chapters in this text, along with many other OT texts, professional journals, and professional organization resources, include evidence that can help guide practice.

In the OT Story, Terry used a combination of interview and observation, both guided by her working hypothesis that Mrs. Munro had cognitive problems that might affect her safe performance at home. She was likely operating based on her understanding of cognitive theories (such as those described in Chapter 55) as well as her own experience with similar clients. As intervention begins, more data are collected, and the OT practitioner gains a sharper clinical image. This clinical image is the result of the interplay between what the OT practitioner expects to see (such as the usual course of the disease) and the client's actual performance. In the OT Story, there was congruence between Mrs. Munro's abilities and problems in performing activities of daily living and Terry's expectations of someone making a good recovery from a stroke.

Mattingly (1994a) made the point that occupational therapists have a "two-body practice" (p. 37). By that, she meant that OT practitioners view a person in two ways: the body as a machine, in which parts may be broken, and the person as a life, filled with personal meanings and hopes. The next form of reasoning, narrative reasoning, provides the OT practitioner with a way to understand a person's illness experience.

Narrative Reasoning

Understanding the meaning that a disease, illness, or disability has to an individual is a task that goes beyond the scientific understanding of disease processes and organ systems. Rather, it requires that practitioners find a way to understand the meaning of this experience from the client's perspective. Mattingly (1994b) suggested that practitioners do this through a form of reasoning called *narrative reasoning*. Narrative reasoning is so named because it involves thinking in story form. Careful attention to the client's perspective provides a window into the client's world, their understanding of their situation, and the impact that it has on their occupations. It is also how therapists enact the ideal of being client centered.

In the OT Story, part of Terry's reasoning was concerned with making decisions in light of what was important to Mrs. Munro. This process of collaboration and empathy has been described as "building a communal horizon of understanding" (Clark et al., 1996, p. 376). Terry gained understanding by listening attentively to Mrs. Munro's stories about her husband and how he loved her cooking. It is apparent that Mrs. Munro's home is more than just a house; it is the place in which she lived with her husband, where he died, and where she still felt his presence. Part of Mrs. Munro's story is that going home is going back to her husband. If the stroke were to prevent that, Mrs. Munro would lose more than her independence; she would lose symbolic connections to her husband. Although a logical case might be made that Mrs. Munro should start

considering a more supportive living environment, Terry understands that for Mrs. Munro, this would not be an acceptable ending. Consequently, Terry worked hard to obtain the support systems that would be necessary for Mrs. Munro to function in her chosen environment, where she will continue her life story.

Often, OT practitioners work with individuals whose life stories are so severely disrupted that they cannot imagine what their future will look like. Mattingly (1994b) believed that in these situations, skillful practitioners help their clients to invent new life stories. This has been referred to as "story-making" (Bonsall, 2012, p. 97), in which therapists help clients "recraft" their "occupational narratives" (Auzmendia et al., 2008, p. 313). To some degree, these stories become visible as the OT practitioner and the client develop goals together. The use of life stories is also apparent when activities are selected for both their healing potential and their particular significance to the person. To do this, one must first solicit occupational stories from the individual (Clark et al., 1996; Hamilton, 2018). With an understanding of clients' past occupational stories, practitioners can help individuals create new stories and new futures for themselves. If Mrs. Munro's symptoms were more severe and she was in a more extended therapy process, Terry might explore Mrs. Munro's interest in cooking as an activity that offered many therapeutic opportunities, such as cooking for others by making special treats, first for other clients and then perhaps for neighbors in exchange for their help with chores. During this process, Mrs. Munro would be regaining not only coordination and dexterity but also her sense of self as a productive person. This narrative aspect of clinical reasoning, which ultimately focuses on the person as an occupational being, provides a link between the founding values of the profession and current practice demands (Gray, 1998).

Pragmatic Reasoning

Pragmatic reasoning is yet another strand of reasoning that goes beyond the practitioner–client relationship and addresses the world in which therapy occurs (Schell, 2018a; Schell & Cervero, 1993). This world is considered from two perspectives: the practice context and the personal context. Everyday issues have been identified over the years that affect the therapy process, including resources for intervention, organizational culture, power relationships among team members, reimbursement practices, and practice trends in the profession (Schell, 2018a; Unsworth, 2005). Studies examining clinical reasoning have confirmed that OT practitioners both actively consider and are influenced by their practice contexts (Schell, 2018a). An example of pragmatic reasoning in the OT Story was Terry's use of immediate resources (the flower vase) in Mrs. Munro's room as a therapy tool. Although Terry had thought of appropriate activities related to self-care, she had to identify practical alternatives quickly when it turned out that Mrs. Munro was already dressed. Practical constraints for Terry included (a) the time it would take to move Mrs. Munro to the clinic, where there might be more resources; (b) the need to get the required information on that day because Mrs. Munro was going home; and (c) the physical constraints of what was available within the room. Terry's invention of a feasible alternative was a product of both her therapeutic imagination and the cues that were provided within her practice setting.

Terry's attention to the influence of team members demonstrates pragmatic reasoning directed to interpersonal and group issues. She knew that the physician had the power to make discharge decisions. She was aware of the pressures on the physician by the third-party payers not only to discharge clients as quickly as possible but also to avoid readmission. Practice requires that practitioners' reason about negotiating their clients' interests within the practice culture. This includes discerning what might be changed and what limitations must be accepted in each situation.

The practitioner's personal situation also is part of the pragmatic reasoning process. Although less readily identified in research, Unsworth (2004) surfaced some examples in her research in which therapists "weighed their own therapy skills against the therapeutic needs of the clients" (p. 36) in deciding whether to refer to others with more expertise. A person's clinical competencies, preferences, commitment to the profession, and life role demands outside work all affect the therapy choices that are considered and thus enter the reasoning process. For instance, if a practitioner does not feel safe helping a client stand or transfer to a bed, the therapist is more likely to use tabletop activities in which the client can participate from a wheelchair. Another OT practitioner might feel uncomfortable interacting with individuals who have depression and, therefore, might be quick to suggest that such clients are not motivated for therapy. A practitioner who has a young family to go home to might opt not to schedule clients late in the day to get home as early as possible. These simple personal issues result in clinical decisions that affect the scope and timing of therapy services. Hooper (2018) suggested that fundamental issues, such as a practitioner's values and general worldview, strongly affect the way in which an individual constructs their reasoning. Such worldviews play an important role in the next kind of reasoning: ethical reasoning.

Ethical Reasoning

All the forms of reasoning that have been described so far help the practitioner to respond to the following questions: What is this person's current occupational situation? What can be done to enhance the person's situation? Ethical reasoning goes one step further and asks: What should be done? Rogers (1983) framed these three questions (here

paraphrased) in her Eleanor Clarke Slagle lecture and went on to state, "The clinical reasoning process terminates in an ethical decision, rather than a scientific one, and the ethical nature of the goal of clinical reasoning projects itself over the entire sequence" (p. 602). In the OT Story, Terry's ethical dilemma is to understand Mrs. Munro's personal wishes and to honor them when developing a therapy plan that realistically addresses Mrs. Munro's limitations. This can be particularly challenging when the pressures of financial realities (such as Mrs. Munro's limited income and the lack of insurance for supported living) come up against concerns for safety or similar therapy concerns. Several OT authors have addressed the ethical aspect of professional reasoning, and Chapter 36 of this text is devoted to the issue of the ethics of the profession. The purpose here is to introduce ethical reasoning as one of the components of professional reasoning in OT.

Interactive Reasoning

The provision of therapy is inherently a communicative process (Schwartzberg, 2002). In OT, practitioners must gain the trust of their clients and of people who are important in the clients' world. This is because OT involves "doing with" as opposed to "doing to" clients (Mattingly & Fleming, 1994, p. 178). A therapist gains this trust by entering the client's life world (Crepeau, 1991) and by using several interpersonal strategies that are designed to motivate clients. These include advocating, collaborating, empathizing, encouraging, instructing, and problem-solving (Taylor et al., 2011), each of which is discussed more in Chapter 28. Once they are in the client's life world, OT practitioners can better understand how to help the individuals resolve performance problems. This form of therapist reasoning is referred to as *interactive reasoning* and is considered important to the OT process (Copley et al., 2008; Taylor, 2020).

It is likely that some reasoning focused on interaction is conscious, as when a practitioner remembers that "I need to be sure to praise the client often because he gets discouraged so easily." Other interpersonal acts might be quite automatic, such as when a therapist touches a person's arm to convey sympathy. It is sometimes easiest to detect the importance of effective interactive reasoning when the therapist makes a mistake or gets an unexpected reaction and is forced to regroup and rebuild the therapy relationship.

A Process of Synthesis in Shared Activity

The preceding section described commonly accepted aspects of professional reasoning separately to illustrate the different parts of the process. Table 25.1 includes examples of the kinds of questions that practitioners seek to answer with the different aspects of professional reasoning. As you read these, keep in mind that you cannot characterize these by watching someone. You must ask practitioners what they were thinking, as one person may perceive something as a purely technical problem requiring a "scientific solution" and thus responds with scientific reasoning, whereas another may frame it as one requiring attention to therapist–client collaboration and focus more on interactive reasoning. It is also likely that individual practitioners may favor some aspects of reasoning over others. It is important to be aware of such biases and actively consider that all aspects of reasoning process have been harnessed to fully define the therapy problem and related therapy actions.

Scientific, narrative, pragmatic, ethical, and interactive reasoning are not separate or parallel processes. The opposite appears to be the case. Virtually, all the research about reasoning in practice suggest that these different forms interact, inform, and overlap with each other (Carrier et al., 2010; Mitchell & Unsworth, 2005). Furthermore, Toth-Cohen (2008) makes the point that the "shared activity" that occurs during the therapy process is an "integral part" of the reasoning process (p. 82).

In the OT Story, Terry's understanding of medical science helped her to know potential impairments and performance problems, but her narrative reasoning helped her to understand the importance to Mrs. Munro of returning home. Put together, these two forms of reasoning help Terry to reach an unspoken understanding that there would be a high risk for depression (which could worsen her client's medical condition) if Mrs. Munro did not return to her home, which means so much to her. Furthermore, the practical constraints associated with the setting and Mrs. Munro's reimbursement prompted Terry to reason about the ethics of suggesting that she return home alone (where she might not be safe), consider more alternative supported living (which she may not want and probably cannot afford), and finally of recommending that she return home with the support of home healthcare and neighbors. Note that not all reasoning results in action—in some cases, deciding not to pursue a particular action (such as Terry's decision not to suggest an assistive living facility for Mrs. Munro) is the best professional action.

Conditional Process

Not only must practitioners blend different aspects of reasoning in order to interact effectively with their clients, but they must also flexibly modify interventions in response to changing conditions and to the context in which the therapy is occurring. Terry showed her flexibility by inventing an activity with the flower vase when her plan to work with Mrs. Munro on bathing and dressing did not pan out. Creighton and colleagues (1995) noticed that OT

practitioners preplanned interventions in a hierarchical manner. They observed that practitioners typically brought several sets of supplies to an intervention session. One set would be directed to the expected level of performance, and the others to a stage higher and a stage lower than the expected performance. This blend of scientific and pragmatic reasoning increased efficiency by anticipating several possible situations that might occur.

On a larger scale, Fleming (1994c) described the ability of skilled OT practitioners to "form an image of future life possibilities for the person" (p. 234). The ability to form these images (or schemata, to use cognitive terms) seems to require a blend of all the forms of clinical reasoning, along with sufficient clinical experience, to have seen various outcomes with former clients. These images help practitioners to select therapeutic activities on a day-to-day basis. For instance, when working with person who has a spinal cord injury, a therapist might suggest a writing or keyboard activity. Not only is this a good activity for increasing coordination but also presages occupations that will enable the client to regain control of their life through writing their own checks, signing their name on legal documents, and using various forms of technology for work and play. If this client were an accountant, these would be powerful images. Conversely, if the client were a professional athlete, the OT practitioner might have to create different activities to allow the client to develop a vision of themselves as a future coach or teacher. The activities used in OT can help to meet specific short-term goals and shape long-term expectations. It is in this way that practitioners help individuals to reengage in their lives by therapeutically using meaningful occupations.

Ecological View of Professional Reasoning

Units I, II, and III contain many chapters that describe how occupational performance is the result of complex transactions among a person's inherent capacities, the person's prior experiences, and the demands of the performance context. Similarly, the professional reasoning process and the resulting therapy actions represent transactions that occur during the actual therapy activity, among the practitioner, client and therapy context (Toth-Cohen, 2008; Unsworth 2012). Schell synthesized these many factors associated with professional reasoning into the Ecological Model of Professional Reasoning (Schell, 2018b), which is described here.

Practitioner reasoning is shaped by both personal and professional perspectives, as shown in Figure 25.1. Each practitioner brings to the therapy situation knowledge and skills that are grounded in life experiences, including personal characteristics such as physical capacities, personality, values, beliefs, and cultural heritage that comprise their

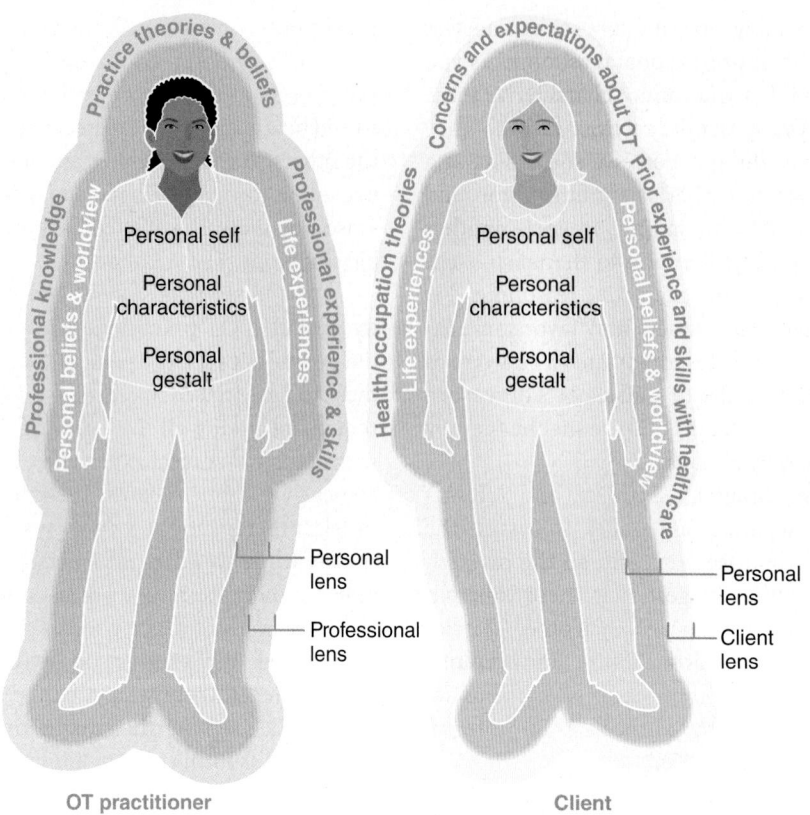

FIGURE 25.1 Personal and professional lenses shape occupational therapists' professional reasoning. OT, occupational therapy.

personal gestalt. These form a *personal self* that consists of the person's embodied characteristics along with their interpretation of the experiences or worldview. These personal factors shape each person's perception and interpretation of all life activities and thus act as a *personal lens* through which each practitioner views all life events. Layered over or entwined with this personal self is the *professional self*, which includes the therapist's professional knowledge from education, experiences from prior clients, and beliefs about what is important to do in therapy along with knowledge of specific technical skills and therapy routines. Thus, a therapist views therapy situations through both a personal lens and a *professional lens*, which, over time, likely merge into the therapist's customary ways of viewing the therapy process. The personal and professional selves act in concert to respond to various problems of practice.

Just as with therapists, clients (also depicted in Figure 25.1) come to therapy with their own life experiences and personal characteristics, cultural heritage, life situations, and performance problems that prompted the need for therapy. Clients may also come with their own theories about what is causing the performance problems, and these theories are influenced by their cultural heritage. They may have past experiences with therapy and healthcare and their own expectations of the therapy process. The therapist and the client come together in a practice context to engage in therapy, as shown in Figure 25.2.

Because this therapy is happening in a finite time and place, it is inherently a process that is embedded in the setting in which it occurs, called here the *practice context*. The practice context includes both physical and sociocultural aspects that influence therapy options. Examples might include outpatient medical setting, a client's home, or a student's classroom. Each of these settings shapes the therapy tools available as well as the rules or social and organizational expectations about what should occur. Other factors in the practice context include the interprofessional team, time, physical resources, social environment, caseload size and characteristics, and payment and discharge options.

The therapist and the client engage in therapy activities together within the practice context. These specific actors, working in a specific context, shape the nature, scope, and trajectory of the therapy process. Thus, professional reasoning is not just what occurs in the therapist's body–mind; it is an ecologic process that comes together in a therapy activity that represents the transaction among the therapist, the client, and the therapy setting (Carrier et al., 2010; Schell, 2018b; Toth-Cohen, 2008; Unsworth, 2011). At various times, different aspects of this system will have a greater influence on what will occur. Reflective therapists are encouraged to be mindful of

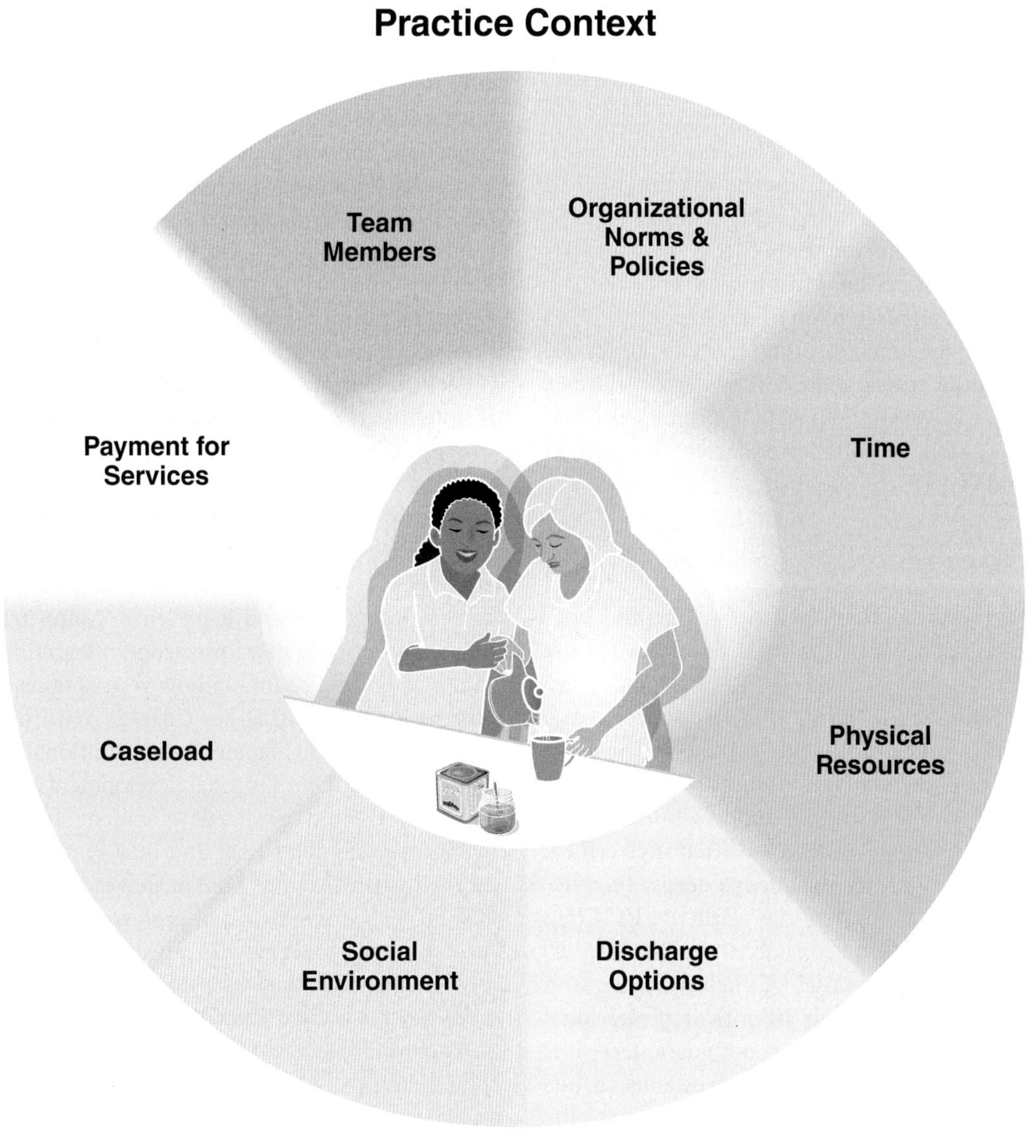

Practice Context

FIGURE 25.2 Schell's Ecological Model of Professional Reasoning. Professional reasoning is an ecological process in which the therapist and the client engage in therapy activities in a specific setting. All of these components transact to shape therapist reasoning, resulting actions with the client and, ultimately, therapy outcomes.

all these factors and their influence on their reasoning and associated therapy actions and therapy outcomes.

Developing Competency and Expertise in Professional Reasoning

Understanding the complexity of professional reasoning helps students and practitioners alike to appreciate why it takes so long to truly become an excellent practitioner.

Research shows that it typically takes a minimum of 10 years for individuals to gain expertise within a given field (Boshuizen & Schmidt, 2000), although some studies in OT show differing expertise levels, showing up as early as 5 years (Rassafiani et al., 2009). Although experience is necessary, experience alone is not sufficient to ensure advancement in professional reasoning skills. Historically, professional reasoning and EBP were viewed as separate processes; however, current evidence suggests that these activities should be viewed as two highly correlated perspectives for understanding how to achieve client goals (Benfield & Johnston, 2020). Quality thinking and decision-making require the practitioner to spiral between professional reasoning and

EBP. Importantly, expert or high-level professional reasoning is found only in those people who also engage in difficult EBP activities (Benfield & Johnston, 2020). Furthermore, high-quality professional thinking is reliant on collecting and reflecting outcomes data. Thus, professional reasoning, at its core, is oriented to quality and the ability to achieve client outcomes. It is the spirit of inquiry and striving to achieve the best outcomes for clients that supports seeking and appraising evidence from a variety of sources. See Figure 25.3 for a representation of this process.

Developing professional reasoning requires purposeful thinking and routine critical reflection by the practitioner, as well as the use of various supports to professional reasoning. In this section, we summarize current research on competency and expertise in professional reasoning.

Competency

Competency is the ability to make good judgments to deliver care in a complex context, with flexibility to modify and adapt services as needed (AOTA, 2021). Competence arises out of the interaction of two different aspects: structure of knowledge and doing. Perhaps, one of the most important professional reasoning tasks is to develop and continually improve valid mental models to guide the therapy process. This is hard work as it requires critical reflection and a willingness to challenge deeply held beliefs and assumptions about how the world works (Chen et al., 2008). Practitioners must establish habits of questioning, reflection, and appraisal of their thinking and decision-making that they apply over their professional lifetimes. Maintaining competency is not guaranteed. It is highly dependent on the person's ability to establish habits of mind and habits of practice in daily professional life (Epstein & Hundert, 2002).

As time passes from entry into the profession, the practitioner must maintain the currency and validity of knowledge to remain competent. How is this done? It requires the integration of knowledge gained from literature, continuing education, and experience, thus transforming their mental model (Bannigan & Moores, 2009; Benfield & Krueger, 2021). The quality of the mental model depends on the routine and frequent performance of specific professional thinking and evidence-based activities. These strategies keep practitioners from over-relying on pattern recognition, which can be prone to errors owing to cognitive biases (Elstein & Schwarz, 2002). For instance, in the OT Story, it is noted that Terry had seen over a hundred people with strokes. In recent years, early medical intervention has changed what used to be the typical course of stroke with the use of specific medications in the acute phase of care. Terry's schema and scripts of a typical stroke survivor may no longer be valid if she had not reshaped them to reflect current knowledge and experience. Competency requires habitually learning new knowledge, integrating it into your thinking, and reflecting on how your actions have affected outcomes (Small, 2020). See Chapter 26 for more information on EBP and Chapter 71 for additional discussion of competency and professional development.

Keep in mind that the development of effective reasoning in practice takes time and may require us to become increasingly insightful about ourselves in order to serve our clients. The actual process of professional reasoning can be overwhelming for a new therapist. Typically, beginners focus on one or two aspects of therapy, as they cannot "hold" either all the complexities in their minds at once or their personal perspectives and even hidden biases are affecting their therapy. In Expanding Our Perspectives, the writer provides a great example of these common responses as she shares a profound experience as a new therapist.

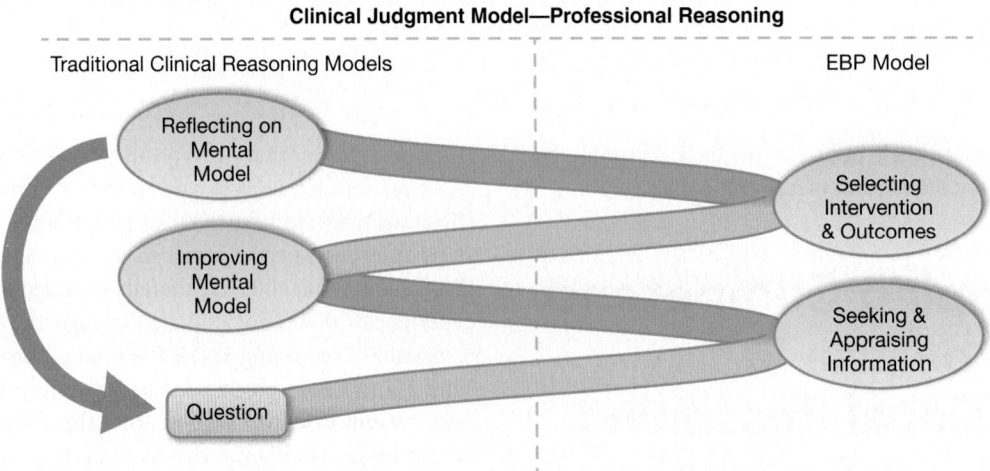

Clinical Judgment Model—Professional Reasoning

Traditional Clinical Reasoning Models | EBP Model

Reflecting on Mental Model

Improving Mental Model

Question

Selecting Intervention & Outcomes

Seeking & Appraising Information

FIGURE 25.3 Improving practitioners' mental models requires ongoing reflection and appraisal of one's own mental model in light of evidence about interventions and outcomes. EBP, evidence-based practice.

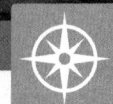

EXPANDING OUR PERSPECTIVES

Novice Professional Reasoning in Practice

Dahlia Castillo

As a new occupational therapist, I was continually overwhelmed with the amount of information to integrate personally and professionally within the therapy process. I struggled with the natural overlap of scientific knowledge, narrative stories, the pragmatics of individuals and situations, ethical considerations, and the interactive and conditional nature of the therapeutic process. My own professional and personal growth became a painful process as I uncovered biases and lacked experience with approaching difficult situations and what basic questions to ask a client. I often felt incompetent, and decision-making for therapy actions was not always client centered.

One example is a 19-year-old named Jay, the victim of a drive-by shooting, with a diagnosis of spinal cord injury that occurred during a transaction for an illicit substance. I thought to myself, "Did he buy the drugs or was he selling the drugs?" I focused on Jay's recovery by keeping my thinking scientific. After the medical chart review, I entered the therapeutic encounter unsure of myself as I gathered information to complete the evaluation with no interest in his story. I did not inquire about or attempt to understand his meaningful occupations. At the same time, I began to wonder if those who shot him might try to shoot me. Irrational fear consumed my 23-year-old self.

Because of this fear, I did not leave the inpatient setting with him. A typical course of action for a person newly diagnosed with a spinal cord injury was to begin outdoor wheelchair mobility as soon as possible. By taking the wheelchair into the community and providing the opportunity to navigate ramps and parking lots to and from buildings close by, people began to value the need for upper body strengthening as well as begin to adjust to the diagnosis. During treatment, I focused on upper body strengthening and independence with self-care, and Jay obediently and politely did everything I asked of him. After 10 days of inpatient rehab, Jay asked me about his roommate Sam, also diagnosed with paraplegia: "I have been inside this hospital for a week and a half and have not been outside once. I love being outside and I heard from Sam that OT takes people outside. Sam got here four days after me and has been outside with you every day. Why don't you take me outside?"

I came to the painful conclusion I was providing inequitable OT services with no regard for the client and what was most meaningful to him. It was not easy for me to admit I was being therapist centered. I often think of how much Jay taught me about my biases, fears, perception of safety, worldviews, and my responsibility to treat all those in my care with dignity and respect in an equitable and ethical manner. I reflect on how this experience helped me understand that professional reasoning is much more than being new or experienced, more than thinking and doing treatment with a client, and more than following a precise protocol or unclear therapeutic process.

Expertise

The development of expertise relies on the routine engagement in critically reflecting on practice, informed by evidence, and assessed in light of outcome measurements (Rousmaniere, 2016).

The conceptualization of expertise is important. Developmental models of expertise are often used to describe typical changes that occur as individuals progress from novice to expert levels. Dreyfus and Dreyfus's (1986) conceptualization of professional expertise has been applied to OT (Slater & Cohn, 1991) and elaborated on over time by several researchers, although, often, the research dichotomizes beginners or novices from experts. Novices enter practice with the knowledge required for competent practice; however, they have more difficulty with accessing and applying it due to their mental models being less rich and complex (Paterson et al., 2006). They rely on rules and formal knowledge, take more time to figure out client problems, and are less sensitive to contextual nuances.

Overall, they are less efficient. In the early years of practice, their mental model increases in complexity, not just from acquiring more knowledge but also from making richer knowledge networks, which are then used in pattern recognition (Paterson et al., 2006). As the person gains experience and reflects on that experience, they become more efficient in finding salient problem spaces and identifying relevant therapy approaches. Expertise is characterized by fluid performance, which is an unconscious, automatic process that is largely intuitive (Benner, 1984). Experts typically have 10 years of reflective practice and have mastered the procedures in their experiential setting. They are highly efficient and accurate in making decisions for routine client problems. These experts often rely on using their tacit knowledge, which can be difficult for them to articulate. More recent theorists describe this level of performance as *routine expertise* (Bohle Carbonell & Dailey-Hebert, 2021). They critique this view of expertise, suggesting an overreliance on automatic behaviors. By not engaging in metacognitive or deliberate practice activities, routine experts may not recognize anomalies or creatively consider practice demands (Gube & Lajoie, 2020).

Newer conceptions describe a higher level of expertise called *adaptive expertise*. The descriptions of adaptive experts include all the skills of the routine expert; however, adaptive experts have mental models, which represent knowledge that is more well connected and more flexible. They can recognize and use new information to meet the goal more effectively (Gube & Lajoie, 2020). Evidence suggests that it is not the amount of knowledge that limits expert performance, but how an individual has organized and connected it (Mylopoulos et al., 2018). This is critical as it indicates that less experienced practitioners who have less knowledge can still exhibit adaptive expertise if they are actively and routinely engaging their professional thinking. The specific professional thinking activities need to include those that are commonly described as deliberate practice: critical reflection on actions, beliefs, and knowledge, with a focus on improving practice knowledge and skills (Ericsson, 2004).

Reflection

Reflection is critical to advancing expertise. Schön (1983) proffered the term *reflective practitioner* to describe how experts think critically about their own experience. Reflection happens in two ways. First, practitioners "reflect in action" (Schön, 1983, p. 49). This involves the practitioners' ability to think in the midst of action and adapt to meet the demands of the situation. Reflection in action most often occurs when the usual approaches are not working. "Reflection on action" (Schön, 1983, p. 61) is the term Schön uses for critical thinking that occurs after the fact. Reflection about practice, identifying what worked and what did not, and being open to alternative conceptions are necessary to support the learning associated with advancing expertise. Further, as they identify process indicators and outcome indicators, adaptive experts use this evidence to develop more nuanced and interconnected mental models that allow for creativity.

Creativity and innovation arise by drawing on different connections to extend practice boundaries while still adhering to their scope of practice (Benfield & Krueger, 2021; Gube & Lajoie, 2020). From this perspective, expertise is relative, and there are always higher levels of skills that they can achieve. Further, flexibility also arises from a deeper, more nuanced understanding of the rules they used to guide their action and their consistent "tuning" of the rules using outcomes data to improve the efficiency of their mental model (Bohle Carbonell & Dailey-Hebert, 2021). As practitioners who value operationalizing the OT process through cocreating meaning with each client, it requires adaptive expertise to develop effective, culturally sensitive interventions. Critically, adaptive expertise is fostered through engaging in critical analysis of practice—analyzing and synthesizing their experiences and knowledge in order to generate new knowledge that guides future performance (Mylopoulos et al., 2018).

Professional Reasoning Supports

So far, we have discussed the development of competence and expertise and the importance of experience and critical reflection as key factors in supporting practice development. In recent decades, there have emerged supports intended to help minimize practice errors and support optimal decision-making.

Clinical decision support systems (CDSSs) are interactive systems that emulate human reasoning in a given domain. They are designed to analyze data to help health professionals make clinical decisions about individual clients by using information and communication technologies, data, documents, knowledge, and models to identify and solve the problem. CDSSs have been used in medicine for several decades to improve medication prescription and dosage and have been shown to be somewhat effective, particularly when they are embedded in systems, such as computerized medical records, to prompt the practitioner (Pearson et al., 2009).

The use of CDSSs in OT is a more recent phenomenon. For example, Danial-Saad and colleagues (2015) demonstrated that novices could make adaptive device recommendations (in this case, pointing devices) comparable to those recommended by assistive technology experts when the novices used a CDSS built to support assistive technology decisions.

Guidelines based on research are another form of support for professional reasoning. Stark and colleagues (2015) proposed clinical reasoning guidelines for recommendations regarding home modifications. In addition, professional organizations publish more comprehensive guidelines that summarize current evidence for OT interventions, such as the *Practice Guidelines—Occupational Therapy Practice Guidelines for Early Childhood: Birth–5 Years* (Frolek Clark & Kingsley, 2020).

Supports to professional reasoning provide important ways for practitioners to both improve their knowledge and reflect upon the validity of their assumptions in light of current evidence. In the next section, we discuss how interprofessional teams can also affect professional reasoning.

Interprofessional Reasoning

Occupational therapists commonly practice in teams. Interprofessional collaborative practice is associated with better quality and coordination of care, fewer errors, and reduced cost, among other benefits (National Academy of Practice, 2019). In medical settings, this may include the patient, physicians, nurses, speech-language pathologists, social workers, and psychologists. In educational settings, team members may include parents, regular and special education teachers, guidance counselors, and school psychologists. In community settings, the team members will vary widely reflecting the practice setting, such as work setting or home modifications. In all these settings, the client is considered a part of the team. Working in teams requires that members bring their individual perspectives to bear on the client's issues. It is a process of sharing knowledge, aligning values, communicating, and establishing shared goals to support quality health outcomes. Thus, it is important to understand how other professions conceptualize their reasoning and practice (Schell et al., in press).

To maximize the benefit of interprofessional teamwork, OT practitioners need to articulate their own professional reasoning and to understand the reasoning of other team members. This can be challenging because of differences in terminology as well as professional or client focus (Young et al., 2018). Successful interprofessional reasoning necessitates that team members must talk about their reasoning. Psychologist Edmonds studied "teaming" and notes that "effective teaming requires everyone to remain vigilantly aware of each other's needs, roles and perspectives. This entails learning to relate to others better and learning to make decisions based on the integration of different perspectives" (2012, p. 2).

Conclusion

Professional reasoning is the process that practitioners use to plan, direct, perform, and reflect on client care. It is an embodied multisensory process that requires complex cognitive activity. Practitioners develop cognitive frames and scripts as they gain experience, forming the basis of professional knowledge and action. Professional reasoning is multifaceted and enables practitioners to understand client issues from different perspectives. Practitioners use the logical processes associated with scientific reasoning to understand the client's impairments, disabilities, and performance contexts and to predict the impact these have on occupational performance. Narrative reasoning helps practitioners to appreciate the meaning of occupational performance limitations to the client and generate therapeutic options to support continued occupational performance. Practitioners use pragmatic reasoning when they address the practical realities associated with service delivery. All these forms of reasoning are undergirded by ethical reasoning to help practitioners select the best therapy action. The process of professional reasoning involves a transaction among the practitioner's personal and professional perspectives, the client's perspectives, and the demands of the practice context that unfolds in therapy activities. Expertise develops as the practitioner gains experience and reflects on that experience for deeper understanding. Sound reasoning habits and the use of reasoning supports promote ongoing expertise.

Acknowledgment

Selected portions of this chapter are from B. A. Schell & J. W. Schell (Eds.), *Clinical and professional reasoning in occupational therapy* (2nd ed., pp. 3–12). Wolters Kluwer.

Lippincott® Connect *For additional resources on the subjects discussed in this chapter, visit Lippincott Connect.*

REFERENCES

American Occupational Therapy Association. (2020). Occupational therapy practice framework: Domain and process (4th ed.). *American Journal of Occupational Therapy*, 74(Suppl. 2), 7412410010. https://doi.org/10.5014/ajot.2020.74S200

American Occupational Therapy Association. (2021). *Standards for continuing competence.* https://www.aota.org/-/media/Corporate/Files/EducationCareers/Standards-for-Continuing-Competence-2021.pdf

Arntzen, C. (2018). An embodied and intersubjective practice of occupational therapy. *OTJR: Occupation, Participation and Health*, 38(3), 173–180. https://doi.org/10.1177/1539449217727470

Auzmendia, A. L., de las Heras, C. G., Kielhofner, G., & Miranda, C. (2008). Recrafting occupational narratives. In G. Kielhofner (Ed.), *Model of human occupation* (4th ed., pp. 313–336). Lippincott Williams & Wilkins.

Bannigan, K., & Moores, A. (2009). A model of professional thinking: Integrating reflective practice and evidence based practice. *Canadian Journal of Occupational Therapy*, 76(5), 342–350. https://doi.org10.1177/000841740907600505

Benfield, A., & Krueger, R. B. (2021). Making decision-making visible—Teaching the process of evaluating interventions. *International Journal of Environmental Research and Public Health*, 18(7), 3635. https://www.mdpi.com/1660-4601/18/7/3635

Benfield, A. M., & Johnston, M. V. (2020). Initial development of a measure of evidence-informed professional thinking. *Australian Occupational Therapy Journal*, 67(4), 309–319. https://doi.org/10.1111/1440-1630.12655

Benner, P. (1984). *From novice to expert.* Addison-Wesley.

Bohle Carbonell, K., & Dailey-Hebert, A. (2021). Routine expertise, adaptive expertise, and task and environmental influences. In M.-L. Germain & R. S. Grenier (Eds.), *Expertise at work: Current and emerging trends* (pp. 39–56). Springer International Publishing. https://doi.org/10.1007/978-3-030-64371-3_3

Bonsall, A. (2012). An examination of the pairing between narrative and occupational science. *Scandinavian Journal of Occupational Therapy*, 19, 92–103. https://doi.org/10.3109/11038128.2011.552119

Boshuizen, H. P. A., & Schmidt, H. G. (2000). The development of clinical reasoning expertise. In J. Higgs & M. Jones (Eds.), *Clinical reasoning in the health professions* (2nd ed., pp. 15–22). Butterworth Heinemann.

Bruning, R. H., Schraw, G. J., & Ronning, R. R. (1999). *Cognitive psychology and instruction* (3rd ed.). Merrill.

Carr, M., & Shotwell, M. (2018). Information processing theory and professional reasoning. In B. A. B. Schell & J. W. Schell (Eds.), *Clinical and professional reasoning in occupational therapy* (2nd ed., pp. 73–104). Wolters Kluwer.

Carrier, A., Levasseur, M., Bédard, D., & Desrosiers, J. (2010). Community occupational therapists' clinical reasoning: Identifying tacit knowledge. *Australian Occupational Therapy Journal*, 57, 356–365. https://doi.org/10.1111/j.1440-1630.2010.00875.x

Chen, D. T., Mills, A. E., & Werhane, P. H. (2008). Tools for tomorrow's health care system: A systems-informed mental model, moral imagination, and physicians' professionalism. *Academic Medicine*, 83(8), 723–732. https://doi.org/10.1097/ACM.0b013e31817ec0d3

Clark, F., Ennevor, B. L., & Richardson, P. L. (1996). A grounded theory of techniques for occupational storytelling and occupational story making. In R. Zemke & F. Clark (Eds.), *Occupational science: The evolving discipline* (pp. 373–392). F. A. Davis.

Cohn, E. S. (1989). Fieldwork education: Shaping a foundation for clinical reasoning. *American Journal of Occupational Therapy*, 43, 240–244. https://doi.org/10.5014/ajot.43.4.240

Copley, J., Turpin, M., Brosnan, J., & Nelson, A. (2008). Understanding and negotiating: Reasoning processes used by an occupational therapist to individualize intervention decisions for people with upper limb hypertonicity. *Disability and Rehabilitation*, *30*, 1486–1498. https://doi.org/10.1080/09638280701654799

Creighton, C., Dijkers, M., Bennett, N., & Brown, K. (1995). Reasoning and the art of therapy for spinal cord injury. *American Journal of Occupational Therapy*, *49*, 311–317. https://doi.org/10.5014/ajot.49.4.311

Crepeau, E. B. (1991). Achieving intersubjective understanding: Examples from an occupational therapy treatment session. *American Journal of Occupational Therapy*, *45*, 1016–1025. https://doi.org/10.5014/ajot.45.11.1016

Danial-Saad, A., Kuflik, T., Weiss, P. L., & Schreuer, N. (2015). Effectiveness of a clinical decision support system for pointing device prescription. *American Journal of Occupational Therapy*, *69*(2), 1–7. https://doi.org/10.5014/ajot.2015.014811

Dougherty, D. A., Toth-Cohen, S. E., & Tomlin, G. S. (2016). Beyond research literature: Occupational therapists' perspectives on and uses of "evidence" in everyday practice. *Canadian Journal of Occupational Therapy*, *83*, 288–296. https://doi.org/10.1177/0008417416660990

Doumanov, P., & Rugg, S. (2003). Clinical reasoning skills of occupational therapists and support staff: A comparison. *British Journal of Therapy and Rehabilitation*, *10*(5), 195–203. https://doi.org/10.12968/BJTR.2003.10.5.13543

Dreyfus, H. L., & Dreyfus, S. E. (1986). *Mind over machine: The power of human intuition and expertise in the era of the computer*. Free Press.

Durning, S. J., Costanzo, M. E., Artino, A. R., Graner, J., van der Vleuten, C., Beckman, T. J., Wittich, C. M., Roy, M. J., Holmboe, E. S., & Schuwirth, L. (2015). Neural basis of nonanalytical reasoning expertise during clinical evaluation. *Brain and Behavior*, *5*(3), Article e00309. https://doi.org/10.1002/brb3.309

Edmonds, A. (2012). *Teaming: How organizations learn, innovate, and complete in the knowledge economy*. John Wiley & Sons.

Elstein, A. S., & Schwarz, A. (2002). Clinical problem solving and diagnostic decision making: Selective review of the cognitive literature. *BMJ*, *324*(7339), 729–732. https://doi.org/10.1136/bmj.324.7339.729

Epstein, R. M., & Hundert, E. M. (2002). Defining and assessing professional competence. *JAMA*, *287*(2), 226–235. https://doi.org/10.1001/jama.287.2.226

Ericsson, K. A. (2004). Deliberate practice and the acquisition and maintenance of expert performance in medicine and related domains. *Academic Medicine*, *79*(10 Suppl), S70–S81. https://doi.org/10.1097/00001888-200410001-00022

Evans, J. S. (2003). In two minds: Dual-process accounts of reasoning. *Trends in Cognitive Science*, *7*(10), 454–459. https://doi.org/10.1016/j.tics.2003.08.012.

Facione, N. C., & Facione, P. A. (2008). Critical thinking and clinical judgment. *Critical thinking and clinical reasoning in the health sciences: A teaching anthology*. 1–13.

Fava, L., & Morton, J. (2009). Causal modeling of panic disorder theories. *Clinical Psychology Review*, *29*(7), 623–637. https://doi.org/10.1016/j.cpr.2009.08.002

Fleming, M. H. (1991). The therapist with the three-track mind. *American Journal of Occupational Therapy*, *45*, 1007–1014. https://doi.org/10.5014/ajot.45.11.1007

Fleming, M. H. (1994a). Conditional reasoning: Creating meaningful experiences. In C. Mattingly & M. H. Fleming (Eds.), *Clinical reasoning: Forms of inquiry in a therapeutic practice* (pp. 197–235). F. A. Davis.

Fleming, M. H. (1994b). Procedural reasoning: Addressing functional limitations. In C. Mattingly & M. H. Fleming (Eds.), *Clinical reasoning: Forms of inquiry in a therapeutic practice* (pp. 137–177). F. A. Davis.

Fleming, M. H. (1994c). The search for tacit knowledge. In C. Mattingly & M. H. Fleming (Eds.), *Clinical reasoning: Forms of inquiry in a therapeutic practice* (pp. 22–33). F. A. Davis.

Friston, K., Schwartenbeck, P., FitzGerald, T., Moutoussis, M., Behrens, T., & Dolan, R. J. (2014). The anatomy of choice: Dopamine and decision-making. *Philosophical Transactions of the Royal Society London B Biological Science*, *369*(1655), 20130481. https://doi.org/10.1098/rstb.2013.0481

Frolek Clark, G., & Kingsley, K. L. (2020). Practice guidelines— Occupational therapy practice guidelines for early childhood: Birth–5 years. *American Journal of Occupational Therapy*, *74*, 7403397010. https://doi.org/10.5014/ajot.2020.743001

Gambrill, E. (2012). *Critical thinking in clinical practice: Improving the quality of judgments and decisions* (3rd ed.). Jossey-Bass.

Gray, J. M. (1998). Putting occupation into practice: Occupation as ends, occupation as means. *American Journal of Occupational Therapy*, *52*, 354–364. https://doi.org/10.5014/ajot.52.5.354

Gube, M., & Lajoie, S. (2020). Adaptive expertise and creative thinking: A synthetic review and implications for practice. *Thinking Skills and Creativity*, *35*, 100630. https://doi.org/10.1016/j.tsc.2020.100630

Hamilton, T. B. (2018). Narrative reasoning. In B. A. B. Schell & J. W. Schell (Eds.), *Clinical and professional reasoning in occupational therapy* (2nd ed., pp. 171–202). Wolters Kluwer.

Higgs, J., & Jones, M. (2019). Multiple spaces of choice, engagement and influence in clinical decision making. In J. Higgs, G. M. Jensen, S. Loftus, & N. Christensen (Eds.), *Clinical reasoning in the health professions* (4th ed., pp. 33–43). Elsevier.

Holm, M. B. (2000). The 2000 Eleanor Clarke Slagle Lecture. Our mandate for the new millennium: Evidence-based practice. *American Journal of Occupational Therapy*, *54*, 575–585. https://doi.org/10.5014/ajot.54.6.575

Hooper, B. (2018). Therapists' assumptions as a dimension of professional reasoning. In B. A. B. Schell & J. W. Schell (Eds.), *Clinical and professional reasoning in occupational therapy* (2nd ed., pp. 51–72). Wolters Kluwer.

Humbert, T. K. (2004). *The use of clinical reasoning skills by experienced occupational therapists* [Order No. 3140036. Doctoral dissertation]. The Pennsylvania State University. Available from ProQuest Dissertations & Theses Global https://libweb.uwlax.edu/login?url=https://www.proquest.com/dissertations-theses/use-clinical-reasoning-skills-experienced/docview/305150204/se-2?accountid=9435

Kinsella, E. A. (2018). Embodied reasoning in professional practice. In B. A. B. Schell & J. W. Schell (Eds.), *Clinical and professional reasoning in occupational therapy* (2nd ed., pp. 105–124). Wolters Kluwer.

Klein, G. (2015). A naturalistic decision making perspective on studying intuitive decision making. *Journal of Applied Research in Memory and Cognition*, *4*(3), 164–168. https://doi.org/10.1016/j.jarmac.2015.07.001

Law, M., & MacDermid, J. (Eds.). (2008). *Evidence-based rehabilitation: A guide to practice* (2nd ed.). SLACK.

Lyons, K. D., & Crepeau, E. B. (2001). The clinical reasoning of an occupational therapy assistant. *American Journal of Occupational Therapy*, *55*, 577–581. https://doi.org/10.5014/ajot.55.5.577

Mattingly, C. (1994a). Occupational therapy as a two-body practice: The body as machine. In C. Mattingly & M. H. Fleming (Eds.), *Clinical reasoning: Forms of inquiry in a therapeutic practice* (pp. 37–63). F. A. Davis.

Mattingly, C. (1994b). The narrative nature of clinical reasoning. In C. Mattingly & M. H. Fleming (Eds.), *Clinical reasoning: Forms of inquiry in a therapeutic practice* (pp. 239–269). F. A. Davis.

Mattingly, C., & Fleming, M. H. (1994). Interactive reasoning: Collaborating with the person. In C. Mattingly & M. H. Fleming (Eds.), *Clinical reasoning: Forms of inquiry in a therapeutic practice* (pp. 178–196). F. A. Davis.

Mitchell, R., & Unsworth, C. A. (2005). Clinical reasoning during community health home visits: Expert and novice differences. *British Journal of Occupational Therapy*, *68*, 215–223. https://doi.org/10.1177/030802260506800505

Motycka, C. A., Rose, R. L., Ried, L. D., & Brazeau, G. (2010). Self-assessment in pharmacy and health science education and professional practice. *American Journal of Pharmaceutical Education*, *74*(5). https://doi.org/10.5688/aj740585

Mylopoulos, M., Kulasegaram, K., & Woods, N. N. (2018). Developing the experts we need: Fostering adaptive expertise through education. *Journal of Evaluation in Clinical Practice*, *24*(3), 674–677. https://doi.org/10.1111/jep.12905

National Academies of Practice. (2019). *State of the science: A synthesis of interprofessional collaborative research.* National Academies of Practice.

Norman, G. (2005). Research in clinical reasoning: Past history and current trends. *Medical Education, 39,* 418–427. https://doi.org/10.1111/j.1365-2929.2005.02127.x

Paterson, M., Higgs, J., & Wilcox, S. (2006). Developing expertise in judgement artistry in occupational therapy practice. *British Journal of Occupational Therapy, 69*(3), 115–123. https://doi.org/10.1177/030802260606900304

Pearson, S. A., Moxey, A., Robertson, J., Hains, I., Williamson, M., Reeve, J., & Newby, D. (2009). Do computerised clinical decision support systems for prescribing change practice? A systematic review of the literature (1990–2007). *BMC Health Services Research, 9,* 154. https://doi.org/10.1186/1472-6963-9-154

Pilecki, B., Arentoft, A., & McKay, D. (2011). An evidence-based causal model of panic disorder. *Journal of Anxiety Disorders, 25*(3), 381–388. https://doi.org/10.1016/j.janxdis.2010.10.013

Rassafiani, M., Ziviani, J., Rodger, S., & Dalgleish, L. (2009). Identification of occupational therapy clinical expertise: Decision-making characteristics. *Australian Occupational Therapy Journal, 56,* 156–166. https://doi.org/10.1111/j.1440-1630.2007.00718.x

Roberts, A. E. (1996). Clinical reasoning in occupational therapy: Idiosyncrasies in content and process. *British Journal of Occupational Therapy, 59,* 372–376. https://doi.org/10.1177/030802269605900807

Rogers, J. C. (1983). Eleanor Clarke Slagle Lectureship—1983; clinical reasoning: The ethics, science, and art. *American Journal of Occupational Therapy, 37,* 601–616. https://doi.org/10.5014/ajot.37.9.601

Rogers, J. C., & Holm, M. B. (1991). Occupational therapy diagnostic reasoning: A component of clinical reasoning. *American Journal of Occupational Therapy, 45,* 1045–1053. https://doi.org/10.5014/ajot.45.11.1045

Rousmaniere, T. (2016). *Deliberate practice for psychotherapists: A guide to improving clinical effectiveness* (1st ed.). Routledge. https://doi.org/10.4324/9781315472256

Saunders, H., Gallagher-Ford, L., Kvist, T., & Vehviläinen-Julkunen, K. (2019). Practicing healthcare professionals' evidence-based practice competencies: An overview of systematic reviews. *Worldviews on Evidence-Based Nursing, 16*(3), 176–185. https://doi.org/10.1111/wvn.12363

Schell, B. A. B. (2018a). An ecological model of professional reasoning. In B. A. B. Schell & J. W. Schell (Eds.), *Clinical and professional reasoning in occupational therapy* (2nd ed., pp. 23–49). Wolters Kluwer.

Schell, B. A. B. (2018b). Pragmatic reasoning. In B. A. B. Schell & J. W. Schell (Eds.), *Clinical and professional reasoning in occupational therapy* (2nd ed., pp. 203–223). Wolters Kluwer.

Schell, B. A. B., & Cervero, R. M. (1993). Clinical reasoning in occupational therapy: An integrative review. *American Journal of Occupational Therapy, 47,* 605–610. https://doi.org/10.5014/ajot.47.7.605

Schell, B. A. B., Doherty, R. F., Thomas, A., & Knab, M. (in press). Clinical and professional reasoning in community-oriented practice. In Michael A. Pizzi & Mark Amir (Eds.), *Interprofessional perspectives on community practice: Promoting health, well-being, and quality of life.* Slack.

Schell, B. A. B., & Schell, J. W. (2018). *Clinical and professional reasoning in occupational therapy* (2nd ed.). Wolters Kluwer.

Schön, D. A. (1983). *The reflective practitioner: How professionals think in action.* Basic Books.

Schwartzberg, S. (2002). *Interactive reasoning in the practice of occupational therapy.* Prentice Hall.

Slater, D. Y., & Cohn, E. S. (1991). Staff development through analysis of practice. *American Journal of Occupational Therapy, 45,* 1038–1044. https://doi.org/10.5014/ajot.45.11.1038

Small, W. (2020). Practical knowledge and habits of mind. *Journal of Philosophy of Education, 54*(2), 377–397. https://doi.org/10.1111/1467-9752.12423

Stark, S. L., Somerville, E., Keglovits, M., Smason, A., & Bigham, K. (2015). Clinical reasoning guideline for home modification interventions. *American Journal of Occupational Therapy, 69,* 6902290030. https://doi.org/10.5014/ajot.2015.014266

Taylor, R. R. (2020). *The intentional relationship: Occupational therapy and use of self* (2nd ed.). F. A. Davis Company.

Taylor, R., Lee, S. W., & Kielhofner, G. (2011). Practitioners' use of interpersonal modes within the therapeutic relationship: Results from a nationwide study. *OTJR: Occupation, Participation, and Health, 31,* 6–14. https://doi.org/10.3928/15394492-20100521-02

Tomlin, G. (2008). Scientific reasoning. In B. A. B. Schell & J. W. Schell (Eds.), *Clinical and professional reasoning in occupational therapy* (pp. 91–124). Lippincott Williams & Wilkins.

Tomlin, G. (2018). Scientific reasoning. In B. A. B. Schell & J. W. Schell (Eds.), *Clinical and professional reasoning in occupational therapy* (2nd ed., pp. 145–169). Wolters Kluwer.

Toth-Cohen, S. (2008). Using cultural-historical activity theory to study clinical reasoning in context. *Scandinavian Journal of Occupational Therapy, 15,* 82–94. https://doi.org/10.1080/11038120701534975

Unsworth, C. A. (2004). Clinical reasoning: How do pragmatic reasoning, worldview and client-centredness fit? *British Journal of Occupational Therapy, 67*(1), 10–19. https://doi.org/10.1177/030802260406700103

Unsworth, C. A. (2005). Using a head-mounted video camera to explore current conceptualizations of clinical reasoning in occupational therapy. *American Journal of Occupational Therapy, 59,* 31–40.

Unsworth, C. A. (2011). Gaining insights to the clinical reasoning that supports an on-road driver assessment. *Canadian Journal of Occupational Therapy, 78,* 97–102. Doi: 10.2182/cjot.2011.78.2.4

Unsworth, C. A. (2012). The evolving theory of clinical reasoning. In E. A. S. Duncan (Ed.), *Foundations for practice in occupational therapy* (5th ed., pp. 209–231). Elsevier/Churchill Livingstone.

Unsworth, C. A. (2021). The evolving theory of clinical reasoning. In E.A.S. Duncan (Ed.), *Foundations for Practice in Occupational Therapy* (6th ed., pp. 178–197). Elsevier.

Unsworth, C. & Baker, A. (2016). A systematic review of professional reasoning literature in occupational therapy. *British Journal of Occupational Therapy, 79*(1), 5–16. doi:10.1177/0308022615599994

Waldmann, M. R., & Hagmayer, Y. (2013). Causal reasoning. In D. Reisberg (Ed.), *The Oxford handbook of cognitive psychology* (pp. 733–752). Oxford University Press. https://doi.org/10.1093/oxfordhb/9780195376746.013.0046

Young, M. E., Thomas, A., Lubarsky, S., Ballard, T. T., Gordon, D., Gruppen, L. D., Holmboe, E., Ratcliffe, T., Rencic, J., Schuwirth, L., Dory, V., & Durning, S. J. (2018). Drawing boundaries: The difficulty in defining clinical reasoning. *Academic Medicine, 93*(7), 990–995. https://doi.org/10.1097/ACM.0000000000002142

Young, M. E., Thomas, A., Lubarsky, S., Gordon, D., Gruppen, L. D., Rencic, J., Ballard, T., Holmboe, E., Da Silva, A., Ratcliffe, T., Schuwirth, L., Dory, V., & Durning, S. J. (2020). Mapping clinical reasoning literature across the health professions: A scoping review. *BMC Medical Education, 20*(1), 1–11. https://doi.org/10.1186/s12909-020-02012-9

Evidence-Based Practice

Integrating Evidence to Inform Practice

Nancy A. Baker, Linda Tickle-Degnen, and Elizabeth E. Marfeo

LEARNING OBJECTIVES

After reading this chapter, you will be able to:

1. Define evidence-based practice (EBP) and how it is integrated into clinical practice.
2. Describe how to organize evidence around clinical tasks.
3. Name the basic steps of EBP.
4. Write answerable questions for different clinical tasks.
5. Identify key methods for searching research literature effectively.
6. Describe how to appraise the clinical relevance and trustworthiness of a research report.
7. Describe how to interpret the results of a study for generalizability and clinical importance.
8. Describe qualities of effective communication about evidence.
9. Describe knowledge translation and implementation.

Introduction

Graff et al. (2006) anonymously describe husband-and-wife clients whom they call Richard and Anne, who are participants in a case study of occupational therapy (OT) for home-living with dementia. In their study, OT is administered by an experienced therapist. For our purposes, we reimagine how a hypothetical novice OT student we call Jaylin might have used current research evidence with clients similar to Richard and Anne. Their case is a compelling example of realistic everyday needs of couples living with dementia. The case study's description of the expert OT's program and the couple's outcome is itself exemplary for demonstrating that a single case study provides useful research evidence for helping to contribute to evidence-based clinical reasoning.

Imagine that Jaylin has been assigned to work with Richard, who has mild-to-moderate dementia and was diagnosed with Parkinson disease 2 years earlier. Richard is Jaylin's first client with a dementia diagnosis. Jaylin discusses Richard with the OT supervisor and her other colleagues to

OT STORY 26.1 RICHARD AND ANNE

Richard is 71 years old, a retired carpenter, living with his wife Anne, a housewife and his primary care partner. Their house has been adapted for safety and has good accessibility. With the couple, Jaylin completes an assessment of Richard's activities of daily living (ADLs), and both of their needs and goals. Jaylin identifies that Richard has problems performing many ADLs, including dressing, and doing tasks around the house. Although he is independently mobile, he has difficulty planning, initiating, sequencing, and completing tasks safely and without confusion and discouraging outcomes.

Anne reports that she supervises or does many of Richard's previous household tasks and is distressed at taking over his enjoyable routines, such as gardening and meal preparation. She is exhausted from the number of hours of supervision and assistance she gives him and does not leave Richard home alone.

Questions

1. How would you prioritize the issues?
2. What resources or tools can be used to make decisions?

receive expert guidance and then looks over Richard's chart. See OT Story 26.1 for Jaylin's OT assessment based upon data from Graff et al. (2006).

Jaylin recognized the need for information or evidence to guide provision of OT services with the couple. The forms of evidence Jaylin used to inform work with Richard were expert opinion, medical records about tests and interventions currently conducted with Richard, information from Richard and his wife Anne, and direct observation of Richard's activity performance. Jaylin did not seek out or use evidence from research studies to inform the practice with Richard, the type of evidence meant in the term *evidence-based practice* (EBP). This chapter describes how evidence from research studies can be put into practice consistently and in a manner that enriches the contributions of OT and the outcomes of clients.

The Evidence-Based Practitioner

Evidence-based practice is a priority within OT practice (Lin et al., 2010). Because EBP has been associated with better outcomes (Shin et al., 2010), it affects daily practice, reimbursement, and policy. The shift to EBP started in the early 1990s. Healthcare practitioners realized that traditional information sources used in practice (textbooks,

experts, and continuing education) were often out of date, ineffective, or just plain wrong (Straus et al., 2011). Initially, EBP focused on finding experimental studies and analyzing them to determine their credibility based on the validity of the study design and scientific rigor. If the experimental evidence was credible, "best evidence," it was used to determine practice. Practitioners placed little emphasis on clinical decision-making (Shin et al., 2010). This definition assumed that evidence was undeniably applicable to a medical situation, so translation from evidence to real world was relatively straightforward. However, because clinicians have struggled with using evidence to make appropriate decisions, a more pragmatic definition of evidence-based practice has emerged (Shin et al., 2010).

This pragmatic approach uses evidence as part of a clinical decision-making process that also takes into consideration the relevance of the evidence to the treatment environment and the individual client's values and circumstances (Mayer, 2010). These latter two areas are as important as the evidence in the decision-making process. Although evidence may support a treatment, if the environment lacks resources, the treatment remains nonviable. In a like manner, even if the evidence supports treatment but does not match a client's values and circumstances, it will not constitute client-centered practice—a cornerstone of OT. Thus, EBP is composed of three equal core components: (a) the current best evidence, (b) the treatment environment, and (c) each client's values and circumstances (Shin et al., 2010), which, in combination with a clinician's expertise, aid in clinical decision-making. Figure 26.1 provides a schematic of the interaction between the client, clinician, evidence, and environment representative of the current thinking about EBP.

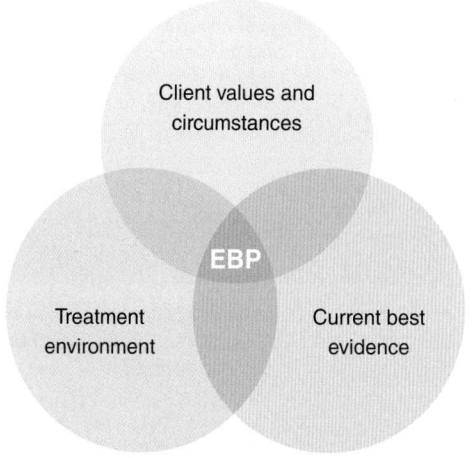

FIGURE 26.1 Interaction between the elements of clinical decision-making in evidence-based practice.

Organizing Evidence Around Central Clinical Tasks

Imagine that you are just about to meet Richard and Anne from the case study. As an evidence-based practitioner, you would use scientific reasoning along with the current best evidence from research studies to support central clinical tasks, such as the selection of appropriate and valid assessment procedures, interventions, and procedures for monitoring clinical progress (Straus et al., 2011). In EBP, research evidence does not replace reasoning that is informed by clinical experience, theory, core values of practice, and ethics. Nor does the use of research evidence replace the clinical use of information derived from observing clients and talking with their family members or from consulting with experts and peers. Evidence-based clinical reasoning involves the use of all forms of evidence in the pursuit of optimal client outcomes. It is the integration of scientific reasoning with professional reasoning that has been matured by clinical experience, validated practice theory, and client-centered values and ethics (Lee & Miller, 2003).

Table 26.1 shows how you, the evidence-based practitioner, could organize the search for and interpret evidence around central clinical tasks, in general, and, specifically, with respect to Richard and Anne. One of the first clinical tasks that the practitioner faces in working with a client is *getting to know the client*. One aspect of getting to know clients is obtaining *background knowledge* about the clinical condition. Background knowledge provides basic information on the clinical nature of a disease (Mayer, 2010). It is often long-standing knowledge, and, therefore, "current best evidence" may be readily available in textbooks or on credible websites. The task of getting to know clients also involves gathering evidence that is descriptive of the experiences and needs of clients living with the disorder in general (e.g., clients who have been research participants in published studies). Expert clinicians who have treated many people with a specific diagnosis may forgo obtaining specific background knowledge because their clinical expertise will already include pertinent information, but a novice clinician, such as Jaylin, should obtain background information before seeing clients. Research designs that would be relevant to this aspect of getting to know the client are **descriptive research**, such as *qualitative studies* and *case series,* and **exploratory research,** such as *cross-sectional studies* and *cohort studies.*

Background knowledge provides the foundation from which to develop treatment strategies, but it must be tempered with information coming from the specific client. Diagnosis, assessing the presence and degree of disorders and their effect on clients' current status with respect to occupational needs and status, is an important part of getting to know clients (Straus et al., 2011). Research on diagnostic studies tests the quality of assessment procedures for

TABLE 26.1   Organizing Evidence Around Clinical Tasks With Richard

Central Clinical Task	Research Evidence	Relevant Research Designs	Use of Evidence for Richard's Case
I. Get to know a client a. *Background*	Typical occupational experiences and needs of clients from populations who can be compared to Richard and Anne	Descriptive and exploratory research 1. Qualitative studies 2. Case series 3. Cohort studies 4. Cross-sectional studies	Generate a discussion with Richard and Anne about his occupational experiences and needs in comparison with the research samples.
b. *Diagnosis*	Quality (e.g., reliability, validity, trustworthiness, usefulness) of occupational assessment procedures	Exploratory research that evaluates assessment tools 1. Cross-sectional studies 2. Case-control studies	Select the best assessment method to identify Richard's and Anne's unique occupational experiences and needs.
II. Choose an effective treatment *Intervention*	Relative effectiveness of different types of treatments designed for this population	Experimental and exploratory research 1. RCTs 2. Quasi-experimental studies 3. *N* of 1 studies 4. Cohort studies	Select, ideally in collaboration with Richard and Anne, potentially beneficial interventions.
III. Estimate the probable outcomes *Prognosis*	Based on factors such as comorbidities, previous and present circumstances identify the outcomes most commonly occurring for these populations.	Exploratory and descriptive research 1. Cohort studies 2. Case-control studies 3. Case series	Assist with planning for discharge, training, and support services necessary for Richard and Anne.

RCTs, randomized clinical trials.

determining an individual client's unique experiences and needs, inclusive of the experiences and needs of primary care partners. High-quality evidence on diagnostic tools ensures that services are relevant and beneficial for the particular situation of clients. Research designs that would be relevant to this task are exploratory research, such as cross-sectional studies and *case-control studies* (Howick et al., 2011).

With respect to Richard, descriptions of the occupational lives of men with mild dementia or similar disorders that can affect cognition could enhance your understanding of possible issues that Richard might face. You could use the information to generate a discussion with Richard about his own life and also with Anne to gather her views and to learn more about her life with Richard. Such a discussion might identify what specific types of in-depth information about Richard and Anne you want to learn in the assessment procedures. After targeting key areas to assess, you could go back to the research literature to find evidence about the **reliability** and **validity** of methods to select the most valuable methods for assessing those areas.

Another central clinical task is that of *choosing an effective treatment* approach and procedure for addressing the client's specific needs and goals. The research evidence that would be relevant to this task includes findings about the relative effectiveness of different types of interventions designed for individuals living with a particular type of personal characteristic or healthcare condition. The task of choosing an effective intervention for clients involves gathering evidence that evaluates the effectiveness or efficacy of a type of intervention in comparison to alternative interventions or no intervention at all. **Effectiveness evidence** is published in studies that use an intervention or treatment research design or procedure. The most relevant research designs are experimental research, such as randomized clinical trials (RCTs), quasi-experimental studies, and *N* of 1 studies (all of which are defined in Table 26.4, later in this chapter), or exploratory research such as cohort studies Centre for Evidence-Based Medicine (CEBM, 2011). With respect to Richard and Anne, you could use effectiveness evidence about interventions designed for individuals living with mild-to-moderate dementia and similar disorders to select an appropriate intervention. In a client-centered approach, this selection involves collaboration with Richard and his wife (Tickle-Degnen, 2002a).

A third central clinical task is *estimating the probable outcomes* based on variables such as the client's age, history, comorbidities, symptoms, and response to treatment, often referred to as prognosis (Moons et al., 2009). This task assists the occupational therapist and client to engage in long-range treatment planning as well as discharge planning, including additional therapies, extended home and community programs, education and training, and accessing resources. Relevant evidence helps track people over time and look for relationships between baseline and long-term outcomes. The most relevant research designs are exploratory research, such as cohort studies and case-control studies, or descriptive research, such as case series CEBM (2011).

For Richard and Anne, it would be important to identify the general prognosis of a client with mild-to-moderate dementia and Parkinson disease. Although it is likely that Richard's functional performance will continue to decline owing to progression of dementia and Parkinson disease, it is also important to identify alterable facilitators and barriers to coping and resilience while living with neurodegenerative changes. The potential for healthy aging with neurodegenerative conditions is a relatively new idea in the healthcare culture (e.g., Tickle-Degnen et al., 2020), a shift that makes it even more imperative that recent literature rather than textbooks or clinical experience be used to estimate prognosis.

The Steps of Evidence-Based Practice

Evidence-based practitioners systematically integrate research evidence into practice by carrying out a series of steps (Lin et al., 2010; Mayer, 2010; Straus et al., 2011).

1. Writing an answerable clinical question
2. Gathering current published evidence that might answer the question
3. Appraising the gathered evidence to determine what is the "best" evidence for answering the question
4. Using the evidence to guide practice for specific clients by collaboratively communicating the results with clients

Step 1: Writing an Answerable Clinical Question

The first systematic step, writing an answerable question, helps the practitioner to focus on the specific type of evidence for a clinical task. The question is written by using key words and terminology that tap into a general body of research literature that may hold an answer to the question and that locates evidence that is relevant to performing a particular clinical task with specific clients. There are two types of questions: background questions and foreground questions (Mayer, 2010; Straus et al., 2011).

Background questions are used to obtain background knowledge and identify descriptive research to understand the nature of the problem. There are two elements to a background question: a question's root (e.g., who, what, when, where) combined with a verb and a disorder, problem, or some aspect of client care (Mayer, 2010). A background question for Richard and Anne is provided in Table 26.2.

TABLE 26.2   Examples of Answerable Questions for Each Type of Clinical Task

Get to Know a Client		Choose an Effective Treatment	Estimate the Probable Outcomes
Background	Diagnosis	Intervention	Prognosis
Example: Answerable Questions			
Root: "What" Verb/adjective: "are common" Problem: "activities of daily living"	P: 71-year-old man with dementia I: Reliable and valid test to evaluate ADLs O: Identify changes in ADL performance	P: 71-year-old man with dementia I: Home-based OT C: Attention control O: Increase the quality of ADLs	P: 71-year-old man with dementia I: Participating weekly in personally valued ADLs O: Age-in-place (home-living) for 3 years following diagnosis
What are common problems in ADLs for people with dementia?	What is a reliable and valid test to identify changes in performance of ADLs in an older man with dementia?	Will home-based OT cause greater increases in the quality of ADL performance than an attention control for an older man with dementia?	How likely is it for a man with dementia who participates weekly in personally valued ADLs age-in-place for 3 years after diagnosis?
Example: Key Terms (MeSH terms)			
Dementia (*neurocognitive disorders; cognitive disorders*) Activities of daily living (*ADLs; daily living activity; chronic limitation of activity*)	Dementia (*neurocognitive disorders; cognitive disorders*) *Test (evaluation)* Activities of daily living (*ADLs; daily living activity; chronic limitation of activity*) Reliable and valid (*psychometrics*)	Dementia (*neurocognitive disorders; cognitive disorders*) Occupational Therapy (*rehabilitation; patient care*) Activities of daily living (*ADLs, daily living activity; chronic limitation of activity*)	Dementia (*neurocognitive disorders; cognitive disorders*) Activities of daily living (*ADLs; daily living activity; chronic limitation of activity*) (*occupation*) Aging-in-place (*Community dwelling; independent living*)

ADLs, activities of daily living; C, comparison; I, intervention; MeSH, Medical Subject Headings; O, outcome; P, patient, population, or problem.

Foreground questions are about current knowledge on the best practice treatment of specific clients. They focus on recent interventions, diagnostic tests, potential client outcomes, and theories about causation (Mayer, 2010). There are three to four elements to a foreground intervention research question (Mayer, 2010; Straus et al., 2011). These are often called PICO questions:

- *Patient, population, or problem.* This element identifies features of the client population of interest, such as the client's clinical condition or diagnosis, gender, ethnicity, age group, and socioeconomic status. Important features are those that identify populations or subpopulations of which the client is a member, ensuring that evidence will be relevant.
- *Intervention of interest.* This can be a specific technique or a general treatment.
- *Comparison treatment.* The best intervention studies examine the effectiveness of one treatment compared to some other treatment. The "some other treatment" does not have to be specified in answerable questions, particularly if the practitioner is not interested if one treatment is better than another, only if the treatment works. Therefore, the comparison treatment may be omitted.

- *Outcomes.* The desired outcomes are results that are applicable to occupational performance. Variables of interest are attributes of clients addressed in OT, such as physical or psychosocial functioning, occupational performance, or satisfaction with outcomes. Models and theories of occupation and OT, such as the Person–Environment–Occupation Model (Law et al., 1996), as well as more general models of health that encompass an OT perspective, such as the International Classification of Functioning, Disability, and Health (World Health Organization [WHO], 2013), provide the language needed to identify occupational variables.

PICO questions are modified when looking for diagnostic or prognostic evidence. For diagnostic/assessment questions, *intervention* will be a diagnostic tool, and outcomes will be the ability of the tool to accurately identify the degree of the problem, distinguish a diagnosis, or determine tool psychometrics. Prognosis, too, requires modifications to the PICO question with interventions becoming *predictor variables* that are expected to alter outcomes and outcomes focusing on long-term participation, health and wellness, and quality of life (see Table 26.2).

Step 2: Gathering Current Published Evidence

Once a clinical question has been written, the practitioner draws on elements of the question to search for and gather evidence. Relevant research is published in various fields: OT, medicine, nursing, physical therapy, education, psychology, sociology, anthropology, and so on. Consequently, search strategies should tap into the research literature of different disciplines.

Each element of an answerable clinical question contains one or more *key terms* for searching the literature. A whole body of literature can be excluded inadvertently simply because the key terms used in a search do not match the terminology used by researchers or catalogers of the research literature. Some of the important terms that OT practitioners use to identify clinical conditions (e.g., sensory integrative disorder) or occupational variables (e.g., occupational performance) are not the most typical terms used to describe research studies in the broader literature. Therefore, it is important to generate a list of synonyms for each key term in each element of the question before beginning the search.

One list of terms that is used by the national databases PubMed and Medline to structure the citations of over thousands of the leading biomedical journals is the U.S. National Medical Libraries *Medical Subject Headings (MeSH)* terminology (U.S. National Library of Medicine, 2017). Freely accessible literature search services such as PubMed (National Center for Biotechnology Information, 2017) provide online tutorials on MeSH, so that evidence-based practitioners can learn how to effectively search the literature with MeSH terms.

Table 26.2 shows examples of questions that you could write with respect to Richard and Anne for each of the clinical tasks. Possible key terms and alternatives that are synonyms and terms that are broader or more specific are listed. For diagnosis ("What is a valid and reliable test to document and identify changes in ADL performance in a man with dementia?"), a combination of *test, activities of daily living, dementia,* and *reliability and validity* yields numerous citations using PubMed, suggesting that this search strategy is effective.

There are numerous free search engines available online for searching the literature as well as clearinghouses for summaries, systematic reviews, and other useful sources of evidence (Lin et al., 2010). One source available to all practitioners is Google Scholar (http://scholar.google.com/), which provides links to full text articles if they are available.

Step 3: Appraising the Evidence

The term *best evidence* is often used in relationship to EBP. Practitioners are encouraged to use best evidence to guide practice. As should be apparent, best evidence is not one

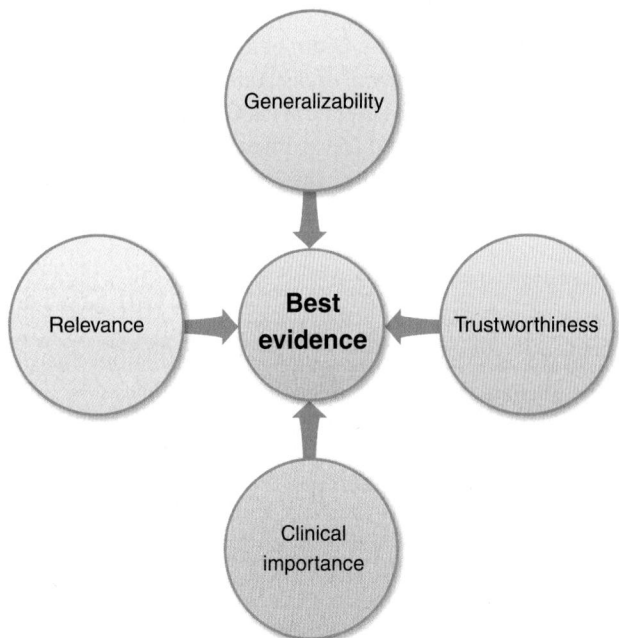

FIGURE 26.2 **Elements of best evidence.**

type of study design or one type of source; it is dependent on the type of question being asked as well as the access to that evidence. Even after a research study has been identified and acquired, it must be appraised to determine whether the study is best evidence for the clinical problem. Evidence that is clinically useful and valuable has the following attributes: (a) it is relevant to the clinical task, (b) it is trustworthy, (c) it has generalizability, and (d) it has clinically important results (Carter et al., 2011; Figure 26.2). There are many excellent resources for guiding the appraisal of research evidence (e.g., Straus et al., 2011).

Appraising the Relevance of a Research Study

The **relevance** of a research study is determined by how well it answers the clinical question and how well its methods fit within constraints and resources of practitioner's context of practice (Tickle-Degnen, 2001, 2002b). Rarely will a search for evidence locate a study or set of studies that directly answers the clinical question. Studies are designed to answer authors' research questions, not your clinical question. The most relevant research study is one that (a) investigates a variable that is the occupational variable of interest or one highly related to that variable, (b) includes research participants who are members of your client's population, and (c) offers clinical methods that are suitable to your context of practice.

To illustrate the process of examining relevance, we return to the citation retrieved for the intervention question in Table 26.2: "Will home-based OT cause greater increase in quality of activities of daily living performance than attention control for an older man with dementia?" One citation was for a paper by Gitlin et al. (2018), which can be retrieved from the *Journal of the American Geriatrics Society*. Examination of the literature via Google Scholar reveals that this article was cited approximately 44 times by important healthcare journals over the 3-year period following its

publication. Study findings were included in a systematic and meta-analytic review of OT interventions for people with dementia (Bennett et al., 2019).

Table 26.3 provides the aim and methods of the Gitlin et al. (2018) research study as applied to determining best evidence. The study tested the effectiveness of the home-based

TABLE 26.3 Evaluation of Gitlin (2018) as "Best Evidence"

	Criteria	Gitlin (2018)
Aim of study	"The goal was to determine whether a home-based activity program (Tailored Activity Program [TAP]-VA) would reduce behavioral symptoms and functional dependence of veterans with dementia and caregiver burden." (p. 339)	
Relevance	Investigates an occupational variable of interest	**Primary outcomes:** Number of behaviors and frequency of their occurrence multiplied by severity of occurrence; Secondary outcomes: Functional dependence, pain, emotional well-being, caregiver burden (time spent caregiving, upset with behaviors) and affect at 4 (primary endpoint) and 8 months
	Study participants are members of your client's population	**Inclusion criteria for veteran subjects:** English-speaking; MMSE score of ≤23 or physician diagnosis of dementia; able to participate in ≥2 self-care activities; not involved in another study; stable medication regimen (psychotropic or anti-dementia meds) ≥60 days prior to study enrollment **Inclusion criteria for caregiver subjects:** English-speaking primary caregivers ≥21 years old; living with the veteran; accessible by telephone; planned to live in an area for 8 months; willing to learn activities; had managed ≥1 behavioral symptoms in the past month; not participating in another study; stable pharmacologic treatment ≥60 days prior to study enrollment
	Clinical methods suitable to your context of practice	**Intervention—TAP-VA program:** Dyads participated in up to eight sessions with OT to customize activities to interests and abilities of veterans and educate caregivers about dementia and use of customized activities. Sessions included assessments of veteran capabilities, executive and physical functioning, fall risk, daily routines, interests and caregivers' routines, employment, readiness, and environments. Reports and follow-up sessions focused on implementing suggested TAP strategies. **Control group:** Caregivers received up to eight telephone-based education sessions with a research team member. Information was provided on relevant topics (home safety, dementia) with no discussion of activity or behavioral symptoms.
Trustworthiness	Type of design that will achieve the stated purpose	Single-blind (interviewer), parallel, randomized, controlled trial; considered strongest evidence for an intervention study; trial registration through clincaltrials.gov best practice for conducting clinical trials
	Methods to enhance trustworthiness	Random assignment: Yes Concealed random allocation: Yes (stratified participants according to caregiver relationship to the veteran (spouse vs. non-spouse) and then randomized within stratum Similar groups at study baseline: Yes (Table 26.1) Follow-up of subjects sufficiently long and complete: Yes (4 and 8 months) Subject's results analyzed in the groups to which they were allocated: Yes Subjects/study personnel blinded: Not complete blinding (Single blinded: trained interviewer masked to group allocation assessed participants; no blinding of participants [i.e., performance bias] nor blinding of outcome assessment [i.e., detection bias]) Groups treated equally apart from the experimental intervention: Yes Attrition less than 20%: No (Total attrition was $n = 57$ [35.6%] caregivers [$n = 26$ TAP-VA; $n = 31$ controls]) p. 342

TABLE 26.3 **Evaluation of Gitlin (2018) as "Best Evidence" (*continued*)**

	Criteria	Gitlin (2018)
Generalizability	*P* value < .05 (significance)	***Statistical tests:*** Descriptive analyses and univariate comparisons between the treatment and control groups using chi-square and Wilcoxon rank-sum tests; primary intention-to-treat analysis to examine the effect of treatment on NPI-C using ANCOVA by calculating adjusted mean differences between groups on the outcome change baseline to 4 months. At 4 months, compared to controls, the TAP-VA group showed reductions in the number of activities needing assistance with (−0.80, 95% CI = −1.41 to −0.20), functional dependence level (4.09, 95% CI = 1.06, 7.13). Caregivers of veterans in TAP-VA reported less behavior-related distress. Benefits did not extend to 8 months.
Clinical importance	Effect size	***Between-treatment and control groups at 4 months:*** Total Number ADL/IADLs needing assist = small effect Level ADL/IADL dependence = small effect # ADLs needing assist = small effect # IADLs needing assist = moderate effect Level ADL dependence = trivial effect Level IADL = trivial effect dependence

ADL, activities of daily living; ANCOVA, analysis of covariance; IADL, instrumental activities of daily living; MMSE, Mini-Mental State Examination. Neuropsychiatric Inventory—Clinician (NPI-C)

Tailored Activity Program to reduce behavioral symptoms and functional dependence of veterans with dementia as well as caregiving burden. Researchers addressed functional outcomes similar to the goals identified by Richard and his wife. Richard's age and severity of disease fall within the research participants' ranges of age and severity of disease. Although the participants are veterans, they are primarily men and the program is individualized to clients, which makes it appropriate for Richard's situation. In addition, caregiving participants in the study are primarily women spouses similar to Anne. Your practice setting has a home-based component, yet it has not implemented a program that specifically customizes activity interventions to the interests and abilities of the client with dementia or educate the care partners about dementia related to that customized activity. The methods of this program are feasible for your practice because they do not require special equipment or knowledge. Overall, the article is relevant to your purposes, and you should continue with your appraisal of the trustworthiness of the findings of the study.

Appraising the Trustworthiness of a Research Study

The relevance of a research study is assessed primarily as a degree of fit between your clinical need, as represented in the clinical question, and the study design. The **trustworthiness** of a research study is assessed primarily as a degree of fit between the research question, or purpose, and methods of the study. A trustworthy study is one for which conclusions are defensible with respect to study design and there are few, if any, alternative plausible explanations—scientific

explanations for the findings beyond the conclusions drawn from the study and its researchers (Carter et al., 2011). Trustworthiness is enhanced when the researcher carefully and rigorously maintains standards of discovery, description, and explanation (Carpenter & Hammell, 2000).

A trustworthy research study (a) uses a study design that will achieve the stated purpose and (b) provides methods to enhance trustworthiness with respect to standards of science. Evidence-based practitioners evaluate the degree to which a descriptive study provides a defensible description of a client or clinical population; an assessment study provides a strong test of reliability, validity, or usefulness of an assessment procedure; an intervention effectiveness study supports the conclusion that outcomes were caused by the intervention and not by other factors.

The first area to assess to determine trustworthiness is whether the best design was used to answer the research question. Table 26.4 provides common types of study designs and their trustworthiness for different clinical tasks. Each type of study is best used for different types of questions; for example, RCTs and other experimental research are the strongest design for answering intervention questions because they are most suited to determining cause and effect. Cross-sectional studies are useful for diagnostic questions because they capture subjects at a single point of time in the diagnostic continuum, allowing for a determination if the instrument can accurately identify a problem or disease. Hierarchies of evidence have been developed to rank the trustworthiness of different study designs. Table 26.5 provides a hierarchy of evidence for the categories of diagnostic, intervention effectiveness, and prognosis evidence.

| TABLE 26.4 | Common Research Study Designs |

Study Design	Definition
Experimental (Test Hypotheses, Identify Cause and Effect)	
RCTs	An intervention study in which subjects are randomly assigned to the experimental treatment group or the control group
Quasi-experimental	An intervention study in which subjects are non-randomly assigned to the experimental treatment group or the control group
N of 1	An intervention study in which a **single subject** is the total population. This subject receives several treatment periods; one period involves the experimental treatment, and the others, alternative or placebo treatments. Usually, the subject receives multiple baseline measurements and multiple outcome measurements to determine if the intervention causes change.
Associative (Identify Risk Factors or Possible Causes; Hypothesis Generating)	
Cohort	A study in which subjects who represent a particular population are measured on suspected risk factors or predictors of outcome(s) of interest and are followed over time to determine (a) the incidence or natural history of the outcome and (b) the relationship between the predictors and the outcome(s).
Case-control	A retrospective study in which subjects with the outcome of interest (cases) are selected and matched to subjects without the outcome of interest (controls). The presence of risk factors or predictors is determined through self-report or chart review, and the relationship between these retrospective predictors and the outcome of interest is determined.
Cross-sectional	A study in which subjects who represent a particular population are measured simultaneously for suspected risk factors or predictors and outcome(s) of interest to determine (a) the prevalence of the outcome and (b) the relationship between the predictors and the outcome(s).
Descriptive (Describe Problem)	
Qualitative	A research paradigm based on the assumption that there are multiple constructed realities and that the purpose of research is to describe and analyze these realities to facilitate the understanding of the phenomena.
Case series (case study)	A study that tracks several patients over the course of a disease. The results are not aggregated and detailed information on the diagnosis, treatment, and outcomes is provided for each individual patient (a case study tracks a single patient in a like manner).

The second area to assess to determine trustworthiness is that of methods used to reduce bias and enhance validity. All studies have some form of bias (see Hartman et al., 2002); nonetheless, some studies are more trustworthy than others because they have addressed these biases and other potential limitations (Carter et al., 2011). There are numerous scales to assess trustworthiness (e.g., Jadad et al., 1996;

Maher et al., 2003). Table 26.6 provides one set of assessment criteria (Straus et al., 2011) that can be used to assess trustworthiness.

Few studies achieve 100% on a trustworthiness scale. A less-than-perfect score does not indicate that you should automatically discard a study. Rather, trustworthiness is a continuous scale from 0% to 100% and each study will lie

| TABLE 26.5 | Hierarchy of Trustworthiness of Study Designs |

Diagnosis	Intervention	Prognosis
I. SR of cross-sectional studies with consistently applied reference standards and blinding II. Cross-sectional study with consistently applied reference standards and blinding III. Nonconsecutive cross-sectional study or studies without consistently applied reference standards IV. Case-control study V. Mechanism-based reasoning	I. SR of RCT or N of 1 studies II. RCT or observational study with dramatic effect III. Non-randomized controlled cohort study IV. Case series, case-control study, or historically controlled study V. Mechanism-based reasoning	I. SR of inception cohort studies II. Inception cohort study III. Cohort study or control arm of RCT IV. Case series, case-control study, or poor-quality prognostic cohort study V. n/a

Hierarchy is represented by the Roman numerals from I (*strongest design*) to V (*weakest design*).
RCT, randomized controlled trial; SR, systematic review.
Adapted from the Centre for Evidence-Based Medicine. (2011). *The Oxford Centre for evidence-based medicine 2011 levels of evidence.* http://www.cebm.net/index.aspx?o=5653

TABLE 26.6 Criteria for Determining Trustworthiness

Diagnosis	Intervention	Prognosis
1. Independent, blind comparison of the new diagnostic test to a reference standard 2. Evaluation of the new diagnostic test on a full spectrum of patients 3. Both reference standard and new diagnostic test obtained on all study subjects	1. Random assignment 2. Concealed random allocation 3. Similar groups at study baseline 4. Follow-up of subjects sufficiently long and complete 5. Subject's results are analyzed in the groups to which they were allocated 6. Subjects/study personnel blinded 7. Groups treated equally apart from the experimental intervention 8. Attrition <20%	1. Baseline data obtained on a defined, representative sample at a common point in their treatment 2. Follow-up of subjects sufficiently long and complete 3. Objective outcome measures applied at follow-up by blinded assessors 4. Adjustments for important prognostic covariates for subgroups with different prognostic outcomes 5. Validation study completed

Source: Data from Straus, S. E., Glasziou, P., Richardson, W. S., & Haynes, R. B. (2011). *Evidence-based medicine* (4th ed.). Churchill Livingstone.

somewhere on that scale. If it is low on the scale, then you have little certainty that the study results represent what might happen to your client; if trustworthiness is high, you can be fairly certain that the study results will reflect what will happen to your client. The more certain you are, the more confident you can be about recommending a particular treatment.

The study by Gitlin and colleagues (2018) was an RCT. The clinical task is to identify intervention effectiveness. RCTs are the best choice to determine cause and effect (see Table 26.4). A review of the study using eight criteria proposed for intervention studies in Table 26.6 suggests that this study has excellent general validity and, therefore, the results are probably trustworthy (see Table 26.4).

Interpreting the Results of a Study: Generalizability and Clinical Importance

Now that you have completed a basic evaluation of relevance and trustworthiness of the study, it is time to examine whether the results can help answer the clinical question. First, results must have **generalizability** from the sample to the population, and second, they must be of **clinical importance.** Clinical importance looks at the practical application of the results. It considers whether the magnitude and scope of the results are sufficient to suggest that using the intervention will produce changes that will improve the outcomes for actual patients in the outcomes tested in the study (see Figure 26.2).

A hallmark of research and the scientific method is to understand general, population-centered truths rather than individual outcomes (Mayer, 2010). However, clinical research cannot be completed on a population because it is not feasible to access every person with the characteristics of interest. Therefore, research is performed on a sample of people who are assumed to be representative of the whole population. Research studies describe the characteristics of the sample (inclusion/exclusion criteria

and demographics) so readers can determine how well the study sample matches a population and how well their clients match the sample. All data generated from a study are sample-specific and represent sample participants but may or may not represent the larger population. If the study is trustworthy, the results are considered to provide a good representation of the sample. How do we know that these trustworthy, sample-specific results can translate to the population?

Inferential statistics determine how confident we should be that sample results can be generalized to the client population. The statistic used to estimate the confidence that sample results can be generalized is the **P value.** The threshold to distinguish between statistically significant results that inspire higher confidence about generalizability versus nonsignificant results that inspire lower confidence is generally set at $P \leq .05$. Essentially, a $P \leq .05$ states "the probability that the results in this study are due to chance is less than 1 in 20. Based on this low probability, we feel somewhat confident that we can generalize the results to the population."

An intervention study finding in which a P value is statistically nonsignificant (e.g., $P > .05$) indicates that we should not feel as confident generalizing the sample results to the population and that the range of possible responses to the intervention is large. This nonsignificant finding does not tell us that the intervention is ineffective. Rather, it tells us that we cannot be sure that the intervention would or would not be effective outside the sample. We must use caution in generalizing nonsignificant results to the population and to our client.

Note that inferential statistics, whether they yield statistically significant or nonsignificant results, tell us only about general tendencies in the population and not about our particular client's responses. However, the results of inferential statistics aid us in our clinical reasoning as we work with the client. We are more likely to feel confident in applying statistically significant results to our client's situation than nonsignificant results.

The results of Gitlin's (2018) study indicated that treatment group dyads did statistically significantly better than people in the control group for behavioral symptoms, functional dependence, pain, and caregiver distress at 4 months. However, the treatment effect did not carry over for outcomes measured at 8 months. Additionally, the outcomes of caregiver depression, burden, and time spent caregiving did not statistically differ across treatment and control groups (Table 26.3). The P values associated with the results suggest that improvements in behavioral symptoms, functional dependence in ADLs/IADLs, and pain among veterans with dementia as well as caregiver distress reductions would also be seen on average in the population, and therefore, we might expect Richard to show improvement with this type of intervention.

Separate from statistical significance is clinical importance. Statistical significance focuses on the ability to generalize results from samples to populations, regardless of how effective those results are. Statistical significance is tied to sample size because it examines the probability that the results represent a true effect. Thus, with a large enough sample, *any* result can be statistically significant and represent a true effect as long as the study was highly controlled and used trustworthy, reliable, and valid assessment procedures. However, this true effect may not be large enough to affect clients in any meaningful way. Best practice guidelines for reporting research results identify the inclusion of effect sizes as a key aspect (Moher et al., 2010). It is important to know that small sample sizes that produce nonsignificant results may actually have produced an effect that would generalize to the population if the study were to be replicated with a larger sample size. The study's sample size might be too small to detect that the effect would generalize to the population (i.e., it does not provide us with enough confidence in the generalizability of the findings).

An *effect size* describes the magnitude of the difference between two treatment effects or the magnitude of the relationship between two variables using some form of a standardized score (Ferguson, 2009). The standardized score eliminates the scale of the original instrument used to measure the variable, which allows effect sizes to be compared between outcome measures or between studies. Often, the numerical effect size is translated into a verbal interpretation, such as "small," "moderate," or "large," to assist clinicians in estimating the magnitude of the effect on treatment (Ferguson, 2009; Tickle-Degnen, 2001).

Another way to determine clinical importance is the **minimal clinically important difference (MCID)**. The MCID is the smallest change in an outcome that will lead to some perceived clinically beneficial improvement. For example, Salaff et al. (2004) identified that MCID for pain intensity for people with chronic musculoskeletal pain owing to arthritis after a 3-month period using a numerical rating scale (NRS) was 2. Thus, a study that reported a change of 2 on an NRS would suggest that the intervention had a clinically important effect on pain intensity. The biggest barrier to using MCID in clinical practice is that clinicians must know the MCID for different outcome measures, and these are not always readily available.

When determining whether to use results, both significance and clinical importance should be considered. A significant result that has large clinical importance clearly has a strong potential to have a positive outcome for a client. Conversely, a nonsignificant result with small clinical importance is unlikely to be worth implementing. Results that are either significant with small clinical importance or are nonsignificant with large clinical importance are potential candidates for use. Clinical reasoning should be used to decide whether to use them (Table 26.7).

Effect sizes calculated for the Gitlin study suggest that the intervention yielded small-to-moderate treatment effects for the ADL and caregiver burden, outcomes you are interested in, when comparing the treatment group with the control group (see Table 26.3). Unfortunately, information to estimate the MCID is not readily available based on the measures used in the study. Therefore, although the results are generalizable from the sample to the population (significant), they may not necessarily yield clinically important differences.

The moderate-to-small effect sizes from this study require the use of clinical reasoning to understand their implications for Richard and other similar clients. On the one hand, the results suggest some short-term, immediate benefits. However, these results were observed 4 months postintervention and did not hold up at the 8-month assessment

TABLE 26.7	Clinical Decision-Making Rubric Based on Generalizability and Clinical Importance of Study Results	
	Clinically Important	**Clinically Not Important**
Statistically significant	Likely to produce meaningful results if it matches your client **(Strong Results)**	Might be worth using; may produce meaningful outcomes for certain clients **(Weak Results)**
Statistically nonsignificant	Moderately worth using; likely to produce meaningful outcomes for certain clients **(Moderate Results)**	Highly unlikely to produce meaningful outcomes **(Negligible Results)**

on a disease process that routinely causes continued deterioration of abilities. Additionally, as the authors mention, many interventions targeting activity engagement require continued active engagement and often modifications over time, which make long-term intervention fidelity challenging to measure. Given the small sample size and potential underpowered statistical calculations, the fact that the participants in this study showed improvements in comparison to a group of similar individuals suggests that this treatment may be more beneficial than the effect sizes indicate. We do not know how Richard would respond as an individual to this type of intervention. This clinical conundrum demonstrates the importance of clinician expertise and client input in the decision-making process. Table 26.8 provides a starting point for the clinical reasoning on how to implement the evidence into practice. From this table, we may decide that the evidence is "moderately worth using" for the case of Richard.

A final test of best evidence is that it should have been replicated; numerous studies should show similar results related to treatment, diagnoses, or prognoses. **Systematic reviews** are frequently cited as the best "best evidence" because they synthesize the results from multiple studies (CEBM, 2011; Lin et al., 2010). A **meta-analysis,** a form of systematic review that includes statistical techniques to combine the results of multiple studies into a single effect size, provides one of the best overall reviews of evidence. The Cochrane Collaboration is one group that has provided numerous high-quality systematic reviews on various

topics (Cochrane Collaboration, 2017). These topics include the effectiveness of cognitive training for people with dementia (Bahar-Fuchs et al., 2019) and the use of mindfulness to reduce stress in family carers (Liu et al., 2018). Although systematic reviews provide overall evidence of the efficacy of a treatment, they may be limited in their use for individual clients. Often, the summaries address a heterogeneous group of subjects or broad treatment plans that reduce their relevance to day-to-day practice. Systematic reviews are best when a topic is well established. They are less effective for new and emerging practices where they may underestimate the effect owing to small sample sizes or unreliable assessment procedures or overestimate it owing to poorly controlled studies with biased assessment procedures. Systematic reviews are excellent sources of articles that deal with a specific sample or treatment topic; evidence-based practitioners can use the reviews to identify and obtain more specific articles for treatments that show an overall effectiveness. Gitlin's study (2018) was included in a meta-analysis of other studies of OT home programs for dementia (Bennett et al., 2019). This meta-analytic study found that Gitlin's beneficial effects of the Tailored Activity Program were replicated by other studies of home programs. This finding provides further evidence that the Gitlin study provides "best evidence" for clinical decision-making with Richard and his wife Anne.

There is one other consideration regarding best evidence. The best evidence is the best that can be found and not "best" in the sense of meeting all of the standards. The

TABLE 26.8 Clinical Reasoning on How to Implement Evidence Into Practice

Trustworthiness Level	Result Level (See Table 26.7)			
	Strong	Moderate	Weak	Negligible
High	Strong recommendation	Moderate recommendation	Moderate recommendation	Weak recommendation
Moderate	Moderate recommendation	Moderate recommendation	Weak recommendation	Do not recommend
Low	Weak recommendation	Weak recommendation	Do not recommend	Do not recommend
Descriptions of Recommendations				
Strong recommendation	This intervention is likely to work for most clients who are similar to the study sample. Most clients would prefer to receive it. Most clients will need few if any decision-making aids to determine to use this intervention if it is consistent with client values and preferences for outcomes			
Moderate recommendation	This intervention is likely to work for many clients who are similar to the study sample. Many clients would prefer to receive this intervention; however, clinicians should provide clients with decision aids to help them make a determination if this treatment is consistent with client values and preferences for outcomes.			
Weak recommendation	This intervention is likely to work for some clients who are similar to the study sample. Some clients would prefer to receive this intervention; however, clinicians should take care when recommending this intervention to clients and provide decision aids and spend time to help them make a determination if this treatment is consistent with client values and preferences for outcomes. Clinicians should be clear that results may be suboptimal.			

possible answer this best evidence delivers may be one about which you can feel a high, moderate, or low degree of confidence. You might not have enough time to gather and evaluate enough evidence to form a confident opinion, which is very likely given, in this scenario, how busy you are as a practitioner in an outpatient clinic. Even with little research evidence about which you feel a modicum of confidence, you may go to the next step of EBP: communication about the evidence with the client, in this case, Richard, and other individuals, such as his wife.

Step 4: Using the Evidence to Guide Practice

By appraising the evidence, you will have identified that a study can potentially be applied to your client; it matches general characteristics and is feasible within your clinical setting. You will also know from your appraisal that study results are generally trustworthy and demonstrate potentially generalizable and clinically important results. This study can now be used as a tool to help develop and implement treatment. However, before you decide to use the results of a study, you must determine whether it matches the values and circumstances of your client (see Figure 26.1) by communicating the evidence to the client to inform decision-making about treatment.

As has been put forward in this chapter, EBP emerges from the core values and ethics of OT (American Occupational Therapy Association, 2020). EBP occurs in a respectful, truthful, and collaborative relationship with clients and with those acting on the clients' behalf. Clients are viewed as active contributors to the therapy process rather than passive recipients of information or services (Law et al., 1995). To be active rather than passive, that is, to act with as much autonomy as possible and the least amount of dependency, clients and those acting on their behalf must be informed. To be an informed client means to know, as best as possible, the meaning of one's occupational status in relationship to one's quality of life, to know the nature and quality of possible OT assessments to be undertaken, to know the quality and probable outcomes of relevant interventions, and to have the means to assess one's own progress toward meaningful outcomes. Once informed, clients and those acting on their behalf can reason and act with the degree of autonomy of which they are capable.

The main goal of communicating about evidence is to inform decision-making (Tickle-Degnen, 2000, 2002b). Wise decisions are ones that are likely to benefit the client and are embraced by them, you (the OT practitioner), and others of importance to the clients, such as other practitioners. Communication that achieves these types of decisions has the following attributes: (a) it has content that accurately represents the research evidence, including its strengths and weaknesses related to relevance and trustworthiness; (b) it involves language that is mutually understandable to all participants; and (c) it encourages an open and mutual discussion of information and ideas rather than a closed-ended or unidirectional delivery of information from one individual to another. Even a small amount of evidence in which you have a small degree of confidence can be helpful in decision-making if it is presented with these qualities in mind.

Communication with Richard and Anne about the ADL program might be as follows: "Programs that help couples living with dementia learn how to better self-manage activities that they find important for their quality of life generally improve the performance of ADLs. However, some people's ADLs improve more than others. Would you be interested in participating in an ADL program?" In this communication, findings are accurately portrayed in past rather than present tense, and pertinent relevant issues are addressed, enabling Richard and Anne to assess the evidence themselves.

One implication of autonomous reasoning and action is that clients can choose to participate or not participate in OT assessments and interventions. Health practitioners may decide to encourage or discourage client participation. EBP is not about the imposition of the will of one individual on the will of the other but rather is a mutual search for and discussion about information that will aid informed, wise decision-making. The practitioner's responsibility is to provide information so that reasoned decision-making is maximized.

Knowledge Translation and Implementation

This chapter has focused on methods to integrate evidence into the treatment of a specific client. There are times when you will want to develop and implement an evidence-based system-wide program that improves or adds to existing evaluation or treatment methods used in your clinic.

Shifting evidence-based interventions from research to practice is very difficult. Studies suggest it takes from 17 to 20 years for an effective treatment to be systematically integrated into practice (Bauer & Kirchner, 2020). Knowledge translation and implementation provide a more systemic method to move research into practice. **Knowledge translation** is "the synthesis, exchange, and application of knowledge by relevant stakeholders to accelerate the benefits of global and local innovation in strengthening health systems and improving people's health" (WHO, 2012, p. 6). Knowledge translation focuses on ways to develop, conduct, and interpret research to enable easier application in clinical practice (Sudsawad, 2007). **Implementation** is an iterative process that focuses on putting to use or integrating evidence-based approaches within a specific clinical or community-based setting (Tabak et al., 2012). Together, knowledge translation and implementation promote the uptake of research and other evidence into practice.

One model of implementation (Damschroder et al., 2009) identifies five actions to integrate treatment into practice. These actions are iterative and circular in practice.

1. *Identification of need.* The key driver of any implementation is the need for the intervention.
2. *Identification of facilitators and barriers to treatment uptake.* Factors to consider include (Damschroder et al., 2009; Thomas & Bussières, 2021):
   - *Individual factors:* knowledge about the intervention, self-efficacy and readiness for the proposed changes, and their identification with the organization proposing the change
   - *Organizational or internal factors:* organizational structure of the site, site culture around norms and values, availability of resources, and overall readiness for change
   - *Systems factors:* healthcare policies and laws shaping how an organization works, interconnectedness of the organization with external organizations, understanding of what other peer institutes are involved in and the competitive pressures related to profit
3. *Development of a clinically useful evidence-based intervention.* There are two considerations when developing a clinically useful evidence-based intervention. First, it must be tailored to the site where it will be used. Research evidence can be adapted to a specific site using opinions by site experts to ensure a match between the intervention and organizational cultures and values and by using site-specific data from electronic health records to identify site characteristics. Second, the intervention should contain characteristics that encourage uptake, such as relative advantage, compatibility, trialability, complexity, observability (Rogers, 2003), good design quality and packaging of the intervention, and reasonable overall cost to implement (Damschroder et al., 2009).
4. *Implementation and evaluation of the intervention.* The proposed intervention should be trialed on a small scale. Once implementation is started, a rapid-cycle problem-solving method such as "Plan–Do–Study–Act" can help lead to success.
5. *Create sustainability.* When trial implementation is completed and the effectiveness of the new method is determined, the intervention needs to become sustainable in the organization.

Knowledge translation and implementation are not easily done by one individual and require collaboration and effort from administrators, clinicians, and other stakeholders, including clients. The process provides a way to ensure that evidence is fully integrated into an organization.

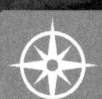

EXPANDING OUR PERSPECTIVES

EBP in Two Middle East Countries

Mehdi Rassafiani

I joined the Department of Occupational Therapy at the University of Social Welfare and Rehabilitation Sciences in Iran in 2008. I taught EBP to Master OT students and was part of a team developing EBP guidelines for a rehabilitation hospital. Then, several years later, I joined Kuwait University, where I was also involved in teaching and practicing EBP.

In those years, I mainly relied on Western countries' resources to teach EBP because there were a limited number of related resources, materials, and published research in Iran and Kuwait. During this experience, I found a number of factors that put limitations on and influenced teaching and practicing of EBP. Two primary factors were underdeveloped at these universities: client-centered practice and student-centered teaching.

EBP is based on the client-centered model where clients are at the center of the teamwork and are involved directly in the process of care. Specifically, clients identify and prioritize their occupational problems at the beginning of the EBP process and discuss and apply the resulting evidence at the end. These two countries have been in the transition process of implementing client-centered practice. Although the OT curriculum for a Bachelor of Science degree (BS) was developed based on the client-centered model, I faced two issues. First, the biomedical model was still dominant in the majority of the settings such as hospitals in both Iran and Kuwait; and second, in the process of teaching and practicing EBP to master's students, some students who were not trained according to the latest BS curriculum found the essence of client-centered practice very challenging. Specifically, one question was frequently raised by these students: what should we do when we are practicing in settings dominated by the biomedical model? Therefore, to answer this challenge, I designed some case studies and discussion groups as well as some materials and resources to fill the gap between the current practice and teaching.

The second factor that put limitations on teaching and practicing EBP was when students had an assignment to

(continued)

EXPANDING OUR PERSPECTIVES (continued)

develop a PICO question based on their experience. Identifying and narrowing down a clinical problem and converting that into a PICO question was very hard for some students who were trained according to the traditional teacher-centered model. These students were less active and relied largely on their teachers to identify and show them how to solve problems. In contrast, within the student-centered model, students reflect on their practice and actively engage in reflection with their peers and teachers. In other words, the students are more active and rely on themselves heavily to identify and solve problems. So, I added some problem-based activities such as group discussions and debates based on their clinical experience to develop PICO questions.

To summarize, in that context, I needed to develop and modify materials, activities, assignments, and resources to allow students to practice identifying clinical questions, finding pertinent research studies, and explaining and discussing the results with clients. Many countries around the world are still working and practicing in the biomedical model and teaching according to the traditional teacher-centered model. Therefore, it is essential to formulate resources, materials, and activities that facilitate understanding and development of these infrastructural skills for EBP.

Conclusion

EBP is an integral part of OT practice. In combination with the treatment environment and client values and circumstances, evidence forms a strong base to achieve best clinical decision-making. To inform the process of decision-making, evidence can be clustered into three types of clinical tasks: getting to know clients, or diagnosis; choosing an effective treatment, or intervention; and estimating probable outcomes, or prognosis. Occupational therapists must develop the skills to identify answerable clinical questions, find and critically appraise research to identify the best evidence for each of the clinical tasks, use their clinical expertise to integrate this best evidence with their clients' values and needs, and implement it within their treatment environment. Critically appraising the evidence involves identifying the relevance, trustworthiness, generalizability, and clinical importance of research. Once the best evidence is determined, occupational therapists must communicate the evidence to clients to ensure collaborative and informed treatment decisions. Without skills in EBP, an occupational therapist will not be competitive in today's healthcare system. EBP takes time and energy; the skills needed are acquired through active learning and practice. Throughout your career as an occupational therapist, you will refine and improve your skills and ensure that you use best evidence to provide best treatments for your clients.

Lippincott® Connect *For additional resources on the subjects discussed in this chapter, visit Lippincott Connect.*

REFERENCES

American Occupational Therapy Association. (2020). Occupational therapy code of ethics and ethics standards. *American Journal of Occupational Therapy, 74*(Suppl. 3), 7413410005p1–7413410005p13. https://doi.org/10.5014/ajot.2020.74S3006

Bauer, M. S., & Kirchner, J. (2020). Implementation science: What is it and why should I care? *Psychiatry Research, 283*, 112376. https://doi.org/10.1016/j.psychres.2019.04.025

Bahar-Fuchs, A., Martyr, A., Goh, A. M., Sabates, J., Clare, L. (2019). Cognitive training for people with mild to moderate dementia. *Cochrane Database Syst Rev. 3*(3), CD013069. doi: 10.1002/14651858

Bennett, S., Laver, K., Voigt-Radloff, S., Letts, L., Clemson, L., Graff, M., Wiseman, J., & Gitlin, L. (2019). Occupational therapy for people with dementia and their family carers provided at home: A systematic review and meta-analysis. *BMJ Open, 9*(11), e026308. https://doi.org/10.1136/bmjopen-2018-026308

Carpenter, C., & Hammell, K. (2000). Evaluating qualitative research. In K. W. Hammell, C. Carpenter, & I. Dyck (Eds.), *Using qualitative research: A practical introduction for occupational and physical therapists* (pp. 107–119). Churchill Livingstone.

Carter, R. E., Lubinsky, J., & Domholdt, E. (2011). *Rehabilitation research: Principles and applications* (4th ed.). Elsevier Saunders.

Centre for Evidence-Based Medicine (CEBM). (2011). *The Oxford Centre for evidence-based medicine 2011 levels of evidence.* http://www.cebm.net/index.aspx?o=5653

Cochrane Collaboration. (2017). *The Cochrane collaboration.* http://www.cochrane.org/

Damschroder, L. J., Aron, D. C., Keith, R. E. et al. (2009). Fostering implementation of health services research findings into practice: a consolidated framework for advancing implementation science. *Implementation Sci, 4*, 50. https://doi.org/10.1186/1748-5908-4-50

Ferguson, C. J. (2009). An effect size primer: A guide for clinicians and researchers. *Professional Psychology: Research and Practice, 40*, 532–538. https://doi.org/10.1037/a0015808

Gitlin, L. N., Arthur, P., Piersol, C., Hessels, V., Wu, S. S., Dai, Y., & Mann, W. C. (2018). Targeting behavioral symptoms and functional decline in dementia: A randomized clinical trial. *Journal of the American Geriatrics Society, 66*(2), 339–345. https://doi.org/10.1111/jgs.15194.

Graff, M. J., Vernooij-Dassen, M. J., Zajec, J., Olde-Rikkert, M. G., Hoefnagels, W. H., & Dekker, J. (2006). How can occupational therapy improve the daily performance and communication of an older patient with dementia and his primary caregiver? A case study. *Dementia, 5*(4), 503–532. https://doi.org/10.1177/1471301206069918

Hartman, J. M., Forsen, J. W., Jr., Wallace, M. S., & Neely, J. G. (2002). Tutorials in clinical research: Part IV. Recognizing and controlling bias. *The Laryngoscope, 112*, 23–31. https://doi.org/10.1097/00005537-200201000-00005

Howick, J., Glasziou, P., Greenhalgh, T., Heneghan, C., Liberati, A., & Moschetti, I. (2011). *OCEBM levels of evidence working group "The Oxford 2011 Levels of Evidence."* http://www.cebm.net/index.aspx?o=5653

Jadad, A. R., Moore, R. A., Carroll, D., Jenkinson, C., Reynolds, D. J. M., Gavaghan, D. J., & McQuay, H. J. (1996). Assessing the quality of reports of randomized clinical trials: Is blinding necessary? *Controlled Clinical Trials, 17,* 1–12. https://doi.org/10.1016/0197-2456(95)00134-4

Law, M., Baptiste, S., & Mills, J. (1995). Client-centered practice: What does it mean and does it make a difference? *Canadian Journal of Occupational Therapy, 62,* 250–257. https://doi.org/10.1177/000841749506200504

Law, M., Cooper, B., Strong, S., Stewart, D., Rigby, P., & Letts, L. (1996). The person-environment-occupation model: A transactive approach to occupational performance. *Canadian Journal of Occupational Therapy, 63,* 9–23. https://doi.org/10.1177/000841749606300103

Lee, C. J., & Miller, L. T. (2003). The process of evidence-based clinical decision making in occupational therapy. *American Journal of Occupational Therapy, 57,* 473–477. https://doi.org/10.5014/ajot.57.4.473

Lin, S. H., Murphy, S. L., & Robinson, J. C. (2010). Facilitating evidence-based practice: Process, strategies, and resources. *American Journal of Occupational Therapy, 64,* 164–171. https://doi.org/10.5014/ajot.64.1.164

Liu, Z., Sun, Y., Zhong, B. (2018). Mindfulness-based stress reduction for family carers of people with dementia. *Cochrane Database of Systematic Reviews.* DOI: 10.1002/14651858.CD012791.pub2

Maher, C. G., Sherrington, C., Herbert, R. D., Mosely, A. M., & Elkins, M. (2003). Reliability of the PEDro scale for rating quality of randomized controlled trials. *Physical Therapy, 83,* 713–721. https://doi.org/10.1093/ptj/83.8.713

Mayer, D. (2010). *Essential evidence-based medicine* (2nd ed.). Cambridge University Press.

Moher, D., Hopewell, S., Schulz, K. F., Montori, V., Gøtzsche, P. C., Devereaux, P. J., Elbourne, D., Egger, M., & Altman, D. G. (2010). CONSORT 2010 explanation and elaboration: Updated guidelines for reporting parallel group randomised trials. *Journal of Clinical Epidemiology, 63,* e1–e37. https://doi.org/10.1016/j.jclinepi.2010.03.004

Moons, K. G. M., Royston, P., Vergouwe, Y., Grobbee, D., & Altman, D. G. (2009). Prognosis and prognostic research: What, why, and how. *BMJ, 338,* 1317–1320. https://doi.org/10.1136/bmj.b375

National Center for Biotechnology Information. (2017). *PubMed.* http://www.ncbi.nlm.nih.gov/pubmed/

National Implementation Research Network. (n.d.). *Active implementation hub.* https://nirn.fpg.unc.edu/

Salaffi, F., Stancati, A., Silvestri, C. A., Ciapetti, A., & Grassi, W. (2004). Minimal clinically important changes in chronic musculoskeletal pain intensity measured on a numerical rating scale. *European Journal of Pain, 8,* 283–291. https://doi.org/10.1016/j.ejpain.2003.09.004

Shin, J., Randolph, G. W., & Rauch, S. D. (2010). Evidence-based medicine in otolaryngology, part 1: The multiple faces of evidence-based medicine. *Otolaryngology—Head and Neck Surgery, 142,* 637–646. https://doi.org/10.1016/j.otohns.2010.01.018

Straus, S. E., Glasziou, P., Richardson, W. S., & Haynes, R. B. (2011). *Evidence-based medicine* (4th ed.). Churchill Livingstone.

Sudsawad, P. (2007). *Knowledge translation: Introduction to models, strategies, and measures.* Southwest Educational Development Laboratory, National Center for the Dissemination of Disability Research. https://ktdrr.org/ktlibrary/articles_pubs/ktmodels/ktintro.pdf

Tabak, R. G., Khoong, E. C., Chambers, D. A., & Brownson, R. C. (2012). Bridging research and practice: Models for dissemination and implementation research. *American Journal of Preventive Medicine, 43*(3), 337–350. https://doi.org/10.1016/j.amepre.2012.05.024

Tickle-Degnen, L. (2000). Communicating with clients, family members, and colleagues about research evidence. *American Journal of Occupational Therapy, 54,* 341–343. Retrieved from http://www.aota.org/Pubs/AJOT_1.aspx

Tickle-Degnen, L. (2001). From the general to the specific: Using meta-analytic reports in clinical decision making. *Evaluation & the Health Professions, 24,* 308–326. https://doi.org/10.1177/01632780122034939

Tickle-Degnen, L. (2002a). Client-centered practice, therapeutic relationship, and the use of research evidence. *American Journal of Occupational Therapy, 56,* 470–473. https://doi.org/10.5014/ajot.56.4.470

Tickle-Degnen, L. (2002b). Communicating evidence to clients, managers, and funders. In M. Law (Ed.), *Evidence-based rehabilitation: A guide to practice* (pp. 221–254). SLACK.

Tickle-Degnen, L., Stevenson, M. T., Gunnery, S. D., Saint-Hilaire, M., Thomas, C. A., Sprague Martinez, L., & Naumova, E. N. (2020). Profile of social self-management practices in daily life with Parkinson's disease is associated with symptom severity and health quality of life. *Disability and Rehabilitation, 43*(22), 3212–3224. https://doi.org/10.1080/09638288.2020.1741035

Thomas, A., & Bussières, A. (2021). Leveraging knowledge translation and implementation science in the pursuit of evidence informed health professions education. *Adv Health Sci Educ Theory Pract, 26*(3), 1157–1171. doi: 10.1007/s10459-020-10021-y.

U.S. National Library of Medicine. (2017). *Medical Subject Headings (MeSH).* http://www.nlm.nih.gov/mesh/meshhome.html

World Health Organization. (2012). *Knowledge translation framework for ageing and health.* https://www.who.int/ageing/publications/knowledge_translation.pdf?ua=1

World Health Organization. (2013). *International classification of functioning, disability, and health.* https://www.who.int/standards/classifications/international-classification-of-functioning-disability-and-health

Additional Resources

American Occupational Therapy Association's Evidence-Based Practice Resources: https://www.aota.org/Practice/Researchers.aspx

https://www.aota.org/-/media/Corporate/Files/Practice/Researcher/EBP%20Resources.ashx

National Implementation Research Network (NIRN). https://nirn.fpg.unc.edu/

Ethical Practice

Regina F. Doherty

"Ethics can be widely described as a moral compass that aids navigation of the often difficult terrain of everyday practice in contemporary health care environments."

—K. JONES-BONOFIGLIO (2020)

LEARNING OBJECTIVES

After reading this chapter, you will be able to:

1. Recognize the ethical issues that occupational therapy practitioners encounter in professional practice.
2. Identify the virtues of health professionals.
3. Understand basic ethics problems, ethical theories, and approaches to ethics.
4. Understand and apply a framework for ethical decision-making.
5. Understand and apply ethical reasoning as a construct within the decision-making process.
6. Identify and know how to access ethics resources.
7. Define moral resilience and integrate tools and strategies to support it in professional practice.
8. Understand effective communication strategies for difficult conversations.

Why Ethics?

Ask yourself the following questions:

- What would I say to a colleague who asked me to change my documentation to indicate that a client is worse than he really is so that the client would qualify for additional services?
- What would I say to a patient who asked me if he could follow me on Instagram while he was undergoing active treatment on the unit where I practice?
- How would I feel if the family of a client with autism told me they were discontinuing his occupational therapy (OT) services because they did not want to comply with the practice's mandatory mask policy?

Ethical questions like these often arise for OT practitioners in their day-to-day practice. They require practitioners to recognize ethical situations and have both the capacity and the willingness to address these situations systematically. In this chapter, ethical issues that arise in OT practice are discussed. This serves as a foundation to aid the reader in understanding, recognizing, and reasoning through ethical dimensions of professional practice.

OT practitioners in all professional roles will encounter ethical problems. Ethics is about reflecting, thinking, critically reasoning, justifying, acting on, and evaluating moral decisions. Ethical problems are often dynamic and complex, requiring additional knowledge, communication with interprofessional colleagues, and consultation with various resources. Consequently, knowledge and understanding of ethical reasoning and ethical decision-making are essential for competent OT practice.

Ethics, Morality, and Moral Reasoning

The terms *ethical* and *moral* are often used interchangeably in professional practice, and although related, they have slightly different meanings. The term *ethics* stems from the Greek word *ethos*, meaning "character." Ethics is a branch of philosophy that involves systemic study and reflection providing language, methods, and guidelines to study and reflect on morality (Doherty, 2021). In contrast, the term *morality* refers to social conventions about right and wrong human conduct and sets the stage for ethical behavior. Values, duty, and moral character guide reasoning and inform ethical decisions (Beauchamp & Childress, 2019). Values are the beliefs or objects a person holds dear (e.g., life). Duties describe an action that is required (e.g., provide food and shelter to care for one's family). Moral character describes traits or dispositions that facilitate trust and human flourishing (e.g., compassion and honesty) (Doherty, 2021).

There are three types of morality: personal or individual, group or organizational, and societal (Glaser, 2005). Personal morality includes individual beliefs and values. Acting in accordance with these values preserves one's integrity. Group morality is the morality of the profession or organization to which an individual belongs. A professional organization, such as the American Occupational Therapy Association (AOTA) or the World Federation of Occupational Therapists (WFOT), maintains collective values that guide group decisions. For occupational therapists, this might be the emphasis on collaborative practice and occupation. Societal morality is the morality of society as a whole. Societal values change over time, and different communities may fight for the protection of different values and rights. Tension often exists between these three realms of morality. It is important to reflect on how these different moralities interrelate because in a pluralistic society, no single vision of morality prevails, making ethical decision-making challenging.

Moral reasoning is a term used to describe the process of reflecting on ethical issues. Moral reasoning is about norms and values, ideas of right and wrong, and how practitioners make decisions in the conditions of complexity and uncertainty (Barnitt, 1993; Doherty, 2021; Higgs & Jensen, 2019). Moral reasoning activates metacognitive thinking that leads to ethically supported actions. It is a manifestation of moral character and mindful reflection (Slater, 2016). We use our moral reasoning to think critically about the meaning and values of a variety of situations including, but not limited to, the therapeutic relationship; the context of practice situations; and the institutional, cultural, and societal influences on the provision of healthcare (Nesbit et al., 2018).

Ethical Implications of Trends in Healthcare and Occupational Therapy Practice

Healthcare systems are increasingly complex. Healthcare policy, as well as demographic and epidemiologic forces, will continue to change the delivery of healthcare services. New technologies, including those used in intensive care, life-sustaining treatment, reproductive medicine, organ/tissue transplantation, artificial intelligence, robotics, genetics, and genomics, have created ethical questions for health professionals, increasing the likelihood of encountering moral distress. Moral distress is an ethical problem that occurs when practitioners know the right thing to do but cannot achieve it because of external barriers or uncertainty about the outcome (Doherty, 2021). Common ethical concerns that OT practitioners encounter in practice are highlighted in Box 27.1 and in Expanding Our Perspectives. Issues that cause moral distress in OT practice with high frequency include those surrounding billing and reimbursement, resource allocation, systemic issues, goals of care, client safety, and upholding professional standards and values (Bushby et al., 2015; Doherty, 2021; Durocher & Kinsella, 2021; Rivard & Brown, 2019; Slater & Brandt, 2016).

Virtues of Health Professionals

Health professionals hold a unique societal role because the public expects them to uphold particular virtues. These include the virtues of integrity, benevolence, competence, kindness, trustworthiness, fairness, conscientiousness,

BOX 27.1 COMMON CAUSES OF MORAL DISTRESS

Common causes of moral distress in OT practice include the following:

- Reimbursement constraints
- Pressures surrounding billing and productivity
- Issues related to client decision-making capacity and safety
- Resource allocation and systemic issues
- Provider competence
- Cultural, religious, and family considerations
- Confidentiality and disclosure
- Vulnerable patient populations
- Upholding professional standards and values
- Balancing benefits and burdens in care
- Practice management
- Conflicting values surrounding goals of care

humility, caring, and compassion (Beauchamp & Childress, 2019; Devettere, 2009; Doherty, 2021; Gawande, 2002; Meindl et al., 2018; Pellegrino, 2002; Purtilo, 2004). First and foremost, OT practitioners (occupational therapists and OT assistants) must cultivate virtuous habits to be benevolent and focus on what is best for the client. Second, the practitioner must be competent. All practitioners are responsible for achieving and maintaining competence in their area of OT practice. They must use evidence to guide practice decisions and participate in continuing education. Third, practitioners must be caring. Care enhances comfort and recovery and is an essential feature of professional practice (Doherty, 2021; Fry & Veatch, 2000). Although most practitioners recognize that caring is inherent in the health professional's role, there are times when professionals interact with challenging clients or families. There may be lack of reciprocity and mutuality caused by the condition itself, such as combativeness resulting from a head injury, which can erode the caring relationship. Finally, practitioners must be compassionate. Compassion is "the recognition, empathic understanding of

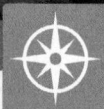

EXPANDING OUR PERSPECTIVES

Dignity of Risk

Aster Harrison, PhD, OTD, OTR/L

Many of the situations that caused me moral distress as a practicing clinician involved conflicts between the rules and norms of healthcare systems and my values as a disabled person and a person who cares deeply about other disabled people. One of the issues that I considered frequently was *dignity of risk*. Dignity of risk means the right for people to choose to take risks. All of us take risks in our daily lives—perhaps talking on the phone while driving a car, riding a bike without a helmet, eating dairy even though it upsets your stomach, or drinking alcohol. People take risks for a wide variety of reasons—including because the risky behaviors can often be pleasurable. Taking risks is also part of how we learn.

In healthcare professions, we also have a value of ensuring patient safety. Preventing harm to patients is part of our professional ethics. In many cases, this is also part of the rules of our workplaces. For example, when I worked in inpatient rehabilitation, we were required to activate bed and wheelchair alarms for all patients, so a light would flash and a noise would sound if they stood up unattended. The goal of this rule was to prevent falls. Fall prevention is a key goal for many hospitals not only because of patient safety, but also because falls are part of hospital quality ratings, and high rates of falls can result in legal consequences, fines, or lost income.

Disabled people, children, older adults, and other persons who are considered by our society to be vulnerable are sometimes prevented from taking risks. This can show up as *paternalism*—overly protecting someone and making decisions for them, instead of letting them make decisions for themselves.

In the hospital setting, many patients would complain about the chair and bed alarms. I remember one patient in particular who really did not want the alarms. Often, the alarms would malfunction and go off every time someone shifted in bed, making it extremely difficult to sleep. This patient was insistent that she needed the alarm off so she could get a good night's rest. She had asked many other hospital workers to disconnect the alarm, but all had said no because of the hospital policy. When she asked me, I informed her of the purpose of the alarms as a fall prevention measure. She remained insistent, so I informed her that she has the right to refuse care—including bed alarms.

Restricted diets were another common area where patients wanted to take risks that the hospital prevented them from taking. For example, a morning cup of coffee is a lifelong pleasurable ritual for many people. I had many patients on restricted diets who were required to thicken their coffee and hated how this changed their sensory experience. Many would request to have their coffee without thickener, and usually this request would be denied. The hospital is worried about patient safety, but they are also worried about lawsuits and financial consequences. As a practitioner in the hospital setting, I often felt the hospital's legal and monetary concerns were prioritized over patients' wishes. Patients have a legal right to refuse care and to go against hospital recommendations, but I rarely witnessed practitioners educating patients about this right or supporting them in exercising this right.

Dignity of risk overlaps with other key concepts in disability ethics, such as bodily autonomy (the right to control what happens to our own bodies) and self-determination. It also relates to the concept of *harm reduction*. Harm reduction frameworks acknowledge that humans will continue to take risks and suggest that rather than demanding people abstain from all risks, we can help them reduce their risks. So, for example, if a patient insists on unthickened coffee

after being informed of the risks and trying it, we might work with the speech therapist on positioning or exercises to lower the risk of drinking unthickened coffee. We may take a harm reduction approach and plan for the patient to have 1 cup of unthickened coffee per day, but to thicken all the rest of their drinks. Similarly, perhaps a patient would agree that while they do not consent to the bed alarm at night, they are willing to keep it on during the day.

As a disabled occupational therapist, I try to bring values of bodily autonomy, self-determination, and harm reduction into my practice. When these values conflict with the policies of my workplace, I remind myself of their importance to summon up my confidence to take a stand. It has also been crucial to seek support from interprofessional colleagues and friends who are also willing to support self-determination and dignity of risk.

---

and emotional resonance with the concerns, pain, distress or suffering of others coupled with motivation and relational action to ameliorate these conditions" (Lown & McIntosh, 2015, p. 3). Compassion serves as a foundation for collaborative, client- and family-centered care. It informs shared decision-making and contributes to positive outcomes for clients, practitioners, and organizations.

Distinguishing among Clinical, Legal, and Ethical Problems in Practice

Practitioners must learn to distinguish ethical questions from other questions that they encounter in the care of clients. Many times, what might appear to be an ethical issue is in fact something else, such as a miscommunication or a clinical or legal issue. For example, a clinical question would be "Can clients with severe dysphagia due to end-stage amyotrophic lateral sclerosis (ALS) eat?" This is a clinical question because there is a factual or diagnostic answer to it. Clients who pass a bedside swallowing evaluation and modified barium swallow (MBS) test are clinically able to eat. If they fail this test but want to continue eating orally, an ethical question could arise. The ethical question would be "Should clients with end-stage ALS who fail an MBS test eat?" This is an ethical question because it raises a values-based question relative to quality of life and the risks and benefits of eating with diminished swallowing capacity.

Legal questions may also arise in patient care decision-making. Law and ethics are related fields; however, they

have different goals and sanctions. Both rely on analytical processes and ground rules for good decision-making; however, laws are legislated and are legally enforceable (Horner, 2003). Laws prescribe what we cannot do. What may be permitted legally might not be justified ethically and vice versa. In the case of clients with ALS, a legal question would be "Do competent clients have the right to refuse medical advice and continue eating orally despite the recommendation of the team?" This example highlights the importance of distinguishing and interpreting the type of question to more critically reason through the problem. Interpretation is a critical step in professional reasoning because how the interprofessional care team understands the situation has great influence on how they will respond to it (Sullivan & Rosin, 2008). See OT Story 27.1.

Reflection and Ethical Practice

Reflective capacity is an essential component of personal and professional development. Reflection on experience promotes the skills and capacities to "discern morally salient features of situations and deliberate about the best act" (Lamb et al., 2021). Recognizing the morally significant features of a situation is one of the first steps in ethical reflection. When reflecting on ethical aspects of practice, practitioners must consider their personal values and how those values might influence their professional work. A value is a belief or an ideal to which an individual is committed (Kanny, 1993). Practitioners, who are aware of their own value positions, critically examine their assumptions, acknowledge biases, and appreciate when values are culturally or socially specific, have a better appreciation of the complexity of moral decisions (McAuliffe, 2014; Thomas et al., 2019).

OT STORY 27.1 CONSIDERING VIRTUES

Victoria is an OT student completing her second Level II fieldwork affiliation in an inpatient rehabilitation setting. She is 8 weeks into her placement and has been enjoying the increased independence and confidence that comes with practice experience and mentorship. Victoria has been primarily assigned to the neurology unit but is working with Tara this week, a covering clinical instructor who practices on the orthopedic unit. She has enjoyed the change of pace and exposure to new diagnoses while working on this unit. Tara and Victoria receive a referral for a newly admitted patient named Joe. Joe was injured in a motor vehicle crash 10 days prior to his admission to the rehab facility. His injuries include open ulna and radius fractures, status post open reduction and internal fixation with skin grafting to cover a soft tissue deficit, a tibia fracture, and a mild concussion.

Tara is excited to treat Joe. The surgical team told her about his upper extremity reconstruction in rounds this morning, requesting a splint to immobilize his forearm. Tara and Victoria go in together to meet Joe. He is sedated and very groggy. Tara introduces herself to Joe and tells him that she needs to make him a splint to protect his forearm where the surgery took place. Joe replies, "I'm too tired." Tara knows that Joe must have this fitted today so that the graft is protected, and so he can begin daily dressing changes to advance his soft tissue healing. Tara communicates the need for the procedure to happen today and tells Joe he can just "chill out" and she and Victoria will do all the work. Joe agrees to the session stating, "Ok I trust you ladies, just get it done and try not to hurt me."

Tara and Victoria begin the splint fabrication, and Victoria is so pleased that she is the student assisting in this intervention session. She has not seen any grafts on her fieldwork experiences so far and finds them a fascinating way

to achieve soft tissue closure. Joe tolerates the session surprisingly well, with very little pain or discomfort at the operative site. When Joe's dressing is removed, Tara turns to Victoria and says, "Wow this is the best graft I have seen! Hold his arm up Victoria, I want to take a picture of it on my phone. It's perfect for my blog." Victoria holds Joe's arm but is immediately uncomfortable with this as Joe is sedated and not aware that the photo is being taken. She feels her uneasiness rise as Tara goes on to take several photos of Joe without his knowledge. She knows that she has a responsibility to do something but is unsure what to do. She broaches the subject by saying, "I know on the neurology unit, we have to get written consent for all photos we take of our clients. Don't you guys have the same policy on this unit?" Tara responds by saying, "Yeah, but no harm done. I'll ask him another time. I'm sure he won't mind. Now can you rotate his arm a little? I want to get a few more images." Victoria is frustrated, and her mind is awhirl thinking of what she should do next.

The case of Victoria highlights the need to call on both character and conduct in professional practice. It also highlights how quickly demands are placed on our reasoning in the practice environment, necessitating us to use our skills of discernment and moral reasoning.

Questions

1. What are the virtues that should guide Victoria in this situation?
2. Victoria is no doubt feeling vulnerable and is at a power differential with Tara. What are the consequences of speaking up versus staying silent in this scenario?
3. How can Victoria best advocate for Joe and uphold the virtue of professional integrity?

Another form of reflection is mindfulness. Mindfulness is a way of tuning in to what is happening in and around us (Schoeberlein & Sheth, 2009). Mindful practice enables practitioners to be present, listen more attentively to clients' distress, recognize their own errors, refine their technical skills, make evidence-based decisions, and recognize the values necessary to act with compassion, competence, presence, and insight (Epstein, 2017; Olson & Kemper, 2014). Mindfulness is an effective way to foster curiosity and reflective capacity, enhance ethical awareness, support clinician well-being, and build moral resilience.

Identifying Different Types of Ethical Problems

When reflecting on ethical dimensions of practice, it is important to distinguish among the different types of ethical problems. An ethical problem is a situation that is believed to

have negative implications regarding cherished moral values and duties *and* that will pose an extremely difficult choice to an individual or group of individuals (Doherty, 2021). It may be manifested by an emotional reaction such as discomfort, anxiety, or anger and is often captured when the practitioner says, "This just doesn't feel right." This "not right" feeling is an emotional response that serves as a trigger to initiate ethical reflection. Being aware of ethical tension or sensing a threat to integrity often drives the need to take moral action and activates the cognitive processes for moral reasoning (Jones-Bonofiglio, 2020; Rushton, 2018). It is through this reflection that professional responsibility is exercised through moral agency, and professional accountability and responsiveness to the patient are manifested through ethical action.

Moral Distress

Moral distress (as defined earlier) results from the conflict of knowing the right thing to do but not being able to achieve it. This cognitive discomfort helps the practitioner realize the potential threat to ethical integrity. Often, multiple stakeholders are involved in the care of the client (e.g., the primary care physician, consulting specialists, rehabilitation practitioners, the organizational administrator, the private insurer, and the family). Moral distress can occur when stakeholders hold different opinions regarding the goals of care, leaving practitioners with no clear course of action.

When conflict arises in the care of patients, the paramount goal should always be patient's welfare. Moral distress must be worked through so that this goal can be achieved (see OT Story 27.2).

Ethical Dilemma

An ethical dilemma is slightly different from a moral distress. A dilemma exists when the individual has obligations to do both X and Y but cannot do both (Horner, 2003). In a true dilemma, there is a strong persuasive argument both for and against a "right" course of action. Each choice, or course of action presented to the moral agent, is morally acceptable in some respects and morally unacceptable in others (Beauchamp & Childress, 2019). In other words, each choice has an element of right and wrong posing a moral conflict. Ethical dilemmas are more complex problems as they often pit values and cherished moral principles against each other (Wells, 2003).

The case of Victoria presented earlier in this chapter is an ethical dilemma. As you will recall, Victoria is the student working with Joe, the patient with post upper extremity reconstruction who was being photographed by Tara, his primary therapist, without his knowledge or consent. It is easy to see that Victoria is experiencing moral distress; however, she also has an ethical dilemma.

Victoria has dual obligations. She has a loyalty to her supervising therapist (and the organization) under whom she is practicing. Tara is a well-respected clinician and has been a resource to Victoria throughout her student affiliation. Victoria wants to honor the student–mentor relationship they have developed. At the same time, she questions whether honoring this relationship is supported because it would disregard the promise she made on entering the OT profession—to above all respect the rights of individuals and refrain from any actions that cause harm (AOTA, 2020). Victoria knows that she also has an obligation to treat her supervisor with respect and discretion. Tara states that she will obtain consent from Joe later. Victoria wonders—does this meet the intent of consent and adequately protect Joe from harm? Can she trust this will happen? Victoria may also be thinking—I am just a student so technically I could just let this go. After all, what if there were repercussions for continuing to insist that Tara not take photos (and delete the ones she has already taken)? Upon reflection, Victoria also realizes that by holding Joe's arm she was an active participant in the session and may be responsible for any consequences of this action. She wonders if she could lose her student affiliation for this. She is feeling angry, anxious, and vulnerable.

Victoria weighs possible courses of action. One option would be to continue to trust Tara's supervisory guidance, allowing her to take the photos and obtain consent from Joe once he is more alert. Perhaps Tara is right; Joe won't mind (and may even be flattered) knowing the photos will be used to educate other therapists. Victoria justifies this action thinking—that would be a "good outcome"—no harm would be done and perhaps even some good would come out of it. By not objecting and deferring to Tara's judgment, Victoria avoids conflict and does not place her student affiliation at risk by bringing the incident to the attention of others.

OT STORY 27.2 EXPERIENCING MORAL DISTRESS

Nakisha works as a certified occupational therapy assistant (COTA) in a skilled nursing facility. She is preparing to treat Padraig who is a 37-year-old male status post traumatic brain injury with diffuse axonal injury. As she begins to enter the room, she overhears Marta, one of the certified nursing assistants on her team say to another colleague, "Do you think he looks okay? I just pretended to bathe him. He was sleeping and will never know the difference. We are short on staff and time today, plus it's such a drag to care for someone who is so out of it."

Questions

1. It is clear that Marta has cheated the patient out of his rightful care. Think about Nakisha's moral distress. If you were in her situation, what would your next step be?

2. What are the clinical, legal, and ethical questions the interprofessional care team faces in this case?

3. What are some alternatives to ensure ethical care for Padraig and restore trust in the interprofessional care team?

4. What ethical principles presented in this chapter can guide Nakisha in this situation?

5. Health professionals that suffer burnout are more likely to take shortcuts. What resources and organizational policies might support Nakisha's moral courage to take action?

Victoria then reasons through another option. In this option, she continues to advocate for Joe and insists that Tara not photograph Joe without his consent. In this way, Victoria upholds her professional responsibility by being both responsive (to the patient's well-being) and by sharing what she knows with her supervisor who is accountable for the action. This action takes both character and courage on Victoria's part as it may cause conflict within the student–mentor relationship. Tara may be upset. She may dismiss Victoria from the case, or Tara may be pleased and she may commend Victoria for her advocacy skills. Either way, if Victoria refrains from further participation in the session, she highlights for Tara that taking photographs without consent is a wrong act (both ethically and legally). This option ensures safety for the client, but it runs the risk of eroding the mentoring relationship, something Victoria greatly values. It also has potential professional repercussions for both Victoria and Tara. The fact is that Victoria cannot choose both options. She must act on one or the other. She has an ethical dilemma.

Moral Theories and Ethical Principles That Apply to Occupational Therapy Practice

Moral theories and ethical principles provide a language for diagnosing, communicating, analyzing, and reflecting on ethical questions. Moral theories and ethical approaches are well-developed, systematic frameworks of rules and principles that provide reasons and ideals for ethical standards. The most commonly used ethical approaches in healthcare are principle-based approaches, virtue- and character-based ethics, utilitarianism, and deontology.

Principle-Based Approach

A principle-based approach to ethics relies on ordinary shared moral beliefs as theoretical content. Principles are duties, rights, or other moral guidelines that provide a logical approach to analyzing ethical issues for a given situation. In case analysis, principles are identified, applied, and compared to weigh one principle against another to guide action. The following principles are commonly used in healthcare (AOTA, 2020; Beauchamp & Childress, 2019; Gillon, 1994):

- **Autonomy.** Autonomy is the ability to act freely and independently on one's own decisions. It is often called the principle of self-determination.
- **Beneficence.** Beneficence refers to actions done on or for the benefit of others.
- **Nonmaleficence.** Nonmaleficence is the duty not to harm others.

- **Fidelity.** Fidelity means being faithful to one's promises or commitments.
- **Justice.** Justice refers to fair and equal treatment. It deals with the proper distribution of benefits, burdens, and resources.
- **Veracity.** Veracity refers to telling the truth.

Virtue-and Character-Based Ethics

Virtues are moral and intellectual dispositions of character and conduct (Lamb et al., 2021). Virtue ethics, derived from Aristotle and Thomas Aquinas, focuses on moral agents and their good character. Using this approach, moral goodness is achieved when behaviors are chosen for the sake of virtue (caring and kindness) rather than obligation.

Utilitarianism

Utilitarianism, derived from the work of Jeremy Bentham and John Stuart Mill, is concerned with actions that maximize good consequences and minimize bad consequences. From this perspective, morally right acts produce the best overall results; that is, the ends justify the means. The ethical action is one whose outcome brings about the most good or the least harm overall (Doherty, 2021). Utilitarianism is often used in public policy development.

Deontology

Deontology is a duty-based moral theory that is based primarily on the work of Immanuel Kant. In this theory, moral rules are universal and never to be broken; consequently, doing one's duty is considered primary, regardless of the consequences. For example, truthfulness is an unconditional Kantian duty. A practitioner would never keep the truth from a client even if the truth would harm the client in some way. From a Kantian perspective, respect for people is a moral imperative; therefore, withholding the truth disrespects the client's right to know.

The Ethical Decision-Making Process

Ethical decision-making is a key component of professional reasoning. It guides client-centered care in day-to-day practice across a wide range of scenarios with an emphasis on moral conduct (Doherty, 2021; VanderKaay et al., 2020). Various ethical decision-making models are available to practitioners. Common aspects of all ethical decision-making models are the need for the practitioners to do the following (Doherty, 2021; Hunt & Ells, 2013; Kornblau & Burkhardt, 2012; Swisher et al., 2005; Swisher & Royeen, 2020; VanderKaay et al., 2020):

1. Recognize and define the ethical question.
2. Gather the relevant data, consider contributing factors, and consult others.
3. Formulate a moral diagnosis and analyze the problem using ethics theory/principles.
4. Problem-solve practical alternatives, weigh options, and decide on an action.

5. Act on a morally acceptable choice.
6. Evaluate and reflect on the process/action/results.

The ethical decision-making process provides a structured and systematic way for practitioners to give due consideration to ethical tensions, reflect on them, generate possible solutions, and make thoughtful choices (see OT Story 27.3). Through this discernment, practitioners actualize their role as moral agents, acting in a way that upholds their responsibility to protect moral values and other aspects of morality. Figure 27.1 outlines qualities and skills that support moral agency.

OT STORY 27.3 APPLYING THE ETHICAL DECISION-MAKING PROCESS

Nicole is an occupational therapist working in an early intervention (EI) setting. She has been working with an interprofessional team of practitioners treating the Suarez family. Their client, Gabriella Suarez, is a 2.5-year-old female status post embolic cerebrovascular accident (CVA).

Gabriella spent more than 3 months in the acute rehabilitation setting because she had lost her ability to perform all occupations, including her ability to speak, eat, and play. The loss of these previously achieved developmental milestones was traumatic to the family, who surrounded this outgoing and loving toddler with support and encouragement throughout her rehabilitation. After weeks of OT and speech therapy, it was determined that Gabriella was ready to be transitioned back to taking food by mouth (since her stroke, she had been receiving nourishment through a gastric tube because she was unable to swallow without aspirating). She was awaiting an MBS test as the final step in this transition.

One afternoon, Nicole arrived to find Gabriella's mother feeding her daughter a cookie. Her initial reaction of joy at the fact that the child was able to enjoy a cookie for the first time in months was quickly overwhelmed by her sobering realization that she had not yet been cleared to eat solid foods. Over the last month, Nicole had become very close to both the child and her mother who were thrilled with this victory. Gabriella smiled, an expression of emotion that Nicole had never seen her exhibit before. This gave the mother great hope, something she had been without for many weeks. Nicole then realized that she was in a tough place when the mother then asked her to "please, please not tell anyone" that she had given her daughter the cookie.

To ensure a professional and caring response to this situation, Nicole must analyze the situation using an ethical decision-making process. This will help guide her thinking and her actions.

Identify the Ethical Question

First, Nicole must identify and reflect on the ethical questions that emerged in the case. This often begins with the question, "What should I do?" In the case of Gabriella and her mother, some questions would be the following: Should Nicole tell the team that the client's mother fed her the

cookie? Should she honor the mother's request not to report the action, knowing that this may cause harm to the child? How can Nicole balance her obligations to the child, the mother, and the EI agency?

Gather the Relevant Data

The next step in ethical analysis is to gather the relevant data, identifying the known facts versus beliefs about the case. It is important to distinguish between the two. Facts are needed to make judicious decisions. Facts regarding medical information and factors such as family context, client preferences, social and cultural considerations, institutional factors, and provider considerations should be confirmed for accuracy. Additional information should be sought if needed. Take a moment and think about the facts and beliefs in this case.

Formulate a Moral Diagnosis and Apply Ethics Principles/Theory to the Case

Once the information has been gathered, a moral diagnosis must be formulated by identifying the type of ethical problem and the ethical principles that apply to the case. If there is more than one problem, they should be ranked in order of importance.

Having considered the ethical questions in the case of Gabriella, Nicole must decide whether the ethical problem is moral distress or ethical dilemma. She decides that she is facing moral distress. Nicole knows the correct course of action requires her to tell the team that the mother has fed the child prior to medical clearance. The relationship that she had with the child and her mother and the mother's emotional plea for her not to tell was a barrier to that disclosure. She was torn with how to best care for Gabriella and show care and concern to the mother. Key ethical principles that relate to this moral distress are beneficence and nonmaleficence. There are other principles and theories that apply; think about which ones as you continue to reason through the case.

Problem-Solve Practical Alternatives and Decide on a Course of Action

Now Nicole must begin to identify practical alternatives and decide what do. She must ask herself, "What is the good or

(Continued)

OT STORY 27.3 APPLYING THE ETHICAL DECISION-MAKING PROCESS (continued)

right thing to do?" She would be wise to seek out resources in her facility and to ask her mentors for guidance in this ethical analysis. She might consult with various stakeholders, such as the interprofessional team, to identify strategies to best educate the family and ensure Gabriella's safety. She could also refer to the AOTA "Occupational Therapy Code of Ethics" (AOTA, 2020a) and "Standards of Practice for Occupational Therapy" (AOTA, 2021b). Generating a list of alternatives enables evaluation of the positive and negative consequences. Once the alternatives have been identified, ethical theory should be applied to support and justify the proposed action.

Nicole brainstormed a list of possible alternatives:

- Ask the mother why she gave Gabriella the cookie and why she does not want other members of the EI team to know. This is an important piece of information to explore. What were the motivating factors behind the mother's decision to give Gabriella the cookie? Did she want to be the first person to reintroduce food to her child? What are the cultural expectations and the meaning of food for the Suarez family?
- Offer support to the mother. She may fear judgment of others or may feel that if the information is revealed, her daughter may suffer consequences of her action causing a delay in her progress.
- Deny the mother's request and inform the team.
- Say nothing to the mother but document the observation in the record. (It is important to note that this alternative is not one that has moral grounding, as it has the potential to cause more harm to all parties involved. It fractures the therapeutic relationship with the family, and although it may alleviate Nicole's anxiety, will only do so temporarily, creating possible future distress.)
- Talk with the mother about the concerns Nicole has related to Gabriella's safety. In a supportive way, this allows the mother to gain better insight into the potential outcomes of her actions and participate in shared decision-making. This conversation may even lead to a joint discussion with other members of the interprofessional care team regarding the mother's understanding of the process for transitioning back to oral feeding. Choice talk and option talk can enhance collaborative goal setting in the best interests of the client and family.
- Describe the situation with the EI nurse without identifying which family was involved.
- Tell the mother that she will not tell the team as long as the mother agrees to not give Gabriella any more food by mouth until medically cleared.

Nicole will need to reason through the alternatives, apply ethical theory to support her actions, and come to a judgment on the best approach. Having virtue, sensitivity to ethical issues, and a process for analyzing ethical questions are important elements in ethical decision-making.

Act on a Morally Acceptable Choice

Now that Nicole has decided on the course of action, she must act on the decision, bridging the gap between knowing what she ought to do and actually doing it. This is where the Aristotelian notion of practical wisdom and moral argument join together with clinical judgment for action. Often, this is the most difficult step because it requires calling on moral courage to take positions that are unpopular or contrary to the interest of others (Aulisio et al., 2000). Moral courage is a skill. It involves facing and overcoming fear to uphold an ultimate good.

Nicole will need courage to talk with Gabriella's mother. She will need to be attentive to the interests and emotions of the mother and remember the ultimate goal, which is to ensure compassionate, quality care for Gabriella.

Evaluate and Reflect on the Process/Action/Results

Finally, Nicole must evaluate the results of her action. Evaluation includes both current and retrospective analysis. This reflection can guide future action by either avoiding or preventing a similar situation or knowing how to act should a similar situation arise in the future. Questions Nicole might ask are as follows:

- What was the most challenging aspect of this situation?
- What have I learned from this case to help improve future patient care?
- What did I learn from the family/team regarding my course of action?
- What have I learned that will contribute to my own moral life and to my virtues as a practitioner?
- How has this case affected me as a care provider? What would I do differently if faced with the same situation again?

Evaluation of the decision-making process in cases such as this one has the potential to change practice, policies, education, or service delivery systems. Evaluation provides the opportunity for personal and professional reflection that can lead to further professional development and greater confidence to respond to future moral distress.

Questions

1. If you were Nicole, which alternative would you have chosen to act on? What character traits or resources might you call upon to uphold your duty to professional integrity in the delivery of client-centered care?
2. How might you use the lessons learned from this case to inform the ethical culture or policies organizationally in the EI agency?

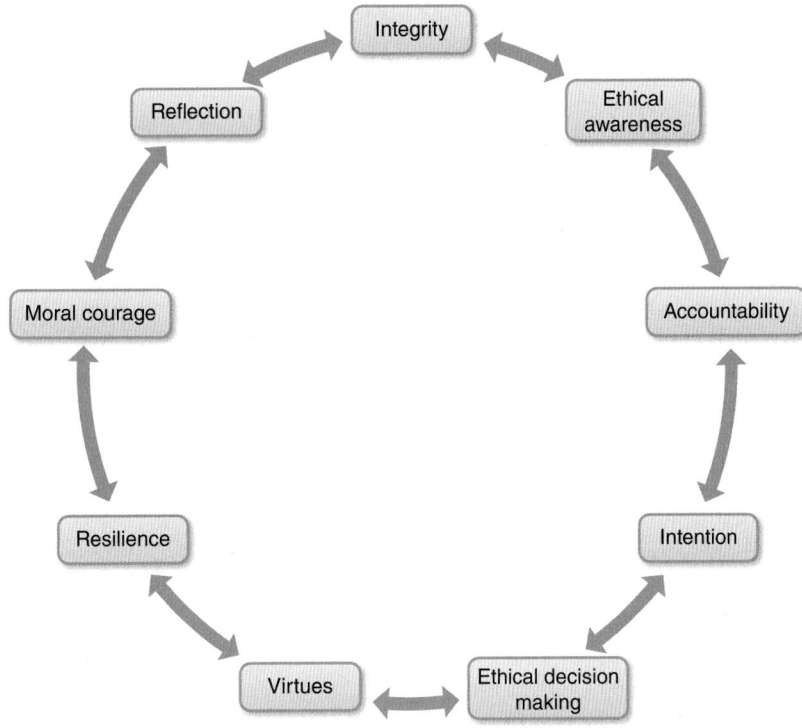

FIGURE 27.1 **Qualities and skills to support moral agency.**

Ethics Resources

Practitioners who face ethical issues must be knowledgeable about the resources that exist to support them in this dimension of their clinical reasoning. Resources are crucial for dealing with the uncertainties related to ethical issues that practitioners encounter at all levels of practice.

Ethics Committees

Ethics committees support practitioners who need assistance in reasoning about ethical dimensions of care. The three primary roles of ethics committees are consultation, education, and policy review and development. Accrediting agencies, such as The Joint Commission in the United States, require that all healthcare organizations have a process to address ethical issues involving patient care and organizational ethics. Ethics committees provide an environment for safe and open discussion of basic moral questions, ease the feelings of staff, provide knowledgeable resources, and empower practitioners and families to make morally justified decisions. Committees serve to help practitioners resolve ethical tensions in keeping with the core competencies for clinical ethics consultation put forth by established organizational guidelines such as the American Society for Bioethics and Humanities and the United Kingdom Clinical Ethics Network.

Effective ethics committees are interprofessional in makeup and have strong institutional support. OT practitioners who are either interested novices or experts in ethics should serve as members of ethics committees because they can bring broad perspectives to ethics discussions, are resources for topics related to values clarification and quality of life, and are skilled in group facilitation. Practitioners in settings without ethics committees should seek counsel in a timely manner from mentors, managers, administrative supports, and professional organizations for appropriate assistance with ethical issues. Other organizational resources such as the office of patient care advocacy (also known as the ombudsman), office of social work, chaplaincy service, and office of legal counsel can also provide guidance with ethical issues.

Institutional Review Boards and Ethical Research Councils

Increased impetus for global research and attention to evidence-based practice have resulted in an increase in the number of OT practitioners involved in research. All practitioners who are involved in research activity have a moral obligation to familiarize themselves with the rules, regulations, and ethical obligations of conducting responsible research. There are many ethical considerations in research (e.g., data integrity and security, conflict of interest, informed consent), but the most compelling pertains to human subjects as research participants.

To ensure an objective review of ethical issues related to human subject research, any institution that receives federal funding is required to have an institutional review board (IRB). An IRB is a panel of diverse individuals, including organization staff and at least one community member, who are responsible for reviewing all research proposals and grants to ensure that adequate protections for research participants are in place. These protections include informed consent, research design and methodology, recruitment, the balance of risks and benefits, and confidentiality. The three fundamental principles that guide the ethical conduct of research involving human participants are respect for persons (autonomy), beneficence, and justice (National Commission for the Protection of Human Subjects of Biomedical and Behavioral Research, 1979). In addition, researchers should consider ethics through "the lens of the whole journey, not just for ethics approvals" (Reid et al., 2021, p. 371).

Codes of Ethics

Codes of ethics are written documents produced by professional associations, organizations, or regulatory bodies that state the commitment to a service ideal, core purpose, or standard of conduct. Codes of ethics are often aspirational, educational, and regulatory in nature (Banks, 2004). The World Federation of Occupational Therapy Code of Ethics is the "overarching global guide to ethical practice" (WFOT, 2016). This code supports OT practitioners in the performance of their professional role. Like many codes, it serves to ensure public trust, safeguard the reputation of the profession, and articulate the values that guide practice.

In the United States, the "Occupational Therapy Code of Ethics" (AOTA, 2020) serves as a guide for professional conduct. Along with the "Standards of Practice for Occupational Therapy" (AOTA, 2021), this document serves as resource to all OT practitioners, educators, students, and researchers encouraging them to attain the highest level of professional behavior. The "Occupational Therapy Code of Ethics" (AOTA, 2020) is a public statement tailored to address the most prevalent ethical concerns of the OT profession. It sets forth aspirational Core Values and outlines Standards of Conduct the public can expect from those in the profession. There are seven AOTA Core Values: altruism, equality, freedom, justice, dignity, truth, and prudence (AOTA, 2020). When practitioners find themselves facing ethical challenges, they should consider these foundational values as guides to ethical practice. Additional information about the code and related documents and the AOTA Ethics Commission can be found at http://www.aota.org.

Regulatory Agencies

Various regulatory bodies, organizations, councils, and health ministries provide oversight for OT practice. In the United States, the AOTA, the National Board for Certification in Occupational Therapy (NBCOT), and state regulatory or licensing boards (SRBs) safeguard and promote public welfare by ensuring that qualifications and standards for professional practice are properly evaluated, applied, and enforced (Doherty & Peterson, 2022). In other countries, oversight takes place through Ministries of Health and Care Professions Councils or is regulated by territory and provincial laws such as Ontario's Regulated Health Professions Act of 1991. Collectively these organizations protect the public by ensuring OT practitioners meet the established standards for education, training, professional competency/behavior, and health. Each has distinct concerns, sanctions, and jurisdiction, but one commonality is their concern for ethical practice.

Licensure or certification is a means of defining a lawful scope of practice. It ensures patient protections and legally articulates the domain of practice for the profession. It also prevents nonqualified individuals from practicing OT or using the title "occupational therapist" or "occupational therapy assistant." Regulatory agencies have the authority to discipline OT practitioners who violate regulations, including the outlined code of conduct. Enforcement procedures, certification violations, and disciplinary actions vary by state, country, and ministry. Typical actions for ethics violations include reprimand, censure, probation, suspension, and permanent revocation of membership/license to practice. The level of regulation varies; therefore, all OT practitioners have the responsibility to understand the regulations under which they work and must be aware of the specific provisions and statutes for their state and country.

Moral Resilience and Clinician Well-Being

OT practitioners experience a variety of ethical challenges throughout their careers. In addition, witnessing trauma, disease, injury, suffering, death, disability, and social injustices can lead to psychological stress for health professionals caring for individuals and families with complex needs (Doherty, 2021). The COVID-19 pandemic heightened these stressors leading to rising rates of anxiety, posttraumatic stress, and burnout in health professionals. The three hallmarks of burnout are

- Emotional exhaustion (being emotionally depleted or overextended)
- Lack of personal accomplishment (feeling one cannot make a difference)
- Depersonalization (characterized by difficulty making personal connections) (Trzeciak & Mazzarelli, 2019)

One way to support clinician well-being and prevent burnout is to build moral resilience. Moral resilience in healthcare has been defined as "the capacity of an individual to sustain or restore their integrity in response to moral complexity, confusion, distress, or setbacks" (Rushton, 2018, p. 112). It provides practitioners with the ability to successfully respond to moral adversity in the workplace. Individual practices such as self-care, ethics education, mindfulness, and engaging in ethical reflection individually and with interprofessional colleagues through activities such as ethics rounds and critical incident debriefings have been found to support moral resilience (Rasoal et al., 2017; Reilly & Jurchak, 2017; Rushton et al., 2021). In addition, organizational ethics supports are key as they contribute to early detection of moral distress, foster feelings of engagement, and promote mindfulness—all of which have the potential to minimize turnover and improve patient outcomes (American Nurses Association, 2019; Bong, 2019; Brigham et al., 2018). Strategies for building moral resilience are highlighted in Box 27.2.

Difficult Conversations

Communication is a fundamental aspect of respectful interactions, therapeutic relationships, and client-centered care (Haddad & Doherty, 2024). The cases of Victoria, Nakisha, and Nicole highlight how difficult conversations are a part of everyday interactions in ethical care delivery. Some of these are with clients, some with families, and some with interprofessional colleagues. Although difficult conversations may be uncomfortable and awkward, practitioners can develop the skill and confidence to improve the quality and outcomes of their communications.

Open communication and empathetic listening are key components to the delivery of compassionate care. The following are suggestions for effective communication:

1. ***Be present.*** Set the stage for the communication by choosing an appropriate environment, modality for the interaction (in-person vs. telehealth), and communication style for the situation. Try to limit distractions and interruptions to be fully present. Establish rapport by making good eye contact and show interest, care, warmth, and responsiveness.

2. ***Use open-ended communication and listen quietly.*** Healthcare practitioners often say too much, which does not allow time for the other person to speak. Talk less and listen without interrupting, judging, or minimizing (Epstein, 2017). Phrases such as "go on" can encourage the person to examine issues at a deeper level (Cameron, 2004).

3. ***Remain focused on the person and the goals of intervention.*** Strive to understand the client's story. What are the connections between the circumstances, beliefs, values, and resources in the client narrative? Ask open-ended questions such as "What is your understanding of the situation?" or "What are your fears?" and "What are your hopes?" This helps you understand another's perspective and can assist both practitioner and client in setting appropriate goals for care (Gawande, 2014; Hinkle et al., 2017; Quill, 2000).

4. ***Be humble.*** If you do not know the answer to a question, say so and assure the person that you will find the answer. Then find the answer and follow up with the person. Share your uncertainty about the case or prognosis.

5. ***Legitimize the losses that the person is experiencing.*** It is important to acknowledge the person's experience. Many clients are not prepared to cope with their newly diagnosed condition. They never expected to be in a compromised state, and their family might not be able to cope with the personal or financial implications of this change. Denial, depression, and anger are common responses to disease and disability. Practitioners need to acknowledge these emotions openly by stating, "What I am hearing you say is that you are angry that you can no longer live alone" or "Let me see if I can summarize what your daughter is trying to say . . . Is that correct?"

6. ***Ensure shared decision-making.*** Questions surrounding new disability, quality-of-life, and end-of-life issues can be especially complex. Shared decision-making is a process in which information is exchanged not *from* professional to patient but *between* professional and patient (Doherty, 2021). OT practitioners are obligated to engage clients in shared decision-making and to fully inform clients of the likelihood of the success or failure of therapeutic interventions. Through this process, health professionals and clients can effectively partner in health decisions.

7. ***Make a team effort.*** In today's complex healthcare environments, the interprofessional care team has a moral obligation to work collaboratively to deliver the

---

BOX 27.2 INDIVIDUAL AND ORGANIZATIONAL SUPPORTS FOR MORAL RESILIENCE

- Education in ethics language, theories, decision-making models, and tools
- A culture of moral accountability and action
- Attention to clinician well-being and healthy self-care practices in individuals and interprofessional teams
- Perspective taking with colleagues, administrators, and clients
- Use of moral distress to inform quality and system improvement initiatives
- Inclusive, participatory decision-making in program planning and resource allocation
- Ethics reflection groups or rounds as opportunities for debriefing, examining differences, and discussion
- Counsel from trusted colleagues, mentors, and employee assistance programs

best care possible. Collective perspectives are foundational to collaborative care delivery. Effective interprofessional teams listen attentively, use understandable communication, provide feedback to others, respond to feedback from others, and address interprofessional conflict (Interprofessional Education Collaborative, 2016). Individuals cannot resolve complex situations and moral distress alone. Effective communication is a lifelong learning process achieved through practice, observation, feedback, and reflection (Kantor & Stadelman, 2020; Shaw et al., 2019).

Conclusion

Ethical issues are ever present in professional practice and will continue to challenge OT practitioners as the fields of medicine, technology, and healthcare delivery evolve. OT practitioners must recognize, critically reason, act, and reflect on ethical issues that arise in their professional roles. OT practitioners who are reflective and knowledgeable in ethical decision-making processes are best prepared to successfully address ethical aspects of practice. Ethical behavior is the responsibility of all OT professionals.

"Moral resilience encompasses the ability to reframe stressful events as opportunities instead of viewing them as threats and to respond in healthy ways."

—Rivard and Brown (2019)

Lippincott® Connect *For additional resources on the subjects discussed in this chapter, visit Lippincott Connect.*

REFERENCES

American Nurses Association. (2019). *A call to action report: Exploring moral resilience toward a culture of ethical practice.* www.nursingworld.org.

American Occupational Therapy Association. (2020). Occupational therapy code of ethics. *American Journal of Occupational Therapy, 74*(Suppl. 3), 7413410005. https://doi.org/10.5014/ajot.2020.74S3006

American Occupational Therapy Association. (2021). Standards of practice for occupational therapy. *American Journal of Occupational Therapy, 75*(Suppl. 3), 7513410050. https://doi.org/10.5014/ajot.2021.75S3004

Aulisio, M. P., Arnold, R. M., & Younger, S. J. (2000). Health care ethics consultation: Nature, goals, and competencies: A position paper from the Society for Health and Human Values-Society for Bioethics Consultation Task Force on Standards for Bioethics Consultation. *Annals of Internal Medicine, 133,* 59–69. https://doi.org/10.7326/0003-4819-133-1-200007040-00012

Banks, S. (2004). *Ethics, accountability, and the social professions.* Palgrave Macmillan.

Barnitt, R. E. (1993). Deeply troubling questions: The teaching of ethics in undergraduate courses. *British Journal of Occupational Therapy, 56,* 401–406. https://doi.org/10.1177/030802269305601104

Beauchamp, T. L., & Childress, J. F. (2019). *Principles of biomedical ethics* (8th ed.). Oxford University Press.

Bong, H. E. (2019). Understanding moral distress: How to decrease turnover rates of new graduate pediatric nurses. *Pediatric Nursing, 45*(3), 109–114. http://www.pediatricnursing.net/issues/19mayjun/

Brigham, T., Barden, C., Dopp, A. L., Hengerer, A., Kaplan, J., Malone, B., Martin, C., McHugh, M., & Nora, L. M. (2018). *A journey to construct an all-encompassing conceptual model of factors affecting clinician well-being and resilience.* NAM Perspectives. Discussion Paper, National Academy of Medicine, Washington, DC. https://doi.org/10.31478/201801b.

Bushby, K., Chan, J., Druif, S., Ho, K., & Kinsella, E. A. (2015). Ethical tensions in occupational therapy practice: A scoping review. *British Journal of Occupational Therapy, 78,* 212–221. https://doi.org/10.1177/0308022614564770

Cameron, M. (2004). Ethical listening as therapy. *Journal of Professional Nursing, 20,* 141–142. https://doi.org/10.1016/j.profnurs.2004.04.012

Devettere, R. J. (2009). *Practical decision making in health care ethics: Cases and concepts* (3rd ed.). Georgetown University Press.

Doherty, R. F. (2021). *Ethical dimensions in the health professions* (7th ed.). Elsevier Saunders.

Doherty, R. F., & Peterson, E. W. (2022). Responsible participation in a profession: Fostering professionalism and leading for moral action. In B. Braveman (Ed.), *Leading and managing occupational therapy services: An evidence-based approach* (3rd ed., pp. 559-591). F. A. Davis.

Durocher, E., & Kinsella, E. A. (2021). Ethical tensions in occupational therapy practice: Conflicts and competing allegiances. *Canadian Journal of Occupational Therapy, 88*(3), 244–253. https://doi.org/10.1177/00084174211021707

Epstein, R. (2017). *Attending: Medicine, mindfulness, and humanity.* Simon & Schuster, Inc.

Fry, S. T., & Veatch, R. M. (2000). *Case studies in nursing ethics.* Jones & Bartlett Learning.

Gawande, A. (2002). *Complications: A surgeon's notes on an imperfect science.* Picador.

Gawande, A. (2014). *Being mortal: Medicine and what matters in the end.* Metropolitan Books.

Gillon, R. (1994). Medical ethics: Four principles plus attention to scope. *BMJ, 309,* 184. https://doi.org/10.1136/bmj.309.6948.184

Glaser, J. W. (2005). Three realms of ethics: An integrating map of ethics for the future. In R. Purtilo, G. M. Jensen, & C. B. Royeen (Eds.), *Educating for moral action: A sourcebook in health and rehabilitation ethics* (pp. 169–184). F. A. Davis.

Haddad, A., & Doherty, R. (2024). *Health professional and patient interaction* (10th ed.). Elsevier.

Higgs, J., & Jensen, G. M. (2019). Clinical reasoning: Challenges and practice in the 21st century. In J. Higgs, G. M. Jensen, S. Loftus, & N. Christensen (Eds.), *Clinical reasoning in the health professions* (4th ed., pp. 3–11). Elsevier.

Hinkle, L. J., Fettig, L. P., Carlos, W. G., & Bosslet, G. (2017). Twelve tips for just in time teaching of communication skills for difficult conversations in the clinical setting. *Medical Teacher, 39,* 920–925. https://doi.org/10.1080/0142159X.2017.1333587

Horner, J. (2003). Morality, ethics, and law: Introductory concepts. *Seminars in Speech and Language, 24,* 263–274. https://doi.org/10.1055/s-2004-815580

Hunt, M. R., & Ells, C. (2013). A patient-centered care ethics analysis model for rehabilitation. *American Journal of Physical Medicine & Rehabilitation, 92,* 818–827. https://doi.org/10.1097/PHM.0b013e318292309b

Interprofessional Education Collaborative. (2016). *Core competencies for interprofessional collaborative practice: 2016 update.* Interprofessional Education Collaborative.

Jones-Bonofiglio, K. (2020). Navigating moral distress. In The International Library of Bioethics (Ed.), *Health care ethics through the lens of moral distress* (Vol. 82, pg. 137-153). Springer. https://doi.org/10.1007/978-3-030-56156-7_10

Kanny, E. (1993). Core values and attitudes of occupational therapy practice. *American Journal of Occupational Therapy, 47,* 1085–1086. https://doi.org/10.5014/ajot.47.12.1085

Kantor, D. P., & Stadelman, A. (2020). Preparing nursing graduates to engage in difficult conversations with patients: The need for faculty to create opportunities to practice communication skills. *AJN American Journal of Nursing, 120*(8), 11. https://doi.org/10.1097/01.NAJ.0000694496.25141.a1

Kornblau, B. A., & Burkhardt, A. (2012). *Ethics in rehabilitation: A clinical perspective* (2nd ed.). Slack.

Lamb, M., Brant, J., & Brooks, E. (2021). How is virtue cultivated? *Journal of Character Education, 17*(1), 81–108. https://oxfordcharacter.org/uploads/files/how-is-virtue-cultivated.pdf

Lown, B. A., & McIntosh, S. (2015). *Recommendations from a conference on advancing compassionate, person- and family-centered care through interprofessional education for collaborative practice.* http://humanism-in-medicine.org/wp-content/uploads/2015/03/TripleCConferenceRecommendations.pdf

McAuliffe, D. (2014). *Interprofessional ethics: Collaboration in the social, health, and human services.* Cambridge University Press.

Meindl, P., Quirk, A., & Graham, J. (2018). Best practices for school-based moral education. *Policy Insights from the Behavioral and Brain Sciences, 5*(1), 3–10. https://doi.org/10.1177/2372732217747087

National Commission for the Protection of Human Subjects of Biomedical and Behavioral Research. (1979). *The Belmont report.* http://www.hhs.gov/ohrp/humansubjects/guidance/belmont.htm

Nesbit, K. C., Jensen, G. M., & Delany, C. (2018). The active engagement model of applied ethics as a structure for ethical reflection in the context of course-based service learning. *Physiotherapy Theory & Practice, 34*(1), 1–12. https://doi.org/10.1080/09593985.2017.1368759

Olson, K., & Kemper, K. J. (2014). Factors associated with well-being and confidence in providing compassionate care. *Journal of Evidence-Based Complementary & Alternative Medicine, 19,* 292–296. https://doi.org/10.1177/2156587214539977

Pellegrino, E. D. (2002). Professionalism, profession and the virtues of the good physician. *The Mount Sinai Journal of Medicine, 69,* 378–384. PMID: 12429956

Purtilo, R. (2004). Professional–patient relationship: III. Ethical issues. In S. G. Post (Ed.), *Encyclopedia of bioethics* (3rd ed., pp. 2150–2158). Macmillan.

Quill, T. E. (2000). Perspectives on care at the close of life. Initiating end-of-life discussions with seriously ill patients: Addressing the "elephant in the room." *JAMA, 284,* 2502–2507. https://doi.org/10.1001/jama.284.19.2502

Rasoal, D., Skovdahl, K., Gifford, M., & Kihlgren, A. (2017). Clinical ethics support for healthcare personnel: An integrative literature review. *HEC Forum, 29,* 313–346. https://doi.org/10.1007/s10730-017-9325-4

Reid, C., Calia, C., Guerra, C., Grant, L., Anderson, M., Chibwana, K., Kawale, P., & Amos, A. (2021). Ethics in global research: Creating a toolkit to support integrity and ethical action throughout the research journey. *Research Ethics, 17*(3), 359–374. https://doi.org/10.1177/1747016121997522

Reilly, K. M., & Jurchak, M. (2017). Developing professional practice and ethics engagement: A leadership model. *Nursing Administration Quarterly, 41*(4), 376–383. https://doi.org/10.1097/NAQ.0000000000000251

Rivard, A., & Brown, C. A. (2019). Moral distress and resilience in the occupational therapy workplace. *Safety, 5*(1), 10. https://doi.org/10.3390/safety5010010

Rushton, C. H. (2018). Integrity: The anchor for moral resilience. In C. H. Rushton (Ed.), *Moral resilience: Transforming moral suffering in healthcare* (pg. 77-103). Oxford University Press.

Rushton, C. H., Swoboda, S. M., Reller, N., Skarupski, K. A., Prizzi, M., Young, P. D., & Hanson, G. C. (2021). Mindful ethical practice and resilience academy: Equipping nurses to address ethical challenges. *American Journal of Critical Care, 30*(1), e1–e11. https://doi.org/10.4037/ajcc2021359

Schoeberlein, D., & Sheth, S. (2009). *Mindful teaching and teaching mindfulness: A guide for anyone who teaches anything.* Wisdom.

Shaw, A. C., McQuade, J. L., Reilly, M. J., Nixon, B., Baile, W. F., & Epner, D. E. (2019). Integrating storytelling into a communication skills teaching program for medical oncology fellows. *Journal of Cancer Education, 34,* 1198–1203, https://doi.org/10.1007/s13187-018-1428-3.

Slater, D. Y. (2016). *Reference guide to the occupational therapy code of ethic and ethics standards* (2nd ed.). AOTA Press.

Slater, D. Y., & Brandt, L. C. (2016). Combating moral distress. In D. Y. Slater (Ed.), *Reference guide to the occupational therapy code of ethics and ethics standards* (2015 ed., pp. 117–123). AOTA Press.

Sullivan, W. M., & Rosin, M. S. (2008). *A new agenda for higher education: Shaping a life of the mind for practice.* Jossey-Bass.

Swisher, L., Arslanian, L. E., & Davis, C. M. (2005). The Realm-Individual-Process-Situation (RIPS) model of ethical decision making. *HPA Resource, 5,* 3–18. https://www.semanticscholar.org/paper/The-Realm-Individual-Process-Situation-(-RIPS-)-of-Lee-Swisher/a83a548c3c59e7c7945ca3f0d4b42207dc46e1a4

Swisher, L. L., & Royeen, C. B. (2020). *Rehabilitation ethics for interprofessional practice.* Jones & Bartlett Learning.

Thomas, Y., Seedhouse, D., Peutherer, V., & Loughlin, M. (2019). An empirical investigation into the role of values in occupational therapy decision-making. *British Journal of Occupational Therapy, 82*(6), 357–366. https://doi.org/10.1177/0308022619829722

Trzeciak, S., & Mazzarelli, A. (2019). *Compassionomics: The revolutionary scientific evidences that caring makes a difference.* Florida, Studer Group, LLC.

VanderKaay, S., Letts, L., Jung, B., & Moll, S. E. (2020). Doing what's right: A grounded theory of ethical decision-making in occupational therapy. *Scandinavian Journal of Occupational Therapy, 27*(2), 98–111. https://doi.org/10.1080/11038128.2018.1464060

Wells, B. G. (2003). Leadership for ethical decision making. *American Journal of Pharmaceutical Education, 67,* 5–8. DOI:10.5688/AJ670103

World Federation of Occupational Therapists. (2016). *The World Federation of Occupational Therapists (WFOT) code of ethics.* https://www.wfot.org/resources/code-of-ethics

Therapeutic Relationships and Person-Centered Collaboration

Applying the Intentional Relationship Model

Carmen Gloria de las Heras de Pablo and Jaime Phillip Muñoz

LEARNING OBJECTIVES

After reading this chapter, you will be able to:

1. Describe the distinct nature of therapeutic relationships in occupational therapy.
2. Outline the evidence supporting therapeutic use of self in occupational therapy.
3. Describe the components of the Intentional Relationship Model (IRM).
4. Define and give examples of interpersonal events.
5. Compare the strengths and weaknesses of the six IRM interpersonal modes.
6. Apply the interpersonal reasoning processes and six IRM modes to practical scenarios.

Introduction: Connecting Through Occupation

Occupation is an innate aspect of human existence (Wilcock, 1993). Human occupation is dynamic. People are constantly transitioning and changing in one way or another. From birth to old age, humans create or experience changes in themselves, in their occupations, and in the environmental spaces where they participate in daily occupations (Hooper & Wood, 2019). Sometimes, when a person's capacity to engage in their world in meaningful and purposeful ways is challenged or becomes obstructed, they may need an expert in doing. Occupational therapists are experts in doing. We collaborate with people to promote their health. We connect with others through purposeful everyday occupations that enhance participation and performance (American Occupational Therapy Association, 2021; Canadian Association of Occupational Therapists, 2013). Doing the work of occupational therapy (OT) requires us to create an alliance with the person (Polatjko et al., 2015). We often are creating these therapeutic relationships just when a person is feeling most challenged to do the things that they want and need to do; the things that have meaning to them and which maintain the fire of their soul

(Mahoney & Egan, 2021). In order to apply our expertise in doing, practitioners need knowledge and skill sets to initiate and sustain therapeutic relationships. This chapter begins by exploring the nature of therapeutic relationships in OT including how and why these relationships in OT can be distinct from those in other health professions. The therapeutic process in OT is then briefly framed as a collaborative process of storytelling and story making (Mattingly, 1991). Finally, the Intentional Relationship Model (IRM) is discussed in detail as an evidence-based approach that practitioners can use to both understand the impact of their own therapeutic use of self and deliberately select interpersonal approaches that facilitate occupational engagement (Taylor, 2020).

The Nature of the Therapeutic Relationship in Occupational Therapy

Is the nature of therapeutic relationships in OT different than in other professions? If so, how? If so, why? The authors of this chapter believe emphatically that therapeutic relationships in OT are indeed distinct. One significant reason for this is that our focus is on human occupation; on doing. Humans engage in diverse sets of occupations, using varied occupational processes in a broad range of distinct contexts (Bailliard & Dickie, 2022). Humans dance, bathe, make tea, keep bees, garden, clean house, cycle, fish, lift weights, create art, cook, play, and work, and we do all these thing in our own ways and for our own reasons. The OT process is one of engaging and enabling each person by learning from them and entering into their unique way of doing and being in the world.

The underlying philosophy of our profession is another reason the nature of therapeutic relationships in OT is distinct. Philosophy is foundational. It underlies what practitioners do and it is the basis for a professional's identity (Taff, 2021). OT's philosophical base helps us explain to ourselves, the people we work with, other professionals, and the public what OT is and how it is distinct from other health professions (Hooper & Wood, 2019). Enduring values and beliefs are core elements of a profession's philosophy. Many influential authors in the professions have explained these elements (Hocking, 2008; Ikiugu & Schultz, 2006; Yerxa, 1983). *In simple terms, the philosophy of OT includes beliefs that humans are occupational beings that may experience occupational dysfunction that can be ameliorated with the therapeutic application of occupations.* Founders of the American OT profession articulated philosophical beliefs about our purpose and practices that specifically addressed therapeutic relationships in the profession (Bing, 1981; Meyer, 1922; Slagle, 1922). One core philosophical belief is person-centeredness. This primary concept compels occupational therapists to seek knowledge about a person and their situation. We do this in collaboration with the person. Knowledge of this nature is necessarily shared knowledge. It is situated in the therapeutic relationship and co-constructed through dialogue (Taff, 2021). A key aspect of OT practice is collaborative problem-solving, and to jointly solve occupational problems a practitioner needs the capacity to build respectful, participatory alliances with others. Peloquin captures the essence of our role when building therapeutic alliances in OT when she says, "We are pathfinders. We enable occupations that heal. We cocreate daily lives. We reach for hearts as well as hands. We are artists and scientists at once. This is our character; this is our genius, this is our spirit" (Peloquin, 2005, p. 617).

Storytelling and Story Making in Occupational Therapy

In order to be such pathfinding, energizing, cocreating, empathic, artistic, practice scholars, occupational therapists need to interact with and relate well to a wide variety of people. We need to elicit their stories. Every person the practitioner meets in OT has a life story. As you read this text, you can look back and think of key chapters in your own life story. You can think in terms of the life story you are in at this present moment, and you can look ahead to chapters you have planned but have not yet experienced. As an occupational therapist, you have the honor and privilege of being part of a person's social context; you enter into their life story, their occupational narratives. These individuals may or may not be experiencing an illness or trauma, but they are people and collectives with occupational needs and concerns.

Many will share stories of transition. You will meet individuals in your practice who have life circumstances you can relate to, but far more may have cultural identities and life experiences that you have no real reference point for. For example, the person you see in therapy may be an older adult transitioning to a life poststroke or a neurodiverse child learning to navigate their school environment. They may be a returning citizen learning to integrate into a community after many years of incarceration or a young man wondering how his life plan will play out after he fractured his neck jumping into the shallow end of the pool during his bachelor's party. Maybe the next person you work with is displaced and dealing with multiple occupational concerns. She is a refugee trying to learn a new language, confused by academic norms in her new elementary school context, and struggling to balance multiple and seemingly contradictory identities in a new country. These individuals each have a story. Eliciting a person's story is a time-tested, effective way to understand human experience (Crepeau & Cohn, 2019; Kleinman, 1980; Mattingly & Garro, 2000).

In therapy, a person tells their story by chaining together events in their life. Their stories are always an interpretation of their experience. Mattingly (1998) states "stories are about someone trying to do something and what happens to her and others as a result" (p. 7). Getting people to tell their story can be a critical aspect of the OT process. Knowing how a person sees their situation can shape the way a practitioner plans and implements interventions. Story making occurs when a practitioner helps move the story from where the person is at today to where they want to be 2 weeks, 2 months, and 2 years from today. Therapy becomes an exercise in visioning and creating the next chapter together (Clark, 1993; Mattingly, 2000). Storytelling and story making are very useful tools in the therapeutic process (Bruner, 1991; Crepeau & Cohn, 2019; Mattingly, 2000). People's stories can be complex. Building therapeutic relationships requires commitment to your craft as a therapist. One needs knowledge and skills to reach for both the hands and the hearts of the people who come to us for care.

Understanding Emotions and Challenging Behaviors Within Therapeutic Relationships

People you meet in your practice will present with a broad array of personalities, dispositions, and interpersonal styles (Taylor et al., 2009). Occupational therapists work with persons and collectives of a wide range of health backgrounds and age, economic, political, cultural, social, and occupational realities. On a daily basis, you may also interact with stakeholders, politicians, community agencies, directors, families, colleagues, and other professionals. This is not an exhaustive list. Every person brings to a relationship their own ways of communicating. Life experiences influence the evolution of people' personalities, disposition to relate to others, and interpersonal styles (Bathel et al., 2018; Fraley & Roisman, 2019).

People, including practitioners themselves, can all face unexpected life events and physical, emotional, psychosocial, social, or economic problems. Some people you meet in practice have never wanted for resources and have experienced multiple opportunities in their lives, whereas others have experienced systemic injustices. People handle the emotions related to their experiences differently. We process and react to life situations, transitions, and challenges in a myriad of ways (Taylor et al., 2009; Van Vieuwenhove & Meganck, 2017). Some experiences can lead to feelings of loss, frustration, anger, despair, or anxiety. As a practitioner, you are likely to interact with people presenting difficult emotions and challenging interpersonal behaviors ranging from being manipulative, demanding, or dependent, to showing frequent hostility, oppositionality, and resistiveness. Some will present with significant passiveness, self-denigrating behaviors, or can be unrealistic about treatment or in denial about their impairments (Taylor et al., 2009). People who

are involved in recovery processes, particularly those making extraordinary efforts to overcome social, cultural, economic, and/or physical barriers, could develop feelings of invalidation, insecurity, uncertainty, helplessness, abandonment, or stigma, and these feelings are often brought into therapy (de las Heras et al., 2019; Kronenberg et al., 2009; Taylor, 2008, 2017, 2020). The occupational therapist's challenge is to connect and collaborate unconditionally.

Therapeutic Use of Self and Collaboration

Collaboration is a process of mutual participation between the person and the practitioner and is a critical element in person-centered care (Yun & Choi, 2019). This process often includes providing choice, involving individuals in decision-making, and encouraging them to actively contribute and to set their own goals for therapy (Parkinson & Brooks, 2021; Santana et al., 2018; Taylor, 2017). Within OT, several qualitative studies using surveys, interviews, and focus groups with practitioners have identified attitudes and behaviors that support therapeutic relationships. These include a sense of connecting with people in helping and caring ways, accommodating the practitioner's interactions to a person's needs, relationship building, trust, motivating others, providing an enabling occupational experience, reciprocity and mutual participation in the therapy process, open communication, and empathy (Cole & McLean, 2003; Eklund, 1996; Eklund & Hallberg, 2001; Guidetti & Tham, 2002; Holland et al., 2018; Jenkins et al., 1994; Rosa & Hasselkus, 1996; Palmadottir, 2006). Taylor et al. (2011) studied 563 practitioners to identify their most preferred strategies for responding to people's personal needs. These included encouraging individuals by reminding them of their strengths, providing positive affirmation, instilling hope and confidence, and collaborating with them by encouraging them to make more decisions during the therapy process. Practitioners also interacted in ways that supported the person's perspectives by gathering feedback before selecting or recommending an activity and by asking the person to recommend their own goals for therapy. Problem-solving, empathizing, and instructing were approaches used less frequently.

These studies suggest that an extensive range of interpersonal skills is necessary to sustain a productive therapeutic relationship. These showed a clear need for increased self-awareness, empathy, and power sharing within the therapeutic relationship and expressed that confidence, self-awareness, and an orientation toward the person's interpersonal needs may lead to improved therapeutic outcomes. The knowledge and skills identified in the studies above require intentionality on the part of the practitioner; they are not automatic. A practitioner must purposefully build these skills, practice them, and critically reflect on the application of these skills or risk losing their authenticity in person-centered practice (Gupta & Taff, 2015; Whalley Hammell, 2013). An evidence-based approach that practitioners can use to both understand the impact of their own therapeutic use of self and deliberately select interpersonal approaches that facilitate occupational engagement is Renée R. Taylor's IRM (2020).

The Intentional Relationship Model

The IRM has benefited our fundamental mission as occupational therapists in different fields of practice. The MOHO-IRM Web (https://moho-irm.uic.edu/) keeps practitioners updated on the IRM model, including highlighted publications and presentation and upcoming conferences specific to the IRM (see also: https://irm.ahs.uic.edu/about-irm/). The following list represents examples of comments made by Latin American and Spanish OT practitioners and students who have participated in IRM workshops with the first author.

- "This whole model is like taking a 'bath of humility.'"
- "It validates who I am as a therapist and as a person at the same time."
- "It helps me grow my interpersonal skills and feel more secure when I relate with clients older than me."
- "Reflective exercises helped me to realize how important is to be open and flexible to the other during therapeutic relationships."
- "Knowing that there is a way to solve interpersonal situations that are challenging for me makes me anticipate that I won't need to avoid them again."
- "The IRM means for me an opportunity for reflection, self-criticism, self-knowledge, flexibility, openness, challenge, reaffirmation."
- "The challenge is to become a versatile therapist, reflecting a true understanding of people's needs."
- "It helps me to maintain relationships inside and outside my job!"

As these statements reflect, the IRM is both a person- and practitioner-centered and an evidence-based conceptual model of practice that is applied across OT with all people in diverse settings and fields. This model has been developed for OT practitioners and students to discover, validate, and improve their natural interpersonal skills and styles they use (or will use) in practice. It offers complementary resources that support practitioners to become more prepared not only for building and maintaining therapeutic relationships but also for taking care of themselves.

Challenging interpersonal events occur often during therapy. Practitioners consider many of these interactions to have a high level of complexity that often feel like they are beyond their interpersonal expertise. They often lack the knowledge

base or intuitive strategies for handling these interactions. The IRM seeks to address these challenges by providing an evidence-based explanation of the therapeutic relationship, an interpersonal reasoning process, and a set of concrete communication skills to help practitioners assume the responsibility of developing a predictable and trusting relationship with people and sustain it irrespective of any difficulties (Taylor, 2019). The IRM is diagrammed in Figure 28.1, which shows the relationship of the central components of the model. These will be briefly described in the following sections. More extensive information is presented in Taylor (2020).

Interpersonal Characteristics

An individual's interpersonal characteristics play a fundamental role during therapeutic relationships. People we see in therapy may experience a diverse range of emotions and a variety of psychological reactions to life events, which can vary significantly in duration and intensity. These impact their psychological, interpersonal, occupational, and health-related behaviors (Taylor, 2020).

In order for practitioners to understand a person's interpersonal characteristics, the IRM calls us to differentiate between *enduring* and *situational interpersonal characteristics*. **Enduring characteristics** are those which come from an individual's personality and reflect their natural interpersonal styles. **Situational characteristics** are emotional and behavioral reactions to immediate stressful personal circumstances or events experienced within the contexts of participation (i.e., problems found in health system's organization or social and physical restrictions to their participation).

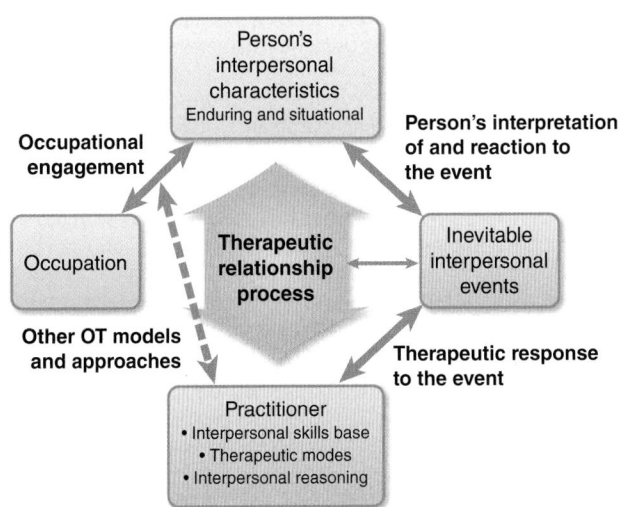

FIGURE 28.1 Model of Intentional Relationship in OT. OT, occupational therapy.

(Adapted from Taylor, R. R., Lee, S. W., & Kielhofner, G. [2011]. Practitioners' use of interpersonal modes within the therapeutic relationship: Results from a nationwide study. *OTJR: Occupation, Participation and Health, 31,* 6–14; Taylor, R. R. [2020]. *The intentional relationship: Occupational therapy and use of self.* F. A. Davis [Figure 3.4]).

Recognizing and understanding these interpersonal characteristics *from an objective but emphatic perspective* is essential for the effective use of self in our profession. It allows us to reason, plan and respond more successfully to a person's needs, especially when facing challenging interpersonal circumstances, thus enabling us to further facilitate their occupational engagement. An extensive discussion of interpersonal characteristics may be found in Taylor (2020).

The IRM defines 14 categories of essential interpersonal characteristics (Taylor, 2020). Definitions and examples of these are provided in Table 28.1.

What Usually Happens in Occupational Therapy: Inevitable Interpersonal Events

According to Taylor (2020, p. 59), an interpersonal event "is a naturally occurring communication, reaction, process, task, or general circumstance that occurs during therapy and that has the potential to detract from or strengthen the therapeutic relationship." These events may have different effects for each person in the relationship. An individual's reactions and interpretations of the interpersonal events during therapy may be experienced differently by the practitioner as each experiences the event based on their own interpersonal skills and interpersonal characteristics (Taylor, 2020).

Given that interpersonal events are inevitable during our relationship with others, one of the primary tasks of a therapist using IRM *is to recognize and respond to these events in a way that leads to repair and strengthening of the therapeutic relationship*. If these events go unnoticed, are deliberately ignored, or are responded to without intentionality, they can threaten both the therapeutic relationship and the person's occupational engagement (Taylor, 2020). The 12 categories of interpersonal events, their definitions, and practice examples are presented in Table 28.2, and see OT Story 28.1 for an example.

The Therapist's Use of Self: The Six Modes

According to the IRM, effective use of self requires practitioners to recognize and cultivate strengths within their personalities and develop less used aspects of their

TABLE 28.1 Interpersonal Characteristics: Definitions and Practical Examples

Communication style
A person's ability to communicate in a clear, well-paced, and detailed yet succinct manner that is appropriate to his or her developmental level and cognitive ability.
María has a hyperverbal communication style, which intensifies when she feels anxious. The first time the practitioner met her she felt overwhelmed, not knowing if asking María a question would increase her anxiety and make interaction more difficult. Next time they met, the practitioner actively listened to her narrative, and carefully linked the content she expressed with meaningful participation experiences, creating a safe space for María to converse.

Tone of voice
A person's voice volume (e.g., low, loud, soft, or shrill) used while speaking, which could indicate emotional states, reactions during interaction, or enduring personal characteristics related to his or her interpersonal style, or physical or sensory conditions.
Moises is a 7-year-old boy who uses a shrill voice volume when he speaks to anyone at home or school. His classmates tease him for this. The school's occupational therapist assessed Moises' circumstances, noticing him becoming withdrawn during school activities in reaction to his classmates' attitudes. His parents told the practitioner Moises was having nasal surgery in a month, but that Moises does not want to return to school until he can speak well.

Body language
A person's nonverbal cues while he or she interacts with others can be exhibited through mannerisms such as posture, eye contact, facial expression, or position of extremities and can be related to a person's interpersonal characteristics.
Mr. Meyer is a 91-year-old man. He lives in a residential facility where he is bedridden. His body posture changes dramatically according to who was on duty to assist him. With one assistant, he becomes very anxious and adopts a stiff posture, which does not allow her to complete hygiene tasks with him. With another assistant, his body is calm and relaxed, which allows her to do her job. These observations were crucial for the OT, who was working with the staff on finding the best ways to relate to the residents.

Level of trust
A person's ability to trust that the practitioner has his or her best interests in mind and that every effort will be made to ensure his or her physical safety and emotional well-being.
Richard is a very talented 40-year-old carpenter. He is reluctant to trust others because of multiple experiences of discrimination related to his sexual orientation. He avoids talking with his occupational therapist. The practitioner asks Richard to collaborate and gives him advice on a home improvement project at his own house. While engaged in this and other related construction tasks, Richard became more relaxed and confident and more spontaneously shared stories with the practitioner.

Need for control
The degree to which a person takes an active versus passive role within the relationship and in determining the course of therapy.
A practitioner worked with William's mother to support her on making small, graded changes in her mothering role, as she had a tendency to prevent her son from making his own decisions. In each meeting, she would try to change the practitioner's plan designed to facilitate her son's autonomy and identity. Slowly mom was able to recognize she was prioritizing her own desires and needs within the plan, as she often did at home with William.

TABLE 28.1	Interpersonal Characteristics: Definitions and Practical Examples (*continued*)

Approach to asserting needs

A person's approach to expressing his or her wishes and needs for support, information, resources, or other requests within the therapeutic relationship.

Victoria has a great capacity to assert her needs. She eagerly works collaboratively with her practitioner on setting her life goals and plans for the future as a mother, worker, and active member of her neighborhood community. When reviewing her goals and the therapy process, she is also able to express when she needs more challenge and less support from the practitioner.

Response to change and challenge

A person's ability to adapt to changes in the therapy plan or environment and his or her approach to occupational therapy tasks and situations that are new or challenging.

Peter is an adolescent who likes structure and plans. He is a member of his school's scout group. When something occurs differently from what he has planned, he needs strong support to face it and to adjust his routine. To maximize satisfaction with his scouting routines, his practitioner advises his scout group guides to offer Peter opportunities to participate in activities he manages well and also to organize periods of time where he participates in a more flexible schedule offering limited choices.

Affect (facial expression)

A person's outward expression of emotion, usually through facial expression, which varies in terms of frequency, intensity, consistency, and fluency.

In conversations with her practitioner, Caroline openly demonstrates a range of emotions reflective of her typical response to the weekly events she goes through with her teenage daughter. She smiles and opens her eyes widely when describing her daughter's improvements. She shows a lost look when her daughter is sad for more than a few days when she seems unable to find her purpose.

Predisposition to giving feedback

A person's ability to provide the therapist with appropriate negative or positive comments about his or her reactions to the therapist and experience of therapy as either helpful or unhelpful.

Liliana is an occupational therapy student completing her last professional affiliation at a hospital. Her supervisor is well recognized for the programs he has developed. During her second formal supervision, Liliana respectfully shared her observations about the possible need to improve one of the key programs he had developed, because of people's decreased motivation to participate in it. Other practitioners joined her and provided evaluative comments about the program.

Response to feedback

A person's ability to maintain perspective when receiving praise from the practitioner or when receiving correction during performance, limits on behavior, or information about his or her strengths and weaknesses.

A community center had been operating for a year when the mayor of the town where it was located sent an order to close the site for noncompliance with regulations of residential/business use. The OT director of the center expressed to him that the error was not theirs but of his office for giving them incorrect information before they rented the house. He did not accept this argument. Giving the circumstances, a group of members of this center drafted a formal letter requesting more time to move.

Response to human diversity

A person's reaction to ways in which he or she may be the same or different from the practitioner in terms of perceived worldview or interpretations of observable characteristics (race, age, ethnicity, gender, and clothing).

Ana is an adolescent with a self-identified gothic lifestyle. She favors gothic fashion, music, and a general outlook on life. Despite her strong beliefs, she is very open to making friends with people having different lifestyles. She also accepts her practitioner, who leads a traditional Jewish lifestyle, but is also open to human diversity. They make a very good team.

Orientation toward relating

A person's need for interpersonal closeness versus professional distance within the therapeutic relationship.

Robert is depressed and has extreme difficulty getting out of his bed. He gets anxious and defensive whenever the practitioner moves closer to him. He covers his head with his bedsheets and positions his body away from her and toward the window.

Preference for touch

A person's observed comfort or discomfort with or expressed reaction to any type of physical touch, whether it be a necessary part of treatment or an expression of caring.

Diane is a young woman who seeks physical connection with people. She jumps over to her practitioner and others to hug them, no matter what they might feel. The practitioner, with a kind and honest attitude, accepts her hugs while at the same time cueing Diane to accommodate the way she does it, so both of them can feel comfortable with the contact.

Interpersonal reciprocity

A person's ability to engage fully in the therapy process and/or show appreciation toward the therapist as a separate but connected partner within the therapy process.

A practitioner works as a consultant with a group of workers from a large company. Her focus is on enhancing their occupational satisfaction and well-being at their work place. She and the workers collaborated on a project designed to create opportunities for participation in valued sports for all employees. As they achieved each step of their project, they would show their gratitude to the practitioner by waiting for him with a cup of coffee to celebrate.

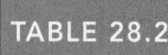

TABLE 28.2 The Inevitable Interpersonal Events of Occupational Therapy: Definitions and Practical Examples

Expression of strong emotion

Observable manifestations of internal feelings that occur with a higher-than-usual level of intensity given a person's cultural context and norms; can be positive or negative expressions.

After being devalued by her teacher in front of her classmates, Rosa ran out of the high school and called her practitioner crying at loud. Sobbing, she stated that she was nothing but a stupid person, that she should not continue studying, and that she was embarrassing her family.

Intimate self-disclosures

Statements or stories that reveal something personal or sensitive about the person making a disclosure; can be related to oneself or to close others.

While naturally conversing with her practitioner, Eileen abruptly changed the subject and revealed that her father had sexually abused her and that she had revenge plans against him.

Power dilemmas

Feelings of stress or conflict that emerge when the person and the practitioner disagree about something. Power dilemmas can manifest overtly or covertly during therapy. They are more likely to occur when people feel a lack or loss of control over their lives.

During a third year OT advanced course class, the OT professor invited students to comment on the readings they would address that day. After listening to his students, the professor, a specialist in the subject, shared his thoughts in detail. During his commentary, a group of students who had not participated in the first activity confronted him arguing the content he was sharing was not accurate. Despite his calm explanations and sharing of evidence substantiating his points, this student group continued defending their position.

Nonverbal cues

Communications that do not involve the use of formal language. Some examples are movement patterns, body posture, and eye contact.

In the context of a home visit, Patrick, an 85-year-old man, took his dental partial off with desperation, moved himself very close to his practitioner's face, and showed him all the defective teeth in his mouth.

Crisis points

Unanticipated, stressful events that cause persons to become absent or distracted from therapy. Examples include natural disasters, a change in the person's health status, or an emergency involving a person's significant others.

Beatriz is still grieving the loss of her father. One day, she presented as unusually active and talkative with her friends at the Church Choir group she belonged to. She got home very late that day. The next morning, her mother called informing the practitioner that Beatriz had a relapse of her affective disorder and had been hospitalized.

Resistance and reluctance

Resistance is a person's passive or active refusal to participate in some or all aspects of therapy for reasons linked to the therapeutic relationship (e.g., unexpressed anger toward the practitioner or situation). Reluctance is disinclination toward some aspect of therapy for reasons outside the therapeutic relationship, such as a person's anxiety about task difficulty or other concerns about performance.

A practitioner works with Bernardo, a 50-year-old man who has spent his life living at home with his mother. The practitioner is challenged to build a therapeutic relationship with Bernardo's five siblings because of their conviction that they hold a status superior to people they hire. At Bernardo's therapy process, the siblings began to openly reject his therapy. They downplayed his efforts when he took initiative to do something he liked. The practitioner observed Bernardo's increasing anxiety caused by his siblings' attitudes and listening to him, she decided on his behalf to discontinue the therapy process.

Boundary testing

A person's behavior that violates or asks the therapist to disclose something or act in ways that the therapist is not comfortable with or that are outside the definition of a professional relationship.

At a meeting with the director of Mental Health Services, a practitioner and one consumer member representing a collective of other service users explained to the director the need for having public community services providing dignifying opportunities for participation. The director responded by questioning the credibility of their arguments and by asking the practitioner her age and the degrees she had earned to make such a request.

Empathic breaks

Any action initiated by the practitioner, or something a practitioner fails to notice or acknowledge, that results in a person feeling disappointed, disillusioned, insignificant, or emotionally injured.

A practitioner was always on time for therapy sessions. One day, the practitioner made a mistake, scheduling two people at the same time. One of them was urged to speak with him. She left in tears and did not come back until the practitioner could reach her and apologize for his mistake.

Emotionally charged therapy tasks and situations

Activities or circumstances that a person feels strongly about because of a past experience, a high level of value for the activity, or because of something embarrassing about the activity.

Cecile is an anthropologist who has schizophrenia. She has worked hard with her practitioner to regain her work position at a well-known university. She and her peers share stories of negative consequence they experienced as a result of their psychiatrists' unethical decisions about their prescribed medications. Cecile decides to use her expertise and begins collecting data directly from peers and families at the waiting rooms, giving the evidence to a lawyer to file a complaint to address the psychiatrists' malpractice. Her practitioner supported her to overcome difficulties that arose during this long process, which eventually ended in a just result for many people.

TABLE 28.2	The Inevitable Interpersonal Events of Occupational Therapy: Definitions and Practical Examples (*continued*)

Limitations of therapy

Restrictions on the available or possible services, time, resources, or nature of the desired relationship with the practitioner.
Luis had chosen the last hour available at a Public Community Services to meet with his practitioner. One day, he asked his practitioner to meet longer because he felt comfortable and secure with him. The practitioner explained to Luis that he could not accommodate his request because he had family responsibilities at that time of the day.

Contextual inconsistencies

Any aspect of a person's interpersonal or physical environment that changes during the course of therapy.
Mary came to the community center on Monday and was clearly emotionally distraught. Spending the entire weekend with her parents made her feel stressed and vulnerable. Her therapist was available for her 10 minutes every Monday morning.

Verbal innuendos

The person says something illusive or oblique that it is meant to serve as a hint about a more direct communication.
Theresa told her practitioner, "I miss your eyeglasses." Her practitioner answered with a question, "What do you mean by that?"

OT STORY 28.1 ROBERTO'S STORY: BECOMING VISIBLE

Roberto is a very talented 45-year-old Chilean artist. He has a young adolescent son. Since he was a young adult, Roberto's family have shunned him and expressed their shame of him for having a mental health diagnosis. His father is a distinguished physician and favors Roberto's brother who followed his father's footsteps into medicine. His mother is a very well-known nurse who prioritizes maintaining her social image. Roberto has always been economically dependent on his parents. His mother manages the family budget and her priorities include social events, clothing, and cosmetics. She refuses to provide resources for art supplies stating these are "wasteful luxuries." Roberto has confided to his OT practitioner that he feels trapped by his own lack of resources and constrained by his family's attitudes. Together they devise a plan to progressively reclaim his most valued life roles as an artist, father, and active citizen. Despite the decades of being excluded, he would also like to find his own space as a member of his family.

After a year of working with his practitioner, Roberto has reentered the vibrant local artist community. Peers willingly shared supplies, space, and resources, allowing Roberto to produce art and participate in exhibits. He also now maintains regular correspondence with his son who lives in Colombia with his mother. Roberto feels he is regaining his identity as a father. The practitioner worked with Roberto's mother, giving her attention, validation, and answering her questions (Empathizing Mode). She encouraged the mother to attend events where Roberto's work was being presented. Roberto's mother was surprised when she realized others loved her son's art and were willing to purchase it. The practitioner helped facilitate a conversation between Roberto and his mother where he successfully negotiated ways she would provide her son resources so that he could produce and sell his art (Collaborating Mode). Just as Roberto was rebuilding his relationship with his mother, she became terminally ill. Roberto dedicated all his time to taking care of his mother at her home until she died.

Roberto asked his practitioner to accompany him to his mother's funeral. He was calm, but very sad. At the funeral, his father and brother stood receiving condolences from friends and family. Per his father's instructions for Roberto "not to interfere," Roberto stood behind them. The practitioner asked Roberto where he wanted to be at that moment and supported his decision when he said he wanted to stand next to his brother. She positioned herself behind him. His father was surprised seeing Roberto take this position. He reacted by addressing the OT practitioner, inviting her to see "how beautiful my wife looks inside the casket." Though uncomfortable seeing death in this context, she did so to show respect. She then used the moment to encourage Roberto's father to see how important it was for Roberto to be included, particularly after caring so lovingly for his mother. The father nodded and acknowledged Roberto belonged. A few minutes later, three physicians came and greeted the father and his other son. One commented: "I didn't know you had another son." The father responded: "Ahh…, no, he is the artist!" Roberto withdrew and broke in tears. The practitioner held his arm and validated his feelings of pain and his reaction. After he calmed down, she invited him to decide what he needed to do at that moment. Roberto decided to return to his position next to his brother with her company until his artist friends came to greet him and pay respects.

Questions

1. Identify the inevitable events that occurred in this context.
2. The story identifies some modes the practitioner used with Roberto's mother. Identify modes the practitioner used with Roberto and those she used with his father.
3. If you were the practitioner, what modes might you consider using with Roberto's brother that could support Roberto's goal of reengaging as a family member?

personalities through honest appraisal of the effects of their behavior on the people they treat (Taylor, 2020). The first step in accomplishing this is through an understanding of the six therapist interpersonal modes.

"A therapeutic mode is a specific way of relating to the client" (Taylor, 2020, p. 82). The IRM identifies six therapeutic modes, each meeting the criteria of unidimensionality (Fan & Taylor, 2016). The six therapeutic modes are *Advocating, Collaborating, Empathizing, Encouraging, Instructing,* and *Problem-Solving*. A brief definition of each mode and a practical example of its use are provided in Table 28.3.

Practitioners naturally tend to use therapeutic modes that are consistent with their own personality characteristics and the way they relate to others in their personal life. As a result, practitioners can vary extensively in terms of the range and flexibility with which they use modes in relating to individuals they treat. A therapeutic mode or set of modes define *a therapist's general interpersonal style* when interacting with a person.

All modes have equal potential to grow the relationship between the practitioner and the person; however, a mode "can [also] have a negative effect on the person's attitude and feelings towards the therapist if it is used too often or inflexibly; when it is not the appropriate time to use it, when it is not consistent with the general personality characteristics of the client or when it is not changed to be more consistent with the interpersonal characteristics of the client" (Taylor, 2020, p. 84). This is why the IRM calls practitioners to intentionally choose and apply a particular therapeutic mode or set of modes based on the interpersonal characteristics of the person and their

TABLE 28.3 The Six Therapeutic Modes: Definitions and Examples

1. Advocating

Ensuring that the person's rights are enforced and resources are secured; may require the practitioner to serve as a mediator, facilitator, negotiator, enforcer, or other type of advocate with external persons and agencies.
Paulina recently immigrated to Spain from Venezuela. She struggles to adjust to a new high school and culture. Her practitioner created a detailed list of occupations in the local community. It included free access libraries, youth clubs, and resources that could meet an adolescent's needs. She also coordinated with Paulina's parents, teacher, and community agencies and worked with Paulina to ensure she knew the routes to get to these resources by herself.

2. Collaborating

Expecting the person to be an active and equal participant in therapy; ensuring choice, freedom, and autonomy to the greatest extent possible.
Sonia is a 75-year-old woman and new to the Community Club for Elders. The practitioner makes time to sit with Sonia and asks for her opinions about the opportunities offered at the Club. She asks Sonia what she would prefer to do first from the various activities and social projects available.

3. Empathizing

Ongoing striving to understand the person's thoughts, feelings, and behaviors while suspending any judgment; ensuring the person verifies and experiences the practitioners understanding as truthful and validating.
Andriy is 6. It is hard for him to stay seated in class or to follow his teacher's directives. He cried and threw his materials against the window when his teacher gave him a time out because he was not behaving like his classmates. The classroom OT took Andriy outside into the hall. He consented to a hug and she held him until he was calm. She invited him to tell her about his feelings, listened carefully, and validated what he was going through at school and at home.

4. Encouraging

Seizing the opportunity to instill hope in a person. Celebrating a person's thinking or behavior through positive comments; conveying an attitude of joyfulness, playfulness, and confidence.
When Argelia doesn't feel confident initiating interactions with her friends, the practitioner smiles at her and gives her a thumbs-up. When Argelia looks back at the practitioner, she moves closer to Argelia, touches her shoulder and says "Let's try!"

5. Instructing

Carefully structuring therapy activities and being explicit with people about the plan, sequence, and events of therapy. Providing clear instruction and feedback about performance; setting limits on a person's requests or behavior as needed.
A practitioner works with a neighborhood council of a poor community on a collective project, "the Common Pot of Food." The program is designed to provide food daily to area residents. The council meets twice a week to plan, collaborate with volunteers, and manage problems. The practitioner teaches different ways of dealing with problematic situations. She often lists step-by-step instructions on a blackboard, and provides handouts with the same instructions in more detail and includes clear examples for problem management.

6. Problem-solving

Facilitating pragmatic thinking and solving dilemmas by outlining choices, posing strategic questions, and providing opportunities for comparative or analytical thinking.
George is someone who expects others to answer his questions and solve his problems and rarely tries to find his own solutions. In his family's culture, only adults are expected to have the right answers and children listen and follow through on their advice. When he asks his practitioner what to do, she gives him paper and pen. She asks him to list three possible actions to address his situation, then supports him to consider the pros and cons of each and choose his best alternative.

reaction to any interpersonal events that may be occurring (Taylor, 2020). Thus, one of the goals in using the IRM is *to become increasingly comfortable using any of six of the modes flexibly and interchangeably* depending on a person's needs. Indeed, some interpersonal events in therapy may require a practitioner to consciously change the way of relating to a person, in IRM terms, to make a *mode shift* (Taylor, 2020).

With the purpose of facilitating an optimal therapeutic relationship between practitioners and the people they work with, Renée R. Taylor and her associates developed IRM theoretical-based assessments called the Clinical Assessment of Modes (CAM). CAM is a valid and reliable tool that comes in different versions. CAM-T is the practitioner version that helps to identify their modes used; CAM-C is a version to elicit from the person in therapy perceptions about their practitioner's mode use; CAM-O is used by a third person to rate a practitioner's modes through observation. The Client Mode Preference Questionnaire measures the extent and type of therapeutic communication that a person would prefer from their practitioner and is most commonly used before therapy begins. The Caregiver Clinical Assessment of Modes (CGCAM-O v2.0) and the Pediatric Clinical Assessment of Modes (PCAM-O v3.0) have

been developed for pediatric practice. All CAM assessments are available in the IRM Clearinghouse, https://irm.ahs.uic.edu/ and updates, listserves and social media specific to the IRM can be accessed through the MOHO-IRM Web https://moho-irm.uic.edu/.

Solving the Puzzle: The Interpersonal Reasoning

Interpersonal reasoning is a dynamic and ongoing six-step process in which practitioners intentionally evaluate and make decisions of the best ways to relate with people under different circumstances, taking into consideration their historic narrative, interpersonal characteristics, occupational needs, and contextual realities. This six-step process is shown in Figure 28.2.

Interpersonal reasoning conveys the use of the practitioner's unique interpersonal abilities, personality strengths, and flexible use of the interpersonal modes. To be effective in this process, the IRM offers practitioners a set of useful and efficient resources to explore their interpersonal skills, their natural relationship style, and the

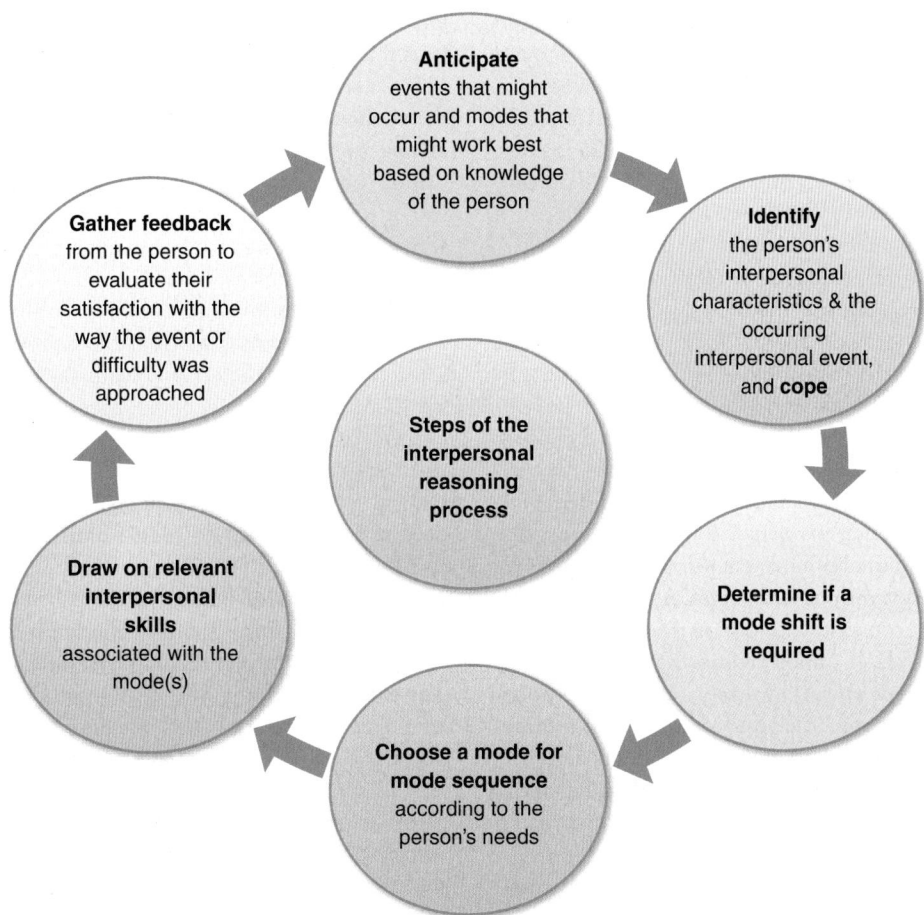

FIGURE 28.2 **The six steps of the interpersonal reasoning process.**

need for improving their interpersonal style with the use of other modes and skills. Each interpersonal mode can be practiced with people seeking OT. When a practitioner reflects on their interpersonal experiences, the six steps of interpersonal reasoning can become habitual and are more easily incorporated into the diverse interpersonal circumstances that arise in therapy. This approach helps practitioners and students gain the discipline, flexibility, and confidence needed to sustain "a mental vigilance toward the interpersonal aspects of therapy in anticipation that a dilemma might occur and a means of reviewing and evaluating options for responding" (Taylor, 2020, p. 179). Expanding Our Perspectives portrays the lived experience of an occupational therapist applying this process in practice. An extensive description and discussion of its six steps can be found in Taylor (2020).

EXPANDING OUR PERSPECTIVES

Developing a Therapeutic Relationship With Carlos

Lucía María Poletti

Carlos is a 58-year-old man I began to work with 5 years ago. He shared a life story that included a career working as an Argentina government official in different positions around the country. He ultimately lost this job as a result of his mental health diagnosis combined with a progressive visual loss. Carlos identified his vision loss as the factor that most restricted his occupational life. After he lost his job, he returned to his hometown and began to live by himself. He managed well enough and moved independently around his neighborhood. This is where he met María. She lived in the streets and had lost the custody of her son because of her homelessness. Carlos had a 19-year-old son who he identified as the most important person in his life, even though he rarely sees him since his marriage ended when his son was still a child.

Carlos and María developed a relationship and soon afterward, Carlos proposed that she live with him. They agreed he would provide shelter, food, and a home for her and her son, and she would help support him with his self-care and home maintenance activities. This agreement was quickly abused by María. She took control of his assets and exerted absolute control of the home. She began a cycle of emotional violence that included depriving Carlos of food, ignoring his personal hygiene needs, disregarding cleaning the home, and even restricting Carlos' freedom to interact with others. It was at this point in his story that I began working with Carlos. The complexity of his situation was clear. Carlos shared that he felt guilty, helpless, and anxious about "my hasty decision of proposing that she live with me." Using an *empathizing mode*, I tried hard to understand and affirm his thoughts and feelings. It was challenging to accept and validate his negative emotions and difficulties without feeling tempted to quickly find a solution.

I noticed Carlos seemed stuck. He constantly ruminated about his decision to invite María into his home. I reflected on whether I too was stalled in the empathizing mode. I wondered if I was being overprotective and whether my listening and validation were not challenging him enough to get him to actively participate in achieving his life goals. After reflection, I shifted into an *instructive mode*. I began setting healthy limits, delivering feedback and expressing disagreements with Carlos regarding his inflexible pattern of complaining and expressing hopelessness. I had to develop skills to share my own point of view and get him to understand other perspectives for considering his situation.

Given the complexity of Carlos's situation, I began using the *advocating mode*. I challenged myself to learn laws that could lead to a "home exclusion" action against María. I learned this was not possible while her son was a minor. Given Carlos' lack of economic resources, I sought advice from state agencies, which could do little. With Carlos' permission, I contacted his son and ex-wife. This was a turning point in Carlos' story. His son and his ex-wife were anxious about being contacted and unaware of Carlos' circumstances. I mainly used the *instructive mode* to help them understand Carlos' situation and learn how to accompany him as a visually impaired person. At the same time, I contacted a private lawyer who was very competent in this subject area, accepted Carlos as a client and worked for free. With Carlos and the lawyer, I mainly used the *collaborative mode* to promote teamwork and making joint decisions toward finding a geriatric institution where Carlos could reside until the judicial process was over.

After 2 years of litigation, Carlos' case was resolved in his favor. The poor sanitary condition of his home prevented Carlos from immediately returning home, but he was excited about the next challenge. Our therapeutic relationship shifted again and this time toward achieving his occupational goal of reconstructing his home.

This process was colored and influenced by a multiplicity of factors that had to be addressed simultaneously. Developing a therapeutic relationship with Carlos gave me the opportunity to know myself better and to make my relational style more intentional and flexible in the face of his circumstances.

Conclusion

This chapter examined the nature of therapeutic relationships in OT and shared evidence defining the characteristics of and processes for therapeutic use of self. Main features of the most current iteration of the IRM were presented, highlighting how using this model has a positive impact on practitioners and can be applied with a diverse range of people in a variety of OT, healthcare, and community contexts. The IRM is a conceptual practice model that deciphers the know-how of therapeutic use of self. It encourages examination of one's interpersonal styles and skills and offers strategies to enrich these. This approach offers a sound explanation of interpersonal reasoning processes defining essential procedures for understanding and responding supportively to individuals according to their needs and interpersonal characteristics. In the words of Renée R. Taylor, "Occupational therapists should strive to understand each person interpersonally, putting one's personal and emotional reactions to individuals to productive use without prejudice or judgment" (Taylor, 2019, p. 537).

Acknowledgments

We are very thankful to Dr. Renée R. Taylor for having written the past editions of this chapter, and for inspiring us through her work to do our best effort on sharing with practitioners the IRM in this important text. We would like to thank all our colleagues and friends from different cultures who collaborated with us sending their reflections and comments. Special thanks to Lucía María Poletti, who shared her lived experience using the IRM in the Expanding Our Perspectives feature in this chapter.

Lippincott® Connect *For additional resources on the subjects discussed in this chapter, visit Lippincott Connect.*

REFERENCES

American Occupational Therapy Association. (2021). Occupational therapy scope of practice. *American Journal of Occupational Therapy, 75*(Suppl. 3), 7513410020. https://doi.org/10.5014/ajot.2021.75S3005

Bailliard, A., & Dickie, V. (2022). Things people do: Toward a comprehensive understanding of human occupations. *Journal of Occupational Science, 29*(1), 1–5. https://doi.org/10.1080/14427591.2022.2057398

Bathel, A. L., Hay, A., Doan, S. N., & Hofmann, S. G. (2018). Interpersonal emotion regulation: A review of social and developmental components. *Behavior Change, 35*(4), 203–216. https://doi.org/10.1017/bec.2018.19

Bing, R. K. (1981). Eleanor Clarke Slagle Lectureship--1981. Occupational therapy revisited: A paraphrastic journey. *American Journal of Occupational Therapy, 35*(8), 499–518. https://doi.org/10.5014/ajot.35.8.499

Bruner, J. (1991). The narrative construction of reality. *Critical Inquiry, 18*, 1–21. http://www.jstor.org/stable/1343711

Canadian Association of Occupational Therapists. (2013). *Enabling occupation II: Advancing an occupational therapy vision for health, well-being, & justice through occupation* (2nd ed.). Author.

Clark, F. (1993). Occupation embedded in a real life: Interweaving occupational science and occupational therapy. *American Journal of Occupational Therapy, 47*, 1069–1078. https://doi.org/10.5014/ajot.47.12.1067

Cole, M. B., & McLean, V. (2003). Therapeutic relationships re-defined. *Occupational Therapy in Mental Health, 19*, 33–56. https://doi.org/10.1300/J004v19n02_03

Crepeau, E. B., & Cohn, E. (2019). Narrative as a key to understanding. In E. B. Crepeau, E. Cohn, & B. Schell (Eds.), *Willard and Spackman's occupational therapy* (13th ed., pp. 142–149). Lippincott Williams & Wilkins.

de las Heras de Pablo, C. G., Llerena, V., & Kielhofner, G. (posthumous). (2019). *The remotivation process: Progressive intervention for people who experience severe volitional challenges (v2.0).* University of Illinois at Chicago: Model of Human Occupation Clearinghouse.

Eklund, M. (1996). Working relationship, participation and outcome in a psychiatric day care unit based on occupational therapy. *Scandinavian Journal of Occupational Therapy, 3*, 106–113. https://doi.org/10.3109/11038129609106693

Eklund, M., & Hallberg, I. R. (2001). Psychiatric occupational therapists' verbal interaction with their clients. *Occupational Therapy International, 8*, 1–16. https://doi.org/10.1002/OTI.128

Fan, C.-W., & Taylor, R. R. (2016). Assessing therapeutic communication during rehabilitation: The clinical assessment of modes. *American Journal of Occupational Therapy, 70*, 7004280010. http://doi.org/10.5014/ajot.2016.018846

Fraley, R. C., & Roisman, G. (2019). The development of adult attachment styles: Four lessons. *Current Opinion in Psychology, 25*, 26–30. https://doi.org/10.1016/j.copsyc.2018.02.008

Guidetti, S., & Tham, K. (2002). Therapeutic strategies used by occupational therapists in self-care training: A qualitative study. *Occupational Therapy International, 9*, 257–276. https://doi.org/10.1002/oti.168

Gupta, J., & Taff, S. D. (2015). The illusion of client-centred practice. *Scandinavian Journal of Occupational Therapy, 22*(4), 244–251, https://doi.org/10.3109/11038128.2015.1020866

Hocking, C. (2008). The way we were: Romantic assumptions of pioneering occupational therapists in the United Kingdom. *British Journal of Occupational Therapy, 71*, 146–155. https://doi.org/10.1177/030802260807100405

Holland, C., Yay, O., Gallini, G., Blanche, E., & Thompson, B. (2018). Relationships between therapist and client actions during sensory integration therapy for young children with autism. *The American Journal of Occupational Therapy, 72*(Suppl 1), 7211515250p1. https://doi.org/10.5014/ajot.2018.72S1-PO4034

Hooper, B., & Wood, W. (2019). The philosophy of occupational therapy: A framework for practice. In B. A. Boyt-Schell & G. Gillen (Eds.), *Willard and Spackman's occupational therapy* (13th ed., pp. 43–55). Wolters Kluwer.

Ikiugu, M. N., & Schultz, S. (2006). An argument for pragmatism as a foundational philosophy of occupational therapy. *Canadian Journal of Occupational Therapy, 73*(2), 86–97. https://doi.org/10.2182/cjot.05.0009

Jenkins, M., Mallett, J., O'Neill, C., McFadden, M., & Baird, H. (1994). Insights into "practice" communication: An interactional approach. *British Journal of Occupational Therapy, 57*(8), 297–302.

Kleinman, A. (1980). *Patients and healers in the context of culture: An exploration of the borderlands between anthropology, medicine and psychiatry.* University of California Press.

Kronenberg, F., Pollard, N., & Sakellariou, D. (2009). *Occupational therapies without borders: Towards an ecology of occupation-based practice* (vol. 2). Elsevier Publications.

Mahoney, W. J. & Egan, B. E. (2021). Focus on the mental and spiritual: Idealism and occupational therapy. In S. D. Taff (Ed.), *Philosophy and occupational therapy: Informing education, research and practice* (pp. 23–31). Slack Incorporated.

Mattingly, C. (1991). The narrative nature of clinical reasoning. *American Journal of Occupational Therapy, 45*(11), 998–1005. https://doi .org/10.5014/ajot.45.11.998

Mattingly, C. (1998). *Healing dramas and clinical plots: The narrative structure of experience.* Cambridge University Press.

Mattingly, C. (2000). Emergent narratives. In C. Mattingly & L. C. Garro (Eds.), *Narrative and the cultural construction of illness and healing* (pp. 181–211). University of California Press.

Mattingly, C. & Garro, L. C. (2000). *Narrative and the cultural construction of illness and healing.* University of California Press.

Meyer, A. (1922). The philosophy of occupational therapy. *American Journal of Physical Medicine and Rehabilitation, 1*, 1–10. PMID: 341715.

Palmadottir, G. (2006). Client-therapist relationships: Experiences of occupational therapy clients in rehabilitation. *British Journal of Occupational Therapy, 69*, 394–401. https://doi.org/10.1177/030802260606900902

Parkinson, S., & Brooks, R. (2021). *A guide to the formulation of plans and goals in occupational therapy.* Routledge.

Peloquin, S. M. (2005). The Eleanor Clarke Slagle Lecture: Embracing our ethos, reclaiming our heart. *American Journal of Occupational Therapy, 59*, 611–625. http://dx.doi.org/10.5014/ajot.59.6.611

Polatjko, H. J., Davis, J. A., & McEwen, S. E. (2015). Therapeutic use of self: A catalyst in the client-therapist alliance for change. In C. H. Christiansen, C. M. Baum, & J. D. Bass (Eds.), *Occupational therapy: Performance, participation and well-being* (4th ed., pp. 81–92). Slack Incorporated.

Rosa, S. A., & Hasselkus, B. R. (1996). Connecting with patients: The personal experience of professional helping. *Occupational Therapy Journal of Research, 16*, 245–260. 10.1177/153944929601600402

Santana, M., Manalili, K., Jolley, R. J., Zelinsky, S., Quan, H., & Lu, M. (2018). How to practice person-centred care: A conceptual framework. *Health Expectations, 21*(2), 429–440. https://doi.org/10.1111/hex.12640

Slagle, E. C. (1922). Training aides for mental patients. *Archives of Occupational Therapy, 1*, 11–18.

Taff, S. D. (2021). *Philosophy and occupational therapy: Informing education, research and practice.* Slack Incorporated.

Taylor, R. R. (2008). *The intentional relationship: Occupational therapy and use of self.* F. A. Davis.

Taylor, R. R. (Ed.). (2017). *Kielhofner's model of human occupation* (5th ed.). Wolters Kluwer.

Taylor, R. R. (2019). Therapeutic relationship and client collaboration: Applying the intentional relationship model. In B. Boyt Shell & G. Gillen (Eds.), *Willard and Spackman's occupational therapy* (13th ed., pp. 527–538). Wolters Kluwer.

Taylor, R. R. (2020). *The intentional relationship: Occupational therapy and use of self.* F. A. Davis.

Taylor, R. R., Lee, S. W., & Kielhofner, G. (2011). Practitioners' use of interpersonal modes within the therapeutic relationship: Results from a nationwide study. *OTJR: Occupation, Participation and Health, 31*, 6–14. https://doi.org/10.3928/15394492-20100521-02

Taylor, R. R., Lee, S. W., Kielhofner, G., & Ketkar, M. (2009). Therapeutic use of self: A nationwide survey of practitioners' attitudes and experiences. *American Journal of Occupational Therapy, 63*, 198–207. PMID: 19432058

Van Vieuwenhove, K., & Meganck, R. (2017). Interpersonal features in complex trauma etiology, consequences, and treatment: A literature review. *Journal of Aggression, Maltreatment and Trauma, 28*(8), 903–928. https://doi.org/10.1080/10926771.2017.1405316

Whalley Hammell, K. R. (2013) Client-centred practice in occupational therapy: Critical reflections. *Scandinavian Journal of Occupational Therapy, 20*(3), 174–181. https://doi.org/10.3109/11038128.2012.75 2032

Wilcock, A. (1993). A theory of the human need for occupation. *Journal of Occupational Science, 1*(1), 11–24. https://doi.org/10.1080/14427591 .1993.9886375

Yerxa, E. J. (1983). Audacious values: The energy source for occupational therapy practice. In G. Kielhofner (Ed.), *Health through occupation: Theory and practice in occupational therapy* (pp. 149– 162). F.A. Davis.

Yun, D., & Choi, J. (2019). Person-centered rehabilitation care and outcomes: A systematic literature review. *International Journal of Nursing Studies, 93*, 74–83. https://doi.org/10.1016/j.ijnurstu.2019.02.012

Group Process and Group Intervention

Moses N. Ikiugu

LEARNING OBJECTIVES

After reading this chapter, you will be able to:

1. Explain a historical overview of how groups and group processes were introduced in occupational therapy (OT) practice.
2. Explain group dynamics using the five-stage development model: forming, storming, norming, performing, and adjournment, and explain these stages from the perspective of complex, dynamical, adaptive systems theory.
3. Discuss group roles and explain how external and internal group dynamics may influence them.
4. Explain group leadership styles.
5. Form an OT group.
6. Create group and session plans.
7. Explain OT group leadership and coleadership based on Cole's (2018) seven-step format.
8. Write a group session report.

Introduction

The use of groups as a tool in therapy came from group techniques in general psychological theory. The prototype of group psychotherapy in occupational therapy (OT) can be traced back to the opening of Jane Addams' Hull House in Chicago in 1889 (Shaffer & Galinsky, 1974). They used a social work group model to help poor immigrants from Europe transition to the American culture. Later, a Boston internist, Joseph Hersey Pratt, ran the first group as a medical intervention (Shaffer & Galinsky, 1974). Participants in the group were poor patients suffering from tuberculosis. Based on the principle of universality, his goal was to help patients share their illness experiences so that they did not feel alone and isolated. He thought that recovering patients could help others feel hopeful through this sharing.

Edward W. Lazell, a psychiatrist, later used this group approach to work with war veterans diagnosed with schizophrenia in 1918 (Shaffer & Galinsky, 1974). At this point, groups and group processes were adopted widely, particularly by psychoanalysts such as Trigant Burrow, Louis Wender, and Paul Schilder. Samuel Slavson introduced the use of activities as part of group therapy to enable children to express their conflicts and pent-up feelings nonverbally. One can argue that Slavson's approach was the precursor for present-day OT groups (Ikiugu, 2007).

The pioneers of OT groups were Fidler and Fidler and Mosey. Fidler and Fidler (1963) developed the *task group model*. The purpose of the task group was to create interpersonal awareness. They proposed that interpersonal, intrapsychic, and environmental factors influence affect, learning, and behavior. They conceptualized OT as a learning laboratory in which these factors could be managed to help service users develop skills for living. In this conceptualization, the purpose of OT task groups was to facilitate self-exploration in the here-and-now using activities to help clients identify stress, conflicts, and problems so that they could learn and change by developing more adaptive behaviors. In this endeavor, they structured groups to help service users understand the relationships among their feelings, thoughts, and behavior and their effect on other people and task performance.

Fidler and Fidler were particular about how task groups would be structured. The group would consist of eight service users and meet for 1.5 hours, 4 times per week. In these meetings, group members worked on a task requiring common effort and consensus among group members. A group task was an activity or process designed to produce an end product or a service for the group members or other people. Examples of group tasks included publishing a hospital newsletter, cooking, gardening, participating in patient councils, and so on.

Mosey (1970) advanced the idea of *developmental groups* designed to evaluate service users and develop social interaction skills. She proposed five types of groups for use in OT. The groups were organized hierarchically based on the service users' level of social skill development.

1. ***Parallel Group***: This was the lowest in the hierarchy. Service users were placed in this type of group if they were at least able to function in the presence of other people, even if they were not able to share roles. People in this type of group did not have a common goal but they were expected to be able to interact verbally and nonverbally with other group members. Therefore, they had to have basic social interaction skills such as saying "please," "thank you," and so on.

2. ***Project Group***: This was the second-lowest type of group in the hierarchy. In this type of group, participants had a shared *short-term* task. An example of a short-term task would be the development of information posters for dissemination to the public as part of a self-advocacy initiative by adults with developmental disabilities supported by a local group home agency. They were expected to be able to share and participate in competitive tasks, seeking assistance when necessary.

3. ***Ego-centric Cooperative Group***: In this type of group, tasks were relatively *long-term*. An example of a long-term task is an antidrug campaign developed by adolescents with emotional and behavioral disorders (EBD) in a mandated day treatment program. Since the adolescents were ordered into the day treatment program by the drug court, the OT practitioner guided them in developing the antidrug campaign as a way of helping them learn through teaching why such drugs were dangerous. The adolescents had to work together to determine what educational materials they needed to develop, the resources they needed for the project, the division of tasks to ensure success, plans for the administration of the project in local high schools, and so on. The project took 3 months to complete. Group members at this level were still focused on self-interest, but now they realized that meeting their needs was predicated on other group members' needs being met. The *self-interest* was therefore *enlightened*. This enlightened self-interest required that group members engage in cooperative and competitive tasks while adhering to group norms, to allow mutual need fulfillment.

4. ***Cooperative Group***: The purpose of a cooperative group was mutual need satisfaction for members. Group members were homogeneous and had shared views and feelings. For this type of group, the satisfaction of group members' needs took precedence over task accomplishment. Members needed to be able to acknowledge their peers' needs and to be willing to try and meet them.

5. ***Mature Group***: This was at the top of the hierarchy in Mosey's model of OT groups. It consisted of members with heterogeneous characteristics, views, values, and needs. In this type of group, the leader and follower roles were delineated, and group members had to be able to follow but also share in the leadership roles. They also had to be able to distinguish between task and socioemotional roles.

Using Mosey's group model, the OT practitioner evaluated service users to determine their social skill mastery and placed them in a group requiring skills at the next developmental level. For example, a person who could function in the presence of other people and had basic social skills but could not work effectively with others was determined to be at the *parallel group* level of social development. The OT practitioner would place such a person in a *project group* where they could learn how to collaborate with other people, even if competitively at times, to complete a short-term project. In recent times, OT practitioners have broadened the use of groups beyond Fidler and Fidler's and Mosey's models. Today, there is a variety of group types including, "activity groups, task groups, directive groups, sensory intervention/modulation groups, psycho-educational groups, community and self-help groups" among others (Zedel & Chen, 2021, p. 279).

Group Process

Human beings naturally exist in groups. We are born into a family that belongs to a community, and the community is part of a larger social entity. As such, human beings are always acting on others and changing them (their values, beliefs, motivations, etc.) in the context of the group to which they belong, and other people in the group act on and change them as well. Thus, as Laing (1969) argued, understanding "a person" is possible only in the context of that person's relationship with others. As social beings, people are always acting on each other. These interactive dynamics that cause mutual change among group members constitute a group process. Because OT aims to create change in service users to enhance their health, well-being, and quality of life (Pizzi & Richards, 2017), these group processes are a very potent means of achieving those changes. As Lewin (1951) observed, it is easier to facilitate therapeutic change in individuals within a group context than individually. In other words, interpersonal processes are the change (or therapeutic) agents in groups. Group members share their experiences, which lightens the burden because of a sense of shared problems (principle of universality), group members get satisfaction from the sense that they are of some help to others (altruism), they gain new useful information, and the group cohesiveness instills a sense of mutual support. These benefits ultimately instill in service users a sense of hope for the future.

Because process denotes dynamism, group process refers to continuous change in both the group as an entity and individual members as agents within that entity. Therefore, group dynamics is a characteristic of the group process. For an OT practitioner to facilitate the group process appropriately to harness its therapeutic power, it is important to understand its dynamics. In this regard, there are many theoretical views of group conceptualization, but one helpful idea might be that of a group as an open, complex, dynamical adaptive system (Gençer, 2019). In this view, groups are understood as consisting of multiple agents dynamically interacting among themselves as the entire group interacts with its environment as well (Uhl-Bien et al., 2007). Through this process, self-organization occurs, leading to the emergence of group characteristics that are different than those of any of the individual group members. This conceptualization may be used to understand the various stages of group development and the behavior of group members during those stages. Understanding the behavior of individuals as well as the group as a whole from a complex dynamical adaptive systems perspective might help a practitioner manage the group with more awareness to ensure the best therapeutic outcomes for group members.

Stages of Group Development

The dynamics can be visualized as occurring through stages of development in a group's lifetime, similar to those of an individual in the life course. Tuckman (1965) and Tuckman and Jensen (1977) developed a stage model of group development that is still used today (Vaida & Şerban, 2021). Initially, the model consisted of four stages: forming, storming, norming, and performing (Tuckman, 1965). Later, based on feedback after the adoption of his model around the world,

he added the fifth stage, adjourning (Tuckman & Jensen, 1977). This model has recently been discussed in the literature as a way of understanding therapeutic processes in OT groups (Carson, 2020; Cole, 2018; Schwartzberg et al., 2008). According to Tuckman and Jensen (1977, see also Vaida & Şerban, 2021), the life of a small group can be defined by the following stages of development:

- *Stage 1. Forming:* Group members have just come together for the very first time. There is ambiguity and tentativeness. They expect the leader to provide clear, detailed directions. At this stage, group members are concerned about defining tasks. They seek approval and a sense of safety from their peers and try to avoid conflict or confrontation. Any content that is likely to be even minimally controversial is avoided. Some group members may have optimism and excitement, but the feeling tone is mostly uncertainty and apprehension. For the group to progress to the next stage, group members need to come to a point where they are willing to leave their comfort zones and take risks. They may need to confront topics that are controversial and not safe.

- *Stage 2. Storming:* As group members try to organize and structure the group tasks, leadership and power struggles begin to emerge, and interpersonal conflicts begin to occur. There are differences in points of view and arguments about what course of action is the correct one. Some group members feel overwhelmed, and many may think that no progress is being made toward accomplishing tasks. Part of the problem is that the roles are not yet clear, and there is not much consensus-building going on. Group members may feel defensive, confused, and resistant to group tasks. They may challenge group leaders and question their wisdom. To move to the next stage, group members have to change their attitude from "testing and proving" (do my leaders and peers know what they are doing?) to "problem-solving" (what is the problem and how do we go about solving it?).

- *Stage 3. Norming:* At this point, the group is evolving into a cohesive entity. There is shared leadership, which demands interpersonal trust. This trust is possible because of agreed-upon norms, procedures, and processes to resolve conflicts and accomplish tasks. There are attempts to reach a consensus in decision-making, and routines are developed to enable the group to set and achieve task milestones. Group members now begin to feel that they belong and they are confident and able to express constructive criticism when warranted. The problem is that group members feel good at this stage and may be afraid that this camaraderie may go away in the near future. To guard against this possible break-up, resistance to any kind of change may emerge.

- *Stage 4. Performing:* This stage is a period of high productivity. There is interdependence among group members who recognize and adapt to meet their peers' needs. The roles are clear, group members know and understand the strengths of their peers, and they are functional and flexible. Everyone understands the group processes. There is empathy for one another and tight bonds form. There is mutual support, group members enjoy their time together and have fun, and there is a general sense of satisfaction. The group experiences peak efficiency at this point, tasks are performed, and there is a lot of progress toward group goals.

- *Stage 5. Adjourning:* Completion of tasks and rapid progress toward goals however means that the group may fulfill its purpose and terminate soon. Awareness of this eventuality creates anxiety and mourning of the impending loss of relationships in which group members have invested so much time and emotions. Group members may become restless. There may be bursts of energy followed by lethargy. The apprehension about termination may constitute a minor crisis, and the group leader needs to manage this stage carefully. One method of managing the stage is preparing group members by guiding reflection on what they have achieved, awarding certificates to recognize accomplishments, and giving group members time to say their goodbyes.

While Tuckman's stages of group development have been used extensively by group facilitators throughout the world (Hingst, 2006; Hurt & Trombley, 2007;), there are other models (Arner et al., 2010; Tuckman & Jensen, 1977; Vaida & Serban, 2021). These include Bass and Ryterband's (1979) model, which focused more on group formation and control rather than its development through stages, and Tubbs's (1978) model, which analyzed group subprocesses and how the group learned from various challenges as it evolved, among others. However, Tuckman's developmental stages have been the most influential in the world of group therapy. His two papers have been cited over 8000 times since he proposed the model (Vaida & Șerban, 2021). Tuckman's stages are also widely used in OT (Cole, 2018; Schwartzberg et al., 2008).

Whether one chooses Tuckman or any of the other models as a theoretical guide, group development can generally be visualized as consisting of three broad stages: introduction, development, and conclusion. Furthermore, there are two things to note about group development in general: First, from the complexity theory perspective, the stages' characteristics can be understood as emerging from the dynamic interactions among group members (system agents) as the entire group interacts with its environmental context. From this perspective, while the stages of development retain the general patterns that can be named as forming, storming, norming, performing, and adjourning, manifestations of those stages depend on slight variations in initial conditions such as how group members are chosen, the environment in which the group is conducted, the purpose of the group, and so on. Those variations can cause big differences in how group members experience and deal with the uncertainties of the forming stage, the conflicts of the storming stage, and so on.

Second, part of the dynamics of group development and how group members negotiate the stages is their roles in the group. Group member roles may fall into the following three categories: task roles, group maintenance roles, and individual roles (Benne & Sheats, 1948; Cole, 2018; Schwartzberg et al., 2008).

- **Task roles** include participation in actions related to the facilitation of successful task performance. They include offering ideas on how to solve problems, asking for and offering opinions, and offering task-related information among others.
- **Group maintenance roles** are related to the maintenance of the group as a functioning unit to complete the task. They include compromising on ideas, encouraging peers to keep going, maintaining harmony in the group, and so on.
- **Individual roles** are oriented toward satisfying individual member needs and may not contribute to group task performance. Examples include blocking group action by disagreeing with all proposed actions without offering alternatives, being overly aggressive, keeping group attention on personal issues. For a complete list of the three categories of roles, see Box 29.1.

Based on the complex dynamical adaptive systems theory, the assumption of group membership roles can also be understood as emerging from the group process. We may think of a group as having a field of energy that creates polarities that organize those roles. Just as we cannot see the magnetic field that creates the polarities of a magnet, we cannot see the field of energy in a group, but we can see its effect through the group membership roles. Consequently, the roles need to be occupied. That is why sometimes you participate in a group and find yourself in the role of the gatekeeper, while in another group, you gravitate toward the harmonizer role. You occupy a position that is empty and consistent with your personality because if a role in a group is vacant, someone will tend to occupy it. Understanding these role dynamics and their function in various stages of group development is very important for an OT practitioner to lead the group effectively.

Finally, the manifestation of the above-discussed group dynamics tends to depend on the type of group members. In highly autonomous groups (e.g., individuals with mental health issues whose conditions have been managed through medication, self-help groups, outpatient therapy groups), the group development and role occupancy are likely to follow the previously described process because group members have a high level of autonomy. For less autonomous groups (e.g., when working with individuals with intellectual disabilities), the practitioner needs to provide the group with more structure, which affects the way group stages manifest. For example, the forming stage

BOX 29.1 GROUP MEMBERSHIP ROLES

Group Task Roles	Group Maintenance Roles	Individual Roles
Initiator/contributor proposes new ideas, goals, procedures, solutions **Information seeker** asks for information or clarifications **Opinion seeker** asks for suggestions and/or clarification of values **Information giver** provides information **Opinion giver** states personal opinions and beliefs **Elaborator** provides suggestions and elaborates on them with examples, provides a rationale for a suggested course of action, etc. **Coordinator** coordinates activities or group members or tries to pull ideas together to make coherent sense **Orienter** keeps the group on task by reminding everybody of the goals and where the group is in relation to the goals **Evaluator/critic** subjects group performance to a standard **Energizer** prods the group to keep going **Procedural technician** takes care of procedural tasks and logistics to expedite group action. **Recorder** records group decisions and activities	**Encourager** commends and praises other group members and accepts their ideas **Harmonizer** attempts to reconcile differences and conflicts **Compromiser** compromises on personal views and ideas by meeting others half-way **Gatekeeper** encourages participation of group members by keeping communication channels open **Standard setter** sets performance standards for the group **Group observer or commentator** keeps tabs on group processes and gives feedback on observations to the group so that the group can periodically evaluate its procedures **Follower** typically assumes the position of the audience and passively follows other group members	**Aggressor** attacks the group activities, may be aggressive and demeaning to other group members by disapproving of their values, actions, and feelings **Blocker** is negative and resistant to group suggestions, stubborn, and comes off as unreasonably oppositional **Recognition seeker** attempts to keep attention on self by constantly boasting on personal achievements among other things **Self-confessor** derails group action by attempting to keep its attention on personal feelings, beliefs, and ideologies **Playboy** is uninvolved and derails the group through cynicism, nonchalance, and other activities unrelated to the group task or group goals **Dominator** tries to be domineering by interrupting others and trying to control the direction of the group process **Help seeker** tries to elicit sympathy from the group through self-depreciation, appearing confused, etc. **Special interest pleader** brings group discourse repeatedly to the personal special interest topic, often using stereotypes of the purported special interest group. This action is typically an attempt to meet an individual need

Adapted from Benne, K. D., & Sheats, P. (1948). Functional roles of group members. *Journal of Social Issues, 4*(2), 41–49. https://doi.org/10.1111/j.1540-4560.1948.tb01783.x

may be mediated by the fact that the uncertainty of group goals not being clear is not a factor. The storming stage may also be different because the clarity of goals makes conflicts about suggested courses of action unnecessary. In general, OT groups are occupation based rather than talking groups. Such groups often require more structure than Benne and Sheat and other psychotherapists conceptualized, and therefore, their developmental process is different.

Group Leadership

Leadership Styles

Group leadership is also a role whose exact nature may emerge from the group process, depending on the group leader's personality, the type of clients in the group, and contextual factors. In assuming leadership roles, group leaders adopt leadership styles according to the group's circumstances. These leadership styles vary from strict control of the group process to letting the group make its own

decisions with little or no interference except when asked for input. In general, three leadership styles are used in therapy groups: democratic (participative), autocratic (authoritarian), and laissez-faire (delegative) (Lewin et al., 1939; Schwartzberg et al., 2008).

- *Democratic style:* In the democratic style, the role of the leader is to build the decision-making process. The group discusses and makes decisions by consensus. The group leader (OT practitioner) acts as a resource person, providing information and other resources as needed, as the group progresses toward its goals and is also a participating member. In other words, the leader participates in the group discussions, providing opinions, suggestions, and key information. This leadership style is appropriate for highly autonomous groups but may not work well for groups with members who have cognitive disabilities. Even for such individuals, however, the leadership style may work with appropriate accommodations. The democratic style is very satisfying for highly autonomous groups, and the product of the group activities is high quality. Group members own and feel pride in both the group process and the outcome.

- *Autocratic style:* For groups with members who have cognitive disabilities or severe mental disabilities, more structure and guidance may be necessary, and such guidance is available in a more autocratic style. In this style, the leader (OT practitioner) makes decisions and gives group members directions. Authoritarian leadership may lead to more efficiency, but group members do not feel a sense of ownership of the group process or the outcome. Therefore, the product may not be of very high quality. Furthermore, the group members may be hostile toward a leader using this leadership style.
- *Laissez-faire style:* In the laissez-faire style, the leader provides the supplies and needed information and leaves the group alone. The term *laissez-faire* means letting things take their course. Therefore, an OT practitioner using this style does not participate in the group. The decision-making power belongs solely to the group members. This leadership style may be appropriate for self-help groups such as a support group for discharged individuals with a history of mental illness or autonomous groups such as college campus student clubs. In these cases, the leader takes more of an adviser role. However, this style may result in frustration if used in a therapeutic setting because in such situations, group members expect more guidance for the group to achieve its goals.

Coleadership

Group coleadership refers to two or more OT practitioners leading a group together. This model is used regularly in psychotherapy, where therapists lead groups in dyads (Luke, 2007; Schwartzberg et al., 2008). There are advantages of coleadership. These include more comprehensive coverage of the group (more group leaders can observe more of what is happening in the group, including dynamics such as transference, and may catch important cues that a single group leader may miss), learning from each other, covering each other's blind spots, and supporting each other. Group members also have a chance to observe the interactions among group leaders and learn from them. This is especially beneficial for multiple gender dyads where practitioners have a chance to model appropriate intergender interactions and cooperation (could be very useful, especially when working with adolescents who are still trying to define their identities in relation to their peers). In this regard, OT practitioners may be able to model appropriate ways of communicating disagreements while treating each other with respect.

Disadvantages of coleadership include the risk of interpersonal conflicts, destructive competition among leaders, and one leader being overdependent on the other. To avoid these possible pitfalls, OT practitioners should meet before every session and discuss their respective roles during the session and what to do if conflicts arise. After every session, the coleaders should meet to debrief the session (discuss what went well, what did not go well, how they feel about the session overall and how they worked together, and the plans for the next session).

Forming a Group

In OT, a significant part of the group session is devoted to group activity designed to help group members learn target skills. Typically, OT practitioners use activity groups, task groups, or social groups (Scaffa, 2019). More specific examples include social skills, independent living, leisure activities, stress management, and assertiveness training groups among others (Stein & Tallant, 2013). A generic group is usually formed (e.g., a social skills group) before the practitioner even knows the identity of individual group members. Service users who need to develop specific target skills (such as social skills) are referred to the group that is already regularly scheduled. A different model of forming groups (Ikiugu, 2007) is proposed in this chapter and outlined in the following sections. In this model, the OT practitioner meets with individual service users, evaluates them, and collaboratively sets individual goals.

Evaluating Individual Service Users

The OT practitioner meets with each service user individually for an interview to determine the individual's occupational participation priorities and suitability for placement in a group. This initial interview can be guided by the American Occupational Therapy Association (AOTA) occupational profile interview (2020). Based on the interview, the practitioner understands the service user's occupational performance issues (perceived occupational participation successes and barriers, interests and values, performance and routines, etc.). Based on this understanding, the practitioner administers standardized occupational participation assessments to create a more precise performance baseline, interprets the assessment results, and collaboratively with the service user formulates goals to improve performance to the service user's satisfaction.

Creating Group Goals

An OT group should be occupation based, person centered, theory based, and evidence based, consistent with the profession's principles and values (AOTA, 2020). To ensure that the group is person centered, the service users' goals are analyzed for similarity in themes, and group goals are developed based on those themes (see examples in Box 29.2). The occupational categories described in the Occupational Therapy Practice Framework (AOTA, 2020) can be used to group service user goals by themes. That way goals are grouped under Activities of Daily Living (ADLs), Instrumental Activities of Daily Living (IADLs), Social Participation, and so on.

Creating a Group Plan

Using the group goals developed based on individual service user goals, a group plan is developed. The plan can be

BOX 29.2 CREATING GROUP GOALS BASED ON INDIVIDUAL SERVICE USERS' GOALS

Service Users' Goals

Participant 1

Within 2 weeks, the service user will demonstrate improved sequencing of the **morning self-care routine, completing brushing teeth and hair, and washing face** with setup and no more than five verbal cues.

Participant 2

In 3 weeks, the service user will rate the perceived performance of **kitchen cleaning** 5/10 or better on the Canadian Occupational Performance Measure (COPM).

Participant 3

Within 2 weeks, the service user will demonstrate improved **social participation**, spontaneously choosing to engage in at least one **leisure activity** once a week for one hour or more with peers at the facility.

Participant 4

Within 1 week, the service user will participate in a chosen **social leisure activity** with supervision and no more than 5 verbal cues

Participant 5

In 2 weeks, the service user will demonstrate competence in using a checklist to complete **brushing teeth and washing hands** with minimal verbal cues.

Common Themes

Theme	Frequency
Basic ADLs (**morning self-care routine, completing brushing teeth and hair, washing face, washing hands**)	2
IADLs (**kitchen cleaning**)	1
Social Participation	2
Leisure participation	2

Therefore, for this group of service users, goals were grouped under 4 themes: Basic ADLs, Instrumental ADLs, Social Participation, and Leisure Participation.

Group Goals (Based on the Above Four Themes)

After this group, each group member will demonstrate improved ability to:

1. Complete the basic ADL routine using cognitive strategies such as checklists
2. Participate in personally meaningful social leisure occupations with desired frequency (combining themes 3 [social participation] and 4 [leisure participation] in one goal).
3. Complete routine IADLs such as cleaning the kitchen at the group home with staff support.

Note: The themes used to formulate the group goals are bolded in the service users' goals to illustrate how they are derived.

created using a group protocol such as the one created by Cole (2018). Creating the plan requires an OT practitioner to choose theoretical conceptual practice models (or frames of reference) to provide group facilitation strategies. The eclectic method (selecting an umbrella and complementary models of practice to ensure comprehensive coverage of group goals) may be useful (Ikiugu, 2007, 2019; Ikiugu & Smallfield, 2010; Ikiugu et al. 2009). A group plan is created using the Intervention Plan Outline (Cole, 2018), the developed group goals, and the chosen theories (see an example in Box 29.3).

BOX 29.3 EXAMPLE GROUP PROTOCOL

Outcome criteria: By the end of this group, each group participant will demonstrate the ability to:

1. Complete all basic ADLs prioritized by service users such as grooming, brushing teeth, hair care, etc. using cognitive strategies such as checklists.
2. Complete IADLs prioritized by service users at the group home with verbal cues.
3. Participate regularly in chosen, personally meaningful leisure occupations with peers.

Method:

Participation in group occupations followed by sharing and discussion

Time and Place of Meeting:

The group will meet at the group home on Tuesday and Wednesday afternoons. Each group session will be one hour long.

Supplies and Cost:

The supplies and cost will be calculated for each group session

Group Title: Skills for Independent and Meaningful Living
Author: MNI, OTR/L
Frame of Reference: The Canadian Model of Occupational Performance will be used to guide this group (Polatajko

(continued)

BOX 29.3 EXAMPLE GROUP PROTOCOL (continued)

et al., 2007). This will entail communicating and modeling empathy in the group, communicating and modeling unconditional positive regard, demonstrating respect for all group members, and encouraging group members to participate in directing the group activities as much as possible. In addition, because participants in this group have cognitive disabilities, the group leaders will be more directive than typical in client-centered interventions. The Ross' Five Stage approach (Ross & Bachner, 2004) will be used to guide the group in addition to client-centered strategies, as is appropriate for a group in which cognitive performance is limited. The Model of Human Occupation (MOHO; Kielhofner, 2008) will be the secondary complementary model of practice. Based on this model, group activities focusing on the interests of group participants (part of the volitional component of the person system) will be identified for use as media in the group process.

Purpose:

This group aims to help group members develop skills necessary for optimal independence and participation in meaningful, enjoyable occupations. Such skills include the optimal performance of basic ADLs, IADLs, and social participation.

Group Membership and Size:

Members of this group will be adults with developmental disabilities, ages 18 to 60. This will be a closed group consisting of 8 members. Group members will have a low to high need for support to live as independently as possible.

Group Goals:

After this group, group members will demonstrate improved ability to:

1. Complete the basic ADL routine using cognitive strategies such as checklists
2. Complete IADLs such as cleaning the kitchen with minimal verbal reminders
3. Participate in personally meaningful social leisure occupations with desired frequency

Rationale, Limitations, and Adaptations:

The participants in this group live in group homes. They have close supervision from the agency staff, but their Quality of Life would improve significantly with optimized independence. Therefore, it is important to work with them to establish support systems that will facilitate their ability to act on their own choices. The above goals are designed to facilitate dignity for group members while recognizing the need to put in place strategies to mitigate any risks to their safety.

Adapted from Cole, M. B. (2018). *Group dynamics in occupational therapy: The theoretical basis and practice application of group intervention* (pp. 300–302). Slack.

Creating Group Session Plans

The total number of sessions for each group can be between two and eight, which may be conducted weekly or twice a week. The number of sessions depends on the number of themes derived from service user goals. In this example, four themes emerged from the analysis of individual service user goals. Therefore, if an OT practitioner plans two sessions for each theme, the total number of sessions would be eight. These eight sessions can be conducted in 4 weeks (two sessions per week) or 8 weeks (one session per week). Group sessions can be planned using Cole's (2018) seven-step format: introduction, activity, sharing, processing, generalizing, application, and summary, which is described in the following section. Each session would be designed to address one of the group themes (e.g., see Box 29.4). The steps will be described in detail in the following section. The objective is to ensure that all individual service user goals are addressed by the time the group concludes.

BOX 29.4 EXAMPLE SESSION PLAN

Group Title: Skills for Independent and Meaningful Living
Session Title: Managing Your Home (Cleaning Kitchen)

Theoretical Conceptual Practice Models:

This session will be facilitated using guidelines from the following theoretical conceptual practice models: the Canadian Model of Occupational Performance and Engagement (CMOP-E), and the Model of Human Occupation (MOHO). The CMOP-E is based on the proposition that service users are the experts in their occupational performance needs. Therefore, OT practitioners have to collaborate with them, communicate empathy, and unconditional positive regard (Polatajko et al., 2007). Using strategies based on this model, the OT practitioner will grade activities to enable all group members to participate irrespective of cognitive level. The practitioner will also use strategies based on the model to encourage group members to engage in the discussions. The MOHO focuses on the importance of innate volition as

BOX 29.4 EXAMPLE SESSION PLAN (*continued*)

a prerequisite for the success of individual occupational participation (Kielhofner, 2008). The model principles guided the creation of group sessions based on group members' goals so that the volition component of the human system (more specifically interests) could be leveraged for optimum client engagement. The environment was structured based on an understanding of the environmental component of the system to ensure that group members received the most positive and empowering feedback.

Format:

- Introduction (10 minutes)
- Activity (25 minutes)
- Sharing (5 minutes)
- Processing (5 minutes)
- Generalizing (5 minutes)
- Application (5 minutes)
- Summary (5 minutes)

Supplies:

- Blank cleaning schedule work-sheets
- Pencils

Description of the Group Activity: In this group session, we will focus on the development of home management skills, specifically kitchen cleaning.

Purpose of the Group Session

The *Occupational Therapy Practice Framework* identifies cleaning, cooking, and laundry tasks as instrumental activities of daily living (IADLs), which are activities that support an individual's daily life within the home environment (AOTA, 2020). This group session will aim to enable individuals to perform home management tasks that they want to perform, specifically cleaning the kitchen successfully. The group members will be provided with resources, including an hourly calendar that they can use to schedule cleaning tasks in their daily routines. Mahoney and Roberts (2009) defined the performance of occupations by adults with developmental disabilities with others such as staff members or volunteers as co-occupations. When participants engaged in co-occupations successfully, they were satisfied and found the occupations to be meaningful. Therefore, to make the group session consistent with the concept of co-occupation, team leaders will facilitate this activity so that group members learn how to perform home management tasks cooperatively with peers.

Goal of the Group Session

By the end of the session, group members will develop a schedule for home management tasks, including cleaning the kitchen after meals, and demonstrate the ability to complete the cleaning task successfully with verbal cues.

Introduction

Ice breaker

Group members will introduce themselves and state their favorite meal and their least favorite cleaning chore. This ice-breaker will be tied to the purpose of the session by introducing the concept of cleaning as part of home management.

Activities

Activity 1: Group members will be given a 1-week calendar template. Group facilitators will assist participants working in subgroups to prepare weekly activities that include making grocery lists for meal ingredients, shopping for groceries, making meals, and cleaning the kitchen after meals.

Activity 2: Group members will discuss and divide cleaning tasks among themselves. They will use the cleaning supplies available at the group home to work together and clean the kitchen. One group member, who the group will nominate, will be responsible for inspecting the kitchen to determine if the cleaning is completed satisfactorily. Another group member will record the steps used by the group to finish the cleaning task so that there is a written protocol that individuals can use later to complete the kitchen cleaning tasks.

Questions to Guide Discussion

Sharing

Would any group member like to share the weekly calendar that you created?

Processing

1. What did you think about today's activities?
2. How do you feel about how the group leaders helped you complete the activities? What was the most helpful about how they helped you with today's activities? What was the least helpful?

Generalizing

1. Please share your experiences in this group session. As you listen to other group members, how do your experiences compare to those of your peers?
2. What have you learned from our discussion today following the group activities?

Application

How will you use the skills you learned today to complete your home cleaning tasks from today?

Summary

Can someone tell me what we did today? What was the first thing we did? Next thing?

1. What was the most important lesson we learned today that we will apply in our lives?

Leading Occupational Therapy Groups

OT groups are designed to help individual service users change their behavior and achieve their therapy goals. Therefore, leadership in such groups should be consistent with the values and best practices in OT (AOTA, 2020); person centered (focus on goals of individual group members); occupation based (the OT practitioner uses occupational participation as a teaching/learning tool to help group members work on their collective goals); theory based (the group planning and intervention strategies should be based on OT theoretical conceptual practice model principles); and evidence based (strategies used to guide the group process should be grounded on the best available research evidence supporting their efficacy). Given the above-described criteria, the OT practitioner may find it best to use a combination of leadership styles as necessary as the group develops to effectively guide the group toward its goals. This dynamic combination of styles would be consistent with the complexity perspective that considers the group's ever-changing internal and external circumstances (Uhl-Bien et al., 2007). Bearing that in mind, in OT groups, group leadership can be understood in the context of Cole's (2018) seven-step format (outlined in the group session plan in Box 29.4).

Step 1: Introduction

As group leaders, OT practitioners are responsible for creating desired therapeutic change using the group process. For this change to occur, they have to create conditions that make the group a safe place (Mills, 2016). If this is the first group meeting, it is in the Tuckman forming stage. Therefore, group members will likely be anxious, apprehensive, and uncertain even though there also may be feelings of optimism and excitement. The role of the leader (OT practitioner) is to set the tone for the group and to create a safe environment. A safe environment is ensured by spelling out the ground rules (e.g., all group discussions must remain confidential, group members must treat each other with respect, and group members' dignity must be respected irrespective of what they disclose during group sessions). At this point, it is also essential that group members introduce themselves. They should be encouraged but not required to share as much as they want about themselves. The group goals are then shared with the members, and an outline of the group sessions is provided. Each subsequent session should begin with an icebreaker followed by the session's goals and how they relate to the overall group and individual group member goals. The introduction part of the first group meeting may be relatively long (10–20 minutes), but the introduction sections should be brief (between 5 and 10 minutes) in subsequent sessions.

Step 2: Activity

The OT practitioner introduces the session's occupation and states how long the activity will take, the target goals and learning outcomes, and the participation expectations. Time must be allowed for sharing and processing because that is where the session lessons are crystallized. Therefore, it is recommended that the occupation should not take more than one-third of the total session time (Cole, 2018). So, if the session is 1 hour long, the time allotted to the occupation should ideally be no more than 20 minutes. However, the exact timing is based on the practitioner's judgment regarding what is doable within the available time.

Step 3: Sharing

Once the occupation is completed, materials and supplies are cleared so that there are no distractions, and group members sit down for sharing and processing. Ideally, group members should sit in a circle so that they can see each other's faces and there are no barriers (such as tables or desks) between them. This setup encourages optimal participation of group members in the discussion. If this is the second session, the group may still be in the Tuckman forming or may have transitioned to the storming stage. If it is in the forming stage, the OT practitioner's role is still to provide assurance to group members by reaffirming confidentiality, the ability to share without ridicule or threat to personal dignity, and so on. If the group is in the storming stage, the practitioner may restate the goals to clarify the group's purpose and mediate any conflicts among group members. As the group progresses through Tuckman's developmental stages in subsequent sessions, the practitioner may provide less structure to the group and allow members to take more ownership of steps three to seven. In Step 3, group members are invited to share what they produced during the occupation step with their peers. Other group members are encouraged to provide feedback as each group member shares. The goal here is for the group members to provide each other with mutual support so that they feel safe to explore what they have learned from the activity. The practitioner relies on therapeutic communication skills throughout the group process, including communicating empathy, unconditional positive regard, appropriate self-disclosure, and confrontation when necessary. The OT practitioner also models empathy for group members and encourages them to communicate empathically with their peers.

Step 4: Processing

In this step, group members are encouraged to share their feelings about the session. This includes feelings about their peers, as well as about the OT practitioner (group leader). The practitioner should specifically seek feedback from group members about how the session was run, what was not too helpful to their participation in the occupation, what was helpful, and what the practitioner can do differently to help improve future sessions. This step is critical because the OT practitioner must understand any underlying anxieties or other feelings that may interfere with full participation in the group process and address them promptly.

Step 5: Generalizing

In this step, the OT practitioner leads the group in drawing out the general principles that emerge from the occupation, sharing, and processing. For example, based on the discussions so far, what are the group members' values, feelings, and lessons learned? Are there any disagreements among group members? What issues seem to stand out in the group? This is the step in which therapeutic change that may be occurring is articulated so that it can be understood cognitively, an essential step for positive therapeutic outcomes. For this generalization to be effective, it is critical that group members communicate directly with each other rather than channel all communication through the practitioner (see Figure 29.1). For example, a group member may state: "In this session, I realized how important it is to have a schedule detailing a routine that includes all the things I want to do every day." Another group member may respond: "I agree. I realized that my activities are quite disorganized, and I do not have a routine that works. I think having a calendar of activities will help with that."

Step 6: Application

Ultimately, any lessons learned are of no use if they are not put into practice to change group members' lives. In this step, the OT practitioner guides the group members in exploring how they can apply the general principles learned in the session in their lives. Consistent with the therapeutic use of relationship principles (Ikiugu, 2007; Mayotte-Blum et al., 2012), the practitioner uses therapeutic immediacy (focus on the here-and-now) and concreteness (specificity) to help group members translate learned principles into actions. The practitioner may state: "Please, tell me how you will use the calendar-making skills to ensure that you perform all your daily activities on time beginning tomorrow morning." Here, the practitioner is using immediacy because the discussion is not about the abstract application of learned skills but rather about specific actions in the approximate here-and-now (tomorrow morning), in a very concrete manner (timely completion of daily activities).

Step 7: Summary

In this concluding step in Cole's (2018) seven-step format, the OT practitioner invites group members to participate in summarizing the day's session. The focus of this summary should be on the substantive lessons learned during sharing, generalization, and application. Examples of guiding questions could be: "What did we learn today about . . .?" "How did we say that we could apply those lessons in our lives?" "Based on what we learned in today's session, what will you do beginning tomorrow morning to improve . . .?"

Group Session Documentation

As is the case with good therapeutic practice in individual therapy, group proceedings must be documented thoroughly and accurately. After each session, the OT practitioner should write a report or what Schwartzberg et al. (2008) refer to as the "Session Evaluation." The session report should, at a minimum, consist of the following details: a list of group members who attended the session, group session (activity/occupation, what was required of group members, how members responded to the activity), analysis (of what was learned by group members, citing evidence to support the stated impressions), and suggestions for what group members should work on in the future. An example of a group session report can be seen in Box 29.5.

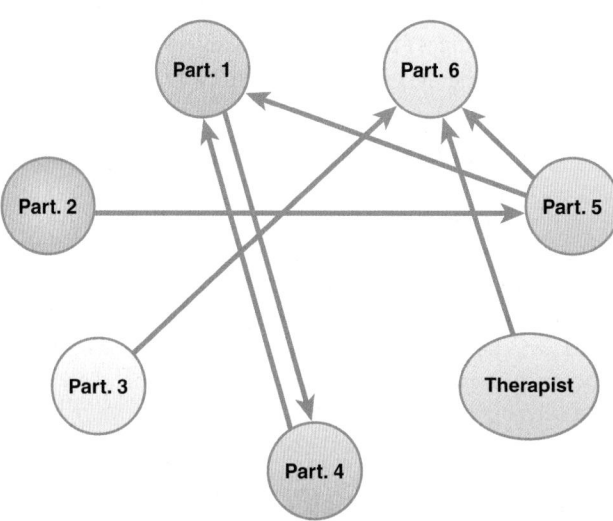

FIGURE 29.1 Seating design and communication patterns in an occupational therapy group during the sharing, processing, application, and summary steps. Part. 1, Part. 2, Part. 3, Part. 4, Part. 5, and Part. 6 stand for participants 1, 2, 3, 4, 5, and 6, respectively.

BOX 29.5 EXAMPLE OF GROUP SESSION DOCUMENTATION

Group Title: Skills for Independent and Meaningful Living
Group Session: Financial Management
Group Activity: Game of Monopoly
Date: 2/19/2020
Group Leader: MNI

In attendance for this session were **R, Ky, Ke, Ka, C, Al,** and **G. H** did not attend the session. **Al** came in a little late and was upset for some reason with **Ky**, who was sitting by **Ke**. She wanted to sit next to **Ke**. Finally, she was placed at her chosen place, and she calmed down. **C** spent a big part of session time in the social worker's office but finally joined the group. He continued making jokes as usual but participated in the group for a short time. The session started with an explanation of the session's purpose, followed by introductions.

Group members were divided into pairs for the activity. The pairs consisted of **Al** and **Ke**, **Ka** and **C**, **R** and **Ky**, and **A** (staff member) and **G**. I played the role of the banker. Group members enjoyed the game of monopoly and were absorbed in it. **Al** loved throwing the dice and moving the piece for her team on the board. Even **G** had a bright smile

on his face during the game. After the game, there was a discussion of some of the positive and negative ways of using money. It was noted that **R** was rather conservative in using monopoly money. He admitted that he was typically cautious with money. **Ke** admitted that she tended to spend more than she had. One of the principles that emerged during generalizing was that investing money, as was practiced during the monopoly game, was a good way of managing money because it ensured that the funds would grow for future use. The session concluded with an examination of how individuals could apply some of the skills they learned during the game in their lives. At the close of the session, my wallet went missing. It was later found that **C** had lifted it out of my pocket.

Analysis

It was clear that group members enjoyed and were involved in the monopoly game. It was also evident that they learned valuable skills through the activity. In a future session, we will focus on specific money management skills. **C**'s behavior of picking pockets will be addressed individually.

Adjournment Process

As the group approaches adjournment (with one or two sessions to go), the OT practitioner should begin preparing members for the conclusion. The preparation should include processing emotions arising out of the anticipated termination of personal relationships that have been developed. Such emotions may include sadness and denial (Vaida & Șerban, 2021). The practitioner should guide the group in reflecting and understanding these feelings, and the members should

discuss life after the group. Group members should celebrate their achievements as a result of participating in the group. In the final session, time should be set aside to discuss what group members have learned during their participation in the group and what this learning means to them (Schwartzberg et al., 2008). Group members' concerns should be addressed while redirecting discussion away from a desire to resist group adjournment. Members can be encouraged to explore resources and support systems on which they can rely upon leaving the group. See OT Story 29.1.

OT STORY 29.1 OCCUPATIONAL THERAPY GROUP FOR A MENTAL HEALTH UNIT IN A SUBACUTE HOSPITAL

My colleague and I were consulted by the rehab department in a subacute rehabilitation hospital and asked to make recommendations for the development of an OT program in their mental health unit. We completed a needs assessment where we interviewed the hospital administrators, OT practitioners and other rehabilitation staff, and the service users in the mental health unit. We also observed the unit and completed an audit of available resources.

Our needs assessment revealed that there were three OT practitioners in the rehabilitation department. The mental health floor was a 15-bed locked unit with 14 double-occupancy and 1 single-bed unit. There were

common areas with comfortable seating, a dining area, and a group activity room. Individuals served in the unit were adults with acute behavioral health needs who were independent in basic ADLs and mobility. Common diagnoses were schizophrenia, anxiety, and depression, with many of them having dual diagnoses. The average length of stay in the unit was 4 to 5 days or longer if there was a weekend preceding discharge.

Group sessions were provided by nurses and a social worker every day. However, our assessment indicated that the following needs were not currently being met: social skill development (including the ability to observe social boundaries), community participation, job skills training, time management, coping skills, and medication management. We recommended that an OT group meeting at least 3 times per week be established to meet these needs.

Questions

1. Based on the information above, would this unit's OT group be open or closed? Please, explain.

2. Use the needs assessment results described above to develop a group plan.
3. Create a group session plan addressing one of the identified needs.
4. Given that service users in this unit stay in the hospital for only 4 to 5 days, what group dynamic factors should the OT practitioner running the group expect?
5. How would the practitioner manage those group dynamics as the group leader?

Conclusion

Groups offer a very potent tool for effective intervention in OT. First, they provide a natural context for therapy because interactions among people are a natural social process (Gençer, 2019). Thus, when OT practitioners use group process as a medium for intervention, they are harnessing a natural human phenomenon because human beings are social animals by nature. Second, groups offer service users an opportunity to experience enhanced self-esteem, feel a sense of belonging by engaging with others with shared experiences, and develop useful life skills (Zedel & Chen, 2021). In addition, there is evidence that group interventions are at least as effective as individual therapy in yielding beneficial therapeutic benefits for service users (Yalom & Leszcz, 2005); see Expanding Our Perspectives. It is also instructive that groups have been a central part of administering intervention in OT throughout the profession's history as discussed earlier (Higgins et al., 2014; Ikiugu, 2007). It is clear that, given that groups offer an effective, natural process of providing therapy by affording an opportunity for social interactions and the use of groups has been central to OT practice historically, OT practitioners should make groups and group processes an integral part of their practice, irrespective of their area of practice. However, to use groups appropriately as therapeutic media, they have to be well planned and administered as discussed in this chapter, so that the therapeutic goals for each service user in the group are achieved.

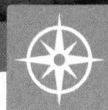 **EXPANDING OUR PERSPECTIVES**

Lisa Mahaffey

Early in my career as a mental health practitioner, I learned about Irvin Yalom's theory suggesting leaders can view the group as a microcosm of the social community in which people act every day (Yalom & Leszcz, 2020). This very simple idea led me to think about how I could use groups more effectively. I began to craft opportunities and spaces where people could engage in valued occupations and within the process of doing, learn from and provide rich feedback to each other. I started by changing my approach. Rather than trying to meet a variety of individual goals, I began using the Model of Human Occupation as a guide to assess the population of people attending the group. I asked questions such as "What are the common roles, and role tasks for the people who typically participate in this group?" "What are the common barriers to those role tasks?" and "What does this population of people typically identify as their long-term occupational outcomes?" I used the answers to create group programs that provided opportunities to explore and address the common barriers to achieving those long-term outcomes. Of course, my group activities always reflected the type of setting I was in, but even in the restricted inpatient setting I was able to create group activities that reflected those long-term outcomes, and we always explored the resources in the community that would help them continue that journey. I found other ways to address individual goals when needed. However, in most cases, the opportunities created for people to interact within the group activities typically allowed for greater progress on individual goals, even if they were not the direct focus.

Why is this switch important? When we are focused on the culmination of individual goals, we miss the socially constructed barriers that are experienced and shared by people in oppressed groups, including people with physical, cognitive, or psychiatric disabilities. For example, I spent some time working in an institution-to-community transitional program for people who were labeled with

(*continued*)

EXPANDING OUR PERSPECTIVES (*continued*)

psychiatric diagnoses, some of whom had lived in institutions for many years. Nearly everyone had common individual goals to complete their ADL and IADL. None of these goals addressed the shared experiences related to institutionalization. Institutionalization strips people of autonomy and negatively affects their ability to identify and solve problems or make even simple decisions (Chow & Priebe, 2013). Many residents experience negative and traumatizing events in these settings because of power structures between workers and residents and within the resident population (Chow & Priebe, 2013). The lack of power and need for self-preservation doesn't allow for developing the skill to recognize, navigate, and mitigate potential safety issues in the community. Having a built-in, often dysfunctional social network doesn't support the development of the skills needed to build social capital, and few people are equipped to understand or navigate the stigma they will face in the community. OT groups that focus on exploring and implementing shared activities are effective.

One example is working together to plan, gather, and prepare healthier food, including sharing sources for inexpensive or free food to manage the small allotments from food benefits. Another example includes creating spaces where members can build interpersonal skills and friendships, build social capital while learning ways to navigate stigmatizing encounters, through planning and participating in community activities, or exploring community resources related to interests. Groups might focus on understanding their rights and working together to implement advocacy activities in the community to fight systematic oppression. All these examples are real-life activities that not only allow for skill development but also

allow participants to build genuine connections that lead to a greater sense of autonomy and empowerment.

Cheryl Mattingly, in her work on clinical reasoning by OT practitioners, identified the two-bodied practice (Mattingly & Hayes Fleming, 1994). OT group intervention embodies this idea. Of course, the group leader must consider some individual goals, watch for group growth and development, and address the dynamics all so well articulated by the author of this chapter. However, the other part of the practitioner's mind can and should be focused on the creation of spaces that allow for safe and supported occupational exploration. These spaces ought to offer opportunities for members to learn together about the social structures that create barriers, and together they take and learn from mitigated risks related to engagement. Rather than directing, group leaders can and should create spaces where they are coaching, recognizing that members benefit from opportunities to set their boundaries and choose to belong on their terms. The two-bodied practice recognizes that intervention is more than fixing people. Group practice can take a population approach that considers the shared experiences of the members, addressing all of the barriers to occupations, sometimes due to impairment, but more often due to barriers in the social, physical, and virtual spaces within which we engage.

References

Chow, W. S., & Priebe, S. (2013). Understanding psychiatric institutionalization: A conceptual review. *BMC Psychiatry, 13*, Article 169. https://doi.org/10.1186/1471-244X-13-169

Mattingly, C., & Hayes Fleming, M. (1994). *Clinical reasoning: Forms of reasoning in a therapeutic practice.* F. A. Davis.

Yalom, I. D., & Leszcz, M. (2020). *The theory and practice of group therapy* (6th ed.). Basic Books.

Acknowledgments

I would like to thank my colleague and Chair of the Occupational Therapy department at the University of South Dakota, Dr. Ranelle Nissen, for allowing me to use OT Story 29.1. Dr. Nissen and I provided the described consultation together. I would also like to thank my graduate assistant, Tori VanVelzen, who assisted with the literature search and double-checked the references. Her assistance in this project is very appreciated.

Lippincott® Connect *For additional resources on the subjects discussed in this chapter, visit Lippincott Connect.*

REFERENCES

American Occupational Therapy Association. (2020). Occupational therapy practice framework: Domain and process—fourth edition. *The American Journal of Occupational Therapy, 74*(Suppl. 2), 7412410010p1–7412410010p87. https://doi.org/10.5014/ajot.2020.74S2001

Arner, C., Batros, J., Belasen, A., Bell, A., Birkhoff, J., Brown, H., Bushe, G., Classetti, P., Dawn, H., DeVreede, G., Drückler, S., Dutko, D., Elbaum, A., Eng, M., Griffin, A., Harkess, C., Harris, D., Hunter, D., Jackson, J., …White, N. (2010). Stages of small-group development revisited. *Group Facilitation: A Research & Applications Journal, 10.* https://www.iaf-world.org/site/sites/default/files/publications/2013%20Issue%2012%20IAF%20GF%20Journal.pdf

Bass, B. M., & Ryterband, E. C. (1979). *Organizational psychology.* Allyn and Bacon.

Benne, K. D., & Sheats, P. (1948). Functional roles of group members. *Journal of Social Issues, 4(2),* 41–49. https://doi.org/10.1111/j.1540-4560.1948.tb01783.x

Carson, N. (2020). *Psychosocial occupational therapy.* Elsevier.

Cole, M. B. (2018). *Group dynamics in occupational therapy: The theoretical basis and practice application of group intervention.* Slack.

Fidler, G. S., & Fidler, J. W. (1963). *Occupational therapy: A communication process in psychiatry.* Macmillan.

Gençer, H. (2019). Group dynamics and behaviour. *Universal Journal of Educational Research, 7*(1), 223–229. https://doi.org/10.13189/ujer.2019.070128

Higgins, S. M., Schwartzberg, S. L., Bedell, G., & Duncombe, L. W. (2014). Current practice and perceptions of group work in occupational therapy. *Group, 38*(4), 317–333. https://doi.org/10.13186/group.38.4.0317

Hingst, R. D. (2006). *Tuckman's theory of group development in a call centre context: Does it still work?* [Conference session]. Fifth Global Conference on Business & Economics, Cambridge, UK. http://eprints.usq.edu.au

Hurt, A. C., & Trombley, S. M. (2007). *The Punctuated-Tuckman: Towards a new group development model* [Conference session]. International Research Conference in the Americas of the Academy of Human Resource Development, Indianapolis, IN. https://files.eric.ed.gov/fulltext/ED504567.pdf

Ikiugu, M. N. (2007). *Psychosocial conceptual practice models in occupational therapy: Building adaptive capability* (1st ed.). Elsevier.

Ikiugu, M. N. (2019). Meaningful and psychologically rewarding occupations: Characteristics and implications for occupational therapy practice. *Occupational Therapy in Mental Health, 35*(1). https://doi.org/10.1080/0164212X.2018.1486768

Ikiugu, M. N., & Smallfield, S. (2010). Ikiugu's eclectic method of combining theoretical conceptual practice models in occupational therapy. *Australian Occupational Therapy Journal, 58*(6), 437–446. https://doi.org/10.1111/j.1440-1630.2011.00968.x

Ikiugu, M. N., Smallfield, S., & Condit, C. (2009). A framework for combining theoretical conceptual practice models in occupational therapy practice. *Canadian Journal of Occupational Therapy, 76*(3), 162–170. https://doi.org/10.1177/000841740907600305

Kielhofner, G. (2008). *Model of human occupation: Theory and application.* Lippincott Williams & Wilkins.

Laing, R. D. (1969). *Self and others.* Penguin Books.

Lewin, K. (1951). *Field theory in social science: Selected theoretical papers* (D. Cartwright, Ed.). Harpers.

Lewin, K., Lippit, R., & White, R. K. (1939). Patterns of aggressive behavior in experimentally created "social climates." *Journal of Social Psychology, 10*(2), 269–299. https://doi.org/10.1080/00224545.1939.9713366

Luke, M. (2007). Group coleadership: A critical review. *Counselor Education and Supervision, 46*(4), 280–293. https://doi.org/10.1002/j.1556-6978.2007.tb00032.x

Mahoney, W., & Roberts, E. (2009). Co-occupation in a day program for adults with developmental disabilities. *Journal of Occupational Science, 16*(3), 170–179. https://doi.org/10.1080/14427591.2009.9686659

Mayotte-Blum, J., Slavin-Mulford, J., Lehamnn, M., Becker-Matero, N., & Hilsenroth M. (2012). Therapeutic immediacy across long-term psychodynamic psychotherapy: An evidence-based case study. *Journal of Counseling Psychology, 99*(1), 27–46. https://doi.org/10.1037/a0026087

Mills, B. (2016). What is group process? Integrating process work into psychoeducational groups. *Georgia School Counselors Association Journal, 23*, 16–24. https://files.eric.ed.gov/fulltext/EJ1140845.pdf

Mosey, A. C. (1970). The concept and use of developmental groups. *American Journal of Occupational Therapy, 24*(4), 272–275. https://psycnet.apa.org/record/1970-21331-001

Pizzi, M. A., & Richards, L. G. (2017). Guest editorial—Promoting health, well-being, and quality of life in occupational therapy: A commitment to a paradigm shift for the next 100 years. *American Journal of Occupational Therapy, 71*, 7104170010p1–7104170010p5. https://doi.org/10.5014/ajot.2017.028456

Polatajko, H. J., Townsend, E. A., & Craik, J. (2007). Canadian model of occupational performance and engagement (CMOP-E). In E. A. Townsend & H. J. Polatajko (Eds.), *Enabling occupation II: Advancing an occupational therapy vision of health, well-being, & justice through occupation* (pp. 22–36). Canadian Association of Occupational Therapists.

Ross, M., & Bachner, S. (Eds.). (2004). *Adults with developmental disabilities: Current approaches in occupational therapy.* American Occupational Therapy Association.

Scaffa, M. (2019). Occupational therapy interventions for groups, communities, and populations. In B. A. Boyt-Schell & G. Gillen (Eds.), *Willard and Spackman's occupational therapy* (13th ed., pp. 436–447). Wolters Kluwer.

Schwartzberg, S. L., Howe, M. C., & Barnes, M. A. (2008). *Groups: Applying the functional group model.* F.A. Davis.

Shaffer, J. B. P., & Galinsky, M. D. (1974). *Models of group therapy and sensitivity training.* Prentice-Hall.

Stein, F., & Tallant, B. K. (2013). Applying the group process to psychiatric occupational therapy part 1: Historical and current use. In D. Gibson (Ed.), *Group process and structure in psychosocial occupational therapy* (pp. 9–25). Routledge.

Tubbs, S. L. (1978). *A systems approach to small group interaction.* Random House.

Tuckman, B. W. (1965). Development sequence in small groups. *Psychological Bulletin, 63*(6), 384–399. https://doi.org/10.1037/h0022100

Tuckman, B. W., & Jensen, M. C. (1977). Stages of small-group development revisited. *Group & Organization Studies, 2*(4), 419–427. https://doi.org/10.1177/105960117700200404

Uhl-Bien, M., Marion, R., & McKelvey, B. (2007). Complexity leadership theory: Shifting leadership from the industrial age to the knowledge era. *The Leadership Quarterly, 18*(4), 298–318. https://doi.org/10.1016/j.leaqua.2007.04.002

Vaida, S., & Șerban, D. (2021). Group development stages: A brief comparative analysis of various models. *Studia Universitatis Babes-Bolyai, Psychologia-Paedagogia, 66*(1), 91–110. https://doi.org/10.24193/subbpsyped.2021.1.05

Yalom, I. D., & Leszcz, M. (2005). *The theory and practice of group psychotherapy* (5th ed.). Basic Books.

Zedel, J., & Chen, S. (2021). Client's experiences of occupational therapy group interventions in mental health settings: A meta-ethnography. *Occupational Therapy in Mental Health, 37*(3), 278–302. https://doi.org/10.1080/0164212X.2021.1900763

Additional Resources

Donohue, M. V. (1999). Theoretical basis of Mosey's group interaction skills. *Occupational Therapy International, 6*(1), 35–51. https://doi.org/10.1002/oti.87

LaForme, A. F. (2012). Group intervention in pediatric rehabilitation. *Physical & Occupational Therapy in Pediatrics, 32*(2), 136–138. https://doi.org/10.3109/01942638.2012.668389

Meyers, S. A., & Anderson, C. M. (2008). *The fundamentals of small group communication.* Sage.

US Department of Health and Human Services: Substance Abuse and Mental Health Services Administration. (2015). *Substance abuse treatment: Group therapy.* https://store.samhsa.gov/product/TIP-41-Substance-Abuse-Treatment-Group-Therapy/SMA15-3991

Professionalism, Communication, and Teamwork

Janet Falk-Kessler

LEARNING OBJECTIVES

After reading this chapter, you will be able to:

1. Understand what it means to be a professional.
2. Understand what types of behaviors are viewed as professional and as unprofessional, and why.
3. Understand the value of teamwork.
4. Be able to distinguish between different types of teams and how they function.
5. Be able to describe the "dos and don'ts" of social media participation.

Introduction

The purpose of this chapter is to review professionalism and collaborative behavior. In this chapter, professionalism encompasses how one presents oneself as a professional and the individual's responsibilities and obligations as a professional and to one's profession.

Professionalism is a concept that has many attributes. It includes behaviors that are on public display; knowledge and skill-based competencies that are continually sought and demonstrated; and overall responsibilities to one's clients, colleagues, profession, and society (Monrouxe et al., 2011). Becoming a professional is a process—one that begins by learning what a professional is and does, enacting the professional role by meeting expectations, and eventually embodying and internalizing professional qualities. Implicit and explicit guidelines, rules, behaviors, and expectations within social contexts contribute to professional development (Monrouxe et al., 2011).

Professionalism reflects the person as well as one's profession. Within medically related professions, professionalism at its core is a belief system that embraces a social contract on healthcare delivery that asserts competency and ethical standards (Wynia et al., 2014). These characteristics echo how professionalism in occupational therapy (OT) has been described (Glennon & Van Oss, 2010; Hordichuk et al., 2015) and served as the foundation for one's behaviors, commitments, collaboration, and teamwork. As one's professionalism develops, one's role as a contributing member of the healthcare team and the OT profession is strengthened. This chapter reviews professionalism as it relates to each of these areas.

Professionalism has been garnering a vast amount of attention in both the public and professional media. Demonstrating professionalism has become a focus within many academic settings, with the emergence of professionalism assessments (Wang et al., 2017; Yuen et al., 2016; Ziring et al., 2015). The development of values, attitudes, and behaviors that mirror one's profession is a process that continually evolves throughout one's career and is in part reflective of a contract between one's discipline and society in general (Cruess & Cruess, 2009; Hordichuk et al., 2015). Maintaining standards of practice, which include maintaining competency, demonstrating evidence-based practice, using appropriate judgment, and abiding by our profession's ethical code, is a professional responsibility (American Occupational Therapy Association [AOTA], 2020a).

Participating in local, state, and national organizations that work to market OT services to various stakeholders—including consumers, third-party payers, and policymakers—and that sponsor continuing education opportunities, provide members with a range of literature, and inform members of legislation as well as other concerns of interest is part of one's professional responsibility. This is further articulated through the core tenets of Vision 2025 (AOTA, 2017), which demands the highest standards of professionalism.

Historically, the transmission of professionalism relied on immersion in a professional environment. Distinct from professional identity, professionalism is defined by behaviors demonstrated in various contexts: with clients, on healthcare teams, and through all modes of communication. Recognizing that each generation brings a different understanding of what professionalism is, many have argued that simply being in professional environments may not be enough to learn the behaviors; instead, it is to be taught within academic and clinical programs (Cruess & Cruess, 2009; Lindheim et al., 2016; Monrouxe et al., 2011; Ziring et al., 2015). These obligations and responsibilities are depicted in Figure 30.1. Moreover, professional expectations may change with time. As professionalism in part reflects the relationship between a profession and its social context, responsibilities may expand. For example, when healthcare biases and occupational justice inequities are recognized, our role as professionals must address these concerns (see Expanding Our Perspectives). The importance of recognizing and taking action against biases have been reinforced by professional organizations (e.g., AOTA, 2020a; Stanley et al., 2020).

Workplace Professionalism and Behavior

In the last few decades, many medical professionals have emphasized and embraced their long-held, traditional values. The "Occupational Therapy Practice Framework" (AOTA, 2020e), with its emphasis on occupational engagement and participation, similarly reminds practitioners of the roots of professional practice and the professional responsibility

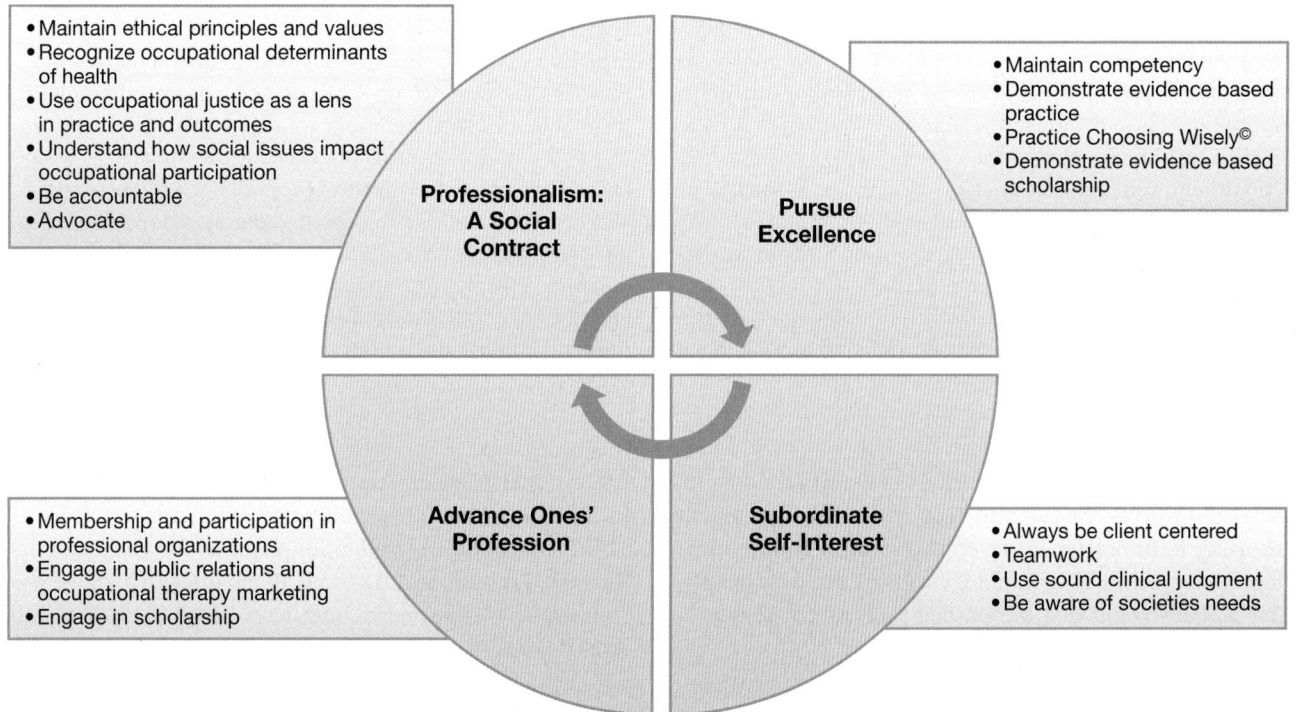

FIGURE 30.1 **Components of professionalism.**

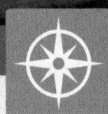

EXPANDING OUR PERSPECTIVES

Professionalism Is a Social Contract

Janet Falk-Kessler

A social contract is not a new idea. While its origins date back thousands of years, current usage frames it as an agreement of reciprocal obligations between groups within society, or groups with society (D'Agostino et al., 2021). In healthcare, patients benefit from ethical obligations, such as beneficence and confidentiality, and practitioners benefit from societal rewards, such as autonomy and self-regulation (Cruess & Cruess, 2020). The social contract framework has been greatly influenced by 20th-century philosopher Rawls (1971), as he positioned his *theory of justice* within the social contract framework, and in doing so promoted its application in a variety of arenas. When applied to healthcare, a just society should emphasize access for all to healthcare as well as recognize and address the social determinants of health (Ekmekci & Arda, 2015). As occupational therapists, addressing the occupational determinants of health can be part of our profession's social contract. In doing so, our ethical obligations include attention to our clients' capability, as discussed by Hammell (2015), to participate in meaningful occupations.

Engagement in occupation, as a determinant of health, is at the core of everything occupational therapists believe and do. To this end, professionalism, which encompasses our knowledge base, our behaviors, and our responsibilities, reveals a belief system to which we are all accountable regardless of practice area. Our loyalty is not only to our clients and our profession but also to the public. To this end, ensuring justice: fairness in access to treatment, utilizing skills and knowledge that are reflective of current evidence, being mindful of occupational justice within treatment settings and post discharge, are a sample of what should dominate an occupational therapist's practice. Thus, what we do must mirror values that are worthy of the public's trust (Wynia et al., 2014).

Recent events, specifically health inequities in the COVID-19 pandemic along with implicit and explicit racial and cultural prejudices, remind us that professionalism is

a social contract. As such, we have an obligation to examine how our prescription of occupation and our desired outcome of enabling fulfilling participation is impacted by biases. To do this, we must start by examining our own implicit biases, which are unconscious attitudes, prejudices, and stereotypes (Byrne & Tanesini, 2015), and how these influence our interactions with our clients and the choices we as professionals make about occupational participation.

Enabling participation requires an occupational justice lens that is focused on treatment and on policy at both the individual and population levels. The way in which we view our various OT roles may need to expand. For example, if a client on an inpatient hospital unit with whom you are working is being discharged home, and you are confident all OT goals have been met and they have the functional ability to engage in occupations of their choice, are you also confident that they will fully participate in their preferred occupations? Is it part of your role to ensure that once discharged, they are able to access their community's offerings? Is following up with your client after they are discharged so that you can identify any barriers to participation part of your role? As a professional with the obligation of ensuring inclusive participation and client-centered practice, it may be necessary to examine and redefine OT's role in all areas of practice. Having the functional ability to engage is not the same as having the opportunity to engage. The OT profession, for which Vision 2025 includes calls for equity, inclusion, diversity, advocacy, and accessibility (AOTA, 2017), appeals for a change in how occupational therapists see their role. It is within the realm of our professional responsibility to identify outcomes beyond abilities. It is also incumbent upon occupational therapists to enable all team members to adopt this approach for treatment and discharge planning. Professionalism, as a social contract, demands advocacy toward a more just environment. Questions to consider are as follows: Are client-centered goals developed within a structured context (hospital environment) enough? If not, should the provider include an additional goal/plan to ensure they are addressing cultural prejudices, health, social, and economic disparities outside of that structured context?

---

to use terminology that reflects these values (Youngstrom, 2002) and affirms one's identity (Fawcett, 2013). The context for using terminology, however, is critical in communication; overly technical terminology with clients, for example, may actually result in a diminished professional presentation (Berman et al., 2016).

Regardless of situation or interaction (e.g., a professor, supervisor, client and/or the client's family, a team meeting, or conference presentation), professionalism is expected.

Professional behavior has become so important that it is included in academic accreditation standards for all levels of OT education (Accreditation Council for Occupational Therapy Education, 2018) and is an integral part of the competencies expected in both level I (AOTA, 2020d) and level II (AOTA, 2020b, 2020c) fieldwork experiences.

Among the many characteristics that shape professionals are values about work, roles, and service recipients. Many believe that values, especially those that revolve around work ethic, cause conflict in academic and employment environments. In recent decades, attention has been paid to differences in work values and expectation that is generationally linked (Lyons & Kuron, 2014; Wiedmer, 2015). How one behaves is rooted in the cultural and societal norms and expectations in which one was raised. It is also shaped by impactful events and experiences. The full impact on the generations, for example, of the COVID-19 pandemic, the MeToo movement, and the Black Lives Matter movement are yet to be fully realized.

When considering the characteristics of different generations, one should not assume that all traits are exhibited by all within one generational cohort or are exhibited consistently regardless of the environment. Nor should one assume these characteristics transcend cultures. Some traits, such as ease with technology, might not translate to professional settings (Hills et al., 2016), and one's identity within a generation, rather than one's birth date, may inform behavior (Campbell et al., 2017; Lyons & Kuron, 2014). But it is nonetheless important to recognize that differences that distinguish cohorts impact both communication and one's perception of professionalism and work ethic, along with one's expectation of the work environment (Anselmo-Witzel et al., 2017; Ozkan, & Solmaz, 2015; Wiedmer, 2015).

Understanding and respecting generational differences, however, is important for two overarching reasons: as a treating professional, when one considers the habits, values, and perceptions of the different generations, one is better prepared for client-centered care. Understanding how an older client might perceive a behavior demonstrated by a young practitioner, for example, is critical to the client–practitioner interaction.

The second consideration regarding generational differences involves one's role as a team member. Because there may be varying perspectives on what constitutes professional and unprofessional behavior, interpersonal conflict between professionals can arise (Johnston, 2006). Furthermore, individuals may acknowledge what is considered unprofessional behavior but rationalize this behavior as not unprofessional when they themselves display it (Aurora et al., 2008). Such individuals have no idea that they are perceived as inappropriate, unreasonable, and even disrespectful. It has been suggested that these behaviors reflect how individuals perceive and understand rules and their expectations of and for themselves (Lake, 2009). As an example, some individuals of more recent generations grew up within home, school, and societal environments that promoted self-esteem, emphasized individualism, and placed little emphasis on social rules. This can result in the expectation of entitlements (Twenge, 2006; Ventriglio & Bhugra, 2016). Many from earlier generations grew up with a respect for authority and the notion that achievement is based on what one has actually accomplished.

Differences in how one perceives work/career values and rewards can also lead to conflict (Lipscomb, 2010). When one considers that professionalism within academia and healthcare is typically defined by those from the Silent or Baby Boomer generations, it is not surprising that those from the more recent generations are unaware that their attitudes and behaviors are viewed as unprofessional. These attitudes and behaviors may be at the root of fieldwork and workplace difficulties rather than knowledge (Langenfeld et al., 2014). See OT Story 30.1.

OT STORY 30.1 JOHN ON FIELDWORK

John Dimet is a graduate student in OT and has just started his first level II fieldwork experience. He has completed all of his coursework. He is 26 years old, having spent the time between undergraduate and graduate school completing his prerequisites, engaging in volunteer work, and working at his aunt's restaurant. Prior to the start of his fieldwork, he sent his supervisor, who he had not yet met, the following e-mail: *Hey Sarah, looking forward to starting on Monday. What time should I arrive, and is there a dress code? JD*

John met his supervisor on Monday at 8 AM as instructed, and they immediately went to morning rounds. His university's fieldwork coordinator had told him that there would be days he would need to arrive at 7 AM so that he could participate in activities of daily living (ADLs) sessions with clients. The site was an inpatient rehabilitation setting with an average length of stay of 4 to 6 weeks.

During the first week, John participated in orientation along with three other OT students and shadowed his supervisor, Sarah Hill. Sarah has 20 years of OT experience plus several specialty certifications. Sarah gave John a schedule of when he was to arrive at 7 AM.

During their weekly supervision session of the second week, Sarah asked John questions about the clinical conditions and functional challenges of the clients seen and pressed him to identify long-term goals for one of the clients. John had very superficial knowledge of the clinical conditions, and when asked about this limitation, John reported that his academic program did not go into depth on every condition. This surprised Sarah, as she was knowledgeable about the academic program's curriculum. John also stated that he hadn't thought about goals for the clients seen, as he thought Sarah would let him know what they were. In addition, Sarah pointed out to John that during the shadowing time, he heard John's

OT STORY 30.1 JOHN ON FIELDWORK (continued)

smartphone vibrate and saw John check its screen. She reminded John that all smartphones are to be off during work hours, but he can use it during his lunch break.

During the third week, John arrived late on 2 days, completely missing morning rounds one day and arriving late to rounds on the second day. She told Sarah that he could get the information missed from one of the other students, and that, if necessary, he can make up the time at the end of the day. He also asked if he really needed to attend rounds every morning, as not much changed from day to day. He suggested that because students have to be at the site at 7 AM twice a week, and on those days, each would attend rounds, whichever student attended rounds can easily text or e-mail the information to those not present. This would make the workday easier for everyone. John added that his commute was close to an hour each way, and a flexible schedule would be very helpful to everyone.

Sarah was troubled with John's professionalism and devoted their next supervision session to review what her concerns were. Sarah and John had very different views on each of the behaviors:

Being Prepared

- Sarah expected students to come to fieldwork prepared, which includes doing research on their own time in any area where they have limited knowledge. They are expected to be ready to discuss OT's role in promoting functional performance and participation and to examine how they might apply evidence-based practice. By not putting in the time to learn, Sarah believes that her student is either unmotivated or simply lazy.
- John assumed it was his supervisor's responsibility to provide him with information about clinical conditions, be told by his supervisor what he needed to do, and if he needed to do anything "extra," he would be given time during the workday to do it. After all, isn't his supervisor a teacher, and as such shouldn't she be giving him the knowledge he needs to have?

Electronic Devices

- Sarah views smartphone use as not just a distraction to patient care but also a demonstration of disrespect to those he needs to interact with.
- John believes he has the ability to multitask, that by keeping his smartphone on vibrate, he is actually showing respect, and that he needs to check it just in case something important is shared. In addition, he does not wear a watch so this is how he knows the time.

Interprofessional Collaboration

- Sarah believes in collaborative teamwork and that participating in morning rounds not only keeps everyone up to date on any changes or progress made by patients but also provides an opportunity to engage with others around patient care. In addition, schedules and their related responsibilities are to be adhered to and not ignored as a matter of convenience.
- John doesn't understand why attendance is required because there are more efficient ways of gathering information. He also doesn't understand why making up the time later in the day isn't an option.

Patient Privacy

- Finally, Sarah is very concerned that John would suggest texting information about patients, as this can easily result in Health Insurance Portability and Accountability Act (HIPAA) violations.
- John views electronic communication as efficient and assures Sarah that it will be shared only with students at the site.

Questions

1. Are you able to relate to John's perspective?
2. Are you able to relate to Sarah's perspective?

What is the underlying issue portrayed in OT Story 30.1? Individuals from two different generations perceive behaviors in very different ways. These perceptions come from experiences specific to their "generational culture." Being from different generational cultures is not an excuse to maintain behaviors and expectations that are viewed by many as unprofessional, nor to hold on to behaviors and expectations that might no longer be appropriate. Although the supervisor in this case example is concerned by what he sees as a combination of laziness and unprofessional behaviors, the younger practitioner believes in efficiency and flexibility while being dependent on his supervisor for knowledge. Both are coming from their own generational context. In practice settings, however, one must remember that the client's needs come first and that most likely, there are generational differences between practitioner and client as well. Therefore, those joining the workforce will succeed if they are aware of how they are perceived and learn to demonstrate all aspects of professionalism that will garner them respect from the multigenerational contexts. Their supervisors will similarly have more satisfying relationships with those they oversee if they, too, understand how to adapt their supervisory styles in order to help the new practitioners adapt and to not blame their supervisees for behaviors shaped by their culture.

Professionalism and Teamwork

Interprofessional models for practice are utilized across varied healthcare settings and with all populations. These models may include collaborative practice and professional networks with the members of each having some degree of shared identity (Reeves et al., 2018). Effective interprofessional teams are distinct from collaborations and networks as members of interprofessional teams share goals, are accountable to each other (Reeves et al., 2018), respect each other's expertise, and focus on their patient's best interest (Cruess et al., 2009). Interprofessional teams in particular enhance client safety and care and are based on the premise that no one person has all the skills and knowledge to meet the client's goals. As a result, competencies have been developed along with healthcare academic programs' accreditation standards to ensure collaborative practice (Interprofessional Education Collaborative [IPEC], 2016). Thus, an important feature of professionalism is one's ability to be an effective team member.

Effective teamwork is often linked with improved client outcomes and improved client safety (Brock et al., 2013; Ndoro, 2014; Zwarenstein et al., 2009), including outcomes in rehabilitation settings (Sinclair et al., 2009). Failures related to the environment's culture and to interpersonal communication can result in treatment errors (Deering et al., 2011). Although improving healthcare is a direct result of improving communication and collaboration (Zwarenstein et al., 2009), there research has not been done to examine teamwork's effect on lessening healthcare inequity (Carey & Taylor, 2021).

Teams are an outgrowth of the knowledge that an individual who functions alone is not as helpful to the client as a team that works well together. The reasoning process, when done in a group, is more effective than when done in isolation (Mercier & Sperber, 2011). This reduces the risk of ignoring information that does not fit within one's belief system and increases access to information from others, which helps decision-making. Being a member of a team does not automatically result in collaboration (Thistlethwaite, 2012), however, and one must be aware that teams can be undermined by power relationships (Baker et al., 2011). Facilitating interprofessional teamwork in clinical sites is critical (Poston et al., 2017), and receiving training in interprofessional teamwork during one's professional education is equally important if not required (Anderson et al., 2016; AOTA, 2015; Boet et al., 2014; Brennan et al., 2014; Brock et al., 2013; House et al., 2016; Ndoro, 2014). Furthermore, interprofessional

education must be competency-based (IPEC, 2016), as it prepares future practitioners for interprofessional teamwork.

Effective teams—whether they are two individuals such as an occupational therapist and an OT assistant or a group of healthcare professionals from varying disciplines—that work well are characterized by communication, respecting and understanding roles, trust and confidence, the ability to overcome adversity as well as personal differences, and collective leadership (Bosch & Mansell, 2015; Nancarrow et al., 2013; Sims et al., 2015). These attributes are developed through shared mental models (Manges et al., 2020), group cohesion, and objective leadership, and can result in increased job satisfaction (Kalisch et al., 2010). In addition, the explicit importance of team meetings, the role of shared objectives in conflict management, and the value of autonomy within the team (Jones & Jones, 2011) are further examples of effective interprofessional teams.

There are multiple compositions of healthcare teams, some of which are comprised of only one discipline, and others that are interprofessional. Practitioners can be members of different teams simultaneously. Unidisciplinary teams are comprised of practitioners of the same discipline and who function in the same role, while intradisciplinary are comprised of practitioners of the same discipline but with different levels of education (Columbia Center for Teaching and Learning, n.d.). For effective client-centered care, interprofessional teams, comprised of individuals from different disciplines, often operate in order to maximize positive outcomes for their clients. These teams include multidisciplinary, interdisciplinary, and transdisciplinary (Figure 30.2). Each is composed of individuals from various professional backgrounds, and each is focused on a common client. It is helpful to consider these teams as a continuum of interprofessional cooperation. Multidisciplinary teams emerged first, with other forms of teams developing as team objectives changed.

Although there are numerous definitions and names for interprofessional teams, there is limited consensus on how each is applied (Flores-Sandoval et al., 2021). For example, multidisciplinary and interdisciplinary are often, inappropriately, used interchangeably. There are however distinctions between them. The names and definitions used in this chapter distinguish between the different types of teams and are based on how the members interact. The names and descriptions used in this chapter are consistent with this book's past editions (e.g., Falk-Kessler, 2018) and reflect moderate consensus in the literature (Flores-Sandoval et al., 2021).

Multidisciplinary Teams

Coordination of care is essential if a patient is to benefit from multiple healthcare services provided by various healthcare professionals (Zwarenstein et al., 2009). The multidisciplinary

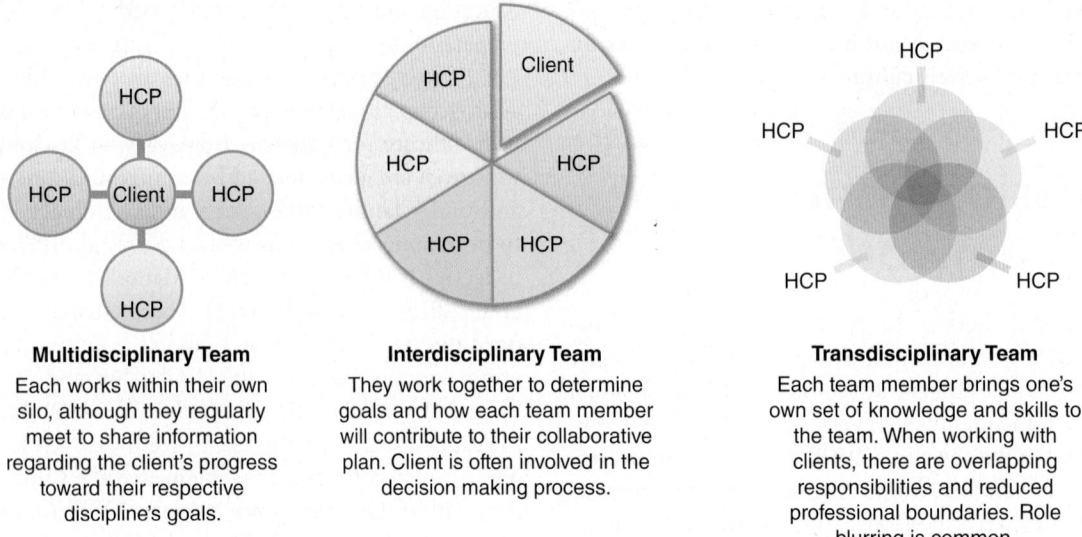

Multidisciplinary Team
Each works within their own silo, although they regularly meet to share information regarding the client's progress toward their respective discipline's goals.

Interdisciplinary Team
They work together to determine goals and how each team member will contribute to their collaborative plan. Client is often involved in the decision making process.

Transdisciplinary Team
Each team member brings one's own set of knowledge and skills to the team. When working with clients, there are overlapping responsibilities and reduced professional boundaries. Role blurring is common.

FIGURE 30.2 **Interprofessional collaboration of healthcare practitioners (HCP).**

team, like all interprofessional teams, is composed of individuals representing professional disciplines that serve the client. In the multidisciplinary team, each professional is responsible for identifying and carrying out their own discipline-related evaluation and intervention. Multidisciplinary teams generally have access to each other's written record, as each typically contributes to chart notes, and so on. If they meet as a group, which is often the case, they share information about their client's progress relative to the discipline-specific goals, and they may coordinate their efforts. For example, they may arrange intervention sessions to be on the same day. Multidisciplinary teams can also provide an opportunity for members to learn from each other. The objective, however, is coordination and cooperation, not necessarily to share goals with a common outcome. Although the expectation is that knowledge of the expertise of other team members will promote cooperation and communication that ultimately benefits the client, each team member functions in a parallel fashion and maintains professional autonomy (Jessup, 2007).

Interdisciplinary Teams

The interdisciplinary team is distinct from the multidisciplinary team. Although similarly composed of members representing and using knowledge and skills of their respective discipline, the team members identify goals and plan intervention collaboratively. They also discuss with each other how their intervention plans will be implemented. Although their skills may complement each other, team members become interdependent as they work toward improving health outcomes for their clients. It is common for interdisciplinary teams to meet as a group with the client, the client's family, and so on. This type of team is further distinguished from the multidisciplinary team in that some

interventions may be jointly carried out, and the client is often involved in the decision-making process (Jessup, 2007).

The benefits of interdisciplinary teams are many (Jessup, 2007; Zwarenstein et al., 2009). They are client-centered, giving clients a role in their care, and team members share their knowledge, which leads to respecting the roles and functions of each other. Because team members share a great deal with each other about how they implement intervention, a synergy develops in how different practitioners in varied disciplines address common and complementary goals. Intervention plans for clients are developed holistically and cost-effectively. Job satisfaction is increased. Ultimately, client care and outcomes are enhanced (see Box 30.1).

There are several potential problems that can also emerge in the functioning of an interdisciplinary team. An overly assertive team member can dominate the meetings, thereby pushing an agenda that was not collaboratively agreed on. A silent or unassertive team member can easily be ignored, with team members assuming the silence means compliance. A hierarchy may develop or a particular team member may assume the leadership simply because of their profession. This can negatively affect decision-making (Jessup, 2007) and promote feelings of being undervalued and disrespected (Baker et al., 2011). The important attributes of trust and mutual respect are keys in ensuring effective teamwork.

Interdisciplinary teams are seen in many settings. In fact, settings have designed specific models of interdisciplinary teams that are deemed effective (Deering et al., 2011; Medlock et al., 2011). Consider, as an example, a day hospital setting serving those with major mental illnesses. An interdisciplinary team may decide that for a particular client with schizophrenia, the goal is to have him be able to live in a group home, participate in chores, and be able to attend a sheltered workshop that prepares packages for shipment.

BOX 30.1 TEAMWORK IN THE TIME OF A PANDEMIC

The importance of effective interdisciplinary teamwork has been critical during the COVID-19 pandemic. To effectively deal with the ever-changing understanding of the COVID-19 virus, intense communication and coordination across disciplines were required so all presented needs could be met. These included increasing bed capacity to care for very ill and highly contagious patients; attention to workforce training in the context of pandemics; changes in staffing patterns; and changes in interpersonal interactions, including practitioner to client (Natale et al., 2020). It also demanded prioritizing infection control in healthcare, corporate, and home settings, which led to diminished social engagement, resulting in significant consequences to physical and mental health (Berlinger et al., 2021). Federal and state regulatory agencies responded to deal with some of these issues.

As an example, the increased use of telehealth required federal and state regulatory agencies to ease limits, if only temporarily, on service provision. In some instances, telehealth services proved to be effective even for "hands-on" professions such as occupational therapy (Gately et al., 2020; Kessler et al., 2021; Klamroth-Marganska et al., 2021; Maeir et al., 2021; Serwe et al., 2017). Despite its increased use, telehealth must be prescribed ethically, with the understanding that not all clients nor all medical conditions can benefit (Chaet et al., 2017). Engaging in telehealth requires team communication and coordination of services continue to be necessary (see Chapter 67).

The COVID-19 pandemic has also shined a light on how a crisis can impact professionalism when economic and available resources came into conflict with healthcare ethics. Although medical teams worked tirelessly to care for the ill, they were also making decisions that would affect all roles and the reallocation of treatment (Ćurković et al., 2020). The outcomes of these teams' decisions influence public trust.

Team members also are aware that he can become nonadherent with medication, has sensory processing issues, has difficulty with following instructions and making decisions, and complains about not seeing his brother often enough. In this team, different professionals address the same objectives and goals collaboratively but through their own profession's lens. For example, the psychiatrist and nurse monitor his medication, whereas the occupational therapist is able to observe if any medication side effects are interfering with function. The occupational therapist is addressing sensory and cognitive impairment while having the recreational therapist monitor changes in leisure function. The social worker is addressing family issues, with the occupational therapist and the nurse attending to activities of daily living (ADLs) issues raised by the brother.

Transdisciplinary Teams

The transdisciplinary team is one that functions without discipline-centered boundaries. Members in these types of teams appear to have blurred roles because many of their role-related functions become interchangeable. As distinguished from interdisciplinary teams, the expertise related to discipline-specific tasks is shared and results in the taking on of each other's responsibilities (Cartmill et al., 2011). This type of team is most efficient and may be cost-effective because, in some examples, fewer professionals interact with a specific client (King et al., 2009).

It has been suggested that there are three key elements for successful and responsible transdisciplinary teamwork. The first is an overall assessment conducted by one professional but observed by all. This type of arena assessment allows each to provide information based on their unique base of knowledge and skill. Next is an ongoing interaction between team members so that each can continuously contribute their knowledge to the plan of care. Perhaps most critical is the third element, which is role release. This allows interprofessional intervention to be carried out by one individual. Ideally and responsibly, this should be done under the direction of and continuous consultation from those responsible for what is being implemented (King et al., 2009).

The transdisciplinary team can be highly effective if used with the right population and in the right manner. A noncompetitive and nonhierarchical environment is important in order to allow for effective intervention. These teams are especially helpful in situations where interprofessional intervention is required, yet it is in the best interest of the client to have only one individual interact. A very good example of effective transdisciplinary teamwork can be seen in a report of a home-visiting program for infants in which the family benefits from the expertise of many professionals but interacts with only one (King et al., 2009). As described by these authors, a home-visiting program for infants with developmental disabilities is established, with the objectives of promoting child development along a series of domains. Rather than overwhelm the caregiver with various visiting professionals, one individual is assigned to each family. Team members learn theories and techniques from each other in order to provide service that spans disciplinary boundaries. The team is responsible for continually appraising and providing input to the professional who visits.

The transdisciplinary team approach is also useful in settings that can benefit from a system-wide approach, in settings with limited resources that do not have access to different professionals, in remote settings where access is limited, or following a crisis or natural disaster. The use of technology can support the functioning of transdisciplinary teams, ensuring a high level of competency.

Paramount for the success of transdisciplinary teams are the same elements identified for interdisciplinary teams: trust, communication, and respect. A major concern of transdisciplinary teamwork can arise when the "agent" for the team is not as skilled or knowledgeable as the team members being represented, resulting in diminished effectiveness of the intervention. Furthermore, if an individual professional providing intervention ceases to obtain ongoing input from fellow team members, the client is at risk for adverse events.

Transdisciplinary approaches have additional ethical and legal concerns. If, on a transdisciplinary team, members assume responsibilities of other professionals, regulatory violations and scope of practice concerns emerge. A team member should never perform actions for which they have not been educated or approved for under their state regulations. This is not the case when there is overlap in assessment and intervention modalities or techniques. Each team member has a responsibility to provide service within his or her scope of practice and request the provision of direct service from another team member when it is necessary to provide service outside of one's scope of practice.

Research Teams

Although much of this section has focused on interprofessional teams in practice settings, there are two important arenas in which interprofessional teams are critical for their success. The first that warrants mention is the research team.

In medically related research, discipline-specific investigators focusing primarily on basic science have carried out investigations. In some circumstances, this is not only appropriate but also necessary. However, having one discipline central to a study can result in outcomes that isolate professions, perpetuate knowledge gaps, and limit information advancement (Bindler et al., 2012). The advantages of interprofessional research include being able to better address the complex issues involved in research, allow for innovative, including more technologically based, approaches (Bindler et al., 2012), and translate results into effective interventions that are functionally and clinically relevant. Like patient-oriented teams, multidisciplinary, interdisciplinary, and transdisciplinary research teams function in distinct ways, with research questions reflecting the nature of the team (Fawcett, 2013). The federal government has placed increased emphasis on interprofessional collaborative research and has set up structures to support the translation and application of basic research to practice-related outcomes (Bindler et al., 2012), although barriers continue to exist that impede translating interprofessional research into clinical practice (Fletcher et al., 2017).

Healthcare Policy Teams

Another area that warrants mention is healthcare policy development. Just as research and intervention address complex needs, healthcare policy deals with issues that are also multifaceted (refer to Box 30.1). From setting healthcare agendas to outlining their implementation in order to improve health service delivery, policymakers need to collaborate on teams to be effective. To ensure this, an interprofessional approach to policy development, just as with clinical care and with research, allows for access to varied sources of information and promotes perspectives that represent different areas of expertise. It has also been suggested that interprofessional team-based learning opportunities facilitate collaboration and enhances the development of effective healthcare policy (Rider et al., 2008).

Scholarship: Presentations and Publications

Two decades ago, Holm (2000), in her Eleanor Clarke Slagle Lecture, called for occupational therapists to acquire evidence to support OT services and to practice based on that evidence (see Chapter 26).

Two of the many reasons to be an evidence-based practitioner are competency and currency. As scientific knowledge continues to amass in an ever-changing healthcare environment, practitioners and educators alike need to embrace and be proficient in interventions proven to be efficacious and cost-effective. Learning from those with a proven scholarly record, such as individuals whose work has appeared in peer-reviewed journals or who are presenting research at conferences or workshops under organizations and/or companies that have met requirements for continuing education, such as AOTA's Approved Provider of Continuing Education, is important. The information learned must be reliable, accurate, and evidence based. It is also incumbent on researchers to address questions pertinent to the practice of OT so that the services provided can be both efficacious and cost-effective. Thus, it is the responsibility of all OT practitioners to participate in learning opportunities based on the most recent knowledge that can be applied to practice.

Presenting and publishing is part of the professional role and provides another venue for sharing information (Table 30.1). When one has an opportunity to present or to publish, it is similarly important to consider the context in which one chooses to present and publish. Again, presenting under the auspices of an approved provider of continuing education enhances credibility.

Presentations take many forms. Within clinical settings, presentations occur in team meetings, at grand rounds, and

TABLE 30.1 **A Sample of Venues for Disseminating Knowledge**

Presentations		Publications	
Professional Venues	**Consumer Venues**	**Peer-Reviewed**	**Non–peer-Reviewed**
Team meeting	Community event	Practice-oriented periodicals[a]	Trade magazines
In-service presentation	Consumer organization	Journals	Practice-oriented periodicals[a]
Grand rounds		Book chapters[a]	Newsletters
Poster session		Websites[a]	News periodicals
Panel discussion			Book chapters[a]
Platform sessions			Self-published books
Workshops			Blogs
Courses			Websites[a]

[a]These venues may or may not be peer reviewed.

at in-service trainings. Some of these settings may appear informal, but presenters must remember that their style of presenting will reflect their integrity and professionalism. In conference settings, a poster session allows the presenter to discuss points of interest to those who review the poster. A paper presentation, which can be anywhere from 20 minutes to 2 hours, is a formal presentation to an audience and typically includes audiovisual technology. Workshop presentations, which are somewhat modeled after a classroom setting, also include audiovisual technology and range from a half-day to a 5-day event. Panel presentations consist of several experts on a single topic in which brief presentations are made to facilitate discussion with the audience.

Each of these presentation types can also be delivered on virtual platforms. Online learning in academic settings has allowed for increased access and flexibility for education, for example, through massive open online courses (MOOCs; Dhawan, 2020). Providing a digital environment for professional conferences has equally allowed for more affordable and increased accessibility to knowledge. However, presenting online has unique challenges that include technical issues, environmental distractions, and effective communication. It is important to understand the challenges associated with presenting using this media (Rapanta et al., 2020).

Although each of these types of presentations allows for the dissemination of information, it is important to be sure that the manner of presenting is professional. There are many guidelines available on *how* to present (e.g., Eggleston, n.d.). Guidelines suggest that presenters should be articulate, focus on the question at hand, and engage the audience, no matter how big or how small. These guidelines also include paying attention to eye contact; avoiding the use of filler words such as "um," "you know," and "like"; and maintaining good posture.

Similarly, there are various types of publication, from traditional, subscription-based journals to digital publications that might not require a subscription. Each type targets different audiences, has varying levels of review and rigor, and has varying levels of perceived value. A publication's value is typically based on the review process used by the journal, along with the journal's quality, reputation, and impact factor. This applies to traditional and digital publications. Digital publications, which are becoming more prevalent, may be open access (OA) publishing venues, such as an institutional OA repository where an author may upload work or work in progress, without any review, and OA journals which may or may not be peer-reviewed and often carry a fee charged to the author (Rowley et al., 2017).

Understanding which media an author publishes in is important to both the writer and to the reader, as it may inform the content's trustworthiness. The peer-review process, valued in scholarly literature, simply refers to a procedure in which a manuscript, once submitted for publication, is reviewed by experts in the field who provide feedback and contribute to the decision of whether the manuscript meets the criteria for publication. Peer review provides a layer of critical evaluation to the publishing process, is often a more challenging route of publication for the writer, and gives the reader a level of trust in the information (Nicholas et al., 2015). Peer-reviewed articles are typically in scientific journals (Farrell et al., 2017) and may or may not be reviewed anonymously (Nobarany & Booth, 2017).

Non-peer review refers to manuscripts that are submitted or invited to be published in books, periodicals, or trade magazines and might be reviewed by an editor rather than go through a longer, more critical process (Jacobs, 2009). Non–peer-reviewed articles are in news or practice-oriented periodicals and trade publications. Non-peer review also includes self-publication, such as blogs and personal websites as well as self-published books. As indicated earlier, publishing in peer-reviewed or non–peer-reviewed media carries different perceived value as a result of the review process. Finally, papers in OA journals, which speed up the time between a paper's acceptance to its publication, may or may not be peer-reviewed.

Professionalism and Social Media: Opportunities and Pitfalls

Social media is a tool that enables individuals and organizations to communicate efficiently and to a wide audience. Hospitals and professional practices use social media to provide information related to medical updates and health information to their patients and the general public (Ficarra, 2011). Consumers use social media sites as a way to assess the quality of their healthcare provider (Rozenblum & Bates, 2013). Because misinformation and disinformation appear on social media outlets, it is important for healthcare providers to ensure that the information they post on social media is factual and evidence-based. It is equally important for consumers, who obtain as well as share information about healthcare on social media, to only use credible sources (Kington et al., 2021). And, if clients are included in social media posts, proper procedures for informed consent must be followed (Bennett & Vercler, 2018).

In addition, professionals have an obligation to understand that their postings on any site can be viewed by unlimited numbers of people without restriction. Once information is posted, it can no longer be controlled, no matter what privacy settings are used.

Relationships and communication are often nurtured through social networks (Bahk et al., 2010), yet behavior on these networks has come under scrutiny. The prevailing concern revolves around postings that include information (e.g., photographs, narratives) about others, which may violate their right to privacy and commitment to their professional environment. Indeed, attention is being paid to how social media and other forms of electronic communication are being used in a variety of academic and work contexts (Ahmed et al., 2020; Gerlich et al., 2010).

Professionalism when using social media is important. Professionalism in part stems from a contract between one's discipline and society, and therefore, how one behaves is a reflection of professionalism. Even accessing social media sites while at work can be unprofessional (Piscotty et al., 2016). Because social media has such a widespread audience and that behavior on social media sites can reflect negatively on one's place of work and on one's profession, policies and guidelines need to be developed and adhered to (Ventola, 2014).

Many have claimed that what they do on their own time is an issue of individual rights and of privacy. Yet, by virtue of being on an Internet site, posted information and photos can be publicly viewed (Langenfeld et al., 2014), and posting information about a client can potentially violate patient privacy (Hader & Brown, 2010). Even posting information about perceived poor medical care related to a family member, can have consequences (Brous & Olsen, 2017).

The Internet allows for efficient communication but also widens the net for who receives the communication. As a result, professionals have an obligation to understand that their postings on any site can be viewed by unlimited numbers of individuals without restriction. Once information is posted, it can no longer be limited to its intended audience no matter what privacy settings are used.

Using social media to seek answers to practice questions may also constitute a breach of ethics. For example, if a student poses a question related to course material to a professional audience, they may unwittingly be sharing proprietary information while circumventing their own need to develop problem-solving behaviors (Newkirk-Turner et al., 2019). Social media users have also posted disrespectful comments about colleagues, clients, and places of work; photos and videos of work-related activities and people; and photos and videos of themselves or their friends engaged in compromising activities. Many of these types of postings have resulted in a wide range of disciplinary actions (Brous & Olsen, 2017; Greysen et al., 2010; Langenfeld et al., 2014; Thompson et al., 2008). In addition to potential violations of HIPAA and Family and Educational Rights and Privacy Act (FERPA), legislative and ethical concerns have been raised. "Friending" patients and clients on Facebook, for example, may impact the therapeutic relationship (Guseh et al., 2009). As stated earlier, inappropriate behaviors, even if subjectively inappropriate, can negatively impact the professional expectations held by the public.

Social media, however, can be an important tool for promoting the profession of OT. Just as it can be used to enhance learning opportunities at the college level (Gerlich et al., 2010), social media has and can be used to share relevant information with peers and to provide learning opportunities about health and wellness to the public (Greysen et al., 2010; McNab, 2009). Positive uses of social media have included using a blog to teach persons with multiple sclerosis about energy conservation, teaching fall prevention strategies to older adults, providing tips on identifying cognitive impairment in daily activities, and identifying the beginning signs of driving impairment. Using Facebook or Instagram to promote professional practice, sharing videos on sites such as YouTube or TikTok that demonstrate an assessment or intervention technique, tweeting about opportunities for community participation on Twitter, and connecting with professionals on chat boards to promote evidence-based research collaboration on a specific topic are also possible uses of social media.

When producing digital content, it is helpful to remember the "dos and don'ts." Table 30.2 provides a checklist for proper online content and conduct.

TABLE 30.2 **Social Media and E-Mail Checklist for the Professional**

YES	NO	For Social Media Sites, Such as Facebook, Instagram, LinkedIn, and Twitter as well as Personal Websites, Blogs, E-mails, and Texts
❑	❑	Did you target the correct audience for your posts?
❑	❑	Is the information you posted factual and backed up by evidence?
❑	❑	Are you in compliance with HIPAA (Health Insurance Portability and Accountability Act) and/or FERPA (Family Educational Rights and Privacy Act) regulations?
❑	❑	Are you in compliance with your workplace's policies?
❑	❑	Are your remarks (and/or status updates) respectful (i.e., Did you avoid making comments that someone might find offensive or hurtful?)?
❑	❑	Did you use proper spelling, grammar, and punctuation in your professional postings? Did you avoid using "text" abbreviations, such as "u" or "r," on sites not limited in character number?
❑	❑	Did you avoid posting photographs or videos of yourself or others that can be considered improper, even if these photographs were taken and posted in non–work-related venues (i.e., Would you want your family, your professors, your boss, or your clients to see these)?
❑	❑	If you posted a photo or video, does it comply with HIPAA, FERPA, and/or additional workplace policies?
❑	❑	Did you send a communication to a colleague that is grammatically and structurally correct?
❑	❑	Did you remember to sign your name on all e-mails so that the recipient can identify you?
❑	❑	Did you remember that whatever you post will be accessible forever, in spite of privacy assurances from websites?
❑	❑	Did you avoid overuse of punctuation marks, all capital letters, and boldface in your content? These may cause the reader to misinterpret your intent or make it difficult to read.
❑	❑	Does your content reflect the appropriate level of formality? For example, did you avoid using the greeting "Hey" in a message to a colleague?

Conclusion

The professional role carries with it a great deal of responsibility. Professionals, whose responsibilities are to their clients, profession, society, are ambassadors for their field. Whether one is at work, with friends, or in the virtual world, how one is perceived as a person may be a reflection of who one is as a professional. The world of OT is an exciting one. Our science is growing, our practice areas are expanding, and our presence is ubiquitous. As an OT professional, you have an opportunity to not only participate in this wonderful profession but also to contribute to its development.

Lippincott® Connect *For additional resources on the subjects discussed in this chapter, visit* Lippincott Connect.

REFERENCES

Accreditation Council for Occupational Therapy Education. (2018). *Accreditation Council for Occupational Therapy Education (ACOTE) standards and interpretive guidelines.* https://acoteonline.org/accreditation-explained/standards/

Ahmed, W., Jagsi, R., Gutheil, T. G., & Katz, M. S. (2020). Public disclosure on social media of identifiable patient information by health professionals: Content analysis of Twitter data. *Journal of Medical Internet Research, 22*(9), Article e19746. https://doi.org/10.2196/19746

American Occupational Therapy Association. (2015). Importance of interprofessional education in occupational therapy curricula. *American Journal of Occupational Therapy, 69*(Suppl. 3), 691341020p1–691341020p14. https://doi.org/10.5014/ajot.2015.696S02

American Occupational Therapy Association. (2017b). Vision 2025. *American Journal of Occupational Therapy, 71,* 7103420010p1. https://doi.org/10.5014/ajot.2017.713002

American Occupational Therapy Association. (2020a). AOTA 2020 occupational therapy code of ethics. *American Journal of Occupational Therapy, 74*(Suppl. 3), 7413410005p1–7413410005p5. https://doi.org/10.5014/ajot.2020.74S3006

American Occupational Therapy Association. (2020b). *Fieldwork performance evaluation (FWPE) for the occupational therapy assistant student* (Rev. ed.). https://www.aota.org/-/media/Corporate/Files/EducationCareers/Fieldwork/Fieldwork-Performance-Evaluation-Occupational-Therapy-Assistant-Student.pdf

American Occupational Therapy Association. (2020c). *Fieldwork performance evaluation (FWPE) for the occupational therapy student* (Rev. ed.). https://www.aota.org/-/media/Corporate/Files/EducationCareers/Fieldwork/Fieldwork-Performance-Evaluation-Occupational-Therapy-Student.pdf

American Occupational Therapy Association. (2020d). *Level I fieldwork competency evaluation for OT and OTA students.* https://www.aota.org/~/media/Corporate/Files/EducationCareers/Educators/Fieldwork/LevelI/Level-I-Fieldwork-Competency-Evaluation-for-ot-and-ota-students.pdf

American Occupational Therapy Association. (2020e). Occupational therapy practice framework: Domain and process—fourth edition. *The American Journal of Occupational Therapy, 74*(Suppl. 2), 7412410010p1–7412410010p87. https://doi.org/10.5014/ajot.2020.74S2001

Anderson, E., Smith, R., & Hammick, M. (2016). Evaluating an interprofessional education curriculum: A theory-informed approach.

Medical Teacher, 38(4), 385–394. https://doi.org/10.3109/0142159X.2015.1047756

Anselmo-Witzel, S., Orshan, S. A., Heitner, K. L., & Bachand, J. (2017). Are generation Y nurses satisfied on the job? Understanding their lived experiences. *The Journal of Nursing Administration, 47(4)*, 232–237. https://doi.org/10.1097/NNA.0000000000000470

Aurora, V., Wayne, D., Anderson, R., Didwania, A., & Humphrey, H. (2008). Participation in and perceptions of unprofessional behaviors among incoming internal medicine interns. *JAMA, 300(10)*, 1132–1134. https://doi.org/10.1001/jama.300.10.1132

Bahk, C. M., Sheil, A., Rohm, C. E., & Lin, F. (2010). Digital media dependency, relational orientation and social networking among college students. *Communications of the IIMA, 10(3)*, 69–78. https://scholarworks.lib.csusb.edu/ciima/vol10/iss3/6/

Baker, L., Egan-Lee, E., Martimianakis, M. A., & Reeves, S. (2011). Relationships of power: Implications for interprofessional education. *Journal of Interprofessional Care, 25(2)*, 98–104. https://doi.org/10.3109/13561820.2010.505350

Bennett, K. G., & Vercler, C. J. (2018). When is posting about patients on social media unethical "Medutainment"? *AMA Journal of Ethics, 20(4)*, 328–335. https://doi.org/10.1001/journalofethics.2018.20.4.ecas1-1804

Berlinger, N., Breznay, J. B., Dubler, N. N., Finger, H., Kirk, T. W., Mukherjee, D., & Weingast, E. G. (2021). *Vaccinated and still isolated: The ethics of overprotecting nursing home residents.* https://www.thehastingscenter.org/vaccinated-and-still-isolated-the-ethics-of-overprotecting-nursing-home-residents/

Berman, J. R., Aizer, J., Bass, A. R., Blanco, I., Davidson, A., Dwyer, E., Fields, T. R., Huang, W.-T., Kang, J. S., Kerr, L. D., Krasnokutsky-Samuels, S., Lazaro, D. M., Schwartzman-Morris, J. S., Paget, S. A., & Pillinger, M. H. (2016). Fellow use of medical jargon correlates inversely with patient and observer perceptions of professionalism: Results of a rheumatology OSCE (ROSCE) using challenging patient scenarios. *Clinical Rheumatology, 35(8)*, 2093–2099. https://doi.org/10.1007/s10067-015-3113-9

Bindler, B., Richardson, K., Daratha, D., & Wordell, D. (2012). Interdisciplinary health science research collaboration: Strengths, challenges, and case example. *Applied Nursing Research, 25(2)*, 95–100. https://doi.org/10.1016/j.apnr.2010.06.004

Boet, S., Bould, M. D., Layat Burn, C., & Reeves, S. (2014). Twelve tips for a successful interprofessional team-based high-fidelity simulation education session. *Medical Teacher, 36(10)*, 853–857. https://doi.org/10.3109/0142159X.2014.923558

Bosch, B., & Mansell, H. (2015). Interprofessional collaboration in health care: Lessons to be learned from competitive sports. *Canadian pharmacists journal : CPJ = Revue des pharmaciens du Canada : RPC, 148(4)*, 176–179. https://doi.org/10.1177/1715163515588106

Brennan, C. W., Olds, D. M., Dolansky, M., Estrada, C. A., & Patrician, P. A. (2014). Learning by doing: Observing an interprofessional process as an interprofessional team. *Journal of Interprofessional Care, 28(3)*, 249–251. https://doi.org/10.3109/13561820.2013.839750

Brock, D., Abu-Rish, E., Chiu, C., Hammer, D., Wilson, S., Vorvick, L., Blondon, K., Schaad, D., Liner, D., & Zierler, B. (2013). Interprofessional education in team communication: Working together to improve patient safety. *BMJ Quality & Safety, 22(5)*, 414–423. https://qualitysafety.bmj.com/content/22/5/414

Brous, E., & Olsen, D. (2017). Lessons learned from litigation. *American Journal of Nursing, 117(9)*, 50–54. https://doi.org/10.1097/01.NAJ.0000524546.50943.9e.

Byrne, A., & Tanesini, A. (2015). Instilling new habits: Addressing implicit bias in healthcare professionals. *Advances in Health Sciences Education: Theory and Practice, 20(5)*, 1255–1262. https://doi.org/10.1007/s10459-015-9600-6

Campbell, S. M., Twenge, J. M., & Campbell, W. K. (2017). Fuzzy but useful constructs: Making sense of the differences between generations. *Work, Aging and Retirement, 3(2)*, 130–139. https://doi.org/10.1093/workar/wax001

Carey, M. J., & Taylor, M. (2021). The impact of interprofessional practice models on health service inequity: An integrative systematic review. *Journal of Health Organization and Management, 35(6)*. Advance online publication. https://doi.org/10.1108/JHOM-04-2020-0165

Cartmill, C., Soklaridis, S., & Cassidy, J. D. (2011). Transdisciplinary teamwork: The experience of clinicians at a functional restoration program. *Journal of Occupational Rehabilitation, 21(1)*, 1–8. https://doi.org/10.1007/s10926-010-9247-3

Chaet, D., Clearfield, R., Sabin, J. E., & Skimming, K. (2017). Ethical practice in telehealth and telemedicine. *Journal of General Internal Medicine, 32(10)*, 1136–1140. https://doi.org/10.1007/s11606-017-4082-2

Columbia Center for Teaching and Learning. (n.d.). *Glossary for healthcare team models.* https://ccnmtl.columbia.edu/projects/sl2/pdf/glossary.pdf

Cruess, R. L., & Cruess, S. R. (2009). Cognitive base of professionalism. In R. L. Cruess, S. R. Cruess, & Y. Steinert (Eds.), *Teaching medical professionalism* (pp. 7–30). Cambridge University Press.

Cruess, R. L., & Cruess, S. R. (2020). Professionalism, communities of practice, and medicine's social contract. *The Journal of the American Board of Family Medicine, 33(Suppl.)*, S50–S56. https://doi.org/10.3122/jabfm.2020.S1.190417

Cruess, R. L., Cruess, S. R., & Steinert, Y. (2009). Core attributes of professionalism. In R. L. Cruess, S. R. Cruess, & Y. Steinert (Eds.), *Teaching medical professionalism* (pp. 285–286). Cambridge University Press.

Ćurković, M., Košec, A., & Ćurković, D. (2020). Medical professionalism in times of COVID-19 pandemic: Is economic logic trumping medical ethics? *Internal Emergency Medicine, 15(8)*, 1585–1586. https://doi.org/10.1007/s11739-020-02446-5

D'Agostino, F., Gerald, G., & Thrasher, J. (2021). Contemporary approaches to the social contract. In E. N. Zalta (Ed.), *The Stanford encyclopedia of philosophy* (Winter 2021 ed.). https://plato.stanford.edu/archives/win2021/entries/contractarianism-contemporary/

Deering, S. J., Johnston, L. C., & Colacchio, K. (2011). Multidisciplinary teamwork and communication training. *Seminars in Perinatology, 35(2)*, 89–96. https://doi.org/10.1053/j.semperi.2011.01.009

Dhawan, S. (2020). Online learning: A panacea in the time of COVID-19 crisis. *Journal of Educational Technology Systems, 49(1)*, 5–22. https://doi.org/10.1177/0047239520934018

Eggleston, S. (n.d.). *Key steps to an effective presentation.* http://www.theegglestongroup.com/writing/keystep1.php

Ekmekci, P. E., & Arda, B. (2015). Enhancing John Rawls's theory of justice to cover health and social determinants of health. *Acta Bioethica, 21(2)*, 227–236. https://doi.org/10.4067/S1726-569X2015000200009

Falk-Kessler, J. (2018). Professionalism, communication & teamwork. In B. Schell & G. Gillen (Eds.), *Willard and Spackman's occupational therapy* (13th ed.). Lippincott, Williams & Wilkins.

Farrell, P. R., Magida Farrell, L., & Farrell, M. K. (2017). Ancient texts to PubMed: A brief history of the peer-review process. *Journal of Perinatology, 37(1)*, 13–15. https://doi.org/10.1038/jp.2016.209

Fawcett, J. (2013). Thoughts about multidisciplinary, interdisciplinary, and transdisciplinary research. *Nursing Science Quarterly, 26(4)*, 376–379. https://doi.org/10.1177/0894318413500408

Ficarra, B. (2011). *Social media: Medical social networking—part 2.* http://healthin30.com/2011/03/social-media-medical-social-networking-part-2/

Fletcher, S., Whiting, C., Boaz, A., & Reeves, S. (2017). Exploring factors related to the translation of collaborative research learning experiences into clinical practice: Opportunities and tensions. *Journal of Interprofessional Care, 31(4)*, 543–545. https://doi.org/10.1080/13561820.2017.1303464

Flores-Sandoval, C., Sibbald, S., Ryan, B.L., & Orange. J. B. (2021). Healthcare teams and patient-related terminology: A review of concepts and uses. *Scandinavian Journal of Caring Science, 35(1)*, 55–66 https://doi.org/10.1111/scs.12843

Gately, M. E., Trudeau, S. A., & Moo, L. R. (2020). Feasibility of telehealth-delivered home safety evaluations for caregivers of clients with dementia. *OTJR: Occupation, Participation and Health, 40*(1), 42–49. https://doi.org/10.1177/1539449219859935

Gerlich, R. N., Browning, L., & Westermann, L. (2010). The social media affinity scale: Implications for education. *Contemporary Issues in Education Research, 3(11)*, 35–41. https://doi.org/10.19030/cier.v3i11.245

Glennon, T., & Van Oss, T. (2010). Identifying and promoting professional behavior: Best practices for establishing, maintaining, and improving professional behavior by occupational therapy practitioners. *Occupational Therapy Practice, 15(17)*, 13–16.

Greysen, S. R., Kind, T., & Chretien, K. C. (2010). Online professionalism and the mirror of social media. *Journal of General Internal Medicine, 25(11)*, 1227–1229. https://doi.org/10.1007/s11606-010-1447-1

Guseh, J. S., II., Brendel, R., & Brendel, D. H. (2009). Medical professionalism in the age of online social networking. *Journal of Medical Ethics, 35(9)*, 584–586. https://doi.org/10.1136/jme.2009.029231

Hader, A. L., & Brown, E. D. (2010). Patient privacy and social media. *AANA Journal, 78(4)*, 270–274. https://www.proquest.com/scholarly-journals/patient-privacy-social-media/docview/749390142/se-2

Hammell, K. W. (2015). Quality of life, participation and occupational rights: A capabilities perspective. *Australian Occupational Therapy Journal, 62(2)*, 78–85. https://doi.org/10.1111/1440-1630.12183

Hills, C., Ryan, S., Smith, D. R., Warren-Forward, H., Levett-Jones, T., & Lapkin, S. (2016). Occupational therapy students' technological skills: Are "generation Y" ready for 21st century practice? *Australian Occupational Therapy Journal, 63(6)*, 391–398. https://doi.org/10.1111/1440-1630.12308

Holm, M. B. (2000). The 2000 Eleanor Clarke Slagle lecture. Our mandate for the new millennium: Evidence-based practice. *American Journal of Occupational Therapy, 54(6)*, 575–585. https://doi.org/10.5014/ajot.54.6.575

Hordichuk, C. J., Robinson, A. J., & Sullivan, T. M. (2015). Conceptualising professionalism in occupational therapy through a western lens. *Australian Occupational Therapy Journal, 62(3)*, 150–159. https://doi.org/10.1111/1440-1630.12204

House, J. B., Sun, J. K., Sullivan, A., & Ross, P. (2016). Introduction to interprofessional education using health professionals. *Medical Education, 50(5)*, 579–580. https://doi.org/10.1111/medu.13021

Interprofessional Education Collaborative. (2016). *Core competencies for interprofessional collaborative practice: 2016 update.* Author.

Jacobs, K. (2009). Professional presentations and publications. In E. B. Crepeau, E. S. Cohn & B. A. Schell (Eds.), *Willard & Spackman's occupational therapy* (11th ed., pp. 411–417). Lippincott Williams & Wilkins.

Jessup, R. L. (2007). Interdisciplinary versus multidisciplinary care teams: Do we understand the difference? *Australian Health Review, 31(3)*, 330–331. http://ezproxy.cul.columbia.edu/login?url=https://search.proquest.com/docview/231778493?accountid=10226

Johnston, S. (2006). See one, do one, teach one: Developing professionalism across the generations. *Clinical Orthopaedics and Related Research, 449*, 186–192. https://doi.org/10.1097/01.blo.0000224033.23850.1c

Jones, A., & Jones, D. (2011). Improving teamwork, trust and safety: An ethnographic study of an interprofessional initiative. *Journal of Interprofessional Care, 25(3)*, 175–181. https://doi.org/10.3109/13561820.2010.520248

Kalisch, B. J., Lee, H., & Rochman, M. (2010). Nursing staff teamwork and job satisfaction. *Journal of Nursing Management, 18(8)*, 938–947. https://doi.org/10.1111/j.1365-2834.2010.01153.x

Kessler, D., Anderson, N. D., & Dawson, D. R. (2021). Occupational performance coaching for stroke survivors delivered via telerehabilitation using a single-case experimental design. *British Journal of Occupational Therapy, 84*(8). 488–496. https://doi.org/10.1177/0308022620988471

King, G., Tucker, M., Desserud, S., & Shillington, M. (2009). The application of a transdisciplinary model for early intervention services. *Infants & Young Children, 22(3)*, 211–223. https://doi.org/10.1097/IYC.0b013e3181abe1c3

Kington, R. S., Arnesen, S., Chou, W. S., Curry, S. J., Lazer, D., & Villarruel, A. M. (2021). Identifying credible sources of health information in social media: Principles and attributes. *NAM Perspectives.* https://doi.org/10.31478/202107a

Klamroth-Marganska, V., Gemperle, M., Ballmer, T., Grylka-Baeschlin, S., Pehlke-Milde, J., & Gantschnig, B. E. (2021). Does therapy always need touch? A cross-sectional study among Switzerland-based occupational therapists and midwives regarding their experience with health care at a distance during the COVID-19 pandemic in spring 2020. *BMC Health Services Research, 21(1)*, Article 578. https://doi.org/10.1186/s12913-021-06527-9

Lake, P. (2009, April 17). Student discipline: The case against legalistic approaches. *The Chronicle of Higher Education, 55*(32), A31, A32. https://www.chronicle.com/article/student-discipline-the-case-against-legalistic-approaches/

Langenfeld, S. J., Cook, G., Sudbeck, C., Luers, T., & Schenarts, P. J. (2014). An assessment of unprofessional behavior among surgical residents on Facebook: A warning of the dangers of social media. *Journal of Surgical Education, 71(6)*, e28–e32. https://doi.org/10.1016/j.jsurg.2014.05.013

Lindheim, S. R., Nouri, P., Rabah, K. A., & Yaklic, J. L. (2016). Medical professionalism and enculturation of the millennial physician: Meeting of the minds. *Fertility and Sterility, 106(7)*, 1615–1616. https://doi.org/10.1016/j.fertnstert.2016.09.047

Lipscomb, V. (2010). Intergenerational issues in nursing: Learning from each generation. *Clinical Journal of Oncology Nursing, 14(3)*, 267–269. https://doi.org/10.1188/10.CJON.267-269

Lyons, S., & Kuron, L. (2014). Generational differences in the workplace: A review of the evidence and directions for future research. *Journal of Organizational Behavior, 35(S1)*, S139–S157. https://doi.org/10.1002/job.1913

Maeir, T., Nahum, M., Makranz, C., Hoba, F., Peretz, T., Nagary, S. N., Silberman, N., & Gilboa, Y. (2021). The feasibility of a combined model of online interventions for adults with cancer-related cognitive impairment. *British Journal of Occupational Therapy, 84(7)*: 430–440. https://doi.org/10.1177/0308022620950993

Manges, K., Groves, P. S., Farag, A., Peterson, R., Harton, J., & Greyson, S. R. (2020). A mixed methods study examining teamwork shared mental models of interprofessional teams during hospital discharge. *British Medical Journal Quality & Safety, 29(6)*, 499–508. https://qualitysafety.bmj.com/content/29/6/499

McNab, C. (2009). What social media offers to health professionals and citizens. *Bulletin of the World Health Organization, 87(8)*, 566. https://doi.org/10.2471/blt.09.066712

Medlock, A., McKee, E., Feinstein, J., Bell, S. H., & Tracy, C. S. (2011). Applying an innovative model of interprofessional team practice: The view from occupational therapy. *Occupational Therapy Now, 13(3)*, 7–9.

https://www.proquest.com/docview/868514514?accountid=10226&parentSessionId=YkDuBv7ePKfGDb%2Fk4E5IlhZnmdb37CBP4q4e4ISYKG0%3D&pq-origsite=summon

Mercier, H., & Sperber, D. (2011). Why do humans reason? Arguments for an argumentative theory. *The Behavioral and Brain Sciences, 34(2)*, 57–111. https://doi.org/10.1017/S0140525X10000968

Monrouxe, L., Rees, C. E., & Hu, W. (2011). Differences in medical students' explicit discourses of professionalism: Acting, representing, becoming. *Medical Education, 45(6)*, 585–602. https://doi.org/10.1111/j.1365-2923.2010.03878.x

Nancarrow, S.A., Booth, A., Arliss, S., Smith, T., Enderby, P., & Roots, A. (2013). Ten principles of good interdisciplinary team work. *Human Resources for Health, 11*, Article 19. https://doi.org10.1186/1478-4491-11-19

Natale, J. E., Boehmer, J., Blumberg, D. A., Dimitriades, C., Hirose, S., Kair, L. A., Kirk, J. D., Mateev, S. N., McKnight, H., Plant, J., Tzimenatos, L. S., Wiedeman, J. T., Witkowski, J., Underwood, M. A., & Lakshminrusimha, S. (2020). Interprofessional/interdisciplinary teamwork during the early COVID-19 pandemic: experience from a children's hospital within an academic health center. *Journal of Interprofessional Care, 34(5)*, 682–686, https://doi.org/10.1080/13561820.2020.1791809

Ndoro, S. (2014). Effective multidisciplinary working: The key to high-quality care. *British Journal of Nursing, 23(13)*, 724–727. https://doi.org/10.12968/bjon.2014.23.13.724

Newkirk-Turner, B. L., Johnson, V. E., & Vaughan-Robinson, L. (2019). Using social media for academic help is dishonest. *The ASHA Leader, 24(5)*, 8–9. https://doi.org/10.1044/leader.FMP.24052019.8

Nicholas, D., Watkinson, A., Jamali, H. R., Herman, E., Tenopir, C., Volentine, R., Allard, S., & Levine, K. (2015). Peer review: Still king in the digital age. *Learned Publishing, 28(1)*, 15–21. https://doi.org/10.1087/20150104

Nobarany, S., & Booth, K. S. (2017). Understanding and supporting anonymity policies in peer review. *Journal of the Association for Information Science and Technology, 68(4)*, 957–971. https://doi.org/10.1002/asi.23711

Ozkan, M., & Solmaz, B. (2015). The changing face of the employees—generation Z and their perceptions of work (a study applied to university students). *Procedia Economics and Finance, 26(2015)*, 476–483. https://doi.org/10.1016/S2212-5671(15)00876-X

Piscotty, R., Martindell, E., & Karim, M. (2016). Nurses' self-reported social media and mobile device use in the work setting. *Online Journal of Nursing Informatics (OJNI), 20*(1). http://www.himss.org/ojni

Poston, R., Haney, T., Kott, K., & Rutledge, C. (2017). Interprofessional team performance, optimized. *Nursing Management, 48(7)*, 36–43. https://doi.org/10.1097/01.NUMA.0000520722.55679.7c

Rapanta, C., Botturi, L., Goodyear, P., Guàrdia, L., & Koole, M. (2020). Online university teaching during and after the Covid-19 crisis: Refocusing teacher presence and learning activity. *Postdigital Science and Education, 2*, 923–945. https://doi.org/10.1007/s42438-020-00155-y

Rawls, J. (1971). *The main idea of the theory of justice. A theory of justice.* Harvard University Press

Reeves S., Xyrichis A., & Zwarenstein M. (2018). Teamwork, collaboration, coordination, and networking: Why we need to distinguish between different types of interprofessional practice. *Journal of Interprofessional Care, 32(1)*, 1–3. https://doi.org/10.1080/13561820.2017.1400150

Rider, E. A., Brashers, V. L., & Costanza, M. E. (2008). Using interprofessional team-based learning to develop health care policy. *Medical Education, 42(5)*, 519–520. https://doi.org/10.1111/j.1365-2923.2008.03078.x

Rowley, J., Johnson, F., Sbaffi, L., Frass, W., & Devine, E. (2017). Academics' behaviors and attitudes towards open access publishing in scholarly journals. *Journal of the Association for Information Science and Technology, 68(5)*, 1201–1211. https://doi.org/10.1002/asi.23710

Rozenblum, R., & Bates, D. W. (2013). Patient-centred healthcare, social media and the internet: The perfect storm? *BMJ Quality & Safety, 22(3)*, 183–186. https://doi.org/10.1136/bmjqs-2012-001744

Serwe, K. M., Hersch, G. I., Pickens, N. D., & Pancheri, K. (2017). Caregiver perceptions of a telehealth wellness program. *American Journal of Occupational Therapy, 71(4)*, 7104350010p1–7104350010p5. https://doi.org/10.5014/ajot.2017.025619

Sims, S., Hewitt, G., & Harris, R. (2015). Evidence of collaboration, pooling of resources, learning and role blurring in interprofessional healthcare teams: A realist synthesis. *Journal of Interprofessional Care, 29(1)*, 20–25. https://doi.org/10.3109/13561820.2014.939745

Sinclair, L. B., Lingard, L. A., & Mohabeer, R. N. (2009). What's so great about rehabilitation teams? An ethnographic study of interprofessional collaboration in a rehabilitation unit. *Archives of Physical Medicine and Rehabilitation, 90(7)*, 1196–1201. https://doi.org/10.1016/j.apmr.2009.01.021

Stanley, M., Forwell, S., Hocking, C., Nayar, S., Rudman, D. L., Prodinger, B., Vera, L. F., Townsend, E., Magalhães, L., Simaan, J., Reid, H., & Pols, V. (2020). A pledge to mobilize against racism. *Journal of Occupational Science, 27(3)*, 294–295. https://doi.org/10.1080/14427591.2020.1793446

Thistlethwaite, J. (2012). Interprofessional education: A review of context, learning and the research agenda. *Medical Education, 46(1)*, 58–70. https://doi.org/10.1111/j.1365-2923.2011.04143.x

Thompson, L. A., Dawson, K., Ferdig, R., Black, E. W., Boyer, J., Coutts, J., & Black, N. P. (2008). The intersection of online social networking with medical professionalism. *Journal of General Internal Medicine, 23(7)*, 954–957. https://doi.org/10.1007/s11606-008-0538-8

Twenge, J. M. (2006). *Generation me: Why today's young Americans are more confident, assertive, entitled—and more miserable than ever before.* Free Press.

Ventola, C. L. (2014). Social media and health care professionals: Benefits, risks, and best practices. *P & T: A Peer-reviewed Journal for Formulary Management, 39(7)*, 491–520. https://www.ncbi.nlm.nih.gov/pmc/articles/PMC4103576/

Ventriglio, A., & Bhugra, D. (2016). Age of entitlement and the young: Implications for social psychiatry. *The International Journal of Social Psychiatry, 62(2)*, 107–109. https://doi.org/10.1177/0020764015602170

Wang, J., He, B., Miao, X., Huang, X., Lu, Y., & Chen, J. (2017). The reliability and validity of a new professionalism assessment scale for young health care workers. *Medicine, 96(25)*, e7058. https://doi.org/10.1097/MD.0000000000007058

Wiedmer, T. (2015). Generations do differ: Best practices in leading traditionalists, boomers, and generations X, Y, and Z. *Delta Kappa Gamma Bulletin, 82*, 51–58. https://www.scinapse.io/papers/2338807891

Wynia, M. K., Papadakis, M. A., Sullivan, W. M., & Hafferty, F. W. (2014). More than a list of values and desired behaviors: A foundational understanding of medical professionalism. *Academic Medicine, 89(5)*, 712–714. https://doi.org/10.1097/ACM.0000000000000212

Youngstrom, M. (2002). The occupational therapy practice framework: The evolution of our professional language. *American Journal of Occupational Therapy, 56(6)*, 607–608. https://doi.org/10.5014/ajot.56.6.607

Yuen, H. K., Azuero, A., Lackey, K. W., Brown, N. S., & Shrestha, S. (2016). Construct validity test of evaluation tool for professional behaviors of entry-level occupational therapy students in the United States.

Journal of Educational Evaluation for Health Professions, 13, 22. https://doi.org/10.3352/jeehp.2016.13.22

Ziring, D., Danoff, D., Grosseman, S., Langer, D., Esposito, A., Jan, M. K., Rosenzweig, S., & Novack, D. (2015). How do medical schools identify and remediate professionalism lapses in medical students? A study of U.S. and Canadian medical schools. *Academic Medicine, 90(7),* 913–920. https://doi.org/10.1097/ACM.0000000000000737

Zwarenstein, M., Goldman, J., & Reeves, S. (2009). Interprofessional collaboration: Effects of practice-based interventions on professional practice and healthcare outcomes. *Cochrane Database of Systematic Reviews,* Article CD000072. https://doi.org/10.1002/14651858.CD000072.pub2

Documentation in Practice

Karen M. Sames

"Escribe lo que no debe ser olvidado."

—ISABEL ALLENDE

LEARNING OBJECTIVES

After reading this chapter, you will be able to:

1. Identify the primary reasons for documentation of occupational therapy (OT) services.
2. Describe the types of clinical, educational, and administrative documentation used in OT practice.
3. Compare and contrast the key features of OT documentation in clinical and educational settings.
4. Identify the components of well-written goals.
5. Write a SOAP note.
6. Identify appropriate documentation methods and approaches that address health literacy and communicate at the level of the intended audience.

Introduction

Occupational therapy (OT) practitioners communicate with many different types of people on a daily basis. They provide instructions for home programs to clients and their caregivers. They inform other professionals on the care team about the client's progress in OT. They write letters to foundations seeking funding for new programs. This chapter addresses the various audiences and types of documentation that OT practitioners may use at some point during their careers.

Audience

How one documents depends greatly on who will read it—one's audience. How a letter to an insurance company is worded might be very different from the way a letter to a parent or physician is worded. Documentation that is read by members of the clinical care team might use more precise anatomical and technical words than would an Individualized Family Service

Plan (IFSP) that is shared with the parents of a 2-year-old. Knowing who will read what is being communicated is an important aspect of effective documentation.

The potential audiences for OT documentation include the following:

- Medical professionals (e.g., doctors, nurses, physical therapists, social workers)
- Education professionals (teachers, principals, etc.)
- Lawyers, judges, and juries
- Accreditation agencies (e.g., The Joint Commission, Department of Education)
- Payers (e.g., managed care and insurance companies, Medicare contractors)
- The client or the client's guardian, caregiver, family member, and/or service provider

Each audience reads documentation through a different lens, depending on the practice setting, educational level, motivation, and cultural background (Sames, 2015). Professional communication requires a level of respect and formality that is not found in informal communication. It uses complete sentences and avoids slang or emotionally charged words. Professional writing uses active voice and is free from bias (Sames, 2015).

Communicating with medical professionals requires the writer to be very precise. Nurses need to know more than that the patient needs assistance with dressing; they need to know how much assistance is required and the nature of the assistance. The physical therapist needs to know how long the client was standing at the sink while working on grooming and hygiene.

When communicating in a school setting, there is a need to focus on the educationally relevant information. The entire team working with the child might not understand medical jargon, so educational terms are more appropriate.

When providing written communication with families, caregivers, and others involved with client care, it is important to include language at their level of understanding and in their preferred method of communication.

Documentation often requires compliance with specific standards. For example, the Individuals with Disabilities Education Act (IDEA) requires that specific items be included in the individualized education program (IEP) and Medicare requires specific documentation elements for outpatient therapy reimbursement. In addition, employers might have policies or procedures that further direct the timing, placement, and word choices of the documentation. Box 31.1 contains some documentation tips that apply to all documentation.

Always remember that people form an impression of your professionalism and intelligence by reading what you write. And it is important to note that what you write can be used as evidence in a court proceeding, whether you are on trial or not (Sames, 2015).

BOX 31.1 DOCUMENTATION TIPS

- Use correct
  - Grammar
  - Spelling
  - Syntax
  - Word choice
  - Literacy level for the reader(s)
- Read spellchecker and grammar checker recommendations carefully; sometimes, it is better to click "Ignore" than to use what they recommend.
- Follow directions carefully.
- Have a dictionary and a writing manual or websites handy.
- Write legibly.
- Proofread, proofread, and proofread again (Sames, 2015).

Describing Clients

Depending on the setting, the person or group receiving OT services may be referred to as the patient, client, resident, participant, student, or by a variety of other terms. This is determined by the practice setting. OT practitioners should use the terminology used by other practitioners in that setting.

Gender

Historically, the pronouns used to describe clients were limited to he/him for those identified on their birth certificate as males and she/her for females. Recently, there is growing recognition that this binary language does not represent the gender identities of all people (Out & Equal, 2020). Practitioners should use the pronouns that the clients themselves use, which means asking the client what their self-identified pronoun is (American Psychological Association [APA], 2020; Out & Equal, 2020). Some people use a gender-neutral pronoun, such as they/them, ze, or xe, whereas others use he/him or she/her (APA, 2020; Out & Equal, 2020). When a person's self-identified pronouns are unknown, APA (2020) recommends using "they." Out & Equal (2020) recommends using the honorific "Mx" rather than "Mr.," "Mrs.," or "Ms." The APA (2020) further recommends using terms like "individuals," "people," or "persons" when referring to a group rather than using "males" and "females."

Disability

There are generally two approaches to terminology related to a person or group's disability: person-first and identity-first (APA, 2020). The person-first approach uses terminology such as "a person with intellectual disability" or "people with mobility impairments" (APA, 2020; Centers for Disease Control and Prevention [CDC], 2020). It recognizes the person ahead of the disability. The identity-first approach places emphasis on the disability. Examples of disability-first terminology include "deaf," "autistic," and "paraplegic." As with gender, in determining which approach to use, it is best to ask the person how they identify themselves or, if that is not possible, to check with advocacy groups associated with the specific disability (APA, 2020). Regardless of the approach, it is best practice to avoid negative or condescending terms like "stroke victim," "alcoholic," or "low functioning" (APA, 2020; CDC, 2020). It is also important to avoid euphemisms such as "special needs" or "handi-capable" (APA, 2020).

Race and Ethnicity

Race refers to physical differences among groups of people and ethnicity refers to shared cultural characteristics such as language or beliefs (APA, 2020). The APA (2020) says that racial and ethnic terms are usually capitalized but not hyphenated, for example, "Black," "Indigenous," or "Asian American." The term "Black" is considered more inclusive than "African American" because it includes people from the Caribbean Islands and people who may have immigrated to the United States but are not American citizens; however, some people prefer to be called "African American." Both terms are acceptable (APA, 2020). When writing about people from Spanish-speaking countries or with Latin American origins, the terms "Hispanic" or "Latinx" may be used (APA, 2020). Note that "Hispanic" is a language-based term and includes people who speak Spanish or have descended from Spanish-speaking people, so it excludes people from Brazil, for example, who speak Portuguese. "Latinx" is geography-based, so it includes people from Latin America (which includes Central and South America and the Caribbean). The terms "Latino" and "Latina" are gendered terms and may or may not be acceptable to all people. Use "Asian" to refer to people who come from Asian countries but use "Asian American" for people of Asian descent (APA, 2020). Indigenous people are referred to in different ways in different parts of the world. In the United States, the term "Native American" is acceptable, whereas in Canada the terms "Indigenous Peoples" or "First Nations People" are used. In Australia, "Aboriginal People" is used (APA, 2020). Whenever possible, name the specific nation, such as "Navajo," "Inuit," or "Maori" (APA, 2020).

The Office of Management and Budget Standards for the classification of Federal Data on Race and Ethnicity (1997) includes five categories of race: (a) American Indian or Native Alaskan, (b) Asian, (c) Black or African American, (d) Native Hawaiian or other Pacific Islander, and (e) White; and it includes two categories for ethnicity: (a) Hispanic or Latino and (b) Not Hispanic or Latino. Medical records, school records, and other legal records have this classification noted in their intake information.

"Race is a social categorization that incorporates biological, social, and cultural characteristics imposed on people for the purpose of making hierarchical, power-based distinctions in social relations." The author continues by stating, "Ethnicity is a social categorization based on shared values, language, and customs that is self-claimed or developed in relation to feelings of belonging to a chosen community" (Wells, 2016, pp.387-400).

Age

For people aged 0 to 12 years, use terms such as "infant," "toddler," or "child" (APA, 2020). For individuals aged 13 to 17 years, use the terms "adolescent" or "youth." For people aged 18 years and over, use "adult" or, when appropriate, "men" or "women" (APA, 2020). "Older adults" is preferred over terms such as "elderly" or "the aged" (APA, 2020).

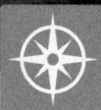

EXPANDING OUR PERSPECTIVES

Ethnocentric Documentation in Practice

Dahlia Castillo

While in OT school, I learned the basics in documentation. Training on the subject primarily occurred on the job. I soon discovered written requirements and formatting differed in every setting. One similarity among settings was accurate descriptions of the client and their meaningful occupations.

Ethnocentrism refers to the evaluation of other cultures according to preconceptions originating in the standards and customs of one's own culture. Living on the US/Mexico border, people speak Spanish, English, or both. 82.9% of people who live in El Paso, Texas, report being Hispanic and 91.8% report being White. We typically refer to each other as being American or Mexican, indicating legal citizenship status. Many cross the border daily, living on one side and working on the other. Others cross occasionally to visit family and for shopping, social gatherings, and other occasions.

For years, initial evaluation narratives began: "Mr. Pena is a 58-year-old Hispanic male diagnosed with left CVA/right hemiparesis referred to OT services to increase independence in ADLs." I would replace the term Hispanic with one of the terms found in the individual's record: American Indian, Native Alaskan, Asian, Black, Hawaiian/Pacific Islander, or White.

One day, Mr. Pena attended a follow-up appointment with a copy of the initial evaluation. He politely asked why I referred to him as Hispanic. Before I could answer, he said: "I am not Hispanic." I apologized quickly saying I did not know he preferred Mexican-American. He shook his head and said: "I am not Mexican-American. I am not Hispanic. I am American. I was born in the US. All my ancestors have lived here all our lives. I grew up south Texas and it became part of the US after the Alamo." He went further to explain that the term "Hispanic was first introduced in the 1970s to encourage cultural assimilation in the US. The term Chicano was for people attempting to keep their cultural heritage. Latino refers to people from Latin American countries. The term Latinx came about to address gender-neutral language from people in academia but Hispanics and Latinos don't like that term. People associate the term Hispanic with Spanish-speaking people. Our friends from Brazil don't speak Spanish so Hispanic, Chicano, or Latino don't work for them." I became aware of some historical context and my own lack of sensitivity that altered my documentation practices permanently.

I began to ask individuals: "Your record indicates you are _____, what is your preference?" The first person I asked preferred Native American, and another preferred Comanche. Next, a preference for African American because their ancestors were from Africa. Then, another person preferred Black because of no known ties to Africa. I met three people of Asian descent who had three different preferences. One preferred Asian, the next preferred Korean American because they were a recent naturalized citizen, and the third person simply preferred American being a fourth-generation Asian. One day, I asked the same question and the woman answered: "I prefer Caucasian. I am about to begin a transition and plan to live as a man for the next six months. Please use the pronouns he/his." The next person indicated they preferred quad and another with an identical diagnosis preferred person diagnosed with tetraplegia. The more I asked, the more preferences I discovered with differences other than race and ethnicity.

Over time, I realized no term is universal to anyone. I became aware of my own cultural biases, ethnocentrism, and lack of sensitivity to individual differences. Initial documentation changed to: "Alexandro Pena is a 58 year old with preferred pronouns of she/her diagnosed with left CVA right hemiparesis referred to OT services to increase independence in ADLs."

Legal and Ethical Considerations

In the United States and other countries, health records are legal documents. Health records can be entered as evidence in any type of legal proceeding involving malpractice, fraud, negligence, or incompetence. OT documentation can be called into court, with or without the occupational therapist being there to explain the documentation, even years after the services were provided. What was written at or near the actual time the event or events in question occurred is stronger evidence than what a person can recall months or years after the event. To remain mindful that all documentation is legal evidence, some people mentally preface their documentation by saying to themselves "Ladies and gentlemen of the jury . . ." before putting pen to paper (Sames, 2015).

Payers can review clinical documentation and client billing records at any time to determine whether fraud has been committed. If documentation is not adequate to support the charges, they can refuse to pay for the services and the OT practitioner who provided the services in question could face a range of penalties (e.g., fines, imprisonment, loss of certification or licensure) (Centers for Medicare & Medicaid Services [CMS], 2021a).

In addition to legal issues of documentation, there are ethical concerns. The American Occupational Therapy Association (AOTA) Code of Ethics (2020a) states in section 3 of the Standards for Conduct of Occupational Therapy Personnel that "Occupational therapy personnel maintain complete, accurate, and timely records of all client encounters" (7413410005p6). Specifically, Standard 3B affirms that OT documentation complies with relevant laws and regulations. Standard 3C states that documentation must be accurate and timely. Standard 3D requires OT practitioners to refrain from participating in any directive to falsify or plagiarize documentation or inaccurate coding (AOTA, 2020a).

Documentation in Clinical Settings

In hospitals, rehabilitation facilities, primary care clinics, outpatient clinics, long-term care, mental health centers, home health, and related settings, similar types of documentation are used although the frequency of documentation may vary. Clinical documentation generally involves reporting and interpreting the clients' responses on assessments and to interventions in a clinical record. Clinical documentation is important for the following reasons:

- Continuity of care within the department
- Communication across shifts, disciplines, departments
- Chronologic record of care
- Legal record
- Reimbursement requirements (Sames, 2015)

It is critical that the objective information reported in the documentation be clearly differentiated from the subjective information or interpretations. All are important. If a practitioner states that a client appeared depressed, that is an interpretation. It is a conclusion drawn from the practitioner's observations. An objective statement should describe what was seen or heard that would logically lead to the conclusion that the client appeared depressed. For example, the practitioner could say, "Client stared at the floor for the entire session. She slouched forward in her chair, responded to questions with one-syllable words, and did not initiate any conversations with peers."

All clinical documentation must be done in compliance with the standards of the setting and the payers as well as standards set by the profession. The essential features of all clinical documentation are as follows (items with an * are automatic in an electronic health record):

- *Date of completion of document
- *Full signature and credentials
- *Type of document
- *Client name and case number
- Acceptable abbreviations and terminology as determined by the facility
- Record storage and disposal policies that comply with federal and state laws and facility procedures
- Confidentiality is protected (AOTA, 2018; Sames, 2015)

The OT practitioner's rationale—the reasons behind the intervention—should be made clear in the documentation. For example, clients with mental health challenges might have problems in living that are not as visible as physical challenges. Whereas people who use wheelchairs might have difficulty with grocery shopping because they cannot reach all the shelves or push the cart while seated in a wheelchair, people with bipolar disorder might have difficulty shopping because of an inability to control impulses to buy everything and talk to everyone in the store. Simply saying a client is working on shopping is not sufficient; the rationale for working on this occupation must be made clear.

Documentation of the Initiation of Occupational Therapy Services

The first type of clinical documentation reflects the first steps in the practitioner–client interaction. In some settings, such as in a long-term care facility, the first step is screening all new admissions to the facility. A screening is used to determine whether the person would benefit from an OT evaluation. In other settings, the first step might be an introduction, or it might be the beginning of the evaluation process.

If the client is seen for a screening or introduction prior to an evaluation, a short note is usually written in the health record summarizing the conversation and/or results of the screening. The OT practitioner writes a short summary and indicates the next step in the intervention process.

Evaluation reports are written by occupational therapists to document the starting point of OT intervention; OT assistants (OTAs) may contribute to the evaluation (AOTA, 2021). Evaluation reports contain an occupational profile, factual data collected during the evaluation process, and an interpretation of the evaluation findings. The report must show the distinct value of OT by documenting which occupations are limited or at risk of being limited (AOTA, 2021, 2018).

The evaluation report content is based on the *Occupational Therapy Practice Framework: Domain and Process*, 4th edition (AOTA, 2020b). Although AOTA recommends that a complete evaluation be conducted and documented for each client, the time constraints of certain settings might require that the occupational therapist abbreviate the evaluation process.

Typically, the evaluation report contains the following:

- Identifying and background information (e.g., client's name, age, diagnoses or conditions, date of referral, date of report, precautions, and contraindications)
- Referral information (date, time, who referred the client and why)
- Evaluation procedures and/or tests used
- Occupational profile
- Findings or results of the evaluation process (occupational analysis)
- An interpretation of the meaning of the findings or results that reflects the occupational needs of the client
- A plan, including goals, frequency, duration, and location of intervention
- Signature and credentials of the occupational therapist (AOTA, 2018; Sames, 2015)

The occupational profile (AOTA, 2018, 2020b, 2020c) is critical for demonstrating the distinct value of OT services. It is a "summary of a client's (person's, group's, or population's) occupational history and experiences, patterns of daily living, interests, values, needs, and relevant contexts" (AOTA, 2020b, p. 21). This information is gathered primarily through interviewing the client or client's surrogate. It will help the occupational therapist understand the client's needs, concerns, and goals and be useful in selecting outcome measures. The AOTA offers a template that every OT practitioner can use to document the occupational profile (AOTA, 2020c). In the United States, the occupational profile is now a requirement when billing for an OT evaluation using Current Procedural Terminology (CPT) evaluation codes (AOTA, 2018).

Occupational analysis is the process of selecting and administering appropriate assessment tools and then using this information, along with the information gathered from the occupational profile, to develop a hypothesis about what is going on with the client and set goals to help the client achieve desired outcomes (AOTA, 2020b).

The initial plan of care is based on the occupational profile and occupational analysis. The occupational therapist, with input from the OTA, and in collaboration with the client, sets short- and long-term goals. Long-term goals describe what the client will do by the time of discharge from OT—the outcome of OT interventions. Short-term goals describe what the client will do in the next 1 to 30 days. If the client will receive OT services for just a couple of days, for example, during a short stay in the acute care hospital before moving on to a transitional care setting, only one set of goals may be developed rather than separate long- and short-term goals. All goals must address performance in areas of occupation, describe observable behavior, be measurable, and be time limited (state target date for when the goal will be met) (Sames, 2015). See Table 31.1 for examples of poorly written goals and how to improve them.

The goals and interventions will help the client create or promote health, establish (habilitate) or restore (rehabilitate or remediate) function, maintain or preserve occupational performance, modify (compensate or adapt) the task or the environment to enable occupational participation, or prevent barriers to performance (AOTA, 202b).

Documentation of Continuing Occupational Therapy Services

In clinical settings, there are two types of notes written to show the client's progress in OT: daily (session) notes and progress reports. The documentation of progress should include more than a list of the activities the client engaged in during the session; it must also show how the client performed, how the client's performance changed since the last intervention session, any functional improvement, adaptive equipment provided, and client or caregiver understanding of any instruction (Sames, 2015).

Daily (contact) notes are usually written at the end of or after each intervention session. The OT practitioner who provided the service writes the daily note. In the United States, although Medicare does not require that notes written by an OTA be cosigned by the occupational therapist, state licensure laws may dictate whether or not a note needs to be cosigned (CMS, 2021b; Sames, 2015). These daily notes and progress reports may be written in narrative, SOAP, or flow-sheet formats.

Progress reports summarize OT interventions at regular intervals between updated plans of care. Medicare requires that the occupational therapist write a progress note at least once every 30 days or 10 treatment days, whichever is less (CMS, 2021b; Sames, 2015).

One of the most common forms of documenting the client's progress is called a SOAP note. It may be used for daily notes or progress reports (Sames, 2015). This note-writing format is used by many medical disciplines, a practice that strengthens communication among professionals. SOAP stands for

Subjective: the subjective experience of the client, what the client says

Objective: the clinician's objective observations and measurements

Assessment: the clinician's interpretation of the meaning of the "O" section

Plan: description of what will happen next (frequency, duration, location)

TABLE 31.1	Examples of Poorly Written Goals and Improved Goals		
Examples of Poorly Written Goals	**Examples of Improved Goals**	**Why the Improved Goal Is Better**	
Increase elbow ROM	By June 1, 2022, Maria will use elbow flexion and extension to fold three T-shirts.	It specifies by when the goal will be met and describes performance in an area of occupation.	
Jamal will dress independently.	Jamal will consistently dress, including shoes and socks, independently by discharge.	It is more specific about what is included in "dressing himself" and specifies by when the goal will be achieved.	
Tsoyushi will use an adapted pencil to write legibly by the end of the year.	By June 15, 2022, Tsoyushi will write two complete, legible sentences within 5 minutes.	It is more specific about the length of the goal and includes a measurement (two legible sentences within 5 minutes).	
By September 13, 2022, Agnes will make toast and tea.	By September 13, 2022, Agnes will prepare toast and tea with no more than one verbal cue.	It includes a measurement.	
Jenny will put six golf tees in each bag, completing each bag in ≤2 minutes, with 90% accuracy on 75% of trials on 3 consecutive days within 2 weeks.	By December 8, 2022, Jenny will package golf tees accurately on 75% of trials.	It is clearer—the original goal had too many measurements, and providing an end date for the goal is clearer than saying within 2 weeks.	

ROM, range of motion.

BOX 31.2 SOAP NOTE

S: "It hurts to reach items on the second shelf. No way could I reach the top shelf. I can't even put my hair in a ponytail."

O: Client reached items on the second shelf of the kitchen cabinet with their right hand, expressing discomfort throughout the range. Client did not attempt to reach items on the top shelf. Client pointed to the anterior aspect of the glenoid fossa when asked where it hurt. Scapular elevation and trunk rotation substituted for part of shoulder flexion and abduction; they never raised their arm above 80°. Client used internal rotation to place items retrieved from the shelf on the counter with no complaints. Client did not use external rotation in replacing objects on shelf, reporting severe pain using that kind of motion. They rated their pain a 9 out of 10.

A: Right shoulder range of motion (ROM) is severely limited and very painful. Limited ROM interferes with household tasks, dressing, hygiene, and grooming.

P: OT 2 times per week, for 45 minutes outpatient sessions to instruct client in use of a reacher, discuss environmental adaptation principles related to placement of objects within comfort zone, and develop a home program to facilitate regaining pain-free ROM.

The most difficult part of writing a SOAP note is separating the objective information from the interpretation of it (assessment). Every statement in the "A" section needs to be supported with evidence in the "S" and the "O" sections (Sames, 2015). Box 31.2 shows an example of a SOAP note. Read about how one OT learned to become a more efficient SOAP note writer in OT Story 31.1.

An updated plan of care is written in settings in which clients are seen for an extended period of time (up to 90 calendar days depending on the setting). This documents the progress that has occurred since the last plan of care was written (or an explanation for lack of progress); updates the short-term goals and sets new ones; and verifies the frequency, duration, and location of continued intervention (AOTA, 2018). The long-term goal, the outcome goal, usually remains the same.

Documentation of Termination of Occupational Therapy Services

Once clients have met their long- and short-term goals or other circumstances require ending OT services, a discontinuation summary (discharge summary) is written (AOTA, 2018; Sames 2015). This summary includes the following:

- Client identification and background information
- Summary of the client's functional status at the initiation of OT services

OT STORY 31.1 AUBREY NEW GRADUATE STRUGGLING WITH DOCUMENTATION

Aubrey is a new graduate working in long-term rehabilitation with patients who have spinal cord and traumatic brain injuries. Writing a SOAP note after each therapy session has been a challenge for them. They wished they had more time to do documentation because it was taking them over 20 minutes per note, but the other occupational therapists take about 5 minutes per SOAP note. The most difficult aspect of documenting the intervention session for Aubrey was the "O" section. They felt they needed to describe everything the client did in the session, so their "O" sections are quite long.

One day, they sat down with a more senior occupational therapist, D'nae, and talked about their concern that they were very slow when documenting. Aubrey asked how D'nae could write a note in 5 minutes or less. D'nae explained that it is not necessary to write a minute-by-minute description of everything that occurred but to focus on those things that most directly address the client's goals, represent the biggest change in the client's behavior, or are unusual in some way. Aubrey argued that if it was not documented, it did not happen, so if they left anything out of their documentation, then they could be accused of not doing something she should have done. D'nae replied that Aubrey needs to document the most important things but not everything, so they need to get comfortable writing a summary, not a blow-by-blow description. They tell Aubrey that if they continue to spend so much time documenting, they would burn out in no time and their productivity would suffer. They encouraged Aubrey to balance the need for completeness with the time and productivity demands of the job.

Aubrey decided to give D'nae's suggestion a try. They found that by being more selective in what they documented, they cut the time it takes to write a SOAP note in half. They asked D'nae to take a look at their notes and give feedback on them. The feedback was very positive and Aubrey is feeling much better about being more efficient in documentation.

Questions

1. What aspects of an initial evaluation are critical to document?
2. What aspects of an intervention session are critical to document?

- Summary of change in functional status at the close of OT services
- Results of outcome measures
- Recommendations for follow-up
- Signature, credentials, and date

According to AOTA (2020b), outcomes of OT intervention can include occupational performance, improvement, enhancement, prevention, health and wellness, quality of life, participation, role competence, well-being, and occupational justice. Outcomes are reflected in subjective and objective data gathered at the end of OT interventions. Subjective data would be based on client reports, and objective data would come from standardized or unstandardized testing and observations (AOTA, 2018, 2020b).

Electronic Health Records

Electronic health records have replaced paper charts in many practice settings. Electronic health records require healthcare providers to enter clinical data into a computerized system. These systems may use desktop, laptop, or tablet computers; smartphones; or other handheld devices (Figure 31.1). Because these systems are electronic, special precautions need to be taken to ensure the security and confidentiality of each client's health record. These systems allow members of the client's healthcare team nearly instant access to updated information about the client's healthcare, test results, medications, and consultation reports.

OT practitioners (and all other healthcare providers) need to log in and log out of the system even if they are going to be away from their computer (or other device) for only a minute or two. No computer can be left unattended while a client's health record is open. When you are logged in, every client record you access, every note you write, and every error you make and correct are recorded under your "signature."

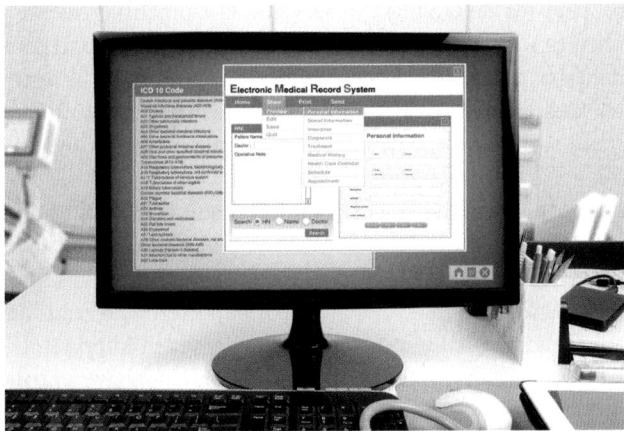

FIGURE 31.1 **Electronic health records require healthcare providers to enter clinical data into a computerized system.**

Documentation of Telehealth

When a client is being treated by an OT practitioner using telehealth technology, documentation is completed in the same way as it would be if the session was conducted in person. One addition to the daily notes would be to indicate that the session was conducted using approved telehealth technology. Individual payers may have additional requirements for documenting and billing for services provided via telehealth.

Documentation in School Settings

Documentation in educational settings in the United States can be very different from clinical documentation, but the same documentation principles apply. Documentation in school systems includes documentation of notice and consent as well as specific documentation depending on the age of the student (Sames, 2015). See Chapter 45 for more details related to OT in education settings.

Documentation of Notice and Consent

According to the IDEA, notice and consent forms are required to communicate with parents or guardians of children being served by the school district. Documents may include notices of team meetings, notice and consent for evaluation or reevaluation, referral for an initial evaluation, procedural safeguards, and a report of an IFSP or IEP meeting (Sames, 2015).

Documentation of Services From Birth Through Age 2 Years

In the United States, services for infants and toddlers are described in Part C of IDEA (Clark & Handley-More, 2017). IFSPs are written to address these services. Each state designates a lead agency (education, health, or human services) to serve the needs of infants and toddlers with special needs to help ready them for school. The lead agency (e.g., school district, health department, or contracted agency) is responsible for creating an IFSP for each child served that is tailored to the specific needs of the child and their family. An IFSP includes the following:

- A summary of the child's present level of performance (physical, cognitive, communicative, social or emotional, and adaptive development)
- Identification of the family's concerns, priorities, and resources
- A summary of expected outcomes (measurable goals)
- Identification of early intervention services needed, including frequency, intensity, and service delivery method
- Identification of other services the child is receiving
- Identification of the child's natural environment (where services will be delivered)
- Date when services will start and the anticipated length of services
- Identification of a service coordinator for the child
- Identification of the steps that will be taken to help the toddler transition to the preschool setting (IDEA, 2017a).

Documentation of Services From Age 3 to 21 Years

The IEP is a document that guides services for a child with disabilities between the ages of 3 and 21 years in the United States (Clark & Handley-More, 2017). The requirements for IEPs are described in Part B of IDEA. IEP services may include both special education and related services. For the purposes of the IEP, OT is considered a related service. As a related service provider, the occupational therapist would contribute to the process of writing and revising the IEP. The IEP is written every year and reviewed at least every 6 months (Sames, 2015).

An IEP must contain the following elements:

- Present level of educational performance
- Annual goals and how they will be measured
- Special education and related services
- Participation with nondisabled children
- Participation in statewide and districtwide tests
- Starting date and location of services
- Transition services (for children aged 14 years and older transitioning to adult programs or work settings)
- Measurement of progress (IDEA, 2017b)

The fundamental difference between an IFSP and an IEP is that IFSPs are more family centered, whereas IEPs are more education focused (Clark & Handley-More, 2017). An IEP must be educationally related. Each state or each school district within a state may establish its own forms for these documents; the federal regulations do not require the use of specific forms. The federal regulations mandate the timetables for completing the documents and the content of the documents (Clark & Handley-More, 2017; Sames, 2015).

Documentation in Emerging Practice Settings

OT practitioners are working in community-based programs such as homeless shelters, prisons, sheltered workshops, home hospice, and summer camps. The clinical approach to documentation might not be appropriate especially if there is no health record in which to enter OT documentation. It is advisable that the OT practitioner develop evaluation, intervention plan, progress, and discontinuation reports that are consistent with the AOTA documentation guidelines (2018) to the greatest extent possible. However, if the OT practitioners are providing services at a community or population level, they may simply provide the agency with periodic consultation reports with a less structured format. Most consultation reports are narrative descriptions of the needs assessment, plan, implementation, and/or outcomes of the OT program.

Because OT practitioners in emerging practice settings are demonstrating the distinct value of OT in new ways, they may use their documentation as a mechanism to demonstrate successful outcomes and benefits of OT services.

Administrative Documentation

OT practitioners in any setting may have to write an incident report, a letter of appeal to a payer source, a grant proposal, or policies and procedures. These types of documentation are administrative because they are necessary for the ongoing administration of OT services. For example, to be paid for delivering OT services, OT practitioners may need to write letters to request funding or to respond to a denial of a payment. Policies and procedures must be written clearly so that all employees of the department understand and follow the departmental standards, ensuring that the department functions well.

Administrative documentation requires the use of terminology that anyone can understand; people who have limited understanding of OT jargon or medical terms may read these documents. Often, the first person who reads an appeal letter will be someone who is trained to interpret insurance company standards but who might not have a medical background.

Box 31.3 shows an example of a section of an evaluation report written for a medical record and how it might be translated in a letter to an insurance company requesting authorization for services.

BOX 31.3 WRITING FOR AN EVALUATION REPORT COMPARED TO A PRIOR AUTHORIZATION REQUEST LETTER

Tatiana is a 16-month-old toddler. Three weeks ago, while under the care of their mother's boyfriend, they were allegedly shaken violently.

Excerpt From Evaluation Report

Tatiana did not focus on or visually track any object in any direction. They did not reach for toys that were quietly placed in front of her, but they did turn her head to localize sounds and flailed her hands in reaction to sound. Their fingers closed around a rattle placed in the palm of their hand. Passive ROM was within normal limits in all extremities. Muscle tone was low. When placed on their stomach, they rolled their head from side to side but did not lift their head. When placed in a sitting position, they were unable to hold their head up or maintain sitting unassisted. Tatiana is fed through a nasogastric tube; therefore, chewing and swallowing were not evaluated at this time. They cried and made other noises but did not form any words. Tatiana will need adaptive seating with head support and OT intervention to maximize their abilities to actively interact with people and her environment.

Excerpt From Prior Authorization Letter

This 16-month-old was diagnosed with shaken baby syndrome resulting in severe head trauma. They have low muscle tone and cannot assume or maintain a seated position unassisted. This child will need adaptive seating and positioning devices to ensure proper positioning of their trunk and limbs and to prevent deformities. Proper positioning is also important for the child's cognitive, social, and physical development. They are functionally blind. In a seated position, they will be better able to localize sound, use their arms and hands, and begin to engage in social interactions. Please refer to the attached list of recommended adaptive positioning devices and their respective costs. In addition, I recommend OT intervention twice a week for 3 months (24 visits) to work on developing the movement, social, and cognitive skills needed to enable participation in daily life activities of typical toddlers.

Conclusion

Individual agencies may opt to develop or purchase their own documentation formats. However, it is critical that whatever documentation formats are chosen conform to federal and state laws; OT documentation, practice, and ethical standards; and the requirements of reimbursement sources. It is the OT practitioner's responsibility to be aware of and comply with all documentation requirements.

Lippincott® Connect *For additional resources on the subjects discussed in this chapter, visit Lippincott Connect.*

REFERENCES

American Occupational Therapy Association. (2018). Guidelines for documentation of occupational therapy. *American Journal of Occupational Therapy, 72*(Suppl. 2), 7212410010. https://doi.org/10.5014/ajot.2018.72S203

American Occupational Therapy Association. (2020a). AOTA 2020 occupational therapy code of ethics. *American Journal of Occupational Therapy, 74*(Suppl. 3), 7413410005. https://doi.org/10.5014/ajot.2020.74S3006

American Occupational Therapy Association. (2020b). Occupational therapy practice framework: Domain and process (4th ed.). *American Journal of Occupational Therapy, 74*(Suppl. 2), 412410010. https://doi.org/10.5014/ajot.2020.74S2001

American Occupational Therapy Association. (2020c). *AOTA occupational profile template.* https://www.aota.org/Practice/Manage/Reimb/occupational-profile-document-value-ot.aspx

American Occupational Therapy Association. (2021). Standards of practice for occupational therapy. *American Journal of Occupational Therapy, 75*(Suppl. 3), 7513410050. https://doi.org/10.5014/ajot.2021.75S3004

American Psychological Association. (2020). *Publication manual of the American Psychological Association* (7th ed.). Author.

Centers for Disease Control and Prevention. (2020). *Communicating with and about people with disabilities.* https://www.cdc.gov/ncbddd/disabilityandhealth/materials/factsheets/fs-communicating-with-people.html

Centers for Medicare & Medicaid Services. (2021a). *Medicare fraud and abuse: Detection, prevention, and reporting.* https://www.cms.gov/Outreach-and-Education/Medicare-Learning-Network-MLN/MLNProducts/Downloads/Fraud-Abuse-MLN4649244.pdf

Centers for Medicare & Medicaid Services. (2021b). *Medicare benefit policy manual: Chapter 15—covered medical and other health services.* https://www.cms.gov/Regulations-and-Guidance/Guidance/Manuals/downloads/bp102c15.pdf

Clark, G. F., & Handley-More, D. (2017). *Best practices for documenting occupational therapy services in schools.* American Occupational Therapy Association.

Individuals with Disabilities Education Act. (2017a). *Sec. 303.344 content of an IFSP.* https://sites.ed.gov/idea/regs/c/d/303.344

Individuals with Disabilities Education Act. (2017b). *Section 1414 (d) (1) (A) individualized education program.* https://sites.ed.gov/idea/regs/c/d/303.344

Out & Equal. (2020). *What's your pronoun? Strategies for inclusion in the workplace.* https://outandequal.org/whats-your-pronoun-strategies-for-inclusion/

Sames, K. M. (2015). *Documenting occupational therapy practice* (3rd ed.). Pearson Prentice Hall.

Wells, S.A. (2016). Health research and issues of race, ethnicity, and culture. In S.A. Wells, R. M. Black, & J. Gupta, *Culture and occupation* (3rd ed., pp. 387–400). AOTA Press.

Safety, Infection Control, and Personal Protective Equipment

Helene Smith-Gabai, Suzanne E. Holm, and John Lien Margetis

LEARNING OBJECTIVES

After reading this chapter, the reader will be able to:

1. Apply infection control practices for the most common infectious conditions based on their transmission routes.
2. Differentiate between standard and transmission-based precautions and the case for each within various healthcare settings.
3. Analyze the role of occupational therapy practitioners in infection control and prevention.

Introduction

Infection control refers to procedures that limit exposure to bacteria, viruses, and other transmissible infectious microorganisms and prevent infection spread within healthcare settings. Infection control practices help protect patients and healthcare staff from infection-related adverse outcomes (Centers for Disease Control and Prevention [CDC], 2020; George, 2018; Torriani & Taplitz, 2010). According to a scoping review by Schwendimann et al. (2018), **healthcare-associated infections (HAIs)** were identified as one of the top three causes of preventable hospital-related adverse events. Infection control practices are considered essential owing to the detrimental effects of infection and the critical nature of some infectious diseases. This chapter covers best practices for infection control precautions, including hand hygiene and **personal protective equipment (PPE)**, reviews the more commonly encountered infectious conditions and transmission methods, and suggests actions if exposed to an infectious pathogen.

Hospital-acquired infections were previously referred to as nosocomial infections, but they have more recently been replaced by the phrase healthcare-associated infections (HAIs) (George, 2018). The most common types of HAIs are related to invasive device use (e.g., catheters, central lines, ventilators) and surgical site infections (CDC, 2021a). Infections are associated with morbidity and mortality rates and are the fourth leading cause of death in the United States (Fairchild et al., 2018). Of the 10 leading causes of death globally, 3 are **communicable diseases**. Specifically, lower respiratory infections rate as the world's most deadly, ranking fourth in 2019, resulting in 2.6 million deaths (World Health Organization [WHO], 2020). That same year in the United States, acute respiratory infections (i.e., pneumonia and influenza) were the ninth leading cause of death, with 49,783 deaths (CDC, 2021b). In 2020, COVID-19 moved into the top 10 causes of global deaths as a communicable disease that disproportionately affected those with chronic and age-related health conditions (e.g., diabetes, obesity) and was the third leading cause of death in the United States (Ahmad et al., 2021; Woolf et al., 2021). In addition, despite declining rates worldwide, communicable diarrheal diseases also remain one of the top 10 causes of death globally (WHO, 2020).

Infection control practices were first adopted in the 1950s in response to an epidemic of nosocomial staph infection (*Staphylococcus aureus*) (Torriani & Taplitz, 2010). In 1996, the CDC first published *Guidelines for Isolation Precautions in Hospitals*, which established Universal Precautions to protect healthcare staff and their patients from infectious diseases such as HIV/AIDS and hepatitis (George, 2018). In 2007, the CDC updated infection control guidelines to include two types of precautions: **standard precautions** and **transmission-based precautions** (George, 2018). Standard precautions are considered wider-ranging and more inclusive than universal precautions. Standard precautions apply to all patients, regardless of suspected or confirmed infection status, serving as the primary manner of reducing HAIs. Transmission-based precautions are implemented when transmission of an infectious organism is inadequately interrupted by standard precautions alone (Siegel et al., 2019).

Infection Prevention and Control Practices

Keeping patients and healthcare workers safe through infection prevention and control policies and practices is a top priority for many hospitals and healthcare facilities (Association for Professionals in Infection Control and Epidemiology, n.d.). According to the American Occupational Therapy Association (AOTA), occupational therapy (OT) is an essential service that can boost a patient's immune system and promote infection prevention through engagement in activity and movement therapies (AOTA, 2020a; Margetis et al., 2021). OT practitioners recognize the value of infection prevention protocols across all practice settings and the importance of education and training in infection control practices for themselves and their patients.

Standard Precautions

In most healthcare settings, *standard precautions* (previously referred to as universal precautions) are uniformly implemented on the principle that all bodily fluids, secretions, skin, and mucous membranes may transmit infectious agents. Standard precautions typically include hand hygiene, glove use, and depending on the anticipated exposure, gown, mask, eye protection, or face shield (Siegel et al.,

---

BOX 32.1 STEPS OF PROPER HAND HYGIENE

1. Wet hands with water and apply enough soap to lather all surfaces.
2. Decontaminate hands by vigorously rubbing all surfaces of hands together, including palmar, interdigital, and dorsal surfaces, for at least 20 seconds.
3. Rinse hands and pat dry with a disposable paper towel or air dryer. Avoid reusable towels to avoid cross-contamination.
4. In facilities without motion or pedal-activated sinks, clinicians may opt to turn off water faucets with a paper towel to minimize the risk of recontaminating hands.

Source: Adapted from Longtin, Y., Sax, H., Allegranzi, B., Schneider, F., & Pittet, D. (2011). Hand hygiene. *New England Journal of Medicine, 364*(13), e24. https://doi.org/10.1056/nejmvcm0903599.

2019). For example, standard precautions for routine OT patient care typically require hand hygiene and gloves. In comparison, standard precautions for providers working in critical care settings where there is a greater risk of exposure to respiratory secretions, blood, or other bodily fluids may require the use of eye and face protection along with the requisite hand hygiene, gowns, and gloves.

Up to 40% of HAIs are attributed to cross-infection from the hands of healthcare workers through direct patient contact or indirectly through contact with contaminated surfaces or equipment (Weber et al., 2010). Therefore, hand hygiene has become an essential job task of all healthcare providers, including OT practitioners working in any healthcare setting (Longtin et al., 2011). Although clinicians often prefer the convenience of alcohol-based hand sanitizers, proper handwashing using soap and water remains superior as hand sanitizers are ineffective against certain types of infections (e.g., *Clostridium difficile*) (CDC, 2002). Additionally, many hand sanitizer manufacturers recommend handwashing between various sanitizer applications. See Box 32.1 and Figure 32.1 for steps for proper hand hygiene.

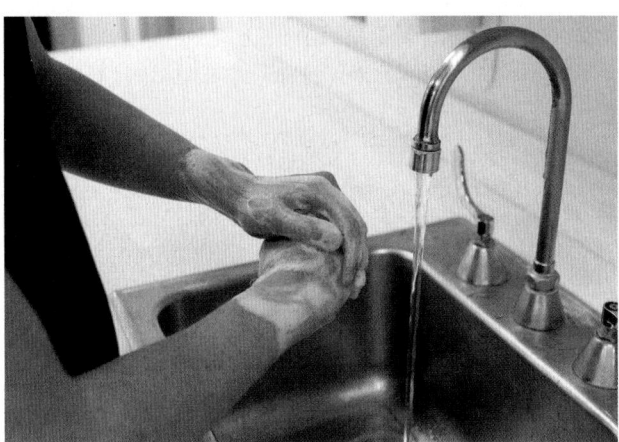

FIGURE 32.1 Handwashing.

Transmission-Based Precautions

Transmission-based precautions typically include contact precautions, droplet precautions, and airborne precautions that can be used alone or in combination, if an infection has multiple transmission modes (Siegel et al., 2019). Transmission-based precaution practices and training may also vary based on institutional guidelines.

Contact Precautions

Contact precautions prevent the transmission of pathogens that spread through direct or indirect patient contact and include wearing a gown and gloves, which are typically discarded after use. Additionally, most facilities prefer to place patients with contact precautions in single-occupancy rooms when possible. OT practitioners should don and doff appropriate PPE (gown and gloves) upon entering and before exiting the patient's room. Figure 32.2 highlights contact precautions.

Droplet Precautions

Droplet precautions prevent transmission of infections that spread via respiratory droplets or mucous membrane contact (Siegel et al., 2019). Additional ventilation or negative pressure is unnecessary because these droplets are typically larger and do not travel long distances. When possible, patients on droplet precautions are placed in single-occupancy rooms. OT practitioners should don a standard surgical mask (not a respirator) upon entry, should dispose of the mask upon exit, and may use eye protection such as goggles or a face shield. See Figure 32.3 for droplet precautions.

Airborne Precautions

Airborne precautions prevent transmission of infections that can travel long distances or remain suspended in the air for extended periods (Siegel et al., 2019). Patients are preferably placed in a single-occupancy **airborne infection isolation room (AIIR)** with special ventilation and

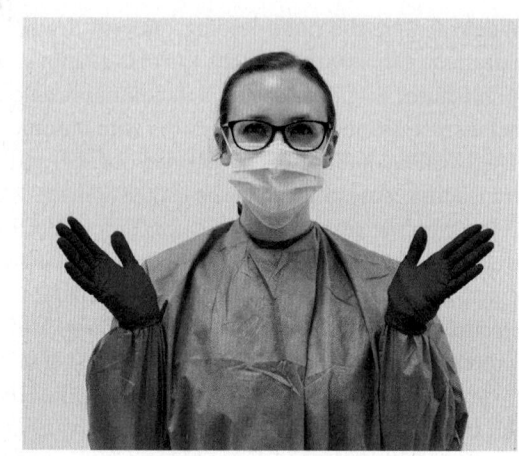

FIGURE 32.3 **Droplet precautions.**

negative pressure capability. When entering or exiting an airborne room, OT practitioners should don/doff appropriate PPE (e.g., gown, gloves, N95 respirator or powered air-purifying respirator [PAPR], face shield, or goggles). Additionally, staff should participate in routine PPE training and fit testing to ensure proper donning/doffing techniques and adequate seal to the N95 respirator or PAPR. Refer to Figure 32.4 for airborne precautions. Refer to Figure 32.5 and Box 32.2 regarding steps for donning an N95 respirator.

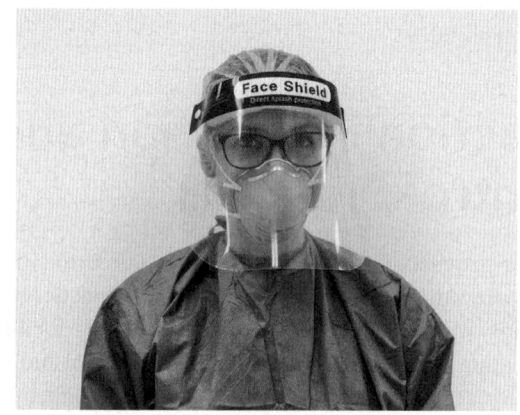

FIGURE 32.4 **Airborne precautions.**

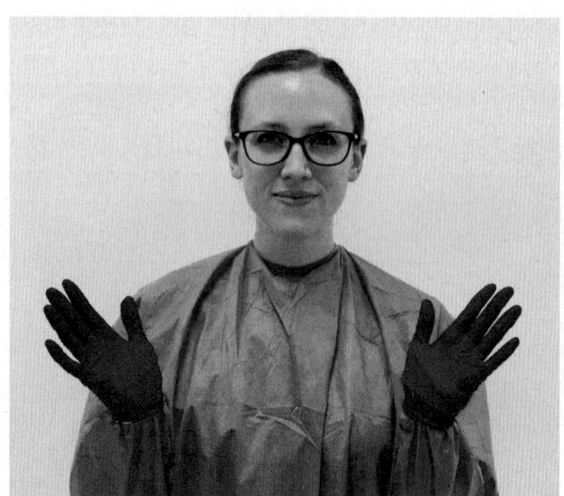

FIGURE 32.2 **Contact precautions.**

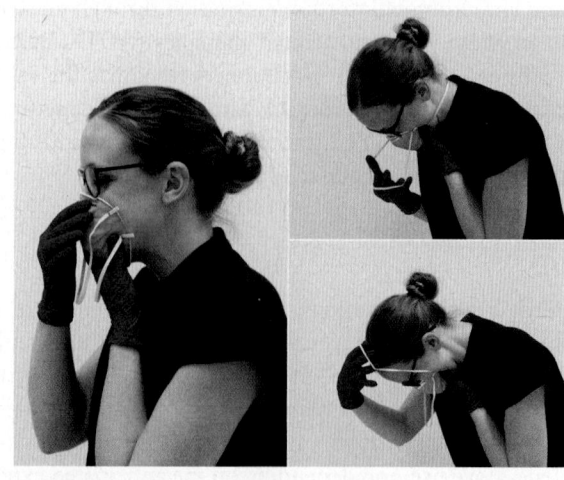

FIGURE 32.5 **N95 donning grid.**

STEPS FOR PROPERLY DONNING AN N95 RESPIRATOR

1. Hold the respirator in the palm of your hand with the straps facing the floor.
2. Place the N95 respirator on your face covering your nose and mouth.
3. Pull the bottom strap up and over top of your head and put it behind your head below your ears.
4. Take the upper strap and put it behind your head toward the crown of your head.
5. Mold the nosepiece of the respirator over the bridge of your nose to obtain a tight seal.
6. Perform a fit check to ensure a good seal against the skin.

*Always follow the manufacturer's instructions for wearing a respirator.

Source: Adapted from Centers for Disease Control and Prevention. (2014). *Donning PPE: Put on N95 respirator.* Retrieved January 25, 2022, from https://www.cdc.gov/vhf/ebola/hcp/ppe-training/n95respirator_gown/donning_09.html

Enhanced Barrier Precautions

Enhanced barrier precautions are between standard and contact precautions (CDC, 2019). Enhanced barrier precautions were established to address a new wave of highly infectious **multidrug-resistant organisms (MDROs)** often found in chronically ill patients who reside in healthcare facilities for extended periods (e.g., long-term care facilities). These precautions are implemented during specific activities with patients with a targeted MDRO and indwelling line or wound, but where contact precautions do not apply (CDC, 2019). Enhanced barrier precautions include wearing PPE, specifically gloves and gowns, during activities where there is close contact with patients, such as dressing, bathing, toileting, hygiene, and transferring. In some cases where patients harbor MDROs such as *Candida auris*, precautions can include mandatory clothing changes, limiting nursing ratios to 1:1, and scheduling therapy sessions at the beginning or end of the day to disrupt the spread of the MDRO (CDC, 2019).

Protective Isolation Precautions

Protective isolation precautions are established for immunocompromised patients, such as patients undergoing hematopoietic stem cell transplantation, those with burns, or patients with neutropenia (Banach et al., 2016; Isolation of Patients, n.d.; Siegel et al., 2019). Protective isolation precautions are intended to reduce the risk of inadvertent HAI spread of pathogens to patients who may have difficulty mounting an adequate immune response. Although practices vary across facilities, appropriate PPE typically includes a combination of standard, droplet, and contact precautions. Notably, in the current post-COVID era, with many

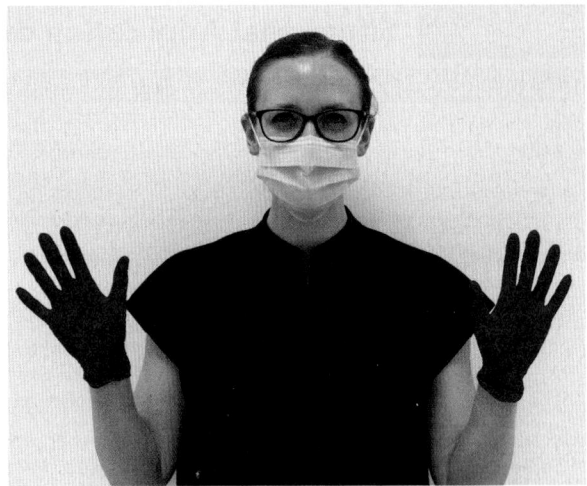

FIGURE 32.6 **Protective precautions.**

healthcare facilities continuing to mask all healthcare providers, OT practitioners should don new PPE (e.g., a standard face mask) when entering a protective isolation room. Protective isolation is sometimes referred to as reverse isolation. Refer to Figure 32.6 for protective precautions and Box 32.3 for CDC recommendations regarding donning and doffing PPE and avoiding cross-contamination.

Creating a positive culture of safety around infection prevention and control is critical. Recommendations for best practices around infection control in everyday situations and environments are outlined in Table 32.1.

CENTERS FOR DISEASE CONTROL AND PREVENTION RECOMMENDATIONS FOR DONNING AND DOFFING PERSONAL PROTECTIVE EQUIPMENT

- Different facilities will have different processes for PPE protocols. Be sure to follow all facility-specific protocols.
- The CDC recommends the following sequence for *donning* PPE: hand hygiene, gown, mask or respirator, eye protection, and gloves.
- The CDC recommends the following sequence for *doffing* PPE: gown and gloves, eye protection, mask or respirator, and hand hygiene.
- When doffing a contaminated gown, grasp the soiled gown *with gloved hands* and pull away from the body to break the ties, gently folding or rolling the gown into an *inside-out* bundle. Once the gown is rolled into a small bundle, peel gloves off and avoid cross-contamination by touching only the inside of the gown/gloves with bare/ungloved hands.
- Perform hand hygiene immediately after removing all PPE.

| TABLE 32.1 | Situational Application of Infection Prevention and Control Practices |

Situational or Environmental Factor	Infection Control Best Practices
Soiled patient care equipment, textiles, and laundry	Handle cautiously to minimize the transfer of microorganisms; wear gloves and perform hand hygiene; follow facility guidelines for bagging and containment.
Contaminated surfaces	Develop procedures for routine cleaning and disinfecting frequently touched surfaces in patient care areas.
Avoid touching mucous membranes (lips, mouth, nasal passages, and eyes or conjunctival membranes)	Exposed mucous membranes are a portal for infectious disease transmission and pathogens; hands are a carrier for the transmission of infections; scrupulous and frequent hand hygiene is needed to reduce auto- or self-inoculation.
Avoid consumption of food and drinks	Prohibit food and drink consumption in areas where exposure to infectious materials is possible or exists. Avoid smoking, makeup application, and handling contact lenses.
Proper disposal of needles and sharps	Use sharps safety devices and needleless or no sharps alternatives; dispose of used sharps in puncture-resistant containers; do not hand-manipulate used needles; watch for sharps in linens, beds, floors, and disposal containers.
Respiratory hygiene and cough etiquette	Cover mouth and nose when sneezing or coughing with a tissue or elbow and instruct others to do the same; dispose of tissues in a no-touch receptacle; perform hand hygiene after contact with respiratory secretions; wear face mask; maintain a separation of > 3 ft.
Additional considerations	Encourage donning masks before exiting hospital room; facilitate handwashing before meals and after toileting; monitor skin integrity and reposition to reduce the risk of skin breakdown; encourage oral care to prevent hospital-acquired pneumonia and other opportunistic infections.

Sources: Centers for Disease Control and Prevention. (2015). *Recommendations for application of standard precautions for the care of all patients in all healthcare settings.* https://www.cdc.gov/infectioncontrol/guidelines/isolation/appendix/standard-precautions.html; Kwok, Y. L., Gralton, J., & McLaws, M. L. (2015). Face touching: A frequent habit that has implications for hand hygiene. *American Journal of Infection Control, 43*(2), 112–114. https://doi.org/10.1016/j.ajic.2014.10.015; and Liao, Y.-M., Tsai, J.-R., & Chou, F.-H. (2015). The effectiveness of an oral health care program for preventing ventilator-associated pneumonia. *Nursing in Critical Care, 20*(2), 89–97. https://doi.org/10.1111/nicc.12037.

Overview of Common Infections and Transmission Mechanisms

In the United States, 1 in 31 hospitalized patients and 1 in 43 nursing home residents have an HAI (CDC, 2018), although that number is likely larger with the recent Coronavirus (COVID-19) pandemic. Even more challenging is the prevalence of multidrug-resistant infections, despite advances in infection prevention strategies.

Whether infection spread is community-acquired (e.g., COVID-19) or hospital-acquired (e.g., ventilator-associated pneumonia), the goal is to slow or stop transmission, interrupting the infection cycle and hindering the pathogen's ability to grow and spread. The minimum infection prevention steps include hand hygiene, respiratory hygiene, the use of PPE, injection and sharp object safety and disposal, and environmental cleaning (Douedi & Douedi, 2021).

For disease or infection to spread, the transfer of infectious agents must occur. Infectious microorganisms include bacteria, fungi, viruses, **protozoa**, and **prions**. Infection transmission routes include direct contact (e.g., touching) and indirect contact. Indirect contact may include

environmental (e.g., contaminated food), **fomite** (e.g., doorknobs, handrails), **vector** (e.g., mosquito), and airborne (e.g., respiratory tract) transmission (Antonovics et al., 2017). Examples of common ways that pathogens may enter or exit the body are through a break in skin or skin contact, inhalation/exhalation through the respiratory tract, exposure to mucous membranes, or the gastrointestinal or genitourinary tract (Antonovics et al., 2017; Fairchild et al., 2018). When the infection cycle is not interrupted, the risk of spreading the disease increases. Sepsis is the condition where an infection spreads from the initial site, enters the person's bloodstream, and results in widespread inflammation, tissue damage, and potentially organ failure and death (Kerrigan, 2017).

Individuals who are at a higher risk for healthcare-acquired infections include those with a compromised immune system (e.g., receiving treatment for cancer, diabetes), those with indwelling catheters, those who are very young or elderly, those who are unvaccinated against common diseases, those who have extended hospital stays, or those treated by healthcare workers who do not wash their hands (Haque et al., 2018).

Various transmissible infections have different characteristics and precautions, highlighted in Table 32.2, along with related special considerations. The table is not exhaustive but includes some of the more commonly encountered conditions. Practitioners should be aware of infections that are less common. Examples include monkeypox and Ebola.

TABLE 32.2 Typically Encountered Infectious Diseases

Organism (Type)	Type and Routes of Transmission	Precautions	Special Considerations
Aspergillus (fungal)	Fungal: enters the body through inhalation; infection can spread from the lungs or sinuses to other organs.	Standard: contact and airborne precautions if copious drainage with infection	A common mold found in the environment. Problematic for persons with weakened immune system, pulmonary disease, infection, or after transplantation
Candida auris (C. auris) (fungal)	Can enter the bloodstream, spreading infection throughout the body via lines, tubes, or central venous catheters	Contact or enhanced barrier precautions	It can spread through person-to-person contact or from contaminated surfaces or equipment. All equipment should be disinfected, and PPE should be worn during activities involving close patient contact.
Carbapenem-resistant enterobacterales (CRE) (bacterial)	Transmitted through skin contact, wounds from injury or surgery, or stool	Contact or enhanced barrier precautions	This multidrug-resistant organism (MDRO) is typically associated with the urinary tract (e.g., retention or catheter). It spreads through person-to-person contact or contact with contaminated medical equipment. Hand hygiene should be performed and all equipment disinfected. PPE should be worn when there is close patient contact. Dedicated equipment is recommended. Toilets and sink drains may be an environmental reservoir for CRE.
Clostridium difficile (C-diff) (bacterial)	Transmitted by coming in contact with an infected person's feces or contaminated surfaces	Contact	Hand hygiene with soap and water is recommended. Alcohol-based foams and gels are not effective to kill spores. PPE (gown and gloves) is recommended. All surfaces should be sanitized with bleach-based products.
	Transmitted through direct contact with breaks in the skin, mucous membranes, exposure to EVD, infected blood or body fluids, parenteral route, or semen of a person recovered from EVD	Contact	EVD can travel to regional lymph nodes and other organs, resulting in multiorgan failure and shock. Wear PPE and avoid direct contact with blood, body fluids, or contaminated surfaces or equipment. Provide dedicated or disposable equipment. A vaccine is available.
Hepatitis (viral)	It is transmitted through different routes depending on the type of hepatitis. Hepatitis A virus (HAV) can be transmitted when ingesting food or water contaminated with HAV stool. Hepatitis B virus (HBV) can be transmitted through a skin puncture or when mucosal linings contact infected bodily fluids, including blood. With hepatitis C virus (HCV), the transmission route is from contact with an infected person's blood (e.g., puncture with a contaminated needle). Hepatitis delta virus (HDV) and hepatitis E virus (HEV) are less common.	Standard, but may have contact precautions if coming in contact with patients who are bowel or bladder incontinent	Avoid eating or drinking in patient care areas. Do not share food or cigarettes or electronic smoking devices with patients or their families. Make sure all open wounds are covered to reduce the risk of exposure. Observe good hand and personal hygiene and PPE protocols. Adhere to facility policies if exposed. This may include reporting exposure to infection control and employee health. Vaccines are available for HAV and HBV, and in most facilities, vaccinations are a condition of employment. The HBV vaccine is effective against HDV.

(continued)

TABLE 32.2 Typically Encountered Infectious Diseases (continued)

Organism (Type)	Type and Routes of Transmission	Precautions	Special Considerations
HIV/AIDS (viral)	Transmission of the human immunodeficiency virus is through contact (HIV) of infected blood or bodily fluids with mucosal linings or skin puncture (i.e., infected blood transfusion, IV drug use, or unprotected sex with someone infected with the virus).	Standard	PPE should be worn if coming in contact with infected blood or bodily fluids. Adhere to facility policies if exposed. Exposure should be reported to infection control and employee health.
Influenza (flu) (viral)	Transmission is generally through inhalation of droplets from someone coughing or sneezing who has the flu. The virus may also be transmitted by touching contaminated surfaces and touching the mouth, nose, or eyes.	Droplet and contact	Respiratory hygiene and cough etiquette should be maintained. A vaccine is available. In many healthcare settings, the annual vaccine is mandated as a condition of employment.
Methicillin-resistant Staphylococcus aureus (MRSA) (bacterial)	Transmission is through direct contact with persons with MRSA or surfaces and devices contaminated with MRSA bacteria.	Contact	PPE should be worn if contacting wounds or bodily fluids. Gloves should be changed and hand hygiene completed after contacting an MRSA-infected wound and before going to another body site (e.g., suctioning trach). Sanitize equipment after use.
Necrotizing fasciitis (bacterial)	Typically caused by group A Streptococcus bacteria; the bacteria enter the body through a break in the skin. It is rarely contagious but is a surgical emergency requiring timely care.	Standard	The bacteria can spread quickly through the body and cause sepsis, which may be fatal. Prompt intervention, including good wound care, is essential.
Pertussis (whooping cough) (bacterial)	It is caused by inhalation of aerosolized Bordetella pertussis bacteria, which attaches to upper respiratory system cilia. Droplets may be transmitted through sneezing, coughing, talking within close breathing space of someone with the infection.	Droplet and standard	This infection is highly contagious. A vaccine is available.
Pneumonia (PNA) (bacterial, viral, fungal)	Transmission can vary based on the organism. PNA can occur through inhalation of toxic substances or aspiration into the lungs (e.g., food, fluids, vomit, secretions).	Standard	There are different types of pneumonia, including community-acquired, nursing home–acquired, hospital-acquired, ventilator-acquired, and aspiration PNA. Some risk factors for PNA include decreased consciousness, intubation, mechanical ventilation, poor oral hygiene, dental disease, and dysphagia. Elevate the head of bed at least 30° to minimize the risk of aspiration PNA. Encourage using incentive spirometry after surgery. Vaccines are available and recommended for adults >65 years.
SARS-CoV-1 and 2 (viral)	Particles are inhaled; however, this virus can also be transmitted through direct contact with the eyes, nose, or mouth.	Contact, droplet, and airborne	Airborne precautions should be in place during aerosol-generating procedures (e.g., during intubation, oral suctioning, and oral care) or any activity that may aerosolize the virus. PPE includes wearing a fitted N95 mask, gown, gloves, face shield, PAPRs, and disposable booties and hairnets in some facilities. Follow facility policies and procedures and CDC guidelines for screening and disease management recommendations. Vaccine is available and highly effective at reducing the severity of illness, although it does not prevent infectious spread between individuals.

Varicella-zoster virus (shingles) (viral)	The varicella-zoster virus (VZV) is usually dormant in persons who previously had chickenpox. Shingles occur when the virus becomes reactivated. VZV can be transmitted through contact with fluid from rash blisters.	Contact and airborne	Practitioners who are immunocompromised, who are pregnant, who never had chickenpox, or who are unvaccinated against chickenpox should NOT work with patients with varicella-zoster. If a person never had chickenpox or the vaccine and is exposed to VZV through someone with shingles, they will develop chickenpox and not shingles. The virus can be reactivated as shingles. Once a shingles rash crusts, the virus is not transmissible. A shingles vaccine is available and recommended for persons >60 years.
Tuberculosis (TB) (bacterial)	Transmitted through inhalation of airborne particles expelled by someone with active TB. Particles may be transmitted through a sneeze, through cough, or while talking.	Airborne	Patients with active TB will be placed in an airborne infection isolation room (AIIR). Therapists should wear a properly fitted N95 respirator before entering the AIIR. Cough etiquette and respiratory hygiene practices should be adhered to. According to CDC guidelines, annual TB skin testing is no longer recommended unless there is exposure or continuing transmission within the healthcare setting.
Vancomycin-resistant enterococci (VRE) (bacterial)	Transmitted through skin contact (e.g., healthcare workers' hands) with persons, equipment, or surfaces contaminated with body fluids infected with VRE	Contact	Special consideration is warranted if working on toileting with patients with VRE. Clean all environmental surfaces thoroughly. Diligent handwashing is essential.
West Nile virus (WNV) (viral)	Transmission to humans is through the bite of infected mosquitoes. In extremely rare cases, it can be transmitted from mother to baby (i.e., pregnancy, delivery, breastfeeding), blood transfusions, or transplantation.	Standard	Possible complications of WNV are meningitis, meningoencephalitis, or encephalitis.

CDC, Centers for Disease Control and Prevention; PAPR, powered air-purifying respirator.

Sources: Centers for Disease Control and Prevention. (2017). *Causes and transmission. Pertussis (whooping cough).* https://www.cdc.gov/pertussis/about/causes-transmission.html; Centers for Disease Control and Prevention. (2019). *Type and duration of precautions recommended for selected infections and conditions. Infection Control.* https://www.cdc.gov/infectioncontrol/guidelines/isolation/appendix/type-duration-precautions.html; Centers for Disease Control and Prevention. (2019). *General information about Candida auris.* https://www.cdc.gov/fungal/Candida-auris/; Centers for Disease Control and Prevention. (2019). *Clinicians: Information about CRE. Healthcare-associated infections.* https://www.cdc.gov/hai/organisms/cre/cre-clinicians.html; Centers for Disease Control and Prevention. (2019). *COVID-19 overview and infection prevention and control priorities in non-US healthcare settings.* https://www.cdc.gov/coronavirus/2019-ncov/hcp/non-us-settings/overview/index.html; Centers for Disease Control and Prevention. (2019). *Transmission.* https://www.cdc.gov/shingles/about/transmission.html; Centers for Disease Control and Prevention. (2019). *Necrotizing fasciitis: All you need to know.* https://www.cdc.gov/groupastrep/diseases-public/necrotizing-fasciitis.html#rarely-contagious; Centers for Disease Control and Prevention. (2021). *Information for healthcare professionals about Aspergillosis. Fungal diseases.* https://www.cdc.gov/fungal/diseases/aspergillosis/health-professionals.html; Centers for Disease Control and Prevention. (2021). *Ebola Virus Disease (EVD) information for clinicians in U.S. healthcare settings.* https://www.cdc.gov/vhf/ebola/clinicians/evd/clinicians.html; Centers for Disease Control and Prevention. (2021). *TB screening and testing of health care personnel.* https://www.cdc.gov/tb/topic/testing/healthcareworkers.htm; Centers for Disease Control and Prevention. (2021). *Transmission. West Nile Virus Home.* https://www.cdc.gov/westnile/transmission/index.html; Hepatitis B Foundation. (2021). *The ABC's of viral hepatitis.* https://www.hepb.org/what-is-hepatitis-b/the-abcs-of-viral-hepatitis/; Johns Hopkins Medicine. (2021). *West Nile Virus. Conditions and Diseases.* https://www.hopkinsmedicine.org/health/conditions-and-diseases/west-nile-virus; Kerrigan, D. A. (2017). *Infectious diseases and autoimmune disorders.* In H. Smit-Gabai & S. E. Holm (Eds.), *Occupational therapy in acute care* (2nd ed., pp. 471–487). AOTA Press; National Institute for Occupational Safety and Health. (2015). *MRSA and the workplace.* https://www.cdc.gov/niosh/topics/mrsa/; National Institute for Occupational Safety and Health. (2016). *Bloodborne infectious diseases: HIV/AIDS, Hepatitis B, Hepatitis C.* https://www.cdc.gov/niosh/topics/bbp/emergnedl.html; Smit-Gabai, H., & Schmitz, M. (2017). The pulmonary system. In H. Smit-Gabai & S. E. Holm (Eds.), *Occupational therapy in acute care* (2nd ed., pp. 278–279). AOTA Press; and World Health Organization. (2020). *Coronavirus disease (COVID-19): How is it transmitted?* https://www.who.int/health-topics/coronavirus#tab=tab_2.

Clinical Reasoning and Leadership in Infection Prevention and Control

In addition to the following guidance from the CDC, OT practitioners may use their professional ethics, clinical reasoning, and leadership to make decisions about infection prevention and control practices. Professional statements and recommendations can be found in resources like the Occupational Therapy Code of Ethics (AOTA, 2020b) and AOTA's statement on disaster response (2017) for guidance and ethical responses during natural disasters and disease threats. Specific to the Code of Ethics (AOTA, 2020b), practitioners may consider these standards of conduct:

- Professional integrity, responsibility, and accountability, principle of justice, Standards A and C; OT personnel must "comply with current federal and state laws, state scope of practice guidelines, and AOTA policies and Official Documents that apply to the profession of occupational therapy" and "inform employers, employees, colleagues, students and researchers of applicable policies, laws, and Official Documents" (p. 5).
- Therapeutic relationship, principle of nonmaleficence, Standard G; OT personnel must ". . . not abandon the service recipient and attempt to facilitate appropriate transitions when unable to provide services for any reason" (p. 6).
- Professional competence, education, supervision, and training, principle of fidelity, Standard E; OT personnel must "take action to resolve incompetent, disruptive, unethical, illegal, or impaired practice in self or others" (p. 8).

Practitioners may want to consider the following recommendations (AOTA, 2020a, 2020c, 2020d; Margetis et al., 2021) when determining the best course of action, especially for limiting disease or infection transmission:

1. Use resources efficiently and accommodate changes in usual standards of care while avoiding the delay of care where it could be detrimental.
2. Advocate to avoid the spread of disease and for access to PPE.

3. Be aware of the scope of practice and assessment of competence, especially if providing care or completing novel tasks.

Healthcare practitioners also need to consider workplace policies and procedures regarding workplace exposures to situations, pathogens, and infectious diseases. Important defenses against infectious diseases include the proper use of vaccines, antibiotics, screening and testing guidelines, and improvements in diagnosing disease (Office of Disease Prevention and Health Promotion, 2021). Practitioners should refer to their facility's Minimum Data Set (MDS) and Occupational Safety and Health Administration (OSHA) standards on PPE regarding recommended action steps following exposure to a pathogen or infectious disease (OSHA, n.d.).

Cultural Implications

As social beings, we have many verbal and nonverbal ways to greet family, friends, colleagues, and strangers, including handshakes, hugs, cheek-kissing, hand-kissing, nose touching, and pressing foreheads and noses together (e.g., Maori tradition of hongi). Social connections may be preserved through noncontact or low-touch greetings, including nodding, smiling, bowing, waving, greeting with folded hands, bumping elbows, foot-shaking, tapping feet, or pressing a hand over one's heart. In epidemics, pandemics, or endemics, people may modify greetings to include no-touch or contactless options to minimize the spread of disease while complying with social distancing and mask-wearing (Dally-Steele & Terry, 2020; Mela & Whitworth, 2014).

Changing greeting practices by avoiding hand contact in medical settings could have positive health benefits. Human hands are a carrier of disease transmission harboring pathogenic microorganisms, with most studies identifying more than 150 bacterial species on the palms alone (Edmonds-Wilson et al., 2015). Healthcare providers are responsible toward their patients and community to model best practices for handwashing and modify greetings to minimize disease transmission (Khichar et al, 2020; Sklansky et al., 2014). See OT Story 32.1.

OT STORY 32.1 MR. ANDERSON: ADDRESSING LIMITED COMMUNICATION AND SELF-CARE PARTICIPATION OWING TO COVID-19

Occupational Profile

Mr. Anderson is a 74-year-old retired schoolteacher, and his leisure occupations include spending time with family, gardening, and table tennis. During retirement, his typical routines include rising early each morning to read his newspaper with a cup of coffee and taking walks in the afternoon with his wife.

Hospital Course and Evaluation

Mr. Anderson tested positive for COVID-19 after developing a cough. He was initially quarantined at home, but he required hospitalization 9 days after initial symptom onset because he became progressively weaker. Upon admission, his blood oxygen saturation (SpO$_2$) was 82% but improved with 10 liters per minute (LPM) of supplemental oxygen. He

OT STORY 32.1 MR. ANDERSON: ADDRESSING LIMITED COMMUNICATION AND SELF-CARE PARTICIPATION OWING TO COVID-19 (*continued*)

was placed in an AIIR with a loud negative pressure intake fan throughout his hospital stay.

Mr. Anderson's initial OT evaluation in the intensive care unit (ICU) revealed disrupted occupational performance and routines with multifocal impairments in body systems and functions. Mr. Anderson had difficulty hearing clinicians through their PPE owing to environmental and personal factors such as the loud negative pressure fan and chemotherapy-induced hearing loss. He required total assistance with activities of daily living (ADLs) and mobility owing to severe ICU-acquired weakness and required ventilatory support through a tracheostomy. He also experienced significant delirium owing to the isolation in the COVID unit and disruption of his sleep/wake cycle.

Patient's Goals

While in intensive care, Mr. Anderson's goals included improving communication with providers and his family using his tablet and laptop computer, increasing independence with ADLs, and improving his mobility to sit in a bedside chair for a few hours each day.

Interventions

OT intervention addressed immediate environmental concerns like Mr. Anderson's difficulty hearing the providers through their masks. OT practitioners provided Mr. Anderson with an augmented communication board and posted signs on his door notifying entering providers of his hearing impairment. Additionally, OT practitioners

worked with engineering to reduce the fan speed (and thus, noise) during provider rounding.

OT practitioners combined Mr. Anderson's goals of getting out of bed and communicating with his family by implementing a mobility schedule for him. He would either ask the nursing staff to transfer him to the chair with the mechanical lift or wait for therapy staff to manually transfer him, strengthening his core and lower extremities, before video-calling his family each day. OT practitioners ensured his electronic devices were accessibly located on his bedside table and provided positioning recommendations to facilitate easier typing given his upper extremity weakness.

During all sessions, OT practitioners wore full protective PPE, including isolation gowns, gloves, and N95 masks. Additionally, all devices and equipment brought into the room were meticulously disinfected following each use to avoid cross-contamination and **iatrogenic** infections in other patients.

In preparation for discharge, the OT practitioner worked with the case manager to identify a post-acute inpatient rehabilitation facility that would meet Mr. Anderson's needs.

Questions

1. What additional precautions would you use with Mr. Anderson?
2. Because Mr. Anderson required an AIIR, in what other ways could his social isolation be decreased, a supportive environment be increased, and his communication be improved?

Conclusion

Many infections and pathogens can pose a risk to patients, caregivers, and other stakeholders in healthcare settings. Owing to the seriousness of infectious diseases and their potential to result in further complications, morbidity, and mortality, all healthcare providers have the responsibility to adhere to infection prevention and control practices. The sequelae of infection may remain long after the initial infection has resolved. For example, a large international survey study of patients with long-COVID revealed that

neurologic and cognitive symptoms, fatigue, and malaise persisted 6 months after infection, affecting their quality of life (Davis et al., 2021; Wilcox & Frank, 2021). Although standard precautions are the basic level of infection control used in all patient care, transmission-based precautions minimize the transmission of known or suspected infections. Practitioners must understand, implement, and model best infection control practices, including hand hygiene and the use of PPE, to maintain barriers to the infection cycle and prevent the spread of infection to themselves and others.

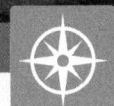

EXPANDING OUR PERSPECTIVES

Safety in All Practice Settings

Lisa Mahaffey

Safety from hospital-based infection is the focus of this chapter, and it is an important one. But it is not the only

safety issue service users face in the healthcare system. After many years working in mental healthcare, I argue that it is time to take a more critical lens when it comes to the role of safety in healthcare decisions. Much of my practice was in hospital-based mental healthcare units, including

(continued)

EXPANDING OUR PERSPECTIVES (*continued*)

units dedicated to supporting people with dementia. These units are crisis intervention units for people at risk for harm because of cognitive or emotional challenges or difficult environmental situations. In units with older adults experiencing mental health disorders and dementia, safety also meant avoiding falls, safety from sharps, and being aware of signs of suicide. In many of these situations, keeping people "safe" often meant using the power afforded to healthcare providers to take away people's right to live in their homes and participate in their neighborhoods and communities, essentially reducing access to valued occupations for their own protection. I know that this same conversation happens all the time in acute care units for people with physical disabilities and even in schools and transitional programs for children and young adults with significant impairments. I would argue that the care teams choosing placement in nursing homes never consider the consequences of keeping people safe.

I live in Illinois, United States, where a significant amount of the long-term care dollars for people with physical, mental, and emotional disabilities continues to go to institutions (Illinois Department of Human Services [IDPH], 2020). This despite the legal right to community-based care established by Title 2 of the Americans with Disabilities Act (ADA, 1990) and upheld by the Olmstead supreme court Decision (Olmstead v L.C., 1999), which determined institutionalization was a form of discrimination. It is true that some people choose nursing home care for good reasons. However, the decision to place people in these facilities for long term is often based on two things: a perceived need to keep people safe and a lack of access to services that would support safe living within the community.

In 2008, the Money Follows the Person (MFP) demonstration project, which was designed to shift long-term care dollars to community-based care, provided researchers with an opportunity to understand the impact of institution-to-community transition (Medicaid.gov, 2022). What is striking are the stories people tell about the harm they experienced in institutional settings. In Illinois for example, statistics indicate that people moving out of nursing homes had three to four more comorbid health conditions than they went in (Hutchings, 2022). Illinois's regulatory body identified thousands of reports of abuse of all kinds in 2019, the latest report available (IDPH, 2020). These reports do not account for deaths owing to COVID-19 in the last 2 years (IDPH, 2022). In addition, studies about long-term institutionalization show serious impacts on executive functions such as decision-making, planning, organization, and other aspects needed for access to self-determination (Chow & Priebe, 2013).

People have the right to the *dignity of risk*. In many ways, the 2020 COVID pandemic elevated the discussion around the right to take risk, and the importance of reasonable, fact-based discussions around risk mitigation, that is,

social distancing and masks. People who are not labeled with illness or disability are afforded the right to take risks. How many people text while driving, forgo helmets on motorcycles, or ignore medical advice? This dignity is often taken away when a person is labeled with a condition considered disabling, especially one that involves perceived difference in cognitive capacity. Dignity of risk means the right to learn from our choices and to experience the consequences. It is the process by which we discover our capacity to do things, and it is how we learn to tolerate discomfort and form our sense of self. It is a human right.

OT practitioners have the skills to evaluate and address the fit between a person's desire and their capacity and the requirements of day-to-day tasks within their culture and environment. In fact, I would argue this is an ethical challenge that requires reconsidering any role we have played in decisions to institutionalize people. We must keep people safe from hospital infections for sure. We must also bring our knowledge and skills to discussions around the right to the dignity of risk, to allow choice for people around where they live and obtain services, and to discussions about the kinds of services and supports that mitigate risk when they choose options that seem "less safe." We must ally with people in the disability community in their efforts to make sure every voice is included when it comes to decision-making regarding where and how people receive their services. Lastly, we must be willing to fill roles in nontraditional settings where our distinct lens can support the creation of alternatives to conjugate living communities that afford people true opportunity to active engagement and a satisfying life.

References

The Americans with Disabilities Act of 1990. (1990). Pub. L. No. 101-336, 104 Stat. 328. http//www.ada.gov/pubs/adastatute08.htm

Chow, W. C., & Priebe, S. (2013). Understanding psychiatric institutionalization: A conceptual review. *Psychiatry, 13,* 169–183. http://www.biomedcentral.com/1471-244X/13/169.

Compliance Assessment Annual Report to the Court. www.dhs.state.il.us/OneNetLibrary/27897/documents/Mental%20Health/Williams/Reports/Williams-Court-Monitor-FY2021-Compliance-Assessment-Report.pdf

Hutchings, G. P. (2022). *Williams vs. Pritzker Case No. C4 673 Court Monitor FY20 2 1 (N.D. Ill.).*

Illinois Department of Human Services. (2020). *Long-term care annual report to the Illinois General Assembly.* https://www.ilga.gov/reports/ReportsSubmitted/1027RSGAEmail2280RSGAAttachLong-TermCareAnnualReport_2020.pdf

Illinois Department of Human Services. (2022). *COVID-19 long-term care data.* https://dph.illinois.gov/covid19/data/long-term-care-data.html

Medicaid.gov. (2022). *Money follows the person.* https://www.medicaid.gov/medicaid/long-term-services-supports/money-follows-person/index.html

Olmstead v. L. C. (Syllabus). 527 U.S. 581 (U.S. Supreme Court June 22, 1999).

Acknowledgments

The authors would like to thank Kelsey Peterson, OTD, OTR/L, and Carnie Lewis, OTD, OTR/L for developing and providing the photographic images featured throughout this chapter.

Lippincott® Connect *For additional resources on the subjects discussed in this chapter, visit Lippincott Connect.*

REFERENCES

Ahmad, F. B., Cisewski, J. A., Miniño, A., & Anderson, R. N. (2021). Provisional mortality data—United States, 2020. *MMWR Morbidity and Mortality Weekly Report 2021*. https://www.cdc.gov/mmwr/volumes/70/wr/mm7014e1.htm

American Occupational Therapy Association. (2017). AOTA's societal statement on disaster response and risk reduction. *American Journal of Occupational Therapy, 71*(Suppl._2), 7112410060p7112410061–7112410060p7112410063. https://doi.org/10.5014/ajot.2017.716S11

American Occupational Therapy Association. (2020a). *The role of occupational therapy: Providing care in a pandemic.* https://www.aota.org/Advocacy-Policy/Federal-Reg-Affairs/News/2020/OT-Pandemic.aspx

American Occupational Therapy Association. (2020b). Occupational therapy code of ethics. *American Journal of Occupational Therapy, 74*(supplement_3), 7413410005. https://doi.org/10.5014/ajot.2020.74S3006

American Occupational Therapy Association. (2020c). *COVID-19 FAQs for practitioners.* https://www.aota.org/Practice/Health-Wellness/COVID19/practitioners-faq.aspx

American Occupational Therapy Association. (2020d). *The advisory opinion for the Ethics Commission: An ethical response to the Covid-19 pandemic.* https://www.aota.org/~/media/Corporate/Files/Practice/Ethics/Advisory/Ethical-Response-to-COVID-19.pdf

Antonovics, J., Wilson, A. J., Forbes, M. R., Hauffe, H. C., Kallio, E. R., Leggett, H. C., Longdon, B., Okamura, B., Sait, S. M., & Webster, J. P. (2017). The evolution of transmission mode. *Philosophical Transactions of the Royal Society of London. Series B, Biological Sciences, 372*(1719), 20160083. https://doi.org/10.1098/rstb.2016.0083

Association for Professionals in Infection Control and Epidemiology. (n.d.). *Who are infection preventionists?* https://apic.org/monthly_alerts/who-are-infection-preventionists/

Banach, D. B., Seville, M. T., & Kusne, S. (2016). Infection prevention and control issues after solid organ transplantation. *Transplant Infections*, 843–867. https://doi.org/10.1007/978-3-319-28797-3_46

Centers for Disease Control and Prevention. (2002). Guideline for hand hygiene in health-care settings: Recommendations of the healthcare infection control practices advisory committee and the HICPAC/SHEA/APIC/IDSA hand hygiene task force. *MMWR Morbidity and Mortality Weekly Report, 51*(No. RR-16). https://www.cdc.gov/mmwr/PDF/rr/rr5116.pdf

Centers for Disease Control and Prevention. (2018). *HAI data.* https://www.cdc.gov/hai/data/index.html

Centers for Disease Control and Prevention. (2019). *Implementation of personal protective equipment (PPE) in nursing homes to prevent spread of novel targeted multidrug-resistant organisms (MDROs).* Healthcare-associated infections (HAIs): Containment Strategy. https://www.cdc.gov/hai/containment/PPE-Nursing-Homes.html

Centers for Disease Control and Prevention. (2020). *Infection control.* https://www.cdc.gov/infectioncontrol/index.html

Centers for Disease Control and Prevention. (2021a). *Data portal.* National Center for Emerging and Zoonotic Infectious Diseases (NCEZID), Division of Healthcare Quality Promotion (DHQP). https://www.cdc.gov/hai/data/portal/

Centers for Disease Control and Prevention. (2021b). *Leading causes of death.* https://www.cdc.gov/nchs/fastats/leading-causes-of-death.htm

Dally-Steele, B., & Terry, R. (2020). *Say hello to the world's new greetings.* https://www.bbc.com/travel/article/20200512-say-hello-to-the-worlds-new-greetings

Davis, H. E., Assaf, G. S., McCorkell, L., Wei, H., Low, R. J., Re'em, Y., Redfield, S., Austin, J. P., & Akrami, A. (2021). Characterizing long COVID in an international cohort: 7 months of symptoms and their impact. *EClinicalMedicine, 38*, 101019. https://doi.org/10.1016/j.eclinm.2021.101019

Douedi, S., & Douedi, H. (2021). Precautions, bloodborne, contact, and droplet. In *StatPearls* [Updated 2021 September 9]. StatPearls Publishing. https://www.ncbi.nlm.nih.gov/books/NBK551555/

Edmonds-Wilson, S. L., Nurinova, N. I., Zapka, C. A., Fierer, N., & Wilson, M. (2015). Review of human hand microbiome research. *Journal of Dermatological Science, 80*(1), 3–12. https://doi.org/https://doi.org/10.1016/j.jdermsci.2015.07.006

Fairchild, S. L., O'Shea, R. K., & Washington, R. D. (2018). *Approaches to infection control Pierson and Fairchild's principles & techniques of patient care* (6th ed., pp. 24–48). Elsevier.

George, A. H. (2018). Infection control and safety issues in the clinic. In H. M. Pendelton & W. Schultz-Krohn (Eds.), *Pedretti's occupational therapy practice skills for physical dysfunction* (8th ed., pp. 141–154). Elsevier.

Haque, M., Sartelli, M., McKimm, J., & Abu Bakar, M. (2018). Health care-associated infections—An overview. *Infection and Drug Resistance, 11*, 2321–2333. https://doi.org/10.2147/IDR.S177247

Isolation of Patients. (n.d.). *The Northern Ireland regional infection prevention and control manual.* https://www.niinfectioncontrolmanual.net/isolation-patients

Kerrigan, D. A. (2017). Infectious diseases and autoimmune disorders. In H. Smit-Gabai & S. E. Holm (Eds.), *Occupational therapy in acute care* (2nd ed., pp. 471–487). AOTA Press.

Khichar, S., Gopalakrishnan, M., Bohra, G. K., Garg, M. K., & Misra, S. (2020). 'Greet with NAMASTE, bye-bye handshake': A behavioural change campaign for infection prevention in the Emergency Department from Jodhpur, India. *Emergency Medicine Journal, 37*(9), 571. https://doi.org/10.1136/emermed-2020-210121

Longtin, Y., Sax, H., Allegranzi, B., Schneider, F., & Pittet, D. (2011). Hand hygiene. *New England Journal of Medicine, 364*(13), e24. https://doi.org/10.1056/nejmvcm0903599

Margetis, J. L., Wilcox, J., Thompson, C., & Mannion, N. (2021). Occupational therapy: Essential to critical care rehabilitation. *American Journal of Occupational Therapy, 75*(2), 7502170010p1. https://doi.org/10.5014/ajot.2021.048827

Mela, S., & Whitworth, D. E. (2014). The fist bump: A more hygienic alternative to the handshake. *American Journal of Infection Control, 42*(8), 916–917. https://doi.org/10.1016/j.ajic.2014.04.011

Occupational Safety and Health Administration. (n.d.). *Personal protective equipment.* https://www.osha.gov/personal-protective-equipment

Office of Disease Prevention and Health Promotion. (2021). *Immunization and infectious diseases.* https://www.healthypeople.gov/node/3527/data-

Schwendimann, R., Blatter, C., Dhaini, S., Simon, M., & Ausserhofer, D. (2018). The occurrence, types, consequences and preventability of in-hospital adverse events—A scoping review. *BMC Health Services Research, 18*(521), 1–13. https://doi.org/10.1186/s12913-018-3335-z

Siegel, J. D., Rhinehart, E., Jackson, M., & Chiarello, L., & the Healthcare Infection Control Practices Advisory Committee. (2019). *2007 guideline for isolation precautions: Preventing transmission of infectious agents in healthcare settings.* https://www.cdc.gov/infectioncontrol/pdf/guidelines/isolation-guidelines-H.pdf

Sklansky, M., Nadkarni, N., & Ramirez-Avila, L. (2014). Banning the handshake from the health care setting. *Journal of American Medicine, 311*(24): 2477–2478. https://doi.org/10.1001/jama.2014.4675

Torriani, F., & Taplitz, R. (2010). History of infection prevention and control. *Infectious Diseases,* 76–85. https://doi.org/10.1016/B978-0-323-04579-7.00006-X

Weber, D. J., Ruala, W. A., Miller, M. B., Huslage, K., & Sickbert-Bennett, E. (2010). Role of hospital surfaces in the transmission of emerging health care-associated pathogens: Norovirus, Clostridium difficile, and Acinetobacter species. *American Journal of Infection Control, 38*(5 Suppl. 1), S25–S33. https://doi.org/10.1016/j.ajic.2010.04.196

Wilcox, J., & Frank, E. (2021). Occupational therapy for the long haul of post-COVID syndrome: A case report. *The American Journal of Occupational Therapy, 75*(supplement_1). https://doi.org/10.5014/ajot.2021.049223

Woolf, S. H., Chapman, D. A., & Lee, J. H. (2021). Viewpoint: COVID-19 as the leading cause of death in the United States. *JAMA Network, 325*(2), 123–124. https://doi.org/10.1001/jama.2020.24865

World Health Organization. (2020). *The top 10 causes of death.* https://www.who.int/news-room/fact-sheets/detail/the-top-10-causes-of-death

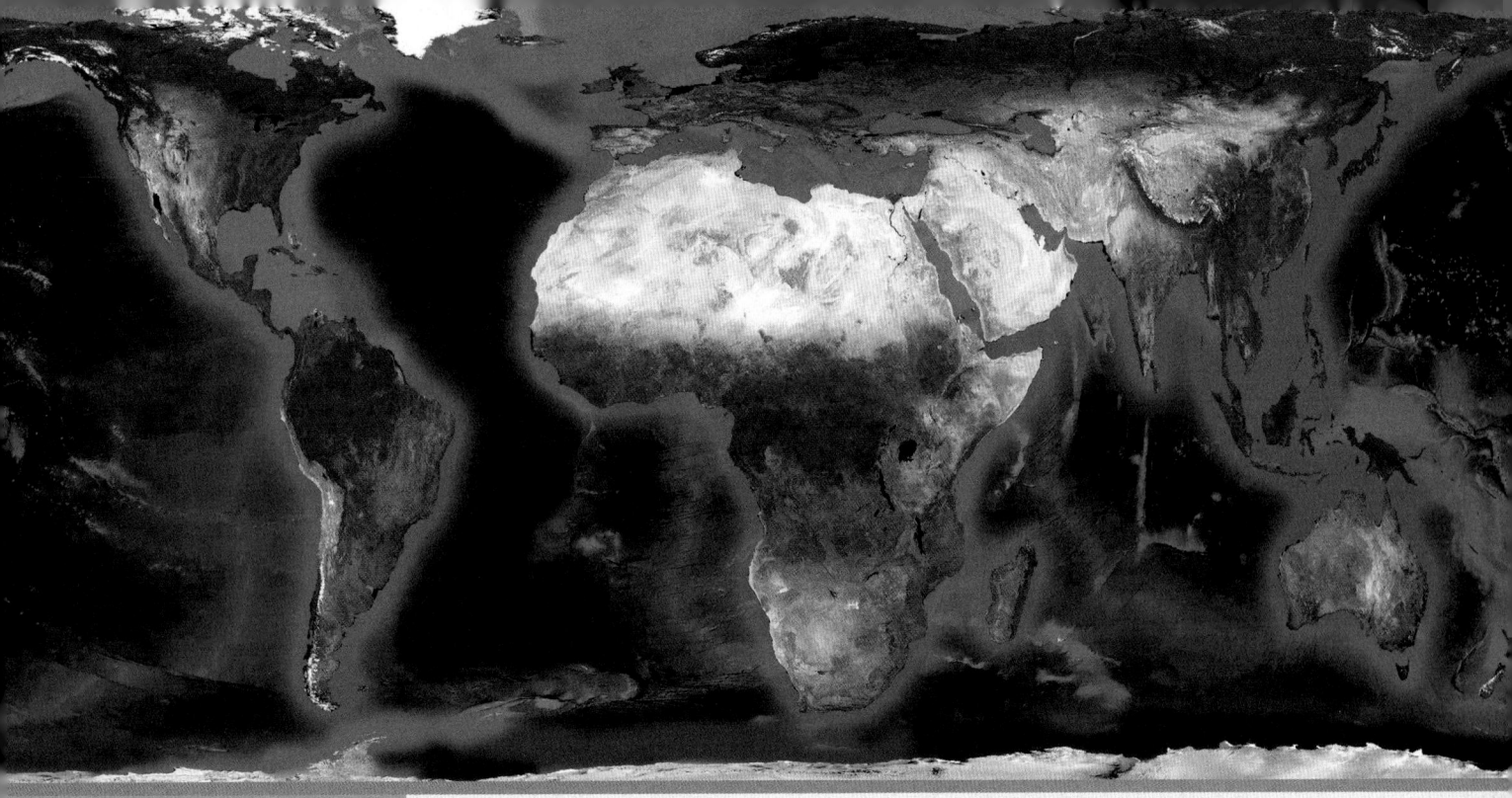

UNIT VI

Broad Conceptual Models for Occupational Therapy Practice

Media Related to Broad Conceptual Models for Occupational Therapy Practice

Readings
- *The Man Who Mistook His Wife for a Hat and Other Clinical Tales:* Neurologist Oliver Sacks tells the stories of individuals afflicted with neurological conditions. He describes patients who have lost their memories, who are no longer able to recognize people and common objects, who have tics and grimaces, whose limbs have become alien to them, and who are gifted with uncanny artistic or mathematical talents. (1998)

Movies
- *Certain Proof: A Question of Worth:* A documentary about three children who are struggling with the public school system in the United States. (2011)

Music
- *The River:* Bruce Springsteen's song of working class life uses the river as a metaphor for a place of refuge and possibilities that were never realized. (1980)
- *Homesick:* Noah Kahan's song about complicated feelings associated with one's hometown. (2022)

Examining How Theory Guides Practice

Theory and Practice in Occupational Therapy

Ellen S. Cohn and Wendy J. Coster

"In theory there is no difference between theory and practice. In practice there is."

—YOGI BERRA

LEARNING OBJECTIVES

After reading this chapter, you will be able to:

1. Compare and contrast the personal and formal theories.
2. Analyze the distinction between tacit and explicit knowledge.
3. Assess assumptions and propositions guiding practice.
4. Critically examine assumptions and propositions of a theory.

Introduction

When occupational therapy (OT) practitioners meet someone seeking OT for the first time, they must quickly figure out why the person or group has come for intervention, what is important to the person or group, what might be helping or interfering with their desired occupations, and what might be the best possible intervention to enable them to achieve their goals. Figuring out what to do requires complex professional reasoning processes that involve ongoing analysis and reflection on the OT practitioner's knowledge, observations, and understanding of the lives of clients and what matters to them.

Note: According to the American Occupational Therapy Association (AOTA, 2020, p. S75), the term *client* refers to *persons* (including those involved in the care of a client), *groups* (a collection of individuals having shared characteristics or common or shared purpose, e.g., family members, workers, students, and those with similar interests or occupational challenges), and *populations* (aggregates of people with common attributes such as contexts, characteristics, or concerns, including health risks) (Scaffa & Reitz, 2014). However, in countries other than the US, the term *client* often refers to persons who are paying for their care directly. In most countries, the term *patient* is used to describe persons who are in hospital or rehabilitation. *Service user* and *person* are terms in general use that describe those in need of OT services. For this chapter, we are using *client* without implying the source of payment for services.

In order to enable clients to achieve their occupational performance goals, OT practitioners must decide which interventions are most likely to achieve these goals. When we propose an intervention that involves particular actions or steps, our reasoning about what to do is guided by our ideas of how change might occur. These ideas include theoretical assumptions and propositions that guide us in what to observe and how to describe, explain, or predict outcomes from the interventions we might use. That is, in addition to client priorities, our experience, and available research evidence, we are guided by theories. The theories that guide professional reasoning are both personal and formal and both tacit and explicit. Whatever their form, theories help practitioners reason about what to assess, how to understand occupational performance problems, how to intervene, and what to expect from the intervention. Often, we need to articulate our reasoning process to others (clients, other professionals, peers, supervisors, policy makers, third-party payers, etc.) to communicate what they may expect from OT intervention.

The purpose of this chapter is to provide a structure to help OT practitioners "unpack" or critically examine the theorizing and theories they use to understand the problems clients present and to guide intervention. Our goal is to help practitioners clarify and evaluate the assumptions and propositions that guide their practice. This analysis is important for several reasons. First, it helps us to determine whether our professional reasoning is sound. Second, critically examining theories help us assess whether each theory is culturally relevant to the population to which the theory is being applied. Then, based on whether we conclude that it is sound or not, we may need to modify our reasoning and potentially the services we provide. Finally, examining our thinking helps us to articulate our professional reasoning to others so we can explain why we are using the assessments we have chosen, how the intervention we are providing works, and what outcomes we expect.

Propositions and Assumptions

To begin our discussion, we make a distinction between two types of ideas that are part of most theories: propositions and assumptions. Propositions are formal statements about causes and effects or the nature of relationships among features of the world. Their distinguishing feature is that it is possible (hypothetically at least) to test them and therefore to prove them false—a characteristic that is referred to in the philosophy of science as "falsifiability" (Popper, 1959). Sometimes, it is possible to test a proposition directly, for example, to test the proposition that a virus causes a particular illness. Other times, evidence accumulates from various sources, and that eventually makes clear that the "old" ideas about the world do not fit with the data as, for example, when scientists challenged the proposition that the sun revolved around the earth. Modern science is built around the posing and testing of hypotheses, which are propositions about how the world "works." In order to make the proposed relationships among the factors explicit, it can be helpful to formulate propositions as "if/then" statements. Table 33.1 presents some examples of propositions, their corresponding if/then statements, and how they might be tested.

In contrast, assumptions are ideas we "believe to be true." They are often ideas we "take for granted." This term is used a little differently in everyday language and in the language of science. In everyday language, we use the term to refer to a wide variety of situations where we have drawn a conclusion without having definite evidence. For example, we might tell our friend we "assume" that Halima took her book because she was the last person we saw reading it. In this situation,

---

TABLE 33.1   **Examples of Propositions With If/Then Statements**

Proposition	If/Then Statement	How It Would Be Tested
Practice of a skill in the context in which it will typically be applied leads to more effective long-term mastery.	If a person practices a skill in the natural context in which it is typically performed, then they will achieve more effective long-term mastery than if the skill is practiced in a contrived context.	A controlled comparison of the transfer of a skill learned under two different conditions: in a typical context and in a laboratory or contrived context
Organization of movement is different when reaching toward a desired object (i.e., a goal) than when simply reaching into space.	If a person reaches a goal, then their movement is organized differently than when he or she reaches into space without a goal.	Kinematic analysis of specific characteristics of reaching movements by the same person under the two different conditions
Sensory defensiveness is a defining characteristic of children with autism.	If a child has autism, then they will display sensory defensiveness.	Use of a structured protocol to examine responses to sensory stimuli in a large sample of children with autism. Calculate the prevalence of sensory defensiveness and compare this rate to that of a sample with a different diagnosis.

although we don't have the evidence on hand to prove our statement, we could readily gather evidence by asking Halima if she has the book. In other words, our conclusion is "falsifiable" and thus more like a proposition. In the language of science, the term *assumption* is applied much more specifically to ideas that really cannot be definitively proven true or false, for example, the idea that people have an inherent drive for mastery of their environment. Evidence can be judged to be more or less consistent with a particular assumption like this, but there is no way to obtain definitive proof.

Because assumptions are so completely accepted, it can be hard at first to recognize when a particular idea is an assumption rather than a proposition that is well supported by evidence. Our assumptions may derive from different sources. Some may have been learned during formal education, for example, from study of the theories of an academic discipline. Others reflect our personal theories and our assumptions derived from our culture and individual life experience. (See Chapter 25 for a more thorough discussion of personal theories.) The distinction between personal and "academic" assumptions is not always clear-cut; often, our preference for a particular formal theory is based on its compatibility with our personal assumptions, which may be linked to our personal and professional interests. For example, we may find it easier to accept theories that emphasize personal control over outcomes because we have a personal assumption that "people are in control of their fates." Table 33.2 gives some examples of how personal and theory-based assumptions might be expressed in the literature or in people's statements regarding their observations.

TABLE 33.2 Examples of How Personal and Theory-Based Assumptions Might Be Expressed

Examples of Assumptions	How the Assumption Might Be Expressed in a Formal Theory	How the Assumption Might Be Expressed in a Personal Theory
Assumptions About Causes		
Behavior is largely controlled by external social influences.	A theory proposes that poor outcomes among youth are due to negative social influences (e.g., unsafe neighborhood, low socioeconomic status)	"You can't blame them, given the kind of neighborhood they grew up in."
Behavior is largely controlled by unconscious motives and conflicts.	A theory proposes that unconscious conflicts stemming from early experiences explain a person's current behavior.	"She's doing that because she's in denial about what happened."
Assumptions About the Nature of the Person		
People are largely aware of and can report accurately on the reasons for their behavior.	A theory proposes that information on motives and goals provided by self-report accurately reflects the real causes of the person's behavior.	"Once we have talked with them, we should have a much better idea of what caused them to do that."
People are largely in control of their own behavior.	A theory proposes that behavior is directed by commitment to personal goals.	"If they really wanted to, they would put in the effort to change that bad habit."
People have an inherent drive to experience sensory stimulation.	A theory proposes that the experiences derived from sensory input are highly rewarding.	"Providing rich sensory experiences for their child is one of the most important things a parent can do."
People have an inherent drive to make sense of their experience.	A theory proposes that people automatically formulate explanations of their experience without being taught to do so.	"There must be a reason why this happened to me."
People are inherently rational.	A theory proposes that given adequate information, people will choose their actions based on an accurate weighing of the pros and cons of various options.	"I don't get it: I explained the importance of doing this, but they're still resisting!"
All people desire to be independent as much as possible.	A theory proposes that being able to do things without the support of others is the greatest indication of success.	"Even though they say they like living in the group home, I'm sure they'd rather live on their own."
Assumptions About Human Development		
There is a universal, optimal sequence to developing competence.	A theory proposes that failure to follow a standard sequence for mastering skills will result in less optimal functioning.	"If we don't focus on fine motor skills first, he will never be able to write well."
There is a timetable of experiences required for optimal development that is universal across cultures.	A theory proposes that if a child does not have certain experiences at a particular time, they will not achieve the same skills as their peers.	"Children need to spend lots of time in free play in order to develop sophisticated social skills."

TABLE 33.2	Examples of How Personal and Theory-Based Assumptions Might Be Expressed (*continued*)	
Examples of Assumptions	**How the Assumption Might Be Expressed in a Formal Theory**	**How the Assumption Might Be Expressed in a Personal Theory**
Assumptions About Knowledge and Learning		
The essence of learning is acquiring more information.	A theory proposes that lack of accurate or sufficiently detailed information explains why people act ineffectively.	"We have a lot of parents who aren't providing the right set of experiences for their child. We should offer a presentation about typical motor development."
The essence of learning is changing the way we think about something.	A theory proposes that people must integrate new information into their existing personal system of knowledge before they can organize new ways to act.	"An interactive teaching session observing how their child solves movement 'problems' will help parents change their approach to supporting their child."
Assumptions About the Impact of Context on Behavior		
The larger cultural context has minimal impact.	A theory proposes that the performance of a skill will be consistent across settings once it is mastered.	"It doesn't matter whether we do the assessment at home or in the clinic."
Behavior can only be fully understood within the person's context.	A theory proposes that sociopolitical and historical influences shape a person's life trajectory.	"We need to remember the economic crisis that was affecting the community at the time this worker's injury occurred."

Our assumptions about the nature of human behavior and corresponding views of reality may shape what we attend to when planning the evaluation process and developing intervention strategies with clients. Our day-to-day practices are rooted in both assumptions and propositions (Hooper, 1997). Often, propositions and assumptions are confounded, viewed as the same things, or confused with each other. Making a distinction between them helps us to identify them more easily, to reflect on how they may influence our reasoning about evaluation and intervention, and to evaluate whether they make sense. If we distinguish our propositions and assumptions, we can then search for relevant evidence to evaluate the propositions, evaluate whether our assumptions are logical and consistent with current knowledge, and reflect on how both the assumptions and propositions are influencing our reasoning and expectations for intervention outcomes. See Expanding Our Perspectives for an example.

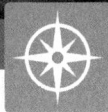

EXPANDING OUR PERSPECTIVES

Challenging Occupational Therapy's Assumptions about Occupation

Karen Whalley Hammell

When I began my OT education in England in the late 1970s, there was little discernable theory informing our profession's practices. Instead, we were guided by a plethora of assumptions about the inherent value of occupation, and in particular, the importance of self-care independence. So when OT's leaders began to articulate the importance to human well-being, not just of self-care, but of productive/work and leisure/play occupations, the horizons of my chosen profession suddenly expanded. Our previous preoccupation with bathing aids and adapted cutlery evolved, with attention now focused on the occupations in which clients might wish to engage after they had bathed and eaten breakfast.

Shortly thereafter, leading occupational therapists declared that *all* occupations could be compartmentalized within three categories of self-care, productivity/work, and leisure/play. They asserted that individuals choose, shape, and orchestrate their engagement in these occupations and that these occupational choices derive from individual volition and rational deliberation. As a White, middle-class, able, straight cis-female raised in the Global North—where the economic and political ideology of neoliberalism reigned (and reigns) supreme—these assumptions all made sense to me. OT's enthusiastic promotion of individualism, independence and self-reliance, and espousals of personal responsibility for one's socioeconomic situation and health fit perfectly with the prevailing myth of meritocracy, which portrays success (in life, in occupations, and in rehabilitation) as the result of individual skill, will, determination and effort. Assumptions were construed as theory, and from my position of privilege, these assumptions all seemed like common sense.

(continued)

EXPANDING OUR PERSPECTIVES (continued)

I was both a full-time carer and an occupational therapist in rural Saskatchewan, Canada, when it first dawned on me that the assumptions portrayed as theory fit neither my own life nor the lives of many of the people with whom I was working. My own occupations could not be classified within the only available categories articulated by our profession's leaders. My most valued occupation—caring—was clearly neither self-care nor leisure; but neither was this experience of loving and doing (or doing loving) "work." Moreover, the expansive range of occupational choices that had been available to me—as the daughter of White, middle-class parents who valued women's education and resisted patriarchy—were prohibited for rural girls raised in fundamentalist religious communities, whose occupations were chosen, shaped, and orchestrated by men.

There is danger in mistaking assumptions for theory. Reflecting on my career, I deeply regret my collusion with OT's "assumptions-as-theories," and the harm I may have caused my clients by my failure to question these ideologically informed and evidence-deficient beliefs. It is obvious to me now that subscribing to the assumption that one's group memberships (such as one's race or class) are irrelevant to one's occupational opportunities, choices, and achievements perpetuates racist and classist explanations for what are, in reality, occupational injustices. Instead of blaming clients who seem to be making "unwise" occupational choices, I now understand these choices to be made, not as a consequence of deficient volition or willpower, but as a response to the inequitable socioeconomic circumstances regulating the availability of opportunities from which occupational choices—wise or otherwise—might be made; and as a result of values and priorities that may differ from my own. Had these understandings arisen earlier in my career, I would have been a better occupational therapist.

Note that some of the examples in Table 33.2 have elements that could be tested or checked for their consistency with the evidence. However, the *broader* assumptions would be hard to prove or disprove. For example, how would one *prove* that all people want to be as independent as possible? This is one reason why it is important to evaluate the evidence supporting your ideas about how to intervene with a client. If you cannot find any evidence, that is one clue that you may be basing your approach on assumptions.

It is important to keep in mind that we all make assumptions; they provide answers to important fundamental questions such as "What is the nature of the person?" or "Am I in control of my fate?" It is not really possible to construct theories without them. However, because assumptions cannot be fully disproved, we need to be cautious in applying them as guides for practice. The propositions of a theory, on the other hand, can be tested so that we can determine whether or not they are accurate guides for achieving desired changes. This systematic testing is what leads to new discoveries and therefore more effective practice.

Cultural Embeddedness of Theories

Theories about human behavior are not value-neutral and cannot be assumed to be culturally universal, although this aspect of the values and assumptions embedded in theories is often not acknowledged explicitly. Currently, the predominant theories in OT have been developed by scholars who live in Western, technologically advanced, relatively wealthy, White-majority countries. As Hammell (2009a) notes, this group actually represents a minority of the world's population. Accordingly, it is important for OT practitioners to critically examine the cultural relevance of the theories underpinning practice. We define cultural relevance as the extent to which a theory's concepts are congruent with the values, circumstance, place, or experiences of a group to which they are applied.

To illustrate, within child development, many theories developed by Western scientists are presented with an implicit assumption that they represent a universal optimal process, pathway, and definition of maturity (Garcia-Coll, 2020). As one example, Piaget's theory, though based on studies that included only his own Swiss children and others of similar background, is often presented in textbooks as a "universal" theory of cognitive development. An important consequence of adopting this assumption is that a child whose behavior on Piagetian tasks does not demonstrate the predicted sequence or timing may be identified as showing delays or impairments. In other words, a value judgment is made that may have real-world consequences. The same child, if assessed on tasks that represent the kind of reasoning common in their own daily life, might appear to have sophisticated thinking skills relative to peers in the same community.

We may slip into a similar assumption of universality as we strive to use "theory-based" and "evidence-based" reasoning to guide the design of OT interventions. These forms of reasoning do assure us that the intervention has an articulated theoretical basis and strong evidence from research to support it. However, the theory being applied may reflect a particular—often Western—set of assumptions, and the evidence may be valid only for people who share that same cultural perspective as the researchers and study participants. Often, we do not know whether the theory or the intervention approach would appear reasonable and appropriate to people living in regions or nations with very different cultural and sociopolitical organization. Caution is especially important when the underlying theory involves cognitive, emotional, or social aspects of occupation and occupational performance because these aspects are most intertwined with our cultural context.

Hammell (2009a, 2009b) has written several papers that examine the assumptions reflected in OT's core beliefs. She argued that many of these core beliefs should be questioned for their appropriateness to represent the occupational lives of the majority of the world's people. For example, the belief that the person can make autonomous decisions about their occupations does not reflect the significant constraints—political, economic, and social—that control what they can do, where, and how. Similarly, the emphasis on what the individual wants and can do is a Western perspective; other cultures might prioritize what the family or community needs and values. See Box 33.1 for some guiding questions to help examine the *contextual relevance* of the proposed theory.

What are the implications of these challenges to core assumptions? Challenge is important for the growth of a profession, but challenges to core beliefs can be uncomfortable and often evoke resistance. However, it is important to remember that all theories are hypothetical: they represent our best explanation of a phenomenon *at the moment*. As such, we must continue to work with our current theories. At the same time, we should stay alert to new ideas being put forward and evaluate whether they help resolve any of our questions or fill a problematic gap. Our theories will evolve, or a new theory will eventually replace a current theory because it offers a better, more accurate, or more complete perspective on important issues.

Tacit and Explicit

Sometimes our reasoning is tacit; that is, implicit or based on information or experiences that we cannot easily put into language. Experienced practitioners have an implicit or tacit understanding of what they do in practice and will make adjustments to the intervention to address the subtle and complex cues observed in the process of intervention. For example, through experience, a therapist might determine that the strength of a muscle "just doesn't seem right" and the therapist then automatically adjusts the activity to compensate for the person's limited strength. Another therapist might instinctively sing a calming, gentle song to soothe a young child who is agitated. The philosopher Polanyi (1966/2009, p. 4) eloquently summarized this process when he noted, "We can know more than we can tell." Tacit reasoning is important to our practice because it allows us to work quickly and effectively at the moment. However, in order to evaluate whether the approach was effective (and if we should continue to use it), we need to be able to translate our tacit or implicit reasoning into clear *explicit* propositions about what we think promoted the desired change for the client. In order to evaluate whether our model of change is logical and is supported by evidence, we need to describe the exact mechanism that we think caused the change. For example, on reflection, we may realize that we asked a client to repeat the same movement numerous times as we increased the task demands because we hypothesized, based on motor learning theory, that "repetition under condition of ever-increasing task demands" will promote change in the movement (Plautz et al., 2000). Then, we could review whether the evidence supports this theoretical proposition.

Theories Vary in Specificity

In OT, authors have used many different terms to define similar concepts (theory, conceptual foundation, frame of reference, paradigm, practice model). Different authors may provide very different definitions of the same terms, which can be confusing. Rather than try to clarify the subtle distinctions across these definitions, this chapter takes a different approach. We suggest that theories can be located along a continuum that reflects their degree of specificity.

> ## BOX 33.1 GUIDING QUESTIONS TO EXAMINE THE *CONTEXTUAL RELEVANCE* OF THE PROPOSED THEORY
>
> - Does the theory's terminology guide us to consider the potential sociopolitical factors that may be relevant to contemporary occupation in a particular context/region/population of the world?
> - Does the theory consider the diversity of ways in which people may participate in occupations?
> - Does the theory emphasize an individualistic or collectivist perspective?
> - Does the theory address the role of context in shaping one's experience of occupation?
> - Do the classifications of occupations reflect the lived experiences of the people in a particular context?
> - Can the theoretical constructs of the theory be translated to a range of languages and cultures?

Broad

One definition of a theory (Merriam-Webster, 2021) is "a plausible or scientifically acceptable general principle or body of principles offered to explain phenomena." This definition is broad, global, and explanatory. A broad theory serves as an "overarching model that helps to explain a large set of findings or observations" (Whyte, 2006, p. 100). A broad or global theory provides a way of organizing or systematizing the elements of the phenomenon being observed and helps us focus our observations and decide what cues to attend to. A broad theory specifies how concepts or factors are related and gives a name to a set of elements that share something in common. However, propositions about change are not specified in precise detail in broad theories. For example, ecological theory tells us to pay attention to the person–environment interaction, but it does not tell us how to intervene to enable the client to participate more satisfactorily in desired occupations. Therefore, broad theories do not provide precise information on how we can intervene to enable change.

In OT, we often use ecological and systems theories, which propose a transactional relation between the mind, the body, and the environment. (See Chapters 34, The Model of Human Occupation; 35, Ecological Models in Occupational Therapy; and 36, Theory of Occupational Adaptation.) We consider the context or environment in its broadest sense (including culture and social aspects) and assume that humans have an innate drive to explore and be competent in their environments. Some broad ecological theories explain the influence of the environment in greater detail than others. These broad theories commonly suggest that in order to explore and be competent in our environments, people need skills and abilities, and we judge our competence by the feedback we receive from the environment. Consequently, in this example, the broad theories help us focus our initial observations of human behavior on the complex transactions among mind, body, and environment.

Several ecological theorists in the field of human development have offered explanations of the transactional relationship between person and environment. Bronfenbrenner (1979), a social scientist, proposed an ecological theory to explain how a person's biology and interactions among ever-changing and multilevel environments are key to human development. Bronfenbrenner proposed that social factors such as families, friends, communities, or institutions can enhance or inhibit development. Gibson's (1979) concept of affordances describes the idea that people's perception of the relationship between objects in the environment and their own personal capabilities enables action. Lawton (1986) proposed the concept of press to explain the idea that the demands of the environment or task impact human performance and suggested that "goodness of fit" between a person's abilities and the demands of the task influences human performance. Numerous theories proposed by occupational therapists (Ecology of Human Performance [Dunn et al., 1994]; Person-Environment-Occupation [Law et al., 1996]; Person-Environment-Occupation Performance [Baum & Christiansen, 2005]; and Model of Human Occupation [Kielhofner, 2008; Kielhofner & Burke, 1980]) are based on these ecological principles (see Chapters 34 and 35). When observing occupational performance, ideas drawn from these ecological theories direct occupational therapists to focus their observations on the person, the environment, and the occupation and how these elements influence each other.

Discrete

Another definition of a theory (Merriam-Webster, 2021) is a "hypothesis assumed for the sake of argument or investigation." This definition describes a discrete theory. Discrete theories often draw on the ideas of broad theories and describe specific causal relationships. These theories may be efforts to identify the specific causes of a problem or may propose how an aspect of intervention leads to therapeutic change. Because discrete theories identify ways in which a phenomenon can be changed or controlled, they help us determine what to do or say in providing interventions and they inform our treatment or intervention theories. A treatment theory helps to narrow the scope of possibilities for change and states how a specific intervention is believed to act. By clearly specifying the mechanisms of action (or mechanisms of change), that is, how specific intervention strategies lead to particular outcomes, treatment theories explicate how change proceeds and the particular conditions under which an intervention achieves the desired results. Consequently, treatment or intervention theories also help us determine what types of clients might benefit from the intervention, how the intervention is best delivered, and what outcomes we might expect.

Both broad and discrete theories make claims about hypothesized relationships. However, these theories are on a continuum in terms of the degree of development and specificity regarding how to intervene, clarity about the essential features, or element of the intervention and evidence to support their propositions. One way to determine where a theory may be on the broad to discrete continuum is to examine the degree to which each causal relationship proposed in the theory is supported by sound evidence. Theories with more developed propositions include clear assertions of the effects of an intervention, the mechanism through which the intervention is believed to exert these effects, and the identification of the components of the intervention that are most responsible for the effects. Because research is conducted to test the hypothesized relationships, theories become more refined and we gain greater clarity about the effectiveness of the various components of an intervention. Box 33.2 provides a simple schematic of the continuum from broad to discrete theories.

BOX 33.2 CHARACTERISTICS OF BROAD AND DISCRETE THEORIES

Broad ➤ Discrete

Broad	Discrete
• Global	• Testable specific postulates about causal relationships
• Explanatory: help explain a large set of findings or observations	• Specify how to behave in intervention, what to say or do, under what conditions changes will occur
• Map out the elements of phenomena being observed	• Explanatory: help explain how intervention works
• Specify what is related to what and gives a name to a set of elements that share something in common	• Predictive: specify what might happen or what to expect as a result of intervention
• Help us focus our initial observations (i.e., what is important to attend to rather than what to do)	• Each particular proposition of the theory is supported by evidence and specified so you can anticipate what the outcome is likely to be.

Where Do Theories Come From?

What prompts someone to propose a new or a revised theory? Recall that theories are an effort to *explain* a particular phenomenon or process and to *organize* information about that phenomenon. Thus, theories, particularly clinical or practice theories, are often developed in response to an observation or experience that the person cannot adequately account for using existing explanations. When we encounter a new phenomenon, we engage in what Swedberg (2012) referred to as "theorizing in the context of discovery": "Theorizing … means an attempt to understand and explain … and it includes everything that precedes the final formulation that is set down on paper or fixed in some other way ('theory')" (p. 14). For example, when Jean Ayres (1972) was working with children in the 1970s, she found that the accepted theories about learning difficulties did not adequately account for the full range of difficulties that she saw in the children she worked with and didn't offer useful guidance for how to intervene. Eventually, after considerable observation and extensive review of current science in relevant areas, this experience led her to develop sensory integration theory and develop a new approach to intervention based on this theory. Sometimes, theory or research in a related field suggests new ways to understand or intervene with clinical problems. For example, Taub et al. (1999) developed constraint-induced movement therapy for people with stroke after observing what they termed "learned non-use" in monkeys who had central nervous system (CNS) damage.

Theories are based on the knowledge available at the time they are first developed. Over time, more evidence will become available about whether or not the propositions of the theory are correct or whether they need to be modified.

For example, evidence may show that a specific feature of the intervention is particularly effective in achieving the desired change and that other features of the intervention may not be necessary. Therefore, it is important for practitioners to remain current in the research related to the theories they are applying in practice. It is also important for practitioners to reflect critically on their own observations, to see whether they fit with current theoretical explanations. If not, like Ayres, they should engage in their own theorizing in the context of discovery.

Cognitive Orientation to Daily Occupational Performance

Let's consider an example of a theory-based intervention. The Cognitive Orientation to Daily Occupational Performance (CO-OP Approach™) intervention was developed by occupational therapists Polatajko et al. (2001) to better meet the needs of children with motor coordination difficulties. At that time, intervention approaches offered to children with mild-to-moderate movement difficulties were primarily impairment oriented, focusing on remediating underlying impairments thought to interfere with functional performance (Mandich et al., 2001a). Dissatisfied with the lack of generalization to skilled action, occupational therapists Helene Polatajko and Angela Mandich turned to literature about growing understanding of motor control and skill learning to develop a highly individualized metacognitive approach to help children master motor skills for real-world performance. The CO-OP Approach™ is an occupation-based, client-centered, metacognitive, performance-based, and evidence-based intervention that combines motor learning principles with other theories that emphasize the role of cognitive processes and goal setting in developing movement skills. The CO-OP Approach™ is an example of a theory-based intervention informed by multiple theoretical perspectives from a range of disciplines, including behavioral and cognitive psychology, education, human movement science, and OT. The original purpose of the intervention was to teach children to use cognitive strategies that support skill acquisition through a process of guided discovery. See OT Story 33.1 for an example of this process.

The CO-OP Approach™ might be an effective intervention to help Alex achieve his goals to play baseball, shuffle playing cards, and type on the computer. The overarching broad assumption of the CO-OP Approach™ is that successful participation in everyday occupation is essential to health and well-being. Figure 33.1 provides a general overview of the key theoretical propositions and essential and structural elements of the CO-OP Approach™. The approach is composed of seven key features: client-chosen goals, dynamic performance analysis, cognitive strategy use, guided discovery, enabling principles, significant other involvement, and intervention format. Table 33.3 presents the if/then statements for the key theoretical propositions.

Based on principles of motor learning and goal setting, the therapist would help Alex to identify goals and discover the relevant aspects of the task, examine how he is currently performing the task, identify where he is getting "stuck," and generate alternative solutions. Bandura (1997) noted that children's actual experiences performing an activity contribute to their self-perceptions and that when children set their own goals, they feel more empowered to work toward achieving their goals. A global strategy is used to provide a consistent framework to help Alex discover task-specific strategies. This structure was based on the problem-solving structure first described by Luria (1976), who drew from Vygotsky's (1967) observation of problem-solving attempts of children, and then further developed by Meichenbaum (1977), a psychologist now known as the founder of cognitive behavioral modification therapy. Meichenbaum adopted a rubric, known as "goal-plan-do-check," originally developed by educators Camp and Bash (1982) for helping boys who acted aggressively to use problem-solving techniques in social situations. In addition to the global problem-solving strategy proposed by Meichenbaum, occupational therapist Angela Mandich (Mandich et al., 2001b), who was a graduate student at the time Polatajko

OT STORY 33.1 ALEX

Alex, a 9-year-old child, has been referred to you, an OT student completing your fieldwork experience in an outpatient private practice for children. Alex is reluctant to try new activities, is beginning to have difficulty keeping up with his peers in school, wanders around the periphery of the playground during recess, and refuses to participate in gym class. The other children have begun to tease Alex, and he has not developed friendships. After observing Alex struggle to complete a variety of fine and gross motor activities, you conduct formal assessments and document delays in both fine and gross motor development. You also complete the Perceived Efficacy and Goal Setting System (PEGS) with Alex to gain insight into his perspectives and concerns. The PEGS is a standardized system designed to enable young children with disabilities to self-report their perceived competence in everyday activities and to set goals for intervention. Alex wants to be able to play baseball, shuffle playing cards, and type on the computer. You are now clear about the outcomes Alex hopes to achieve but need to determine how to best intervene to help Alex achieve his goals in an effective and efficient manner. Your supervisor asks you to explain the "theoretical rationale" of the intervention you propose for Alex. Your supervisor wants to know what you think the "mechanisms of action" are for the intervention.

Before reading further, take a moment to think about and write down your ideas about the following questions.

Questions

1. Why might Alex have trouble developing friendships?
2. Why might Alex be reluctant to try new activities?
   Go back and review your explanations for why Alex might have trouble developing friendships and be reluctant to try new activities.
3. Which ideas are testable (i.e., are propositions)?
4. How might you test the propositions?
5. Which are more like assumptions?
6. Can you identify the sources of some of your assumptions?
7. Before reading further, take another moment to think about this question:
8. Are your ideas about Alex's challenges with friendships and new activities based on personal theories or some formal theories that you may have learned in your studies to date?
9. Identify in writing the personal theories that guided your reasoning about Alex.
10. Identify in writing the formal theories (either broad or discrete) that guided your reasoning about Alex.
11. How would your thinking change if you learned that Alex was a refugee who had escaped from a war zone with his mother and sister?

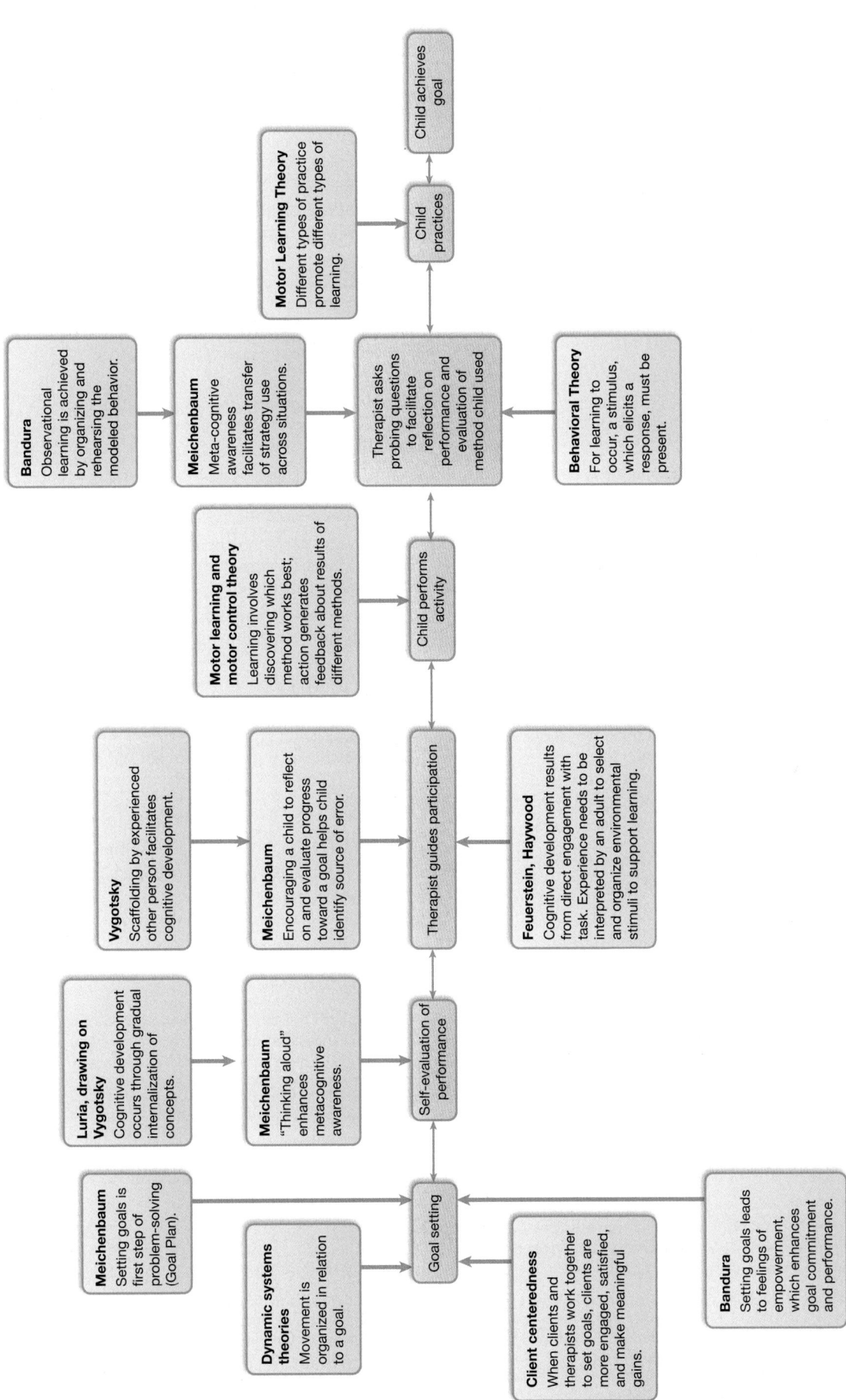

FIGURE 33.1 Theoretical propositions and key features of the Cognitive Orientation to Daily Occupational Performance (CO-OP Approach™).

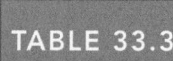

TABLE 33.3	Theoretical Propositions and If/Then Statements of the CO-OP Approach™
Intervention Feature	**If/Then Statements From Key Theories**
Essential Elements: Key Elements to Be Considered in the CO-OP Approach™	
Goal setting: client-chosen, occupation-based goals	If a movement is directed toward a goal, then that movement will be organized uniquely in relation to that goal.
	If the person is collaboratively engaged in setting a goal, then his or her problem-solving process in relation to that goal will be facilitated.
	If the person is collaboratively engaged in setting a goal, then he or she will experience increased self-efficacy.
	If the person's self-efficacy is increased, then his or her motivation and commitment to the goal will be enhanced.
Dynamic performance analysis: dynamic (ongoing), analytical process of identifying performance problems that engages both the practitioner and the client; initially led by the therapist and then becomes collaborative	If a person can identify performance problems and where the performance is breaking down, then this information can be used to guide the person to discover, learn, and apply strategies to support performance.
Cognitive strategy use: goal-directed and consciously controlled cognitive processes that facilitate or support performance and skill acquisition. Strategies may be global (general) or domain (task) specific.	If a person engages in talking aloud while attempting to solve a problem (cognitive scaffolding), then awareness of his or her performance will be enhanced.
	If a person develops strategies to address the challenges/sources of error, then using the strategies will develop competence in the desired activity.
	If a person engages in talking aloud while attempting to solve a problem, then the problem-solving process will be facilitated.
	If a person engages in self-evaluation of performance, he or she will develop a structure for self-monitoring (check) and evaluating performance.
Guided discovery: Practitioner asks logical and sequential questions that guide client to discover a concept, rule, principle, or action to support performance that was not previously known.	If a more experienced person guides and supports (scaffolds) a learner who is attempting to solve a problem, then the learner's problem-solving capacity (cognitive development) will be enhanced.
	If the therapist asks appropriate questions, then the child's ability to identify effective strategies will be enhanced.
	If an adult models the thinking process to be mastered and if the child repeats the steps of that process aloud, then the child's learning of the process will be enhanced.
Enabling principles based on learning and motor behavior: instructional and feedback methods that promote learning, facilitate goal attainment, promote generalization and transfer	If the child performs an activity, then he or she will receive meaningful feedback about the results of a particular approach to the activity.
	If the therapist engages the child in "thinking out loud" about his or her performance, then the child's ability to evaluate the effectiveness of his or her strategies will be enhanced.
Structural Elements: Key Elements That Are Preferred or Suggested, May Be Altered to Meet Specific Needs of Person, Practice Setting, or Other Factors	
Parent or support person involvement: Important people in the client's life are aware of and use guided discovery and enabling principles outside the intervention environment.	If people important to the client's real-world performance can use guided discovery and enabling principles in a range of environments, then the client will continue skill development beyond the intervention environment.
Intervention format: Setting, number of intervention sessions, and sequence of sessions may vary. Sessions may be group or individual, delivered in person or by telerehabilitation.	If the intervention includes the essential elements specified by the CO-OP Approach™, then the number and sequence of sessions may vary to meet client needs.

Sources: Based on Polatajko, H., McEwen, S., Dawson, D. R., & Skidmore, E. R. (2017). Cognitive orientation to daily occupational performance. In M. Curtin, M. Egan, & J. Adams (Eds.), *Occupational therapy for people experiencing illness, injury or impairment: Promoting occupation and participation* (7th ed., pp. 636–647). Elsevier and Skidmore, E., McEwen, S., Green, D., van den Houten, J., Dawson, D., & Polatajko, H. (2017). Essential elements and key features of the CO-OP Approach™. In D. Dawson, S. McEwen, & H. Polatajko (Eds.), *Cognitive orientation to daily occupational performance in occupational therapy: Using the CO-OP approach to enable participation across the lifespan.* AOTA Press, The American Occupational Therapy Association, Incorporated..

and her colleagues were developing the CO-OP Approach™, identified eight domain-specific strategies directly related to specific task performance problems. Mandich proposed that task knowledge and cognitive strategies specific to the performance challenges were necessary "mechanisms of action" to support children's competence in their desired occupations. Informed by principles of mediated learning described by educators Feuerstein and colleagues (1986) and Haywood (1988), the occupational therapist structures the environment by asking probing questions to facilitate Alex's awareness and reflection on his performance. Once Alex identifies a helpful strategy, the therapist uses questions to help Alex think about how he might apply or generalize the strategy to other situations.

Figure 33.2 provides a conceptual mapping of what the practitioner actually does to implement the CO-OP Approach™ in a way that reflects the theoretical propositions. We could actually test the propositions of the theory by observing the therapist's actions and Alex's responses. For example, to test the proposition related to goal setting, we could observe the therapist asking Alex to identify three skills that he needs, wants, or is expected to do at school, home, or when playing. We could determine whether Alex increases his efforts to catch a small ball after setting a goal focused on ball catching.

The intervention process is dynamic and continuously changes over time as we learn more and reflect on our initial propositions. As we continue to work with Alex to achieve his goals, we are constantly reflecting on and examining our intervention approaches to determine whether they are effective. If the approach is not effective, we must be open to changing or adapting the approach. We might discover that, for Alex, verbalizing the strategies to prompt the motor movement is only effective when there are no other distracters in the immediate context. Based on this ongoing examination of the intervention, we might modify the context as distracting stimuli emerged as an important element influencing Alex's performance. We might also discover the CO-OP Approach™ works well with Alex, but that does not mean that we stop reflecting on the propositions because the research evidence is constantly evolving and our understanding of the causal relationships may also change. For example, Batte and Polatajko (2006) analyzed videotapes of children during the CO-OP Approach™ and other intervention approaches to determine the role of practice in skill acquisition. Because the CO-OP Approach™ is a cognitive-based intervention, the children who received the CO-OP Approach™ spent more intervention time discussing performance. The children who received other interventions had more practice time than the children receiving the CO-OP Approach™. Yet, the children who received the CO-OP Approach™ showed significantly greater gains in performance, illustrating that strategy use, in addition to practice, is an important "mechanism of action"

in the CO-OP Approach™. Such research evidence helps us clarify what to do in the intervention process. As the research evolves, the theoretical propositions also evolve (Miller et al., 2001). Therefore, the question we must always ask is "Is there a basis to what I'm doing in the intervention that is supported by theory and evidence?"

Occupational Therapy Task-Oriented Approach

Let's consider another scenario and another theoretical approach, the Occupational Therapy Task-Oriented Approach for people who have had stroke, developed by occupational therapists Virgil Mathiowetz and Julie Bass-Haugen (1994). The Occupational Therapy Task-Oriented Approach is another example of a theory and evidence-based intervention informed by multiple theoretical perspectives from a range of disciplines. During the early 1990s, many researchers began to question the assumptions and propositions of theories of motor development (Thelen & Ulrich, 1991) and motor behavior change (Jongbloed et al., 1989; Sabari, 1991). Therapists were using interventions based on assumptions such as (a) the CNS is hierarchically organized, (b) normal movement can be facilitated by providing specific patterns of sensory input, and (c) recovery from brain damage follows a predictable sequence. Clients were not making desired changes, and practitioners were searching for a better understanding of the challenges clients presented. Therapists and clients were particularly dissatisfied that retraining of normal movement patterns did not result in carryover to functional daily living skills.

The Occupational Therapy Task-Oriented Approach includes assumptions and propositions from broad OT theories, a systems model of motor control, an ecological approach to perception and action, and dynamic systems theory. This multidisciplinary approach represents understanding of motor control and learning from the neuropsychological, biomechanical, and behavioral sciences. An overarching assumption of the Occupational Therapy Task-Oriented Approach is that movement is organized around a goal and influenced by the environment. Movement emerges as an interaction among many systems, each contributing to motor control.

The term *task-oriented approach* was first proposed by a physical therapist at a professional conference focused on contemporary management of motor control problems (Horak, 1991). Occupational therapists revised the task-oriented approach to consider task performance in relation to a person's valued activities in their culture and community. The inclusion of performance in the Occupational Therapy Task-Oriented Approach is based on Trombly's (1995) proposition that a person must be able to do the

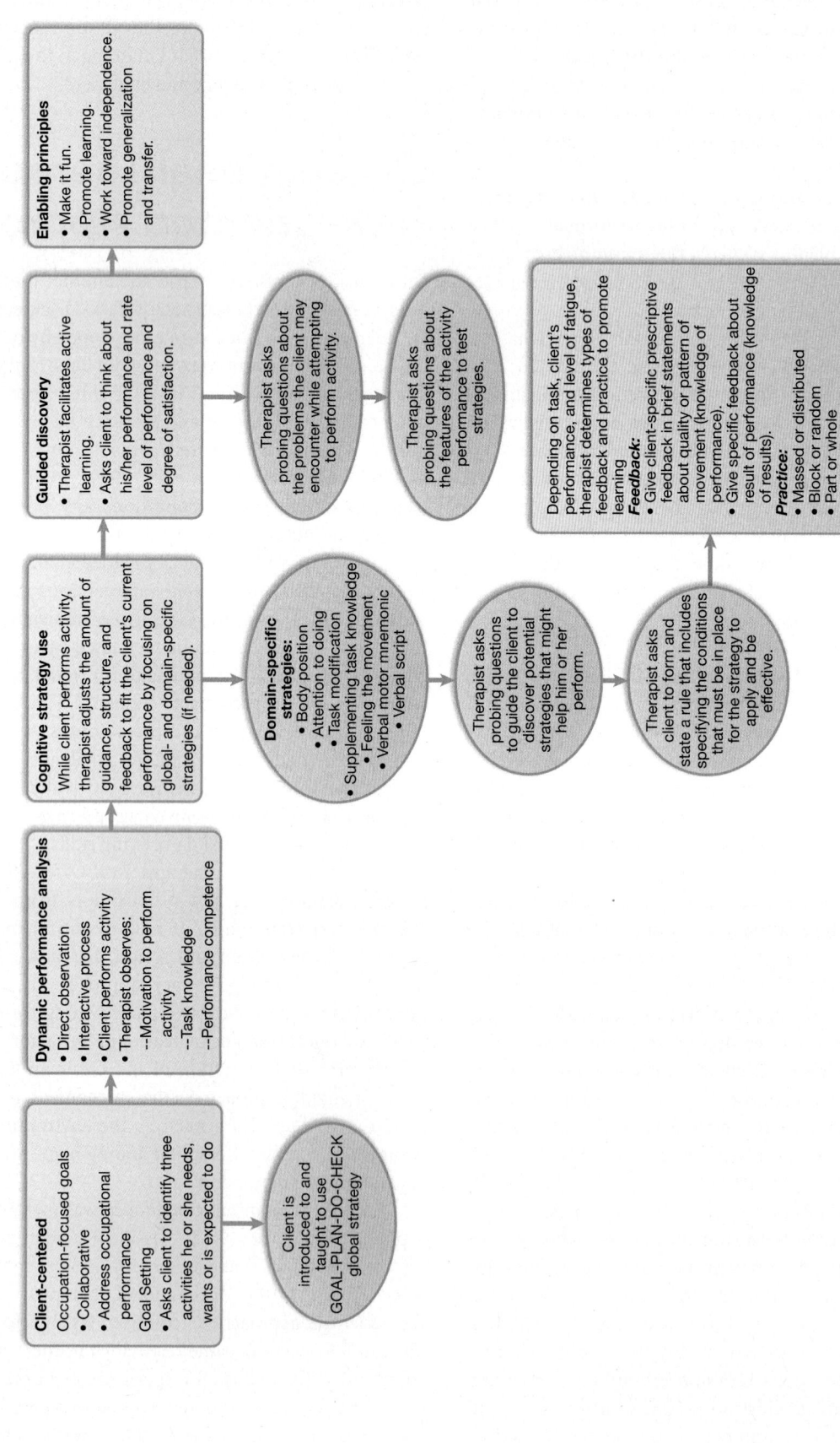

FIGURE 33.2 Conceptual mapping of practitioner's actions.

Client-centered
Occupation-focused goals
• Collaborative
• Address occupational performance
Goal Setting
• Asks client to identify three activities he or she needs, wants or is expected to do

Client is introduced to and taught to use GOAL-PLAN-DO-CHECK global strategy

Dynamic performance analysis
• Direct observation
• Interactive process
• Client performs activity
• Therapist observes:
--Motivation to perform activity
--Task knowledge
--Performance competence

Cognitive strategy use
While client performs activity, therapist adjusts the amount of guidance, structure, and feedback to fit the client's current performance by focusing on global- and domain-specific strategies (if needed).

Domain-specific strategies:
• Body position
• Attention to doing
• Task modification
• Supplementing task knowledge
• Feeling the movement
• Verbal motor mnemonic
• Verbal script

Therapist asks probing questions to guide the client to discover potential strategies that might help him or her perform.

Therapist asks client to form and state a rule that includes specifying the conditions that must be in place for the strategy to apply and be effective.

Depending on task, client's performance, and level of fatigue, therapist determines types of feedback and practice to promote learning
Feedback:
• Give client-specific prescriptive feedback in brief statements about quality or pattern of movement (knowledge of performance).
• Give specific feedback about result of performance (knowledge of results).
Practice:
• Massed or distributed
• Block or random
• Part or whole

Guided discovery
• Therapist facilitates active learning.
• Asks client to think about his/her performance and rate level of performance and degree of satisfaction.

Therapist asks probing questions about the problems the client may encounter while attempting to perform activity.

Therapist asks probing questions about the features of the activity performance to test strategies.

Enabling principles
• Make it fun.
• Promote learning.
• Work toward independence.
• Promote generalization and transfer.

activities and tasks that support their engagement in meaningful occupations. As research and theories have evolved, the Occupational Therapy Task-Oriented Approach continues to evolve and become more discrete as new research helps us refine the specific mechanisms of action (Bass-Haugen et al., 2008; Mathiowetz, 2011; Preissner, 2010).

As we examine the Occupational Therapy Task-Oriented Approach, consider OT Story 33.2 and how a practitioner working with Maria following a stroke might adopt the Occupational Therapy Task-Oriented Approach to inform their reasoning related to evaluation and intervention.

The OT practitioner also uses the Occupational Therapy Task-Oriented Approach to guide Maria's intervention. The emphasis of intervention is on enabling clients to successfully engage in tasks and activities associated with the occupations clients are expected to, need to, or want to fulfill; purposeful and meaningful tasks are the primary intervention modality. The practitioner believes that the Occupational Therapy Task-Oriented Approach might be an effective intervention to help Maria achieve her goals to cook and return to weaving with her granddaughters. The overarching assumptions of the Occupational Therapy Task-Oriented Approach are presented in Box 33.3.

Figure 33.3 provides a general overview of the key theoretical propositions and features of the Occupational Therapy Task-Oriented Approach. Table 33.4 presents if/then statements for the key theoretical propositions outlined in Figure 33.3.

BOX 33.3 ASSUMPTIONS OF OCCUPATIONAL THERAPY TASK-ORIENTED APPROACH

- Personal and environmental systems, including the CNS, are heterarchically organized.
- Functional tasks help organize behavior.
- Occupational performance emerges from the interaction of persons and their environment.
- Experimentation with various strategies leads to optimal solutions to motor problems.
- Recovery is variable because patient factors and environmental contexts are unique.
- Behavioral changes reflect an attempt to compensate to achieve task performance.

CNS, central nervous system.

Following an assessment of Maria's performance in relation to desired tasks and activities, the therapist and Maria will consider whether to develop compensatory approaches for challenging tasks or attempt to remediate skills necessary for successful task completion. Based on dynamical systems theory, the therapist continuously analyzes the critical control parameters—personal and environmental variables—that may have the potential to impact task

---

OT STORY 33.2 MARIA

Maria, a 72-year-old homemaker and weaver, had a right middle cerebral artery stroke with resulting left-sided weakness and decreased balance 3 weeks ago. She lives with her daughter, son-in-law, and their two daughters, ages 11 and 13 years outside of Quito, Ecuador. Maria loves to cook traditional Ecuadorian food for her family and has been teaching her granddaughters the value of merging the physical and spiritual worlds through weaving. She is eager to regain function so she can return to these important occupations within her family. How will occupational therapists use theory to guide their reasoning about the best possible intervention for Maria?

The occupational therapist begins the evaluation by focusing on Maria's daily life and living situation. First, the therapist interviews Maria to understand the activities that she wants or must do in the future. The therapist then proceeds to collaborate with Maria to identify her priorities and goals for intervention. This emphasis on Maria's priorities reflects the theoretical proposition that clients who are actively engaged in their treatment are more likely to achieve their goals and have better outcomes. These initial evaluation

and goal-setting processes are also supported by propositions from client-centered perspectives: When clients and therapist work together to achieve goals, clients are more engaged, are satisfied, and make meaningful gains.

After discussing what's important to Maria and her goals for OT, Maria and the occupational therapist decide to make llapingachos, traditional Ecuadorian fried potato omelets, in the OT department kitchen in the rehabilitation clinic. As Maria cuts a boiled potato, the occupational therapist notices that Maria is able to place her left arm on the table to stabilize the bowl as she puts the cut-up pieces of potatoes in the bowl with her right hand. Maria and the therapist discuss how Maria might use her left hand to assist with weaving tasks.

Questions

1. How does the Task-Oriented Approach to intervention guide the therapists' reasoning about what to do in the intervention session?
2. How might the therapist determine whether the Task-Oriented Approach is culturally relevant for Maria?

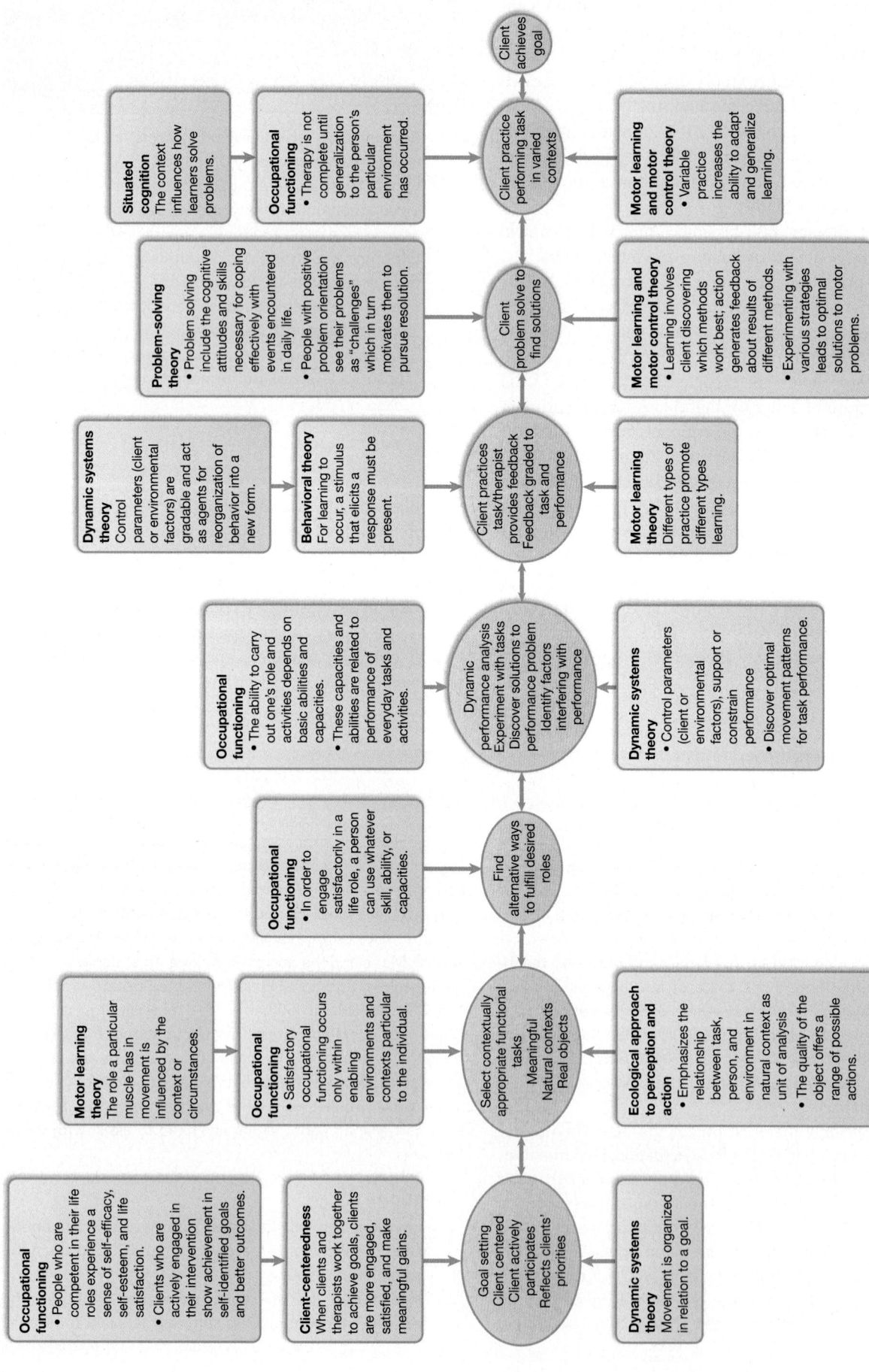

FIGURE 33.3 General overview of Occupational Therapy Task-Oriented Approach.

TABLE 33.4	Theoretical Propositions and If/Then Statements of the Occupational Therapy Task-Oriented Approach	

Intervention Feature	If/Then Statements From Key Theories	Evidence to Support Proposition
Goal setting: client guides selection of tasks for intervention • Client centered • Intervention reflects client's priorities. • Elicit active participation of client	If the client sets goals for intervention, then they will be more engaged in intervention and achieve desired outcomes.	Law et al. (1995) Law and Mills (1998) Siegert and Taylor (2004) Trombly (1995)
Functional and meaningful tasks	If the task is functional and meaningful to the client, then the quality of movement during execution of the task will be better.	Lin et al. (1997) Wu et al. (2001)
Natural context (if rehabilitation setting, should simulate real-life setting as much as possible)	If the intervention is provided in a natural context, then clients will develop more flexible movement patterns for the task and context.	Bernstein (1967) Burgess (1989) Gillen and Wasserman (2004)
Real objects	If a person uses real objects, rather than rote exercise without objects, then the quality of movement will be better.	Mathiowetz and Wade (1995) Nelson et al. (1996) Wu et al. (2000)
Help clients adjust task performance limitations	If clients can find alternative ways to perform associated tasks, then they will be able to continuously engage in desired occupations.	Trombly (1995)
Dynamic performance analysis • Experiment with functional tasks to discover efficient strategies for optimal solutions to performance problems. • Identify salient client or environmental factors interfering with effective and efficient task performance.	If the client experiments with functional activities, then they will discover the most effective and efficient way to perform the task. If a client factor (e.g., strength, sensation) is critical to occupational performance of the desired task and there is potential to change that factor, then remedial techniques should be used. If a client, after a stroke, has active wrist and finger extension in the involved extremity, then the client is likely to benefit from constraint-induced movement therapy (CIMT). • If a client has active extension of the wrist >10° starting at neutral, some active abduction of the carpometacarpal (CMC) joint of thumb and 10° of active extension in elbow flexion, then the client is likely to benefit from modified constraint-induced therapy (mCIT). If remediation is unlikely, then adaptive and compensatory approaches should be used.	Bonaiuti et al. (2007) Flinn (1995) Gillen (2002) Van Peppen et al. (2004)
Adapt task to promote optimal performance	Changing task and environmental characteristics can elicit changes in the client's movement forms and patterns.	Davis and Burton (1991)
Client practices task and therapist provides feedback to facilitate learning. • Feedback graded to task and performance	If the therapist provides graded feedback for the type of task and client performance, then the client will learn the task. If the feedback is gradually tapered, then the client will learn how to use his or her own feedback mechanisms to monitor and evaluate his or her own performance.	Crutchfield and Barnes (1993)
Problem-solve with client	If the client can break down the task and problem-solve on his or her own, then he or she will be more likely to generate solutions in other contexts and environments.	D'Zurilla and Nezu (2007) Elliott (1999)
Practice performing tasks outside of therapy context • Follow-up	If the client uses abilities discovered in therapy in varied contexts, then abilities will become more automatic.	Gillen and Wasserman (2004) Trombly (1995)

performance. A review of available evidence will support the practitioner's reasoning regarding the probability of changing a control parameter to support performance. The dynamic systems perspective that proposes that movement is organized in relation to a goal echoes the propositions informed by other theoretical perspectives. Together, these theoretical perspectives inform the practitioner's actions with Maria. It is possible to test these propositions, and numerous researchers have conducted studies to demonstrate support for these propositions (e.g., see Trombly et al., 1998).

At first glance, the CO-OP Approach™ and the Occupational Therapy Task-Oriented Approach appear quite similar because both approaches are based on the proposition that if people are engaged in the process of setting goals for intervention based on their values and preferences, they will engage in more effective problem solving and be more motivated to engage in the intervention activities. Guided practice with specific feedback is another common feature of the two approaches. Yet, the CO-OP Approach™ is informed by metacognitive theories, whereas the Occupational Therapy Task-Oriented Approach is derived from motor learning and behavioral control theories; thus, the discrete propositions are different; intervention strategies, the resulting therapist actions, and expected outcomes might differ. Baking cookies and a cake provide a useful metaphor for capturing this distinction. We might use the ingredients of flour, sugar, and butter in preparing both cake and cookies. Yet, in order to achieve our goal or desired outcome, we need to use the appropriate amount or dose of ingredients, perhaps select among different forms of the ingredients, add other unique ingredients, and introduce the ingredients in a particular order or sequence. In contrast to baking, OT is a complex and dynamic process, and the outcome being sought is unique to each client. This complexity requires a unique approach for each client that is constructed and continually revised through the application of the therapist's professional reasoning. In order to ensure that interventions are optimally suited to each client's capacities and effective to achieve the client's goals, therapists must continually articulate and examine the assumptions and propositions underlying their actions and be prepared to revise their approach when desired outcomes are not achieved or the evidence does not support the reasoning.

Conclusion

Within OT, some of our interventions and treatment theories are more developed than others. As we develop a more refined understanding of the causal relationships represented in our intervention theories and deconstruct how the intervention works, we can be more precise in our intervention. We can also articulate the basis of what we are doing more clearly to others. Thus, for example, we can explain to Maria how the activities she is engaging in during an intervention session relate to achieving the goals she has set for herself or explain to the supervisor why we expect CO-OP Approach™ to be more effective for Alex than the simple practice of desired skills with feedback. It is our professional responsibility to continually examine the assumptions and theoretical propositions guiding our intervention approaches so that we can improve practice and achieve desired outcomes for clients.

Lippincott® Connect *For additional resources on the subjects discussed in this chapter, visit* Lippincott Connect.

REFERENCES

American Occupational Therapy Association. (2020). Occupational therapy practice framework: Domain and process (4th ed.). *American Journal of Occupational Therapy, 74*(Suppl. 2), 7412410010. https://doi.org/10.5014/ajot.2020.74S2001

Ayres, A. J. (1972). *Sensory integration and learning disorders.* Western Psychological Services.

Bandura, A. (1997). *Self-efficacy: The exercise of control.* W. H. Freeman.

Bass-Haugen, J., Mathiowetz, V., & Flinn, N. (2008). Optimizing motor behavior using the occupational therapy task-oriented approach. In M. V. Radomski & C. A. T. Latham (Eds.), *Occupational therapy for physical dysfunction* (6th ed., pp. 598–617). Lippincott Williams & Wilkins.

Batte, M., & Polatajko, H. J. (2006). CO-OP vs. practice for children with developmental coordination disorder: A question of strategy [Unpublished dissertation]. University of Toronto, Canada.

Baum, C. M., & Christiansen, C. H. (2005). Person-environment-occupation-performance: An occupation-based framework for practice. In C. H. Christiansen, C. M. Baum, & J. Bass-Haugen (Eds.), *Occupational therapy: Performance, participation, and well-being* (pp. 242–266). SLACK.

Bernstein, N. (1967). *The coordination and regulation of movements.* Pergamon Press.

Bonaiuti, D., Rebasti, L., & Sioli, P. (2007). The constraint induced movement therapy: A systematic review of randomized controlled trials on the adult stroke patients. *Europa Medicophysica, 43,* 139–146. PMID: 17525700.

Bronfenbrenner, U. (1979). *The ecology of human development: Experiments by nature and design.* Harvard University Press.

Burgess, M. K. (1989). Motor control and the role of occupational therapy: Past, present, and future. *American Journal of Occupational Therapy, 43,* 345–348. https://doi.org/10.5014/ajot.43.5.345

Camp, B. W., & Bash, M. S. (1982). *Think aloud: Increasing social and cognitive skills—A problem solving program for children: Primary level.* Research Press.

Crutchfield, C. A., & Barnes, M. R. (1993). *Motor control and motor learning in rehabilitation.* Stokesville.

Davis, W. E., & Burton, A. W. (1991). Ecological task analysis: Behavior theory into practice. *Adapted Physical Activity Quarterly, 8,* 154–177.

Dunn, W., Brown, C., & McGuian, M. (1994). The ecology of human performance: A framework for considering the effect of context. *American Journal of Occupational Therapy, 48,* 595–607. https://doi.org/10.5014/ajot.48.7.595

D'Zurilla, T., & Nezu, A. (2007). *Problem-solving therapy: A positive approach to clinical intervention* (3rd ed.). Springer.

Elliott, T. R. (1999). Social problem-solving abilities and adjustment to recent-onset spinal cord injury. *Rehabilitation Psychology, 44,* 315–332. https://doi.org/10.1037/0090-5550.44.4.315

Feuerstein, R., Hoffman, M., Jensen, M., Tzuriel, D., & Hoffman, D. (1986). Learning to learn: Mediated learning experiences and instrumental enrichment. *Special Services in Schools*, 3, 48–82. https://doi.org/10.1300/J008v03n01_05

Flinn, N. (1995). A task-oriented approach to the treatment of a client with hemiplegia. *American Journal of Occupational Therapy*, 49, 560–569. https://doi.org/10.5014/ajot.49.6.560

Garcia-Coll, C. (2020). Globalization, culture, and development: Are we ready for a paradigm shift? *Human Development*, 64, 245–249. https://doi.org/10.1159/000512903

Gibson, J. J. (1979). *The ecological approach to visual perception*. Houghton Mifflin.

Gillen, G. (2002). Improving mobility and community access in an adult with ataxia. *American Journal of Occupational Therapy*, 56, 462–466. https://doi.org/10.5014/ajot.56.4.462

Gillen, G., & Wasserman, M. (2004). Mobility: Examining the impact of environment on transfer performance. *Physical and Occupational Therapy in Geriatrics*, 22, 21–29. https://doi.org/10.1080/J148v22n04_03

Hammell, K. W. (2009a). Sacred texts: A skeptical exploration of the assumptions underpinning theories of occupation. *Canadian Journal of Occupational Therapy*, 76(1), 6–13. https://doi.org/10.1177/000841740907600105

Hammell, K. W. (2009b). Self-care, productivity, and leisure, or dimensions of occupational experience? Rethinking occupational "categories". *Canadian Journal of Occupational Therapy*, 76(2), 107–114. https://doi.org/10.1177/000841740907600208

Haywood, H. C. (1988). Bridging: A special technique of mediation. *The Thinking Teacher*, 4, 4–5.

Hooper, B. (1997). The relationship between pretheoretical assumptions and clinical reasoning. *American Journal of Occupational Therapy*, 51, 328–338. https://doi.org/10.5014/ajot.51.5.328

Horak, F. B. (1991). Assumptions underlying motor control for neurologic rehabilitation. In M. J. Lister (Ed.), *Contemporary management of motor control problems: Proceeding of the II STEP conference* (pp. 11–27). Foundation for Physical Therapy.

Jongbloed, L., Stacey, S., & Brighton, C. (1989). Stroke rehabilitation: Sensorimotor integrative treatment versus functional treatment. *American Journal of Occupational Therapy*, 43, 391–397. https://doi.org/10.5014/ajot.43.6.391

Kielhofner, G. (2008). *The model of human occupation: Theory and application* (4th ed.). Lippincott Williams & Wilkins.

Kielhofner, G., & Burke, J. P. (1980). A model of human occupation, part 1. Conceptual framework and content. *American Journal of Occupational Therapy*, 54, 572–581. https://doi.org/10.5014/ajot.34.9.572

Law, M., Baptiste, S., & Mills, J. (1995). Client-centered practice: What does it mean and does it make a difference? *Canadian Journal of Occupational Therapy*, 62, 250–257. https://doi.org/10.1177/000841749506200504

Law, M., Cooper, B., Strong, S., Stewart, D., Rigby, P., & Letts, L. (1996). The person-environment-occupation model: A transactive approach to occupational performance. *Canadian Journal of Occupational Therapy*, 63, 9–23. https://doi.org/10.1177/000841749606300103

Law, M., & Mills, J. (1998). Client-centered occupational therapy. In M. Law (Ed.), *Client-centered occupational therapy* (pp. 1–18). SLACK.

Lawton, M. P. (1986). *Environment and aging* (2nd ed.). Plenum Press.

Lin, K., Wu, C., Tickle-Degnen, L., & Coster, W. (1997). Enhancing occupational performance through occupationally embedded exercise: A meta-analytic review. *Occupational Therapy Journal of Research*, 17, 25–47. https://doi.org/10.1177/153944929701700102

Luria, A. R. (1976). *Cognitive development: Its cultural and social foundations*. Harvard University Press.

Mandich, A., Polatajko, H. J., Macnab, J. J., & Miller, L. T. (2001a). Treatment of children with developmental coordination disorder: What is the evidence? *Physical and Occupational Therapy in Pediatrics*, 20, 51–68. PMID: 11345512.

Mandich, A. D., Polatajko, H. J., Missiuna, C., & Miller, L. T. (2001b). Cognitive strategies and motor performance in children with developmental coordination disorder. *Physical and Occupational Therapy in Pediatrics*, 20(2–3), 125–143. PMID: 11345507.

Mathiowetz, V. (2011). Task-oriented approach to stroke rehabilitation. In G. Gillen (Ed.), *Stroke rehabilitation* (pp. 80–99). Elsevier Mosby.

Mathiowetz, V., & Bass-Haugen, J. (1994). Motor behavior research: Implications for therapeutic approaches to CND dysfunction. *American Journal of Occupational Therapy*, 48, 733–745.

Mathiowetz, V. G., & Wade, M. (1995). Task constraints and functional motor performance of individuals with and without multiple sclerosis. *Ecological Psychology*, 7, 99–123.

Meichenbaum, D. (1977). *Cognitive behaviour modification*. Plenum Press.

Merriam-Webster. (2021). Theory. In *Merriam-Webster.com dictionary*. https://www.merriam-webster.com/dictionary/theory

Miller, L. T., Polatajko, H. J., Missiuna, C., Mandich, A. D., & Macnab, J. J. (2001). A pilot trial of a cognitive treatment for children with developmental coordination disorder. *Human Movement Science*, 20, 183–210. https://doi.org/10.1016/s0167-9457(01)00034-3

Nelson, D. L., Konosky, K., Fleharty, K., Webb, R., Newer, K., Hazboun, V. P., Fontane, C., & Licht, B. C. (1996). The effects of an occupationally embedded exercise on bilaterally assisted supination in persons with hemiplegia. *American Journal of Occupational Therapy*, 50, 639–646. https://doi.org/10.5014/ajot.50.8.639

Plautz, E. J., Milliken, G. W., & Nudo, R. J. (2000). Effects of repetitive motor training on movement representations in adult squirrel monkeys: Role of use versus learning. *Neurobiology of Learning and Memory*, 74, 27–55. https://doi.org/10.1006/nlme.1999.3934

Polanyi, M. (2009). *The tacit dimension*. University of Chicago Press. (Original work published 1966)

Polatajko, H. J., Mandich, A. D., Missiuna, C., Miller, L. T., Macnab, J. J., Malloy-Miller, T., & Kinsella, E. A. (2001). Cognitive orientation to daily occupational performance (CO-OP): Part III—the protocol in brief. In C. Missiuna (Ed.), *Children with developmental coordination disorder: Strategies for success* (pp. 107–123). Haworth Press.

Popper, K. (1959). *The logic of scientific discovery*. Basic Books.

Preissner, K. (2010). Use of the occupational therapy task-oriented approach to optimize the motor performance of a client with cognitive limitations. *American Journal of Occupational Therapy*, 64, 727–734. https://doi.org/10.5014/ajot.2010.08026

Sabari, J. S. (1991). Motor learning concepts applied to activity-based intervention with adults with hemiplegia. *American Journal of Occupational Therapy*, 45, 523–530. https://doi.org/10.5014/ajot.45.6.523

Scaffa, M. E., & Reitz, S. M. (Eds.). (2014). *Occupational therapy in community-based practice settings* (2nd ed.). F. A. Davis.

Siegert, R. J., & Taylor, W. J. (2004). Theoretical aspects of goal-setting and motivation in rehabilitation. *Disability and Rehabilitation*, 26, 1–8. https://doi.org/10.1080/09638280410001644932

Swedberg, R. (2012). Theorizing in sociology and social science: Turning to the context of discovery. *Theory and Society*, 41(1), 1–40. http://www.jstor.org/stable/41349133

Taub, E., Uswatte, G., & Pidikiti, R. (1999). Constraint-induced movement therapy: A new family of techniques with broad application to physical rehabilitation. *Journal of Rehabilitation Research and Development*, 6, 237–251. PMID: 10659807.

Thelen, E., & Ulrich, B. D. (1991). Hidden skills: A dynamic systems analysis of treadmill stepping during the first year. *Monographs of the Society for Research in Child Development*, 56, 1–98. PMID: 1922136.

Trombly, C. A. (1995). Occupation: Purposefulness and meaningfulness as therapeutic mechanisms. *American Journal of Occupational Therapy*, 49, 960–972. https://doi.org/10.5014/ajot.49.10.960

Trombly, C., Radomski, M. V., & Davis, E. S. (1998). Achievement of self-identified goals by adults with traumatic brain injury: Phase I. *American Journal of Occupational Therapy, 52,* 810–818. https://doi.org/10.5014/ajot.56.5.489

Van Peppen, R. P., Kwakkel, G., Wood-Dauphinee, S., Hendriks, H. J., Van der Wees, P. J., & Dekker, J. (2004). The impact of physical therapy on functional outcomes after stroke: What's the evidence? *Clinical Rehabilitation, 18,* 833–862. https://doi.org/10.1191/0269215504cr843oa

Vygotsky, L. S. (1967). Play and its role in the mental development of the child. *Soviet Psychology, 5,* 6–18.

Whyte, J. (2006). Using treatment theories to refine the designs of brain injury rehabilitation treatment effectiveness studies. *Journal of Head Trauma Rehabilitation, 21,* 99–106. PMID: 16569984.

Wu, C., Trombly, C. A., Lin, K., & Tickle-Degnen, L. (2000). A kinematic study of contextual effects on reaching performance in persons with and without stroke: Influences of object availability. *Archives of Physical Medicine and Rehabilitation, 81,* 95–101. https://doi.org/10.1016/s0003-9993(00)90228-4

Wu, C., Wong, M., Lin, K., & Chen, H. (2001). Effects of task goal and personal preference on seated reaching kinematics after stroke. *Stroke, 32,* 70–76. https://doi.org/10.1161/01.str.32.1.70

The Model of Human Occupation

Kirsty Forsyth and Catana Brown

LEARNING OBJECTIVES

After reading this chapter, you will be able to:

1. Describe the personal factors addressed by the Model of Human Occupation (MOHO) and articulate how each concept affects occupational life.
2. Explain the environmental factors that are addressed by MOHO and articulate how each concept affects occupational life.
3. Identify dimensions of doing that MOHO uses to describe and examine a person's engagement in occupations.
4. Outline the steps of therapeutic reasoning in MOHO.
5. Articulate how change occurs in occupational therapy and identify client actions and therapeutic strategies that lead to change.
6. Analyze how MOHO can be applied to clients with various diagnoses across the life course in different practice contexts.

Introduction

The Model of Human Occupation (MOHO) (Kielhofner, 2008; Taylor, 2017) is an approach to occupational therapy (OT) practice that is occupation focused (Fisher et al., 2017), theory driven (Elenko et al., 2000), client centered (Law, 1998), and evidence based (Law et al., 1997). The MOHO was introduced 30 years ago by three practitioners seeking to articulate an approach to occupation-based intervention. They described MOHO as a theory to guide thinking about clients and the therapy process (Kielhofner, 1980a, 1980b; Kielhofner & Burke, 1980; Kielhofner et al., 1980). Evidence indicates that MOHO is the most widely used occupation-based model in practice worldwide (Taylor, 2017). Developed in the 1980s, MOHO has undergone four decades of research and refinement and promotes an occupation-focused practice and a clearer professional identity.

Overview of the Model of Human Occupation

The MOHO emerged at a time when the field was just beginning to rediscover the importance of occupation as an outcome and means of intervention.

In the 1970s, when MOHO was being formulated as an approach to practice, Dr. Kielhofner recognized that a practice focused on understanding and reducing impairment was not enough. The impetus for developing MOHO was the recognition that many factors beyond motor, cognitive, and sensory impairments contribute to difficulties in everyday occupation. These include occupational barriers posed by the physical and social environment, difficulties in choosing and finding meaning in occupations, and the challenge of maintaining positive involvement in life roles and routines. The MOHO was developed to address these factors.

Consequently, the MOHO concepts address (a) the motivation for occupation, (b) the routine patterning of occupations, (c) the nature of skilled performance, and (d) the influence of environment on occupation. These concepts serve as a framework for gathering data about a client's situation, enable therapists to identify the client's occupational strengths and limitations, and help therapists and clients plan and implement a course of OT. The MOHO is appropriate for clients with a wide range of impairments (physical, mental, cognitive, and sensory) throughout the life course.

Core Concepts of the Model of Human Occupation

The MOHO explains how occupations are chosen, patterned, and performed (Kielhofner, 2008). The MOHO is concerned with how people participate in daily occupations and achieve a sense of competence and identity (Figure 34.1). The model begins with the idea that a

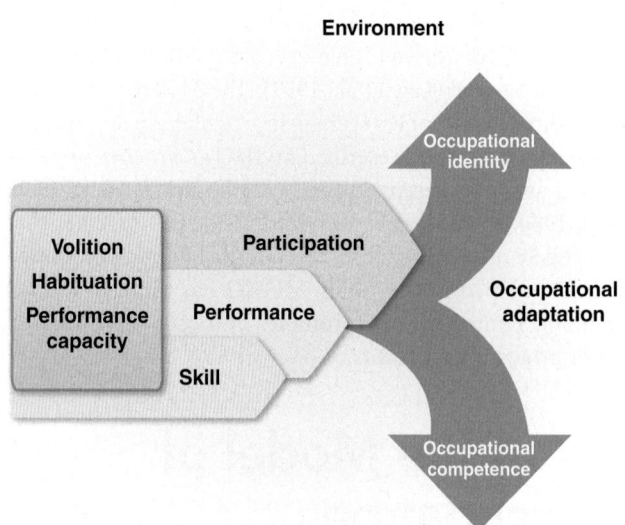

Environment

FIGURE 34.1 **Model of human occupation concepts.**

person's characteristics and his or her environment are linked together when someone is engaged in an occupation. Moreover, the model asserts that motives, patterns of performance, and skills are maintained and changed through engagement in occupations. The MOHO understands OT as a process in which practitioners support client engagement in occupations in order to shape the clients' choices, their routine ways of doing things, and their skills.

Model of Human Occupation Concepts Related to the Person

To explain how occupations are chosen, patterned, and performed, MOHO conceptualizes people as composed of three interacting elements: volition, habituation, and performance capacity. The sections that follow discuss these elements.

Volition

Volition refers to the process by which people are motivated toward and choose occupations. The concept of volition asserts that all humans have a desire to engage in occupations and that this desire is shaped by previous experiences. Volition occurs in a cycle of anticipating possibilities for doing, choosing what to do, experiencing what one does, and subsequent interpretation of the experience. These thoughts and feelings are influenced by underlying personal factors, for example, how capable and effective one feels (called *personal causation*), what one holds as important (called *values*), and what one finds enjoyable and satisfying (called *interests*).

Personal causation refers to thoughts and feelings about one's abilities and effectiveness as they engage in everyday occupations. These include, for example, recognizing one's strengths and weaknesses, feeling confident or anxious when faced with an occupation, and reflecting on how well one did after doing something.

Values are beliefs and commitments about what is good, right, and important to do. They include thoughts and feelings about activities that are worth doing, beliefs about the proper way to complete those activities, and the meanings that are ascribed to the things one does. Values specify what is worth doing, how to perform, and what goals or aspirations deserve commitment.

Interests are developed through the experience of pleasure and satisfaction derived from occupational engagement (Matsutsuyu, 1969). Therefore, the development of interests depends on available opportunities to engage in occupations.

Volition has a pervasive influence on occupational life. Volition guides choices of what to do and determines the experience of doing. It shapes how people make sense of what they have done. Volition is also central to the OT process. All therapy requires that clients make choices to do things; therefore, it *must* engage clients' volition. Moreover, how clients experience what they do in therapy (a function of volition) to a large extent determines therapy outcomes.

Habituation

Habituation refers to a process whereby people organize their actions into patterns and routines. Through repeated action within specific contexts, people establish habituated patterns of doing. These patterns of action are governed by habits and roles, which shape how people go about the routine aspects of their lives.

Habits involve learned ways of doing things that unfold automatically. Habits operate in cooperation with context, using and incorporating the environment as a resource for doing familiar things. They influence how people perform routine activities, use time, and behave. For instance, habits shape how people intuitively go about self-care each morning, organize the weekly routine, and complete a familiar task.

Roles provide a cultural script for one's identity and provide a set of responsibilities and obligations that are associated with that identity. People see themselves as students, workers, and parents and recognize that they should behave in certain ways to fulfill these roles. Much of what people do is done as a spouse, parent, worker, or student. People learn how to acquire each of these roles successfully through the expectations that others have for a role and the social environment in which each role is located. Thus, through interaction with others, people internalize an identity and a way of behaving that is associated with each role they have internalized.

Habits and roles make up how people routinely interact with their physical and social environments. When habituation is challenged by impairments and/or environmental circumstances, people can lose a great deal of what has given life familiarity and consistency. One of the major tasks of therapy may be to reconstruct habits and roles so that the person can more routinely participate in life occupations within the everyday environment.

Performance Capacity

Performance capacity refers to a person's underlying mental and physical abilities and how those abilities are used and experienced in occupational performance. The capacity for performance is affected by the status of musculoskeletal, neurologic, cardiopulmonary, and other bodily systems that are called on when a person does things. Biomechanical, motor control, cognitive, and sensory integration approaches to practice address these aspects of performance capacity that can be observed, measured, and modified (Bundy & Lane, 2020; Dirette & Gutman, 2021).

The MOHO recognizes the importance of approaches that address physical and mental capacities for occupational performance, and it is typically used in conjunction with such models. The MOHO stresses the importance of also paying attention to how people experience impairments. This includes paying attention to how people's bodies feel to them and how they perceive the world when they have impairments.

Model of Human Occupation Concepts Concerning the Environment

The MOHO stresses that all occupation results from an interaction of the person (volition, habituation, and performance capacity) with the characteristics of the physical and social environment. The *environment* can be defined as the particular physical, social, cultural, economic, and political features within a person's context that influence the motivation, organization, and performance of occupation. There are several dimensions of the environment that may have an impact on an individual's occupational life. For example, people encounter different physical spaces, objects, and people as well as expectations and opportunities for doing things. At the same time, the larger culture, economic conditions, and political factors also exert an influence. Accordingly, the environment includes the following dimensions:

- The objects that people use when they do things
- The spaces within which people do things
- The tasks that are available, expected, and/or required of people in a given context and that provide a set of social norms and conventions for engaging in recognizable occupations (such as "studying," "cleaning the house," or "playing cards")
- The social groups (e.g., family, friends, coworkers, neighbors) that make up the context and the expectations those social groups hold
- The surrounding culture, political, and economic forces

Objects and spaces together comprise the physical environment. The social environment includes both tasks and social groups.

The things that people do and how they think and feel about these things reflect a complex interplay of motives, habits and roles, and abilities with the dimensions of the environment noted previously. Political and economic conditions determine what resources people have for doing things and what occupational roles are available to them. Social injustices such as poverty, discrimination, and excessive incarceration constrain what people can do. Culture shapes the formation of ideas about how one should perform and what is worth doing. The demands of a task can determine the extent to which a person feels confident or anxious. The match of objects and spaces to the capacity of the individual influences how the person performs. In these and a myriad of other ways, the environment has an impact on what people do and how they think and feel about their doing. In turn, people also choose and modify their environments. For instance, people select environments that match and allow them to realize their values and interests.

Dimensions of Doing

As Figure 34.1 shows, MOHO identifies three levels at which we can examine a person's engagement in occupations: occupational participation, occupational performance, and occupational skill.

Occupational participation refers to engaging in work, play, or activities of daily living (ADLs) that are part of one's sociocultural environment and that are desired and/or necessary to one's well-being. This is the highest "level" of conceptualizing engagement in occupations. Examples of occupational participation are volunteering for an organization, working in a full- or part-time job, regularly getting together with friends, doing self-care, maintaining one's living space, and attending school. Each area of occupational participation involves a cluster of related tasks that one does. For example, participating to maintain one's living space may include paying the rent, doing repairs, and cleaning. Doing a task related to participation in a major life area is referred to as *occupational performance*.

During occupational performance, we carry out discrete purposeful actions. For example, making tea is a culturally recognizable task in many cultures. To do so, one *gathers* together tea, kettle, and a cup; *handles* these materials and objects; and *sequences* the steps necessary to brew and pour the tea. These actions that make up occupational performance of a task are referred to as *skills*. Skills are goal-directed actions that a person uses while performing (Forsyth et al., 1998). In contrast to *performance capacity*, which refers to underlying ability (e.g., range of motion and strength), skill refers to the actions *within* an occupational performance, such as reaching or sequencing. There are three types of skills: motor skills, process skills, and communication and interaction skills. Detailed taxonomies of each of the three types of skills have been developed (Bernspang & Fisher, 1995; Doble, 1991; A. Fisher & Kielhofner, 1995; Forsyth et al., 1998, 1999). See Chapter 26 for more detail on performance skills.

Occupational Identity, Competence, and Adaptation

Over time, what people do creates their occupational identity. This identity, generated from experience, is the cumulative sense of who people are and who they wish to become as occupational beings. The degree to which people are able to sustain a pattern of doing that enacts their occupational identity is referred to as *occupational competence*. These two essential elements of occupational adaptation entail the creation of an occupational identity and the ability to enact this identity in various circumstances.

The Process of Change and Therapy

A basic premise of MOHO is that all change in OT is driven by clients' occupational engagement. The term *occupational engagement* refers to clients' doing, thinking, and feeling under certain environmental conditions in the midst of therapy or as a planned consequence of therapy.

When clients engage in tasks in therapy or as a result of therapy, volition, habituation, and performance capacity are all involved in some way. For example, a client may be (a) drawing on performance capacity to exercise skill in occupational performance, (b) evoking old habits that shape how the occupational performance is done, (c) enacting or working toward acquiring a role, (d) experiencing a level of satisfaction and enjoyment (or dissatisfaction) with occupational performance, (e) assigning meaning and significance to what is done (i.e., what this means for the client's life), or (f) feeling able (or unable) when doing an occupation.

Each of these aspects of what the client does, thinks, and feels shapes the change process. For this reason, practitioners using MOHO are mindful of their clients' volition, habituation, performance capacity, and environmental conditions in the midst of therapy and how these elements are interacting as the therapy unfolds. To help practitioners think about the process of occupational engagement, MOHO identifies the nine dimensions of occupational engagement shown in Table 34.1. These nine dimensions provide a basic structure for thinking about how clients achieve change and for planning how therapy goals will be achieved. This process is discussed in the next section.

Using the Model of Human Occupation in Practice

Using MOHO in practice involves thinking with its concepts—a process referred to as *therapeutic reasoning*. Therapeutic reasoning refers specifically to the use of MOHO concepts in thinking about clients' needs throughout the OT process (American Occupational Therapy Association, 2020). The therapeutic reasoning process has six steps:

1. Generating questions about the client
2. Gathering information on and with the client
3. Using the information gathered to create a theory-based explanation of the client's situation
4. Generating goals and strategies for therapy
5. Implementing and monitoring therapy
6. Determining outcomes of therapy

| TABLE 34.1 | Dimensions of Client Occupational Engagement |

Dimensions of Occupational Engagement	Definition
Choose/decide	Anticipate and select from alternatives for action.
Commit	Decide to undertake a course of action to accomplish a goal or personal project, fulfill a role, or establish a new habit.
Explore	Investigate new objects, spaces, social groups, and/or occupational forms/tasks; do things with altered performance capacity; try out new ways of doing things; and examine possibilities for occupational participation in one's context.
Identify	Locate novel information, alternatives for action, and new feelings that provide solutions for and/or give meaning to occupational performance and participation.
Negotiate	Engage in a give-and-take approach with others that creates mutually agreed-upon perspectives and/or finds a middle ground between different expectations, plans, or desires.
Plan	Establish an action agenda for performance or participation.
Practice	Repeat a certain performance or consistently participate in an occupation with the intent of increasing skill, ease, and effectiveness of performance.
Reexamine	Critically appraise and consider alternatives to previously held beliefs, attitudes, feelings, habits, or roles.
Sustain	Persist in occupational performance or participation despite uncertainty or difficulty.

Practitioners generally move back and forth between these steps over the course of therapy. Each step is briefly discussed in the subsequent section.

Generating Questions

Practitioners must come to understand their clients in order to plan and implement therapy. This understanding begins with asking questions about their clients (Table 34.2). The MOHO concepts allow a practitioner to generate these questions systematically. That is, the major concepts of the theory (environmental impact, volition, habituation, performance capacity, participation, performance, skills, occupational identity, and occupational competence) orient the practitioner to be concerned about certain things when learning about a client. For example, practitioners using MOHO would ask what their clients' thoughts and feelings are in relation to personal causation, values, and interests. Moreover, they would ask about their clients' roles and habits and how these affect the clients' routines. These questions would, of course, be tailored to the clients' circumstances.

| TABLE 34.2 | Model of Human Occupation (MOHO)-Based Therapeutic Reasoning Questions |

MOHO Concept	Questions
Occupational identity	• What is the person's sense of who he or she has been, is, and wishes to become in relation to family life, school, friendships, hobbies, and interests? • What is the family's sense of who this person has been, is, and what do they wish him or her to become? How does this affect the person's occupational identity?
Occupational competence	• To what extent has this person sustained a pattern of satisfying occupational participation over time? • Does this person feel that he or she can do the things he or she needs to do in school, with friends, and in the community? • To what extent has this person's life sustained patterns of occupational participation over time that reflect his or her occupational identity?
Participation	• Does the person currently engage in work, play, and ADLs that are part of his or her sociocultural context and that are desired and/or necessary for his or her well-being?
Performance	• Can this person do the occupations that are part of the work, play, and ADLs that make up, or should make up, his or her life? • Can the person do the occupations that are expected of his or her roles?
Skill	• Does the person exhibit the necessary communication/interaction, motor, and process skills to perform what he or she needs and wants to do?

(continued)

TABLE 34.2	Model of Human Occupation (MOHO)-Based Therapeutic Reasoning Questions (*continued*)

MOHO Concept	Questions
Environment	• Does the family support the person in developing the necessary volition, habituation and communication/interaction, motor, and process skills needed for participation? • What impact do the opportunities, resources, constraints, and demands (or lack of demands) of the environment have on how this person thinks, feels, and acts? • How do the opportunities, resources, constraints, or demands provided by spaces, objects, occupations/tasks, and social groups affect the person's skill, performance, and participation?
Volition	• What is this person's view of his or her personal capacity and effectiveness? • What does this person think is important? • What are this person's interests? What does this person enjoy doing?
Habituation	• What routines does this person participate in, and how do routines influence what he or she does? • What are the roles with which this person identifies with, and how do they influence what he or she routinely does?

ADLs, activities of daily living.

Gathering Information

To answer the questions generated in the first step, practitioners must gather information on and with the client. Practitioners may take advantage of naturally occurring opportunities to gather information. For example, a practitioner might learn about a client's personal causation by observing the client's emotional reaction when attempting to learn a challenging new task. Practitioners may also use structured MOHO assessments. Some MOHO assessments will capture comprehensive information on several aspects of the person and the environment. Some MOHO assessments attempt to capture more in-depth information on one aspect of MOHO, such as assessments that focus on volition. A wide range of MOHO-based assessments has been developed; they are summarized in Table 34.3. Thus, practitioners using MOHO have a range of choices when they decide which assessment(s) to use. Some OT services have developed assessment protocols to indicate service response to assessment needs. For another look at assessments needed for MOHO, see Expanding Our Perspectives.

TABLE 34.3	Model of Human Occupation (MOHO) Assessments Summary	

MOHO Assessment	Method of Administration	Description
Active in Children Health Integrating Evidence Valuing Experience (ACHIEVE) Assessment (Forsyth et al., 2012)	Questionnaire, interview, or observation	The assessment can be administered by mail or over the telephone and is completed by the child's teacher with a separate rating scale for the parent or guardian. It affords an opportunity for teachers or parents to share their view of how the child is participating in everyday activities. It asks for information on the frequency of their child's engagement in home, community, and school activity and then asks MOHO-orientated questions as to why this engagement is positive or negative.
Assessment of Communication and Interaction Skills (ACIS) (Forsyth et al., 1998)	Observation	Gathers information about the communication and interaction skills that a person displays while engaged in an occupation across the domains of physicality, information exchange, and relations. Used to generate goals for therapy related to communication/interaction skills and to assess outcomes/changes in skill.
Assessment of Motor and Process Skills (AMPS) (A. G. Fisher, 2003)	Observation	Gathers information about the motor and process skills that a person displays while engaged in an occupation. Used to generate goals for therapy related to motor and process skills and to assess outcomes/changes in skill.
Assessment of Occupational Functioning-Collaborative Version (AOF-CV) (Watts et al., 1999)	Interview and/or client self-report	Yields qualitative information and a quantitative profile of the impact of a client's personal causation, values, roles, habits, and skills on occupational participation. Used to inform intervention.
Child Occupational Self Assessment (COSA) (Keller et al., 2005)	Client self-report	Children and youths rate their occupational competence for engaging in 25 everyday activities in the home, school, and community and the importance of those activities. Used to generate goals and assess outcomes/change in competence and values.

TABLE 34.3 Model of Human Occupation (MOHO) Assessments Summary (*continued*)

MOHO Assessment	Method of Administration	Description
Interest Checklist (Matsutsuyu, 1969)	Client self-report	Checklist that indicates strength of interest and past, present, and future engagement in 68 activities. Used to inform intervention.
Model of Human Occupational Screening Tool (MOHOST) (Parkinson et al., 2006)	Observation, interview(s), and/or chart review	Information gathered assesses impact of volition, habituation, skills, and environment on client's occupational participation. Used to generate goals and assess outcomes or changes in participation.
National Institutes of Health Activity Record (Frust et al., 1987; Gerber & Frust, 1992)	Client self-report	Self-report "log" records information in half-hour intervals throughout the day on perceptions of competence, value, enjoyment, difficulty, and pain experienced when engaging in various occupations in that time period. Used to inform intervention and assess outcomes or change in participation.
Occupational Circumstances Assessment Interview and Rating Scale (OCAIRS) (Forsyth et al., 2005)	Interview	Interview yields information to assess values, goals, personal causation, interests, habits, roles, skills, readiness for change, and environmental impact on participation. Used to generate goals and assess outcomes or changes in participation.
Occupational Performance History Interview-II (OPHI-II) (Kielhofner et al., 2004)	Interview	Detailed life history interview that yields (a) scales measuring competence, identity, and environmental impact and (b) a narrative representation/analysis of the life history. Used as an in-depth, comprehensive assessment to generate goals, inform intervention, and build the therapeutic relationship.
Occupational Therapy Psychosocial Assessment of Learning (OT PAL) (Townsend et al., 1999)	Observation or interview	This assessment evaluates a student's volition (the ability to make choices), habituation (roles and routines), and environmental fit within the classroom setting. The manual includes reproducible assessment and data summary forms.
Occupational Questionnaire (OQ) (Smith et al., 1986)	Client self-report	Self-report "log" records information in half-hour intervals throughout the day on perceptions of competence, value, and enjoyment experienced when engaging in various occupations in that time period. Used to inform intervention and assess outcomes or change in participation.
Occupational Self Assessment (OSA) (Baron et al., 2006)	Client self-report	Clients rate their occupational competence for engaging in 21 everyday activities and the importance of those activities. Allows clients to set priorities for change. Used to generate goals and assess outcomes or changes in competence and values.
Pediatric Interest Profiles (PIP) (Henry, 2000)	Client self-report	Assessment includes three age-appropriate scales (some with line drawings) for children and adolescents to indicate participation, interest, and perceived competence in various play and leisure activities. Used to generate goals and assess outcomes or changes in participation.
Pediatric Volitional Questionnaire (PVQ) (Basu et al., 2002)	Observation	Guides a systematic observation of a child across multiple environments to assess volition and the impact of the environment on volition. Used as an in-depth assessment of volition to generate goals and assess outcomes or change in volition.
Residential Environment Impact Survey (REIS) (G. Fisher et al., 2008)	Observation or interview	Assesses how well the home environment is meeting the needs of the residents as a whole. Ratings in 24 areas provide a summary of the data and a structure for generating recommendations to enhance the qualities of the environment. The intent of this assessment tool is to not only assess the residential environment but also determine the impact of the environment on the residents and make recommendations to improve the quality of life for the residents and the work life of the staff.
Role Checklist (Oakley et al., 1985)	Client self-report	Checklist provides information on past, present, and future role participation and the perceived value of those roles. Used to inform intervention and assess outcomes or changes in role performance.
Short Child Occupational Profile (SCOPE) (Bowyer et al., 2006)	Observation, interview(s), and/or chart review	Information gathered assesses impact of volition, habituation, skills, and environment on child's or adolescent's occupational participation. Used to generate goals and assess outcomes or changes in participation.

(continued)

| TABLE 34.3 | Model of Human Occupation (MOHO) Assessments Summary (*continued*) | |

MOHO Assessment	Method of Administration	Description
School Setting Interview (SSI) (Hemmingson et al., 2005)	Interview	Interview works with students to gather information on student–environment fit and identify the need for accommodations. Used to generate goals, inform intervention, and assess outcomes or changes in student–environment fit.
Volitional Questionnaire (VQ) (de las Heras et al., 2003)	Observation	Guides a systematic observation of a client across multiple environments to assess volition and the impact of the environment on volition. Used as an in-depth assessment of volition to generate goals and assess outcomes or change in volition.
Worker Role Interview (WRI) (Braveman et al., 2005)	Interview	Interview yields information to rate the impact that volition, habitation, and perceptions of the environment have on psychosocial readiness for the worker role or return to work. Used to generate goals and assess outcomes or changes in psychosocial readiness for work.
Work Environment Impact Scale (WEIS) (Moore-Corner et al., 1998)	Interview	Interview works with client to assess environmental impact on participation in the worker role and to identify needed accommodations. Used to generate goals and inform intervention.

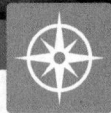

EXPANDING OUR PERSPECTIVES

Developing the Best Assessments for the Clients

Masataka Shikata

As a professional, I provide OT to clients at an older adult care facility in Japan. Community-dwelling clients who require long-term care are provided with meals, bathing, recreation, interaction with others, exercise, and hobbies. I was expected to gather information about the interests, values, roles, habits, and performance capacities of the clients and facilitate the client's participation in occupation by modifying environments and providing counsel and opportunities for engagement. Practices based on MOHO are useful for providing such services. A number of MOHO-based assessments have been developed and can be used, regardless of language and culture. However, I sometimes experienced difficulties in implementing these assessments in my setting and desired a more suitable assessment for my facility's clients.

Time limitation was one consideration. To serve all clients with a limited number of therapists made it difficult to allocate sufficient time on each client. Time constraints implied that we had to conduct the evaluation in an extremely short time frame. Another concern was the attitude of the surrounding individuals. At the facility, the clients, family members, and other professionals often demanded a biomechanical approach to prevent long-term frailty; therefore, conducting lengthy interviews was difficult. However, from a MOHO perspective, I wanted a self-report method for assessing occupational identity, specifically for the older adult. Japan has one of the world's most aged populations, and the number of clients who use senior citizen facilities is increasing every

year. Understanding occupational identity is a useful perspective to support clients as occupational beings. I also hoped that the self-report assessment would provide an opportunity for the clients to reflect on themselves as occupational beings.

I believed that a self-report assessment that could overcome time limitations and efficiently gather information on occupational identity for therapy was needed. Therefore, I conducted a study to investigate the state of the occupational identity of clients at my facility using qualitative study methods. Using the concepts of occupational identity obtained through the study, I developed an occupational identity questionnaire draft. In addition, we asked occupational therapists who provide services to older adults who require care in the community to participate in the data collection. Through this process, we developed the Occupational Identity Questionnaire.

This self-report assessment allows the therapist to obtain a relatively rapid understanding of the occupational identity by having the client fill out the questionnaire in advance. The OT can then ask additional questions during the following session. The questionnaire also allows us to identify the past benefits and current challenges our clients face regarding the occupational identity of older adults.

I believe that the existing assessments are absolutely useful. However, I realized that it is not always optimal to apply existing assessments to all clients in all settings. In some cases, I believe that it is useful to develop assessments that resolve such constraints and collect the necessary information from the client. By developing new assessments, I hope to aid the therapists who face similar problems and provide better services to clients.

Creating a Theory-Based Understanding of the Client

The information that the practitioner gathers to answer questions about a client is used to create a theory-based understanding of that client. In this step, the practitioner uses MOHO theory as a framework for creating an explanation of that particular client's situation to guide the next step of generating goals and strategies for therapy.

As part of creating an explanation of clients' circumstances, practitioners identify problems or challenges that need to be addressed in therapy as well as strengths that can be drawn on in therapy. Problems and challenges may be a function of volition, habituation, performance capacity, or the environment.

Generating Measurable Goals and Strategies

This step involves creating therapy goals (i.e., identifying what will change as a result of therapy), deciding what kinds of occupational engagement will enable the client to change, and determining what kind of therapeutic strategies will be needed to support the client to change.

Goals (Table 34.4) indicate the kinds of changes that therapy will aim to achieve. Change is required when the client's characteristics and/or environment are contributing to occupational problems or challenges. For instance, if a client feels ineffective, therapy would seek to enable the client to feel more effective, or if a client has too few roles, development of new roles would become the focus of therapy. In this way, identifying challenges or problems in the third step allows one to select the goals in the fourth step.

The next element in this step is to identify how the goals will be achieved. This involves indicating what occupational engagement on the part of the client will contribute to achieving these goals and how the practitioner will support the client. The previous section on change offered nine dimensions of occupational engagement, and these serve as a framework for thinking in this step. The MOHO also identifies key therapeutic strategies that practitioners will use, as listed in Box 34.1.

The fifth edition of *Kielhofner's Model of Human Occupation: Theory and Application* (Taylor, 2017) provides a comprehensive resource, the Therapeutic Reasoning Table, for this component of the therapeutic reasoning process. It identifies a wide range of problems and challenges that correspond to the concepts of MOHO along with types of changes that would be warranted. The table also indicates what types of occupational engagement could contribute to achieving those changes and what type of support from the practitioner could facilitate change. Table 34.5 shows one small section from this Therapeutic Reasoning Table related to personal causation.

TABLE 34.4	**Model of Human Occupation (MOHO)-Based Therapy Goals: Examples**
MOHO Concept	**Measurable Goal**
Volition	Within [time frame], [client] will be *able to identify* (number of) occupations that are significant to his or her occupational life (or roles) and are consistent with his or her current skills and abilities [action] within [setting] independently [degree] Within [time frame], [client] will *make the choice* to engage in (name occupation) having *identified* this as significant to his or her (successful performance of/or as a step in the progress toward) his or her performance as a (name role) [action] within [setting] with minimal support [degree]
Habituation	Within [time frame], [client] will be able to *identify* the responsibilities for roles that are valuable and meaningful to the person [action]; this will be achieved with minimal support [degree] within [setting] Within [time frame], [client] will be able to *practice* and develop a habit pattern that will support achievement of a single occupation [action]; this will be achieved with minimal support [degree] within [setting]
Skill	Within [time frame], [client] will be able to perform within (name the occupation) using (name skills) [action] within [setting], independently [degree] Within [time frame], [client] will be able to perform in (name the occupation) using adapted techniques to support lack of skill [action] within [setting], independently [degree]
Performance capacity	Within [time frame], [client] will be able to incorporate damaged or estranged parts of the body into completion of occupations [action], within [setting] independently [degree] Within [time frame], [client] will be able to manage symptoms while engaged in (name the occupations) [action] within [setting] independently [degree]
Environment	Within [time frame], [client] will be able to *perform* in (name the occupation) [action] within his or her physical and social home environment [setting], independently [degree] Within [time frame], [client] will be able to *perform* in the occupation using adapted objects or new objects [action] within [setting], independently [degree]

Source: Adapted from Kielhofner, G. (2008). *A model of human occupation: Theory and application* (4th ed.). Lippincott Williams & Wilkins.

BOX 34.1 THERAPEUTIC STRATEGIES IDENTIFIED BY THE MODEL OF HUMAN OCCUPATION

- **Validating:** Attending to and acknowledging the client's experience
- **Identifying:** Locating and sharing a range of personal, procedural, and/or environmental factors that can facilitate occupational performance
- **Giving feedback:** Sharing your understanding of the client's situation or ongoing action
- **Advising:** Recommending intervention goals/strategies
- **Negotiating:** Engaging in a give-and-take approach with the client

- **Structuring:** Establishing parameters for choice and performance by offering client alternatives, setting limits, establishing ground rules
- **Coaching:** Instructing, demonstrating, guiding, verbally and/or physically prompting
- **Encouraging:** Providing emotional support and reassurance in relation to engagement in an occupation
- **Providing physical support:** Using one's body to provide support for a client to complete an occupational form/task

TABLE 34.5 Excerpt From the Therapeutic Reasoning Table Showing a Problem/Challenge Related to Personal Causation and Corresponding Intervention Goals and Strategies

Problem/Challenge	Goal	Client Occupational Engagement	Therapeutic Strategies to Support the Client
• Feelings of lack of control over occupational performance leading to anxiety (fear of failure) within occupations	• Reduce client's anxiety and fear of failure in occupational performance (e.g., "The client will complete a simple three-step meal in 20 min without verbalizing anxiety or concern."). • Build up confidence to face occupational performance demands (e.g., "The client will identify and participate in three new leisure activities with minimal support in 1 week.").	• *Reexamine* anxieties and fears in the light of new performance experiences. • *Choose* to do relevant and meaningful things that are within performance capacity. • *Sustain* performance in occupational forms tasks despite anxiety.	• *Validate* how difficult it can be to do things that provoke anxiety. • *Identify* client's strengths and weaknesses in occupational performance. • Give *feedback* to client about match/mismatch between choice of occupational forms/tasks and performance capacity. • Give *feedback* to support a positive reinterpretation of his or her experience of engaging in an occupation. • *Advise* client to do relevant and meaningful things that match performance capacity.

Source: Adapted from Kielhofner, G. (2008). *A model of human occupation: Theory and application* (4th ed.). Lippincott Williams & Wilkins.

Implementing and Monitoring Therapy

To implement therapy means not only following the plan of action that was set out in the previous step but also monitoring how the therapy process unfolds. This monitoring process might confirm the practitioner's understanding of the client's situation or require the practitioner to reformulate the client's situation. The monitoring process also can confirm the usefulness of therapy and whether a change to the goals and/or plan is required. When things do not turn out as expected, the practitioner returns to earlier steps of generating questions, selecting methods to gather information, formulating the client's situation, setting goals, and establishing plans.

Collecting Information to Assess Outcomes

Determining therapy outcomes is an important final step in the therapy process. Typically, therapy outcomes are documented by examining the extent to which goals have been achieved and readministering structured assessments that were administered initially. Both of these approaches are valuable in documenting outcomes. Assessing outcomes by examining goal attainment is helpful in reflecting on the extent to which the therapeutic reasoning process resulted in good decisions for therapy. Using structured MOHO assessments also allows one to compare change across different clients or when different strategies are used. In this way, they can contribute to evidence-based therapy.

Evidence to Support Using the Model

The MOHO has been developed through the efforts of an international community of practitioners and scholars. It is supported by a substantial evidence base of well over 400 articles and chapters that present theoretical, applied, or research aspects of the model (Lee et al., 2008). The MOHO is taught in most OT programs and is highly influential in current occupation-based practice (Wong & Fisher, 2015). For example, the MOHO was identified as the predominant model used by occupational therapists in forensic mental health (Taylor et al., 2022),

Other examples of recent use of the MOHO are listed here.

Descriptive and Predictive Studies

- A scoping review examined the association between volition and participation among people with acquired disabilities (Harel-Katz & Carmeli, 2019). Only two studies specifically addressed the two constructs and did find that volition, or having confidence in one's ability and interest in an activity, was related to greater participation.
- A study was undertaken to examine constructs from MOHO, specifically occupational competence and occupational identity, and their relationship to recovery in schizophrenia (Tan et al., 2020). The study found that personal recovery predicted occupational competence, and occupational identity was predicted by depressive symptoms and hope. The study also found that managing finances, concentration, and taking care of self were performance items that participants most wanted to improve.
- A scoping review examined occupational priorities at the end of life using the MOHO to organize themes (Morgan et al., 2022). The review found that even when

participation is difficult, people prioritize continued engagement in valued occupations. Influence and control over participation become increasingly important as the disease progresses.

Assessment

- The Planning to Make Meals Performance Measure was developed using the MOHO (Schmelzer et al., 2022). A study examining the construct validity of the measure found that it was significantly correlated with the Food Skills Confidence Measure and the Cooking Skills Confidence Measure.
- There are many studies examining translations of MOHO assessments, including a study exploring the validity and reliability of the traditional Chinese version of the Occupational Self-Assessment (Pan et al., 2020) and a Turkish version (Pekçetin et al., 2018) validation of the Icelandic version of the Assessment of Work Performance (Skúladóttir et al., 2021), and psychometric properties of the Finnish translation of the Assessment of Communication and Interaction Skills (Fan et al., 2020).

Intervention

- Individual Placement and Support (IPS) is a widely used evidence-based vocational rehabilitation model for individuals with serious mental illness. In a prospective cohort study, the MOHO was used to enhance IPS, and a MOHO assessment, the Worker Role Interview (WRI), was used as a predictor of success in the program (Prior et al., 2020). The enhanced IPS program had a 63% success rate, which is higher than comparable studies of standard IPS, and the WRI found that motivational and habitual factors were useful in determining who would benefit most from the intervention.
- A small randomized controlled trial found that a home modification intervention based on MOHO found improvements in competence of occupational performance and time spent in ADLs and rest (Jo & Kim, 2022).
- Investigators examined the efficacy of a peer-play intervention informed by the MOHO for improving executive function in children with learning disabilities (Esmaili et al., 2019). The randomized controlled trial found that the intervention was effective for improving executive function, but it did not change perceived occupational values and competence.

OT Stories 34.1 and 34.2 illustrate how the MOHO is used throughout the OT process.

OT STORY 34.1 COLLECTING INFORMATION AND CREATING A THEORY-BASED UNDERSTANDING OF STEPHEN

Stephen is in his mid-30s and lives with his parents. He is very close to his supportive parents and younger brother who live in the same city. He described himself as a helpful son, supportive brother, loyal friend, and devoted dog owner. He enjoys the outdoors and sports, and he is currently unemployed.

Background

Stephen did well academically at school but became unwell and was diagnosed with schizophrenia in his final year of university. He left without completing his degree. Throughout this period, Stephen worked part time in various jobs: retail, hospitality, and caregiving. He also volunteered in a local day center for the older adult. Throughout his 20s, Stephen's mental health was poor with regular long admissions to hospital. He became socially withdrawn, spending time only with family members and health professionals; he rarely participated in swimming and running, which had previously been his daily occupations. During this period, Stephen's family helped him find several temporary jobs in retail and catering, all of which he left owing to deterioration in his mental health.

Recently, Stephen's mental health has improved, which he attributes to an improved medication regime. He is engaging in sporting activities and is keen to return to employment. In the past, he attended an OT prevocational training project where he participated in office administration tasks. His goal was to return to employment. He gradually built confidence and on discharge from the project and went on to a college course. He attained a vocational qualification in office administration but had been unable to secure employment.

The OT service provides an evidence-based vocational MOHO rehabilitation program, based on supported employment, where service users are supported to find a job quickly and rehabilitation is focused on maintaining the job ("place then train") as opposed to prevocational training ("train then place"). More information about the service is contained in *The WORKS: Occupational Therapy and Evidence Based Vocational Rehabilitation* (Prior et al., 2011). The service operates a self-referral system, and Stephen contacted the service with the goal of returning to paid employment.

Generating Questions

The occupational therapist was initially interested to explore Stephen's perceptions of his past, present, and future worker roles, including the following:

* What work activities does Stephen enjoy and value, and how able does he feel doing these activities (volition)?

* How are his present roles and routines impacting his engagement in work or impacting on work (habituation)?
* What level of support is offered in a social and physical work environment?
* Stephen had not reported any specific challenges in motor, process, or communication and interaction skills, and therefore, early reflection on questions did not relate to these areas.

Gathering Information

The occupational therapist used the WRI (Braveman et al., 2005) to identify psychosocial and environmental factors that may potentially impact Stephen's ability to obtain employment. The Work Environment Impact Scale (WEIS) (Moore-Corner et al., 1998) was selected by the occupational therapist to complement information gathered through the WRI to better understand the impact that previous work environments have had on Stephen's participation in his worker role.

Creating a Theory-Based Understanding of the Client

The following occupational formulation was created from the assessment findings.

* ***What is Stephen's occupational identity?*** Stephen is a son, brother, friend, and dog owner. He is a regular runner and swimmer. Stephen recognizes himself as an unemployed person who is seeking work.
* ***What is Stephen's occupational competence?*** Stephen enjoys and feels competent in all roles he is currently pursuing. He reported a tendency to underestimate his abilities; the standards he applies to his own work performance usually exceed those of his colleagues and managers. This has interfered with Stephen's personal causation in relation to work and has led him to doubt his competence in previous work roles. However, given improvements in mental health and his strong work ethic, he is confident that he will succeed in a worker role.
* ***What are the occupational issues Stephen is having difficulty with?*** Stephen reported frustration in his lack of success in applying for work. Previous worker roles had all been in entry-level jobs, and he had no aspirations for career development beyond attaining a paid job. Stephen described a lack of enjoyment of previous worker roles in hospitality and retail; in particular, he found the fluctuating demands of the role difficult to manage with high levels of noise and stress at busy times contrasting with lack of routine tasks in quiet periods. There was limited opportunity for Stephen to work with any autonomy in organizing his tasks. All the positions he had previously

OT STORY 34.1 COLLECTING INFORMATION AND CREATING A THEORY-BASED UNDERSTANDING OF STEPHEN (*continued*)

held were temporary, low-paid entry-level jobs and had offered little reward. Stephen has previously had poor relationships with colleagues and managers and has felt stigmatized because of his mental health condition. Stephen's life at the time of assessment lacked structure and routines; his roles as a family member, friend, and dog owner were important but demanded little time.

- *What are the positive occupational issues for Stephen?* Stephen has a strong commitment to being in paid employment. He has a clear understanding of the expectations of work roles he has held in the past. He has a strong supportive network of family and friends. They are very encouraging and had in the past used contacts to secure employment on his behalf.
- *Why is Stephen unable to work or having challenges engaging in work?* Previous worker roles Stephen has held were mainly in retail and hospitality and were a poor fit with his interest in office administration. His current methods for seeking employment have been unsuccessful, and he has been unable to adjust his strategies. His current routine lacks structure because of the absence of a worker role, and Stephen is concerned that he will find adjusting to the greater demands of a worker role challenging. Stephen has experienced difficulty in unsupportive relationships with coworkers and managers in past worker roles and is concerned this may occur in the future.

Generating Therapy Goals and Strategies

The following goals were jointly generated:

- *Within 2 weeks,* Stephen (with the support of the occupational therapist) will identify jobs that match his interests and preferred working style using online and paper-based career planning material at the therapy clinic.
- *Within 4 weeks,* Stephen's (with the support of the occupational therapist) assistant will develop a résumé and begin applying for jobs in his local library.
- *Within 6 weeks,* Stephen will independently spend time daily identifying, researching, and applying for jobs at home, in the job center, and in the library.
- *Within 6 weeks,* Stephen and the occupational therapist will investigate potential opportunities for unpaid internship in positions relevant to preferred worker role.

The therapist used the format featured in Table 34.4 to create a clear goal structure for Stephen. For example, the first goal indicates the following:

- The time frame as "2 weeks"
- The degree (or amount of assistance) as "with the support of the occupational therapist"

- The action as "identify jobs that match his interests and preferred working style using online and paper-based career planning materials"
- The setting as "the therapy clinic"

The goals also include examples of occupational engagement that will help Stephen achieve the change necessary to obtain these goals. For example, the occupational engagement in the first goal is "identify."

Implementing and Monitoring Therapy

The intervention plan includes the therapeutic strategies (in italics) that will support Stephen's achievement of his goals.

- Stephen and the occupational therapist worked together and explored a range of employment options and *negotiated* which types of worker roles offered the best fit with his interests and working styles.
- The occupational therapist *coached* Stephen on how to use career planning material and *encouraged* him to discuss his future worker roles with his natural social support network of family and friends.
- The OT assistant *coached* Stephen and assisted in *structuring* how to build a résumé and complete application forms.
- The therapist regularly met with Stephen to review his increasing work routine; during these sessions, the occupational therapist offered *advice* and *encouragement* and *gave feedback*.
- Initially, the occupational therapist *identified* opportunities and barriers for establishing a work routine for Stephen and offered support by *structuring* increasing participation. As he became more confident and independent, the occupational therapist offered *encouragement*.
- The occupational therapist and Stephen identified a relevant unpaid internship opportunity; they then met with the manager of the workplace to *negotiate* and *structure* a placement of gradually increasing demand.
- The occupational therapist and Stephen discussed the social environment of the work placement in advance of commencing the internship. Stephen was anxious about establishing new relationships with coworkers. The therapist listened to Stephen's concerns based on previous negative experience and demonstrated respect by *validating* his perspective. The therapist *coached* Stephen in strategies for meeting and conversing with new people at work. Stephen chose not to disclose his mental health condition to coworkers and so role-playing allowed Stephen to practice tricky conversations.
- The therapist offered advice to Stephen and his manager about managing mental health and well-being in the workplace.

(*continued*)

OT STORY 34.1 COLLECTING INFORMATION AND CREATING A THEORY-BASED UNDERSTANDING OF STEPHEN (*continued*)

- The therapist regularly communicated with Stephen's wider mental health team to share information, feedback progress, and ensure compatibility of care plans and objectives.

Collecting Information to Assess Outcomes

After 3 months, Stephen was established in his internship—working 2.5 days per week, totaling 16 hours. He was also regularly applying for similar paid roles and had secured two interviews. The occupational therapist chose to assess outcomes to date. The assessment strategy was *Goal attainment* (i.e., review of initial goals):

- Stephen and the occupational therapist worked together, establishing that Stephen had gained the greatest levels of satisfaction in administrative roles; this had been his chosen course of study at college.
- Stephen has a résumé that he tailors and shares with local employers, and he regularly applies for relevant available jobs, recently securing two interviews.

- Stephen has established a work routine of activities related to applying for employment.
- The occupational therapist secured an unpaid internship at a local leisure center where Stephen gradually built up his routine from 3 half days per week to 2 full days and 1 half day. The manager of the leisure center is very positive about Stephen as a worker and has provided an excellent reference. The manager would be willing to appoint Stephen if a post was available.

Questions

1. Using Table 34.3, are there any other assessments that you think would be helpful for providing additional information for helping Stephen obtain and maintain employment?
2. In the past, Stephen had difficult relationships with managers and colleagues. It appears that Stephen's relationship with his current manager is a good one. Using the MOHO, what intervention strategies might you put in place to prepare Stephen for future interpersonal challenges at work?

OT STORY 34.2 COLLECTING INFORMATION AND CREATING A THEORY-BASED UNDERSTANDING OF JOHN

John is a 7-year-old boy who is a third grader in elementary school, a son, a grandson, a brother, a friend, a swimmer, and a bike rider. He wants to be a computer engineer like his dad when he grows up. He is described by his family as a lovable, endearing boy and, by his schoolteacher, as chaotic, disorganized, and worried.

Background

John lives at home with his two parents and his brother. John has been referred for a specialist assessment by his elementary schoolteacher who was concerned about his awkward movement within the classroom, distractibility, and laborious handwriting. These issues have been long standing; the strategies tried within the school have not been helpful, and the challenges persist. The teachers within John's school had already tried some of the strategies from *Inclusive Learning and Collaborative Working: Teachers Ideas in Practice* (CIRCLE Collaboration, 2009b). This is a resource based on what teachers have found helpful when supporting children with additional support needs. They had identified supports and strategies from the motor skill section, namely, task breakdown, hand-over-hand support, modeling, and additional verbal instructions. There is a concern that if the issues are

not resolved, John will not be able to keep up with his class peers in terms of academic performance. Following a discussion between John's class teacher and the headmaster, it was decided that it would be appropriate to refer John for an OT assessment.

Generating Questions

The occupational therapist started with an intention to understand what was important to John, his teacher, and his family. The therapist wanted to use the MOHO as a framework for understanding how the issues raised on the referral affected John's engagement and participation in everyday occupations. Therefore, the therapist asked the following questions:

- What is important to John (his values), and what motivates him to participate in occupations at school?
- How do John's distractibility and awkward movement impact his ability to fulfill his responsibilities, maintain his routines, interact with others, and organize activities?
- What is John's view of his abilities and his limitations?
- How does John's occupational performance vary in different environments (home and school)?

OT STORY 34.2 COLLECTING INFORMATION AND CREATING A THEORY-BASED UNDERSTANDING OF JOHN (*continued*)

Gathering Information

When John was referred to a local therapy facility, the therapists chose an assessment pattern that would provide information for the previous questions.

Before Attendance at the Therapy Clinic

The Active in Children Health Integrating Evidence Valuing Experience (ACHIEVE) Assessment (Forsyth et al., 2012) was administered by mail and was completed by John's mother and teacher. It affords an opportunity for John's mother/teacher to share their view of how their child is participating in everyday activities. As the teacher indicated on the referral form that John's movement was awkward, the ACHIEVE Assessment also included a Developmental Coordination Disorder Questionnaire (DCDQ) (Wilson et al., 2000), which is a brief questionnaire designed to screen for coordination disorders in children aged 5 to 15 years.

During Therapy Clinic

The therapist reviewed and verified the findings of the ACHIEVE Assessment (Forsyth et al., 2012) with parent. In addition, the Movement Assessment Battery for Children (ABC) (Henderson & Sugden, 1992) was administered. This assessment identifies, describes, and guides the treatment of motor impairment. It is used to assess children's motor skills disabilities and determine intervention strategies. The Standardized assessment of handwriting, *The Handwriting File* (Alston & Taylor, 1988), was completed to understand if John's writing skill was significantly slower than would be expected of a child of his age.

After the Therapy Clinic

The Short Child Occupational Profile (SCOPE) (Bowyer et al., 2006) was rated by the therapist using information gathered from the other assessments as well as during an observation of John's participation within the classroom. This allowed for "triangulation" between the parents' view, the teacher's view, and the therapist's view on how different personal and environment factors impacted John's participation. This provides a range of views to build a comprehensive understanding of John.

Creating a Theory-Based Understanding of the Client

The following occupational formulation was created from the assessment findings.

- **What was important to John, his family, and his teacher?** John stated, "Writing is not my thing," and wanted to be

able to keep up with his friends and not feel his cheeks getting hot and feeling panicky about being the last to complete writing tasks. John's mother wanted him to be able to write better and not find it so difficult to do this. John's teacher wants John to be less clumsy, less distractible, and, for his writing, to be less laborious.

- **What is John good at, and what does he enjoy?** Comparing teacher and parent assessments, John performs more consistently in activities at home than at school. John has many areas of strength, including home and community activities; for example, able to get dressed/undressed, able to ride a bike, able to take part in social events. John's teacher reports that John enjoys math and physical education.

- **Why does John have these strengths?** Despite concerns, John can achieve 26 letters per minute (normative performance is 28 letters per minute for a 7-year-old) *when focused*. John's mother, teacher, and therapists identified that John has structured routines at both home and school. His mother, teacher, and therapists agree that John mostly understands responsibilities, has appropriate social skills, and has a supportive school and home environment matched to his abilities and skills.

- **What does John find challenging?** John does not have any areas of challenge at home. John was, however, observed in the classroom to have challenges using learning materials effectively (e.g., pens, pencils, crayons, rules, glue sticks, scissors) and being able to make effective shapes or letters and writing within a school context.

- **Why does John have these challenges?** Parents were concerned about John's motor skill development; however, from their point of view, there are no other health concerns. Indeed, John's teacher reported he has challenges navigating around his physical school environment. Although the DCDQ indicates challenges in fine motor or handwriting and general coordination within school and the Movement ABC was within the 9th percentile (which is suggestive of being at risk of movement difficulties with manual dexterity and balance), it is likely that these scores have been significantly impacted by John's distractibility or lack of attention. John was observed to be *highly* distractible during both the therapy clinic and classroom. This is further supported by John's handwriting being normative for his age group when formally tested—when he was focused in a quiet environment. Moreover, John's teacher reports that John has significant challenges in the area of organizational ability in school (i.e., extremely poor concentration throughout written tasks, lack of effort in writing tasks, following through on instructions),

(*continued*)

which was consistent with the therapist's observation. The impact on John's confidence in school was noticeable in the classroom (i.e., having confidence in abilities, enjoyment or having satisfaction in school activities, and not trying despite challenges). This was consistent with John giving up easily within the therapy clinic, although he was competitive when performing against a timer.

Generating Therapy Goals and Strategies

Although the initial referral from the teacher was framed as challenges in movement and coordination, the assessment process identified that the main areas of occupational change to target in therapy were the following:

- Improvement in the use of learning materials through developing organizational skills and increased confidence for tasks completed within the classroom

The joint measurable goal shared between therapy and education was therefore:

- Within 4 weeks, John will be able to confidently use learning materials (such as books, writing utensils) through organizing objects and maintaining concentration within his classroom independently.

A meeting was arranged between the therapist, the parent, and the teacher to exchange strategies that worked for John at home and resulted in John performing better within the home environment (i.e., routine praise for completing activities regardless of outcome or speed), making eye contact with John before sharing instructions, and creating an environment with limited distractions when completing homework. The parent, teacher, and occupational therapists, therefore, identified strategies—from *Intervention Descriptions: Occupational Therapy* (CIRCLE Collaboration, 2009c)—of (a) modifying the school environment, (b) recreating volition, and (c) process skill building.

Implementing and Monitoring Therapy

The philosophy of the school therapist was to empower those around a child to provide therapeutic supports to allow for a more consistent approach to supporting a child's occupational participation. The understanding of John was shared with the teacher through the use of the *Collaborative Communication Chart* (CIRCLE Collaboration, 2009a) and *Therapy Manual: Occupational Therapy* (CIRCLE Collaboration, 2009d). This chart was created by therapists and teachers as a structured set of language to support consistent communication. This provided a common language for the therapist and teacher to discuss strategies that John could

use to improve his organizational skills and concentration in the classroom.

The following was agreed as the intervention package:

- John was given a pencil grip.
- John's desk was moved to a front corner of the classroom from his current position in the center of the class to reduce distractions. He was also provided with a bigger desk that would have adequate space for work materials and support materials.
- John was provided with a range of objects that provide sensory feedback during writing (i.e., rubber grips, weighted pencils, weighted wristbands).
- John's teacher provided praise on completion of activities and displayed work alongside others to show its equal value.
- John's teacher created writing tasks where John could write about strong interests.
- John's teacher made him more aware of when he was feeling enjoyment during writing tasks.
- John's teacher facilitated positive feedback on his writing by his friends in the classroom.
- John's teacher was positive about any perceived failure to support task perseverance despite challenges.
- John's teacher was more aware of John disengaging from his writing task; and when she noticed disengagement, she supported John to use his concentration strategies to ensure continued focus.
- John's teacher made eye contact with John before providing instruction on his writing task.
- John was provided with strong routines for setting up and clearing away his workstation space on a daily basis.
- John was provided with a timer and taught how to use it to work in 10-minute increments.
- The therapist and John collaborated to make a checklist for materials and for checking task completion that John could then reference independently at the beginning and end of each class work period.

The teacher was encouraged to contact the therapist if there were any concerns or insurmountable challenges during the intervention period. Otherwise, the intervention was provided solely by the teacher.

Collecting Information to Assess Outcomes

The expected therapeutic change in John's occupational participation was within school. A reassessment after 4 weeks was arranged, and the following review was completed.

- Goal attainment (i.e., review of joint therapy or educational goal)

OT STORY 34.2 COLLECTING INFORMATION AND CREATING A THEORY-BASED UNDERSTANDING OF JOHN (continued)

- ACHIEVE Assessment (Forsyth et al., 2012)
- SCOPE (Bowyer et al., 2006)

John reached his 4-week goal of being able to perform within the classroom more confidently. This was supported by his teacher reporting improved confidence and organizational skills. He was observed to use his self-monitored strategies. She also reflected that John was "calmer" and more "focused" within the classroom and less disruptive. Classroom observations using the SCOPE also revealed improved scores for confidence and organizational ability. Most importantly, John stated that he felt less panicked

when writing tasks were assigned, and his posture and demeanor were more relaxed. He proudly showed his workstation to the therapists as his space.

Questions

1. Why was it important to include John's mother in the assessment process, when John's challenges were all school related?
2. Consider the therapeutic strategies listed in Box 34.1. How would you classify each of the interventions that were provided for John?

Conclusion

This chapter provided an overview of the concepts and practice resources of MOHO. Two cases were used to demonstrate how MOHO concepts are used to guide the process of therapeutic reasoning. As the cases illustrate, therapists can use MOHO to support a client-centered and occupationally focused practice. This chapter was able to demonstrate only a small fraction of the theoretical, empirical, and practical resources that are available under this model. Anyone who wishes to use MOHO is encouraged to take advantage of those resources.

Acknowledgments

The authors would like to thank Brent Braveman for reviewing this edition of the chapter and acknowledge the following for contributing to the 13th edition of the chapter: Renée R. Taylor, Jessica M. Kramer, Susan Prior, Lynn Ritchie, and Jane Melton.

Lippincott® Connect For additional resources on the subjects discussed in this chapter, visit Lippincott Connect.

REFERENCES

Alston, J., & Taylor, J. (1988). *The handwriting file* (2nd ed.). LDA.

American Occupational Therapy Association. (2020). Occupational therapy practice framework: Domain and process (4th Edition). *American Journal of Occupational Therapy, 74*(Suppl. 2), 7412410010p1–7412410010p87. https://doi.org/10.5014/ajot.2020.74S2001

Baron, K., Kielhofner, G., Iyenger, A., Goldhammer, V., & Wolenski, J. (2006). *The occupational self assessment (OSA; Version 2.2)*. Model of Human Occupation Clearinghouse.

Basu, S., Kafkes, A., Geist, R., & Kielhofner, G. (2002). *The pediatric volitional questionnaire (PVQ; Version 2.0)*. Model of Human Occupation Clearinghouse.

Bernspang, B., & Fisher, A. (1995). Differences between persons with a right or left cerebral vascular accident on the assessment of motor and process skills. *Archives of Physical Medicine and Rehabilitation, 75*, 1144–1151. https://doi.org/10.1016/s0003-9993(95)80124-3

Bowyer, P., Ross, M., Schwartz, O., Kielhofner, G., & Kramer, J. (2006). *The short child occupational profile (SCOPE; Version 2.1)*. Model of Human Occupation Clearinghouse.

Braveman, B., Robson, M., Velozo, C., Kielhofner, G., Fisher, G., Forsyth, K., & Kerschbaum, J. (2005). *The worker role interview (WRI; Version 10.0)*. Model of Human Occupation Clearinghouse.

Bundy, A. C., & Lane, S. J. (2020). *Sensory integration: Theory and practice*. F.A. Davis.

CIRCLE Collaboration. (2009a). *Collaborative communication chart*. City of Edinburgh Council, Queen Margaret University, and NHS Lothian.

CIRCLE Collaboration. (2009b). *Inclusive learning and collaborative working: Teachers' ideas in practice*. City of Edinburgh Council, Queen Margaret University, and NHS Lothian.

CIRCLE Collaboration. (2009c). *Intervention descriptions: Occupational therapy*. City of Edinburgh Council, Queen Margaret University, and NHS Lothian.

CIRCLE Collaboration. (2009d). *Therapy manual: Occupational therapy*. City of Edinburgh Council, Queen Margaret University, and NHS Lothian.

de las Heras, C. G., Lierena, V., & Kielhofner, G. (2003). *Remotivation process: Progressive intervention for individuals with severe volitional challenges (Version 1.0)*. Department of Occupational Therapy, University of Illinois at Chicago.

Dirette, D. P., & Gutman, S. A. (2021). *Occupational therapy for physical dysfunction* (8th ed.). Wolters Kluwer.

Doble, S. (1991). Test-retest and inter-rater reliability of a process skills assessment. *Occupational Therapy Journal of Research, 11*, 8–23. https://doi.org/10.1177/153944929101100102

Elenko, B. K., Hinojosa, J., Blount, M.-L., & Blount, W. (2000). Perspectives. In J. Hinojosa & M.-L. Blount (Eds.), *The texture of life: Purposeful activities in occupational therapy* (pp. 16–35). American Occupational Therapy Association.

Esmaili, S. K., Mehraban, A. H., Shafaroodi, N., Yazdani, F., Masoumi, T., & Zarei, M. (2019). Participation in peer-play activities among children with specific learning disability: A randomized controlled trial. *American Journal of Occupational Therapy, 73*(2), 7302205110p1–7302205110p9. https://doi.org/10.5014/ajot.2018.028613

Fan, C. W., Keponen, R., Piikki, S., Tsang, H., Popova, E. S., & Taylor, R. (2020). Psychometric evaluation of the Finnish translation of the Assessment of Communication and Interaction Skills (ACIS-FI). *Scandinavian Journal of Occupational Therapy, 27*(2), 112–121. https://doi.org/10.1080/11038128.2018.1483425

Fisher, A. G. (2003). *Assessment of motor and process skills* (5th ed.). Three Star.

Fisher, A., & Kielhofner, G. (1995). Skill in occupational performance. In G. Kielhofner (Ed.), *A model of human occupation: Theory and application* (2nd ed., pp. 113–137). Lippincott Williams & Wilkins.

Fisher, G., Arriaga, P., Less, C., Lee, J., & Ashpole, E. (2008). *The residential environment impact survey (REIS; Version 2.0)*. Model of Human Occupation Clearinghouse.

Fisher, G., Parkinson, S., & Haglund, L. (2017). The environment and human occupation. In R.L. Taylor (Ed.), *Kielhofner's model of human occupation* (5th ed., pp. 91–106). Wolters Kluwer Health/Lippincott Williams and Wilkins.

Forsyth, K., Deshpande, S., Kielhofner, G., Henriksson, C., Haglund, L., Olson, L., Skinner, S., & Kulkarni, S. (2005). *The Occupational Circumstances Assessment Interview and Rating Scale (OCAIRS; Version 4.0)*. Model of Human Occupation Clearinghouse.

Forsyth, K., Lai, J., & Kielhofner, G. (1999). The assessment of communication and interaction skills (ACIS): Measurement properties. *British Journal of Occupational Therapy, 62*, 69–74. https://doi.org/10.1177/030802269906200208

Forsyth, K., Salamy, M., Simon, S., & Kielhofner, G. (1998). *Assessment of communication and interaction skills (Version 4.0)*. Model of Human Occupation Clearinghouse.

Forsyth, K., Whitehead, J., Owen, C., & Gorska, S. (2012). *A users guide to the Active in Children Health Integrating Evidence Valuing Experience (ACHIEVE) assessment*. Queen Margaret University.

Frust, G., Gerber, L., Smith, C., Fisher, S., & Shulman, B. (1987). A program for improving energy conservation behaviors in adults with rheumatoid arthritis. *American Journal of Occupational Therapy, 41*, 102–111. https://doi.org/10.5014/ajot.41.2.102

Gerber, L., & Frust, G. (1992). Scoring methods and application of the activity record (ACTRE) for patients with musculoskeletal disorders. *Arthritis Care and Research, 5*, 151–156. https://doi.org/10.1002/art.1790050307

Harel-Katz, H., & Carmeli, E. (2019). The association between volition and participation in adults with acquired disabilities: A scoping review. *Hong Kong Journal of Occupational Therapy, 32*(2), 84–96. https://doi.org/10.1177/1569186119870022

Hemmingson, H., Egilson, S., Hoffman, O., & Kielhofner, G. (2005). *School setting interview (SSI; Version 3.0)*. Swedish Association of Occupational Therapists.

Henderson, E., & Sugden, D. (1992). *The movement assessment battery for children*. Psychological Corporation.

Henry, A. D. (2000). *The pediatric interest profiles: Surveys of play for children and adolescents* [Unpublished manuscript]. Model of Human Occupation Clearinghouse, Department of Occupational Therapy, University of Illinois.

Jo, Y. J., & Kim, H. (2022). Effects of the model of human occupation-based home modifications on the time use, occupational participation and activity limitation in people with disabilities: A pilot randomized controlled trial. *Disability and Rehabilitation. Assistive Technology, 17*(2), 127–133. https://doi.org/10.1080/17483107.2020.1768306

Keller, J., Kafkes, A., Basu, S., Federico, J., & Kielhofner, G. (2005). *A user's guide to child occupational self assessment (COSA; Version 2.1)*. University of Illinois, Chicago.

Kielhofner, G. (1980a). A model of human occupation: 2. Ontogenesis from the perspective of temporal adaptation. *American Journal of Occupational Therapy, 34*, 657–663. https://doi.org/10.5014/ajot.34.10.657

Kielhofner, G. (1980b). A model of human occupation: 3. Benign and vicious cycles. *American Journal of Occupational Therapy, 34*, 731–737. https://doi.org/10.5014/ajot.34.11.731

Kielhofner, G. (2008). *A model of human occupation: Theory and application* (4th ed.). Lippincott Williams & Wilkins.

Kielhofner, G., & Burke, J. (1980). A model of human occupation: 1. Conceptual framework and content. *American Journal of Occupational Therapy, 34*, 572–581. https://doi.org/10.5014/ajot.34.9.572

Kielhofner, G., Burke, J., & Heard, I. C. (1980). A model of human occupation: 4. Assessment and intervention. *American Journal of Occupational Therapy, 34*, 777–788. https://doi.org/10.5014/ajot.34.12.777

Kielhofner, G., Mallison, T., Crawford, C., Nowak, M., Rigby, M., Henry, A., & Walens, D. (2004). *Occupational Performance History Interview-II (OPHI-II; Version 2.1)*. Model of Human Occupation Clearinghouse.

Law, M. (1998). *Client-centered occupational therapy*. SLACK.

Law, M., Cooper, B. A., Strong, S., Stewart, D., Rigby, P., & Letts, L. (1997). Theoretical contexts for the practice of occupational therapy. In C. Christiansen & C. Baum (Eds.), *Occupational therapy: Enabling function and well-being* (2nd ed., pp. 73–102). SLACK.

Lee, S. W., Taylor, R., Kielhofner, G., & Fisher, G. (2008) Theory use in practice: A national survey of therapists who use the Model of Human Occupation. *American Journal of Occupational Therapy, 62*, 106-117. https://doi.org/10.5014/ajot.62.1.106

Matsutsuyu, J. (1969). The interest checklist. *American Journal of Occupational Therapy, 23*, 323–328.

Moore-Corner, R. A., Kielhofner, G., & Olson, L. (1998). *A user's guide to Work Environment Impact Scale*. Model of Human Occupation Clearinghouse.

Morgan, D. D., Taylor, R. R., Ivy, M., George, S., Farrow, C., & Lee, V. (2022). Contemporary occupational priorities at the end of life mapped against Model of Human Occupation constructs: A scoping review. *Australian Occupational Therapy Journal*. Advance online publication. https://doi.org/10.1111/1440-1630.12792

Oakley, F., Kielhofner, G., & Barris, R. (1985). An occupational therapy approach to assessing psychiatric patients' adaptive functioning. *American Journal of Occupational Therapy, 39*, 147–154. https://doi.org/10.5014/ajot.39.3.147

Pan, A. W., Chung, L., Chen, T. J., & Hsiung, P. C. (2020). The study of the validity and reliability of the Occupational Self-Assessment-traditional Chinese version. *Hong Kong Journal of Occupational Therapy, 33*(1), 18–24. https://doi.org/10.1177/1569186120930300

Parkinson, S., Forsyth, K., & Kielhofner, G. (2006). *A user's manual for the model of human occupation screening tool (MOHOST; Version 2.0)*. University of Illinois, Chicago.

Pekçetin, S., Salar, S., İnal, Ö., & Kayıhan, H. (2018). Validity of the Turkish Occupational Self Assessment for elderly individuals. *OTJR: Occupation, Participation and Health, 38*(2), 105–112. https://doi.org/10.1177/1539449217743457

Prior, S., Forsyth, K., & Ritchie, L. (2011). *ActiVate collaboration: Occupational therapy & evidence based vocational rehabilitation*. Queen Margaret University, NHS Lothian.

Prior, S., Maciver, D., Aas, R. W., Kirsh, B., Lexen, A., van Niekerk, L., Irvine Fitzpatrick, L., & Forsyth, K. (2020). An enhanced individual placement and support (IPS) intervention based on the Model of Human Occupation (MOHO): A prospective cohort study. *BMC Psychiatry, 20*(1), 361. https://doi.org/10.1186/s12888-020-02745-3

Schmelzer, L., Stanger, H., & Hughes, R. (2022). The development and validation of the planning to make meals performance measure. *OTJR: Occupation, Participation and Health, 42*(2), 105–114. https://doi.org/10.1177/15394492211063172

Skúladóttir, E. B., Fenger, K., Bejerholm, U., & Sandqvist, J. (2021). Translation and validation of Assessment of Work Performance (AWP) into the Icelandic language and culture. *Work, 69*(4), 1305–1316. https://doi.org/10.3233/WOR-213551

Smith, N. R., Kielhofner, G., & Watts, J. (1986). The relationship between volition, activity pattern, and life satisfaction in the elderly. *American Journal of Occupational Therapy, 40*, 278–283. https://doi.org/10.5014/ajot.40.4.278

Tan, B. L., Zhen Lim, M. W., Xie, H., Li, Z., & Lee, J. (2020). Defining occupational competence and occupational identity in the context of recovery in schizophrenia. *The American Journal of Occupational Therapy, 74*(4), 7404205120p1–7404205120p11. https://doi.org/10.5014/ajot.2020.034843

Taylor, J., Mynard, L., & Farnworth, L. (2022). Occupational therapists experiences using the model of human occupation in forensic mental health. *Occupational Therapy in Mental Health, 38*, 67–85. https://doi.org/10.1080/0164212X.2021.1974325

Taylor, R. T. (2017). *Kielhofner's model of human occupation: Theory and application* (5th ed.). Lippincott Williams & Wilkins.

Townsend, S., Carey, P.D., Hollins, N.L., Helfrich, C., Blondis, M., Hoffman, A., Collins, L., Knudson, J., & Glackwell, A. (1999). *The Occupational Therapy Psychosocial Assessment of Learning (OT PAL; Version 2.0)*. Model of Human Occupation Clearinghouse.

Watts, J. H., Hinson, R., Madigan, M. J., McGuigan, P. M., & Newman, S. M. (1999). The assessment of occupational functioning—Collaborative version. In B. J. Hempill-Pearson (Ed.), *Assessments in occupational therapy in mental health* (pp. 183–193). SLACK.

Wilkeby, M., Pierre, B. L., & Archenholtz, B. (2006). Occupational therapists' reflection on practice within psychiatric care: A Delphi study. *Scandinavian Journal of Occupational Therapy, 13*, 151–159. https://doi.org/10.1080/11038120500380570

Wilson, B. N., Kaplan, B. J., Crawford, S. G., Campbell, A., & Dewey, D. (2000). Reliability and validity of a parent questionnaire on childhood motor skills. *American Journal of Occupational Therapy, 54*, 484–493. https://doi.org/10.5014/ajot.54.5.484

Wong, S. R., & Fisher, G. (2015). Comparing and using occupation-focused models. *Occupational Therapy in Health Care, 29*, 297–315. https://doi.org/10.3109/07380577.2015.1010130

Ecologic Models in Occupational Therapy

Catana Brown

LEARNING OBJECTIVES

After reading this chapter, you will be able to:

1. Outline the historical foundations of ecologic models and how these concepts contributed to the development of occupational therapy ecologic models.
2. Evaluate the role of the environment in understanding occupational performance.
3. Compare and contrast the similarities and differences among the four ecologic models described in this chapter (Ecology of Human Performance, Person–Environment–Occupation, and Person–Environment–Occupational Performance, Canadian Model of Occupational Performance and Engagement).
4. Analyze and apply the ecologic models (Ecology of Human Performance, Person–Environment–Occupation, Person–Environment–Occupational Performance, Canadian Model of Occupational Performance and Engagement) and their concepts to occupational therapy practice.
5. Distinguish the five intervention strategies: establish/restore, adapt/modify, alter, prevent, and create.

Introduction

Models provide occupational therapy (OT) practitioners with a representation along with language to help the practitioner understand and explain practice. OT practitioners are ultimately concerned with what the person wants or needs to do, in other words, occupational performance and participation. Before intervention begins, the OT practitioner must first identify barriers and facilitators to performance and participation. This is where the ecologic models are helpful. These models provide the profession with a greater appreciation for the role of the environment.

In the 1990s, different groups of occupational therapists working independently created four separate models that emphasized the importance of considering the environment in OT practice:

• The Ecology of Human Performance (EHP) model, developed by Dunn et al. (1994)

- The Person–Environment–Occupational Performance (PEOP) model, developed by Christiansen and Baum (1997)
- The Person–Environment–Occupation (PEO) model, developed by Law et al. (1996)
- The Canadian Model of Occupational Performance (CMOP), developed by the Canadian Association of Occupational Therapists (1997); in 2013, the CMOP became the CMOP-E to indicate OT extends beyond occupational performance to include occupational engagement (Townsend & Polatajko, 2013)

These **ecologic models** share many similarities and a few distinctions. The four dynamic models consider occupational (task) performance as a primary outcome of interest to occupational therapists. In addition, all the models indicate that occupational performance is determined by the person, environment (context), and occupation (task). However, the developers of these models were concerned that the construct of environment was not receiving adequate attention and that the tendency to focus on person factors neglected the influence of the environment on occupational performance. Therefore, the ecologic models were developed so that along with consideration for the person and occupation, OT practice includes assessments and interventions that focus on the environment.

Overview of the Ecologic Models

The ecologic models were built on social science theory, earlier OT models, and the disability movement. Each of the ecologic models draws heavily on social science theories that describe person–environment interactions (Bronfenbrenner, 1979; Csikszentmihalyi, 1990; Gibson, 1979; Lawton, 1986) as well as earlier models in OT, such as the Model of Human Occupation (Kielhofner & Burke, 1980) and Occupational Adaptation (Schkade & Schultz, 1992).

Perhaps most importantly, the ecologic models in OT were influenced by the disability rights movement. Healthcare practice is dominated by a focus on impairment in the person and interventions that are designed to fix that impairment. Individuals with disabilities challenged this perspective. People in the independent living movement pointed out that environmental barriers are typically the greatest impediment to a successful and satisfying life (DeJong, 1979; Shapiro, 1994). Furthermore, individuals with psychiatric disabilities revealed that the power of stigma and subsequent discrimination interfere with full participation in community life (Chamberlin, 1990; Deegan, 1993).

The disability movements advocated for civil rights for individuals with disabilities and promoted self-determination and empowerment. The ecologic models embrace the values of the disability movement. This is reflected in both the emphasis on the environment as a significant barrier and facilitator of participation and occupational performance and the adoption of principles of client-centered practice.

The disability rights movement was also instrumental in impacting broader disability and health-related models. For example, the social model of disability distinguishes between the concepts of impairment and disability (Oliver, 1996). Impairment is a condition of the body that is not standard, whereas a disability is a restriction from participation caused by physical or social barriers. When the first *International Classification of Functioning, Disability and Health* was adopted in 2001, it provided a unifying framework for classifying the consequences of disease. The document's presentation of disability was important in that disability was not a feature of the individual but instead an interaction of the person and the environment (Schneidert et al., 2003).

Core Concepts of the Ecologic Models

Person

The EHP, PEO, PEOP, and CMOP-E models have similar definitions of the **person**. The holistic view of the person acknowledges the mind, body, and spirit. Variables associated with the person include values and interests, skills and abilities, and life experiences. Values and interests help determine what is important, meaningful, and enjoyable to the person. Skills and abilities include cognitive, social, emotional, and sensorimotor skills as well as abilities such as reading and knowing how to post on Instagram. Life experiences form the person's history and personal narrative. In CMOP-E, spirituality is emphasized as the essence of the person and the source from which determination and meaning happen.

The person influences and is influenced by the environment. For example, a person's family and friends contribute to the development of their particular values and interests. A child might develop a love of reading because of the availability of books in the home and parents who read to the child, and having a child in the home might cause the parents to be more concerned about having healthy foods at home and creating a safe physical environment.

Environment

The *environment* is also described similarly across the four models. The environment is where occupational performance takes place and consists of physical, cultural, and social characteristics. The EHP model also includes the temporal environment, and the CMOP-E includes the institutional environment. The physical environment is the most tangible. It includes built and natural features, large elements such as the terrain or buildings, and small objects such as tools. The cultural environment is based on shared experiences that determine values, beliefs, and customs. The cultural environment includes, but is not limited to, ethnicity, religion, and national identity. For example, individuals may also adopt values and beliefs from the culture of their family, profession, organizations or clubs, and peer group.

The social environment is made up of many layers. It includes close interpersonal relationships, such as family and friends. Another layer includes work groups or social organizations to which the individual belongs. A larger layer consists of political and economic systems, which can have a profound effect on the daily life of people with disabilities. These systems make decisions related to the rights of people with disabilities, availability of services, and financial benefits, such as Social Security Disability and Health Insurance. This larger layer of the social environment is comparable to the institutional environment in CMOP-E. The temporal environment is made up of time-oriented factors associated with the person (developmental and life stage) and the task (when it takes place, how often, and for how long).

Occupational performance cannot be understood outside the context or environment. The environment can create barriers to performance and enhance occupational performance. For example, a well-organized and familiar grocery store that provides foods that are culturally familiar and consistent with the person's likes might be described as an adaptive environment. Conversely, the grocery store might be a barrier if the person is overwhelmed by too many choices, cannot find the items they are looking for, and is anxious when the store is crowded.

Occupation or Task

One difference in the four models is found in the concepts related to *occupations* or *tasks*. The PEO, PEOP, and CMOP-E use the term *occupation*, whereas EHP uses *task*. The developers of EHP were intentional about the selection of the term *task* because a primary purpose of the model was to facilitate interdisciplinary collaboration. It was felt that the term *task* would be more accessible to other disciplines. Tasks are defined as objective representations of all possible activities available in the universe. Although this was not explicitly expressed in the early writings of EHP, occupations exist when the person and context factors come together to give meaning to tasks (Dunn et al., 2003).

In CMOP-E, occupation is composed of three purposes: self-care, productivity, and leisure, which form the link between the person and the environment. In comparison, the PEO and PEOP models describe a series of nested concepts that make up occupations. In PEO, activities are the basic units of tasks. Tasks are purposeful activities, and occupations are self-directed tasks that a person engages in over the life course. The PEOP model involves actions, which are observable behaviors; tasks, which are combinations of actions with a common purpose; and occupations, which are goal-directed, meaningful pursuits that typically extend over time. For example, chopping vegetables might be the observable behavior or activity, embedded within the task of preparing soup, which falls under the larger occupation of cooking dinner for the family.

Occupational Performance

Occupational performance is the outcome that is associated with the confluence of the person, environment, and occupation factors. The degree to which occupational performance is possible depends on the goodness of fit of these factors. The structures of the models are depicted in slightly different ways. In PEO, a Venn diagram is used to illustrate the meeting of person, environment, and occupation variables (Figure 35.1). The space in which the three circles come together is occupational performance. PEOP is similar; however, there are four circles instead of three (Figure 35.2). Person and environment touch but do not overlap. Occupation and performance are two separate circles that overlay person and environment. These circles come together to form occupational performance and participation. In EHP, the person is embedded inside the context, with tasks floating all around (Figure 35.3). The performance range includes the tasks that are available to the person because of the existing environmental supports and his or her own skills, abilities, and experiences. In EHP, the person is embedded in their environment that determines the occupational performance possibilities, and in PEOP, the person and environment remain separate until occupational performance occurs. In CMOP-E, occupational performance and engagement connect the person and environment, with occupation as the core domain of interest for OT (Figure 35.4). Engagement was added to the CMOP to emphasize that the OT focus is on the broadest sense of participation, which goes beyond diversion to encompass full involvement in the occupation.

In all of the models, the performance range or occupational performance area is constantly changing as the other variables change. The area of occupational performance increases or the performance range expands when the person acquires new skills. Likewise, expansion occurs when stigma is decreased, physical barriers are removed, additional social supports are acquired, or schedules are accommodated. Unfortunately, people with disabilities are often faced with limited personal capacities and multiple environmental barriers. The role of the occupational therapist is to change this dynamic so that more occupations are available to the person and that there is an increased possibility for satisfying and effective performance of the available occupations.

Using the Ecologic Models in Practice

Evaluating the Client

OT practice begins by identifying what occupations or tasks the person wants or needs to perform. Using a top-down approach, the targeted area of occupational performance is identified first by the client or family. This is followed by an assessment of barriers and facilitators that affect occupational performance.

Some examples of environmental assessments are presented here because they tend to be overlooked in OT practice. Informal questions that address all aspects of the ecological models are available in Box 35-1.

All aspects of the environment (physical, social, cultural, and temporal) should be evaluated to determine relevant environmental influences. For example, several standardized assessments are available to assess the physical environment of the home for older people at risk of falling (Romli et al., 2018). The Child and Adolescent Social Support Scale measures the person's perceived

---

BOX 35.1 CLINICAL QUESTIONS RELATED TO CONSTRUCTS OF THE ECOLOGIC MODELS

Person

Skills (cognitive, social, psychological, sensory, motor)
- What are the person's inherent strengths?
- What are potential areas of cognitive, social, or sensorimotor impairment?

Life skills
- What life skills has the person learned, and what skills has the person not learned?
- What life skills has the person mastered, and what skills are problematic?

Interests
- What does the person like to do?

Experiences
- What are the life experiences that contribute to or interfere with occupational performance?
- What are the major life events for the person?
- What are the themes in the person's life story?

Environment/Context

Culture
- What cultural groups does the person identify with?
- What values does the person derive from these cultural groups?
- Are the beliefs and expectations of these cultural groups accepting of the person?

Social
- Are friends and family available to provide support?
- What providers are involved?
- How does public policy influence the person's ability to engage in tasks or occupations?

Physical
- What aspects of the home environment facilitate or interfere with performance?
- Does the person have access to the natural and built environments in their community?

Temporal
- Is the person able to engage in occupations that are consistent with the person's developmental or life phases?
- Does the person have too much time or not enough time to perform important tasks or occupations?

Occupation or Tasks

- What does the person want or need to do?
- What occupations or tasks come together to create roles or identity for the person?
- What occupations or tasks give meaning to the person's life?

Performance or Performance Range

- Which tasks or occupations fall inside or outside the performance range?
- Are there factors related to the person, environment/context, or occupation that interfere with performance?

Therapeutic Intervention

- What intervention approach would be the most efficient and have the most desirable outcomes?
- Is there evidence to support the intervention approach?
- Which intervention approach does the service recipient want?

PEO model

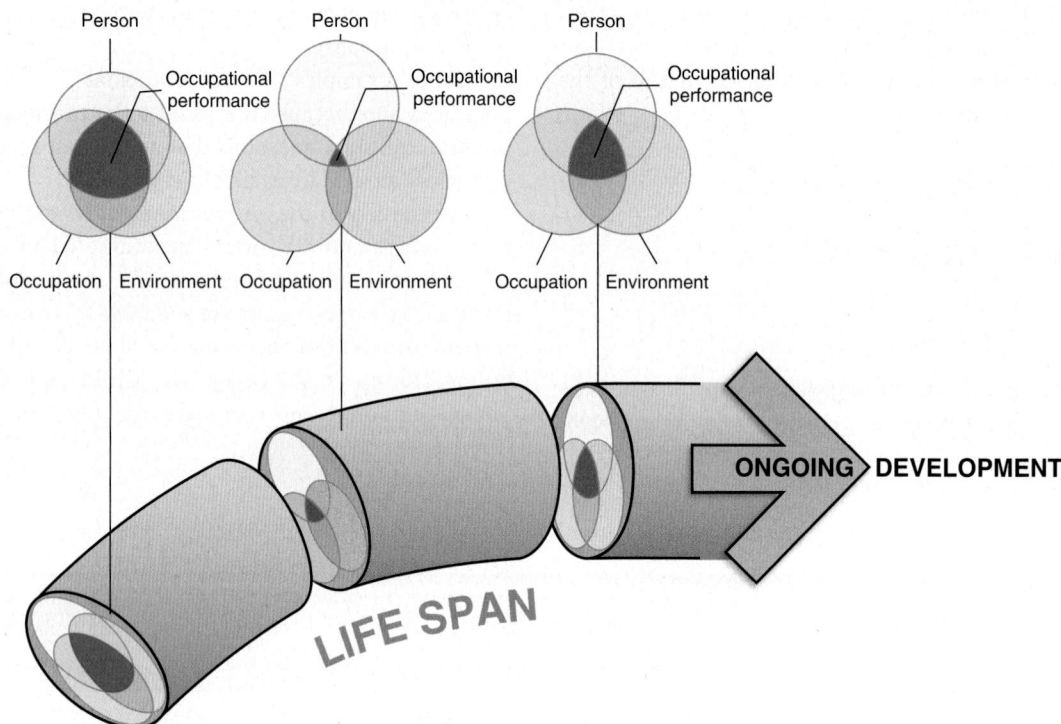

FIGURE 35.1 Person–Environment–Occupation (PEO) model.

(Reprinted with permission from Law, M., Cooper, B., Strong, S., Stewart, D., Rigby, P., & Letts, L. [1996]. The person-environment-occupation model: A transactive approach to occupational performance. *Canadian Journal of Occupational Therapy, 63*, 9–23.)

PEOP model

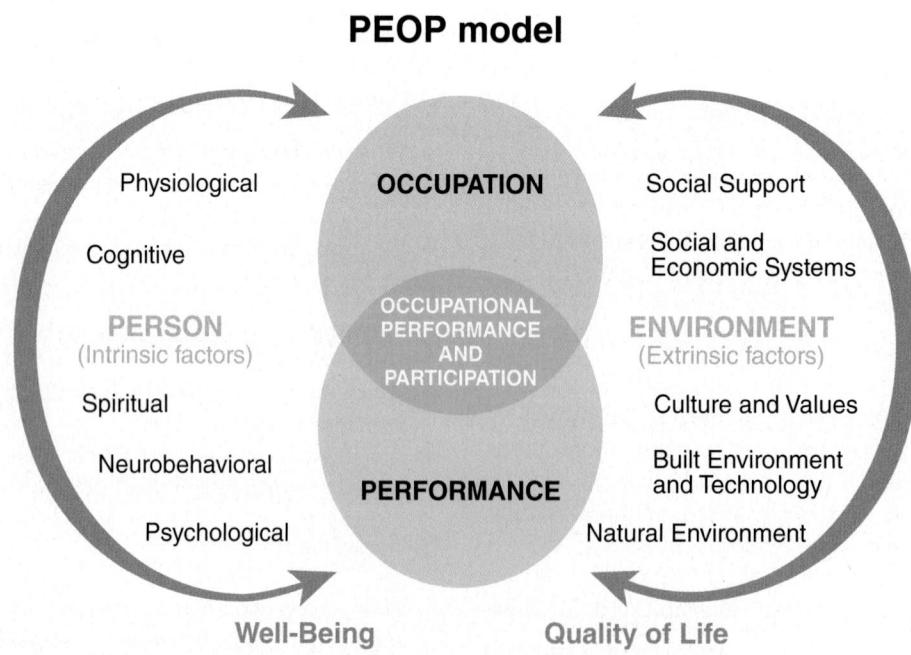

FIGURE 35.2 Person–Environment–Occupation Performance (PEOP) model.

(Reprinted with permission from Christiansen, C., Baum, C., & Bass-Haugen, J. [Eds.]. [2005]. *Occupational therapy: Performance, participation, and well-being* [3rd ed.]. Slack.)

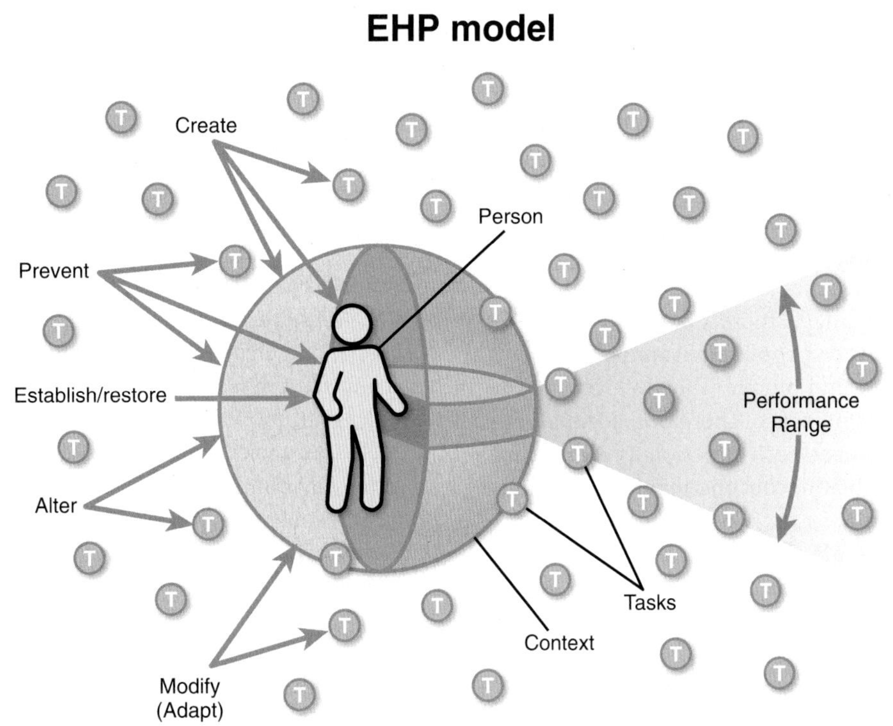

EHP model

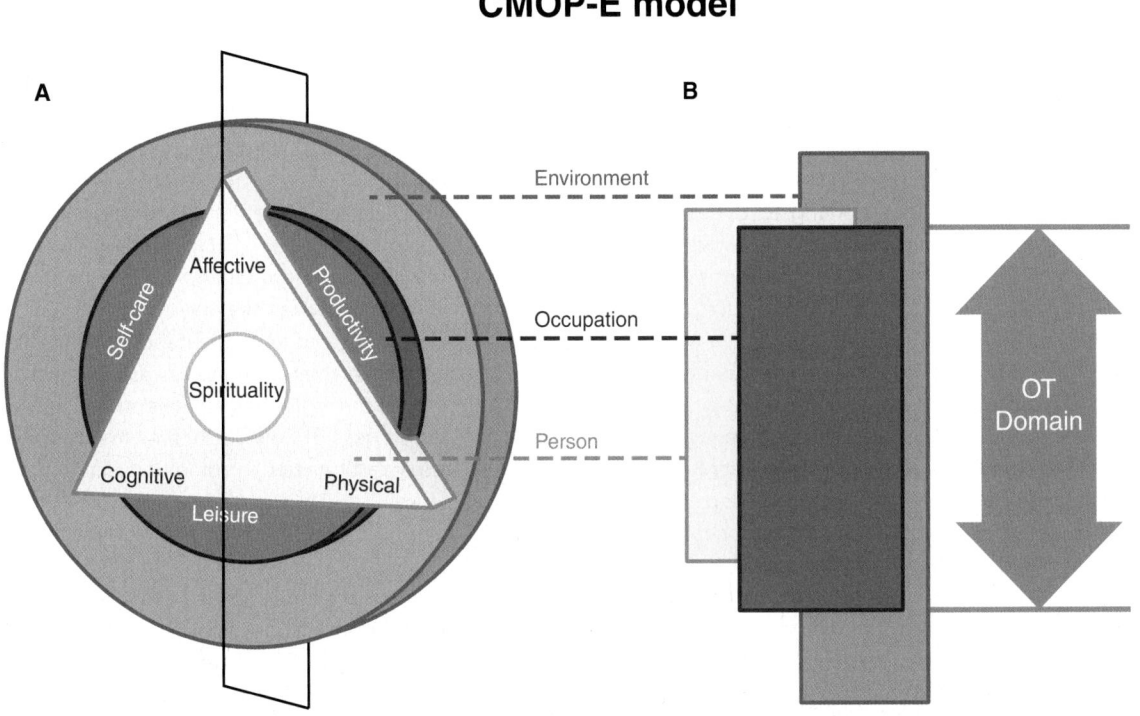

FIGURE 35.3 Ecology of Human Performance (EHP) model.

(Reprinted with permission from Dunn, W., McClain, L. H., Brown, C., & Youngstrom, M. J. [2003]. The ecology of human performance. In E. B. Crepeau, E. S. Cohn, & B. A. B. Schell [Eds.], *Willard & Spackman's occupational therapy* [10th ed., pp. 223–226]. Lippincott William & Wilkins.)

CMOP-E model

FIGURE 35.4 Canadian Model of Occupational Performance and Engagement (CMOP-E). OT, occupational therapy.

(Reprinted with permission from Polatajko, H. J., Townsend, E. A., & Craik, J. [2007]. Canadian Model of Occupational Performance and Engagement (CMOP-E). In E. A. Townsend & H. J. Polatajko [Eds.], *Enabling occupation II: Advancing an occupational therapy vision of health, well-being, & justice through occupation* [p. 23]. CAOT.)

social support received from peers, parents, and teachers (Malecki & Demary, 2002). The Everyday Discrimination Scale examines the frequency of discriminatory experiences in daily life and is associated with health disparities (Williams & Mohammed, 2013). Occupational therapists can use the Modified Occupational Questionnaire to assess the meaningfulness of time use (Scanlan & Bundy, 2011). The Work Environment Impact Scale evaluates aspects of the work environment that can impact work participation and satisfaction (Moore-Corner et al., 1998). The relationships between people, environments, and occupations are dynamic and unique. They interact continually and across time and space. Therefore, occupational therapists should approach each situation as ever changing and distinct. Evaluating occupational performance in real-life contexts allows for a more authentic assessment process. For example, the Test of Grocery Shopping Skills is administered in an actual grocery store (Brown et al., 2009). See Expanding Our Perspectives for more information.

Developing an Intervention Plan

Once barriers and facilitators to occupational performance are identified, the occupational therapist can develop a plan of intervention. One consideration in intervention planning involves the target of intervention, which can be the person, environment, occupation, or some combination. Using an ecologic model requires an intentional effort on the part of the occupational therapist to consider the environment as extensively as they consider the person. There is a tendency for occupational therapists to consider environmental interventions only when it is determined that a person focused intervention is no longer feasible. However, it may be equally or more efficient and effective to change the environment or find a person–environment match at the outset of treatment. For example, a study that compared a remediation versus a compensatory approach for young children with cerebral palsy found both approaches equally effective (Law et al., 2012).

Ecologic models provide a framework for practice but do not provide specific guidelines or theory about intervention techniques. However, the selection of interventions

---

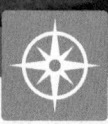

EXPANDING OUR PERSPECTIVES

Whose Context, Skills, and Knowledge?

Ellie Fossey

I began my OT career in the 1980s—a time when the articulation of ecologic models in OT were in their infancy. I nevertheless learned to consider the importance of the environment—in particular its physical features such as steps, ramps, and rails when working to overcome barriers to engagement in occupations in individuals' home environments. Likewise, I learned about the importance of welcoming and supportive environments to facilitate therapeutic group interventions.

One of my early experiences as an occupational therapist was of being asked to provide skills training for a group of clients deemed to lack skills in managing their finances. I was working in a community mental health service located in London, England, that provided treatment and support for adults experiencing mental health issues who lived in the inner city. The majority of the people attending this service were unemployed and received welfare payments or lacked secure income. For this group, I initially planned that we would talk about spending patterns so that I could better understand the budgeting skills that needed to be taught or practiced. These were challenging discussions—this was not because the group members were unwilling or unable to identify the nature of their financial difficulties. Rather the discussions were challenging because I was confronted with the restricted choices and control over their financial situations available

to the group, and my own limited experience and knowledge of how one might survive on their income. I also came to view "life skills" differently as group members shared their knowledge and strategies for living on very restricted incomes, such as where to obtain necessities like food and warm clothing cheaply or free, how to share costs, and how to reduce expenditure on electricity, transport, and so on.

This practice experience taught me that the skills and knowledge are contextual; that our assumptions about capabilities and constraints related to activity and participation may not align with the day-to-day realities of individuals' lives; and that an understanding of the barriers faced by people in their own lives is essential to finding relevant and useful solutions. Furthermore, this group raised my awareness of how social and structural barriers can restrict full participation in community life and opened my eyes to valuing lived experience–based knowledge, the power of peers sharing their knowledge, and its potential to create different solutions to the troubles and struggles that beset people in their everyday lives.

Using a theoretical model provides a lens or perspective for framing and understanding issues in practice. Ecologic perspectives call us to place greater emphasis in practice on attending to the range of physical, cultural, social, economic, and political barriers and facilitators to participation in community life; this has the potential to advance working collaboratively with people whose lives have been directly affected in striving to identify and eliminate barriers that prevent full participation.

should be faithful to the values of the ecologic models. Mostly, this means that the practice models that are used to guide intervention cannot be limited to person and occupational factors but must address the environment as well. The association of ecologic models with disability rights means that occupational therapists should also be involved at the systems level, supporting a policy that promotes full participation in all aspects of community life.

Implementing the Intervention

Additional terms that are included in the EHP model are five different intervention strategies: (a) establish/restore, (b) adapt/modify, (c) alter, (d) prevent, and (e) create. These interventions were spelled out so that occupational therapists would consider the full range of options. In particular, the articulation of intervention choices was designed to encourage occupational therapists to use more interventions directed at the environment.

- *Establish/restore* interventions target the person, rather than the environment, and are aimed at developing and improving skills and abilities so that the person can perform tasks (occupations) in context. For example, increasing range of motion so that an individual can better manage self-care tasks and teaching someone how to use a microwave oven for meal preparation involve establish/restore strategies.
- *Adapt/modify* interventions change the environment or task to increase the individual's performance range. Using assistive devices, such as an adapted car for driving or a built-up handled spoon for eating, is intervention that changes the typical environment. Changes to the physical environments are most common in OT; however, it is important to consider interventions that target the social, cultural, and temporal environments as well. Adapt/modify strategies can include providing education about disabilities to students in an elementary school classroom so that the child with special needs will be more accepted, or adapting work schedules to enable employees with disabilities to commute outside peak hours. These are adapt/modify strategies because the social and temporal environments are, respectively, being changed.

- *Alter* interventions do not change the person, task, or environment but are designed to make a better fit. Occupational therapists may overlook alter interventions because it does not appear that they are "doing" anything. However, alter interventions can be very effective because they take advantage of what is already naturally occurring. Making a good match requires that the occupational therapists have strong skills in activity analysis and environmental assessment. Examples of alter interventions include moving from a two-story house with stairs to a ranch home for a person with limited endurance and matching a person's skills with a particular job.
- *Prevent* interventions are implemented to change the course of events when a negative outcome is predicted. Prevention can use interventions that change the person (establish/restore), change the environment (adapt/modify), or make a better match (alter); but prevent interventions occur before the problem develops. For example, teaching at-risk parents skills in facilitating developmentally appropriate play is a prevent strategy, as is using a special cushion in a wheelchair to prevent pressure injuries.
- *Create* interventions do not assume that a problem has occurred or will occur but are designed to promote and enrich performance in context. Similar to the prevent strategies, create interventions can use establish/restore, adapt, or alter approaches. Setting up a study space within a quiet area with adequate lighting is an example of a create intervention. A sensory garden in a senior residence promotes occupational engagement and enriches the living environment.

Assessing the Outcome

The dynamic nature of the ecologic models acknowledges that situations are constantly changing, indicating that regular reevaluation should occur. If desired occupational performance goals are not achieved, then the occupational therapist should reexamine barriers and facilitators and determine whether a different intervention approach is warranted.

The OT Story 35.1 on the Asbury Café demonstrates the ecologic model in practice.

OT STORY 35.1 THE ASBURY CAFÉ

The Asbury Café is an employment program developed by the author. The Asbury Café operates every Wednesday night at a local church in the United States. Five individuals with serious mental illness are employees of the café. A meal is served at a reasonable cost for church members, neighbors, and friends. An occupational therapist oversees the running of the café, assisted by volunteers and college students. It is an example of a program that uses the principles of the ecologic models to promote work participation for people with psychiatric disabilities. However, that is just one of the aims of the program, which, on a larger scale, aspires to make changes in social and cultural environments to reduce the stigma associated with serious mental illness. People with serious mental illness are frequently depicted in the media as dangerous, peculiar, and in need of care and protection. Although serious mental illness is not uncommon, many people do not disclose their diagnosis because of the associated stigma. The Asbury Café provides an opportunity for people with and without mental illness to come together and interact in a positive environment (Figure 35.5).

(continued)

OT STORY 35.1 THE ASBURY CAFÉ (continued)

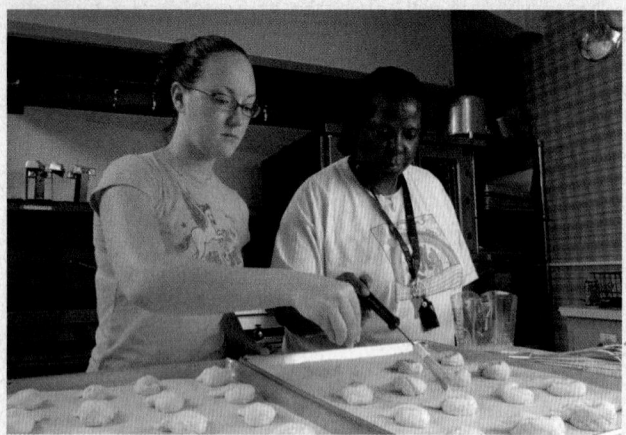

FIGURE 35.5 Jess and Janet at the Asbury Café.

(Photo courtesy of C. Brown.)

The first aim of the program is to provide employment to individuals with psychiatric disabilities. Individuals who are referred by the vocational team to this worksite are typically individuals who have less work experience, have more overt symptomatology, and need more extensive adaptations to the work environment. No formal assessments are completed; however, extensive skilled observation and task analysis are used to match employees with tasks and to make adaptations to the task and environment.

The second purpose of the Asbury Café is to reduce the stigma associated with serious mental illness by promoting positive social interactions between people with and without mental illness.

The Asbury Café demonstrates how OT can have an impact outside a traditional service setting. The café is true to the values of the ecologic models, which emphasize client-centered practice and full participation in community life. The program enhances occupational performance in the areas of work and social interaction by providing interventions targeting the person, environment, and occupation. The program itself is designed to change the stigmatizing social and cultural environment that is currently so pervasive for people with serious mental illness.

Target Area of Occupational Performance: Work

Ecologic Model Components	Interventions
Person Factors	
Individuals with serious mental illness often have cognitive impairments that slow information processing and interfere with learning of the job tasks.	*Establish/restore:* Provide simple instructions with demonstration, models, and regular feedback. *Alter:* Match worker with café task that best meets the person's interests and abilities. *Adapt:* Pair workers so that one with stronger skills can model, help focus, and provide feedback to the worker with developing skills.
Psychiatric symptoms such as anxiety and auditory hallucinations can make it more challenging to focus on work tasks.	*Establish/restore:* Teach the worker individual strategies to use when feeling anxious (e.g., deep breathing) or experiencing hallucinations (e.g., talk aloud to others). *Adapt:* Allow for frequent breaks, set up an environment of acceptance and support, use the environment to create distractions from hallucinations or worries.
Environmental Factors	
Fewer job opportunities are available to the employees of the café in the neighborhoods where they live, and typical worksites do not offer the limited schedule needed and desired by current employees.	*Adapt:* The full Asbury Café program is an adapt strategy. Supervisors and volunteers have experience in mental health services. Employees at the café are individuals who need more extensive supports for successful work performance.
Employees at the café do not have cars, and no public transportation is available to the work location.	*Adapt:* Although this is not ideal, the mental health center provides transportation.
Occupation	
The major occupation is work in the area of meal preparation, serving, and cleanup. Each task has many subcomponents.	*Alter:* Over time, the best matches become known; and individual workers assume responsibility for their tasks. They are able to perform these tasks without assistance or oversight. *Adapt:* The tasks are often adapted so that there are fewer steps or one task is done by two or three people so that the full task is not too difficult for an individual.

OT STORY 35.1 THE ASBURY CAFÉ (continued)

Target Area of Occupational Performance: Social Interaction

Ecologic Model Components	Interventions
Person Factors	
Many of the customers at the café have limited exposure to individuals with serious mental illness.	*Alter:* Employees with mental illness are assigned work tasks so that they have opportunities to interact directly with the café customers (taking money, serving meals). Employees with mental illness are also assigned work tasks that require regular contact with church staff. This provides an opportunity for real work relationships to develop.
Environmental Factors	
US culture tends to portray individuals with serious mental illness as dangerous, unpredictable, and in need of protection. Yet, the church is an environment that is open to accepting diverse individuals and welcomes the program.	*Establish/restore:* Educational opportunities are provided through the church in the form of lectures, articles in the newsletter, and presentations by consumers of the mental health center to provide accurate information to potential café customers about serious mental illness. *Adapt:* The program director and volunteers create an environment that models positive interactions with individuals with serious mental illness (e.g., avoiding distinguishing between those who do and do not have mental illness; in addition to working alongside one another, also socializing together during breaks).
Occupation	
Eating together socially.	*Alter:* The Asbury Café provides a naturally occurring opportunity for people to socialize in a natural setting. The café workers, supervisor, and volunteers eat during the time when the customers are eating so that there are more times for interaction.

Evidence to Support Using the Ecologic Models

The ecologic models are broad conceptual frameworks, making them difficult to study in their entirety. However, research indicating a relationship between environment and occupational performance, studies of environmental assessments, and efficacy studies of environmental interventions provide support for the ecologic models. This section provides examples of these types of research.

Research examining the relationship between the environment and occupational performance has implications for rehabilitation. For example:

- Neighborhood characteristics affect social participation for older adults such that greater population density was associated with more attendance in sports and social clubs and greater social cohesion was associated with greater attendance of nonreligious organizations (Hand & Howrey, 2019).

- Environmental features affect participation for individuals with mobility impairments. Negative attitudes, physical barriers, and inadequacy of systems, services, and policies affect participation in multiple areas, such as participation in education, employment, and healthcare (Wong et al., 2017).

- A study of factors related to sleep disruption in schizophrenia classified factors into person, environment, and occupation domains. The environment domain included sensory intrusions, bedding quality, and roommates (Chang et al., 2021).

- A large multisite study found racial disparities in poststroke functional recovery with Hispanic patients having the lowest levels of recovery. The study suggests that work is needed to ameliorate these disparities (Simmonds et al., 2021).

Other research that is useful to occupational therapists examines environmental assessments.

- One study supported the reliability and validity of the Participation and Sensory Environment-Questionnaire—Home Scale, which is intended to evaluate the sensory features of the home environment (Bevans et al., 2020).

- A study was undertaken to assess the cross-cultural adaptation and validity of an Italian version of the Craig Hospital Inventory of Environmental Factors, which assesses environmental barriers that interfere with participation for people with disabilities (Miniera et al., 2020).
- The use of a mobile app was studied as a way of assessing the home environment in three dimensions for the purpose of developing home modifications (Guay et al., 2021).

There are several examples of research that support the efficacy of OT intervention with an ecologic basis.

- A systematic review of home-based OT for people with dementia found 10 studies that resulted in improved activities for daily living (ADLs) or instrumental ADLs (IADLs) performance using compensatory techniques, such as home modifications, task simplifications sensory cues, and the promotion of daily changes (Raj et al., 2021).
- A study explored the application of the Matching Person and Technology model for increasing satisfaction with assistive technology for paralympic athletes (Teixeira & Alves, 2021). Important factors to consider included safety, comfort, and effectiveness of the devices.
- One study of a peer-mediated intervention in which typically developing children are trained to deliver the intervention found that the approach was effective in helping children with autism generalize their play performance from a dyad to a triad social environment (Kent et al., 2020).

These studies provide just a few examples of this rapidly growing body of research. The research evidence suggests that occupational therapists are now more informed about the role of the environment as it relates to occupational performance and better prepared to provide relevant and useful assessments and interventions using an ecologic approach.

Conclusion

OT practice is aimed at promoting occupational performance. Ecologic models provide a framework for understanding the multiplicity of factors that must be taken into account in assessing and providing interventions to enhance occupational performance. These models require that the occupational therapist use a client-centered approach and always consider the importance of the environment in the OT process.

Lippincott® Connect *For additional resources on the subjects discussed in this chapter, visit Lippincott Connect.*

REFERENCES

Bevans, K. B., Piller, A., & Pfeiffer, B. (2020). Psychometric evaluation of the Participation and Sensory Environment Questionnaire-Home Scale (PSEQ-H). *The American Journal of Occupational Therapy, 74*(3), 7403205050p1–7403205050p9. https://doi.org/10.5014/ajot.2020.036509

Bronfenbrenner, U. (1979). *The ecology of human development: Experiments by nature and design.* Harvard University Press.

Brown, C., Rempfer, M., & Hamera, E. (2009). *The test of grocery shopping skills.* AOTA Press.

Canadian Association of Occupational Therapists. (1997). *Enabling occupation: An occupational therapy perspective.* CAOT Publications ACE.

Chamberlin, J. (1990). The ex-patients' movement: Where we've been and where we're going. *Journal of Mind and Behavior, 11*(3 & 4), 323–336. https://www.jstor.org/stable/43854095

Chang, Y. C., Chang, M. C., Chang, Y. J., & Chen, M. D. (2021). Understanding factors relevant to poor sleep and coping methods in people with schizophrenia. *BMC Psychiatry, 21*(1), 373. https://doi.org/10.1186/s12888-021-03384-y

Christiansen, C., & Baum, C. (Eds.). (1997). *Occupational therapy: Enabling function and well-being* (2nd ed.). Slack.

Csikszentmihalyi, M. (1990). *Flow: The psychology of optimal experience.* Harper & Row.

Deegan, P. E. (1993). Recovering our self of value after being labeled. *Journal of Psychosocial Nursing, 31*(4), 7–11. https://doi.org/10.3928/0279-3695-19930401-06

DeJong, G. (1979). Independent living: From social movement to analytic paradigm. *Archives of Physical Medicine and Rehabilitation, 60,* 435–446.

Dunn, W., Brown, C., & McGuigan, A. (1994). The ecology of human performance: A framework for considering the impact of context. *American Journal of Occupational Therapy, 48,* 595–607. https://doi.org/10.5014/ajot.48.7.595

Dunn, W., McClain, L. H., Brown, C., & Youngstrom, M. J. (2003). The ecology of human performance. In E. B. Crepeau, E. S. Cohn, & B. A. B. Schell (Eds.), *Willard & Spackman's occupational therapy* (10th ed., pp. 223–226). Lippincott William & Wilkins.

Gibson, J. J. (1979). *The ecological approach to visual perception.* Houghton Mifflin.

Guay, M., Labbé, M., Séguin-Tremblay, N., Auger, C., Goyer, G., Veloza, E., Chevalier, N., Polgar, J., & Michaud, F. (2021). Adapting a person's home in 3D using a mobile app (MapIt): Participatory design framework investigating the app's acceptability. *JMIR Rehabilitation and Assistive Technologies, 8*(2), e24669. https://doi.org/10.2196/24669

Hand, C. L., & Howrey, B. T. (2019). Associations among neighborhood characteristics, mobility limitation and social participation in late life. *The Journals of Gerontology, 74,* 546–555. https://doi.org/10.1093/geronb/gbw215

Kent, C., Cordier, R., Joosten, A., Wilkes-Gillan, S., & Bundy, A. (2020). Can I join in? Multiple case study investigation of play performance generalisation for children with autism spectrum disorder from dyad to triad. *Australian Occupational Therapy Journal, 67,* 199–209. https://doi.org/10.1111/1440-1630.12635

Kielhofner, G., & Burke, J. P. (1980). A model of human occupation, Part 1. Conceptual framework and content. *American Journal of Occupational Therapy, 34,* 572–581. https://doi.org/10.5014/ajot.34.9.572

Law, M. C., Cooper, B., Strong, S., Stewart, D., Rigby, P., & Letts, L. (1996). The person-environment-occupation model: A transactive approach to occupational performance. *Canadian Journal of Occupational Therapy, 63,* 9–23. https://doi.org/10.1177/000841749606300103

Law, M. C., Darrah, J., Pollock, N., Wilson, B., Russell, D. J., Walter, S. D., Rosenbaum, P., & Galuppi, B. (2012). Focus on function: A cluster randomized controlled trial comparing child-versus context-focused intervention for young children with cerebral palsy. *Developmental Medicine and Child Neurology, 53,* 621–629. https://doi.org/10.1111/j.1469-8749.2011.03962.x

Lawton, M. P. (1986). *Environment and aging* (2nd ed.). Plenum Press.

Malecki, K. C., & Demary, K. M. (2002). Measuring perceived social support: Development of the Child and Adolescent Social Support Scale (CASSS). *Psychology in the Schools, 39,* 1–18. https://doi.org/10.1002/pits.10004

Miniera, F., Berardi, A., Panuccio, F., Valente, D., Tofani, M., & Galeoto, G. (2020). Measuring environmental barriers: Validation and cultural adaptation of the Italian Version of the Craig Hospital Inventory of Environmental Factors (CHIEF) Scale. *Occupational Therapy in Health Care, 34*(4), 373–385. https://doi.org/10.1080/07380577.2020.1834174

Moore-Corner, R. A., Kielhofner, G., & Olson, L. (1998). *Work Environmental Impact Scale (WEIS) Version 2.0.* The University of Illinois Chicago.

Oliver, M. (1996). *Understanding disability: From theory to practice.* St. Martin's Press.

Raj, S. E., Mackintosh, S., Fryer, C., & Stanley, M. (2021). Home-based occupational therapy for adults with dementia and their informal caregivers: A systematic review. *American Journal of Occupational Therapy, 75*(1), 7501205060. https://doi.org/10.5014/ajot.2020.040782

Romli, M. H., Mackenzie, L., Lovarini, M., Tan, M. P., & Clemson, L. (2018). The clinimetric properties of instruments measuring home hazards for older people at risk of falling: A systematic review. *Evaluation & The Health Professions, 41*(1), 82–128. https://doi.org/10.1177/0163278716684166

Scanlan, J. N., & Bundy, A. C. (2011). Development and validation of the modified occupational questionnaire. *American Journal of Occupational Therapy, 65*(1), e11–e19. https://doi.org/10.5014/ajot.2011.09042

Schkade, J. K., & Schultz, S. (1992). Occupational adaptation: Toward a holistic approach to contemporary practice, Part I. *American Journal of Occupational Therapy, 46,* 829–837. https://doi.org/10.5014/ajot.46.9.829

Schneidert, M., Hurst, R., Miller, J., & Ustün, B. (2003). The role of environment in the International Classification of Functioning, Disability and Health (ICF). *Disability and Rehabilitation, 25*(11–12), 588–595. https://doi.org/10.1080/0963828031000137090

Shapiro, J. P. (1994). *No pity: People with disabilities forging a new civil rights movement.* Three Rivers Press.

Simmonds, K. P., Luo, Z., & Reeves, M. (2021). Race/ethnic and stroke subtype differences in poststroke functional recovery after acute rehabilitation. *Archives of Physical Medicine and Rehabilitation, 102*(8), 1473–1481. https://doi.org/10.1016/j.apmr.2021.01.090

Teixeira, G., & Alves, A. (2021). Occupational therapy intervention in paralympic sport: A look at low-cost assistive technology for wheelchair rugby. *Disability and Rehabilitation. Assistive Technology, 16*(4), 432–437. https://doi.org/10.1080/17483107.2020.1839577

Townsend, E. A., & Polatajko, H. J. (2013). *Enabling occupation II: Advancing an occupational therapy vision for health, well-being, & justice through occupation* (2nd ed). CAOT Publications ACE.

Williams, D. R., & Mohammed, S. A. (2013). Racism and health I: Pathways and scientific evidence. *American Behavioral Scientist, 57.* https://doi.org/10.1177/0002764213487340

Wong, A. W. K., Ng, S., Dashner, J., Baum, M. C., Hammel, J., Magasi, S., Lai, J.-S., Carlozzi, N. E., Tulsky, D. S., Miskovic, A., Goldsmith, A., & Heinemann, A. W. (2017). Relationships between environmental factors and participation in adults with traumatic brain injury, stroke, and spinal cord injury: A cross-sectional multi-center study. *Quality of Life Research, 26,* 2633–2645. https://doi.org/10.1007/s11136-017-1586-5

Theory of Occupational Adaptation

Lenin C. Grajo and Angela K. Boisselle

LEARNING OBJECTIVES

After reading this chapter, you will be able to:

1. Articulate occupational adaptation as an internal, normative human process that results from the transaction of the person and the occupational environment.
2. Discuss the four core concepts of occupational adaptation—person, occupational environment, press for mastery, and occupational participation—as they relate to everyday life.
3. Apply the five essential elements of occupational adaptation in assessment and intervention.
4. Analyze how the concepts and theory of occupational adaptation can be used in daily clinical practice and research.
5. Identify ways the theory of occupational adaptation can be understood and used in more culturally humble and inclusive ways in daily practice.

Introduction

In 1987, Dr Janette Schkade, Dr Sally Schultz, and several faculty members began developing the theory of occupational adaptation (OA) as a theoretical framework to guide the Doctor of Philosophy in Occupational Therapy program at Texas Woman's University. Drawing from two foundational concepts—occupation and adaptation—Schkade and Schultz were influenced by the rich historical literature in occupational therapy (OT) (Schultz, 2014). Some of the historical underpinnings of the theory (Grajo, 2017, p. 288) included the use of occupation to facilitate adaptation (Meyer, 1922/1977); human's need to master the environment (Reilly, 1962); occupation as a way to achieve competency, mastery, and motivation (Florey, 1969; Llorens, 1970; White, 1959); the importance of self-initiated occupation (Yerxa, 1967); and different perspectives and definitions of adaptation, competence, and resilience as a result of doing, active involvement, and choice (Fidler, 1981; Fidler & Fidler, 1978; Fine, 1991; Kielhofner, 1977; King, 1978; Kleinman & Bulkley, 1982; Nelson, 1988).

The theory of OA was first introduced in a two-part publication in the *American Journal of Occupational Therapy* (Schkade & Schultz, 1992; Schultz & Schkade, 1992). It was first published in the eighth edition of *Willard & Spackman's Occupational Therapy* (1988). OA has been referred to in Willard and Spackman's book as a frame of reference (eighth and ninth editions,

1988 and 1998, respectively); a theory derived from occupational behavior perspectives (ninth and tenth editions, 1998 and 2003, respectively); as a conceptual basis for practice (11th edition, 2009); and as an occupational performance theory of practice (12th edition, 2014).

Between 1993 and 2015, the OA theory has been cited at least 74 times in published research articles as a primary influence in the understanding of the process of adaptation in humans, both in quantitative and qualitative studies (Grajo et al., 2018), and more work using the theory continues to emerge. After several brainstorming and consultation sessions with Dr Sally Schultz, the first author published this reconceptualization for the first time in 2017 (Grajo, 2017). There have been many scholarly discussions about what concepts are the "soul and at the core" of the theory and whether the reconceptualization became an oversimplification of the theory when several complex concepts of the theory were not retained in the 2017 and succeeding revisions. We let the emerging literature and a systematic analysis of how the theory of OA is applied and used by educators, clinicians, and researchers become the primary guide and impetus for reconceptualization. We also believe in diversity in thought and welcome evidence in the use of the more complex concepts of the theory from the seminal work of Drs Schkade and Schultz.

We believe that the reconceptualization has allowed more educators, scholars, clinicians, and students to better appreciate the theory's concepts. More importantly, the work from this reconceptualization has made way for OA as an important concept to now be better represented and recognized in key documents of the profession:

> Occupational adaptation, or the client's effective and efficient response to occupational and contextual demands (Grajo, 2019), is interwoven through all of these (occupational therapy) outcomes. (*Occupational Therapy Practice Framework*, 4th ed.; American Occupational Therapy Association [AOTA, 2020], p. 26)
>
> . . . participation in meaningful occupations is a determinant of health and leads to adaptation. (Philosophical base of occupational therapy; AOTA, 2017, p. 1)

In this chapter, we use numbered boxes labeled "Making OA a More Inclusive Theory in Practice." The use of these boxes signifies our continued commitment to reconceptualize and evolve the theory of OA, to decolonize a theory developed from Western perspectives, and to encourage reflection and action on how perspectives from the theory can be used for a more culturally humble and inclusive practice.

Overview of Occupational Adaptation

This chapter presents a reconceptualization of Schkade and Schultz's (1992) theory as presented in two previous works (Grajo, 2017, 2018). The reconceptualization aims to

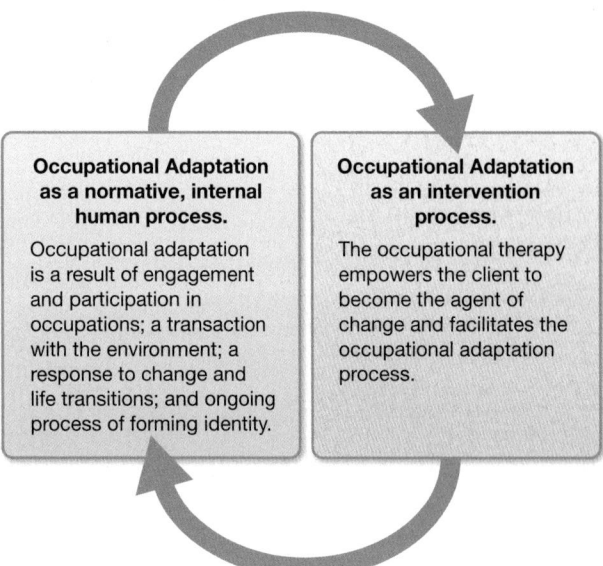

FIGURE 36.1 Summary of the principles of the theory of occupational adaptation.

facilitate easier understanding and use of the theory in daily practice, education, and research. The **occupational adaptation** (OA) theory can be summarized in two interrelated principles (Figure 36.1):

1. OA is a normative, internal human process.
2. OA is an intervention process that can guide an occupational therapist's critical thinking and clinical reasoning within the therapeutic process and relationship.

A major disruption in the normative process in humans (principle 1) as a result of illness, disease, or disability; a major life transition; or an alteration of typical human development may be a basis for seeking OT intervention (principle 2). The goal of OT intervention (principle 2) is to facilitate the OA process in the person (principle 1).

Core Concepts: Occupational Adaptation as an Internal Normative Process

A scoping review of literature (Grajo et al., 2018) identified four concepts to define OA. OA is a product of: engagement and participation in occupations; a transaction with the environment; a manner of responding to change, altered situations, and life transitions; and a manner of forming identity. Figure 36.2 illustrates a summary of these definitions of OA as a normative process.

Four main concepts (also termed as *constants* by Schkade & Schultz, 2003) are essential in understanding this normative process.

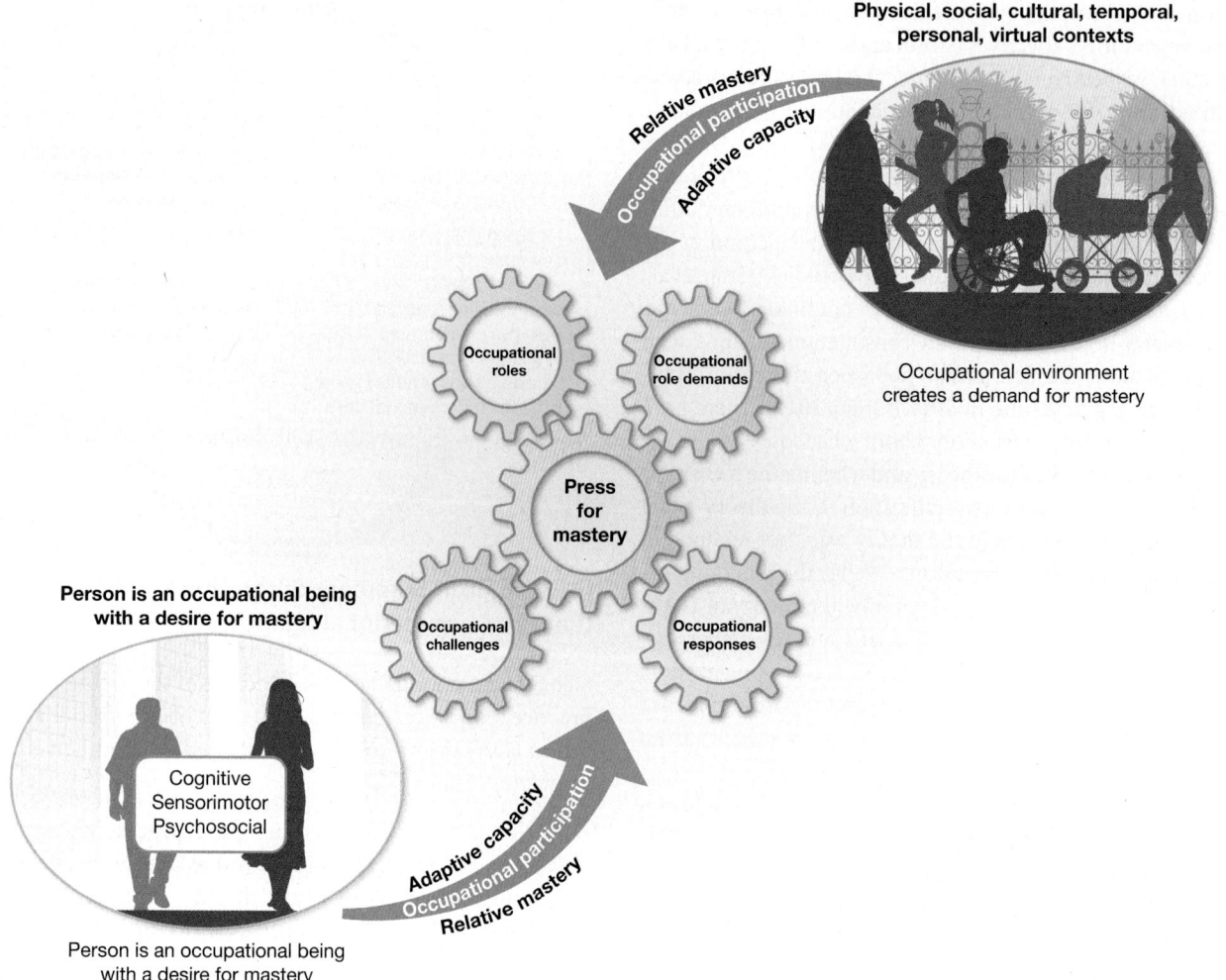

FIGURE 36.2 A reconceptualization of Schkade and Schultz's occupational adaptation process illustration. (Adapted from Grajo, L. [2017]. Occupational adaptation. In J. Hinojosa, P. Kramer, & C. Royeen [Eds.], *Perspectives in occupation* [2nd ed., pp. 287–311]. F. A. Davis.)

Person

The person is an occupational being with an inherent *desire to master* occupations through transactions with the environment (Grajo, 2017). Three-person systems, in typical human development, enable the person to perform and participate in occupations:

1. Cognitive (i.e., neurologic and processing abilities)
2. Sensorimotor (i.e., integrated sensory, perceptual, and motor capacities)
3. Psychosocial systems (i.e., emotional, social, behavior-related abilities) (Schkade & Schultz, 1992)

Occupational Environment

The occupational environment includes settings and contexts that influence occupational performance and participation. More broadly, contexts are the environmental and personal factors that influence engagement and participation in occupations (AOTA, 2020). The occupational environment creates a *demand for mastery* from the person. Circumstances and personal factors (e.g., limited time, norms, cultural expectations, social background) and aspects of the built environment and expectations by society may all create various forms and levels of demand for mastery from the person. These conditions require the person to behave, perform, and participate in life in ways that may facilitate or hinder the OA process.

Occupational Participation

A revision to the "Philosophical base of occupational therapy" as stated previously in this chapter emphasized the influence of occupational participation in a person's adaptation process. Occupational participation is the mechanism for OA as an internal, normative process to manifest because it leads to increased adaptation. Increased adaptation leads to improved occupational participation. Occupations have three important properties: (a) they require active engagement, (b) they serve a purpose or are meaningful to the individual, and (c) they are goal oriented (i.e., they produce a tangible or intangible product as a result of participation) (Grajo, 2017; Schkade & Schultz, 1992).

Press for Mastery

When the person and the occupational environment transact during occupational participation, the *press for mastery* manifests. The situational element of the press for mastery is observed when the person perceives a demand for mastery (asserted by the occupational environment), analyzes the skill demands of the occupation (cognitive, sensorimotor, and psychosocial demands), and assesses personal desire for mastery of the occupation. The press for mastery manifests as a series of simultaneously or concurrently occurring processes, dependent on the occupation's features, factors within the person, and the complexities of the occupational environment and contexts for occupational participation (Figure 36.3). These processes include the following:

1. ***Occupational roles.*** These are person-defined sets of behaviors based on society's expectations and are heavily influenced by culture and context (AOTA, 2020, p. 42).
2. ***Occupational challenges.*** Based on the person's current abilities, desire for mastery of the occupation and the environment, and assessment of the level of

demand for mastery from the environment, certain occupational challenges may surface. Some occupational challenges may be easy to overcome, whereas others may hinder the OA process and cause a temporary or persistent occupational dysadaptation.
3. ***Role demands or expectations.*** Occupational roles assert a combination of internal and/or external role demands. The person perceives internal role demands (e.g., a single father perceives the need to work two jobs to provide for the family). The occupational environment creates external role demands (e.g., some cultures may dictate that mothers spend more time with children than at work).
4. ***Occupational responses.*** During transaction with the environment and participation in occupations, the person evaluates the level of occupational challenge, roles expected by society or assumed by the person, and role demands. The person then identifies how to respond to these challenges, roles, and role demands or expectations. This configuration of response is referred to as an *adaptation gestalt*. The adaptation gestalt allows the person to assess how to respond to the challenge so as to achieve mastery and competence in occupational participation. Based on cognitive, sensorimotor, and psychosocial abilities, the person may choose an existing response that previously worked, develop a new response, or modify an existing response as necessary to meet the occupational challenge.

The Adaptation Gestalt

The adaptation gestalt is an assessment of the amount and level of cognitive, sensorimotor, and psychosocial capacities needed to respond to occupational challenges, roles, and role demands and perform an occupation with a level of mastery and competence (Schkade & Schultz, 1992). Occupations require different levels of skills and demands from the person systems. Some occupations may require higher cognitive skills (e.g., studying for a final exam), higher psychosocial skills (e.g., making new friends), or higher sensory and motor abilities (e.g., completing a 60-minute upper body workout). A pie chart (Figure 36.4) can be used to visualize a configuration of the adaptation gestalt (Schultz & Schkade, 1997). Depending on the occupational performance demands, the gestalt may be modified as needed so that specific person systems occupy bigger proportions of the pie at different points in time as necessary. The pie chart configuration also helps determine a person's skills, strengths, and challenges. Experiences by the person based on occupations performed and challenges encountered form variations of the adaptation gestalts. When transacting with the occupational environment, the person identifies a configuration of the gestalt that will enable optimal participation in occupations with mastery and competence.

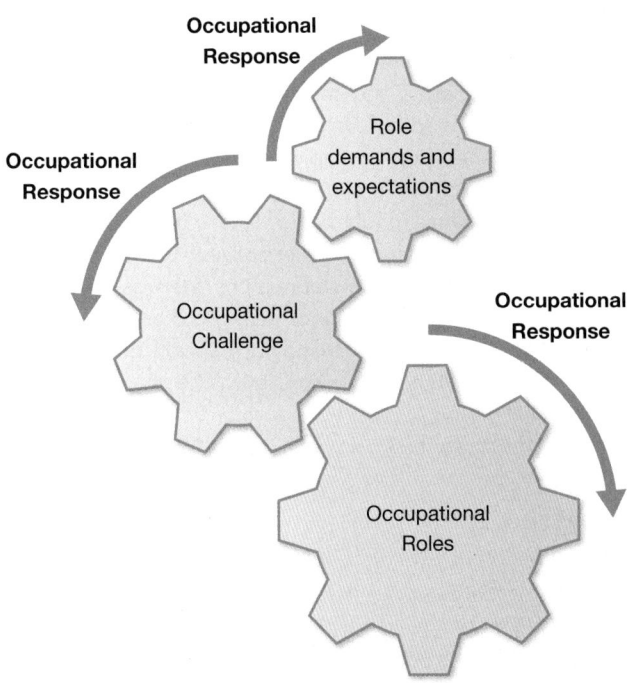

FIGURE 36.3 **Press for mastery.**

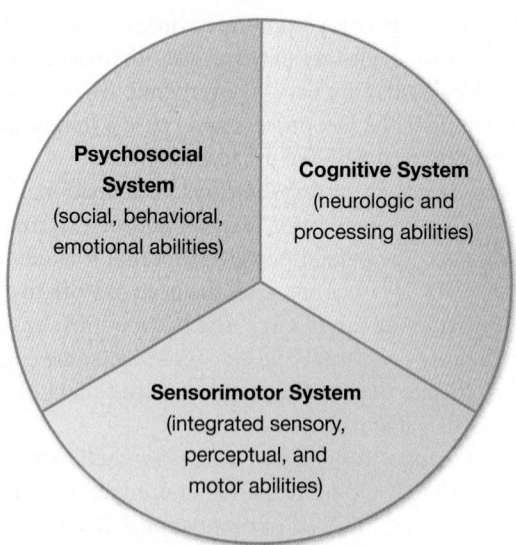

FIGURE 36.4 **The adaptation gestalt.**

The case of Bobbye provides an overview of how to apply the four core concepts of the OA theory (OT Story 36.1).

Adaptive and Dysadaptive Responses

Schkade and Schultz (2003) described complex and layered adaptive response subprocesses. The adaptive response subprocesses can be understood as an iterative process of identifying, producing, evaluating, and modifying occupational responses to occupational challenges so that the person can participate in occupations with mastery and competence. Experience heavily influences these iterative adaptive response subprocesses.

- Occupational responses may be described as *adaptive*: *Adaptive responses* overcome or help manage the occupational challenge and promote mastery and competence in the occupation.

OT STORY 36.1 OCCUPATIONAL ADAPTATION AS A NORMATIVE PROCESS

Bobbye is a 35-year-old transgender woman who recently completed gender-affirming surgery. Before her transition, she was married to Diane. They divorced 5 years ago and remain friends. Together, they have a 6-year-old daughter. Bobbye works as a marketing and public relations specialist at a pediatric hospital. She enjoys photography, live music, and art. Diane has expressed difficulty with Bobbye's transition, but has been supportive. Some family members and co-workers have responded negatively by discontinuing communication. Bobbye's employer is a strong ally for LGBTQ rights.

Let us try to understand Bobbye's OA process: *Bobbye is undergoing life and identity challenges as she navigates the coming out and transition processes.*

Desire for mastery: Bobbye (person) has a desire to master occupations and life roles that she truly values. She wants to continue to provide support to her family and be a good employee at the hospital while also exploring her evolving identity and new romantic and intimate relationships.

Demand for mastery: Bobbye's ex-partner demands that they maintain current partner roles as related to child-rearing and financial support. Likewise, their family, friends, and employer would like for Bobbye to continue current roles; however, some family members asserted that they want to see Bobbye "dressing and acting like the father he should be to his daughter" during family gatherings.

Press for mastery: Bobbye is experiencing shifts in her sense of self/identity while navigating her occupational roles and demands.

- *Important occupational roles:* Parent, family member, friend, coworker
- *Role expectations/demands:* Continue participating in occupations to fulfill the occupational demands related

to the occupational roles of family member, friend, and coworker
- *Possible occupational challenges:* Adapting to new roles as a parent and navigating new romantic relationships, psychosocial issues, and ongoing identity navigation issues related to negative external responses from family, friends, and/or co-workers

Bobbye may demonstrate adaptive responses that will promote mastery and competence or, conversely, react negatively to the press for mastery, leading to decreased relative mastery and competence.

- ***Adaptive occupational responses:*** She may seek assistance from friends and family members for support in meeting the needs of her daughter; she can potentially seek assistance from therapists, support group, or social media group or explore strategies to manage psychosocial stress, such as meditation or listening to music.
- ***Dysadaptive occupational responses:*** She may isolate herself and experience depression, feelings of inadequacy and helplessness, and feelings of guilt for being her authentic self while trying to maintain co-parenting and cordial relationship with Diane. She may no longer feel satisfied in personal relationships with those who do not support the transition.

Questions

1. In what ways have Bobbye's role demands and expectations changed owing to her transitioning to a woman?
2. Describe personal factors that may be concerning for her during the transition.
3. What examples of adaptive and dysadaptive responses might one expect from Bobbye as she navigates dating and romantic relationships?

An important consideration in understanding adaptive responses is that these responses are specific to the person. Some responses may be adaptive to some (e.g., going shopping when stressed or exercising when faced with an anxiety-triggering challenge), whereas for others, it may be dysadaptive (e.g., spending too much while shopping or over-exercising to the point of injury). Central in understanding adaptive responses is the understanding of the unique contextual factors of the person and that a dysadaptive response for one person may be an adaptive response for another.

- Other occupational responses may be described as *dysadaptive*: When a person exhibits *dysadaptive responses,* they do not overcome the occupational challenge and the person may feel "stuck" and unable to perform occupations and transact with the occupational environment with mastery and competence.

Throughout growth and development, the person produces, evaluates the effectiveness of, and modifies adaptive and dysadaptive responses to enable them to participate in daily occupations (see Box 36.1).

Relative Mastery and Adaptive Capacity: Assessing Occupational Adaptation

Two terms have been used in the OA theory to describe how to evaluate the normative process of OA and when occupational adaptiveness is demonstrated. They are *relative mastery* and *adaptive capacity*.

Relative Mastery. Relative mastery has three components (Grajo, 2017; Schkade & McClung, 2001):

- *Effective participation* in occupations is assessed based on how well people achieve their occupational engagement and participation goals.
- *Efficiency* is assessed by the extent to which a person uses available personal resources and resources in the occupational environment appropriately (e.g., appropriate use of time, energy, task objects and materials, social supports).
- *Satisfaction* refers to the extent to which people are content with their occupational performance and the congruence between occupational participation and performance expectations. Satisfaction is measured

based on satisfaction with self and satisfaction by other significant people with a person's performance.

Adaptive Capacity. *Adaptive capacity* can be understood using the analogy of using "tools in a toolbox" (Grajo, 2017). Adaptive capacity can be defined as the person's ability to perceive the need to change, modify, or refine responses to occupational challenges in the environment (Schkade & Schultz, 2003). When faced with difficulties in life and when participating in occupations that may pose challenges, does the person have enough tools in the toolbox to meet the challenge? Can the person develop new tools or modify existing tools to overcome the occupational challenge?

A major life transition or the experience of illness or disability may impact a person's relative mastery and adaptive capacity and, therefore, the OA process. When life events during transitions make the person unable to assume important roles and perform occupations, and when the person feels overwhelmed by role demands and responsibilities or is unable to use appropriate tools or strategies for occupational or task performance, a persistent state of occupational dysadaptation may occur (Grajo, 2018). In these cases, an occupational therapist may need to support and assist the person (the client) to reestablish important roles, resume participation in meaningful occupations, and facilitate the OA process (see Box 36.2).

Evaluating relative mastery and adaptive capacity must be situated with consideration of the intersectionality of the person. *Intersectionality* is defined as the examination of race, sex, class, national origin, sexual orientation, and how the combination of these factors play out when the person is in various settings (Delgado & Stefancic, 2017). Measuring factors such as "reasonable attainment of a goal," "independence," "without assistance from a caregiver," "satisfaction with performance," and "meaningfulness of an occupation" must be assessed within the contextual and intersecting factors unique to the individual. For example, in some cultures, it is a noble culturally sanctioned responsibility for family members to provide care and assistance to family members with a disability. In this case, the notion of "independence in self-care" must be assessed with careful consideration of these culture-specific factors and meanings.

Using the Model in Practice: Occupational Adaptation as an Intervention Process

Occupational therapists may use the OA theory to guide them in facilitating therapeutic process and relationship with clients. The OA-guided intervention is not protocol based. It is not a collection of techniques, or a series of action steps (Schkade & Schultz, 2003). The OA-guided intervention uses critical and clinical reasoning skills to assist the therapist in assessment and intervention. Establishing a meaningful therapeutic relationship is critical in OA-guided intervention. The intervention has five essential elements, as shown in Figure 36.5 (adapted from Grajo, 2017, 2018; Schultz, 2014).

Evaluating the Client: Using Holistic and Participation Approaches to Assessment

Based on the OA theory, assessments should measure both the static outcomes and the impact of intervention on the client's engagement in personally meaningful life roles (Schultz, 2014). An OA-guided occupational therapist uses a combination of standardized and nonstandardized assessments to create a holistic picture of the client. The occupational therapist assists the client in

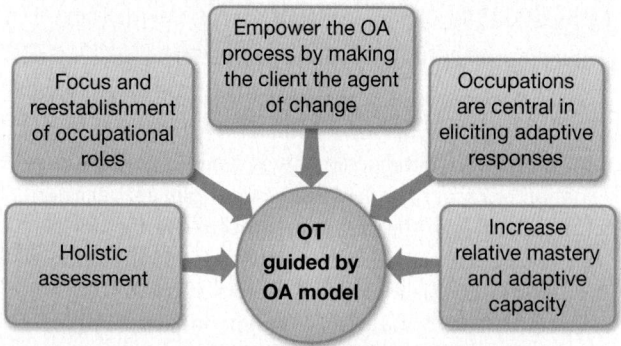

FIGURE 36.5 Essential elements of occupational adaptation (OA)-guided intervention. OT, occupational therapy. (Adapted from Grajo, L. [2018]. Occupational adaptation as a normative and intervention process—New perspectives on Schkade and Schultz's professional legacy. In L. C. Grajo & A. K. Boisselle [Eds.], *Adaptation through occupation: Multidimensional perspectives*. SLACK.)

creating an *occupational profile* to identify strengths and weaknesses and meaningful occupational roles. Norm-referenced assessments can be used in combination with patient report–type instruments that assess perceptions of roles, participation in occupations, and observational assessments of occupational performance and participation (Grajo, 2018). The OA-guided occupational therapist must evaluate the client's effectiveness, efficiency, and satisfaction with occupational performance (relative mastery) and the client's ability to assess and use a variety of tools and responses to overcome challenges (adaptive capacity). Factors that may influence occupational participation and the adaptive process must also be carefully considered.

Developing an Intervention Plan: Reestablishing Important Occupational Roles

Life roles provide the context for expressing competence in occupational functioning (Schkade & McClung, 2001). A focus on reestablishing roles rather than developing performance skills is critical in OA-guided intervention (Schkade & Schultz, 2003). When intervention focuses on improving a client's occupational adaptiveness based on personally important roles, the client can better participate in occupations and improve performance skills (Grajo, 2018; Schultz, 2014). Fulfillment of roles provides meaning and satisfaction in life.

Implementing the Intervention: The Client Is the Agent of Change

The OA-guided intervention focuses on making the client the agent of change in the therapeutic process. The occupational therapist must use the therapeutic relationship to help facilitate the client's OA process. This can be done in a variety of ways:

- ***Learning when to push and when to hold back:*** The occupational therapist must assume the role of a facilitator rather than an instructor. Instead of telling the client what to do, how to do, and what strategies to use in task performance and participation in occupations, the occupational therapist can use a series of questions and probing statements to facilitate the process. The occupational therapist must also learn how to provide clients with opportunities to experience performance challenges and problem-solve. The therapist then supports the client in identifying ways to solve the occupational challenges instead of providing answers.

BOX 36.3 MAKING OA A MORE INCLUSIVE THEORY IN PRACTICE: THE CLIENT AS THE AGENT OF CHANGE

The element of the client "as the agent of change" can be rooted in theoretical perspectives of self-determination and empowerment. These tenets of "self-determination" and "empowerment" are rooted in many seminal legal and political contexts (Freeman, 1999) that need to be understood within many specific cultural perspectives. This is a central tenet of occupational therapy practice that can sometimes be overlooked: being client centered. But even the notion of "client-centered practice" is a Western assumption (Dirette, 2018). Dirette further asserted that "choice is a concept of the middle class. For people who are oppressed by poverty, racism, and gender bias, choices are often shaped by the oppressors" (p. 3).

It is the goal of occupational therapy practice and the use of the theory of OA to enable clients to make their own choices, determine their optimal levels of function, independence, and participation. However, the occupational therapist must also understand many cultural and contextual factors that may facilitate or hinder the client from being the agent of one's own change. Some clients may defer decision-making related to outcomes of therapy or goals of therapy to a caregiver, partner, or other family members. The occupational therapist can consider these as still part of empowering the client and their significant others as agents of change in the therapeutic process.

OA, occupational adaptation.

- *Facilitating the use of occupations:* The occupational therapist must allow the client to self-initiate and choose occupations that they want to work on rather than prescribing or identifying goals and tasks that the client needs to complete. When using occupations to facilitate the OA process, the occupational therapist must let the client be in charge of setting the levels of difficulty (grading or modifying the task difficulty) to make occupations less or more challenging.
- *Facilitating the occupational environment:* The occupational therapist must involve the client in identifying ways of making the occupational environment supportive of masterful and competent occupational participation. The occupational therapist must be skillful in identifying contextual and environmental factors that may facilitate or hinder the OA process. The transaction with the occupational environment (as manifested in the press for mastery) is situation dependent. Aldrich and Heatwole-Shank (2018) asserted that the OA process could be seen as occurring within the person–environment relationship where both the individual and social factors play a role in shaping solutions to a problematic situation. Whereas Aldrich and Heatwole-Shank believe that OA cannot be an intervention outcome, Schkade and Schultz (2003) asserted that facilitated and self-initiated transactions with the occupational environment can provide mechanisms for the internal OA process to improve. This is likewise emphasized in the fourth edition of the OT Practice Framework, asserting that OA is interwoven in the different outcomes of intervention (AOTA, 2020; see document for a full list of OT intervention outcomes).

The occupational therapist must also be cognizant of a tendency to become a "fixer" for the client. Innate in occupational therapists is the desire to help clients in all aspects of living. By focusing on the client as the agent of change, the therapist must creatively learn how to navigate the therapeutic relationship to avoid assuming a "fixer" role (see Box 36.3).

Occupations Are Central in Eliciting Adaptive Responses

When clients feel "stuck" and in a state of occupational dysadaptation, the OT can use occupations to help clients get "unstick" (Grajo, 2018). Two types of intervention can be used to elicit adaptive responses (Schkade & Schultz, 1992): *occupational readiness* and *therapeutic occupations.* Occupational readiness interventions are based on preparatory activities or performance skill-building approaches. This is because limitations in body function need to be addressed to prepare the client for occupations. This may include reducing spasticity or edema and addressing strength limitations or cognitive deficits. However, the occupational therapist must not only rely on occupational readiness methods alone but should also move right away to facilitating client's participation in actual therapeutic occupations (originally termed *occupational activities*). The occupational therapist guided by OA must try to move away from occupational readiness to occupation-based interventions using simulated tasks, materials, and tools in an environment that resembles the context for natural occupational participation (Grajo, 2018).

Assessing the Outcome: Increase in Relative Mastery and Adaptive Capacity

The OA-guided therapist consistently assesses the client's relative mastery and adaptive capacity during the therapeutic process. Successful OT intervention empowers the normative process of OA in the client and an increase in relative mastery and adaptive capacity. Successful OA-guided OT intervention also facilitates the transfer and generalization of skills. When the client is able to use adaptive responses to occupational challenges in similar situations and/or when the client is able to develop new or modified occupational responses when presented with new challenges or situations, then we know that the client has attained relative mastery and adaptive capacity (see OT Story 36.2).

OT STORY 36.2 OCCUPATIONAL ADAPTATION TO FACILITATE OCCUPATIONAL PARTICIPATION

Joaquin is a 16-year-old adolescent with spina bifida who lives in a two-bedroom apartment in California with five members of his family (father, uncle, aunt, and two teenage cousins). Joaquin's father is his primary caregiver, and they share one of the bedrooms. His mother lives in El Salvador, taking care of his maternal grandmother. Except for him, all members of his household work for a local pistachio farm. He has multiple pieces of adaptive equipment, most of which are not used because of a lack of space. During the home health evaluation, he informed the occupational therapist that he performs many activities of daily living (ADLs), such as eating, dressing, grooming, and homework in bed, because there is no room for his wheelchair in his bedroom. He also expressed frustration when attempting to video chat with his girlfriend with his father in the room.

Analysis of Joaquin's Occupational Adaptation and the Role of the Occupational Therapist

Joaquin is going through life challenges owing to his current living situation, the limited space and accessibility of the built environment (his apartment), and the lack of privacy. He is supported physically and psychosocially by his family and girlfriend.

Desire for mastery: Joaquin (person) wants to be able to perform basic daily activities in a different manner so that he does not have to do activities in bed. He mentions he would like to be more like his friends. In particular, he wishes to have more privacy when spending time with his girlfriend at home.

Demand for mastery: Joaquin and his father are not particularly concerned about him being able to do everything independently. He accepts the fact that he needs assistance with certain things such as transfers or dressing but wants to do many ADLs and occupations in a different manner than he is currently doing.

Press for mastery: Joaquin's participation in occupations at home offers unique challenges related to sensorimotor and psychosocial abilities for engagement within the small physical environment and the social and cultural contexts in which he is living.

- *Important occupational roles:* Family member and boyfriend

- *Role expectations/demands:* Joaquin wishes to participate in occupations that are typical of his age as an adolescent. His family wishes that he is provided with an opportunity to participate in self-care and school-related occupations in a manner that maximizes independence.
- *Occupational challenges:* Difficulties with multistep tasks, for example, due to low endurance and decreased strength. He is also at risk for sensorimotor challenges owing to the lack of sensation and movement in his trunk and lower extremities, resulting in potential pressure injuries due to excessive time spent in bed.

Joaquin may respond to the press for mastery adaptively and dysadaptively:

- *Adaptive occupational responses:* He may seek assistance from other family members when his father is not available; potentially identify ways to do occupations differently or tasks in smaller chunks and steps or with a modified environmental setup in his room.
- *Dysadaptive occupational responses:* He may be frustrated by the lack of space. He may also feel guilt about burdening his family because of the inability to do things on his own.

Potential Need for OT Programming Guided by Occupational Adaptation

The occupational therapist can facilitate Joaquin's adaptive functioning so that he can fulfill important occupational roles and participate in occupations with satisfaction within the occupational environment.

Questions

1. What strategies can the occupational therapist use to assess Joaquin's relative mastery in occupational participation?
2. What strategies can the occupational therapist use to empower Joaquin to be an agent of change?
3. Identify three occupational readiness and three therapeutic occupations that the occupational therapist can use in intervention to facilitate Joaquin's occupational participation.

Evidence to Support Using Occupational Adaptation

The theory of OA has been used to guide the exploration of the lived experiences of disability, life transition, and altered life situations that disrupt the normative OA process. Examples of such exploration include understanding the OA process in adults with multiple sclerosis (Lexell et al., 2011), adults with stroke (Williams & Murray, 2013), adults with, posttraumatic stress disorder (Lopez, 2011), adults with acquired brain injuries (Parsons & Stanley, 2008), adults with traumatic brain injuries (Hoogerdijk et al., 2011), and those experiencing changes owing to the aging process (Moyers & Coleman, 2004). Studies based on the OA theory have also been conducted with women who immigrated to a new country (Nayar & Stanley, 2015), Filipino OT educators (Cabatan et al., 2020), and caregivers of people with multiple sclerosis (Motaharinezhad et al., 2021).

The OA theory has also been used to guide intervention in a variety of setting with a variety of populations, including adolescents with limb deficiencies (Pasek & Schkade, 1996), adults with stroke (Dolecheck & Schkade, 1999; Gibson & Schkade, 1997; Johnson & Schkade, 2001), adults with hip fractures (Buddenberg & Schkade, 1998; Jackson & Schkade, 2001), community-dwelling older adults (Spencer et al., 1999), older adults with physical disabilities (Bontje et al., 2004), adults with psychiatric illness (Adami & Evetts, 2012; Whisner et al., 2014), and children with reading difficulties (Grajo & Candler, 2016). Settings where such studies have been conducted include schools (Orr & Schkade, 1997), prison and court systems (George-Paschal & Bowen, 2019; Stelter & Whisner, 2007), and training programs for dementia care teams (McKay et al., 2021). Several assessments based on the OA theory have been developed and are currently being validated. See Table 36.1 for a summary of OA-guided assessments.

Despite mounting evidence supporting the use of the OA theory (Grajo et al., 2018; Johansson et al., 2018), Grajo et al. (2018) suggested that there is a need for more rigorous randomized controlled studies on the clinical effectiveness of interventions based on the OA theory.

TABLE 36.1 OA-Guided Assessments

Assessment and Authors	Purpose and Intended Population
Relative Mastery Measurement Scale (George et al., 2004)	Assessment designed to measure efficiency, effectiveness, and satisfaction with performance for persons facing occupational challenges
Occupational Adaptation Practice Guide (Boone & George-Paschal, 2017)	A critical reasoning tool based on the theory of occupational adaptation used for client evaluation and treatment planning
Looking Into Family Experiences (LIFE) Assessment (Honaker et al., 2012)	Occupation-based assessment completed in collaboration with the caregiver(s) and occupational therapist to evaluate family occupations and perceived satisfaction with performance of those occupations
The Inventory of Reading Occupations–Adult version (IRO-Adult) (Grajo & Gutman, 2019)	An assessment of functional literacy of adults aged 18 years and older. The IRO-Adult is a two-part self-report and/or interview-based instrument that can be used to develop a Functional Literacy profile of adults.
Kindergarten Readiness Inventory (K-READI) (Alonzi-Gold & Grajo, 2021)	Kindergarten readiness screener for children aged 3.10 to 5.11 years on the autism spectrum focused on five areas: school activities of daily living, school activities, basic concepts, social participation, and school behavior
Occupational Therapy Pediatric Inventory of Cognitive Skills (OT-PICS) (Dumas & Grajo, 2021)	An assessment for school-aged children used to evaluate functional cognitive skills used in play, self-care, and participation in education
Adaptation Process in Academia Questionnaire (APA-Q) (Cabatan et al., 2020)	A 199-item instrument used to assess educators' adaptation process in their academic roles and role demands

EXPANDING OUR PERSPECTIVES

Is the Theory of Occupational Adaptation Truly Acultural?

Moses Ikiugu

As the chapter authors aptly point out, one of the key assumptions right from the conception of the OA model of practice was that because the internal adaptation process is individual, the process is acultural (Schkade & Schultz, 1992; Schultz & Schkade, 1992). In other words, it should be valid for application in any culture. The question however, is this really the case? A closer examination would suggest that indeed this is not the case. Even though the emphasis of the model is the internal, individualized adaptation process, it is clear that the Western assumption of an independent individual, who is adapting by managing and shaping the environment, is still implied. That is why two of the key constructs for the assessment of relative mastery are efficiency (judicious use of time and resources) and individual satisfaction with performance.

In many cultures, the abovementioned assumptions would not hold true. For example, in the ubuntu philosophical stance of many of the African cultures, social connectivity is even more important than using time efficiently (Coetzer et al., 2018). I can personally attest to this from my own experience. I started practice in mental health in Kenya, East Africa. When we interacted with clients and their families, the use of time was not so much of a priority because we understood that it was not that important in that culture. What was more important was making meaningful connections with not only the client but also family members. Social relationships take time to build. Therefore, time spent just talking may be seen, according to the OA model, as inefficient use of time. As Coetzer et al. observed in the South African context, when we worked with clients, we understood that due to their illness, "their interconnectedness to others" was lost and "the broad generic aim of" rehabilitation was "an attempt to reduce the impact of clients' impairment and associated disability." Of course, one of the indicators of relative mastery according to the model is satisfaction by significant other people with the clients' performance. However, this is not the same as the need to feel that sense of connectedness that comes from the metaphysical sense that we exist because of others around us.

The same case applies to an efficient use of resources to complete occupations as an indicator of relative mastery. Again this notion is based on the Western Judeo-Christian perspective of resources provided by the environment as ours by right to use (Hayashi, 2002). The implied attitude here would be contrary to the cultural view of many from the East, who do not see a separation between themselves and the environment. In that cultural view, we are an extension of the environment that contains and nurtures us. So, rather than using resources for the purpose of accomplishing tasks so that we can achieve a personal sense of mastery, someone from that cultural perspective would instead see satisfaction as resulting from a respectful symbiotic relationship with the environment where the environment nurtures the individual and the person in return takes care of that environment.

Given the abovementioned cultural limitations of the model, what would make it more inclusive? May be instead of saying that the internal adaptation process is acultural, we could begin from the premise that the process is individual, but the way in which it unfolds is determined by the cultural context of the individual. For example, for a person in the South (Africa and related regions), the notion of relative mastery can be revised to emphasize the sense of social connectivity consistent with the worldview of these more collectivist cultures. From that cultural perspective, relative mastery may be defined as performance with satisfaction of co-occupations that restore the social connectedness that may have been lost due to illness. Intervention programming could be more group rather than individual based, and the more family members and other important people in the client's community are involved in the intervention groups, the better. For someone from a more Eastern cultural perspective, relative mastery may be defined by not only using resources to complete occupations without waste but also doing something to give back (take care of the environment so that it continues to be nurturing). OT programming that focuses on immersion into the environment as much as possible would probably be preferable.

In summary, clearly, the OA theoretical model is a good guide to person-centered, occupation-based intervention. However, it might be challenging to apply across cultures because of the Western-based assumptions of centrality of the individual in therapy and the need to master usage of resources in the environment rather than viewing the person/environment transaction as symbiotic. Making those assumptions explicit may improve the model applicability by giving therapists from multiple cultures permission to modify the definition of key constructs for better application in their unique cultural contexts.

Conclusion

The OA theory presents a way of understanding mechanisms of occupational participation in the context of the person–environment relationship. The theory provides guidance for OT assessment and intervention. As an internal human process, with concepts grounded and supported by theoretical underpinnings in the history of OT, it is important to understand the factors and mechanisms that may facilitate or disrupt this normative process. As an intervention model, the OA theory is not a manner of doing OT but rather a way of thinking about understanding specific actions and steps that the occupational therapist can take to support the client. The OA theory can be used with other frames of reference or specific intervention approaches (e.g., cognitive models, motor learning theories, sensory processing approaches, specific rehabilitation techniques, cognitive-behavioral approaches) to provide a holistic approach to intervention.

Lippincott® Connect *For additional resources on the subjects discussed in this chapter, visit Lippincott Connect.*

REFERENCES

Adami, A. M., & Evetts, C. (2012). A natural approach in mental health practice: Occupational adaptation revealed. *Occupational Therapy in Mental Health, 28*, 170–179. https://doi.org/10.1080/0164212X.2012.679589

Aldrich, R., & Heatwole-Shank, K. (2018). An occupational science perspective on occupation, adaptation, and participation. In L. C. Grajo & A. K. Boisselle (Eds.), *Adaptation through occupation: Multidimensional perspectives*. SLACK.

Alonzi-Gold, D., & Grajo, L. C. (2021). The content validity and clinical utility of the Kindergarten Readiness Inventory (K-READI): A screening tool of school readiness for children on the Autism Spectrum. *Journal of Occupational Therapy, Schools, & Early Intervention, 14*(1), 75–89. https://doi.org/10.1080/19411243.2020.1822257

American Occupational Therapy Association. (2017). Philosophical base of occupational therapy. *American Journal of Occupational Therapy, 71*, 7112410045p1. https://doi.org/10.5014/ajot.2017.716S06

American Occupational Therapy Association. (2020). Occupational therapy practice framework: Domain and process (3rd edition). *American Journal of Occupational Therapy, 74*(Suppl 2), 7412410010p1–7412410010p87. https://doi.org/10.5014/ajot.2020.74S2001

Bontje, P., Kinébanian, A., Josephsson, S., & Tamura, Y. (2004). Occupational adaptation: The experiences of older persons with physical disabilities. *American Journal of Occupational Therapy, 58*, 140–149. https://doi.org/10.5014/ajot.58.2.140

Boone, A. E., & George-Paschal, L. A. (2017). Feasibility testing of the occupational adaptation practice guide. *British Journal of Occupational Therapy, 80*(6), 368–374. https://doi.org/10.1177/0308022616688018

Buddenberg, L. A., & Schkade, J. K. (1998). A comparison of occupational therapy intervention approaches for older patients after hip fracture. *Topics in Geriatric Rehabilitation, 13*, 52–68. http://ovidsp.ovid.com/ovidweb.cgi?T=JS&PAGE=reference&D=ovftc&NEWS=N&AN=00013614-199806000-00008.

Cabatan, M. C., Grajo, L. C. & Sana, E. (2020). Occupational adaptation as a lived experience: The case of Filipino occupational therapy

academic educators. *Journal of Occupational Science, 27*(4), 510–524. https://doi.org/10.1080/14427591.2020.1741020

Coetzer, R., Yeats, G., Balchin, R., & Schmidt, K. (2018). I am who I am through who we are: The potential role of ubuntu in neurorehabilitation. *Panamerican Journal of Neuropsychology, 12*(2). https://www.redalyc.org/journal/4396/439655913012/html/

Delgado, R., & Stefancic, J. (2017). *Critical race theory: An introduction*. New York University Press.

Dirette, D. P. (2018). Decolonialism in the profession: Reflections from WFOT. *The Open Journal of Occupational Therapy, 6*(4), Article 1. https://doi.org/10.15453/2168-6408.1565

Dolecheck, J. R., & Schkade, J. K. (1999). Effects on dynamic standing endurance when persons with CVA perform personally meaningful versus non-meaningful tasks. *OTJR: Occupation, Participation and Health, 19*, 40–54. https://doi.org/10.1177/153944929901900103

Dumas, C. M., & Grajo, L. C. (2021). The content validity and inter-rater reliability of the Occupational Therapy Pediatric Inventory of Cognitive Skills (OT-PICS): An assessment tool of functional cognition in children. *Occupational Therapy in Health Care*, 1–17. Advance online publication. https://doi.org/10.1080/07380577.2021.197

Fidler, G. (1981). From crafts to competence. *American Journal of Occupational Therapy, 35*, 567–573. https://doi.org/10.5014/ajot.35.9.567

Fidler, G., & Fidler, J. (1978). Doing and becoming: Purposeful action and self-actualization. *American Journal of Occupational Therapy, 32*, 305–310. https://doi.org/10.5014/ajot.64.1.142

Fine, S. (1991). Resilience and human adaptability: Who rises above adversity? *American Journal of Occupational Therapy, 45*, 493–503. https://doi.org/10.5014/ajot.45.6.493

Florey, L. (1969). Intrinsic motivation: The dynamics of occupational therapy theory. *American Journal of Occupational Therapy, 23*, 319–322.

Freeman, M. (1999). The right to self-determination in international politics: Six theories on search of a policy. *Review of International Studies, 25*, 355–370. https://www.jstor.org/stable/20097605

George, L. A., Schkade, J. K., & Ishee, J. H. (2004). Content validity of the relative mastery measurement scale: A measure of occupational adaptation. *OTJR: Occupation, Participation and Health, 24*(3), 92–102. https://doi.org/10.1177/153944920402400303

George-Paschal, L., & Bowen, M. (2019). Outcomes of a mentoring program based on occupational adaptation for participants in a juvenile drug court program. *Occupational Therapy in Mental Health, 35*(3), 262–286. https://doi.org/10.1080/0164212X.2019.1601605

Gibson, J., & Schkade, J. (1997). Occupational adaptation intervention with patients with cerebrovascular accident: A clinical study. *American Journal of Occupational Therapy, 51*, 523–529. https://doi.org/10.5014/ajot.51.7.523

Grajo, L. (2017). Occupational adaptation. In J. Hinojosa, P. Kramer, & C. Royeen (Eds.), *Perspectives on human occupation: Theories underlying practice* (2nd ed., pp. 287–311). F. A. Davis.

Grajo, L. (2018). Occupational adaptation as a normative and intervention process—New perspectives on Schkade and Schultz's professional legacy. In L. C. Grajo & A. K. Boisselle (Eds.), *Adaptation through occupation: Multidimensional perspectives* (pp. 83-104). SLACK.

Grajo, L. (2019). Theory of occupational adaptation. In B. E. B. Schell & G. Gillen (Eds.), *Willard and Spackman's occupational therapy* (13th ed., pp. 633-642). Lippincott Williams & Wilkins.

Grajo, L., & Candler, C. (2016). An occupation and participation approach to reading intervention (OPARI) part II: Pilot clinical application. *Journal of Occupational Therapy, Schools and Early Intervention, 9*, 86–98. https://doi.org/10.1080/19411243.2016.1141083

Grajo, L., & Gutman, S. (2019). *The inventory of reading occupations–Adult version*. https://www.ot.wustl.edu/about/resources/ot-for-literacy-1687

Grajo, L., Boisselle, A., & DaLomba, E. (2018). Occupational adaptation as a construct: A scoping review of literature. *The Open*

Journal of Occupational Therapy, 6(1), 2. https://doi.org/10.15453/2168-6408.1400

Hayashi, A. (2002). Finding the voice of Japanese wilderness. *International Journal of Wilderness, 8*(2), 34–37. http://weaj.jp/blog/wp/wp-content/uploads/2021/07/Aug-02-IJW-Hayashi.pdf

Honaker, D., Rosello, S. S., & Candler, C. (2012). Test-retest reliability of family L.I.F.E. (Looking into Family Experiences): An occupation-based assessment. *American Journal of Occupational Therapy, 66*(5), 617–620. https://doi.org/10.5014/ajot.2012.004002

Hoogerdijk, B., Runge, U., & Haugboelle, J. (2011). The adaptation process after traumatic brain injury: An individual and ongoing occupational struggle to gain a new identity. *Scandinavian Journal of Occupational Therapy, 18*, 122–132. https://doi.org/10.3109/11038121003645985

Jackson, J., & Schkade, J. (2001). Occupational adaptation model versus biomechanical-rehabilitation model in the treatment of patients with hip fractures. *American Journal of Occupational Therapy, 55*, 531–537. https://doi.org/10.5014/ajot.55.5.531

Johansson, A., Fristedt, S., Boström, M., & Björklund, A. (2018). The use of occupational adaptation in research: A scoping review. *Occupational Therapy in Health Care, 32*(4), 422–439. https://doi.org/10.1080/07380577.2018.1526433

Johnson, J., & Schkade, J. (2001). Effects of an occupation-based intervention on mobility problems following a cerebral vascular accident. *Journal of Applied Gerontology, 20*, 91–110. https://doi.org/10.1177/073346480102000106

Kielhofner, G. (1977). Temporal adaptation: A conceptual framework for occupational therapy. *American Journal of Occupational Therapy, 31*, 235–242.

King, L. J. (1978). 1978 Eleanor Clarke Slagle Lecture: Toward a science of adaptive responses. *American Journal of Occupational Therapy, 32*, 429–437.

Kleinman, B., & Bulkley, B. (1982). Some implications of a science of adaptive responses. *American Journal of Occupational Therapy, 36*, 16–19. https://doi.org/10.5014/ajot.36.1.15

Lexell, E. M., Iwarsson, S., & Lund, M. L. (2011). Occupational adaptation in people with multiple sclerosis. *OTJR: Occupation, Participation and Health, 31*, 127–134. https://doi.org/10.3928/15394492-20101025-01

Llorens, L. (1970). Facilitating growth and development: The promise of occupational therapy. *American Journal of Occupational Therapy, 24*, 93–101.

Lopez, A. (2011). Posttraumatic stress disorder and occupational performance: Building resilience and fostering occupational adaptation. *Work, 38*, 33–38. https://doi.org/10.3233/WOR-2011-1102

Motaharinezhad, F., Mehraban, A., Lajevardi, L., Ghahari, S., & Salimi, Y. (2021). A qualitative exploration of occupational adaptation in caregivers of people with multiple sclerosis. *Occupational Therapy in Health Care, 35*(1) 1–15, https://doi.org/10.1080/07380577.2020.1843103

McKay, M. H., Pickens, N. D., Medley, A., Cooper, D., & Evetts, C. L. (2021). Comparing occupational adaptation-based and traditional training programs for dementia care teams: An embedded mixed-methods study. *The Gerontologist, 61*(4), 582–594. https://doi.org/10.1093/geront/gnaa160

Meyer, A. (1977). The philosophy of occupation therapy. *American Journal of Occupational Therapy, 31*, 639–642. (Original work published 1922)

Moyers, P. A., & Coleman, S. D. (2004). Adaptation of the older workers to occupational challenges. *Work, 22*, 71–78.

Nayar, S., & Stanley, M. (2015). Occupational adaptation as a social process in everyday life. *Journal of Occupational Science, 22*, 26–38. https://doi.org/10.1080/14427591.2014.882251

Nelson, D. (1988). Occupation: Form and performance. *American Journal of Occupational Therapy, 42*, 633–641. https://doi.org/10.5014/ajot.42.10.633

Orr, C., & Schkade, J. (1997). The impact of classroom environment on defining function in school-based practice. *American Journal of Occupational Therapy, 51*, 64–69. https://doi.org/10.5014/ajot.51.1.64

Parsons, L., & Stanley, M. (2008). The lived experiences of occupational adaptation following acquired brain injury for people living in a rural area. *Australian Occupational Therapy Journal, 55*, 231–238. https://doi.org/10.1111/j.1440-1630.2008.00753.x

Pasek, P. B., & Schkade, J. K. (1996). Effects of a skiing experience on adolescents with limb deficiencies: An occupational adaptation perspective. *American Journal of Occupational Therapy, 50*, 24–31. https://doi.org/10.5014/ajot.50.1.24

Reilly, M. (1962). Occupational therapy can be one of the greatest ideas of 20th century medicine (1961 Slagle Lecture). *American Journal of Occupational Therapy, 16*, 1–9. https://doi.org/10.1177/000841746303000102

Schkade, J. K., & McClung, M. (2001). *Occupational adaptation in practice: Concepts and cases.* SLACK.

Schkade, J. K., & Schultz, S. (1992). Occupational adaptation: Toward a holistic approach for contemporary practice, part 1. *American Journal of Occupational Therapy, 43*, 829–837. https://doi.org/10.5014/ajot.46.9.829

Schkade, J. K., & Schultz, S. (2003). Occupational adaptation. In P. Kramer, J. Hinojosa, & C. B. Royeen (Eds.), *Perspectives in human occupation: Participation in life* (pp. 181–221). Lippincott Williams & Wilkins.

Schultz, S. (2014). Theory of occupational adaptation. In B. A. B. Schell, G. Gillen, & M. E. Scaffa (Eds.), *Willard & Spackman's occupational therapy* (12th ed., pp. 527–540). Lippincott Williams & Wilkins.

Schultz, S., & Schkade, J. K. (1992). Occupational adaptation: Toward a holistic approach for contemporary practice, part 2. *American Journal of Occupational Therapy, 46*, 917–925. https://doi.org/10.5014/ajot.46.10.917

Schultz, S., & Schkade, J. K. (1997). Adaptation. In C. Christiansen & C. Baum (Eds.), *Occupational therapy: Enabling function and wellbeing* (2nd ed., pp. 458–481). SLACK.

Spencer, J., Hersch, G., Eschenfelder, V., Fournet, J., & Murray-Gerzik, M. (1999). Outcomes of protocol-based and adaptation-based occupational therapy interventions for low-income elders on a transitional unit. *American Journal of Occupational Therapy, 53*, 159–170. https://doi.org/10.5014/ajot.53.2.159

Stelter, L., & Whisner, S. (2007). Building responsibility for self through meaningful roles: Occupational adaptation theory applied in forensic psychiatry. *Occupational Therapy in Mental Health, 23*, 69–84. https://doi.org/10.1300/J004v23n01_05

Whisner, S. M., Stelter, L. D., & Schultz, S. (2014). Influence of three interventions on group participation in an acute psychiatric facility. *Occupational Therapy in Mental Health, 30*, 26–42. https://doi.org/10.1080/0164212X.2014.878527

White, R. (1959). Motivation reconsidered: The concept of competence. *Psychological Review, 66*, 297–333. https://doi.org/10.1037/h0040934

Williams, S., & Murray, C. (2013). The lived experiences of older adults' occupational adaptation following a stroke. *Australian Occupational Therapy Journal, 60*, 39–47. https://doi.org/10.1111/1440-1630.12004

Yerxa, E. (1967). Authentic occupational therapy (1966 Slagle Lecture). *American Journal of Occupational Therapy, 21*, 1–9.

The Kawa (River) Model

Michael K. Iwama and Asako Matsubara

LEARNING OBJECTIVES

After reading this chapter, you will be able to:

1. Describe the cultural nature of theory in occupational therapy.
2. Name the main components of a river and explain their symbolic meaning in the Kawa model.
3. Briefly explain two reasons why the Kawa model was developed.
4. Identify at least three ways the Kawa model addresses issues of diversity, equity, and inclusion.
5. Apply the Kawa model to your own life.
6. Explain how occupational therapists can use the Kawa model in practice.

Introduction

Occupational therapy (OT) conceptual models are created by people; therefore, the models are cultural artifacts. Many of our theoretical materials carry the forms and structure, language, behavioral norms, expectations, and explanations of occupation as constructed and discussed by occupational therapists in the English-speaking regions of the world. As cultural artifacts, these models contain common assumptions about the group's social norms, beliefs, values, and ideals. Autonomy, ability, individual agency, and an ontology that regards the environment as a separate entity to the self are a few examples of cultural assumptions that are tacitly understood and often taken for granted when examining and considering OT theory. Imbued with these culturally approved qualities, models can serve as useful, powerful guides, and explanations of contemporary OT among those who share similar spheres of experience with the models and their authors.

Models, however, can be used unwittingly as agents of confusion, and even oppression when they are applied to people who abide in different cultural contexts and have different spheres of shared experience from the model's origins. For example, when individualist expectations guided by models that favor independence and autonomy in daily living tasks are applied to people who abide in a collectivist and interdependent social ethic,

OT can become confusing and even harmful to clients[1] and the community to which they belong. When culturally narrowed, OT can become comparatively undiversified, inequitable, and exclusive.

In this chapter, the authors introduce and explain the Kawa (Japanese for "river") model of OT (Iwama, 2006). This relatively new model represents a number of historical firsts in our profession. The Kawa model is the first substantial theoretical work in OT to originate outside of the English-speaking world. And it is the first major conceptual model to be raised from practice, through qualitative research methods, by practitioners, for practitioners.

Diversity, Equity, and Inclusion: The Basis for the Kawa Model

In this postmodern age of information (Castells, 1997), matters of social justice, equity, diversity, and inclusion continue to emerge as important considerations for health and well-being in society. OT theory and models, and the practices they explain and inform are cultural products that can carry significant influence on matters of equity and inclusion for our diverse clientele. Concerns on matters of diversity, equity, and inclusion in OT models can include the following:

- Cultural norms and imperatives imbedded in OT models and their implications
- Sociocultural construction of the model's concepts and their meanings
- Matters of privilege and power conveyed implicitly or explicitly by the model's structure and application
- Status of the client and of their narrative (of daily life experiences)

Conceptual Models as Cultural Artifacts

OT models implicitly convey the underlying norms of the social and cultural contexts in which they were formed. These norms are largely invisible to those who abide in or share similar experiences with the status quo of a particular location and time. A significant challenge facing the profession of OT in this current era is mitigating the exclusionary and inequitable features of our practices and the theories that guide

and explain them. North American OT models may reflect the worldviews and lifestyle expectations of North American, middle-class, affluent, and individual-centric lifestyles, in which people, as a matter of right, choose and engage in activities that enhance their personal health and well-being. Such OT models also carry within their concepts, structure, and application the culture of the profession of contemporary OT. Although these priorities resonate well and appear reasonable and achievable to many, the same should not be assumed for clients who are situated outside of these familiar North American cultural norms. Gaps can appear between the current culture of OT and the cultures of diverse clients.

The cultural myopia that can occur when applying models universally across cultural boundaries of meaning are mitigated when the client's narrative of their daily life experience becomes the central "model" of interest for everyone concerned about the client. This shift in power from the professional over to the client can be enabled and mediated through the application of client-centric frameworks such as the Kawa model. Rather than leading all clients to fit a single, universal model, each client's unique daily life narrative becomes the model around which OT revolves.

The Sociocultural Construction of Occupational Therapy Models, Concepts, and Their Meanings

OT clients located outside of Western, English-speaking nations where the concept of *occupation* as occupational therapists have constructed it originated, often lack a word in their language (and experience) to accurately comprehend and apply the concept of occupation. *Sagyou* is the Japanese term officially assigned to stand for *occupation*. Sagyou represents a kind of work activity that is particularly difficult, often repetitive, and unpleasant to perform. And it has remained in place, unchanged for over 60 years since OT was imported into Japan in the last century. For the Japanese, who have been described as a collectivist or group-oriented society, where interdependence and dependence are normal social behavior patterns, the existing language of OT models that are anchored to individual-centric, agentic, ableist (Campbell & Kumari, 2009) ideals of the Western world is exclusive and difficult to comprehend. The more specialized concepts/constructs that a particular model employs, the more sophisticated the principles are that bind them and the narrower and more exclusive the applicability can become. The implicit value in these models that emphasizes the experiences of individualism, agency, self-determinism, and occupation potentially create challenges and difficulties for clients and occupational therapists situated outside of the Western social landscapes. These challenges are in terms of the value and relation to relevant culture (Iwama, 2003).

The Kawa model addresses this issue by viewing the client as the "theorist (of their own model/narrative)." Rather

---

[1] According to the American Occupational Therapy Association (AOTA, 2020, p. S75), the term *client* refers to *persons* (including those involved in care of a client), *groups* (a collection of individuals having shared characteristics or common or shared purpose, e.g., family members, workers, students, and those with similar interests or occupational challenges), and *populations* (aggregates of people with common attributes such as contexts, characteristics or concerns, including health risks. However, in countries other than the US, the term *client* often refers to persons who are paying for their care directly. In most countries, *patient* is used to describe persons who are in hospital or rehabilitation. *Service user* and *person* are terms in general use that describe those in need of OT services. For this chapter, we are using *client* without implying the source of payment for services.

than trying to force the client's unique narrative and concepts of daily living through the universal language and concepts constructed onto someone else's cultural reality, the client exercises power over their own story to construct the concepts and explain the relations (principles) that connect those concepts together. The Kawa model offers a solution to these fundamental issues of diversity, equity, and inclusion by making the client's narrative the primary theory that guides the OT process that follows.

Privilege and Power Reflected in a Model's Structure and Application

Applying theoretical materials and protocols universally and uncritically across cultural boundaries of meaning can mirror a familiar pattern of privilege and power that was deemed to be normal and common practice in past colonial times. A familiar practice of employing a single (grand) narrative or model to oversee, filter, and interpret the client's (unique) narrative of their priorities and experiences of everyday life can solidify a power status and dynamic that sets the relationship and decision-making behaviors between the health professional and the client. In such cases, the client can be vulnerable to becoming a passive recipient of OT intervention, with less involvement and responsibility in setting priorities and goals for their treatment. However, each person's life journey is unique and is informed by the culture in which they live. The Kawa model puts the client's unique narrative of their daily living realities in their own culture at the center of the client's and occupational therapist's concerns.

Situating the Client and Their Narrative of Day-to-Day Life

Often the client's narrative gets filtered through or brought into alignment with the concepts and language of a given model or theoretical framework. In some cases, a client may not recognize their own narrative after it has been filtered and processed through a given universal model or framework and its specialized concepts and principles. This inequitable practice, as benign as it may appear on the surface, can subordinate the client to the therapist and render their narrative secondary to the ideals and norms privileged in the theoretical framework or model. Instead of *doing* OT *with* the client through a partnering dynamic, this practice of subordinating the client and their narrative to the grand narrative of a given model can reduce OT to be something we *do to* the client, unwittingly.

If occupational therapists value the principles of equity—that each client is unique and therefore has different circumstances and needs—then a critical review and adjustment of such practices is imperative. If occupational therapists want to maintain their focus on client-centered practice, then they must find ways to elevate and understand

the client's unique narrative and make that narrative central to OT, forming the rationale for the OT process that follows.

Overview of the Kawa Model

The Kawa model was developed by a Canadian occupational therapist (of Japanese heritage), and a group of Japanese OT practitioners and students. They sought to create a culturally safe (Ramsden, 2000) and relevant model of practice that was easily understood and used by occupational therapists and their diverse clientele. Although the model was raised from Japanese social contexts, the metaphor that the model is based on—a river to explain each person's life journey—can be related to and utilized by many clients and occupational therapists situated in varying cultural contexts around the world.

The original Kawa model from 2006 comprises four basic constructs that interact to form a river (Iwama, 2006):

- Water (life force, occupation)
- River Walls including the sides and floor (immediate and ambient environment)
- Rocks (difficulties, problems, and challenges)
- Driftwood (personal factors)

Each of these elements interplays to determine the volume and flow rate of the river from moment to moment at any point along its journey. Applying this metaphor to the client's life journey, the client and their occupational therapist search between the hard structures of the river (rocks, river walls, driftwood) for channels of water (strengths) that are flowing well or have the potential for better flow. The client is the expert of their experience and view of daily life. The occupational therapist is an expert in encouraging greater flow in their client's lives and partnering with them to move toward their potential. In this 2023 update, we have included two additional constructs, spaces and ambient environment, which will be described later in the chapter.

The Kawa model places the client and their unique daily life narrative as the central focus of interest and concern. By elevating and centralizing the client and their unique experience, told by the client in their own words and on their terms, the OT process can become truly client centered.

With the Kawa model, the client metaphorically becomes a *theorist* who builds a model to explain their daily life realities and experiences. The client names the concepts and explains the principles that connect their concepts in a manner that makes sense to them. The occupational therapist becomes a *student* of the *theorist's* (client's) model, asking questions and engaging in a dialogue to enable an accurate understanding of the client's model. The occupational therapist then thoughtfully considers what OT has to offer (to restore and/or enhance life flow) before partnering with the client to set the objectives for meaningful intervention, support, and mobilization of resources.

The model was originally cast as a *culturally relevant* work, primarily intended to support equitable OT practice in Japan (Iwama, 2006). Since the model has been used and taught in many languages and cultural spaces, the original Japanese concepts have been adapted by occupational therapists and clients to their respective languages and diverse cultural contexts. The Kawa model has been published in seven languages (with Arabic [Iwama & Baksh, in press] being the most recent production), is taught in more than 700 OT and health professional educational programs around the world, and it is used in practice across six continents.

Development of the Kawa Model

Faced with the challenges of comprehending and applying OT models across cultural boundaries of meaning, as described in the previous section, a group of Japanese occupational therapists and clients led by Dr. Iwama embarked on a mission to develop a new, *culturally neutral* (Lape et al., 2019) conceptual model of OT practice. Through a process of (modified) qualitative research, the team was organized into focus groups to explore and gather their cultural experiences and views toward matters of OT, health, and what constitutes well-being in everyday life for Japanese citizens (Iwama, 2006). A number of guiding questions were established to direct group discussions around how OT in Japan was culturally situated and informed. Focus groups were asked to share their culturally situated views concerning what they felt was essential to their lives, including their explanations of wellness and their definitions and understanding of illness, health, and disability. They were prompted to articulate and discuss what they and their clients lived for, and what they felt was essential to life, fulfillment, and to the *collectivist* Japanese ethos of "belonging" (Lebra, 1976). Through this process, the participants were encouraged to redefine *occupation* from their own (East Asian) cultural perspectives and realign the purposes of OT to matters that Japanese people deemed to be of essential importance to their lives and world.

For a detailed explanation of the qualitative research that was conducted in producing the Kawa model, please see Chapter 6 of Iwama, M. (2006). *The Kawa Model: Culturally relevant occupational therapy* (260 pp.). Elsevier/Churchill Livingstone.

At an early stage of the research, it became apparent that there were fundamental differences in how *self* and *environment* were imagined and represented in established (Western) models compared to the actual lived experiences of the research group participants. For a model to effectively explain *self* and *environment*, the central placement of a distinctly defined self that was adjacent to but separate from the environment, which is commonly seen in conventional (Western) models, was nonexistent. Further deliberation by the group revealed comprehensions of *self* and *environment* (or context) that were more diffuse and inseparably integrated by the Japanese than by their Western counterparts. For the Japanese research participants, their concept of *self*, *environment*, *well-being*, and *disability* could not be explained by linear diagrams or by boxes or categories set in a logical sequence.

The group's first attempt at illustrating their view of these concepts is shown in Figure 37.1. Captured in this early diagram was the interconnectedness of all elements and phenomena in the frame of life experience. It shows

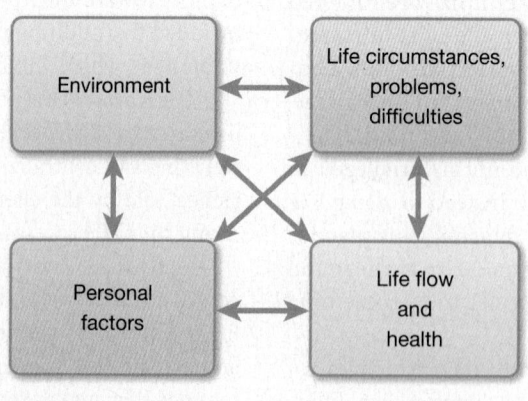

FIGURE 37.1 Early conceptualization of the Kawa model before the river metaphor was applied.

that states of well-being and disability are neither entirely located internally (in the body) nor externally (in the environment). Here, the self and environment are inextricably connected in a manner in which a change in one or more components would effect a change in the greater whole.

In order to capture and better represent a conceptualization of a diffuse self that is amorphous, interdependent with, and inseparable from other elements in the environment, the initial box and arrow diagram was put aside for an alternate framework (Figure 37.2). The research participants decided to employ a metaphor of nature (a river or *kawa* in Japanese) to better explain the dynamic intercourse and fluid nature of the model. The use of such a metaphor contrasted dramatically with the familiar mechanical and systems metaphors frequently employed in the construction of conventional, modern, and conceptual models.

Some Philosophical Insights Into the Kawa Model

How we construct the world and situate the self in relation to it has fundamental implications for how we make sense of *occupation*. If individuals are viewed as one part of an all-encompassing universe, the decentralized selves will tend to regard and value people's actions and doings in a broader context of an integrated and diffuse universe. The value and appropriateness of people's actions and doings tend to be determined by their meanings and implications for the collective/community that they belong to. Rather than interpreting the value and meaning of an occupation through the ethos of individual agency and self-satisfaction, the value and meaning of the same occupations are appreciated through the collective/community ethos of *belonging* (Lebra, 1976). Issues of health and well-being are appreciated

and located in the broader context of an integrated, diffuse universe. OT intervention shaped by this alternative worldview extends beyond treating the individual to include issues and factors situated equally in the environment.

By centralizing and focusing on the client's narrative of their daily living realities as seen, felt, and interpreted through their perspective and lived experience, the Kawa model neutralizes any bias that individualist or collectivist worldviews (ontologies) might exert upon the attending occupational therapist's comprehension of the client's occupational state. After all, it is the client's biases that will be affirmed in their narrative, translated through the river metaphor.

The underlying ontology of the Kawa framework is *harmony*—a state of individual or collective being in which the client, either an individual or the community, is in balance with the surrounding context and circumstances. In the Kawa model, the essence of such harmony is conceptualized as flowing water, which stands for "life energy" or "life flow." Western occupational therapists often equate the water channels in the *kawa* as *occupations*. The purpose of OT, then, is to help clients enhance and balance their life flow by enabling and supporting their occupations.

Core Concepts of the Kawa Model

Life can be understood as a complex, profound journey that flows through time and space, like a river (Figure 37.3). An optimal state of well-being in one's life (or river) can be metaphorically portrayed by an image of deep, powerful, and unimpeded flow. Aspects of the environment and circumstances, like certain hard structures and the spaces around them found in a river, can influence and affect the quality

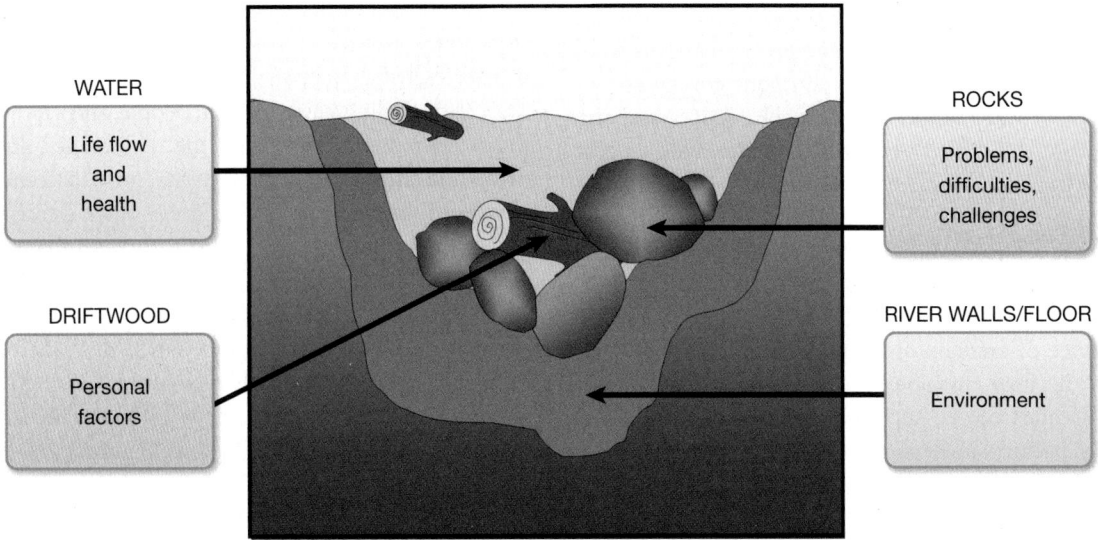

FIGURE 37.2 **Cross-section of a river: The four original concepts of the Kawa model.**

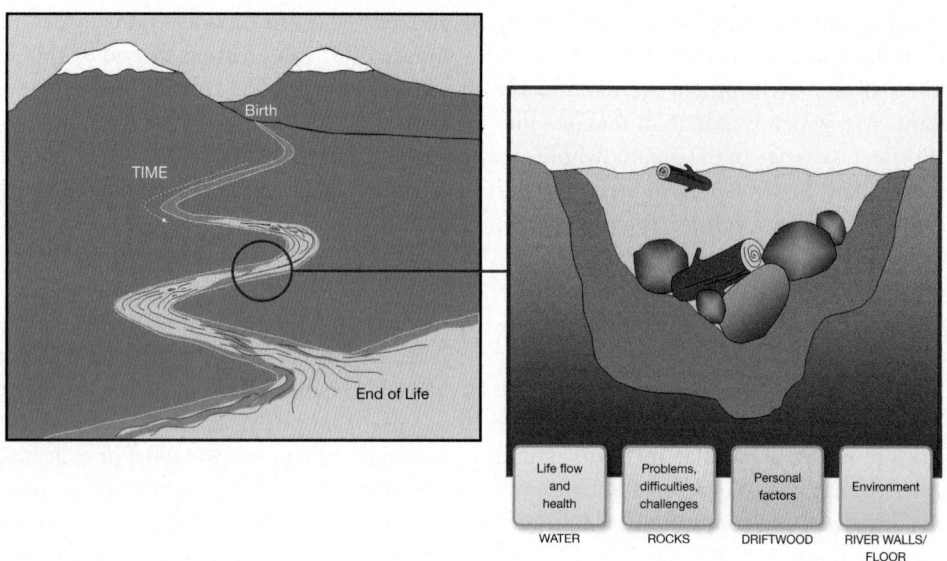

FIGURE 37.3 **Life is like a river, beginning up in the hills and flowing and meandering over varied terrains until it enters the sea.**

and characteristics of that flow. Rocks (life circumstances), river walls (environment), driftwood (personal factors) and the spaces between them are all inseparable parts of a river that determine its boundaries, shape, flow rate, and overall quality (Figure 37.8). OT's purpose, then, is to enable and enhance life flow by enhancing harmony between all elements that form the overall context.

The basic framework of the Kawa model now comprises six fundamental concepts. Through the course of the OT process, the client may choose to modify these concepts, as well as add their own, to personalize and increase the value of their narrative. These concepts are merely symbolic structures that the client can use to reveal, organize, and communicate their narrative of daily living experiences. If a cross-sectional view of a river was taken and examined at any point along its journey, the frame would reveal the original four components of the model (water, river wall, rocks, and driftwood) arranged in a unique configuration. The two new components of the model—spaces and the distal environment—have been added to illuminate aspects of the river that were tacitly regarded to be important facets of the river metaphor. By naming the spaces, opportunities, strengths, occupations, and "good points" of the client could be acknowledged and validated. Further, the addition of a deeper layer of the river walls acknowledges the presence and influence of ambient environmental factors that contribute to the flow character of the river. Socioeconomic status and catastrophes, such as wars and diaspora, and pandemics, political and religious conditions, are some examples of distal environmental factors that can exert influence on the river's flow. The interrelations and interactions of these components determine the rate and quality of the water flow at each particular spot and instance in the river.

水 Mizu (*Water*): Life Energy, Life Flow, and Occupation

Water is perhaps the most important component in the Kawa model. Water metaphorically represents a person's or collective's *life energy* or *life flow* (Figure 37.4). Without the presence of water, a river ceases to be. And water is the only element that touches, interacts with, and connects all of the other elements of the river. Some OT practitioners in North America, the United Kingdom, and Australia have anecdotally reported their practice of relating water in the model with the construct of *occupation*—as Western occupational therapists socially construct (Berger & Luckmann, 1966) and define it. Fluid, pure, spiritual, filling, cleansing, and renewing are only some of the characteristics and functions commonly associated with this object and phenomenon of nature. Just as people's lives are shaped and bounded by their surrounding environment, people, and circumstances, the river's water flow touches the rocks, sides, and debris/driftwood and all other elements that form its context. Water envelopes, defines, and effects these other elements of the river in a similar way to which the same elements effect the water's volume, shape, and flow rate.

When life energy or the water flow weakens, the client, whether individual or collective, can be described as unwell or in a state of disharmony. When it stops flowing altogether, as when the river dries up or flows into a vast ocean, the *end of life* is symbolically arrived at (see Figure 37.3).

Just as water is fluid, malleable, and adopts the shape of its container, indigenous and collective-oriented people often regard their social and physical environs as a primary shaper of the individual self. For those who share a

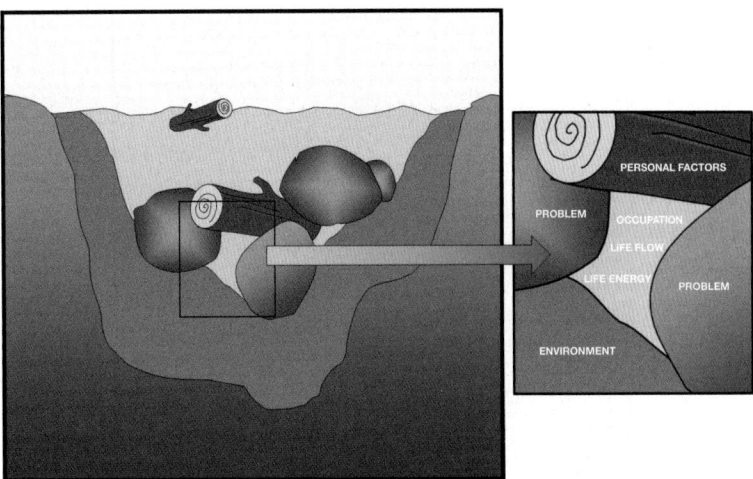

FIGURE 37.4 *Water:* Each channel of flow within the river represents occupation, life flow, and the potential for better flow. Each channel is bounded by other river components (water, rocks, driftwood, walls/floor). Changes to any or all components change the channel as well as the river. The occupational therapist views each component as potential focal points for OT intervention.

worldview that regards the self as being inseparably connected and embedded with the surrounding social, physical, and spiritual environment, the interdependent self is deeply influenced and even determined by the surrounding social context, at a given time and place, in a similar way to which water in a river, at any given point along its path, will vary in form, flow direction, rate, volume, and clarity.

Within the Kawa model, a person's state of well-being coincides with life flow. Just as there are constellations of interrelated factors/structures in a river that affect its flow, a rich combination of internal and external circumstances and structures in a client's life context can determine their life flow. OT's overall purpose in this context is to enhance life flow, regardless of whether it is interpreted at the level of the individual, institution, organization, community, or society.

川底 Kawa Zoko (*River Walls*): Proximal/Immediate Environment and Distal/Ambient Environment

In the Kawa model, the river's sides and floor (commonly referred to as "River Walls") represent the client's environment. These are perhaps the most important determinants of a person's life flow in a collectivist social context because of the primacy accorded to the environmental context in determining the construction of self, experience of being and subsequent meanings of personal action (Lebra, 1976). In the Kawa model, the river walls represent the person's *immediate* and *ambient* environments. These are shown as two layers that comprise the river's sides and floor (see

Figure 37.5); the proximal layer referring to the immediate environment, and the deeper, distal layer referring to the ambient environment. In the original Kawa model, the proximal and distal river walls were treated as a singular construct. In an attempt to clarify and better organize the complex environmental factors affecting life flow, the then singular concept of the river walls was reconceptualized into two categories: the proximal/immediate environment and the distal/ambient environment.

Proximal/Immediate Environment

The proximal/immediate environment corresponds symbolically to the person's social and physical contexts. This is the environmental layer that is immediate to and touching the other elements of the river. The social contexts of the river walls represent mainly those who share a direct social relationship with the subject. In the Kawa model, the social environment is not limited to other human beings. The river walls can represent other important social elements of a person's life, such as pets (e.g., cats, hedgehogs, dogs) and people who are deceased. Because the model is a framework used to bring the client's narrative forward, the client determines who comprises their rivers walls in their "Kawa."

Depending upon which social frame is perceived as being most important in a given instance and place, the river walls and bottom can represent family members, workmates, friends in a recreational club, classmates, and so on. In certain non-Western societies like those of Japan, social relationships are regarded to be the central determinant of individual and collective life flow (Lebra, 1976). The physical context refers to the physical environment surrounding the person. This can include the home, workplace, and built

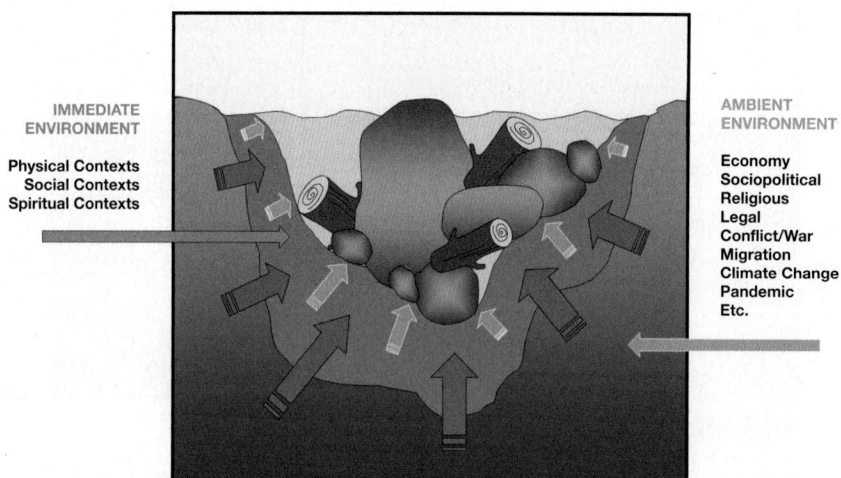

FIGURE 37.5 **River walls:** Two layers of river walls and floor represent the immediate (proximal) and ambient (distal) environment.

and natural environments. A foreboding set of stairs in the home or workplace, the lack of a ramp as an intermediate between road pavement and sidewalk, or even a heavy door separating where one is presently situated and where one would like to go qualify as the *immediate* physical environment of the river's walls.

Aspects of the surrounding social and physical frame on the subject can affect the overall flow (volume and rate) of the Kawa. Harmonious social relationships can enable and complement life flow. Increased flow can have an agentic effect upon difficult circumstances and problems as the force of water displaces rocks in the channel and even create new conduits to flow through. Conversely, a decrease in flow volume can exert a compounding, negative effect on the other elements that take up space in the channel (Figure 37.3). If there are obstructions (rocks and driftwood) in the watercourse when the river walls are thick and constricting, the flow of the river can become increasingly compromised. As can be readily imagined, the rocks in this river can directly butt up against the river walls and bottom, compounding and creating larger impediments to the river's usual flow.

Distal/Ambient Environment: A New Development of the Kawa Model

The second, deeper (distal to the river's water) layer that symbolizes the ambient environment is a recent reconceptualization of the river walls. The original concept that translated the client's physical and social environmental factors was reorganized into two categories to better organize and clarify the multiple, complex elements that comprise the river walls. This deeper layer represents the "macro" factors that may not be as close to the person as the elements of the immediate environment. Yet these distal factors and conditions impose upon and influence the overall flow of the river. Ambient environmental elements can

be, but are not limited to, cultural, moral, and philosophical norms (such as the Confucian Ethic, faith practices and expectations, cultural behavioral norms and expectations, and caste systems); static or fluid geopolitical conditions (such as democracies, dictatorships, socialist government systems, political invasion, and occupation); macroeconomic conditions (such as recession and stock market fluctuations); social oppression (such as racism, homophobia, ageism, and ableism); natural catastrophes and changes (such as earthquakes, tsunamis, floods, and climate change); human-made catastrophe (such as climate change, global pandemic, war, and diaspora); and any such macrophenomena that exert an indirect force on the flow of a person's/community's life.

Problems and issues concerning the environment are shown in the Kawa metaphor as thickening of the river walls. When the walls thicken, the volume of water in the river becomes constrained. The thickening walls encroach upon the normal channels of flow, and the relative impact of the other structures in the river channel, such as rocks and driftwood, will typically increase. Conversely, changes and improvements to the social and physical environment can have the effect of increasing the volume of flow in a person's river. As the walls recede, the river's capacity for better and stronger flow is enabled.

岩 Iwa (*Rocks*): Difficulties, Problems, and Challenges

Rocks of different size and numbers represent discrete circumstances that can impede one's *life flow*. They are life circumstances and factors perceived by the client to be problematic and difficult to remove. Every rock, like a life circumstance, has a unique quality, varying in size, density, shape, color, and texture (Figure 37.6). Most rivers, like people's lives, have such rocks or other debris that can impede flow. Large rocks, by themselves or in combination with other rocks, jammed directly or indirectly against other hard objects of the river, such as the river walls and sides (environment), or driftwood (personal factors), can effectively impede and alter the river's flow and course. A client's current rocks may have been there since childhood or some earlier time, such as with congenital conditions. They may appear instantaneously, as in sudden illness or embodied injury, and even by catastrophes generated or originated outside of the body, in the environment.

In the context of a flowing river, rocks do not exist solitarily or in isolation. Each rock is touched by water (life flow, occupation), river walls (social and physical environment), and whatever driftwood are drawn to it by the water current. Also, rocks (life circumstances, problems, and challenges) can appear alongside other rocks.

Once the client's perceived rocks are known (including their relative size and situation), the therapist can help to identify potential areas of intervention and strategies to enable better life flow. The broader contextual definition of disabling circumstances necessarily brings into play the client's surrounding environment. Though often limited by narrower, medically oriented and defined interventions in hospital institutions, OT intervention should include treatment strategies that expand beyond the client to include their social network and policies or social structures of the surrounding institution or society that ultimately plays a part in creating and setting the disabling context.

The concepts and the contextual application of the Kawa model are by natural design flexible and adaptable. Each client's unique river takes its important concepts and configuration from the situation of the client in a given time

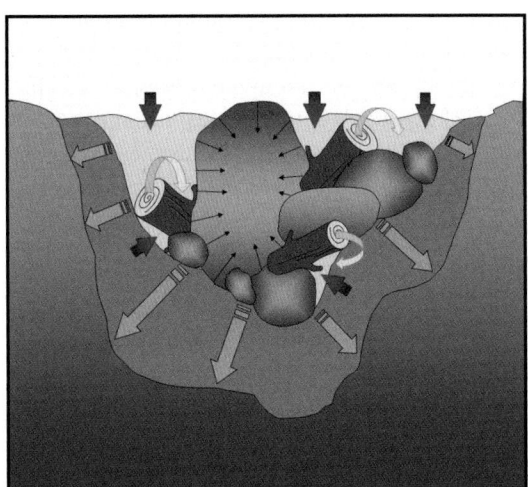

FIGURE 37.6 *Rocks, driftwood, and spaces:* **Rocks constitute problems, challenges, and difficulties in the flow of life's journey. Driftwood represents the person's embodied attributes and resources. The blue arrows indicate the construct of spaces.**

and place. The definition of problems and circumstances is broad—as broad and diverse as the clients' worlds of meanings. In turn, this conceptualization of people and their circumstances foreshadow the broad outlook and scope of OT interventions in particular cultural contexts.

The client, be it an individual or a collective, identifies specific rocks, their number, magnitude, quality, and situation in the river. As with all other elements of the model, if the client is unable to express their own river, family members, or a community of people connected with the issues may lend assistance and perspective. A common occurrence when examining the client's river is to see that rocks do not always appear in isolation. When a rock appears in the client's river, other rocks of varying sizes and shapes seem to spontaneously catch and accumulate driftwood, debris, and whatever the river sends down to this current section.

Rocks constitute problems, challenges, and difficulties in the flow of life's journey. The adaptive aim here is to decrease the number of rocks, decrease their size, and look for ways in which the water can find a way around and past these obstructions to *life flow*.

流木 Ryuboku (*Driftwood*): Personal Factors

Driftwood in a river can be observed to have varying effects upon its flow. Driftwood in some sections of a river can take on a neutral status when seen to be floating along with the current, suspended in the water flow and not touching or affecting the other components of the river. Driftwood can take on a negative value when it becomes caught between the hard surfaces of other structures, such as rocks of varying sizes and shapes, the river walls, and other driftwood (see Figure 37.6). The same driftwood can be mobilized to collide with, move, erode the surfaces of, and even destroy obstructions that appear in the river.

In the context of the Kawa model, driftwood represents the person's embodied attributes and resources (personal factors) that can positively or negatively affect the client's circumstances and life flow. Driftwood can metaphorically represent values (such as honesty and thrift), character (optimism, stubbornness), personality (reserved, outgoing), knowledge and experience (advanced school diploma, military service), special skill (carpentry, public speaking, drawing, playing a musical instrument), and special relationships (family, friends, pets). Driftwood can also include material assets (wealth, special equipment).

Like driftwood in a river, these factors are transient in nature and can carry a certain quality of fate/karma or coincidence/serendipity. Driftwood can appear to be inconsequential in some instances and significantly obstructive in others, particularly when it settles in among rocks and the river walls, compounding the impediment to the river's flow.

On the other hand, they can collide with the same structures, nudge obstructions out of the way, and even erode the surfaces of river walls and rocks to expand or create new channels of flow. For example, a client's religious faith and sense of divine-inspired confidence can be positive factors in persevering to erode or move rocks out of the way.

A person who self-identifies as being determined and headstrong may feel frustrated by their sudden inability to participate in prioritized occupations. This may be metaphorically shown by a piece of driftwood getting caught between some rocks, compounding the impediment to flow. If the tendency toward being determined and headstrong can be redirected and focused on a particular occupation or therapeutic activity, the same piece of driftwood can be mobilized to act adaptively on the surrounding structures and effect larger and new channels of flow.

In another example, receiving a monetary gift or donation to acquire specialized assistive equipment can be a piece of (favorable, positive) driftwood that collides against existing flow impediments and opens a greater channel for one's life to flow more strongly. In another instance, a vocational counselor may be commissioned to assist in pushing away a large rock of unemployment.

Driftwood is a part of everyone's river and often comprises the intangible components carried within each unique person or community that can determine their life flow. Astute therapists pay particular attention to these components of a client's or community's assets and circumstances and consider their real or potential effect on the client's life flow.

罅 Sukima (*Spaces*): The Magnificent Promise of Occupational Therapy

In the Kawa model, spaces are the channels along and through which the client's life flows (see the blue arrows in Figure 37.6). These channels of life flow are considered strengths—positive and adaptive opportunities that are bounded by structures and objects that have appeared in the client's life flow. As the client's life flow narrative becomes clearer, attention shifts to the spaces between the rocks, snagged driftwood, and river walls and bottom. These spaces are the existing channels through which the client's life is flowing. Regardless of the channel's size, they carry possibilities and potential for greater, stronger flows ahead, downriver. They can inspire hope in the client for better days ahead.

For some occupational therapists, these channels of flow are synonymous with *occupation* and *occupational priorities*. By understanding what makes up the borders of a channel (rocks, driftwood, walls), the client can, in collaboration with the occupational therapist, assemble a meaningful, comprehensive, intervention plan directly relevant and tailored to their situation. Rather than focusing primarily on the client's narrowly defined embodied pathology, the Kawa and its components can serve as a guide to a more comprehensive, holistic view of the client that naturally takes their environments and occupations into deeper, interrelated consideration. The weight of importance placed upon these spaces through which the client's life evidently flows qualifies the Kawa model as *strengths based*.

Water (life energy and flow) naturally coursing through these spaces can work to erode the rocks and river walls and bottom that define its boundaries, transforming them into larger conduits for life flow. This effect reflects the latent healing potential that each client naturally holds within their self and context. Thus, OT in this perspective retains its hallmark of purposeful activity and working with the client's abilities and resources. It also directs OT intervention toward all elements that comprise the context that surrounds and supports the client's occupations.

Life circumstances rarely occur in isolation. By changing one aspect of the client's world, all other aspects of their river changes. The Kawa model compels the occupational therapist to view and treat issues within a holistic framework, seeking to appreciate the clients' identified issues within their integrated, inseparable contexts of daily life. Occupations are therefore regarded in wholes, including the meaning of the activity to self and to the community to which the individual inseparably belongs.

和 Wa (*Harmony*): The Essence of Inclusive Human Occupation

The aim and end point of the Kawa model is *harmony:* a state of balance between self, circumstances, and all elements of nature. The force and determination of the river is to find reservoirs of deep, unimpeded flow. Some OT conceptual frameworks and models frame the process of occupational adaptation as a struggle between a distinct and separate self, juxtaposed against a distinct and separate environment that at times can present challenges of congruence and accommodation. As such, there can be a tendency toward wanting to break down or remove the obstructions from the linear path forward. In the Kawa metaphor of the river depicting the life journey, this may be imagined as rocks obstructing the water flow being obliterated or moved completely out of the water's path. However, nature can show us a more realistic, less catastrophic alternative for facing obstructions. A constant flow/pressure of water (occupations) against the obstruction can move it, erode its surfaces (thus decreasing the magnitude of the obstruction), and find ways to flow around and past it.

What has been described through the river metaphor and its components is the underlying ontology of the Kawa framework. The Kawa model's central point of reference is not the individual but rather *harmony*—a state of individual or collective being in which the subject is constantly seeking balance with the surrounding context. Here, the essence of such harmony is conceptualized as life energy or life flow. OT's purpose is to help the client and community enhance and balance this flow.

In this constant search for harmony there is coexistence, a balanced synergy between all of the elements of a person's life or river. This approach to OT naturally leads to several guiding questions: How can one come to terms with one's circumstances? How can harmony between the elements (of which the *self* is merely one element) be realized? How, and in what ways, can occupational therapists and their clients work together to achieve this construction of well-being?

Using the Kawa Model in Practice

By using the Kawa model, occupational therapists are partnering with their clients to stem further obstructions of life energy/flow and looking for every opportunity in the broader context of person and environment to enhance the flow. The Kawa is merely a metaphor; a vehicle of communication that carries potential to be an effective medium of mutual understanding and respect between client and therapist. Through the river metaphor, the client's narrative is brought into consciousness, validated, and centralized to be the focal point and guiding framework for the OT that follows. The occupational therapist then thoughtfully considers what OT has to offer (to restore and/or enhance life flow) before working with the client(s) to set the objectives for meaningful intervention, support, and mobilization of resources. Once the constructed model is explained and mutually understood, both theorist (client) and student (occupational therapist) can discuss intervention objectives and priorities, as well as the desired outcomes and how those will be measured.

The Kawa model is not a universal, one-size-fits-all, grand narrative. As such, there is not one correct or recommended way for the model to be used. The primary aim is to access and comprehend the client's account of their daily life experience and help them find and enact ways to *flow* better. In other words, the model performs like an instrument to uncover, organize, and mutually comprehend the client's unique daily life narrative. On these premises, the occupational therapist uses their own intuition, professional reasoning, and creativity in applying the Kawa model.

Despite the Kawa model's use in diverse settings around the world, there is still a dearth of academic publications that describe and explain where and how the Kawa model is being used. The following information is largely anecdotal, reporting on how practitioners in different parts of the world have applied the Kawa model and have found it to be effective.

The Kawa model is reportedly used in practice in three basic ways.

1. As an assessment to map the client's experience of daily life
2. As a therapeutic modality
3. As a mental framework to support the occupational therapist's holistic regard of the client

Assessment to Map the Client's Experience of Daily Life

Mapping the client's narrative of daily life is perhaps the most popular application of the Kawa model. Through direct interaction with the occupational therapist, the client expresses their daily life narrative verbally or/and figuratively through a drawing or material representation of their river (Figure 37.7). In North America, where independence, autonomy, and self-determinism are considered familiar and normal, the client drawing or producing a diagram of a river to depict their life experience and outlook is often seen. Most often, the therapist asks the client to produce a diagram or picture of a river to show how the client views their life flow. The four basic starting components of the river (water rocks, driftwood, and walls) and their meanings are explained in everyday, casual language. The therapist then asks the client to think about their river and how it is flowing. Adequate time is given for the client to reflect and construct their narrative through the river metaphor. Sometimes, the instruction to draw a river is assigned as homework to be discussed at the next treatment session.

It is important to stress that the aim of this process is to comprehend and value what the client reports about their experience of daily life. Any move to *correct* the client's narrative or to force it to comply with an external narrative such as a universal conceptual model or framework is

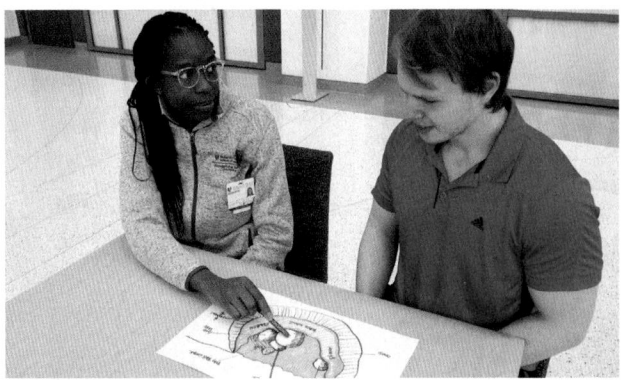

FIGURE 37.7 An OT practitioner reviews a Kawa model with a client.

discouraged. The therapist should try to be a *student* of the client's narrative to encourage its production and expression. The full benefit of the Kawa model is not in how the concepts or protocol comply with some expected ideal or universal standard but rather in the client's explanations of the items that they disclose in their rivers. As Glaser and Strauss (1967) suggested in their seminal work on the grounded theory method of qualitative research—to "trust emergence" is suggested in the use of the Kawa model. Trust that the client will produce and uncover a theory of their daily life experience and its basic concepts and the principles that connect the concepts together.

As with any request to reveal personal information, it is normal for clients to hesitate in discussing their private and personal matters. River narratives early in the treatment course are often sparse in content—as if a fog has shrouded the river, preventing accurate and deeper analysis. Also, clients may not be accustomed to such reflection and contemplation and discussions around their selves. The therapist should treat the client's narrative with utmost care and empathy and work with only those items in their rivers that their clients feel safe to divulge. Over time, as mutual trust develops between client and therapist, it is common to see the river narratives fill with pertinent, deeper, and more complete information.

This common application of the Kawa model is outlined in Teoh and Iwama's (2015) guide to applying the Kawa model (The Kawa Model Made Easy). The authors of this chapter stress that the application protocol suggested in this manual is merely one way for how the Kawa model can be applied. Users are encouraged to adapt and change the protocol to suit their diverse clients and local cultural contexts.

Figure 37.8 and the following steps outline one common example for how the Kawa model is employed in medical settings.

Step 1: Appreciating the Client in Context

This is the initial step where the occupational therapist begins interacting with the client. Mutual rapport and trust for the therapeutic relationship are being established, and the Kawa model is being employed as a guide to explore how the person's daily life is flowing. Questions and discussion revolve around the components of the Kawa model: (water) "How are things going for you, these days?"; (rocks) "What kinds of difficulties and problems stand in your way these days?"; (river walls) "Can you tell me about where you live and how that is for you?" "Can you tell me about your workplace?" "Who are the important people in your life? and How are those relationships going?"; (spaces/channels) "What is going well for you these days?" "What types of activities and things do you enjoy doing?"; (driftwood) "Do you have any special abilities or skills?" "How would you describe your personality/character?" "What would your family and close friends say about you that is positive, including what they think you're good at?"

Further, the occupational therapist may choose to use the river metaphor to explain their role (as an occupational therapist and "life-flow enabler") and aim to help the client's life to "flow" better, using a multifaceted approach that includes the environment.

Step 2: Clarifying the Context

This step brings the client's narrative of their daily life experiences into greater clarity. The occupational therapist begins to affirm the client's narrative, which is uncovered through use of the river metaphor and its basic concepts. Specific questions are asked of the client to ensure that their narrative is fully comprehended. Doing so can validate the client's reported experience and may elevate their sense of trust and confidence in their occupational therapist and the

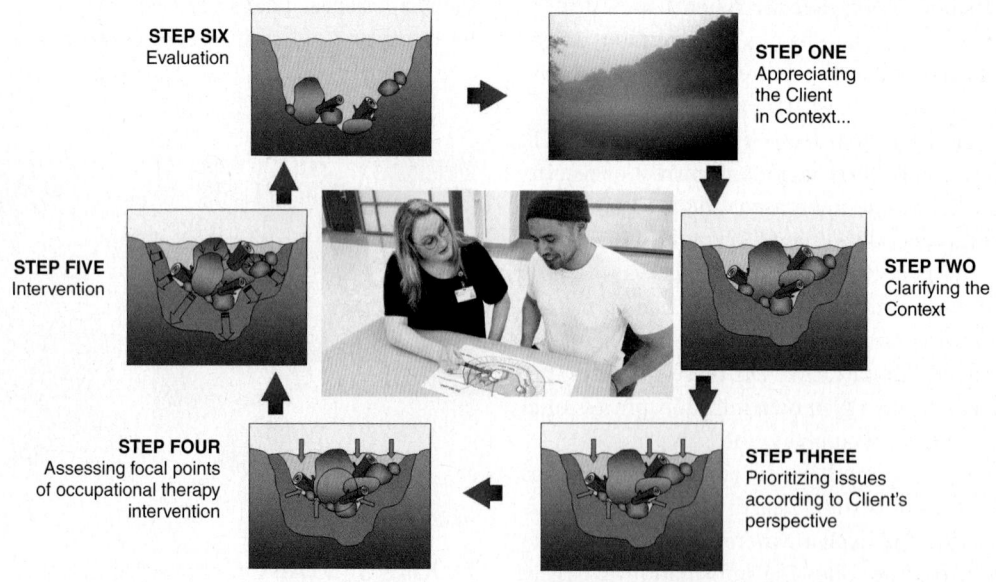

STEP SIX Evaluation

STEP ONE Appreciating the Client in Context...

STEP FIVE Intervention

STEP TWO Clarifying the Context

STEP FOUR Assessing focal points of occupational therapy intervention

STEP THREE Prioritizing issues according to Client's perspective

FIGURE 37.8 **Typical flow of Kawa model application in the medical setting.**

therapeutic process. At this step, the many parts of the client's daily life experience are clarified and regarded as occurring concurrently in a manner in which all of the river/life components are interrelated. Occupational therapists have often reported that it is not uncommon for clients to express that the occupational therapist is the first and only one in their healthcare experience to want to understand what the client is experiencing in day-to-day life. "Finally, someone really understands me and my situation; everyone else seems to be focused on the diagnosis but not on me and how my illness has turned my daily life and sense of well-being upside-down."

Validating the client's experience of daily living is the starting point for improving life flow. It can encourage the client to take greater power of their situation and invest in decreasing the impediments that stand in the way of better life flow.

Step 3: Prioritizing Issues According to Client's Perspective

Now that the client's river is clarified and validated, a mutual, deep, exploratory dive into the river is possible. Both client and occupational therapist can now look for channels of water that exist in the frame. In between, the hard structures of the river are channels of occupation and hope. Channels of water (life flow and occupations) signify potential for greater flow. Closer examination of these channels may reveal the (social and physical) environmental factors, self attributes, and particular difficulties/problems that form the boundaries around (and constrain) each course of occupation and life flow.

Once the inventory of water channels is completed, the client is asked to rank each channel according to personal importance and value. These channels are referred to by many occupational therapists as the client's occupational priorities.

Step 4: Assessing Focal Points of OT Intervention

Each of the prioritized channels is considered carefully by the therapist and client. Each channel is then named by the client for the occupation, strength, or area of life flow that it represents. Each of the named channels is then assessed extensively for components and characteristics that comprise it. The same is then done for the characteristics of each of the elements that form a part of the border around each channel. Typically, detailed characteristics of the named occupation (water channel or spaces), the immediate and ambient environment (river walls), the client's personal factors (driftwood), and their difficulties and problems (rocks) are produced.

The information gathered about the client's river flow at this stage is predominantly subjective. More information about the client's capacity for engagement and participation in the occupational priorities identified in Step 3 can be gathered through selection and employment of relevant objective assessments. The Kawa model can be useful in mapping the client's unique occupational issues, in turn pointing to appropriate and relevant assessments and OT intervention.

For each of these elements, the client and therapist can discuss and determine therapeutic activities required to modify the magnitude of the element. Some examples of questions that are often asked in this frame are as follows: "How can we make the flow of this channel stronger?" "How can we decrease the size of this obstruction?" "Will increasing the water flow of this channel result in eroding back the surface of these hard structures?" "Can increasing this occupation (water channel) push this rock out of the way?" "Can the water surge push/mobilize this driftwood to push that rock to the side; or the driftwood, itself, float away?"

It is important to keep in mind that interventions to all involved elements may not be necessary. A change in just one component is often enough to increase water flow through a particular channel. Eroding back the surface of a river wall (immediate environment) may trigger a surge of water flow through a particular space. The ensuing surge may move or change other obstructing elements, resulting in greater overall flow. The ontology on which the Kawa model is situated regards all elements in nature to be inseparably connected and in continuous flux. Changing one part of the river will change the overall river. The serendipitous way in which nature moves toward equilibrium and harmony has a way of inspiring hope and showing its truth that "things will get better."

Step 5: Intervention

At this stage, the planned OT interventions agreed upon by the client and occupational therapist are conducted.

Step 6: Evaluation

Has OT been demonstrably effective in enabling the client's occupational performance? Has OT made a positive difference in the client's life flow? Is the client's river flowing better? Are there new channels that have appeared? Does the client feel that their experience of health and well-being have improved through OT? What areas of the client's occupational engagement need further and sustained attention? At this step, the occupational therapist is considering what evaluation procedures can be applied in the client's situation to measure progress and success. In addition to standard tests, the occupational therapist may want to repeat the Kawa model procedure that was introduced to the client in an earlier session. Comparing and contrasting recent Kawa model assessments with previous assessments may illuminate changes in the client's life flow and engagement in daily life activities.

Therapeutic Modality

The Kawa model has been reported anecdotally to be used as a therapeutic modality. Keeping in mind that the model is primarily a metaphor for life flow, the model can be employed by occupational therapists in a number of creative ways. Some occupational therapists have reported (to the author) that the Kawa model is helpful in mental health practice—particularly in instances where the occupational therapist and clients are working on matters of insight (upriver); self-awareness and identity (current river); and future planning (downriver). Instead of relying on verbal and written communication alone to address these complex, personal topics, the Kawa metaphor in drawing or craft form offers another medium for the client to communicate their perspectives, thoughts, and feelings. Conversely, therapists have occasionally applied the model in reverse; to communicate the purpose and plan for OT in a way that both therapist and client can mutually understand.

The Kawa model appears to be useful for helping clients organize their thoughts regarding their future lives in a holistic way that also takes into account their experiences (wisdom) and strengths/attributes. "Are there things that we can do now regarding your social environment (river walls), abilities and skills (driftwood), and occupations (water/spaces) to ensure that the big rocks you anticipate running into downriver won't constrain your river flow too much?" Note, however, that not all rivers that clients have seen are the same; see Expanding Our Perspectives.

 EXPANDING OUR PERSPECTIVES

The Kawa Model From a South African Perspective

Chantal Christopher

What if our experiences of rivers were different? What if my river did not resemble the one in your head, let alone the one on a Kawa Model template? The universality of the river metaphor may be messy and contested as a result of the experience of the river and life itself (particularly in majority of world countries). For me, the practitioner and academic, I understand that the river may be bound up in concepts of land reparations/settler colonialism. It, in all probability, is enmeshed within apartheid's legacy, where often people of color did not have access to water (the river) as it was out of their power. The river was dammed for other people's use, aqueducted for the landowner's business, or far away from the land that people of color were forced to reside on. This experience of having the "river's life force" inaccessible becomes part of the outer walls in a life story, shaping occupational consciousness, inherited occupations, and narrowed occupational choice. In this scenario, this background, perhaps intergenerational, becomes the foreground. The ugliness and existential pain need to be held by the OT practitioner, as a listener and practitioner, whether in Chicago's south side, or Tower Hamlets-London, or the favelas of Rio de Janeiro. *Take-home message:* Our positionalities and perspectives inform our lives and "rivers."

The "river" in eThekwini/Durban South Africa and the riverbanks have become sites of nonsanctioned informal settlements, where homes were built precariously on flood plains and therefore become part of survival and urban life on the one hand and death and destruction on the other. Figure A shows a rich tableau of homes that were rebuilt partially after devastating floods, while children who were out of school walked through the litter-strewn riverbanks. Would the resultant upheaval, loss, grief and trauma,

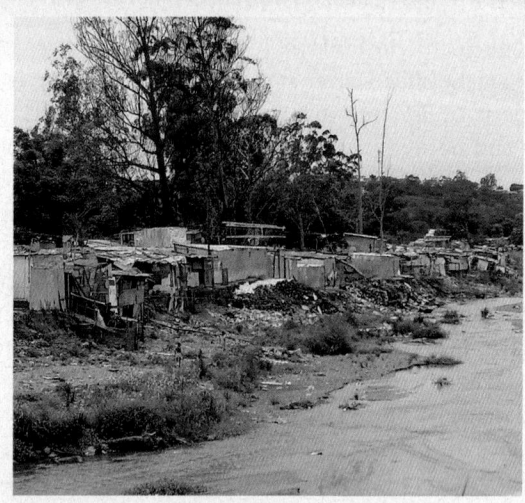

FIGURE A. How will this river cross-section look? (Varsity Drive settlement—eThekwini-Durban, KwaZulu—Natal, South Africa)

survival, and continued danger, form part of the children's internal river archetype? I present these anecdotes in order to emphasize Iwama's point within this chapter that "The Kawa model can be instrumentally described as a way to raise the client's narrative of their experience of everyday life and make it the center of everyone's concern. Through the river metaphor, the client's narrative is brought into consciousness, validated, and centralized to be the focal point and guiding framework for the occupational therapy that follows." The river is not always pretty, it is not always clean, it encompasses a thousand rivers in the one narrator, and the single story is more likely a censored story and or a composite—a crashing together of many rivers—if a level of trust has been built. *Take-home message:* Look for the messiness and nuance, guard against template-like analysis.

As a community health activist and an OT practitioner, I find that the Kawa model offers a method to raise the consciousness and understanding of the narrator and the practitioner at the same time. I believe that if used judiciously, in culturally responsive ways, it allows a witnessing of life and for insight into the phenomenon that fractures the possibilities of life.

This Kawa requires a reading in terms of cultural, sociopolitical, and historical, lenses. Without careful exploration and journeying together, the nuances and opportunities—the Spaces—will be lost. Figure B, a photo of the same river in Figure A, on the same day, offers me and hopefully you a visual prompt. Without a bulldozer that can carefully, skillfully, and methodically clear away the debris, the landscape has little chance to recover, the person will continue to survive in harsh conditions. *Take-home message:* Sometimes be a bulldozer. Some phenomena will require advocacy and speaking back to systemic injustices to comprehensively change the flow, but in the face of seemingly long-term efforts, we realize that perhaps this will change many Kawas.

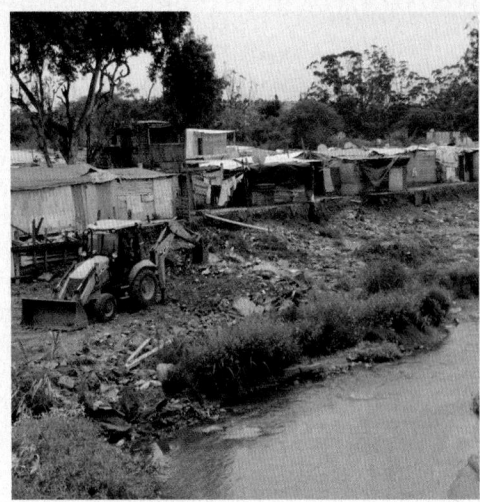

FIGURE B. **A bulldozer clears the riverbanks. Who is the bulldozer? (Varsity Drive settlement-eThekwini-Durban, KwaZulu—Natal, South Africa)**

Mental Framework to Enable Holistic Appreciation of the Client

Many occupational therapists have anecdotally reported that they use the Kawa model mainly as a mental framework to ensure that they maintain a holistic view of their clients. Some occupational therapists working in medical institutions may find it difficult to implement an occupation-centric model that is based on a metaphor of nature. The Kawa model supports a holistic and comprehensive regard for their clients inseparably connected to their environs that expand beyond the boundaries of

intervention plans that center on specific, embodied pathology. Experienced healthcare professionals understand that fixing or curing an embodied abnormality or impairment does not necessarily restore the client's full well-being. Occupational therapists are committed to continue helping people manage their embodied health problems, while also committing to helping people manage the consequences of those pathologies on their occupations and patterns of daily living activity. Our focus on the client isn't limited to the rocks (problems, difficulties) in their rivers but also encompasses the river walls (environment), driftwood (personal factors), and spaces (occupation and hope).

See OT Story 37.1 for an example of the Kawa model in practice.

OT STORY 37.1 OCCUPATIONAL THERAPY TO RESTORE THE HARMONIOUSLY FLOWING KAWA AGAIN

Kei is a 72-year-old single woman, the youngest of three siblings, who lives with her parents. She worked as an elementary school teacher for about 30 years, and after her parents passed away, she lived independently. Nine years ago, she was diagnosed with Parkinson disease and continued to live independently until this year when she lost consciousness and had a fall. As a result of falling, she fractured her cervical vertebrae. For 1 month, she managed to live in her home but gradually began to have difficulty walking. Subsequently, she was admitted to the hospital. Orthopedic surgery for her cervical spine was performed and rehabilitation was started; however, severe orthostatic

hypotension was observed and medical treatment was given. As her blood pressure gradually stabilized, she was transferred to a rehabilitation hospital and rehabilitation was resumed.

At the time of admission, she needed assistance with self-care except for eating and had difficulty sitting or standing for long periods of time due to the residual effects of orthostatic hypotension. Voluntary movement of the extremities was possible, but muscle strength and endurance, as well as hand and finger dexterity, were also diminished. Cognitive function was intact, with an MMSE score of 29/30. OT was planned to enable her to live independently in the

(continued)

OT STORY 37.1 OCCUPATIONAL THERAPY TO RESTORE THE HARMONIOUSLY FLOWING KAWA AGAIN (*continued*)

community at home as she did before the injury, with the goal of reacquiring her activities of daily living, instrumental activities of daily living, and hobbies, and improvement of upper extremity function. Given these clear markers of embodied, medically defined issues, the occupational therapist is interested in understanding and acting on the consequences of these embodied "pathologies" on Kei's experience of daily life. An interview guided by the Kawa Model was conducted to better understand Kei's situation holistically and to identify, select, and prioritize tasks for OT intervention.

Because Kei reported that drawing the river was difficult for her to do alone, her OT practitioner offered to support her through the process. As she interacted with her therapist to draw the Kawa, she had an opportunity to reflect on her life and remembered that she had enjoyed painting, sewing, and eating out with friends when she was an elementary school teacher. She also recounted her struggles when she was diagnosed with Parkinson disease, the depression she suffered, and the loneliness she felt when she took care of her parents. The cross-section of the Kawa at the time of her admission showed not only her physical and psychological condition at the time but also her personality tendencies and beliefs.

Using the river drawings and her accompanying narrative as common points of mutual understanding and communication, her therapist discussed the proposed OT program with her. In OT, she practiced ADL, IADL, and therapeutic activities using handicrafts. ADL were practiced independently at an early stage, and IADL, such as washing, cleaning, and cooking, were practiced in the hospitalized environment. Therapeutic activities included various handicrafts in which she was interested. Her occupational therapist, together with the physical therapist on her care team, supported and encouraged Kei to strengthen her walking to the level required for Kei to resume shopping from home. In addition, she confirmed the support she could receive from her siblings in her recovery. Kei's occupational therapist conferred with the social worker on the team about necessary home improvements as well as medical services she would be receiving at home. Kei was then discharged from the hospital and returned to her home. After she left the hospital, her river cross-section showed a smoother and easier flowing, as she expressed feeling optimistic and full of hope for her life going into the future.

Questions

1. What purposes can the occupational therapist use the Kawa model for?
2. When drawing a cross-section of the Kawa in Kei's situation, what information can each component of the model reveal?
3. How can the occupational therapist use the information obtained by the Kawa model to support Kei's return to the community?

Evidence to Support Using the Kawa Model

Perhaps owing to its roots in practice, the Kawa model has only recently begun to appear in the OT academic literature and theoretical discourse. The strongest evidence to support the Kawa model's use continues to be anecdotal—mainly by practitioners outside of North America who have discovered its practical utility and relevance to local practice. The authors believe that the model's simplicity and practicality, as well as the relevance of the river metaphor that the model is based on, account for its steady growth of acceptance and popularity. A selection of papers demonstrating the Kawa model's potential to support efficacy of OT in the field is presented below.

The theme for many studies was that the Kawa model facilitated communication and collaboration and enhanced understanding between therapists and their clients. A qualitative study in which the Kawa model was used for individuals with multiple sclerosis found that the model facilitated occupation-based practice (Carmody et al., 2007). The Kawa model was used in another qualitative study to examine the experiences of fathers with a history of substance use (Garramone et al., 2021). Fathers described their river flows as ever changing and identified drugs as a rock that affected their relationships with the families. In a study of parents that lost a child to drug overdose, the Kawa model was helpful for understanding the unique experiences of grieving parents (Weis et al., 2019). The Kawa model helped therapists better appreciate the struggles associated with interpersonal relationships for their clients with schizophrenia (Yeh et al., 2016).

Several studies found that implementation of the model could improve practice situations. For example, the model has been used to facilitate collaboration among rehabilitation team members (Lape & Scaife, 2017; Lape et al., 2019). These studies found that the Kawa model provided a method for team members to problem solve and identify ways to improve their team flow. Occupational therapists practicing in mental health found that use of the Kawa model improved their client interactions and interest in practice (Paxson et al., 2012). A scoping review of the Kawa model indicates it is useful for gathering client-centered qualitative information and for building therapeutic relationships (Ober et al., 2022).

Conclusion

The evolution of OT theory and practice, like people's lives, can be seen to flow like a river. It is in constant flux—changing in form, content, and direction, from moment to moment. As the world changes, people's construction of and understanding of health and well-being also change. The power of OT flowing to the future hinges largely on its relevance to the day-to-day experiences and needs of a vast, diverse clientele. To effectively align OT's offerings to people and their communities, access to their narratives is essential. The Kawa model's main purpose and value is found in its utility and effectiveness in raising and comprehending the client's unique narrative of their everyday life to make it the central standard around which culturally relevant OT can revolve.

As OT continues to cross cultural boundaries in the wake of unbridled technological progress and globalizing social media, there is a pressing need to proceed beyond merely adapting its form and technologies to meet the requirements of its varied target practice contexts. Occupational therapists around the world and the communities they serve may need to critically examine current OT ideology, epistemology, and theory and to participate in innovating culturally safe variations and approaches that reflect and meet the needs of OT's diverse clientele. The Kawa model is an early example of such innovation.

The Kawa model is not a grand narrative. All claims for the model being universal in its applicability are dismissed, making the model amenable to alteration by occupational therapists in conceptual and structural ways to match the specific social and cultural contexts of their diverse clients. Although the model may appear to favor Japanese cultural contexts, the Kawa model should not be viewed as culturally exclusive. The utility of this model for varying populations depends on the river metaphor's relevance to each client's real world of meanings. Following the model's introduction outside of Japan, groups of practitioners in diverse cultural locations around the world have begun to use the model, adapting it freely to suit the cultural requirements and unique features of their practice. The Kawa model is a novel postmodern theoretical product bringing the well-being needs of a diverse clientele into alignment and harmony with OT's magnificent promise.

Lippincott® Connect *For additional resources on the subjects discussed in this chapter, visit* Lippincott Connect.

REFERENCES

American Occupational Therapy Association. (2020). Occupational therapy practice framework: Domain and process, 4th edition. *American Journal of Occupational Therapy, 74*(Suppl. 2), 7412410010. https://doi.org/10.5014/ajot.2020.74S2001

Berger, P. L., & Luckmann, T. (1966). *The social construction of reality: A treatise in the sociology of knowledge.* Anchor Books.

Campbell, F., & Kumari, A. (2009). *Contours of ableism: The production of disability and ableness.* Palgrave Macmillan. ISBN 978-0-230-57928-6

Carmody, S., Nolan, R., Chonchuir, N., Curry, M., Halligan, C., & Robinson, K. (2007). The guiding nature of the Kawa (river) model in Ireland: Creating both opportunities and challenges for occupational therapists. *Occupational Therapy International, 14*(4), 221–236. https://doi.org/10.1002/oti.235

Castells, M. (1997). *The power of identity, the information age: Economy, society and culture Vol. II.* Blackwell. ISBN 978-1-4051-0713-6.

Garramone, P., Knis-Matthews, L., Brandeis, P., Kret, M., Sliwa, L., & Leva, A. (2021). Against the current: Exploring the experiences of five fathers with a history of substance use. *Occupational Therapy in Mental Health, 37*(4), 332–356. https://doi.org/10.1080/0164212X.2021.1980174

Glaser, B., & Strauss, A. (1967). *The discovery of grounded theory: Strategies for qualitative research.* Sociology Press.

Iwama, M. (2003). The issue is…toward culturally relevant epistemologies in occupational therapy. *The American Journal of Occupational Therapy, 57*(5), 217–223. https://doi.org/10.5014/ajot.57.5.582

Iwama, M. (2006). *The Kawa Model: Culturally relevant occupational therapy* (260 pp.). Elsevier/Churchill Livingstone.

Iwama, M., & Baksh, H. (in press). *Namudhaj Alnahr Aleilaj Amahni Almurtabit Bialthaqafati* [Arabic version of the Kawa Model: Culturally relevant occupational therapy]. Princess Nourah bint Abdul Rahman University Press, Riyadh, Kingdom of Saudi Arabia.

Lape, J., Lukose, A., Ritter, D., & Scaife, B. (2019). Use of the Kawa Model to facilitate interprofessional collaboration: A pilot study. *Internet Journal of Allied Health Sciences and Practice.* https://doi.org/10.46743/1540-580X/2019.1780.

Lape, J., & Scaife, B. (2017). Use of the Kawa Model for teambuilding with rehabilitative professionals: An exploratory study. *Internet Journal of Allied Health Sciences and Practice.* https://doi.org/10.46743/1540-580X/2017.1647.

Lebra, T.-S. (1976). *Japanese patterns of behavior* (295 pp.). University of Hawaii Press.

Ober, J.L., Newbury, R.S., & Lape, J.D. (2022). The dynamic use of the Kawa Model: A scoping review. *Open Journal of Occupational Therapy, 10*(2), 1–12. https://doi.org/10.15453/2168-6408.1952

Paxson, D., Winston, K., Tobey, T., Johnston, S., & Iwama M. (2012). The Kawa model: Therapists' experiences in mental health practice. *Occupational Therapy in Mental Health, 28*(4), 340–355. https://doi.org/10.1080/0164212X.2012.708586

Ramsden, I. (2000). Cultural safety/Kawa Whakaruruhau ten years on: A personal overview. *Nursing Praxis in New Zealand, 15*(1), 4–12. https://doi.org/10.36951/NgPxNZ.2000.001

Teoh, J. Y., & Iwama, M. K. (2015). *The Kawa model made easy: A guide to applying the Kawa model in occupational therapy practice* (2nd ed.). https://www.kawamodel.com/v1/2016/08/06/the-kawa-model-made-easy-download/

Weis, A., Kugel, J., Javaherian, H., & De Brun, J. (2019). Life after losing an adult child to a drug overdose: A Kawa perspective. *Open Journal of Occupational Therapy, 7*(3), 1–14. https://doi.org/10.15453/2168-6408.1488

Yeh, E., Huang, L.-J., & Wu, C. (2016). Activity participation and restriction for community clients with schizophrenia through the Kawa model perspective. *American Journal of Occupational Therapy, 70*(4 Suppl. 1), 1. https://doi.org/10.5014/ajot.2016.70S1-PO6113

The Model of Occupational Wholeness

An Emerging Theory in Occupational Therapy

Farzaneh Yazdani

LEARNING OBJECTIVES

After reading this chapter, you will be able to:

1. Describe the basic components of the Model of Occupational Wholeness: Doing, Being, Belonging, Becoming, Contextual Factors, Meaning-Making, and Choice-Making.
2. Indicate the negative and positive contextual factors.
3. Draw a helpee's actual and ideal triangles.
4. Analyze a client's narrative using the Model of Occupational Wholeness.
5. Discuss the potential use of the Model of Occupational Wholeness in various settings and for different people.

Introduction

Life and occupational balance have been the foci of a variety of disciplines including occupational therapy (OT) for decades. The concept of balance has traditionally been used to weigh up the separate demands of life and work or to identify different roles concerning life balance (Khateeb, 2021). The concept of balance has also been used to distinguish between different types of activities when addressing occupational balance. Literature shows that the concepts of life and occupational balance are used in a number of ways when referring to the words *occupation* and *balance*. By way of explanation, scholars use the word *balance* quantitatively when adopting (referring to) a "time use" approach or qualitatively when assigning value to different aspects of life or types of occupation (Christiansen & Matuska, 2006; Wagman et al., 2012; Westhorp, 2003, 2011; Yazdani et al., 2016).

The central construct of the Model of Occupational Wholeness (MOW) is occupational wholeness (OW). The model emerged from a series of studies in occupational balance, including those by Yazdani et al. (2016, 2018). These studies explored the concepts of life and occupational balance from the perspectives of OT practitioners, practice educators, academics, and scholars in the field of OT. Study participants used terms such as *harmony, integration, satisfaction,* and *contentment* to explain what occupational balance and/or life balance meant to them. The findings of these studies also showed that, regardless of the types of activities and aspects of life and work, people do things in relation to who they are, who they wish to be, and what makes them feel connected to people, places, and things and their own values. These findings led to conceptualizing balance as a point (position, place) between what may be considered as being, becoming, and belonging. The findings also led to the creation of the concept of life balance and later the MOW.

The concepts of being, doing, becoming (Wilcock, 1993), and belonging (Hammell, 2014; Wilcock, 1993) have been discussed previously within the occupational science literature. Wilcock (1993) believes that human beings have a biological need to do. Doing is seen as a part of being, and people engage in doing to meet their needs (Wilcock, 1993). The MOW expands upon the concepts of doing, being, and becoming to include life balance.

Knowledge of chaos theory (Duke, 1994), choice theory (Glasser, 1975), needs theories (Deci & Ryan, 2009), and the theories of occupational science (Wilcock, 2006), cognition (Whitfield & Davidson, 2016), and learning (McInerney et al., 2011) were also employed in conceptualizing the MOW.

Models of practice assist OT practitioners in organizing their thinking throughout the therapeutic process as well as in establishing a theoretical framework in research. Occupational therapists may find it difficult to operationalize being, doing, becoming, and belonging. The MOW is proposed as a framework that occupational therapists can utilize to organize their thoughts throughout the therapeutic process.

Occupational wholeness (OW), therefore, was coined to explain what people experience as life balance and/or occupational balance from their own perspective. It refers to a sense of wholeness through Doing. An individual feels well integrated and whole if there is a positively meaningful combination of Doing that satisfies their need for Being, Belonging, and Becoming. For instance, a person who spends some of their time taking care of themselves physically and psychologically such that it is perceived as good enough by them and does some activities that help them feel they are moving forward in their life and toward their aims for their future, in addition to spending a satisfying length of time and amount of energy being with others who matter to them, would feel in one piece, a whole!

As life changes and people go through different stages of their life, individuals move toward or grow distant from a sense of Wholeness. OW is dynamic, and a sense of OW is achieved through being in this process. Being aware of the journey toward achieving a sense of OW is accompanied by a sense of satisfaction.

It is essential for OT practitioners who use the MOW to be aware of cultural differences in language, views, values, and ideals when translating the MOW terminology and framework. They need to ensure the translation is understandable and linguistically reflects the cultural beliefs of the clients. These considerations are crucial to developing a mutual understanding of an individual's narrative (Jiang, 2000).

Core Concepts of the Model of Occupational Wholeness

The subjective experience of well-being is the special focus of the MOW. The MOW helps people in rethinking and replanning their life in order to promote a sense of OW. A sense of wholeness occurs in the interaction of Being, Belonging, and Becoming within an individual's Context. Doing is the means by which these complex interactions are formed. *Occupational wholeness* refers to an individual's sense of being whole through their Doings.

Occupational Wholeness

The concept of OW refers to one's sense of Being a Whole through their Doings. An individual feels well integrated and whole if there is a positively meaningful combination of *Doings* that satisfies their need for *Being, Belonging*, and *Becoming*. According to the MOW, the sense of OW is associated with a sense of contentment and satisfaction with life, the world, and self-fulfillment. The MOW aims to enhance people's self-awareness about their situation in relation to their sense of Being, Belonging, Becoming, Doings, and Context. Life is a journey that consists of developmental stages, circumstances, and mishaps that may cause resultant dissatisfaction and unhappiness; in other words, a disruption to a sense of OW.

Being

The MOW adheres to the concept of *occupational being* introduced by Del Fabro Smith et al. (2011), which refers to the sense of *Being* as "who we understand ourselves to be," at present. A sense of Being starts with a need for survival and expands to a need for autonomy, competence, and affiliation (Vansteenkiste et al., 2020). The interaction of individuals with their context, explicitly and implicitly, contributes to the formation and development of their sense of Being: an individual's perception of who they are, their capacities, their similarities to and differences from others, and what they potentially can and cannot do. Individuals shape their sense of Being by choice-making, meaning-making, and reflecting on what they choose to do or not do.

Belonging

Expansion of the sense of Being outside the self for the purpose of building relationships with people and creating an affiliation with places, objects, and concepts forms a sense of *Belonging*. According to Rogers (1951), belonging is a subjective experience, a need for connection with others, and a positive regard. Belonging is indeed a subjective experience, and it does not necessarily depend on physical proximity or sharing space with others (Allen, 2020; Yazdani, Nazi, et al., 2021; Yazdani, Rezaee, et al., 2021).

A sense of Belonging consists of various elements, such as sharing, identification, similarities, closeness, and trust. One may develop a superficial sense of belonging to others as a result of sharing physical spaces and shared time together. This is the lowest level of belongingness. The deeper levels are accompanied by deeper emotions and thoughts that relate or connect people together. A reciprocal sense of relatedness and connectedness between people enhances the sense of Belonging. People can also have a sense of Belonging to places, ideas, and concepts, although these targets of belonging have no capacity to reciprocate. For instance, an individual may develop a sense of belonging to a particular place such as a building, but the same building has no capacity to exchange a sense of belonging with that individual.

Becoming

Becoming is developed as an extension of Being, when humans' need for exercising autonomy and competence is linked to the future. Becoming is the dynamic process that moves humans beyond the present (Hitch et al., 2014). A future sense of Being is demonstrated in people's sense of Becoming and includes their hopes, aspirations, and plans. While becoming is about change, it is also about maintaining an optimal situation. Van Huet and colleagues (2013) refer to this kind of becoming as managing and maintaining a situation. Choice-making and meaning-making are inseparable factors when it comes to context and future planning. Physical, virtual, social, organizational, political, geographical, and even temporal factors strongly contribute to the meaning of Becoming.

Doings (Doing/Not Doing)

Doings (Doing/Not Doing) refers to the ways in which people meet their needs for Being, Belonging, and Becoming (the 3Bs), and they are central to the concept of OW. Together, Doing and Not Doing in the MOW terminology are called *Doings,* and they require the element of intention. Doing is essential for the formation and development of the 3Bs. Similar to Wilcock's (2006) conceptualization of Doing, the MOW uses *Doing* as equivalent to occupation. Cutchin et al. (2008) state that Doing refers to actions that are clearly physical, not sedentary or mental activity. The MOW also considers Doing to be external as opposed to internal activities, such as thoughts. In other words, Doing is neither the implicit process behind actions nor is it about involuntary human actions, such as breathing, seeing, and hearing. Doing, as the core component of OW, is voluntary (as opposed to reflexive) and intentional. Not Doing, when intentional, is equally a means for meeting the needs of the 3Bs. To meet the 3B needs, Doings have a purpose. There are two aspects to be considered in addressing Doings as purposeful action.

Purpose is necessary for Doings, although, as Hitch et al. (2014) pose, "whose purpose" needs to be considered for Doing: the individual themselves or the observer? The MOW response is that, regardless of whether this purpose is identified by the doer or by someone external to them, purpose is necessary for human acts to be considered as human *Doings.* Most Doings have a purpose by nature, even though people may have different perspectives on the purpose of some of their Doing/Not Doing. Consider a person with dementia when they eat without thinking of its purpose. A lack of cognitive capacity may have caused confusion in the person's thinking. However, eating by nature has a purpose for survival.

Meaningfulness may be associated with a positive, negative, or even neutral emotional value. The word *meaningful* is widely used in literature as a positive value and, therefore, as a drive for Doing. The MOW, however, puts emphasis on the different ways a phenomenon, act, or event is explained and assigned a meaning. According to the MOW, meaningfulness may signify a positive or negative value, and both of these may motivate or demotivate Doings. Meaning-making is a crucial element in motivation/demotivation toward an action.

Doings–Being–Belonging–Becoming Interactions

OW is illustrated using the three sides of a triangle to demonstrate the links between the components of Being, Belonging, and Becoming, creating an Occupational Wholeness Triangle (see Figure 38.1). Each of the 3Bs impacts the others. Harmony, or lack of it, around what people Do/Not Do toward meeting the 3Bs informs their sense of OW. When Doings that meet the needs of one of the 3B components also meet one or both of the other 3Bs, the person feels less stretched or distressed, which encourages harmony. However, it is rare that all human Doings are at all times in harmony in relation to meeting the 3B needs. In fact, most of the time, life requires people to prioritize one or two components over the other(s). A problem can arise when meeting one component competes with meeting the other components over a long period of time.

Context

All Doings occur within a Context that refers to a person's total environment (Hitch et al., 2014) that embraces the spaces they occupy, the time they spend in each space, and the other people in their environment. Time and space together create the environment where Being, Belonging, and Becoming form. Although human needs for the 3Bs stay the same at all times, there are differences in the degree and extent of their influence on life. The way people make meaning and attribute value to their needs, and the way those needs are met, vary in different places and at different times.

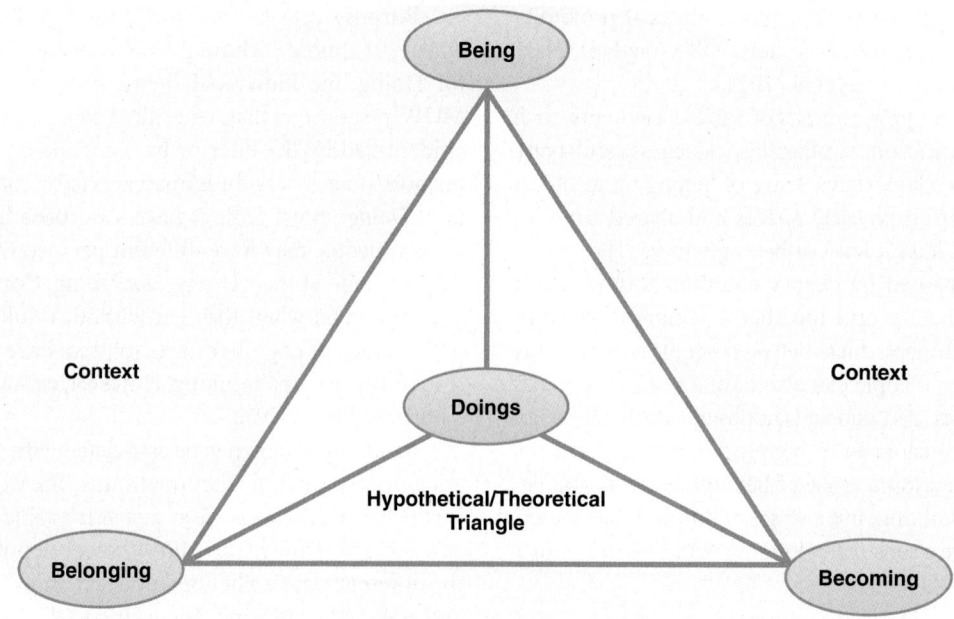

FIGURE 38.1 Occupational Wholeness is illustrated by a triangle of Being, Belonging, and Becoming (3Bs) that surrounds the Doings that meet the needs of the 3Bs.

People's Doings to meet their needs are influenced by the environment they live in. Various factors, especially other people in a person's Context, can affect their feelings, thinking, and Doings in a positive or negative way. Contextual roles such as *Expecting* and *Demanding* may be positive or negative depending on their intensity, the way they are interpreted by the individual, and the authority with which they are issued. *Encouraging, Facilitating,* and *Supporting* are considered positive and *Restricting, Blocking,* and *Opposing* are negative contributors to an individual's Doings and their overall sense of OW. Table 38.1 presents the contextual roles of Ramina, who is introduced in OT Story 38.1.

TABLE 38.1 Contextual Roles With Definitions and Examples Based on Ramina

Contextual Role	Definition	Example
Expecting	Belief about something that influences Doings	Ramina thinks that her parents are expecting her to help her aunt
Demanding	Insisting or requiring certain Doings	Ramina's parents require her to visit her aunt and help her with her hospital appointment
Encouraging	Instilling hope and confidence for Doings	Ramina's tutors told her that they believe with some reorganization she can manage her assignment as she has been successful before when she had some issues during the final assignment period
Facilitating	Make Doings easier	Ramina's tutor arranged for her to receive a recorder and be granted extra time to prepare for her assignment
Supporting	Bear part or all of the weight to make Doings happen	Ramina's classmates offered to do the typing for her and help her with library searching and so on
Restricting	Put a limit on, control Doings	Ramina's bathroom faucets were designed for a right-handed person only
Blocking	Prevent Doings	Ramina's parent stopped their financial support that made it almost impossible for her to go to cafés and restaurants even if she wanted to
Opposing	Causing conflict in Doings or compete with Doings	Ramina's parents blocked her mobile phone number, and she could not check on her dog

OT STORY 38.1 UNFOLDING RAMINA'S STORY THROUGH THE MOW TERMINOLOGY

Ramina, age 34, is a master's student in political science. She lives alone in a one-bedroom flat that she has rented and lived in since the beginning of her coursework. Ramina used to walk every day for about a mile, drink a coffee at the nearby café, and meet friends once a week at a local restaurant. She spends 5 hours a day on her studies, either by attending lectures or in the library. She regularly talks to her parents on the phone and enjoys receiving news about her little dog that she left with them when she moved to the city.

Ramina was in a car crash recently that led to fractures in her right arm and three of her fingers. She is right handed, and this has caused some difficulties in managing her day-to-day life. She has not been able to use her right hand effectively for about 8 weeks. While receiving OT services, her occupational therapist suggested a MOW-based intervention to her. She has observed Ramina's disappointment with her situation, including worries about her assignments and anger with her family who she believes have contributed to her problems. The change in Ramina's life and her dissatisfaction with it led her therapist to consider Ramina eligible for a MOW-based intervention plan.

The therapist explained to Ramina that her dissatisfaction and unhappiness with her situation could be looked at through the lens of the MOW. Ramina showed interest by saying that she was keen to do anything that might help her find a way to stop feeling miserable about herself. The therapist started with introducing the MOW philosophy and principles and familiarized Ramina with MOW terminology. This made Ramina interested in learning more about the MOW. "It's what I need right now," she said. Soon the therapist and Ramina started to discuss what Ramina could and could not do since she has been discharged from the hospital to identify her state of Doing in relation to her 3B needs. Ramina understood that her ideal situation needed to be modified as it felt impossible to achieve what she had planned to do before her accident. They agreed that not only did her actual Doings change due to her impairment but also her ideals need to be reviewed in light of her new circumstances.

Ramina was not able to shower daily or take a walk owing to the longer time that she needed to spend on her self-care, which affected her Sense of Being. She could not use the computer easily to do her education-related activities. She had planned to achieve A grades in her assignments, and she felt that she was not able to achieve this anymore, which affected her Sense of Becoming. She was angry with her parents as they had asked her to visit her aunt to help her with her hospital appointment, and Ramina's car accident occurred on the way to her aunt's place. She believed that her aunt has always brought bad luck to her life and that her parents making her go and visit was unkind of them. Ramina had stopped calling her parents, and they became upset and blocked her number, so she had no news about her dog anymore. Ramina had to stop going to cafés and restaurants as her parents stopped their financial support after she called and shouted at them and accused them of being the cause of her problems. She missed her friends and their gathering at the local restaurant. All of this affected her Sense of Belonging.

Ramina's course tutors had shown understanding toward her, and her classmates had offered to share their notes with her, accompany her to the library, and assist her with searching for material and typing. But Ramina had made a choice not to ask for help from classmates, and instead, she learned to use a recorder and the voice options for searching for material on the computer. This meant to her that she could stay independent. While Ramina's positive meaning for making use of these resources to stay independent motivated her to learn more about and use them (Do), it also made her refuse her friends' offers (Not Do). Ramina has assigned a negative meaning to her parents request for visiting her aunt as "unkind" and the accident as an event that was caused by her aunt's bad luck for her that meant it was out of her control. This had a negative significant meaning that motivated her to stop contacting her parents.

Questions

1. What do you consider as a rationale for introducing the MOW to Ramina?
2. How can you link Ramina's meaning-making and choice-making in her response to her accident and its consequences?
3. What do you think are the consequences of Ramina's meaning-making and choice-making on her sense of belonging?

Illustrating the Model of Occupational Wholeness

The MOW is illustrated by using four triangles: Hypothetical, Actual, Ideal, and Tailored (see Figure 38.2), which are described as follows:

- *Hypothetical/Theoretical Triangle (HT)* represents all available Doings.
- *Actual Triangle (AT)* shows what helpees currently Do or Not Do to meet their 3Bs.
- *Ideal Triangle (IT)* shows the helpee's ideals for meeting their 3Bs.

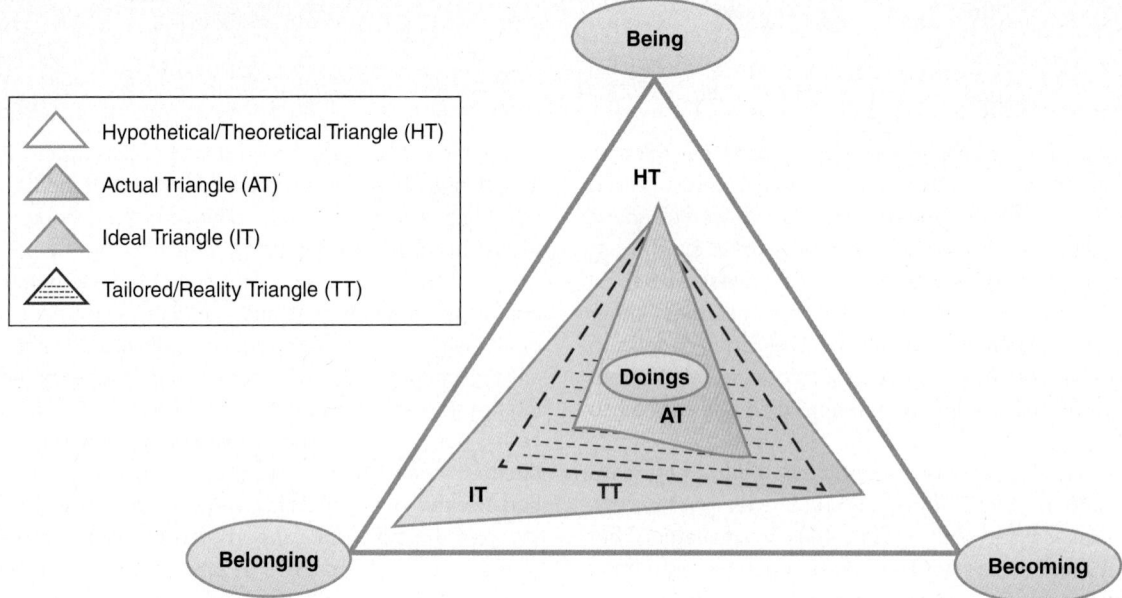

FIGURE 38.2 The Model of Occupational Wholeness is illustrated with four triangles: Hypothetical/Theoretical, Actual, Ideal, and Tailored/Reality.

• *Tailored/Reality Triangle (TT)* represents the changes that the helper and helpee agree on, plan, and implement together.

The angles formed by the triangles indicate the 3Bs; the center shows the Doings. The triangles are surrounded by contextual factors, which can be negative or positive contributors to motivation for action and Doing. The AT and IT demonstrate the following two main points:

1. The congruence/incongruence between the two triangles
2. The harmony or lack of it in Doings that meet or could meet the 3Bs

The four triangles are used to unfold the helpee's story and formulate the change.

People may assign positive or negative meaning to incongruence and lack of harmony in their lives. Positive meanings and attribution of values to an incongruence or lack of harmony contribute to a more positive sense of OW, satisfaction with self and life, and subjective experience of well-being. However, this does not necessarily mean that it is the best objective situation for the person in terms of their health. In other words, a lack of congruence and harmony, particularly if significant and for a long time, has its own negative consequences on one's health. Here are two examples (see OT Story 38.2 and 38.3) to illustrate the positive and negative assignment of meaning and attribution of value to incongruence of AT and IT and lack of harmony in meeting the 3B needs.

OT STORY 38.2 PURYA'S POSITIVE MEANING-MAKING

Purya is a young father of two children. Purya and his wife used to work full time. Purya had applied for training to improve his computer skills that would help with his promotion at work. Purya's wife has become very ill and lost her job recently, and this meant Purya had to give up the computer training. His employer, however, facilitated extra hours of work for Purya and agreed to delay his training. He has become his wife's carer, and his responsibilities for his children's care have increased. He sleeps very little as taking care of children has taken all his time when he is not at work. He has not been in contact with any friends or family members for about 3 months. He values socializing and visiting his family and not being able to do so has made him unhappy. He used to go swimming every weekend, but currently, he has had to give that up too.

His relationships with his children and wife are only at a very basic level, and they have hardly any time to enjoy the things they used to do together. For a person like Purya with a strong belief in family life, stopping his weekly outdoor activities together is hard. Purya feels he has no choice but instead to continue this way of life for at least another 3 months with a hope that his wife's health will get better and she will find a job soon after. He thinks this is a period of time that is part of life for him and his family to learn from, and if they can cope and manage it, they will have a better future.

Purya's AT and IT show a huge incongruence (see Figure 38.3). However, the way he has assigned a positive meaning to his situation and has attributed what he is doing as worthwhile has made him feel more accepting and given

OT STORY 38.2 PURYA'S POSITIVE MEANING-MAKING (*continued*)

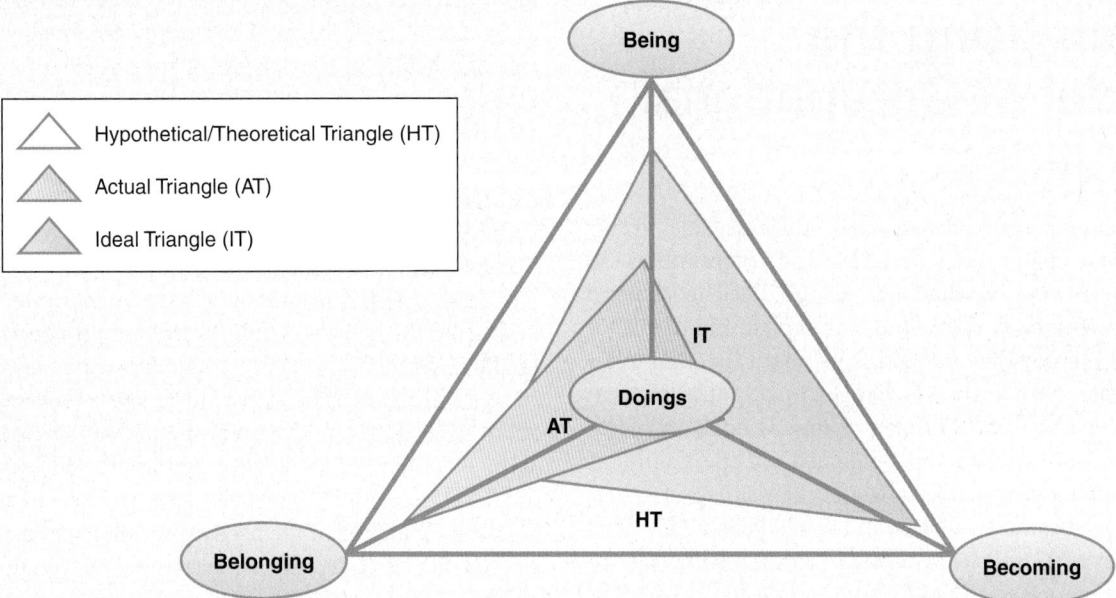

FIGURE 38.3 Illustration of Purya's triangles and change plan.

him hope for the future. Although he feels more tired and has started showing sleep problems, his positive thinking and feelings about his family's situation and being realistic about the fact that his wife's health will improve and the difficulties will be over have helped him cope with this situation.

Questions

1. Imagine that Purya assigns a negative meaning to his situation. For instance, a punishment from the universe for his previous mistakes. How do you think this meaning-making would impact his motivation for his Doings and his physical/mental well-being?
2. What do you think about the role of hope in Purya's motivation for his Doings?
3. Can you identify different values that Purya considers for different Doings, and explain how you think Purya has come to a decision about managing them?

OT STORY 38.3 RIERO'S NEGATIVE MEANING-MAKING

Riero, age 56, had a stroke 18 months ago that led to a left hemiplegia. He has been visiting a physiotherapist, and his gait is almost back to normal. His hand function, however, still shows some limitations, although he is able to manage all his self-care independently. Riero's stroke had little impact on his performance as a teacher and he continued his work. But he stopped socializing with friends and family as he felt embarrassed by his awkward walking, even though it is hardly noticeable by others. Riero felt lonely and believed his friends did not try enough to encourage him to join gatherings since his stroke. He feels forgotten by his family, even though Riero himself was the one who stopped communicating. He rarely attends the public places that he used to love visiting, like the local library and meadows. He recently joined an online support group for people after a stroke. He feels unhappy as he feels he has no choice now that he has left his friends and family for a relatively long time. Riero feels he has lost his happiness as his life is incomplete without the people and places that mattered to them. He believes that this situation and lack of communication between himself and his friends and family are irreversible and that he has no control over the situation.

Questions

1. Identify negative meanings that Riero has given to different events in his life.
2. How does the role of context influence the way Riero assigns meaning to these different events in his life?
3. How do you think negative meaning-making would impact Riero's motivation for Doings, sense of being, belonging, and becoming?

Role and Process of Occupational Therapy When Using the Model of Occupational Wholeness

Developmental life changes and unforeseeable events can impose change on individuals and communities. To maintain a sense of wholeness, people need to respond to these changes by rethinking and replanning their Doings and the way they *feel* and *think* about them. In other words, they need to make changes in response to what happens in their life. At times, change is not possible or is difficult, and therefore, people need to cope. Coping is a form of changing people's view of their situation—their dreams, ideals, wants, wishes, and so on. People may need help to explore and learn, decide, and make choices toward change, especially in difficult circumstances such as illness and losses.

Occupational therapists working with individuals or groups of people need to identify whether their clients are eligible for a MOW-based intervention. Eligible clients are those who implicitly or explicitly show signs of dissatisfaction or feel unhappy about the following:

- Themselves or their life in general
- Their doings
- One, two, or all three senses of Being, Belonging, and Becoming
- The contextual factors that they believe affect their feelings, thinking, and Doings

Role of Occupational Therapy in the Model of Occupational Wholeness

The MOW can be conceptualized as a coaching model that aims to promote the well-being of people who are eligible for a MOW-based intervention. Coaching is about improving an individual's self-awareness of possibilities through unlocking their innate potential (Du Toit & Reissner, 2012). According to coaching theories and models that aim to develop self-awareness, an individual must have access to an empowering process that enhances their learning and development (Du Toit & Reissner, 2012; Lord et al., 2008). In the context of the MOW, the occupational therapist coaches their client to create a narrative of change that would enhance their OW.

The MOW strategy to facilitate effective change is achieved through developing a *narrative* that shows what is happening and what could potentially happen. The occupational therapist is called the *helper,* and the person who receives the helping service is called the *helpee.* The helper is the person who assists the individual who has identified they have a problem and is ready to ask for help/assistance in their learning and development process. The role of a helper in the context of the MOW is to collaborate, accompany, or coach. The word *helpee* is used to indicate the person's acceptance and readiness to go through the process of seeking assistance for rethinking and replanning their life. The level and nature of help is, however, identified and agreed upon between the occupational therapist and the client.

After entering helpees in a MOW-based intervention, evaluating the helpees' readiness for change is the first step in the intervention. Helpees who are ready to start the *change process* are those with a higher level of self-awareness about what they can or cannot do and with a clearer idea about what they value, idealize, and wish to do or not do to meet their needs for Being, Belonging, and Becoming. These people have identified the need for seeking help that is considered the first step of self-awareness and readiness for change. Helpees with little or no readiness for change need to be prepared for the change process before they can enter the MOW-based intervention. Through a collaborative relationship, the helper applies two main sets of strategies: empowering the person and changing the context so that it is enabling in order to facilitate the change that they plan together. Empowering a helpee is about emphasizing with clients/helpees and encouraging them to consider their capacities, knowledge, and skills that contribute to thinking, feeling, and Doings. Enabling involves identifying and employing facilitating resources, acknowledging the context, and encouraging and advocating social support.

Evaluating the Client and Developing an Intervention Plan

The MOW intervention starts from the point where the helper and helpee discuss the helpee's readiness for change. Developing the helpee's narrative and drawing Actual, Ideal, and consequently Tailored Triangles forms the structure of a MOW-based intervention. The Tailored Triangle is an indicator of the change that helper and helpee agree on, plan, and implement together. The change process consists of identifying where change is needed and how it can be achieved. The helpee's feelings, thinkings, and Doings and their interrelationships are explored to determine where change is needed and how it should proceed. Two crucial elements of sustainability of change are practice and reflection. The helper, therefore, needs to use strategies to assist the helpee in practicing and reflecting on the consequences of the changes on their 3Bs, their sense of OW, their satisfaction with themselves, their life, and their subjective experience of well-being.

To guide the helper's thinking and reasoning process, the MOW principles, which are described in the next section, should be applied throughout a helper–helpee encounter. Although the occupational therapist adheres to these principles, they need to borrow compatible strategies from other disciplines in the helping process.

Implementing the Intervention

The helpers use two main approaches throughout the intervention by:

1. Empowering helpees through encouragement and educating them to acquire the knowledge and skills that facilitate change
2. Refining the Context through enhancing opportunities and supportive resources and facilitating positive contextual contributors that provide enabling circumstances for the helpee's Doings

The MOW intervention relies heavily on the helper–helpee relationship and the narrative they create together. Therefore, strategies to develop the helper–helpee relationship are fundamental. The model of Intentional Relationships by Taylor (2008, 2020) is presented in an accessible textbook with scenarios and examples that apply to MOW-based occupational therapists to increase their knowledge and enhance their skills in developing and maintaining a helper–helpee relationship.

Drawing Triangles

Drawing triangles is a way to visualize at least part of the helpee's narrative, which facilitates self-awareness and helps specify what within the helpee's narrative is picked up to inform the change process. The helper and helpee then decide about the incongruence and disharmony between their AT and IT and agree on a Tailored Triangle (see Figure 38.4). Helpees need to determine the positively and negatively influencing aspects of the people within their Context and understand how they might affect the change process. The helper and helpee then discuss what they see that needs to be changed from both of their perspectives.

Asking Questions

The following questions are helpful in guiding the next step:

- How does the helpee feel about the situation?
- How does the helpee explain the situation, their own role, and the contextual roles of others in what is happening?
- What are the helpee's views on incongruence and disharmony?
- What does the helpee think about their ability to make change in the situation?
- What does the helpee predict as an outcome of change?
- What does the helpee expect from themselves and their context through the process of change?

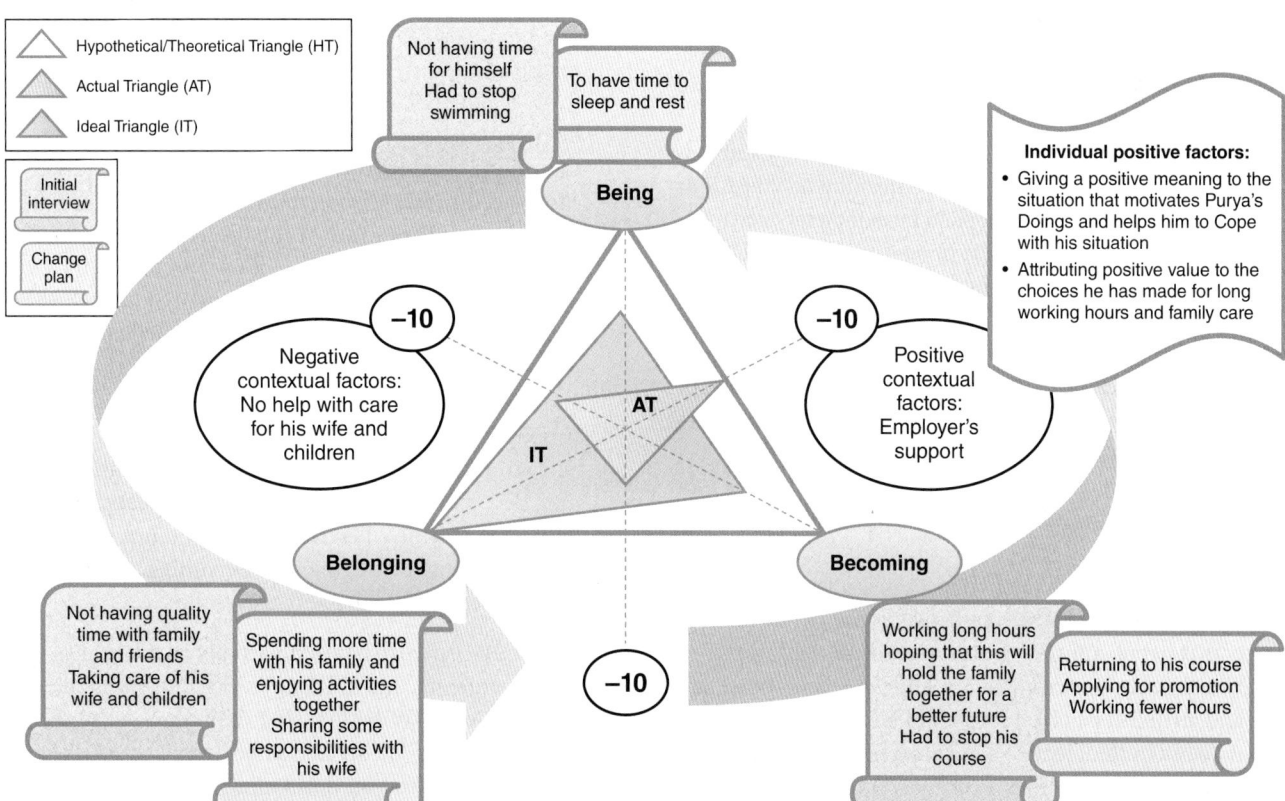

FIGURE 38.4 The helper and helpee investigate the incongruence between the helpee's actual and ideal triangles and agree on a Tailored Triangle (TT).

Finding answers to these questions enables the helper and helpee to identify and prioritize the problems.

Model of Occupational Wholeness Principles

To guide the helper's thinking and reasoning process, the MOW principles should be applied throughout a helper–helpee encounter.

1. The things people Do/Not Do contribute to meeting one, two, or more of their 3B needs.
   - The things people Do/Not Do that help to meet one of the 3Bs may conflict with meeting another need.
   - Choices people make for their Doings can have positive and negative consequences for their health and well-being.
   - An exaggerated and/or long-term skewed profile of Doings that is insufficient for meeting all 3B needs will lead to a decreased sense of OW and can potentially lead to health issues.
2. People's choices are limited by their personal capacities and by the resources of their Context.
   - People may make a choice to meet one 3B need, although this may overshadow the other needs.
   - There are realities of life, such as human capacities, contextual opportunities, outside demands, and occupational complexities, that limit human choices.
3. People not only make choices but also make and assign meanings to their choices.
   - Everyone encounters contextual and personal obligations that restrict options, opportunities, and choices.
   - A positive meaning-making of an obligation is healthier than not finding any meaning in obligations or considering obligations to be completely negative.
   - People attribute positive or negative values to their Doings and the meaning they have assigned to those Doings.
   - Positive meaning-making and attribution of positive values to Doings contribute to a sense of self-fulfillment, life satisfaction, and subjective well-being.
4. Occupational choices and meaning-making are not made just by individuals; they are also made in a social context.
   - Positive subjective experiences of a situation can help reduce the negative impact of some of the Doings that people must do because of social obligations.
5. Congruence between the IT and AT, their meanings, and attributions of values should be analyzed and evaluated in both objective and subjective ways.
   - Each individual has a unique profile representing combinations of Doings.

- The level of incongruence changes throughout one's life.
- A Tailored Triangle needs to be planned to help people achieve the best possible congruence.
- Long-term, skewed triangles can potentially impact health and well-being.
- The issues of time, stage of life, duration of events, and the meanings and values assigned to skewed situations are significant in relation to the degree of effect they have on life, health, and well-being.
- Although incongruence between a helpee's actual situation and their ideal situation is natural, a significant incongruence that is intensive and long term can put a helpee's health at risk.
- To feel well integrated, contented, and whole, people need to meet all their 3B needs to some extent.
- Harmony among *Doings* that serve the 3Bs is necessary for health and well-being.

6. The significance of self-awareness is important because OW might not be brought into consciousness automatically. In the context of subjective experience of well-being and health, it is necessary to help people become aware of the link between what they Do/Not Do and how their *Doings* within their context are associated with their needs of Being, Belonging, and Becoming. In other words, the sense of OW is achieved through the person's recognition of their Doings and the effects produced by them.
7. The aim of intervention is to raise the helpee's self-awareness about thinking, feeling, and Doings in relation to their Being, Belonging, and Becoming and their contextual factors. Through self-awareness, the helpee may be able to make changes toward meeting their needs and approaching a sense of wholeness. The *change* is the intervention in the MOW.
8. Changes in one or more of the helpee's 3Bs impact the others and their overall sense of OW. Although the outcome can be predicated to some extent, it never can be absolute because there are always unseen factors or interactions of factors that would influence the change and, consequently, the outcome.
9. If people have difficulty in making positive meanings and attributing positive values to their situation, they may become dissatisfied with themselves and/or their lives. This may be when their *Doings* do not meet their needs of Being, Belonging, and Becoming, or when the 3Bs are not in harmony with each other.

The MOW can also be used partially in relation to one or two components, and OT Story 38.4 illustrates the application of the MOW by focusing on Laura's sense of belonging and its impact on her subjective well-being. The intervention was based on developing a narrative through Laura's art piece as her Doing.

OT STORY 38.4 LAURA'S SENSE OF BELONGING

Laura is a painter from a family of Portuguese immigrants that lives in England. She feels she has become distanced from a Portuguese identity, but she does not feel entirely British either. This was an emotionally challenging situation for her as she felt she had to choose between the two, which provoked discomfort and, at times, anxiety in her. Through her artwork, Laura and her helper developed a narrative that empowered Laura to rethink her sense of Belonging. She discovered that she can choose and embrace values from both her family and the community she lives in. Laura realized that she had a choice and practiced her autonomy by taking control over what she wanted to feel connected to. Figure 38.5 shows Laura's AT before and after the MOW-based intervention, indicating the changes in her sense of being and belonging through her painting.

The painting in Figure 38.6A was painted before Laura's MOW intervention; she showed people shaded to match the colors of their homes. After the MOW intervention, her painting shown in Figure 38.6B shows the outcome of her

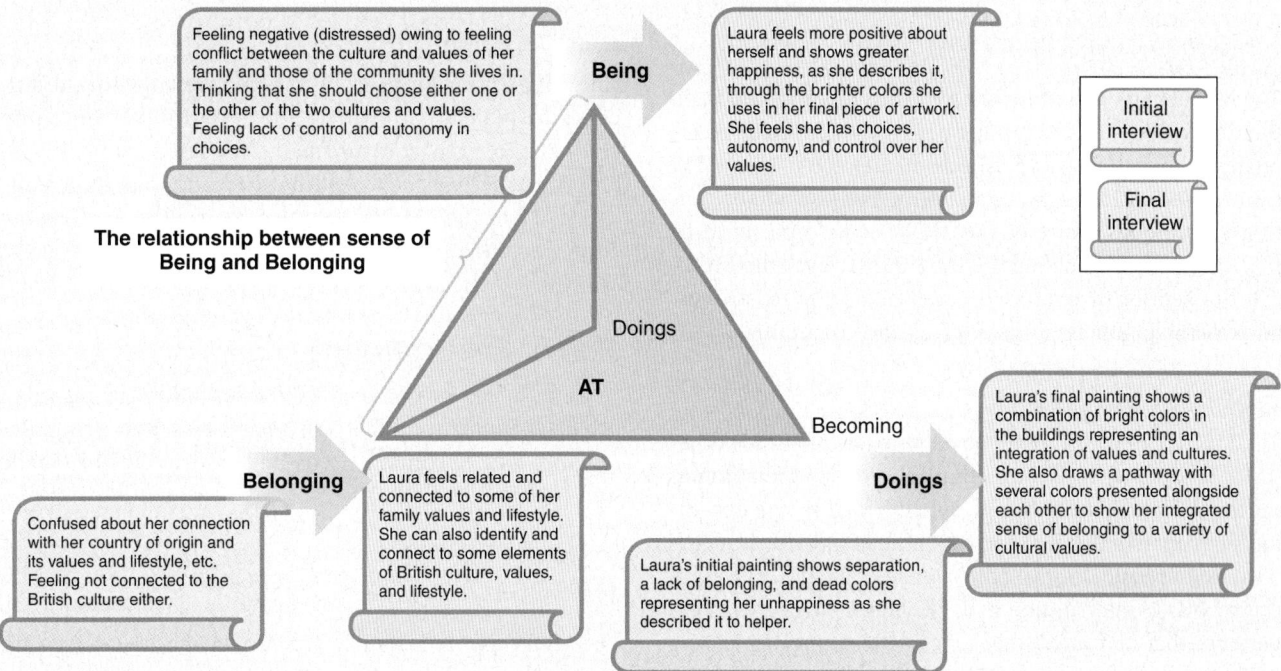

Being

Feeling negative (distressed) owing to feeling conflict between the culture and values of her family and those of the community she lives in. Thinking that she should choose either one or the other of the two cultures and values. Feeling lack of control and autonomy in choices.

Laura feels more positive about herself and shows greater happiness, as she describes it, through the brighter colors she uses in her final piece of artwork. She feels she has choices, autonomy, and control over her values.

Initial interview

Final interview

The relationship between sense of Being and Belonging

Doings

AT

Becoming

Belonging

Confused about her connection with her country of origin and its values and lifestyle, etc. Feeling not connected to the British culture either.

Laura feels related and connected to some of her family values and lifestyle. She can also identify and connect to some elements of British culture, values, and lifestyle.

Doings

Laura's final painting shows a combination of bright colors in the buildings representing an integration of values and cultures. She also draws a pathway with several colors presented alongside each other to show her integrated sense of belonging to a variety of cultural values.

Laura's initial painting shows separation, a lack of belonging, and dead colors representing her unhappiness as she described it to helper.

FIGURE 38.5 Laura's Actual Triangle showing her Being and Belonging relationship before and after the intervention. Gray scrolls show Laura's initial interview, and gold scrolls show her final interview.

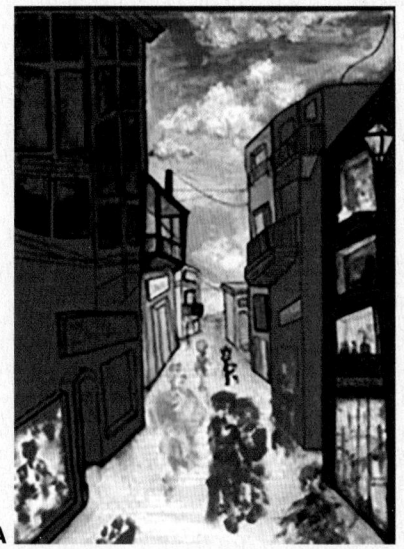
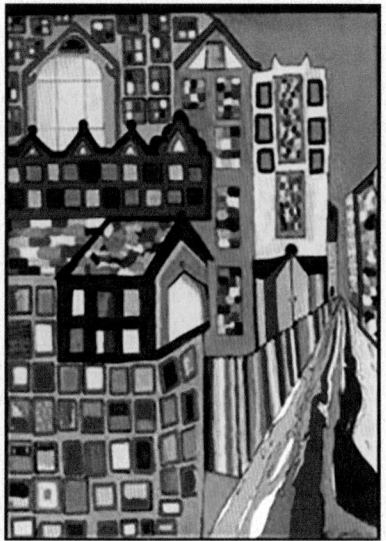

A   B

FIGURE 38.6 Laura's paintings (A) before and (B) after working with the Model of Occupational Wholeness.

(continued)

journey with a narrative she made with her helper that shows a road with all different colors going in the same direction and a city full of blended colors to illustrate an integrated sense of Belonging, bringing different lifestyles, cultures, and values together.

Questions

1. How would you explain the changes in Laura's sense of autonomy in choice-making in the beginning and at the end of the intervention?
2. How would you explain the impact of changes on Laura's sense of autonomy in choice-making on her sense of belonging?

Practice Settings

The MOW can be used for a wide range of populations, either individually or as a group, as long as their problems are related to one, two, or all aspects of their OW. The MOW can be used in inpatient, community, and educational settings. A unique feature of the MOW is its capacity to be implemented at a public level. At a public level, the MOW can be used for promoting the well-being, life satisfaction, and overall happiness of individuals and communities.

Hospital Setting

The MOW can be used in hospital settings, alongside other services patients receive, to rethink and replan their Doings during their hospitalization to aid with well-being. Becoming a patient in a hospital bed can limit an individual's sense of autonomy and control (their sense of Being). Hospitalization brings interruption in day-to-day Doings. It is an experience that may affect the sense of Belonging, depending on the period of time spent in the hospital, the regularity of visitors, and whether hospital facilities provide a connection to the outside world, such as a TV room. Hospitalization changes the way people connect and relate to others in and out of the hospital. Meaning-making determines the individual's thinking and feeling about an experience and hence the way that experience affects their sense of Being, Belonging, and Becoming. The effect of hospitalization on the sense of Becoming may be more complicated, and this depends on how a patient assigns meaning to it. For instance, an operation may aim to improve a person's function and, ultimately, enhance their Doings. Even if it causes interruptions to employment or education, it may be associated with hope for the future and perhaps a better sense of Becoming.

The MOW can also be used in discharge planning, when a patient needs to rethink and replan for their Doings considering the outcome of their hospitalization.

Educational Setting

The MOW can be used as a reflective tool to aid students to plan for university life. The MOW can equip students to take control, make educated choices, and identify whether they need help throughout their educational life. The MOW can also be used to explore the contextual factors in educational settings that affect Doings and the 3Bs.

Public Engagement

A unique feature of the MOW is its utility in planning projects to enhance public self-awareness about Being, Belonging, and Becoming needs and potentially the public well-being.

Assessing the Outcomes

The MOW uses reflection in order to review the changes and their impact of different components of the OW. The details of the reflective exercises and scoring triangles are beyond the scope of this chapter but are available in the book, *The model of occupational wholeness: Re-thinking, Re-planning.* (Yazdani, 2023).

The Occupational Wholeness Questionnaire (OWQ) may be used before and after the intervention as a reflection tool to aid with identifying the changes in overall sense of OW and in each component. Other assessment tools, such as Satisfaction with Life Scale (Diener et al., 1985), may be used to assess the changes in the person's life satisfaction and subjective well-being that, according to the MOW, are associated with a sense of OW. Further research is needed to investigate the usability of the OWQ in different settings and with different population and its sensitivity for measuring the changes on OW, being, belonging, and becoming.

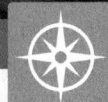

EXPANDING OUR PERSPECTIVES

The UnDoings of Occupational Wholeness: Understanding Substance Use as an Occupation

Jane A. Davis

As a student occupational therapist in the early 1990s, I did not learn about working with people living with substance use disorders; it was just a diagnosis in a book. Thus, when, after graduation, I found myself practicing as the first sole occupational therapist in a general hospital behavioral health inpatient unit in the United States, half dedicated to working with people living with substance use disorders, I was on my own to figure out my place. At the time, I did not know other occupational therapists who worked in this area, so I leaned on my unit colleagues to learn from them, many with lived experience, to understand the current views on substance use and addiction treatment.

The unit offered an abstinence-based program for women who were pregnant and ordered by the court to attend inpatient treatment. As a young occupational therapist who was brought up in a privileged, supportive family and community environment, their stories were in stark contrast to my reality. As such, I felt that it was most appropriate to act as a facilitator of resources, information, and conversations, so I created psychoeducation and life skills groups, as was typical at that time in mental health, facilitating discussions on various topics. I also applied my burgeoning occupational lens in offering individual sessions on activity scheduling and routines and child development.

In the ensuing years, I have reflected on my experiences working with these women and the many things I learned from them. My occupational lens, which has become much stronger, has led me to view substance use as an occupation that is linked to a constellation of other occupations. Although most would not conceptualize these occupations as holding positive meaning, these occupations, in their totality, not only constituted the Doings of the women with whom I worked but also the Being, Belonging, and Becoming; it was through engaging in their repertoire of occupations, dominated by those related to substance use, that they found their OW.

Many of these women lived in a context of understanding about themselves and their society that differed greatly to my own. As the program was founded on an abstinence philosophy, the women were immediately expected to rid themselves of their past repertoire, along with their sense of Being, Belonging, and Becoming, or OW. Although one could argue that this extreme change was needed to work toward well-being and for the well-being of their unborn child, I now view this process of complete unDoing as an implosion of their OW, without consideration of the significance of their past occupational repertoire and engagement in their lives. This perspective is not arguing for substance use as a lifestyle or while pregnant; instead, it speaks to the need for occupational therapists to consider how diverse occupational repertoires, often very different from our own, may compose a sense of OW for an individual, and that listening to and respecting the occupational lives of our clients may provide a structure for them to come to a point of readiness to explore their new sense of OW.

Evidence to Support Using the Model of Occupational Wholeness

The concept of OW was developed based on the author's research in investigating the concept of occupational balance (Yazdani et al., 2016, 2018). Later, the MOW was introduced in Yazdani and Bonsaksen (2017), and since then, a group of scholars from different countries has applied the MOW with their clients to explore its utility. Although some of these works have not been yet published in international journals, they have been disseminated locally where and when possible by these scholars. The development of the OWQ was one of the strategies that the author applied

for testing the MOW components. The first version of this questionnaire was tested and published by Bonsaksen and Yazdani (2018, 2020). Since then, further investigation has led to OWQ version II. The process of developing the questionnaire is reported in the OW book (Yazdani, 2023).

Mehdi Rezaee has applied the MOW in working with a client in a university well-being service. The client was diagnosed with anxiety and depression. Mehdi is a PhD holder and academic in the field of mental health, and, according to him, the MOW provided him with a means for enhancing his client's self-awareness about the huge incongruence between her AT and IT that seemed to feed into her depression (Yazdani, 2023).

Sarah Kufner from Germany applied the MOW in assisting a young autistic girl called Hannah who was unhappy about her life. Together, they developed her narrative

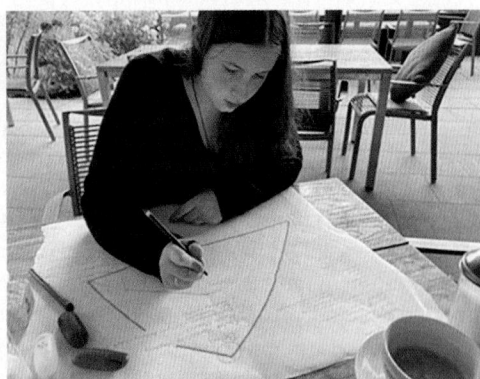

FIGURE 38.7 Hannah drawing her Model of Occupational Wholeness triangles.

using the triangles and identified the changes that could be made to aid Hannah to meet her 3B needs (Figure 38.7). According to Sarah, using strategies to facilitate trust and empowering Hannah to self-explore in a safe environment was the most effective part of the MOW intervention. Hannah said to Sarah that she started feeling more positive with the changes they had made in her Doings. She also said to Sarah that she found the MOW-based intervention a positive experience as it focused on what mattered to her.

Nadine Scholz-Schwärzler from Germany applied the MOW in an educational setting to address a team's dissatisfaction with their job. She said that using the triangles brought them together and facilitated a sense of Belonging when the team realized they have similarities in what has created the gap between their two Triangles.

A group of scholars also applied a MOW-based survey to investigate the perceived impact of the COVID-19 first isolation measure at the very beginning of the pandemic on their sense of Being, Belonging, and Becoming. The findings signified the difference between social participation and a sense of Belonging. During the pandemic isolation measures, even though people were restricted in their social engagement, gatherings, and participation, their sense of Belonging was perceived as strong. Making connections with people whom they had not been in touch with for a long time, taking care of others, providing support to each other, and developing a sense of cohesion against a common problem were among the contributing factors to people's perception of a stronger sense of Belonging (Yazdani, Nazi, et al., 2021; Yazdani, Rezaee, et al., 2021).

Conclusion

The MOW provides an assessment tool in the form of a drawing to explore the concepts of OW, Being, Belonging, Becoming, Doings, and Context in the ideal and actual situation of the person. To explain the link between these components and how they contribute to an overall sense of OW,

the MOW posits some principles. These principles not only are the means in unfolding people's narrative but also guide the intervention plan. The MOW intervention is strongly based on the helper and helpee relationship and the narrative they create together. Therefore, the occupational therapist in the role of helper requires a great knowledge of themselves, people, and skills in developing and maintaining a helper–helpee relationship. The MOW is in its very early stages of development, and so far, the MOW scholars have used it in educational, community, and public engagement projects. The next step for the MOW is to produce evidence to improve its applicability in a variety of settings and with different populations.

Lippincott® Connect *For additional resources on the subjects discussed in this chapter, visit Lippincott Connect.*

REFERENCES

Allen, K. A. (2020). *The psychology of belonging.* Routledge.

Bonsaksen, T., & Yazdani, F. (2018). Sociodemographic factors associated with the Norwegian occupational wholeness questionnaire scales. *Ergoscience, 13*(1), 21–27. https://doi.org/10.2443/skv-s-2018-54020180103

Bonsaksen, T., & Yazdani, F. (2020). The Norwegian occupational wholeness questionnaire (N-OWQ): Scale development and psychometric properties. *Scandinavian Journal of Occupational Therapy, 27*(1), 4–13. https://doi.org/10.1080/11038128.2018.1426783

Christiansen, C. H., & Matuska, K. M. (2006). Lifestyle balance: A review of concepts and research. *Journal of Occupational Science, 13*(1), 49–61. https://doi.org/10.1080/14427591.2006.9686570

Cutchin, M. P., Aldrich, R. M., Bailliard, A. L., & Coppola, S. (2008). Action theories for occupational science: The contributions of Dewey and Bourdieu. *Journal of Occupational Science, 15*(3), 157–165. https://doi.org/10.1080/14427591.2008.9686625

Deci, E. L., & Ryan, R. M. (2009). Self-determination theory: A consideration of human motivational universals. In P. J. Corr & G. Matthews (Eds.), *The Cambridge handbook of personality psychology* (pp. 234–240). Cambridge University Press.

Del Fabro Smith, L., Suto, M., Chalmers, A., & Backman, C. L. (2011). Belief in doing and knowledge in being mothers with arthritis. *OTJR: Occupation, Participation and Health, 31*(1), 40–48. https://doi.org/10.3928/15394492-20100222-01

Diener, E., Emmons, R. A., Larsen, R. J., & Griffin, S. (1985). The satisfaction with life scale. *Journal of Personality Assessment, 49*(1), 71–75. https://doi.org/10.1207/s15327752jpa4901_13

Duke, M. P. (1994). Chaos theory and psychology: Seven propositions. *Genetic Social and General Psychology Monographs, 120*(3), 265–265. https://www.scinapse.io/papers/6805653

Du Toit, A., & Reissner, S. (2012). Experiences of coaching in team leading. *International Journal of Mentoring and Coaching in Education, 1*(3), 177–190. https://doi.org/10.1108/20466851211279448

Glasser, W. (1975). *Reality therapy: A new approach to psychiatry* (Ser. Perennial library). Harper & Row.

Hammell, K. (2014). Belonging, occupation, and human well-being: An exploration: Appartenance, occupation et bien-être humain: Une étude exploratoire. *Canadian Journal of Occupational Therapy, 81*(1), 39–50. https://doi.org/10.1177/0008417413520489

Hitch, D., Pepin, G., & Karen, S. (2014). In the footsteps of Wilcock, part one: The evolution of doing, being, becoming, and belonging. *Occupational Therapy in Health Care, 28*(3), 231–246. https://doi.org/10.3109/07380577.2014.898114

Jiang, W. (2000). The relationship between culture and language. *ELT Journal, 54*(4), 328–334. https://doi.org/10.1093/elt/54.4.328

Khateeb, F. R. (2021). Work life balance—A review of theories, definitions and policies. *Cross Cultural Management Journal*, 27–55. https://seaopenresearch.eu/Journals/articles/CMJ2021_I1_3.pdf

Lord, P., Atkinson, M., & Mitchell, H. (2008). *Mentoring and coaching for professionals: A study of the research evidence.* National Foundation for Educational Research.

McInerney, D. M., Walker, R. A., & Liem, G. A. D. (2011). *Sociocultural theories of learning and motivation: Looking back, looking forward.* Information Age Pub.

Rogers, C. (1951). *Client-centered therapy.* Houghton Mifflin.

Taylor, R. R. (2008). *The intentional relationship: Occupational therapy and use of self.* F. A. Davis Company.

Taylor, R. R. (2020). *The intentional relationship: Occupational therapy and use of self* (2nd ed.). F. A. Davis.

van Huet, H., Innes, E., & Stancliffe, R. (2013). Occupational therapists perspectives of factors influencing chronic pain management. *Australian Occupational Therapy Journal, 60*(1), 56–65. https://doi.org/10.1111/1440-1630.12011

Vansteenkiste, M., Ryan, R. M., & Soenens, B. (2020). Basic psychological need theory: Advancements, critical themes, and future directions. *Motivation and Emotion, 44*(1), 1–31. https://doi.org/10.1007/s11031-019-09818-1

Wagman, P., Håkansson, C., & Björklund, A. (2012). Occupational balance as used in occupational therapy: A concept analysis. *Scandinavian Journal of Occupational Therapy, 19*(4), 322–327. https://doi.org/10.3109/11038128.2011.596219

Westhorp, P. (2003). Exploring balance as a concept in occupational science. *Journal of Occupational Science, 10*(2), 99–106. https://doi.org/10.1080/14427591.2003.9686516

Whitfield, G., & Davidson, A. (2016). *Cognitive behavioural therapy explained.* Taylor & Francis.

Wilcock, A. (1993). A theory of the human need for occupation. *Journal of Occupational Science, 1*(1), 17–24, https://doi.org/10.1080/14427591.1993.9686375

Wilcock, A. (2006). *An occupational perspective of health* (2nd ed.). SLACK Incorporated.

Yazdani, F. (2023). *The model of occupational wholeness: Re-thinking, Re-planning.* Taylor & Francis.

Yazdani, F., & Bonsaksen, T. (2017). Introduction to the model of occupational wholeness. *ErgoScience, 12*(1), 32–36. https://doi.org/10.2443/skv-s-2017-54020170104

Yazdani, F., Harb, A., Rassafiani, M., Nobakht, L., & *Yazdani*, N. (2018). Occupational therapists' perception of the concept of occupational balance. *Scandinavian Journal of Occupational Therapy, 25*(4), 288–297. https://doi.org/10.1080/11038128.2017.1325934

Yazdani, F., Nazi, S., Kavousipor, S., Karamali Esmaili, S., Rezaee, M., & Rassafiani, M. (2021). Does Covid-19 pandemic tell us something about time and space to meet our being, belonging and becoming needs? *Scandinavian Journal of Occupational Therapy*, 1–10. https://doi.org/10.1080/11038128.2021.1994644

Yazdani, F., Rezaee, M., Rassafiani, M., Roberts, D., Abu-Zurayk, W., & Amarlooee, M. (2021). The COVID-19 pandemic may force the world to reflect on the pre-pandemic style of life. *International Journal of Travel Medicine and Global Health, 9*(3), 124–131. https://doi.org/10.34172/ijtmgh.2021.21

Yazdani, F., Roberts, D., Yazdani, N., & Rassafiani, M. (2016). Occupational balance: A study of the sociocultural perspective of Iranian occupational therapists. *Canadian Journal of Occupational Therapy, 83*(1), 53–62. https://doi.org/10.1177/0008417415577973

Recovery Model

Skye Barbic and Krista Glowacki

LEARNING OBJECTIVES

After reading this chapter, you will be able to:

1. Describe contemporary perspectives on recovery in the mental health field.
2. Identify elements or components of the recovery process.
3. Integrate various frameworks or models of the recovery process.
4. Summarize approaches to measure recovery systematically in practice.
5. Apply recovery-oriented principles in occupational therapy practice.

Introduction

> The concept of recovery is rooted in the simple and yet profound realization that people who have been diagnosed with mental illness are human beings and can live fulfilling and meaningful lives. The goal is to become the unique, awesome, never to be repeated human being that we are called to be. Those of us who have been labeled with mental illness are not de facto excused from this fundamental task of becoming human. In fact, because many of us have experienced our lives and dreams shattered in the wake of mental illness, one of the most essential challenges that face us is to ask who can I become and why should I say yes to life. (Deegan, 1996, p. 92)

This opening quote is by Patricia Deegan (1996), who is widely credited with coining the term "recovery" to describe the phenomena whereby people come to live rich and meaningful lives while experiencing mental illness. As a person with lived experience of mental illness, Deegan provides a powerful real-life example of how recovery can unfold within a life situation characterized by despair, isolation, and deprivation. Deegan has poignantly described how mental health service providers have the power to be either insensitive and hardened or enabling and supportive of the journey that people with mental illness experience and embark on in determining "who to become" and in "saying yes to life." Indeed, becoming familiar with the range of Deegan's early writings and speeches might be considered foundational knowledge for occupational therapists learning about recovery (see, e.g., Deegan, 1988, 1990, 1996, 2001).

In this chapter, the reader is introduced to recovery as it is evolving in the field of mental health. **Multiple perspectives on recovery are**

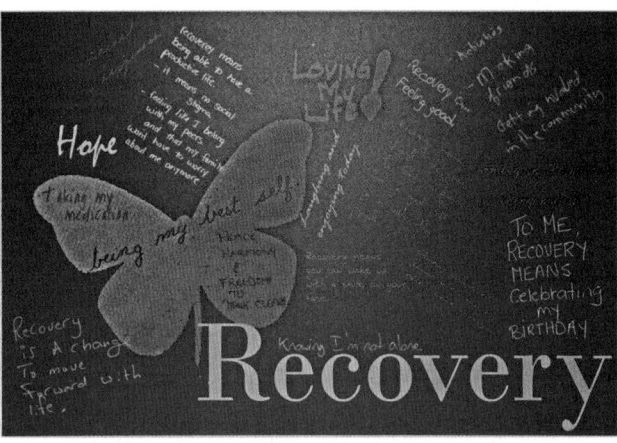

FIGURE 39.1 Recovery-oriented services create a vision of recovery that includes the voices of people served.

presented, but particular emphasis is placed on the perspectives of people with lived experience of mental illness (Figure 39.1). The recovery construct is not free of debate in the mental health field. Understanding the history surrounding recovery can position occupational therapists to better evaluate their own practice and to contribute to the ongoing evolution of the recovery vision and emerging science. This chapter includes the definitions of recovery, conceptual frameworks, and models of recovery and also includes a discussion of recovery in practice that reviews recovery intervention programs and issues related to evaluation. The final section of this chapter provides an overview of the relationship between recovery and occupational therapy (OT).

Overview of the Model: Defining Recovery

Recovery as a Personal Life Journey

In this chapter, **recovery** is defined as a process experienced by people with mental illness whereby they come to a life that is defined less by illness and pathology and defined more by a personal sense of purpose, agency and control, and active participation in valued and meaningful activities (Noordsy et al., 2002). The understanding of recovery as a *process* is important; it denotes an ongoing personal life journey, rather than an endpoint, or final outcome. As with everyone's life journey, it suggests that there will be ups and downs, high points and low points, and successes and failures. Yet the overarching expectation is that the journey of recovery will provide opportunities for greater well-being, positive growth, and community participation.

Slade (2009) refers to this as *personal recovery* acknowledging the process. Deegan stresses that service providers are not responsible for making people recover, but they can play an important role by creating conditions that will invite people to engage in the recovery journey and to help navigate the difficulties in the recovery process that will inevitably present (Deegan, 1988, 1996).

The U.S. Substance Abuse and Mental Health Services Administration (SAMHSA) describes four dimensions that support a person's recovery journey:

1. ***Health***: Overcoming or managing one's disease(s) or symptoms—for example, abstaining from use of alcohol, illicit drugs, and nonprescribed medications if one has an addiction problem—and, for everyone in recovery, making informed, healthy choices that support physical and emotional well-being
2. ***Home***: Having a stable and safe place to live
3. ***Purpose***: Conducting meaningful daily activities, such as a job, school, volunteerism, family caretaking, or creative endeavors, and the independence, income, and resources to participate in society
4. ***Community***: Having relationships and social networks that provide support, friendship, love, and hope

The dimensions resonate clearly with OT, where health is understood within the context of what is important and meaningful to a person. These dimensions also highlight that recovery is an ongoing process and requires regular evaluation of how personal, environmental, and occupational factors influence the recovery trajectory of a person. Finally, perhaps the most important point for consideration is that these dimensions are relevant to most people, regardless of whether a person is diagnosed with a mental illness or not. Del Vecchio (2012) describes the journey of recovery as highly personal, which may occur via many pathways and is characterized by continual growth and improvement in one's health and wellness.

As definitions of recovery emerge across research, practice, and policy, so too do reflections about what it means to be "recovery-oriented" as a health practitioner and how "recovery" can be influenced by culture and community. Some countries and health organizations have clear principles and guidelines about what it means to be recovery-oriented. These guidelines can provide a shared language about recovery to support clinical practice/policy and can provide a benchmark against which to measure service alignment with evidence-informed recovery-oriented practices (Mental Health Commission of Canada [MHCC], 2016). However, in order to be applicable, these guidelines and definitions must apply to the context of use in which occupational therapists and other service providers work. Considerations for culture, history, equity, and inclusion are critical to ensure the terms and their applications are meaningful to the diverse clients, families, and communities that occupational therapists have the privilege to work with.

Clinical/Medical Versus Personal Recovery

Outside of North America, recovery has gained international prominence as a guiding vision for the development of mental health services and systems. Yet, despite its influence, confusion persists, and there is no guarantee that discussions about recovery in mental health will start from a shared agreement about its meaning. One reason for the confusion is that definitions of recovery have emerged from many different sources, and the definitions can be very personal.

Clinical Recovery

Definitions of recovery that have emerged from mental health professionals have tended to focus on the improvement of the mental illness, measured by the reduction of symptoms and the need for intensive treatment services. Slade (2009) refers to this as a definition of "recovery as cure," whereas others refer to the medical model and recovery described as an endpoint of illness. Davidson and Roe (2007) suggest that *clinical interpretations* are perhaps best described as "recovery from mental illness," whereas *personal interpretations* are best described as "being in recovery." The ongoing confusion between personal and medical definitions of recovery has historical roots. OT Story 39.1 illustrates divergent views on the meaning of recovery and expectations regarding participation in occupations for persons with mental illness.

Personal Recovery

What can be referred to as *personal recovery* emerges from people with lived experience and, as discussed in previous sections of this chapter, is an ongoing journey and process rather than an end goal. Davidson and Roe (2007) acknowledge *personal interpretations* as "being in recovery." The assumptions underlying personal recovery—that people with mental illness can be largely in control of managing their illnesses, that effective illness management strategies exist outside the realm of the authority of mental health professionals, and that people with mental illness can enjoy a life of inclusion in their communities—have been largely overlooked and, at worst, depreciated. Davidson et al. (2010), in their study of the historical roots of the recovery movement, pointed out that although other branches of healthcare have largely accepted that people who experience chronic forms of disease or significant disability should not "put their lives on hold until the illness resolves" (p. 4), this notion has not received the same broad acceptance in the mental health service arena.

Recovery as a Citizenship Movement

Another perspective on recovery, perhaps of increasing relevance in today's culture, is the argument that definitions of recovery have been highly individualistic and ultimately unable to integrate the influence of exceptional levels of disadvantage and marginalization that characterize the social

OT STORY 39.1 "THE PEOPLE WE SERVE ARE TOO SICK TO WORK"

Shandra, an occupational therapist, works for a community mental health program that is focused on helping people with serious mental illness (SMI) to live successfully in the community. At their annual retreat, the agency set aside time to discuss practices related to employment and other vocational or productive activities. Shandra examined the employment and productive participation of the people receiving services and informed the team that fewer than 15% of the 90 people served identified any regular involvement in productive activities, such as work, school, or volunteering. During the ensuing discussion, team members made comments such as "the people we serve are too sick to work," "we don't have the time or resources to focus on work—that isn't our job," "no one I work with has said they want to work," and "work will make their symptoms flare up." The team encouraged Shandra to follow up on her interest in employment and productivity but left the discussions without any firm plans for follow-up.

Questions

1. Evaluate the service response to the issue of employment and productivity with respect to contemporary perspectives on recovery.
2. Shandra decides to give some thought to how she might respond to this discussion, so that she can facilitate a shift to more recovery-oriented services. What might she say to challenge the idea that addressing employment and productivity is not within the scope of the service?
3. The OT Story does not reflect the voices of people with mental illness. How might Shandra engage their involvement in this discussion about employment and productivity?
4. How is the language of Shandra's colleagues stigmatizing for people with mental illness? How might she address her concern of this language with her colleagues?

position of people with mental illness. From this perspective, it is argued that people with mental illness in their recovery process encounter injustices embedded within social structures, such as discrimination, oppressive public policies, and social segregation. Social perspectives on recovery highlight the extent to which the daily lives of people with SMI are characterized by conditions of social and economic poverty, marginalization, and stigma. There is evidence to support that these social and financial strains will have a negative impact on the recovery process (Mattsson et al., 2008; Pelletier et al., 2015). Marginalization can be amplified in some cultural groups. A systematic review of Asian Americans, Black Americans, and Latinx Americans found that public stigma led to service barriers, and families in these groups were more likely to conceal mental illness (Misra et al., 2021).

From this social perspective, recovery is conceptualized as a civil rights movement focused on securing full citizenship rights and responsibilities for people with mental illness.

Drawing from the "build back better" approach to post-disaster recovery, scholars such as Whalley Hammell (2021) imagine a post-COVID-19 recovery world that considers dual attention to recovery and to environmental vulnerabilities. Whalley Hammell argues that:

> Occupational therapy for a post-COVID-19 world; an occupational therapy that takes seriously the premise that occupations and people are inseparable from their environments; a profession that no longer colludes in individualizing problems that are inherently social or in depoliticising the systemic social and economic inequalities that create stress and illness; an occupational therapy that no longer promotes the values of neoliberal ableism; and an occupational therapy dedicated to expanding people's just and equitable opportunities to engage in meaningful occupations that contribute positively to their own wellbeing and the wellbeing of their communities. (p. 444)

The Definition Matters

The definition of recovery does matter—a great deal. With recovery being adapted as a guiding vision for mental health services in many jurisdictions, the definition selected will ultimately influence how human and material resources are distributed, how success in the system will be evaluated, and what kinds of service activities and supports will be expected. The choice of definition is the foundation from which communication can take place.

The perspective of personal recovery offers an important opportunity for a fundamental transformation in the mental health service arena toward an integrated system that is able to address illness, health, well-being, and citizenship in a synergistic fashion. In response to this challenge, efforts have been directed to describing how the concepts and ideals of personal recovery can be translated to reform service delivery and service systems, avoiding the very real risk that conflicting perspectives on recovery will lead to the conclusion that only small tweaks are required or, worse, that recovery-oriented practices are already in place. Without clear guidelines for what recovery services look like, it is easy for systems to pay lip service to the philosophy of recovery. However, Tondora and Davidson (2006) and Davidson et al. (2007) have advanced practice guidelines to direct the development of recovery-oriented services and to identify what people in recovery should expect from the mental health service system. In some countries, evidence-based guidelines for recovery-oriented practice exist such as in Canada (MHCC, 2016). Moreover, Barbic (2016) has advanced practice by working with people with lived experience to conceptualize recovery as a linear continuum and map the types of evidence-based services that a person could consider.

Recovery Frameworks or Models

To date, no single theory or conceptual model of recovery has been universally accepted and used, but the mental health field is replete with systematic efforts to capture critical elements of an overarching framework for recovery.

OT STORY 39.2 RECOVERY IN THE COMMUNITY

Priyanka, an occupational therapist, works for an assertive community treatment (ACT) team that focuses on helping people with SMI to live successfully in the community. In preparation for their staff meeting, Priyanka's manager asks her to present to her team about the types of services OT can provide for a person in recovery.

Questions

1. In preparation for this presentation, Priyanka decides to meet with some of her clients to ask them what their recovery journey looks like. If recovery can be mapped as a continuum from low to high, what might Priyanka's clients say to describe what high (optimal) recovery looks like? What might low levels of recovery look like?

2. What types of OT assessments are available to evaluate Priyanka's clients as they move along their recovery journey from low to high?

3. What types of evidence-based OT interventions exist to support Priyanka's clients along the recovery journey?

4. What can Priyanka tell their team about the value of OT services to support individuals receiving ACT services?

Empirically constructed conceptualizations of the personal recovery process incorporate a common understanding of the components or elements of the recovery process and the phases and tasks central to the process. See OT Story 39.2.

Elements of the Recovery Process

Based on an analysis of published qualitative accounts of recovery, Davidson (2005) identified and described elements that appear common to the experience of the recovery process, including:

- Renewing hope and commitment
- Redefining self
- Incorporating illness
- Being involved in meaningful activities
- Overcoming stigma
- Assuming control
- Becoming empowered
- Exercising citizenship
- Managing symptoms
- Being supported by others

The elements provide an understanding of the nature of the personal transformations that are experienced in the recovery process. The renewal of hope provides the individual with a growing sense that the future holds possibilities. The individual develops a growing sense that the illness need not be the defining feature of their identity; there are other stories about the self that are waiting to be explored and developed. A transition from passive acceptance

of circumstances to a growing sense of control and personal agency occurs. The illness experience is not ignored but becomes integrated into this broader view of the self and the self in the world. The sense of personal agency, or self-determination, is extended to developing a personal understanding of the illness that supports these processes of growth and change and the development of strategies to manage the illness experience. The critical elements include actions that connect the individual to living a full life in the broader community.

The 10 components of recovery identified in the *National Consensus Statement on Mental Health Recovery* by the SAMHSA (2006) have similarities to those proposed by Davidson (2005) but are written more from a perspective that guides mental health service delivery and the design of service systems (Box 39.1). The components highlight important elements of the mental health service system, such as peer support. At its core, the recovery process reflects a release of strengths and a growth of abilities, capacities, and possibilities that should be valued and nurtured by others. All of the components are interdependent and act synergistically toward the goal of recovery (Figure 39.2). The consensus statement concludes with a powerful statement that recovery benefits not only the individual in recovery but also society. See OT Story 39.3.

Leamy and colleagues undertook a systematic review and modified narrative synthesis on personal recovery and used it to create a conceptual framework for recovery (Leamy et al., 2011). A total of 87 distinct studies and 10 elaborating papers were included, and the studies were conducted in 13 countries, including the United States ($n = 50$), the United

OT STORY 39.3 LEARNING TO TAKE THE BUS

This is a true story told from the perspective of the fieldwork supervisor who oversaw the student's experience.

Lenora attends a community support program in a medium-sized city in the Midwestern United States. Several years ago, the program underwent major changes, adopting many recovery-oriented principles and services. Rachel is doing her level II fieldwork at the program and received a referral for Lenora from her case manager. After conducting the Canadian Occupational Performance Profile, Rachel learns that Lenora is interested in learning how to ride the bus from home to the community support program. However, there's a problem. Lenora currently lives with her parents who tend to be very protective and drive her to the program when she plans to attend. Lenora knows that her parents will be opposed to her taking the bus. Before moving forward, Rachel sets up a meeting with Lenora and her parents. Lenora is very uneasy about the meeting, but Rachel and Lenora role-play the scenario so that Lenora

can gain confidence in asserting her desire to be more independent. Although they still have reservations, the parents become supportive based on Lenora's enthusiasm and Rachel's assurance that she will work with Lenora until both are convinced that she can manage the trip on her own. After several trial runs, Lenora learns to ride the bus to the community support program and eventually is able to take the bus to additional locations. She talks about how this experience was a major turning point in her life and uses the word "empowered" to describe her newfound sense of freedom.

Questions

1. What elements of the recovery process are illustrated by this story?
2. What if Lenora's parents remained opposed to the idea? How might you have handled the situation as Lenora's occupational therapist?

BOX 39.1 NATIONAL CONSENSUS STATEMENT ON MENTAL HEALTH RECOVERY: THE 10 FUNDAMENTAL COMPONENTS OF RECOVERY

1. *Self-direction:* Consumers lead, control, exercise choice over and determine their own path of recovery by optimizing autonomy, independence, and control of resources to achieve a self-determined life. By definition, the recovery process must be self-directed by the individual, who defines his or her own life goals and designs a unique path toward those goals.
2. *Individualized and person-centered:* There are multiple pathways to recovery based on an individual's unique strengths and resiliencies as well as his or her needs, preferences, experiences (including past trauma), and cultural background in all of its diverse representations. Individuals also identify recovery as being an ongoing journey and an end result as well as an overall paradigm for achieving wellness and optimal mental health.
3. *Empowerment:* Consumers have the authority to choose from a range of options and to participate in all decisions—including the allocation of resources—that will affect their lives, and they are educated and supported in so doing. They have the ability to join with other consumers to collectively and effectively speak for themselves about their needs, wants, desires, and aspirations. Through empowerment, an individual gains control of his or her own destiny and influences the organizational and societal structures in his or her life.
4. *Holistic:* Recovery encompasses an individual's whole life, including mind, body, spirit, and community. Recovery embraces all aspects of life, including housing, employment, education, mental health and healthcare treatment and services, complementary and alternative health services, addictions treatment, spirituality, creativity, social networks, community participation, and family supports as determined by the person. Families, providers, organizations, systems, communities, and society play crucial roles in creating and maintaining meaningful opportunities for consumer access to these supports.
5. *Nonlinear:* Recovery is not a step-by-step process but one based on continual growth, occasional setbacks, and learning from experience. Recovery begins with an initial stage of awareness in which a person recognizes that positive change is possible. This awareness enables the consumer to move on to fully engage in the work of recovery.
6. *Strengths-based:* Recovery focuses on valuing and building on the multiple capacities, resiliencies, talents, coping abilities, and inherent worth of individuals. By building on these strengths, consumers leave stymied life roles behind and engage in new life roles (e.g., partner, caregiver, friend, student, employee). The process of recovery moves forward through interaction with others in supportive, trust-based relationships.
7. *Peer support:* Mutual support—including the sharing of experiential knowledge and skills and social learning—plays an invaluable role in recovery. Consumers encourage and engage other consumers in recovery and provide each other with a sense of belonging, supportive relationships, valued roles, and community.
8. *Respect:* Community, systems, and societal acceptance and appreciation of consumers—including protecting their rights and eliminating discrimination and stigma—are crucial in achieving recovery. Self-acceptance and regaining belief in one's self are particularly vital. Respect ensures the inclusion and full participation of consumers in all aspects of their lives.
9. *Responsibility:* Consumers have a personal responsibility for their own self-care and journeys of recovery. Taking steps toward their goals may require great courage. Consumers must strive to understand and give meaning to their experiences and identify coping strategies and healing processes to promote their own wellness.
10. *Hope:* Recovery provides the essential and motivating message of a better future—that people can and do overcome the barriers and obstacles that confront them. Hope is internalized but can be fostered by peers, families, friends, providers, and others. Hope is the catalyst of the recovery process. Mental health recovery not only benefits individuals with mental health disabilities by focusing on their abilities to live, work, learn, and fully participate in our society but also enriches the texture of American community life. America reaps the benefits of the contributions individuals with mental disabilities can make, ultimately becoming a stronger and healthier nation.

Kingdom ($n = 20$), Australia ($n = 8$), and Canada ($n = 6$). This includes the analysis of published qualitative accounts of recovery originally published by Davidson (2005).

Based on the review and analysis, Leamy's team (2011) identified and described characteristics of the recovery journey present in all studies:

- Recovery is an active process
- Individual and unique process
- Nonlinear process
- Recovery as a journey
- Recovery as stages or phases
- Recovery as a struggle

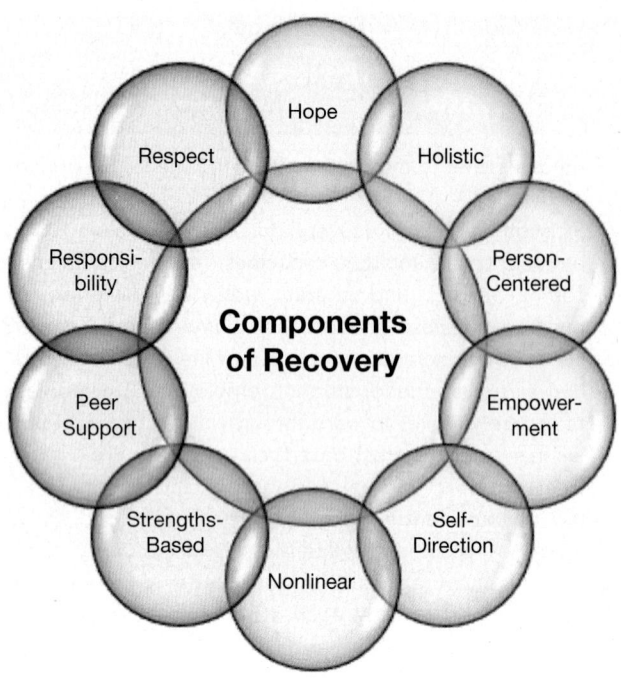

FIGURE 39.2 **A synergistic model of recovery.**

- Multidimensional process
- Recovery is a gradual process
- Recovery as a life-changing experience
- Recovery without cure
- Recovery is aided by supportive and healing environment
- Recovery can occur without professional intervention
- Trial and error process

Leamy et al. (2011) also identified and described categories of the recovery process using the acronym CHIME:

> *Connectedness*: Includes peer-support and support groups, relationships, support from others, and being part of a community
>
> *Hope and optimism about the future:* Includes belief in the possibility of recovery, motivation to change, hope-inspiring relationships, positive thinking and valuing success, having dreams and aspirations
>
> *Identify:* Includes dimensions of identity, rebuilding/redefining positive sense of identity, overcoming stigma
>
> *Meaning in life:* Includes the meaning of mental illness experiences, spirituality, quality of life, meaningful life and social roles/goals, rebuilding life
>
> *Empowerment:* Includes personal responsibility, control over life, focusing on strengths

Stage and Task Models of Recovery

There have been several efforts to understand how the recovery process unfolds and how the various defined elements of the process are related to each other over time. These have led to the development of several stage models of the process, largely developed empirically from persons in recovery (see Andresen et al. [2003] for an integrated review of several stage models).

One such model was developed by people with lived experience of mental illness who are considered leaders across the United States in their roles as members of a Recovery Advisory Group (Ralph, 2005). They described a six-stage model of the recovery process:

1. *Anguish,* described as an experience of despair related to the accepted label of "mentally ill"
2. *Awakening,* reflecting the beginning sense that things can change
3. *Insight* or the growing understanding and personalization of possibilities of change
4. *Action planning,* reflecting the increase in doing toward well-being and meaning
5. *Determined commitment to become well,* describing the growing resolution for action and self-determination
6. *Well-being and empowerment,* an experience of belief in the self to help the self and others.

A particularly helpful feature of the model is the inclusion of specific domains of change—four internal (occurring within the self) and four external (responses or actions)—and descriptions of changes that occur in these domains across the six stages.

Another example of a linear model of recovery is that developed from the Canadian Personal Recovery Outcome Measurement study led by Barbic (2016). In this model, a set of indicators are hypothesized to reflect a person's journey of recovery from low to high. The model summarizes a hierarchy of items that describe basic requirements for recovery (such as safety, resources, hope), moderate needs (energy, goals, purpose), and high needs (contribution to the community, intimacy, peace of mind). The model has also been used to guide the development of a 30-item measure of personal recovery called the Canadian Personal Recovery Outcome Measure (C-PROM) (Barbic, 2016).

Although stage models advance our understanding and provide empirical support for the recovery process, they are inherently problematic. If we are to conceptualize recovery as an individual and nonlinear process, then how can defining moments of the recovery process be ordered in any sort of generalizable way? In addition, outside forces such as stigma, discrimination, and marginalization might interfere with a staged process. The field will need to evaluate how stage models capture the range of expressions of recovery, and perhaps a staged approach needs to be considered iterative in which a person can move back and forth between stages throughout their journey of recovery.

In contrast to stage models, Slade (2009) proposed a model of recovery based on the tasks that people are engaged in over the course of the recovery process. The tasks are highly consistent with empirically derived elements of recovery, account for recovery as both an internal process and a process that is positioned within a larger social environment, and are only loosely ordered, acknowledging considerable individual variability. The four tasks include:

1. Developing a positive identity
2. Framing the mental illness
3. Self-managing the illness
4. Developing valued social roles

As shown in Table 39.1, each of these tasks requires personal work ranging from changing one's own self-perception to the development of expertise and supports needed to manage the mental illness within the broader context of one's life.

Recovery in Practice

Recovery-oriented practice is not considered the domain of any one discipline or professional group. Rather, efforts to instill a recovery-oriented vision in our mental health systems have depended on all providers to consider their own practice with respect to the evolving understanding of recovery processes. The relationship between recovery and OT is reciprocal. OT can contribute to the growing knowledge and evidence base of recovery, and recovery concepts can inform OT practice.

Many occupational therapists have actively contributed to efforts to realize the vision of recovery in the mental health services sector. They work in diverse settings such as community treatment teams to promote recovery-oriented principles. Occupational therapists have served as study leads and investigators on research advancing our understanding of recovery. Occupational therapists have been hired to serve as recovery facilitators to assist mental health

organizations in achieving the difficult transformation to recovery-oriented care. Occupational therapists have worked in close collaboration with groups of individuals with lived and living experience to advocate for and implement structures that ensure their meaningful involvement in creating recovery-oriented practices, services, and systems.

Of particular interest in this chapter, however, is the consideration of how the distinct knowledge and practice base of the OT profession might contribute to the ongoing evolution of recovery. From this perspective, the question engages occupational therapists in considering how their particular focus on their domain of concern—occupation—can advance recovery knowledge and practice. The connection between occupation and recovery is explicit, given that participation in personally and socially meaningful activities and roles has been considered a critical element of the recovery process. Davidson and colleagues (2010) in their history of the roots of the recovery movement express that participation in the everyday but meaningful activities of daily life is not the outcome of recovery but rather the foundation of recovery. Consistent with OT theory and practice, the authors contend that the recovery process can be positively influenced by the actual doing of activities, particularly when supported by others in their engagement in occupations. Lamenting the loss of attention to activity-based approaches within the mental health service system with the closure of psychiatric hospitals, they suggest, "There currently are glimmers of hope that the recovery movement may bring about a bit of renaissance of OT and science within psychiatry" and state they would "heartily welcome such a development, and suggest that the recovery movement would have much to learn from this discipline" (Davidson et al., 2010, p. 237). The remainder of this section describes how occupational therapists have or could advance their expertise in the area of occupation to further the vision of recovery.

Contextualizing care planning in a person's goals is increasingly becoming best practice on most community mental health teams. Increased research has focused on the importance of recovery plans to be strengths focused. Xie (2013) highlights that strengths-based approaches to recovery planning move the focus away from the deficits of people with mental illnesses (consumers) and to the strengths and resources of the person receiving services. The implications of this approach have been shown to improve outcomes such as client engagement, functioning, satisfaction with care, and quality of life (Lyons et al., 2000; Rapp & Goscha, 2012; Rust et al., 2009).

An important systematic review of other occupation- or activity-based interventions examines the extent to which these interventions lead to positive changes in areas of community integration and normative life roles for adults with SMI (Gibson et al., 2011). The study considered a range of

TABLE 39.1 Slade's Task Model of Recovery

Task	Personal Work Involved
Developing a positive identity	Developing a multifaceted view of a valued sense of self
Framing the mental illness	Making sense of the illness experience as an important challenge to be negotiated within the context of important broader life experiences
Self-managing the illness	Developing expertise in controlling the experience of mental illness
Developing valued social roles	Connecting to others and the broader world through personally and socially valued activities

interventions from training in social skills to instrumental activities of daily living (IADLs) and life skills training and role development. Not all interventions were developed specifically by occupational therapists (e.g., supported employment and education and neurocognitive training), but all interventions were considered within the OT scope of practice. The review suggested that the evidence for social skills training was strong, whereas the evidence supporting the effectiveness of neurocognitive training paired with skills training across domains of occupational performance and training in life skills and IADLs was only moderate. The review provides a valuable summary of evidence-based, occupation-focused interventions and perhaps offers a prototype for how a range of seemingly disparate interventions might be organized conceptually within the framework of recovery.

People with mental illness frequently experience profound disruptions in both their performance of important occupations and their experience of these occupations. Descriptions of the nature of these disruptions are being advanced by the profession with a view to connecting the experience of occupations closely with intervention and support approaches. For example, an individual whose occupational patterns are characterized by an exceptional lack of involvement might best be characterized as disengagement or difficulties associated with emotional detachment, or it might be more characterized by deprivation or exceptional levels of disadvantage with respect to opportunities (Krupa et al., 2009). In the former case, the individual in recovery and the therapist might work together to identify and build sources of meaning in occupation, whereas in the latter, they might assertively organize opportunities and resources of occupation. Developing ways to talk directly about occupation is important for the evolution of recovery as a guiding vision for mental health service delivery. It can provide a way to describe people who experience mental illness as social and community beings rather than focusing on illness and pathology. Rebeiro Gruhl (2008) suggests that the occupational issues facing people with SMI need to be conceptualized as an issue of occupational injustice, highlighting that social and structural issues constrain and restrict their occupational lives and that this needs to be reconciled if the recovery vision in mental health is to be realized. These highlight the importance of advocacy as a fundamental element of OT practice within a recovery framework.

For a personal reflection on recovery, see "Expanding Our Perspectives" section.

EXPANDING OUR PERSPECTIVES

Recovery Is a Choice I Make Every Day

Erin Connor

Developing and Implementing Recovery Interventions

I was 15 years old the first time I wrote a poem about wanting to die. My journal at that age was filled with all the typical teenage angst, but if you looked closer you would be able to see that I was in a lot of emotional pain. Unfortunately, I was also exceptionally good at hiding it, a lovely gift that I developed out of self-preservation and desperately needing to be liked. I will spare you the details of how I came to be suicidal before I even learned how to drive, but I will say that anyone who knew me outwardly at that stage of my life would have been shocked to learn this truth about me.

My journey toward recovery has brought me a richness of experiences of life that on my good days I feel lucky to have had and on my not so good days makes me feel targeted and incapable. I have lived with Depression and post traumatic stress disorder (PTSD) most of my life, although I was not always aware that this is what was happening. I was very convinced for many years that I was just broken and that if I did not find some way to hide that from others, I was doomed to a life of loneliness. So, I plastered on a great big smile, got exceptionally good at telling people what they wanted to hear, and steered my life in the direction of helping others. Because if I were helping others, then no one would look at all the things that were wrong with me.

I remember very vividly this intense conversation I had with my mother when I was about 21 years. I had been working in a residential treatment facility for troubled youth, and it had started to tug at all the things I had been burying for many years for fear that those parts of me were unlovable. I was trying to explain to her that I did not want to go to a family friends' gathering because I did not feel like I fit in with the people who were going. She could not understand what I meant. I insisted louder and louder that I did not fit there, that I did not fit anywhere. My mother turned to me and said "Honey, you fit in EVERYWHERE." I realized then I had worked so hard at my bubbly and perky exterior that even my own mother was convinced that I was that person. I broke down and told her everything, and she was amazing. She listened, she held me, she shared some of her own experiences. It was rough . . . but it was also an immense relief.

I finally realized that I had to make my own choice to let someone else in, to take the risk that they could tolerate the parts of me that I decided were not acceptable. It was humbling to realize that the person who was standing in

EXPANDING OUR PERSPECTIVES (*continued*)

my way was me the whole time. The experience of acknowledging my mental health issues, accepting my diagnoses, and making the choice to get myself help was deeply empowering. It was also scary to accept that this would be a lifelong learning experience for me. Recovery for me is not about an endgame state of perpetual happiness. It is not a hierarchy of skills that once I have attained means I am all better. Every time I get arrogant enough to say I am "fully recovered," the

universe has a curveball to remind me to stay grounded in my self-awareness. Recovery is a choice I make every day. Honesty is a choice I make every day. Intimacy is a choice I must make every day. Sometimes, I choose healthy things, sometimes I do not. It has only been through allowing myself to be open and vulnerable; to risk someone finding out that I am not always the best version of myself that has allowed real Recovery to be possible. You have to choose to love yourself.

Various intervention approaches and strategies have been developed in response to the growing understanding of the recovery process. Evidence demonstrating the effectiveness of these strategies is emerging. Generally, these intervention approaches attempt to operationalize key elements of recovery-oriented practice. The *Recovery Workbook* (Spaniol et al., 1994) takes individuals with mental illness through a series of activities meant to increase their awareness of recovery, increase their knowledge about and control of psychiatric conditions, understand the importance of stress, build a meaningful and enjoyable life and personal supports, and begin to develop sustained plans of action. A pilot research study, using a randomized controlled trial design, evaluated the effectiveness of a modified version of the workbook that shortened the 30 weekly sessions to 12 sessions. Findings suggested that participants experienced positive changes in perceived levels of hope, empowerment, and general measures of recovery (Barbic et al., 2009). The well-known *Wellness Recovery Action Plan* (Copeland, 1997) engages people with mental illness in activities designed to identify and implement personalized wellness strategies and raise awareness of benefits of peer support. A large-scale study using randomized controlled trials demonstrated positive changes in experiences of psychiatric symptoms, increased levels of hopefulness, and enhanced quality of life (Cook et al., 2012).

The Illness Management and Recovery intervention program uses a series of activities based on five practices for teaching illness self-management, including psychoeducation, behavioral training focused on integrating medications into daily routines, relapse prevention planning, coping skills training, and social skills training to enhance social support (Gingerich & Mueser, 2005). A randomized controlled trial of the intervention program suggested that participants experienced improvements in illness self-management, as evaluated by both self and clinician ratings (Levitt et al., 2009). Evidence exists to support an OT-based intervention called "Action Over Inertia" (Krupa et al., 2010) that aims to allow individuals with mental illness to increase their activity engagement and community participation. To date, the authors have shown evidence for

the intervention based on how peoples' time-use patterns have changed to be more reflective of patterns associated with health and well-being (Edgelow & Krupa, 2011).

Peer-support services are a vital component of recovery-oriented intervention. Peer support occurs when people with a lived experience of mental illness provide help and support to others with a shared experience of mental illness (Shalaby & Agyapon, 2020). In recent years, the encouragement of informal support has evolved to systems employing peer-support providers in specific positions within systems of care. Peer-support providers may assume positions such as case manager, group leader, or personal care provider. Research indicates there are benefits for service recipients and providers alike related to quality of life, empowerment, and wellness.

In another example, organizations arising from people with a lived experience are providing de-medicalized and self-determined acceptance of what is typically pathologized in the majority culture. The Hearing Voices Movement, which began in Holland (Higgs, 2020), is a loose, grassroots organization with local chapters that aims to change perception of voice-hearing, reduce stigma, and provide spaces for people to share personal experiences. Hearing Voices Groups are sessions with different formats and leadership but all provide peer support related to acceptance of living with the experience of hearing voices (Hearing Voices, n.d.).

Physical Activity and Recovery

Physical activity can play an important role for health outcomes and to promote some of the characteristics of personal recovery discussed earlier in this chapter. Exercise (a subset of physical activity that is structured, planned, and done for the purpose of maintaining or improving health and/or fitness) has been shown to improve quality of life (Schuch et al., 2016) as well as reduce symptoms for people living with depression (Morres et al., 2019). Individuals with mental illness have a life expectancy of 12 to 15 years less than the general population and are at a higher risk of developing chronic conditions, such as diabetes and heart disease; exercise reduces this risk (Richardson et al., 2005; Rosenbaum et al., 2014). If done with others, physical activity can provide opportunity for social interaction and the development of social skills. It can also provide opportunity for people to set and achieve goals, to engage in meaningful and purposeful activity, and to provide structure to the day. Such opportunities can promote confidence and a sense of achievement, which can help to promote recovery and improve mental health (Craft, 2013).

When considering physical activity in the context of mental health and recovery, it is important to consider behavioral factors. For people with mental illness engaging in physical activity, a literature review identified common barriers inclusive of low mood, lack of energy, fatigue, and lack of motivation (Glowacki et al., 2017). The top facilitators identified include others' attitude and emotional support and ongoing support for engagement in physical activity. For healthcare providers promoting physical activity to individuals with mental illness, barriers identified were the barriers faced by clients related to their mental illness (e.g., low mood), a lack of training on how to promote physical activity, and lack of resources (Glowacki, Weatherson, et al., 2019). Facilitators include training on physical activity and knowing the health benefits of engaging in activity.

To support healthcare providers and individuals with depression (and anyone experiencing low mood) to collaboratively consider exercise and physical activity in recovery, "The Exercise and Depression Toolkit" was developed using a systematic phased approach (Glowacki, Arbour-Nicitopoulos, et al., 2019). This includes literature reviews, interviews with stakeholders, an expert panel meeting, and final toolkit development. The toolkit has had an international reach, and preliminary evaluation indicates the toolkit is acceptable for use in practice, has positive innovation attributes, is easy to use, and is well-liked by healthcare providers (Glowacki et al., 2021). The toolkit is free and available for download at www.exerciseanddepression.ca.

Evaluating Recovery

The complexity of the recovery process extends to design and methodological issues related to research and evaluation. If, for example, recovery is an ongoing process, how can any meaningful outcome associated with recovery be conceptualized and evaluated? How can we reconcile the notion of recovery as a process experienced and owned by people with mental illness within a healthcare system (and research funding system) that highly values controlled trials, researcher objectivity, and quantified results?

People with mental illness have long been concerned that innovations in practice and advances in research have largely occurred without their input and voice. The popular slogan "Nothing about us without us" became a sort of rallying call against a mental health system that did not, in any meaningful way, include the voices of the people it served. The understanding of recovery as a personal journey experienced and owned by people with mental illness has advanced this movement because it has relied on first-person narratives of the lived experience. This has led to a greater understanding of the value of the experiential knowledge of people who live with mental illness and has subsequently contributed to the growth of valued, formal peer-support services in the mental health system and the development of research relationships with people in recovery that engage them to a varying extent—from seeking their perspectives to involving them as partners in research (Figure 39.3).

Advances in the conceptual development of recovery are providing a foundation for advancing evaluation. A wide array of measures to evaluate individual recovery have now been developed and been subject to psychometric testing. Most measures are self-report measures, such as the Recovery Process Inventory (Jerrell et al., 2006), which asks people with mental illness to rate themselves on six dimensions (anguish, connection to others, confidence or purpose, others' care or help, living situation, and hope). Many of these measurement tools are available electronically on the Web and are not subject to restrictive copyright rules (see, e.g., Barbic, 2016; Campbell-Orde et al., 2005).

In addition to generic measures of recovery, such as the Recovery Assessment Scale (Corrigan et al., 2004) and the Recovery Quality of Life Scale (Keetharuth et al., 2017), evaluation can be designed to focus on particular elements of the recovery

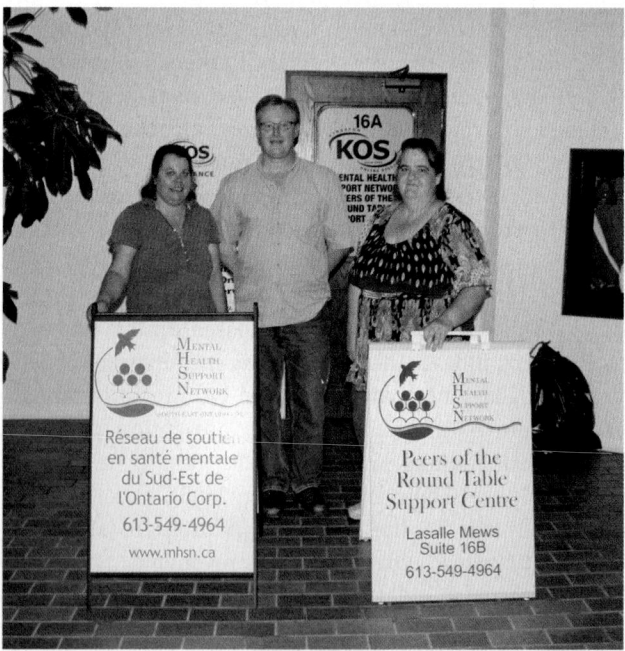

FIGURE 39.3 Peer involvement including formal peer-support services is a critical element of a recovery-oriented service system.

process. For example, it is widely accepted that a fundamental shift in agency occurs in the recovery process whereby individuals with mental illness move from attitudes and behaviors that reflect passivity, internalized stigma, the absence of expectations, and helplessness to positions of control and a growing sense of expectations for the self in the larger world. With this in mind, evaluators may choose to focus on the changing sense of empowerment within the recovery process and use established measures such as the Empowerment Scale (Rogers et al., 1997)—a self-report scale developed by individuals with mental illness, which operationalizes the many dimensions of empowerment in 28 items reflecting five factors of self-efficacy and self-esteem, power and powerlessness, community activism, righteous anger, and optimism toward the future.

Another outcome important to personal recovery is time use. The Illness Management Recovery (IMR) scale (Salyers et al., 2007) has a specific item that asks people about time use. Occupational therapists are familiar with many other time-use assessments, including diaries and time logs. Targeting time use is an outcome of important consideration for occupational therapists working in mental health (Eklund et al., 2009). "Time" has a common unit that most people clearly understand, and how people spend their time meaningfully to achieve health and well-being has been developed by occupational therapists as a concern for public health (Gewurtz et al., 2016). Depending on the chosen definition of recovery, meaningful time use is an important target for OT treatment, is easily measured, and can be a common metric of the value added of OT as a healthcare intervention for diverse populations in diverse settings. Assessment tools, such as the Occupational Performance History Interview, have been developed to engage individuals in telling their occupational stories in a way that can build on the individual's lived experiences and reveal strengths and potential opportunities (Ennals & Fossey, 2009). Similarly, assessment tools that measure time use help to capture the actual occupational patterns of people with mental illness to facilitate collaborative planning (Eklund et al., 2009).

Other tools such as the Profile of Occupational Engagement (Bejerholm et al., 2006) can help with the interpretation of occupational patterns by considering how elements of well-being and health are being experienced through occupation. For example, occupational patterns might be explored with respect to the extent to which they provide the individual with structure and routine, provide a good level of satisfaction, and provide opportunities for social interactions and access to a range of community environments. Occupational therapists have used the evidence-based practice of psychoeducation to explicitly inform people with mental illness and their support networks about the link between activity, occupation, and recovery. Figure 39.4 provides an example of a handout used in one such initiative, Action Over Inertia, which addresses the activity-health needs of people with SMI. Initial testing of Action Over Inertia

has suggested that it may be effective in enabling people to make meaningful changes in their occupational patterns (Edgelow & Krupa, 2011; Krupa et al., 2010). However, it should be noted that the role of OT in recovery has rarely been explicitly tested in recovery interventions. Although the guiding principles of recovery are much in line with OT's values and scope, future evidence is needed to support the unique evidence-based role of the profession practicing in this new model of care.

Measures also exist to capture recovery-orientation or providers and systems. For example, the Recovery Self-Assessment (RSA) tool has been used to engage services in adopting a recovery-orientation (O'Connell et al., 2005) and the Recovery Knowledge Inventory (RKI) (Bedregal et al., 2006) is commonly used to assess provider attitudes and knowledge about recovery and recovery-orientation. These measures have been leveraged in several parts of the world to support professional development and standards development (Mental Health Commission of New Zealand, 2001; MHCC, 2016). Threats to recovery-oriented care have been documented recently by Parker and colleagues (2017). These include staff burnout and external pressure to accept clients who are "not ready" for recovery. Parker and colleagues recommend active vigilance to maintain a focus on recovery and rehabilitation and that leadership focus on adapting services to the emergent needs of people receiving mental health services. The development and implementation of meaningful recovery-standards can inform a person-centered learning health system, in which recovery indicators are articulated, data are routinely collected, and evidence is systematically embedded and applied to clinical practice, processes, and policies. This can allow for continuous innovation and improving outcomes and experiences for clients and families accessing care.

Conclusion

The core values, assumptions, and philosophy of OT are remarkably consistent with those embraced within contemporary perspectives on personal recovery. However, it is important to remember that occupational therapists practice within a health service delivery system in which major challenges and obstacles to implementing a recovery-oriented vision exist. It would be unreasonable to think that occupational therapists have somehow not been influenced by these obstacles and that their practice has always been recovery-oriented within a larger system that has had such difficulty with this transformation. For example, Davidson and colleagues (2006) identified several concerns about recovery that emerged during efforts to transform a state mental health system. These concerns include such difficulties as practicing from the assumption that recovery is possible for only a selection of people with mental illness; difficulties with orienting professional expertise to practice

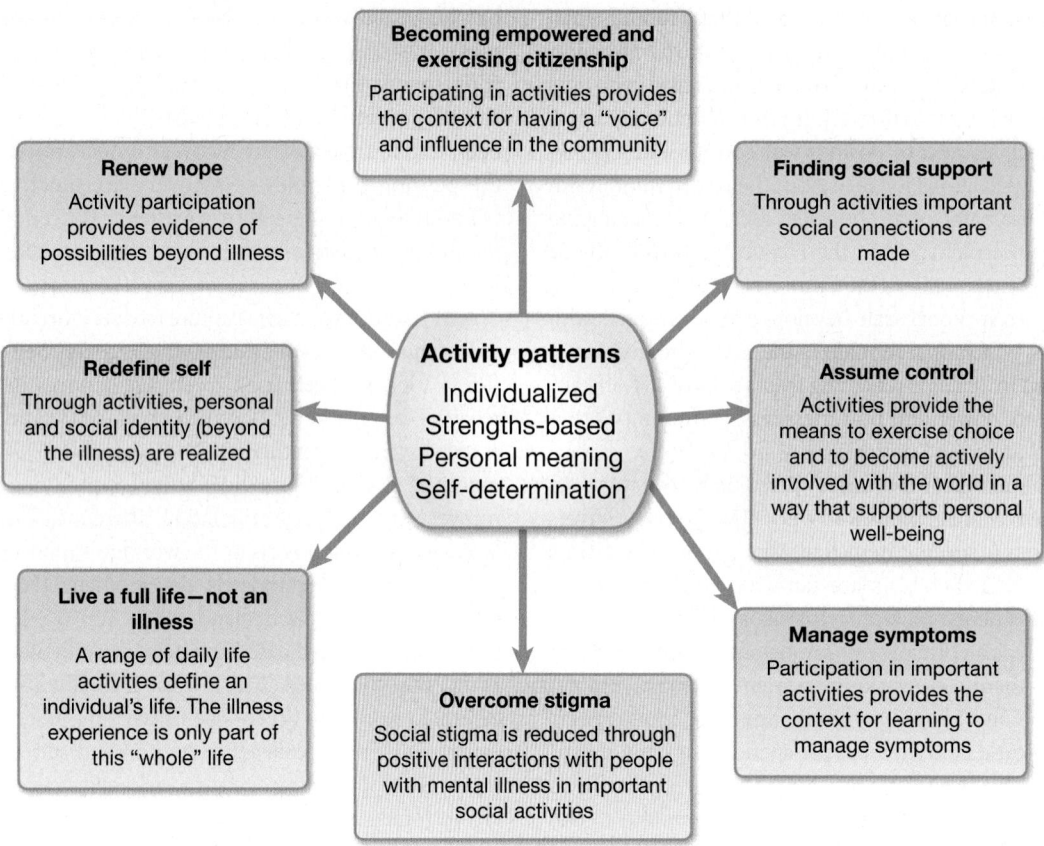

FIGURE 39.4 **The recovery benefits of activity participation.**

(Adapted from Krupa, T., Edgelow, M., Chen, S.-P., Mieras, C., Almas, A., Perry, A., Radloff-Gabriel, D., Jackson, J., & Bransfield, M. [2010]. *Action over inertia: Addressing the activity-health needs of individuals with SMI.* Canadian Association of Occupational Therapists. Reprinted with permission.)

that is assertively supportive of self-determination, personal agency, and control; and difficulties with refining practice to actively develop evidence-based approaches and interventions that will enable recovery.

Occupational therapists need to acknowledge the challenges of maintaining a recovery-oriented practice in rapidly evolving health and social systems. As best practices and policies emerge, it is critical for occupational therapists to offer leadership to advocate for the rights of all people with mental illness to have access to meaningful occupations that are developmentally, culturally, and personally relevant.

Lippincott® Connect *For additional resources on the subjects discussed in this chapter, visit* Lippincott Connect.

REFERENCES

Andresen, R., Oades, L., & Caputi, P. (2003). The experience of recovery from schizophrenia: Towards an empirically validated stage model. *Australian and New Zealand Journal of Psychiatry, 37,* 586–594. https://doi.org/10.1046/j.1440-1614.2003.01234.x.

Barbic, S. (2016, April). *Development and testing of the Personal Recovery Outcome Measure (PROM) for people with mental illness.* Paper presented at the Canadian Association of Occupational Therapists, Banff, Canada.

Barbic, S., Krupa, T., & Armstrong, I. (2009). A randomized controlled trial of the effectiveness of a modified recovery workbook program: Preliminary findings. *Psychiatric Services, 60,* 491–497. https://doi.org/10.1176/ps.2009.60.4.491

Bedregal, L. E., O'Connell, M., & Davidson, L. (2006). The recovery knowledge inventory: Assessment of mental health staff knowledge and attitudes about recovery. *Psychiatric Rehabilitation Journal, 30,* 96–103. https://doi.org/10.2975/30.2006.96.103.

Bejerholm, U., Hansson, L., & Eklund, M. (2006). Profiles of occupational engagement in people with schizophrenia (POES): The development of a new instrument based on time-use diaries. *British Journal of Occupational Therapy, 69,* 58–69. https://doi.org/10.1177/030802260606900203

Campbell-Orde, T., Chamberlin, J., Carpenter, J., & Leff, H. S. (2005). Measuring the promise: A compendium of recovery measures (Vol. 2). http://www.power2u.org/downloads/pn-55.pdf

Cook, J. A., Copeland, M. E., Jonikas, J. A., Hamilton, M. M., Razzano, L. A., Grey, D. D., Floyd, C. B., Hudson, W. B., Macfarlane, R. T., Carter, T. M., & Boyd, S. (2012). Results of a randomized controlled trial of mental illness self-management using wellness recovery action planning. *Schizophrenia Bulletin, 38,* 881–891. https://doi.org/10.1093/schbul/sbr012

Copeland, M. E. (1997). *Wellness recovery action plan.* Peach Press.

Corrigan, P. W., Salzer, M., Ralph, R. O., Sangster, Y., & Keck, L. (2004). Examining the factor structure of the recovery assessment scale. *Schizophrenia Bulletin, 30,* 1035–1041. https://doi.org/10.1093/oxfordjournals.schbul.a007118

Craft, L. L. (2013). Potential psychological mechanisms underlying the exercise and depression relationship. In P. Ekkekakis, D. B. Cook, L. L. Craft, S. N. Culos-Reed, J. L. Etnier, M. Hamer, K. A. Martin Ginis, J. Reed, J. A. J. Smits, & M. Ussher (Eds.), *Routledge handbooks: Routledge handbook of physical activity and mental health* (pp. 161–168). Routledge/Taylor & Francis Group.

Davidson, L. (2005). Recovery in serious mental illness: Paradigm shift or shibboleth. In L. Davidson, C. Harding, & L. Spaniol (Eds.), *Recovery from severe mental illnesses: Research evidence and implications for practice* (pp. 5–26). Centre for Psychiatric Rehabilitation, Boston University.

Davidson, L., O'Connell, M., Tondora, J., Styron, T., & Kangas, K. (2006). The top ten concerns about recovery encountered in mental health system transformation. *Psychiatric Services, 57*, 640–645. https://doi.org/10.1176/ps.2006.57.5.640

Davidson, L., Rakfeldt, J., & Strauss, J. (2010). *The roots of the recovery movement in psychiatry: Lessons learned.* Wiley-Blackwell.

Davidson, L., & Roe, D. (2007). Recovery from versus recovery in serious mental illness: One strategy for lessening confusion plaguing recovery. *Journal of Mental Health, 16*, 459–470. https://doi.org/10.1080/09638230701482394

Davidson, L., Tondora, J., O'Connell, M., Kirk, T., Jr., Rockholz, P., & Evans, A. (2007). Creating a recovery-oriented system of behavioral health care: Moving from concept to reality. *Psychiatric Rehabilitation Journal, 31*, 23–31. https://doi.org/10.2975/31.1.2007.23.31

Deegan, P. (1988). Recovery: The lived experience of rehabilitation. *Psychosocial Rehabilitation Journal, 11*(4), 11–19. https://doi.org/10.1037/h0099565

Deegan, P. (1990). Spirit breaking: When the helping professions hurt. *The Humanistic Psychologist, 18*, 301–313. https://doi.org/10.1080/08873267.1990.9976897

Deegan, P. (1996). Recovery as a journey of the heart. *Psychiatric Rehabilitation Journal, 19*, 91–97. https://doi.org/10.1037/h0101301

Deegan, P. (2001). Recovery as a self-directed process of healing and transformation. *Occupational Therapy in Mental Health, 17*, 5–21. https://doi.org/10.1300/J004v17n03_02

del Vecchio, P. (2012). *SAMHSA working definition of recovery updated.* Substance Abuse and Mental Health Services Administration. https://blog.samhsa.gov/2012/03/23/defintion-of-recovery-updated/#.Wa3l07pFwrE

Edgelow, M., & Krupa, T. (2011). Randomized controlled pilot study of an occupational time-use intervention for people with serious mental illness. *American Journal of Occupational Therapy, 65*, 267–276. https://doi.org/10.5014/ajot.2011.001313

Eklund, M., Leufstadius, C., & Bejerholm, U. (2009). Time use among people with psychiatric disabilities: Implications for practice. *Psychiatric Rehabilitation Journal, 32*, 177–191. https://doi.org/10.2975/32.3.2009.177.191

Ennals, P., & Fossey, E. (2009). Using the OPHI-II to support people with mental illness in their recovery. *Occupational Therapy in Mental Health, 25*, 138–150. https://doi.org/10.1080/01642120902859048

Gewurtz, R., Moll, S., Letts, L., Larivière, N., Levasseur, M., & Krupa, T. (2016). What you do every day matters: A new direction for health promotion. *Canadian Journal of Public Health, 107*, e205–e208. https://doi.org/10.17269/cjph.107.5317

Gibson, R. W., D'Amico, M., Jaffe, L., & Arbesman, M. (2011). Occupational therapy interventions for recovery in the areas of community integration and normative life roles for adults with serious mental illness: A systematic review. *American Journal of Occupational Therapy, 65*, 247–256. https://doi.org/10.5014/ajot.2011.001297

Gingerich, S., & Mueser, K. T. (2005). Illness management and recovery. In R. E. Drake, M. R. Merrens, & D. W. Lynde (Eds.), *Evidence-based mental health practice: A textbook* (pp. 395–424). Norton.

Glowacki, K., Arbour-Nicitopoulos, K., Burrows, M., Chesick, L., Heinemann, L., Irving, S., Lam, R., Macridis, S., Michalak, E., Scott, A., &

Taylor, A. (2019). It's more than just a referral: Development of an evidence-informed exercise and depression toolkit. *Mental Health and Physical Activity, 17*, 100297. https://doi.org/10.1016/j.mhpa.2019.100297

Glowacki, K., Duncan, M., Gainforth, H., & Faulkner, G. (2017). Barriers and Facilitators to physical activity and exercise among adults with depression: A scoping review. *Mental Health and Physical Activity, 13*, 108–119. https://doi.org/10.1016/J.MHPA.2017.10.001

Glowacki, K., Weatherson, K., & Faulkner, G. (2019). Barriers and facilitators to health care providers' promotion of physical activity for individuals with mental illness: A scoping review. *Mental Health and Physical Activity, 16*, 152–168. https://doi.org/10.1016/j.mhpa.2018.10.006

Glowacki, K., Zumrawi, D., Michalak, E., & Faulkner, G. (2021). Evaluation of health care providers' use of the 'Exercise and Depression Toolkit': A case study. *BMC Psychiatry, 21*, 243. https://doi.org/10.1186/s12888-021-03248-5

Hearing Voices Network. (n.d.). *Hearing voices groups.* https://www.hearing-voices.org/hearing-voices-groups/

Higgs, R. N. (2020). Reconceptualizing psychosis: The Hearing Voices Movement and social approaches to health. *Health and Human Rights, 22*(1), 133–144. https://www.ncbi.nlm.nih.gov/pmc/articles/PMC7348419/

Jerrell, J. M., Cousins, V. C., & Roberts, K. M. (2006). Psychometrics of the recovery process inventory. *The Journal of Behavioral Health Services and Research, 33*, 464–473. https://doi.org/10.1007/s11414-006-9031-5

Keetharuth, A., Brazier, J., Connell, J., Carlton, J., Taylor Buck, E., Ricketts, T., & Barkham, M. (2017). *Development and validation of the Recovering Quality of Life (ReQoL) outcome measures.* http://www.eepru.org.uk/article/development-and-validation-of-the-recovering-quality-of-life-reqol-outcome-measure/

Krupa, T., Edgelow, M., Chen, S.-P., Mieras, C., Almas, A., Perry, A., Radloff-Gabriel, D., Jackson, J., & Bransfield, M. (2010). *Action over inertia: Addressing the activity-health needs of individuals with serious mental illness.* Canadian Association of Occupational Therapists.

Krupa, T., Fossey, E., Anthony, W. A., Brown, C., & Pitts, D. (2009). Doing daily life: How occupational therapy can inform psychiatric rehabilitation practice. *Psychiatric Rehabilitation Journal, 32*, 155–161. https://doi.org/10.2975/32.3.2009.155.161

Leamy, M., Bird, V., Le Boutillier, C., Williams, J., & Slade, M. (2011). Conceptual framework for personal recovery in mental health: Systematic review and narrative synthesis. *The British Journal of Psychiatry, 199*(6), 445–452. https://doi.org/10.1192/bjp.bp.110.083733

Levitt, A. J., Mueser, K. T., DeGenova, J., Lorenzo, J., Bradford-Watt, D., Barbosa, A., Karlin, M., & Chernick, M. (2009). Randomized controlled trial of illness management and recovery in multiple-unit supportive housing. *Psychiatric Services, 60*, 1629–1636. https://doi.org/10.1176/ps.2009.60.12.1629

Lyons, J. S., Uziel-Miller, N. S., Reyes, F., & Sokol, P. T. (2000). Strengths of children and adolescents in residential settings: Prevalence and associations with psychopathology and discharge placement. *Journal of the American Academy of Child and Adolescent Psychiatry, 39*, 176–81. https://doi.org/10.1097/00004583-200002000-00017

Mattsson, M., Topor, A., Cullberg, J., & Forsell, Y. (2008). Association between financial strain, social network and five-year recovery from first episode psychosis. *Social Psychiatry and Psychiatric Epidemiology, 43*, 947–952. https://doi.org/10.1007/s00127-008-0392-3

Mental Health Commission of Canada. (2016). *Guidelines for recovery-oriented practice.* https://www.mentalhealthcommission.ca/sites/default/files/MHCC_RecoveryGuidelines_ENG_0.pdf

Mental Health Commission of New Zealand. (2001). *Recovery competencies for New Zealand mental health workers.* http://www.maryohagan.com/resources/Text_Files/Recovery%20Cometencies%20O%27Hagan.pdf

Misra, S., Jackson, V. W., Chong, J., choe, K., Tay, C., Wong, J., & Yang, L. H. (2021). Systematic review of cultural aspects of stigma and mental illness among racial and ethnic minority groups in the United States: Implications for interventions. *American Journal of Community Psychology, 68*, 486–512. https://doi.org/ajcp.12516.

Morres, I. D., Hatzigeorgiadis, A., Stathi, A., Comoutos, N., Arpin-Cribbie, C., Krommidas, C., & Theodorakis, Y. (2019). Aerobic exercise for adult patients with major depressive disorder in mental health services: A systematic review and meta-analysis. *Depression and Anxiety, 36*(1), 39–53. https://doi.org/10.1002/da.22842.

Noordsy, D., Torrey, W., Mueser, K., Mead, S., O'Keefe, C., & Fox, L. (2002). Recovery from severe mental illness: An intrapersonal and functional outcome definition. *International Review of Psychiatry, 14*, 318–326. https://doi.org/10.1080/0954026021000016969

O'Connell, M. J., Tondora, J., Croog, G., Evans, A. C., & Davidson, L. (2005). From rhetoric to routine: Assessing perceptions of recovery-oriented practices in a state mental health and addiction system. *Psychiatric Rehabilitation Journal, 28*, 378–386. https://doi.org/10.2975/28.2005.378.386

Parker, S., Dark, F., Newman, E., Korman, N., Rasmussen, Z., & Meurk, C. (2017). Reality of working in a community-based, recovery-oriented mental health rehabilitation unit: A pragmatic grounded theory analysis. *International Journal of Mental Health Nursing, 26*, 355–365. doi:10.1111/inm.12251

Pelletier, J. F., Corbière, M., Lecomte, T., Briand, C., Corrigan, P., Davidson, L., & Rowe, M. (2015). Citizenship and recovery: Two intertwined concepts for civic-recovery. *BMC Psychiatry, 15*, 37. https://doi.org/10.1186/s12888-015-0420-2

Ralph, R. (2005). Verbal definitions and visual models of recovery: Focus on the recovery model. In R. O. Ralph & P. W. Corrigan (Eds.), *Recovery in mental illness: Broadening our understanding of wellness* (pp. 131–145). American Psychological Association.

Rapp, C., & Goscha, R. (2012). *The strengths model: A recovery-oriented approach to mental health services* (3rd ed.). Oxford University Press.

Rebeiro Gruhl, K. (2008). Strengths and challenges to practice: Reconciling occupational justice issues as a prerequisite to mental health recovery. In E. A. McKay, C. Craik, K. H. Lim, & G. Richards (Eds.), *Advancing occupational therapy in mental health practice* (pp. 103–117). Blackwell.

Richardson, C. R., Faulkner, G., McDevitt, J., Skrinar, G. S., Hutchinson, D. S., & Piette, J. D. (2005). Integrating physical activity into mental health services for persons with serious mental illness. *Psychiatric Services, 56*(3), 324–331. https://doi.org/10.1176/appi.ps.56.3.324

Rogers, E. S., Chamberlin, J., Ellison, M. L., & Crean, T. (1997). A consumer-constructed scale to measure empowerment among users of mental health services. *Psychiatric Services, 48*, 1042–1047. https://doi.org/10.1176/ps.48.8.1042

Rosenbaum, S., Tiedemann, A., Sherrington, C., Curtis, J., & Ward, P. B. (2014). Physical activity interventions for people with mental illness: A systematic review and meta-analysis. *Journal of Clinical Psychiatry, 75*, 964–974. https://doi.org/10.4088/JCP.13r08765

Rust, T., Diessner, R., & Reade, L. (2009). Strengths only or strengths and relative weaknesses? A preliminary study. *The Journal of Psychology, 143*, 465–476. https://doi.org/10.3200/JRL.143.5.465-476

Salyers, M. P., Godfrey, J. L., Mueser, K. T., & Labriola, S. (2007). Measuring illness management outcomes: A psychometric study of clinician and consumer rating scales for illness self-management and recovery. *Community Mental Health Journal, 43*, 459–480. https://doi.org/10.1007/s10597-007-9087-6

Schuch, F. B., Vancampfort, D., Rosenbaum, S., Richards, J., Ward, P. B., & Stubbs, B. (2016). Exercise improves physical and psychological quality of life in people with depression: A meta-analysis including the evaluation of control group response. *Psychiatry Research, 241*, 47–54. https://doi.org/10.1016/j.psychres.2016.04.054

Shalaby, R. A. H., & Agyapong, V. I. O. (2020). Peer support in mental Health: Literature review. *JMIR Mental Health, 7*(6), e15572. https://doi.org/10.2196/15572

Slade, M. (2009). *Personal recovery and mental illness: A guide for mental health professionals.* Cambridge University Press.

Spaniol, L., Koehler, M., & Hutchinson, D. (1994). *Recovery workbook: Practical coping and empowerment strategies for people with psychiatric disability.* Centre for Psychiatric Rehabilitation, Boston University.

Substance Abuse and Mental Health Services Administration. (2006). *National consensus statement on mental health recovery.* U.S. Department of Health and Human Services. http://store.samhsa.gov/shin/content//SMA05-4129/SMA05-4129.pdf

Tondora, J., & Davidson, L. (2006). *Practice guidelines for recovery-oriented behavioural health care.* Connecticut Department of Mental Health and Addiction Services.

Whalley Hammell, K. (2021). Building back better: Imagining an occupational therapy for a post-COVID-19 world. *Australian Occupational Therapy Journal, 68*(5), 444–453. https://doi.org/10.1111/1440-1630.12760

Xie, H. (2013). Strengths-based approach for mental health recovery. *Iran Journal of Psychiatry and Behavioral Sciences, 7*(2), 5–10. https://www.ncbi.nlm.nih.gov/pmc/articles/PMC3939995/

Health Promotion Theories

S. Maggie Reitz and Janet V. DeLany

LEARNING OBJECTIVES

After reading this chapter, you will be able to:

1. Substantiate the role of occupational therapy (OT) in promoting health, well-being, and quality of life (QOL).
2. Reflect how health determinants and health disparities influence OT practice.
3. Differentiate theories of health behavior and health promotion that can be used to inform OT practice.
4. Integrate OT theories with health behavior theories to frame occupation-based health promotion practices.
5. Apply theory to the development of occupation-based OT health promotion interventions in interdisciplinary health promotion practice.
6. Examine the evidence available related to OT health promotion and health behavior interventions.
7. Demonstrate how health promotion can and should be used throughout OT practice to maximize health, well-being, and QOL in individuals, groups, and populations.

Introduction

Health promotion activities have long been engaged in by a small portion of occupational therapy (OT) practitioners (American Occupational Therapy Association [AOTA], 1982, 1987, 1991, 2001, 2006, 2010, 2015, 2020a) and have been seen as an appropriate role for the profession for decades (AOTA, 2020b; Brunyate, 1967; Finn, 1972; Jaffe, 1986; Johnson, 1986; Kaplan & Burch-Minakan, 1986; Reitz, 1992, 2010; West, 1967, 1969; Wiemer, 1972). Health and wellness were identified as one of the major practice areas in the AOTA's Centennial Vision (Baum, 2006). In addition, health promotion was included as an important part of the remaining five identified practice areas, which include children and youth; productive aging; mental health; rehabilitation, disability, and participation; and work and industry. The terms **well-being** and quality of life (QOL) also have a prominent place in Vision 2025—"occupational therapy maximizes health, well-being, and QOL for all people, populations, and communities through effective solutions that facilitate participation in everyday living" (AOTA, 2017b, p. 1).

Health and wellness as well as QOL were identified as possible outcomes of OT intervention in the AOTA (2008) *Occupational Therapy Practice Framework*, hereafter referred to as the Framework. Well-being was added as a potential outcome of OT services in the third edition of the Framework (AOTA, 2014). **Health management** was added to the most recent Framework (AOTA, 2020d, p. 3) "as a general occupation category" and is defined as "occupation focused on developing, managing, and maintaining routines for health and wellness by engaging in self-care with the goal of improving or maintaining health, including self-management, to allow for participation in other occupations" (p. 77). For more information on health management, see Chapter 50.

Within this chapter, OT's potential to enhance the health of clients through the use of occupation-based health promotion interventions will be detailed in the hope of encouraging greater involvement in this important area of practice. Clients can be individuals, groups such as families, or populations (AOTA, 2020d).[*] This information will be provided through a lens of theory-driven practice, based on the assumption that ethical OT practice is theory-based, occupation-based, and evidence-driven/informed (AOTA, 2020b, 2020c, 2021). The objective is to demonstrate how health behavior and health promotion theories can be blended with occupation-based theories to support and strengthen OT's role in health promotion, thereby maximizing the health and well-being of the society we serve.

Definitions of Health, Health Promotion, Well-Being, and Quality of Life

Definitions of health promotion and the focus of health promotion interventions vary across the many disciplines that engage in this type of practice; however, the definition of health is generally agreed on. The following definition of health from the World Health Organization (WHO) is probably the most frequently cited. **Health** is "the complete state of physical, mental and social well-being and not just the absence of disease or infirmity" (WHO, 1947, p. 29). **Health promotion** is the use of discipline-specific

techniques to assist people in achieving their health-related goals, while being mindful of underlying and secondary conditions. **Occupational therapy–directed health promotion**, based on the constructs of the Ecology of Human Performance (EHP) by Dunn et al. (1994), can be described as the client-centered use of occupations, adaptations to context, or alteration of context to maximize individuals', groups', families', communities', and populations' pursuit of health and QOL. Health promotion is a process that can vary in length, intensity, and audience. For example, it can include providing a specific short-term standardized intervention such as a fall prevention program or more complex, community-wide initiatives such as providing access to clean water or developing a community garden or co-op in an urban or rural food desert. A **food desert** is a geographic area where inhabitants "lack access to affordable fruits, vegetables, whole grains, low-fat milk, and other foods that make up the full range of a healthy diet" (Centers for Disease Control and Prevention [CDC], 2017, para. 2).

Health promotion is a process of maximizing health through structured interventions, whereas *wellness* is the outcome of health promotion and ultimately is the responsibility of the individual, family, community, or society (Reitz & Scaffa, 2010). The Framework uses a definition provided by Schell and Gillen, which reads, "the individual's perception of and responsibility for psychological and physical well-being as these contribute to overall satisfaction with one's life situation" (AOTA, 2020d, p. 84), whereas well-being is defined as being content with one's life including physical, mental, and social aspects (AOTA, 2020d).

In recent years, especially within the field of gerontology, there has been an increased focus on well-being and QOL. **Quality of life** is the self-appraisal of the client's life satisfaction, hope, sense of self, health, function, and socioeconomic status (SES) (AOTA, 2020d). Health-related quality of life (HRQOL) is a more specific type of QOL that considers "an individual's or group's perceived physical and mental health over time" (CDC, 2021, para. 1).

Social Determinants of Health

In a US national government report entitled Healthy People 2030, social determinants of health (SDOH) are described within five broad categories: economic stability, education access and quality, healthcare access and quality, neighborhood and built environment, and social and community context (U.S. Department of Health and Human Services [USDHHS], n.d.-c). These five determinants are shown in Figure 40.1, together with the mission of Healthy People 2030 and the overarching goals for the next decade for improving health of the nation.

---

[*]According to the AOTA (2020d, p. S75), the term *client* refers to *persons* (including those involved in care of a client), *groups* (a collection of individuals having shared characteristics or common or shared purpose, e.g., family members, workers, students, and those with similar interests or occupational challenges), and *populations* (aggregates of people with common attributes such as contexts, characteristics, or concerns, including health risks). However, in countries other than the United States, the term *client* often refers to persons who are paying for their care directly. In most countries, *patient* is used to describe persons who are in hospitals or rehabilitation. *Service user* and *person* are terms in general use that describe those in need of OT services. For this chapter, we are using *client* without implying the source of payment for services.

Social Determinants of Health

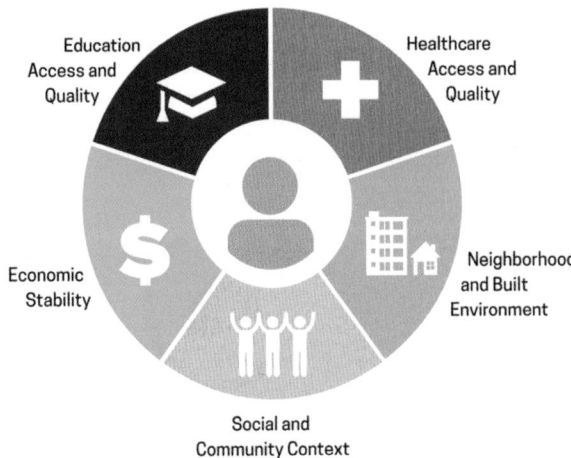

FIGURE 40.1 The five domains of the social determinants of health. (From Healthy People 2030, U.S. Department of Health and Human Services, Office of Disease Prevention and Health Promotion. Retrieved July 1, 2022, from https://health.gov/healthypeople/objectives-and-data/social-determinants-health)

The foundational principles of Healthy People 2030 (n.d.-a, para. 4) appear verbatim:

- The health and well-being of all people and communities is essential to a thriving, equitable society.
- Promoting health and well-being and preventing disease are linked efforts that encompass physical, mental, and social health dimensions.
- Investing to achieve the full potential for health and well-being for all provides valuable benefits to society.
- Achieving health and well-being requires eliminating health disparities, achieving health equity, and attaining health literacy.
- Healthy physical, social, and economic environments strengthen the potential to achieve health and well-being.
- Promoting and achieving health and well-being nationwide is a shared responsibility that is distributed across the national, state, tribal, and community levels, including the public, private, and not-for-profit sectors.
- Working to attain the full potential for health and well-being of the population is a component of decision-making and policy formulation across all sectors.

Healthy People 2030 is a framework available for usage by federal, state, and local governments; nonprofits; health and education professionals; and businesses to address and assess outcomes of programs and policies that aim to improve the health and well-being of populations living in the United States (USDHHS, n.d.-a). If a community or population has not already identified a health need, then a review of the objectives identified in this report may be of assistance to start the conversation. A roadmap to put the Healthy People 2030 principles into action is detailed in Figure 40.2.

The WHO, through a document entitled *Ottawa Charter for Health Promotion* published in 1986, identified eight prerequisites for health. These prerequisites include the following (WHO, 1986, p. 1): education, food, income, peace, shelter, social justice and equity, stable ecosystem, and sustainable resources.

OT practitioners should consider the impact of these SDOH on their clients at the individual, group, and population levels when conducting occupational profiles. A core question to ask is: What keeps clients from safely and successfully participating in life tasks that they need and want to do? Successful health promotion programs should address the prerequisites and determinants of health that are applicable to the individual, group, and population levels, based on their self-determination, which is influenced by geopolitics, geographical location, and other contextual features.

Occupational Deprivation and Health Disparity

Access to meaningful, valued, and safe occupations, or occupational enrichment (Molineux & Whiteford, 2011), is an important contributor to health. Lack of access to meaningful, valued, and safe occupations can result in occupational deprivation, which in turn can have a significant negative impact on the health of individuals, families, and communities. **Occupational deprivation**, which is the lack of access to engagement in an array of occupations that have meaning to the individual, family, or community, can result in ill health (Wilcock, 2006) and cascading occupational injustice. Examples of the potential relationships between occupational deprivation and health determinants are depicted in Table 40.1.

From a health promotion perspective, occupational deprivation is one of the unfortunate results of health disparities. The hallmarks of health disparity are inequality, discrimination, and limitations placed on a group of people, which then create negative effects on the health of persons in that group (Box 40.1). The impact of decades of limited access to robust SDOH and resulting occupational deprivation is readily apparent in an analysis of the Baltimore unrest (Moore & Green, 2021), families in war-torn and drought-stricken countries (Biven, 2015; Garcia-Ruiz,

How can I use Healthy People 2030 in my work?

Healthy People addresses public health priorities by setting national objectives and tracking them over the decade. Join us as we work to improve health and well-being nationwide.

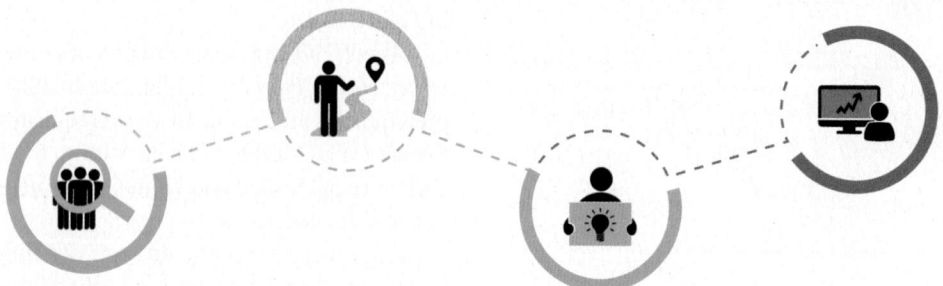

1. Identify needs and priority populations

» Browse objectives to learn about national goals to improve health

» See how national goals align with your priorities

» Consider focusing on groups affected by health disparities

Use this information to make the case for your program, secure resources, and build partnerships.

2. Set your own targets

» Find data related to your work

» Use national data to set goals for your program

Healthy People 2030 establishes objectives and targets for the entire United States, but setting local targets contributes to national success.

3. Find inspiration and practical tools

» Explore critical public health topics relevant to your work

» Learn about successful programs, policies, and interventions

» Look for evidence-based resources and tools your community, state, or organization can use

4. Monitor national progress — and use our data as a benchmark

» Check for updates on progress toward achieving national objectives

» Use our data to inform your policy and program planning

» See how your progress compares to national data

Visit **health.gov/healthypeople/tools-action** to get started using Healthy People 2030 — and use **#HP2030** to share your successes on social media!

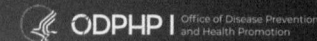

FIGURE 40.2 How can I use Healthy People 2030 in my work? (From Healthy People 2030, U.S. Department of Health and Human Services.)

TABLE 40.1 Occupational Deprivation and Health Impacts

Occupational Deprivation	Relationship to Health Determinants (USDHHS, n.d.-c)
Children with congenital sensory and motor challenges who do not have opportunities to play with peers on accessible playgrounds	• Biology and genetics • Social environment • Physical environment
Youth living in migrant camps with limited opportunities to access various positive group occupations with peers turn to unhealthy habits to cope with boredom and isolation	• Individual behavior • Social environment • Physical environment
Working parents' limited access to healthcare and/or educational services because of lack of proof of citizenship	• Health services • Social environment
Older adults who cannot negotiate exit from house become imprisoned in own home	• Social environment • Physical environment
Men and women of color and those with political or religious beliefs that differ from ones that are locally accepted are at increased risk for incarceration, with minimal access to healthcare, intervention programs, and community re-entry supports because of fear and persecution	• Political institutions • Legal institutions

2015), and the stark disparities in access to vaccines from COVID-19 as well as morbidity and mortality rates (Abuelezam, 2020; Bhatia et al., 2022; Schmidt et al., 2021; Webb Hooper et al., 2021). Although there has been progress toward improving the overall US population health, disparities in health indicators remain across populations and geographic areas, as displayed in Box 40.2 (USDHHS et al., 2020).

Persistent health disparities exist in the United States in terms of life expectancy because of geographic location, race, SES, and educational level, and also because of policies that perpetuate discriminatory institutional structures based on race, gender, sex, ability status, and immigrant status. For example, in a 10-mile area in Atlanta, Georgia, there is a 10- to 12-year discrepancy in life expectancy (Virginia Commonwealth University Center on Society and Health, 2017). Similarly, there is a 14-year gap in life expectancy

between neighborhoods in Baltimore, Maryland, that are two miles apart (Pietella, 2010). This geographic disparity follows racial and SES divisions and institutional discriminatory policies as well. Such factors must be considered in program or intervention planning. Because many of the areas in Atlanta and Baltimore with lower life expectancy also are areas lacking healthy options for food (i.e., food deserts),

BOX 40.1 HEALTH DISPARITIES DEFINED

Health disparity is a particular type of health difference that is closely linked with social, economic, and/or environmental disadvantage. Health disparities adversely affect groups of people who have systematically experienced greater obstacles to health based on their racial or ethnic group; religion; socioeconomic status; gender; age; mental health; cognitive, sensory, or physical disability; sexual orientation or gender identity; geographic location; or other characteristics historically linked to discrimination or exclusion (USDHHS & The Secretary's Advisory Committee on National Health Promotion and Disease Prevention Objectives for 2020, 2010, p. 28).

BOX 40.2 DISPARITIES IN HEALTH INDICATORS

- Infant mortality
- Life expectancy
- Cardiovascular disease
- Cancer
- Diabetes
- Chronic obstructive pulmonary disease (COPD)
- HIV/AIDS
- Healthcare access and utilization
- Health insurance
- Disability
- Mental health
- Preventive health services such as cervical and colorectal cancer screening
- Smoking
- Obesity
- Substance use
- Suicide
- Homicide
- Unintentional injuries

U.S. Department of Health and Human Services, Health Resources & Services Administration, & Office of Health Equity. (2020). *Health equity report 2019–2020: Special feature on housing and health inequalities* (p. 187). Author.

plans for the individual or group to address the high rates of obesity or heart disease must consider the barriers within the environmental context in addition to specific client factors. The AOTA's Societal Statement on Health Disparities stresses that OT practitioners should intervene when clients (both individuals and communities) face limitations to participation because of inequalities by advocating for access to services and health promoting occupations (AOTA, 2013).

Each of the examples in Table 40.1 can be the beginning of a negatively reinforcing relationship leading to additional threats to health as occupational deprivation increases. For example, youth living in rural areas with limited access to age-appropriate group occupations because of geographic location can move from using tobacco and abusing alcohol to exploring controlled substances. This in turn could lead to a driving under the influence (DUI) conviction, a manslaughter charge, theft, or an arrest for the use of illegal drugs, any of which could result in a period of incarceration, which then can result in decreased access to various self-chosen occupations and an acceleration of health problems. Death from an accidental overdose could be another outcome, as rural communities face a disproportionate impact from the opioid epidemic (Allen et al., 2019).

While the opioid epidemic stretches across the United States, certain populations are at greater risk. A study of opioid-involved deaths in rural and metropolitan areas between 1999 and 2017 indicated that mortality rates increased for certain racial/ethnic groups (Lippold & Ali, 2020). Although the largest increase occurred in white non-Hispanics in rural areas (13.6% per year), there was also an increase in black non-Hispanics in medium-to-small metropolitan areas (11.3% per year). Interdisciplinary, multipronged, targeted, culturally sensitive strategies to address opioid abuse are needed (Lippold & Ali, 2020). One example of such an initiative was implemented in Morris County, Minnesota, through a newly launched Controlled Substance Care Team. The team worked with patients to taper, maintain current usage levels, or discontinue their use of opioids. Members of the team included a social worker, nurse, two physicians, and a pharmacist. Evaluation of results indicated the strategy was successful, with 483 patients being tapered off of controlled substances, as well as a decrease in the number of distributed prescriptions (Au-Yeung et al., 2019). Occupational therapists participating in a study of their professional experiences with individuals suspected of or already abusing opioids noted the importance of and need for interdisciplinary teams to enhance intervention outcomes (McCombie & Stirling, 2018).

In addition to interdisciplinary strategies to reduce the impact of health disparities and occupational deprivation, education of health professionals and policy changes are often also required. In January 2018, the Report of the

Ad Hoc Committee on Opioid Abuse was submitted to the AOTA Representative Assembly (Robinson et al., 2018). AOTA released a continuing education article on opioid guidelines for OT in August 2018, which was one of the recommendations of the Ad Hoc Committee. The authors of the article stressed the importance of evidence-based interdisciplinary intervention for chronic pain (Rowe & Breeden, 2018). In order to participate in interdisciplinary work, it is helpful to be aware of theories and models of health across disciplines.

Health Promotion and Health Behavior Models and Theories

Health promotion interventions beyond those typically offered to individuals or families are most often conducted by interdisciplinary teams or in close consultation with other disciplines. Thus, an understanding of frameworks and theories commonly used in health promotion is important in enhancing communication and understanding. The PRECEDE–PROCEED framework and two health behavior theories will be briefly introduced—the Health Belief Model (HBM) and the Stages of Change Model. Prior to using any of these or other theories or framework, additional knowledge should be sought through reading, mentoring, continuing education, or working toward a specialized doctoral degree.

PRECEDE–PROCEED: A Framework for Planning Health Promotion Programs

The acronym PRECEDE–PROCEED is a shorthand way of referring to a model designed to support program planning. PRECEDE refers to Predisposing, Reinforcing, and Enabling Constructs in Educational/Environmental Diagnosis and Evaluation. PROCEED refers to Policy, Regulatory, and Organizational Constructs in Educational and Environmental Development. The PRECEDE–PROCEED model is not a theory but rather a planning framework comprising eight phases. These phases are helpful for guiding ethical health promotion interventions at the community or population level (Green & Kreuter, 2005; National Cancer Institute [NCI], 2005). The originators share OT's value of client-centered care by communicating the importance of the community or population as decision-makers. Community engagement starts immediately in the PRECEDE portion of the framework in which the community guides the health promotion experts in the selection of the priority health concern that is to be addressed. In the next group of steps called the PROCEED section, health promotion and health behavior models such as the HBM are used to guide the specific details of the chosen intervention. The PROCEED portion of the framework also details the evaluation process of the intervention.

The phases of the PRECEDE–PROCEED framework (Green & Kreuter, 2005; NCI, 2005) and potential actions for each phase are described in Table 40.2. This is an introductory table; additional reading on the framework would

be required before using it to plan or evaluate a health promotion program. Based on a scoping review study of models, Pashmdarfard and colleagues (2020) determined that the PRECEDE–PROCEED was one of two models that could be used to enhance the quality of OT clinical education and to access the efficacy of health promotion programs. As an example, the PROCEED portion of the framework was used to develop a weight management program for young adults from disadvantaged backgrounds (Walsh et al., 2014). OT Story 40.1 describes how this planning model can be used with other theories to design a healthy weight intervention.

TABLE 40.2　PRECEDE–PROCEED Planning Framework

Phase	Description	Potential Change Strategies
PRECEDE		
1. Social assessment and situational analysis	Engaging the community in identifying current social problems and their vision of an improved quality of life	• Review available data on the status of the prerequisites of health in the community • Share data at meetings with community stakeholders; conduct focus groups with community members to elicit their priorities for interventions and identify community capacities that can be tapped • Formalize relations with a community-identified group or institute a community board
2. Epidemiological assessment	Reviewing health and health-related data that are linked to the social health concerns identified in Phase 1	• Review summary of data and data sources with local stakeholders. Identify need for additional data or sources for data
3. Educational and ecological assessment	Identifying the predisposing factors, enabling factors, and reinforcing factors linked to the identified social problem	• Review summary of data and data sources with stakeholders and government leaders if none are on the board • Identify need for additional data or sources for data
4. Administrative and policy assessment and intervention alignment	Identifying potential policy and fiscal, political, and societal barriers to initiate and maintain program; developing and securing needed policy changes and additional resources	• Review findings with stake holders and local government leaders
PROCEED		
5. Implementation	Launching and conducting the program	• Facilitate a culturally relevant kickoff for the program with stakeholders
6. Process evaluation	Evaluating success of continued community involvement and utilization of community resources	• Review program implementation as it is occurring and solicit feedback from stakeholders and participants
7. Impact evaluation	Evaluating short-term progress toward goals of program such as access to resources and gaining of skills, knowledge, and community acceptance	• Collect data from participants through previously planned strategy (e.g., post portion of a pretest posttest plan, focus group)
8. Outcome evaluation	Evaluating long-term achievement of goals of program related to quality of life and health indicators	• Continue to collect data from participants through previously planned strategy • Review and share current social and epidemiological data with community board to determine if there were changes in desired quality of life and health indicators

Adapted from National Cancer Institute. (2005). *Theory at a glance* (2nd ed., p. 42, Table 10). National Institutes of Health. http://www.cancer.gov/theory.pdf

OT STORY 40.1 LEARNING HEALTHY WEIGHT MANAGEMENT HABITS FOR A LIFETIME

Parents and school officials raised concerns about the increased obesity among the female high school students. In response, Antonella, an occupational therapist, working with a health educator, met with female student representatives from each of the classes to discuss the issue, the root causes, and students' potential interest in designing and participating in a weight management program. Collaborating with the female high school students, Antonella and the health educator developed a successful weight management program based on the theories shown in Table 40.6. The program includes occupation-based activities such as learning complicated line or group dances, healthy cooking classes that emphasize portion control, and a lecture series on dress-for-success for all body types with a culminating fashion show. Each of these activities focused on establishing skills (the Ecology of Human Performance [EHP] construct) and self-efficacy (the Health Belief Model [HBM] construct) as well as social support to live a healthy life. A series of outings also were taken to local healthy fast-food restaurants to sample healthier alternatives to fried food and red meat with the goal of permanently altering locations

(EHP construct) of after-school meals to foster continued healthy food choices. The use of nondieting strategies was incorporated into the education portion of the program based on the work of Cole and Horacek (2009) who used the PRECEDE–PROCEED framework to develop an intuitive eating approach to weight management.

Based on Antonella's success, she has been asked to replicate the program with middle school boys and girls. The health educator with whom Antonella developed the program has retired and is no longer available to assist.

Questions

1. Given the retirement of the health educator, does Antonella have the knowledge, skills, and resources to adapt, promote, implement, and evaluate the current program for the new population?
2. What are the implications of using the currently chosen theories with the new population?
3. Is there a place for developmental theory or other theory to guide Antonella in adaptations to the programs for the new populations?

Health Belief Model

The HBM is one of the first and most widely used models to explore and facilitate health behavior change. It was originated by public health social psychologists in the 1950s (NCI, 2005). OT practitioners frequently recommend that their clients change occupational behaviors to promote their occupational health and well-being. This model explores the way people examine and balance competing factors when deciding whether to adopt the health recommendations. The constructs of the model are described together with strategies to promote behavior change related to each specific construct in Table 40.3. Various health promotion programs can be designed using these constructs.

TABLE 40.3 Health Belief Model

Concept	Definition	Potential Change Strategies
Perceived susceptibility	Beliefs about the chances of getting a condition	• Define what population(s) are at risk and their levels of risk • Tailor risk information based on an individual's characteristics or behaviors • Help individuals develop an accurate perception of their own risks
Perceived severity	Beliefs about the seriousness of a condition and its consequences	• Specify the consequences of a condition and recommended action
Perceived benefits	Beliefs about the effectiveness of taking action to reduce risk or seriousness	• Explain how, where, and when to take action and what the potential positive results will be
Perceived barriers	Beliefs about the material and psychological costs of taking action	• Offer reassurance, incentives, and assistance; correct misinformation
Cues to action	Factors that activate "readiness to change"	• Provide "how to" information, promote awareness, and employ reminder systems
Self-efficacy	Confidence in one's ability to take action	• Provide training and guidance in performing action • Use progressive goal setting • Give verbal reinforcement • Demonstrate desired behaviors

Reprinted from National Cancer Institute. (2005). *Theory at a glance* (2nd ed., p. 14). National Institutes of Health. http://www.cancer.gov/theory.pdf

The basis of this model is the balancing of threats (i.e., perceived susceptibility and perceived severity) with barriers of taking the recommended action (e.g., time, financial cost) and the potential benefits. When the individual, family, or community believes the threat outweighs the cost of action, then change will occur (NCI, 2005). Other components of the model include self-efficacy and cues to action. A cue to action can be a roadside poster featuring an adult carrying a child with text advertising "I got my kid vaxxed." The poster cue to action more likely will result in parents seeking vaccines for their children if they perceive doing so reduces risks, provides greater benefit than not vaxxing them, and contributes to their ability to care for their children (e.g., self-efficacy).

Transtheoretical Model of Change/Stages of Change Model

The originators of this model first investigated why some people were better able to quit smoking than others (Prochaska & DiClemente, 1982, 1983). Their work led to the development of a model that can be used to study people's readiness for change—ceasing a poor health habit such as smoking or starting a good health habit such as

exercise. Literature regarding the model refers to it as either the *transtheoretical model of change* or the *stages of change model*. According to the proponents of the model, there are potentially five stages that individuals go through as they change a health-related behavior. These stages include precontemplation, contemplation, decision, action, and maintenance (NCI, 2005). As this model is based on cognitive processes, it would benefit from integration with OT models that address personal, social, and environmental factors. The components of this model are presented in Table 40.4 and discussed in greater detail in other sources (NCI, 2005; Reitz et al., 2010) and in Table 40.5.

Core Concepts of Health Promotion Models

Quintuple Aim

The Quintuple Aim is built upon earlier Triple Aim and Quadruple Aim frameworks. The Triple Aim included the objectives of improving population health, enhancing the healthcare experience, and reducing cost (Berwick et al., 2008). Concern for the personal well-being of health

TABLE 40.4 • Stages of Change Model

Stage	Definition	Potential Change Strategies
Precontemplation	Has no intention of taking action within the next 6 months	Increase awareness of need for change; personalize information about risks and benefits
Contemplation	Intends to take action within the next six months	Motivate; encourage making specific plans
Preparation	Intends to take action within the next 30 days and has taken some behavioral steps in this direction	Assist with developing and implementing concrete action plans; help set gradual goals
Action	Has changed behavior for less than 6 months	Assist with feedback, problem-solving, social support, and reinforcement
Maintenance	Has changed behavior for more than 6 months	Assist with coping, reminders, finding alternatives, and avoiding slips/relapses (as applicable)

Reprinted from National Cancer Institute. (2005). *Theory at a glance* (2nd ed., p. 15). National Institutes of Health. http://www.cancer.gov/theory.pdf

TABLE 40.5 • Comparison of Theories to Support Occupation-Based Health Promotion

Theory	Focus	Key Constructs
Ecology of Human Performance (Dunn et al., 1994)	How performance range can be maximized through skill, habit, or role development and/or modification of the environment	• Establish or restore • Adapt • Alter • Prevent • Create
Health Belief Model (National Cancer Institute [NCI], 2005)	How individuals or communities balance the threat posed by a health problem with the benefits of avoiding the threat, the cost to avoid the threat, and other factors that influence the decision to act	• Perceived susceptibility • Perceived severity

(continued)

TABLE 40.5	Comparison of Theories to Support Occupation-Based Health Promotion (*continued*)		
Theory	**Focus**	**Key Constructs**
		• Perceived benefits • Perceived barriers • Cues to action • Self-efficacy
Occupational Adaptation (Schultz, 2009)	How the ability to use adaptive capacities to solve problems, experience relative mastery, and enhance occupational performance can be enhanced	• Adaptive capacity • Adaptation energy • Adaptive response • Relative mastery
Model of Human Occupation (Kielhofner, 2009)	How individuals and communities develop performance capacity to perform habitual occupations to support participation and occupational adaption	• Volition • Habituation • Performance capacity • Occupational adaptation • Occupational competency • Occupational identity
Stages of Change Model (Prochaska & DiClemente, 1982, 1983)	Identification of when individuals or communities are ready to change a problem behavior, their current stage of change, and the optimal matching of intervention to current stage of change	• Precontemplation • Contemplation • Decision • Action • Maintenance • Relapse

Adapted from National Cancer Institute. (2005). *Theory at a glance* (2nd ed., p. 45, Table 11). National Institutes of Health. http://www.cancer.gov/theory.pdf

professionals resulted in the development of the Quadruple Aim, which then added improving the health provider experience to the Triple Aim (Bodenheimer & Sinsky, 2014). Recently, a fifth aim was aided—enhancing health equity—resulting in the Quintuple Aim (Nundy et al., 2022). The Quintuple Aim should serve as a helpful framework along with health promotion and OT theories to ensure programs are comprehensive while protecting the health professionals who are involved.

Health Promotion and OT

The development of noteworthy documents has helped to support and communicate OT's contribution to health promotion. A sample of these documents is listed in Box 40.3. The AOTA, through the statement "Occupational Therapy in the Promotion of Health and Well-Being" (AOTA, 2020c), describes the role of OT in health promotion not only for individuals but also for families, communities, and populations. The philosophical link and match of occupational values to national and international policies on health promotion are reviewed to provide the context for a series of examples of potential assessments, interventions, and strategies. Examples and case studies are provided for each of the three levels of prevention (i.e., primary, secondary, and tertiary) and with various clients (i.e., individuals, groups, and populations). These are excellent sources of ideas for potential interventions at the person and policy levels.

The AOTA, the World Federation of Occupational Therapists (WFOT), and other national OT associations, through publication of documents, also advocate for access

BOX 40.3 SAMPLING OF OCCUPATIONAL THERAPY DOCUMENTS RELATED TO HEALTH PROMOTION

- "AOTA's Societal Statement on Disaster Response and Risk Reduction" (AOTA, 2017a)
- "AOTA's Societal Statement on Health Disparities" (AOTA, 2013)
- "AOTA's Societal Statement on Health Literacy" (AOTA, 2017c)
- "AOTA's Societal Statement on Livable Communities" (AOTA, 2016)
- "AOTA's Societal Statement on Youth Violence" (AOTA, 2018a)
- "Occupational Therapy in the Promotion of Health and Well-Being" (AOTA, 2020c)
- "World Federation of Occupational Therapists' (WFOT) Position Paper: Community Based Rehabilitation" (WFOT, 2004)
- WFOT Position Paper: Occupational Therapy in Disaster Risk Reduction" (WFOT, 2016)

to prerequisites for health, including access to meaningful occupations in the community. For example, the document entitled *AOTA's Societal Statement on Livable Communities* (AOTA, 2016) informs the public, students, and new practitioners about the profession's support for access to services, establishment of policies, and implementation of design features that will allow older adults to age in place and individuals with varying abilities to fully engage in the community and reach their full occupational potential. The WFOT (2004), through the *Position Paper on Community Based Rehabilitation*, also advocates for equal access to the right of occupational engagement of individuals with disabilities and their families.

Health Literacy

Health literacy is an essential aspect of ensuring clients' abilities to participate in their own health management. **Health literacy** has been defined as the "the degree to which individuals have the capacity to obtain, process, and understand basic health information and services needed to make appropriate health decisions" (USDHHS & Health Resources and Services Administration, 2019, para. 1). Thus, health literacy includes reading literacy but also considers numeracy abilities such as calculating sliding scale dosage for diabetes or interpreting risk of disease as well as ability to advocate for self by discussing health with healthcare providers. Limited health literacy is most prevalent in medically underserved groups, low SES communities, minority populations, and older adults (USDHHS & Office of Disease Prevention and Health Promotion [ODPHP], 2008). The AOTA's Societal Statement on Health Literacy states that OT practitioners have a responsibility to promote health by developing programs and associated materials that are "understandable, accessible, and usable by the full spectrum of consumers" and tailored to person factors and context (AOTA, 2017c, pp. 1–2). Attention to health literacy can help facilitate self-management skills associated with enhanced participation in the instrumental activity of daily living of health management and maintenance.

Addressing and promoting health literacy is critical because of the poor health outcomes such as higher mortality, longer hospital stays, and increased visits to emergency room associated with lower health literacy as was noted in the Netherlands (Heijmans et al., 2015). In the last US national survey in 2003, only 12% of those surveyed had proficient health literacy (e.g., were able to use a table to calculate employee share of health insurance costs) and 35% had basic or below basic health literacy levels (e.g., read instructions and determine what they can and cannot drink prior to a medical test).

Promoting health literacy is a common goal shared across public health and healthcare professionals across the globe. As stated in its constitution, the vision of the International Health Literacy Association is to promote "health literacy for all in a world where people and societies can act to improve health and quality of life" (IHLA, 2022, p. 2).

The Agency for Healthcare Research and Quality (AHRQ) has developed the Health Literacy Universal Precautions online resource to encourage all professionals working in healthcare to assume that all patients might have difficulty understanding and accessing health information and services. There are multiple resources available to assess health literacy levels of clients. These include screenings such as the vital signs and the Rapid Estimate of Adult Literacy in Medicine (REALM), organizational assessments, intervention recommendations, and training resources available at their website (AHRQ, 2017). Practitioners can ensure adequate client understanding by using techniques such as teach back, show me, verbal rehearsal, and providing clear, concise materials at appropriate reading levels. Refer to Chapter 23 for examples of effective educational methods for use with clients.

OT Frameworks and Models to Guide Practice

Program Planning and Implementation: Needs Assessment, Intervention, and Evaluation

The process of developing appropriate interventions and programs to promote health, prevent injury, or occupational performance limitations should follow several basic steps. OT practitioners must (a) understand the role of OT in health promotion and prevention and the potential to assist in making meaningful change, (b) identify the clients' (clients can be individuals, groups, or communities) needs and wants, (c) select an appropriate theory to guide reasoning and joint decision-making, (d) develop an intervention based on available evidence, (e) ethically implement the intervention (AOTA, 2020b), and (f) evaluate the program for improvement and effectiveness during and after the program is completed.

This process mirrors the evaluation and intervention process outlined in the Framework (AOTA, 2020d). The individual or community needs assessment is equivalent to the occupational profile. For health promotion, the target individuals, group, or population should share enough in common so that the program will address their common needs. Part of this initial needs assessment should include client and key informant priorities, a review of health and health disparities data to assist with prioritization of key areas, identification of limitations in occupational performance or participation, and assets. An appropriate theory should guide interventions to address identified problems and assets. OT models and theories and health promotion theories can be used together to design interventions, including prevention, that enhance health and well-being programming and care.

It is helpful to note the meaning of common terms in the public health arena that are related to assessment of effectiveness. In OT, the term *evaluation* is typically used to denote the initial analysis of occupational performance (based on a variety of assessments), and the term *reevaluation* is typically used for subsequent checks during the course of care, culminating in the evaluation of outcomes achieved (AOTA, 2020d). In public health and other health disciplines, the first process is referred to as a *needs assessment*. Then, the term *evaluation* is used for methods to assess program or intervention effectiveness at several different time points, including during a program (i.e., formative/process evaluation), immediately following the program (i.e., impact evaluation), and finally toward evaluation of whether the program met broader goals geared to QOL and well-being over time (i.e., outcome evaluation).

For another perspective on program planning and implementation, see Expanding Our Perspectives.

Integrating OT With Health Promotion and Health Behavior Frameworks and Models to Guide Practice

Weighing which health promotion or health behavior theory to integrate with an OT model to guide the occupation-based health promotion process is a central part of the decision-making when determining the occupation and health needs to be addressed and how to address them. There are a variety of factors to consider in the selection of a health promotion theory; first and foremost must be the ease with which the theory and its constructs can be translated into lay language or the language of the cultural group requesting the intervention or assistance. Second is whether there is evidence that this theory has been useful in developing programs or evaluating health promotion interventions.

There are various health behavior theories as well as OT theories available to guide health promotion interventions as well as research that can inform interdisciplinary health promotion efforts. Health behavior theories generally lack an essential occupation perspective, whereas OT theories often can be strengthened through the application of constructs from one or more health behavior theories.

EXPANDING OUR PERSPECTIVES

The Importance of Including the Target Population

Sabrina Salvant

I was fortunate to attend an occupational therapy (OT) program that allowed me to attain my master's in occupational therapy and in public health as I was interested in working at the population level using the social determinants of health as my guide. Early in my career, I focused on developing programs relying heavily on population-based data and research and using public health and health education models and frameworks as the basis for occupation-based program development. Over time, I found that interest, outreach, and sustainability were constant challenges. Program participation was strong initially, but waned quickly. To develop the programs, I conducted needs assessment and analyzed the issues impacting the population's occupational performance. I looked at context, including environmental and social context, and assessed personal agency and motivation for program participation. Looking back, I realized that I never included the target population in

planning and developing, nor implementing the program that addressed their occupational performance needs.

I learned that including the target population throughout the process (inception to completion) helped me to get buy-in and allowed me to discover the barriers and supports that either impeded or increased success. I developed allegiances with change agents, program champions, and key influencers in the community and enlisted the community to develop sustainability plans that ensured the program would survive even after I was no longer involved. I learned to do needs assessments looking at root causes that were creating occupation dysfunction within the communities. This helped me methodically develop results-driven strategic plans and initiatives over time. I learned how to do program evaluation and continuous quality improvement—all leading to my increased ability to excel in project management. I now approach each population, project, or group with fresh eyes ready to learn and partner with them to create custom programs that address the needs of their persons, groups, and populations.

Pyatak et al. (2015) used social cognitive theory, the transtheoretical model, and the social ecological theory combined with Lifestyle Redesign® principles regarding meaningful occupation to help inform the theoretical framework for a manualized intervention for diabetes called REAL (Resilient, Empowered, Active Living with Diabetes).

A selection of the available theories to use in health promotion intervention and research that were introduced earlier is described in Table 40.5 together with a selection of OT theories. Table 40.6 provides an example of the use of a blended theory approach to developing a healthy weight program for high school girl students. Although pragmatic blending of theories can strengthen health programs, this work should be extended beyond simple evaluation of program outcomes in order to facilitate the creation of new, more powerful theories from the initial constituent theories, thus leading to broader benefit.

Using the AOTA Practice Framework and PRECEDE–PROCEED to Reduce Dating and Partner Violence on Campus

The PRECEDE–PROCEED framework has the potential to work well with the Framework (AOTA, 2020d) as well as other OT theories in order to develop occupation-based health promotion programs. The development of a potential dating etiquette program designed to decrease dating and partner violence among adolescents and young adults illustrates this possibility.

The need for programs to reduce dating/partner violence is important, especially for high school– and college-age students in the United States. Most intimate partner violence (IPV) happens in adolescence and young adulthood. Approximately one-quarter of women and 14% of men in the United States have experienced severe IPV (Smith et al., 2017). Based on this knowledge, an OT student and a health education student approached the student government association (SGA) at their university with a request for funds to develop a program to increase awareness of IPV (see OT Story 40.2).

Occupational therapists can pair the Framework (AOTA, 2020d) and the OT models with the PRECEDE–PROCEED framework to design and implement health promotion programs with an interdisciplinary team, including community members to develop and evaluate:

- A family wellness program at a county prison for incarcerated parents and their children
- A community-based independent living program for homeless LGBTQ+ youth
- An integrated arts program for exploited women
- A community-based cooking co-op for people with diabetes

Using the Health Belief Model

The impact and relationship of these constructs can be shown through a description of the potential roles of a health educator and an OT practitioner on an interdisciplinary smoking cessation program development team. Health educators have the background knowledge and expertise to ensure the perceived severity (e.g., ill health,

TABLE 40.6 Use of Multiple Frameworks and Theories in a Health Promotion Intervention to Reduce Obesity

Step	Models to Partially Apply	Objective	Healthy Weight Example
1	PRECEDE portion of PRECEDE–PROCEED	Apply structure to work with community to identify occupation and health needs	Parents and school officials raise concerns regarding an increase in obesity rates among high school students
2	Health Belief Model	Determine level of threat (i.e., perceived seriousness and susceptibility weighed against benefits), relevant cues to action, and self-efficacy	Conduct separate groups prior to program development with parents, school employees, students, and local pediatricians to discuss culturally relevant cues to actions and approaches
	Stages of Change	Determine readiness for change	Develop mechanisms to identify and recruit students in the precontemplation, contemplation, and preparation stages
	Ecology of Human Performance	Determine which skills need to be established or restored through appropriate occupation-based intervention, which context or tasks be adapted or context altered to prevent harm; and determine what programs or initiatives warrant being created	Assess environmental supports by identifying what foods are available for meals and snacks; observe meal and snack time behaviors of students; and conduct formative or process evaluations with student participants to modify program as needed to ensure needed skills and knowledge are being obtained
3	PROCEED portion of PRECEDE–PROCEED	Plan and implement program evaluation to include process, impact, and outcomes evaluations	Involve student leaders, parents, and school officials in program evaluation planning

OT STORY 40.2 DEVELOPING A PROGRAM TO REDUCE IPV ON A COLLEGE CAMPUS

Serena, an occupational therapy (OT) student, along with Olivia, a health education student, approached their student government association (SGA) and shared that fellow students were concerned about campus safety. They had been asked by their respective student organizations to take the lead in developing a solution (Phase 1). Serena and Olivia also shared with the SGA the data that showed the incidence of intimate partner violence (IPV) both on their campus and other campuses as well as reports from the literature of health impacts of such violence that had been gathered and vetted by the leadership of both student groups (Phases 2 and 3). Meeting with the SGA, requesting funds, and meeting with the vice president of student affairs, which preceded the request for funds, were parts of Phase 4. An evaluation plan for the program was shared with the SGA, which included process, impact, and outcome evaluation (Phases 6, 7, and 8).

The program was developed to meet the needs of the specific student group using recommendations from the CDC Division of Violence Prevention (Niolon et al., 2017). During implementation, process measures were used to assess whether the program was being administered according to the protocol. Impact assessments immediately following the educational program included a pre-/post-knowledge/awareness survey results from attendees as well as the number of total attendees reached by the program.

The outcome evaluation at one year indicated an increase in IPV reported to campus security. This was expected because the program goal was to increase awareness of IPV; an increase in reported IPV did not necessarily mean that IPV incidence had increased but rather that there was an increase in reporting of incidences. The second-year outcome report showed that reported IPV levels had decreased from the first-year post-program levels. The program was considered as one of the factors that had resulted in this decrease; thus, funding to sustain the program was earmarked in the student affairs budget.

Question

1. Based on an examination of their disciplines' curricula and standards of practice, outline the distinct perspectives that Serena and Olivia can contribute to the program.

---

death, decreased life course) and susceptibility are appropriately represented in the program without causing undue fear. Although both health educators and occupational therapists can be familiar with barriers to behavior change, occupational therapists can add a perspective in terms of establishing new habits to support health decisions while extinguishing unhealthy habits through an occupation lens. For example, an OT practitioner may suggest highlighting additional negative aspects of smoking related to social consequences that could increase the level of perceived seriousness (e.g., social ostracization secondary to co-workers complaining of tobacco odor and frequency of smoking "breaks," marginalization of smokers because of smoking bans). Occupational therapists, using knowledge of biology, psychology, and sociology, and discipline-specific knowledge of habits, can use an occupation-based approach to move smokers from the immediate gratification of smoking to the delayed gratification of the health and social benefits derived from a nonsmoking lifestyle.

Implementing a peer or buddy occupation-based strategy could strengthen the likelihood of a person taking a positive health action. In order to successfully stop smoking, a change in social occupations and friends is often needed to prevent relapse. When first stopping smoking, for example, it is best to avoid social and physical contexts that reinforce smoking such as happy hours at an outside bar that permits smoking (i.e., barrier). The buddy strategy pairs successful ex-smokers (i.e., a cue to action) with individuals desiring to stop smoking. Through the use of an instrument, such as the activity checklist, alternate activities and identification of a new peer group of nonsmokers could be identified. Completing and describing a drawing or three-dimensional sculpture analysis of their smoking habits, using the constructs of the Kawa model (Iwama, 2006), to their buddy may help self-identify additional barriers (i.e., rocks and driftwood) and supports for change (i.e., river walls and bottom; driftwood).

The HBM has been used to help explain the poor results from the use of a curriculum for parents of children with sickle cell disease (Drazen et al., 2014). In this program, parents were not following the recommendations for caring for their children, which was explained as possibly because of lack of perception of serious risk for the children rather than disinterest in the program. In another example of HBM theory in research, a multidisciplinary research team investigated factors associated with older adult decisions to discuss their fall risks with health professionals using HBM to guide development of the survey questions (Lee et al., 2013). Other researchers have used it to explore occupation-based health behaviors such as college students' eating habits (Deshpande et al., 2009) and weight management (James et al., 2012). OT researchers have used the HBM to guide the program design of a community-based physical activity program for preschool children (Hight et al., 2021) and as the framework for an educational program for parents on neuroplasticity and home programs (Hines et al., 2020).

Using the Transtheoretical Model of Change

There are two aspects of the transtheoretical model of change that are particularly helpful to OT health promotion practice. One is the belief that relapse can be part of the normal cycle of behavior change. Therefore, neither the OT practitioner nor the client should give up hope. The second is the belief that specific strategies can be matched to each of the stages. For example, *consciousness raising* is a process that is well-matched for moving someone from the precontemplation to the contemplation stage. OT practitioners can be helpful in moving someone closer to smoking cessation through consciousness raising. For example, if a smoker reports concerns about walking to the corner store for milk, the OT practitioner, besides offering energy conservation strategies, also can suggest that they may be less out of breath walking if they stopped or decreased the number of cigars smoked. A grandparent complaining about only seeing their grandchild who has asthma outside in mild weather because of their tobacco habit could provide an opening about habit patterns and successful strategies to modify behaviors using the constructs of habits and volition from the Model of Human Occupation (MOHO; Taylor, 2017).

This model has contributed to the design and success of various health behaviors at the individual and group levels. For example, a program for children with fibromyalgia used a pain outcome measure based on the stages of change model that measured adolescents' motivation to change and accept responsibility for pain control by engaging in an intensive program of physical therapy, OT, and psychotherapy rather than medication (Sherry et al., 2015). Another example is a faith-based community weight loss program (Kim et al., 2008) named WORD (wholeness, oneness, righteousness, deliverance).

Evidence to Guide Health Promotion Practice

In addition to incorporating theory, OT health promotion interventions should be based on evidence. Several systematic reviews are available in a special issue of the *American Journal of Occupational Therapy* focused on the impact of health promotion on the health and well-being of community-dwelling older adults (AOTA, 2018b). Although randomized trials are seen by many as the most important level of evidence, by their nature, they require tight control over all aspects of the program development and evaluation. Generally, to be effective at a community level, programs must also go through translation studies to evaluate if they will still produce results in "real-world" settings. Other programs may begin from an even stronger client-centered perspective by using a participatory action research approach that arises from community needs and champions and incorporates the researcher as a mentor for the community team.

Evidence-Based Occupational Therapy Health Promotion Practices

The Well Elderly Study (Clark et al., 1997, 2001) and falls prevention initiatives (e.g., Clemson et al., 2004) are examples of health promotion interventions that have been evaluated through randomized controlled trials. In addition, researchers have used mixed methods (Mulry et al., 2017) and other techniques (Persch et al., 2015; Suarez-Balcazar et al., 2016) to investigate the impact of OT health promotion practice.

The Well Elderly Study in California demonstrated through a randomized clinical trial design that a preventive OT intervention (i.e., Lifestyle Redesign®) resulted in measurable benefits in health, function, and QOL (Clark et al., 1997), and these results were sustained after a 6-month follow-up (Clark et al., 2001). The Well Elderly Trial 2 was conducted over a 5-year period for the purpose of replicating and assessing the effectiveness and cost-effectiveness of Lifestyle Redesign® among a more ethnically and economically diverse group of older adults from a greater number of sites around Los Angeles than in the first well-elderly trial. "The primary goal of the intervention was to enable the elders to develop a sustainable and customized healthy lifestyle in their daily context" (Clark & Jackson, 2010, para. 2). Results indicated that the intervention had a greater impact on measures of mental well-being (e.g., vitality, social function, life satisfaction) at statistically significant levels than on physical, health, and well-being measures (Clark et al., 2012). Lifestyle Redesign® was found to be a cost-effective intervention for use in ethnically diverse urban communities (Clark & Jackson, 2010; Clark et al., 2012). Recently, the Lifestyle Redesign® program was successfully used with 45 patients with chronic pain to improve patient function, self-efficacy, and QOL (Simon & Collins, 2017).

A mixed methods study continued research on the *Let's Go* community mobility program using the Person-Environment-Occupation-Performance (PEOP) model's fit between intrinsic (personal) and extrinsic (environmental) factors using group and individual sessions in a 4-week period (Mulry et al., 2017). Content included participants identifying desired occupations and supports as well as barriers for community mobility. Significant improvement in participation, confidence, and community mobility was found at 4 weeks and 6 months post program. This program addressed the needs of marginalized older adults to promote wellness, participation, and QOL. Although the authors referenced only PEOP, it is easy to see an application with the HBM from the language used to describe the study (i.e., benefits, barriers, and self-efficacy).

Persch and colleagues (2015) discussed multiple research-based interventions that support healthy habits for children in the areas of sleep, physical activity, and nutrition. They advocated that OT practitioners are well-situated via their expertise in activity analysis to apply healthy habit interventions within a variety of school settings. Suarez-Balcazar and colleagues (2016) researched a 16-week program on healthy habits for Latino families who had at least one child with a disability. They partnered with a local community organization for the program that included goal setting and action planning around, physical activity, and identification of barriers in community using concepts associated with the social ecological theory and MOHO. Although only 28% of the family goals were met at the conclusion of the study, researchers noted that all 17 families achieved at least one of the average three goals they had set. In addition, all families in the study reported they were planning to continue to address their other unmet goals.

Other Examples of Occupational Therapy Health Promotion in Action

Although there are many examples of OT health promotion activities, the link of the program development to theory is not always explicit. A small sampling of initiatives is provided here to show the potential for the role of OT in the promotion of health via research, program development, and program evaluation. Each initiative is linked to a potentially supporting health promotion theory, either identified by the developer of the program or suggested by the authors.

AOTA's National School Backpack Awareness Day

One initiative for children and youth is the AOTA's National School Backpack Awareness Day (Jacobs et al., 2011), which happens annually in September with the express goal of having students wear their backpack over both shoulders and to monitor the weight they carry. The programs feature fun activities to ensure that the students understand their potential susceptibility for an injury, the potential seriousness of

an injury (two constructs from the HBM), and proper wearing techniques. Self-efficacy is enhanced when students perform the correct techniques, receive feedback about their ability to perform the task HBM constructs), and experience firsthand the benefits (HBM construct).

Powerful Tools for Caregivers via Telehealth

In recent years, technology has improved to allow virtual face-to-face meetings, and, as a result, telehealth has become an increasing popular option, especially for those with limited access to services (AOTA, 2018c). An existing caregiver program offered at many US Area Agencies on Aging, called Powerful Tools for Caregivers, was piloted using a synchronous, face-to-face telehealth approach (Serwe et al., 2017). Qualitative data collected via focus group following the program reflected positive participant experiences with attending the program this way; however, learning to use the technology was challenging for some participants. This study exemplifies how OT practitioners working in the field of health promotion can effectively use their skills to advance use and research of existing evidence-based programs. Since this study, the use of telehealth in OT has expanded as a method to maintain health (Jensen, 2021) and access to OT services (Cason & Test, 2021) during the COVID-19 pandemic. For more information on providing OT services via telehealth, see Chapter 67.

CarFit

CarFit is a program developed jointly by AOTA, AARP (formerly the American Association of Retired Persons), and the American Automobile Association (AAA) to assess the fit between older drivers and their vehicles. Stav (2010) linked CarFit to theoretical constructs from the HBM and the Person-Environment-Occupation (PEO) Model (Law et al., 1996). CarFit sessions are offered in the community often in between rush hours when older adults are more typically running errands. The evaluations are scheduled in 30-minute increments to ensure that the 12-step checklist can be completed without rushing.

The primary purpose of the program is for older adults to gain information about the fit between their body and their car while sitting in their car (PEO constructs). Adjustments needed for mirrors, steering wheels, and seats can be made immediately, and other recommendations for additional adaptations are provided as needed. Participants are educated about the findings that proper seating and alignment of mirrors decrease risk for a crash (HBM construct) because of increased visibility. At the end, participants walk around the car and reenter and can reassess the increased visibility leading to self-efficacy (HBM construct). The social atmosphere and encouragement in a group of peers acts as a socio-structural facilitator.

People With Disabilities in Refugee Camps

In collaboration with nongovernmental organizations (NGOs), OT can promote the health and occupational needs of people with disabilities in refugee camps. Understanding the QOL of refugees with disabilities and how these refugees are perceived by the others in the camp are an essential first steps. Programs that are sensitive to local customs, that are participatory, that build on strengths and capacities, and that address nutritional issues, security concerns, employment and income needs, healthcare access, education, vocational training, and resettlement options are a catalyst for improving the health and well-being of these individuals (Abdi & Matthews, 2015). Theoretical models such as the MOHO, the Kawa model, and concepts associated with occupational injustice can provide structure for developing such programs.

Conclusion

Occupation can be prescribed to promote health and well-being of individuals, families, and communities. However, this prescription must be unique and designed to be culturally relevant, client-centered, and based on theory and the most current evidence available. Using a blend of theories drawn from health behavior and OT has the potential to strengthen OT health promotion program design and success. The prescription or intervention then must be evaluated to determine if outcomes are achieved, whether the prescription or program needs to be modified, and whether the theoretical foundation needs to evolve. It is expected that new theories and models will develop across health disciplines, and that as interdisciplinary practice grows, the use of a blending approach will become more prevalent.

Acknowledgments

The authors would like to thank Kay Graham for his contribution to the previous edition of this chapter.

Lippincott® Connect *For additional resources on the subjects discussed in this chapter, visit Lippincott Connect.*

REFERENCES

Abdi, S., & Matthews, B. (2015). The Dadaab refugee camps and the voices of people with disabilities. In N. Rushford & K. Thomas (Eds.), *Disasters and development: An occupational therapy perspective* (pp. 111–118). Elsevier.

Abuelezam, N. N. (2020). Health equity during COVID-19: The case of Arab Americans. *American Journal of Preventative Medicine, 59*(3), 455–457. https://doi.org/10.1016/j.amepre.2020.06.004

Agency for Healthcare Research and Quality. (2017). *AHRQ health literacy universal precautions toolkit* (2nd ed.). https://www.ahrq.gov/ professionals/quality-patient-safety/quality-resources/tools/literacy-toolkit/index.html

Allen, S. T., O'Rourke, A., White, R. H., Schneider, K. E., Kilkenny, M., & Sherman, S. G. (2019). Estimating the number of people who inject drugs in a rural county in Appalachia. *American Journal of Public Health, 109*(3), 445–450. https://doi.org/10.2015/AJPH.2018.304873

American Occupational Therapy Association. (1982). *1982 Member data survey.* Author.

American Occupational Therapy Association. (1987). *1986 Member data survey: Interim report #1.* Author.

American Occupational Therapy Association. (1991). *1990 Member data survey: Summary report.* Author.

American Occupational Therapy Association. (2001). *AOTA 2000-member compensation survey.* Author.

American Occupational Therapy Association. (2006). *AOTA 2006 workforce and compensation report.* Author.

American Occupational Therapy Association. (2008). Occupational therapy practice framework: Domain and process, 2nd edition. *American Journal of Occupational Therapy, 62,* 625–683. https://doi .org/10.5014/ajot.62.6.625

American Occupational Therapy Association. (2010). *2010 Occupational therapy compensation and workforce study.* Author.

American Occupational Therapy Association. (2013). AOTA's societal statement on health disparities. *American Journal of Occupational Therapy, 67,* S7–S8. https://doi.org/10.5014/ajot.2013.67S7

American Occupational Therapy Association. (2014). Occupational therapy practice framework: Domain and process, 3rd edition. *American Journal of Occupational Therapy, 68,* S1–S48. https://doi .org/10.5014/ajot.2014.682006

American Occupational Therapy Association. (2015). *2015 AOTA salary and workforce survey.* Author.

American Occupational Therapy Association. (2016). AOTA's societal statement on livable communities. *American Journal of Occupational Therapy, 70,* S1–S2. https://doi.org/10.5014/ajot.63.6.847

American Occupational Therapy Association. (2017a). AOTA's societal statement on disaster response and risk reduction. *American Journal of Occupational Therapy, 71,* 7112410060. https://doi.org/10.5014/ ajot.2017.716S11

American Occupational Therapy Association. (2017b). Vision 2025. *American Journal of Occupational Therapy, 71,* 1. doi: 10.5014/ajot.2017.713002

American Occupational Therapy Association. (2017c). AOTA's societal statement on health literacy. *American Journal of Occupational Therapy, 71,* 7112410065p1–7112410065p2. https://doi.org/10.5014/ ajot.2017.716S14

American Occupational Therapy Association. (2018a). AOTA's societal statement on youth violence. *American Journal of Occupational Therapy, 72*(Suppl. 2), 1–2, 7212410090. https://doi.org/10.5014/ ajot.2018.72S209

American Occupational Therapy Association. (2018b). Special issue on productive aging for community-dwelling older adults. *American Journal of Occupational Therapy, 72*(4), 263–265. https://doi .org/10.5014/ajot.2010.005165

American Occupational Therapy Association. (2018c). Telehealth in occupational therapy [Position paper]. *American Journal of Occupational Therapy, 72*(Suppl. 2), S1–S18, 7212410059. *https://doi .org/10.5014/ajot.2018.72S219*

American Occupational Therapy Association. (2020a). *2019 workforce and salary survey: Executive summary.* Author.

American Occupational Therapy Association. (2020b). AOTA 2020 occupational therapy code of ethics. *American Journal of Occupational Therapy, 74*(Suppl. 3), 7413410005. https://doi.org/10.5014/ ajot.2020.74S3006

American Occupational Therapy Association. (2020c). Occupational therapy in the promotion of health and well-being. *American*

Journal of Occupational Therapy, 74, 1–14. 7403420010. *https://doi .org/10.5014/ajot.2020.743003*

American Occupational Therapy Association. (2020d). Occupational therapy practice framework: Domain and process (4th ed.). *American Journal of Occupational Therapy, 74*(Suppl. 2), 7412410010. https://doi.org/10.5014/ajot.2020.74S2001

American Occupational Therapy Association. (2021). Standards of practice for occupational therapy. *American Journal of Occupational Therapy, 75*(Suppl. 3), 7513410050. https://doi.org/10.5014/ajot.2021.75S3004

Au-Yeung, C., Blewett, L. A., & Lange, K. (2019). Addressing the rural opioid addiction and overdose crisis through cross-sector collaboration: Little Falls, Minnesota. *American Journal of Public Health, 109*(2), 260–262. *https://doi.org/10.2105/AJPH.2018.304789*

Baum, M. C. (2006). Presidential address, 2006: Centennial challenges, millennium opportunities. *American Journal of Occupational Therapy, 60*, 609–616. https://doi.org/10.5014/ajot.60.6.609

Berwick, D. M., Nolan, T. W., & Whittington, J. (2008). The Triple Aim: Care, health, and cost. *Health Affairs, 27*(3), 759–769. https://doi .org/10.1377/hlthaff.27.3.759

Bhatia, G., Dutta, P. K., Canipe, C., & McClure, J. (2022). COVID-19 vaccination tracker. *UpToDate.* https://graphics.reuters.com/world-coronavirus-tracker-and-maps/vaccination-rollout-and-access/

Biven, J. (2015). Drought: Slow-onset disaster and its burden upon families. In N. Rushford & K. Thomas (Eds.), *Disasters and development: An occupational therapy perspective* (pp. 167–176). Elsevier.

Bodenheimer, T., & Sinsky, C. (2014). From Triple Aim to Quadruple Aim: Care of the patient requires care of the provider. *Annals of Family Medicine, 12*(6), 573–576. https://doi.org/10.1370/afm.1713

Brunyate, R. W. (1967). From the president: After fifty years, what stature do we hold? *American Journal of Occupational Therapy, 21*, 262–267. https://pubmed.ncbi.nlm.nih.gov/6066211/

Cason, J., & Test, L. A. (2021). *School-age telehealth: Practice considerations and resources for occupational therapy practitioners.* AOTA.

Centers for Disease Control and Prevention. (2017). *Food deserts.* http://www.cdc.gov/Features/FoodDeserts/

Centers for Disease Control and Prevention. (2021). *Health related quality of life (HRQOL).* https://www.cdc.gov/hrqol/index.htm#:~:text=Health%2Drelated%20quality%20of%20life%20(HRQOL)%20is%20an%20individual's,and%20mental%20health%20over%20time

Clark, F., Azen, S. P., Carlson, M., Mandel, D., LaBree, L. Hay, J., Zemke, R., Jackson, J., & Lipson, L. (2001). Embedding health-promoting changes into the daily lives of independent-living older adults: Long-term follow-up of occupational therapy intervention. *The Journal of Gerontology, 56B*, 60–63. https://doi.org/10.1093/geronb/56.1.p60

Clark, F., Azen, S. P., Zemke, R., Jackson, J., Carlson, M., Mandel, D., Hay, J., Josephson, K., Cherry, B., Hessel, C., Palmer, J., & Lipson, L. (1997). Occupational therapy for independent-living older adults: A randomized controlled trial. *Journal of the American Medical Association, 278*, 1321–1326. https://doi.org/10.1001/jama.1997.03550160041036

Clark, F., & Jackson, J. (2010). *Well Elderly II clinical trial results: Effectiveness and cost-effectiveness of the Lifestyle Redesign intervention in community settings.* http://www.wfot.org/wfot2010/program/pdf/1457.pdf

Clark, F., Jackson, J., Carlson, M., Chou, C., Cherry, B. J., Jordan-Marsh, M., Knight, B. J., Mandel, D., Blanchard, J., Granger, D. A., Wilcox, R. R., Lai, M. Y., White, B., Hay, J., Lam, C., Marterella, A., & Azen, S. P. (2012). Effectiveness of a lifestyle intervention in promoting the well-being of independently living older people: Results of the well elderly 2 randomised controlled trial. *Journal of Epidemiology and Community Health, 66*, 782–790. https://doi.org/10.1136/jech.2009.099754

Clemson, L., Cumming, R. G., Kendig, H., Swann, M., Heard, R., & Taylor, K. (2004). The effectiveness of a community-based program

for reducing the incidence of falls in the elderly: A randomized trial. *Journal of the American Geriatrics Society, 52*, 1487–1494. https://doi .org/10.1111/j.1532-5415.2004.52411.x

Cole, R. E., & Horacek, T. (2009). Applying PRECEDE–PROCEED to develop an intuitive eating nondieting approach to weight management pilot program. *Journal of Nutrition Education and Behavior, 41*, 120–126. https://doi.org/10.1016/j.jneb.2008.03.006

Deshpande, S., Basil, M. D., & Basil, D. Z. (2009). Factors influencing healthy eating habits among college students: An application of the health belief model. *Health Marketing Quarterly, 26*, 145–164. https://doi.org/10.1080/07359680802619834

Drazen, C. H., Abel, R., Lindsey, T., & King, A. A. (2014). Development and feasibility of a home-based education model for families of children with sickle cell disease. *BMC Public Health, 14*, 116. https://doi .org/10.1186/1471-2458-14-116

Dunn, W., Brown, C., & McGuigan, A. (1994). The ecology of human performance: A framework for considering the effect of context. *American Journal of Occupational Therapy, 48*, 595–607. https://doi .org/10.5014/ajot.48.7.595

Finn, G. (1972). The occupational therapist in prevention programs. *American Journal of Occupational Therapy, 26*, 59–66. https://pubmed.ncbi.nlm.nih.gov/5014201/

Garcia-Ruiz, S. (2015). Community-based rehabilitation in Columbia's armed conflict. In N. Rushford & K. Thomas (Eds.), *Disasters and development: An occupational therapy perspective* (pp. 129–146). Elsevier.

Green, L. W., & Kreuter, M. W. (2005). *Health promotion planning: An educational and ecological approach* (4th ed.). McGraw-Hill.

Heijmans, M., Waverijn, G., Rademakers, J., van der Vaart, R., & Rijken, M. (2015). Functional, communicative, and critical health literacy of chronic disease patients and their importance for self-management. *Patient Education and Counseling, 98*, 41–48. https://doi.org/10 .1016/j.pec.2014.10.006

Hight, J., O'Brien, S. P., & Schneck, C. M. (2021). Promoting population health in local communities: Parental perceptions of an embedded movement and physical activity program for a preschool population. *The Open Journal of Occupational Therapy, 9*(3), 1–11. https://doi .org/10.15453/ 2168-6408.1841

Hines, D., York, K., & Kaul, E. (2020). Basic research: Optimizing compliance with home programming through neuroplasticity education among parents of children receiving outpatient OT. *American Journal of Occupational Therapy, 74* (Suppl. 1), *1.* https://doi.org/10.5014/ajot.2020.74S1-PO3133

International Health Literacy Association. (2017). *International Health Literacy Association Constitution and bylaws.* Retrieved March 16, 2022, from https://i-hla.org/

Iwama, M. K. (2006). *The Kawa model: Culturally relevant occupational therapy.* Elsevier.

Jacobs, K., Wuest, E., Markowitz, J., & Hellman, M. (2011). Get packing: Planning your own National School Backpack Awareness Day event. *OT Practice, 16*(13), 11–14. https://eds.p.ebscohost.com/eds/detail/detail?vid=1&sid=a161ceb6-ef52-4af6-9be5-8db59d48e3a

Jaffe, E. (1986). Nationally speaking—The role of occupational therapy in the disease prevention and health promotion. *American Journal of Occupational Therapy, 40*, 749–752. https://doi.org/10.5014/ajot

James, D. C. S., Pobee, J. W., Oxidine, D., Brown, L., & Joshi, G. (2012). Using the health belief model to develop culturally appropriate weight-management materials for African American women. *Journal of the Academy of Nutrition and Dietetics, 112*, 664–670. https:// doi.org/10.1016/j.jand.2012.02.003

Jensen, M. (2021, January). *Workplace wellness: Helping clients meet physical, mental, and emotional challenges on the job during COVID-19.* AOTA.

Johnson, J. A. (1986). *Wellness: A context for living.* Slack.

Kaplan, L. H., & Burch-Minakan, L. (1986). Reach out for health: A corporation's approach to health promotion. *American Journal of Occupational Therapy, 40*, 777–780. https://10.5014/ajot.40.11.777

Kielhofner, G. (2009). *Conceptual foundations of occupational therapy* (4th ed.). F. A. Davis.

Kim, K. H., Linnan, L., Campbell, M. K., Brooks, C., Koenig, H. G., & Wiesen, C. (2008). The WORD (wholeness, oneness, righteousness, deliverance): A faith-based weight-loss program utilizing a community-based participatory action research approach. *Health Education & Behavior, 35,* 634–650. hhttps://doi.org/10.1016/j .cct.2014.11.009

Law, M., Cooper, B., Strong, S., Stewart, D., Rigby, P., & Letts, L. (1996). The person-environment-occupation model: A transactive approach to occupational performance. *Canadian Journal of Occupational Therapy, 63,* 9–23. https://pubmed.ncbi.nlm.nih.gov/6066217/

Lee, D. C. A., Day, L., Hill, K., Clemson, L., McDermott, F., & Haines, T. P. (2013). What factors influence older adults to discuss falls with their health care providers? *Health Expectations, 18,* 1593–1609. https://doi.org/10.1111/hex.12149

Lippold, K., & Ali, B. (2020). Racial/ethnic differences in opioid-involved overdose deaths across metropolitan and non-metropolitan areas in the United States, 1999−2017. *Drug and Alcohol Dependence, 212,* 108059. *https://doi.org/10.1016/j.drugalcdep.2020.108059*

McCombie, R. P., & Stirling, J. L. (2018). Opioid substance abuse among occupational therapy clients. *Occupational Therapy in Mental Health, 34*(1), 49–60. https://doi.org/10.1080/0164212x.2017.1360827

Molineux, M. L., & Whiteford, G. E. (2011). Prisons: From occupational deprivation to occupational enrichment. *Journal of Occupational Science, 6,* 124–130. https://doi.org/10.1080/14427591.1999.9686457

Moore, W., & Green, E. L. (2021). *Five days: The fiery reckoning of an American city.* One World.

Mulry, C. M., Papetti, C., De Martinis, J. D., & Ravinsky, M. (2017). Facilitating wellness in urban-dwelling, low-income older adults through community mobility: A mixed methods study. *American Journal of Occupational Therapy, 71,* 7104190030p1–7104190030p7. https://doi.org/10.5014/ajot.2017.025494

National Cancer Institute. (2005). *Theory at a glance* (2nd ed.). National Institutes of Health. http://www.cancer.gov/theory.pdf

Niolon, P. H., Kearns, M., Dills, J., Ramo, K., Irving, S., Armstead, T., & Gilbert, L. (2017). *Preventing intimate partner violence across the lifespan: A technical package of programs, policies, and practices.* National Center for Injury Prevention and Control, Centers for Disease Control and Prevention.

Nundy, S., Cooper, L. A., & Mate, K. S. (2022). The Quintuple Aim for health care improvement: A new imperative to advance health equity. *JAMA, 327*(6), 521–522. https://doi.org/10.1001/jama.2021.25181

Pashmdarfard, M., Arabshahi, K. S., Shafaroodi, N., Mehraban, A. H., Parvizi, S., & Haracz, K. (2020). Which models can be used as a clinical education model in occupational therapy? Introduction of the models: A scoping review study. *Medical Journal of the Islamic Republic of Iran, 34,* 76. https://www.ncbi.nlm.nih.gov/pmc/articles/PMC7711038/

Persch, A. C., Lamb, A. J., Metzler, C. A., & Fristad, M. A. (2015). Healthy habits for children: Leveraging existing evidence to demonstrate value. *American Journal of Occupational Therapy, 69,* 6904900010p1.

Pietella, A. (2010). *Not in my neighborhood: How bigotry shaped a great American city.* Ivan R. Dee.

Prochaska, J. O., & DiClemente, C. C. (1982). Transtheoretical therapy: Toward a more integrative model of change. *Psychotherapy: Theory, Research and Practice, 19,* 276–288. https://doi.org/10.1037/h0088437

Prochaska, J. O., & DiClemente, C. C. (1983). Stages and processes of self-change of smoking: Toward an integrative model of change. *Journal of Counseling and Clinical Psychology, 51,* 390–395. https://doi.org/10.1037//0022-006x.51.3.390

Pyatak, E. A., Carandang, K., & Davis, S. (2015). Developing a manualized occupational therapy diabetes management intervention: Resilient, empowered, active living with diabetes. *OTJR: Occupation, Participation and Health, 35,* 187–194. https://doi .org/10.1177/1539449215584310

Reitz, S. M. (1992). A historical review of occupational therapy's role in preventive health and wellness. *American Journal of Occupational Therapy, 46,* 50–55. https://doi.org/10.5014/ajot.46.1.50

Reitz, S. M. (2010). Historical and philosophical perspectives of occupational therapy's role in health promotion. In M. E. Scaffa, S. M. Reitz, & M. A. Pizzi (Eds.), *Occupational therapy in the promotion of health and wellness* (pp. 1–21). F. A. Davis.

Reitz, S. M., & Scaffa, M. E. (2010). Public health principles, approaches, and initiatives. In M. E. Scaffa, S. M. Reitz, & M. A. Pizzi (Eds.), *Occupational therapy in the promotion of health and wellness* (pp. 70–95). F. A. Davis.

Reitz, S. M., Scaffa, M. E., Campbell, R. M., & Rhynders, P. A. (2010). Health behavior frameworks for health promotion practice. In M. E. Scaffa, S. M. Reitz, & M. A. Pizzi (Eds.), *Occupational therapy in the promotion of health and wellness* (pp. 46–69). F. A. Davis.

Robinson, M. L., Costa, D. M., Mattila, A., McCombie, R. P., & Yeager, J. (2018). *Report of the Ad Hoc committee on drug opioid abuse to the representative assembly.* American Occupational Therapy Association.

Rowe, N. C., & Breeden, K. L. (2018). *Opioid guidelines and their implications for occupational therapy.* CE-Article-August-2018.pdf (aota .org)

Schultz, S. (2009). Occupational adaptation. In E. B. Crepeau, E. S. Cohn, & B. A. B. Schell (Eds.), *Willard & Spackman's occupational therapy* (11th ed., pp. 462–475). Lippincott Williams & Wilkins.

Schmidt, H., Weintraub, R., Williams, M. A., Miller, K., Buttenheim, A., Sadecki, E., Wu, H., Doiphode, A., Nagpal, N., Gostin, L. O., & Shen, A. A. (2021). Equitable allocation of COVID-19 vaccines in the United States. *Nature Medicine, 27,* 1298–1307. https://doi .org/10.1038/s41591-021-01379-6

Serwe, K. M., Hersch, G. I., Pickens, N. D., & Pancheri, K. (2017). Caregiver perceptions of a telehealth wellness program. *American Journal of Occupational Therapy, 71,* 7104350010p1. https://doi.org/10.5014/ajot.2017.025619

Sherry, D. D., Brake, L., Tress, J. L., Sherker, J., Fash, K., Ferry, K., & Weiss, P. F. (2015). The treatment of juvenile fibromyalgia with an intensive physical and psychosocial program. *The Journal of Pediatrics, 167,* 731–737. https://doi.org/10.1016/j.jpeds.2015.06.036

Simon, A. U., & Collins, C. R. (2017). Lifestyle Redesign® for chronic pain management: A retrospective clinical efficacy study. *American Journal of Occupational Therapy, 71,* 7104190040. https://doi .org/0.5014/ajot.2017.025502

Smith, S. G., Chen, J., Basile, K. C., Gilbert, L. K., Merrick, M. T., Patel, N., Walling, M., & Jain, A. (2017). *The National Intimate Partner and Sexual Violence Survey (NISVS): 2010–2012 State Report.* National Center for Injury Prevention and Control, Centers for Disease Control and Prevention. https://www.cdc.gov/violenceprevention/pdf/ipv-technicalpackages.pdf

Stav, W. (2010). CarFit: An evaluation of behavior change and impact. *British Journal of Occupational Therapy, 73,* 589–597. https://doi.org/10.4276/030802210X12918167234208

Suarez-Balcazar, Y., Hoisington, M., Orozco, A. A., Arias, D., Garcia, C., Smith, K., & Bonner, B. (2016). Benefits of a culturally tailored health promotion program for Latino youth with disabilities and their families. *American Journal of Occupational Therapy, 70,* 7005180080p1. https://doi.org/10.5014/ajot.2016.021949

Taylor, R. R. (2017). *Kielhofner's model of human occupation* (5th ed.). Wolters Kluwer.

U.S. Department of Health and Human Services. (n.d.-a). *Healthy people 2030: Framework. Healthy People 2030* | health.gov

U.S. Department of Health and Human Services. (n.d.-b). *How can I use Healthy People 2030 in my work.*

U.S. Department of Health and Human Services. (n.d.-c). *Social determinants of health. Healthy People 2030* | health.gov

U.S. Department of Health and Human Services, & Health Resources & Services Administration. (2019). *Health literacy.* Official web site of the U.S. Health Resources & Services Administration (hrsa.gov).

U.S. Department of Health and Human Services, Health Resources & Services Administration, & Office of Health Equity. (2020). *Health equity report 2019–2020: Special feature on housing and health inequalities.* Author.

U.S. Department of Health and Human Services, & Office of Disease Prevention and Health Promotion. (2008). *America's health literacy: Why we need accessible health information.* https://health.gov/communication/literacy/issuebrief/

U.S. Department of Health and Human Services, & The Secretary's Advisory Committee on National Health Promotion and Disease Prevention Objectives for 2020. (2010). *Phase I report: Recommendations for the framework and format of Healthy People 2020* [Internet]. Section IV: Advisory Committee findings and recommendations [cited 2010 January 6]. http://www.healthypeople.gov/sites/default/files/PhaseI_0.pdf

Virginia Commonwealth University Center on Society and Health. (2017). *Mapping life expectancy.* http://www.societyhealth.vcu.edu/work/the-projects/mapsatlanta.html

Walsh, J. R., White, A. A., & Kattelmann, K. K. (2014). Using PRECEDE to develop a weight management program for disadvantaged young adults. *Journal of Nutrition Education and Behavior, 46,* 1–9. https://doi.org/10.1016/j.jneb.2013.11.005

Webb Hooper, M., Nápoles, A. M., & Pérez-Stable, E. J. (2021). No populations left behind: Vaccine hesitancy and equitable diffusion of effective COVID-19 vaccines. *Journal of General Internal Medicine, 36,* 2130–2133. https://doi.org/10.1007/s11606-021-06698-5

West, W. (1967). The occupational therapist's changing responsibility to the community. *American Journal of Occupational Therapy, 21,* 312–316.

West, W. (1969). The growing importance of prevention. *American Journal of Occupational Therapy, 23,* 226–231. https://pubmed.ncbi.nlm.nih.gov/5008166/

Wiemer, R. (1972). Some concepts of prevention as an aspect of community health. *American Journal of Occupational Therapy, 26,* 1–9.

Wilcock, A. A. (2006). *An occupational perspective of health* (2nd ed.). Slack.

World Federation of Occupational Therapists. (2004). *WFOT position paper: Community based rehabilitation.* http://www.wfot.org/ResourceCentre.aspx Community-Based-Rehabilitation.pdf

World Federation of Occupational Therapists. (2016). *WFOT position paper: Occupational therapy in disaster risk reduction.* http://www.wfot.org/ResourceCentre.aspx Occupational-Therapy-in-Disaster-Risk-Reduction-DRR.pdf

World Health Organization. (1947). Constitution of the World Health Organization. *Chronicle of the World Health Organization, 1*(1), 29–40. http://apps.who.int/gb/bd/PDF/bd47/EN/constitution-en.pdf?ua=1

World Health Organization. (1986). *The Ottawa charter for health promotion.* http://www.who.int/hpr/NPH/docs/ottawa_charter_hp.pdf

CHAPTER 41

Principles of Learning and Behavior Change

Christine A. Helfrich

LEARNING OBJECTIVES

After reading this chapter, you will be able to:

1. Identify and describe the four theories of learning: behavioral, social cognitive, constructivist, and motivational.
2. Compare the essential elements and assumptions of each theory of learning.
3. Explain how different theories of learning contribute to occupational therapy intervention.
4. Analyze a learning need and synthesize information to select the most appropriate strategy.

Introduction

Think of the many things you may have taught different people. Perhaps you taught a younger sibling how to share toys, a friend how to navigate a bus or subway system, grandparents how to keep track of their medicines, a classmate how to organize information and prepare for an important test, a son or daughter how to overcome a fear or anxiety, and yourself a new leisure activity or how to use a new cell phone. Did you teach everyone the same way? What did you consider about *how* to teach the person? Why did you teach the skill or behavior *in a particular way*? What *strategies* did you use? *What beliefs about how people learn guided you in your selection of strategies?* In your efforts to teach others, you have likely developed a beginning set of beliefs about how people learn best. Hopefully, you have also begun to notice that different strategies work best for different people and/or different situations.

This chapter presents an overview of selected theories of learning. In general, learning theories provide a conceptual framework to explain how and why changes in performance occur (Driscoll & Burner, 2021). Learning theories have provided the foundation for many occupational therapy (OT) theories and frames of reference such as cognitive disabilities and the Model of Human Occupation. It is important to understand the basic concepts of learning when using theoretical approaches that are considered unique to OT. Four different overall ways of thinking about and conceptualizing theories of learning are reviewed in this chapter: behavioral, social cognitive, constructivist, and motivational.

Why Should Occupational Therapists Study Theories of Learning?

Svinicki (2004) identified several reasons to study theories of learning. Many of these are relevant to occupational therapists and relate to general ideas about how theory guides practice; however, the following two are particularly salient:

- *Theory enhances practitioners' effectiveness and ability to solve problems.* The primary goal of OT is to help people function in their daily occupations. Interventions may be designed, suggested, and implemented in many different ways. Practitioners who understand different perspectives on how people learn are likely to be more effective at presenting a range of interventions that match their clients' learning needs and learning styles.[1] And when problems do arise, it is important to be able to analyze why the intervention may not be working. Understanding theories of learning will help you to solve problems that emerge during intervention and generate new approaches with your client when an intervention strategy is not effective.
- *Theory promotes individualized and creative interventions.* Each client with whom you work will have different values, interests, needs, abilities, and preferred ways of learning. Understanding theories of learning will help you design interventions that respond to each client's unique strengths and limitations.

In addition to the above listed reasons to study theories of learning, theories of learning serve several other purposes. At perhaps the most basic level, they provide us with a way to organize vast amounts of knowledge that are used in practice. Theory helps us to put our knowledge together, to organize otherwise random knowledge into a cohesive set of ideas that explain some phenomenon—in this case, learning. Theories of learning enable us to see how interesting and complex even the most seemingly simple things can be. This does not mean that theory makes things more complicated. Rather, theory helps us to see that there is usually more to any teaching–learning situation than meets the eye. Theories of learning reflect beliefs about how people think and how they store and use information (Svinicki, 2004). According to Hergenhahn (1976):

> Since most human behavior is learned, investigating the principles of learning will help us understand why we behave as we do. An awareness of the learning process will not only allow greater understanding of normal and adaptive behavior, but will also allow greater understanding of the circumstances that produce maladaptive and abnormal behavior. (p. 12)

Therefore, in any intervention situation, OT practitioners need to understand the reason or reasons that contribute to challenges with learning or behavior change in order to identify the strategies for success. For another perspective on the importance of understanding theories of learning, see Expanding Our Perspectives.

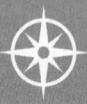

EXPANDING OUR PERSPECTIVES

The Need for Understanding Theories of Learning

Mariel Pellegrini

During my studies as an occupational therapist in Argentina, in the mid-1980s, my training was solid in the knowledge of intervention techniques and strategies for different types of clients. But I had no training on how to teach these to the people I was working with.

Usually, I intuitively tried different ways of explaining how to dress, how to organize your daily meal, how to teach a craft, and how to teach to look both ways when crossing the street. Most probably because of my life story,

family experiences, learning styles, and problem-solving, I had developed that intuition of being able to explain and teach. In all innocence, I thought that just by being an occupational therapist, I magically developed these skills. Since the beginning of my profession I have worked in mental health, and these strategies were organized based on the needs of the assisted client. But years later, working in community spaces with populations in situations of social vulnerability but without a diagnosis of disability, I began to question my beliefs about how people learn. On what was my style of teaching occupational doing based? Was there really a choice of strategies based on something more than my own intuition and empirical experience?

---

[1]According to the American Occupational Therapy Association (AOTA, 2020, p. S75), the term *client* refers to *persons* (including those involved in care of a client), *groups* (a collection of individuals having shared characteristics or common or shared purpose (e.g., family members, workers, students, and those with similar interests or occupational challenges), and *populations* (aggregates of people with common attributes such as contexts, characteristics or concerns, including health risks). However, in countries other than the United States, the term *client* often refers to persons who are paying for their care directly. In most countries, *patient* is used to describe persons who are in hospital or rehabilitation. *Service user* and *person* are terms in general use that describe those in need of OT services. For this chapter, we are using *client* without implying the source of payment for services.

At that time, in addition to clinical work, I was working as a professor at the university, a role that I have enjoyed for more than 27 years, which made me study learning theories. These taught me the theoretical bases for the development of teaching strategies in the classroom, but also for my role as an occupational therapist. Driscoll and Burner (2021) argue that learning theories provide a conceptual framework to explain how and why changes in performance occur. Therefore, it is important to understand the basic concepts of learning when we work as occupational therapists.

This chapter identifies several reasons to study theories of learning. Many of these are relevant to occupational therapists and relate to general ideas about how theory guides practice. However, in my experience, there is not enough training about them in occupational therapy degrees. As the director of an OT program in Argentina, these theories are currently included in the undergraduate training for the development of the professional reasoning of the future occupational therapist. Zabalza (2022) says that the objective of teaching is not to produce learning but to produce conditions for learning. Taking this to the field of OT, professionals must create the conditions for learning, but the one who learns is the client. It is essential to closely observe the client's experience of learning. This requires that the professional knows what actually happens from the perspective of the learner and chooses which learning theory provides more customer-focused strategies.

Models of Learning and Behavior Change

What is learning? How do we know when someone is learning? Under what conditions does learning occur? Why does learning occur? What does the learner do to cause the learning? What are the outcomes of learning? The answer to all of these questions is "it depends." It depends because different learning theories attribute different causes, reasons, actions, and circumstances to learning. The challenge for the therapist in choosing the most appropriate theory to treat a person is to consider the unique individual, task, and environment for every situation.

Behavioral Theory

Behavioral theory focuses on how observable, tangible behaviors are learned in response to some environmental stimulation (Martin & Pear, 2019). Behavioral theorists focus on observable events rather than on mental processes. For example, how does a child learn to take turns while playing a game with friends? How might a person with a developmental disability learn to respond appropriately in a conversation? And how would a person learn to propel and navigate a wheelchair in an urban community? In these examples, the observable events are the child waiting for and taking their turn during a game of kickball, a person waiting for a conversation partner to finish speaking before providing new information, and a person successfully navigating curbs and crowds in a wheelchair. The overall emphasis in behavioral theories of learning is on the relationship between an environmental stimulus and a behavioral response and on how learning is indicated by an observed change in behavior.

Essential Elements and Assumptions of Behavioral Learning Theory

Behaviorists use the term *conditioning* to explain changes in behavior rather than learning because behavioral theory asserts that a person's behavior is conditioned by events in the environment. A behavior is gradually shaped, changed, and molded as it reflects the environment's response to the behavior. There are several key terms that you will notice in most types of behavioral theory: **conditioning** (a behavior modification process that increases or decreases the likelihood of a behavior being performed), **stimulus** (verbal, sensory, or environmental input that prompts a behavior), **response** (the reaction to the stimulus), **fading** and **shaping** (strategies to develop closer and closer approximations of a behavior), **chaining** (a stepwise process for teaching a multistep task), **reinforcement** (a stimulus that causes a behavior to be strengthened and performed again [positive or negative reinforcement]), **punishment** (an aversive stimulus that causes a behavior to decrease in frequency), and **extinction** (the process of reducing the frequency of a behavior by withholding reinforcement).

Behavioral Intervention Approaches: Classical and Operant Conditioning, Positive and Negative Reinforcement, Punishment, and Extinction

There are several types of interventions that are designed to strengthen or increase behavior, whereas others are designed to decrease or eliminate behavior.

- In classical conditioning, there is an unconditioned stimulus and a conditioned stimulus. The conditioned stimulus brings about the conditioned response. The response is automatic and involuntary. For example, consider John, a 77-year-old man attending a community behavioral health center. An example of classical conditioning would be if the community center was playing old songs (stimulus) that reminded John of past experiences with friends. This could make John feel comfortable and pleasant (response) and cause John to want to attend the center more often.

- In operant conditioning, a response is *followed by* a reinforcing stimulus. The response is *voluntary*. The organism has control over whether it emits the response. *Operant conditioning* would occur if after John went to the community center (response), he received praise and enthusiasm (reinforcing stimulus) and then attended the center more regularly as a result.

- *Positive reinforcement* is the presentation of a reinforcer (stimulus) immediately following a behavior that causes the behavior to be more likely to reoccur. Different types of reinforcement may include consumable (i.e., food), manipulative (i.e., toy to play with), social (i.e., positive feedback or attention), activity (i.e., swinging or bouncing on lap or watching television), and possession (i.e., money or tokens). The reinforcer must be appealing to the individual for it to be effective.

- *Negative reinforcement* occurs when the removal of a stimulus immediately after a response causes the response to be strengthened or to increase in frequency. For example, Norre is required to attend a social skills group and participate. They are asked to leave the group every time they say "pass" to answering a question. Norre soon realizes that if they keep saying "pass," they will be sent out of the group and not be asked to return. In this case, removal of the aversive stimulus of attending the group causes Norre to increase their refusal to participate, and the response is strengthened.

- *Punishment* is the presentation of an aversive stimulus contingent on a response that reduces the rate of that response. Such an approach is common in the legal arena, as for example, when an individual commits a crime or breaks a law, they are fined or imprisoned each time the misbehavior occurs. It should be noted that punishment is often confused with negative reinforcement.

- *Extinction* is the process of reducing the frequency of a behavior by withholding reinforcement. Extinction can be challenging to enact because it may be difficult to know which reinforcer is the one actually reinforcing the undesirable behavior. For example, a child who hits other children and is given a time-out for that behavior may actually be receiving positive reinforcement (in the form of social contact) for that behavior from the adult giving the time-out. When trying to extinguish a behavior, you may also see an extinction burst or spontaneous recovery. An extinction burst occurs when the behavior being extinguished gets worse before it gets better. For example, an individual who is diagnosed with diabetes and told they

must eliminate all sweets from their diet, goes out to a dessert buffet every night for a week before starting the new diet. *Spontaneous recovery* occurs when the behavior being extinguished reappears after a delay, even though typically it is not as severe. An example of this is a child who has stopped taking other's toys and then begins to do so again, seemingly for no reason. Often, spontaneous recovery can be linked to a stressful or anxiety-producing event for the individual. Reimplementing the behavioral strategies that extinguished the behavior initially can usually be done quite quickly and successfully.

Reinforcement Schedule, Differential Reinforcement, Stimulus Discrimination, and Stimulus Generalization

Behaviors are changed by being reinforced. The frequency and type of reinforcement determine the reinforcement schedule.

- *Reinforcement schedule.* Each type of reinforcement used to change a behavior is delivered on a schedule. A reinforcement schedule indicates which instances of behavior, if any, will be reinforced. There are two main types of reinforcement schedules: (a) Continuous reinforcement reinforces every instance of the behavior and is most often used at the beginning of treatment. (b) Intermittent reinforcement only reinforces certain demonstrations of the behavior and is more effective at maintaining the desired response. Intermittent reinforcement can be delivered using one of the following four types of reinforcement schedules: (a) *ratio schedules*: reinforcement is based on the number of behaviors required, (b) *interval schedules*: reinforcement is based on the passage of time between behaviors occurring, (c) *fixed schedules*: the requirements for reinforcement are always the same, and (d) *variable schedules*: the requirements for reinforcement change randomly. It is easiest for someone to change their behavior initially when they know when they will receive their next reinforcement; however, variable reinforcement is more effective at maintaining behavior change. For example, if the goal is for Gavin to get to school on time every day, you would begin by giving them positive reinforcement *each* day they arrived on time (*continuous*). Once they were arriving on time consistently, you might reward them each time they arrived 3 days in a row (*ratio*) or every fourth day (*interval*) they arrived on time. Once either or both of these patterns were achieved, you would provide random reinforcement (*variable schedule*) for their on-time arrival to school.

- *Differential reinforcement* teaches individuals to discriminate between desired and undesired behavior and can be used to increase or decrease behavior. There are four types of differential reinforcement. Differential reinforcement at low rates (DRL) and differential reinforcement of zero responding (DRO) involve the simple decrease or absence of behavior (i.e., decreases or stops talking out in class). Differential reinforcement of incompatible responding (DRI) and differential reinforcement of alternative behavior (DRA) involve adding an incompatible or alternative behavior to replace the original behavior (e.g., eating a lollipop instead of sucking one's thumb [DRI], going to a needle exchange program instead of sharing needles to use heroin [DRA]). Note: Harm reduction programs use forms of differential reinforcement by reinforcing less harmful behaviors that replace more harmful behaviors.

- *Stimulus discrimination* learning is the procedure by which an individual can learn to emit a behavior under certain conditions instead of others. For example, children learn to raise their hands to be called on in the classroom if they wish to speak, whereas at the family dinner table, they wait for a pause in the conversation to speak (without raising their hands).
- *Stimulus generalization*, in contrast, occurs when a behavior becomes more probable in the presence of one stimulus as a result of being reinforced in the presence of another similar stimulus. For example, a child who has been abused by their father may generalize their response to being fearful of all men and demonstrate this fear by avoiding males in general.

Behavioral Techniques: Fading, Shaping, and Chaining

Whereas different types of reinforcement are used to increase or decrease specific behaviors, fading, shaping, and chaining are behavioral methods used to teach skills that involve more than one step.

- *Fading* occurs when prompts or cues that guide the performance of a complex behavior are gradually withdrawn. A prompt is a stimulus (physical, verbal, or visual) introduced to control the desired behavior during the early part of a learning program. For example, when Mariana is learning how to swing a golf club, the instructor will first provide hand-over-hand guidance to show Mariana how to hold and swing the club, then will move to using only verbal cues, and next will use fewer and fewer verbal cues until eventually Mariana is swinging the club on her own.
- *Shaping* occurs by reinforcing successively closer approximations to the target behavior while extinguishing preceding approximations of the behavior. For example, when baby Jennifer is learning how to talk and says "Je" when first attempting to say their own name, their parents reinforce the behavior with smiles and verbal praise. With practice, Jennifer next refers to themself as "Jen," then "Jen-fer," and finally as "Jennifer." As Jennifer's pronunciation improves, their parents provide smiles and verbal praise for each improved pronunciation while no

longer reinforcing previous versions. For example, once Jennifer learns to say "Jen-fer," they are no longer praised for referring to themself as "Je."

Both fading and shaping involve a gradual change. Fading involves a gradual change in stimulus while the response stays the same. Shaping uses the same stimulus to establish a gradual change in the response.

- *Chaining* is used to teach a complex behavior by reinforcing the performance of each part of the behavior separately, but in order, until the individual can complete the entire sequence.

There are three types of chaining: (a) *Forward chaining* begins with reinforcing the first step and then adding sequential steps while fading the prompts/reinforcers for previous steps as they are learned. Forward chaining is the natural way that you would teach yourself a task that you had to read directions for, such as setting up a new computer system. (b) *Backwards chaining* begins with reinforcing the final step of the complex behavior and then the second-to-last step, and so on, until the behavior is learned. For example, Raisa recently had a cerebrovascular accident (CVA) and needs to learn to feed themself again. You would prepare their food, cut it into pieces, and place their fork correctly in their hand, and then they would complete the last step: placing the food in their mouth—a natural reinforcement. The advantage of backwards chaining is that it is a natural reinforcer because the task is already completed and sometimes there is less frustration (Figure 41.1).

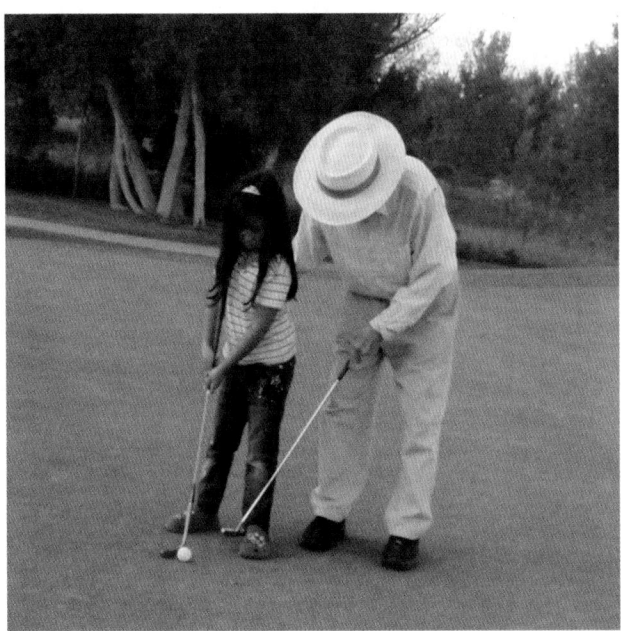

FIGURE 41.1 **A great uncle uses backwards chaining to teach his young niece to golf by first reinforcing the final step of putting the golf ball into the hole.**

(c) *Total task training* occurs when the individual is asked to attempt to do all the steps from the beginning to the end. Prompting may be provided along the way, and reinforcement is provided following the last step. This method often instills confidence when an individual is relearning a previously learned skill or learning a skill he or she may consider insulting to be taught yet may be necessary for safety or independence evaluations (i.e., bathing, cooking).

Behavior Modification: Assessment and Treatment

There are four phases of a successful behavioral modification program: (a) screening, (b) baseline, (c) treatment, and (d) follow-up. Behavioral assessment can be carried out throughout the whole behavioral modification program or during each phase of the program.

Three sources of getting information for the baseline assessment include indirect assessment, direct assessment, and functional assessment.

- *Indirect assessment* includes interviews, questionnaires, role-playing, consulting with other professionals, and client self-monitoring.
- *Direct assessment* records the characteristics of behaviors that are observed, including (a) topography: form of a particular response; (b) amount: frequency and duration of the behavior; (c) intensity: force or magnitude; (d) stimulus control: a certain behavior occurs in the presence of certain stimuli; (e) latency: the time between the occurrence of a stimulus and the beginning of a response; and (f) quality of behavior.
- *Functional assessment* is used to identify the cause of a problem behavior. There are several approaches to completing a functional assessment, including (a) questionnaires; (b) observations: observe and describe the antecedents and immediate consequences of the behavior in natural settings; and (c) functional analysis: directly assesses the effects of controlling variables on the problem behavior. In functional analysis, environmental events are systematically manipulated to test their roles as antecedents or as consequences in controlling and maintaining specific behaviors.

Social Cognitive Theory

The social learning and social cognitive theories of learning are outgrowths of behavioral theories. Theorists such as Piaget and Bandura were dissatisfied with the limits of behavioral theory because they believed that there was more to learning than just the interaction of a person with the environment. They developed theories of learning that integrated *social* and *cognitive* processes with behavioral processes. Although there are individual variations and areas of focus, in general, social cognitive theory explains learning

as occurring in a social context, that is, the "where, what, when, with whom, how often, and under what circumstances" aspects of our lives and is now referred to primarily as social cognitive theory (Ormrod, 2020). Humans learn by observing others, cognitively processing observations, storing those observations and thoughts, and then using them, sometimes at a much later time. This is an important contrast with behavioral theorists, who view learning as an observable change in behavior at a specific point in time. Social cognitive theorists disagree and say that *learning can occur even in the absence of an observable change in behavior* (Ormrod, 2020). Social and cognitive processes such as observation, storing observations in memory, self-assessment, and self-appraisal promote learning. The interactions between a person, behavior, and the environment are emphasized.

Four major assumptions are inherent to social cognitive theory (Ormrod, 2020).

1. ***People can learn by observing others and the consequences that result.*** For example, people observe the behavior of models and the outcomes that result from such behavior.
2. ***Learning can occur without an observable change in behavior.*** For example, people observe a behavior and store it in memory for future use: It may be demonstrated later or never at all.
3. ***Cognition plays important roles in learning.*** For example, people adjust their behavior on the basis of anticipated (positive or negative) consequences or the observation of the outcome of a behavior demonstrated by others.
4. ***People can have considerable control over their actions and environments.*** For example, people can modify themselves or the environment to influence the outcome of their behavior (Ormrod, 2020).

Modeling

It is important for a person to observe skills and behaviors via models and to note the reinforcement that models receive for behaviors. Models can be live (a person with whom the learner has actual contact), symbolic (a pictorial or abstract representation of behavior, such as through television or other media), or verbal instructions (a written description of expected behavior). Whatever the source, the modeled behavior serves as information for the observer/learner. A person can also learn through vicarious reinforcement, which is when they observe the reinforcement that another person received and change their behavior accordingly. Other determining factors include how much attention gets paid to the model; how competent, prestigious, or powerful the model is; and how the model is rewarded. It is also important for the model to be relevant to the observer's situation in some way (Ormrod, 2020).

Bandura (1986) identified four conditions that are necessary for modeling to occur. Because people can learn by observing others, it is important that they pay attention to the behavior. Retention is more likely to occur when the learner consciously attends to the behavior, rehearses it in their own mind, and develops personal verbal or visual ways to represent the information. Motor reproduction is necessary to replicate modeled behaviors; thus, it is important to separate motor limitations from the ability to learn a behavior. Finally, to demonstrate effective modeling, the learner must be motivated. For example, it is important for children to see role models that look like them in order to imagine themselves being successful. When a Latinx girl encounters only White OT practitioners during her treatment sessions, it is more difficult for her to see the possibility of becoming an OT practitioner herself. However, when she participates in therapy in the clinic and sees other children of color who are further along in their progress than her and sees practitioners who look like her, she can imagine herself achieving those same accomplishments.

Self-Efficacy

Perceived self-efficacy refers to one's beliefs about their ability to learn or complete a skill or behavior (Bandura, 1977). The emphasis is on the person's beliefs and how those beliefs influence their performance. For example, a person might believe that a particular action performed or executed by a person in general will produce a certain outcome. However, this is different from the person's belief that they have the ability to perform the action and that it will result in a successful outcome. A person's efficacy expectations also influence the person's persistence with different occupations. "Efficacy expectations determine how much effort people will expend and how long they will persist in the face of obstacles and aversive experiences. The stronger the perceived self-efficacy, the more active the efforts" (Bandura, 1977, p. 194).

Typically, a person's self-efficacy is developed over time and through four sources of information: (a) the person's previous successes and failures, (b) messages from others about their potential success, (c) their physiological state when performing a skill, and (d) the successes and failures of others (Ormrod, 2020).

Efficacy expectations have three important dimensions: magnitude, generality, and strength (Bandura, 1977). Magnitude involves the level of difficulty for a task—for example, making a sandwich versus making an elaborate dinner. Generality involves the degree to which a person's perceived self-efficacy for one task transfers to another—for example, maneuvering a wheelchair around the OT clinic versus maneuvering a wheelchair in a busy urban community. Strength refers to the degree to which people believe they can be successful—for example, being very confident about one's success in taking a virtual college class versus being only slightly confident about participating in an online discussion group.

Constructivist Theory

Constructivism, or "discovery" learning, explains the process where people seek, find, and integrate information for themselves. *Constructivism* speaks to the role of the client being responsible for their own learning, rather than the focus being on the teacher or therapist providing instruction (Fosnot, 20005). A constructivist would assert that individual differences in the learning process are to be expected; that "everyone's construction of the world is unique even though we share a great many concepts" (Svinicki, 2004, p. 14). Although there are several "traditional" methods of providing information, such as through imparting information or finding information in books or on the Internet, this does not necessarily indicate or result in learning, according to constructivism. There must be interaction with the information. For constructivists, the learner must access information, use this information to alter or modify existing knowledge and understanding, and integrate the new information with previous information to *create* a new understanding that is relevant to themself (Marlowe & Page, 2005).

There are some basic assumptions about the teaching–learning process that are common to constructivism.

1. ***Learners must be active participants in their learning.***
2. ***Learners are capable of creating their own knowledge*** through interaction with the human and nonhuman environment.
3. ***Learners develop the ability to think critically to solve problems*** when they participate in this type of learning environment.
4. ***Active participation in the learning environment enhances critical thinking and problem-solving abilities.*** When actively engaged in constructing their own knowledge, people gather information and develop strategies at the same time (Marlowe & Page, 2005).

According to Bruner (1961), a constructivist approach fosters intellectual potency, meaning that when people seek and find information for themselves, that information is more meaningful, relevant, and powerful for them. First, people organize information they find for themselves so that it is more efficiently and effectively retrieved for future use. Constructivists call this a *conservation of memory*. Second, because the learners "own" the information, this approach fosters intrinsic motivation. Rather than settling into a pattern in which learners conform to what the instructor wants them to learn, learners discover for themselves. This promotes motivation to learn. Third, the only way to improve one's ability to think, question, and discover is to do it actively and repeatedly—to engage in the process. Constructivism fosters people's learning the process of discovery.

Motivational Theory

Motivational theories view change as coming from within the person and rely on their desire to make a change. The transtheoretical model (TTM) of intentional change was built on multiple theories of psychotherapy to identify an individuals' readiness to change and uses stages of change and processes to facilitate one's progress toward goals. The theory, developed by examining how people change both in and out of various forms of psychotherapy, proposes that a person may progress through six stages of behavior change: precontemplation, contemplation, preparation, action, and maintenance and termination (Prochaska & Norcross, 2018). The TTM proposes that effective interventions address an individual's *present stage of change*. This model has two essential elements that will be discussed. The six integrated stages of change and the various processes that facilitate a person's movement from one stage to the next. The six are listed here. Although the stages might appear to be linear, occurring in a step-by-step progression from one stage to the next, they occur in a spiral manner as people experience relapses or other setbacks as they work to change behaviors. In fact, relapse is common and expected. Relapse can occur back to *any* stage; however, the subsequent progress usually is easier for the individual.

- *Precontemplation.* The stages of change begin with precontemplation. Here, a person demonstrates a behavior that is perceived *by others* as needing to be changed. These behaviors are often harmful or destructive (e.g., a substance use or addiction, poorly controlled anger or stress, or general health and wellness issues). The person might be unaware or minimally aware of their problem and has no intention to change it in the foreseeable future. Strategies are not effective at this point because the person lacks awareness to engage in or benefit from change.
- *Contemplation.* In the contemplation stage, the person is likely to be aware of their problem and is thinking about overcoming it, but is not yet ready to take action.
- *Preparation.* In the preparation stage, the person demonstrates both intention to change *and* small changes in their behavior.
- *Action.* In the action stage, the person is committed to making the change and is involved in change behaviors on a regular basis. The person is putting forth great energy to modify behaviors, the environment, or their experiences to effect serious change.
- *Maintenance.* In the maintenance stage, the person puts forth considerable effort to maintain the change, working to sustain accomplishments and prevent relapse.
- *Termination.* The final or termination stage occurs when the person no longer experiences temptation to return

to the behavior or needs to focus on maintenance activities. It is important to note that treatment most often ends prior to termination, which partially explains the need for individuals to return to treatment (Prochaska & Norcross, 2018).

The processes of change explain how to promote the shifts between stages. Individuals at different stages of change require different strategies to make progress. For example, Helfrich and colleagues (2012) demonstrated that, even though they are not ready to change, people in the precontemplation stage of change may move to the contemplation stage through the process of *being exposed to treatment interventions*. The process of introducing the possibility of change may allow an individual to risk changing. People who have progressed to the contemplation stage may benefit from consciousness-raising strategies that help them to get information about their problem and themselves, by being encouraged to express their feelings about their problems through various dramatic relief strategies such as role-playing, and by environmental reevaluation to assess how their behavior affects their physical and social surroundings (e.g., perhaps a person's smoking deters family or friends from visiting or there are stains and cigarette burns on the person's furnishings). Strategies such as values clarification exercises to enhance self-reevaluation, or how we think and feel about ourselves, can be helpful for moving to the preparation stage. Making a real commitment to change, believing in the ability to change, and using techniques such as personal goal setting to enhance self-liberation or will power can be helpful during the action stage. Several processes are important in the maintenance stage, such as fostering helping relationships and social supports that encourage the person to be open and honest about their problems; avoiding things that elicit the problem behavior and substituting alternatives (stimulus control and counterconditioning); and reinforcement management, rewarding oneself for making changes. Social liberation helps to promote change across various stages through advocacy, empowerment, and social change mechanisms (Prochaska & Norcross, 2018). See OT Story 41.1, for a practice example.

Motivational interviewing (MI) is another clinical process (technique) that encourages people to consider and implement change. "Motivational interviewing is a collaborative conversation style for strengthening a person's own motivation and commitment for change" (Miller & Rollnick, 2013, p. 12). The spirit of MI includes (a) partnership, (b) acceptance, (c) compassion, and (d) evocation. The processes used during MI, which are both sequential and recursive, include (a) engaging, (b) focusing, (c) evoking, and (d) planning (Miller & Rollnick, 2013). Box 41.1 summarizes the processes of MI.

OT STORY 41.1 OLIVIA: BEHAVIOR CHANGE

Olivia, a 55-year-old Black woman, has been overweight her entire life. Over the years, she has tried many different diets and has joined (and quit) numerous exercise programs and groups. After a recent episode of chest pain, Olivia's healthcare provider strongly recommended that she participate in organized nutrition, exercise, and overall health promotion activities.

- How might you help Olivia to understand and reflect on her challenges with health and wellness issues over the years through the transtheoretical perspective?
- What stage might she be at currently?
- How might you help her move from one stage to the next?
- How might you work to minimize any setbacks to the process and remedy those setbacks when they occur?
- How would each theory of learning presented in this chapter be helpful with this case?

Strategies might include the following:

- The OT practitioner would first work with Olivia to help her understand the processes of change. Their work together would include helping Olivia to understand how change occurs, the spiraling nature of change, and the natural, to-be-expected gains and setbacks that occur. The OT practitioner would use counseling and discussion to encourage Olivia's conscious reflection on her behavior and recognition of the different stages of change. Olivia's current stage could be seen as preparation.
- Olivia would be presented with the behaviors she has demonstrated that have contributed to her weight gain and interfered with her weight loss. She would also be presented with the health consequences of those behaviors. With support, as needed, from the therapist, Olivia would go to the health library and identify the long-term results of not addressing these concerns.
- A variety of intervention strategies, such as personal goal setting, developing social supports, creating a self-reward system for positive change or progress, and evaluation and reevaluation of progress, could be introduced using motivational interviewing techniques. As Olivia applied

and practiced these strategies in her life, she could come back to the occupational therapist to problem-solve and revise those that did not work as well as update her self-reward system for those that were successful.

- The OT practitioner would recommend that Olivia participate in a group based on social learning principles so that she could benefit from hearing others' strategies. This type of group would also help to build her self-esteem as she shared her own accomplishments and strategies with others as well. After the group sessions, Olivia would meet individually with the OT practitioner to identify one or two new strategies that she heard to try each week. Olivia would develop a plan, with coaching, as needed from the occupational therapist, to go out and try the new strategy.
- Olivia would also be encouraged to view earlier obstacles or setbacks to change as typical and predictable. When setbacks do occur, the OT practitioner would reinforce the importance of conscious understanding of the spiraling nature of progress, the success of identifying setbacks when they occur, the opportunity to prevent any setback from spiraling too far down, and a return to strategies that were successful in the past or continuing to develop new strategies. The OT practitioner would reinforce the ongoing nature of change and progress.

Questions

1. After Olivia attends the exercise group that you recommended, she tells you that she was the only Black person there. She has also shared with you in the past that her mother was also overweight. You suddenly realize that while you have been trying to use social cognitive theory with her, she does not have any relevant role models for this situation. What can you do to help her find some?
2. If each person constructs their own learning and therefore there is no "objective reality," what challenges would that present to an OT practitioner who advocates a constructivist perspective on learning in working with Olivia? What opportunities does it provide? How would you address her goals in a group setting?

BOX 41.1 PROCESSES OF MOTIVATIONAL INTERVIEWING

1. *Engaging involves both establishing a helpful connection and a working relationship.* Engaging with the client is essential before change can take place.
2. *Focusing is the process of developing and maintaining specific direction in the conversation about change.* Guiding the client back to the difficult topic of change facilitates progress.
3. *Evoking involves eliciting the client's own motivation for change.* Clients respond better to their own words and reasons for making a change.
4. *Planning which encompasses both developing commitment to change and formulating a concrete plan of action.* The therapist listens for the client to begin identifying solutions and strategies for change and then collaborates with them to develop a concrete plan.

BOX 41.2 SIX THEMES OF CHANGE TALK

1. *Desire:* Verbs include *want*, *like*, and *wish*. These tell you something that the person wants (i.e., I *wish* I could lose some weight).
2. *Ability:* The prototypical verb is *can* (*could*). These show you what the person perceives as within their ability (i.e., I *could* probably cut down a bit).
3. *Reasons:* There are no particular verbs here, but words used always express specific reason for a certain change (i.e., This pain keeps me from playing the guitar!).
4. *Need:* Marker verbs include *need*, *have to*, *got to*, *should*, *ought*, and *must*. These tell you some necessity (i.e., I *must* quit smoking. I *should* wear a mask in crowded indoor spaces).
5. *Commitment:* Most used verbs are *will*, *intend to*, and *going to*. These can be presented with strong or lower level of commitment (i.e., I *will* go to Alcoholics Anonymous [AA] group once a month).
6. *Taking steps:* Reporting recent specific action (step) toward change (i.e., I quit drinking for a couple of weeks but then started again).

There are five key communication skills that are suggested to implement these principles of MI: (a) asking open questions, (b) affirming, (c) reflective, (d) summarizing, and (e) providing information and advice with permission. In addition, the therapist should always be listening for *change talk* and to elicit the possibility of change talk during conversation with the client. Box 41.2 describes the six themes of change talk.

The key to success for this model is the careful, systematic, and close fit between the person, the stage, and the process. According to Prochaska et al. (1992), "efficient self-change depends on doing the right things (processes) at the right time (stages)" (p. 1110). Table 41.1 summarizes the stages and processes of change as outlined by Prochaska and Norcross (2018).

Using the Models in Practice

Occupational Therapy and Behavioral Theory

Behavioral theories emphasize observable behavior, rewarding and reinforcing desirable behavior, and reducing problematic behaviors. Clients who might benefit from intervention approaches that are grounded in behavioral theories of learning include people who have difficulty planning and organizing activities, those who have problems with memory and/or attention, those who have deficits in sequencing activities, and those who demonstrate inappropriate social behaviors.

OT practitioners use behavioral theory to understand human learning and guide their intervention by analyzing a complex behavior that needs to be learned (e.g., a child's need to take turns when they play) and sequence that behavior from simple to complex. Sometimes the process of *learning* a new behavior also involves *extinguishing* a problem behavior. Intervention would consist of opportunities for the person to participate in increasingly complex behaviors, using behavioral principles such as reinforcement, shaping, and chaining. Progress would be measured by observing the client's occupational performance and their ability to complete increasingly complex behaviors necessary for occupational performance.

For instance, some strategies that could help a child develop sharing and turn-taking skill include praising appropriate behavior (to provide positive reinforcement for sharing), not giving attention every time they take toys from others (to decrease the negative reinforcement for the undesired behavior), using a sticker chart to document sharing (to gradually shape appropriate behavior), and providing

---

TABLE 41.1 Stages and Processes of Change

Stage	Process (How to Promote Change)
Precontemplation	Strategies are not effective because the person lacks awareness to engage in or benefit from change.
Contemplation	Consciousness-raising strategies to learn about problem, role-play strategies to express feelings, and assessment of how behavior affects physical and social environment
Preparation	Values clarification exercises to promote reevaluation of feelings or self-perception.
Action	Goal-setting strategies and techniques
Maintenance	Development of social supports, substitution of alternatives to problem behavior, avoidance of experiences that elicit the problem behavior, and rewarding oneself for making changes
Termination	Support changed behavior and return to treatment if needed.

rewards for good sharing, such as letting them stand first in line to go to the playground. Box 41.3 provides an alternative perspective to turn taking using a development approach. For another example of behavioral theory in use, see Box 41.4.

Occupational Therapy and Social Cognitive Theory

Social cognitive theories emphasize the importance of learning essential skills for living in a social context. Clients who might benefit from intervention approaches grounded in social cognitive theories of learning include people who have the ability to attend to their environment in some way. In other words, although social cognitive theory relies on modeling and self-efficacy, only individuals with the most severe limitations in social awareness might not benefit from these approaches.

An occupational therapist might use a self-assessment such as the Occupational Self-Assessment (Baron et al., 2006) to identify the client's priorities and goals. The practitioner would provide multiple opportunities for the client to develop or relearn skills through activities such as role-play, observation, problem-solving, and practice in real-life situations. Clients observe models that serve to

---

BOX 41.3 DEVELOPMENTAL PERSPECTIVE ON TURN TAKING

There are many different meanings attributed to the concept of turn taking in childhood. Everyone wants a chance at a turn. It is their opportunity to participate in the activity or social interaction.

Looking through a developmental lens, let's look at how turn taking evolves. As an infant, turn taking begins by imitation within the context of relationship (Wittmer, 2012). The baby takes turns with their primary caregiver in long strings of interaction, also known as circles of communication (Greenspan et al., 1998). What allows for these circles of communication? The flow of affect. Affect is an internalized sensation that is interconnected with the sensory and motor systems. Affect is expressed through motor action. If affect is organized and managed, there is a continuous flow between the two or more people within the interaction/relationship. If affect is disorganized or dysregulated, the child, or adult for that matter, becomes focused on sustaining themselves and there is no room for the other person within the relationship because they are not feeling the desire for relating.

Anyone can be taught to wait their turn; however, as OT practitioners, we want the opportunity to provide a meaningful experience to the child. We need to determine if the child is developmentally ready for turn taking. We need to ensure that the child can imitate, is engaged, and is reciprocal within relationship, which is the first phase of turn taking. Therefore, if we behaviorally teach turn taking when a child is not yet engaged nor reciprocal in relating, it will not generalize to other opportunities. It is likely to cause frustration for the child and the therapist because the child isn't developmentally ready for turn taking. What can we do to support turn taking from a developmental and meaningful perspective? Begin with enticing the child into relating with you while you two are working within your session. Once there is a back and forth or multiple circles of communication, then elaborate into a simple game and begin to label your turn. Have the child experience the feeling of getting a turn. Then, you can grab a turn for yourself. Is the child able to manage you taking a turn? The child has to be developmentally ready. If the child is accepting of you getting a turn, comment about how you like getting a turn also. If the child isn't feeling as if they have not had enough turns, speak to the possibility of you getting a turn as in "I hope to have a turn." Then, hopefully the child will invite you to a turn. If the child is ignoring the need for their peer to take a turn, you might question with playful use of your affect and highlight "You get ALL the turns and your friend gets NONE?" This will help the child make meaning of the situation.

When considering a behavioral perspective, the idea of meaning-making is simply not acknowledged. When thinking developmentally, we ensure the individual is making meaning of the social cue necessary for turn taking. Turn taking requires commitment to relationship (see Figure 41.2).

Lois Gold, OTR/L, OTD—Private Practitioner, Miami, FL

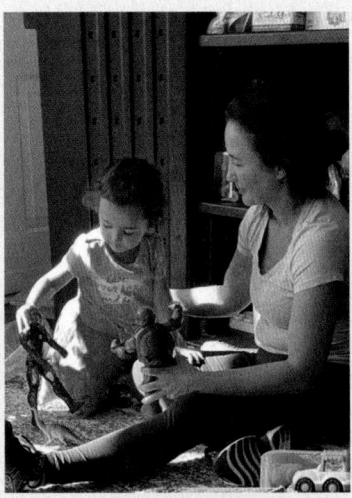

FIGURE 41.2 During an OT session, a mother and child work on the development of reciprocal turn taking. OT, occupational therapy.

BOX 41.4 USING BEHAVIORAL THEORY IN PRACTICE

Gonzalo is a 19-year-old client diagnosed with schizophrenia. He attends a day hospital three times a week. He comes with a bag full of cartoons that he has drawn at his house. He is observant; he always carries his cartoon bag with him. He has difficulty participating in conversations because of his sensitivity to delusional constructs in conversations. The therapist's intervention is based on behavioral theories and uses progressive instructions, modeling, and physical cues. All the necessary steps are identified and sequenced so that Gonzalo can place his bag of drawings on a chair next to him. As a modeling technique, the therapist progressively uses her own bag on the chair next to her and Gonzalo. In this way, the client progressively places his bag on the same chair used by the therapist, freeing his hands to start drawing in the occupational therapy workshop. A series of progressive instructions are used with gradual modeling of behavior according to the needs and physical cues of Gonzalo, such as pointing to where the bag was and showing his proximity to it. This helps him to improve his participation, to gradually carry out painting and ceramic activities, and to move in the environment. In conclusion, a direct sequence chain is used to model management in space, the use of objects, materials, and tools. The prompts and reinforcements are progressively removed as Gonzalo is able to initiate and complete the task and move autonomously in the environment.

elicit and promote learning and behavior change. The client sets goals that are informed by their perceived self-efficacy, and the therapist strives to identify tasks that are challenging but not overwhelming.

Often, a person's self-perceptions and beliefs about their ability to be successful with an occupation influence the person's decision about whether to participate in that occupation. For example, a person who believes that she has good interview skills will be more likely to respond to a job advertisement even though she might not have direct experience with the type of work that needs to be done. A person who did not have that sense of effectiveness might be less likely to pursue the job. Intervention strategies to promote a person's perceived self-efficacy in the job interview situation described here would include determining with the person that she had all the requisite skills to be successful, using peer role models so that the person could practice or "try on" the essential skills and behaviors, having the person practice interview skills, providing feedback on specific successes, and encouraging the person to evaluate their skills in a personal way rather than comparing these skills to someone else's. These theories all emphasize the importance of an individual's participation in meaningful occupations as both the foundation and result of motivation and self-efficacy (Figure 41.3).

Occupational Therapy and Constructivist Theory

Within the constructivist approach, clients actively direct what needs to be learned and how the learning will occur. Clients who might benefit from intervention approaches grounded in constructivist theories of learning include people who have some ability to direct their own learning but may need help with mastery at a particular developmental level. Clients help to determine the resources that will enhance their learning. Independent thinking, collaborative problem-solving, and using past experience to reframe and revise new learning are all important.

A practitioner who uses a constructivist approach in the teaching–learning process emphasizes skills and activities such as asking questions, exploring independently, identifying problems, brainstorming, and generating individual solutions to problems. The practitioner emphasizes the client's essential role in the process and sees their role as facilitating the client's progress. The practitioner views the therapy process as recognizing, embracing, respecting, and encouraging people to develop individual meanings in order to promote and enhance the client's knowledge and skill. In many ways, the practitioner takes a "back seat"

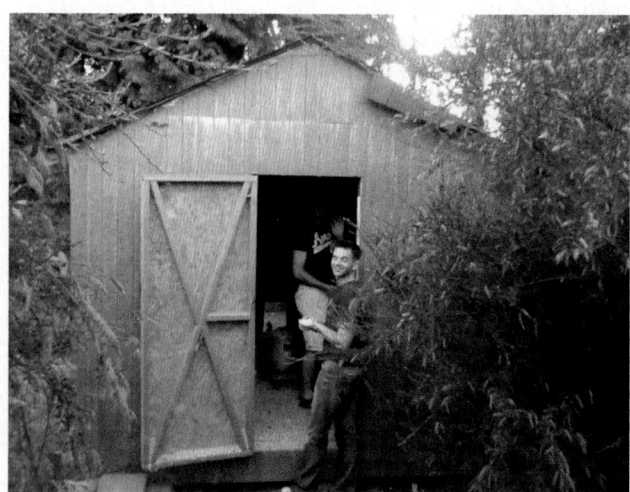

FIGURE 41.3 A couple who work in finance and value sustainability successfully build their own chicken coop to raise chickens and sell eggs, demonstrating self-efficacy and Prochaska's "action" stage of change.

as the client pursues learning; the practitioner's role is to address problems that arise. The OT practitioner does not provide "the intervention" but instead works to facilitate the person developing their own strategies to identify, address, and solve problems. The practitioner is alert to major issues but is neither prescriptive nor directive (Lederer, 2001) (Figure 41.4). For an example of using constructivist theory in practice, see Box 41.5.

Occupational Therapy and Motivational Theory

Motivational theories view learning and behavior change as coming from within the learner. Clients who might benefit from these approaches are those who either need or want to make a change in their lives and might need some assistance with the process. Clients for whom this approach is often effective are those who need to make a change, but do not think they need to, or do not feel ready to change. Examples include people with behaviors that are harmful to themselves or others such as substance abuse or partner abuse. An individual may be at risk for significant loss (e.g., job, children, or home) or incurring unfavorable consequences (e.g., financial, health, or legal) if a change is not made.

An OT practitioner would first evaluate the client to determine their goals and stage of change and then use MI to facilitate their movement through the various stages. Clients may be an individual, group, organization, or a population. The role of the practitioner is primarily as a facilitator and guide (similar to that in constructivism). The control needs to reside within the client, or treatment will not be successful. Thus, using this approach requires the

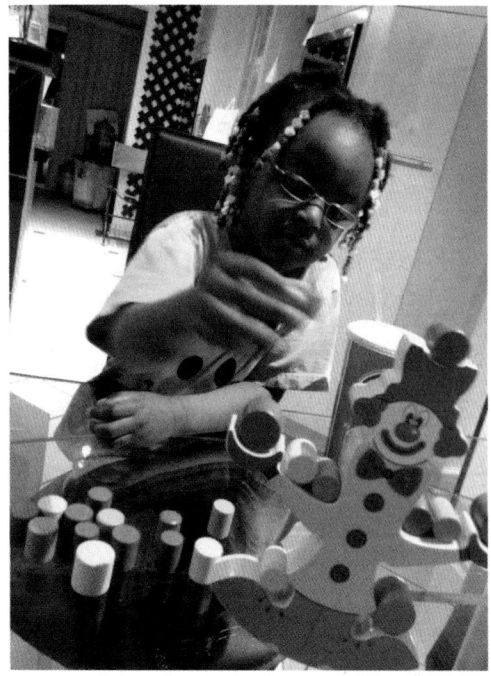

FIGURE 41.4 **A young girl actively participates in her own learning by exploring principles of balance through play with blocks of different sizes and weights.**

practitioner to "let go" of being an expert, meet the client where they are, and be willing to work at the client's pace. The practitioner's role in motivational treatment focuses on addressing the issues of motivation and self-efficacy to learn, whereas in constructivism the role is facilitation of learning.

BOX 41.5 USING CONSTRUCTIVIST THEORY IN PRACTICE

In a neighborhood community kitchen, a group of women prepare food daily for families who lack food security. Two days a week, at the end of the lunch hour, an occupational therapist offers two workshops. One is a health management workshop and the other is a community toy library. In both, the therapist uses the teaching and learning process of constructivism so the participants have an active role in their own learning and knowledge development.

In the health management workshop, strategies are used that facilitate each client discovering and creating their own knowledge. For example, the therapist and client brainstorm about health issues to work on together, jointly determine the priority among the identified issues, and choose one of the issues to focus on. Then the therapist starts by asking the participant what they know or think about that topic. In this way, knowledge is built from

a critical discussion, gathered information, and shared central concerns of each topic are addressed.

Similar processes are used in the toy library; first with a workshop for the construction and recycling of games and toys and second with a family game workshop. Different games and toys are suitable at various ages; so the therapist discusses child development with the parents, and they determine the risks of toys according to age (size, materials, and care). After that information is gathered, the toys are built or refurbished communally. During the family game workshop, the therapist stays in the background as a facilitator of the discovery of knowledge and not as a prescriber of behavior. In this way, with the application of the constructivist theory of learning, the autonomy and sustainability of the community program are guaranteed, strengthening community empowerment.

Evidence to Support Using the Models

There is a long history of evidence demonstrating the efficacy of each of the learning theories discussed in this chapter within the field of psychology; however, the effectiveness of these approaches within OT is less robust. This section will highlight a few studies to illustrate the diversity of theoretical application with the hope of encouraging others to continue the pursuit of evidence-based outcome studies.

Behavioral Theory

• Howe and Wang (2013) completed a systematic review of the use of behavioral interventions used by occupational therapists with children in the treatment of feeding disorders. They found behavioral techniques were effective across a wide range of children with a variety of feeding disorders.
• Giles and Wilson (1988) and Giles et al. (1997) described programs to help retrain people who had sustained severe brain injuries and needed help with washing and dressing: basic self-care behaviors. Practitioners used a specific set of instructions to gradually add skills to each person's repertoire (shaping) and eventually teach the entire behavior.
• Katzmann and Mix (1994) presented a case report of a 34-year-old woman with viral encephalitis. The woman had difficulty processing written and verbal information and had great difficulty with various complex self-care tasks. The practitioners' used techniques such as prompting with step-by-step instructions, shaping, and verbal or physical cues. The practitioners used forward chaining by cueing the woman with directions or providing physical assistance for a step that needed to be completed and gradually removed the cues as she initiated and completed the task independently.

Social Cognitive Theory

• Kramer et al. (2018) demonstrated that youth with intellectual and developmental disabilities transitioning from high school to adulthood who completed e-mentoring, with a peer mentor, experienced sustained changes in self-determined behavior and had significant goal attainment during *Project TEAM*. Peer mentors guided youth through the problem-solving process and shared examples from their lives where they identified and resolved physical, social, or sensory environmental barriers.
• Helfrich et al. (2012) described a life skills intervention in the community for individuals who were homeless

using *situated learning*. Situated learning theory, which is derived from social cognitive learning theory (Lave & Wenger, 2003), posits that behavior results from interaction between the person and the situation. The learner is placed in contexts that allow for simulated and actual application to everyday situations, whereas peers enhance the learning experience with feedback. In social situations, individuals gain motivational support from others and access both expertise and collaborative thinking, increasing opportunities to acquire and apply new knowledge. This approach allowed group participants functioning at a variety of levels to benefit from others' experiences with the life skills being taught.

Constructivist Theory

• Lund et al. (2019) demonstrated that when mental health service users in Sweden were able to explore their process of making lifestyle changes, they were able to successfully break a cycle of perceived failure and create a more balanced lifestyle.
• Sullivan et al. (2021) found that when OT students had the opportunity to use self-direction with simulated learning modules to learn MI skills, their self-confidence increased significantly.

Motivational Theories

• In a meta-analysis of 39 studies, Norcross and Wampold (2011) found the transtheoretical approach and the integration of the stages and processes of change attest to the value of stage-matched interventions. Those beginning in the preparation and action stages do better than those beginning in the precontemplation or contemplation stages.
• Building on the tradition of integrating various theoretical perspectives, Park et al. (2019) proposed a framework for understanding impairment and the change processes involved in reducing work disability and improving return to work (RTW) outcomes using the Model of Human Occupation and MI.

Conclusion

Behavioral, social cognitive, constructivist, and motivational theories of learning have great relevance and use for OT practitioners. Table 41.2 summarizes the four different theories of learning that were presented in this chapter and highlights their relevance to OT practice. The information presented in this chapter can be used to influence how you think about the learning needs of patients and clients, to reinforce the importance of designing optimal learning environments, to contribute to your ongoing professional development, and to promote your clients' abilities to achieve their goals.

TABLE 41.2 Summary Table

Theory	Major Emphases	Application to Occupational Therapy Practice
Behavioral	• Learned behavior as an observable event (not a mental process) • Behavior is conditioned by the environment. • Environmental response alters subsequent behaviors.	• Analyze and sequence behaviors from simple to complex. • Measure progress as the person completes increasingly complex behaviors. • Use strategies including reinforcement, shaping, and rewards.
Social cognitive	• Integrates behavior, social, and cognitive processes • Learning occurs in a social context. • Learning may occur without observable behavior change. • People regulate and adjust their own behavior. • Self-efficacy is developed over time and through experience. • Efficacy expectations are influenced by the difficulty of the task, how well completing a task transfers to other situations, and the degree to which a person believes that he or she will be successful.	• Emphasize client learning essential skills for living. • Use role-play, peer observation, role modeling, problem-solving, and real-life practice activities to promote learning. • Encourage the client to identify the problem, set goals, develop a plan, and evaluate outcomes. • Tasks should be challenging but not overwhelming and should be transferable to other situations.
Constructivist	• Learner is an active participant in their own learning. • Learner creates/constructs knowledge through past experience and interaction with the environment. • Self-constructed knowledge has great meaning and relevance for the learner. • Self-constructed knowledge promotes the learner's motivation for learning.	• Client actively directs what is to be learned and how learning will occur. • Use strategies including brainstorming, individual problem-solving, independent exploration, and asking questions. • Occupational therapist facilitates but does not direct the learning process.
Motivational	• Learning and change occur in a spiral fashion. It is not linear. • A person's readiness (desire) for change will influence the outcomes. • Relapses are common and to be expected.	• Intervention processes must match behavior stage. • Intervention processes become increasingly active, self-directed, self-motivated, and self-monitored.

Acknowledgments

The author would like to thank Perri Stern for her contributions to the previous edition of this chapter.

Lippincott® Connect *For additional resources on the subjects discussed in this chapter, visit* Lippincott Connect.

REFERENCES

American Occupational Therapy Association (AOTA). (2020). Occupational therapy practice framework: Domain and process, 4th edition. *American Journal of Occupational Therapy, 74*(Suppl. 2), 7412410010. https://doi.org/10.5014/ajot.2020.74S2001

Bandura, A. (1977). Self-efficacy: Toward a unifying theory of behavioral change. *Psychological Review, 84,* 191–215. https://doi.org/10.1037//0033-295x.84.2.191

Bandura, A., & National Institute of Mental Health. (1986). *Social foundations of thought and action: A social cognitive theory.* Prentice-Hall.

Baron, K., Kielhofner, G., Iyenger, A., Goldhammer, V., & Wolenski, J. (2006). *The occupational self-assessment (OSA) (Version 2.2).* Model of Human Occupation Clearinghouse, Department of Occupational Therapy, College of Applied Health Sciences, University of Illinois at Chicago.

Bruner, J. S. (1961). The act of discovery. *Harvard Educational Review, 31,* 21–32.

Driscoll, M. P., & Burner, K. (2021). *Psychology of learning for instruction* (4th ed.). Pearson Education.

Fosnot, C. T. (Ed.). (2005). *Constructivism: Theory, perspectives, and practice* (2nd ed.). Teachers College Press.

Giles, G. M., Ridley, J. E., Dill, A., & Frye, S. C. (1997). A consecutive series of adults with brain injury treated with a washing and dressing retraining program. *American Journal of Occupational Therapy, 51,* 256–266. https://doi.org/10.5014/AJOT.51.4.256

Giles, G. M., & Wilson, J. C. (1988). The use of behavioral techniques in functional skills training after severe brain injury. *American Journal of Occupational Therapy, 42,* 658–665. https://doi.org/10.5014/ajot.42.10.658

Greenspan, S. I., Wieder, S., & Simons, R. (1998). *The child with special needs: Encouraging intellectual and emotional growth.* Perseus Books.

Helfrich, C. A., Chan, D. V., Simpson, E., & Sabol, P. (2012). Readiness-to-change cluster profiles among adults with mental illness who were homeless participating in a life skills intervention. *Community Mental Health Journal, 48,* 673–681. https://doi.org/10.1007/s10597-011-9383-z

Hergenhahn, B. R. (1976). *An introduction to theories of learning.* Prentice-Hall.

Howe, T.-H., & Wang, T.-N. (2013). Systematic review of interventions used in or relevant to occupational therapy for children with feeding difficulties ages birth–5 years. *American Journal of Occupational Therapy, 67*(4), 405–412. https://doi.org/10.5014/ajot.2013.004564

Katzmann, S., & Mix, C. (1994). Improving functional independence in a patient with encephalitis through behavior modification shaping techniques. *American Journal of Occupational Therapy, 48,* 259–262. https://doi.org/10.5014/ajot.48.3.259

Kramer, J., Hwang, I., Helfrich, C., Samuel, P., & Carrellas, A. (2018). Evaluating the social validity of Project *TEAM*: A problem-solving intervention to teach transition age youth with developmental disabilities to resolve environmental barriers. *International Journal of Disability, Development and Education, 65,* 57–75. https://doi.org/10.1080/1034912X.2017.1346237

Lave, J., & Wenger, E. (2003). *Situated learning: Legitimate peripheral participation.* Cambridge University Press.

Lederer, J. M. (2001). The application of constructivism to concepts of occupation using a group process approach. *Occupational Therapy in Health Care, 13,* 81–93. https://doi.org/10.1080/J003v13n01_06

Lund, K., Argentzell, E., Bejerholm, U., & Eklund, M. (2019). Breaking a cycle of perceived failure: The process of making changes toward a more balanced lifestyle. *Australian Occupational Therapy Journal, 66*(5), 627–636. https://doi.org/10.1111/1440-1630.12604

Marlowe, B. A., & Page, M. L. (2005). *Creating and sustaining the constructivist classroom* (2nd ed.). Corwin Press/Sage.

Martin, G., & Pear, J. J. (2019). *Behavior modification: What it is and how to do it* (11th ed.). Taylor & Francis.

Miller, W. R., & Rollnick, S. (Eds.). (2013). *Motivational interviewing: Helping people change* (3rd ed.). Guilford Press.

Norcross, J. C., & Wampold, B. E. (2011). Evidence-based therapy relationships: Research conclusions and clinical practices. *Psychotherapy, 48*(1), 98. https://doi.org/10.1037/a0022161

Ormrod, J. E. (2020). *Human learning: Principles, theories and educational applications* (8th ed.). Pearson.

Park, J., Gross, D. P., Rayani, F., Norris, C. M., Roberts, M. R., James, C., Guptill, C., & Esmail, S. (2019). Model of human occupation as a framework for implementation of motivational interviewing in occupational rehabilitation. *Work, 62*(4), 629–641. https://doi.org/10.3233/WOR-192895

Prochaska, J. O., DiClemente, C. C., Norcross, J. C. (1992). In Search of the Structure of Change. In Klar, Y., Fisher, J.D., Chinsky, J.M., Nadler, A. (Eds.), *Self Change.* Springer. https://doi.org/10.1007/978-1-4612-2922-3_5

Prochaska, J. O., & Norcross, J. C. (2018). *Systems of psychotherapy* (9th ed.). Oxford University Press Academic US.

Sullivan, A., Albright, G., & Khalid, N. (2021). Impact of a virtual role-play simulation in teaching motivational interviewing communication strategies to occupational therapy students for readiness in conducting screening and brief interventions. *Journal of Higher Education Theory and Practice, 21*(2). https://doi.org/10.33423/jhetp.v21i2.4117

Svinicki, M. D. (2004). *Learning and motivation in the postsecondary classroom.* Anker.

Wittmer, D. (2012). The wonder and complexity of infant and toddler peer relationships. *Young Children, 67*(4), 16–23. https://openlab.bmcc.cuny.edu/ece-209-lecture-fall-2019-longley/wp-content/uploads/sites/77/2020/01/Wittmer-2012.pdf

Zabalza, M. (2022). *Coreografías Didácticas en Educación Superior* (p. 157). NARCEA.

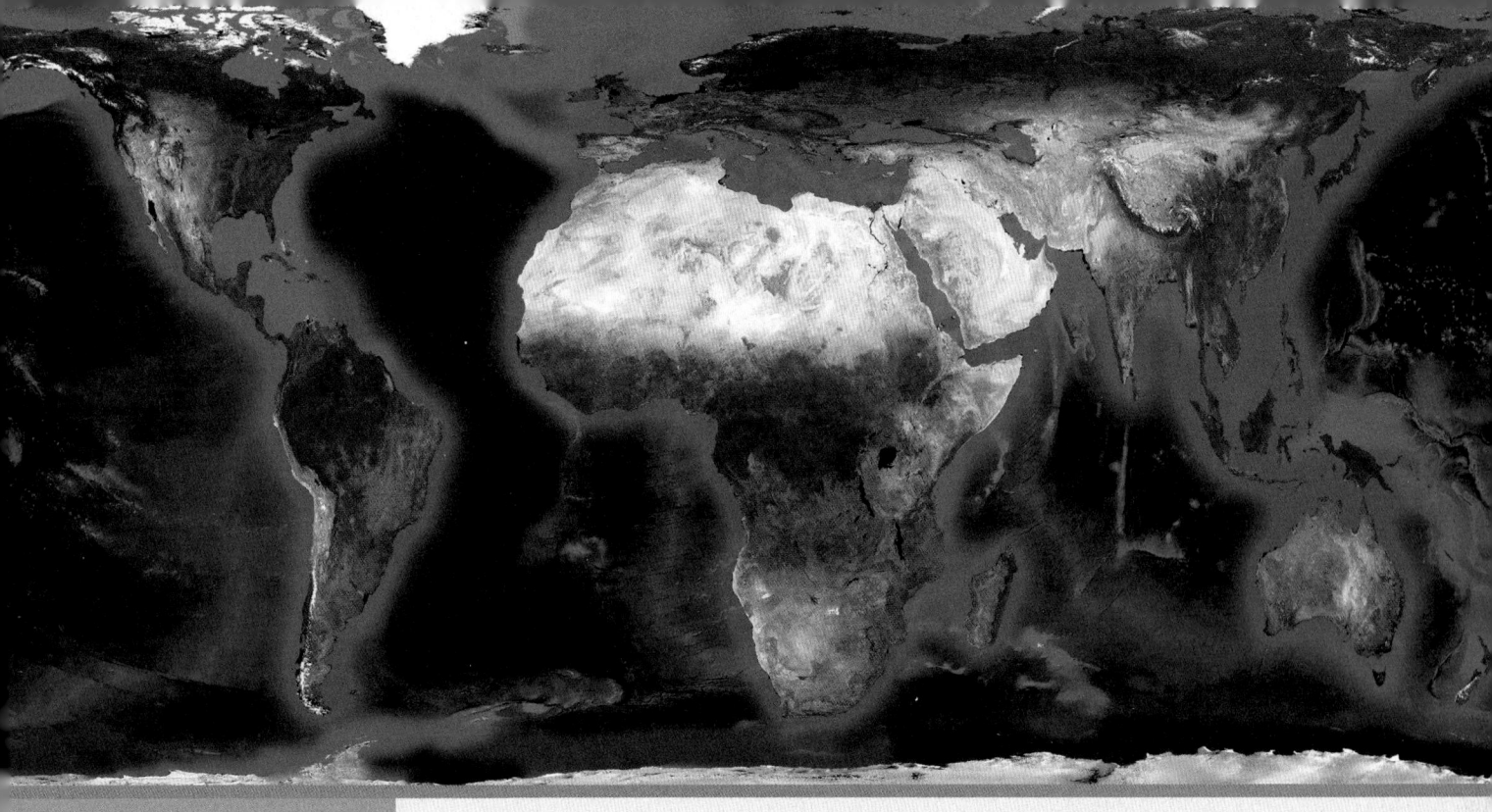

UNIT VII

Evaluation, Intervention, and Outcomes for Occupations

Media Related to Evaluation, Intervention, and Outcomes for Occupations

Readings
- *Working: People Talk About What They Do All Day and How They Feel About What They Do:* Studs Terkel's oral history project is a compelling look at jobs and the people who do them. It features over 100 interviews with everyone from a gravedigger to a studio head and provides an enduring portrait of people's feelings about their working lives. (1997)

Movies
- *Mad Hot Ballroom:* This movie looks inside the lives of 11-year-old New York City public school kids who journey into the world of ballroom dancing. Told from the students' perspectives as they strive toward the final citywide competition, the film chronicles the experiences of students at three schools in different sociocultural neighborhoods. (2005)

Art and Theater
- *Theatre for All:* The mission of this organization in the United States is to empower people with disabilities, nurture community connections, and overturn stereotypes through performing arts. They provide theater education and opportunities for people with disabilities. (theatreforall.org)
- *Typhlological Museum:* This museum in Madrid, Spain, is defined as a museum to be seen and touched. It takes its name from the Greek word *typhlós* that means blind.
- *Feel Florence:* This website and app features a section called "Without barriers" that covers accessible experiences in Florence, Italy. (feelflorence.it)

CHAPTER 42

Introduction to Evaluation, Intervention, and Outcomes for Occupations

Glen Gillen and Barbara A. Boyt Schell

LEARNING OBJECTIVES

After reading this chapter, you will be able to:

1. Understand classification systems used to discuss areas of occupation.
2. Appreciate the complexity of occupation and the potential difficulties in applying these classification systems.

Categories of Occupation

As occupational therapists, we consider the many types of occupations in which clients engage across the course of the day. These occupations fall under the category of activities and participation in the World Health Organization's (WHO, 2001) *International Classification of Functioning, Disability, and Health* (ICF). The WHO (2001) defines **activity** as "the execution of a task or action by an individual" and **participation** as "involvement in a life situation" (p. 123). Furthermore, they define the term **activity limitations** as "difficulties an individual may have in executing activities" and **participation restrictions** as "problems an individual may experience in involvement in life situations" (WHO, 2001, p. 123). Within the ICF, the domains for the Activities and Participation component are presented as a single list that covers the full range of life areas. Examples of included areas are mobility, self-care, domestic life, interpersonal interactions, major life areas (e.g., education, work, and economic life), communication, etc.

Occupational therapy (OT) classification systems typically sort the broad ranges of activities or occupations into categories called **areas of occupation**. There is no standardized classification system, and these areas of occupation have been categorized and classified in a variety of ways. On the one hand, the Canadian Occupational Performance Measure (Law, 2019), which is a standardized measure of occupational performance, uses a three-category system of self-care, productivity, and leisure. On the other hand, the American Occupational Therapy Association (AOTA, 2020a) categorizes these areas of occupation as nine kinds of life activities in which people, populations, or organizations engage. Because the AOTA categories for the areas of occupation are used as the basis for the major chapters in this unit, they are briefly described here, using the AOTA Practice Framework (AOTA, 2020a) as the primary source. Readers are referred to the chapters themselves for more in-depth definitions and discussions about each category of occupations.

Activities of Daily Living

Activities of daily living (ADLs) are activities that focus on caring for one's body and which are directed toward basic survival. Examples include bathing, grooming, dressing, swallowing/eating, feeding, functional mobility, sexual activity, personal device care, etc.

Instrumental Activities of Daily Living

Instrumental activities of daily living (IADLs) are groupings of activities that are also necessary for daily life but that go beyond basic bodily care and survival. They typically involve a broader context, including family and community. A variety of activities are categorized as IADL, including child-rearing, pet care, financial management, religious and spiritual activities, meal preparation, shopping, and home management (see Figure 42.1).

Education

Educational occupations are focused on formal and informal learning. Examples include formal educational participation (academic, nonacademic, extracurricular, and vocational participation), informal personal educational needs or interest explorations, and informal personal education participation.

Work

The category of work includes productive activities such as work and volunteer activities. It includes employment interests and pursuits, employment seeking and acquisition, job performance, retirement preparation and adjustment, volunteer exploration, and volunteer participation (see Figure 42.2).

Play and Leisure

Play and leisure are activities that are characterized by enjoyment or diversion, and which typically arise out of interests and motivation of the person, as opposed to social obligation or survival requirements. This grouping encompasses play exploration and play participation, and it includes both leisure exploration and participation (see Figure 42.3).

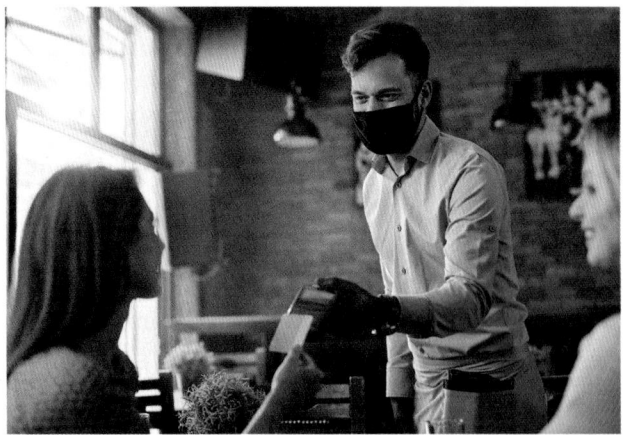

FIGURE 42.2 **Work is one of the many categories of occupation.**

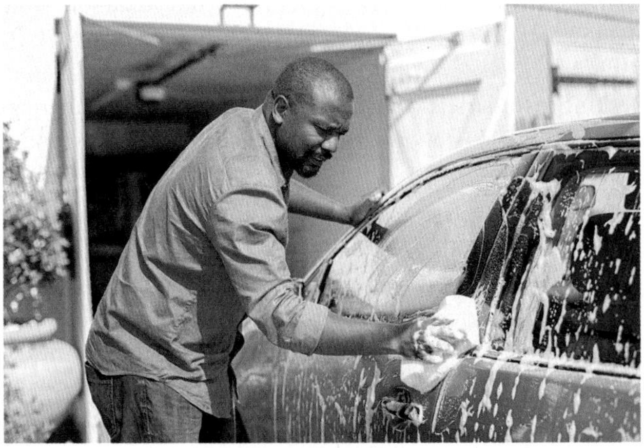

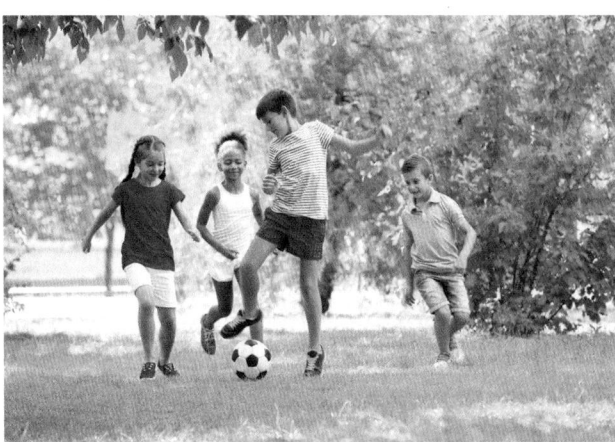

FIGURE 42.1 **Washing a car on the weekend is an IADL.**

FIGURE 42.3 **The category of play and leisure includes exploration and participation.**

Rest and Sleep

The activities associated with rest and sleep are more recently included in the AOTA Practice Framework, in recognition of the role they play in supporting all other occupational functioning. Beyond rest and sleep, this area of occupation also includes sleep preparation and sleep participation. Examples include bedtime routines, ability to manage cues for waking such as the use of wake-up signals, as well as the management of the physical environment for comfort and safety. Occupations in this category may include negotiating the needs and requirements of others within the social environment such as sleep partners and children.

Health Management

Activities related to developing, managing, and maintaining health and wellness routines, including self-management, with the goal of improving or maintaining health to support participation in other occupations. Examples include medication management, nutrition management, physical activity, social and emotional health promotion and maintenance, communication within the healthcare system, personal care device management, and symptom and condition management.

Social Participation

Social participation refers to the interweaving of occupations to support desired engagement in community and family activities, those involving peers and friends, and intimate partner relationships.

Cautions About Categorization

Personal Perspectives

An important consideration when using any classification system to guide evaluation and intervention is to fully understand the way that the person engaging in the occupation perceives the particular activity. For instance, making a meal may be considered work to a busy parent who sees it as part of his or her "job" as a parent to feed the family. Individuals who live by themselves or who take responsibility for this occupation as a part of family chores may consider meal preparation an IADL. Others may classify meal preparation as a leisure activity because it may help them to relax or decrease their stress levels. A chef in a restaurant is most likely to classify meal preparation as work. Finally, meal preparation may be considered under the heading of Social Participation. Examples include participating in a weekly

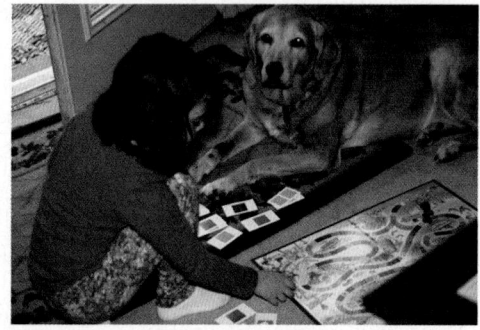

FIGURE 42.4 In this picture, the child is hard at work playing . . . but is the dog resting or playing? Or both? Or perhaps engaged in child care?

neighborhood soup kitchen to serve meals to the homeless or being part of a group of friends or family engaged in making a holiday feast. Care of pets is another of many other examples to consider. Depending on one's perspective, this may be considered as an IADL, as part of leisure/play, or as work for someone employed as a part-time dog walker (Figure 42.4).

Occupational Blends Versus Categories

Some occupational scientists suggest that rather than trying to classify occupations into discrete categories, it might be more helpful to consider the relative mix within a particular activity. For example, someone who loves his or her job may have parts of the job that really feel like work, parts that are fun and feel like play, and parts that feel like IADL, such as using a calendar to coordinate work and home life. Indeed, in her paper "Work and Leisure: Transcending the Dichotomy," Primeau (1996) cites the work of Csikszentmihalyi (1975) who was an early challenger of the work versus leisure dichotomy: "One way to reconcile this split is to realize that work is not necessarily more important than play and play is not necessarily more enjoyable than work" (p. 202). Thus, client-centered care relies in part on the practitioner seeking to understand clients' particular perspective on their daily occupations in order to avoid incorrect assumptions.

Attention to Scope and Detail

In her discussion of using broad categories to classify occupations, Hasselkus (2006) expressed concern that we as OT practitioners " . . . risk losing sight of the unique contexts and individual small behaviors of everyday life and everyday occupation that make up those sweeping categories" (p. 629). However, a positive aspect of having a variety of classification systems is that it serves as a reminder to OT practitioners to inquire and evaluate a person's occupational engagement as a whole. Too often, OT may be overfocused on an occupation of particular interest in that setting. For instance, in medical rehabilitation, there is a strong focus on self-care retraining. We need to always reflect that our scope is much greater and holistic. As far back as 1995, Radomski reminded us that "there is more to life than putting on your pants" (p. 487). Likewise, in school-based practice, the need in the United States to justify services to be educationally related does not preclude the importance of appreciating that children engage in a range of occupations during a school day in addition to the activities they do with their families.

Client Values and Choice

It is of critical importance to understand the value that our clients place on chosen occupations. Although self-care may be important and valued by many clients, exclusive focus on this area of occupation may not serve our clients well in terms of giving them the ability to engage in occupations that are considered quality-of-life changers. For one client, this may be focused on regaining the ability to drive, for another to be able to interact with grandchildren, for another to access e-mail via the Internet, and for another to feed himself or herself independently. The OT profession has discussed the importance of client-centered care and client-centered assessment for more than two decades. A continued emphasis on this aspect of care will assure that we are truly collaborating with our clients and placing our therapy focus on meaningful client-chosen occupations regardless of how they might be classified.

Considering Culture

Related to client values and choice is the consideration of the cultural beliefs and background of our clients to assure relevance of the occupations they are being engaged in (AOTA, 2020b). To prepare practitioners to develop cultural humility and awareness, AOTA (2020b) recommends that OT curriculums address:

- Recognition of one's own stereotypes and biases, with reflection on their impact on practice.

- Self-awareness of one's own cultural background and identities and how they influence one's attitudes, values, priorities, health behaviors, occupations, and participation.
- Knowledge of social determinants of health, health disparities, and health inequities and their institutionally situated resistance to change
- The importance of curiosity surrounding cultural hypotheses and testing of those hypotheses as well as general knowledge about similarities and differences across cultures.

Orchestrating Life

Finally, practitioners must not only consider specific occupations and engagement in occupations but also understand how clients orchestrate their engagement over time and within various environments (Molineux, 2007). Many of our clients are required to engage in multiple occupations at the same time, alternating back and forth between occupations based on changing priorities. They must organize and sequence occupations into a routine, which is satisfactory to themselves and those important to them. This may require that they balance participation in an array of occupations in a variety of familiar and unfamiliar contexts.

No Simple Hierarchies

The chapters that follow in this unit place specific focus on evaluating and intervening to maximize participation in specific categories of areas of occupation. Readers are cautioned that the order of presentation of these topics does not represent a hierarchy. New practitioners may wrongly assume that basic ADL are foundational skills and that clients must gain competence in these before tackling other areas. However, both clinical experience and current research suggest that other activities such as making a hot beverage or hand-washing dishes may be much easier as compared to upper body grooming and total body dressing, depending on the patterns of performance skill abilities and limitations that a client presents with (Fisher & Jones, 2012).

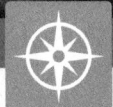

EXPANDING OUR PERSPECTIVES

Occupations from the Asian Perspective

Asako Matsubara

Occupations—as activities that are meaningful and purposeful, are as plentiful and unique as the stars in the sky. Occupations change with the changing times, and new occupations are born in concert with the development of technology and

societal transformations. Different generations of people know different occupations, and the meanings and ways to perform the same tasks differ according to culture. I continue to learn new occupations from my clients in the clinical setting regularly even though I have practiced occupational therapy for more than two decades. Our clients are often our "teachers" who teach us about their occupations and their meanings to us. Occupational therapists must listen

(continued)

EXPANDING OUR PERSPECTIVES (*continued*)

carefully to their clients and observe their behavior through evaluation and treatment.

The meaning of occupations for the client is greatly influenced by culture. Iwama (2006) relates the *East Asian Cosmological Myth*, as "All elements of the universe being subsumed into one inseparable whole." In Buddhist terminology, there is the word "Jitaichinyo," which suggests that "unrelated life does not exist in this world; everyone (everything) connects deeply." Also, in collectivist countries, especially in Asia, the "good of the group" may be prioritized over any "good for the individual." In Japanese culture, for example, clients may be compelled to select and carry out occupations related to their age and roles that are encouraged and required of the social surroundings. Occupations that meet the approval and blessing of the client's own social environment (including loved ones and the family) can often take priority over their own personal wishes. According to Iwama (2006), "in individual-centered societies, the prime mover is located within the self, while in collective-oriented society, the prime mover is located towards the periphery of the self into the domain of the collective" (p. 44). It is often observed in "collective-oriented" societies like Japan that the intention of the family is prioritized over the intention of the individual. In Japanese clinical practice, when clients are discharged from the hospital, "what the family wants the person to do" is also as important as "what the client want [*sic*] to do."

For Japanese occupational therapists abiding in a "collectivist" culture, the definition of the (individual) client is regularly broadened to include the service user, the family, and surrounding (physical and social) environment, and this is very important to choose occupations for the intervention. As an occupational therapist, I am convinced that understanding the meaning of occupations and sharing experience of them, taking into account the subject's culture, can be the basis for a real client-centered occupational therapy.

Conclusion

In summary, the domain of OT is best described as "achieving health, well-being, and participation in life through engagement in occupation" (AOTA, 2020a, p. S5). Knowledge gained from this unit should give the readers a range of therapy options to help our clients engage in their chosen occupations, maximize our clients' ability to participate fully, and assure satisfaction with the care we provide.

Lippincott® Connect *For additional resources on the subjects discussed in this chapter, visit* Lippincott Connect.

REFERENCES

American Occupational Therapy Association (AOTA). (2020a). Occupational therapy practice framework: Domain and process (4th ed.). *American Journal of Occupational Therapy, 74*(Suppl. 2). https://doi.org/10.5014/ajot.2020.74S2001

American Occupational Therapy Association. (2020b). Educator's guide for addressing cultural awareness, humility, and dexterity in occupational therapy curricula. *American Journal of Occupational Therapy, 74*(Suppl. 3), 7413420003. https://doi.org/10.5014/ajot.2020.74S3005

Csikszentmihalyi, M. (1975). *Beyond boredom and anxiety: Experiencing flow in work and play.* Jossey-Bass.

Fisher, A. G., & Jones, K. B. (2012). *Assessment of motor and process skills: Development, standardization, and administration manual* (7th ed., Rev ed.). Three Star Press.

Hasselkus, B. R. (2006). The world of everyday occupation: Real people, real lives. *American Journal of Occupational Therapy, 60,* 627–640. https://doi.org/10.5014/ajot.60.6.627

Iwama, K. M. (2006). *The Kawa model: Culturally relevant occupational therapy.* Churchill Livingstone.

Law, M. (2019). *Canadian occupational performance measure* (5th ed.). Canadian Association of Occupational Therapists.

Molineux, M. (2007). The occupational careers of men living with HIV infection in the United Kingdom: Insights into engaging in and orchestrating occupations. *Australian Occupational Therapy Journal, 54,* 85. https://doi.org/10.1111/j.1440-1630.2007.00654.x

Primeau, L. A. (1996). Work and leisure: Transcending the dichotomy. *American Journal of Occupational Therapy, 50,* 569–577. https://doi.org/10.5014/ajot.50.7.569

Radomski, M. V. (1995). There is more to life than putting on your pants. *American Journal of Occupational Therapy, 49,* 487–490. https://doi.org/10.5014/ajot.49.6.487

World Health Organization (WHO). (2001). *International classification of functioning, disability, and health.* Author.

Analyzing Occupations and Activities

Barbara A. Boyt Schell, Glen Gillen, and Doris Pierce

LEARNING OBJECTIVES

After reading this chapter, you will be able to:

1. Differentiate between activity and occupation and correctly identify them in daily life and in practice.
2. Describe how activity analysis is used in occupational therapy.
3. Complete an activity analysis using the *Occupational Therapy Practice Framework* Activity Analysis Guide.
4. Describe how to analyze personal factors that support or impede performance.
5. Appreciate the degree to which occupation-based practice depends on the practitioner's focus on the client's experience and subjective interpretation of the occupations in which the client engages.
6. Describe a broad analysis of occupational performance when beginning treatment with a new client.
7. Complete an analysis of occupational performance, using the provided analysis structure.
8. Describe analysis of a single occupational experience during intervention.
9. Complete an occupational analysis, using the provided analysis format.
10. Describe analysis of the client's orchestration of their full occupational pattern.
11. Complete an analysis of the orchestration of an occupational pattern, using the provided guide.

Introduction

Think about all the things you will do today. Perhaps you started your day with a bath or shower. Did you do that? Or do you prefer to bathe at night? Are you someone who prefers to bathe less often? Where was the place where you bathed? Did you have to go very far to get to the bathing area? Was it inside or outside? Did you have to carry your supplies or are they stored in the bathing area? Was it a private place or were others bathing at the same time? If you did bathe or shower, did you wash your hair? If you washed your hair, did you shampoo it once or twice? Did you apply a conditioner? Did you wash your hair before or after you washed the rest of your body? Were you standing in a shower, sitting in a tub, leaning over a basin, or wading in a river? How hot was the water? Did your arms get tired? Were you afraid while you bathed? Did you dry your hair with a towel or just comb it and let it dry? Or did you style your hair with a hair dryer? Did you use a pick, comb, brush, wrap, or something else? What physical functions would you say are critical to doing your hair? What mental functions? Now that you think about it, what do you take for granted about bathing? Do you think this is the same for others?

Answering questions such as these is part of the daily thinking processes that occupational therapy (OT) practitioners consider when they go about planning and implementing care for their clients.[*] Whether the attention is on self-maintenance activities, such as bathing and hair care, or on work activities, such as driving a bulldozer or planting crops, practitioners require systematic frameworks to understand exactly what each person wants or needs to do. Application of these systematic frameworks is called activity analysis and occupational analysis. Activity analysis is a structured approach to considering *a general idea* of how something is usually done. Occupational analysis is systematically analyzing what and how a person *actually experiences* what that person is doing.

OT practitioners analyze activities to understand their component parts, the context in which the activity commonly occurs, their possible meaning to clients, and their therapeutic potential. For instance, a therapist who sees a lot of clients from a local chicken-processing factory could do an activity analysis to better understand what it usually involves. If the assembly line work typically involves reaching up to get the poultry item and then placing it in a container before sending it down the line, then the therapist may wish to create a simulated portion of that activity in the outpatient clinic that uses the same sorts of containers at the same work height.

When beginning intervention with a new client, the occupational therapist may complete a broad analysis of that client's occupational performance. The therapist draws on an occupational profile of the client and selected assessments to establish the client's desired intervention outcomes and collaboratively set goals.

Practitioners observe and analyze a client's specific occupational experiences in order to gain an appreciation of performance strengths, potential problems, and how the context affects the performance. Using the example of

the chicken plant, a practitioner may observe a particular worker who is very short to see what specific aspects of the usual factory routine are aggravating a back or hand condition. In a different therapy situation, the therapist may be interested to see how a client manages money. Observing the client while shopping may reveal no problems related to the physical manipulation of money but an inability to calculate money (acalculia). The problems of money management may be worse when the person has no calculator available to compensate. Such a problem can interfere with household management, grocery shopping, or online shopping and banking. Occupational analysis is used to design therapeutic interventions that will enable clients to engage or reengage in those occupations that have particular meaning and value to them.

Practitioners also analyze how clients orchestrate their occupations across a day, a week, or longer. Occupational orchestration is an individual's sequencing and completion of daily occupations within an understanding of their broader occupational pattern. This may include attention to habits and routines and the interface of these with the needs and expectations of others. For example, making up an agenda for the next meeting of the pastoral care committee of the church or cooking dinner for the family may each be very feasible for an individual to perform. However, performing these tasks in a timely and effective manner while working full time and caring for other family needs requires skillful planning and coordination of multiple occupations. For some OT clients, orchestration is an important skill gap that can be addressed in intervention.

The analytic processes practitioners bring to their work are at the core of OT practice. This chapter describes the differentiation of activity and occupation and how these two core concepts of the profession are used to analyze and employ activities and occupations throughout the therapeutic process.

Distinguishing Between Activity and Occupation: Essential Differences in Two Key Concepts of Occupational Therapy

The Dissimilar Historical Roots of Activity and Occupation

At its inception, OT incorporated two distinctly different primary concepts that have remained in tension ever since (Pierce, 2001). Growing out of the moral treatment and arts and crafts

---

[*]According to the American Occupational Therapy Association (AOTA, 2020, p. S75), the term *client* refers to *persons* (including those involved in care of a client), *groups* (a collection of individuals having shared characteristics or common or shared purpose, e.g., family members, workers, students, and those with similar interests or occupational challenges), and *populations* (aggregates of people with common attributes such as contexts, characteristics, or concerns, including health risks). However, in countries other than the United States, the term *client* often refers to persons who are paying for their care directly. In most countries, *patient* is used to describe persons who are in hospital or rehabilitation. *Service user* and *person* are terms in general use that describe those in need of OT services. For this chapter, we are using *client* without implying the source of payment for services.

movements, OT valued the curative effects of working with one's hands, using those experiences to return persons with disabilities to independence and productivity. Additionally, the importance of engaging in health habits and routines was believed to be critical for invalid recovery, and handicrafts were seen as ideal to promote healthy activity (Quiroga, 1995). This attention to engaging patients in occupations formed the basis of OT. This perspective is also at the root of occupational science and is reflected in the field's strong emphasis on occupation-based practice (see Chapter 9).

From its early years, OT also adopted the tenets of scientific management (Creighton, 1992). Developed by Frederick Taylor just as assembly lines began reconfiguring factory labor, industrial efficiency theory used meticulous analyses of workers' physical movements to refine manufacturing workflow and increase profit. In France, this approach was first applied in the rehabilitation of veteran amputees. Within OT, this fine-grained perspective on human action is called activity analysis.

While deeply contrasting, the concepts of occupation and activity have lasted over OT's history. They are both essential to the profession. Problems arise, however, when occupation and activity are not separately defined, are used interchangeably, or are even combined as subsets of each other across a hierarchy of scale, importance, temporal size, breadth, or degree to which the individual defines them. To use a common cliché, the two concepts are apples and oranges. They are completely different. It is not logical to consider the subclasses of each other (Russell, 1989). So, to understand what **activity analysis** and **occupational analysis** can offer to practice, first we must differentially define occupation and activity.

Definitions of Occupation and Activity

In science, it is typical to have multiple definitions of important theoretical ideas. In professions, this normal but somewhat confusing condition is often resolved by committees that synthesize a variety of definitions into an official definition that is regularly updated. The profession's understanding of activity has been refined over many years. Beginning in the 1980s, the American Occupational Therapy Association (AOTA) published three successive versions of *The Uniform Terminology of Occupational Therapy,* which provided Payer with definitions of the profession's key concepts. Then, that document evolved into four successive versions of the *Occupational Therapy Practice Framework (OTPF): Domain and Process,* most recently published in 2020 (AOTA). These efforts to craft comprehensive compilations of all of the profession's concepts accelerated our understanding of the concept of activity.

Present-day activity analysis generally uses the structure of the OTPF to guide a detailed breakdown of all aspects of an activity (Hersch et al., 2005; Thomas, 2015). The

structured simplicity of activity analysis seems to fit well with the fast pace and productivity pressures of the healthcare industry. Although activity analysis is in some ways the easier of the two approaches, it may not offer the practice excellence of an occupational analysis, especially within the complex lives of diverse clients in less medical settings, such as schools, industry, and community health.

In this chapter, we will use Pierce's (2001) definitions of activity and occupation because they most clearly differentiate between these concepts.

> An ***activity*** is an idea held in the minds of persons and in their shared cultural language. An activity is a culturally defined and general class of human actions. The commonsense meanings of activities, such as play or cooking, enable us to communicate about generalized categories of occupational experiences in a broad, accessible way. An activity is not experienced by a specific person: it is not observable as an occurrence; and it is not located in a fully existent temporal, spatial, and sociocultural context. (Pierce, 2001, p. 139)

The following definition of occupation is grounded in the long history of OT's exploration of the therapeutic applications of occupation. It was shaped through occupational science research into infant–toddler play that used the video methods of Jane Goodall (Pierce, 2000, 2005; Pierce et al., 2009). Occupational science, which emerged from OT in the 1980s, is dedicated to building OT's knowledge base through the study of occupation and continues to flourish today (Clark et al., 1991; Pierce, 2014). Occupational science has influenced OT to define best practice as occupation-based and client-centered (see Chapter 9).

> An ***occupation*** is a specific individual's personally constructed, nonrepeatable experience. That is, an occupation is a subjective event in perceived temporal, spatial, and sociocultural conditions that are unique to that one-time occurrence. An occupation has a shape, a pace, a beginning and an ending, a shared or solitary aspect, a cultural meaning to the person, and an infinite number of other perceived contextual qualities. (Pierce, 2001, p. 139)

To summarize most simply, an occupation is the nonrepeatable experience of a specific person, but an activity is a cultural idea that generally describes a particular type of doing. For example, "fishing" is an activity idea, a general notion with which we can communicate about trying to catch a fish. In the United States, many people will think of fishing as standing on a bank with a pole and a baited hook, but others may think of fly fishing or deep-sea fishing. A man who has worked in the Chinese commercial fishing industry will think of fishing in yet another way. Still, everyone is using the same idea of fishing. An activity idea is general, cultural, and flexible.

To demonstrate how different the activity idea of fishing is from an occupational experience of fishing, imagine a young mother named Christa taking her 6-year-old daughter, Ellie, to a Michigan pay lake (a privately owned lake stocked with fish where you pay to participate) on a sunny May afternoon to learn to fish. Ellie is hungry when they arrive, so they carry their picnic basket along, get their poles and bait, and settle on a bench beside the pond. Since the fish are not really biting, they hold their poles while they eat their sandwiches. Suddenly, Ellie's bobber starts jumping, the sandwiches go flying, and Christa pulls Ellie's fish out of the water, but she slips into the lake herself, which frightens Ellie into crying. The lake owner runs over and pulls Christa out and everything is OK (except the sandwiches). That is the nonrepeatable and subjective occupational experience of Christa and Ellie fishing. To know whether they decided they loved fishing or were so discouraged they would never fish again, you would have to ask them!

The General Context of Activity Versus the Specific Context of Occupation

The differentiation of activity and occupation is further clarified by considering the distinct contrast between their contextual elements. Jean Lave (1988), an anthropologist, refers to these differences as *arenas*, which are the general **context** of an activity idea, and *settings*, which are the actual **environment** of an occurring occupation. Think of context as the spatial, temporal, social, and cultural surround, or conditions, of an activity or an occupation. An activity idea is a cultural concept, and thus, a person of a particular culture will have learned the wide repertoire of activity ideas of that culture, each of which includes these contextual aspects. To return to our earlier example, when fishing is mentioned to the Chinese commercial fisherman, he would generally expect to see Chinese ships of different sizes, Chinese workers, a large river or the ocean, and work that is returned to, day after day. Beginning in childhood, we stock our view of the world with activity ideas that fit the culture in which we live. Notice also that the context of an activity idea is relatively flexible and open. It contains a range of contextual possibilities. In the Chinese commercial fishing example, the loosely flexible aspects of context are many, including the type of ship and body of water, the length of the activity, the number and responsibilities of the people involved, and how well-paid the fishermen might be.

Now, consider the context of an occupational experience. There is very little flexibility there. "An occupation has a shape, a pace, a beginning and an ending, a shared or solitary aspect, a cultural meaning to the person, and an infinite number of other perceived contextual qualities" (Pierce, 2001, p. 139). Further, the conditions under which an occupation occurs are those perceived by the person experiencing, or authoring, that nonrepeatable occupation. The best way to know what a person is perceiving in the context of their occupations is **interviewing**, which is a vital skill of

occupation-based practice. Of course, in serving persons for whom interviews are not practical, such as those who are too young or are too cognitively impaired to respond articulately, the therapist will need to access that occupational experience through observation.

Returning to Christa and Ellie's fishing experiences, 6-year-old Ellie might describe some of the contexts of her experience this way. "We were at a huge lake with big poles and wiggly worms, and we just sat there forever and ate peanut butter and jelly until I finally caught a fish and Mommy fell in the lake! It was scary." In contrast, Christa might describe her occupation like this. "I took Ellie to this tiny little pay lake. My grandfather used to take me there when I was a kid, so the whole time, I was just flooded with memories of him. They gave us these little poles that I swear were the same poles we used 30 years ago. We were only there a few minutes before Ellie caught a fish. I slipped in up to my knees and could hardly get that little fish into our net for laughing so hard. It was a special day." Both reports are accurate because they are provided by the persons who had the experiences. This complete acceptance that a person having an experience is the truest interpreter of the meaning and context of that experience honors OT's deep roots in respect for the life meanings of the individual client.

Co-occupation

What Christa and Ellie were doing is a special type of occupation that is called a co-occupation (Pierce, 2009; Zemke & Clark, 1996). "Co-occupation is a dance between the occupations of one individual and another that sequentially shapes the occupations of both persons" (Pierce, 2009, p. 273). Examples that are often given for co-occupation are two people playing tennis or a breast-feeding mother and child. The individuals are having different occupational experiences, but their experiences are intertwined by affecting each other. The concept of co-occupation emerged from the examination of play theories as occupational science began. Parten's Play Scale (Brassard & Boehm, 2008; Parten, 1932) describes different types of social play: "unoccupied, solitary, parallel, associative, and cooperative" (Pierce, 2009, p. 203). It is important to acknowledge that, although co-occupations can be symmetrical, as in the tennis example, a co-occupation does not require the two individuals to share the same intent, or even the same space, time, or affect. It requires only the sequential interaction of their occupational experiences. Not all co-occupations are so closely matched as those of a pair of tennis players. For example, engaging in the co-occupation of teaching-learning requires at least two persons but could include more. Here is a possible occupational sequence for teaching-learning: a teacher explains a concept to a class of 10 students, the students discuss the concept in class, the teacher gives an assignment on the concept, the students complete the assignment, then they are all back in the classroom together to consider a different concept, and so on across the time-frame of the course. Unlike the tennis players, the teacher and the students do not complete their interactive sequence of occupational experiences together, in the same place and time, or for the same reasons. A practitioner's recognition of the co-occupations of their clients, especially those that occur frequently, can provide powerful insights into the client's occupational pattern.

Relationships Between Activity and Occupation

A part of the difficulty in differentiating between activity and occupation may be due to the fact that, although they are not at all the same, they do influence each other. We use activity ideas, or culturally shaped expectations for how something is generally done, to guide us as we anticipate and then carry out any occupation. Our expectations for the occupational experience come from the activity idea that guides us as we begin. Our experience may turn out to be close to the activity idea we had, or it can be disappointingly unlike what we expected.

Further, a single occupational experience often draws on multiple activity ideas. As an example, an occupational experience that a person might describe as "driving home today" could include the activity ideas of driving, listening to a podcast, eating fast food, and thinking about work. All of the activity ideas simultaneously guide the person's experience. They are not subparts of the occupational experience. The driving does not stop so the driver can listen to the podcast or take a bite of food. The occupation is a blend of activity expectations and a multitasking experience.

Activity and occupation are also related through repetition and routine. The more times a person experiences a type of occupation, such as woodworking, the more developed and accurate their activity idea about woodworking will be. That is, the occupational experiences build and fill out the activity idea. The activity ideas of experts are excellent guides to engaging in the occupation in which a person has expertise. On the other hand, the activity ideas of novices do not fit as well with the occupation and require the person to monitor and adjust their experience to compensate for the unexpected, since aspects of their activity ideas will not be as accurate. When a person does the same type of occupation on a regular basis, such as driving home from work, the activity idea becomes so refined that using it to guide that occupation requires very little conscious problem-solving or adjustment.

Activity Analysis in Practice

Activity Analysis in the Design of Treatment

In activity analysis, the practitioner considers an activity in the abstract or general sense, as it might typically be done within a given culture (Pierce, 2001; Polatajko et al., 2000). Practitioners do this sort of activity analysis for at least two reasons. First, the practitioner may wish to anticipate possible areas of concern in working with clients with different kinds of health conditions or occupational performance challenges. Second, practitioners often need to generate activities that may support the acquisition of performance skills relevant to a client's occupational goals (AOTA, 2020). Many familiar activities are commonly used to shape interventions: such as eating, cooking, dressing, bathing, word processing, work tasks, and gross motor play. Most age-appropriate activities can be effectively designed or graded to fit a specific client's needs for occupation-based experiences that will help the client to develop functional capacities, recover from an impairment, or learn an adaptive approach. See OT Story 43.1.

OT STORY 43.1 CULTURAL DIFFERENCES IN MEANINGFUL OCCUPATIONS

Carly Goldberg

Living and working in New York City, I have always been aware of and exposed to a variety of cultures. However, working as a new-ish acute care occupational therapist, cultural values and routines weren't always at the forefront of my mind when working with patients and assessing for the best discharge recommendation. Everybody gets dressed, and eats and bathes, right? Within the first 5 years of my career, our hospital developed an international program. This initiative worked with other countries without strong rehabilitation fields, mostly those countries throughout the Middle East, and clients were brought to our hospital for medical care, specifically for the rehabilitation services we offered. A big draw for these clients in coming to New York was the intense PT and OT program. We had to shift to an inpatient rehab mentality while still working as acute care therapists.

The OT department soon came to realize we had to re-evaluate how we provided care. Everything from how the day was structured, to who provided the therapy, and the content of the sessions needed to be addressed. This was

(continued)

OT STORY 43.1 CULTURAL DIFFERENCES IN MEANINGFUL OCCUPATIONS (*continued*)

way more than just the length of our sessions, or even the language barrier. Cultural context is a huge part of meaningful occupation. The International Services department always had interpreters available, but the approach to care was more difficult to get right. One of the biggest challenges was understanding priorities. Even though everyone does, indeed, get dressed and eat and bathe, it wasn't as important for our international patients to do those things for themselves. These patients were prepared to be in NY for an extended stay, and all of them came with family who stayed at the hospital with them at all times. Spouses, adult children, or staff often completed basic ADLs for our patients, and it was difficult to treatment plan for those patients who did not have the same motivation to address these activities.

Additionally, the whole concept of using occupations as both a means and an end shifted when we had to understand a novel set of occupations. "Therapeutic use of self" meant something different when understanding and respecting a completely different culture. Some patients were requesting male therapists. Others would not participate in therapy before noon. The basics we took for granted in the acute care setting needed to be re-addressed. Our hospital eventually hired a Middle Eastern OT and a PT in order to specifically be more culturally responsive. Not only was this OT able to speak the language and understand the nuances of the culture, but it was also helpful for the entire OT staff

to learn more about another culture, as well as appreciate some of the cultural norms to which we needed to be more sensitive.

We learned to understand that while toileting independently might be of importance regardless of culture, it was often not a priority for our clients who preferred receiving assistance over working on this as an activity within therapy. Although the inpatient rehab unit had a full OT gym, complete with taxi cab and mini market, the privacy of a bedside session was valued over using the gym with other patients and family present. It was through my experience with this population that I learned that it was not just about the activities we address in OT, but the context in which they occur during our intervention as well as in real life. The environment cannot be separated from the activity. In acute care, by nature of the setting, you are never performing an activity in its natural environment, but as an acute care therapist, being able to understand the context—whether physical or cultural—is a key piece of OT's role in one's rehabilitation.

Questions

1. What could the institution have done to better prepare therapists to work with individuals from a different culture.
2. What could OT education programs do to better prepare therapists to work with individuals from a different culture.

Here are examples of how activity analysis can be used to design interventions. If practitioners think about what is typically involved in bathing or showering for people in the culture that they typically serve, it is possible to anticipate likely problems for someone with partial paralysis (e.g., difficulty stepping over the tub wall, risk of fall, inability to reach the faucets, balance issues in lowering into a traditional Japanese hot spring), or difficulty remembering how to sequence activities (e.g., applying soap before wetting the body, beginning to dry off before rinsing off soap). Alternatively, while at a toy store or hardware store, the practitioner might notice and mentally consider how various toys or objects lend themselves to helping individuals develop or improve various skills or bodily capacities. For example, the practitioner might analyze how video games can be used to challenge postural control, eye–hand coordination, motor planning, endurance, self-confidence, and problem-solving. If the practitioner serves a largely Hispanic client population, it would be useful to learn about the activities that are often included in the holiday celebrations of that culture, such

as the preparation of special foods. Having these activity ideas in the practitioner's mental "toolbox" makes it easier to generate therapy possibilities for working with clients. See Expanding Our Perspectives.

Activity analyses can also be applied to groups of people (e.g., members of a choir or workers in a plant), organizations (e.g., the local recreation center), and populations (e.g., homeless urban campers, middle school students, or older adults in a community). This chapter focuses primarily on the analysis of activity and occupation at the individual level because most OT intervention occurs in a one-on-one interaction between the therapist and the client. Applications to groups build on these core analytic approaches. Other chapters later in the text provide illustrations of how occupational analysis can be used in relation to groups, organizations, and populations. See Chapter 22 for examples.

Activity Analysis and Theory

OT practitioners draw on their education, knowledge of activities, and professional experience when analyzing

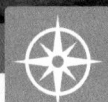

Melding Cultures and Occupations in a Blended Family

Joan Wagner

When choosing to build a family through international adoption there is the awareness of choosing a different culture for your child than the culture of their birth country. My children were babies when I brought them to the United States from Ethiopia. They had spent the first months of their lives being cared for by people who looked like them with the same dark hair and similar skin tone. The smells, tastes, and sounds were already forming a sense of culture and familiarity even at their young ages. I don't have the same skin color or hair texture as my children. I didn't cook with the same spices one of my children had become accustomed to. I don't know how to sing lullabies in the only language they had heard. In my mind, I was giving something to my children, a loving home. I knew I was also taking something from them, the culture of their birth country. In addition to learning how to parent, I felt a great responsibility to expose my kids to some of their Ethiopian roots. Fortunately, there are a few families in my community who are from Ethiopia, and they taught me a great deal. We ate Kik Alicha with injera every Friday night for dinner. We dressed in traditional Ethiopian fashion and attended Christmas celebrations at an Ethiopian church. We attended music and dance performances by Ethiopian artists, and I read Ethiopian children's books to my kids.

My kids are now in their teens. They're into TikTok, basketball, oversized hoodies, and pizza. They have fully embraced the American culture and that makes sense. I exposed my kids to their Ethiopian heritage, but our family, their friends, and our day-to-day life experiences are influenced by our current environment. This is their story, and my hope is that one day when they reconnect with their Ethiopian roots there will be some familiarity.

---

activities (Neistadt et al., 1993). This analysis may be so automatic that it is often ignored or unappreciated, becoming another aspect of the tacit nature of the reasoning process used by practitioners (Mattingly & Fleming, 1994; Schell & Cervero, 1993). Practitioners analyze activities from the perspective of practice theories to understand problems in performance and intervention strategies that may be appropriate from that theoretical perspective. Their analysis is also based on access to particular activities and the degree to which they are willing to engage in trial and error or experimentation to understand activities more fully (Schell, 2018). As part of activity analysis, practitioners may consider the use of the activity as viewed through different theoretical lenses. For instance, a therapist who is working with a population of people with biomechanically related impairments (i.e., hand injuries, back injuries) may emphasize in analyzing an activity the typical strength, range of motion, and endurance required to complete it. Alternatively, someone who is concerned about supporting interpersonal skills in clients with mental illnesses may look primarily at the complexity of social interactions that the activity typically demands (Davidson, 2003). By using the principles of a particular practice theory that seems well fit to the needs of anticipated clients, OT practitioners analyze activities as they think about performance strengths and problems addressed by the particular theory. The potential therapeutic intervention should be consistent with the theory and will likely entail the grading and adaptation of the occupations chosen by the client. Box 43.1 presents a format for the analysis of activities.

Activity Analysis While Working With Clients

Activity analysis is also a way of thinking about activities during intervention. Practitioners must perform quick analyses while working with clients. In addition, OT practitioners may also think about activities for their therapeutic potential, for instance, by sizing up new games, cooking gadgets, technology, and other objects or activities. The goal of activity analysis is to understand as much as possible about an activity, including the particular skills required to do it competently and its relation to participation in the world at large (Cynkin, 1995). It is this knowledge of activities, their properties, and their potential cultural meanings that sensitize practitioners to the occupations of their clients and helps them to know what activities to suggest to their clients. Through activity analysis, practitioners gain an understanding of the therapeutic potential of a wide range of activities. Because practitioners routinely analyze activities, they develop the capacity to quickly analyze a wide range of activities for their therapeutic or evaluation potential.

The OTPF Activity Analysis Guide

Like most approaches to activity analysis today, the activity analysis format provided here is based on the organization of the Occupational Therapy Practice Framework (OTPF) (AOTA, 2020). The OTPF is a primary official document of the AOTA and exerts a wide influence on practice. It is designed to reflect OT's dedication to supporting the health and participation of people in society. The following OTPF Activity Analysis Guide (Box 43.1) can be used to guide any practitioner though a full activity analysis that rests on the structure of the OTPF. Box 43.2 offers a demonstration of the use of the Guide in an analysis of the activity of a child taking a nap at preschool.

BOX 43.1 THE *OCCUPATIONAL THERAPY PRACTICE FRAMEWORK (OTPF)* ACTIVITY ANALYSIS GUIDE

What is the activity? (Give it a common name.)

Activity Type. Select one: "activities of daily living (ADLs), instrumental activities of daily living (IADLs), health management, rest and sleep, education, work, play, leisure, social participation." (OTPF, Exhibit 1, p. 7)

Activity Subtype. Choose a subtype under the activity type. See OTPF, Tables 2 and 3, pp. 30–36. For example, the activity subtypes of rest and sleep are rest, sleep preparation, and sleep participation.

Context: Environmental Factors (See OTPF, Table 4, pp. 36–39 for examples and details to support description of each of the following environmental factors.) Natural environment and human-made changes to the environment; products and technology; support and relationships; attitudes; services, systems, and policies.

Context: Personal Factors (See OTPF, Table 5, p. 39 for examples and details to support description of each of the following personal factors.) Age; sexual orientation; gender identity; race and ethnicity; cultural identification and cultural attitudes; social background, social status, and socioeconomic status; upbringing and life experiences; habits and past and current behavioral patterns; individual psychological assets; education; profession and professional identity; lifestyle; other health conditions and fitness.

Performance Patterns of a Person or Group/Population (See OTPF, Table 6, pp. 40–42 for examples and details to support description of each of the following performance patterns.) Habits (person only), routines (person or group/population), roles (person or group/population), rituals (person or group/population).

Performance Skills of a Person or Group/Population (See OTPF, Tables 7 and 8, pp. 43–50 and for examples and details to support description of each of the following performance skills for a person or a group.) Motor skills, process skills, social interaction skills.

Client Factors of a Person, Group, or Population (See OTPF, Table 9, pp. 51–54 for examples and details to support description of each of the following client factors.) Values, beliefs, and spirituality; body functions (specific mental functions; global mental functions; sensory functions; neuromuscular and movement-related functions; muscle functions; movement functions; cardiovascular, hematologic, immunologic, and respiratory system functions; voice and speech functions; digestive, metabolic, and endocrine system functions; genitourinary and reproductive functions; skin and related structures functions); body structures.

BOX 43.2 TAKING A NAP AT PRESCHOOL: AN ACTIVITY ANALYSIS EXAMPLE

Activity and Activity Subtype

- Rest and Sleep, Sleep Preparation, and Sleep Participation

Context: Environmental Factors

- Natural environment and human-made changes to the environment—group of preschool children and teacher(s), typically a ground floor classroom with adjoining children's bathroom, tile floor with a 12-foot circular rug in the center. Against exterior walls: windows, hallway door, toyboxes, play kitchen, tables, child-level sink, storage cupboards, stack of sleep matts, cubbies, bulletin board. Nap at 12:00 pm, immediately following lunch. Sounds of other children settling for naps.
- Products and technology—Nap matt, covers if cool weather.
- Support and relationships—Teacher(s), other students.

- Attitudes—Expectation of independence in preparing for nap and maintaining sleep or quiet during naptime.
- Services, systems, and policies—Private pay or government-supported preschool program.

Context: Personal Factor

- Age—2 to 5 years
- Upbringing and life experience—Experience/lack of experience with preschool will be a factor
- Habits and past and current behavioral patterns—Current sleep and classroom habits will be important
- Individual psychological assets—Ability to transition between classroom activities, follow directions, self-calm, screen out movement and noise from other children
- Education—Preschool experience or inexperience
- Profession and professional identity—NA

- Other health conditions and fitness—Mobility or assistance requirements to move sleep matt and to lie supine at floor level

Performance Patterns of a Person

- Habits—Current sleep and classroom habits will affect performance, habit of smoothly entering naptime
- Routines—Ability to follow and transition smoothly between the sequence of classroom activities
- Roles—Student, classmate
- Rituals—Same sequence every school day to prepare for and enter sleep at naptime, may include soothing nursery music

Performance Patterns of a Group or Population

- Routines—Classroom of children need ability to follow and transition smoothly between the sequence of classroom activities
- Roles—Students, classmates, all children tolerate and show social support to other children who may have difficulty falling asleep
- Rituals—Same sequence every school day to prepare for and enter sleep at naptime, may include soothing nursery music

Performance Skills for a Person

- Motor skills—Walking/mobility skills to navigate through classroom and around classmates, hand coordination to carry sleep matt and covers, ability to spread sleep matt and covers in location with adequate space, motor planning to transition from upright to prone or supine on matt, sufficient hand coordination and body awareness to pull cover over self, younger children likely to require assistance
- Process skills—Understand directions and how to unfold matt and covers, use spatial and body awareness, ability to self-calm and remain quiet, tolerance of noise and movements of other children, younger children likely to require assistance
- Social interaction skills—Accept and follow directions given by teacher, dampen or cease play interactions with others in preparation for sleep, respect personal space

of other children, maintain quiet so others can nap, younger children likely to require assistance

Performance Skills for a Group

- Motor skills—Full class requires walking/mobility skills sufficient to navigate through classroom and around each other, hand coordination to carry sleep matts and covers without colliding with each other, ability to spread sleep matt and covers in location with adequate space, motor planning to transition from upright to prone or supine on matt, sufficient hand coordination and body awareness to pull cover over self, younger children likely to require assistance
- Process skills—Full class understands directions and how to unfold matt and covers, use spatial and body awareness, ability to self-calm and remain quiet, tolerance of noise and movements of other children, younger children likely to require assistance
- Social interaction skills—Full class accepts and follows directions given by teacher, dampens or ceases play interactions with others in preparation for sleep, respects interpersonal space, maintains quiet so others can nap, younger children likely to require assistance

Client Factors of a Person, Group, or Population

- Values, beliefs, and spirituality—Young child's (or children's) desire to exhibit good behavior, comply with directions, show age-appropriate independence, demonstrate respect for teacher and classmates, value opportunity to rest
- Body functions (specific mental functions; global mental functions; sensory functions; neuromuscular and movement-related functions; muscle functions; movement functions; cardiovascular, hematologic, immunologic, and respiratory system functions; voice and speech functions; digestive, metabolic, and endocrine system functions; genitourinary and reproductive functions; skin and related structures functions)—Young child's (or children's) age-appropriate and typically capable body functions or adaptation and assistance required
- Body structures—Young child's (or children's) age-appropriate and typically capable body structures or adaptation and assistance required

Analysis of Personal Factors That Support or Impede an Activity

OT practitioners may also analyze selected activities from a **micro perspective** in terms of how the presence, absence, or impairment of body functions supports or limits engagement. Árnadóttir (2021) suggests that the therapist can use

this analysis to consider potential errors that may occur due to client conditions, indicating the effect of neurobehavioral deficits on task performance. Subsequently, the therapist can hypothesize about the impaired body functions that caused the error (Árnadóttir, 1990). This approach suggested by Árnadóttir can be expanded to include musculoskeletal impairments, psychological impairments, and so forth (Table 43.1). See Unit VIII for an in-depth discussion of personal factors.

TABLE 43.1   An Analysis of Personal Factors That Support or Impede an Activity

Activity to Be Analyzed: *Morning Self-Care*

Body Function	Support for Effective and Efficient Engagement in Activity	Impairments of Body Function Potentially Impeding Activity
Praxis	Understands the concept of a morning routine, knows how to use pertinent objects (comb, razor, socks, etc.), is able to organize and sequence the steps of the task and to plan movements	Apraxia: uses the comb to brush teeth; improperly sequences the steps of dressing (socks on top of shoes); unable to plan movements related to donning pants, resulting in clumsy and inefficient movements
Visuospatial processing	Judges depth and distance, orients clothing properly to body, differentiates foreground from background such as finding a bar of white soap on a white sink	Spatial relations impairment: spills toothpaste when attempting to squeeze it on to the brush, dons shirt backward, unable to differentiate sleeves from the body of shirt
Arousal/attention	Alert, stays on task, disregards irrelevant environmental stimuli, attends to stimuli in both the right and left attentional fields	Arousal/attention deficits: falls asleep, gets distracted by television and stops dressing before completing the task, does not attend to clothing hanging on the left side of the closet
Motor control	Controls posture to stand at the sink, bends to retrieve shoes from the floor, reaches into the closet for a shirt, coordinates movements to brush teeth	Impaired motor control: leans to the left while standing at the sink, loses balance while bending or reaching for clothing, trembles while reaching for brush, cannot reverse movements for efficient toothbrushing
Affect	Motivated to engage in tasks, able to tolerate frustrations that arise, show affect appropriate to situation and task	Affective disturbance: requires coaxing and encouragement to participate in and continue morning care, easily frustrated and terminates task, moods shift rapidly during performance

Sources: Data from Árnadóttir, G. (1990). *The brain and behavior: Assessing cortical dysfunction through activities of daily living.* Elsevier/Mosby; and Árnadóttir, G. (2021). Impact of neurobehavioral deficits on activities of daily living. In G. Gillen (Ed.), *Stroke rehabilitation: A function-based approach* (5th ed., pp. 556–592). Elsevier/Mosby.

Occupational Analysis in Practice

What Is Occupational Analysis?

In occupational analysis, practitioners are concerned with understanding the specific situation of the client and therefore must understand the specific occupations the client wants or needs to do in the actual context in which occupations are performed. In contrast to activity analysis, occupational analysis *places the person in the foreground* by considering the particular person's life experiences, values, interests, and goals. Occupational analysis attends to the *actual* body functions and structures, the *actual* performance skills within an *actual* performance setting, including physical and social contexts along with the demands of the occupation itself. These considerations shape the practitioner's efforts to help the person reach their goals through carefully designed evaluation and intervention. Practitioners vary the scope of the occupational analysis depending on the nature of the client's concerns, occupational performance challenges, health problems, and the nature of the intervention setting (see Figure 43.1).

The AOTA's OTPF (2020) describes different types of OT interventions, most of which would be accomplished by engaging the client in occupations that are designed to meet their goals. Often, intervention takes the form of participation in aspects of that client's life that are important to them and are presenting challenges of different kinds, such as problems in carrying out activities of daily living (ADLs), completing tasks at school or work, or engaging in play or leisure. Occupational therapists also sometimes use education or training to assist the client in understanding and mastering valued occupations. The therapist may also advocate for a client's needs, or help the client develop the important skill of advocating for their own needs. Some interventions are preparatory to engagement in occupation, such as using a sensory strategy to regulate arousal before the client engages in a stressful work assignment. Therapists also support their clients' occupations through services such as the recommendation, fitting, or set up of an orthotic brace, wheelchair, or other assistive technology devices.

Through the Eyes of the Client

Over and over again, practitioners must remind themselves that meaning is individually constructed and interpreted and is central to human existence (Bruner, 1990; Frankl, 1959; Hasselkus, 2002; Peloquin, 2005, 2007). A practitioner is obligated to understand the meaning of occupations

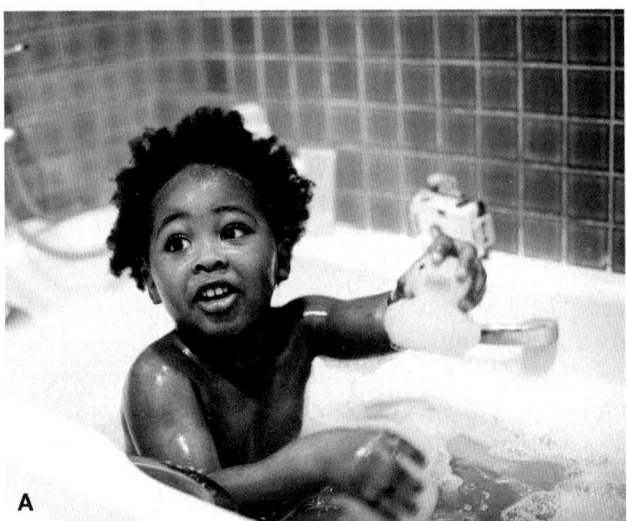
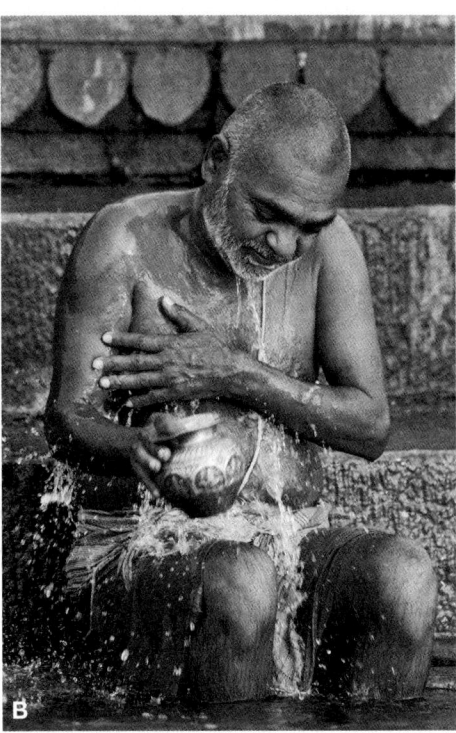

FIGURE 43.1 Bathing: Analyze these two very different examples of bathing. **A:** A toddler enjoys bath time. **B:** A man takes a ritual bath in the river Ganga in the holy city of Varanasi, India.

from the client's perspective. To do so requires empathy, experience, and professional-level interview and observation skills. For example, a therapist may want to use cooking in a weekly skills group for older adults in an assisted living setting. Beyond considering goals for the group, group members' current skills, and the time and space where the group will cook, it is also important for the OT practitioner to choose a cooking project to best fit the meanings they may hold for the clients. Baking Christmas cookies in December may call up fond memories for some group members. Others, however, who have not grown up in an American Christian tradition may feel excluded by this choice. The meanings of occupations are defined, not by the therapist, but by the individuals experiencing them.

As this example illustrates, the different experiences, values, and beliefs of clients make the interpretation of meaning a particularly complex aspect of practice. This challenge is exacerbated by potential cultural and socioeconomic differences between practitioners and their clients, which can make it more challenging for practitioners to fully understand the experiences of their clients and the meanings they ascribe to their occupations (Crepeau, 1991; Kielhofner & Barrett, 1998; Payne et al., 2001). See also Chapters 14, 15, 17, and 59 which address culture, socioeconomics, place, and spirituality, respectively. It is the practitioner's responsibility to develop therapeutic relationships that foster an understanding of clients and their world (Crepeau & Garren, 2011; Peloquin, 1995). See also Chapter 28, which addresses person-centered collaboration and the

therapeutic relationship. Occupational analysis is a tool that can help practitioners to achieve this understanding.

In contrast to the consideration of activities for their therapeutic implications, occupational analysis is a highly individualized process because it is embedded in the particular perspective of the person, the person's occupational performance, and the performance context. Occupational analysis occurs when attempting to understand the person as an occupational being in concert with identifying occupational performance skills and barriers to effective performance (Coster, 1998; Fisher & Jones, 2014; Hocking, 2001; Polatajko et al., 2000; Trombly, 1995; Trombly Latham, 2014). Client-centered evaluation models examine the ability of a person to engage in a valued occupation and the transaction among actual performance, activity demands, and context (Law, 1998).

The concept of **role** has had an influence on the development of theory within the profession. For instance, the Model of Human Occupation, developed in the 1980s, uses role as a way of articulating how individuals see themselves and the multiple aspects of a person's life (see Chapter 34). The concept of role has been translated into assessments such as the Role Checklist and Worker Role Interview. In sociological and psychological theories, roles are seen as social positions (Hagedorn, 2000; Jackson, 1998a). Roles can be thought of as normative models shaped by the culture. For example, role articulates cultural expectations for what constitutes a "good" mother, father, or student, and the activities people in these positions should perform. Importantly, such expectations can differ radically from one cultural group to another.

Jackson (1998a, 1998b) argued that our concern should be with the occupations individuals engage in, not their roles, because the concept of role is problematic from several perspectives. First, roles may overlap. For example, it is often impossible to distinguish children's "student" roles from their "friend" roles. When someone is cleaning up the kitchen after a meal, is it in the role of father, mother, child, church volunteer, or busboy? Our concern must be with the occupation, the person's ability to engage in the occupation, and the meaning the person ascribes to it, not the role to which the activity is often connected. Second, although the concept of role provides a shorthand way of understanding the occupational world of an individual, Jackson (1998a) contended that this approach is risky because inherent in the concept of role are the power issues embedded in many cultural models. For example, who decides what a "good mother" is? Who says the mother is the one to clean up the dinner dishes for the family?

Still, role is not easy to ignore because it is such a widely held concept. For example, Trombly Latham (Trombly, 1995; Trombly Latham, 2014) uses role as an organizing construct; however, she cautions that roles should be considered from the definitional perspective of the individual rather than from the normative expectations of society. But how does one get to this definitional perspective except through understanding the occupations the individual attaches to a particular role? By focusing on occupations people engage in, we can see what people do, what the occupation means to them, how they feel about their performance, and how they organize their occupations to meet their needs and the needs of the people around them. Jackson's (1998a, 1998b) cautions about the use of roles are important because it is easy to unconsciously slip into normative expectations or use one's personal experience to frame expectations for clients. Practitioners bring unarticulated personal assumptions to the therapy process (see Chapter 25). The concept of role was not selected as an organizing construct for this chapter because we want to focus on those occupations that are most important to an individual, regardless of which role or roles that person might attribute to them.

Although occupational analysis is used in all occupation-based interventions, the analysis itself can be done at different degrees of detail or breadth, as well as for different reasons. In the following section, three distinct types of occupational analysis are described: a broad analysis of occupational performance when beginning treatment with a new client, an analysis of a single occupational experience that occurs during intervention, and analysis of the client's orchestration of their full occupational pattern.

Beginning Occupation-Based Intervention: Analysis of Occupational Performance

To begin intervention with a client, the therapist completes the Analysis of Occupational Performance (Box 43.3). This broad analysis draws on the occupational profile, observations of occupational engagement, and identified assessments to develop hypotheses about the case and collaboratively set goals and desired outcomes that are custom fit to the values and priorities of the client. The type of outcomes identified in the OTPF (AOTA, 2020) includes occupational performance, improvement in occupational performance, enhancement of occupational performance, prevention of risk and ill health, health and wellness, quality of life, participation in desired occupations, role competence, well-being, and occupational justice.

Occupational Analysis During Intervention

Once the client and therapist set goals for intervention, OT practitioners will observe individuals as they engage in occupations that are selected to contribute to their progress toward desired occupations. This may range from observing a student in the classroom or on the playground, a person working in an office or factory, an older adult in a leisure setting or an assisted living facility, or a person living at a shelter. In all of these situations, the practitioner's attention is on the dynamic transaction of the person's occupational performance within the performance context. It should be noted that at times close facsimiles of performance environments are used by practitioners. This may be true for example by practitioners working in facilities where the occupational therapy area only resembles a gymnasium style room. Although the practitioner must be concerned with the quality of the results, the major focus is on the process of engagement. Thus, practitioners become adept at carefully observing skills associated with occupational performance. These performance skills are the smallest observable units of occupational performance, goal-directed actions a person carries out one by one during naturalistic and relevant daily life task performances (Fisher & Jones, 2014). See Chapter 52 for an in-depth discussion of performance skills. See Table 43.2 for an occupational analysis format and example.

Analysis of the Client's Orchestration of the Full Occupational Pattern

Orchestration, a musical term, implies a rhythmic, harmonious composition of daily life that has habitual or routine components but is also responsive to changes in demands from day to day (Larson, 2000). Every person, every client, manages the flow of their occupations across a broad pattern of time. We must constantly reevaluate, and make decisions about, the arrangement of our occupations over the day, the week, the month, the year, and even over a lifetime. In orchestrating our occupations, we consider, not only their temporal sequence, but also the spatial, social, and experiential aspects of those occupations. We think

BOX 43.3 ANALYSIS OF OCCUPATIONAL PERFORMANCE

"Occupational performance is the accomplishment of the selected occupation resulting from the dynamic transaction among the client, their contexts, and the occupation. In the analysis of occupational performance, the client's ability to effectively complete desired occupations is identified. The client's assets and limitations or potential problems are more specifically determined through assessment tools designed to analyze, measure, and inquire about factors that support or hinder occupational performance. The analysis of occupational performance involves one or more of the following:

Multiple methods often are used during the evaluation process to assess the client, contexts, occupations, and occupational performance. Methods may include observation and analysis of the client's performance in specific occupations and assessment of specific aspects of the client or their performance. The approach to the analysis of occupational performance is determined by the information gathered through the occupational profile and influenced by models of practice and frames of reference appropriate to the client and setting. The analysis of occupational performance involves one or more of the following:

- Synthesizing information from the occupational profile to determine specific occupations and contexts that need to be addressed
- Completing an occupational or activity analysis to identify the demands of occupations and activities on the client
- Selecting and using specific assessments to measure the quality of the client's performance or performance

deficits while completing occupations or activities relevant to desired occupations, noting the effectiveness of performance skills and performance patterns
- Selecting and using specific assessments to measure client factors that influence performance skills and performance patterns
- Selecting and administering assessments to identify and measure more specifically the client's contexts and their impact on occupational performance." (AOTA, 2020, pp. 22–23)

"The occupational therapist synthesizes the information gathered through the occupational profile and analysis of occupational performance. This process may include the following:

- Determining the client's values and priorities for occupational participation
- Interpreting the assessment data to identify supports and hindrances to occupational performance
- Developing and refining hypotheses about the client's occupational performance strengths and deficits
- Considering existing support systems and contexts and their ability to support the intervention process
- Determining desired outcomes of the intervention
- Creating goals in collaboration with the client that address the desired outcomes
- Selecting outcome measures and determining procedures to measure progress toward the goals of intervention, which may include repeating assessments used in the evaluation process."

From American Occupational Therapy Association. (2020). Occupational therapy practice framework: Domain and process (4th ed.). *American Journal of Occupational Therapy, 74*(Suppl. 2), 7412410010. https://doi.org/10.5014/ajot.2020.74S200

TABLE 43.2   Occupational Analysis Format and Example

Occupational Analysis	Example of Occupational Analysis
Briefly describe the client, including name, age, gender, diagnosis or specific limitations, general goals, cultural background, and any aspects of client values, beliefs, or spirituality that bear on the occupation being analyzed.	Maksym is a 20-year-old male with autism who is a super senior in his local high school. He emigrated to the United States from Ukraine with his family in 2021. He has difficulty with interpersonal communication, independent problem-solving, and working without supervision. He is painfully shy. His English skills are good, but his accent adds to communication difficulties. Maksym's goals include independent living skills, early work experiences, and social inclusion in his community. He regularly attends Catholic church services with his family. On Sundays, he works after the service as a volunteer janitor, with on-site support available from the youth minister. He lives in a small apartment above the garage of his family home. He is learning to drive.
Briefly describe the occupation.	The occupation is hosting friends to play video games. Maksym invited two male friends from his high school transition program to his apartment to play video games after school. It is a short walk from the school to his apartment. He provided two frozen pizzas, pop, and packaged cookies during the visit. After arriving, Maksym and his friends began drinking pop and taking turns playing video games. Maksym started baking the pizzas at about 4:30 pm. The two guests were picked up by family members at 9 pm. Maksym has never had visitors before, but he occasionally cooks simple foods in his family kitchen with his mother's support. In his own apartment, he has previously prepared for himself cereal, toaster waffles, cold cut sandwiches, and frozen pizzas.

(continued)

| TABLE 43.2 | Occupational Analysis Format and Example (*continued*) |

Occupational Analysis	Example of Occupational Analysis
Describe the tools, materials, and equipment actually used. Note the symbolism/meaning of the objects to this person.	Maksym's mother helped him to prepare for the visit by driving him to the grocery to shop for the food and by giving him suggestions for finishing up the cleaning of his apartment. Before leaving for school on the day of the visit, Maksym checked to make sure his favorite video game had two working controllers, put the pop in the fridge, placed paper plates and napkins on the kitchen bar, set the pizza cutter and two oven mitts beside the stove, and poured two large packages of cookies into a big bowl and set the bowl of cookies inside a cupboard so he could bring them out after the pizza was eaten. During the visit, his friends said they had fun, and they greatly enjoyed the food, although the pizza was somewhat burned. They ate at the coffee table, in front of the television. Maksym cleaned up the kitchen/living room area after his guests had left, with prompting from his mother.
Describe the actual physical environment in which the occupation will be performed. Consider how the physical environment supports or impedes performance. Include key aspects, such as the following: • Does this occur in a natural or built environment? • What are the major natural or built structures? • How do structures, furnishings, and equipment affect the person's performance? • What is the light level and does it change? How does lighting affect performance? • Describe the kind and level of noise and how it affects performance. • Describe any other features that affect the person's performance (e.g., smell, humidity, texture, temperature). • In addition to the context just described, where else does this person engage in this occupation? Briefly describe all additional contexts, with emphasis on how they are different from the first one described.	Maksym's apartment above the garage is reached by one flight of outdoor stairs. His kitchen/living room area is small but efficient, well-lit, and quiet. He does not have a table, but there is eating space on the kitchen bar or at the coffee table in front of the couch, which faces the television. Maksym stores groceries in cupboards above the kitchen counters or in the refrigerator/freezer. The pizza cutter is kept in a drawer to the left of the stove. The sink is directly behind Maksym as he faces his work counter. Due to the small size of his kitchen, all objects are within reach of his countertop work surface. His kitchen is lit by a fluorescent fixture. Maksym occasionally helps his mother with cooking family meals and has some experience with cleaning as a janitor at his church.
Describe the social and cultural demands as the person engages in this occupation using the categories listed below. • Describe other people involved in the occupation. What is their relationship to each other? What do they expect from each other? • Describe the rules, norms, and expectations of this person while engaged in this occupation. • Describe the cultural and symbolic meanings that this person and their significant others ascribe to this occupation. • Consider all the other social contexts in which the occupation might be performed. How do the rules, expectations, and meanings vary from this setting?	Maksym felt the visit was a great success and plans to do it again. They enjoyed the video games, an activity with limited requirements for conversation and eye contact. It was especially important to Maksym that he provided his friends "cool" American foods, rather than the ethnic Ukrainian foods he usually eats with his family. Having friends over for the first time is an important milestone in Maksym's desire to live independently and be socially included in his community.
List the sequential steps (no more than 15) of the occupation as the person does it. Include any timing requirements, such as waiting for glue to dry, bread to rise, etc. • How much flexibility exists in the sequence and timing of the steps of this occupation? • Does this occupation typically occur or reoccur at a specific time of day? When and with what frequency (i.e., daily, weekly, monthly)?	For Maksym, the sequential steps of this occupation were planning for the visit, grocery shopping with assistance from his mother, cleaning up his apartment before the visit, preparing for the visit before school, serving pop to his friends, playing video games, baking the two pizzas, getting out the cookies after the pizzas were gone, and cleaning up after his friends left. Maksym did not get the pizza out of the oven in time: he will need to learn to use the kitchen stove timer. The sequence had little flexibility except during the time the guests were present, at which time Maksym moved between playing video games, interacting with friends, baking pizza, and offering his friends food and drink.

TABLE 43.2 Occupational Analysis Format and Example (*continued*)

Occupational Analysis	Example of Occupational Analysis
Using the OTPF, or other published list of skills, identify 5–10 skills critical to this person's occupational performance. • Consider skills which demand from the person movement, cognition, sensory, and emotional perception as well as communicative and social actions. • Consider skills typically demanded from the applicable environment (physical, social, and virtual).	Examples of the skills that Maksym required, and that were most pertinent to his goals of independent living, early work experiences, and social inclusion in his community, include: choosing groceries; sequencing the shopping, cleaning, visiting, food prep, and clean-up; pacing his video game playing, social interactions, and food preparation; using the oven and pizza cutter appropriately; handling hot pizza safely; following frozen pizza directions; initiating baking the pizza and serving the cookies; noticing/responding to the pizza overcooking; regulating social behaviors; and transitioning between playing video games, preparing pizza, and serving guests.
Consider the underlying capacities of the person that are required when doing this occupation in the contexts just identified. • Briefly list the body structures (anatomical parts of the body) the person uses. • Briefly list the essential body functions (physiological and psychological).	Examples of required body structures include all extremities and trunk, including bones, joints, muscle, tendon, eyes, and central and peripheral nervous systems. Examples of body functions include arousal, working memory, sustained attention, praxis, visual acuity, interpreting spatial relationships, problem-solving, tactile feedback, active joint range of motion, muscle strength, and postural alignment and control.
List potential safety hazards for this person while performing this occupation. Consider cognitive and judgment problems, diminished sensation, etc.	Potential hazards include inserting and removing the pizzas from a hot oven on time; tolerating a multi-hour social interaction without becoming over-stimulated.
How much flexibility exists for this person to do this occupation in different ways? How willing is the person and key stakeholders to consider doing it differently? Consider the following: • Person-based variables (e.g., personal context, impairments) • External contextual variables (physical, social, temporal, virtual, cultural)	Maksym looks forward to having his friends over again to play video games and may begin to increase his frequency of entering social situations in the community. Now that he has expanded his cooking experience to include frozen pizza, he plans to explore other frozen prepared foods he can cook without assistance in his apartment.
List three ways to make the occupation easier in relation to an identified personal or contextual variable.	This occupation can be made less challenging regarding social skill development by repeating the same planned visit with the same friends and the same foods and playing video games; ordering pizza instead of baking it; offering premade foods instead of preparing foods; hosting family members to play video games instead of friends; or inviting only one friend.
List three ways to make the occupation more challenging in relation to an identified personal or contextual variable.	This occupation can be made more challenging regarding social skill development via inviting additional or less well-acquainted friends; hosting friends for a special occasion such as a birthday; hosting a mixed-gender group of friends; or baking pizzas at a church event.

Source: Adapted from American Occupational Therapy Association. (2020). Occupational therapy practice framework: Domain and process (4th ed.). *American Journal of Occupational Therapy, 74*(Suppl. 2), 7412410010. https://doi.org/10.5014/ajot.2020.74S200

about our needs and aspirations, the meanings to us of desired occupations, our usual routines, our abilities, and our resources. The skills of orchestration mature in synch with other aspects of typical development. To be most beneficial, they require experience and attentive judgment. For the clients of OT, the ability to orchestrate this complex pattern can be especially challenging, due to impairments, unexpected life disruptions, environmental constraints, lack of resources and supports, or oppressive systems. Analyzing a client's occupational orchestration may not be required in every case, but it will be especially important for clients who are having difficulty orchestrating over a single day or are facing critical challenges and decisions in regard to a longer occupational pattern. See Table 43.3 Guide to Analysis of Orchestration of Occupational

Pattern for guidance in completing this type of occupational analysis.

Conclusion

Activity analysis and occupational analysis are foundational to OT. To implement these analyses effectively, and within a best practice occupation-based approach, it is essential to understand the difference between an activity idea and an occupational experience and to appreciate the centrality of personal meaning to occupation. With that awareness as a basis, this chapter prepares OT personnel to implement two types of activity analysis and three forms of occupational analysis in service to their clients (Box 43.4).

TABLE 43.3	Guide to Analysis of Orchestration of Occupational Pattern
Occupations	Identify the occupations that are central to the person's identity. List these occupations.
Meaning	• How meaningful are these occupations to the individual? • How central are the occupations to the person's identity? • How important are the occupations to the individual? • How important is the occupation to others in the person's social world (family, friends, coworkers, etc.)?
Purpose	What purpose(s) does each occupation serve in the individual's life (e.g., self-maintenance, health, support to family, support to friends or others, contribution to community, play or leisure, work)?
Level of Skill and Efficiency	For each occupation, does the individual believe they are able to do this occupation at an appropriate level of skill within the expected timelines? • If not, what are the problems/concerns from the individual's perspective? • If not, what are the problems/concerns from the perspective of people in the individual's social world?
Routines	Identify the pattern in which the individual engages in these occupations. • What occupations occur daily? • What occupations occur weekly? • What occupations occur monthly and annually? • Describe a typical day. • Describe a typical week.
Organization of Routines	To what extent is the daily and weekly pattern of occupations routinized (patterns of behavior that are observable, regular, repetitive, and provide structure for daily life; routines and occupations with established sequences)? • Is the individual satisfied with this level of organization? If not, why not? • To what extent do these routines meet the expectations of family, friends, and coworkers? • Are these expectations reasonable given the person's physical and emotional capacities, and expectations from the context, family, friends, and employers? • Describe the degree to which these routines are disorganized, stable, or rigid.
Adaptability to Promote Participation	To what extent are the occupations and/or routines flexible based on • Individual-based variables: personal context, impairments, openness to change? • Expectations from social environment (family, friends, coworkers)? • Environmental adaptability (potential to change physical environment to promote increased participation)?
Needs	Describe the extent to which the occupational routine is sufficient to meet the person's needs and the needs of those in their social world. This might include attention to occupational deprivation or overload. Describe the changes required to meet the individual's needs: • Changes in the individual (skill development) • Changes in the social environment (expectations for performance) • Changes in the occupation (adapting or grading to promote more effective performance)

BOX 43.4 HOW ACTIVITY ANALYSIS AND OCCUPATIONAL ANALYSIS INFORM PRACTICE

Practitioners analyze activity in the abstract for the following reasons:

• To understand the therapeutic potential of a wide range of activities
• To determine the impact of personal factors (including health conditions) on performance
• To determine the impact of contextual factors on performance
• To identify ways to foster improved performance through grading or adaptation
• To identify activities that lend themselves to

Improving client performance through acquiring new skills or learning adaptive strategies

Restoring a skill or client factor that impacts performance skills

Prevention of future problems by changing or adapting activity demands or performance context

Practitioners analyze the occupational experiences of their clients to:

• Begin intervention with a broad examination of the client's occupations and collaboratively set meaningful client goals
• Evaluate the quality of current performance of an occupation targeted by, or used therapeutically in, intervention
• Examine a client's effectiveness in orchestrating their occupations across time

Lippincott® Connect *For additional resources on the subjects discussed in this chapter, including videos of occupations that can be analyzed, visit Lippincott Connect. See* **Appendix II, Table of Assessments** *for more information on Role Checklist and Worker Role Interview.*

REFERENCES

American Occupational Therapy Association. (2020). Occupational therapy practice framework: Domain and process (4th ed.). *American Journal of Occupational Therapy, 74*(Suppl. 2), 7412410010. https://doi.org/10.5014/ajot.2020.74S200

Árnadóttir, G. (1990). *The brain and behavior: Assessing cortical dysfunction through activities of daily living.* Elsevier/Mosby.

Árnadóttir, G. (2021). Impact of neurobehavioral deficits on activities of daily living. In G. Gillen (Ed.), *Stroke rehabilitation: A function-based approach* (4th ed., pp. 556–592). Elsevier/Mosby.

Brassard, M., & Boehm, A. (2008). *Preschool assessment: Principles and practices.* Guilford Press.

Bruner, J. (1990). *Acts of meaning.* Harvard University Press.

Clark, F. A., Parham, D., Carlson, M. E., Frank, G., Jackson, J., Pierce, D., Wolfe, R. J., & Zemke, R. (1991). Occupational science: Academic innovation in the service of occupational therapy's future. *American Journal of Occupational Therapy, 45,* 300–310. https://doi.org/10.5014/ajot.45.4.300

Coster, W. (1998). Occupation-centered assessment of children. *American Journal of Occupational Therapy, 52,* 337–344. https://doi.org/10.5014/ajot.52.5.337

Creighton, C. (1992). The origin and evolution of activity analysis. *American Journal of Occupational Therapy, 46,* 45–48. https://doi.org/10.5014/ajot.46.1.45

Crepeau, E. B. (1991). Achieving intersubjective understanding: Examples from an occupational therapy treatment session. *American Journal of Occupational Therapy, 45,* 1016–1025. https://doi.org/10.5014/ajot.45.11.1016

Crepeau, E. B., & Garren, K. R. (2011). I looked to her as a guide: The therapeutic relationship in hand therapy. *Disability and Rehabilitation, 33,* 872–881. https://doi.org/10.3109/09638288.2010.511419

Cynkin, S. (1995). Activities. In C. B. Royeen (Ed.), *AOTA self-study series: The practice of the future: Putting occupation back into therapy* (Module 7; pp. 1–52). American Occupational Therapy Association.

Davidson, L. (2003). *Living outside mental illness: Qualitative studies of recovery in schizophrenia.* New York University Press.

Fisher, A. G., & Jones, K. B. (2014). *Assessment of motor and process skills: User manual* (8th ed.). Three Star Press.

Frankl, V. E. (1959). *Man's search for meaning: An introduction to logotherapy.* Pocket Books.

Hagedorn, R. (2000). Glossary. In R. Hagedorn (Ed.), *Tools for practice in occupational therapy: A structured approach to core skills and processes* (pp. 307–312). Churchill Livingstone.

Hasselkus, B. R. (2002). *The meaning of everyday occupation.* SLACK.

Hersch, G., Lamport, N., & Coffey, M. (2005). *Activity analysis: Application to occupation.* SLACK.

Hocking, C. (2001). Implementing occupation-based assessment. *American Journal of Occupational Therapy, 55,* 463–469. https://doi.org/10.5014/ajot.55.4.463

Jackson, J. (1998a). Contemporary criticisms of role theory. *Journal of Occupational Science, 5,* 49–55. https://doi.org/10.1080/14427591.1998.9686433

Jackson, J. (1998b). Is there a place for role theory in occupational science? *Journal of Occupational Science, 5,* 56–65. https://doi.org/10.1080/14427591.1998.9686434

Kielhofner, G., & Barrett, L. (1998). Meaning and misunderstanding in occupational forms: A study of therapeutic goal setting. *American Journal of Occupational Therapy, 52,* 345–353. https://doi.org/10.5014/ajot.52.5.345

Larson, E. A. (2000). The orchestration of occupation: The dance of mothers. *American Journal of Occupational Therapy, 54,* 269–280. https://doi.org/10.5014/ajot.54.3.269

Lave, J. (1988). *Cognition in practice: Mind, mathematics and culture in everyday life.* Cambridge University Press.

Law, M. (Ed.). (1998). *Client-centered occupational therapy.* SLACK.

Mattingly, C., & Fleming, M. H. (1994). *Clinical reasoning: Forms of inquiry in a therapeutic practice.* F. A. Davis.

Neistadt, M. E., McAuley, D., Zecha, D., & Shannon, R. (1993). An analysis of a board game as a treatment activity. *American Journal of Occupational Therapy, 47,* 154–160. https://doi.org/10.5014/ajot.47.2.154.

Parten, M. (1932). Social participation among preschool children. *Journal of Abnormal and Social Psychology, 27,* 243–269. https://doi.org/10.1037/h0074524

Payne, R. K., DeVol, P., & Dreussi Smith, T. (2001). *Bridges out of poverty: Strategies for professionals and communities* (Rev. ed.). aha! Process.

Peloquin, S. M. (1995). The fullness of empathy: Reflections and illustrations. *American Journal of Occupational Therapy, 49,* 24–31. https://doi.org/10.5014/ajot.49.1.24

Peloquin, S. M. (2005). Embracing our ethos, reclaiming our heart. *American Journal of Occupational Therapy, 59,* 611–625. https://doi.org/10.5014/ajot.59.6.611

Peloquin, S. M. (2007). A reconsideration of occupational therapy's core values. *American Journal of Occupational Therapy, 61,* 474–478. https://doi.org/10.5014/ajot.61.4.474

Pierce, D. (2000). Maternal management of the home as an infant/toddler developmental space. *American Journal of Occupational Therapy, 54,* 290–299. https://doi.org/10.5014/ajot.54.3.290

Pierce, D. (2001). Untangling occupation and activity. *American Journal of Occupational Therapy, 55,* 138–146. https://doi.org/10.5014/ajot.55.2.138

Pierce, D. (2005). The usefulness of video methods for occupational therapy and occupational science research. *American Journal of Occupational Therapy, 59,* 9–19. https://doi.org/10.5014/ajot.59.1.9

Pierce, D. (2009). Co-occupation: The challenges of defining concepts original to occupational science. *Journal of Occupational Science, 16*(3), 273–287. https://doi.org/10.1080/14427591.2009.9686663

Pierce, D. (2014). *Occupational science for occupational therapy.* SLACK.

Pierce, D., Myers, C., & Munier, V. (2009). Informing early intervention through an occupational science description of infant-toddler interactions with home space. *American Journal of Occupational Therapy, 63,* 273–287. https://doi.org/10.5014/ajot.63.3.273

Polatajko, H. J., Mandich, A., & Martini, R. (2000). Dynamic performance analysis: A framework for understanding occupational performance. *American Journal of Occupational Therapy, 54,* 65–72. https://doi.org/10.5014/ajot.54.1.65

Quiroga, V. A. (1995). *Occupational therapy: The first 30 years 1900–1930.* American Occupational Therapy Association.

Russell, B. (1989). My mental development. In P. A. Schilpp (Ed.), *The philosophy of Bertrand Russell* (pp. 1–20). Open Court.

Schell, B. A. (2018). Pragmatic reasoning. In B. A. B. Schell & J. W. Schell (Eds.), *Clinical and professional reasoning in occupational therapy* (pp. 203–224). Wolters Kluwer.

Schell, B. A., & Cervero, R. M. (1993). Clinical reasoning in occupational therapy: An integrative review. *American Journal of Occupational Therapy, 47,* 605–610. https://doi.org/10.5014/ajot.47.7.605

Thomas, H. (2015). *Occupational and activity analysis* (3rd ed.). SLACK.

Trombly, C. A. (1995). Occupation: Purposefulness and meaningfulness as therapeutic mechanisms. 1995 Eleanor Clarke Slagle Lecture. *American Journal of Occupational Therapy, 49,* 960–972. https://doi.org/10.5014/ajot.49.10.960

Trombly Latham, C. A. (2014). Conceptual foundations for practice. In M. V. Radomski & C. A. Trombly Latham (Eds.), *Occupational therapy for physical dysfunction* (7th ed., pp. 1–20). Lippincott Williams & Wilkins.

Zemke, R., & Clark, F. (1996). *Occupational science: The evolving discipline.* F. A. Davis.

CHAPTER 44

Activities of Daily Living and Instrumental Activities of Daily Living

Jennifer S. Pitonyak and Kirsten L. Wilbur

LEARNING OBJECTIVES

After reading this chapter, you will be able to:

1. Describe the purposes of an occupational therapy evaluation of activities of daily living (ADLs) and instrumental activities of daily living (IADLs).
2. Recognize that ADL and IADL are defined by diverse sociocultural influences and in relation to varied client outcomes beyond independence.
3. Given a case, identify client and contextual factors that may influence the evaluation plan.
4. Develop client-centered goals that will guide the intervention process.
5. Explain the most common approaches to ADL and IADL intervention.
6. Describe the role of client and caregiver education in intervention for ADL and IADL.
7. Grade intervention activities to progress clients toward increased participation in ADL and IADL.

Introduction

This chapter focuses on the occupational therapy (OT) process for occupations that are classified as activities of daily living (ADL) and instrumental activities of daily living (IADL) in the *Occupational Therapy Practice Framework: Domain and Process*, 4th edition (OTPF) (American Occupational Therapy Association [AOTA], 2020). Dysfunctions in ADL and IADL are termed *activity limitations* in the *International Classification of Functioning, Disability, and Health* (ICF) framework (World Health Organization, 2002). Evaluation of and intervention for barriers to ADL and IADL are central to individuals' participation in meaningful occupation. Individuals may value ADL and IADL as meaningful in and of themselves and as prerequisite tasks to engagement in education, work, play, leisure, social participation, and other forms of occupation.

Definition of Activities of Daily Living and Instrumental Activities of Daily Living

Conceptually, the term activities of daily living could apply to all activities that individuals perform routinely. In the OTPF, however, ADL are defined more narrowly as "activities oriented toward taking care of one's own body" (AOTA, 2020, p. 30), which include eight activity categories: bathing/showering, toileting and toilet hygiene, dressing, eating and swallowing, feeding, functional mobility, personal hygiene and grooming, and sexual activity. **Instrumental activities of daily living** are defined as "activities that support daily life within the home and community" (AOTA, 2020, p. 30). IADL include 11 activity categories: care of others, care of pets and animals, child-rearing, communication management, driving and community mobility, financial management, home establishment and management, meal preparation and cleanup, religious and spiritual expression, safety and emergency maintenance, and shopping.

Although the OTPF's (AOTA, 2020) definitions of ADL and IADL are consistent with those of the National Center for Health Statistics (2009), other healthcare practitioners or OT practitioners outside the United States might use other terms to refer to these same ADL and IADL concepts or use the same terms but define them differently. For example, some define ADL more broadly, referring to activities performed in daily life (e.g., Archenholtz & Dellhag, 2008). Other terms that are used to refer specifically to functional mobility and personal care are *basic ADL* and *personal ADL* (AOTA, 2020). The term *instrumental activities of daily living* appears outside the OT literature in a less consistent way (Chuang et al., 2020). Related to defining ADL and IADL, international OT scholars have pointed out that categorizations of occupation, such as in the OTPF, are based on Western, white theories about occupation that tend to emphasize individualism rather than collectivism in occupation. For example, Whalley Hammell (2009, 2014) urges the field of OT to rethink traditional categories of occupation that may be simplistic, value laden, decontextualized, and lack subjectivity, and to move toward a conceptualization of occupation as restorative, facilitating belonging and connectedness, providing purpose through doing, and fostering hope for the future.

Conceptualizations of IADL vary considerably (Pashmdarfard & Azad, 2020). For example, the Nottingham Extended ADL Scale includes leisure activities, tasks that fall outside the OTPF definition of IADL (das Nair et al., 2011). Further, the authors of a recent systematic review (Pashmdarfard & Azad, 2020) located five articles appraising assessments of IADL. In translating their findings to practice in their home country of Iran, they noted that while most of the available assessment measures are performance-based, none of the measures were originally developed within the cultural context of Iran (Pashmdarfard & Azad, 2020). As such, it is crucial to understand that daily activities are defined in variable ways, and that more widely used definitions and measures of ADL and IADL will not be culturally relevant for all clients.

However, this chapter does focus on the evaluation and intervention of occupational performance specifically related to ADL and IADL as defined by the OTPF. It is essential to have a fundamental understanding of the OT process before reading this chapter; the process is described in Chapter 18. The reader should be aware that ADL and IADL, although often a primary focus of OT practice, do not typically represent the full complement of occupational performance tasks needed for satisfying and meaningful participation in individual and societal roles. Evaluation and intervention should always begin with a comprehensive occupational profile (AOTA, 2020). Intervention should address all of the client's priorities, which will typically extend beyond ADL and IADL, although the rest of this chapter focuses exclusively on ADL and IADL.

Evaluation of ADL and IADL

Evaluation refers to the overall process of gathering and interpreting data needed to plan intervention, including developing an evaluation plan, implementing the data collection, interpreting the data, and documenting the evaluation results (AOTA, 2015). Assessment refers to the specific method or tools that are used to collect data, which is one component of the evaluation process (AOTA, 2015). Standardized assessment methods are referred to as *assessment tools* or *instruments*. The evaluation is carried out by an occupational therapist. An OT assistant may participate in administering selected assessments under the supervision of an occupational therapist who is responsible for interpreting assessment data for use in intervention planning. In addition to standardized assessment methods, it is critical that the occupational therapist also use methods such as interview and observation in order to best capture subjectivity in the purpose and meaning of ADL and IADL occupations for each client (Pitonyak et al., 2021; Whalley Hammell, 2009, 2014).

The ADL/IADL evaluation is discussed in two stages in this chapter: (1) planning the evaluation, which includes selecting specific assessment methods; and (2) implementing the evaluation, which includes gathering assessment data, making critical observations, generating hypotheses, and performing ongoing revision of the evaluation plan until adequate data have been collected. Keep in mind that ADL and IADL evaluation is only one part of a more comprehensive OT evaluation.

Planning the Evaluation: Selecting the Appropriate ADL and IADL Assessment Methods

Occupational therapists can choose from various ADL and IADL assessment methods designed to meet the varied needs of clients and intervention settings. Selecting an appropriate assessment method will facilitate optimal intervention planning and can be initiated by following these steps:

1. Identify the overall purpose(s) of the evaluation.
2. Have clients identify their needs, interests, and perceived difficulties with ADL and/or IADL as part of the occupational profile.
3. Further explore the purpose and meaning of ADL/IADL engagement for the client as it fits with their personal and cultural contexts.
4. Estimate client factors that affect occupational performance and/or the evaluation process.
5. Identify how context may affect ADL/IADL evaluation.
6. Consider aspects of assessment methods, particularly features of assessment tools.
7. Integrate the information from steps 1 to 6 to select optimal ADL and IADL assessment methods.

Although these steps appear to follow a linear progression, in practice, the steps become integrated because the occupational therapist continually blends knowledge and experience with information from and about the client.

Step 1: Identify the Purpose of the ADL/IADL Evaluation

ADL and IADL may be evaluated for different purposes. At the level of individual client care, evaluation may be done to assess occupational performance problems to plan OT intervention or to facilitate decision-making concerning discharge environment, competency, conservatorship, and/or involuntary commitment. The occupational therapist must determine how the information will be used so that appropriate and sufficient data are obtained.

Evaluation to Plan and Monitor OT Interventions. When an evaluation is conducted to plan OT intervention, certain types of data are needed to establish a client's baseline performance (Dunn, 2017). First, barriers and supports to occupational performance need to be identified so that the intervention plan can focus on enabling participation and performance. Second, data are needed

about underlying impairment in client factors and performance skills. For example, the inability to perform cooking might be caused by low vision, poor endurance, or decreased motivation to cook. OT intervention to increase engagement in cooking is different for each of these causes. In order to create an intervention plan that both enables participation and performance of ADL or IADL and establishes and restores functional skills necessary for ADL or IADL, data about occupational performance need to be integrated with data about the client's performance patterns and skills, client factors, activity demands, and contexts (Dunn, 2017). Third, the OT evaluation should provide practitioners with possibilities for modifying the client's activity performance. Information about the activity demands and context should include consideration of which aspects might be modifiable to support performance and which features cannot be changed. The potential to change performance patterns and skills or client factors must also be assessed. Interventions that involve skill acquisition are feasible for some clients, depending on the cause of the problem. For example, a child with impaired balance secondary to cerebral palsy may have the potential to increase balance to support participation across several ADL and IADL, whereas a person with similar deficits from Parkinson disease might not because the disorder is progressive. All three types of data (performance impairments, underlying causes, and potential for change) are needed to devise adequate intervention plans.

Evaluation to Facilitate Decision-Making About Eligibility or Discharge Environment. Clients may also be referred for evaluation of ADL and IADL to facilitate decision-making about eligibility for OT services or discharge environment. The ability to care for oneself and one's home can make the difference between independent and supported or assisted living. Supported living represents a continuum of options that includes in-home services (e.g., chore services), assisted living centers, group homes, supervised apartments, long-term care facilities, and more. Varied levels of support are offered within these settings to maintain or enhance daily living skills. When ADL and IADL are evaluated to inform eligibility or discharge decisions, the evaluation may be less comprehensive than those for planning individual interventions. For example, in response to the passage of the Improving Medicare Post-Acute Care Transformation (IMAPCT) Act of 2014 (Pub. L. 113-185), OT researchers have advocated the inclusion of functional cognition screening as a component of discharge evaluation (Giles et al., 2017). Traditional cognitive screening tools may not identify impairments in functional cognition (executive functions) that are often associated with ADL and IADL performance problems (Giles et al., 2017). Rather, performance-based testing such as the Menu Task (MT) may better predict performance in post-discharge settings (Edwards et al., 2019).

A somewhat similar evaluation objective occurs when OT practitioners are asked to make recommendations regarding legal competence for independent living. This usually involves competence in caring for oneself or managing one's property. Guardianship is a legal association in which a protected individual's personal affairs are managed by one or more people or an agency. Conservatorship is a legal relationship, like guardianship, but is limited to managing the protected individual's financial affairs and property (Moye, 2005). Evaluation may also be requested in conjunction with involuntary commitments to psychiatric facilities to appraise the influence of psychiatric status on daily living. When competence is used in the legal sense, the capacity to make judicious or responsible decisions usually takes precedence over the capacity to perform activities. Individuals who have the ability to procure services and supervise caregivers in managing their personal care and living situation are viewed as competent, even though they might not be able to perform these activities themselves. Thus, OT evaluations that are conducted with guardianship, conservatorship, or involuntary commitment in mind must take into account the decisional capacities and supervisory skills needed by clients.

Step 2: Have Clients Identify Their Needs, Interests, and Perceived Difficulties With ADL/IADL

Once the purpose of the ADL/IADL evaluation has been determined, the occupational therapist must identify the specific activities to be evaluated. This is *one* component of the occupational profile, which will also encompass other aspects of occupational performance, including education, play, leisure, work, and social participation (AOTA, 2020). Developing the client's occupational profile is a crucial step in a client-centered evaluation as it identifies the ADL and IADL problems of concern to the *client* (AOTA, 2020; Law & Baum, 2017) and the meaning of these occupations in their daily life (Whalley Hammell, 2009). Meaning for an individual client will vary in relationship to diverse identity attributes as well as contextual influences (Pitonyak et al., 2021; Whalley Hammell, 2009). It is easy to make assumptions about a client's priorities based on both clinical and personal experience and values; however, it is important to remember that unique circumstances may affect clients' ADL or IADL priorities for intervention. Clients' perception of their ADL and IADL problems, needs, and goals can be gathered through a semistructured interview process or through a more formal assessment, such as the Canadian Occupational Performance Measure (COPM) (Law et al., 2014), Occupational Performance History Interview II (Kielhofner et al., 2004), or Perceived Efficacy and Goal Setting System (Vroland-Nordstrand et al., 2015).

Step 3: Further Explore the Purpose and Meaning of ADL/IADL Engagement for the Client

The purpose and meaning of ADL and IADL occupation varies for individuals, groups, and populations. Accepted categorizations of occupation are not always inclusive of the diverse ways in which individuals engage in what is defined as ADL/IADL occupation (Whalley Hammell, 2009). For example, negotiating social services (affordable housing, accessible transportation, etc.) is a part of the daily routine for some persons with disabilities that is not encompassed in usual definitions of ADL and IADL activities (Magasi, 2012). In order to understand the process of negotiating social services and what activities this entails, the practitioner may need to engage in interprofessional collaboration with a case manager, social worker, or others who support clients in this process. Therefore, before ADL/IADL occupations are evaluated, the OT practitioner needs to collaborate with the client to identify the form, function, and meaning of ADL/IADL occupations. For example, meal preparation for a middle school student might consist of making cereal for breakfast and packing a lunch, whereas meal preparation for a homemaker feeding a family of five involves many food preparation tasks and a very different set of skills. Assessment tools may define activities differently, so it is important to select an instrument that is congruent with activities as defined by the client. For example, in assessing feeding, clients are rated "independent" on the Barthel Index if they can feed themselves, which includes cutting up food and spreading butter on bread (Mahoney & Barthel, 1965). Clients are rated as "needing assistance" if they can get food from the plate to the mouth but need help cutting food into bite-sized pieces. The Katz Index of ADL, however, does not include preparation of food on the plate (e.g., cutting and spreading butter on bread) in the operational definition of feeding, so clients are rated independent if they can get food from the plate to the mouth, even if they cannot cut food or butter bread (Katz et al., 1963). Many adolescents and adults would be dissatisfied with their feeding performance if their food had to be cut by another person, so the Katz Index of ADL would not be an appropriate measure for these individuals.

OT practitioners also need to consider relevant performance parameters when planning an evaluation. Performance parameters include independence, safety, and adequacy. Operational definitions of acceptable ADL and IADL performance should include attention to all relevant parameters in order to establish appropriate baseline data and intervention outcomes.

Level of Independence. Although clients often wish to be independent in ADL and IADL, practitioners should not make this assumption because some level of assistance, either verbal or physical, might be acceptable. For example, many clients who undergo total hip replacements must follow movement precautions for 2 months that make it challenging to don shoes and socks independently without adaptive equipment. A person who lives with others might prefer to have temporary assistance rather than purchasing and using adaptive equipment. As long as they have someone who is willing and able to assist, a goal for assisted lower extremity dressing is perfectly appropriate, and intervention may focus on making sure that the client and caregiver can complete the task together while adhering to total hip precautions. Independence is the performance parameter that is the focus of most assessment tools, so occupational therapists can select from various assessment tools that measure independence.

Safety. Many assessment tools address safety indirectly by specifying that performance be completed in a safe manner in order to be rated as independent (e.g., the Kettle Test; Hartman-Maeir et al., 2009). Some tools do not address safety directly (e.g., the Katz Index of ADL; Katz et al., 1963), and a few rate safety separately from independence (e.g., the Performance Assessment of Self-Care Skills; Chisholm et al., 2014). When safety is a particular concern (e.g., with clients who have cognitive deficits that impair judgment), a separate measure of safety can be more effective for documenting progress toward goals and making it clear in the OT documentation that safety has been addressed.

Adequacy. Clients may have criteria regarding the efficiency of task performance and the acceptability of the outcome of the performance, and these should be considered in selecting assessment tools. For example, a client might be safe and independent in lower body dressing but deem their performance inefficient because it takes them an hour to complete the task and they end up too exhausted to work.

Or a client might be independent and safe in feeding themself but find their performance outcome unacceptable because they drop food onto their clothing at each meal and do not wish to wear a bib, especially when eating with others. An assessment tool that measures only independence and safety makes it hard to justify intervention in either of these examples because both clients were safe and independent. There are, however, occupational performance needs that warrant intervention; that is, decreasing the time needed to complete lower body dressing or eliminating food spilled on clothing during eating. Adequacy parameters to consider in ADL and IADL performance include perceived difficulty, pain, fatigue, dyspnea (shortness of breath), societal standards, satisfaction, aberrant behaviors, and past experience with the activity. Practitioners must keep in mind that independence might not be the only important performance parameter to assess in the OT evaluation. See Expanding Our Perspectives.

Step 4: Estimate the Client Factors That Affect ADL/IADL and the Evaluation Process

One purpose of the ADL/IADL evaluation is to identify supports and hindrances to occupational performance. However, some estimate of underlying impairment prior to the evaluation can help the occupational therapist to select the assessment methods that will be most effective in identifying and documenting occupational performance problems and any underlying impairments. Occupational therapists use their knowledge of pathology and how it affects occupational performance when selecting assessment tools. For example, some instruments rely on self-report, which is a very efficient way to gather information about a wide range of activities. However, self-reported measures could be inaccurate if the client has cognitive deficits (e.g., a person

---

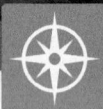

EXPANDING **OUR PERSPECTIVES**

Dining Etiquette in Bangladeshi Culture

Mary Devadas

Arif was referred to OT after his parents noticed he was not meeting the same milestones as his cousins. His parents described him as being "slower" than his cousins and noted that he uses his left hand during mealtime. Arif's OT evaluation showed that he demonstrated poor utensil use and at times switched hands. Overall, he demonstrates a left-hand preference; however, his parents discourage him from using his left hand, saying the left hand is "unclean," specifically for eating. The evaluation also highlighted that Arif could not drink from a

straw, stab food with a fork, or scoop food with a spoon without significant spillage.

Dining etiquette in Bangladeshi culture does not require the use of utensils. Instead, paratha (a flatbread) is used to scoop up the food, and children are encouraged to drink from an open cup instead of a straw or sippy cup. According to cultural norms of the Global North, Arif has delays in self-feeding skills; however, in Bangladeshi cultural norms, his left-hand preference is the area of concern. OT is rooted in culture and norms of the Global North, and consequently many of the assessment tools may be inappropriate for other cultures. Therefore, occupational therapists, wherever they practice, need to consider culture as a part of the therapeutic process.

with Alzheimer disease), distorted thought functions (e.g., a person with schizophrenia), or little experience with the disorder (e.g., a teenager who sustained a spinal cord injury with tetraplegia just 5 days earlier). Additionally, insight into clients' underlying problems will be enhanced by actually seeing the client attempt to perform tasks rather than relying on a description of the problem. For example, a client who has had a stroke might report that they are unable to reach items stored above chest height with their affected hand, but the OT practitioner gains valuable information for intervention planning by observing the client reaching into cabinets and using skilled observation to see if the movement problem is caused by limitations in movement of the scapula, glenohumeral joint, or elbow or some combination of the three.

Knowledge of underlying pathology and anticipated impairments also enables occupational therapists to select appropriate assessment tools that are designed for specific diagnostic groups, focusing on activities that are more commonly problematic for that population. For example, the Arthritis Impact Measurement Scale was developed for adults with rheumatic diseases and includes not only measures of ADL and IADL performance but also symptoms that are commonly experienced by people with arthritis during or following activities, such as pain and fatigue (Meenan et al., 1992).

Step 5: Identify How Context May Affect ADL/IADL Evaluation

In this step, the occupational therapist considers context and its impact on the evaluation of ADL and IADL. This may include environmental factors and personal factors, and their influence on client performance. Environmental factors include physical, social, and attitudinal components, and personal factors are the unique features of the client that are not a part of their health condition (AOTA, 2020). Contextual influences on occupational performance are complex and numerous, such as policy and systems components, and go beyond the focus of this chapter. However, practitioners must consider how context may affect ADL and IADL evaluation.

Environmental Factors. Practitioners may observe clients performing occupational tasks under natural or clinical conditions. Timing, lighting, the presence of technology, and the human-made design of the environment are examples of components that may impact ADL/IADL evaluation. Natural conditions, which can often be met in long-term care settings and home-based care, provide the most accurate assessment of clients' performance (Rogers et al., 2003). Although the therapy setting will dictate where an assessment takes place, the influence of the environment on activity performance should be considered so that valid conclusions about performance can be drawn (Bottari

et al., 2006). OT clinics are designed to promote function with adaptive features, which may make it easier for clients to perform activities in the clinic than in their own homes (Holm & Rogers, 2017). Conversely, performance might be more difficult for some tasks because clients are unfamiliar with the clinic setting. For example, Provencher et al. (2012) examined the impact of familiar and unfamiliar settings on cooking task assessment in frail older adults and found that the home setting may produce more accurate assessment results, particularly when the client has executive functioning problems. Similarly, Provencher et al. (2013) found that older adults' process skills during IADL were typically higher in their homes than in clinic settings. In contrast, driving is an IADL with a critical safety component, and although on-road assessments are considered to be the most accurate, driving simulators offer a safe alternative for gathering data to determine whether or not the client is appropriate to assess on city streets (Bédard et al., 2010).

The OT evaluation also occurs in a social context. Practitioners must oversee activity performance during assessment, and their very presence can affect the manner and adequacy of the activities performed. The practitioner's presence especially affects the client's ability to initiate participation in ADL or IADL because the structure of the assessment process itself prompts clients to engage in the tasks. If initiation of task performance is impaired, the practitioner must supplement performance measures from a structured therapy session. For example, the Independent Living Scale includes a subscale for initiation (Ashley et al., 2001). Alternatively, family members might be asked, for example, to keep track of the number of days the client completed pet care responsibilities without being asked. Clients' occupational performance might be impacted by the differences in social context between clinic and natural environments. For example, a client with a spinal cord injury who must be skilled in directing a personal care attendant during ADL might give directions effectively to a rehabilitation aide who is familiar with caring for people with similar needs but might not give detailed enough instructions for an employee in the home who has less experience. Conversely, a client who requires a setup to feed themselves will be more independent at home than in the clinic if they live in a family where meals are routinely set up for the entire family by a caregiver who does all the cooking.

Personal Factors. Clients will come with varied experience with ADL and IADL based on personal context. Typically, ADL practice begins in childhood, and the societal expectation is that adolescents and adults have a wide range of experience with these activities and can perform them adequately. However, a similar expectation does not hold for IADL, where people have more options. Clients may not have developed proficiency in all IADL activities. Some might have no experience in planning and preparing meals, doing the laundry, or managing finances. Children with developmental disabilities often experience delays in the acquisition of ADL and IADL skills and might lack experience that a typically developing child would have at a given age. Clients' activity performance history is essential for understanding their current performance level. An activity limitation is interpreted differently for a client who has had no or little prior experience performing the activity than for one who had been doing it effectively prior to OT intervention.

Step 6: Consider Features of Assessment Tools

The occupational therapist must be familiar with available assessments and consider what tasks are included in the assessment, how tasks are defined, the psychometric properties, the type of data to be collected, and the method of data collection.

Tasks Assessed. Tasks that are included in an ADL or IADL assessment should be consistent with clients' priorities, and the operational definition of effective performance should fit clients' needs and address all parameters of importance. For example, many assessment instruments measure independence, but if clients would also like to complete tasks independently without experiencing shortness of breath or pain, occupational therapists might want to use a dyspnea or pain scale in conjunction with the independence measure.

Types of Assessments and Data. Some assessments are not standardized; that is, the individual therapist designs the assessment and decides the type of information to gather. Results of nonstandardized assessments are often reported using qualitative data; that is, the salient characteristics of clients' activity performance are observed or obtained through client or caregiver narratives. Clients' status is documented by simply describing their performance. Nonstandardized assessments lack testing of psychometric properties, such as reliability, validity, or sensitivity to change in a client's status (Dunn, 2017); however, they are useful for capturing each client's unique ways of performing ADL/IADL. Standardized assessments use a uniform approach that makes the assessment more reliable when it is used for reassessment or by multiple therapists. For example, the term *moderate assistance* could be interpreted in several ways, but if it is operationally defined as "the patient requires more help than touching, or expends between 50% and 74% of the effort" (UB Foundation Activities, 2002, p. III-7), agreement among therapists using the instrument is likely to be higher. There is variability in the extent to which the psychometric properties of standardized assessments have been established. Some assessments have been extensively studied and include a wide range of

psychometric statistics to support the reliability and validity of the tool. When possible, it is best to use an assessment with established psychometric properties (Dunn, 2017). Standardized measures that reduce observed behavior to a number also make it efficient for reporting data in documentation. However, loss of qualitative data can make it difficult for the reader to get a clear understanding of the client's limitations. Standardized assessments are at risk of bias, particularly when a normative group differs from the client's demographics and identities. Often, documentation includes quantitative assessment data accompanied by some qualitative data to provide a more comprehensive picture of client performance. A brief case, presented in Table 44.1, compares qualitative and quantitative data from two children. See Chapter 20 for more information on types of assessments.

It is possible to rely entirely on qualitative data to document a client's baseline status, which is needed to determine whether or not progress is made in OT; however, this can be difficult and time-consuming. For example, if Aiden's and Brody's occupational therapists had to document the status of *all* ADL and IADL as presented in Table 44.1, the evaluation report would take a great deal of time to write and to read. Additionally, the OT practitioner who is documenting qualitative data should be very careful to distinguish between *observations* and *clinical judgments* (subjective interpretations about the observations). The statements listed in Table 44.1 are observations. A statement of clinical judgment is interpretive, and several plausible interpretations could be made from the more objective observations. For example, the OT practitioner could conclude that Brody has weak trunk muscles that interfere with balance. This conclusion should be presented as a hypothesis, not as an observation, because Brody's inability to maintain balance while dressing could be the result of other factors, such as impaired vestibular and proprioceptive input that interferes with his ability to detect when he is starting to fall to one side.

A quantitative assessment measure is a more efficient way to document progress, although it might not provide the reader with complete information. For example, although Aiden and Brody have the same quantitative score on the WeeFIM™, the qualitative information enables readers to see that there are very different underlying problems. Occupational therapists can document key qualitative data to support their evaluation and intervention plan, but most observations are simply used by therapists for planning intervention, whereas quantitative data are recorded in documentation (Gateley & Borcherding, 2017).

Data about ADL and IADL performance can be gathered by report or through direct observation. Reported data about the client's abilities and limitations in performance can be gathered from the client, the caregiver, and/or another health professional. The OT practitioner poses questions about ADL and IADL performance in oral or written

TABLE 44.1	Comparison of Descriptive and Quantitative Data from a Dressing Assessment of Two Children

Aiden	Brody
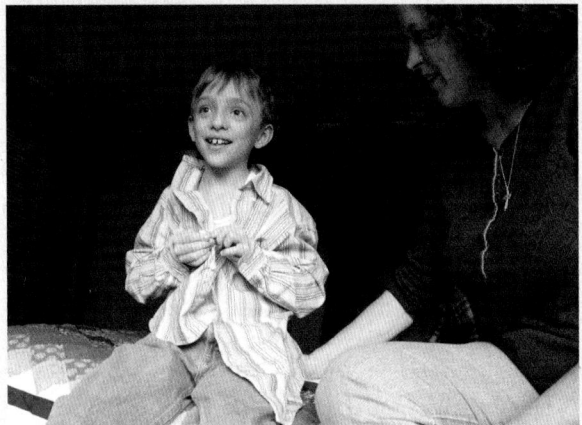	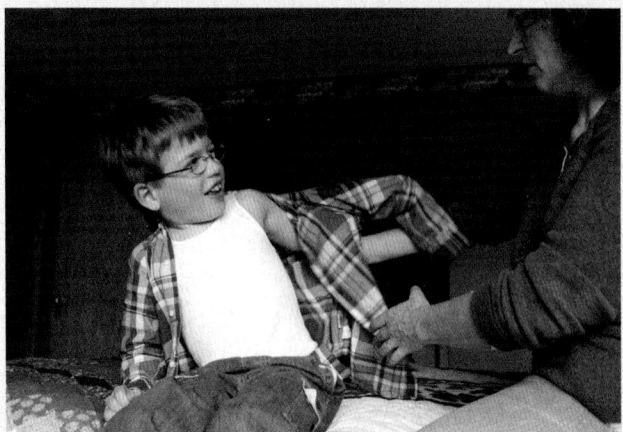

Client Description

Aiden is a 7-year-old child who sustained a traumatic brain injury. Before his injury, he was able to dress himself independently.	Brody is a 7-year-old child with cerebral palsy affecting the right side of his body. His parents have been helping him dress prior to this assessment.

Descriptive Data from Observing Dressing

• Well-coordinated and smooth movements of both upper extremities (UEs) when manipulating clothing • Maintenance of appropriate posture, sitting unsupported on the bed • Reached all areas of his body (behind, overhead, feet) without loss of balance • Frequently stopped midtask to verbalize thoughts, which were disjointed and difficult to follow • Made repeated (total of five) attempts to get his left arm in a sleeve turned inside out; did not attempt to self-correct or respond to verbal directions to turn the sleeve right side out. The practitioner turned the sleeve right side out after giving three verbal cues and gesturing toward the sleeve. • Aiden left the dressing task to look out of the window when he heard a plane and continued to talk about the plane when asked to return to the dressing task. • Aiden returned to the task when the practitioner physically guided him to the bed and placed one of his arms in the sleeve. He then completed putting the shirt on his other arm on his own. • When asked to button his shirt, he completed two of six buttons, which were misaligned. When asked how well his shirt was buttoned, he looked down at himself and said, "It's perfect" and then skipped out of the room saying that he wanted to watch TV.	• Started to put left (stronger) UE in his shirtsleeve first; responded immediately to verbal cue to dress the right side of the body first • Wavering of trunk when using both UEs to position the shirt. Practitioner steadied Brody's trunk to prevent him from falling forward when he pulled the shirt across his back. He could not get the shirt far enough around to reach the sleeve. The practitioner moved the shirt so he could reach it with the left arm. • Left UE movements were smooth and well coordinated. • Right UE movement was minimal, and he could not use his hand for fine tasks, such as buttoning. Several attempts were required to complete the bottom three buttons with the left hand, and the practitioner had to complete the top three. • Putting on his shirt took 15 minutes. Brody reported he felt "pretty tired" at the end. He was focused during the task, even when his little brother ran into and out of the room. • Brody followed instructions consistently and made five attempts to help solve problems encountered along the way, for example, suggesting he wear pullover shirts that do not have buttons. • When asked which arm he will dress first when he tries the task tomorrow, Brody responded, "My right arm."

Quantitative Data Based on the WeeFIM™

Upper Body Dressing = 4	Upper Body Dressing = 4

format, using interviews or questionnaires, respectively. Although the questioning is frequently done face to face, either format can be done without physical interaction. Interviews may be conducted over the telephone. Questionnaires may be completed while the client is waiting for an appointment or can be mailed out in advance of a session. Gathering data via report can be done informally; that is, the practitioner develops the questions to be asked or through

the use of a standardized protocol such as the COPM (Law et al., 2014), the Occupational Self-Assessment (Baron et al., 2006), or the Child Occupational Self Assessment (Keller et al., 2005). Although self-report is an efficient way to measure ADL and IADL, it is not always consistent with actual performance (Brown & Finlayson, 2013; Goverover et al., 2009; Rogers et al., 2003), and the occupational therapist should select performance-based assessments when the client's accuracy is in question. Additionally, gathering data about selected ADL or IADL through both self-report and performance-based measures can provide the occupational therapist with valuable insight into the accuracy of the client's self-awareness regarding supports and hindrances to their occupational performance.

In some situations, clients might be unable to respond on their own, so caregivers or other proxies can be queried on behalf of clients. The usefulness of information from caregivers or proxies depends on their familiarity with the client's ADL and IADL. For example, if the proxy has not observed a client bathing recently, the information might be based more on opinion than on concrete knowledge of bathing performance. In addition, there are known biases in the reporting tendencies of caregivers and proxies (Cohen-Mansfield & Jensen, 2007). Caregivers and proxies can readily observe evaluation parameters such as independence, safety, and aberrant activity behaviors. Some evaluation parameters, however, are subjective, so clients are the only appropriate respondents (e.g., values, satisfaction with performance, and activity-related pain; Garratt & Pond, 2014).

Assessment data can also be gathered through direct observation of ADL and IADL, which gives the

practitioner more information about how the client performs a task. Observation of performance, however, requires more time and material resources and is therefore more costly. Direct observation of performance can also be done in a nonstandardized way or through use of a standardized assessment. The constraints of practice settings, often imposed by third-party payers or limited funding, can place restrictions on the time an occupational therapist has available for evaluation. Occupational therapists must be strategic in selecting ADL and IADL assessments that will provide information relevant to the client and can be generalized to other tasks so that the practitioner does not have to observe all meaningful ADL and IADL that may be addressed in OT. For example, if a client requires assistance with cooking because of an inability to transport food and cooking equipment safely while using a walker, the occupational therapist can reasonably project, without having to observe performance, that the same client will require assistance in doing laundry because laundry also requires the transportation of task objects.

Selected standardized ADL and IADL assessments are listed in Table 44.2. The assessments that are included in Table 44.2 are readily available and are either commonly

TABLE 44.2 **Summary of Selected Activities of Daily Living (ADL) and Instrumental Activities of Daily Living (IADL) Instruments**

Title	Areas Addressed	Population	Method	Learning to Use the Assessment
ADL-focused Occupation-based Neurobehavioral Evaluation (A-ONE)	Feeding, dressing, grooming and hygiene, transfers and mobility, and communication	16 years and older with central nervous system dysfunction	Observation of ADL	Training required to rate reliably (Árnadóttir, 1990, 2011)
Assessment of Motor and Process Skills (AMPS)	125 calibrated ADL and IADL activities; client and therapist select two or three for assessment	Children (age >2 years) and adults	Identify two to three ADL or IADL tasks for observation.	Training required. Software for scoring and required rater calibration available only through course. Course information and extensive reference list are available from the Center for Innovative OT Solutions Website: https://www.innovativeotsolutions.com/tools/amps
Barthel Index	10 ADL skills	Adults	Based on "best evidence," observation, self- or proxy-report	Test items and guidelines for administering can be found at https://www.sralab.org/sites/default/files/2017-07/barthel.pdf
Canadian Occupational Performance Measure (COPM)	Measures performance and satisfaction in self-care (ADL and some IADL), productivity (some IADL and work), and leisure	Children and adults	Self-report using a semistructured interview; five most important problems rated for performance and satisfaction	Training and purchase information (paper manual, electronic PDF, and the COPM App) is available at: http://www.thecopm.ca/

TABLE 44.2	**Summary of Selected Activities of Daily Living (ADL) and Instrumental Activities of Daily Living (IADL) Instruments (*continued*)**			
Title	**Areas Addressed**	**Population**	**Method**	**Learning to Use the Assessment**
Functional Independence Measure (FIM™)	18 activities, 13 ADL tasks, and 5 communication and social cognition skills (no IADL)	Adolescents and adults	Observation of ADL	Training is recommended for interrater reliability. Training often provided by employer. Also available from the Uniform Data System for Medical Rehabilitation: http://www.udsmr.org
Goal-Oriented Assessment of Lifeskills (GOAL)	Assesses functional motor abilities needed for daily living using seven common occupational tasks	Children ages 7 to 17 years	Observation of intervention targets	Available for purchase at Pearson Assessments: http://www.pearsonassessments.com
Independent Living Scale (ILS)	Assesses information/performance and comprehension on 68 items in five areas: memory and orientation, managing money, managing home and transportation, health and safety, and social adjustment	Adolescents and adults with cognitive impairment	Observation of functional activities	Available for purchase at Pearson Assessments: http://www.pearsonassessments.com
Instrumental Activities of Daily Living (IADL) Scale	Eight IADL tasks	Adults	Self- or proxy-report	The instrument is available at https://nursing.ceconnection.com/ovidfiles/00000446-200804000-00023.pdf
Kohlman Evaluation of Living Skills (KELS)	13 living skills in five areas: self-care, safety and health, money management, community mobility and telephone, and employment and leisure	Adults	Observation and self-report of task performance	Manual included in test kit describes testing procedures. The KELS can be purchased from the AOTA: https://myaota.aota.org/shop_aota/search.aspx#q=KELS&sort=relevancy
Pediatric Evaluation of Disability Inventory (PEDI)	Measures functional abilities in self-care, mobility, and social function. The PEDI is a normed test.	Children 6 months to 7+ years	Report of parent, clinician, or educator	Manual includes detailed instructions and cases to practice scoring the PEDI. Available for purchase at Pearson Assessments: http://www.pearsonassessments.com
Performance Assessment of Self-Care Skills (PASS)	26 tasks, including ADL and home management IADL tasks; different protocols for both client's home- and clinic-based.	Adults	Observation of independence, safety, and adequacy	Validity, reliability, and standardized procedures are described in the manual. The PASS is available through: http://www.shrs.pitt.edu/ot/about/performance-assessment-self-care-skills-pass
WeeFIM™ II	Measures 18 items in self-care, mobility, and cognition	Children from 6 months to 7 years	Observation, interview, or both	Training information at https://www.udsmr.org/products-pediatric-rehab

used in practice or research or provide a unique approach to assessment (e.g., the Independent Living Scale measures task initiation; Ashley et al., 2001). Resources with more information about the assessments, including learning to use them, are also provided. The IADL instruments that were selected include a range of activities.

Step 7: Integrate the Information from Steps 1 to 6 to Select the Optimal ADL/IADL Assessment Methods

After establishing the purpose of the evaluation and the client's priorities and gathering some preliminary information

about the client and supports and barriers to their occupational performance, assessment methods can be selected that are client centered, yield appropriate data, are reliable and valid, and are feasible to administer. Occupational therapists should engage in best practice by considering the evidence regarding the selection and use of assessments, for example, the reliability of instruments and the validity for a given practice situation. Perhaps the best data-gathering strategy is to use a combination of methods and sources, relying on the convergence of data for the best profile of clients' activity abilities and limitations. Planning an effective ADL and IADL evaluation is best illustrated by OT Story 44.1, which follows the seven steps for selecting an ADL/IADL assessment tool.

OT STORY 44.1 EVALUATION OF A CLIENT WITH MORBID OBESITY AND RESPIRATORY FAILURE

Mrs. Gomez is a 59-year-old cisgender woman with a history of morbid obesity (5 ft tall and 376 lb). She was admitted to a hospital with difficulty breathing secondary to an allergic reaction. She went into respiratory arrest and required a tracheostomy and mechanical ventilation for 3 weeks. After 1 month in acute care, Mrs. Gomez was transferred to a rehabilitation hospital where she participated in OT for ADL and IADL training and physical therapy (PT) for mobility training. She was dependent in all areas of ADL and IADL on admission and made considerable gains in function before her discharge home 3 months after her initial hospitalization. At discharge, she was ambulating short distances (up to 50 ft) independently with a rolling walker. She had an extra wide wheelchair for limited community outings (e.g., doctor's appointments), but the chair did not fit in her home. She continued to require supplemental oxygen. Mrs. Gomez was referred for home-based services, including skilled nursing, nutritional counseling, home health aide (3 days a week, 2 hours each day), PT, and OT.

Occupational Profile

Mrs. Gomez lives with her husband of 30 years. He works full time but is physically able and willing to assist his wife when he is home. Mr. and Mrs. Gomez have two grown children and two school-age grandchildren who live in the area. Before hospitalization, Mrs. Gomez was independent in ADL and IADL. She had primary responsibility for cooking, light housekeeping, and laundry. She worked 20 hours a week at the public library. Mrs. Gomez had several close friends she enjoyed meeting for lunch or shopping, especially bargain hunting at flea markets. She and her husband also frequently attended their grandchildren's sports

events in a nearby town. The following considerations were used to select appropriate ADL and IADL assessments for Mrs. Gomez:

1. **Identify the overall purpose(s) of the evaluation.** The purpose is to plan and monitor OT intervention, so baseline data need to be effective for determining progress toward goals.
2. **Have clients identify their needs, interests, and perceived difficulties with ADL and/or IADL as part of the occupational profile.** Mrs. Gomez's primary goal is to regain her independence in ADL, IADL, and leisure. She identified ADL and IADL, including driving, as priorities because she is concerned about being a burden on her husband. She reported that her biggest difficulties are with lower body ADL (unable to reach) and with all IADL (fatigue, shortness of breath, limited reach, and mobility). She has frequent medical appointments and lives in a rural area, and she hates relying on others for getting to and from appointments.
3. **Further explore the purpose and meaning of ADL/IADL engagement for the client as it fits with their personal and cultural contexts.** The "problem activities" that Mrs. Gomez identified were briefly discussed in more detail. The ADL were completed in the typical fashion. She reported that sexual activity is not currently a priority, but she would like to address it later, once she had sufficient energy for and independence in other ADL/IADL.
4. Additionally, Mrs. Gomez reported adequacy parameters, including the ability to complete ADL and IADL in a timely manner and regain the ability to sustain activity

OT STORY 44.1 EVALUATION OF A CLIENT WITH MORBID OBESITY AND RESPIRATORY FAILURE (*continued*)

without fatigue or shortness of breath. Priorities for Mrs. Gomez include the following:

- Transporting laundry from bedroom to kitchen (top-loading washer) and out to the clothesline (no dryer).
- Cooking complete dinners, including accessing the refrigerator, oven, stovetop, cooking utensils, dishwasher, and sink. A sample dinner would include fish, rice, steamed green beans, and a salad.
- Driving and riding in her minivan.
- Accessing all areas of her one-story home except the basement, including home office for doing finances and using the computer, linen closets, and so forth.

5. *Estimate the client factors that affect occupational performance and/or the evaluation process.* Mrs. Gomez's primary occupational performance problems are caused by her obesity, which limits her reach and ability to move and causes fatigue and dyspnea. Cognition and perception do not appear to be factors that interfere with function on review of her rehabilitation records and the initial interview.

6. *Identify how context may affect ADL/IADL evaluation.* Contextual features that support the evaluation process include the following:
   - The assessment will occur in Mrs. Gomez's home, her natural environment.
   - There is a ramp into the home, providing access to the yard and driveway.
   - Mrs. Gomez has years of experience with all of the tasks she wished to return to.

Contextual features that are barriers to the evaluation process include the following:

- Clutter in the home that presents a safety issue, restricting mobility and access.
- Use of supplemental oxygen, with the unit in the bedroom and a very long tube that she has to manage as she moves around the house.
- The evaluation will occur midweek. The therapist is alone with the client whose weight presents a safety concern to the therapist when guarding her during new tasks.
- Mrs. Gomez has private insurance, which requires that the OT evaluation be completed in one visit.

7. *Consider features of assessment tools.* This step is included in the discussion of step 7.

8. *Integrate the information from steps 1 to 6 to select the optimal ADL and IADL assessment methods.* The time limit of one visit (approximately 60–75 minutes) has a significant impact on which assessments are selected.

The occupational therapist decided to start with the COPM based on the following considerations:

- The COPM has well-established psychometric properties and assesses both ADL and IADL and leisure (Law et al., 2014).
- The COPM relies on self-report; however, Mrs. Gomez is cognitively intact and has been learning to live with her disability for the past 3 months. One advantage of self-report is that it does not pose safety hazards. For example, the occupational therapist gets a baseline performance and satisfaction rating on driving her car (including getting in and out) without having to attempt the task with Mrs. Gomez.
- Mrs. Gomez felt stress about burdening her husband. The COPM will help the occupational therapist prioritize ADL and IADL to reduce caregiver burden.
- The COPM included a satisfaction measure, which reflects some of the adequacy parameters that Mrs. Gomez identified (e.g., if she can dress independently but it takes her 45 minutes, she would give that a low satisfaction score).
- The COPM can be completed in about 20 minutes.

After the COPM, the occupational therapist selects the Functional Independence Measure (FIM™) subtests of transfers, lower body dressing, and grooming. Other FIM™ tasks are not observed because Mrs. Howard reported no difficulty with them (including feeding, toileting, and upper body dressing) or because of time constraints (e.g., bathing). The FIM™ is an appropriate measure because of the following reasons:

- Mrs. Gomez reports that she requires physical assistance for lower body dressing and getting out of bed (included in FIM™ transfer subtest), and the scale is believed to have adequate sensitivity in levels of physical assistance to document progress.
- The occupational therapist has discharge FIM™ scores from the rehabilitation center, so performance in the clinic and at home can be compared using the same tool to examine the impact of the home context on performance and aid in problem-solving for intervention.
- These tasks can all be completed in 25 minutes.

Two additional parameter measures are used to supplement the FIM™. Lower body dressing and grooming are timed, which requires no additional assessment time. Dyspnea will be measured after each of the three subtasks, using a 100-mm visual analog scale where 0 = "no shortness of breath," 50 mm = "moderate shortness of breath," and 100 mm = "severe shortness of breath" (Lansing et al., 2003). Completion of the dyspnea scales

(continued)

OT STORY 44.1 EVALUATION OF A CLIENT WITH MORBID OBESITY AND RESPIRATORY FAILURE (continued)

requires little additional time, fitting into the 25 minutes allowed for the FIM™.

At this point, Mrs. Gomez needs a rest, although the occupational therapist wants to include some observation of IADL in the evaluation. While Mrs. Gomez rests, the therapist uses the walker to do an informal accessibility assessment for several key areas in the home (e.g., dresser, closet, personal computer, kitchen appliances, and cabinets). Although standardized home assessments are available, the occupational therapist uses a nonstandardized approach because Mrs. Gomez's walker requires additional room for accessibility and the therapist needs to focus on a few key areas because time is limited. The occupational therapist also begins some intervention by making a list of suggestions to make Mrs. Gomez's environment more accessible and reviewing them with Mrs. Gomez so she can enlist a friend or family member in modifying the environment to enhance performance. The informal assessment of context and review with Mrs. Gomez is completed in 15 minutes.

At this point, Mrs. Gomez and her occupational therapist are about 1 hour into the initial evaluation. The therapist would like to observe Mrs. Gomez perform a simple cooking task and also assess her potential to return to driving by having her get in and out of her car, including folding and storing the walker. However, Mrs. Gomez is fatigued, and

15 minutes is not enough time for both. Mrs. Gomez has a minivan that requires a significant step up. Given her level of fatigue with lighter activities and concerns about safely guarding someone of her size, the occupational therapist opts to have Mrs. Gomez make a cup of tea, deferring the car assessment to another session. The kettle is placed in a low cabinet to assess her ability to retrieve it. The tea is in an over-counter cabinet. The therapist gathers qualitative data, times the task, and uses the visual analog scale to measure dyspnea on completion. The task takes less than 10 minutes. After the assessment, Mrs. Gomez settles into her favorite chair to enjoy her cup of tea.

Questions

1. What are some examples of how the therapist implemented ADL and IADL evaluation with Mrs. Gomez in order to maximize generating assessment data despite the time constraints?
2. What adequacy parameters of ADL and IADL performance are important to Mrs. Gomez and how did the therapist assess these parameters?
3. What prior assessment data informed the therapist's professional reasoning and decision to have Mrs. Gomez make a cup of tea rather than get in and out of her car?

Implementing the Evaluation: Gathering Data, Critical Observation, and Hypothesis Generation

Gathering Data and Critical Observation

Once occupational therapists develop an evaluation plan, they must carry it out. The thoughtful and deliberate selection of appropriate assessment methods described previously is key in making the data gathering run smoothly. A few additional considerations about the actual implementation of the evaluation warrant discussion. The OT practitioner who is conducting an evaluation should do the following:

- *Collect all equipment and supplies* needed for carrying out the evaluation plan, making sure assessment test kits are complete and organized and that necessary equipment and supplies are available, including clients' personal items (e.g., clothing from home).
- *Schedule evaluation sessions in the best environment available and at the most appropriate time of day.* For

example, a client in an inpatient rehabilitation center would find it more comfortable to dress in their room than in a curtained-off area in a busy clinic and may find it more meaningful and motivating to dress early in the day.
- *Be sensitive to individual needs for modesty,* which can vary greatly among clients. Many ADL are personal tasks that are typically done alone, including dressing, bathing, and toileting. Assessment for potential impairment in sexual activity should be included in ADL evaluation but must be handled with sensitivity.
- *Structure the optimal environment.* For example, the practitioner might wish to have family members present during an interview to gain their perspectives about a client's abilities or needs, whereas having several family members observing a performance-based assessment of cooking might be distracting to the client and interfere with the evaluation process.
- *Bring appropriate tools to record data.* A well-planned evaluation session will reveal a lot of information about a client. Standardized assessments often come with forms for recording data. The practitioner might also want to jot down relevant observations, for example, noting that a client complained of shoulder pain when putting a shirt on overhead or that a client's grocery list included

primarily nonnutritious foods. If possible, practitioners should record directly into the client's health record to reduce the time needed for completing the evaluation report.

During the evaluation, the practitioner should engage in critical observation, which can be framed by questions the practitioners ask themselves throughout the process, such as the following:

- *What are some of the possible underlying causes of the occupational performance problems that are being observed or reported?* For example, various factors may limit a client's ability to reach the clothes in their closet, including upper extremity weakness, impaired passive range of motion (ROM), poor coordination, diminished standing balance, or a clothes rod that is out of reach for the client's height. Observations made as the client tries to get clothes from the closet can provide clues to the underlying causes that will aid the occupational therapist in making sound intervention decisions, as shown in Figure 44.1.
- *What changes might need to be made in the initial evaluation plan based on the data from the first assessments?* For example, a cooking assessment might reveal mild cognitive deficits that were not apparent during initial interactions with a client, so the occupational therapist may add a cognitive assessment to the evaluation plan.
- *Are there discrepancies in the assessment data that were collected?* Discrepancies need to be clarified and reconciled and can provide valuable insight into the nature of the client's ADL and IADL problems. For example, a practitioner might observe during performance testing that a client can execute bed-to-wheelchair transfers, yet the client might insist that they cannot. The inconsistency might arise because, although the client performs the transfer independently with the practitioner present, they feel insecure about their abilities and will not transfer on their own. In this example, the use of different data sources identified a performance discrepancy between skill and habit that would not have been apparent from the use of one source alone.

Hypothesis Generation

The evaluation data that are obtained through questioning, observing, and testing methods must be analyzed, synthesized, and integrated into a cohesive problem statement (Gateley & Borcherding, 2017). This integration of data is accomplished through diagnostic or scientific reasoning, a component of professional reasoning (Tomlin, 2018) that occurs as a kind of internal dialogue about the interpretation of the data. Evidence supporting one interpretation is weighed against evidence rejecting that interpretation, and the interpretation that has the most compelling evidence is selected. If the evidence fails to sufficiently support one interpretation over another, more evaluative data are collected

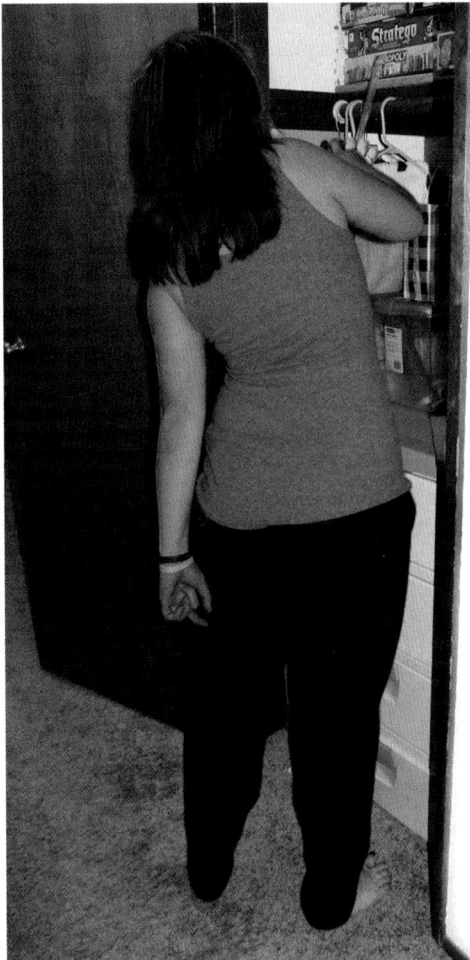

FIGURE 44.1 Observations made during reach: lateral flexion of the trunk suggests that the client is compensating for an inability to raise the arm, which could be from limited passive range of motion or decreased strength. The height of the closet rod relative to the client's size should require only about 50% of typical shoulder flexion. Balance does not appear to be an issue because the client appears stable even while shifting her center of gravity toward the left as she reaches.

to supplement the reasoning process. This process is best illustrated through an example based on the cases presented in Table 44.1. Aiden and Brody had the same dressing scores on the WeeFIM™, a quantitative ADL assessment, but the occupational therapist's clinical interpretation of the descriptive data will lead to very different assumptions about the problems that are causing dressing impairments for the two children. Before reading on, take a minute to reflect on the different observations reported in Table 44.1 and consider the following for both Aiden and Brody:

- What are the underlying factors that interfere with each child's ability to dress independently?

- What are their strengths, that is, what skills support each one's dressing performance?
- What observed behaviors led to your conclusions about each child's strengths and challenges?

For Aiden, limited attention, impaired awareness of occupational performance hindrances, and inconsistent response to feedback seemed to be underlying problems that limited his ability to dress independently. This is a hypothesis or clinical judgment rather than an objective observation because constructs such as attention and awareness of deficits cannot be directly observed and must be inferred from specific behaviors. At the same time, Aiden's physical capabilities seemed to be an asset and supported performance in many ways. Compare the observations and clinical judgments made by the occupational therapist about Aiden to those made about Brody. In both cases, the children required verbal cueing and occasional physical assistance; however, descriptive data led the occupational therapist to a very different hypothesis about Brody's dressing limitations. The underlying problems for Brody were physical impairments, for example, impaired sitting balance, incoordination of the right upper extremity, and decreased endurance. Behaviors that supported performance included attention to task, follow-through with feedback, the ability to recall adaptive strategies, and engagement in active problem-solving. Generating hypotheses about the nature of the occupational performance problem is crucial for planning effective intervention, which must address the underlying problem. For example, adaptive equipment could be provided to help Brody reach his feet independently or to compensate for limited right-hand function during buttoning; however, this equipment would be of no help to Aiden and would likely impede performance by distracting him from the task.

Through this process, the occupational therapist arrives at a cohesive understanding of the ADL and IADL performance of the client, factors that are interfering with performance, and appropriate therapeutic actions given the nature of the client's problems. This understanding is presented to clients or their proxies for verification and collaborative decision-making concerning the therapeutic action to be implemented.

Establishing Clients' Goals: The Bridge Between Evaluation and Intervention

The OTPF includes creating goals in collaboration with the client as part of the synthesis of the evaluation process and as the first component of the intervention plan (AOTA,

2020), so establishing client goals serves as a transition from evaluation to intervention. Synthesizing evaluation results into an effective intervention plan is a complex professional reasoning task and can be overwhelming for the student or new OT practitioner. The process of planning and implementing interventions is much easier for practitioners who have reasonable, attainable, and measurable goals or outcomes. The following section is designed to guide novice practitioners in the professional reasoning used for establishing effective client goals.

Establishing goals requires analysis of the evaluation results in conjunction with additional factors that influence outcomes, such as the client's self-awareness and ability to learn, prognosis, time allocated for intervention, discharge disposition, and ability to follow through with new routines or techniques. The next section focuses on using performance parameters to establish meaningful goals for clients that have a clearly identified behavior; that is, what the client is expected to *do*. The behavior must be observable and include an appropriate *assist level*; that is, a characteristic of the behavior that is measurable, for example, "independently" or "without pain" (Gateley & Borcherding, 2017).

Identifying Appropriate Goal Behaviors

A comprehensive evaluation examines ADL and IADL performance across a variety of performance parameters. Four of these performance parameters—value, level of difficulty, safety, and fatigue and dyspnea—are particularly relevant to consider in order to identify goals for intervention that target realistic and appropriate client behaviors.

Value

Occupational therapists should select goal behaviors (i.e., ADL and IADL tasks) that reflect the values defined by the client during the evaluation. The value that clients place on given activities influences their motivation for participation in any intervention aimed at improving performance for that activity (Doig et al., 2009; Jack & Estes, 2010). Because many OT interventions require the acquisition of new skills through practice, motivation can greatly influence the ultimate functional outcome. Clients who put little value on the activity that is being addressed during an intervention might appear uncooperative and are unlikely to follow through with programs outside of direct intervention that are necessary for improving skill in that activity.

Clients' self-awareness of ADL and IADL performance problems can have an impact on identifying goals and their relative value. Clients with cognitive deficits and poor self-awareness may not value ADL or IADL goals if they perceive they are already independent, efficient, and effective in their performance of those tasks. Doig et al. (2009, 2016) found that the process of collaborative goal setting with clients with traumatic brain injury and their significant others actually facilitated clients' self-awareness and increased their participation in OT. OT practitioners who work with children may also face challenges in collaborative goal setting, although young school-age children with neurodevelopmental disabilities were able to engage effectively in setting goals with support of an assessment instrument that measured their perceived competence in various physical tasks (Vroland-Nordstrand et al., 2015). Clients with good insight into their occupational performance challenges may be more easily engaged in collaborative goal setting, but OT practitioners must carefully attend to the complex issues that can impact clients' priorities.

ADL and IADL are often highly valued by both children and adults because of the dependency on others that accompanies role dysfunction (Vroland-Nordstrand et al., 2015). However, OT practitioners should be careful not to assume that ADL and IADL are immediate priorities. Some people, especially those with severe activity limitations, might need or want to accept assistance from others in ADL so that they can focus on improving other areas of occupational performance. This was the case with Mr. Fritz, a 32-year-old, cisgender man with a recently sustained spinal cord injury resulting in C6 tetraplegia. He was married, had three small children, and was self-employed as a tax accountant, and the family depended on Mr. Fritz's income. The ADL outcomes were initially established for Mr. Fritz, but self-care retraining was met with resistance and frustration. Further discussion of the intervention outcomes revealed that Mr. Fritz was anxious to return to work and wanted to focus on computer skills. Although he did want to be independent in self-care eventually, he felt it was best for him to return to work to minimize the financial burden on his family. His wife was able and willing to help him, and they both felt that self-care retraining could be delayed until the family business was again operational. With intervention outcomes refocused on activities most valued by Mr. Fritz—namely computer access and home mobility—he became highly motivated to participate in therapy.

Clients' values should drive long-term goals, but OT practitioners may need to help clients focus on ADL initially when they have identified priorities for more complex occupational performance areas (e.g., IADL, work, or leisure) that may be difficult to treat effectively early in the intervention process (Doig et al., 2016). Self-care training often helps clients develop capacities and problem-solving skills that can later be applied to activities that are more complex, particularly when dealing with severe disorders of sudden onset (e.g., stroke and traumatic injuries). For example, suppose Mr. Fritz could not work from a home office and wanted to focus on driving to get to work—a realistic long-term goal for someone with C6 tetraplegia.

Initiating intervention with driver training, however, would be impractical because Mr. Fritz lacked the prerequisite functional mobility skills early in his rehabilitation. The ADL training—involving bathing, dressing, transferring, and wheelchair mobility—can facilitate the development of functional mobility skills. Such training, therefore, would logically precede driver training. If Mr. Fritz had been in this situation, his needs may have been met through a referral to social services for assistance with financial planning to help the family manage until he could return to work. The OT practitioner would have also needed to educate Mr. Fritz about the commonalities among skills needed for both self-care and driving. This plan would simultaneously recognize Mr. Fritz's valued roles and progress him to the desired outcome in the most efficient way possible.

When the most valued activities and roles are beyond the client's potential skill level, the OT practitioner helps the client refocus priorities, so goals are realistic and achievable. If Mr. Fritz were the owner and cook of a small restaurant, for example, it is unlikely that he would meet the essential job requirements of a short-order cook even if the kitchen were adapted for wheelchair accessibility because the activities require bilateral hand function and must be done quickly. It is possible, however, that he could perform the activities of a restaurant owner, including managing personnel and finances, operating the cash register, and seating customers. In this and similar situations, OT practitioners use their expertise in activity analysis and functional adaptation to assist clients in creating a realistic yet meaningful life for themselves and help them establish achievable goals to progress them to that vision (Doig et al., 2009, 2016).

Difficulty

The perceived ease with which a client completes an activity and the projected difficulty that will remain after intervention are important considerations in selecting goal behaviors (Esposito et al., 2014). The OT practitioner, who is skilled in activity analysis and has knowledge of pathology and impairment, must determine the prognosis for functional difficulty. This prognosis must then be communicated to clients so that decisions about acceptable levels of difficulty can be made collaboratively. Clients set intervention priorities, in part, by weighing the projected level of difficulty within the context of value—that is, how much difficulty they are willing to tolerate to be independent in an activity. The frequency with which an activity is performed should also be considered in establishing goals for ADL and IADL that are likely to remain difficult for a client to perform. In general, a higher level of proficiency is needed for activities that need to be done routinely, whereas a lower level of proficiency may be acceptable for activities that are done only occasionally.

For example, James is a 7-year-old boy with spina bifida, resulting in paralysis from the waist down. He has a neurogenic bladder and requires regular intermittent catheterization. He identified self-catheterization as a critical task for fulfilling his role as a student because he does not want to have help with this personal task from school personnel. James will need to be able to self-catheterize independently and efficiently for this task to fit into his school day. The occupational therapist believes that James will be capable of achieving independence with little difficulty after a period of practice. The goal is agreed on, and intervention begins. Another client, Amy, also has spina bifida, but it affects her upper extremities as well as her trunk and lower extremities. Unlike James, the spinal cord damage is incomplete, so she can usually empty her bladder without self-catheterization. On occasion, however, she has episodes of urinary retention, requiring catheterization within about 1 hour of experiencing symptoms. Amy would also like to be independent in self-catheterizing at school, so she does not need help from school personnel. The occupational therapist thinks that independent self-catheterization using safe and clean technique is a reasonable goal for Amy, but it will always be difficult because of her impaired hand function and difficulty positioning herself so that she can see and reach to insert the catheter. Amy will need to go to the nurse's office to transfer to a bed. Despite the difficulty, Amy opts to work on this goal. Because she has to catheterize herself so infrequently, she believes that her skill level will be adequate for meeting her needs.

Safety

The degree of risk inherent in the person-task-environment transaction must also be considered when establishing client goals. The IADL tasks tend to pose more safety risks, for example, working with sharp or hot objects while cooking, driving, or operating snow blowers or lawn mowers for home maintenance. However, some ADL can also pose safety risks for people, such as bathing, managing medications, or using safe-sex practices during sexual activity. Oftentimes, intervention is effective in reducing safety risks to an acceptable level; however, if the occupational therapist believes that performance cannot be effectively modified to meet safety standards, then those tasks may not be appropriate goals.

In North America, safe driving has received increasing attention in the healthcare literature as the number of older drivers, many with health-related impairments, continues to increase. Occupational therapists are often the health professionals who evaluate and treat this important IADL (Korner-Bitensky et al., 2010). Because of the potentially grave consequences of unsafe driving, occupational therapists must develop the skills to identify when it is appropriate to pursue driving goals and when safety precludes a return to driving and intervention should focus on driving cessation and goals that address alternative transportation methods, such as using public transportation (Kartje, 2006).

Understanding and implementing "safer-sex" practices to prevent sexually transmitted diseases may be an important safety-related goal for clients that is often not addressed by OT practitioners. Clients with cognitive deficits that may impair decision-making (e.g., developmental disability, traumatic brain injury, or mental health disorders) may benefit from education about the potential health threats associated with unprotected sex. Clients with physical disabilities may require adaptations for safer-sex tasks, such as applying condoms.

Fatigue and Dyspnea

Fatigue, the sensation of tiredness that is experienced during or following an activity, and dyspnea, difficult or labored breathing, can interfere with activity performance (Seo et al., 2011; Van Heest et al., 2017) and both are likely to be exacerbated by activity performance. The occupational therapist uses activity analysis to take into account the effort required to perform a task and its typical duration. In addition, the client's entire daily routine must be examined so that the energy demands of one activity can be weighed in relation to the client's other activities (Mathiowetz et al., 2001). Assisting clients to examine the physical demands of their preferred activities can help them to prioritize activities so that appropriate goals can be established. Similar to budgeting money, clients must be encouraged to look at their "energy dollars" and decide how they wish to spend them. The OT practitioner contributes to this decision-making process by bringing valuable information about options for activity adaptation that can reduce the energy demands of activities, thereby saving clients' energy for other tasks.

For example, Ms. Saito, a 67-year-old, transgender woman lived alone in an apartment in a retirement community. Her sister and brother-in-law also resided in the community as well as many close friends. She has had multiple sclerosis for many years, with some weakness and spasticity, but she remained independent in her ADL until a recent exacerbation required hospitalization. Increased fatigue and decreased strength resulted in the need for physical assistance with dressing and bathing and the use of a wheelchair for mobility. The retirement community required residents to manage their own ADL and prepare breakfast and a light evening snack. A hot meal was provided at midday. The OT practitioner explained to Ms. Saito that although independence in ADL and simple meal preparation were reasonable goals, completing her ADL would likely be time-consuming and fatiguing, leaving her limited energy for other activities. Ms. Saito was enthusiastic about beginning therapy, indicating that she was willing to engage in fewer IADL and leisure activities in order to be independent in tasks that would enable her to remain in the retirement community with family and friends.

A different scenario played out with Ms. McKay, a divorced, 34-year-old, cisgender woman who also had multiple sclerosis. Like Ms. Saito, she had a recent exacerbation that caused a functional decline, and achieving independence in ADL was likely to expend much of her daily energy. Ms. McKay had been working full time as a programmer for a local radio station and was the mother of two young children. She perceived her role as a self-carer to be important, along with those of worker and mother. However, when it became apparent that independence in ADL would leave her with little energy for performing work and parenting roles, she decided not to establish goals for independence in ADL, opting instead to hire a personal care attendant for assistance so she could focus on work and parenting goals.

Identifying an Appropriate Degree of Performance

OT goals must include a measurable outcome that indicates how well or at what level the identified behavior will be done, sometimes referred to as the *degree of performance* (Kettenbach, 2009). Independence is the most common degree of performance; however, several performance parameters can also provide effective goals, especially when the client is independent, but occupational performance deficits remain that warrant intervention. For example, this would be the case when a client can open jars independently, but it is painful and results in deforming forces to the hand joints.

Independence

Independence is the performance parameter most commonly focused on in OT interventions (Bonikowsky et al., 2012), and it becomes the level of assist, the measurable part of the goal (Gateley & Borcherding, 2017). Across all ages and disabilities, the goal is generally to increase the level of independence (Clarke et al., 2009; Eyres & Unsworth, 2005; Legg et al., 2006; Pillastrini et al., 2008). Independence in activity performance includes three phases: initiation of a task, continuation of a task, and completion of a task. The most common OT goals focus on the completion of the task, which implies that initiation and continuation of the task occurred. For example, a goal might be "Client will be independent in feeding their cats 3/3 meals a day by December 12, 2023" or "Client will require moderate assistance for bed to/from wheelchair transfers in 1 week."

Initiation is an aspect of activity performance that is frequently overlooked when goals are established, in part because it is difficult to evaluate and treat. The very presence of the OT practitioner may be a cue to initiate a task. Adults are typically expected to initiate ADL and IADL independently. Expectations for children also exist, depending on the children's age and skills and the division of task responsibilities among family members. Impairments in activity initiation may occur as a result of many diseases and disorders, such as attention-deficit disorder, dementia, depression, schizophrenia, brain injury from trauma or stroke, multiple sclerosis, and Parkinson disease. Family members generally find it frustrating to have to cue ("constantly nag") a client with impaired initiation for each aspect of a daily routine. The occupational therapist may write an independence goal that includes initiation, such as "Client will initiate and complete bathing independently three to seven times a week by November 30, 2023." In this example, measuring progress toward the goal would require the client or a proxy to record the number of times in a week that the client initiated bathing without cueing or assistance from another person.

Safety

Although some goals may not be feasible at all because of safety concerns, other times, it is possible to improve a person's safe performance of ADL/IADL, so safety becomes a part of the goal. Because safety is a quality of the person-task-environment transaction, it cannot be observed or treated in isolation from independence (Jennings et al., 2017). Goals related to safety are typically linked to independence outcomes; that is, independent performance is assumed to be safe (Bonikowsky et al., 2012; Tamaru et al., 2007) because an occupational therapist could not ethically create a goal for independent performance that was not deemed to be safe. Although OT practitioners agree that safety is an intervention priority, there is less consensus about specific activity behaviors that are safe or unsafe. Many behaviors fall into a questionable zone, where some would rate them as safe, whereas others perceive them as unsafe, for example, standing to pull up pants during dressing. In determining acceptable risk for setting independence goals, it is useful to consider clients' comfort level with risk; their ability to analyze the risks associated with a particular activity and devise a plan for managing them; and, most important, their ability to implement the plan expeditiously despite impairments. At times, the goal for level of independence in activity performance might need to be sacrificed for safety.

A comparison of two clients with bilateral lower extremity fractures sustained in separate car crashes who are learning independent transfers illustrates this point: Roberto and Harlan were both recently injured. Each is non-weight-bearing on both lower extremities, and each is learning to transfer with a transfer board. Roberto demonstrates good judgment and a realistic perception of his skills. The occupational therapist has determined that the following goal is realistic: "Client will be independent in transfers with a transfer board from wheelchair to/from bed within three therapy sessions." Through training, Roberto learns to execute a safe transfer with the transfer board while keeping weight off his fractured legs. After a couple of sessions, his goal of independence in transferring from wheelchair to bed and back is met. Harlan's injuries are similar to Roberto's, but he also incurred a mild brain injury. Although Harlan's motor skills are comparable to Roberto's, Harlan has difficulty recalling the steps for a safe transfer and forgets to keep weight off his lower extremities, which could interfere with fracture healing. The occupational therapist considers safety when setting a goal for Harlan by aiming for a lower level of independence, for example, "Client will require supervision and verbal cues for transfers from wheelchair to/from bed using a transfer board while adhering to weight-bearing precautions within six therapy sessions." The degree of independence and the time frame in Harlan's goal were adjusted to reflect his capacity for safe transfer performance.

In some situations, it may be better to establish client goals in which the goal behavior is directly related to safety rather than being assumed in the degree of independence indicated. Goals can be aimed at the occupational performance level, that is, the IADL "safety and emergency maintenance" (AOTA, 2020; Jennings et al., 2017), for example, the goal might be "Client will verbally describe correct responses to a minimum of 10 potential home emergencies with 100% accuracy within 3 weeks." Safety goals may also be aimed at developing safe habits; for example, "Client will pause when entering a room and scan for obstacles on the floor 100% of the time to reduce fall risk during functional mobility by June 1, 2023."

Adequacy

Several aspects of activity performance contribute to the adequacy or quality of the behavior stated in the goal, which can also be reflected in the goal as the degree to which the behavior is expected to be done. In addition to independence, these performance parameters may be crucial components of meaningful goals, especially for clients who are independent and safe with their performance but who feel dissatisfied with the process or some other aspect of the outcome. Goals with measurable adequacy parameters can be used to justify OT even if clients are independent in tasks. Six adequacy parameters can be used as measurable outcomes: pain, fatigue and dyspnea, duration, societal standards, satisfaction, and aberrant task behaviors. Some of these parameters may be interdependent within a single client. For instance, pain might lead to changes in duration of activity performance (e.g., the activity takes longer) as well as the ability to meet normative standards and personal satisfaction. A goal should include only one measurable parameter so that it is clear what has changed in documenting progress toward goals.

Pain. Pain, either during or following an activity, can negatively influence engagement in ADL or IADL even if the activity is completed independently (Covinsky et al.,

2009; Dudgeon et al., 2006; Liedberg & Vrethem, 2009). The source of pain and the prognosis for it must be carefully considered in establishing goals and selecting an intervention approach. Both the evaluation and goals must include an index of pain so that intervention remains focused on achieving the projected level of independence while simultaneously reducing the presence of pain. For example, the goal might be "Client will prepare a simple meal (soup, sandwich, and beverage) independently with a maximum pain level of 2 cm on a 10-cm visual analog scale 4/5 times within 2 weeks."

Fatigue and Dyspnea. Fatigue and dyspnea can influence the actual task behaviors that are selected for client goals, as described earlier in this section, but when fatigue or dyspnea can be reduced through task adaptation or conditioning, goals can be established that use these performance parameters as performance criteria outcomes. The initial evaluation should include baseline data for comparison. For example, a goal might be "Client will complete morning care routine (shower, grooming, dressing) with a maximum score of 12 on the Borg Rate of Perceived Exertion Scale 75% of the time by July 28, 2023." As long as the Borg Scale (Centers for Disease Control and Prevention, 2015) was used during the initial evaluation, a lower number (meaning less exertion) can be used in a goal to indicate progress toward becoming less fatigued during ADL or IADL tasks. Dyspnea can be monitored in a similar way, using a visual analog scale or numerical rating scale (Gift & Narsavage, 1998). Diagnosis is important to consider when goals are formulated relative to fatigue and dyspnea. Overexertion can exacerbate symptoms or even the disease process itself for conditions such as cardiac disease and multiple sclerosis. Prognosis is another important consideration in setting goals that measure fatigue or dyspnea. Clients with chronic obstructive pulmonary disease are likely to become worse; therefore, goals must be reasonable to achieve through activity adaptations and might need to accommodate a decline in function. A client with paraplegia secondary to spinal cord injury, by contrast, experiences fatigue from having to use the smaller muscles of the upper extremity for wheelchair mobility to compensate for the larger lower extremity muscles previously used for walking. Endurance is likely to improve significantly as upper extremity strength and muscle endurance increases with use, and more ambitious goals for reducing fatigue could be appropriate.

Duration. The length of time that is required to complete activities is typically thought of as a reflection of efficiency, which may be affected by many types of impairments, including poor endurance, impaired coordination, and cognitive deficits such as reduced attention for tasks. Although measuring performance time may be relatively simple, interpreting time data in a meaningful way is often difficult.

The duration of ADL/IADL depends highly on the nature of the activity and the task objects that people choose to use in performing the activity. Most of us spend more time dressing when we are going out to dine in an elegant restaurant than we do when we are going to a neighborhood diner. Therefore, it is difficult to establish meaningful time norms for ADL and IADL, but duration is often a parameter that clients wish to incorporate into their OT goals when they are frustrated by slow performance.

Establishing acceptable time frames for ADL goals must be done collaboratively with clients and their significant others. Occupational therapists should also consider safety and independence parameters when establishing goals with time frames. Clients may be at increased risk when they rush through activities or even when they attempt them at a typical pace. For example, clients with swallowing deficits might need to eat more slowly than people without such deficits to avoid choking. People with poor fine motor coordination or sensory deficits might need to slow down when using sharp knives to improve control of the knives and prevent injury. In these examples, setting goals to decrease the duration of performance would be inappropriate because it could result in unsafe performance.

Societal and cultural standards also need to be taken into consideration in establishing outcomes for activity duration. In the United States, timeliness is highly valued, and efficient performance in community skills is expected. Shoppers might become irritated when they are standing in a checkout line behind a customer who takes 5 minutes to identify and count currency, even though in other cultures, this delay might go unnoticed. A person living in America who has cognitive or visual impairments that interfere with the ability to count currency might wish to decrease the time required for this activity to reduce embarrassment when shopping. The goal, then, needs to include an efficiency measure to reflect this performance parameter, for example, "Client will independently complete a simple cash transaction (select appropriate currency and count change) in less than 1 minute within 3 weeks to support participation in shopping."

Societal Standards. Performance standards, determined by the society and culture in which the client lives, are likely to exist in terms of both the end result and the process through which it is achieved. The line between acceptable and unacceptable performance is likely to be wide rather than narrow and may vary considerably, depending on characteristics such as age, gender, and cohort (generation) membership.

Societal standards exist for neatness, for example. A client might dress safely and independently, but if clients select clothing with multiple patterns or their appearance is disheveled (the end product), then dressing might not meet societal standards. If the client is a teenager, such an appearance might be considered acceptable. However, if the client is a public relations manager going to the office, it could well put the client's job in jeopardy. Identifying societal standards might seem subjective and difficult, but the use of measurable indicators of societal standards is critical for effective goals and can justify intervention. A goal for a client who eats rapidly, putting food in their mouth when it is still full, might include a measure of societal standard, such as "When eating during a social event, the client will demonstrate appropriate pacing as evidenced by completing a meal in no less than 15 minutes and swallowing each bite before putting additional food in his mouth by April 8, 2023."

Satisfaction. In addition to societal standards, clients have their own standards of acceptable performance, which also need to be incorporated into goals (Doig et al., 2016; Eklund & Gunnarsson, 2008). Setting goals with satisfaction measures requires collaboration with clients because personal standards will vary greatly from person to person. Mr. Balouris, for example, is always losing things. He never seems to know where his wallet and keys are, and he is always searching for something. Nonetheless, items seem to turn up, and he sees no reason to go to the trouble of organizing his apartment better to help him keep track of his belongings. Mr. Johnson, however, has always been meticulously neat and could put his hands on items the minute he wanted them. Recently, he sought medical attention for memory problems. He complained that he needed to search for items because he failed to put them in their usual places. He was particularly concerned about his memory problem because of a family history of Alzheimer disease. He was referred to OT to learn strategies to help him remember where items are placed. Objectively, Mr. Johnson's performance is similar to that of Mr. Balouris; however, Mr. Johnson is dissatisfied with his performance, which he views as impaired.

Client satisfaction can be measured quickly and easily with a visual analog scale or numerical scale, such as the 10-point scale that is used in the COPM (Law et al., 2014) that can be easily incorporated into goals to reflect specific conditions for performance, for example, "Client will be independent in locating items needed for ADL and IADL in the home with a satisfaction rating of at least 8/10 within 3 weeks to support participation in ADL and IADL."

Aberrant Task Behaviors. Goals and interventions may also address any aberrant task behaviors that interfere with activity performance (Ashley et al., 2001). Aberrant task behaviors vary widely and include unwanted motor behavior such as athetoid or ballistic movements and behavioral responses such as skin-scratching or hitting caregivers. Exploration of the underlying cause of the aberrant task behavior facilitates the establishment of realistic goals and the selection of effective intervention strategies. Goals are aimed at eliminating or diminishing aberrant task behavior typically by replacing it with more functional behaviors in the context of ADL and IADL tasks; for example, for a client with tongue thrusting during eating, a goal might be "Client will use tongue lateralization to form a bolus during eating, within 2 months, in order to support safe and adequate oral intake." Tongue lateralization is incompatible with tongue thrust and would indicate a reduction of that behavior. Goals focused on performance inconsistent with aberrant behaviors are preferable than those that simply reflect a reduction in those behaviors.

Additional Considerations for Setting Realistic Client Goals

The occupational therapist uses performance parameters to identify goal behaviors and degrees of performance, but several additional factors that can affect goal achievement must also be considered. The process of setting goals is complex and must be based not only on clients' hopes but also on what changes are realistic (Doig et al., 2016). Several contextual factors must be considered, such as physical and social environment, financial resources, time available for intervention, and the client's past experience and learning ability. The prognosis for recovery, given the client's disability, can also affect goal achievement.

Prognosis for Impairments

The client's potential for improvement in performance skills and patterns and client factors must be examined within the context of any existing disease or disorder and resulting impairments (Egan & Dubouloz, 2014). First, the practitioner must consider precautions or contraindications pursuant to the diagnosis that could preclude the use of certain intervention strategies. For example, compare two clients whose endurance significantly limits their performance. Mrs. Tanaka has chronic fatigue syndrome, a disorder that may worsen if she becomes overfatigued. An aggressive program to increase endurance is contraindicated for her, so alternative intervention strategies should be explored, and goals for increasing endurance for ADL must be reasonable, given Mrs. Tanaka's potential for exacerbation of her disease. Conversely, Mr. Krull is deconditioned from inactivity resulting from major depressive illness and would like to increase his endurance to support participation in heavy home maintenance tasks, such as mowing the lawn and finishing an addition on his house. A rigorous activity program to increase endurance is not contraindicated and would help to increase Mr. Krull's participation in IADL.

Second, the prognosis for improvement in impairments, given the client's diagnosis, must be considered. Increasing impairment is expected in progressive disorders, such as muscular dystrophy and Alzheimer disease. Goals must be established with potential declines in mind so that the goals are realistic.

OT practitioners must consider various impairments separately, however, because progressive diseases might affect bodily structures and functions differently. For example, Jorge, a teenage boy who has muscular dystrophy, has significant muscle weakness in the trunk and all four extremities with limitations in pelvic and ankle passive ROM that preclude maintaining an optimal position for functioning from his wheelchair. His muscle strength is expected to decline, even with intervention. His passive ROM restrictions are secondary to the muscle weakness and not a direct result of the disease process. Gains can be expected in passive ROM with intervention, despite the overall prognosis. In turn, increased passive ROM can enhance function by improving Jorge's position in the wheelchair.

Stable or diminishing impairments may be anticipated in many disorders and after injury. Pharmacologic intervention, for example, may improve impairments associated with depression so that OT intervention can be focused on transferring gains made in mental and psychological capacities into ADL and IADL performance.

Typically, clients of any age with brain injuries from trauma or stroke can expect some spontaneous return of body functions in the early stages of recovery. Projected intervention goals should take into account the typical improvements for this diagnosis. Predicting "typical improvements" takes time and experience to develop, and the novice practitioner might find it helpful to consult with more experienced clinicians to facilitate the ability to set realistic goals.

Experience

Information gathered in the evaluation about a client's past and recent experience with an activity is important to consider when setting goals. Recent experience may facilitate progress in reestablishing independence in an activity because the client is learning a new way to do the activity rather than developing a new skill.

For example, Mrs. McCarthy needs to relearn cooking skills following a stroke. She uses a wheelchair for mobility and has minimal use of her right (dominant) hand. Her cognitive skills are intact, and she can easily follow a recipe. Furthermore, she demonstrates good problem-solving skills in adapting cooking activities to improve her performance. Miranda, a 19-year-old woman with spastic hemiplegia secondary to cerebral palsy, like Mrs. McCarthy, has limited use of one hand and uses a wheelchair for mobility. Miranda wants to cook simple meals and bake cookies. Her intervention will require more time and guidance than Mrs. McCarthy's intervention because Miranda has to learn basic cooking skills along with the activity adaptations to compensate for her impairments.

Many clients are faced with learning new activities, particularly skills needed to manage new impairments, such as performing self-catheterization, donning pressure garments, or learning to operate assistive technology. Whenever a skill is unfamiliar to a client, additional intervention time and education will be needed for basic skill acquisition and should be incorporated into the goal and the intervention plan.

Client's Capacity for Learning and Openness to Alternative Methods

The client's capacity for learning and openness to using alternative methods for task completion must be evaluated because intervention often requires learning new methods of completing activities (Flinn, 2014). Clients with limited learning capacity resulting from cognitive or affective impairments can still learn new skills if appropriate teaching approaches are used and the duration of the intervention is adequate (Davis, 2005). Some clients might resist intervention that incorporates adaptive equipment if they do not want to use a special device to do a task that most people do without a device (Lund & Nygård, 2003). Clients with a good capacity for learning and openness to alternative methods may be able to address more task deficits because of increased intervention options and the reduced time required for learning. It is important to view capacity for learning on a continuum; clients can fall between the extremes, and capacity might be better for some tasks than for others.

Clients' capacity for learning may also change as they progress through the rehabilitation process, particularly for clients with a new disability. The focus of learning should progress from more directive, therapist-initiated learning to client-initiated learning, where the client is more autonomous in identifying goals and directing his or her own learning (Greber et al., 2007; Jack & Estes, 2010). Autonomous learning strategies enable clients to solve problems long after therapy has ended and enables them to develop their own adaptive strategies. The ability to be an independent problem solver can be learned, so occupational therapists should structure intervention activities that promote self-directed learning whenever possible (Greber et al., 2007).

Projected Follow-Through With Program Outside of Direct Intervention

Efforts to contain healthcare costs have led to increasingly shorter lengths of stay in hospitals and rehabilitation centers and a reduction in outpatient and home health visits. Clients are expected to take an active role in their therapy programs and to supplement formal interventions with home programs (Novak et al., 2009). Goals therefore need to be established with some estimate of the client's capacity to follow through with a self-directed program because this may influence the success of an intervention (Radomski, 2011).

Several of the performance parameters that were previously described can give the OT practitioner guidance in this area. Clients have more motivation for programs aimed at activities that they highly value than at those that they do not value, making a client-centered approach critical for success (Doig et al., 2009, 2016). In addition, performance parameters such as difficulty, fatigue, pain, and satisfaction must be considered so that self-directed programs are manageable for the client. Manageability of the program must be determined by clients in consultation with the OT practitioner and should take into consideration clients' daily activities and responsibilities, tolerance for frustration, and perseverance.

Many clients require some assistance to practice activities, and the OT practitioner must be sure that these resources are available; for example, someone to set up an activity or provide assistance. Impairments can affect a client's ability to initiate or persevere with activities, so assistance may be needed for initiation and follow-through in the home program. OT practitioners need to interact with and educate caregivers about their critical role and home programs must accommodate caregiver needs.

Time for Intervention

The projected timeline for OT may be influenced by multiple factors, including the client's functional prognosis, motivation for improvement, and finances. In the United States, third-party payers vary in their reimbursement allowances for therapy visits, which can impact access to services and intervention outcomes (Arango-Lasprilla et al., 2010). Ongoing changes in Medicare impact services across settings such as outpatient rehabilitation (Simpson et al., 2015). OT goals must be tailored to meet a client's needs as much as possible within the time allotted. Nonetheless, it must also be recognized that best practice takes into account *all* the client's needs. OT practitioners need to be aware of their professional responsibility to clients to request intervention extensions and to support these requests through detailed documentation and to appeal payment denials for needed services (Gateley & Borcherding, 2017). They must also establish intervention timelines that meet the needs of the client, rather than the needs of the facility, which may benefit from providing services that extend beyond the client's needs or tolerance level.

Expected Discharge Context and Resources

Clients' expected discharge environments must be considered in establishing goals and selecting interventions that will be relevant to the environment in which clients will ultimately perform tasks (Law & Dunbar, 2007; Nakanishi et al., 2010). The expected environment is critical for clients who require assistance from others after discharge; that is, it is important to determine whether there are people who are willing and able to provide needed assistance. Clients' needs vary broadly in terms of the type and duration of assistance required. Some clients need only supportive services, such as help with shopping or housecleaning. Those with significant activity limitations and intact cognition might require considerable physical assistance but can be left alone once ADL have been completed, they have eaten, and they are mobile in their wheelchairs. Clients with cognitive impairments do not always need physical assistance but might need verbal cueing to initiate or sustain activities or to perform them in a safe manner. This assistance might be specific to certain tasks (e.g., when cooking or interacting with small children) or it may need to be constant. Inadequate support in the client's expected environment may necessitate a change in the discharge plan. Some families or friends might be able to provide the level and type of assistance needed, whereas others may not.

The physical environment must also be considered in setting realistic goals (Gitlin et al., 2001). For example, Mr. Feng has reached his goal of independence in bathing during his hospital-based rehabilitation. He requires a transfer tub seat, a handheld shower hose, and a grab bar to bathe safely without help (Figure 44.2). The OT practitioner wants to order this equipment for him. However, Mr. Feng reports that he must shower in a 4 × 4 ft shower stall because the only bathtub is on the second floor and he cannot manage stairs. His shower will not accommodate the transfer tub bench that he requires for safe transfers and balance during showering. An alternative bathing goal should have been established at the beginning of intervention so that Mr. Feng's program focused on developing skills he could use at home, such as sponge bathing at the sink.

The adaptability of the discharge environment must also be explored before setting goals. A house that is high above the street on a small lot with 21 steps to the front door makes the installation of a properly graded ramp impossible. Wall grab bars cannot be installed on some fiberglass tub surrounds, making a safety rail placed on the side of the bathtub the only feasible option regardless of where the client really needs the most support.

Established functional goals must also be achievable within the client's available resources, including property and financial resources. For example, clients living in rental units might be unable to make structural alterations as desired because they do not own the unit. Some individuals may benefit from equipment or devices that they cannot afford and are not covered by their third-party payer. This situation can result in a practice dilemma for the occupational therapist.

Last, all of the various places in which a client expects to function after discharge must be explored if activities are likely to be performed in more than one place. Clients in a hospital-based setting may be focused primarily on returning home, but most people do not confine themselves to a single environment. Adaptations for toilets, such as raised

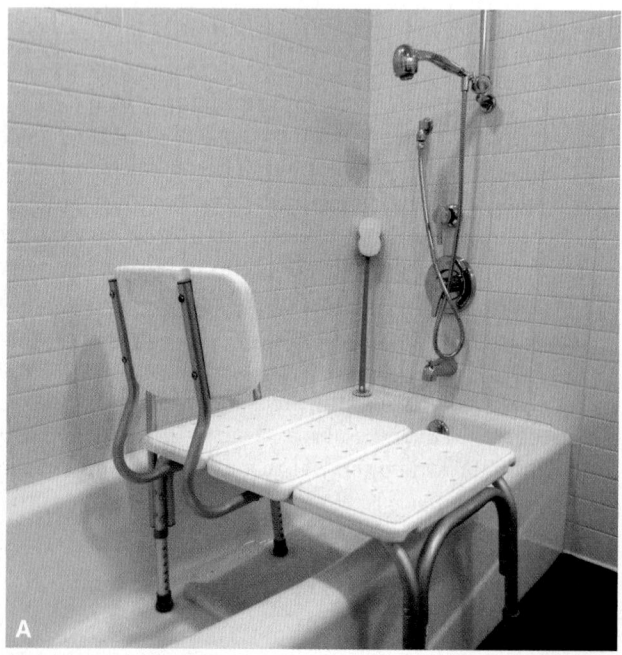
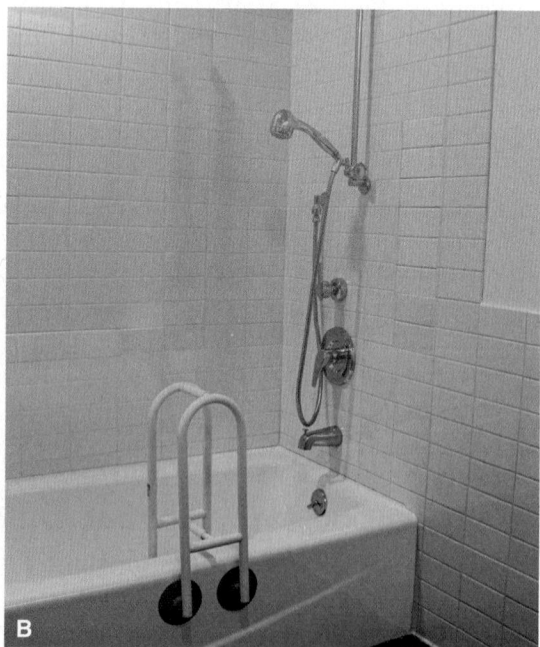

FIGURE 44.2 A transfer tub seat requires more space than Mr. Feng's small bathroom and shower can accommodate. Knowing the client's discharge environment can help practitioners determine interventions that will be successful after discharge.

toilet seats and toilet armrests, are commonly used for people with limited mobility. Home adaptations are easily made, but clients are often in environments that have not been adapted, such as public buildings, friends' homes, airplanes, hotels, and portable toilets at the local fair. If clients are likely to be in these environments, their goals should address their ability to perform tasks in varied settings.

Interventions for ADL and IADL Impairments

Interventions for ADL and IADL problems are based on clients' goals and involve selecting intervention approaches and activities, carrying out the intervention, and reviewing the intervention to ensure that it is effective in progressing clients toward their goals.

Planning and Implementing Intervention

Five approaches to intervention are described in the OTPF: create/promote, establish/restore, maintain, modify, and prevent (AOTA, 2020). Although all of these approaches can be used to support or enhance ADL and IADL performance, modify and establish/restore are the most commonly used in practice and will be the focus of intervention discussed in this chapter. Both modify and establish/restore approaches need to be combined with client and/or caregiver education to ensure carryover of the program to function in everyday life (Grajo & Boisselle, 2021). OT practitioners select specific intervention activities for clients that are guided by a range of theory-guided approaches, sometimes referred to as *frames of reference*. Specific OT approaches are beyond the scope of this chapter, but examples can be found in Unit VI, Broad Conceptual Models for Occupational Therapy Practice. The following subsection focuses on broader intervention approaches and related strategies and includes a discussion of client and caregiver education and strategies for grading activities to progress clients to the established goals.

Selecting an Intervention Approach

The OT practitioner considers several variables when deciding whether it is more appropriate to focus on compensating for a client's deficits through adaptation or restoring underlying skills needed to reach goals or a combination of both (Buzaid et al., 2013). These considerations are addressed in the sections that follow.

Modify. Activity performance can be enhanced through modifications that compensate for limitations rather than restore previous capacities. This is often necessary when

restoration is not an option. For example, a client with a complete C5 tetraplegia will not regain hand function regardless of the restorative approach used, so compensation is needed for successful participation in ADL and IADL. Even for clients for whom restoration is possible, a modified approach might be more appropriate if time limitations or client motivation would lead to less-than-optimal outcomes. Compensatory strategies may also be warranted when some, but not full, restoration of function is achieved. Generally, compensatory strategies require less intervention time for achieving functional outcomes compared with restorative strategies, although skilled intervention is warranted for selection and training in appropriate devices (Zanatta et al., 2017).

There are three general intervention strategies for compensation, which may be used alone or in combination: modify the activity or task method, modify the task objects, or modify the environment. Examples of these three intervention strategies for selected ADL and IADL are included in Table 44.3.

- *Modify the Task Method.* The task objects and contexts are unchanged, but the method of performing the task is altered to make the task feasible given the client's impairments. Many one-handed techniques for tasks that are normally done with two hands use this strategy, such as one-handed shoe tying (Figure 44.3) and one-handed typing techniques. Another example is minimizing tremors or ataxia by having a client stabilize their forearms on tabletops, armrests, or walls to improve hand coordination when performing a range of ADL (Gillen, 2000).

  To master an altered task successfully, clients require the capacity to learn. The necessary level of learning capacity depends on the complexity of the method that is to be learned (Grajo & Boisselle, 2021). OT practitioners should also attend to the level of automaticity clients may wish to achieve for specific ADL and IADL. People often rely on automatic processing for well-learned tasks, which means they require little direct attention. Automatic processing of routine tasks frees the individual for other things, such as planning one's workday while getting ready in the morning or chatting with a child during meal preparation. Practice is a necessary component of all learning and is especially crucial for clients who wish to develop or return to automatic performance of ADL or IADL. Clients benefit from follow-through with a training program that includes the practice and repetition needed to meet adequacy parameters, such as reducing difficulty and duration of performance and increasing satisfaction.

- *Modify the Task Objects or Prescribe Assistive Devices.* The objects that are used for the task may be adapted to facilitate performance. For example, handles can be built up on utensils for clients with decreased active finger ROM or training in the use of memory aids

TABLE 44.3	Examples of the Three Approaches to Modifying Tasks to Compensate for Impairments		
Task	**Modify the Task Method**	**Modify the Task Objects**	**Modify the Task Environment**
Bathing	Substitute washing at sink for someone unable to get in/out of the tub safely even with adaptive equipment.	Use a bath mitt and soap on a rope so that a person who cannot retrieve objects does not drop them.	Install grab bars and a transfer tub seat to enable a client to remain seated during bathing.
Grooming	Client stabilizes small containers with the ulnar digits and unscrews lids with the radial digits to compensate for loss of the use of one hand.	An extended handle is added to a razor so that a woman can shave her legs without bending forward.	A daily schedule is posted in the bathroom for a client with impaired attention to improve adherence to a daily grooming routine.
Toileting	Use an alarm watch to encourage regular emptying of the bladder.	Use a toilet aid to extend the range of reach for toilet hygiene.	Install a bidet to eliminate the need for manipulating toilet paper for hygiene.
Dressing	Learn to dress the affected side first to compensate for loss of use of one side of the body.	Use a sock aid to put socks on without having to reach the feet.	Lower clothing racks or replace a high dresser with a low one to increase access to clothes.
Feeding	Serve different food items (e.g., meat, starch, vegetable) in consistent places on the plate for someone who is blind.	Use a built-up handled utensil to compensate for diminished prehension in the hand.	Have a second grader with an attention disorder eat with a few friends in a small room rather than the loud and busy cafeteria.
Sexual activity	Identify alternate erogenous zones for a person without sensation in the genital area.	Use a vibrator for satisfying a female partner for a male partner with erectile dysfunction.	Provide bed rails or overhead trapeze to facilitate repositioning during sexual activity in bed.
Transfers	Sit first in the car seat before swinging the legs in rather than entering by leading with the leg.	Use a sliding board to eliminate the need for the lower extremities to support body weight.	Rearrange furniture to allow the wheelchair to be positioned near to the bed or a favorite chair.
Child care	Use safe lifting techniques when lifting a child out of a crib or onto a changing table.	Add a handle to a baby bottle to reduce finger grip needed to hold and position the bottle.	Install a wall-mounted changing table that allows for easy wheelchair access.
Caregiving for an adult	Change from showers to sponge baths to reduce the need for multiple transfers during morning care.	Use of a slip sheet to reduce friction when repositioning a person in bed.	Add high contrast stickers to the bottom of the tub to make the bottom visible and reduce fear of bathing for an adult with dementia.
Cooking	Sit at the kitchen table to chop vegetables to conserve energy.	Use a cutting board with aluminum nails to hold vegetables for cutting or peeling.	Install a mirror above the stove to enable a wheelchair user to see items cooking.
Driving	Enter the vehicle by sitting first then swinging the legs in.	Provide hand controls to compensate for paralysis of the legs.	Restrict driving to daylight or low-volume hours.
Shopping	Shift to online shopping to reduce the need for community mobility.	Purchase a walker basket for carrying items.	Request assistance from a grocery store employee to help reach items.

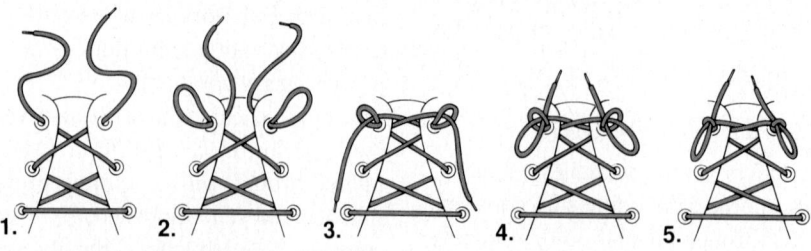

1. Lace laces in usual way.
2. Put both lace ends back through the holes they exited until the loops formed are small.
3. Put the lace ends through the opposite loops and pull to tighten loops, allowing just enough room to put the lace end back through the loop.
4. Put lace ends back through the loops, forming another loop.
5. Pull on these loops alternately to tighten.

FIGURE 44.3 One-handed shoe-tying method.

(e.g., checklists, cue cards, and electronic devices) may help clients who have difficulty initiating tasks (Gillen, 2009; specifically, Chapter 9). For some task adaptations, the task method does not change much, so the need for learning may be minimal. When this is the case, the need for practice is also reduced, and performance can improve quickly. Examples of simple adaptations include utensils with enlarged or extended handles, a cutting board with nails to stabilize food while cutting, and elastic shoelaces. Some adaptations, however, require more extensive training; for example, learning to drive with hand controls.

The prescription of assistive devices must take into account the client's capabilities and willingness to use the device as well as the features of the device. For example, a sock aid can help a client with poor sitting balance to reach her feet without leaning forward, which could throw her off balance. However, if the client's balance deficit is secondary to hemiplegia and she also has poor use of one hand, it will be very difficult or impossible for her to get the sock onto the sock aid, which typically requires both hands (Figure 44.4). Figure 44.5 depicts the number of decisions that an OT practitioner makes when selecting an adapted spoon, a very simple type of adaptive equipment.

One disadvantage of adapting task objects is that the adapted item must be available to clients whenever or wherever they engage in the task. This may pose a problem, depending on the task and the adaptation. Clients who rely on phone alerts to remember appointments have their adaptation within a device they would normally have with them throughout the day. If a client requires built-up utensils for eating, however, and wishes to eat at a restaurant, the utensils must be taken along. This is cumbersome, and some clients find it embarrassing.

Finally, some clients find that the use of adaptive equipment reduces satisfaction with task performance. To enhance personal satisfaction with task performance, they might be willing to cope with the increased difficulty of doing a task without adapted tools. For example, a man with multiple sclerosis, who finds that using a wheelchair for outdoor mobility reduces fatigue, may opt to walk if his desire to be ambulatory in public outweighs his desire to save energy.

- *Modify the Task Environment.* Modification of the environment itself may facilitate task performance (Carnemolla & Bridge, 2020; Szanton et al., 2019). Typically, when the environment is modified, the demand for learning and practice is less than that required for learning an alternative method or using adapted task objects. Environmental modifications are often fixed in place so that clients do not need to remember to bring along the necessary adaptations and the adaptations cannot be easily displaced (e.g., dropped out of reach). The task

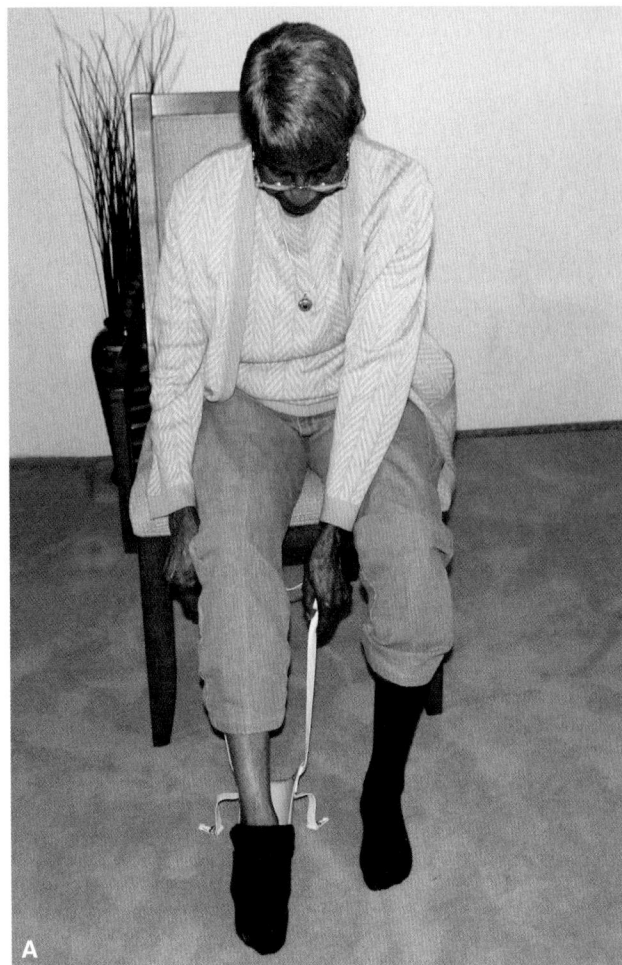

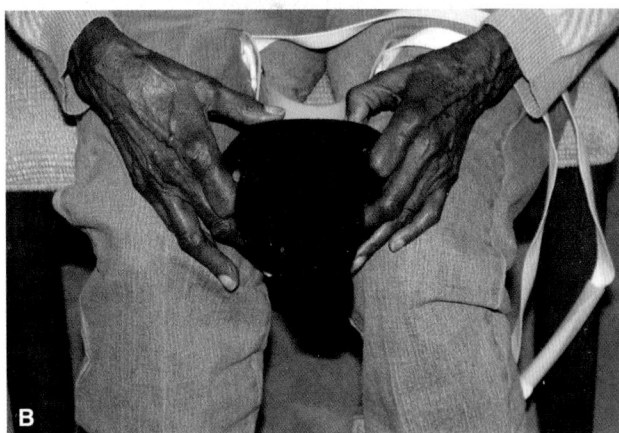

FIGURE 44.4 **A:** A sock aid is useful for people with limited reach, for example, from limited balance or range of motion. **B:** However, the client needs to have the use of both hands to get the sock onto the device, which could make it impractical for some clients.

method is often unchanged, or only minimally changed, so that clients can rely on previous experience. Examples include installing a wheelchair ramp, increasing available light, labeling cupboard doors to compensate for cognitive

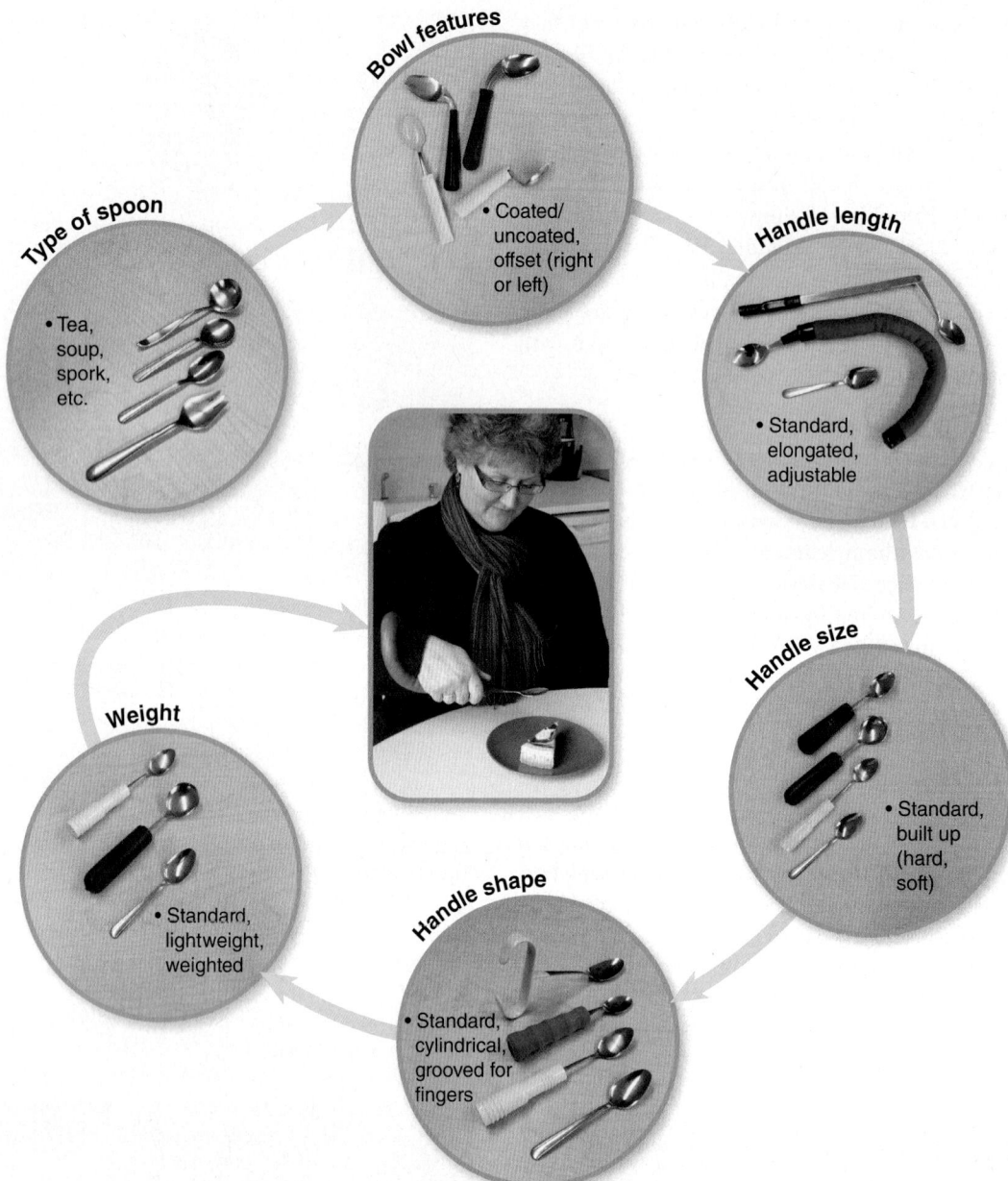

FIGURE 44.5 Potential decisions for prescribing an adapted spoon, a simple assistive device.

deficits, and installing a toilet seat frame (Figure 44.6) or provide modifications to a client's positioning equipment during sexual activity to maintain hip flexion after a total hip arthroplasty (Mohammed, 2017). Environmental control systems and now smart home technology are also environmental modifications that enable people to operate home electronics (e.g., computer, phone, lights, stereo, and television) and even open doors by using an accessible switch, user display, and a processor (Novaria et al., 2021).

The biggest drawback of environmental modifications is that clients might become limited in terms of performance context. They must do the task in the modified environment or in one that has been similarly modified because the modifications are not easily transportable and might be

custom designed for a specific setting. However, interprofessional practice between OT providers and architects in the area of community mobility and universal design holds promise for expanding the accessibility of built environments (AOTA, 2015; Welu & Naber, 2020).

Establish/Restore. An establish or restorative approach typically focuses intervention at the impairment level with the aim of restoring or establishing the capacities that are needed for functional tasks (AOTA, 2020), such as strength, endurance, ROM, short-term memory, visual scanning, and interests (Buzaid et al., 2013). More information about specific techniques can be found in the chapters in Unit V, Core Concepts and Skills. Regardless of the underlying theories or techniques used, one must always

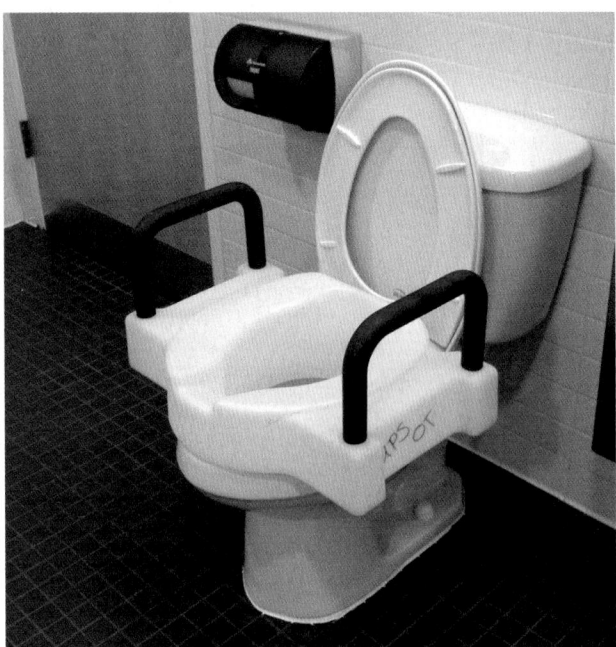

FIGURE 44.6 A toilet frame used to help the individual move between sitting and standing and to increase stability during transfers.

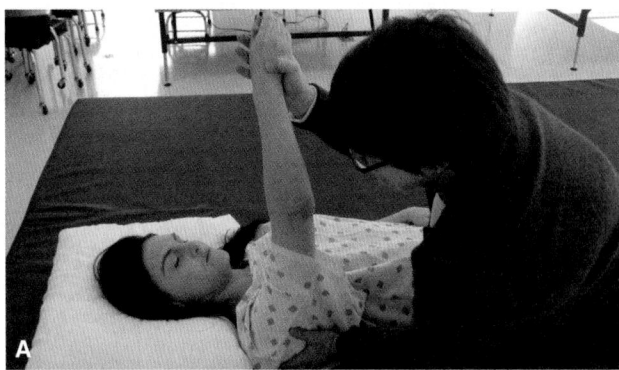

establish the link between the impairment and the resulting activity limitations. Careful documentation of the evaluation contributes to interprofessional collaboration by assisting other providers and third-party payers to understand the connection between the intervention and the established occupation-based outcomes (Gateley & Borcherding, 2017). Clients must be educated about the relationship between the capacities they are addressing in therapy and the occupations they support so that they understand how the intervention will ultimately lead to improved performance. Intervention must include opportunities to transfer new performance skills into everyday activities; for example, hanging laundry or pinning pictures on a bulletin board is a treatment activity that requires a client to use increased shoulder active ROM in a functional context (Figure 44.7). Table 44.4 includes additional examples.

Intervention that is aimed at establishing or restoring capacities is often most efficient for clients who have a few impairments that affect many tasks, and those impairments are expected to improve. For example, Mr. Stapinski, a 47-year-old, cisgender male, had circumferential burns to both upper extremities.

The resulting bilateral restrictions in elbow flexion prevented him from completing most ADL because he could not reach his face, head, or trunk. Tasks could be easily adapted by using long-handled devices, but extended tools would have been needed for many ADL tasks (e.g., eating utensils, toothbrush, comb, brush, and bath sponge). Because people with burns can usually regain passive ROM with stretching, scar management, and exercise, intervention aimed at increasing Mr. Stapinski's elbow flexion was

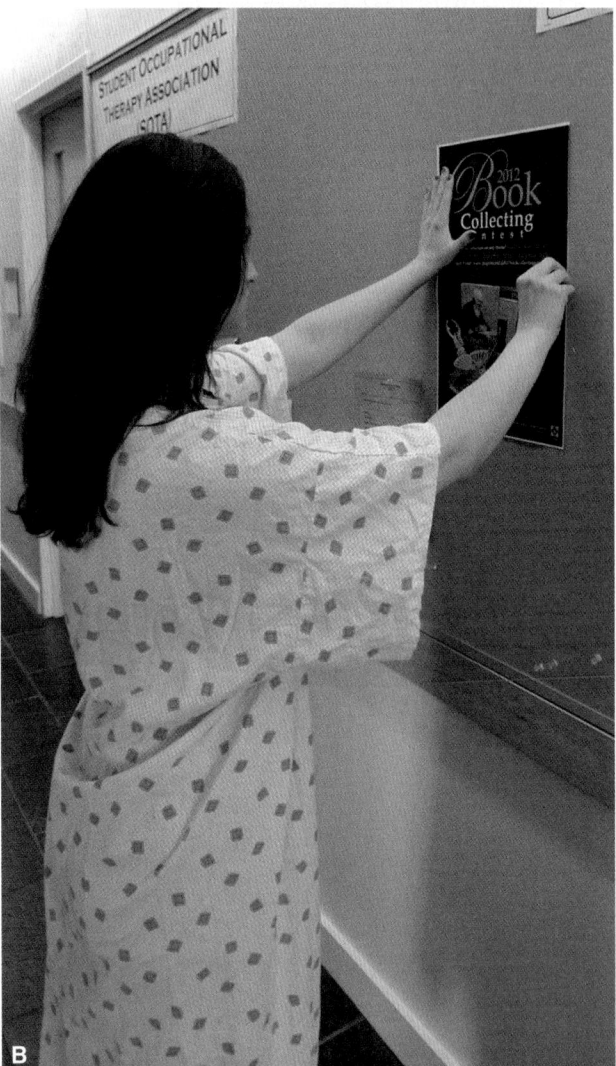

FIGURE 44.7 Stretching to restore passive range of motion (PROM) may be an effective treatment for improving reach **(A)**, but practitioners should be sure to incorporate PROM gains into occupation-based activities **(B)**.

most efficient. Adapting selected task objects improved his ADL performance in the short term; however, restoring Mr. Stapinski's capacity to flex his elbows enhanced function across many different tasks.

| TABLE 44.4 | Occupation as Means: Integrating an Establish/Restore Approach Into Functional Tasks |||

Impairment	Preparatory Activity to Reduce Impairment	Task to Integrate Gains Made Into ADL/IADL	Functional Outcomes
Impaired grip strength	Hand putty exercises	Cooking task with light resistance (e.g., stirring Jell-o) that progresses to more resistive tasks (e.g., brownies then cookies)	Increased ability to grasp task objects firmly (e.g., opening containers, doors, pulling up pants)
Decreased upper extremity muscle endurance	Using an arm ergometer	Wheelchair mobility, increasing time and difficulty (e.g., progress from flat surfaces to ramps)	Increased ability to engage in sustained upper extremity work (e.g., propelling a wheelchair, shampooing hair, washing windows)
Dyspnea	Practice diaphragmatic and pursed-lip breathing seated, doing nothing else.	Incorporate breathing techniques into seated ADL, progressing to standing and moving.	Ability to minimize dyspnea by improving oxygen intake during ADL and IADL
Hyperresponsiveness to tactile stimuli	Provide tactile desensitization activities	Progress from bathing in a tub to a shower, which provides a stronger stimulus.	Ability to tolerate tactile stimuli in everyday tasks including dressing, brushing teeth, and interacting with others
Anxiety in new situations	Practice progressive relaxation in a quiet place to reduce anxiety.	Use progressive relaxation in community outings with the therapist.	Ability to function effectively in new situations without experiencing excessive anxiety (e.g., job interview, cultural events, travel)

ADL, activities of daily living; IADL, instrumental activities of daily living.

For clients with some types of impairments, carefully selected and graded intervention activities can restore or establish capacities while simultaneously permitting the practice of the meaningful occupations. Clients with limited endurance resulting from deconditioning could do aerobic exercise to increase cardiopulmonary endurance, shifting to meaningful activities when an adequate increase in cardiopulmonary capacity is achieved. Instead, an intervention that graded the intensity and duration of daily activities could be as effective in increasing cardiovascular fitness while enabling the client to participate in desired tasks. For example, an individual with a spinal cord injury may benefit from graded interventions focused on increasing endurance to maximize sexual participation (Mohammed, 2017). Similarly, children and adults may engage more effectively in play or leisure activities that incorporate the necessary repetitive movements compared to a rote exercise (Melchert-McKearnan et al., 2000). Practice and participation in ADL and IADL programs also give clients with a new disability an opportunity to become familiar with their altered bodies (Guidetti et al., 2007) and may be more effective in overall outcomes, particularly in IADL (Orellano et al., 2012).

Depending on performance impairment, intervention time needed to establish or restore underlying skills may be longer than that required for compensatory approaches. This increased time must be considered, particularly for clients who have limited reimbursement for OT. In addition, clients must recognize that the rehabilitation period might be longer and that follow-through with a home program is vital if gains are to be made. Telehealth offers a possible means of follow-up with clients to support adherence with a home program and performance of health management

and maintenance activities among persons with chronic conditions (Arif et al., 2014; Schepens Niemiec et al., 2021).

Integrating Intervention for Impairments and Activity Limitations. A carefully crafted intervention plan may include both modify and establish/restore approaches to enable a client to be more functional through the use of compensatory strategies while at the same time working to restore underlying capacities (Buzaid et al., 2013). It is critical that the OT practitioner reduce the use of compensatory strategies as clients make gains in skill performance when using the two approaches.

For example, Mr. Stapinski, whose burns resulted in bilateral limitations in elbow flexion, might benefit from using utensils with extended handles to feed himself independently during the 2 to 3 weeks that it takes to increase his elbow flexion sufficiently for him to feed himself without these utensils. The extended handles should be fabricated to require him to flex fully within his available range and should be shortened as gains in passive ROM are made so that the new range is used whenever he feeds himself.

Whenever OT practitioners anticipate that task or environmental adaptations will be temporary, they must consider the cost in relation to the anticipated time the adaptations will be needed and the potential benefit to clients. Thermoplastic extensions can be added to the handles of regular utensils rather than prescribing the more costly commercially available utensils with elongated handles. Safety concerns, of course, supersede cost considerations. Using a collapsible lawn chair in the shower would be an inexpensive alternative to a shower chair, but it would not provide adequate stability for most clients.

Education of the Client or Caregiver

Instructional Methods. Various instructional methods are available for client and caregiver education (Greber et al., 2007), and methods should be selected that best meet the person's needs. When a facility has a client population with similar goals, group instruction can be an efficient method for education that also provides learning through peer interaction and problem-solving.

Individualized instruction is more appropriate for many clients and caregivers because the personal nature of many ADL is not conducive to group instruction. One-on-one client or caregiver education gives the OT practitioner immediate feedback from the person as the session progresses, so the amount and focus of learning can be adjusted accordingly. Similarly, parent and caregiver coaching using the Family Activity Adaptation Model (FAAM) (Osei & Dimitropoulou, 2019) that incorporates a teach-coach-review proccss is showing promise with early intervention involving intensive treatments (Eckberg Zylstra & Sidhu, 2021).

A vast array of media are available to facilitate the client's or caregiver's learning process. Written materials may be developed specifically for a client or caregiver, or published materials can be used if they meet the client's needs. Digital audio and visual recorders are usually available on the client's or caregiver's phone, and custom-made videos can be an effective teaching tool. The Internet contains a wealth of information about various disorders that is specifically geared toward clients and caregivers, or practitioners can develop and upload customized educational content to accessible sites, such as YouTube, as long as client confidentiality is maintained. Healthcare professionals, including occupational therapists, are using teleconferencing for educational purposes, for example, to engage in occupation-based coaching for parents of children with autism and cerebral palsy to increase children's participation in daily activities (Little et al., 2018; Osei & Dimitropoulou, 2021).

Care must be taken to assess the match between client and caregiver skills and the educational content. For example, adults living in developed countries have mean reading skills that range from fifth to eighth grade, so written materials should be designed with these literacy levels in mind in order to improve clients' learning (McKenna & Scott, 2007). When working with older adults, there is evidence to support the effectiveness of using narrative formats (Koops van't Jagt et al., 2016). More information on client education can be found in Chapter 41.

COMMENTARY ON THE EVIDENCE

Client Learning

Finding the Best Educational Strategies for Client Learning

As individual therapy time in the United States has been reduced by third-party reimbursement plans, client and caregiver education has played a more important role in intervention. Many studies have demonstrated the effectiveness of different and varied educational programs. For example, patient education programs have been effective in improving self-management and reducing pain and disability for people with rheumatoid arthritis (Siegel et al., 2017), reducing the impact of fatigue in people with chronic conditions (Van Heest et al., 2017), and increasing fall threats knowledge and fall prevention behaviors in older adults (Schepens et al., 2011). Eklund and colleagues (2004) compared a health education program for people who have visual impairment with traditional individualized intervention and reported that participants in the health education program had higher perceived security for several ADL and IADL. Researchers typically describe the educational programs used in their studies, and the educational methods reported vary significantly. Although there is ample research to support the efficacy of patient education programs on client outcomes, few studies were found that compared varied educational approaches for clients to identify best practice in this area. For example, research on group intervention that includes active participation, collaborative problem-solving, and learning tasks that relate to a current, relevant problem seem to be more effective in equipping clients with tools needed to meet challenges in the future (Eklund & Dahlin-Ivanoff, 2006). A systematic review looking at health literacy among older adults found strong evidence for the use of narrative formats and/or multiple-feature revisions (textual and visual characteristics) for the comprehensibility of health-related documents (Koops van't Jagt et al., 2016). Learning is a complex process, and factors such as motivation and authenticity of training should be addressed in planning learning experiences (Schepens et al., 2011). Many educational programs are aimed at changing clients' habits, such as engaging in home exercise programs or incorporating energy conservation techniques into daily activities, which require behavioral approaches for supporting the development of new habits and follow-up studies to examine program effectiveness (Mathiowetz et al., 2007). Future research should also examine the impact of varied impairments on the effectiveness of education, for example, problems with initiation, attention, or executive function. Gathering additional evidence will enable practitioners to become even more effective in helping clients to reach their goals (see Chapters 33 and 53).

Caregiver Training. Caregiver training may be implemented to maximize a client's functional outcome (Buzaid et al., 2013; Chard et al., 2009; DiZazzo-Miller et al., 2017) while minimizing the efforts of the caregiver (Dooley & Hinojosa, 2004). For example, Alex had a stroke and required minimal physical assistance with verbal cues for wheelchair transfers. Alex's partner was physically fit but had no experience assisting a person with transfers. One day, Alex's partner decided to help Alex move from the hospital bed to the chair. The partner had seen it done but did not know some of the important strategies, so they both fell onto the bed. No one was hurt but Alex's partner was distraught as they thought that they would not be able to care for Alex at home and Alex would have to go to a nursing home. The partner was open to transfer training from the OT practitioner and delighted to find that by using specific physical and verbal techniques, they could easily and safely assist Alex. In this example, caregiver training increased the client's level of independence and the probability that Alex could go home at discharge.

Like clients, caregivers have varied learning styles, capacities, and experience. In many situations, the caregiver is a family member who is still coping with the emotional impact of having a family member with a disability, whether a new parent with a child with cerebral palsy or the spouse of someone who has had a stroke. Caregivers experiencing emotional stress have impaired learning and memory (Mackenzie et al., 2009) and often need more time and repetition to process information accurately. In other cases, caregivers have been providing care for years and bring a wealth of caring expertise to the OT session. The OT practitioner should work collaboratively with all caregivers but may move into a more consultative role with experienced caregivers who can articulate problems and engage actively in problem-solving based on prior learning (Toth-Cohen, 2000). When caregivers must assist clients physically, their physical capacity for providing this assistance also warrants evaluation, and training must match their physical capacity.

When caregivers are helping to carry out an intervention program, the goals and general intervention strategies should be made clear to them (McKenna & Scott, 2007). Likewise, caregivers view communication as a primary method for receiving to assist with decision-making and advocacy (Harper et al., 2021). Caregivers are often pivotal in motivating clients. Spurring clients on who have disorders that impact motivation, such as depression, can be particularly challenging. Helping caregivers to understand that disinterest and lack of motivation are a part of the disorder, and providing concrete strategies for managing the "getting going" phase of the home program will foster its success (Resnick, 1998). For clients with behavior problems, such as the reactions that may accompany autism or Alzheimer disease, teaching caregivers behavior management strategies that prevent or defuse potentially volatile situations can be invaluable to their success as caregivers.

When caregivers need to provide physical assistance, they should be trained in using proper body mechanics, especially during transfers or bed mobility and for wheelchair positioning. Hinojosa and Rittman (2009) found that caregivers with greater educational needs were more likely to have sustained a physical injury, suggesting that caregiver education may reduce the risk of injury. Taking care of the caregiver is frequently overlooked in OT, but it is an essential component of the person-task-environment transaction, particularly when it is anticipated that the client will require assistance over a long period of time.

Grading the Intervention Program

It is important to progress the client continually toward established intervention goals and to set new goals as initial goals are met. The specific means of grading intervention when a restoration approach is being implemented depends on the impairments and the intervention strategies that are being used (Grabanski & Janssen, 2021). If the intervention plan blends establish/restore and modify/adapt approaches, the program can be graded by reducing the amount of task and environmental adaptations as clients' capacities are restored.

Grading Task Progression From Easier to Harder. One means of grading an intervention program is to begin with easier ADL or IADL tasks and progress to more difficult ones. Task difficulty will be relative to a client's activity limitations and underlying impairments. For example, paying bills might be relatively easy for a client with tetraplegia to perform once the use of a writing tool is mastered, whereas lower extremity dressing is much more difficult. Conversely, a client with an acquired brain injury who has significant cognitive impairment but relatively preserved motor skills is likely to find lower extremity dressing to be relatively easy but money management extremely difficult.

Increasing Complexity Within the Task. Rather than progressing only from easier to harder activities, intervention may also be graded by increasing the complexity within an activity or by progressing from simple to more complex ways of doing it. Cooking skills might extend from simple preparations such as cold sandwiches to more complex, multiple-course dinners. Even seemingly simple tasks can often be graded. A sock-donning intervention, for example, might be scaled from using looser ankle socks to tighter knee socks and finally to tight antiembolic hose.

Same Task in Varied Performance Environments. A critical part of a graded intervention program involves progression from the intervention environment to the real-life environment. This can involve transfer from a clinic to a home setting or the more subtle dynamics associated with the transfer of help from the OT practitioner to the natural caregiver. The client who is independent in donning a jacket while sitting on a mat table in the clinic might be unable to do so when sitting on a chair with a back or when standing. Providing practice in increasingly demanding performance environments can facilitate the generalization of skills, thereby enhancing the client's functional flexibility.

Therapist-Facilitated to Client-Facilitated Problem-Solving.

Clients with permanent disabilities or chronic diseases must develop problem-solving skills in order to meet new challenges in their lives after discharge from OT services. Initially, when facing a new task or becoming familiar with a changed body or mind, therapists may use explicit instruction or demonstration to help clients learn new approaches to ADL and IADL. Intervention can be graded by engaging the client in problem-solving, for example, by asking a client who is a new wheelchair user to come up with strategies for traveling after completing more direct training in community mobility in a familiar setting. See OT Story 44.2 for an example of intervention planing for Diego who is diagnosed with COVID-19.

OT STORY 44.2 INTERVENTIONS FOR ADL IMPAIRMENTS RESULTING FROM COVID-19 INFECTION

Diego is a 43-year-old, cisgender, male, with no past medical history who in March 2020 was diagnosed with COVID-19 at a community health clinic. Diego is from El Salvador and communicates using Spanish predominantly, however has some fluency in English. He was managing well at home until 9 days after his diagnosis, when he began experiencing shortness of breath and went to the emergency department. He was initially placed on 2 liters per minute (LPM) nasal cannula (NC) supplemental oxygen. A few hours later, he was transitioned to 50 LPM, 50% fraction of inspired oxygen via high-flow NC and admitted to the intensive care unit (ICU), where he was ultimately intubated because of hypoxemic respiratory failure. Diego remained hospitalized for 42 days and required mechanical ventilation, proning, and sedation for the first 27 days. Despite maximal medical intervention, Diego needed to be placed on femorally cannulated venous-venous extracorporeal membrane oxygenation as a result of refractory hypoxemia (Mannion & Sullivan, 2021).

On hospital Day 35, Diego underwent surgical tracheostomy and placement of a percutaneous endoscopic gastrostomy (PEG) tube. After weaning off sedation, his neurologic examination was notable for diffuse weakness, with his right side more affected than his left. He was diagnosed with myopathy and unspecified cerebrovascular disease resulting from COVID-19 infection. He received OT and PT services twice per week during the last 15 days of his hospitalization. He continued to require a high level of medical care and was transferred to a long-term acute care hospital (LTACH) for medical management and rehabilitation.

Upon evaluation, it was noted that Diego had the following precautions for therapy consideration: contact and isolation precautions because of respiratory infection, Stage 2 occipital wound, heart rate parameter <150 beats per minute (BPM), oxygen (O_2) saturation parameter ≥90%, and multiple lines (i.e., tracheostomy, PEG, peripherally inserted central catheter in his right upper extremity, rectal tube, indwelling urinary catheter, cardiac telemetry, and peripheral O_2 monitoring). A video-based Spanish interpreter was used for the evaluation via an iPad provided by the LTACH.

Diego was found to be alert and oriented to person, place, and month and year and grossly oriented to situation. He was tearful and verbalized feeling anxious about the transition out of the hospital. He performed grooming and upper body ADL tasks at bed level with maximal assistance and required total assistance for all other ADLs. Because of the aspiration risk, he was unable to eat anything by mouth and received all of his nutritional needs via the PEG tube. He tolerated sitting at the edge of the bed with one person assisting; however, his heart rate elevated to 152 BPM, and he was significantly fatigued afterward, requiring return to supine.

Further assessment results indicated impaired ability to perform self-care activities, decreased hand strength, and decreased fine motor control compared to age-matched norms. Primary barriers to performance were identified as strict isolation precautions; tracheostomy; impaired hemodynamic response to activity; language barrier; pressure wound to occiput; impaired body functions; fluctuating anxiety; and the psychosocial effects of prolonged hospitalization, sedation, and isolation (Mannion & Sullivan, 2021).

Occupational Profile

Diego lives in the city of Chicago with his mother and brother in a single-level apartment with two flights of stairs to enter. They had no previous experience using durable medical equipment. Diego emigrated to the United States from El Salvador approximately 15 years ago. He works as a porter 5 to 6 days per week. He has an active role in his community church, and prayer is a strong source of spiritual strength. Diego enjoys exercising, spending time outside, and playing the guitar. He was independent in all basic ADLs and IADLs before admission. Diego's family was very involved and willing to provide as much assistance as Diego needed; however, Diego stated that he was not comfortable with family assistance for personal care (Mannion & Sullivan, 2021).

Intervention Plan and Goals

The occupational therapist collaborated with Diego and established client-centered goals with strong consideration

OT STORY 44.2 INTERVENTIONS FOR ADL IMPAIRMENTS RESULTING FROM COVID-19 INFECTION (continued)

of Diego's supporting and inhibiting factors: Diego' values, roles, and routines; and his estimated length of stay. The occupational therapist also used standardized assessment scores for enhanced objectivity and measurability when formulating the following goals:

- Perform ADL routines independently
- Demonstrate improved hand strength and fine motor control for self-feeding and simulated violin playing
- Complete medication management with minimal assistance from family (Mannion & Sullivan, 2021).

Intervention

Diego participated in 1:1, in-person, OT treatment sessions 3 days/week for 5 weeks. The occupational therapist used a video interpreter via the facility-issued iPad for all intervention sessions.

Activity modification, use of compensatory treatment strategies, and client-caregiver education were integral to Diego's care. During the initial phase of Diego's intervention, treatment focused on improving independence with ADL routines, including grooming, bathing, dressing, and toileting initially emphasizing a modify/adapt approach. With increased time out of bed, Diego's vital signs stabilized, and his cardiopulmonary endurance improved, resulting in increased ability to participate in seated ADL routines. Diego progressed to transfers using a rolling walker for toileting and was able to complete bathing and dressing while seated. Blocked practice for grooming, bathing, and dressing, as well as overall activity tolerance exercises, energy conservation strategies, and positioning were also incorporated. Diego progressed to modified independent ADL routines (Mannion & Sullivan, 2021).

Diego had bilateral upper extremity (BUE) weakness, with the proximal joints being weaker than the distal joints, resulting in difficulty with self-feeding. The occupational therapist provided Diego with proximal stabilization at the elbows, a right-wrist cockup splint, built-up spoon, and scoop dish. By modifying the task objects, Diego was able to feed himself 20% of his meal with increased time and moderate assistance. The occupational therapist reassessed Diego's BUE strength biweekly with manual muscle testing and a manual dynamometer to ensure appropriate gradation of exercises.

As Diego's strength and skills improved, he was able to feed himself at a modified independent level by rehab Day 22 and perform self-feeding without adaptations by rehab Day 32.

Using a variety of instructional methods, the occupational therapist educated Diego and his family members on potential adaptive equipment and its use, as well as medication management. The occupational therapist introduced Diego and his family members to different types of medication management systems to compensate for his ongoing short-term memory impairments. Diego verbalized his preference to use his smartphone and with the occupational therapist's assistance Diego was able to use a smartphone app to track and manage his medication without making errors.

Outcomes

Diego participated in 5 weeks of inpatient OT, PT, and speech therapy. Diego demonstrated improvement on all outcome measures and met his stated long-term goals. At discharge, he was able to complete basic ADLs at a modified independent level and used a rolling walker for functional transfers. He was able to self-feed all meals independently and simulate playing the guitar at a seated level for up to 5 minutes. His family verbalized understanding of adaptive equipment recommendations and plan of care for community reentry. On rehab Day 36 he was discharged home with orders for home health services to include OT, PT, and speech therapy (Mannion & Sullivan, 2021).

Questions

1. Identify the ADL/IADL the therapist modified and determine if the modification is the result of modifying the task object, modifying the task method, or modifying the task environment.
2. Describe the role of caregiver education in intervention to assist Diego with medication management.
3. Describe how you would grade the intervention activities to progress Diego toward independence in playing the guitar.

Source: Medical data for this OT Story was adapted from Mannion, N., & Sullivan, N. (2021). Occupational therapy for functional impairments resulting from COVID-19 infection: A case report. *American Journal of Occupational Therapy, 75*(Suppl. 1), 7511210040. https://doi.org/10.5014/ajot.2021.049215

Intervention Review: Reevaluation to Monitor Effectiveness

The ADL and IADL are evaluated on entry to OT to provide a measure of the client's baseline performance status. Regardless of the extent and length of the intervention, reevaluation of ADL and IADL performance is needed to ascertain whether the intervention is resulting in improvement, whether the intervention should be continued or changed, or whether maximal benefit from OT has been achieved and activity performance has reached a plateau (AOTA, 2020). OT practitioners routinely engage in informal review of interventions by observing clients' performance during intervention and considering the actual or potential impact of their performance on established goals.

Periodically, a more formal intervention reevaluation is needed to objectively measure clients' progress toward goals and to document progress in clinical records. The best strategy for reevaluation is to readminister the same assessments done in the initial evaluation, which enhances the possibility of detecting change in the client's performance attributable to intervention. If the reevaluation assessments vary from a prior evaluation, the potential for detecting change is reduced. For example, if ADL performance is assessed initially by self-report but is reassessed with a performance-based measure, differences in level of assistance may reflect an actual change in performance or simply differing views of the client and the therapist.

Conclusion

This chapter described the OT process for clients with ADL and IADL performance problems. Performance parameters of value, independence, safety, and adequacy were reviewed, and their relevance to the selection of specific assessment methods was described. Occupational therapists should establish objective baseline measures through the use of standardized ADL and IADL assessments whenever possible; however, the realities of the intervention setting may also require the use of nonstandardized assessment methods. Developing objective goals that address all relevant performance parameters is a crucial first step in implementing intervention by providing a "road map" for guiding client care. General approaches that occupational therapists use to increase participation in ADL and IADL include modifying the task or environment, establishing or restoring underlying impairments, and providing client and caregiver education. Grading activities effectively will maximize clients' progress toward goals. Specific intervention activities vary significantly according to the clients' ages and disabilities and are beyond the scope of this chapter. Readers should use this chapter to guide them in the overall process of ADL and IADL intervention and refer to sources that focus on specific client populations and service delivery models when selecting specific intervention activities.

Acknowledgments

Jennifer Pitonyak thanks Dr. Anne Birge James for inviting her to coauthor the previous edition of the ADL/IADL chapter for *Willard & Spackman's Occupational Therapy, 13th edition,* and acknowledges the contributions and continued influences of Dr. Margo B. Holm and Dr. Joan Rogers on the thinking in this chapter. Both authors also wish to thank clients, students, and colleagues who posed for photographs.

Lippincott® Connect *For additional resources on the subjects discussed in this chapter, visit Lippincott Connect. See* **Appendix II, Table of assessments** *for more ADL and IADL Assessments.*

REFERENCES

American Occupational Therapy Association. (2015). Standards of practice for occupational therapy. *American Journal of Occupational Therapy, 69,* Article e6913410057. https://doi.org/10.5014/ajot.2015.696S06

American Occupational Therapy Association. (2020). Occupational therapy practice framework: Domain and process (4th ed.). *American Journal of Occupational Therapy, 74*(Suppl. 2), 7412410010. https://doi.org/10.5014/ajot.2020.74S2001

Arango-Lasprilla, J. C., Ketchum, J. M., Cifu, D., Hammond, F., Castillo, C., Nicholls, E., Watanabe, T., Lequerica, A., & Deng, X. (2010). Predictors of extended rehabilitation length of stay after traumatic brain injury. *Archives of Physical Medicine and Rehabilitation, 91,* 1495–1504. https://doi.org/10.1016/j.apmr.2010.07.010

Archenholtz, B., & Dellhag, B. (2008). Validity and reliability of the instrument Performance and Satisfaction in Activities of Daily Living (PS-ADL) and its clinical applicability to adults with rheumatoid arthritis. *Scandinavian Journal of Occupational Therapy, 15,* 13–22. https://doi.org/10.1080/11038120701223165

Arif, M. J., El Emary, I. M., & Koutsouris, D. D. (2014). A review on the technologies and services used in the self-management of health and independent living of elderly. *Technology and Health Care, 22,* 677–687. https://doi.org/10.3233/THC-140851

Árnadóttir, G. (1990). *The brain and behavior: Assessing cortical dysfunction through activities of daily living.* Mosby Elsevier.

Árnadóttir, G. (2011). Impact of neurobehavioral deficits on activities of daily living. In G. Gillen (Ed.), *Stroke rehabilitation: A function-based approach* (3rd ed., pp. 456–500). Mosby Elsevier.

Ashley, M. J., Persel, C. S., & Clark, M. C. (2001). Validation of an independent living scale for post-acute rehabilitation applications. *Brain Injury, 15,* 435–442. https://doi.org/10.1080/02699050118777

Baron, K., Kielhofner, G., Iyenger, A., Goldhammer, V., & Wolenski, J. (2006). The occupational self-assessment (version 2.2). Model of Human Occupation Clearinghouse.

Bédard, M., Parkkari, M., Weaver, B., Riendeau, J., & Dahlquist, M. (2010). Brief report—Assessment of driving performance using a simulator protocol: Validity and reproducibility. *American Journal of Occupational Therapy, 64,* 336–340. https://doi.org/10.5014/ajot.64.2.336

Bonikowsky, S., Musto, A., Suteu, K. A., MacKenzie, S., & Dennis, D. (2012). Independence: An analysis of a complex and core construct in occupational therapy. *British Journal of Occupational Therapy, 75,* 188–195. https://doi.org/10.4276/030802212X13336366278176

Bottari, C., Dutil, E., Dassa, C., & Rainville, C. (2006). Choosing the most appropriate environment to evaluate independence in everyday activities: Home or clinic? *Australian Occupational Therapy Journal, 53,* 98–106. https://doi.org/10.1111/j.1440-1630.2006.00547.x

Brown, C. L., & Finlayson, M. L. (2013). Performance measures rather than self-report measures of functional status predict home care use in community-dwelling older adults. *Canadian Journal of Occupational Therapy, 80,* 284–294. https://doi.org/10.1177/0008417413501467

Buzaid, A., Dodge, M. P., Handmacher, L., & Kiltz, P. J. (2013). Activities of daily living: Evaluation and treatment in persons with multiple sclerosis. *Physical Medicine and Rehabilitation Clinics of North America, 24,* 629–638. https://doi.org/10.1016/j.pmr.2013.06.008

Carnemolla, P., & Bridge, C. (2020). A scoping review of home modification interventions—Mapping the evidence base. *Indoor and Built Environment, 29,* 299–310. https://doi.org/10.1177/1420326X18761112

Centers for Disease Control and Prevention. (2015). *Perceived exertion (Borg Rating of Perceived Exertion Scale).* https://www.cdc.gov/physicalactivity/basics/measuring/exertion.htm

Chard, G., Liu, L., & Mulholland, S. (2009). Verbal cueing and environmental modifications: Strategies to improve engagement in occupations in persons with Alzheimer's disease. *Physical & Occupational Therapy in Geriatrics, 27,* 197–211. https://doi.org/10.1080/02703180802206280

Chisholm, D., Toto, P., Raina, K., Holm, M., & Rogers, J. (2014). Evaluating capacity to live independently and safely in the community: Performance Assessment of Self-care Skills. *British Journal of Occupational Therapy, 77,* 59–66. https://doi.org/10.4276/030802214X13916969447038

Chuang, I. C., Hsu, W. C., Chen, C. L., Wu, Y. R., Chiau, H. Y., & Wu, C. Y. (2020). Psychometric evaluation of an ICF-based instrumental activities of daily living assessment with older adults with cognitive decline. *American Journal of Occupational Therapy, 74,* Article e7406205050. https://doi.org/10.5014/ajot.2020.039354

Clarke, C. E., Furmston, A., Morgan, E., Patel, S., Sackley, C., Walker, M., Bryan, S., & Wheatley, K. (2009). Pilot randomized controlled trial of occupational therapy to optimize independence in Parkinson's disease: The PD OT trial. *Journal of Neurology, Neurosurgery, & Psychiatry, 80,* 976–978. https://doi.org/10.1136/jnnp.2007.138586

Cohen-Mansfield, J., & Jensen, B. (2007). Adequacy of spouses as informants regarding older persons' self-care practices and their perceived importance. *Families, Systems, & Health, 25,* 53–67. https://doi.org/10.1037/1091-7527.25.1.53

Covinsky, K. E., Lindquist, K., Dunlop, D. D., & Yelin, E. (2009). Pain, functional limits, and aging. *Journal of the American Geriatric Society, 57,* 1556–1561. https://doi.org/10.1111/j.1532-5415.2009.02388.x

das Nair, R., Moreton, B. J., & Lincoln, N. B. (2011). Rasch analysis of the Nottingham Extended Activities of Daily Living Scale. *Journal of Rehabilitation Medicine, 43,* 944–950. https://doi.org/10.2340/16501977-0858

Davis, L. A. (2005). Educating individuals with dementia: Perspectives for rehabilitation professionals. *Topics in Geriatric Rehabilitation, 21,* 304–314. https://doi.org/10.1097/00013614-200510000-00007

DiZazzo-Miller, R., Winston, K., Winkler, S. L., & Donovan, M. L. (2017). Family Caregiver Training Program (FCTP): A randomized controlled trial. *American Journal of Occupational Therapy, 71,* Article e7105190010. https://doi.org/10.5014/ajot.2017.022459

Doig, E., Fleming, J., Cornwell, P. L., & Kuipers, P. (2009). Qualitative exploration of a client-centered, goal-directed approach to community-based occupational therapy for adults with traumatic brain injury. *American Journal of Occupational Therapy, 63,* 559–568. https://doi.org/10.5014/ajot.63.5.559

Doig, E., Prescott, S., Fleming, J., Cornwell, P., & Kuipers, P. (2016). Reliability of the Client-Centeredness of Goal Setting(C–COGS) scale in acquired brain injury rehabilitation. *American Journal of Occupational Therapy, 70,* 7004290010. https://doi.org/10.5014/ajot.2016.017046

Dooley, N. R., & Hinojosa, J. (2004). Improving quality of life for persons with Alzheimer's disease and their family caregivers: Brief occupational therapy intervention. *American Journal of Occupational Therapy, 58,* 561–569. https://doi.org/10.5014/ajot.58.5.561

Dudgeon, B. J., Tyler, E. J., Rhodes, L. A., & Jensen, M. P. (2006). Managing usual and unexpected pain with physical disability: A qualitative analysis. *American Journal of Occupational Therapy, 60,* 92–103. https://doi.org/10.5014/ajot.60.1.92

Dunn, W. (2017). Measurement concepts and practices. In M. Law, C. Baum, & W. Dunn (Eds.), *Measuring occupational performance: Supporting best practice in occupational therapy* (3rd ed., pp. 17–28). SLACK.

Eckberg Zylstra, S., & Sidhu, A. (2021). Use of a caregiver coaching model for implementation of intensive motor training for hemiplegic cerebral palsy: A case study. *The Open Journal of Occupational Therapy, 9*(3), 1–11. https://doi.org/10.15453/2168-6408.1839

Edwards, D. F., Wolf, T. J., Marks, T., Alter, S., Larkin, V., Padesky, B. L., Spiers, M., Al-Heizan, M. O., & Giles, G. M. (2019). Reliability and validity of a functional cognition screening tool to identify the need for occupational therapy. *American Journal of Occupational Therapy, 73*(2), e7302205050p1–7302205050p10. https://doi.org/10.5014/ajot.2019.028753

Egan, M., & Dubouloz, C.-J. (2014). Practical foundations: For practice: Planning, guiding, documenting and reflecting. In M. V. Radomski & C. A. Trombly Latham (Eds.), *Occupational therapy for physical dysfunction* (7th ed., pp. 24–49). Lippincott Williams & Wilkins.

Eklund, K., & Dahlin-Ivanoff, S. (2006). Health education for people with macular degeneration: Learning experiences and the effect on daily occupation. *Canadian Journal of Occupational Therapy, 73,* 272–280. https://doi.org/10.2182/cjot.06.004

Eklund, K., Sonn, U., & Dahlin-Ivanoff, S. (2004). Long-term evaluation of a health education programme for elderly persons with visual impairment. A randomized study. *Disability and Rehabilitation, 26,* 401–409. https://doi.org/10.1080/09638280410001662950

Eklund, M., & Gunnarsson, A. B. (2008). Content validity, clinical utility, sensitivity to change and discriminant ability of the Swedish Satisfaction with Daily Occupations (SDO) instrument: A screening tool for people with mental disorders. *British Journal of Occupational Therapy, 71,* 487–495. https://doi.org/10.1177/030802260807101106

Esposito, F., Gendolla, G. H., & Van der Linden, M. (2014, May). Are self-efficacy beliefs and subjective task demand related to apathy in aging? *Aging & Mental Health, 18*(4): 521–530. https://doi.org/10.1080/13607863.2013.856865

Eyres, L., & Unsworth, C. A. (2005). Occupational therapy in acute hospitals: The effectiveness of a pilot program to maintain occupational performance in older clients. *Australian Occupational Therapy Journal, 52,* 218–224. https://doi.org/10.1111/j.1440-1630.2005.00498.x

Flinn, N. A. (2014). Learning. In M. V. Radomski & C. A. Trombly Latham (Eds.), *Occupational therapy for physical dysfunction* (7th ed., pp. 394–411). Lippincott Williams & Wilkins.

Garratt, S., & Pond, D. (2014). Person-centred comprehensive geriatric assessment. In R. Nay, S. Garratt & D. Fetherstonhaugh (Eds.), *Older people: Issues and innovations in care* (p. 223). Elsevier.

Gateley, C., & Borcherding, S. (2017). *Documentation manual for writing SOAP notes in occupational therapy* (4th ed.). SLACK.

Gift, A. G., & Narsavage, G. (1998). Validity of the numeric rating scale as a measure of dyspnea. *American Journal of Critical Care, 7,* 200–204. https://doi.org/10.4037/ajcc1998.7.3.200

Giles, G. M., Edwards, D. F., Morrison, M. T., Baum, C., & Wolf, T. J. (2017). Health policy perspectives—Screening for functional cognition in postacute care and the Improving Medicare Post-Acute Care Transformation (IMPACT) Act of 2014. *American Journal of Occupational Therapy, 71,* Article e7105090010. https://doi.org/10.5014/ajot.2017.715001

Gillen, G. (2000). Improving activities of daily living performance in an adult with ataxia. *American Journal of Occupational Therapy, 54,* 89–96. https://doi.org/10.5014/ajot.54.1.89

Gillen, G. (2009). *Cognitive and perceptual rehabilitation: Optimizing function.* Mosby Elsevier.

Gitlin, L. N., Corcoran, M., Winter, L., Boyce, A., & Hauck, W. W. (2001). A randomized, controlled trial of a home environmental intervention: Effect on efficacy and upset in caregivers and on daily function of persons with dementia. *Gerontologist, 41,* 4–14. https://doi.org/10.1093/geront/41.1.4

Goverover, Y., Chiaravalloti, N., Gaudino-Goering, E., Moore, N., & DeLuca, J. (2009). The relationship among performance of instrumental activities of daily living, self-report of quality of life, and self-awareness of functional status in individuals with multiple sclerosis. *Rehabilitation Psychology, 54*, 60–68. https://doi.org/10.1037/a0014556

Grabanski, J. L., & Janssen, S. L. (2021). Occupational selection, analysis, gradation, and adaptation. In D. P. Dirette & S. A. Gutman (Eds.), *Occupational therapy for physical dysfunction* (8th ed., p. 33). Wolters Kluwer.

Grajo, L. C., & Boisselle, A. K. (2021). The teaching and learning process. In D. P. Dirette & S. A. Gutman (Eds.), *Occupational therapy for physical dysfunction* (8th ed., pp. 44–51). Wolters Kluwer.

Greber, C., Ziviani, J., & Rodger, S. (2007). The four-quadrant model of facilitated learning (part 2): Strategies and applications. *Australian Occupational Therapy Journal, 54*, S40–S48. https://doi.org/10.1111/j.1440-1630.2007.00663.x

Guidetti, S., Asaba, E., & Tham, K. (2007). The lived experience of recapturing self-care. *American Journal of Occupational Therapy, 61*, 303–310. https://doi.org/10.5014/ajot.61.3.303

Harper, A. E., Terhorst, L., Moscirella, M., Turner, R. L., Piersol, C. V., & Leland, N. E. (2021). The experiences, priorities, and perceptions of informal caregivers of people with dementia in nursing homes: A scoping review. *Dementia, 20*(8), 1–20. https://doi.org/10.1177/14713012211012606

Hartman-Maeir, A., Harel, H., & Katz, N. (2009). Kettle Test—A brief measure of cognitive functional performance: Reliability and validity in stroke rehabilitation. *American Journal of Occupational Therapy, 64*, 592–599. https://doi.org/10.5014/ajot.63.5.592

Hinojosa, M. S., & Rittman, M. (2009). Association between health education needs and stroke caregiver injury. *Journal of Aging and Health, 21*, 1040–1058. https://doi.org/10.1177/0898264309344321

Holm, M. B., & Rogers, J. C. (2017). Measuring performance in instrumental activities of daily living. In M. Law, C. Baum, & W. Dunn (Eds.), *Measuring occupational performance: Supporting best practice in occupational therapy* (3rd ed., pp. 305–331). SLACK.

Improving Medicare Post-Acute Care Transformation (IMAPCT) Act of 2014, Pub. L. No. 113-185, 128 Stat. *1952 etseq.* (2014).

Jack, J., & Estes, R. I. (2010). Documenting progress: Hand therapy treatment shift from biomechanical to occupational adaptation. *American Journal of Occupational Therapy, 64*, 82–87. https://doi.org/10.5014/ajot.64.1.82

Jennings, L. A., Palimaru, A., Corona, M. G., Cagigas, X. E., Ramirez, K. D., Zhao, T., Hays, R. D., Wenger, N. S., & Reuben, D. B. (2017). Patient and caregiver goals for dementia care. *Quality of Life Research, 26*(3), 685–693. https://doi.org/10.1007/s11136-016-1471-7

Kartje, P. (2006, October). Approaching, evaluating, and counseling the older driver for successful community mobility. *OT Practice, 11*(19), 11–15. https://higherlogicdownload.s3-external-1.amazonaws.com/AOTA/OTP%2019%20Oct%2023%202006.pdf?AWSAccessKeyId=AKIAVRDO7IEREB57R7MT&Expires=1680629071&Signature=w3eFkKjaJPzkXNc27scNNhRcX1M%3D

Katz, S., Ford, A. B., Moskowitz, R. W., Jackson, B. A., & Jaffe, M. A. (1963). Studies of illness in the aged. The index of ADL: A standardized measure of biological and psychosocial function. *Journal of the American Medical Association, 185*, 914–919. https://doi.org/10.1001/jama.1963.03060120024016

Keller, J., Kafkes, A., Basu, S., Federico, J., & Kielhofner, G. (2005). The child occupational self assessment (version 2.1). Model of Human Occupation Clearinghouse.

Kettenbach, G. (2009). *Writing patient/client notes: Ensuring accuracy in documentation* (4th ed.). F. A. Davis.

Kielhofner, G., Mallinson, T., Crawford, C., Nowak, M., Rigby, M., Henry, A., & Walens, D. (2004). Occupational performance history interview II (OPHI-II) (version 2.1). Model of Human Occupation Clearinghouse.

Koops van't Jagt, R., Hoeks, J. C. J., Jansen, C. J. M., de Winter, A. F., & Reijneveld, S. A. (2016). Comprehensibility of health-related documents for older adults with different levels of health literacy: A systematic

review. *Journal of Health Communication, 21*(2), 159–177. https://doi.org/10.1080/10810730.2015.1049306

Korner-Bitensky, N., Menon, A., von Zweck, C., & Van Benthem, K. (2010). Occupational therapists' capacity-building needs related to older driver screening, assessment, and intervention: A Canadawide survey. *American Journal of Occupational Therapy, 64*, 316–324. https://doi.org/10.5014/ajot.64.2.316

Lansing, R. W., Moosavi, S. H., & Banzett, R. B. (2003). Measurement of dyspnea: Word labeled visual analog scale vs. verbal ordinal scale. *Respiratory Physiology & Neurobiology, 3*, 77–83. https://doi.org/10.1016/S1569-9048(02)00211-2

Law, M., Baptiste, S., Carswell, A., McColl, M. A., Polatajko, H., & Pollock, N. (2014). *The Canadian occupational performance measure* (5th ed.). Canadian Association of Occupational Therapists.

Law, M., & Baum, C. (2017). Measurement in occupational therapy. In M. Law, C. Baum, & W. Dunn (Eds.), *Measuring occupational performance: Supporting best practice in occupational therapy* (3rd ed., pp. 1–16). SLACK.

Law, M., & Dunbar, S. B. (2007). Person-environment-occupation model. In S. B. Dunbar (Ed.), *Occupational therapy models for intervention with children and families* (pp. 27–49). SLACK.

Legg, L., Drummond, A., & Langhorne, P. (2006). Occupational therapy for patients with problems in activities of daily living after stroke. *Cochrane Database of Systematic Reviews, (4)*, 1–47. https://doi.org/10.1002/14651858.CD003585.pub2

Liedberg, G. M., & Vrethem, M. (2009). Polyneuropathy, with and without neurogenic pain, and its impact on daily life activities—A descriptive study. *Disability and Rehabilitation, 31*, 1402–1408. https://doi.org/10.1080/09638280802621382

Little, L. M., Pope, E., Wallisch, A., & Dunn, W. (2018). Occupation-based coaching by means of telehealth for families of young children with autism spectrum disorder. *American Journal of Occupational Therapy, 72*, Article e7202205020. https://doi.org/10.5014/ajot.2018.024786

Lund, M. L., & Nygård, L. (2003). Incorporating or resisting assistive devices: Different approaches to achieving a desired occupational self-image. *OTJR: Occupation, Participation and Health, 23*, 67–75. https://doi.org/10.1177/153944920302300204

Mackenzie, C., Wiprzycka, U., Hasher, L., & Goldstein, D. (2009). Associations between psychological distress, learning, and memory in spouse caregivers of older adults. *Journals of Gerontology Series B: Psychological Sciences & Social Sciences, 64B*, 742–746. https://doi.org/10.1093/geronb/gbp076

Magasi, S. (2012). Negotiating the social service systems: A vital yet frequently invisible occupation. *OTJR: Occupation, Participation and Health, 32*, S25–S33. https://doi.org/10.3928/15394492-20110906-03

Mahoney, F. I., & Barthel, D. W. (1965). Functional evaluation: The Barthel Index. *Maryland State Medical Journal, 14*, 61–65. https://doi.org/10.1037/t02366-000

Mannion, N., & Sullivan, N. (2021). Occupational therapy for functional impairments resulting from COVID-19 infection: A case report. *American Journal of Occupational Therapy, 75*(Suppl. 1), 7511210040. https://doi.org/10.5014/ajot.2021.049215

Mathiowetz, V. G., Matuska, K. M., Finlayson, M. L., Luo, P., & Chen, H. Y. (2007). One-year follow-up to a randomized controlled trial of an energy conservation course for persons with multiple sclerosis. *International Journal of Rehabilitation Research, 30*, 305–313. https://doi.org/10.1097/MRR.0b013e3282f14434

Mathiowetz, V., Matuska, K. M., & Murphy, M. E. (2001). Efficacy of an energy conservation course for persons with multiple sclerosis. *Archives of Physical Medicine and Rehabilitation, 82*, 449–456. https://doi.org/10.1053/apmr.2001.22192

McKenna, K., & Scott, J. (2007). Do written education materials that use content and design principles improve older people's knowledge? *Australian Occupational Therapy Journal, 54*, 103–112. https://doi.org/10.1111/j.1440-1630.2006.00583.x

Meenan, R. F., Mason, J. H., Anderson, J. J., Guccione, A. A., & Kazis, L. E. (1992). AIMS2: The content and properties of a revised and expanded Arthritis Impact Measurement Scales Health Status Questionnaire. *Arthritis and Rheumatism, 35*, 1–10. https://doi.org/10.1002/art.1780350102

Melchert-McKearnan, K., Deitz, J., Engel, J. M., & White, O. (2000). Children with burn injuries: Purposeful versus rote exercise. *American Journal of Occupational Therapy, 54*, 381–390. https://doi.org/10.5014/ajot.54.4.381

Mohammed, A. (2017). Addressing sexuality in occupational therapy. *OT Practice, 22*(9), CE1–CE7. https://higherlogicdownload.s3-external-1.amazonaws.com/AOTA/0fdec3b1-5de6-321a-4536-5703661d4415_file.pdf?AWSAccessKeyId=AKIAVRDO7IEREB57R7MT&Expires=1680629285&Signature=Q38w0rRb70o14w02EYq4TFTDLIs%3D

Moye, J. (2005). Guardianship and conservatorship. In T. Grisso (Ed.), *Evaluating competencies: Forensic assessments and instruments* (2nd ed., pp. 309–390). https://www.springer.com/gp/book/9780306473432

Nakanishi, M., Sawamura, K., Sato, S., Setoya, Y., & Anzai, N. (2010). Development of a clinical pathway for long-term inpatients with schizophrenia. *Psychiatry and Clinical Neurosciences, 64*, 99–103. https://doi.org/10.1111/j.1440-1819.2009.02040.x

National Center for Health Statistics. (2009). *Limitations in activities of daily living and instrumental activities of daily living, 2003-2007.* http://www.cdc.gov/nchs/health_policy/ADL_tables.htm

Novak, I., Cusick, A., & Lannin, N. (2009). Occupational therapy home programs for cerebral palsy: Double-blind, randomized, controlled trial. *Pediatrics, 124*, e606–e614. https://doi.org/10.1542/peds.2009-0288

Novaria, G. A., Fairman, A. D., Morris, L. L., & Ding, D. (2021). Smart home technology: Harnessing the potential of mainstream devices. *OT Practice, 26*(9), 10–13. https://www.aota.org/-/media/corporate/files/secure/publications/otp/2021/otp-volume-26-issue-9-2021-smart-home-technology.pdf

Orellano, E., Colón, W. I., & Arbesman, M. (2012). Effect of occupation- and activity-based interventions on instrumental activities of daily living performance among community-dwelling older adults: A systematic review. *American Journal of Occupational Therapy, 66*, 292–300. https://doi.org/10.5014/ajot.2012.003053

Osei, E., & Dimitropoulou, K. (2019). Use of the family activity adaptation model (FAAM) to coach caregivers and children with hemiplegic cerebral palsy in development of bimanual hand use. *AOTA 2019 annual meeting.* New Orleans.

Osei, E., & Dimitropoulou, K. (2021). Telehealth use of the family activity adaptation model (FAAM) to coach caregivers and children with hemiplegic cerebral palsy in development of bimanual hand use. *AOTA 2021 annual meeting.* On-line.

Pashmdarfard, M., & Azad, A. (2020). Assessment tools to evaluate activities of daily living (ADL) and instrumental activities of daily living (IADL) in older adults: A systematic review. *Medical Journal Islam Republic Iran, 34*(33). https://doi.org/10.34171/mjiri.34.33

Pillastrini, P., Mugnai, R., Bonfiglioli, R., Curti, S., Mattioli, S., Maioli, M. G., Bazzocchi, G., Menarini, M., Vannini, R., & Violante, F. S. (2008). Evaluation of an occupational therapy program for patients with spinal cord injury. *Spinal Cord, 46*, 78–81. https://doi.org/10.1038/sj.sc.3102072

Pitonyak, J. S., Souza, K., Umeda, C., & Jirikowic, T. (2021). Using a health promotion approach to frame parent experiences of family routines and their significance for health and well-being. *Journal of Occupational Therapy, Schools, & Early Intervention.* https://doi.org/10.1080/19411243.2021.1983499

Provencher, V., Demers, L., Gagnon, L., & Gélinas, I. (2012). Impact of familiar and unfamiliar settings on cooking task assessments in frail older adults with poor and preserved executive functions. *International Psychogeriatrics, 24*(5), 775–783. https://doi.org/10.1017/S104161021100216X

Provencher, V., Demers, L., Gélinas, I., & Giroux, F. (2013). Cooking task assessment in frail older adults: Who performed better at home and in the clinic. *Scandinavian Journal of Occupational Therapy, 20*, 374–385. https://doi.org/10.3109/11038128.2012.743586

Radomski, M. V. (2011). More than good intentions: Advancing adherence with therapy recommendations. *American Journal of Occupational Therapy, 65*, 471–477. https://doi.org/10.5014/ajot.2011.000885

Resnick, B. (1998). Motivating older adults to perform functional activities. *Journal of Gerontological Nursing, 24*, 23–30. https://doi.org/10.3928/0098-9134-19981101-08

Rogers, J. C., Holm, M. B., Beach, S., Schulz, R., Cipriani, J., Fox, A., & Starz, T. W. (2003). Concordance of four methods of disability assessment using performance in the home as the criterion method. *Arthritis Care & Research, 49*, 640–647. https://doi.org/10.1002/art.11379

Schepens, S. L., Panzer, V., & Goldberg, A. (2011). Research scholars initiative—Randomized controlled trial comparing tailoring methods of multimedia-based fall prevention education for community-dwelling older adults. *American Journal of Occupational Therapy, 65*, 702–709. https://doi.org/10.5014/ajot.2011.001180

Schepens Niemiec, S. L., Vigen, C. L. P., Martínez, J., Blanchard, J., & Carlson, M. (2021). Long-term follow-up of a lifestyle intervention for late midlife, rural-dwelling Latinos in primary care. *American Journal of Occupational Therapy, 75*, Article e7502205020. https://doi.org/10.5014/ajot.2021.042861

Seo, Y., Roberts, B. L., LaFramboise, L., Yates, B. C., & Yurkovich, J. M. (2011). Predictors of modifications in instrumental activities of daily living in persons with heart failure. *Journal of Cardiovascular Nursing, 26*, 89–98. https://doi.org/10.1097/JCN.0b013e3181ec1352

Siegel, P., Tencza, M., Apodaca, B., & Poole, J. L. (2017). Effectiveness of occupational therapy interventions for adults with rheumatoid arthritis: A systematic review. *American Journal of Occupational Therapy, 71*, Article e7101180050. https://doi.org/10.5014/ajot.2017.023176

Simpson, A. N., Bonilha, H. S., Kazley, A. S., Zoller, J. S., Simpson, K. N., & Ellis, C. (2015). Impact of outpatient rehabilitation Medicare reimbursement caps on utilization and cost of rehabilitation care after ischemic stroke: Do caps contain costs? *Archives of Physical Medicine and Rehabilitation, 96*, 1959–1965. https://doi.org/10.1016/j.apmr.2015.07.008

Szanton, S. L., Xue, Q.-L., Leff, B., Guralnik, J., Wolff, J. L., Tanner, E. K., Boyd, C., Thorpe, R. J., Bishai, D., & Gitlin, L. N. (2019). Effect of a biobehavioral environmental approach on disability among low-income older adults: A randomized clinical trial. *JAMA Internal Medicine, 179*, 204–211. https://doi.org/10.1001/jamainternmed.2018.6026

Tamaru, A., McColl, M. A., & Yamasaki, S. (2007). Understanding "independence": Perspectives of occupational therapists. *Disability and Rehabilitation, 29*, 1021–1033. https://doi.org/10.1080/09638280600929110

Tomlin, G. (2018). Scientific reasoning and evidence in practice. In B. A. B. Schell & J. W. Schell (Eds.), *Clinical and professional reasoning in occupational therapy practice* (2nd ed., pp. 145–169). Lippincott Williams & Wilkins.

Toth-Cohen, S. (2000). Role perceptions of occupational therapists providing support and education for caregivers of persons with dementia. *American Journal of Occupational Therapy, 54*, 509–515. https://doi.org/10.5014/ajot.54.5.509

UB Foundation Activities. (2002). *IRF-PAI training manual.* III-7. https://www.cms.gov/Medicare/Medicare-Fee-for-Service-Payment/InpatientRehabFacPPS/downloads/irfpai-manualint.pdf

Van Heest, K. N. L., Mogush, A. R., & Mathiowetz, V. G. (2017). Effects of a one-to-one fatigue management course for people with chronic conditions and fatigue. *American Journal of Occupational*

Therapy, 71, Article e7104100020. https://doi.org/10.5014/ajot.2017.023440

Vroland-Nordstrand, K., Eliasson, A.-C., Jacobsson, H., Johansson, U., & Krumlinde-Sundholm, L. (2015). Can children identify and achieve goals for intervention? A randomized trial comparing two goal-setting approaches. *Developmental Medicine and Child Neurology, 58,* 589–596. https://doi.org/10.1111/dmcn.12925

Welu, J., & Naber, A. (2020). Occupational therapy and public space design: Why it matters and how to get started. *OT Practice, 25*(9), 10–12. https://www.aota.org/-/media/corporate/files/secure/publications/otp/2020/otp-volume-25-issue-9-september-home-2020.pdf

Whalley Hammell, K. R. (2009). Self-care, productivity and leisure, or dimensions of occupational experience? Rethinking occupational "categories." *Canadian Journal of Occupational Therapy, 76,* 107–114. https://doi.org/10.1177/000841740907600208

Whalley Hammell, K. R. (2014). Belonging, occupation, and human well-being: An exploration. *Canadian Journal of Occupational Therapy, 81*(1), 39–50. https://doi.org/10.1177/0008417413520489

World Health Organization. (2002). *Towards a common language for functioning, disability, and health: ICF.* https://cdn.who.int/media/docs/default-source/classification/icf/icfbeginnersguide.pdf

Zanatta, E., Rodeghiero, F., Pigatto, E., Galozzi, P., Polito, P., Favaro, M., Punzi, L., & Cozzi, F. (2017). Long-term improvement in activities of daily living in women with systemic sclerosis attending occupational therapy. *British Journal of Occupational Therapy, 80,* 417–422. https://doi.org/10.1177/0308022617698167

CHAPTER 45

Education in the United States

Susan M. Cahill

LEARNING OBJECTIVES

After reading this chapter, you will be able to:

1. Identify educational settings in which an occupational therapy practitioner may provide services in the United States.
2. Outline the occupational therapy process within educational settings.
3. Explain key requirements of occupational therapy services under guiding legislation such as the Individuals with Disabilities Education Improvement Act, Every Student Succeeds Act, and Section 504 of the Rehabilitation Act.
4. Describe multitiered occupational therapy services.
5. Compare and contrast an Individualized Family Service Plan (IFSP), an Individualized Education Program (IEP), and an Individualized Transition Plan (ITP).
6. Describe the importance of educational expectations and standards in relation to intervention planning.
7. Explain quality indicators for occupational therapy practice in schools.

Occupational Therapy in Educational Settings

In the United States, occupational therapists and occupational therapy assistants (i.e., OT practitioners) work in a variety of educational settings. These may include public schools, charter schools, private schools, alternative schools, vocational schools, and university settings. Across these settings, practitioners work with children and adolescents, generally from birth through age 21 in a variety of contexts. For example, an OT practitioner might work with infants and families on play skills and sleep routines in a 0 to 3 center and with young children on kindergarten readiness skills in a preschool. OT practitioners might work in the classroom and in the cafeteria with children in middle school, or in a simulated apartment and at worksite with adolescents in high school. OT practitioners might also work with college age students who are learning to live away from their families for the first time on budgeting, managing multiple role expectations (e.g., student and worker), and developing effective performance patterns to alleviate stress and anxiety. Approximately 23% of occupational therapists and 19% of OT assistants (OTAs) who are members of the American Occupational Therapy Association (AOTA) identify schools/early intervention as their primary work setting (AOTA, 2020a).

The primary focus of this chapter is on occupational performance within school settings in the United States. The reader is encouraged to consider the wide variety of educational settings that may benefit from the skills and expertise of an OT practitioner. These types of OT services may be innovative and preventive and may increase the occupational performance of individuals in various ways. For example, OT practitioners might develop a literacy program for students in underserved communities (Arnaud & Gutman, 2021), work with an interprofessional team to address students' diabetes-related health management concerns at school (Polo & Cahill, 2017), or train school cafeteria workers to promote mental health through established programs such as Every Moment Counts' *Comfortable Cafeteria* (Bazyk et al., 2018). In addition, OT practitioners might work with colleges and university disability service teams to develop programming (e.g., time management skills, job skills, and life skills), consult on access issues, and provide direct services to address performance and participation with young adult students (Dirette, 2019).

Legislation Guiding Practice

In the United States, practice across educational settings is guided by federal legislation, with the focus on occupational performance and participation in the student role. Although the occupation of education is the primary focus in early intervention and school settings, OT practitioners also address sleep and rest, social participation, play and leisure, activities of daily living (ADLs) (e.g., toileting, toilet hygiene, feeding and eating) and instrumental activities of daily living (IADLs) (e.g., meal preparation, driving and community mobility), work, and health management (see Unit VII). The Individuals with Disabilities Education Improvement Act (2004) specifically addresses services for infants and children with delays and disabilities in early intervention and schools that receive public funds. Similarly, Every Student Succeeds Act (ESSA) (2015) provides for services for students in kindergarten through 12th grade through consultation and school-wide systems of support (i.e., multitiered systems of support [MTSS] to address learning, social emotional, and behavioral needs) in publicly funded schools. The requirements of Section

504 of the Rehabilitation Act (1973) as well as the Americans with Disabilities Act (ADA) of 1990 (Pub. L. 101-336) must be met by every type of educational setting, including private schools, community colleges, and universities. Section 504 supports reasonable accommodations for individuals with a disability, a history of a disability, or a perceived disability if accommodations are needed to allow the individual to participate in educational settings. The ADA is a civil rights act and provides protection to individuals with disabilities similar to those provided to individuals on the basis of race, color, sex, national origin, age, and religion. Furthermore, the ADA supports the right of individuals with disabilities to have equal opportunities to live, learn, work, and play within society. See Table 45.1 for an overview of legislation.

Since 1975, the key goals of IDEA 2004 (originally the Education for All Handicapped Children Act [EHA]) have remained the same. However, in recent years there has been a significant shift away from trying to reduce the effects of disability and tolerating minimal progress to using a strengths-based approach and holding appropriately ambitious expectations for students regardless of disability status (Wehmeyer, 2022). The role of OT under the IDEA 2004 has shifted to include a focus on students' strengths and abilities and the contextual factors that support and limit performance and participation across different learning environments.

The IDEA 2004 has four parts, A to D; however, this chapter primarily addresses parts B and C. (Part A addresses the general provisions of the IDEA, and Part D addresses research and training.) Under Part C of the IDEA 2004, OT can be a primary service for infants and toddlers from birth through 2 years of age who are eligible for early intervention services (Myers & Cason, 2020). Part B of the IDEA 2004 identifies OT as a related service for children ages 3 through 21 years old for whom the team determines the service is *necessary* for students to benefit from their special education program. Two key concepts of Part B of IDEA 2004 are a free appropriate public education (FAPE) in the least restrictive environment (LRE) (see Box 45.1 for definition of key terms found within the IDEA 2004). IDEA 2004 allows each state and local education agency (LEA) some flexibility in how the federal legislation will be implemented if the FAPE and LRE provisions are not compromised. There are differences across states and local school districts regarding the specifics of how services are provided.

The purpose of IDEA 2004 is "to ensure that all children with disabilities have available to them a FAPE that emphasizes special education and related services designed to meet their unique needs and prepare them for further education, employment and independent living" (§ 300.1). Occupational therapy practitioners in the public school setting provide services within this structure and are generally a related (i.e., supportive) service to the educational program (i.e., specially designed instruction).

TABLE 45.1	Legislation Guiding OT Services in Educational Settings in the United States	

Legislation	Purpose	Role of the OT Practitioner
Part B of the Individuals with Disabilities Education Improvement Act (IDEA) of 2004	To provide for a free appropriate public education (FAPE) in the least restrictive environment (LRE). (Part B of IDEA 2004 is applicable only for students [ages 3–21 years] who receive special education services through their or public school setting.)	To collaborate with the Individualized Education Program (IEP) team to determine the student's needs and then to provide services as outlined in the IEP to support student performance relevant to the educational environment.
Part C of the Individuals with Disabilities Education Improvement Act (IDEA) of 2004	To enhance the development of infants and toddlers with developmental delays and disabilities and to foster the capacity of families to meet the needs of their infants and toddlers. (Part C of IDEA 2004 is applicable only for infants and toddlers [ages 0–2 years] with documented delays and disabilities] who receive early intervention services through their State.)	To collaborate with the family and interdisciplinary team to determine the child's needs and then to provide services as outlined in the Individualized Family Service Plan (IFSP) to support development and participation in the natural environment.
Every Student Succeeds Act of 2015	All students who attend kindergarten-12th grade. The focus of ESSA is on academic achievement and ensuring that students meet educational outcomes through school/district accountability measures.	To collaborate with school teams to provide universal, targeted, and intensive interventions to address all students' learning and mental health in the educational environment.
Section 504 of the Rehabilitation Act	Students who have a disability, a history of a disability, or a perceived disability that affects access to the curriculum or learning environment at school (i.e., early childhood settings, K-12 schools, community colleges, and universities). Students who receive a 504 plan typically do not have other types of plans (e.g., IEP in place). Students who meet the definition of "individual with a disability" are defined as those individuals who have a physical or mental impairment that substantially limits one or more major life activities.	To collaborate with the 504 team to provide the accommodations and adaptations that the student needs to access the curriculum and school environment.
Americans with Disabilities Act (ADA)	The ADA ensures equal opportunity for individuals with disabilities in employment, state and local government services, public accommodations, commercial facilities, and transportation. Thus, it is a civil rights legislation that supports participation in the educational setting by students who have a disability.	To provide support through consultation and monitoring to ensure that students with disabilities have access to and can participate in the educational setting. It often involves working with environmental adaptations, accommodations, and the use of assistive devices.

BOX 45.1 COMMON TERMS IN THE INDIVIDUALS WITH DISABILITIES EDUCATION ACT 2004

Early intervening services: academic and behavior support to succeed in general education but is not part of special education

Free appropriate public education (FAPE): special education and related services provided at public expense that meets the standards of the state education agency (SEA)

General education: the environment, curriculum, and activities that are available to all students

General education curriculum: the same curriculum as for children without disabilities

Individualized Education Program (IEP): a commitment of services that ensures that an appropriate program is developed that meets the unique educational needs of children ages 3 to 21 years

Individualized Family Services Plan (IFSP): a commitment of services that ensures that an appropriate program is developed that meets the unique developmental and preeducational needs of children 0 to 3 years old and their families

Least restrictive environment (LRE): the environment that provides maximum interaction with nondisabled peers and is consistent with the needs of the child/student

Related services: transportation and such developmental, corrective, and other supportive services (including speech-language, audiology, psychological, and physical and occupational therapy services) needed to help the child benefit from special education

Special education: specially designed instruction at no cost to parents to meet the unique needs of a child with a disability

IDEA 2004 also allows for the provision of early intervening services (EIS) for students receiving a general education who need additional academic or behavioral support (§ 300.226). Schools often provide EIS through MTSS. The purpose of MTSS is to address students' learning and behavioral concerns early and to prevent the need for more intensive services later (Cahill & Bazyk, 2020). Key elements of MTSS include high-quality and evidence-based instructional methods, continuous monitoring of students' progress, universal screening, and progressively more intensive services as they are needed (Jimerson et al., 2015).

The ESSA of 2015 names OT practitioners as specialized instructional support personnel (SISP). Under ESSA, OT practitioners are expected to consult with other educational personnel (e.g., teachers, administrators, other SISP) to support the academic achievement of all students. The ESSA definition of SISP is included in Box 45.2.

Occupational Therapy Process in Educational Settings

A variety of factors affect the OT process in educational environments. Services that are provided in educational settings are often influenced by collaborative interprofessional teams. Collaboration has been shown to increase the team's capacity to meet students' needs and result in positive outcomes for students (Shepherd et al., 2019). The child and their family are also important partners on the educational team and should be equally involved in all aspects of planning and decision-making. Working collaboratively as part of a team provides a framework to ensure that all strengths and needs specific to participation across educational settings are addressed.

BOX 45.2 FEDERAL DEFINITION OF SPECIALIZED INSTRUCTIONAL SUPPORT PERSONNEL

ESSA defines Specialized Instructional Support Personnel as, "(i) school counselors, school social workers, and school psychologists; and (ii) other qualified personnel, such as school nurses, speech-language pathologists, and school librarians, involved in providing assessment, diagnosis, counseling, educational, therapeutic, and other necessary services including related services as that term is defined in section 602 of the Individuals with Disabilities Education Act (20 U.S.C 1401) as part of a comprehensive program to meet students needs" (ESSA 2015, Sec. 8002).

Decision-Making

Occupational therapists collaborate with school teams to make decisions about placement, services, and accommodations and modifications. Effective and efficient decision-making is based on an ethical and systematic approach to problem-solving. Problem-solving is a collaborative and data-driven process used to identify and prioritize a student's academic or behavioral concerns and select interventions to improve the student's outcomes (Cahill, 2019). The problem-solving cycle is similar to the OT process (AOTA, 2020b) and is shown in Figure 45.1. Educational teams have access to a variety of tools that support a systematic process of decision-making and team problem-solving (e.g., School Setting Interview [SSI] and McGill Action Planning System [MAPS]). Additionally, school-based practitioners may encounter ethical dilemmas unique to practicing in educational settings. This may include a mismatch between the Occupational Therapy Code of Ethics (AOTA, 2020c) and special education law or non-OT practitioners writing services on the Individualized Education Plan (IEP) without collaborating with the occupational therapist and more (Reed & Polichino, 2019). School-based practitioners should be aware of when educational legislation and priorities may conflict with the Occupational Therapy Code of Ethics and then negotiate any incongruences.

Educational Teams

Multiple teams collaborate to make decisions in educational settings. Collaboration takes place when individuals with diverse experiences and expertise come together

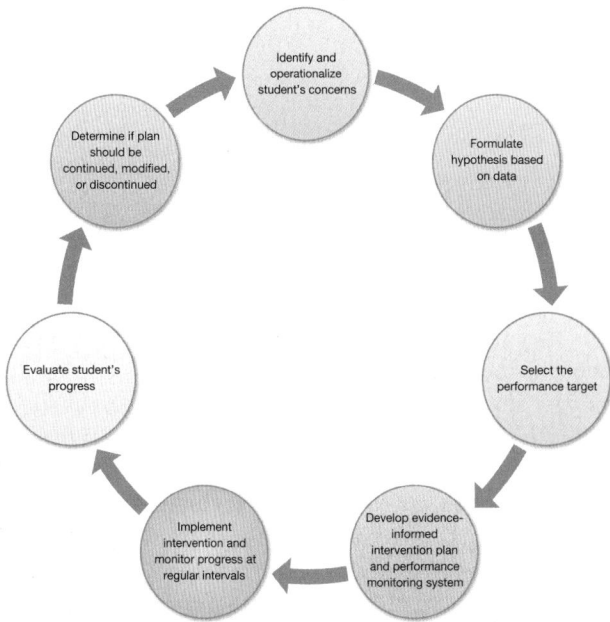

FIGURE 45.1 **Problem-solving cycle.**

to focus on the needs of the child in the educational setting (Hanft & Shepherd, 2016). Collaborative teams share a common goal and operate with mutual trust and respect (Shepherd et al., 2019). Families bring expertise on the child's personal context, developmental history, and daily habits and routines. Families should be viewed as equal team members and involved whenever educational decisions are made about a child. The types of teams most commonly seen in educational settings are the Individualized Family Service Plan (IFSP) team for children 0 to 3 years and the Individualized Education Program (IEP) team. These teams function to make educational decisions to benefit the child or student. Other common teams are evaluation teams (for determining whether a student has an educational disability), Individualized Transition Plan (ITP) team (for adolescents who receive special education to address postsecondary outcomes), and problem-solving teams (for making decisions regarding students receiving interventions through multitiered systems of support). IDEA 2004 requires both the IFSP and IEP teams to include the family and qualified professionals who are knowledgeable about the child's needs.

In public schools, IEPs teams are comprised of general and special education teachers, related service providers (e.g., occupational therapists, physical therapists, and speech-language pathologists), psychologists, social workers, counselors, families (i.e., parents and caregivers), the student when possible, and different community members as needed. If a decision is being made about OT involvement in a child's educational program, then an occupational therapist must be involved in the collaborative process. The focus of the team decision-making process must be on student outcomes and performance with an emphasis on participation in the general education environment as appropriate.

Students as Members of the Team

Students should be at the center of all educational decisions made by collaborative school teams. Students are not required to attend IEP meetings under IDEA (2004) until they are 14 or 16 years old, depending on the requirements of their state. However, it is best practice to invite younger students to participate in the IEP process as soon as it is appropriate. Students provide valuable insights to teams about their learning styles, personal strengths, and preferences (Biegun et al., 2020). Including students in IEP meetings fosters self-determination skills (Biegun et al., 2020) and results in improved learning outcomes (Cavendish et al., 2017). Participation in the IEP process should be graded based on the student's age, abilities, and comfort level.

Evaluation Requirements in the Schools

Referral

The referral process in schools is different from other practice settings and varies based on each school district or LEA. Families, teachers, and other individuals may make a referral for special education if they suspect that a child has disability that affects their learning and ability to benefit from the general education program. An OT evaluation can be included in the initial referral or added later. However, most public schools use problem-solving teams to address concerns about student performance in general education before a referral to special education is made. Some schools have an established process for providing pre-referral interventions through MTSS. The purpose of MTSS is to identify students who are having difficulty making progress in general education and then to provide them with services to address their learning and behavioral needs. The provision of MTSS falls under the role of SISP. Most MTSS frameworks use three levels:

- *Tier 1:* Universal screening, supports and instruction; for example, using a school-wide mechanism to screen students for mental health concerns
- *Tier 2:* Differentiated instruction and more intensive interventions provided in a small group; for example, identifying activities to support the development of literacy skills for first-grade students who did not attend formal preschool or kindergarten
- *Tier 3:* Intensive interventions provided in a small group or on an individual basis (Cahill & Bazyk, 2020).

Occupational therapy practitioners work with teams to identify common learning needs demonstrated by students in general education and develop interventions to support the general development of students and the typical acquisition of skills. The interventions may be delivered by other SISP or members of the school community. If the MTSS interventions are not successful, the student is often referred to special education. Occupational therapists should not conduct an evaluation unless the proper referral channels are followed, and permissions are obtained.

In other educational settings, the referral process may be less formal. For example, in some college and university settings, a referral might come through the center for disability access (e.g., a student access concern). Occupational therapists who work in such settings might need to develop a referral system to ensure that the process meets the needs of the client(s). If a physician referral is required by a state practice act, then the occupational therapist must comply with this requirement regardless of the setting.

Evaluation

In public schools in the United States, multidisciplinary evaluation teams collaborate to determine whether a student has an educational disability, document the student's educational needs, and develop the IEP. Evaluations are only conducted after obtaining consent from the student's parent or legal guardian, and teams conduct evaluations even if students have a known developmental disability (e.g., cerebral palsy) or medical condition (e.g., traumatic brain injury) (Cahill & Bazyk, 2020). Occupational therapists are often part of this team. However, if the occupational therapist is not involved in the initial evaluation process, the team may request an OT evaluation at any time after determining that the student is eligible for special education. If the occupational therapist works in a state where the OT practice act requires a physician referral for services, then such a referral may be necessary before starting the evaluation. If a physician refers a student for an OT evaluation,

this referral does not guarantee services in a school setting. The occupational therapist in the public school must first ensure that the student is eligible for special education and related services and then collaborate with the team to determine if services are necessary for the student to benefit from the education program.

The occupational therapist in the school setting focuses the evaluation on what is needed for effective and efficient student role performance and participation in meaningful and purposeful school occupations. Based on the student's educational needs and program, the OT evaluation addresses the student's areas of strengths and concerns related to the occupation of education, as well as ADL, IADL, work, play/leisure, sleep and rest, health management, and social participation (Table 45.2). For example, in infant and toddler programs, sleep and rest are critical occupations; driving and community mobility are critical occupations for high school; and financial management and meal preparation are critical occupations for transition

TABLE 45.2 Examples of Critical Occupations in Educational Contexts

Occupations	Critical Occupations for Children	Critical Occupations for Adolescents and Young Adults
Activities of daily living	Performs feeding, toileting, toilet hygiene, managing shoes and clothing, functional mobility	Performs feeding, toileting, toilet hygiene, managing shoes and clothing, functional mobility
Instrumental activities of daily living	Cares for classroom pets, evaluates and responds to safety situations (e.g., disembarking the school bus and crossing the street)	Performs communication management, driving and community mobility, financial management, meal preparation and cleanup, safety, shopping, home establishment and maintenance
Health management	Manages emotions, expresses needs effectively, seeks activities that support health, adheres to hydration and dietary recommendations, uses and cares for personal care devices	Performs social and emotional health promotion and maintenance, symptom and condition management, communication with healthcare system, medication management, physical activity, nutrition, personal care device management
Rest and sleep	Identifies need to relax, reduces involvement in taxing activities, engages in relaxation	Identifies need to relax, reduces involvement in taxing activities, engages in relaxation, engages in routines that promote restful sleep, determines when and how much to sleep, sleep participation in independent living situations (e.g., dorm room)
Education	Performs and participates in the academic (e.g., math, reading, writing), nonacademic (e.g., lunch, recess, after-school activities), prevocational, and vocational activities	Performs and participates in the academic (e.g., math, reading, writing), nonacademic (e.g., lunch, recess, after-school activities), and vocational activities. Identifies topics of interest and how to obtain information and skills
Work	Develops interests, aptitudes, and skills necessary for engaging in prevocational or volunteer activities for transition to community life on completion of high school	Identifies and selects work opportunities, seeks employment, performs jobs, manages relationships with co-workers, responds to feedback on performance
Play/leisure	Identifies and engages in age-appropriate toys, games, and leisure experiences; participates in art, music, sports, and after-school activities	Participates in independent and group play and leisure activities, balances play/leisure with participation in other occupations
Social participation	Interacts with peers, teachers, and other educational personnel during academic and nonacademic educational activities including extracurricular and preparation for work activities	Interacts with peers, teachers, other educational personnel, and community members during educational and work activities

programs and college and university settings. As in all other practice settings, the occupational therapist is responsible for the administration of assessment tools and procedures, the interpretation and documentation of results, and the communication of evaluation results with other team members. However, if an OTA is part of the team, they may contribute to any part of the process under the supervision of the occupational therapist in alignment with their state's practice act.

The evaluation process in schools involves gathering and interpreting information to identify the client's strengths and needs. Evaluation of students is dynamic and ongoing and often continues during intervention. According to IDEA 2004, the evaluation determines whether a child has a disability and the nature and extent of the special education program and related services that the child needs (§ 300.15). IDEA 2004 does not require use of specific types of assessment tools or procedures. Rather, it requires that a variety of tools and strategies be used to gather relevant "functional and developmental information" related to enabling the child to "be involved in and progress in the general education curriculum" (§ 300.304[1]). In addition, the evaluation should help to determine how the disability affects the child's participation across school contexts and activities. The occupational therapy evaluation includes two parts, the occupational profile and the analysis of occupational performance (AOTA, 2020b).

Occupational Profile

The occupational profile (AOTA, 2021) is used to understand the student's educational history, preferences, values, interests, and needs. It is developed by gathering data from the student, family, and educational staff. The OTA, community providers, and others who know the student well may also contribute to this process. Often, the development of the occupational profile occurs over time. Information from the occupational profile can highlight the critical occupations that the student needs or wants to

engage in at school and whether they are experiencing satisfaction with their performance (Cahill, 2020). Questions to guide occupational profile development are included in Box 45.3.

Tools such as MAPS (O'Brien et al., 1989) include questions that can assist in occupational profile development. For example, the MAPS consists of seven specific questions that support the planning process and identification of team-generated outcomes for students with disabilities (O'Brien et al., 1989). The questions include the following:

1. What is the student's history?
2. What are your dreams for the student?
3. What are your fears for the student?
4. Who is the student? (one-word statements that describe the student)
5. What are the student's strengths, gifts, and abilities?
6. What are the student's needs?
7. What would the student's ideal day at school look like and what must be done to make it happen?

MAPS can be used with students of all ages. However, planning sessions may take 2 hours or more and may not be practical in all educational settings. Transition teams often use MAPS when setting priorities for postsecondary outcomes (Haines et al., 2018). The entire team (parents, students, therapists, and teachers) and other invited members (siblings, other family members, or community members) provide input to answer each question. The questions provide a strong foundation from which to develop the student's program, including any OT services. The process focuses on the value of integrating the student in neighborhood schools and in general education classes to develop friendships and ensure high-quality education for the child. By the time the team members are addressing question 6 ("What are the student's needs?"), they have the background to be able to establish both short- and long-term goals. These goals are then used to guide a discussion regarding the student's ideal day and how to get there.

BOX 45.3 OCCUPATIONAL PROFILE QUESTIONS FROM THE OCCUPATIONAL THERAPY PRACTICE FRAMEWORK (ADAPTED FOR THE EDUCATIONAL SETTING)

1. Who is the student?
2. Why was the student referred to special education and/or for an OT evaluation in the schools?
3. In what occupations does the student feel successful, and what barriers are affecting success, causing concerns, or putting the student at risk?
4. What are the student's values and interests?
5. What is the student's educational history?
6. What are the student's typical performance patterns and how have they changed over time?
7. Besides student, what are the child's other life roles?
8. What aspects of the context or environment support occupational engagement? What aspects of the context or environment pose barriers to occupational engagement? What are the student's priorities?
9. What are the family's and educational staff's priorities and desired target outcomes?

Analysis of Occupational Performance

The analysis of occupational performance provides information to the occupational therapist about "the dynamic transaction among the client, their contexts, and the occupation" (AOTA, 2020b, p. 22). The evaluation process should be individualized and begin with observing how the student performs critical activities and occupations in the educational context and across school environments (Cahill, 2020).

Occupational performance may be assessed through standardized and nonstandardized tools. Additional information may be collected through teacher, student, and caregiver report. After the occupational therapist understands the expectations associated with the student's critical activities and occupations and has assessed occupational performance and participation, performance skills are considered. The occupational therapist will focus on the performance skills that present the most significant limitations to

successful engagement. There may be overlap across professional disciplines regarding specific skills assessed (e.g., motor skills with physical therapy, process skills with psychology, and social interaction skills with speech-language pathology), but the input of an occupational therapist is needed to make the connection between these skills, context/environmental factors, and performance. If the occupational therapist suspects that performance skill limitations are caused by client factor deficits, client factors may then be assessed (Cahill, 2020). Performance patterns (e.g., habits and routines) should be considered during every evaluation. Performance patterns can be assessed through observation, student interview, or caregiver or teacher report (Cahill, 2020). Table 45.3 and Appendix II list some of the assessments and procedures that are used in educational settings.

Many of these assessment tools must be completed with input from all team members, including the student and family. Ideally, the assessments should address the student's strengths and concerns as well as contextual factors

TABLE 45.3 Examples of Common Assessment Tools Used in Educational Settings[a]

Focus	Assessment Tool
Collecting Occupational Profile Information and Establishing Goal Areas	
Student's perspectives regarding social well-being, activity preferences, and activity performance	Children's Assessment of Participation and Enjoyment (CAPE) and the Preferences for Activities of Children (PAC) (King et al., 2004)
Student's performance priorities, level of satisfaction with performance, and desired goal areas	Canadian Occupational Performance Measure (COPM) (Law et al., 2005)
Questions that support the planning process and identification of team-generated outcomes	McGill Action Planning System (O'Brien et al., 1989)
Student's perspectives about how competent they feel performing tasks and activities and the satisfaction with their performance	Child Occupational Self-Assessment (Kramer et al., 2014)
Analysis of Occupational Performance	
Performance completing school activities in different school environments that affect academic and social outcomes	School Function Assessment (Coster et al., 1998)
Performance completing schoolwork tasks	School AMPS (Fisher et al., 2007)
Performance during social interactions	Evaluation of Social Interaction (ESI) (Fisher & Griswold, 2010)
Performance during simulated school activities	Miller Function & Participation Scales (Miller, 2006)
Performance during simulated life skills activities	Goal-Oriented Assessment of Life Skills (GOAL) (Miller et al., 2013)
Performance Skills	
Gross and fine motor skills performance	Bruininks-Oseretsky Test of Motor Proficiency (Bruininks & Bruininks, 2005)
Handwriting skills performance	Evaluation Tool of Children's Handwriting (Amundson, 1995)
Social skills performance	Social Skills Improvement System SSIS Rating Scales (Gresham & Elliott, 2008)
Client Factors	
Processing vulnerabilities within each sensory system across multiple school environments and at home	Sensory Processing Measure (SPM) (Parham et al., 2021)
Visual perception	Motor-Free Visual Perception Test (Colarusso & Hammill, 2015)
Visual-motor integration	Beery-Buktenica Developmental Test of Visual-Motor Integration (Beery & Buktenica, 2010)
Selecting Accommodation	
Student-environment fit and the need for accommodations	School Setting Interview (Hemmingsson et al., 2005)

[a]This is not an exhaustive list nor is it an endorsement of any one assessment.

that may affect student performance and outcomes. The assessments also help the occupational therapist identify strengths and challenges specific to the student's performance patterns and activity demands.

OT Story 45.1 describes the process of developing an occupational profile and conducting an analysis of occupational performance with Sophia, a fifth-grade student with Down syndrome. Findings from such an evaluation would

OT STORY 45.1 DEVELOPING AN OCCUPATIONAL PROFILE AND CONDUCTING AN ANALYSIS OF OCCUPATIONAL PERFORMANCE WITH SOPHIA, A 10-YEAR-OLD STUDENT WITH DOWN SYNDROME

Background

Sophia is a 10-year-old student with Down syndrome. She has received clinical and school-based OT in the past. Sophia and her family recently moved, and the team in her new school district decided to complete an evaluation to determine her educational needs.

Occupational Profile

Once parental consent was obtained, the occupational therapist gathered data for the occupational profile by meeting with Sophia to complete the Children's Assessment of Participation and Enjoyment (CAPE) and the Preferences for Activities of Children (PAC) (King et al., 2004), talking to Sophia's mom on the phone and reviewing Sophia' past educational records.

Analysis of Occupational Performance

Over the course of 2 weeks, the occupational therapist observed Sophia during several 15-minute increments. The occupational therapist wanted to understand how Sophia engaged in occupation throughout the school day and in different contexts.

Sophia was observed in two of her academic courses, art class, lunch period, and in the hallway during a transition period. During the observation, the occupational therapist paid attention to Sophia's overall performance with different activities (e.g., opening containers and cleaning up after lunch, copying assignments from the white board, constructing a sculpture of clay, joking with peers in the hallway, and putting items away in her locker). The occupational therapist also observed Sophia's motor, process, and social interaction skills as outlined in the Occupational Therapy Practice Framework (AOTA, 2020b) and considered how aspects of the environment facilitated or limited Sophia's success with different activities.

The occupational therapist completed the School Function Assessment (Coster et al., 1998) with input from team members who knew Sophia well (i.e., two teachers, the speech-language pathologist, and the paraeducator who aids in the bathroom).

Summary

The occupational therapist summarized the following findings and recommendations to the educational team:

	Strengths	Barriers to Performance
Performance with Everyday School Activities	Sophia enjoys and feels successful playing computer games, going to the library, doing crafts, and being with her friends. Sophia is able to travel to different classes, maintain and change positions, engage in recreational movement, go up/down stairs, and use the computer without assistance. Sophia communicates with her teachers and classmates and loves to tell jokes. She remembers and follows classroom routines and follows a series of instructions to complete projects using a checklist.	Sophia does not enjoy writing stories or engaging in individual physical activities (e.g., running laps in physical education class). Sophia needs frequent assistance when using materials (e.g., taking off and replacing caps on pens and markers, shaping clay, cutting off and applying tape, erasing pencil marks, using paper clips, and collating papers to put into a folder); setup and cleanup (e.g., remove and replace lids on food storage containers during lunch, opening milk cartons, and opening sealed bags); eating (i.e., using a napkin to wipe face and hands), and hygiene (i.e., wipes nose, obtains toilet paper from roll or dispenser, wipes self after toileting).
Contextual Factors Influencing Performance	Even though she has been at her new school for a relatively short period of time, Sophia has established close relationships with three peers and identifies Emma as her best friend. Sophia likes her teachers and paraeducator. The paraeducator is available to assist Sophia in the bathroom, at lunch, and during academic and special area (e.g., art) classes. One of Sophia's parents drives her to/from school each day and her teenage sisters sometimes assist her with homework.	Although the paraeducator is available for assistance, time is divided between Sophia and three other students. The sinks, stall locks, and toilet paper dispensers at this school are different from Sophia's last school. Sophia's lunch is packed in airtight reusable containers. Classrooms frequently don't have facial tissue.

Questions

1. In what ways could an occupational therapy practitioner address Sophia's performance with using materials in art class?

2. In what ways could an occupational therapy practitioner address Sophia's performance with setup/cleanup and eating during lunch?

be included in a written report and shared with the evaluation team to help establish Sophia's educational needs, goals, special education program, and related services.

Intervention

Occupational therapy services address a student's performance based on the evaluation results to support the student's participation in the curriculum, access to the school contexts, and participation in extracurricular activities (Figures 45.2 and 45.3). Intervention services should be

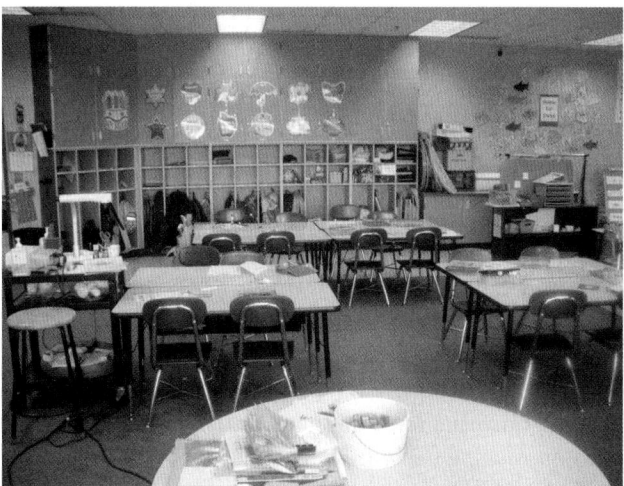

FIGURE 45.2 Occupational therapists may work with teachers to help design a classroom to support student participation.

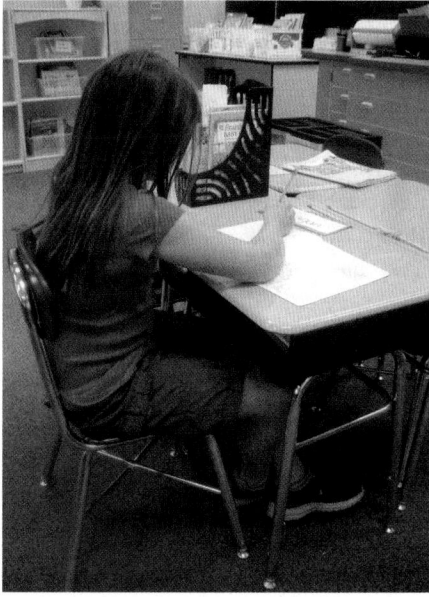

FIGURE 45.3 Occupational therapy works with classroom staff to support proper positioning in the classroom.

contextually based and provided within the context or environment where the student typically spends their time and where the occupation, activity, or skill will usually be performed (e.g., integrated into the student's classroom environment). Interventions should emphasize maximizing the student's strengths.

Factors That Influence Occupational Therapy in Educational Settings

In addition to legislation, a variety of factors affect the planning and implementation of occupational therapy interventions within educational settings. These include unique educational expectations and standards, whether the setting uses a caseload or workload model, and the research evidence supporting intervention.

Educational Expectations and Standards

Each educational setting is driven by expectations and standards. School culture, or the values, beliefs, and traditions shared by members of the school community (e.g., administrators, teachers, students, other educational personnel, and families) help to shape expectations for everyone who identifies as part of that community. Though the concept of school culture is not new, it is often overlooked when planning interventions and new initiatives. Awareness of different aspects of a school's culture may help the occupational therapist prioritize intervention strategies and provide insights into how to best collaborate with the team. Some aspects of school culture that should be considered include attitudes about risk taking, trust, openness, leadership, parent relationships, shared values, and student achievement; habits and routines related to communication, socialization, and decision-making; collegial awareness; and organizational history (Gruenert & Whitaker, 2015). Ideally schools will have a collaborative school culture that values professional development and student achievement, and challenges ineffective practices (Gruenert & Whitaker, 2015).

In addition to expectations associated with school culture, each educational setting is guided by academic standards. It is important to be aware of academic standards so that interventions can be embedded in naturally occurring learning activities. For example, each state and territory in the United States has adopted early learning standards and development guidelines (ELGs) (National Center on Early Childhood Quality Assurance, 2017) for infants and toddlers. Occupational therapy practitioners that work under Part C of IDEA 2004 and in early childhood education settings (e.g., preschools) should be familiar with ELGs. The Common Core standards are used to guide literacy, language arts, and math outcomes for students in kindergarten through 12th grade and are designed to prepare students for success after high school completion (National Governors Association Center for Best Practices & Council of Chief State School Officers, 2010). Schools may also adopt standards related to other academic subject areas (e.g., science and technology) and other aspects of student development (e.g., social emotional learning and character development). Finally, colleges and universities have defined educational outcomes for each program of study.

Caseload or Workload Model

Another factor that influences occupational therapy in educational settings is the service delivery model used in the school or LEA. There are two common service delivery models, one based on caseloads and one based on workloads. The more traditional caseload model is based on the number of students receiving OT services as specified on IEPs, without much consideration to the time spent on other related duties (e.g., performing evaluations for students not yet identified as having an educational disability) or responsibilities (e.g., serving on a school-wide curriculum committee) (Cahill & Bazyk, 2020; Garfinkel & Seruya, 2018). A workload model is based on all of the direct and indirect services performed by the practitioner to benefit students and the school community (Cahill & Bazyk, 2020). The workload model is thought to provide more flexibility and opportunities for practitioners to collaborate with team members, attend meetings, serve on committees, and provide MTSS services (Cahill & Bazyk, 2020). Practitioners who would like to adopt a workload approach should understand their state guidelines, their school or district's formula for determining caseload, and consider ways to gain administrative support (Seruya & Garfinkel, 2020). Time studies and careful documentation of workload responsibilities and student outcomes may be used to advocate for a workload approach (Cahill & Bazyk, 2020; Seruya & Garfinkel, 2020).

Multitiered Systems of Support. As mentioned earlier, MTSS are used by many school districts to provide just-in-time services (i.e., services provided at the first sign of need and before concerns progress or fully develop) to students who are in general education in kindergarten through 12th grade. Occupational therapy practitioners may be involved in each level of MTSS. A workload model might best facilitate their participation. MTSS are implemented systematically and as part of core instruction. MTSS use differentiated instruction and universal design for learning (UDL) strategies. Team-based problem-solving, data collection, and progress monitoring are key aspects of effective MTSS (Cahill & Bazyk, 2020). Response to intervention (RtI) and positive behavioral intervention supports (PBIS) are frameworks often used to provide MTSS.

IDEA 2004 provides an opportunity for school districts to use up to 15% of special education funds for EIS (also known as *pre-referral interventions* or *whole-school approaches*) (Cahill, 2007). EIS are provided to students, not in special education, who need "additional academic and behavioral support to succeed in a general education environment" (§ 300.226). These services are for students "kindergarten through 12th grade (with particular emphasis on kindergarten through grade 3) who are not currently identified as needing special education or related services, but who need additional academic and behavioral support to succeed in a general education environment" (CFR, § 300.226[a]).

All MTSS services should be evidence-based and focused on improving student outcomes. This model generally uses a three-tiered approach to support (Figure 45.4). The role of OT at each tier varies across school districts. Under MTSS, occupational therapy practitioners may provide professional development to other school staff, serve as case managers, develop classroom-level programs, assist with universal screening, and participate in data-based decision-making (Cahill, 2019). OT Story 45.2 provides an illustration of how an occupational therapist might be involved in MTSS.

If the EIS (i.e., tiers 1–3) are not effective, a student is then referred to a special education team for evaluation. The evaluation team determines whether the special education process, as outlined in the IDEA 2004, should be initiated or whether the student should be referred for some other type of support, such as a 504 plan.

College and University Settings. A workload model may also be desirable in other educational systems such as community colleges, colleges, and universities, so that a range of OT services may be provided. Occupational therapy practitioners may work with campus disability service centers to provide direct services to students and support to faculty (e.g., incorporating principles of universal design in instruction). Occupational therapists might develop programs that focus on skill acquisition to promote occupational engagement in the classroom or in independent and group living situations; goal setting and attainment strategies; self-assessment of learning styles and strengths and barriers; study skills and test taking strategies; occupational balance; professional behaviors and time management; and mental health promotion and prevention (Keptner & McCarthy, 2020).

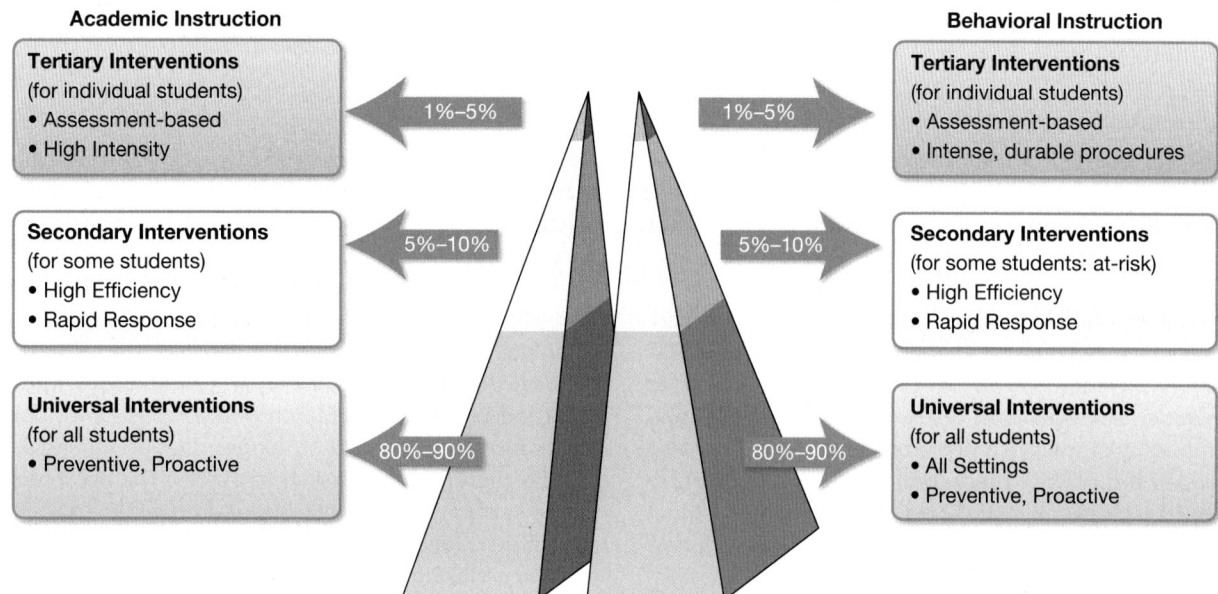

FIGURE 45.4 Multi-tiered system of support (MTSS): A school-wide system for student success that includes both academic and behavioral instruction. (Used with permission from https://www.pbis.org/pbis/what-is-pbis).

OT STORY 45.2 MTSS TO SUPPORT MASON'S EDUCATIONAL PROGRAM

Background

Mason is a 10-year-old boy in fifth grade. He was referred to the school's problem-solving team (i.e., assistant principal, school psychologist, occupational therapist, reading specialist, and general education teacher) by his general education teacher at the beginning of the third quarter. The teacher shared with the problem-solving team that Mason had difficulty with work completion and organization. Mason did not meet expectations on first and second quarter report cards in reading and English/language arts (ELA). His teacher reported that Mason frequently looked frustrated in class and was concerned that if he continued to struggle, he would stop trying and not be prepared for middle school. The teacher shared that Mason's strengths included having many friends, listening to stories, answering comprehension questions, and math skills.

Tier 2

After viewing some of Mason's work products and a brief discussion, the problem-solving team determined that one reason Mason was not meeting expectation was because he frequently turned in half-completed assignments. They also noted that Mason's assignments frequently included misspellings and grammatical errors. They hypothesized that Mason might need short-term support with time management and developing habits associated using classroom

resources (e.g., word wall and dictionary) and recommended him for tier 2 services. One of the tier 2 supports used at the school was a study hall group led by the occupational therapy assistant (OTA). The study hall group was designed by OT and the OTA to address common concerns experienced by general education students preparing to enter middle school (e.g., managing long-term projects and allowing enough time for homework after school).

The team worked with Mason's teacher to develop a plan to address his concerns. Mason's parents were informed of the intervention plan and gave permission for Mason to receive tier 2 services provided by the OTA. The plan included temporarily extending assignment due dates, allowing Mason to bring home in-class assignments to finish as homework, and inviting him to attend a weekly 30-minute-long "study hall" with the OTA and a small group of students with similar concerns for 6 weeks. In the group, the OTA worked with Mason and the other students to estimate how long it would take them to complete different types of assignments, use a calendar to plan timelines for different assignments, and develop a checklist for items every fifth grader should review before turning in an assignment. The OTA also worked with the group of students to develop habits around using classroom resources that would support their performance (e.g., bringing the dictionary and grammar "cheat sheet" to their desk before independent work time, drafting an assignment

(continued)

OT STORY 45.2 MTSS TO SUPPORT MASON'S EDUCATIONAL PROGRAM (continued)

and circling words that might be misspelled, looking up the words in the dictionary after the first draft was completed, revising words that were misspelled, reviewing other checklist items, and correcting the assignment as needed).

The team also set up a continuous progress monitoring system to track Mason's progress with the intervention plan. The team tracked the total number of reading and ELA assignments Mason had per week for 6 weeks, as well as the number of assignments that were fully completed and the frequency of spelling and grammatical errors. They also developed a quick self-check form (three visual scales) for Mason to indicate how confident he felt using classroom resources and the checklist, how satisfied he was with how long it took him to complete assignments, and how satisfied he was with the quality of his final work product. Mason completed the self-checks in class on days when he did not attend the study hall group. The teacher saved all of Mason's assignments and his self-checks and gave them to the reading specialist at the end of the week. The reading specialist summarized the progress monitoring data for the team to review after the 6-week intervention.

Six-Week Review Meeting

After 6 weeks of the intervention, the problem-solving team met to review Mason's progress monitoring data. The team discovered that Mason's frequency of missing assignments reduced significantly from 5 per week to zero per week. The frequency of misspelled words was also reduced and so were basic grammatical errors, like punctuation. Mason's self-checks indicated that he felt increased confidence using classroom resources and the checklist and that he was more satisfied with the quality of his work. However, his satisfaction with the amount of time it took him to complete assignments was not much improved. The occupational therapist shared the OTA's observations with the team and explained that Mason worked consistently during the group study hall and no longer needed reminders to use the checklist or classroom resources. The occupational therapist also reported that Mason frequently asked what certain questions on assignments meant and that he had a hard time making inferences about what he read. Mason's teacher confirmed that even though he was more successful with turning in assignments and had less spelling and grammatical errors, that the quality of his work was not at the same level as his peers.

Questions

1. Should the occupational therapist recommend continuing or discontinuing Mason's tier 2 intervention? What other interventions or referrals might be needed at this time?

2. What strategies or interventions could be introduced to address Mason's satisfaction with the amount of time it takes him to complete his assignments?

EXPANDING OUR PERSPECTIVES

Occupational Therapy in Higher Education

Karen M. Keptner, PhD, OTR/L

Education is seen as a vehicle for social inclusion and a social determinant of health (Whiteford, 2017; Wilcock & Hocking, 2015). Successful performance in educational spaces can be enhanced by providing appropriate supports, including occupational therapy. However, lack of visibility in secondary settings influences the role that OT has in transition services (Eismann et al., 2017; Kardos & White, 2005) and also limits the availability of OT on campuses of higher education. As a unique support on campus, the role of OT is highlighted by the following example:

Julie is a first-year law student who was recently diagnosed with ADHD. She explains that through most of her schooling she did well, but felt "stressed" a lot, but she still got good grades. Once she got to law school, her ability to manage that bit of "stress" and the demands of being a law student became overwhelming. She finally sought support and was diagnosed with ADHD. When she was interviewed by an occupational therapist, she stated "everything makes sense now—I am so happy to have you here to help me figure out how to understand my strengths and my ADHD and how I can change what I am doing to be successful."

Since 2014, I have dedicated much of my time and energy to promoting OT in a higher education space. I envisioned OT on the campus of Cleveland State University in Cleveland, Ohio. As part of that process, I started collecting information about the occupational needs of students (Keptner, 2019; Keptner & Rogers, 2019) and provided a 5-week group intervention that focused on occupations with university freshmen (Keptner et al., 2016). Those students who participated in this targeted intervention exhibited improved occupational performance and satisfaction in self-identified areas (Keptner et al., 2016). Over the years, I have nurtured relationships on campus with Office of Disability Services, Office of Institutional Equity, and in offices that support first-generation, low-income, and foster youth. It was in these collaborative relationships and showing the value of OT through "doing" that I developed interventions to target both skill development and health promotion.

A credit-bearing course sequence that I developed addresses occupational skill development. In addition to the course, OT students at Cleveland State are now offering limited OT intervention as part of a level I fieldwork opportunity in the fall and spring semesters. This level I work is facilitated by staff in the OT program, but follow-up care is provided by an occupational therapist who has been hired on campus. As the visibility of OT has grown, I have been asked to consult in various programs on campus that service students who need additional supports, such as those who have experienced foster care.

For OT professionals wishing to work on campuses, a group of OT professionals from around the globe have joined forces to support each other and advocate for this as a recognized practice area in occupational therapy. We are called OT-U. #ot_u #otu

References

Eismann, M. M., Weisshaar, R., Capretta, C., Cleary, D. S., Kirby, A. V., & Persch, A. C. (2017). Centennial topics—Characteristics of students receiving occupational therapy services in transition and factors related to postsecondary success. *American Journal of Occupational Therapy, 71,* 7103100010. https://doi.org/10.5014/ajot.2017.024927

Kardos, M., & White, B. P. (2005). The role of the school-based occupational therapist in secondary education transition planning: A pilot survey study. *American Journal of Occupational Therapy, 59,* 173–180. https://doi.org/10.5014/ajot.59.2.173

Keptner, K. M. (2019). Relationship between occupational performance measures and adjustment in a sample of university students. *Journal of Occupational Science, 26*(1), 6–17. https://doi.org/10.1080/14427591.2018.1539409

Keptner, K. M., & Rogers, R. (2019). Competence and satisfaction in occupational performance among a sample of university students: An exploratory study. *Occupational Therapy Journal of Research: Occupation, Participation, and Health, 39*(4). 204–212. https://doi.org/10.1177/1539449218813702

Whiteford, G. (2017). Participation in higher education as social inclusion: An occupational perspective. *Journal of Occupational Science, 24*(1), 54–63. https://doi.org/10.1080/14427591.2017.1284151

Wilcock, A. A., & Hocking, C. (2015). *An occupational perspective on health* (3rd ed.). Slack.

Development of the Individualized Plan

Once the evaluation has been completed, the IFSP, IEP, or ITP team collaborates to design the child or student's educational program. IFSPs are plans that include the child and family needs and are used in early intervention (age 0–3 year services) programs. IEPs are programs that address the needs of students in preschool through high school. ITPs are developed by the time a student turns 16 years and reflect the student's skills and aptitudes and guides teams to discuss and prepare the student for postschool programs (i.e., work, higher education, and adult day health) (Figure 45.5). When developing the IFSP, IEP, or ITP, the team, which includes the parents and the student (whenever appropriate), first reviews the evaluation results and writes a summary of the student's educational performance, called *present levels of academic achievement and functional performance.* The present levels describe the student's strengths and areas of concern in relation to the expectations of the general education curriculum. The team then develops the student's *goals and objectives* based on the data summarized in the present levels and the agreed-on outcomes that the team has identified.

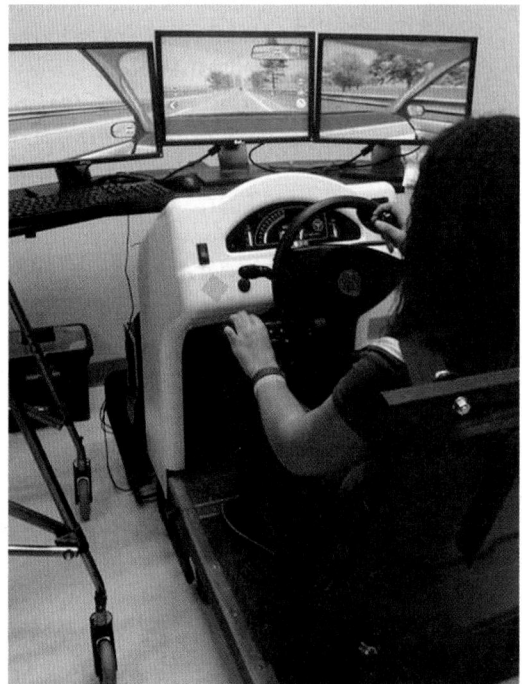

FIGURE 45.5 School-based therapists can support transition planning through activities such as adaptive driving.

Different settings have different requirements for how goals and objectives are written. Under the IDEA 2004, it is ideal for goals and objectives to be developed as a team. After the goals and objectives have been developed, the team discusses which professional(s) should address particular goals (e.g., teacher and occupational therapist or maybe occupational therapist and speech-language pathologist), when they will be addressed (e.g., during physical education, during art, and when walking in the hall), and where they will be addressed (e.g., in the general education classroom, in the cafeteria, and on the playground). Each of these decisions is made based on the student's needs, not the personal preferences of professionals.

The Occupational Therapy Intervention Plan

Once the team has developed the educational program and determines that a student would benefit from receiving OT services to reach anticipated outcomes, the occupational therapist develops a specific OT intervention plan. The intervention plan addresses the occupational performance areas that are affecting the student's ability to fully participate in the educational environment. The IFSP, IEP, or ITP goals may be the goals on the intervention plan. However, if the goals were written collaboratively, then the OT intervention plan may have OT-specific goals.

As in other settings, the occupational therapist considers motor skills, process skills, and social interaction skills when determining student needs. Additionally, the occupational therapist considers performance patterns, such as habits and routines, the activity demands in the school setting, and the entire school context when determining student needs. With occupational performance as the core, a variety of conceptual frameworks for practice and frames of references guide OT interventions in educational settings.

Service Delivery

Planning Intervention

When planning the intervention implementation, occupational therapists must consider the LRE requirement of IDEA 2004: "to the maximum extent appropriate, children with disabilities are to be educated with children who are not disabled . . . removal of these children from the general educational environment occurs only when the nature or severity of the disability is such that education in regular classes with the use of supplementary aids and services cannot be achieved satisfactorily (Least Restrictive Environment)" (§ 300.114[a][2][i]). Occupational therapy should

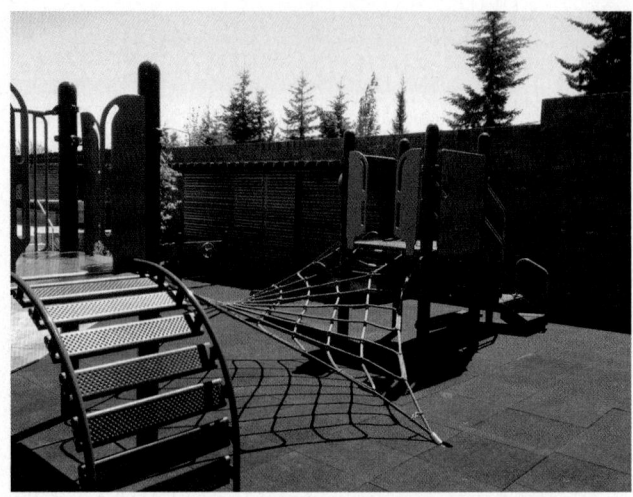

FIGURE 45.6 Occupational therapists support student participation on the playground and may be involved in playground design.

be contextually based and embedded in the student's typical context and environments to the extent possible. It is appropriate to provide occupational therapy services in general and special education classrooms, cafeterias, bathrooms, playgrounds (Figure 45.6), and during transition periods (e.g., on/off bus and in the hallway during passing periods).

Service Delivery Categories

Service delivery happens in many ways within educational settings. IDEA 2004 defines four different categories for service delivery:

1. Specially designed instruction
2. Related services
3. Supplemental aids and services
4. Services on behalf of the child

In most educational settings, OT practitioners provide related services, supplemental aids and services, and services on behalf of the child. Depending on the rules and regulations in a particular state, an occupational therapist might provide specially designed instruction. For example, a student with typical cognition but significant motor delays (e.g., muscular dystrophy, spina bifida, and cerebral palsy) might require more support than just accommodations or adaptations to participate within their educational setting.

The term *indirect services* is used to describe situations where the OT practitioner does not work directly with the student. In the terms of IDEA, these can be viewed as related services, but some districts document these services as supplemental aids and services (especially if provided in the general education setting) or services on behalf of the child when they are provided around a specific need

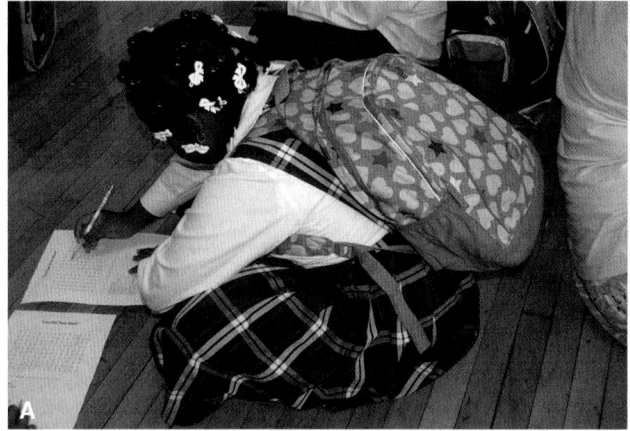

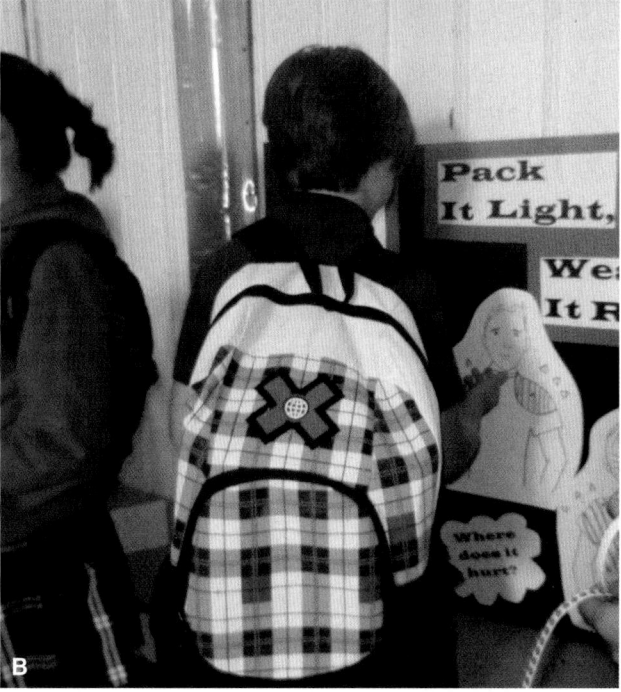

FIGURE 45.7 **A and B:** Participating in the American Occupational Therapy Association's (AOTA) backpack campaign in the schools may prevent future injury for some students. (Photos courtesy of Karen Jacobs, EdD, OTR/L, CPE, FAOTA.)

of a specific student. Some system supports, information sharing, and accommodations may be provided to general education students as part of MTSS, particularly if they are designed to benefit the majority of general education students. Occupational therapy practitioners in the schools can help other stakeholders in the schools better understand students' unique health needs, such as why it is important not to overweight school backpacks (Figure 45.7A and B).

For some students, a greater intensity of services may be needed. These services are often referred to as *direct services* and may include the OT practitioner working directly with

the student. The goal is to provide services *in context* (e.g., in the classroom, lunchroom, and during recess) whenever possible. Removing a student from the educational setting to go to a therapy room (or any other space) should be done only if the skill cannot be addressed in context and only for a short period of time, because removing the child from the typical context is considered a more restrictive environment. When this is necessary, an LRE option of service delivery should be implemented as soon as possible. Often, services are provided out of context for very brief periods of time to help a child learn a new skill (e.g., a technique for donning a coat). But once the skill is learned in a 1:1 setting, the student should practice and refine the skill as part of the natural school routine (e.g., near their locker at the end of the school day). Regardless of the type of service delivery provided by the practitioner, *team supports* should be considered (Hanft & Shepherd, 2016).

Interagency Collaboration

Another important aspect of OT service delivery in educational settings includes collaboration between school personnel and staff from any clinic a child might be attending as well as collaboration with other agencies. Interagency collaboration is particularly necessary if the OT practitioner is providing services to students who use assistive technology or have a transition plan. Such collaboration is important for other educational settings as well. For example, if a student with a disability who is attending university needs specialized adaptive equipment to fully participate, the Department of Vocational Rehabilitation might help with the procurement of such device.

Documentation and Intervention Review

Inherent in service delivery in any setting is the documentation of services. Documentation serves as a communication tool to the students and families regarding the individualized program. Additionally, all decision-making about OT intervention in the schools should be evidence-informed and based on student outcome data to the maximum extent possible. IDEA 2004 requires that the IFSP, IEP, or ITP be reviewed at least annually, with regular updates to the family regarding the student's progress. These updates regarding student progress on IEPs/ITPs must be at least at the same intervals as general education report cards. However, the occupational therapist should consistently (more often than quarterly) review the intervention plan to ensure that the student is progressing toward targeted outcomes. If necessary, the OT intervention plan or even the IFSP, IEP, or ITP might need to be modified before the annual review.

Additional Practice Considerations

Services in schools continue to evolve based on the unique, changing occupational needs of the students and the system. Occupational therapy practitioners with their unique skills in activity analysis and their awareness of the interaction among the client, occupation, and environment are well equipped to collaborate and partner with many other professionals in the schools to support participation and performance. Some practice considerations resulting from changing occupational needs in education include quality indicators, student mental health, health management, telehealth, and school leadership.

Quality Indicators

Coordinating and managing the delivery of OT in the schools in the United States is complex and requires compliance with federal legislation and state and local policies, as well as astute professional reasoning (Laverdure & Polichino, 2019). Occupational therapy practitioners working in the schools often receive little oversight by supervisors and are evaluated with tools designed for measuring teacher performance (Laverdure & Polichino, 2019). Supervisors evaluating the effectiveness of OT services should be familiar with the Occupational Therapy Practice Framework (4th ed., AOTA, 2020b), Code of Ethics (AOTA, 2020c), and Quality Indicators for School-based Practice (Laverdure et al., 2019). Quality indicators are criteria used to measure the quality of provided services, identify areas that require additional development, and track changes over time. The Quality Indicators for School-based Practice include seven key principles and over 25 quality indicators (Box 45.4) with objective criteria that define exemplary, proficient, and developing professional behaviors (Laverdure et al., 2019; Laverdure & Swinth, 2022).

Student Mental Health

Occupational therapy has strong roots in mental health and addressing psychosocial needs of children and youth. There has been an increased emphasis on building the capacity of school-based OT practitioners to provide mental health services to students (Bazyk et al., 2015, 2020). The increased awareness of developmental trauma and the impact on the student's behavior as well as the ability to engage, learn, and/or interact with others increases the need for service providers in the schools who understand the unique needs of this population (AOTA, 2018). Occupational therapy practitioners are well positioned to provide trauma-informed care (Lynch et al., 2021) and help school teams address the mental health and psychosocial needs of students. See Chapter 69.

Practitioners in the schools may collaborate with school counselors or school psychologists to address mental health across MTSS and in special education. Bazyk (2011) lays a foundation for this work in her book, *Mental Health Promotion, Prevention, and Intervention With Children and Youth*. In addition, Bazyk started the *Every Moment Counts* mental health promotion initiative (www.everymoment-counts.org) to help all children and youth achieve a positive state of mental health. Every Moment Counts includes evidence-based ready-to-use resources for practitioners to address mental health when embedding services, working with students during recess (e.g., Refreshing Recess), at lunchtime (e.g., Comfortable Cafeteria, including modifications for middle school students), and throughout the school day (e.g., Calm Moment Cards and Making Leisure Matter).

Health Management

With the emphasis on health in the Occupational Therapy Practice Framework (4th ed., AOTA, 2020b) and the necessity of health management skills for students with chronic conditions, OT practitioners may work as part of the team to support student engagement in this occupation (Cahill et al., 2016; Polo & Cahill, 2017). Occupational therapy practitioners play important roles in addressing health management in a variety of settings, including in schools and communities and at home. In each setting, intervention may focus on education about symptom and condition management, medication management, social and emotional health promotion and maintenance, personal care device management, physical activity, nutrition management, and communication with the healthcare team (e.g., school nurse) (AOTA, 2020b). For more information on health management, see Chapter 50.

Telehealth

School-based OT practitioners quickly adapted to using telehealth as the main form of service delivery during the global COVID-19 public health emergency (Niblock, 2021). The successful use of telehealth requires that OT practitioners have competence using software and web-based meeting systems, demonstrate interprofessional collaboration with school personnel and e-helpers (Niblock, 2021), and apply principles of ethical, procedural, interactive, and conditional reasoning (Jackson, 2021). Nearly all traditional hands-on services provided by OT practitioners can be achieved through telehealth, including evaluation (Jackson, 2021), establishing rapport and intervention (Little & Wallisch, 2021), supporting self-regulation (Watling & Anderson, 2021), and coaching and supporting caregivers and other professionals (Wallisch & Little, 2021). This form of service delivery can be more cost-effective for school districts by decreasing travel time as well. Additionally, telehealth may help address the shortage of school-based

BOX 45.4 QUALITY INDICATORS FOR EFFECTIVE SCHOOL PRACTICE

Occupational therapy practitioners should:

- Demonstrate knowledge of children's developmental and learning characteristics
- Demonstrate knowledge of current research related to school-based practice
- Promote wellness and safety
- Advocate for access to occupational therapy service
- Demonstrate knowledge of federal, state, and local policies that impact occupational therapy service delivery
- Demonstrate knowledge of structure of educational settings and related agencies
- Demonstrate knowledge of special education process and curriculum standards
- Adheres to the Code of Ethics
- Demonstrate knowledge of licensure mandates and professional documents that drive practice
- Support school-wide screening, early intervening services and response to intervention
- Determine students' strengths and needs related to participation in school activities and contexts
- Select and administer assessment tools and procedures

- Demonstrate theoretical foundations of school occupational therapy and how it relates to the curriculum and students' needs
- Use student data to make decisions and participate in IEP development
- Document student progress throughout the school year
- Embed interventions into students' typical contexts
- Use various types of service delivery
- Adapt environments to facilitate student access and participation
- Promote environments that value all types of diversity
- Educate school teams and families
- Collaborate and partner with all members of the school team, family, and community members
- Provide supervision to occupational therapy students and other professionals
- Evaluate and apply evidence
- Produce accurate and defensible written documentation
- Evaluate and document effectiveness of occupational therapy
- Demonstrate effective time management and prioritization skills
- Participate in program evaluation

Adapted from: Laverdure, P., & Swinth, Y. (2022, March). *Quality indicators in school occupational therapy practice.* https://drive.google.com/drive/folders/1etGA05OQmAI1LQAERdOxmA6oaCs2U5dk

practitioners in some areas. As with any other OT services, school-based practitioners using telehealth need to attend to ethical considerations specific to this service delivery method. See Chapter 67.

School Leadership

School-based practitioners are seeking leadership positions in the schools. Although this can be challenging because of different state requirements, occupational therapists are well suited for this role in the schools. Many occupational therapists lead SISP teams, and some others have been successful obtaining other positions such as case manager and program coordinator. Occupational therapy practitioners should continue to advocate for school leadership opportunities by seeking representation on school-wide committees and teams, mobilizing with other practitioners who share common goals, and looking for opportunities to share OT's unique value and skill set with administrators and other leaders in education (Schefkind, 2019).

Outcomes

Occupational therapy practitioners provide services in educational settings to support goals and participation in

the LRE (Cahill & Bazyk, 2020). Practitioners address all areas of student role development and performance and begin with engagement in meaningful occupations and activities (Figure 45.8). Integrated or contextually based services provide opportunities to address needs where they happen. Research related to OT and school outcomes

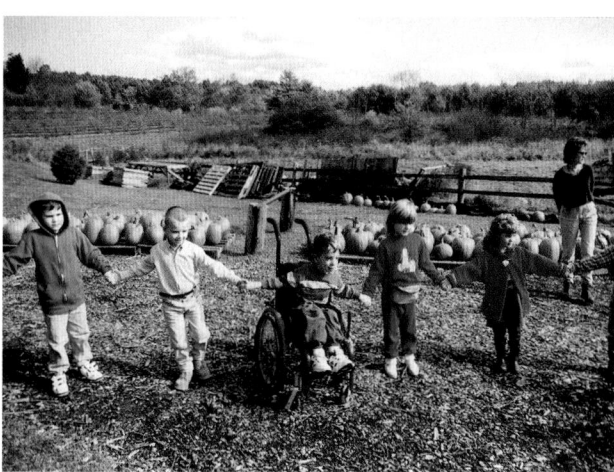

FIGURE 45.8 **A functional outcome for a child in a preschool setting is participation with classmates during a field trip to pick pumpkins.**

" COMMENTARY ON THE EVIDENCE

School-Based Practice

The Individuals with Disabilities Education Act (IDEA) 2004 requires that OT practitioners use "scientifically based instructional practices, to the maximum extent possible" (§ 601[c][5][E]). This requirement is congruent with OT in any setting and is applicable to all professionals who provide services in public schools. Occupational therapy practitioners should use research evidence to examine the assumptions that guide their practice. To increase the breadth and depth of the evidence, a culture of inquiry needs to be established among school-based practitioners. Occupational therapy school leaders who value evidence-based practice should consider collaborating with universities to provide targeted professional development opportunities to increase skills and confidence with finding and applying evidence to practice (Cahill et al., 2015). In addition, Frolek Clark et al. (2019) edited *Best Practices for Occupational Therapy in Schools* (2nd ed.); this book provides information on all aspects of school practice in the United States and the latest research on a variety of related different topics. Systematic reviews related to interventions within the scope of OT to improve children's academic participation school-based practice (see, e.g., Grajo et al., 2020) and AOTA Practice Guidelines (see, e.g., Cahill & Beisbier, 2020) are also available.

The following table provides *examples* of evidence and implications for decision-making that can be used by school-based OT practitioners.

Performance Area	Evidence Source	Implications for Decision-Making
ADL	Beisbier and Laverdure (2020)	• Engagement in self-care activities and routines improves participation and performance of functional life skills of children with disabilities. • Collaborative goal setting, instruction, and feedback improves self-care participation, performance, and satisfaction.
IADL	Beisbier and Laverdure (2020) Cahill et al. (2020)	• Training in interactive virtual pedestrian environment and at street-side locations, along with widely available video and internet programs on pedestrian safety are effective in supporting the development of safety skills in children. • On-the-road training and self-evaluation exercises, video-based hazard perception training, and coaching practices are effective for teaching driving skills. • Productive occupations, life skills training, and graded activities are effective in addressing psychosocial and mental health outcomes associated with IADL participation.
Education	Grajo et al. (2020)	• Literacy stations and embedded creative discussions increase positive attitudes toward reading and improve children's self-concept as a reader. • Combining sensorimotor and therapeutic practice using a manualized program (e.g., Write Start, Handwriting Without Tears, and Size Matters) during usual classroom routines improves handwriting.
Work	Le et al. (2021)	• Video modeling improves participation in work for autistic adolescents and adults with a spectrum of different cognitive abilities.
Play/Leisure	Laverdure and Beisbier (2021)	• Contextual modifications (painting of playground surfaces, provision of small and large equipment, school policy changes) increase play among school-age children.
Social Participation	Beisbier and Laverdure (2020) Laverdure and Beisbier (2021)	• Organized recess activities, class game time, and coach training improve student participation during recess. • Active coaching, modeling, and guided play during recess increase engagement for autistic children. • Manualized social participation interventions over extended periods of time increase peer engagement, social awareness, communication, and motivation for autistic children.
Health management	Beisbier and Laverdure (2020)	• Education and skills training using cognitive behavioral strategies and provided during small group activities is effective for children and youth with health concerns.

is growing and evidence-informed practice should be the norm. When evidence is not available to support practice, OT practitioners should systematically collect data to guide decision-making about the use and continuation of certain interventions. See Commentary on the Evidence for more information.

Conclusion

Occupational therapy practitioners provide services to address educational needs across various settings. Practitioners who work in the schools collaborate with educational teams to determine student needs and targeted outcomes. Occupational therapy intervention in schools focuses on occupational performance in the student role and within the educational environment. Practitioners also provide services that are directed to the needs of the educational staff, parents, or system. Intervention strategies should be evidence-informed and decision-making should be data-driven.

Acknowledgments

The author would like to acknowledge Yvonne Swinth, PhD, OTR/L, FAOTA for her contributions to this chapter.

Lippincott® Connect *For additional resources on the subjects discussed in this chapter, visit Lippincott Connect.*

REFERENCES

American Occupational Therapy Association. (2018). AOTA's societal statement on stress, trauma, and posttraumatic stress disorder. *American Journal of Occupational Therapy, 72*(Suppl. 2), 7212410080. https://doi.org/10.5014/ajot.2018.72S208

American Occupational Therapy Association. (2020a). *AOTA 2019 workforce and salary survey: Executive summary.* Author.

American Occupational Therapy Association. (2020b). Occupational therapy practice framework: Domain and process (4th ed.). *American Journal of Occupational Therapy, 74*(Suppl. 2), 7412410010. https://doi.org/10.5014/ajot.2020.74S2001

American Occupational Therapy Association. (2020c). Occupational therapy code of ethics. *American Journal of Occupational Therapy, 74*(3), 7413410005p1–7413410005p13. https://doi.org/10.5014/ajot.2020.74S3006

American Occupational Therapy Association. (2021). The association—Improve your documentation and quality of care with AOTA's updated occupational profile template. *American Journal of Occupational Therapy, 75*(2), 7502420010. https://doi.org/10.5014/ajot.2021.752001

Americans with Disabilities Act of 1990, 42 U.S.C.A. § 12134 (1990).

Amundson, S. (1995). *Evaluation tool of children's handwriting: ETCH examiner's manual.* OT Kids.

Arnaud, L. M., & Gutman, S. A. (2021). Supporting literacy participation for underserved children: A set of guidelines for occupational therapy practice. *Journal of Occupational Therapy, Schools, & Early Intervention,* 1–20. https://doi.org/10.1080/19411243.2021.1934234

Bazyk, S. (2011). *Mental health promotion, prevention, and intervention with children and youth: A guiding framework for occupational therapy.* AOTA Press.

Bazyk, S., Demirjian, L., Horvath, F., & Doxsey, L. (2018). The comfortable cafeteria program for promoting student participation and enjoyment: An outcome study. *The American Journal of Occupational Therapy, 72*(3), 7203205050p1–7203205050p9. https://doi.org/10.5014/ajot.2018.025379

Bazyk, S., Demirjian, L., LaGuardia, T., Thompson-Repas, K., Conway, C., & Michaud, P. (2015). Building capacity of occupational therapy practitioners to address the mental health needs of children and youth: A mixed-methods study of knowledge translation. *The American Journal of Occupational Therapy, 69*(6), 6906180060p1–6906180060p10. https://doi.org/10.5014/ajot.2015.019182

Bazyk, S., Pataki, K., & DeBoth, K. (2020). Building capacity of occupational therapy students to address the mental health needs of children and youth during a level II fieldwork in a school setting. *Journal*
of Occupational Therapy, Schools, & Early Intervention, 13(4), 443–461. https://doi.org/10.1080/19411243.2020.1776186

Beery, K., & Buktenica, N. (2010). *Beery-Buktenica developmental test of visual-motor integration* (6th ed.). WPS Services.

Beisbier, S., & Laverdure, P. (2020). Occupation-and activity-based interventions to improve performance of instrumental activities of daily living and rest and sleep for children and youth ages 5–21: A systematic review. *The American Journal of Occupational Therapy, 74*(2), 7402180040p1–7402180040p32. https://doi.org/10.5014/ajot.2020.039636

Biegun, D., Peterson, Y., McNaught, J., & Sutterfield, C. (2020). Including student voice in IEP meetings through use of assistive technology. *Teaching Exceptional Children, 52*(5), 348–350. https://doi.org/10.1177/0040059920920148

Bruininks, R., & Bruininks, B. (2005). *Bruininks-Oseretsky test of motor proficiency* (2nd ed.). Pearson.

Cahill, S. (2007). A perspective on response to intervention. *School System Special Interest Section Quarterly, 14*(3), 1–4.

Cahill, S. (2019). Multi-tiered systems of support. In G. Frolek Clark, J. E. Rioux, & B. E. Chandler (Eds.), *Best practices for occupational therapy in schools* (2nd ed., pp. 211–217). AOTA Press.

Cahill, S. (2020). Evaluation, interpretation and goal writing. In J. O'Brien & H. Miller-Kuhanek (Eds.), *Occupational therapy for children and adolescents* (8th ed., pp. 181–197). Elsevier.

Cahill, S., & Bazyk, S. (2020). School-based occupational therapy. In J. O'Brien & H. Miller-Kuhanek (Eds.), *Occupational therapy for children and adolescents* (8th ed., pp. 627–658). Elsevier.

Cahill, S. M., & Beisbier, S. (2020). Practice guidelines—Occupational therapy practice guidelines for children and youth ages 5–21 years. *American Journal of Occupational Therapy, 74*, 7404397010. https://doi.org/10.5014/ajot.2020.744001

Cahill, S. M., Egan, B. E., & Seber, J. (2020). Activity- and occupation-based interventions to support mental health, positive behavior, and social participation for children and youth: A systematic review. *American Journal of Occupational Therapy, 74*, 7402180020. https://doi.org/10.5014/ajot.2020.038687

Cahill, S. M., Egan, B. E., Wallingford, M., Huber-Lee, C., & Dess-McGuire, M. (2015). Results of a school-based evidence-based practice initiative. *American Journal of Occupational Therapy, 69*, 6902220010. https://doi.org/10.5014/ajot.2015.014597

Cahill, S. M., Polo, K. M., Egan, B. E., & Marasti, N. (2016). Interventions to promote diabetes self-management in children and youth: A scoping review. *The American Journal of Occupational Therapy, 70*(5), 7005180020p1–7005180020p8. https://doi.org/10.5014/ajot.2016.021618

Cavendish, W., Connor, D. J., & Rediker, E. (2017). Engaging students and parents in transition-focused individualized education programs. *Intervention in School and Clinic, 52*(4), 228–235. https://doi.org/10.1177/1053451216659469

Colarusso, R., & Hammill, D. (2015). *Motor-free visual perception test* (4th ed.). WPS Services.

Coster, W., Deeney, T., Haltiwanger, J., & Haley, S. (1998). *School function assessment (SFA).* The Psychological Corporation.

Dirette, D. P. (2019). Disability services for students in postsecondary education: Opportunities for occupational therapy. *The Open Journal of Occupational Therapy, 7*(2), Article 1. https://doi.org/10.15453/2168-6408.1609

Education for All Handicapped Children Act of 1975, Pub. L. No. 94-142, 20 U.S.C., § 1401, Part H, § 677 (1975).

Every Student Succeeds Act of 2015, Pub. L. No. 114-95 § 114 Stat. 1177 (2015).

Fisher, A. G., Bryze, K., Hume, V., & Griswold, L. A. (2007). *School AMPS: School version of the assessment of motor and process skills* (2nd ed.). Three Star Press.

Fisher, A. G., & Griswold, L. A. (2010). *Evaluation of social interaction.* Three Star Press.

Frolek Clark, G., Rioux, J. E., & Chandler, B. E. (Eds.). (2019). *Best practices for occupational therapy in schools* (2nd ed.). AOTA Press.

Garfinkel, M., & Seruya, F. M. (2018). Therapists' perceptions of the 3:1 service delivery model: A workload approach to school-based practice. *Journal of Occupational Therapy, Schools, and Early Intervention, 11,* 273–290. https://doi.org/10.1080/19411243.2018.1455551

Grajo, L. C., Candler, C., & Sarafian, A. (2020). Interventions within the scope of occupational therapy to improve children's academic participation: A systematic review. *The American Journal of Occupational Therapy, 74*(2), 7402180030p1–7402180030p32. https://doi.org/10.5014/ajot.2020.039016

Gresham, F., & Elliott, S. (2008). *Social skills improvement system SSIS rating scales manual.* Pearson.

Gruenert, S., & Whitaker, T. (2015). *School culture rewired: How to define, assess, and transform it.* ASCD.

Haines, S. J., Francis, G. L., Shepherd, K. G., Ziegler, M., & Mabika, G. (2018). Partnership bound: Using MAPS with transitioning students and families from all backgrounds. *Career Development and Transition for Exceptional Individuals, 41*(2), 122–126. https://doi.org/10.1177/2165143417698123

Hanft, B., & Shepherd, J. (2016). *Collaboration and teamwork: Essential to school-based occupational therapy* (2nd ed.). AOTA Press.

Hemmingsson, H., Egilson, S., Hoffman, O., & Kielhofner, G. (2005). *The school setting interview.* University of Illinois at Chicago.

Individuals with Disabilities Education Act Amendments of 1990, Pub. L. No. 101-476, 20 U.S.C. §1400–1485, 104 Stat. 1142 (1990).

Individuals with Disabilities Education Act Amendments of 1997, Pub. L. No. 105-117, 20 U.S.C. 1400 et se, 111 Stat. 37 (1997).

Individuals with Disabilities Education Improvement Act of 2004, Pub. L. No. 108-446, 20 U.S.C. § 1400 et seq, 118 Stat. 2647 (2004).

Jackson, D. (2021). Telehealth evaluation and assessment in schools. In American Occupational Therapy Association (Ed.), *Telehealth and occupational therapy in schools* (pp. 51–78). AOTA Press.

Jimerson, S., Burns, M., & VanDerHeyden, A. (2015). From RtI to MTSS: Advances in the science and practice of assessment and intervention. In S. Jimerson, M. Burns, & A. VanDerHeyden (Eds.), *Handbook of response to intervention: The science and practice of multi-tiered systems of support.* Springer.

Keptner, K. M., Harris, A., Mellyn, J., Neff, N., Rassie, N., & Thompson, K. (2016). Occupational therapy services to promote occupational performance, performance satisfaction, and quality of life in university freshmen: A pilot study. *Occupational Therapy in Mental Health, 32*(2), 185-202. https://doi.org/10.1080/0164212X.2015.1135094

Keptner, K. M., & McCarthy, K. (2020). Mapping occupational therapy practice with postsecondary students: A scoping review. *The Open Journal of Occupational Therapy, 8*(1), 1–17. https://doi.org/10.15453/2168-6408.1617

King, G., Law, M., King, S., Hurley, P., Hanna, S., Kertoy, M., Rosenbaum, P., & Young, N. (2004). *Children's Assessment of Participation and Enjoyment (CAPE) and Preferences for Activities of Children (PAC).* Harcourt Assessment.

Kramer, J., ten Velden, M., Kafkes, A., Basu, S., Federico, J., & Kielhofner, G. (2014). *Child Occupational Self-Assessment (v 2.2).* University of Illinois at Chicago.

Laverdure, P., & Beisbier, S. (2021). Occupation-and activity-based interventions to improve performance of activities of daily living, play, and leisure for children and youth ages 5 to 21: A systematic review. *The American Journal of Occupational Therapy, 75*(1), 7501205050p1–7501205050p24. https://doi.org/10.5014/ajot.2021.039560

Laverdure, P., McCann, M., McLoone, H., Moore, L., & Reed, L. (2019). Developing quality indicators for school practice. *Journal of Occupational Therapy, Schools, & Early Intervention, 12*(1), 38–50. https://doi.org/10.1080/19411243.2018.1496871

Laverdure, P., & Polichino, J. (2019). Best practice for occupational therapy practitioners as school administrators. In G. Frolek Clark, J. E. Rioux, & B. E. Chandler (Eds.), *Best practices for occupational therapy in schools* (2nd ed., pp. 61–68). AOTA Press.

Laverdure, P., & Swinth, Y. (2022, March). *Quality indicators in school occupational therapy practice.* https://drive.google.com/drive/folders/1etGA05OQmAI1LQAERdOxmA6oaCs2U5dk

Law, M., Baptiste, S., Carswell, A., Mccoll, M. A., Polatajko, H., & Pollock, N. (2005). *Canadian occupational performance measure. Assessment (Vol. Fourth).* Canadian Association of Occupational Therapists.

Le, T., Rodrigues, B., & Hess, L. G. (2021). Video modeling use in work occupations for people with autism: A systematic review. *The American Journal of Occupational Therapy, 75*(3). https://doi.org/10.5014/ajot.2021.041921

Little, L., & Wallisch, A. (2021). Implementing interventions in schools through telehealth. In American Occupational Therapy Association (Ed.), *Telehealth and occupational therapy in schools* (pp. 123–146). AOTA Press.

Lynch, A., Ashcraft, R., & Tekell, L. (2021). *Trauma, occupation, & participation.* AOTA Press.

Myers, C. T., & Cason, J. (2020). Early intervention services. In J. O'Brien & H. Miller-Kuhanek (Eds.), *Occupational therapy for children and adolescents* (8th ed., pp. 601–626). Elsevier.

Miller, L. J. (2006). *Miller function & participation scales manual.* Harcourt Assessment.

Miller, L. J., Oakland, T., & Herzberg, D. (2013). *Goal-oriented assessment of life skills manual.* Western Psychological Services.

National Center on Early Childhood Quality Assurance. (2017). Early learning standards. https://childcareta.acf.hhs.gov/sites/default/files/public/075_1707_state_elgs_web_final_0.pdf

National Governors Association Center for Best Practice, & Council of Chief State School Officers. (2010). *Common core standards state initiative.* Author.

Niblock, J. (2021). Best practice in providing telehealth to support participation in schools. In American Occupational Therapy Association (Ed.), *Telehealth and occupational therapy in schools* (pp. 27–50). AOTA Press.

O'Brien, J., Forest, M., Snow, J., Pearpoint, J., & Hasbury, D. (1989). *Action for inclusion: How to improve schools by welcoming children with special needs into regular classrooms.* Inclusion Press.

Parham, L. D., Ecker, C., Kuhaneck, H., Henry, D., & Glennon, T. (2021). *Sensory processing measure-2 manual* (2nd ed.). WPS Services.

Polo, K. M., & Cahill, S. M. (2017). Interprofessional collaboration to support children with diabetes. *The Open Journal of Occupational Therapy, 5*(3), 3. https://doi.org/10.15453/2168-6408.1338

Reed, K., & Polichino, J. (2019). Best practices in ethical reasoning for school occupational therapy practitioners. In G. Frolek Clark, J. E. Rioux, & B. E. Chandler (Eds.), *Best practices for occupational therapy in schools* (2nd ed., pp. 27–34). AOTA Press.

Rehabilitation Act of 1973, 29 U.S.C. § 504 (1973).

Schefkind, S. (2019). Best leadership practices through everyday advocacy. In G. Frolek Clark, J. E. Rioux, & B. E. Chandler (Eds.), *Best practices for occupational therapy in schools* (2nd ed., pp. 71–78). AOTA Press.

Seruya, F. M., & Garfinkel, M. (2020). Caseload and workload: Current trends in school-based practice across the United States. *American Journal of Occupational Therapy, 74,* 7405205090. https://doi.org/10.5014/ajot.2020.039818

Shepherd, J., Hanft, B., & Read, J. S. (2019). Best practice in collaborating on school and community teams. In G. Frolek Clark, J. E. Rioux, & B. E. Chandler (Eds.), *Best practices for occupational therapy in schools* (2nd ed., pp. 93–100). AOTA Press.

Wallisch, A., & Little, L. (2021). Coaching and supporting caregivers via telehealth. In American Occupational Therapy Association (Ed.), *Telehealth and occupational therapy in schools* (pp. 147–171). AOTA Press.

Watling, R., & Anderson, J. (2021). Supporting student self-regulation in telehealth. In American Occupational Therapy Association (Ed.), *Telehealth and occupational therapy in schools* (pp. 79–122). AOTA Press.

Wehmeyer, M. L. (2022). From segregation to strengths: A personal history of special education. *Phi Delta Kappan, 103*(6), 8–13. https://doi.org/10.1177/00317217221082792

Work

Julie Dorsey, Holly Ehrenfried, Denise E. Finch, and Lisa A. Jaegers

LEARNING OBJECTIVES

After reading this chapter, you will be able to:

1. Define work in the context of occupational therapy (OT), including theoretical foundations, and discuss opportunities within the profession.
2. Describe work participation across the life course, including the varied meaning and value of work for persons, groups, and populations.
3. Consider the impact of social determinants of health on work and work-related outcomes, including disparities in marginalized communities.
4. Discuss various work-related evaluation and assessment methods including the development of the occupational profile and job analysis.
5. Analyze client-centered, work-related intervention approaches and evidence for work and nonwork-related injury, illness, and disease.
6. Identify common settings, reimbursement/payment systems, and legislation related to work participation.
7. Articulate the distinct role of OT as part of the interprofessional team for work-related practice.

Introduction

What do you want to be when you grow up?
What is your major?
Where do you work?

It is very likely that you have been asked these questions many times in your life and that you often have asked these questions of others. Remember that you are reading this textbook as part of your work—as a student learning about occupational therapy (OT) or a practitioner expanding your knowledge to support and enhance your work.

Work as an occupation is defined in the Occupational Therapy Practice Framework (OTPF) as employment interests and pursuits, employment seeking and acquisition, job performance and maintenance, retirement preparation and adjustment, volunteer exploration, and volunteer participation (American Occupational Therapy Association [AOTA], 2020a).

Participation in work contributes to an individual's sense of identity and development of meaning and purpose in life. It adds structure and routine to the day, provides valuable opportunities for making social connections and contributions to society, and allows us to seek financial security. The conditions in the places where people live and seek to engage in work participation are called as **social determinants of health**. These are highly important aspects to be considered during assessment and goal setting (U.S. Department of Health and Human Services [USDHHS], 2020). Awareness of social determinants such as racial disparities, gender divides, educational barriers, healthcare accessibility, and gaps in built environment are critical to considering barriers and facilitators to work-related activities of daily living (ADL) and health outcomes (Ahonen et al., 2018; USDHHS, 2020). Furthermore, work participation as an occupation is a human right, central to occupational justice, and fundamental to OT practice (Bailliard & Aldrich, 2016).

OT practitioners are distinctly qualified to work with individuals, groups, and populations across the life course and across settings to address the occupation of work (AOTA, 2020a). OT practitioners are specifically trained to analyze and address the complex and dynamic interactions of individuals, their occupations, and the contexts that support or hinder occupational performance. This training and perspective are crucial to facilitating work performance and engagement.

Work holds different meanings for different people and at different phases, stages, or times in their lives. Consider the following scenarios:

- An autistic 17-year-old is working with an OT practitioner to explore career interests.
- A 28-year-old is taking time away from paid work to work at home and raise a family.
- A 54-year-old who is the primary financial contributor in the family and experiences a mental health challenge.
- A 67-year-old who recently retired is looking for new ways to contribute to the community.
- A 35-year-old manufacturing worker with a work-related injury.

Although these situations are different in terms of what the OT process would involve, they have common issues related to occupational participation that are explored in this chapter. It is essential for OT practitioners to understand how individuals value work participation and to take these values into account throughout the OT process while also recognizing work within the context of the employer and the broader culture in a region or country.

Within OT practice, work can be used both as means and as ends to achieve occupational performance goals. For example, an artist who experienced a stroke and is receiving OT services in an inpatient rehabilitation unit may enjoy painting at an easel to practice weight shifting and weight bearing, visual scanning, and impulse control. Returning to work may not directly be addressed within the OT plan of care because the emphasis may be on safely returning home. Rather, work can be used as a meaningful occupation to engage the individual in addressing underlying problem areas. However, that same artist may bring specific concerns about returning to work when seeking outpatient services.

In other situations, OT practitioners may address an individual's underlying skills needed for work participation, the work environment, and work demands as part of stay-at-work or return-to-work treatment plans. OT practitioners are responsible for addressing work as means and/or ends across all practice settings and populations. Even if work participation is not the primary emphasis of a treatment plan, it is a meaningful occupation and warrants specific attention.

OT practitioners are responsive to the dynamic needs of their clients[1] within the broader context of a changing society and a modern, global economy. In workplaces, there is a rise in workers with chronic physical, mental health, and other conditions that impact work participation and engagement, such as obesity, diabetes, opioid and other substance abuse, autism spectrum disorders, trauma, general aging, anxiety, cancer, and mild traumatic brain injury (mTBI). These populations present opportunities for OT practitioners to provide direct and indirect services in the form of preventing injuries, facilitating workplace health and well-being, advocating for clients' needs, recommending workplace accommodations, and other services. Population health interventions such as the National Institute for Occupational Safety and Health's (NIOSH) Total Worker Health® (Hudson et al., 2019; Jaegers, 2015) and opportunities within primary care (AOTA, 2020b) can be valuable strategies for addressing the needs of these growing populations.

Additional considerations and trends in workplaces include the following:

- Increased use of technology and flexible workstation locations especially as necessitated by the global COVID-19 pandemic (e.g., accessing more documents electronically, Web conferencing programs to allow for virtual meetings

---

[1]*Note:* According to the American Occupational Therapy Association (AOTA, 2020, p. S75), the term *client* refers to *persons* (including those involved in care of a client), *groups* (a collection of individuals having shared characteristics or common or shared purpose, e.g., family members, workers, students, and those with similar interests or occupational challenges), and *populations* (aggregates of people with common attributes, such as contexts, characteristics or concerns, including health risks). However, in countries other than the United States, the term *client* often refers to persons who are paying for their care directly. In most countries, *patient* is used to describe persons who are in hospital or rehabilitation. *Service user* and *person* are terms in general use that describe those in need of OT services. For this chapter, we are using *client* without implying the source of payment for services.

and working from home or other remote locations, home computer workstations, working in varied locations for access to sufficient internet, automation, robotics)

- Staffing shortages in many areas of work for various reasons (e.g., extended pandemic related unemployment benefits, childcare issues, job skills gaps)
- Trauma in the workplace associated with frontline workers, including healthcare workers, during the global pandemic
- Increased acceptance and interest in workplace health and wellness initiatives by employers (e.g., safe patient-handling initiatives, incentives for participating in fitness programs, on-site wellness programs)
- Shifts toward more active work environments (e.g., desk exercise programs, sit–stand stations, walking meetings)
- Trends in building design, such as "green" buildings through various certification programs, that can impact the worker (e.g., large windows for passive solar and lighting benefits that result in excessive glare for workers)
- Focus on work in underserved and marginalized populations through a lens of occupational justice (e.g., community reentry for incarcerated individuals, low-income individuals, migrant workers, BIPOC, LGBTQ+ individuals, and individuals who are homeless as well as services for veterans)

The Occupational Therapy Process

The evaluation portion of the OT process includes the occupational profile and analysis of occupational performance, or needs assessment, community profile, and review of secondary data at the group and population level (AOTA, 2020a). Building rapport with the client through interview and discussion leads to the answering of important questions related to why the client is seeking services. At the individual level, the occupational profile also reveals concerns related to engagement in occupations (including specific work tasks and occupations outside work); occupational history (including prior work history); performance in roles, routines, and habits (including related to work); supports and barriers to occupational engagement (including those at work); and priorities and preferred outcomes to target (AOTA, 2020a). At the group and population level, the needs assessment or community profile informs program development, implementation, and evaluation; advocacy; and policy to address health promotion (Centers for Disease Control and Prevention [CDC], 2016). Listening to the voices of workers in a participatory way assists with understanding root issues, potential solutions, and where to focus efforts on workplaces changes. Participatory action and community-based participatory approaches

have been effective methods for increasing worker, administrative, and employer input for promoting worker engagement and upper-level support (Cherniack & Punnett, 2019). Examples of formal work evaluation tools are available through AOTA at https://www.aota.org/community/special-interest-sections/work-and-industry.

Service provision by OT practitioners includes direct and indirect services, consultation, advocacy, and education and training (AOTA, 2020a). Work-related interventions commonly address factors affecting work participation. The approaches fall into the following basic categories: create, promote, establish, restore, maintain, modify, compensate, adapt, or prevent (AOTA, 2020a).

Theoretical Foundations and Models to Guide Practice

There is a broad spectrum of OT practice areas related to work. Work is an occupation that spans nearly all populations, practice settings, and social–ecological levels (e.g., individual, group, organization, community, and population). The primary goal of work-related OT practice is to promote participation and engagement in work activities. This includes identifying work opportunities, seeking and acquiring work, job performance, retirement preparation and adjustment, as well as volunteer exploration and participation (AOTA, 2020a, pp. 33–34). Work as an occupation is a primary aspect of individual, group, and population health; personal being; and sense of ability (AOTA, 2020a). Lack of work or an overabundance of work can be detrimental to health. Individuals who are deprived of the opportunity to engage in occupations that they find meaningful have a reduced sense of well-being (Durocher et al., 2014).

Conversely, individuals who are overworked may experience serious adverse health issues, and this situation can even result in death (Eguchi et al., 2016). To address the occupation of work, a conceptual framework to guide practice, research, and knowledge acquisition was developed that highlights the broad scope of work, including preparation, accommodation, and adaptation; health promotion, wellness, and disease prevention; injury prevention and ergonomics; rehabilitation and return to work; and evaluation and practitioner education (Jaegers et al., 2015). The importance of science-driven and practice-informed evidence (Hinojosa, 2013) is stressed throughout the framework for advancing knowledge and ensuring the use of efficacious interventions in work-based practice.

Although much of work-related OT practice focuses on individual- and organizational-level interventions, the health of human populations (e.g., the workforce, the population of unemployed individuals, and the aging population of workers) is also addressed through various service delivery approaches. Population or community health is the outcome of efforts across the wide array of social determinants of health (Kindig, 2017), including health systems and services, employment, housing, transportation, education, social environment, public safety, and the physical environment (National Academies of Sciences, Engineering, and Medicine, 2017). OT practitioners seek to reduce disparities that have consequences on health factors that affect a person's ability to participate in work-related activities and must be cognizant of health inequities surrounding their practice. It is also important to consider factors concerning occupational and social justice and underserved populations to be inclusive and provide a holistic approach. OT practitioners also consider approaches of service delivery appropriate for groups, communities, and populations in the context of work. They serve roles as direct providers of interventions including group sessions and through telehealth methods (AOTA, 2020a). They provide indirect, consulting services to businesses for workplace environmental design and ergonomics and serve as advocates and health and wellness leaders for health promotion (AOTA, 2020a).

Several models and theories can be used to guide the OT process in the area of work. *General systems theory* is useful in shaping our understanding of the complex interactions of the various parts within a system. Concepts from systems theory are the basis for multiple models within OT, including the following occupation-based models:

- Person–Environment–Occupation (PEO) (Law et al., 1996)—see Chapter 35
- Model of Human Occupation (Kielhofner, 2009)—see Chapter 34

These models can provide a foundation for evaluation and interventions to address the occupation of work because they provide practitioners with a holistic perspective from which to view the client. For example, a practitioner using the PEO model may structure an ergonomic assessment of an individual at their computer workstation by evaluating the person (e.g., posture, stress levels, height of person, habits and routines), the environment (e.g., height of desk, lighting, noise levels, supervisor support and social environment), and the occupation (e.g., specific work tasks, repetition and frequency of tasks). Once a mismatch is identified, an intervention plan can target the specific area(s) of the person, environment, and occupation.

There are also *health promotion models* that can guide the OT process in the area of work (see Chapter 40). Behavior change models such as the Transtheoretical Model (describes stages of person-level change) and Health Belief Model (explains health-related beliefs that are predictors to change) help practitioners identify and understand the various factors that can lead to behavior changes

in the workplace. The social–ecological model considers complexities among individual, interpersonal, community, and policy interactions. At the population level, theories and models such as Diffusion of Innovations Theory, Social Marketing approach, and the PRECEDE-PROCEED Model can guide practitioners on how to facilitate more widespread changes within a workplace, employment system, or community (Rimer & Glanz, 2005). OT practitioners select a model/theory/framework based on what needs to be understood and addressed through the OT process.

Overview of Legislation Related to Work

There are many relevant pieces of legislation that influence OT practice in the area of work. Several pieces of key legislation are discussed in the online materials to provide context for the chapter including what qualifies as a disability under the Americans with Disabilities Act (ADA).

The term *disability* may take on many meanings to various stakeholders when considering the rights and needs of people experiencing disability. The World Health Organization (WHO, 2008) describes three dimensions of disability:

- Impairment in a person's body structure or function, or mental functioning; examples of impairments include loss of a limb, loss of vision, or memory loss.
- Activity limitation, such as difficulty seeing, hearing, walking, or problem-solving
- Participation restrictions in normal daily activities, such as working, engaging in social and recreational activities, and obtaining healthcare and preventive services

Furthermore, these disability dimensions interact with environmental and personal context factors that then influence how individuals experience disability (WHO, 2008).

Efforts to address disability and the associated environmental and contextual factors vary between countries and may include laws, policies, and programs. In the United States, the Americans with Disabilities Act of 1990 was the first comprehensive civil rights law to address the needs of people with disabilities. Related to work, the ADA prohibits discrimination in employment and mandates reasonable accommodations in the workplace for people with physical and mental disabilities who meet the prerequisite job requirements and who can perform the essential functions of the job with or without modification. The ADA was amended in 2008 (Americans with Disabilities Act Amendments Act—ADAAA) to clarify the definition of disability to make it simpler for individuals seeking protection and to shift the focus to *discrimination* versus the disability.

The ADAAA (2008) defines a person with a disability as follows:

1. "Has a physical or mental impairment that substantially limits one or more major life activities" (29 C.F.R. § 1630.2[g][1][i])
2. "A record of a physical or mental impairment that substantially limited a major life activity" (29 C.F.R. § 1630.2[g][1][ii])
3. "Is regarded as having a disability or substantially limiting impairment" (29 C.F.R. § 1630.2[g][1][iii])

Promoting Work Participation and Engagement

In a person's life course, there is an ebb and flow of occupational transitions related to work. An **occupational transition** is "a major change in the occupational repertoire of a person in which one or several occupations change, disappear, and/or are replaced by others" (Jonsson, 2010, p. 212). For example, life changes can occur as a result of a family change, such as a parent choosing to place their career on hold in order to care for a child and then facing new preparations for returning to the paid workforce. Work participation may also be influenced by work or nonwork injury, disease, or disability. Individuals with a disability may need accommodations or adaptations to the physical and/or operational aspects of a job in order to fully engage in work activities. There can be obstacles to performing and accessing work that may lead to occupational imbalance, alienation, marginalization, and deprivation (Durocher et al., 2014). Additionally, in recent times mental health is being exceptionally challenged through unforeseen experiences.

Adaptation describes methods for adjusting the "current context or activity demands to support performance" (AOTA, 2020a, p. 64). Adaptations are applied at the person, group, and population level to compensate for, enhance, or provide cues to facilitate performance. As an example, at the person level, a person experiencing low vision may be recommended to adjust computer monitor display settings and lighting to improve visual contrast as adaptations to word processing tasks. At the group level, equipment or physical aspects of work may be adjusted to improve access, usability, and ability to work. Adaptations can also address workplace practices, for example, to facilitate an inclusive office culture and environment for individuals who are transitioning gender (Human Rights Campaign, 2017). These workplace changes may include policy and guidelines, everyday work practices, access to facilities, and employee education. At the population level, policies may guide the prevention and response to workplace violence, injury risk exposure, and equity in benefits and opportunities for advancement.

OT practitioners provide services to promote work participation and engagement in the following areas and each will be described in more detail later within this chapter:

- Health promotion and wellness
- Ergonomics, injury prevention, and workplace modifications
- Rehabilitation and return to work/ stay at work
- Work transitions

Understanding Work Through Job Analysis

Regardless of the service provision area or focus, a key component of the OT process is the practitioner's ability to understand work through job analysis.

In OT, occupation-based analysis (client specific) and activity analysis (generic) are used to analyze the demands of an activity or occupation in order to understand the performance patterns, performance skills, and client factors that are required to perform it (AOTA, 2020a, p. 20). **Job analysis** is a form of activity analysis that is specific to work tasks and includes the process of gathering and analyzing data related to job task requirements or demands, the environment, and human capacities needed to complete job functions. Performance skills are particularly valuable when analyzing task requirements because they enhance our ability to identify critical components related to cognitive, social, and physical performance requirements.

Job analysis can be generic (i.e., related primarily to measuring and recording job activities and demands), problem or occupation based (i.e., addresses work activities and demands related to a specific person, group, or population), or related to identification of ergonomic risk factors. For working adults with injuries, disability, or disease, as well as those who seek jobs or volunteer positions, job analysis can be an important part of the OT evaluation process because it informs decision-making related to interventions and outcomes to promote work participation. The scope and type of job analysis vary depending on the needs of the individual, group, or population as well as work environment factors, reimbursement or referral sources, and OT service settings.

Job analysis is a broad term used by a number of professionals, including employers, vocational rehabilitation professionals, ergonomists, safety professionals, and OT practitioners. For OT practitioners, the most frequently used types of evaluations are the following:

- Occupation-based or problem-based job analysis
- Functional job demands (FJDs) or functional job analysis
- Musculoskeletal disorder (MSD) ergonomic risk assessment

Each of these types of job analysis is described in Table 46.1, and risk assessments for musculoskeletal disorders are shown in Table 46.2.

TABLE 46.1 Types and Uses of Job Analyses

Type of Job Analysis	Purpose and Uses
Occupation-based or problem-based job analysis Evaluation and intervention related to a specific client for rehabilitation, accommodation, and/or modification	• Identify primary or essential tasks to be completed • Assess the required physical, cognitive, social, and performance skills demands related to client's strengths and weaknesses • Measure specific environmental factors related to the client's needs, such as lighting, chair height, work surface height, or the weight and size of objects handled • Based on client needs/status, assess relevant environmental factors • Gather person- or group-specific information regarding client factors, roles, habits, routines, and performance skills that may influence performance • Analyze client capacities and performance relative to job demands
Functional analysis Measurement/evaluation of job requirements for hiring, job matching or other evaluation (e.g., post-offer testing, ADA-related job accommodation and modification decisions, functional job descriptions)	• Gather and analyze information related to required job functions for job or job category rather than for a specific person • Identify required knowledge, background, and qualifications • With the employer/employee, identify essential/marginal functions of job and time spent in those functions • Identify the required physical, cognitive, social, and performance skills job demands • Analyze and measure environmental factors such as lighting, flooring types, noise, workbench heights, tools, box sizes and weights, etc. • Formats vary and may be determined by employer or reimbursement source
Musculoskeletal Disorder Risk Assessment (also called Ergonomic Risk Assessment and Risk Analysis) Injury prevention and health and wellness promotion	• Using risk assessment tools, measure risk factor exposures, such as force, repetition, sustained postures, awkward postures, extreme temperatures, vibration, contact stress, and job stress • Gather additional data such as injury patterns in the worker and group or population health information • The results can help to identify effective interventions to resolve or reduce symptoms, vary work methods, modify the work environment or work organization, or redesign a job task or work area. A number of MSD risk assessments are available to evaluate jobs tasks (Table 46.2).

ADA, Americans with Disabilities Act; MSD, musculoskeletal disorder.

TABLE 46.2 Selected Musculoskeletal Disorder Risk Assessment Tools

Assessment Tool	Purpose and Application	Source
The Revised NIOSH Lifting Equation	Evaluates lifting loads to identify potential risk of back injury; uses a formula to identify the maximum acceptable load for a lifting task	https://www.cdc.gov/niosh/docs/94-110/pdfs/94-110.pdf?id=10.26616/NIOSHPUB94110
Rapid Upper Limb Assessment (RULA)	Used to evaluate upper extremity postures that are not highly repetitive or forceful	http://www.rula.co.uk/
WISHA Hazard Zone Checklist	Screens to review movements or postures that are a "regular and foreseeable part of the job" and identify related risk factors	https://lni.wa.gov/safety-health/_docs/HazardZoneChecklist.pdf
Quick Exposure Checklist	Provides a risk factor score that considers exposures to multiple body parts, tasks performed, duration, work cycles, and worker perceptions	https://lni.wa.gov/safety-health/_docs/QECReferenceGuide.pdf

(continued)

TABLE 46.2	Selected Musculoskeletal Disorder Risk Assessment Tools (*continued*)	
Assessment Tool	**Purpose and Application**	**Source**
Computer Workstations eTool	This online checklist and evaluation resource provides information to evaluate computer workstations, related equipment setup and the work process. It also provides recommendations for improving ergonomics.	https://www.osha.gov/etools/computer-workstations/checklists
NIOSH Generic Stress Questionnaire	This 22-module subjective questionnaire gathers information from workers including their health, perceived demands and workload, conflict, and job satisfaction.	https://www.cdc.gov/niosh/topics/ workorg/detail088.html
Body picture pain diagram	Collects subjective symptom information; consists of an outline of a full body, anterior and posterior views. Clients are asked to mark the location of the pain or discomfort on the body chart and then describe the qualities of the pain.	https://www.cdc.gov/niosh/docs/97-117/pdfs/97-117.pdf
Observation-Based Posture Assessment: Review of Current Practice and Recommendations for Improvement	Describes observational approach for assessing work postures and provides related evidence	https://www.cdc.gov/niosh/docs/2014-131/

NIOSH, National Institute for Occupational Safety and Health; WISHA, Washington Industrial Safety and Health Act.

Job analysis data are useful when planning interventions and outcomes for individuals, groups, or populations experiencing challenges with sustaining, returning to, or gaining work participation. The purpose is to assess work activities and their related barriers and facilitators to performance that help to identify needs to be addressed through OT interventions. At the group or population level, job analysis may be considered in a community needs assessment where interviews, observations, and data are used to identify needed interventions. At the individual level, examples include injured workers; young adults with disabilities transitioning from school into the workforce; adults with mental illness; and adults with disease or disability such as a traumatic brain injury (TBI), low vision, and multiple sclerosis. Job analysis data can also be used to assist special populations such as older workers, prison personnel, farmers, volunteers, and those preparing for retirement to remain healthy at work or sustain participation.

For person-specific environmental and ergonomic interventions, careful attention to the effect of client factors helps to identify mismatches and potential modifications. These factors include strength, range of motion, pain, sensory functions, and mental functions on occupational performance and role competence. It is also important to pay attention to specific job demands such as work schedules, sequencing of tasks, cognitive and social demands, equipment used, equipment set up, body postures, and physical demands.

Job analysis services may be part of many OT service settings that provide work-related OT services including the following:

- Business and industrial environments
- Acute care and rehabilitation facilities
- Outpatient clinics
- Community-based settings such as mental health centers
- Sheltered or supported workshops
- Schools and universities
- Vocational programs
- U.S. Military Vocational Rehabilitation and Education Divisions (AOTA, 2017)

Requests for a job analysis may come from the employer, the medical or rehabilitation team, the vocational rehabilitation team, the workers compensation insurance company, long-term disability insurance carrier, or the individual client. The source of the referral will often determine the payment source as well. Reimbursement sources include private pay by the employer or individual client, various insurance companies, or vocational rehabilitation.

Prior to scheduling the job analysis, it is helpful to determine the desired outcome in order to select the most appropriate analysis format (e.g., problem based, FJDs, or MSD risk assessment), to gather tools required to conduct the analysis and to estimate the time needed. Regardless of the source, it is important to contact the referral source and employer's human resources representative to discuss and agree on the purpose of the analysis, the desired outcome, how the analysis will be conducted, and the data and report format.

A conversation with the individual about the job analysis and expected outcomes facilitates a client-centered approach that addresses the needs of multiple stakeholders including the employee, employer, the payer, and referring source. Employers may also require adherence to specific security, safety, and/or confidentiality procedures related to documentation, data collection, access to the worksite, and completion of the job analysis.

Preparation for a job analysis includes assembling the equipment needed to gather the desired data such as the following:

- Camera/video recorder
- Measuring tape
- Goniometer
- Push/pull force gauge
- Scale
- Pinch/grip gauge
- Light meter
- Pedometer or other device to measure walking distance
- Stopwatch
- Borg exertion scale (Borg, 1982)
- Forms (e.g., outline for data collection, risk assessment, task and tool measures)

Gathering Data

OT practitioners can gather job analysis data in a number of ways to obtain comprehensive and accurate data regarding the job requirements and environment. Some methods of data collection include the following:

- **On-site observation** can be time intensive and requires ½ hour to 4 or more hours of observation depending on the type of job analysis required and complexity of the job. Typically, this includes talking to the supervisor(s) and employee(s) to identify the individual tasks to be evaluated, observing completion of job tasks, measuring the work area and equipment, and recording the information.
- **Videotape and photos** obtained by the OT practitioner, the employer, or other stakeholders provide visual information that can depict or clarify job tasks and features of the job that may be difficult to describe. Videos are particularly helpful when analyzing specific motion patterns or complicated jobs. Videos and photos can also serve as a record of what components of a job were analyzed.
- **Remote observation** of the job site via synchronous, real-time electronic media, such as robots, Facetime, and Skype
- **Production and job description** information from the employer
- **Generic job demands data** for specific jobs and job categories are available through O*NET, an online job description database sponsored by the U.S. Department of Labor. It provides generic job descriptions for over 1,000

occupations in a wide variety of job categories (O*NET, 2017). Data from O*NET can be used to review job demands for a specific job category, assist with job searches, create plans for skill training, and structure more detailed job analyses.

- **Self-report/daily task log by worker** describes the workday pattern, including tasks, how long tasks take to complete, nonscheduled and scheduled breaks, and other factors that may influence tasks. For example, in some jobs, workload may increase around the holidays owing to increased number of orders.
- **Symptom log by worker** tracks work activities for several days with a focus on identifying patterns of activity that may influence symptoms such as pain, fatigue, and stress.
- **Review of injury records** for MSD injury includes the type and frequency of injury and provides useful information to target risk assessments and injury prevention programming.

Reporting formats vary widely and could include a combination of FJDs, physical demand analyses, and MSD ergonomic risk assessments. The ideal scenario is to complete a job analysis at the work setting, but when an on-site visit is not possible, job analysis may occur via simulation in the clinic using actual parts or tools from the worksite when available through use of client and employer job descriptions and via video/photographs. These methods may be sufficient for some individual-level treatment planning and interventions. However, the use of remote technology or media to capture critical job information for detailed job analysis, in lieu of physical presence at the worksite, has not been studied extensively at this time. Table 46.3 provides examples of data that may be collected.

Risk Factors

When conducting job analyses, it is essential to have an understanding of the various factors that can impact health and well-being.

Physical Workplace Factors

Musculoskeletal disorders can result from both work- and nonwork-related task demands. With some exclusions, MSDs are considered work related if "an event or exposure in the work environment either caused or contributed to the resulting condition or significantly aggravated a preexisting injury or illness" (Bureau of Labor Statistics [BLS], 2016, para. 1). The NIOSH (2017) further defines MSD-type injuries as "Disorders of the muscles, nerves, tendons, ligaments, joints, cartilage or spinal discs that

- are caused by sudden or sustained physical exertion
- are not the result of any instantaneous non-exertion event (e.g., slips, trips, or falls)
- range in severity from mild/occasional to intense/chronic pain."

TABLE 46.3   **Job Analysis Data Collection: Categories of Information and Examples**

Data Category	Examples of Data
Job title and brief description	• Assembler I: assembles electronic components while seated at a workbench • Customer service representative: answers customer calls while seated at a computer; uses computer to search for solution and enters data to record interaction
Shift and breaks	• Full time, Monday through Friday 8:00 AM to 4:30 PM • Four 10-h days with one 30-min lunch and two 15-min breaks
Number of people who complete the job	• One person completes this job per shift. • Eight people complete this task on first shift. • Four people work in a "cell" and rotate between tasks every 2 h.
Tasks (brief description, frequency, and duration)	• Assembles parts 5.5 h • Completes setup 15 min for every new part (2 to 4 times per shift) • Uses phone while typing on computer 4 h per shift • Computer work requires about 50% typing, 5% number pad use, and 45% mouse use.
Physical demands (e.g., postures, actions and motions) and motor performance skills	• Body movements required to drive a truck or operate a machine • Sustained grip or bent back posture • Lifts 30 lb 2 times per hour from floor to 50" high shelf • Uses two hands to manipulate small parts and tools to assemble device • Pushes 50 lb box along conveyor
Cognitive demands (e.g., attention, memory, judgment) and process performance skill requirements (e.g., initiates, gathers, searches)	• Task requires short-term memory to recall a three-item customer order or instructions. • Long periods of attention are required during a data analysis task. • Manage and enact safety protocols in event of emergency. • Work task requires searching for gathering of appropriate materials prior to completing task.
Interpersonal and social interaction skills	• Work task requires interaction with 10–20 coworkers for 75% of the day vs. works alone with only intermittent coworker interaction each day. • Conducts 30–50 sales calls using phone-based verbal interactions • Initiates conversation with coworkers to complete shared work task • Responds to inquiries from subordinates to address problems in workflow
Physical environment (layout, tools, equipment, temperature, vibration, lighting, noise, stairs, heights, indoor/outdoor footing/flooring)	• Soldering tool, tweezers, workbench, adjustable tool, parts weighing <1 lb • Boxes of parts weighing 25 lb are 10 in high, 20 in wide, and 30 in long • Computer, computer screen, keyboard, mouse, phone, adjustable chair • Space is indoors and temperature controlled. • Overhead lighting or task lighting (light meter) • Environment is noisy.
Other physical skills (e.g., visual acuity, hearing acuity)	• Requires color vision to distinguish differences in wire colors • Machine for quality testing emits "beep" when part passes inspection
Worker, group, or population demographics	• Number of male/female workers • Age range • Socioeconomic status • May include health, illness or disease related information, lifestyle, habits and routines of a group or population of workers • Injury rates for industry, job type, or specific worker population

Musculoskeletal disorders include diagnoses such as low back pain, lateral epicondylitis, carpal tunnel syndrome (CTS), and neck pain (NIOSH, 2016b). The presence of risk factors does not mean that an injury will definitely occur; however, injury risk is associated with the intensity, duration, and frequency of exposure to risk factors, such as the following:

- Force (weight, grip, pinch, push/pull)
- Awkward postures (body positions that are potentially damaging such as working with the arms overhead, extreme wrist deviations, or twisting of the spine)
- Static postures (defined by duration of sustained position)
- Repetition (variable definitions based on work cycle or actual number of movements during a period of time)
- Contact stress/compression (typically refers to external compression of the tissue from a sharp edge, tool handle or surface)
- Vibration
- Lack of rest and recovery time
- Extremes in temperature

Research conducted to understand the dose–response relationship between certain types of physical risk factors and the risk of developing an MSD is ongoing. Home activities and demands such as lifting children, computer use, woodworking, playing video games, and yard work may also expose individuals to physical risk factors. Therefore, clinical reasoning should be guided by careful analysis of evidence, understanding the job demands, as well as consideration of nonwork tasks demands and client factors. Assumptions such as "they do repetitive work so that must be why they have wrist pain" should be avoided. For example, Fan et al. (2015) found that hand force was strongly associated with the prevalence of CTS, whereas repetition as a single risk factor and wrist posture were not. This information can guide employers and employees to more closely examine forceful hand exertions and possible modifications to reduce the frequency, duration, and/or intensity of hand force during work and nonwork activities to reduce the intensity of or prevent CTS.

Psychosocial Workplace Factors

Job stress is a concern relative to the overall health of workers, and stress occurs when the requirements of the job do not match the "capabilities, resources and needs of the worker" (NIOSH, n.d.). In the publication "Stress at Work," NIOSH (n.d.) reports that coping style and personality are personal factors that may influence how workers manage job stress; however, there are a number of workplace conditions that are believed to affect most people. To address work organization and psychosocial risk factors, risk assessments, surveys, and other tools that provide information regarding work organization and psychosocial conditions should include the following (NIOSH, n.d.):

- High physical, mental, or emotional demands
- Machine pacing or time pressure

- Shiftwork
- Low participation in decision-making
- Badly designed, inadequate, or faulty equipment
- Poor communication
- Low social support
- Social/physical isolation
- Role ambiguity or role conflict
- Job insecurity

External events may also affect the psychosocial work environment and health of the worker. For example, for healthcare workers, the COVID-19 pandemic altered work routines and job expectations. Frontline healthcare workers and women were found to be at higher risk of experiencing anxiety and depressive symptoms (Vindergaard & Benros, 2020). Therefore, surveys to understand the experience of the worker, the psychosocial environment of work and data concerning work organization, can help inform interventions to promote health and wellness in the workplace and identify potential areas of modification to facilitate work participation.

Personal Factors and Health Behaviors

Personal risk factors refer to individual characteristics such as age, body mass index (BMI), gender, smoking, and other activities or medical conditions. In addition, social determinants of health such as family conflict or caring for a child with a disability, income, food insecurity, and limited access to affordable housing or healthcare, may alter the clients' ability to fully engage in work. These factors may place some workers at higher risk of job burnout, absence from work, and lower job productivity. Whereas some factors may be local, larger-scale events such the COVID-19 pandemic can also influence clients' health and well-being. For example, a systematic review conducted by Vindergaard and Benros (2020) found that frontline healthcare workers caring for COVID-19 patients experienced higher rates of depressive symptoms, psychological distress, and sleep difficulties. They also reported that the general public experienced higher levels of anxiety and depression owing to the pandemic. These data accentuate the need for broad evaluation of person and client factors, including mental health, in order to better meet the needs of workers. Occupational therapists can use a variety of mental health assessment tools to evaluate the needs of their clients and resources can be found in Chapter 63.

Interactions Between Risk Factors

The interactions between personal risk factors, physical risk factors in job tasks, psychosocial risk factors, such as high workloads and tight deadlines, along with the impact of social determinants of health are complex. This inherent complexity makes the determination of what causes specific work injuries difficult. With this in mind, the degree to which each type of factor contributes to the injury and the determination as to work relatedness is as much a legal matter managed by the workers' compensation laws as a medical diagnosis issue. The difficulty of identifying a single risk factor as the cause of an injury is apparent in a study conducted by Fan et al. (2015) where in a sample of approximately 3,000 US workers, CTS was associated with age (>35 years), female gender, obesity, prior upper extremity disorder, participating in recreational hand activities, and other medical conditions such as diabetes. In another study of 60 workers with low back pain, Govindu and Babski-Reeves (2014) reported that both direct and interactive effects of physical risk factors and psychosocial and personal risk factors influenced ratings of low back pain severity. The findings from these studies suggest selecting intervention approaches incorporating solutions to address potential contributions of personal, psychosocial, and physical risk factors as well as considering social determinants of health could provide a more holistic approach to worker health and injury management and injury prevention. Consideration of personal factors, physical and social environments, and activities and tasks is an inherent part of OT practice.

Focus Areas of Occupational Therapy in Work-Related Practice

Health Promotion and Wellness

Health promotion is a process for enabling individuals to increase their control over, and ultimately improve, their health (Smith et al., 2006) and includes wellness and chronic disease prevention. Workers in the United States typically spend more than one-third of their day on the job, and effective workplace health programs and policies have the potential to benefit quality of life among workers (CDC, 2020). This time use is consistent with many other industrialized countries, though there is some variance depending on factors such as culture and economic status of the country (Global Change Data Lab, 2022). For example, workers in China spend one hour more on average and workers in Belgium spend one hour less on average (Global Change Data Lab, 2022). The US average usual weekly hours is 38.6, and around the world, work hours range from 29.4 hours (Netherlands) to 47.6 hours (Columbia) (Organisation for Economic Cooperation and Development, 2019). OT practitioners seek health outcomes as a result of the OT process and utilize wellness participation and engagement as a means to achieve mental, physical, and social well-being (NIOSH, 2014). According to the OTPF (AOTA, 2020a; Hettler, 1984, p. 1117), wellness is "an active process through which individuals [or groups or populations]

become aware of and make choices toward a more successful existence." According to WHO, there are two main focal concerns of wellness: (a) an individual's realization of their fullest physical, psychological, social, spiritual, and economic potential and (b) the fulfillment of an individual's expectations in family, workplace, community, place of worship, and other settings (Smith et al., 2006). Wellness practices can be individual, but they are often practiced in workgroups or at the workplace level to address the needs of organizations. Chronic disease prevention practices address the health epidemic surrounding heart disease, stroke, and related conditions such as hypertension, diabetes, and obesity (CDC, 2017).

With the passage of the Affordable Care Act, improving the health of employees and promoting wellness have become increasingly important to employers as a way to reduce private health insurance costs and work-related injury claims and related costs. Poor worker health can be costly to employers. For example, workers who had a BMI in obesity class III (BMI ≥40) had an elevated rate of lost work time, lost workdays, and higher medical claim costs when compared with workers at their recommended weight (Ostbye et al., 2007). Additionally, mental health affected by stress and leading to illness such as depression are associated with higher rates of disability and unemployment and with negative job performance (Centers for Disease Control and Prevention [CDC], 2018).

The health and well-being of workers is of interest to OT practitioners because it influences engagement in occupations and in particular work participation. OT practitioners view workers from a holistic perspective, and they can contribute significantly to the health and wellness of individuals, groups, and populations in work environments by working with employers and employees to identify areas of concern, determine possible strategies, and implement solutions to create a fully engaged and capable workforce. The OT practitioner may provide indirect services as part of a planning team as a consultant or manager or provide direct services. Some examples include the following:

- OT practitioners working in a mental health setting can address an employee's return to work, identify areas of performance challenges, and work with clients to implement strategies and work modifications to ease transition and promote successful work engagement. To improve return-to-work program outcomes for individuals with mental health disorders, work with employers may include education and training of employees and managers. This could include learning about various mental health disorders and recovery to avoid stereotypes and bias in the workplace, the ADA, reasonable accommodations, and work modifications. OT has been shown to increase long-term depression recovery and to increase probability of long-term return to work (Hees et al., 2013). OT practitioners are well prepared to discuss strategies to help such individuals address their mental health in both the acute and outpatient settings and can teach strategies to facilitate a successful return to work without negatively impacting self-care and leisure occupations.

- To facilitate wellness at work, OT practitioners may also be involved in developing or providing training for employers and employees to address a variety of topics such as smoking cessation, suicide prevention, stress management, and sleep. As a consultant, the OT provider would work with the employer's human resources, employee health, or health and safety team to conduct a needs assessment, identify evidence to support the content, and plan the delivery of the training.
- Aging workers are another group of focus for employers and OT practitioners. Increasing numbers of older workers are in the workplace as a result of longer life courses and improved health as well as a financial need to work past the traditional retirement age. The perception exists among some employers that older workers are more costly than younger workers because of higher absenteeism, higher wages, higher pensions, and increased use of healthcare and other benefits (Taskforce on the Aging of the American Workforce, 2008). This can negatively impact employability of older workers owing to stereotypes and discrimination. In contrast, some employers report that older workers have greater knowledge of the job tasks they perform than their younger colleagues, willingly learn new tasks quickly, bring experience and resilience to work, and are able to keep up with the physical demands of their jobs (Munnell et al., 2006; Vasconcelos, 2015).
- OT practitioners can serve the older adult demographic by educating and assisting employers in making the workplace more "friendly" to the aging worker and working directly with individuals to consider adaptive strategies, promote health, and prevent the risk of injury and illness. Interventions may include teaching adaptive strategies and improving work capacity, such as by addressing changes in physical strength, vision and hearing deficiencies, fall risk, and other age-related changes. The OT practitioner can also advocate in the workplace for universal design and age-friendly procedures that are beneficial to the older adult and most employees of the organization.

Population-level interventions for the workplace such as the NIOSH Total Worker Health® (Jaegers, 2015; Schill, 2017) can be valuable strategies for addressing the needs of workers. Total Worker Health® is a holistic approach to workplace health protection and health promotion that encourages participatory methods for hazard assessment, understanding the intersection of risk factors in the work system, and mitigation of risks. Many projects informed by TWH have shown efficacy for this strategy including improved safe patient handling equipment use (Dennerlein et al., 2017) and work–life balance (Hammer et al., 2016).

Strategies using TWH have been described for addressing hearing health, fatigue among retail workers, sedentary work, and tobacco prevention (NIOSH, 2019). One example of a wellness intervention is the Total Worker Health® initiative that spans company-wide participation for where a participatory team identifies problems and solutions regarding the balance among work, leisure, and family life (group) (AOTA, 2017). Understanding the challenges and facilitators to implementing programs through process and impact evaluation are critical to continuously informing adjustments to workplace interventions. Program evaluation is 2-fold: Understanding (a) the extent to which the program was implemented as intended (process evaluation) and (b) the efficacy or effectiveness of the program (impact evaluation) (Steckler & Linnan, 2002).

Ergonomics, Work Injury Prevention, and Workplace Modifications

The problem of workplace injuries is significant, with MSD injuries accounting for 30% of cases involving days out of work in 2019 (BLS, 2020a). To reduce the risks for injuries and illness including MSDs and maximize work performance, employers look to **ergonomics** to improve the fit between the work and the worker (International Ergonomics Association [IEA], 2017). Based on this concept, ergonomics is often considered part of workplace safety. In the United States, workplace safety is the purview of the OSHA (n.d.-b) through the U.S. Department of Labor, which guides safe work practices through standards, training, and outreach. Their work is informed by the NIOSH (2016a), which supports the transfer of research to occupational safety and health practices. Both the OSHA and NIOSH websites provide excellent resources related to workplace safety, ergonomics, and injury prevention programming.

Although often associated with safety, the field of ergonomics is broad and its concepts are applied to both the design and redesign of tasks and environments. The field of ergonomics is compatible with OT and provides useful information regarding anthropometrics, human capacity, equipment design, space design, and organizational structure to consider when working with clients to improve occupational performance. The IEA defines ergonomics as follows:

> Ergonomics (or human factors) is the scientific discipline concerned with the understanding of interactions among humans and other elements of a system, and the profession that applies theory, principles, data and methods to design in order to optimize human well-being and overall system performance. Practitioners of ergonomics and ergonomists contribute to the design and evaluation of tasks, jobs, products, environments and systems in order to make them compatible with the needs, abilities and limitations of people. (IEA, 2017)

Occupational therapists are well suited to evaluate work tasks and environments including conducting ergonomic and MSD risk assessments with background in anatomy and physiology, psychology, client factors, environmental factors, and occupational performance. Job analysis in the form of MSD ergonomic risk assessments is used to identify injury risk factors related to a particular job or task, develop programs to prevent work injuries, or identify specific ergonomic problems and solutions for an individual worker.

Anthropometrics provides critical ergonomic information to assist in determining changes to improve the match between the work, worker, and the environment. **Anthropometry** is a field of science that studies and defines the physical measures of a person's size (e.g., overall height and weight, length of extremities, height in sitting and standing, size of head) and functional capacities (e.g., range of motion, strength, and aerobic capacity). In the workplace, this information is used to design tasks, tools, machines, and personal protective equipment (PPE) to maximize the fit and usability of equipment to promote safety and injury prevention (NIOSH, 2018). Gathering data from a wide variety of populations is important because individual dimensions and capacities vary greatly depending on geographic location, personal factors, and gender. The NIOSH gathers data from specific populations, such as firefighters and emergency medical technicians (EMTs), to create profession-specific databases to use in the design of job-specific tools and work environments. Such anthropometric data inform ergonomics and are useful to OT practitioners when conducting ergonomic assessments, selecting work equipment such as chairs and tools, and working as part of an ergonomics team to design new or suggest modifications to existing work environments, tools, and tasks. Another design approach that is beneficial when considering the fit between the worker and the work environment is universal design. When universal design features are included in work environments, they can increase accessibility for all populations.

As OT practitioners, we may refer to environmental interventions as modifications, adaptations, or accommodations to the environment or adaptation on the part of the person. The language of ergonomic interventions refers to these types of changes as engineering controls, administrative/work practice controls, and PPE.

- *Engineering controls* are changes to equipment or physical demands of the job that result in the reduction or removal of potential injury risk factors. These include, for example, providing a tool with a small grip span for persons with smaller hands, providing a pneumatic lifting device to assist with lifting heavy boxes, or redesigning machinery to reduce the force necessary to turn a lever. These types of controls could also include simple changes such as adjusting the height of a computer screen to improve head position or reducing the reaching distance required to pick up a part. When possible, implementation of engineering controls that "design out" the potential risk factor are preferable over other types of controls.

- *Administrative and work practice controls* refer to changes in task sequences or assignments in an effort to reduce exposure to strenuous or high-demand job tasks. Job rotation, reducing the speed of work, or implementing more breaks may provide needed changes to alter exposure to or increase recovery time from highly repetitious or difficult tasks. These types of controls also include training workers to complete tasks in a particular way that may reduce stress to the body such as how to adjust a chair or set up a computer workstation properly.

- *Personal protective equipment controls* refer to equipment that employees wear, such as safety glasses to prevent chemicals or metal shards from contacting the eye and earplugs to protect the ears from loud noises. Examples of PPE controls include antivibration gloves, splints, N95 respirator, and back belts issued to the worker to use during their job performance. It is important to note that the evidence to support use of these devices to prevent injuries is scant or mixed. For example, a rigid wrist splint may reduce bending at the wrist but increase stress to the wrist flexor and extensor muscles or shoulder if the person is pushing against the splint or adjusting their shoulder to compensate for the limited wrist movement. Therefore, the use and potential complications of using PPE devices need to be carefully reviewed prior to implementation. As another example, during the COVID-19 pandemic, the use of N95 respirators was essential on many job sites. Fit testing is required and this can be complicated by facial hair. When facial hair is part of a religious practice, there are many factors for the employee to consider.

Ergonomic interventions can be provided at the individual and group levels. Group-level interventions can include ergonomic training for occupational health and safety personnel, ergonomic teams, employees, or target jobs that are associated with higher rates of injury, turnover, and worker discomfort complaints. The desired outcomes include reducing injury rates, improving worker satisfaction, and preventing injury. The NIOSH (2017) provides resources to create and implement effective ergonomics programs to prevent or reduce the incidence of workplace injuries. OT practitioners can design and provide worker-centered education and training to reduce ergonomic risk factors through improved postures, changes in work setup to reduce reach/effort, and changes in work technique. Training workers to complete stretching programs, rotate work tasks, and manage stress may also be useful. Although these types of programs often address cumulative type MSD injuries, workers may also experience acute injuries, such as TBI from a fall or blunt force incident. OT practitioners have built evidence-based interventions to prevent falls and reduce injuries and deaths from falls from ladder and building surfaces (Kaskutas et al., 2016).

At the individual level, multifaceted interventions can be helpful in addressing ergonomic concerns and return to work. For example, workplace modifications including ergonomics and graded return to work as part of coordinated care planning among healthcare professionals, including OT practitioners, were effective in reducing time out of work and improving functional status (Lambeek et al., 2010). Similarly, in a review of factors affecting return to work following injury or illness, Cancelliere and colleagues (2016) found that stakeholder participation, work modification/accommodation, and return-to-work coordination were associated with positive return-to-work outcomes. Furthermore, in a systematic review conducted by Nevala and colleagues (2015), self-advocacy, changes in work schedules, work organization, and transportation availability promoted employment among people with disabilities. OTs have the skills to provide or contribute to interventions such as self-advocacy, ergonomic modification, work modification and accommodations, and graded return to work promote work participation.

Computer Workstation Ergonomics. Many websites and handouts provide good basic information about ergonomic guidelines for computer workstations. For more detail, the American National Standards Institute/Human Factors and Ergonomics Society (ANSI/HFES) standard 100-2007: Human Factors Engineering of Computer Workstations (HFES, 2007) provides detailed workstation design standards related to seating, posture, computer equipment, workstations, and lighting. The standards serve as a resource for ergonomics for the office environment. Several guiding principles of interest can be found in Table 46.4. Opportunities to vary work postures throughout the day are also suggested. Healthy work postures for computer work can be seen in Figures 46.1 and 46.2.

The frequency of use, style or design, and location of keyboards, mouse input devices, computer screens, desks, and chairs influence the users' accessibility, work postures, and activity demands. There are a number of computer workstation assessment and screening tools available to assess the ergonomic factors of office workstations, such as the Rapid Office Strain Assessment (ROSA; Sonne et al., 2012) and the Computer Workstation eTool (OSHA, n.d.-a), which is an online problem-solving tool that provides suggestions on how to select and arrange various workstation components.

Although ergonomic guidelines and screening tools serve as a general reference, person-specific evaluation of performance and selection of modifications to the computer workstation equipment or tasks may be necessary to accommodate individual needs. For example, an individual with right elbow pain that increases while holding the mouse with the wrist in extension may benefit from placing

TABLE 46.4 Work Posture Guidelines for Computer Users

Body Part	Work Posture Guidelines
Upper extremity	• Shoulders relaxed • Minimal shoulder abduction and flexion • Elbow bent midrange at about 90° • Wrist flexion and extension at <30°
Lower extremity	• Hip angle 90° or slightly more • Knee angle at 90° or slightly more • Feet on the floor or foot rest
Head and back	• Head aligned over shoulders • Natural curves of spine maintained

Equipment	Suggested Features/ Placement
Keyboard/mouse platform—seated	• Adjustable between 22 and 28.5 in from the floor to the front edge of the platform • Place keyboard at about elbow height.
Keyboard/mouse platform—standing	• Adjustable between 37.4 and 46.5 in from floor to front edge of platform • Place keyboard at about elbow height.
Computer screen	• Place the computer screen at least 20 in from the eyes. • Position monitor so the top line of the screen falls below the horizontal gaze (eye level) of the user.
Chairs	• 4.5 in adjustment capacity within the recommended range of 15–22 in as measured from the floor to the top of the seat • Rounded front seat edge • Adjustable lumbar support

the mouse at elbow height, to the left side of the keyboard, or from using a different style input device (Figure 46.3). Additionally, some workstations are shared by multiple users who have varied needs. In these cases, workstations should be designed with flexible and adaptable features (e.g. adjustable height desk and movable footrest) so that each user can customize the workstation during their shift. This includes mobile workstations, or "computers on wheels," used in some settings such as hospitals and medical offices.

Ergonomics in Non-office Work Environments. People work in a wide array of environments, such as general manufacturing of parts for cars using power tools, lifting devices computers, and other equipment; laboratories that require use of microscopes and pipettes; warehouses where workers lift and handle boxes or parts; food service

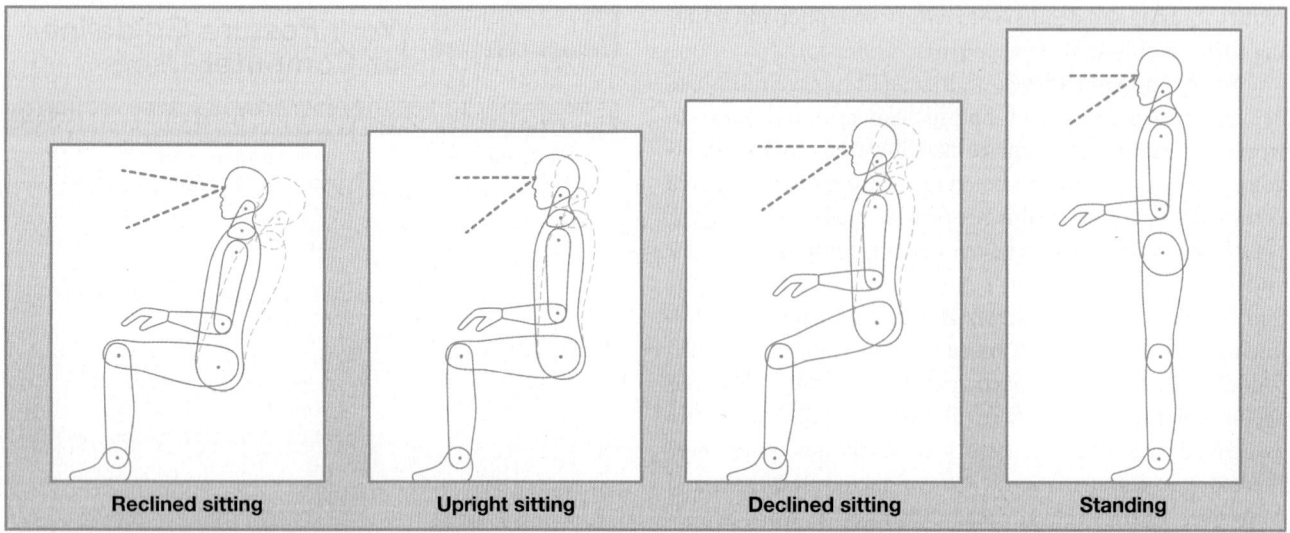

Reclined sitting   Upright sitting   Declined sitting   Standing

FIGURE 46.1 **Healthy working positions.**

(Reprinted from Occupational Safety and Health Administration. (n.d.-a). *Computer workstations eTool: Good working positions.* https://www.osha .gov/SLTC/etools/computerworkstations/positions.html)

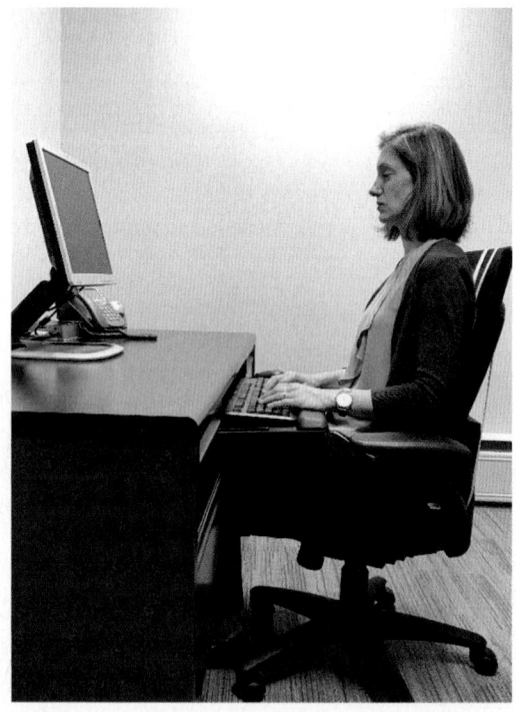

FIGURE 46.2 **Seated computer workstation position. Person seated with arms relaxed and near side of body. Keyboard positioned at about elbow height. Top of screen is slightly below eye level. Back and feet supported.**

settings such as cafeterias and restaurants; and healthcare facilities such as hospitals, nursing homes, and clinics. Each of these environments has unique workspaces, tools, equipment, and work demands.

The design of workplace tools and equipment has an impact on user comfort, postures, and the degree of effort required to complete a task. Poorly designed tools, workplaces, and tasks can expose workers' bodies to stresses and strains that contribute to musculoskeletal injury (NIOSH, 2016b). Worker-centered ergonomic programs, along with changes to tools, workplaces, tasks, and routines can help reduce musculoskeletal stressors and injuries. Ergonomic changes may address the underlying task, tool, equipment, or job design features (engineering controls) that create injury risk. Reducing risk exposures may also be controlled by changing work routines to limit high-risk or problem tasks (administrative controls) or changing work methods such as altering lifting technique or using a stronger position such as gripping rather than pinching when holding a tool.

Back injuries are a significant concern for many workers. For example, in 2016, nursing assistants, stock clerks, and laborers accounted for the highest percentage of back injuries that resulted in time out of work (BLS, 2018). Changes to the workplace, such as reducing the size and weight of a box, placing heavier items on middle shelves, and using a mechanical device to move objects and people are examples of changes that can help reduce injury risk exposure or modify a job for an individual with a back injury or limited capacity for lifting.

In the healthcare setting, careful analysis of patient lifting and transfers in emergency rooms, operating rooms, patient rooms, and therapy rooms can identify areas of concern related to body postures, unpredictable patient movements, and unanticipated events that put the person(s) involved in the transfer, including the patient, at risk of injury. Decision-making processes to help healthcare personnel identify when help (e.g., another person or device) is needed for transferring or repositioning a patient and selecting appropriate assistive devices are some

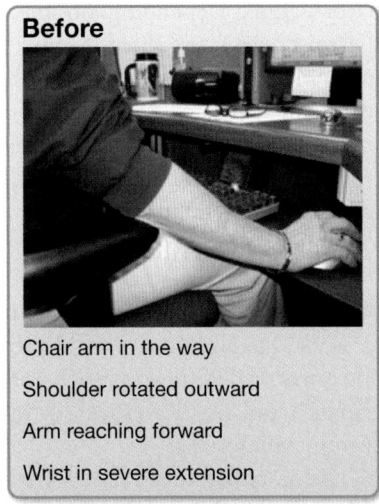
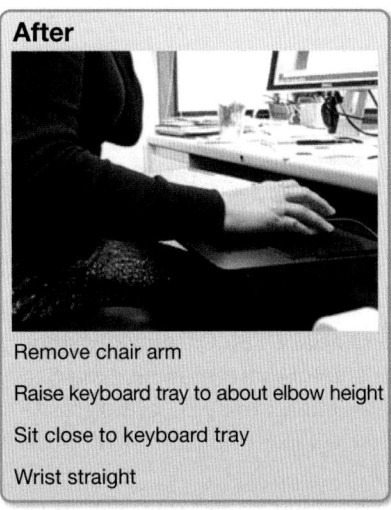

Before	After
Chair arm in the way	Remove chair arm
Shoulder rotated outward	Raise keyboard tray to about elbow height
Arm reaching forward	Sit close to keyboard tray
Wrist in severe extension	Wrist straight

FIGURE 46.3 Before and after ergonomic solutions. This individual experienced right elbow pain that increased when holding the mouse with the wrist in extension.

solutions to reduce injury risk. This is especially important in the context of the trend of increasing weight of patients (e.g., bariatrics) and the resultant impact on those in patient care roles.

In manufacturing and construction environments, highly repetitive, forceful tasks using tools such as knives and screwdrivers may place strain on wrist and forearm muscles, causing injury. Changing the tool handle size or shape, reducing vibration, and keeping tools sharp can help reduce exposure to risk factors and strain on the arm. Ergonomic assessment tools as well as task- and industry-specific suggestions for ergonomic changes are available through a variety of OSHA and NIOSH publications. A list of these resources and others can be found in Table 46.5.

TABLE 46.5 Ergonomics and Injury Prevention Program Resources

Resources	Content Examples
Ergonomic Guidelines for Manual Materials Handling (https://www.cdc.gov/niosh/docs/2007-131/pdfs/2007-131.pdf)	• Data gathering process • Assessment tools such as NIOSH lifting equation and materials handling checklist • Ergonomic suggestions • Guidelines for materials handling techniques
Safe Patient Handling and Mobility (SPHM) (https://www.cdc.gov/niosh/topics/safepatient/)	• Patient handling hazards • Patient handling ergonomics • Additional resources and tools
Guidelines for Nursing Homes: Ergonomics for the Prevention of Musculoskeletal Disorders (https://www.osha.gov/sites/default/files/publications/ final_nh_guidelines.pdf)	• Identifying management support • Decision-making trees for patient transfers and repositioning • Suggestions for assistive devices related to patient handling, housekeeping, kitchen tasks, and laundry
Guidelines for Retail Grocery Stores: Ergonomics for the Prevention of Musculoskeletal Disorders (https://www.osha.gov/Publications/osha3192.pdf)	• This resource reviews ergonomic hazards of work activities related to shelf stocking, stockrooms cashiering, bagging, produce handling, deli work, and baker work. • Suggestions include workstation design for cashiers and cake-decorating stations, using sharp tools, and rearranging work routines for difficult tasks.
A Guide to the Selection of Non-powered Hand Tools (https://www.cdc.gov/niosh/docs/2004-164/)	• Ergonomic hazards related to hand tools • Ergonomics for hand tool design

NIOSH, National Institute for Occupational Safety and Health.

Rehabilitation and Return to Work/Stay at Work

When a person experiences an injury, illness, or disease, the OT practitioner is a key provider of rehabilitation services to facilitate readiness for return to work. Rehabilitation after a hand injury such as tendon laceration involves treatment activities to address ADL such as self-care, scar remodeling, active range of motion, strengthening, and overall functional use of the hand for activity performance. For individuals who experienced a TBI, OT provides a holistic approach to help with motor skill retraining, executive function, and coping skills and a variety of related treatment approaches to assist with rehabilitation and work preparation.

Return to work focuses on multilevel aspects of work participation (e.g., individual preparation, workplace policy, and environmental adaptation) that are impacted by changes in work status owing to a personal need such as taking care of a family member experiencing terminal cancer, being unemployed owing to a job layoff, or being unable to work owing to an injury or illness. Return to work also affects veterans moving from active duty to civilian work, wounded warriors, individuals incarcerated and transitioning to the community, and many others who experience a major change in their participation in work.

Work-Related Injuries. Interrupted or altered participation in work for individuals affected by work injuries across the United States is significant. In 2019, approximately 2.7 million workers in private industry experienced a work injury that required time out of work, a job transfer, or restriction of work activities (BLS, 2021). OT practitioners involved in work programs may perform their duties in a variety of settings, such as outpatient clinics, hospitals, office settings, manufacturing environments, and warehouses. OT practitioners need not confine their services to specially designed "occupational medicine" clinics to address work issues with their clients. Work should be addressed with all clients who want to work with the goal of improving the match between work demands and the worker's capacities for effective participation and engagement.

Acute Injury Management. When an individual is injured on the job and referred by a healthcare provider for OT, the occupational therapist performs an initial evaluation that includes an occupational profile. This portion of the evaluation includes identifying what the client needs and wants to do, barriers and facilitators related to occupational engagement including work, and occupational history.

Occupational performance analysis related to completion of work tasks, use of tools, and other activity demands is completed to identify factors related to effective participation. Depending on the specific diagnosis, the therapist evaluates client factors, such as muscle functions, movement-related functions, and sensory functions (e.g., pain or thermal awareness). For work participation issues, information about the job demands may be obtained from the client, job description or a job analysis, if available. Information of interest includes physical demands of the job, method of injury, length of time on the job, and current work status. An intervention plan is developed in conjunction with the client, keeping in mind the goal of returning to work. Interventions are selected to meet the targeted outcomes related to work, such as being able to lift, sustain grip on a tool, reach overhead, or working at a computer for 45-minute intervals.

As described in the OTPF (AOTA, 2020a), a variety of intervention types may be used, including occupations and activities, interventions to support occupations, education and training, advocacy, group interventions, and virtual interventions. Examples of these types of interventions include addressing hand coordination to improve keyboarding with an individual who has had a stroke and wants to return to work in an office environment, fabricating an orthotic device for a client who sustained a distal radius fracture, educating a client on proper positioning when lying down so back pain can be minimized, and advocating for a client to obtain reasonable light duty restrictions to avoid aggravation of symptoms while working on a light duty job. When the client's primary reason for attending therapy is beginning to resolve, the OT practitioner may need to consider work conditioning or work hardening as methods to return the client back to employment if the client's physical abilities do not match the physical demands required to perform their job.

An accurate understanding of job demands provides key information when selecting and creating occupation-based interventions and recommending environmental modifications, such as ergonomic changes to reduce the impact of injury or facilitate resolution of the injury. Although a full job analysis may not be necessary, a focused review of symptom-aggravating tasks can yield useful information.

Work Hardening and Work Conditioning. Clients are typically ready to participate in a work-conditioning or work-hardening program when the client factors such as swelling, acute inflammation, or trauma that limit occupational performance in the acute OT intervention phase have resolved or are under control. See OT Story 46.1. **Work conditioning** is an approach to restore the performance of a worker recovering from an injury or illness; the focus is on restoring the musculoskeletal and cardiovascular systems and promoting safe work performance (AOTA, 2017). Work conditioning is typically performed using work simulation 3 to 5 days per week, 2 to 4 hours per day. **Work hardening** is

OT STORY 46.1 ANN: ADDRESSING RIGHT WRIST PAIN, ANXIETY

Ann (she/her) is a right hand–dominant 40-year-old single parent with two children aged 14 and 12 years who is experiencing pain on the ulnar side of her right wrist that is present at rest and increases with work and daily activity. She has been an ultrasound sonographer in a busy obstetrician-gynecologist office for the past 10 years. During the COVID-19 pandemic, limited staffing in her department has occurred as a result of employee sickness, resignations, and terminations. Consequently, she is required to work 10+ extra hours per week, through her lunch, and perform patient scans faster to meet the volume of patients per day. She began experiencing pain in her ulnar wrist 10 months ago that she initially ignored because she could not get time off work to seek medical intervention. When pain became constant, she went to employee health and was referred to an orthopedic hand surgeon. She was diagnosed with flexor carpi ulnaris (FCU) tendonitis and was placed on light duty and sent to OT. Employee health also requested an ergonomic assessment. In development of the occupational profile, she expressed increasing levels of anxiety owing to working in a healthcare environment and fear of acquiring COVID and giving it to her sons. She is also anxious her injury will prevent her from returning to her job and she will be unable to support family. She has been unable to sleep and has been short tempered. When asked about leisure participation, she states she has not been participating in any leisure activity other than watching television and taking occasional walks during the pandemic.

Upon observation, the client stands while using her right hand to grasp the ultrasound transducer while reaching across the patient's abdomen to perform the scan. The shoulder is positioned in 60 degrees abduction and the wrist is in 30 to 40 degrees of flexion while exerting force to depress the tissue. The position can be maintained up to 45 minutes in duration. The patient is lying supine on a standard patient examination table that is adjustable for height via a foot pedal. Photographs of Ann from the side and posterior reveal a right trunk–side bend and shoulder depression with left upper–extremity abduction to operate the machine.

Questions

1. What should you consider during Ann's occupational performance analysis?
2. How can you get information about Ann's work requirements, work setup, and work techniques?
3. Why is it important to look at all tasks and not just work tasks?
4. What should be considered in relation to Ann's level of anxiety related to work stress and effects of working during a pandemic?

When analyzing the work environment and occupational performance related to work tasks, it is important to consider what may be stressing the injured tissue, including work and nonwork activities. By visiting Ann in her work environment, you see how she interacts with the space and equipment as well as note the location of devices and implements in the scanning room. Steps to follow may include the following:

1. Speaking with Ann about her job and what she does, work hours, breaks, work routine, types of equipment she uses and how often she uses it, and a description of her discomfort: Discuss off-work activity to determine if there are other activities aggravating or contributing to her condition.
2. Observing Ann performing her job duties: can take photos of Ann (with their permission) and then show her the photos so she can see her posture.
3. Taking relevant measurements of Ann's work area: Using a tape measure, document the height of all relevant areas.
4. Reviewing your recommendations with Ann and following up with a written report to her employer and referring provider as needed: Consider the organization's policies around return to work (e.g., light duty, full duty) as well as any information sharing guidelines governed by the OT practitioners' facility, the employer, workers' compensation laws, and HIPAA.

---

similar to work conditioning; however, there are several key differences: Work hardening is multidisciplinary and may include psychology, vocational rehabilitation, physical therapy, and OT. Work-hardening strategies may include counseling, coaching, work simulation, cardiovascular conditioning, and ergonomic assessment. It is typically performed 5 days per week. Completing occupation-based activities is an important predictor of success in an occupational rehabilitation program (Hardison & Roll, 2017), and this is often achieved through the use of work simulation activities.

Typically, work hardening has been viewed as an intervention for individuals seeking to return to work who have physical limitations resulting from a musculoskeletal injury such as a back or shoulder injury. However, *cognitive work hardening* is a return-to-work intervention strategy for individuals with mental health problems, particularly depression. It is a relatively recent arrival in the area of work rehabilitation and an appropriate area for OT practitioners to exercise their skills. **Cognitive work hardening** uses graded work tasks to simulate a person's actual work tasks and/or the cognitive demands of the person's job to develop the cognitive skills required for job performance (Wisenthal & Krupa, 2013). The tasks usually include concentration, memory, multitasking, and planning, which are often impaired as a result of illnesses such as depression or injuries such as concussion or head injury. Cognitive work hardening is an excellent choice for a worker experiencing a mental health condition and whose job has high cognitive demands. The intervention strategies may address stress management, how to address interpersonal issues, following a work schedule, learning effective communication strategies, organizational skills, pacing, and focusing on mental stamina for returning to work. An example of this would be a client who has been diagnosed with depression who begins a cognitive work–hardening program by participating in an initial evaluation to determine their current status. The OT practitioner interviews the client and establishes a collaborative treatment plan to return the client to work. The emphasis of the program will be to arrive on time each day, participate in all activities, and discuss any issue that arises. The program will increase in intensity each day depending on how the client did the previous day. Activities will simulate the client's job and will either increase in length or difficulty each day. For example, if the worker assembles light switches, the OT practitioner may be able to get actual product from the employer to use in the clinic or could use another hand assembly task. The client may assemble for 10 minutes one day and 20 minutes the next day depending on how the client is progressing. The OT practitioner will give positive feedback when it is relevant and will discuss ways of dealing with negative feedback with the client so the client can strategize for handling negative comments in the workplace.

Functional Capacity Evaluation. A **functional capacity evaluation (FCE)** is a clinical evaluation to determine an individual's capacity to perform work activities related to their participation in employment (Soer et al., 2008). An FCE can be performed by a variety of professionals, but OT practitioners are distinctly qualified to perform FCEs because of their training to evaluate an individual's ability to perform activities, analyze activity (job analysis), and measure the environment using a wide variety of methods.

FCEs are usually performed in a clinic. They can be several hours in duration or extend up to 2 consecutive days. FCEs can be classified as either generic or job specific. A generic FCE assesses worker capacities compared to physical demands (in the United States, these are described by the U.S. Department of Labor, 2014) and provides a complete view of all the physical abilities of the client, such as lifting, carrying, pushing, pulling, bending, sitting, crawling, kneeling, reaching, and grasping.

The generic FCE typically does not compare the client's abilities to the targeted job's physical or cognitive demands; rather, it documents the client's abilities as related to a list of general physical or cognitive demands. Thus, it typically does not determine whether the client can return to a specific job. The information gleaned from a generic FCE can be utilized to make disability determinations for clients who are unable to work and may be used for workers' compensation and

disability settlement determinations. **Cognitive FCEs** are a growing area and occupational therapists are well suited to conduct these detailed evaluations. Through cognitive FCE, the cognitive capacity of the worker is evaluated as related to job demands.

With job-specific FCEs, there is a targeted job for the client. A FJD should be obtained to identify specifics about the job, such as weight capacities, distances, and frequencies of tasks. The FCE tests only those areas required for the job and determines whether the client's abilities match the required job demands. The written report will give a recommendation as to whether the client can perform the job duties. Job-specific FCEs have been shown to have a high predictive validity in relation to recommendations to return to the previous job or to change jobs in individuals with nonspecific low back pain (Cheng & Cheng, 2010) and with patients with a specific injury (e.g., distal radius fracture) than patients with a nonspecific injury (Cheng & Cheng, 2011).

At the conclusion of an FCE, a report is written to detail the results of the evaluation, including a review of the medical history; musculoskeletal or cognitive assessment; description of job duties; summary of strengths and limitations, any inconsistency in performance, and pain behaviors; and detailed results of the FCE including the maximum safe abilities to perform tasks. The report may also list suggested accommodations or modifications to increase the chances of a successful return-to-work process.

Post-offer Pre-employment Testing. Employers want to hire individuals who can safely perform the physical demands of the job. A *post-offer test* is one way an employer can identify whether an applicant who has been offered the job is physically capable of performing the job. By hiring an employee who is physically capable of performing the job, it may be less likely the employee will sustain a work-related injury. The post-offer test can be developed based on the FJD and the physical demands identified; a job-specific test can be developed that simulates the most physically demanding job tasks. The test should be validated by having workers who perform the job take the test and give feedback regarding whether it adequately simulates the job demands. The test should be an accurate reflection of the job—not easier or more difficult than the actual job. OT practitioners can develop a post-offer test utilizing their skills at analyzing activities.

Nonwork-Related Injury, Illness, and Conditions. Injuries affecting a person's capacity to work are not always a cumulative type of musculoskeletal injury or sustained on the job. For example, an individual can fall at home or sustain a fracture while walking on ice, injure their back working in the garden, or experience a mental health challenge that interferes with completing work tasks. The end results are the same, and the client may or may not be able to return to work.

Illnesses, injuries, and disorders such as depression, anxiety, substance use, cancer, stroke, and concussion as well as the normal aging process can affect an individual's ability to perform the physical, social, and/or cognitive demands of a job. Whether the occupation of work is disrupted by an acute injury (e.g., TBI, spinal cord injury), the side effects of disease or illness (e.g., cancer, depression), progressive disorders (e.g., amyotrophic lateral sclerosis [ALS], multiple sclerosis), or the normal aging process, it is important to consider the barriers and facilitators to work participation in conjunction with the person, their capacities and skills, required work tasks, and the work environment. OT practitioners can address the factors that limit work participation at the level of the person through individualized interventions. To address environmental and task-oriented concerns, a job analysis can be particularly valuable. The data can be used to plan and select interventions, identify outcomes, and strategize for workplace accommodations.

In 2019, nearly 11% of the US population aged 18 years and older reported symptoms of anxiety disorder or depression (Terlizzi & Schiller, 2021). The global COVID-19 pandemic has exacerbated this problem with an estimated additional 76.2 million cases of anxiety disorders globally in 2020 (25.6% increase) and an additional 53.2 million cases of major depressive disorder globally in 2020 (increase of 27.6%; Santomauro et al., 2021). Just as physical disorders disrupt physical work abilities, mental health disorders can disrupt a client's ability to attain, keep, or return to work. Symptoms may be present with or in the absence of physical challenges such as pain, movement limitations, or injuries that impact physical work abilities. Work performance may be affected by changes in concentration, emotional regulation, stamina, time management, memory, alertness, and skills related to managing stress.

Client factor assessments may include those that address anxiety, depression, substance use, cognitive function, and pain. Client performance assessments may include those related to specific work tasks, as well as motor, process and social performance skills, health management skills, and time management. The findings can then be reviewed along with job analysis results and workplace environment factors to identify areas of intervention, including work modification and accommodation. Suggestions may include modifying break schedules or work start times, using electronic organizers, lighting changes and noise abatement, setting up support from others, and identifying and reducing triggers that exacerbate symptoms. Work conditioning, transitional return to work, job shadowing, and use of virtual support are viable interventions to help clients learn or relearn skills needed to sustain work participation.

The American Cancer Society (2022) estimated there will be 1.9 million new cancer cases in 2022. In addition, Sung et al. (2021) estimated a worldwide cancer incidence

of 19.3 million cases. A systematic review investigated the effects and characteristics of intervention studies on breast cancer survivors in which the goal was to return to work (Hoving et al., 2009). The results indicated that there were no methodologically sound intervention studies specific to breast cancer and return to work; the researchers suggested that evidence from general return-to-work interventions should be applied to breast cancer survivors, developed further, and evaluated. Issues that frequently occur among breast cancer patients were identified as fatigue, diminished physical work capacity and psychosocial functioning, cognitive limitations, difficult mobility, difficulty managing stress and anxiety, difficulty coping with new self-image, and changed attitude toward work (Hoving et al., 2009). OT and return-to-work planning for the breast cancer survivor must be carefully considered and discussed with the patient and the physicians involved in the medical care. An example is as follows: a 42-year-old female patient status post right axillary radiation and chemotherapy for metastatic breast cancer has been referred to OT for strengthening and conditioning owing to fatigue. The evaluation reveals not only fatigue limiting her performance of a full workday as an elementary school teacher but also peripheral neuropathy in her fingers as a side effect of the chemotherapy drugs. The neuropathy decreases her sensation in her hands, limiting her ability to type on a computer, write with a pen, and write on a dry-erase board in class, and causes her to drop objects. The fatigue is addressed through promotion of a walking program up to 20 minutes each day, journaling to keep track of fatigue patterns, and monitoring fatigue because it is related to medications. The neuropathy proves to be a very limiting factor in the return-to-work process, but the OT practitioner teaches her how to compensate by using her eyes to type and use voice recognition software on her computer and smartphone. She uses a pop socket on her phone and a lanyard for her keys so she does not drop them. The patient made a successful return to work and utilized combination of adaptive strategies and accommodations provided by her employer.

Mild TBI such as concussion and mild stroke can impact one's ability to participate in work. When individuals of working age sustain a concussion, return to work may be compromised owing to impairment in a variety of cognitive, physical, and social interaction capacities. Participation in a job requires cognitive functioning of varying intensities and durations. When a cognitive workload is not matched to the person's abilities, they may jeopardize their safety in the workplace and be determined unfit to perform their job. Executive functioning is often impaired in mTBI, including shifting, planning, and strategy use as well as emotional regulation, attention, and decision-making. Even when awareness is intact, deficits in executive functioning can significantly impact daily life activities, including leisure, employment, and overall initiation (Erez et al., 2009).

Project CAREER is an example of a program in which OT addresses TBI and concussions in college-aged students experiencing cognitive impairments that may lead to barriers in work participation and engagement (Jacobs et al., 2015). This program is active on three college campuses across the United States and uses cognitive support technology (e.g., iPads) to assist with career planning and vocational support including transitioning from college to a workplace.

The percentage of working age people with mild stroke has risen and evidence indicates that even mild stroke impacts cognition, executive functioning, and daily functioning, which affects participation, quality of life, and return to work (Fride et al., 2015). The effects of mild stroke can produce similar executive function deficits as mTBI that may not be recognized in the acute hospital setting. Individuals with mild stroke are typically independent in self-care, do not have motor impairment, have no speech issues, and are therefore discharged with little to no rehabilitation services. Those with minor symptoms who have problems returning to work might benefit from cognitive screening and cognitive rehabilitation. In addition, cognitive screen of the patients with mild to moderate stroke should receive more attention so they can be better supported in returning to work from very early onset by learning to compensate (van der Kemp et al., 2019).

Executive function deficits are commonly missed in the acute care environment, resulting in individuals being unable to successfully return to work. OT in acute care is focused on rehabilitating functional ADL and home independence, which may deflect attention from performance skills that are necessary to successfully return to work. That is, although the emphasis on ADL is important for the overall functioning of the individual, it can fail to address how an injured or ill individual such as a stroke survivor will be able to complete activities within the complex social context of everyday life (Wolf et al., 2009). Early intervention of cognitive deficits may be neglected after a neurologic injury in favor of motor and sensory interventions (Johansson, 2011). The need for cognitive training, especially in executive function, is needed when preparing people to succeed in employment postinjury (Wong et al., 2019).

Executive function deficits can impair an individual's ability to perform their job when prior to the mTBI they had no job performance issues. For example, Ben is a 52-year-old man who fell on the ice and hit his head resulting in a concussion. He is a waiter and prided himself in his ability to take multiple orders and customer requests and not have to write things down. After the concussion, he returned to work and realized he was unable to remember multiple meal orders and was confusing customer requests and making mistakes. His employer was getting frustrated with his work and started disciplinary proceedings for his poor work skills. He recognized his problems, went to

a healthcare provider, and eventually was referred to OT where an evaluation revealed high-level executive function deficits in ability to memorize, multitask, and pay attention to details. He was able to educate his employer and participate in an OT program to eventually return to work at his previous level of function.

Addressing Work With Individuals With Disabilities. OT practitioners play an important role in addressing work with individuals with disabilities such as intellectual disability, autism spectrum disorder, behavioral disorders, and chronic physical and mental health illnesses. Preparation for work occurs under a variety of circumstances and at any point in time from childhood to adulthood. However, much of this work occurs in the school system for individuals up to age 21 years and within the community (college, trade schools, on-the-job training, sheltered workshops) for adults. It is imperative that the needs of this population are addressed because there are poorer employment outcomes for adults with disabilities for all age groups and education levels. In the United States and throughout the world, people with disabilities have lower rates of employment (BLS, 2020b) and often have lower mean annual wages compared with those without disabilities. Although 66% of people with serious mental illness indicate that they would like to be employed, less than 15% actually are (Bond et al., 2015). People with disabilities are more likely to be employed part time despite needing full-time work for financial reasons (BLS, 2020b). OT practitioners are distinctly qualified to address the needs of adolescents and adults with disabilities as related to work participation and engagement.

Career Interests, Job Exploration, and Job Matching. Adolescents and adults with disabilities may need support in identifying potential jobs that match their interests, skills, and abilities. OT practitioners can assist with investigating career interests, performing job analysis based on the essential functions of the job, and recommending reasonable accommodations to promote job placement and success. Many career interest assessment tools are available, including the O*NET's Interest Profiler (National Center for O*NET Development, 2017), and such tools can be a valuable first step in client-centered job exploration.

"Job matching is the collaborative, data-based decision-making process used by transition teams to determine the best fit between an individual's abilities and preferences and the job's environmental and occupational demands" (Persch, Cleary, et al., 2015, p. 271). The Vocational Fit Assessment (VFA) was designed to "assess job demands, identify the pros and cons of each potential job match, and identify areas of need that are suitable for intervention" (Persch, Gugiu et al., 2015). This can be a useful tool for occupational therapists because it is based on job analysis for multiple subscales (e.g., cognitive abilities, communication skills, interpersonal skills, safety, self-determination) and can be used as an outcome measure.

Community-Based Work. OT practitioners may work with people with disabilities through agencies that provide work opportunities and support within the community. This is often referred to as a *supported employment model* in which OT practitioners are part of an interdisciplinary team. In the United States, the Workforce Innovation and Opportunity Act (Pub. L. No. 113-128) of 2014 (WIOA) defines **supported employment** as "competitive integrated employment, including customized employment, or employment in an integrated work setting in which individuals are working on a short-term basis toward competitive integrated employment, that is individualized and customized consistent with the strengths, abilities, interests, and informed choice of the individuals involved, for individuals with the most significant disabilities" (Govinfo, 2021). Examples of supported employment opportunities include the following:

- Sheltered workshops
- Individual placement—place and support
- Enclaves
- Mobile work crews
- Entrepreneurial business employment
- Transitional employment
- Supported jobs

WIOA is designed to increase access to the employment, education, training, and support services necessary for employment success. Among other goals, WIOA aims to improve services to individuals with disabilities, and this presents many opportunities for OT practitioners. Additional information related to supporting individuals with disabilities can be found at https://www.doleta.gov/WIOA/Overview.cfm.

Work Transitions

Work transitions occur across the life course and with changes in life situations. Some transitions may be employee initiated (e.g., change from full time to part time, move to a different employer, change in job roles after an injury or illness), whereas others may be employer initiated (e.g., change in roles and responsibilities, shift in work schedule, loss of job). Other transitions may relate to anticipated or unanticipated life events, such as preparing for retirement or adjusting to changing abilities or circumstances. OT practitioners can be an important part of preparation for and adjustment and adaptation to these transitions. This section includes some examples of common work transitions.

Transitional Work Programs. **Transitional work** is a process performed at the client's actual job location and uses the client's job duties to assist in a safe gradual return-to-work process following an illness or injury. The OT practitioner works closely with the client's employer, healthcare provider, and perhaps worker's compensation insurance representatives to arrange appointments at the client's job. After gaining a thorough understanding of the job by performing a job analysis, the OT practitioner selects job tasks with frequencies and durations the client can perform on the job and makes recommendations for modifications in the job. The OT practitioner then obtains approval from the client's healthcare provider to initiate an adapted work program based on the information about the client's physical or mental abilities; the physical, cognitive, and social demands of the job; and the employer's level of cooperation. After the client returns to work performing the modified job duties, they are closely monitored by the employer and OT practitioners. Work duties are graded up or down based on how the client is tolerating the job duties. The process is continued until the client achieves full, unrestricted duty; however, if this is not possible, the OT practitioner can make recommendations for accommodations or alternative job placement.

School-to-Work Transition. Society values work performance and engagement, and work for individuals with disabilities is often considered the next step after secondary school completion, especially if postsecondary education is not a goal. In the United States, students covered under the Individuals with Disabilities Education Improvement Act of 2004 (IDEA; Pub. L. No. 108-446) have individualized education plans (IEPs) that address developmental, academic, and social challenges in the role of student. IDEA Part B mandates that transition from adolescence to adulthood must begin to be addressed by 16 years of age, as related to training, education, employment, and independent living skills when appropriate (U.S. Department of Education, n.d.).

OT practitioners may be part of the interdisciplinary transition team when students have an IEP that includes OT (see Chapter 45). However, this is an underserved area because data from the National Longitudinal Transition Study-2 found that only 7.5% of eligible students with disabilities actually receive OT services during the transition years (Eismann et al., 2017). OT practitioners need to advocate for their important role in school-to-work transition in order to facilitate work participation and engagement for people with disabilities. OT practitioners can use a person-centered approach to assist in

- Identifying appropriate and meaningful work opportunities through person-centered job matching to address interests, preferences, skills, and abilities
- Evaluating motor, process, and communication and interaction skills as relevant to work participation
- Building work-related skills (e.g., establishing a timely morning routine specific to preparing for a workday—appropriate clothing, packing lunch)
- Modifying or adapting work tasks to match the skills of the student (e.g., use of assistive technology, flexible work schedule, on-the-job supports)

- Promoting workplace communication skills, social behaviors, and social inclusion (e.g., ability to receive feedback from a supervisor, managing interactions with coworkers)
- Addressing environmental and social supports in the desired work environment as well as in the student's family and community
- Promoting self-determination and advocacy during the transition period
- Addressing ADL and instrumental ADL skills that are important for work participation, such as self-care, community mobility, laundry, shopping, medication management, and money management
- Implementing other direct, consultative, and/or advocacy-related interventions and approaches.

Other Work Transitions. The process outlined earlier for individuals with disabilities seeking work transition opportunities is applicable to many people and their life situations. For example, the population of aging adults can benefit from work OT to explore interests and needs for transition from work to retirement, volunteer, and other work participation activities. Exploration of a current career and ideas for reinvention or encore are often of interest to individuals who seek to retire but want to continue using their skills in a new way (Arbesman, 2015).

Transitions also occur with life changes such as the following:

- ***Post-active military duty:*** Historically, OT practitioners have strong foundations in mental and physical rehabilitation services for soldiers in times of war. Challenges to

occupational performance identified by young veterans include engagement in relationships, educational pursuits, physical health activities, quality sleep, driving, and community mobility (Plach & Sells, 2013).
- ***Progressive diseases:*** Individuals who experience chronic progressive symptoms from diseases such as multiple sclerosis, Parkinson disease, or ALS face many changes to their daily activities including work. Supportive work-related interventions described by individuals diagnosed with multiple sclerosis included being aware of symptoms and how to deal with them at work, decreasing anxiety, educating and influencing their employer, adjusting to change in confidence, and having access to skilled professional support (Bronwyn et al., 2014).
- ***Post-incarceration:*** The majority of people incarcerated in prisons or held in jails will return to the community, and typically their main goal for transition is employment, despite many social, societal, and policy challenges. See Expanding Our Perspectives for examples. Exploration of vocational interests among incarcerated women shows the need for considering personality traits with career interests and potential barriers to reentry (Washington et al., 2019).
- ***Unemployment:*** The complexities in unemployment among individuals who are motivated to work span a variety of social and political issues. It is important to consider individuals' lived experiences and related events when they are expressing that they are "doing all the right things" to become reemployed but still feeling "stuck" across occupational arenas (Laliberte Rudman & Aldrich, 2016).

✦ EXPANDING OUR PERSPECTIVES

Intersections of Justice System Involvement and Provision of OT Services

Lisa Jaegers, Clover Hutchinson, and Christine Hayes Picker

The issue is...

Over 110 million people in the United States have a criminal history. In other words, one in three people have been justice-involved, potentially affecting their family and social circle (U.S. Department of Justice, 2020). People with a record of incarceration are citizens in US society, neighbors, and community members and are often missed or not seen in OT literature, education, or research. Employment has been shown to reduce rearrests and support community living (Ramakers et al., 2017). Resources for OT practitioners to explore work performance and roles with consideration of nonsanctioned occupations (Kiepek et al., 2019)—activities sometimes related to unlawful or

culturally unaccepted behavior that may support the person's survival, such as stealing, selling illegal drugs, or sex work—are typically limited in scope. As a practitioner, you will have clients who have been directly or indirectly affected by incarceration and it will affect their lived experience and occupations.

Consider these stories...

When reading these examples, take note of the feelings you experience that may or may not negatively affect your provision of skilled OT. Reflect on why you feel this way, and how you may work through these feelings to provide unbiased, ethical, holistic care, as you would for people with other lived experiences.

Igor is a 25-year-old Russian American male referred to outpatient department for multiple flexor tendon laceration to his dominant hand. He describes his occupation as, "supplier." Igor was angry and demanding of the therapist during his visits. Although Igor's attendance was inconsistent and his compliance with the home programs

EXPANDING OUR PERSPECTIVES (continued)

was low, he would regularly threaten to sue the surgeon to voice his displeasure with his perceived poor outcome. His behavior annoyed the occupational therapist who often expressed to coworkers, "why should I give him the best treatment if that would allow him to return to his job as a drug dealer; and why should his therapy be paid through Medicaid?"

Jerry, a 40-year-old Black man from St. Louis, released from prison after serving 24 years, is working with an occupational therapist from Saint Louis University's OT Transition and Integration Services (OTTIS; Jaegers et al., 2020) to address employment, housing, and health. Jerry does not have any community-based work experience but has prison experience in manufacturing and food service. Jerry has struggled to find full-time, permanent employment owing to his incarceration history but has obtained part-time work through a temp agency. He struggles with finding and applying for jobs online and has missed several doses of his medication owing to being preoccupied with his job search.

How do you feel about working with the clients in these stories?

What can we do?

As individuals, we can question our potential fears, apprehensions, or personal judgment of the client and consider our level of comfort in providing unbiased care.

We can seek mentorship and guidance if feelings of apprehension are affecting our focus on the client. For those who feel comfortable working with clients who have a history of incarceration or choose to engage in nonsanctioned occupations, we can listen to those who are questioning their level of comfort and offer a safe space to work through their biases.

References

Jaegers, L. A., Skinner, E., Conners, B., Hayes, C., West-Bruce, S., Vaughn, M. G., Smith, D. L., & Barney, K. F. (2020). Evaluation of the jail-based occupational therapy transition and integration services program for community reentry. *The American Journal of Occupational Therapy, 74*(3), 7403205030p7403205031–7403205030p7403205011. https://doi.org/10.5014/ajot.2020.035287

Kiepek, N. C., Beagan, B., Rudman, D. L., & Phelan, S. (2019). Silences around occupations framed as unhealthy, illegal, and deviant. *Journal of Occupational Science, 26*(3), 341–353. https://doi.org/10.1080/14427591.2018.1499123

Ramakers, A., Nieuwbeerta, P., Van Wilsem, J., & Dirkzwager, A. (2017). Not just any job will do: A study on employment characteristics and recidivism risks after release. *International Journal of Offender Therapy and Comparative Criminology, 61*(16), 1795–1818. https://doi.org/10.1177/0306624x16636141

U.S. Department of Justice. (2020). *Survey of State Criminal History Information Systems, 2018.* https://www.ojp.gov/pdffiles1/bjs/grants/255651.pdf

Interprofessional Teams and Relationships

OT practitioners will interact with many other professionals who have similar goals in addressing work participation and engagement. These professionals work in variety of settings, including schools, community agencies, therapy clinics, medical provider offices, vocational rehabilitation agencies, insurance companies, and business organizations. Understanding the complementary and distinct roles of other professionals is important to facilitate desired outcomes in any setting. An example of an OT practitioner working collaboratively with other professionals to return an injured worker back to their job might include the following scenario. An occupational health physician has referred a patient to OT for acute injury management of right lateral epicondylitis. The patient's symptoms have resolved after several weeks of treatment, but in direct communication with the physician, both agreed the patient may be at risk of reinjury owing to possible musculoskeletal risk factors present during performance of the job. The certified case manager contacts the human resource manager at the patient's employer and requests the ability of the occupational therapist to assess the patient's work area to determine if there are potential areas of concern to compromise a successful return to work and to make recommendations to reduce exposure to the risk factor. The human resource manager is pleased with the suggestion, and the occupational therapist meets with the plant manager and the employee's direct supervisor to obtain information about the job. It is determined there are several risk factors the employer should address prior to the worker returning to the job, such as moving items closer to the worker, reducing the weight of certain boxes, and sharpening several tools. The interprofessional collaboration between all disciplines assured a successful return to work for the patient.

The online resources summarize common professionals with whom OT practitioners may collaborate and highlights their distinct and complementary roles in addition to further information to complement this chapter.

Lippincott® Connect *For additional resources on the subjects discussed in this chapter, visit Lippincott Connect.*

REFERENCES

ADA Amendments Act (ADAAA) of 2008, Pub. L. No. 110-325, 122 Stat. 3553 (2008).

Ahonen, E. Q., Fujishiro, K., Cunningham, T., & Flynn, M. (2018). Work as an inclusive part of population health inequities research and prevention. *American Journal of Public Health, 108*(3), 306–311. https://doi.org/10.2105/AJPH.2017.304214

American Cancer Society. (2022). *Risk of dying from cancer continues to drop at an accelerated pace.* https://www.cancer.org/latest-news/facts-and-figures-2022.html

American Occupational Therapy Association. (2017). Occupational therapy services in facilitating work participation and performance. *American Journal of Occupational Therapy, 71,* 7112410040p1–7112410040p13. https://www.aota.org/$/media/Corporate/Files/Secure/Practice/OfficialDocs/Statements/off

American Occupational Therapy Association. (2020a). Occupational therapy practice framework: Domain and process—Fourth Edition. *The American Journal of Occupational Therapy, 74*(Suppl. 2), 7412410010p1–7412410010p87. https://doi.org/10.5014/ajot.2020.74S2001

American Occupational Therapy Association. (2020b). The role of occupational therapy in primary care. *The American Journal of Occupational Therapy, 74*(Suppl. 3), 7413410040p1–7413410040p16. https://doi.org/10.5014/ajot.2020.74S3001

Americans with Disabilities Act of 1990, Pub. L. No. 101-336, 104 Stat. 328, 42 U.S.C. § 12101 (1990).

Arbesman, M. (2015). Finding new work and reinventing oneself. In L. A. Hunt & C. E. Wolverson (Eds.), *Work and the older person: Increasing longevity and well-being* (pp. 125–134). SLACK.

Bailliard, A., & Aldrich, R. (2016). Occupational justice in everyday occupational therapy practice. In D. Sakellariou & N. Pollard (Eds.), *Occupational therapies without borders: Integrating justice with practice* (pp. 83–94). Elsevier.

Bond, G., Kim, S. J., Becker, D. R., Swanson, S. J., Drake, R. E., Krzos, I. M., Fraser, V. V., O'Neill, S., & Frounfelker, R. L. (2015). A controlled trial of supported employment for people with severe mental illness and justice involvement. *Psychiatric Services, 66,* 1027–1034. https://doi.org/10.1176/appi.ps.201400510

Borg, G. (1982). Psychophysical bases of perceived exertion. *Medicine and Science in Sports and Exercise, 14,* 377–381. https://doi.org/10.1249/00005768-198205000-00012

Bronwyn, J., Sweetland, J., Riazi, A., Cano, S. J., & Playford, E. D. (2014). Staying at work and living with MS: A qualitative study of the impact of a vocational rehabilitation intervention. *Disability and Rehabilitation, 36*(19), 1594–1599. https://doi.org/10.3109/09638288.2013.854842

Bureau of Labor Statistics. (2016). *Occupational safety and health definitions.* https://www.bls.gov/iif/oshdef.htm

Bureau of Labor Statistics. (2018, August 28). *The Economics Daily, Back injuries prominent in work-related musculoskeletal disorder cases in 2016.* https://www.bls.gov/opub/ted/2018/back-injuries-prominent-in-work-related-musculoskeletal-disorder-cases-in-2016.htm

Bureau of Labor Statistics. (2020a). *Injuries, illnesses, and fatalities. Fact sheet: Occupational injuries and illnesses resulting from musculoskeletal disorders.* https://www.bls.gov/iif/oshwc/case/msds.htm

Bureau of Labor Statistics. (2020b). *Persons with a disability: Labor force characteristics summary.* https://www.bls.gov/news.release/pdf/disabl.pdf

Bureau of Labor Statistics. (2021). *Employer-reported workplace injuries and illnesses, 2020.* https://www.bls.gov/news.release/osh.nr0.htm

Cancelliere, C., Donovan, J., Stochkendahl, M. J., Biscardi, M., Ammendolia, C., Myburgh, C., & Cassidy, J. D. (2016). Factors affecting return to work after injury or illness: Best evidence synthesis of systematic reviews. *Chiropractic & Manual Therapies, 24,* 32. https://doi.org/10.1186/s12998-016-0113-z

Centers for Disease Control and Prevention. (2016). *Workplace health model.* https://www.cdc.gov/workplacehealthpromotion/model/index.html

Centers for Disease Control and Prevention. (2017). *Workplace health promotion.* https://www.cdc.gov/workplacehealthpromotion/index.html

Centers for Disease Control and Prevention. (2018). *Mental health in the workplace.* https://www.cdc.gov/workplacehealthpromotion/tools-resources/pdfs/WHRC-Mental-Health-and-Stress-in-the-Workplac-Issue-Brief-H.pdf

Cheng, A. S. K., & Cheng, S. W. C. (2010). The predictive validity of job-specific functional capacity evaluation on the employment status of patients with nonspecific low back pain. *Journal of Occupational and Environment Medicine, 52,* 719–724. https://doi.org/10.1097/JOM.0b013e3181e48d47

Cheng, A. S. K., & Cheng, S. W. C. (2011). Use of job-specific functional capacity evaluation to predict the return to work of patients with a distal radius fracture. *American Journal of Occupational Therapy, 65,* 445–452. https://doi.org/10.5014/ajot.2011.001057

Cherniack, M. G., & Punnett, L. (2019). A participatory framework for integrated interventions. In H. L. Hudson, J. A. S. Nigam, S. L. Sauter, L. C. Chosewood, A. L. Schill, & J. Howard (Eds.), *Total worker health* (pp. 107-124). American Psychological Association.

Dennerlein, J. T., O'Day, E., Mulloy, D. F., Somerville, J., Stoddard, A. M., Kenwood, C., Teeple, E., Boden, L. I., Sorensen, G., & Hashimoto, D. (2017). Lifting and exertion injuries decrease after implementation of an integrated hospital-wide safe patient handling and mobilisation programme. *Occupational and Environmental Medicine, 74,* 336–343. https://doi.org/10.1136/oemed-2015-103507

Durocher, E., Gibson, B. E., & Rappolt, S. (2014). Occupational justice: A conceptual review. *Journal of Occupational Science, 21,* 418–430. https://doi.org/10.1080/14427591.2013.775692

Eguchi, H., Wada, K., & Smith, D. R. (2016). Recognition, compensation, and prevention of karoshi, or death due to overwork. *Journal of Occupational and Environmental Medicine, 58,* e313–e314. https://doi.org/10.1097/jom.0000000000000797

Eismann, M. M., Weisshaar, R., Capretta, C., Cleary, D. S., Kirby, A. V., & Persch, A. C. (2017). Characteristics of students receiving occupational therapy services in transition and factors related to postsecondary success. *American Journal of Occupational Therapy, 71,* 7103100010p1–7103100010p8. https://doi.org/10.5014/ajot.2017.024927

Erez, A. B. H., Rothschild, E., Katz, N., Tuchner, M., & Hartman-Maeir, A. (2009). Executive functioning, awareness, and participation in daily life after mild traumatic brain injury: A preliminary study. *American Journal of Occupational Therapy, 63,* 634–640. https://doi.org/10.5014/ajot.63.5634

Fan, Z. J., Harris-Adamson, C., Gerr, F., Eisen, E. A., Hegmann, K. T., Bao, S., Silverstein, B., Evanoff, B., Dale, A.M., Thiese, M.S., Garg, A., Kapellusch, S. B., Merlino, L., & Rempel, D. (2015). Associations between workplace factors and carpal tunnel syndrome: A multi-site cross sectional study. *American Journal of Industrial Medicine, 58,* 509–518. https://doi.org/10.1002/ajim.22443

Fride, Y., Adamit, T., Maeir, E., Assayag, B., Bornstein, N. M., Korczyn, A. D., & Katz, N. (2015). What are the correlates of cognition and participation to return to work after first ever mild stroke? *Topics in Stroke Rehabilitation, 22*(5), 317–325. https://doi.org/10.1179/1074935714Z.0000000013

Global Change Data Lab. (2022). *Our world in data.* https://ourworldindata.org/time-use-living-conditions

Govindu, N. K., & Babski-Reeves, K. (2014). Effects of personal, psychosocial and occupational factors on low back pain severity in workers. *International Journal of Industrial Ergonomics, 44,* 335–341. https://doi.org/10.1016/j.ergon.2012.11.007

Govinfo. (2021). *Public Law 113-128 Workforce Innovation and Opportunity Act.* https://www.govinfo.gov/content/pkg/PLAW-113publ128/pdf/PLAW-113publ128.pdf

Hammer, L. B., Johnson, R. C., Crain, T. L., Bodner, T., Kossek, E. E., Davis, K. D., Kelly, E. L., Buxton, O. M., Karuntzos, G., Chosewood, L. C., & Berkman, L. (2016). Intervention effects on safety compliance and citizenship behaviors: Evidence from the Work, Family, and Health Study. *Journal of Applied Psychology, 101*(2), 190–208. https://doi.org/10.1037/apl0000047

Hardison, M. E., & Roll, S. C. (2017). Factors associated with success in an occupational rehabilitation program for work-related musculoskeletal disorders. *American Journal of Occupational Therapy, 71,* 7101190040p1–7101190040p8. https://doi.org/10.5014/ajot.2016.023200

Hees, H. L., de Vries, G., Koeter, M. W., & Schene, A. H. (2013). Adjuvant occupational therapy improves long-term depression recovery and return-to-work in good health in sick-listed employees with major depression: Results of a randomised controlled trial. *Occupational and Environmental Medicine, 70,* 252–260. https://doi.org/10.1136/oemed-2012-100789

Hettler, W. (1984). Wellness—The lifetime goal of a university experience. In J. D. Matarazzo, J. A. Herd, N. E. Miller, & S. M. Weiss (Eds.), *Behavioral health: A handbook of health enhancement and disease prevention* (pp. 1117–1124). Wiley.

Hinojosa, J. (2013). The evidence-based paradox. *American Journal of Occupational Therapy, 67,* e18–e23. https://doi.org/10.5014/ajot.2013.005587

Hoving, J. L., Broekhuizen, M. L., & Frings-Dresen, M. H. (2009). Return to work of breast cancer survivors: A systematic review of intervention studies. *BMC Cancer, 9,* 117. https://doi.org/10.1186/1471-2407-9-117

Hudson, H. L., Nigam, J. A. S., Sauter, S. L., Chosewood, L. C., Schill, A. L., & Howard, J. (Eds.). (2019). *Total worker health.* American Psychological Association.

Human Factors and Ergonomics Society. (2007). *ANSI/HFES 100-2007: Human factors engineering of computer workstations.* Author.

Human Rights Campaign. (2017). *Transgender inclusion in the workplace: Recommended policies and practices.* https://www.hrc.org/resources/transgender-inclusion-in-the-workplace-recommended-policies-and-practices

Individuals with Disabilities Education Improvement Act of 2004, Pub. L. No. 108-446, 20 U.S.C. 1400 et seq. (2004).

International Ergonomics Association. (2017). *Definition and domains of ergonomics.* https://iea.cc/about/what-is-ergonomics/

Jacobs, K., Rumrill, P., Hendricks, D., Elias, E., Leopold, A., Sampson, E., Nardone, A., Chen, H., & Stauffer, C. (2015). Project CAREER: Interprofessional support to transition college students with traumatic brain injuries to employment. *American Journal of Occupational Therapy, 69,* 6911510217p1. https://doi.org/10.5014/ajot.2015.69S1-PO6106

Jaegers, L. (2015). Total Worker Health™: An opportunity for integrated occupational therapy practice. *Work and Industry Special Interest Section Quarterly, 29,* 1–4. https://www.aota.org/publications/sis-quarterly/sis-quarterly-issues

Jaegers, L., Finch, D., Dorsey, J., & Ehrenfried, H. (2015). Supporting occupational therapy practice in work & industry: Hot topics. *Work & Industry Special Interest Section Quarterly, 29,* 1–4. https://www.aota.org/publications/sis-quarterly/sis-quarterly-issues

Johansson, B. B. (2011). Current trends in stroke rehabilitation. A review with focus on brain plasticity. *Acta Neurologica Scandinavica, 123,* 147–159. https://doi.org/10.1111/j.1600-0404.2010.014

Jonsson, H. (2010). Occupational transitions: Work to retirement. In C. H. Christiansen & E. A. Townsend (Eds.), *Introduction to occupation: The art and science of living* (2nd ed., pp. 211–230). Pearson Education.

Kaskutas, V., Buckner-Petty, S., Dale, A. M., Gaal, J., & Evanoff, B. A. (2016). Foremen's intervention to prevent falls and increase safety communication at residential construction sites. *American Journal of Industrial Medicine, 59,* 823–831. https://doi.org/10.1002/ajim.22597

Kielhofner, G. (2009). *Conceptual foundations of occupational therapy practice* (4th ed.). F. A. Davis.

Kindig, D. (2017). Population health equity: Rate and burden, race and class. *JAMA, 317,* 467–468. https://doi.org/10.1001/jama.2016.19435

Laliberte Rudman, D., & Aldrich, R. (2016). "Activated, but stuck": Applying a critical occupational lens to examine the negotiation of long-term unemployment in contemporary socio-political contexts. *Societies, 6*(3), 28. https://doi.org/10.3390/soc6030028

Lambeek, L. C., van Mechelen, W., Knol, D. L., Loisel, P., & Anema, J. R. (2010). Randomised controlled trial of integrated care to reduce disability from chronic low back pain in working and private life. *BMJ, 340,* c1035. https://doi.org/10.1136/bmj.c1035

Law, M., Cooper, B., Strong, S., Stewart, D., Rigby, P., & Letts, L. (1996). The person-environment-occupation model: A transactive approach to occupational performance. *Canadian Journal of Occupational Therapy, 63,* 9–23. https://doi.org/10.1177/000841749606300103

Munnell, A. H., Sass, S. A., & Soto, M. (2006). *Employer attitudes towards older workers: Survey results.* https://ideas.repec.org/p/crr/crrwob/wob_3.html

National Academies of Sciences, Engineering, and Medicine. (2017). *Communities in action: Pathways to health equity.* The National Academies Press. https://doi.org/10.17226/24624

National Center for O*NET Development. (2017). *O*NET interest profiler.* https://www.mynextmove.org/explore/ip

National Institute for Occupational Safety and Health. (2014). *National occupational research agenda.* Proposed national Total Worker Health™ agenda for public comment. http://www.cdc.gov/niosh/docket/review/docket275/pdfs/NationalTWHAgendaFinalDraft9_5_14.pdf

National Institute for Occupational Safety and Health. (2016a). *About NIOSH.* https://www.cdc.gov/niosh/about/default.html

National Institute for Occupational Safety and Health. (2016b). *Musculoskeletal disorders and ergonomics.* https://www.cdc.gov/workplacehealthpromotion/health-strategies/musculoskeletal-disorders/index.html

National Institute for Occupational Safety and Health. (2017). *Elements of ergonomics programs.* https://www.cdc.gov/niosh/topics/ergonomics/ergoprimer/default.html

National Institute for Occupational Safety and Health. (2018). *Anthropometry.* https://www.cdc.gov/niosh/topics/anthropometry/default.html

National Institute for Occupational Safety and Health. (2019). *Publications and reports: Workplace solutions.* https://www.cdc.gov/niosh/twh/publications.html

National Institute for Occupational Safety and Health. (n.d.). *Publication No. 99-101: Stress at work.* https://www.cdc.gov/niosh/docs/99-101/pdfs/99-101.pdf

Nevala, N., Pehkonen, I., Koskela, I., Ruusuvuori, J., & Anttila, H. (2015). Workplace accommodation among persons with disabilities: A systematic review of its effectiveness and barriers or facilitators. *Journal of Occupational Rehabilitation, 25,* 432–448. http://link.springer.com/article/10.1007/s10926-014-9548-z

Occupational Safety and Health Administration. (n.d.-a). *Computer workstations eTool: Good working positions.* https://www.osha.gov/SLTC/etools/computerworkstations/positions.html

Occupational Safety and Health Administration. (n.d.-b). *OSHA law & regulations.* https://www.osha.gov/law-regs.html

O*NET. (2021). *The O*NET resource center.* https://www.onetcenter.org/overview.html

Organisation for Economic Cooperation and Development. (2019). *Average usual weekly hours worked – averages.* https://www.oecd-ilibrary.org/employment/data/hours-worked/average-usual-weekly-hours-worked-averages_data-00306-en

Ostbye, T., Dement, J. M., & Krause, K. (2007). Obesity and workers' compensation: Results from the Duke Health and Safety Surveillance System. *Archives of Internal Medicine, 167,* 766–773. https://doi.org/10.1001/archinte.167.8.766

Persch, A. C., Cleary, D., Rutkowski, S., Malone, H., Darragh, A., & Case-Smith, J. (2015). Current practices in job matching: A project SEARCH perspective on transition. *Journal of Vocational Rehabilitation, 43,* 259–273. https://doi.org/10.3233/JVR-150774

Persch, A. C., Gugiu, P. C., Onate, J. A., & Cleary, D. S. (2015). Development and psychometric evaluation of the Vocational Fit Assessment (VFA). *American Journal of Occupational Therapy, 69,* 6906180080p1–6906180080p8. https://doi.org/10.5014/ajot.2015.019455

Plach, H. L., & Sells, C. H. (2013). Occupational performance needs of young veterans. *American Journal of Occupational Therapy, 67,* 73–81. http://doi.org/10.5014/ajot.2013.003871

Rimer, B. K., & Glanz, K. (2005). *Theory at a glance: A guide for health promotion practice* (2nd ed.). U.S. Department of Health and Human Services, National Institutes of Health, National Cancer Institute.

Santomauro, D., Mantilla Herrera, A. M., Shadid, J., Zheng, P., Ashbaugh, C., Pigott, D. M., Abbafati, C., Adolph, C., Amlag, J. O., Aravkin, A. Y., Bang-Jensen, B. L., Bertolacci, G. J., Bloom, S. S., Castellano, R., Castro, E., Chakrabarti, S., Chattopadhyay, J., Cogen, R. M., Collins, J. K., … Ferrari, A. J.; COVID-19 Mental Disorders Collaborators. 2021. Global prevalence and burden of depressive and anxiety disorders in 204 countries and territories in 2020 due to the COVID-19 pandemic. *Lancet, 398,* 1700–1712. https://www.thelancet.com/action/showPdf?pii=S0140-6736%2821%2902143-7

Schill, A. L. (2017). Advancing well-being through Total Worker Health®. *Workplace Health & Safety, 65,* 158–163. https://doi.org/10.1177/2165079917701140

Smith, B. J., Tang, K. C., & Nutbeam, D. (2006). WHO health promotion glossary: New terms. *Health Promotion International, 21,* 340–345. https://doi.org/10.1093/heapro/dal033

Soer, R., van der Schans, C. P., Groothoff, J. W., Geertzen, J. H., & Reneman, M. F. (2008). Towards consensus in operational definitions in functional capacity evaluation: A Delphi survey. *Journal of Occupational Rehabilitation, 18,* 389–400. https://doi.org/10.1007/s10926-008-9155-y

Sonne, M., Villalta, D. L., & Andrews, D. M. (2012). Development and evaluation of an office ergonomic risk checklist: ROSA—Rapid Office Strain Assessment. *Applied Ergonomics, 43,* 98–108. https://doi.org/10.1016/j.apergo.2011.03.008

Steckler, A., and Linnan, L. (2002). *Process evaluation for public health interventions and research.* Jossey-Bass

Sung, H., Ferlay, J., Siegel, R., Laversanne, M., Soerjomataram, I., & Jemal, A. (2021, February). *Global cancer statistics 2020: GLOBOCAN estimates of incidence and mortality worldwide for 36 cancers in 185 countries.* https://acsjournals.onlinelibrary.wiley.com/doi/10.3322/caac.21660

Taskforce on the Aging of the American Workforce. (2008). *Report of the taskforce on the aging of the American workforce.* https://www.doleta.gov/reports/FINAL_Taskforce_Report_2_27_08.pdf

Terlizzi, E. P., & Schiller, J. S. (2021, March). *Estimates of mental health symptomatology, by month of interview: United States, 2019.* National Center for Health Statistics. https://www.cdc.gov/nchs/data/nhis/mental-health-monthly-508.pdf

U.S. Department of Education. (n.d.). Building the legacy: IDEA 2004. http://idea.ed.gov/explore/view.html

U.S. Department of Health and Human Services. (2020). *Healthy People 2030.* Retrieved December 7, 2021, from https://health.gov/healthypeople/objectives-and-data/social-determinants-health

U.S. Department of Labor. (2014). *Work capacity evaluation musculoskeletal conditions.* http://www.dol.gov/owcp/dfec/regs/compliance/OWCP-5c.pdf

Van der Kemp, J., Kruithof, W. J., Nijboer, T. C. W., van Bennekom, C. A. M., van Heugten, C., & Visser-Meily, J. M. A. (2019). Return to work after mild-to-moderate stroke: Work satisfaction and predictive factors. *Neuropsychological Rehabilitation, 29*(4), 638–653. https://doi.org/10.1080/09602011.2017.1313746

Vasconcelos, A. F. (2015). Older workers: Some critical societal and organizational challenges. *Journal of Management Development, 34,* 352–372. https://doi.org/10.1108/JMD-02-2013-0034

Vindergaard, N., & Benros, M. E. (2020) COVID-19 pandemic and mental health consequences: Systematic review of the current evidence. *Brain, Behavior, and Immunity, 89,* 531–542. https://doi.org/10.1016/j.bbi.2020.05.048

Washington, S. E., Katz, I., & Jaegers, L. A. (2019). Vocational interests of women incarcerated and perceived barriers of societal prison reentry. *Annals of International Occupational Therapy.* https://doi.org/10.3928/24761222-20191018-01

Wisenthal, A., & Krupa, T. (2013). Cognitive work hardening: A return-to-work intervention for people with depression. *Work, 45,* 423–430. https://doi.org/10.3233/WOR-131635

Wolf, T., Baum, C., & Connor, L. T. (2009). The changing face of stroke: Implications for occupational therapy. *American Journal of Occupational Therapy, 63*(5), 621–625. https://doi.org/10.5014/ajot.63.5.621

Wong, A. W., Chen, C., Baum, C. M., Heaton, R. K., Goodman, B., & Heinemann, A. W. (2019). Cognitive, emotional, and physical functioning as predictors of paid employment in people with stroke, traumatic brain injury, and spinal cord injury. *American Journal of Occupational Therapy, 73*(2), 7302205010p1-7302205010p15. https//doi.org/10.5014/ajot.2019.031203

World Health Organization. (2008). *International classification of functioning, disability and health: ICF.* WHO Press.

Play and Leisure

Anita C. Bundy and Sanetta Henrietta Johanna du Toit

LEARNING OBJECTIVES

After reading this chapter, you will be able to:

1. Compare and contrast play and leisure as meaningful occupations.
2. Describe play and leisure as reflections of identity.
3. Evaluate existing assessments to determine which, if any, characteristics of play and leisure they reflect.
4. Distinguish between interventions in which play and leisure are means to meet other goals and those for which play and leisure are the targeted outcomes of intervention.
5. Evaluate the benefits associated with interventions promoting play and leisure using Hammell's (2009) categories (engagement in doing; belonging, connectedness, contribution; restoration; life continuity and hope).
6. Assess the environment and other contexts for factors that promote, or detract from, play and leisure.
7. Synthesize the state of existing research demonstrating the effectiveness of interventions to promote play and leisure and that using play and leisure as means to meet other objectives.

Introduction

Arguably, play and leisure comprise some of the most meaningful occupations in which people of all ages and abilities engage. Nonetheless, occupational therapy (OT) practitioners have a long, but ambivalent, relationship with both occupations (Parham, 2008), focusing instead on increasing functional independence. Although founders of the profession (Saunders, 1922; Slagle, 1922; Ziegler, 1924) believed that the "play spirit" was essential to a worthwhile life, even Slagle and Robeson (as cited in Kielhofner, 2009, p. 21) spoke of play as a means to an end. They wrote,

> Let our minds be engaged with the spirit of fun and competitive play and leave our muscles, nerves and organs to carry on their functions without conscious thought—then our physical exercise will be correspondingly more beneficial and we can readily picture the effect exerted on the mood of the sullen, morose patient by the genial glow which suffuses the body following active exercise.

In time, occupational therapists came to believe that a "[mechanistic paradigm] would bring OT recognition as an efficacious medical service and increase its scientific respectability" (Kielhofner, 2009, p. 31). Thus, when they were considered at all, play and leisure were second-class occupations relegated to discretionary time. Only people who could not engage in productive occupations—the very young, the older people, and people in untoward circumstances—could claim discretionary time legitimately. But, as Hammell (2009) cautioned, "Placing occupations in a hierarchy easily justifies placing the doers of those occupations in a similar hierarchy" (p. 108).

A single voice in the wilderness, Reilly (1974) guided her students to explore play in OT in a scholarly way. She offered *Play as Exploratory Learning*, the first textbook on the subject in the field. Nonetheless, in this text, only Reilly explored play itself. In the Preface, she wrote,

> [*Play as Exploratory Learning*] is divided into two parts. Each part is an aspect of an heuristic approach to the phenomenon of play. Part One [Reilly's portion] searches for the most general questions about external and internal reality that play can answer; Part Two [student contributions] applies specific play questions to the behavior of disabled people. What the reader should realize is *that the theoretical approach of Part One is not applied in Part Two* [emphasis added]. The heuristic strategies, it needs also to be said, grew from the remedial setting in which occupational therapists use play. As an applied field, occupational therapy is not obliged to hold any allegiance to a specific science of theoretical methodology. The graduate student contributors in Part Two used play as a master's thesis theme . . . and drew upon their abundant clinical experiences acquired in rehabilitation clinics. Both the strengths and weaknesses of the contributors are that they were under no compulsion to make their data fit a particular scientific methodology or theoretical foundation. (p. 10)

Prominent publications in OT, such as the *Willard and Spackman* text, largely ignored play and leisure for a long time. Up to the third edition of Willard and Spackman's *Occupational Therapy* textbook, there is no mention of play *or* children (Willard & Spackman, 1963). In the third edition, the word *leisure* is included in a table of aspects to consider when working in geriatrics. In the fifth edition, play is discussed as a treatment modality (i.e., medium) and reference is made to play behavior (Willard et al., 1978). The fifth edition does not mention leisure. However, it *does* include the word *recreation* in the index, referring readers to "play." Finally, for the first time in the eighth edition, Susan Knox contributed a seven-page chapter devoted to play and leisure (Willard et al., 1993). Perhaps unsurprisingly, the majority of studies of play and leisure in OT, even now, describe the consequences of impairment to children or adults, often comparing their play or leisure with that of typically developing peers.

In the early 1990s, scholars in OT and occupational science (e.g., Bundy, 1993; Canadian Association of Occupational Therapy, 1996; Parham, 1996; Primeau, 1996; Suto, 1998) began to reclaim play and leisure as significant domains of human occupation. More recently, Lynch and colleagues (Lynch & Moore, 2016; Ray-Kaeser & Lynch, 2017) explicitly challenged occupational therapists to consider play for the sake of play. Researchers and theorists linked play and leisure as occupations to life satisfaction, quality of life and mental health for individuals of all ages, with and without disability (Goltz & Brown, 2014; Hess & Bundy, 2003; King et al., 2013; Parham, 2008; Pereira & Stagnitti, 2006; Rodríguez et al., 2008). Importantly, some authors, both within and outside occupational science, described differences in play and leisure of autistic individuals,[1] without pathologizing them (e.g., Conn, 2015; Fahy et al., 2020; Seija Kangas et al., 2012). Others (e.g., Wang et al., 2012) suggested that engaging in leisure may provide a "buffer" against disability. Thus, play and leisure are important concerns of OT (e.g., Parham, 2008; Wilcock, 2007). In fact, Parham (2008) felt that play was so important that we should describe a rhetoric of "play as health."

Contributing to a regained status of play and leisure, occupational scientists applied a broader lens to these occupations. Lynch et al. (2016) explored sociocultural influences on infant play in Irish homes. Graham et al. (2014) studied the ways in which parents expanded the concept of play for their children with severe cerebral palsy. Gerlach et al. (2014) explored how Indigenous children's play is shaped by historical, political, and economic structures. Ramugondo (2012) examined intergenerational play in one South African family, revealing both persistence and change. Angelou et al. (2022) expanded on the concept of intergenerational leisure by facilitating more opportunities for meaningful engagement between university students and older adults within residential aged care facilities, when students become neighbors and live in close proximity of older residents.

The Inherent Qualities of Play and Leisure

Play and leisure have much in common; however, they are not synonymous. Neither does the age of participants distinguish them. That is, play is not an occupation solely of children and leisure of adults. Nonetheless, because play is an important contributor to development, it is often associated only, but incorrectly, with childhood. Similarly, the restorative and self-expressive outcomes of leisure mean that it is often, but equally incorrectly, considered only an adult occupation.

---

[1]In this chapter, we have chosen to use identity-first language (e.g., autistic children) rather than people-first language (e.g., child with autism).

Play and leisure, like many other constructs within OT, have multiple definitions but there is no consensus on either term (Hurd & Anderson, 2010). And, although single, all-purpose definitions, responsive to the needs of the entire profession, may not be required (Hurd & Anderson, 2010; Parham, 2008), we argue an understanding of the value of play and leisure and the role they have in an individual's life would support practitioners' assessment and promotion of play and leisure.

Defining Play

The American Occupational Therapy Association's Occupational Therapy Practice Framework (OTPF, 4th ed.; AOTA, 2020) defined play in much the same way we propose here: as intrinsically motivated, internally controlled, freely chosen activities that may include suspension of reality, exploration, humor, risk taking, contests, and celebrations. Similarly, drawing from Parham and Fazio (2008), the OTPF defines leisure as nonobligatory activity that is intrinsically motivated and engaged in during discretionary time.

Expanding on Neumann's (1971) work, Bundy and colleagues proposed three traits that define play and separate it, along a continuum, from nonplay: *internal control, intrinsic motivation*, and *suspension of reality* (Skard & Bundy, 2008). Neumann argued that, like play and nonplay, each trait comprises a continuum. A transaction would be play if a greater presence of some traits offset the lesser presence of others (see Figure 47.1). Skard and Bundy (2008) further argued that intrinsic motivation, internal control, and suspension of reality were sufficient to capture most of the traits that scholars commonly attribute to play.

In further defining play, Skard and Bundy (2008) placed a frame around the scale shown in Figure 47.1. Drawing from Bateson's (1972) work, the frame represents cues that, like a picture frame, separate play from "reality." **Play** can therefore be defined as a transaction characterized by relative intrinsic motivation, relative internal control, and suspension of reality that is framed in such a way as to separate it from "real life."

Defining Leisure

Bundy et al. (2018) similarly defined leisure by its traits. They applied a variation of Skard and Bundy's model, describing a continuum of engagement in leisure ranging from "distracted" to "absorbed" (i.e., totally engaged). They further associated total engagement with self-actualization. As with play, Bundy et al. proposed that control, motivation, and disengagement from unnecessary constraints of reality, collectively, determine leisure. They also indicated that each element of leisure reflects a continuum; that is, they

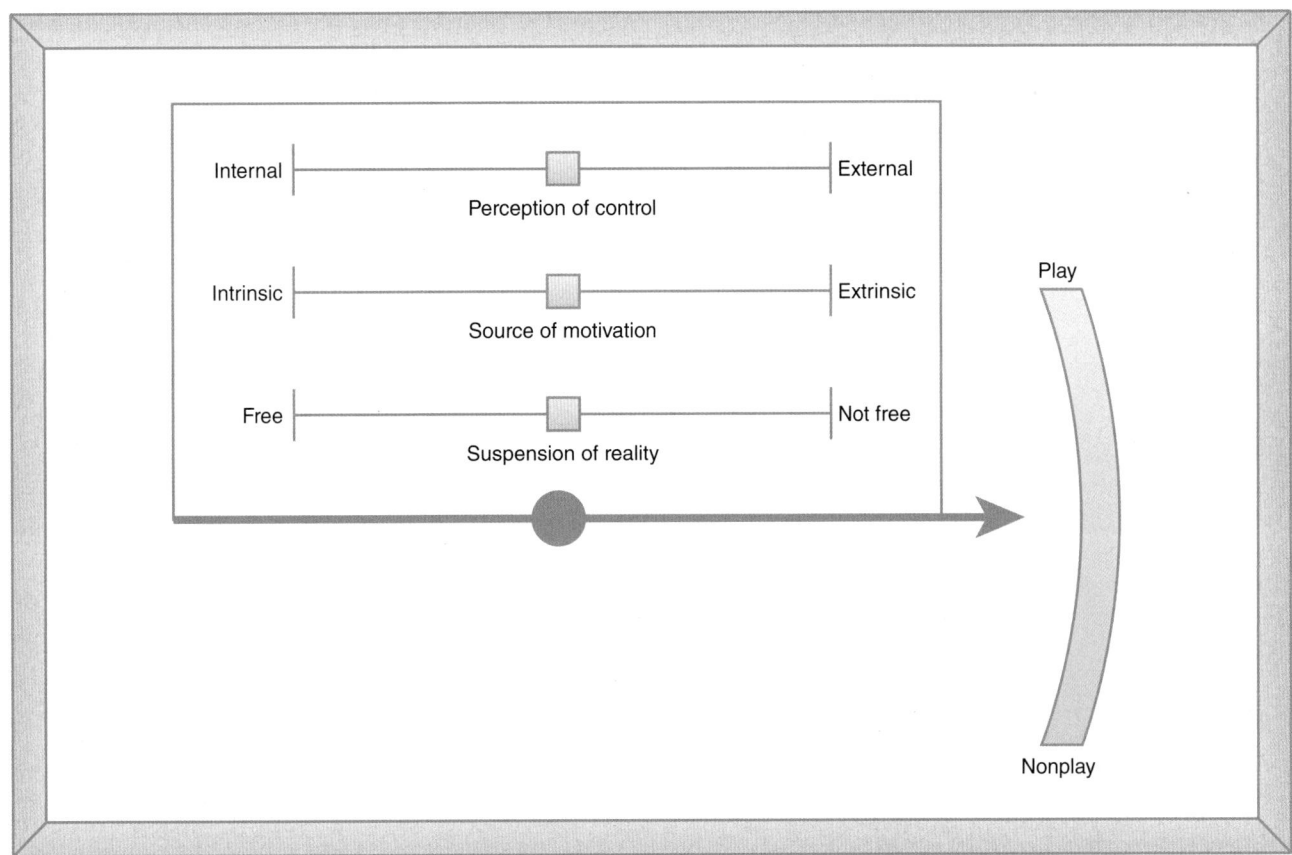

FIGURE 47.1 **Elements of play.**

are not all-or-none phenomena. The elements of leisure also are mutually influencing. That is, individuals engaging in an activity in which they feel little control are unlikely to be able to disengage from the constraints of real life. The summative contributions of "control," "motivation," and "disengagement from the constraints of real life" to leisure are illustrated in Figure 47.2.

Although similar, the elements that define leisure are somewhat different from those defining play. Unlike play, motivations for leisure are as often extrinsic as intrinsic. However, if the motivation is extrinsic, it must be self-determined (i.e., performed for one's own long-term gain [e.g., exercise] or for another's benefit [e.g., knitting a sweater for a grandchild or doing home repairs for an adult child]; Losier et al., 1993; Mannell et al., 1988). Thus, **leisure** can be defined as a transaction in which one becomes totally engaged and that is characterized by relative internal control, a high level of motivation (intrinsic or *self-determined extrinsic*), and disengagement from unnecessary constraints of reality; it is often framed in such a way as to clearly indicate it as leisure (see "Framing" section).

Considering Play and Leisure as Occupations

Earlier we said that play and leisure are not synonymous, although they share many of the same traits. We also said that, although age of a participant does not distinguish play from leisure, outcomes might. Development is commonly associated with play, whereas restoration and self-expression are associated with leisure. Some activities can be play *or* leisure, depending on how it is perceived and the meaning attached to it.

Considering play and leisure by the characteristics that distinguish them from other occupations, allows two individuals to consider the same activity as play or nonplay, leisure or nonleisure. A highly skilled individual might consider soccer to be a cherished play or leisure activity, whereas an individual with developmental coordination disorder might find soccer the furthest thing from play or leisure. The highly skilled individual feels in control of her body and the ball and loves the feeling of engaging in the sport. She wants to win the game (extrinsic motivation), but she enjoys playing even when her team loses. When playing soccer, she is free, for a short time, from the everyday tasks she left behind (e.g., homework, cooking dinner). She is completely engaged.

Because of the personalized nature of play and leisure experiences, the same activity can serve different purposes (Hammell, 2009; Jonsson, 2008). For example, some people enjoy reading for intellectual stimulation, whereas others seek relaxation and restoration. Understanding the motivation for a play or leisure activity is key to client-centered practice. For example, singing in a choir may be deemed involvement in a cultural activity, but it also could be performed primarily for socialization with choir members. Or, both socialization and the cultural aspects may be equally important. Understanding the motivations fulfilled by being a choir member facilitates replacement of that activity should that be necessary.

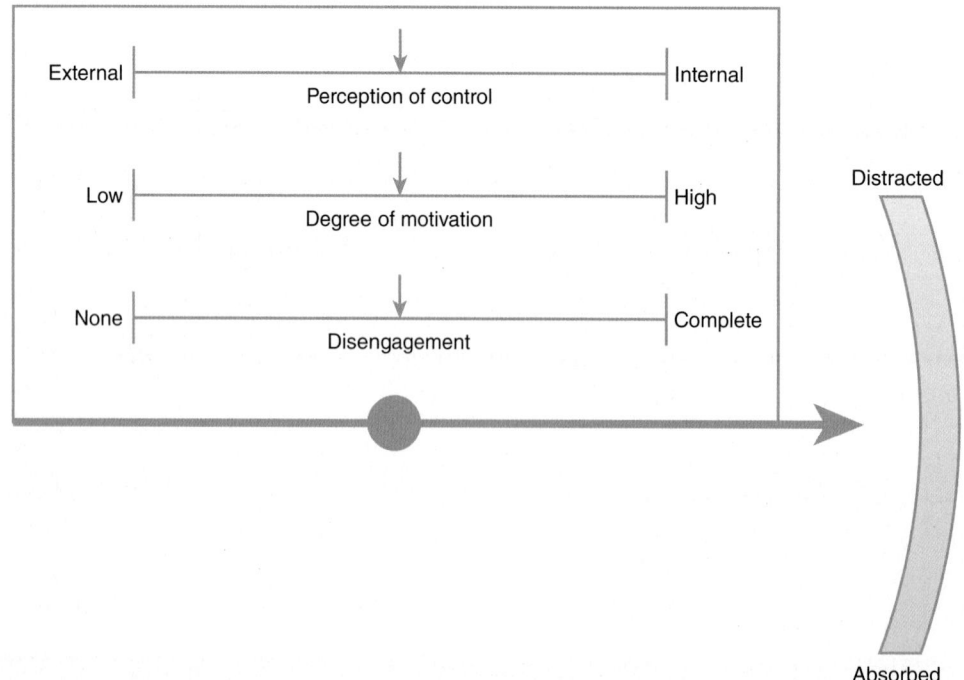

FIGURE 47.2 Summative contribution of the elements to total engagement in leisure.

When is an activity considered play but not leisure, or vice versa? Admittedly, this may be of more interest theoretically than practically, but surely the way practitioners think about play and leisure influences the way we assess and promote them. We propose that aspects of motivation, suspension of reality, and framing distinguish play from leisure. Although each of these elements is equally important to both play and leisure, they can look quite different in the two.

Motivation

Most theorists agree that intrinsic motivation is a defining feature of play and often of leisure. Drawing from Rubin et al. (1983), Parham (2008) described the meaning of intrinsic motivation in play as "motivated by the experience of the play itself, not by the promise of rewards that are external to the play" (p. 5). The sources of intrinsic motivation are individually determined and varied. They commonly include, for example, mastery (e.g., White, 1959), social interaction, sensation (e.g., Caillois, 1979), and the pleasure of being a cause (e.g., Sutton-Smith, 1997). Of course, play may also have extrinsic motivators (e.g., the desire to win or gain praise), but the driving force must be intrinsic for a transaction to be played.

In contrast, some authors (Losier et al., 1993; Mannell et al., 1988) have found that intrinsic motivation and self-determined extrinsic motivation are equally correlated with leisure satisfaction. Although not specifically discussing leisure, Ryan and Deci (2017) described such activity as having integrated regulation (i.e., the goals of the activity, although extrinsic, are fully assimilated within the self). Although self-determined extrinsic motivators are undoubtedly powerful drivers for leisure, they seem less associated with play. What do you think are the differing motivations of the dad, grandmother, and daughter/granddaughter in Figure 47.3?

As occupations and identities evolve across the life course, individuals' motivations for engaging in play and leisure also change. For example, Passmore and French (2003) categorized leisure of adolescents according to whether activities met an intrinsic need for achievement, social interaction, or time-out. They associated achievement leisure with engagement in competitive and challenging pursuits, like team sports and music performances. Achievement leisure could also include creative activities like drawing. Achievement activities require regular commitment and organization. Social leisure activities (e.g., visiting friends, eating out, chatting/texting online) involve friends and social experiences and fulfill a need for belonging. Time-out leisure encompasses relaxing and calming. Time-out leisure (e.g., listening to music, watching television, or keeping a diary) has low demand, can be undertaken alone, and includes time for reflection.

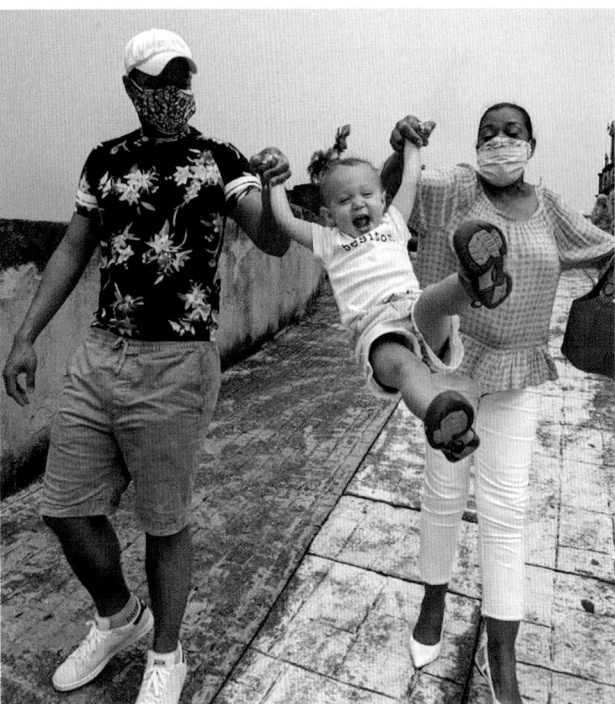

FIGURE 47.3 Is it play or leisure? And what are the motivations for each?

Suspension of Unnecessary Constraints of Reality

Albeit by slightly different names, the bottom continua in the scales shown in Figures 47.1 and 47.2 refer to freedom from unnecessary constraints of reality. In defining play, we name that element suspension of reality, whereas in defining leisure, we refer to "disengagement" as a release from everyday reality. Neumann (1971) described suspension of reality by noting that a player is free to determine the degree to which a transaction resembles objective reality. A child swinging on a backyard swing could choose to "just swing"—the fun being in the sensation or from swinging as high as possible. Alternatively, the child could choose to "become a superhero"—flying to save a "victim" from "sure death." The choice is the child's. Pretending is a common form of suspending reality. Players can be whoever they choose, pretend an object is something it is not or pretend to be doing something they are not. Playful joking, teasing, mischief, and clowning are other ways of stepping outside of reality (Skard & Bundy, 2008).

We argue that, although both play and leisure depend on being free from unnecessary constraints of everyday life, the presence of pretend, playful joking, clowning, mischief, and teasing distinguishes play from leisure. Further, although pretending may be more common in children, adults also pretend (see Figure 47.4). When taking a self-report version of the Test of Playfulness, many of the German adult participants in Weigl and Bundy's (2013)

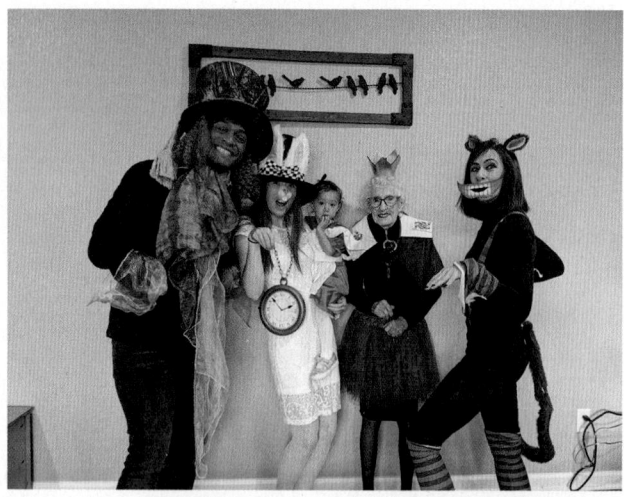

FIGURE 47.4 Although pretending may be more common in children, adults also play.

study revealed that they pretended in the context of everyday activities like choir practice. Glynn and Webster (1992) found that flights of playful joking and banter were not only common in the workplace but also contributed to productivity. And more than one longstanding cartoon (e.g., *Rose Is Rose* by Pat Brady and *Foxtrot* by Bill Amend) depict adults and adolescents pretending. Cartoons are only funny because readers readily identify with the characters (see, e.g., Box 47.1). "Zipho" assumed an alter ego every day when he went off to work, pretending changed his entire outlook on life. We argue that playful clowning, joking, teasing, mischief, and pretend are common in both adults and children and are characteristic of play but not of leisure.

Framing

Framing is the use of cues to separate play transactions from "real life." Cues reveal how a player wishes to be viewed and treated by others (Bateson, 1972). A child on all fours entering the kitchen barking gives a clear cue that he is a "puppy" and his parents should interact with him accordingly. A father, exaggerating his motions, roaring and chasing after

his child, likewise gives cues that he is a "monster" and his child should run away in mock fear. Of course, that father must alter his cues in response to the reactions of his child. Otherwise, the play may turn to nonplay. Importantly, overt cues do not accompany all pretending. Although Zipho (see Box 47.1) pretended overtly—changing his clothing to support a make-believe role—many adults pretend more in their imaginations than in actions.

Framing also happens outside of pretend play. Rules, for example, are a frame that distinguish what is allowed in a game and what is not (Caillois, 1979). Of course, players can renegotiate the rules. By changing what is allowed in the game, they change the frame.

The ability to frame play is critical to being a good playmate. Cordier et al. (2010a, 2010b) found that children with attention-deficit/hyperactivity disorder (ADHD) tended to have difficulty with framing. They suggested that responding to play cues reflects empathy. Later, Wilkes-Gillan and colleagues developed an intervention in which they successfully taught cue-reading skills to children with ADHD (Wilkes et al., 2011; Wilkes-Gillan et al., 2014a, 2014b, 2015, 2016a, 2016b, 2017). Kent and colleagues (2018, 2020a, 2020b, 2020c) extended their intervention to autistic children who also have difficulty giving and reading cues.

Framing is important to some types of leisure as well as play. Caillois (1979, cited in Henricks, 2010, p. 180) wrote about indicators of collective affiliation where play becomes "a special world isolated from everyday affairs." These indicators are seen, for example, in the uniforms of sporting teams or other organized groups (e.g., scouting, cheerleading). Even solitary runners and bicyclists often don "uniform" clothing as a cue about how others should view them. Caillois (1979) described these indicators of group membership in reference to games and play, but we argue that such cues are more related to leisure (as we define it) than play. Adults assuming a theatrical role also give cues about how other cast members and the audience should interact with them (see Figure 47.5). Arguably, those cues are about collective membership. Not all leisure is clearly framed as such. Some individuals performing self-determined

BOX 47.1 PRETENDING ENABLES ALTERNATE REALITIES

Suspending reality through pretend provides unique opportunities to take on roles and embrace identities not otherwise possible, especially for members of marginalized groups as demonstrated by the main character in The Script's music video *Superheroes* (https://www.youtube.com/watch?v=WIm1GgfRz6M). This father (whom we shall refer to as Zipho) supports his daughter financially by working in a garbage dump. But every morning, he leaves home dressed in a suit and tie. Zipho travels to the dump, changes his clothing,

works all day, changes back to his suit and tie, and returns home to his daughter. When Zipho and his daughter go out together in the evening, he wears his suit and tie. Dressing up allows Zipho to pretend to have a role he believes will make his daughter proud. When he can, Zipho rescues a discarded toy from the rubbish he sorts, cleans it, and presents it to his daughter. They share make-believing that his business is doing well, and he can afford to spoil her with gifts. One might ask, "Which is the real Zipho and which is the pretend Zipho?"

Play and Leisure as Statements of Identity

Because play and leisure activities are freely chosen, they make important statements about the identities of participants (Kelly, 1982; Neulinger, 1974; Scraton & Holland, 2006). In fact, Plato is credited with having said that you could learn more about a person in an hour of play than in a year of conversation. Theorists and researchers clearly link occupation and selfhood in general (Eakman et al., 2018) and leisure and identity in particular. Families from some parts of the world decorate their homes with mementos of leisure experiences (Csikszentmihalyi & Halton, 1981; Rockwell-Dylla, 1992). Some of the most compelling photographs of children are taken while they play. Mementos make statements of accomplishments, selfhood, and things that bring great joy. When at risk of losing valued play or leisure unintentionally, individuals also risk losing important reflections of themselves.

Because of their importance and healing properties, play and leisure may counter some negative effects of adverse personal circumstances, thus preserving identity. Numerous individuals described the importance of play to children facing crises imposed by war, weather, COVID-19 (Moore et al., 2020), and other untoward circumstances (e.g., Casey et al., 2017). Similarly, Pereira and Stagnitti (2006) indicated that older adults displaced by immigration found traditional leisure activities associated with their culture of origin to be very important. In OT Story 47.1 (adapted from Bundy et al., 2018), we relay an account of an OT assessment and intervention with leisure at the heart. This intervention went a long way to preserving identity.

The link between identity and play, which is both logical and theoretical, is not as well supported as that between identity

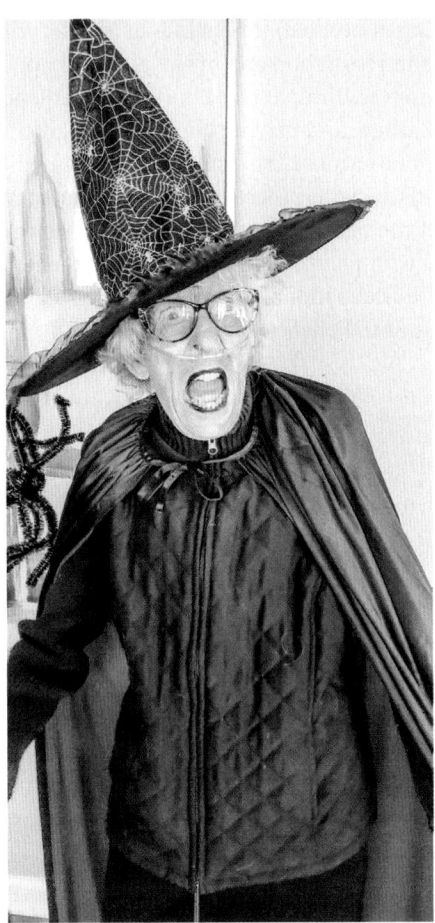

FIGURE 47.5 Adults in a theatrical role give cues about how others should interact with them.

extrinsically motivated leisure may not don a uniform or give other cues that their activity is separate from real life, a father making repairs to his adult child's home, for example, or a grandmother knitting a scarf for her granddaughter.

OT STORY 47.1 SARAH: THE SAILING GRANDMOTHER

At age 74, following a stroke, Sarah was depressed not only because she had lost physical capability but also because her children wanted her to go into a long-term care setting to receive "the kind of care they felt she needed." Sarah chose instead to attend a Day Therapy Center where the occupational therapist completed an assessment of her leisure using an interest checklist supplemented by interview. The therapist, learning that, as a child, Sarah and her family had been avid sailors, developed an intervention plan that included an adapted sailing program called Sailability. Sarah flourished. She became a "sailing grandmother," won a championship race, and was featured in a local newspaper. These achievements were turning points in her recovery. Sarah did not have the strength or movement to handle the sails, but she said, "I'm the captain. I choose who rolls the sails and tell them how to do it. You have to think or you might hit another boat." Sailing renewed her identity and self-confidence. Sailability kept her independent and mentally alert. She went every week. Clearly, leisure, for Sarah, not only reflected identity but also contributed to a renewed identity.

Questions

1. How might Sarah's identity have changed if she had gone into the retirement village as her children wanted?
2. How might you help Sarah's children to think differently about Sarah's choice of the Day Therapy Center over a retirement village?

and leisure. Little research addresses that link (Sutton-Smith, 1997). Sutton-Smith described three modern, largely individualistic, rhetorics of play that help us understand potential links. Of course, because these rhetorics are focused on individuals, they may apply best in Western cultures.

Sutton-Smith termed the first of these three rhetorics "progress." Theories reflecting a progress rhetoric value play because it promotes development, particularly of skills and abilities. Parham (2008) explicitly named the progress rhetoric as dominant in pediatric OT. However, although skills and abilities are a piece of one's identity, they are only one piece. Unfortunately, viewing play through a progress lens devalues play as an occupation. Further Sutton-Smith suggested that theories reflecting a progress rhetoric promote adult control of children's play: "to stimulate it, negate it, exclude it, or encourage limited forms of it" (p. 49). Thus, embracing play primarily as a means of promoting skill development may unintentionally detract from, as much as promote, the development of identity.

Sutton-Smith (1997) also described a rhetoric of the self that reflects the experiences and characteristics of play. The definition of play we propose in this chapter falls largely within this rhetoric, which also commonly frames OT interventions (Parham, 2008). Some theories that fall within a rhetoric of the self, define play as freely chosen, intrinsically motivated, and controlled by players. If this is true, then play is a relatively pure reflection of players' identities. When players engage in activity they enjoy for its own sake, they learn about who they are—and they tell others. As they modify the play, they also modify their identities.

Sutton-Smith (1997) termed the third of the rhetorics applicable here "the imaginary." Freedom from unnecessary constraints of reality, an important characteristic of the definition of play we propose here, comprises an element of the imaginary. According to Sutton-Smith, in fantasy, children do more than replicate the real world, and they fabricate another world, one "that is much more vivid than mundane reality" (p. 158). Sutton-Smith further claimed that childhood fantasies help children understand how to react emotionally to the experience of living in the world. This, we believe, is an important tie between fantasy play and the development of identity.

The Benefits of Play and Leisure

Hammell (2004b, 2009) indicated that all occupations (defined here as anything people do with their time) should be classified by the intrinsic needs they meet, in other words, by their benefits. Hammell categorized those intrinsic needs as (a) engagement in doing; (b) belonging, connecting, and contributing; (c) restoration; and (d) life continuity and hope for the future. Similarly, Pierce (2001a, 2003, 2014) labeled restoration, pleasure, and productivity as the motivations

for engaging in occupations, including leisure. Productivity, pleasure, and restoration are interrelated and not categories unto themselves. Thus, horseback riding, needlepoint, playing with Barbies, and playing Nintendo are all occupations that foster one or more intrinsic needs. Notably, the connection of pleasure with process, rather than outcome, is reminiscent of the definition of play. Categorizing occupations associated with play and leisure by their benefits is appealing because occupational therapists often need a reminder of the enormous benefits of play and leisure.

Benefits of Engagement in Doing

Hammell (2009) cited her own earlier work (Hammell, 2004a, 2004b) and that of Laliberte-Rudman et al. (2000), Nagle et al. (2002), and Ville et al. (2001), indicating that having something meaningful and purposeful to wake up and do contributed to self-perceptions of capability and value and to other indicators of well-being. Similarly, Atler (2014) indicated that the interrelated nature of productivity, pleasure, and restoration, and the understanding that pleasure is associated with process rather than only the outcome of an experience, directs what individuals *do* every day in order to meet their needs (see Figure 47.6).

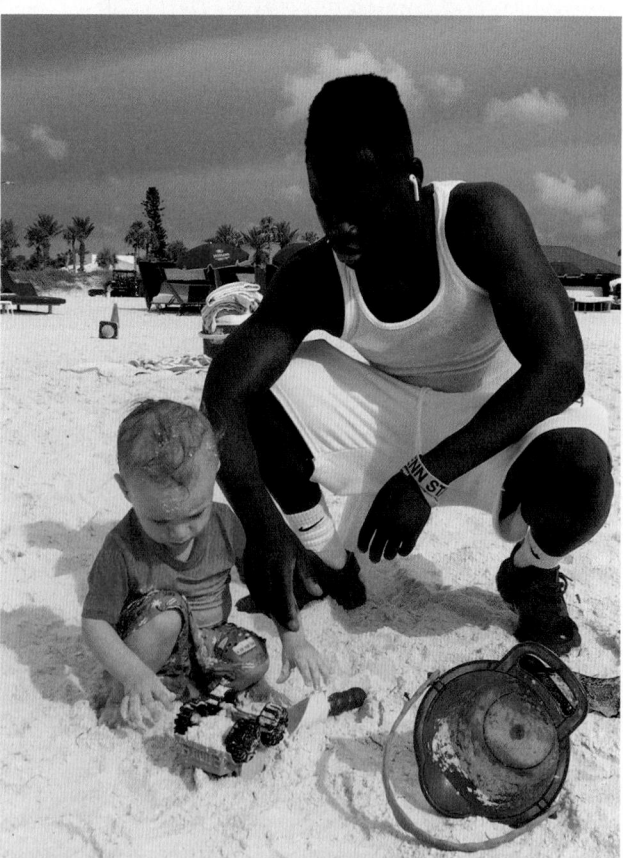

FIGURE 47.6 **Doing is a hallmark of play between children and adults.**

Doing is certainly a hallmark of play. In fact, a cursory look at the major OT texts that describe play (i.e., Parham & Fazio, 2008; Reilly, 1974) reveals that large portions of both describe doing associated with play. Most of the assessments cited in *Play in Occupational Therapy for Children* (Parham & Fazio, 2008) address doing, most notably the skills children use in play and the activities children at various ages prefer. Similarly, the five chapters about play in practice in *Play as Exploratory Learning* (Reilly, 1974) describe doing and the assessment of doing in play.

Whether motivated intrinsically or by self-determined extrinsic sources (Ryan & Deci, 2017), doing is an important aspect of leisure. As with play, many assessments of leisure that occupational therapists use examine activities people enjoy doing. Further, based on a longitudinal study of Swedish workers transitioning to retirement, Jonsson (2011) distinguished between free time as fully engaging and "killing time." In contrast to time-killing occupations, Jonsson viewed doing meaningful occupations as significant to enhancing personal well-being.

Benefits of Belonging, Connecting, and Contributing

Observation of play and leisure almost always reveals a social side (Figure 47.7). In their synthesis of qualitative research, Eakman et al. (2018) indicated that belonging and helping are two important aspects of the social meaning of occupation. Other authors (e.g., Ryan & Deci, 2017), although not writing specifically about play or leisure, made clear that feeling connected is necessary to intrinsic motivation. In turn, intrinsic motivation is a hallmark of play and, very commonly, of leisure.

Although social interaction is clearly an important motivator for play, most research and theory in OT related to social play deal with the acquisition and relative competence of social skills in children, especially children with

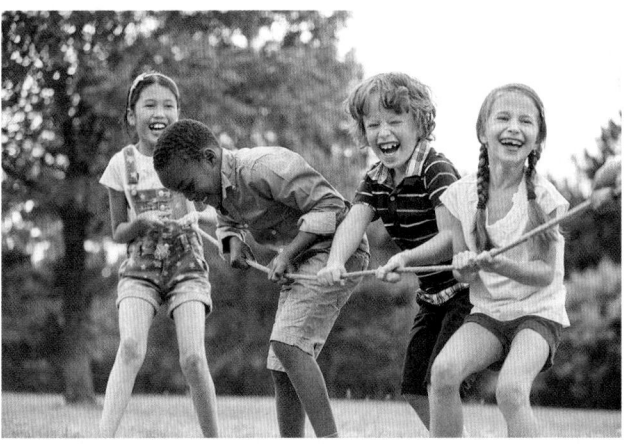

FIGURE 47.7 Play and leisure almost always are social events.

disabilities (see, e.g., Parham, 2008). Some works in the last decade are exceptions (e.g., Gerlach et al., 2014; Graham et al., 2014; Lynch et al., 2016; Powrie et al., 2015, 2020; Ramugondo, 2012). Based on a systematic review of qualitative research exploring the meaning of leisure (which also included play) for children and young people with physical disabilities, Powrie et al. (2015) argued persuasively that friendship is a universal trait, being more important than the activity itself. What is more, when young people played alone, they usually did not experience fun *or* leisure.

The social benefits of leisure are important across the life span and regardless of severity of disability. Social isolation and loneliness in older adults are risks for poor mental health (Cacioppo et al., 2006), poor physical health (Buchman et al., 2010; Perissinotto et al., 2012), and cognitive decline (Sundström et al., 2020). Factors that contribute to a decline of older adults' social networks include retirement, death of a spouse/friends, living alone, reduced community access, and, more recently, COVID-19 pandemic's stay-at-home orders (Beer et al., 2016; Courtin & Knapp, 2017; Gardiner et al., 2018; Goll et al., 2015; Nicholson, 2012; Strutt et al., 2021). In fact, feeling connected through support networks ensures that older adults are more likely to cope during and after events such as pandemics and natural disasters (Cadigan & Koh, 2008; Kim & Zakour, 2017; Rooney & White, 2007).

Raber et al. (2010) identified that older adults with dementia who were experiencing decline in abilities continued to embrace opportunities for connectedness and belonging. When allowed to engage as an observer, rather than join physically, Raber's participants contributed to activities by providing feedback and advice to others. The adapted doing of older adults with dementia included relying on others engaged in the activity to initiate and provide structure. Doing for these participants required connectedness and co-occupation of two or more people (Pierce, 2009).

Parents and professionals often wonder about the best playmates, social contacts, and school placements for children. This may be particularly relevant to children and young people with disabilities. Do children benefit more from contact with others who share similar impairments or those who are typically developing? The answer is never simple and likely varies from child to child and context to context.

Several authors (Jessup et al., 2013, 2010; Powrie et al., 2015, 2020) reflected on the value of comparing oneself against similar others. In a qualitative study of disabled adolescents, Powrie et al. (2015) indicated that:

> Leisure in segregated settings, such as camps and sports teams, generally provided a sense of camaraderie and connectedness with others with disabilities. Participants could be themselves, and there was a sense of shared understanding and acceptance, without the negative interactions they experienced in other settings. (p. 1008)

However, when comparing results among schools in a playground-based cluster trial, Grady-Dominguez and colleagues (2021) found that autistic children and children with intellectual disability enrolled in a mainstream primary school had more play gains than children with similar impairments attending a special school. Grady-Dominguez et al. concluded that staff beliefs about disability and play were major contributors to the findings.

Benefits of Restoration

Restoration is an important benefit of leisure, although it is less readily associated with the busy doing of play. Pierce (2001a) described restoration as a subjective "experience that restores our energy levels and ability to continue to engage in our daily lives" (p. 253). She believed restoration was the most neglected and poorly understood dimension of occupation. Leisure can be highly restorative, especially for clients who are "very disorganized, depleted, or discouraged" (Pierce, 2001a, p. 254). Waking restoration is highly individualized and could include such quiet-focus leisure activities as reading, listening to music, knitting, and viewing art; it might also include activities that yield solitude: being in nature, a solitary physical workout, or prayer and meditation (Pierce, 2001a).

Benefits of Life Continuity and Hope for the Future

Hammell (2009) indicated that continuity and hope for the future are especially important to people enduring life crises. Importantly, leisure may contribute to continuity and hope, thus providing a "buffer" against some aspects of disability (Coleman & Iso-Ahola, 1993; Fabrigoule et al., 1995; Kleiber et al., 2002; Sörman et al., 2013; Wang et al., 2012). Leisure that reflects hope for the future allows people to become who they want to be, despite changing circumstances and altered abilities (Hammell, 2007). In a critical interpretative synthesis, Du Toit and colleagues (2018) cautioned that occupational deprivation will prevail for residents living with advanced dementia unless every resident is viewed holistically as a person with a past, present, and future that includes opportunities for growth and engagement. And, in a systematic review of qualitative research exploring the meaning of leisure for children and young people with physical disabilities, Powrie et al. (2015, 2020) provided evidence that the benefits of life continuity and hope for the future associated with leisure apply to children and young people as well as adults. Children and young people "described how leisure allowed them to experience fulfillment by proving their abilities, demonstrating their potential, countering assumptions about their abilities, and showing that there is more to their identity than being disabled" (Powrie et al., 2015, p. 1006).

Previous researchers (Atchley, 1989, 1993; Kelly, 1993) suggested that individuals maintain a core set of leisure

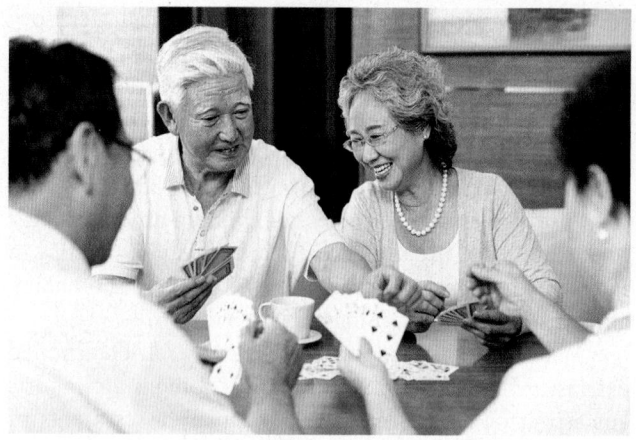

FIGURE 47.8 Many maintain a core set of leisure activities across the life course.

activities across the life course. Some of these activities are learned early in life and derive their meaning from culture and the influence of significant others (Csikszentmihalyi & Kleiber, 1991; Iso-Ahola et al., 1994; McGuire et al., 2004) (Figure 47.8). For example, Pöllänen and Hirsimäki (2014) revealed that persons with dementia in residential care found pleasure in craft-related reminiscence, especially when they had enjoyed crafting earlier in life. Craft activities led to shared experiences and talking about crafts in general, promoting social interaction and higher quality reciprocal language.

Numerous researchers (Chung, 2004; Lape, 2009; Pöllänen & Hirsimäki, 2014; Warchol, 2006; Wood et al., 2005) promoted life stories for identifying former interests and previously enjoyed activities with nursing home residents. In-depth examination of the benefits of previous leisure can facilitate participation in new activities, when necessary. However, *thorough analysis into the benefits one derived from previous activity* is required. For example, individuals who enjoyed fishing because it allowed them to be outdoors probably would not find a similar themed Wii game to be a good replacement. And reading sports magazines would not be a good replacement for participating in sport for individuals whose primary motivations were social or physical.

Combining Benefits: Doing and Social

Most play and many leisure activities involve doing in a social situation. Thus, participants may reap benefits associated with both (Figure 47.9). Opportunities for shared doing support reciprocity, the feeling that, overall, what people receive is similar to what they give (Goodman, 1984). Particularly in the case of older individuals, feeling as though one is giving to another is often the most important motivator for

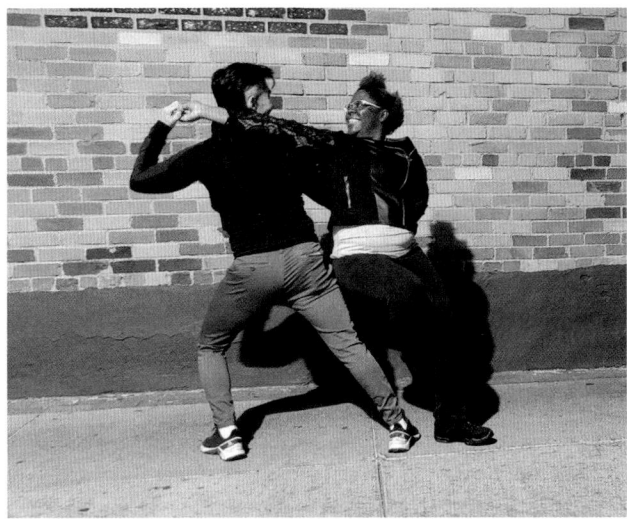

FIGURE 47.9 Leisure allows people to become who they want to be.

leisure engagement (Allen & Chin-Sang, 1990; Havighurst, 1979; Jacobson & Samdahl, 1998; Lawton, 1993). Without reciprocity, a state of indebtedness develops (Goodman, 1984). Indebtedness alters a relationship and prohibits the experiences of control, choice, comfort, and freedom characteristic of leisure.

Shared doing does not have to be with other *people*. At the turn of the century, people with AIDS experienced social isolation because of prejudice. In a small-scale study, Allen et al. (2000) explored pet ownership, finding that not only did participants receive unconditional love, but they also engaged in daily walks and social events with other pet owners. Pet ownership offered both "normalized" experiences and a reason to care for themselves (i.e., hope for the future), as this quote illustrates: "He keeps me from giving up" (p. 276).

Environmental Influences

Context includes a wide array of interrelated variables critical to control, choice, comfort, and freedom—hallmarks of play and leisure. Traits of the physical and social environments can promote or diminish those important variables (AOTA, 2020). More than two decades ago, Bronson and Bundy (2001) correlated scores on the Test of Playfulness (ToP) and the Test of Environmental Supportiveness (TOES) in children. Later, Bundy et al. (2009) demonstrated a statistical method for adjusting ToP scores to reflect supportiveness of the environment. That is, Bundy et al. showed that a low ToP score of a child playing in an unsupportive environment could be increased systematically to estimate what that child's score would be if she played in a supportive environment. Similarly, a high ToP score of a child playing

in a supportive environment could be decreased to estimate what that child's score would be if he played in an unsupportive environment.

The TOES considers four factors: attitudes and practices of caregivers; supportiveness of playmates; configuration, accessibility, and sensory qualities of the play space; and characteristics of play objects. For an environment to be supportive, the four elements must enable players to get what they seek in their play (i.e., to achieve their motivations). Adults in a play environment are always caregivers. That is, they enforce rules, keep children safe, and, by their words and actions, set a tone regarding the importance of play. Adult caregivers exert a marked influence on children's play. In support of the importance of attitudes and practices of caregivers, and as noted above, Grady-Dominguez et al. (2021) concluded that staff beliefs about play were major contributors to autistic children's play on the school playground. And Thomson (2014) named a paper describing the play of typically developing children on British school playgrounds, *Adulterated Play*.

In addition to being caregivers, therapists, parents, and other adults often have opportunities to assume a playmate role. To succeed in the playmate role, they must play as equals, lose themselves in the play, and follow the child's lead. Although all of these things can be difficult for adults who worry about being taken seriously, the rewards of being a good playmate are unequivocal. The best way to know children well and help them learn who they are and who they can become, is to play with them.

The physical environment is also critical to promoting play and leisure. Open spaces are important to play and leisure for many people regardless of age or ability. Many adults enjoy walking, hiking, skiing, fishing, hunting, and other outdoor activities, experiencing the exhilaration of physical activity and the solace of nature or the joy of doing these things together. Numerous researchers (e.g., Brussoni et al., 2015; Engelen et al., 2013; Sandseter & Kennair, 2011) have associated children's outdoor play with a variety of positive developmental, physical, and mental health outcomes. Despite this, researchers (e.g., Lynch et al., 2020; Sterman et al., 2016, 2019, 2020) identified numerous difficulties ensuring disabled children have opportunities for outdoor play. Further, parents', educators', and other caregivers' fears have resulted in unnecessary restrictions to children's outdoor play, which, in turn, may contribute to sedentary lifestyles and difficulties with coping and other aspects of mental health. In Expanding Our Perspectives, we relay the story of a 7-year-old girl and how her mother, a play expert, promoted her daughter's engagement in risky play—and the benefits both received.

Numerous researchers have examined the effect of environmental characteristics on traits related to play and leisure in older adults. Nursing homes with group living, social isolation, regimentation of daily routines, and too

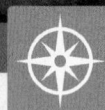

EXPANDING OUR PERSPECTIVES

Risky Play: Provide a Scaffold and Trust the Child

Ellen Beate Sandseter

"Risky" play[2] has many benefits, including players learning what they can do. Too often we forget the benefits and instead focus on our fears for children' safety or that we will be blamed should even a minor accident happen. Ellen Beate Sandseter, a prominent researcher of children's risky play, provided the following true story of her young daughter's mastering climbing a tall tree.

Up in the mountains where we have our cabin, there is a tall pine tree. It is about 10–15 meters (40–50 feet) high. My son, Simen (10 years), had been playing in the tree for many years—climbing it, building a tree house and jumping down from the branches. His little sister, Sara (3 years younger), had been watching this all the time, and tried to do the same as Simen. The branches were too high for her to reach at the start, but when she was about 5 years old, she was able, with some help from a ladder, to get up to the lowest branch and start climbing the tree. At first, she stopped when she reached the first branch. Then, the next time she climbed up to the second branch. After some months of playing in the tree she dared and managed to reach the third branch, and as time went on, she was able to get higher and higher up in the tree. She worked progressively in her play to increase her climbing skills as well as gaining more courage and risk management skills to handle the risk involved in climbing. I watched her competence and confidence grow, both climbing up and down the tree. Sara had watched her older brother managing to get to the top of the tree. A pine tree has very thick and strong branches at the top, and Simen was able to stand up on the top branches—sticking up from the top of the tree.

One day when I was painting the shed behind the cabin, I suddenly heard Sara, at that time 7 years old, shouting: "Mom, mom! Come look at me! I am at the top of the tree!" I walked to the other side of the cabin, where the pine tree was, and saw Sara standing on the top branches—sticking up from the top of the tree. I shouted to her: Just stand there and wait a little. I want to take a picture!" I went inside the cabin, grabbed my camera, went out and took a picture. Then I walked back to the shed and continued painting.

How did she get down from the tree? I don't know. But she got down safely. I was very relaxed that she would manage to get down by herself—having watched her progressively and step-by-step learning how to climb both up and down the tree.

The lesson? Provide a scaffold and trust the child (e.g., go paint the shed).

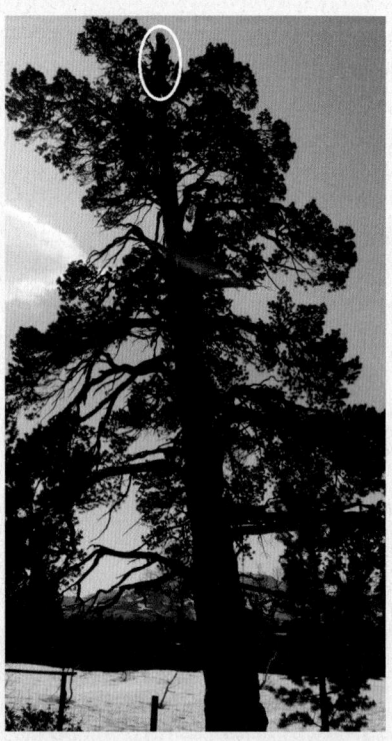

Sara reaches the top of the tall tree.

much unobligated time are often associated with loss of autonomy, control, roles, and privacy (Burack et al., 2012; Lee et al., 2002; Thomas et al., 2014). Several researchers (Causey-Upton, 2015; Cohen-Mansfield, 2005; Morgan-Brown et al., 2011) found that residents typically spend up to 69% of their day inactive (Dionigi, 2017; Raymore et al., 1999). Despite active aging, successful aging and healthy aging agendas pushed by policy makers, health professionals, academics, and aged care organizations continue to provide/repetitive, time-killing activities (Dionigi, 2017; Raymore et al., 1999) that negatively impact well-being (Power, 2010; Thomas, 1996).

The situation is dire for residents living with dementia in institutional settings. Nursing home staff and healthcare workers, in general, expect that older adults with dementia

---

[2]We define risky play in the way that Sandseter (2009) defined it, as thrilling and exciting forms of play that involve a risk of physical injury.

will experience increased difficulty making decisions and retaining control of their lives resulting in what Swaffer (2015) termed Prescribed Disengagement™. Despite research indicating that engagement in leisure pursuits is the factor that most strongly impacts well-being within residential care (Thomas et al., 2013) and that lack of meaningful activity was more disabling to older people with moderate dementia than the decrease in their abilities (Raber et al., 2010), staff expectations of residents with dementia are low and meaningful activity is lacking, leaving many residents trapped in a constant state of inactivity, isolation, and helplessness.

And, finally, although they intend to create meaningful leisure experiences, some adult day programs fail to do so (Tse & Linsey, 2005). Getting participants "out of the house" and "occupied" is not enough. True involvement in leisure reflects the characteristics specified above. The extent to which those traits are present is individually determined.

Causey-Upton (2015) challenged occupational therapists to advocate for vulnerable client groups. Access to resources and prejudice associated with disability constitutes a form of social injustice. An occupational justice approach focuses on individuals' rights to engage in play and leisure. Therefore, it is paramount for occupational therapists to support the right to play and leisure for all clients, including those who are frail and disabled.

Influence of COVID-19 on Play and Leisure

Although relatively little research exists on the effects of the COVID-19 pandemic on play and leisure, there seems to be general agreement on two interrelated factors: First, during the height of the pandemic, adults and children spent more time engaged in virtual play, social media, and screen time and less time engaged in physical activity and socializing (Araújo et al., 2020; Barr & Copeland-Stewart, 2021; Dunton et al., 2020). Second, decreased income and increased fear of contagion led to greater stress for parents, which, in turn, contributed to emotional distress and lowered self-regulation in children (Thibodeaux-Nielsen et al., 2021). Both factors caused concern about potential long-term negative effects.

Concerns about screen time began in the mid-20th century when television viewing became widespread; those concerns intensified with the appearance of computer games and game consoles in the 1980s and 1990s and mobile devices in the mid-2000s. Worries about screen time stem from a displacement theory: what are people missing out on when they spend time on screens—and what are the consequences? Nonetheless, even before COVID-19, researchers found benefits of screen time, especially virtual game playing for adults: stress relief (Reinecke, 2009), cognitive skill development (Barr, 2017), combating loneliness (Kaye et al., 2017), and dealing with trauma and improving well-being (Colder Carras et al., 2018).

With the onset of COVID-19 and dramatic increases in screen time, researchers (e.g., Barr & Copeland-Stewart, 2021) found primarily positive effects on well-being: decreased anxiety and increased coping, stress relief, and escape from worries (e.g., about health and politically motivated injustices). Participants also reported feeling stimulated cognitively, a sense of agency and normality, and having opportunities to socialize. The only negative they reported was the perception that playing games was a waste of time.

Although much of the research described above was with adults, some researchers have studied children. Thibodeaux-Nielsen et al. (2021) found that children's self-initiated, COVID-themed pretend play weakened the adverse association between parental stress and children's distress, suggesting that pretend play can help protect children from the harmful effects of adversity. And, as Thibodeaux-Nielsen et al. indicated, although the idea that play helps children cope with stress is not new, the notion that virtual environments can serve that purpose *is* new. Further, Quinones and Adams (2020) found that virtual environments can provide young children with opportunities for social pretend as revealed in their study of two 7-year-old girls who engaged in multiple kinds of virtual dramatic play.

COVID-19 severely impacted normal leisure and play routines. Not only did it expand online activity and increase sedentary behavior, it also made people reconsider and modify certain activities (see OT Story 47.2).

OT STORY 47.2 COVID-19: OPPORTUNITY OR THREAT TO LEISURE

Ivy Lai is third-year student at the University of Sydney. Ivy was born in Vancouver but spent most of her summer vacations in Hong Kong with her grandparents. She decided to study in Australia so she could visit her family in Hong Kong more regularly before embarking on her professional career.

Ivy lives with cerebral palsy and uses bilateral crutches to support her mobility; for longer outings, she uses a wheelchair. Ivy identified shopping as her most valued leisure activity. Not only does shopping provide her momentary escape when she is experiencing stress, making her feel "refreshed

(continued)

OT STORY 47.2 COVID-19: OPPORTUNITY OR THREAT TO LEISURE (*continued*)

and happy" in new clothes, but it also provides her with a link to other young people. Sharing fashion trends creates a "sense of belonging" and provides her with a way to initiate conversations when she is in an unfamiliar social setting. Shopping is part of her weekly routine, and she usually meets up with friends on Saturdays. When she compares shopping in the three countries, she highlights how the social and physical contexts differ. She finds Canada the best set up to support people with a disability—more spacious shopping precincts, very accessible, and well signposted. When shopping in Hong Kong, the whole day centers around the outing as everything is close—places to eat, shop, and enjoy other activities, such as ice skating. Moreover, shopping areas stay open late; most people spend time together after work as it does not take long to travel home afterward. Ivy found shopping in Sydney especially challenging because of limited shopping hours and crowded shopping precincts. COVID-19 motivated Ivy to engage in online shopping (Figure 47.10). She bought fewer clothes, but ordered flowers, purchased a digital piano, and acquired exercise equipment (a yoga mat and dumbbells) to engage in a Zoom™ exercise group with fellow students.

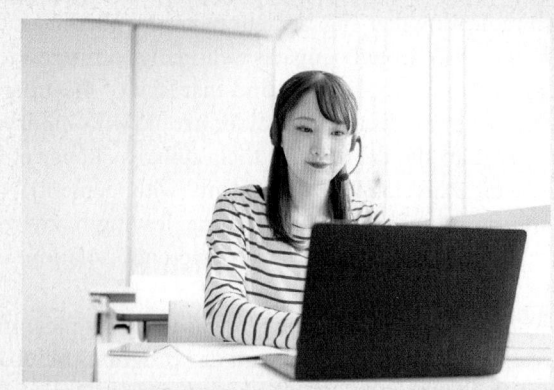

FIGURE 47.10 Ivy enjoyed online shopping during the pandemic.

Questions

1. The combination of COVID-19 and living in Sydney curtailed Ivy's engagement in her favorite leisure activity. How do you think Ivy's identity was affected by that loss?
2. Ivy also experienced some silver linings to COVID-19. How do you think her identity changed in positive ways as a result?

Evaluation of Play and Leisure

Best practice in OT means that evaluation begins with clients (often including family members and other caregivers) and practitioners collaboratively identifying what clients *want* to do (AOTA, 2020) and the extent to which they *actually* engage in desired activities (Coster, 1998). Broadly, evaluation of play and leisure addresses how context, environment, and client strengths facilitate or inhibit engagement. Further, best practice suggests that evaluation takes place in everyday life settings using a top–down approach (AOTA, 2020).

Logically, assessments of play and leisure would parallel their respective definitions. We defined play and leisure using the characteristics that separate them from other occupations. Nonetheless, although some assessments explicitly capture the characteristics of play, Hammell's (2009) occupational categories (i.e., doing, belonging, restoration, and life continuity) offer a somewhat more inclusive way of thinking about assessments of play and leisure.

Evaluation of Play

Play is a multifaceted and complex phenomenon. In practice, although play is a lifelong occupation, therapists are more likely to evaluate play in children than in adults. Hammell's (2009) category "engagement in doing" seems to capture the content of most existing play assessments for children. Although there are some relatively new assessments of adult playfulness (e.g., Román-Oyola et al., 2019; Shen et al., 2014a, 2014b; Waldman-Levi & Bundy, 2016), those that occupational therapists have developed (e.g., Román-Oyola et al., 2019; Waldman-Levi & Bundy, 2016) tend to be about how adults facilitate the play of children.

We purport that a complete OT assessment of play would comprise the five aspects listed below. However, although play is multifaceted, generally it is neither necessary nor practical to evaluate each aspect for any individual. Thus, practitioners must consider carefully which are most important in a given situation and choose assessments that reflect those aspects. Such choices require practitioners to carefully evaluate the items of an assessment.

Factors of a complete play assessment include the following:

1. The player's capacity to play (i.e., skills used in play or types of play, reflecting skills)
2. What players do (i.e., play activities)
3. How players approach play (i.e., playfulness)
4. The supportiveness of the environment
5. The motivations for play (i.e., why players choose particular play activities)

Capacity to Play

Probably because of the importance attached to learning through play, most children's play assessments focus on skills. Assessments such as Knox's Revised Preschool Play Scale (Knox, 2008) and Linder's (2008) Transdisciplinary Play-Based Assessment provide reliable and valid data comparing the skills of a particular child with those of peers. Stagnitti (2007) developed an assessment of pretend play, the Child-Initiated Pretend Play Assessment (CHIPPA) that seems to fall into this category because examiners use it to determine level of pretend play, a reflection of cognitive development. Any of these assessments can be useful for planning intervention to promote development, but they do not tell us much about play itself or how to promote it. Historically, assessments of the capacity to play take the form of taxonomies—largely based on Piaget's (1962) stages of cognitive play and Parten's (1932) stages of social play—and focused on indoor play of very young children and with the purpose of assessing social or cognitive development, more than play. The Tool for Observing Play Outdoors (TOPO; Loebach & Cox, 2020) is a new typology for evaluating both play behaviors (i.e., types) and supportiveness of the environment (see also comments below). Digital play, bio play (play with plants and wildlife), restorative play, expressive play (e.g., performance), and nonplay are categories of the TOPO along with the more common types: physical play, exploratory play, imaginative play, and play with rules. The TOPO was primarily designed for research, but the authors indicated that it can also be used for extended observation of individual children.

What Players Do

Assessments such as Henry's (2008) Pediatric Interest Profiles (PIP) and, to a lesser extent, the Children's Assessment of Participation and Enjoyment (CAPE) and the Preferences for Activities of Children (PAC) (King et al., 2004) offer reliable and valid ways of assessing *what* players do. All concentrate on factors such as interest, intensity, enjoyment, and context. The various versions of the PIP (Kid Play Profile and Preteen Play Profile) focus exclusively on play activities, whereas the CAPE and PAC extend beyond play to include a range of activities children do outside of school. A version of the PIP, the Adolescent Leisure Interest Profile, includes activities that may be classified as play or leisure. Scores for the various versions of the PIP offer comparisons with preferences of peers, although this information may be somewhat outdated, and not all activities are relevant to all geographic locations or cultures. These assessments provide descriptive data about individual children that can be useful for planning interventions. However, it can be difficult to interpret the meaning of scores from any of these interest-checklist-type assessments. Is it better to have a lot of preferred activities or just a few in which one is intensely engaged? And, how important is it that preferred activities match a child's skills (Clifford & Bundy, 1989)?

The Approach to Play

So far as we know, the ToP (Skard & Bundy, 2008) is the only observational assessment that targets children's approach to play. In the ToP, Skard and Bundy applied operational definitions of the characteristics of play (i.e., intrinsic motivation) to players themselves, arguing that these traits also characterized playful people. They further argued that playfulness is relevant to many occupations—not only to play. The ToP scores offer a comparison of playfulness across children of a range of ages and abilities. And although Skard and Bundy offered a means to compare individual ToP scores with those of a large data set, the meaning of relative amounts of playfulness is not yet clear. Importantly, some researchers (e.g., Hess & Bundy, 2003; Saunders et al., 1999) linked playfulness to coping, which may provide insight about the importance of playfulness.

Two other child assessments of playfulness are of note. The Children's Playfulness Scale (CPS; Barnett, 1991) is completed by a caregiver who knows the child well. The Child Self-Report Playfulness Scale (SCRP; Fink et al., 2020) is a promising new approach to the measurement of dispositional playfulness in young children. A few adult assessments of playfulness also exist (Román-Oyola et al., 2019; Shen et al., 2014a, 2014b; Waldman-Levi & Bundy, 2016). All are self-report assessments. The ToP is occasionally used with adults as a self-report measure (e.g., Weigl & Bundy, 2013).

Supportiveness of the Environment

Assessments such as the TOES (Skard & Bundy, 2008), the TOPO (Loebach & Cox, 2020), and the Young Children's Participation and Environment Measure (YC-PEM) by Khetani and colleagues (Khetani et al., 2013, 2015) take very different approaches to evaluating environmental supportiveness. The TOES is set in the context of a player's motivations for play (i.e., what players seem to be seeking). In administering the TOES, practitioners determine the extent to which four environmental components (playmates, caregivers, play objects, and space) promote or detract from players' abilities to meet their motivations for play. The TOES is best used as a tool for consultation with adults seeking to promote play by optimizing the supportiveness of the play environment. One use of the TOPO is to assess the quality of the play environment—either outdoors or indoors. TOPO authors defined quality of environmental support by examining types of play that occur in the space. YC-PEM items allow practitioners to assess the effect of environmental features (e.g., physical layout, sensory qualities, adult supports, peer relationships) on participation of young children at home, in daycare/preschool, and in the community. Play is an important aspect of participation for young children in all of these settings

Motivations for Play

Numerous researchers and theorists (e.g., Csikszentmihalyi, 1975a, 1975b, 1990; Ryan & Deci, 2017; Ziviani et al., 2012) studied motivation and wrote about ways of capturing and understanding it. The work of these authors applies to play and beyond. As described, knowledge of the source of motivation for play forms the basis for the TOES. However, so far as we know, there are no formal assessments for determining a child's motivations for particular play activities. Practitioners must glean information about motivation through observation and interview. To do so, they seek answers to questions such as: What does the child get from particular play activities? What play activities bring the child great joy? In what kinds of activities does the child become totally immersed?

Evaluation of Leisure

As with play, we know of no assessments of leisure that parallel our definition (i.e., the characteristics that separate leisure from other occupations). To structure our discussion of assessment, we use Hammell's (2009) categories of the benefits of leisure: (a) engagement in doing; (b) belonging, connecting, and contributing; (c) restoration; and (d) life continuity and hope for the future. Importantly, Hammell warned against prescribing how clients *should* use their time to obtain a balance between self-care, leisure, and productive occupations. Clients are the only ones who can determine a balance that ensures their priorities and needs are met.

A range of assessments are available to support leisure assessment. Honoring client-centered assessment, we recommend the following, much of which, in addition to (and occasionally instead of) standardized assessment, requires interviewing clients and sometimes caregivers:

- Collaborating to identify meaningful activities that clients consider leisure
- Examining motivations for/benefits sought in leisure
- Examining the degree of control participants can and want to experience and the form they want that control to take
- Gaining an understanding of personal, environmental, and contextual factors that impact leisure choices and participation

Many self-report checklists query clients' interests in activities commonly associated with leisure as well as factors such as intensity and enjoyment. Clients describe any activities that they engage in presently or have done previously and those that are potential future pursuits. These include the Modified Interest Checklist by Kielhofner and Neville (Taylor, 2017), the Occupational Performance History Interview–Second Version (OPHI-II) by Kielhofner et al. (Taylor, 2017), and the Activity Card

Sort (ACS) (2nd edition) by Baum and Edwards (2008). However, because the lists are predetermined, unless supplemented by interview, they may provide limited insight. Further, being physically able to do a particular leisure activity, even if it was once highly valued, does not ensure full engagement or feelings of belonging, hope, or restoration in the present.

When clients are unable to self-report on opportunities and experiences they find meaningful, the Assessment Tool for Social and Occupational Engagement (ATOSE) by Morgan-Brown and Chard (2014) can be useful. In addition, in institutional settings, tools such as the Residential Environmental Impact Scale (REIS) that employ observation and interview can guide assessment (Fisher et al., 2014).

Importantly, when leisure is the primary occupation, the focus of assessment should be on the process and not the outcome (Fenech & Collier, 2017). Identifying personal strengths, abilities, preferences, and resources is particularly important (Townsend & Polatajko, 2007; Townsend & Wilcock, 2004). Functional outcomes are secondary to creating moments of shared joy and the sense of belonging (Du Toit et al., 2018; Hitch et al., 2014).

Play and Leisure in Intervention

Play and leisure are meaningful, lifelong occupations (AOTA, 2020). Thus, improved play or leisure is an important outcome in its own right. However, perhaps because of cultural and remaining professional beliefs that play and leisure are not as important as other occupations, they rarely seem to be explicit goals of intervention. Not surprisingly, few rigorously designed studies in OT have tested the effectiveness of interventions for promoting play and leisure.

In contrast, many OT practitioners (e.g., Blanche, 2008; Lynch et al., 2018; Munier et al., 2008; Stagnitti et al., 2012) use play as a means to achieve performance-related intervention goals. As Pierce (2001b) indicated, a careful blend of pleasure, productivity, and restoration is likely to increase clients' motivation to participate in intervention.

Play and Leisure as Outcomes

Only very recently have OT researchers used rigorous research designs to examine the effectiveness of interventions for increasing play and related skills in children. The research in leisure is even less well developed than that in play.

Play Interventions

Two basic types of OT interventions focusing on play have been the subject of rigorous research conducted in Australia. These include: (a) modeling and facilitated play and (b) loose parts intervention and risk reframing.

Modeling and Facilitated Play. Wilkes-Gillan and colleagues (Barnes et al., 2017; Cantrill et al., 2015; Wilkes-Gillan et al., 2015, 2016a, 2017) engaged children with ADHD and a familiar playmate in direct and indirect interventions to increase play and social skills. The researchers demonstrated maintained effectiveness 18 months after the intervention concluded with children with ADHD; one year after the intervention was completed, parents of still reported on its appropriateness (Allan et al., 2018). More recently, members of that same research group (Kent et al., 2018, 2020a, 2020b) extended the intervention to autistic children, also finding positive results.

The Australian researchers' intervention described just above was based on Cordier's earlier studies (Cordier et al., 2009, 2010a, 2010b, 2010c) of the patterns of play deficit common in children with ADHD. Later analysis suggested that autistic children experienced similar difficulties in play, making a variation of the intervention equally appropriate for that group.

The intervention, conducted as randomized controlled trials, involved video and therapist modeling and engaging the children in facilitated play to help them respond appropriately to playmates' cues. Parents carried out a home program using a video story of an alien whose earthling friends helped him see that he would have more fun if his playmate was also having fun.

Loose Parts Intervention and Risk Reframing. In the second group of Australian-based studies, Bundy and colleagues (Bundy et al., 2015, 2017; Bundy, Naughton, et al., 2011; Engelen et al., 2013) placed recycled materials with no obvious play value (i.e., loose parts) on school playgrounds for children to play with at recess (Figure 47.11). Simultaneously, Niehues and colleagues conducted small-group interventions with parents and school staff to help them reconsider the value of manageable risk taking in play (Niehues et al., 2013, 2015, 2016; Spencer et al., 2016). Participating children (who were typically developing) in the first trial had increased physical activity at recess. Time spent playing also increased, but the change was not statistically significant. More recently, the team applied the same interventions to autistic children and children with intellectual disability, targeting coping and quality of play on the playground (Bundy et al., 2015; Grady-Dominguez et al., 2019, 2020, 2021). They found wide variability in outcomes by school, attributing those to school culture.

Other Interventions to Promote Play. Using less rigorous research designs, OT researchers reported the results of other interventions designed to influence play—with varying results. Sonday and Gretschel (2016) used qualitative methodology to examine the effects, which were marked, of powered wheelchairs on the play of two children with physical disabilities. Four papers

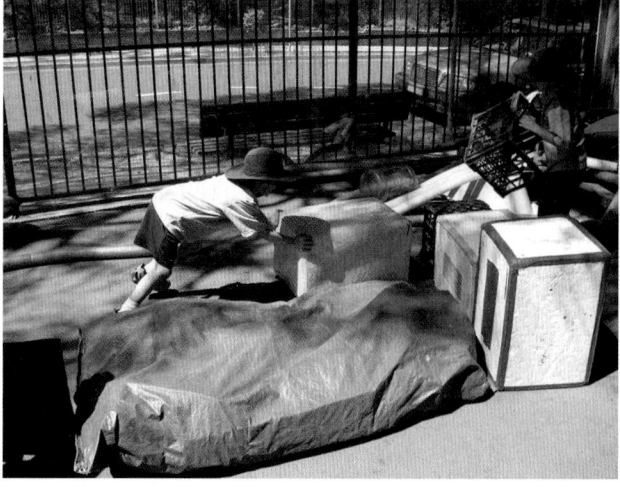

FIGURE 47.11 **Loose parts promote play as well as physical activity.**

reported findings from single group, pretest–posttest studies (Bundy, Naughton, et al., 2011; Keen et al., 2007; O'Connor & Stagnitti, 2011; Stagnitti et al., 2012). Two additional papers reported findings from a pretest–posttest study and compared child and parent outcomes at multiple points (Fabrizi & Hubbell, 2017; Fabrizi et al., 2016). Notably, all but one of these studies (Bundy, Naughton, et al., 2011) occurred in a natural setting (i.e., home, school or community-based play group). Two studies (Bundy, Kolrosova, et al., 2011; Keen et al., 2007) were parent interventions; one was with parents of children with varying disabilities and one with parents of autistic children. Two studies (Fabrizi & Hubbell, 2017; Fabrizi et al., 2016) focused on the children but included parents as part of the playgroup intervention.

Fabrizi and colleagues (Fabrizi & Hubbell, 2017; Fabrizi et al., 2016) found increases in child playfulness across playgroup types. However, they did not find increases in parent competence or participation. In a hospital-based group intervention, Bundy, Kolrosova, et al. (2011) failed to find increases in child playfulness but, in interviews, parents reported positive changes in interactions among family members. Keen et al. (2007) employed a combined workshop and home-based format (Stronger Families). Although parents reported changes in communication and symbolic behaviors, those were not supported by evaluator-scored observation. Both Keen et al. (2007) and Stagnitti and colleagues (O'Connor & Stagnitti, 2011; Stagnitti et al., 2012) targeted symbolic play in young autistic children in a small-group, school-based direct interventions that involved adults modeling play scripts. They did not find increases in pretend play. However, they reported increased social interaction and language and decreased social disconnection; they also found relationships between language and pretend play.

Leisure Interventions

OT research exploring interventions to promote leisure is sketchy. Practitioners frequently use adapted procedures to enhance leisure. Among occupational therapists who reported using leisure assessments to plan their intervention, 11% focused on developing ways to adapt leisure activities to match clients' skills (Turner et al., 2000). However, most support for effectiveness is anecdotal. We know of no empirical research to support effectiveness.

In a textbook focusing on OT interventions for the older people, Bundy and Clemson (2009) described the intervention for an older woman who reported that cooking for her family, once her primary leisure, was no longer satisfying after she had a stroke. The occupational therapist intervened by teaching adapted procedures the client could use to compensate for mild weakness and abnormal muscle tone in her affected arm (e.g., sliding pans onto and off the cooktop rather than lifting them). Instead of focusing intervention on performance skills and remediation of motor control, the practitioner used the client's preferred leisure activity of cooking as a means to enable her to regain the experience of leisure.

Use of electronic media as an outcome is an area in which occupational therapists could expand practice. Technology provides older adults living in nursing homes with opportunities to engage in meaningful activities that promote overall well-being (Budak et al., 2021; Neal et al., 2020). In a scoping review, Neal et al. (2020) found that technology is most meaningful when it promotes human-to-human interaction. However, technology is often two-dimensional and rigid, whereas virtual reality can be flexible and person specific. For example, *Tovertafel*[TM] (magic table) is a dynamic, creative games console (Le Riche, 2017) containing a projector, infrared sensors, a loudspeaker, and a processor. *Tovertafel*[TM] projects interactive games onto a table so that older adults living with dementia can engage in playful, meaningful activity, alone or with others.

Researchers from other disciplines (e.g., Stendal et al., 2011; Vizenor, 2014) explored how virtual worlds contribute to opportunities for leisure participation of people with disabilities. For older adults, Moyle et al. (2018) found that Virtual Reality Forests had a positive effect on residents living with moderate dementia, as they experienced pleasure and a greater level of alertness during the experience. Studies are needed to specifically explore the role of technology as an OT intervention to promote play and leisure.

Play and Leisure as a Means for Meeting Other Goals

Practitioners using play or leisure as a means for meeting other goals are likely doing so to engage their clients fully in therapy. People learn skills through practice, and clients are more likely to keep practicing when it is fun. There are few

rigorous studies of play and hardly any of leisure as a medium, but the effectiveness of this approach is an emerging area of research.

Play as a Medium

In two rounds of the Sydney Playground Project, Bundy and colleagues implemented loose parts and risk-reframing interventions to increase physical activity and coping skills (Bundy, Naughton et al., 2011, 2015, 2017; Engelen et al., 2013; Grady-Dominguez et al., 2019, 2020, 2021). Because improving play also was a target of this intervention, we described it in the section on play as an outcome. Play is also characteristic of sensory integration interventions (Bundy & Lane, 2020; Figure 47.12).

In reasonably large-scale surveys of occupational therapists working with young children, Couch et al. (1998) and, more recently, Miller Kuhaneck and colleagues (2013) and Lynch and colleagues (Lynch et al., 2018) found that therapists regarded play primarily as a motivator to entice children to participate in interventions to meet performance goals. Several correlational studies suggest that engaging in play may enhance developmental skill acquisition (Harris & Reid, 2005), school readiness (Long et al., 2006), coping (Hess & Bundy, 2003; Saunders et al., 1999), and social interaction and language (Keen et al., 2007; O'Connor & Stagnitti, 2011; Stagnitti et al., 2012). Two groups of researchers studying interventions for burn patients (one a randomized controlled trial and one a single case study) found that play activities were as effective or more effective than exercise for reducing pain (Melchert-McKearnan

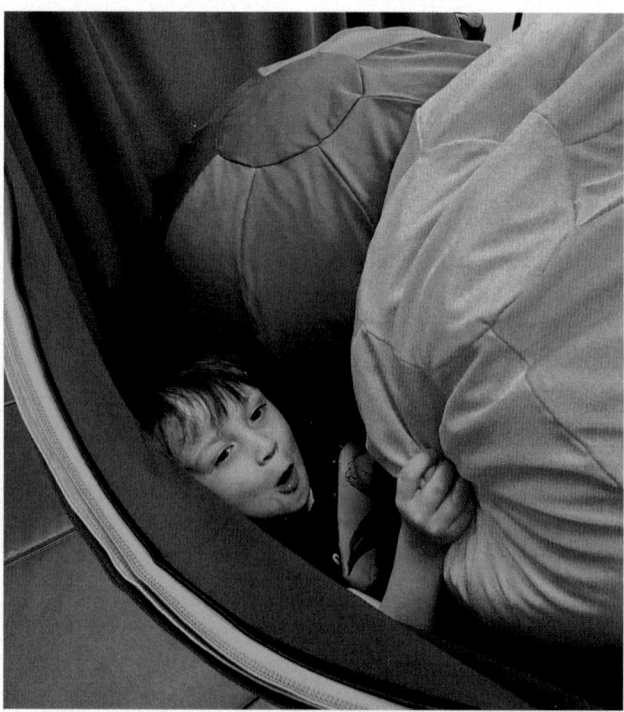

FIGURE 47.12 **Play is characteristic of sensory integration interventions.**

et al., 2000; Omar et al., 2012) and distress (Melchert-McKearnan et al., 2000) and increasing hand function (Omar et al., 2012) and engagement in, and enjoyment of therapy (Melchert-McKearnan et al., 2000).

Leisure as a Medium

In a review of eight primarily cross-sectional studies investigating the effect of engaging in leisure activities on depression or self-esteem in older adults, Fine (2001) concluded that participation had a positive effect on mental health. However, only one of the three most rigorous studies revealed a statistically significant effect on mental health, and in that study, relaxation had a greater effect than participation in active leisure (Bensink et al., 1992).

We often rely on traits associated with leisure to promote participation in intervention to help clients gain or regain movement, especially when they experience discomfort or pain on moving. OT Story 47.3 describes an intervention where leisure was the medium. The case demonstrates how interest, motivation, and creativity supported a marine in improving strength and range of motion in his injured hand.

OT STORY 47.3 LEISURE AS A MEANS OF MEETING OTHER GOALS

Arthur is a 26-year-old US marine stationed at Fort Worth, Texas, and attending outpatient rehabilitation services. He damaged his right (preferred) hand in a motor vehicle crash. He was in the back seat, resting his elbow on the window frame with his hand gripping the roof. As a result of the accident, he experienced an arthrodesis of the interphalangeal joints of his right hand. Hand function was the target of the OT intervention. Although range of motion had improved, Arthur still experienced challenges with grip and strength. He found sessions with TheraPutty™ and hand-exercise equipment distressing and painful. Thus, the occupational therapist suggested that they make a gift for Arthur's girlfriend using different colors of grated soap, course sea salt, and dried lavender to create bath salts. (Arthur had often mentioned that his girlfriend was angry with him for not making sure the driver had been sober on the night of the accident.) Grating different shapes and sizes of soap and cutting and drying lavender sprigs improved his grip strength and provided him with profound satisfaction when he presented his girlfriend with the end product.

Questions

1. Why do you think the gift, which had many of the same demands as TheraPutty™ and hand-exercise equipment, was a more effective intervention for Arthur?
2. What characteristics of leisure were captured in creating the gift?

COMMENTARY ON THE EVIDENCE

In a class lecture in the 1990s, Jeanne Pretorius, a lecturer at the University of the Free State in South Africa, dubbed leisure the "stepchild of occupational therapy" (Pretorius, 1993). About the same time, Bundy (1993) published a paper in the *American Journal of Occupational Therapy* addressing the problem of play and leisure: Despite being primary, lifelong occupations, neither was important enough to devote resources to developing valid and reliable assessments on which to base interventions. Almost a decade later, Turner et al. (2000) surveyed 103 therapists: 75% reported using leisure assessments to plan interventions and 35% said that they used leisure activity in intervention to promote their clients' future leisure participation. Nonetheless, we uncovered no rigorous research examining the effectiveness of such interventions.

Play has fared better—but only slightly. In 1998 and again in 2015, researchers (Couch et al., 1998; Lynch et al., 2018; Miller Kuhaneck et al., 2013) surveyed occupational therapists working with preschool-age children. All respondents in both surveys regarded play primarily as a motivator to entice children to participate in intervention to elicit improvement in other areas. Nonetheless, so far as we know, there are no rigorous studies of play as a medium. There are a handful of rigorous studies done by two groups of Australian-based researchers—Wilkes-Gillan, Cordier and colleagues (Allan et al., 2018; Barnes et al., 2017; Cantrill et al., 2015; Kent et al., 2018, 2020a, 2020b, 2020c; Wilkes-Gillan et al., 2011, 2015, 2016a, 2016b, 2017), and Bundy and colleagues (Bundy, Naughton et al., 2011, 2015, 2017; Engelen et al., 2013; Grady-Dominguez et al., 2019, 2020, 2021)—promoting play as an outcome. Several other groups have attempted to promote play using somewhat less rigorous research designs with varying results.

A quarter of a century later, we have made some, but not nearly enough, progress in promoting play and leisure as primary, lifelong occupations. As proponents of social and occupational justice, we have a duty to ensure access to non–income-generating ("nonproductive") occupations that support engagement in doing, belonging, connecting, and contributing; restoration; life continuity; and hope for the future.

Conclusion

We end this chapter as we began it. Play and leisure comprise some of the most meaningful occupations in which people of all ages and abilities engage. And, as Plato is credited with saying, "You can learn more about a person in an hour of play than in a year of conversation." What better arguments could there be for focusing practice and research on these important occupations?

Lippincott® Connect *For additional resources on the subjects discussed in this chapter, visit Lippincott Connect.*

REFERENCES

Allan, N., Wilkes-Gillan, S., Bundy, A., Cordier, R., & Volkert, A. (2018). Parents' perceptions of the long-term appropriateness of a psychosocial intervention for children with attention deficit hyperactivity disorder. *Australian Occupational Therapy Journal, 65*, 259–267. https://doi.org/10.1111/1440-1630.12460

Allen, J. M., Kellegrew, D. H., & Jaffe, D. (2000). The experience of pet ownership as a meaningful occupation. *Canadian Journal of Occupational Therapy, 67*, 271–278. https://doi.org/10.1177/000841740006700409

Allen, K. R., & Chin-Sang, V. (1990). A lifetime of work: The context and meanings of leisure for aging black women. *The Gerontologist, 30*, 734–740. https://doi.org/10.1093/geront/30.6.734

American Occupational Therapy Association. (2020). Occupational therapy practice framework: Domain and process (4th ed). *American Journal of Occupational Therapy, 74*(Suppl. 2), 7412410010p1–7412410010p87. https://doi.org/10.5014/ajot.2020.74S2001

Angelou, K., MacDonnell, C., Low, L. F., & Du Toit, S. H. J. (2022). Promoting meaningful engagement for residents with dementia through intergenerational programs: A pilot study. *Journal of Aging and Mental Health, 13*, 1–10. doi: 10.1080/13607863.2022.2098910

Araújo, L. A., Veloso, C. F., Souza, M. C., Azevedo, J. M., & Tarro, G. (2020). The potential impact of the COVID-19 pandemic on child growth and development: A systematic review. *Jornal de Pediatria (Rio J), 97*(4), 369–377. https://doi.org/10.1016/j.jped.2020.08.008

Atchley, R. C. (1989). A continuity theory of normal aging. *The Gerontologist, 29*, 183–190. https://doi.org/10.1093/geront/29.2.183

Atchley, R. C. (1993). Continuity theory and the evolution of activity in later adulthood. In J. R. Kelly (Ed.), *Activity and aging* (pp. 5–16). Sage.

Atler, K. (2014). The daily experiences of pleasure, productivity and restoration profile: A measure of subjective experiences. In D. Pierce (Ed.), *Occupational science for occupational therapy* (pp. 187–199). Slack.

Barnes, G., Wilkes-Gillan, S., Bundy, A., & Cordier, R. (2017). The social play, social skills and parent–child relationships of children with ADHD 12 months following a RCT of a play-based intervention. *Australian Occupational Therapy Journal, 64*, 457–465. https://doi.org/10.1111/1440-1630.12417

Barnett, L. (1991). The playful child: Measurement of a disposition to play. *Play and Culture, 4*, 51–74. http://psycnet.apa.org/record/1991-20176-001

Barr, M. (2017). Video games can develop graduate skills in higher education students: A randomised trial. *Computers & Education, 113*, 86–97. https://doi.org/10.1016/j.compedu.2017.05.016

Barr, M., & Copeland-Stewart, A. (2021). Playing video games during the COVID-19 pandemic and effects on players' well-being. *Games and Culture*, 1–18. https://doi.org/10.1177/15554120211017036

Bateson, G. (1972). Toward a theory of play and phantasy. In G. Bateson (Ed.), *Steps to an ecology of the mind* (pp. 14–20). Bantam.

Baum, C. M., & Edwards, D. (2008). *ACS: Activity card sort.* AOTA Press.

Beer, A., Faulkner, D., Law, J., Lewin, G., Tinker, A., Buys, L., Bentley, R., Watt, A., McKechnie, S., & Chessman, S. (2016). Regional variation in social isolation amongst older Australians. *Regional Studies, Regional Science, 3*, 170–184. https://doi.org/10.1080/21681376.2016.1144481

Bensink, G. W., Godbey, K. L., Marshall, M. J., & Yarandi, H. N. (1992). Institutionalized elderly. Relaxation, locus of control, self-esteem. *Journal of Gerontological Nursing, 18*, 30–36. https://doi.org/10.3928/0098-9134-19920401-08

Blanche, E. I. (2008). Play in children with cerebral palsy: Doing with—Not doing to. In L. D. Parham & L. S. Fazio (Eds.), *Play in occupational therapy for children* (2nd ed., pp. 375–393). Mosby.

Bronson, M., & Bundy, A. C. (2001). A correlational study of the test of playfulness and the test of environmental supportiveness. *Occupational Therapy Journal of Research, 21*, 241–259. https://doi.org/10.1177/153944920102100403

Brussoni, M., Gibbons, R., Gray, C., Ishikawa, T., Sandseter, E. B., Bienenstock, A., Chabot, G., Fuselli, P., Herrington, S., Janssen, I., Pickett, W., Power, M., Stanger, N., Sampson, M., & Tremblay, M. (2015). What is the relationship between risky outdoor play and health in children? A systematic review. *International Journal of Environmental Research and Public Health, 12*, 6423–6454. https://doi.org/10.3390/ijerph120606423

Buchman, A. S., Boyle, P. A., Wilson, R. S., James, B. D., Leurgans, S. E., Arnold, S. E., & Bennett, D. A. (2010). Loneliness and the rate of motor decline in old age: The rush memory and aging project, a community-based cohort study. *BMC Geriatrics, 10*, 77. https://doi.org/10.1186/1471-2318-10-77

Budak, B., Atefi, G., Hoel, V., Laporte Uribe, F., Meiland, F., Teupen, S., Felding, S., & Roes, M. (2021). Can technology impact loneliness in dementia? A scoping review on the role of assistive technologies in delivering psychosocial interventions in long-term care. *Disability and Rehabilitation Assistive Technology*, 1–13. https://doi.org/10.1080/17483107.2021.1984594

Bundy, A. C. (1993). Assessment of play and leisure: Delineation of the problem. *American Journal of Occupational Therapy, 47*, 217–222. https://doi.org/10.5014/ajot.47.3.217

Bundy, A. C., & Clemson, L. M. (2009). Leisure. In B. Bonder (Ed.), *Functional performance in older adults* (3rd ed., pp. 290–306). F. A. Davis.

Bundy, A. C., Du Toit, S., & Clemson, L. (2018). Leisure. In B. Bonder & V. D. Bello-Haas (Eds.), *Functional performance in older adults* (4th ed., pp. 295–311). F. A. Davis.

Bundy, A. C., Engelen, L., Wyver, S., Tranter, P., Ragen, J., Bauman, A., Baur, L., Schiller, W., Simpson, J. M., Niehues, A. N., Bapp, G., P., Jessup, G., & Naughton, G. (2017). Sydney playground project: A cluster-randomized trial to increase physical activity, play, and social skills. *The Journal of School Health, 87*, 751–759. https://doi.org/10.1111/josh.12550

Bundy, A. C., Kolrosova, J., Paguinto, S.-G., Bray, P., Swain, B., Wallen, M., & Engelen, L. (2011). Comparing the effectiveness of a parent group intervention with child-based intervention for promoting playfulness in children with disabilities. *Israeli Journal of Occupational Therapy, 20*, e95–e113. http://www.jstor.org/tc/accept?origin=/stable/pdf/23470291.pdf

Bundy, A. C., & Lane, S. J. (Eds.) (2020). *Sensory integration: Theory and practice* (3rd ed.). F. A. Davis.

Bundy, A. C., Naughton, G., Tranter, P., Wyver, S., Baur, L., Schiller, W., Bauman, A., Engelen, L., Ragen, J., Luckett, T., Niehues, A., Stewart, G., Jessup, G., & Brentnall, J. (2011). The Sydney playground project: Popping the bubblewrap—Unleashing the power of play: A cluster randomized controlled trial of a primary school playground-based intervention aiming to increase children's physical activity and social skills. *BMC Public Health, 11*, 680–688. https://doi.org/10.1186/1471-2458-11-680

Bundy, A. C., Waugh, K., & Brentnall, J. (2009). Developing assessments that account for the role of the environment: An example Using test of playfulness and test of environmental supportiveness. *Occupational Therapy Journal of Research, 29*, 135–143. https://doi.org/10.3928/15394492-20090611-06

Bundy, A. C., Wyver, S., Beetham, K. S., Ragen, J., Naughton, G., Tranter, P., Norman, G., Villeneuve, M., Spencer, G., Honey, A., Simpson, J., Baur, L., & Sterman, J. (2015). The Sydney playground project—Levelling the playing field: A cluster trial of a primary school-based intervention aiming to promote manageable risk-taking in children with disability. *BMC Public Health, 15*, 1125. https://doi.org/10.1186/s12889-015-2452-4

Burack, O. R., Reinhardt, J. P., & Weiner, A. S. (2012). Person-centered care and elder choice: A look at implementation and sustainability. *Clinical Gerontologist, 35*, 390–403. https://doi.org/10.1080/07317115.2012.702649

Cacioppo, J. T., Hughes, M. E., Waite, L. J., Hawkley, L. C., & Thisted, R. A. (2006). Loneliness as a specific risk factor for depressive symptoms: Cross-sectional and longitudinal analyses. *Psychology and Aging, 21*, 140–151. https://doi.org/10.1037/0882-7974.21.1.140

Cadigan, R., & Koh, H. (2008). Disaster preparedness and social capital. In I. Kawachi, S. V. Subramanian, & D. Kim (Eds.), *Social capital and health* (pp. 273–285). Springer.

Caillois, R. (1979). *Man, play and games.* Schocken Books.

Canadian Association of Occupational Therapy. (1996). Occupational therapy and children's play. *Canadian Journal of Occupational Therapy, 63*, 1–20. https://doi.org/10.1177/000841749606300201

Cantrill, A., Wilkes-Gillan, S., Bundy, A., Cordier, R., & Wilson, N. J. (2015). An eighteen-month follow-up of a pilot parent-delivered play-based intervention to improve the social play skills of children with attention deficit hyperactivity disorder and their playmates. *Australian Occupational Therapy Journal, 62*, 197–207. https://doi.org/10.1111/1440-1630.12203

Casey, T., Chatterjee, S., Assi, M., Maharjan, S., Wirunrapan, K., & Gupta, S. (2017, September). *Unleashing the power of play in situations of crisis.* Paper presented at the 20th international play association triennial world conference, Calgary, Alberta, Canada.

Causey-Upton, R. (2015). A model for quality of life: Occupational justice and leisure continuity for nursing home residents. *Physical & Occupational Therapy in Geriatrics, 33*, 175–188. https://doi.org/10.3109/02703181.2015.1024301

Chung, J. C. (2004). Activity participation and well-being of people with dementia in long-term—Care settings. *OTJR: Occupation, Participation and Health, 24*, 22–31. https://doi.org/10.1177/153944920402400104

Clifford, J. M., & Bundy, A. C. (1989). Play preference and play performance in normal boys and boys with sensory integrative dysfunction. *Occupational Therapy Journal of Research, 9*, 202–217. https://doi.org/10.1177/153944928900900402

Cohen-Mansfield, J. (2005). Nonpharmacological interventions for persons with dementia. *Alzheimer's Care Quarterly, 6*, 129–145. https://doi.org/10.1017/S104161021800039X

Colder Carras, M., Kalbarczyk, A., Wells, K., Banks, J., Kowert, R., Gillespie, C., & Latkin, C. (2018). Connection, meaning, and distraction: A qualitative study of video game play and mental health recovery in veterans treated for mental and/or behavioral health problems. *Social Science & Medicine, 216*, 124–132. https://doi.org/10.1016/j.socscimed.2018.08.044

Coleman, D., & Iso-Ahola, S. E. (1993). Leisure and health: The role of social support and self-determination. *Journal of Leisure Research, 25*, 111–128. https://doi.org/10.1080/00222216.1993.11969913

Conn, C. (2015). "Sensory highs", "vivid rememberings" and "interactive stimming": Children's play cultures and experiences of friendship in autistic autobiographies. *Disability & Society, 30*, 1192–1206. https://doi.org/10.1080/09687599.2015.1081094

Cordier, R., Bundy, A., Hocking, C., & Einfeld, S. (2009). A model for play-based intervention for children with ADHD. *Australian Occupational Therapy Journal, 56*, 332–340. https://doi.org/10.1111/j.1440-1630.2009.00796.x

Cordier, R., Bundy, A., Hocking, C., & Einfeld, S. (2010a). Comparison of the play of children with attention deficit hyperactivity disorder by subtypes. *Australian Occupational Therapy Journal, 57*, 137–145. https://doi.org/10.1111/j.1440-1630.2009.00821.x

Cordier, R., Bundy, A., Hocking, C., & Einfeld, S. (2010b). Empathy in the play of children with attention deficit hyperactivity disorder. *OTJR: Occupation, Participation and Health, 30*, 122–132. https://doi.org/10.3928/15394492-20090518-02

Cordier, R., Bundy, A., Hocking, C., & Einfeld, S. (2010c). Playing with a child with ADHD: A focus on the playmates. *Scandinavian Journal of Occupational Therapy, 17*, 191–199. https://doi.org/10.1080/11038120903156619

Coster, W. (1998). Occupation-centered assessment of children. *American Journal of Occupational Therapy, 52*, 337–344. https://doi.org/10.5014/ajot.52.5.337

Couch, K. J., Deitz, J. C., & Kanny, E. M. (1998). The role of play in pediatric occupational therapy. *American Journal of Occupational Therapy, 52*, 111–117. https://doi.org/10.5014/ajot.52.2.111

Courtin, E., & Knapp, M. (2017). Social isolation, loneliness and health in old age: A scoping review. *Health & Social Care in the Community, 25*, 799–812. https://doi.org/10.1111/hsc.12311

Csikszentmihalyi, M. (1975a). *Beyond boredom and anxiety: Experiencing flow in in work and play.* Jossey-Bass.

Csikszentmihalyi, M. (1975b). Play and intrinsic rewards. *Humanistic Psychology, 15*(3), 41–63. https://doi.org/1177/002216787501500306

Csikszentmihalyi, M. (1990). *Flow: The psychology of optimal experience.* HarperPerennial.

Csikszentmihalyi, M., & Halton, E. (1981). *The meaning of things: Domestic symbols and the self.* Cambridge University Press.

Csikszentmihalyi, M., & Kleiber, D. A. (1991). Leisure and self-actualization. In B. L. Driver, P. J. Brown, & G. L. Peterson (Eds.), *Benefits of leisure* (pp. 91–102). Venture.

Dionigi, R. (2017). Leisure and recreation in the lives of older people. In M. Bernoth & D. Winkler (Eds.), *Healthy ageing and aged care* (pp. 204–220). Oxford University Press.

Dunton, G. F., Do, B., & Wang, S. D. (2020). Early effects of the COVID-19 pandemic on physical activity and sedentary behavior in children living in the U.S. *BMC Public Health, 20*, 1351. https://doi.org/10.1186/s12889-020-09429-3

Du Toit, S. H. J., Shen, X., & McGrath, M. (2018). Meaningful engagement and person-centered residential dementia care: A critical interpretive synthesis. *Scandinavian Journal of Occupational Therapy, 26*, 343–355. https://doi.org/10.1080/11038128.2018.1441323

Eakman, A. M., Rumble, M., Atler, K. A., Gee, B. M., Romriell, B., & Hardy, N. (2018). A qualitative research synthesis of positive subjective experiences in occupation from the Journal of Occupational Science (1993–2010). *Journal of Occupational Science, 25*, 346–367. https://doi.org/10.1080/14427591.2018.1492958

Engelen, L., Bundy, A. C., Naughton, G., Simpson, J. M., Bauman, A., Ragen, J., Baur, L., Wyver, S., Tranter, P., Niehues, A., Schiller, W., Perry, G., Jessup, G., & van der Ploeg, H. P. (2013). Increasing physical activity in young primary school children—It's child's play: A cluster randomised controlled trial. *Preventive Medicine, 56*, 319–325. https://doi.org/10.1016/j.ypmed.2013.02.007

Fabrigoule, C., Letenneur, L., Dartigues, J. F., Zarrouk, M., Commenges, D., & Barberger-Gateau, P. (1995). Social and leisure activities and risk of dementia: A prospective longitudinal study. *Journal of the American Geriatrics Society, 43*, 485–490. https://doi.org/10.1111/j.1532-5415.1995.tb06093.x

Fabrizi, S., & Hubbell, K. (2017). The role of occupational therapy in promoting playfulness, parent competence, and social participation in early childhood playgroups: A pretest posttest design. *Journal of Occupational Therapy, Schools and Early Intervention, 10*, 346–365. https://doi.org/10.1080/19411243.2017.1359133

Fabrizi, S. E., Ito, M. A., & Winston, K. (2016). Effect of occupational therapy–led playgroups in early intervention on child playfulness and caregiver responsiveness: A repeated-measures design. *American Journal of Occupational Therapy, 70*, 700220020p1–700220020p9. https://doi.org/10.5014/ajot.2016.017012

Fahy, S., Delicâte, N., & Lynch, H. (2020). Now, being, occupational: Outdoor play and children with autism, *Journal of Occupational Science, 28*, 114–132. https://doi.org/10.1080/14427591.2020.1816207

Fenech, A., & Collier, L. (2017). Leisure as a route to social and occupational justice for individuals with profound levels of disability. In D. Sakellariou & N. Pollard (Eds.), *Occupational therapies without borders: Integrating justice with practice* (2nd ed., pp. 126–133). Elsevier.

Fine, J. (2001). The effect of leisure activity on depression in the elderly: Implications for the field of occupational therapy. *Occupational Therapy in Health Care, 13*, 45–59. https://doi.org/10.1080/J003v13n01_04

Fink, W., Mareva, S., & Gibson, J. L. (2020). Dispositional playfulness in young children: A cross-sectional and longitudinal examination of the psychometric properties of a new child self-reported playfulness scale and associations with social behaviour. *Infant and Child Development, 29*, e2181. https://doi.org/10.1002/icd.2181

Fisher, G., Forsyth, K., Harrison, M., Angarola, R., Kayhan, E., Noga, P., & Irvine, L. (2014). *Resident Environment Impact Scale (REIS) (Version 4.0 user's manual).* University of IL at Chicago Department of Occupational Therapy, The MOHO Clearinghouse.

Gardiner, C., Geldenhuys, G., & Gott, M. (2018). Interventions to reduce social isolation and loneliness among older people: An integrative review. *Health & Social Care in the Community, 26*(2), 147–157. https://doi.org/10.1111/hsc.12367

Gerlach, A., Browne, A., & Suto, M. (2014). A critical reframing of play in relation to Indigenous children in *Canada. Journal of Occupational Science, 21*, 243–258. https://doi.org/10.1080/14427591.2014.908818

Glynn, M. A., & Webster, J. (1992). The adult playfulness scale: An initial assessment. *Psychological Reports, 71*, 83–103. https://doi.org/10.2466/pr0.1992.71.1.83

Goll, J., Charlesworth, G., Scior, K., & Stott, J. (2015). Barriers to social participation among lonely older adults: The influence of social fears and identity. *PLoS ONE, 10*(2), e0116664. https://doi.org/10.1371/journal.pone.0116664

Goltz, H., & Brown, T. (2014). Are children's psychological self-concepts predictive of their self-reported activity preferences and leisure participation? *Australian Occupational Therapy Journal, 61*, 177–186. https://doi.org/10.1111/1440-1630.12101

Goodman, C. C. (1984). Natural helping among older adults. *The Gerontologist, 24*, 138–143. https://doi.org/10.1093/geront/24.2.138

Grady-Dominguez, P., Bundy, A. C., Ragen, J., Wyver, S., Villeneuve, M., Naughton, G., Tranter, P., Eakman, A., Hepburn, S., & Beetham, K. (2019). An observation-based instrument to measure what children with disabilities do on the playground: A Rasch analysis. *International Journal of Play, 2*, 79–93. https://doi.org/10.1080/21594937.2019.1580340

Grady-Dominguez, P., Ihrig, K., Lane, S., Aberle, J., Beetham, K., Ragen, J., Spencer, G., Sterman, J., Tranter, P., Wyver, S., & Bundy, A. (2020). Reframing risk: Working with caregivers of children with disabilities to promote risk-taking in play. *International Review of Research in Developmental Disabilities, 59*, 1–45. https://doi.org/10.1016/bs.irrdd.2020.09.001

Grady-Dominguez, P., Ragen, J., Sterman, J., Spencer, G., Tranter, P., Villeneuve, M., & Bundy, A. (2021). Expectations and assumptions: Examining the influence of staff culture on a novel school-based intervention to enable risky play for children with disabilities.

International Journal of Environmental Research and Public Health, 18(3), 1008. https://doi.org/10.3390/ijerph18031008

Graham, N., Truman, J., & Holgate, H. (2014). An exploratory study: Expanding the concept of play for children with severe cerebral palsy. *British Journal of Occupational Therapy, 77*, 358–365. https://doi.org/10.4276/030802214X14044755581781

Hammell, K. W. (2004a). Dimensions of meaning in the occupations of daily life. *Canadian Journal of Occupational Therapy, 71*, 296–305. https://doi.org/10.1177/000841740407100509

Hammell, K. W. (2004b). Quality of life among people with high spinal cord injury living in the community. *Spinal Cord, 42*, 607–620. https://doi.org/10.1038/sj.sc.3101662

Hammell, K. W. (2007). Reflections on . . . a disability methodology for the client-centred practice of occupational therapy research. *Canadian Journal of Occupational Therapy, 74*, 365–369. https://doi.org/10.2182/cjot.07.003

Hammell, K. W. (2009). Self-care, productivity, and leisure, or dimensions of occupational experience? Rethinking occupational "categories." *Canadian Journal of Occupational Therapy, 76*, 107–114. https://doi.org/10.1177/000841740907600208

Harris, K., & Reid, D. (2005). The influence of virtual reality play on children's motivation. *Canadian Journal of Occupational Therapy, 72*, 21–29. https://doi.org/10.1177/000841740507200107

Havighurst, R. J. (1979). The nature and values of meaningful free-time activity. In R. W. Kleemeier (Ed.), *Aging and leisure* (pp. 309–344). Arno Press.

Henricks, T. S. (2010). Caillois's "Man, Play, and Games": An appreciation and evaluation. *American Journal of Play, 3*, 157–185. https://files.eric.ed.gov/fulltext/EJ1070247.pdf

Henry, A. (2008). Assessment of play and leisure in children and adolescents. In L. D. Parham & L. S. Fazio (Eds.), *Play in occupational therapy for children* (2nd ed., pp. 95–191). Mosby.

Hess, L. M., & Bundy, A. C. (2003). The association between playfulness and coping in adolescents. *Physical & Occupational Therapy in Pediatrics, 23*, 5–17. https://doi.org/10.1080/J006v23n02_02

Hitch, D., Pépin, G., & Stagnitti, K. (2014). In the footsteps of Wilcock, part one: The evolution of doing, being, becoming, and belonging. *Occupational Therapy in Health Care, 28*, 231–246. https://doi.org/10.3109/07380577.2014.898114

Hurd, A. R., & Anderson, D. M. (2010). *The park and recreation professional's handbook.* Human Kinetics.

Iso-Ahola, S. E., Jackson, E. L., & Dunn, E. (1994). Starting, ceasing, and replacing leisure activities over the human life-span. *Journal of Leisure Research, 26*, 227–249. https://doi.org/10.1080/00222216.1994.11969958

Jacobson, S., & Samdahl, D. M. (1998). Leisure in the lives of old lesbians: Experiences with and responses to discrimination. *Journal of Leisure Research, 30*, 233–255. https://doi.org/10.1080/00222216.1998.11949828

Jessup, G., Bundy, A. C., & Cornell, E. (2013). To be or to refuse to be? Exploring the concept of leisure as resistance for young people who are visually impaired. *Leisure Studies, 32*, 191–205. https://doi.org/10.1080/02614367.2012.695388

Jessup, G., Cornell, E., & Bundy, A. C. (2010). The treasure in leisure activities: Fostering resilience in young people who are blind. *Journal of Visual Impairment & Blindness, 104*, 419–430. https://doi.org/10.1037/0003-066X.55.5.469

Jonsson, H. (2008). A new direction in the conceptualization and categorization of occupation. *Journal of Occupational Science, 15*, 3–8. https://doi.org/10.1080/14427591.2008.9686601

Jonsson, H. (2011). The first steps into the third age: The retirement process from a Swedish perspective. *Occupational Therapy International, 18*, 32–38. https://doi.org/10.1002/oti.311

Kaye, L. K., Kowert, R., & Quinn, S. (2017). The role of social identity and online social capital on psychosocial outcomes in MMO players. *Computers in Human Behavior, 74*, 215–223. https://doi .org/10.1016/j.chb.2017.04.030

Keen, D., Rodger, S., Doussin, K., & Braithwaite, M. (2007). A pilot study of the effects of a social-pragmatic intervention on the communication and symbolic play of children with autism. *Autism, 11*, 63–71. https://doi.org/10.1177/1362361307070901

Kelly, J. R. (1982). Leisure in later life: Roles and identities. In N. J. Osgood (Ed.), *Life after work* (pp. 268–292). Praeger.

Kelly, J. R. (1993). Theory and issues. In J. R. Kelly (Ed.), *Activity and aging* (pp. 5–16). Sage.

Kent, C., Cordier, R., Joosten, A., Wilkes-Gillan, S., & Bundy, A. (2018). Peer-mediated intervention to improve play skills in children with autism spectrum disorder: A feasibility study. *Australian Occupational Therapy Journal, 65*(3), 176–186. https://doi.org/ 10.1111/1440-1630.12459

Kent, C., Cordier, R., Joosten, A., Wilkes-Gillan, S., & Bundy, A. (2020a). The play differences of children with autism spectrum disorder (ASD) within sibling and nonsibling peer dyads. *American Journal of Occupational Therapy, 74*(4_Suppl._1), 7411515329p1. https://doi .org/10.5014/ajot.2020.74S1-PO2109

Kent, C., Cordier, R., Joosten, A., Wilkes-Gillan, S., & Bundy, A. (2020b). Can I learn to play? Randomized control trial to assess effectiveness of a peer-mediated intervention to improve play in children with autism spectrum disorder. *Journal of Autism and Developmental Disorders, 51*(6), 1823–1838. https://doi.org/10.1007/s10803-020-04671-5

Kent, C., Cordier, R., Joosten, A., Willkes-Gillan, S., & Bundy, A. (2020c). Can I join in? Multiple case study investigation of play performance generalisation for children with autism spectrum disorder from dyad to triad. *Australian Occupational Therapy Journal, 67*, 199–209. https://doi.org/10.1111/1440-1630.12635

Khetani, M., Coster, W., Law, M., & Bedell, G. (2013). *Young children's participation and environment measure*. CanChild.

Khetani, M. A., Graham, J. E., Davies, P. L., Law, M. C., & Simeonsson, R. J. (2015). Psychometric properties of the young children's participation and environment measure. *Archives of Physical Medicine and Rehabilitation, 96*, 307–316. https://doi.org/10.1016/j.apmr.2014.09.031

Kielhofner, G. (2009). *Conceptual foundations of occupational therapy practice* (4th ed.). F. A. Davis.

Kim, H., & Zakour, M. (2017). Disaster preparedness among older adults: Social support, community participation, and demographic characteristics. *Journal of Social Service Research, 43*, 498–509. https://doi.org/10.1080/01488376.2017.1321081

King, G., Law, M., King, S., Hurley, P., Hanna, S., Kertoy, M., Rosenbaum, P., & Young, N. (2004). *Children's Assessment of Participation and Enjoyment (CAPE) and Preferences for Activities of Children (PAC)*. Harcourt Assessment.

King, G., Law, M., Petrenchik, T., & Hurley, P. (2013). Psychosocial determinants of out of school activity participation for children with and without physical disabilities. *Physical & Occupational Therapy in Pediatrics, 33*, 384–404. https://doi.org/10.3109/01942638.2013.791915

Kleiber, D. A., Hutchinson, S. L., & Williams, R. (2002). Leisure as a resource in transcending negative life events: Self-protection, self-restoration, and personal transformation. *Leisure Sciences, 24*, 219–235. https://doi.org/10.1080/01490400252900167

Knox, S. (2008). Development and current use of the revised Knox Preschool Play Scale. In L. D. Parham & L. S. Fazio (Eds.), *Play in occupational therapy for children* (2nd ed., pp. 55–70). Mosby.

Laliberte-Rudman, D., Yu, B., Scott, E., & Pajouhandeh, P. (2000). Exploration of the perspectives of persons with schizophrenia regarding quality of life. *American Journal of Occupational Therapy, 54*, 137–147. https://doi.org/10.5014/ajot.54.2.137

Lape, J. (2009). Using a multisensory environment to decrease negative behaviors in clients with dementia. *OT Practice, 14*(9), 9–13.

Lawton, M. P. (1993). Meanings of activity. In J. R. Kelly (Ed.), *Activity and aging* (pp. 25–41). Sage.

Lee, D. T., Woo, J., & Mackenzie, A. E. (2002). A review of older people's experiences with residential care placement. *Journal of Advanced Nursing, 37*, 19–27. https://doi.org/10.1046/j.1365-2648.2002.02060.x

! e Riche, H. (2017). *Playful design for activation: Co-designing serious games for people with moderate to severe dementia to reduce apathy* [Unpublished dissertation]. Delft University of Technology, Delft, Netherlands.

Linder, T. (2008). *Transdisciplinary play-based assessment* (2nd ed.). Paul Brookes.

Loebach, J., & Cox, A. (2020). Tool for observing play outdoors (TOPO): A new typology for capturing children's play behaviors in outdoor environments. *International Journal of Environmental Research and Public Health, 17*, 5611. https://doi.org/10.3390/ijerph17155611

Long, D., Bergeron, J., Doyle, S. L., & Gordon, C. Y. (2006). The relationship between frequency of participation in play activities and kindergarten readiness. *Occupational Therapy in Health Care, 19*, 23–42. https://doi.org/10.1080/J003v19n04_03

Losier, G. F., Bourque, P. E., & Vallerand, R. J. (1993). A motivational model of leisure participation in the elderly. *The Journal of Psychology, 127*, 153–170. https://doi.org/10.1080/00223980.1993.9915551

Lynch, H., Hayes, N., & Ryan, S. (2016). Exploring socio-cultural influences on infant play occupations in Irish home environments. *Journal of Occupational Science, 23*, 352–369. https://doi.org/10.1080/14 427591.2015.1080181

Lynch, H., & Moore, A. (2016). Play as an occupation in occupational therapy. *Journal of the Association of Occupational Therapists, 79*(9), 519–520. https://doi.org/10.1177/0308022616664540

Lynch, H., Moore, A., Edwards, C., & Horgan, L. (2020). Advancing play participation for all: The challenge of addressing play diversity and inclusion in community parks and playgrounds. *British Journal of Occupational Therapy, 83*, 107–117. https://doi.org/10.1177/0308022619881936

Lynch, H., Prellwitz, M., Schulze, C., & Moore, A. H. (2018). The state of play in children's occupational therapy: A comparison between Ireland, Sweden and Switzerland. *British Journal of Occupational Therapy, 81*, 42–50. https://doi.org/10.1177/0308022617733256

Mannell, R. C., Zuzanek, J., & Larson, R. (1988). Leisure states and "flow" experiences: Testing perceived freedom and intrinsic motivation hypotheses. *Journal of Leisure Research, 20*, 289–304. https://doi.org/10 .1080/00222216.1988.11969782

McGuire, F. A., Boyd, R., & Tedrick, R. T. (2004). *Leisure and aging: Ulyssean living in later life* (2nd ed.). Sagamore.

Melchert-McKearnan, K., Deitz, J., Engel, J. M., & White, O. (2000). Children with burn injuries: Purposeful activity versus rote exercise. *American Journal of Occupational Therapy, 54*, 381–390. https://doi .org/10.5014/ajot.54.4.381

Miller Kuhaneck, H., Tanta, K. J., Coombs, A. K., & Pannone, H. (2013). A survey of pediatric occupational therapists' use of play. *Journal of Occupational Therapy, Schools and Early Intervention, 6*, 213–227. https://doi.org/10.1080/19411243.2013.850940

Moore, S. A., Faulkner, G., Rhodes, R. E. Brussoni, M., Chulak-Bozzer, T., Ferguson, L. J., Mitra, R., O'Reilly, N., Spence, J. C., Vanderloo, L. M., & Tremblay, M. S. (2020). Impact of COVID-19 virus outbreak on movement and play behaviors of Canadian children and youth: A national survey. *International Journal of Behavioral Nutrition and Physical Activity, 17*, 85. https://doi.org/10.1186/s12966-020-00987-8

Morgan-Brown, M., & Chard, G. (2014). Comparing communal environments using the assessment tool for occupation and social engagement: Using interactive occupation and social engagement as outcome measures. *British Journal of Occupational Therapy, 77*, 50–58. https://doi.org/10.4276/030802214X13916969446994

Morgan-Brown, M., Ormerod, M., Newton, R., Manley, D., & Fitzpatrick, M. (2011). Social and occupational engagement of staff in two Irish nursing homes for people with dementia. *Irish Journal of Occupational Therapy, 39*, 11–17. https://www.researchgate.net/ publication/220023008_Social_and_occupational_engagement_of_ staff_in_two_Irish_nursing_homes_for_people_with_dementia

Moyle, W., Jones, C., Dwan, T., & Petrovich, T. (2018). Effectiveness of a virtual reality forest on people with dementia: A mixed methods pilot study. *The Gerontologist, 58*(3), 478–487. https://doi.org/10.1093/geront/gnw270

Munier, V., Myers, C. T., & Pierce, D. (2008). Power of object play for infants and toddlers. In L. D. Parham & L. S. Fazio (Eds.), *Play in occupational therapy for children* (2nd ed., pp. 219–249). Mosby.

Nagle, S., Cook, J. V., & Polatajko, H. J. (2002). I'm doing as much as I can: Occupational choices of persons with a severe and persistent mental illness. *Journal of Occupational Science, 9,* 72–81. https://doi.org/10.1080/14427591.2002.9686495

Neal, I., Du Toit, S. H. J., & Lovarini, M. (2020). The use of technology to promote meaningful engagement for adults with dementia in residential aged care: A scoping review. *International Psychogeriatrics, 32,* 913–935. https://doi.org/10.1017/S1041610219001388

Neulinger, J. (1974). *The psychology of leisure: Research approaches to the study of leisure.* Charles C. Thomas.

Neumann, E. A. (1971). *The elements of play.* MSS Information.

Nicholson, N. (2012). A review of social isolation: An important but underassessed condition in older adults. *The Journal of Primary Prevention, 33*(2–3), 137–152. https://doi.org/10.1007/s10935-012-0271-2

Niehues, A. N., Bundy, A., Broom, A., & Tranter, P. (2015). Parents' perceptions of risk and the influence on children's everyday activities. *Journal of Child and Family Studies, 24,* 809–820. https://doi.org/10.1007/s10826-013-9891-2

Niehues, A. N., Bundy, A., Broom, A., & Tranter, P. (2016). Reframing healthy risk taking: Parents' dilemmas and strategies to promote children's well-being. *Journal of Occupational Science, 23,* 449–463. https://doi.org/10.1080/14427591.2016.1209424

Niehues, A. N., Bundy, A., Broom, A., Tranter, P., Ragen, J., & Engelen, L. (2013). Everyday uncertainties: Reframing perceptions of risk in outdoor free play. *Journal of Adventure Education & Outdoor Learning, 13,* 223–237. https://doi.org/10.1080/14729679.2013.798588

O'Connor, C., & Stagnitti, K. (2011). Play, behaviour, language and social skills: The comparison of a play and a non-play intervention within a specialist school setting. *Research in Developmental Disabilities, 32,* 1205–1211. https://doi.org/10.1016/j.ridd.2010.12.037

Omar, M. T. A., Hegazy, F. A., & Mokashi, S. P. (2012). Influences of purposeful activity versus rote exercise on improving pain and hand function in pediatric burn. *Burns, 38,* 261–268. https://doi.org/10.1016/j.burns.2011.08.004

Parham, L. D. (1996). Perspectives on play. In R. Zemke & F. A. Clark (Eds.), *Occupational science: The evolving discipline* (pp. 71–80). F. A. Davis.

Parham, L. D. (2008). Play and occupational therapy. In L. D. Parham & L. S. Fazio (Eds.), *Play in occupational therapy for children* (2nd ed., pp. 3–39). Mosby.

Parham, L. D., & Fazio, L. S. (Eds.). (2008). *Play in occupational therapy for children* (2nd ed). Mosby.

Parten, M. B. (1932). Social participation among preschool children. *Journal of Abnormal Psychology, 27,* 243–269. https://doi.org/10.1037/h0074524

Passmore, A., & French, D. (2003). The nature of leisure in adolescence: A focus group study. *British Journal of Occupational Therapy, 66,* 419–426. https://doi.org/10.1177/030802260306600907

Pereira, R. B., & Stagnitti, K. (2006, July). *The relationship between leisure experiences and health in an ageing Italian community in Australia.* Paper presented at the 14th world federation of occupational therapists congress, Sydney, Australia.

Perissinotto, C. M., Stijacic Cenzer, I., & Covinsky, K. E. (2012). Loneliness in older persons: A predictor of functional decline and death. *Archives of Internal Medicine, 172*(14), 1–7. https://doi.org/10.1001/archinternmed.2012.1993

Piaget, J. (1962). *Play, dreams, and imitation in childhood.* W.W. Norton.

Pierce, D. (2001a). Occupation by design: Dimensions, therapeutic power, and creative process. *American Journal of Occupational Therapy, 55,* 249–259. https://doi.org/10.5014/ajot.55.3.249

Pierce, D. (2001b). Untangling occupation and activity. *American Journal of Occupational Therapy, 55,* 138–146. https://doi.org/10.5014/ajot.55.2.138

Pierce, D. (2003). *Occupation by design: Building therapeutic power.* F. A. Davis.

Pierce, D. (2009). Co-occupation: The challenges of defining concepts original to occupational science. *Journal of Occupational Science, 16,* 203–207. https://doi.org/10.1080/14427591.2009.9686663

Pierce, D. (2014). *Occupational science for occupational therapy.* Slack.

Pöllänen, S. H., & Hirsimäki, R. M. (2014). Crafts as memory triggers in reminiscence: A case study of older women with dementia. *Occupational Therapy in Health Care, 28,* 410–430. https://doi.org/10.3109/07380577.2014.941052

Power, G. A. (2010). *Dementia beyond drugs: Changing the culture of care.* Health Professions Press.

Powrie, B, Copley, J., Turpin, M., Ziviani, J., & Kolehmainen, N. (2020). The meaning of leisure to children and young people with significant physical disabilities: Implications for optimizing participation. *British Journal of Occupational Therapy, 83,* 67–77. https://doi.org/10.1177/0308022619879077

Powrie, B., Kolehmainen, N., Turpin, M., Ziviani, J., & Copley, J. (2015). The meaning of leisure for children and young people with physical disabilities: A systematic evidence synthesis. *Developmental Medicine and Child Neurology, 57,* 993–1010. https://doi.org/10.1111/dmcn.12788

Pretorius, J. (1993). *Recreation, the stepchild of occupational therapy.* Recreation lecture (ABT114). University of the Free State.

Primeau, L. A. (1996). Work and leisure: Transcending the dichotomy. *American Journal of Occupational Therapy, 50,* 569–577. https://doi.org/10.5014/ajot.50.7.569

Quinones, G., & Adams, M. (2020). Children's virtual worlds and friendships during the COVID-19 pandemic. *Video Journal of Education and Pedagogy, 5,* 1–18. https://doi.org/10.1163/23644583-bja10015

Raber, C., Teitelman, J., Watts, J., & Kielhofner, G. (2010). A phenomenological study of volition in everyday occupations of older people with dementia. *British Journal of Occupational Therapy, 73,* 498–506. https://doi.org/10.4276/030802210X12892992239116

Ramugondo, E. L. (2012). Intergenerational play within family: The case for occupational consciousness. *Journal of Occupational Science, 19,* 326–340. https://doi.org/10.1080/14427591.2012.710166

Ray-Kaeser, S., & Lynch, H. (2017). Occupational therapy perspective on play for the sake of play. In V. Stancheva-Popkostadinova, S. Besio, & D. Bulgarelli (Eds.), *Play development in children with disabilities* (pp. 155–165). De Gruyter Open Poland. https://doi.org/10.1515/9783110522143-014

Raymore, L. A., Barber, B. L., Eccles, J. S., & Godbey, G. C. (1999). Leisure behavior pattern stability during the transition from adolescence to young adulthood. *Journal of Youth and Adolescence, 28,* 79–103. https://doi.org/10.1023/A:1021624609006

Reilly, M. (1974). An explanation of play. In M. Reilly (Ed.), *Play as exploratory learning: Studies of curiosity behavior* (pp. 117–149). Sage.

Reinecke, L. (2009). Games and recovery: The use of video and computer games to recuperate from stress and strain. *Journal of Media Psychology Theories Methods and Applications, 21,* 126–142.

Rockwell-Dylla, L. A. (1992). *Older adults' meaning of environment: Hospital and home* [Unpublished masters thesis]. University of Illinois at Chicago.

Rodríguez, A., Látková, P., & Sun, Y.-Y. (2008). The relationship between leisure and life satisfaction: Application of activity and need theory.

Social Indicators Research, 86, 163–175. https://doi.org/10.1007/s11205-007-9101-y

Román-Oyola, R., Vazquez-Gual, C., Dasta-Valentin, I., Diaz-Lazzarini, G., Collazo-Aguilar, G., Yambo-Martinez, C., Bundy, A., Lane, S., & Bonilla-Rodriguez, V. (2019). Development of the Scale of Parental Playfulness Attitude (PaPA) during the co-occupation of play. *American Journal of Occupational Therapy, 73*, 7311500050. https://doi.org/10.5014/ajot.2019.73s1-po8016

Rooney, C., & White, G. W. (2007). Consumer perspective: Narrative analysis of a disaster preparedness and emergency response survey from persons with mobility impairments. *Journal of Disability Policy Studies, 17*, 206–215. https://doi.org/10.1177/10442073070170040301

Rubin, K., Fein, G., & Vandenberg, B. (1983). Play. In P. H. Mussen (Ed.), *Handbook of child psychology: Socialization, personality and social development* (Vol. 4, pp. 693–774). Wiley.

Ryan, R. M., & Deci, E. L. (2017). *Self-determination theory: Basic psychological needs in motivation, development, and wellness.* Guilford Press.

Sandseter, E. B. H. (2009). Characteristics of risky play. *Journal of Adventure Education and Outdoor Learning, 9*, 3–21. https://doi.org/10.1080/14729670802702762

Sandseter, E. B. H., & Kennair, L. E. O. (2011). Children's risky play from an evolutionary perspective: The anti-phobic effects of thrilling experiences. *Evolutionary Psychology, 9*, 257–284. https://doi.org/10.1177/147470491100900212

Saunders, E. B. (1922). Psychiatry and occupational therapy. *Archives of Occupational Therapy, 1*, 99–114.

Saunders, I., Sayer, M., & Goodale, A. (1999). The relationship between playfulness and coping in preschool children: A pilot study. *American Journal of Occupational Therapy, 53*, 221–226. https://doi.org/10.5014/ajot.53.2.221

Scraton, S., & Holland, S. (2006). Grandfatherhood and leisure. *Leisure Studies, 25*, 233–250. https://doi.org/10.1080/02614360500504693

Seija Kangas, S., Määttä, K., & Uusiautti, S. (2012). Alone and in a group: Ethnographic research on autistic children's play, *International Journal of Play, 1*, 37–50. https://doi.org/10.1080/21594937.2012.656920

Shen, X. S., Chick, G., & Zinn, H. (2014a). Playfulness in adulthood as a personality trait: A reconceptualization and a new measurement. *Journal of Leisure Research, 46*, 58–83. https://doi.org/10.1080/00222216.2014.11950313

Shen, X. S., Chick, G., & Zinn, H. (2014b). Validating the Adult Playfulness Trait Scale (APTS): An examination of personality, behavior, attitude, and perception in the nomological network of playfulness. *American Journal of Play, 6*, 345–369.

Skard, G., & Bundy, A. C. (2008). Test of playfulness. In L. D. Parham & L. S. Fazio (Eds.), *Play in occupational therapy for children* (2nd ed., pp. 71–94). Mosby.

Slagle, E. C. (1922). Training aides for mental patients. *Archives of Occupational Therapy, 1*, 11–19. https://doi.org/10.1192/bjp.69.284.127

Sonday, A., & Gretschel, P. (2016). Empowered to play: A case study describing the impact of powered mobility on the exploratory play of disabled children. *Occupational Therapy International, 23*, 11–18. https://doi.org/10.1002/oti.1395

Sörman, D. E., Sundström, A., Rönnlund, M., Adolfsson, R., & Nilsson, L.-G. (2013). Leisure activity in old age and risk of dementia: A 15-year prospective study. *The Journals of Gerontology, 69*, 493–501. https://doi.org/10.1093/geronb/gbt056

Spencer, G., Bundy, A., Wyver, S., Villeneuve, M., Tranter, P., Beetham, K., Ragen, J., & Naughton, G. (2016). Uncertainty in the school playground: Shifting rationalities and teachers' sense-making in the management of risks for children with disabilities. *Health, Risk & Society, 18*, 301–317. https://doi.org/10.1080/13698575.2016.1238447

Stagnitti, K. (2007). *The child initiated pretend play assessment.* Co-ordinates Publications.

Stagnitti, K., O'Connor, C., & Sheppard, L. (2012). Impact of the Learn to Play program on play, social competence and language for children aged 5–8 years who attend a specialist school. *Australian Occupational Therapy Journal, 59*, 302–311. https://doi.org/10.1111/j.1440-1630.2012.01018.x.

Stendal, K., Balandin, S., & Molka-Danielsen, J. (2011). Virtual worlds: A new opportunity for people with lifelong disability? *Journal of Intellectual & Developmental Disability, 36*, 80–83. https://doi.org/10.3109/13668250.2011.526597

Sterman, J. J., Naughton, G. A., Bundy, A. C., Froude, E., & Villeneuve, M. A. (2019). Planning for outdoor play: Government and family decision-making. *Scandinavian Journal of Occupational Therapy, 26*, 484–495. https://doi.org/10.1080/11038128.2018.1447010

Sterman, J. J., Naughton, G. A., Bundy, A. C., Froude, E., & Villeneuve, M. A. (2020). Mothers supporting play as a choice for children with disabilities within a culturally and linguistically diverse community. *Scandinavian Journal of Occupational Therapy, 27*, 373–384. https://doi.org/10.1080/11038128.2019.1684556

Sterman, J., Naughton, G., Froude, E., Villeneuve, M., Beetham, K., Wyver, S., & Bundy, A. (2016). Outdoor play decisions by caregivers of children with disabilities: A systematic review of qualitative studies. *Journal of Developmental and Physical Disabilities, 28*, 931–957. https://doi.org/10.1007/s10882-016-9517-x

Strutt, P. A., Johnco, C. J., Chen, J., Muir, C., Maurice, O., Dawes, P., Siette, J., Botelho Dias, C., Hillebrandt, H., & Wuthrich, V. M. (2021). Stress and coping in older Australians during COVID-19: Health, service utilization, grandparenting, and technology use. *Clinical Gerontologist, 44*, 1–13. https://doi.org/10.1080/07317115.2021.1884158

Sundström, A., Adolfsson, A. N., Nordin, M., Adolfsson, R., & Anderson, N. (2020). Loneliness increases the risk of all-cause dementia and Alzheimer's disease. *The Journals of Gerontology, 75*, 919–926. https://doi.org/10.1093/geronb/gbz139

Suto, M. (1998). Leisure in occupational therapy. *Canadian Journal of Occupational Therapy, 65*, 271–278. https://doi.org/10.1177/000841749806500504

Sutton-Smith, B. (1997). *The ambiguity of play.* Harvard University Press.

Swaffer, K. (2015). Dementia and prescribed Disengagement™. *Dementia, 14*, 3–6. https://doi.org/10.1177/1471301214548136

Taylor, R. R. (2017). *Kielhofner's model of human occupation: Theory and application.* Wolters Kluwer Health.

Thibodeaux-Nielsen, R. B., Palermo, F., White, R. E., Wilson, A., & Dier, S. (2021). Child adjustment during COVID-19: The role of economic hardship, caregiver stress, and pandemic play. *Frontiers in Psychology, 12*, Article 716651. https://doi.org/10.3389/fpsyg.2021.716651

Thomas, C., Du Toit, S. H. J., & van Heerden, S. M. (2014). Leadership: The key to person-centred care. *South African Journal of Occupational Therapy, 44*, 34–39. http://www.scielo.org.za/pdf/sajot/v44n3/09.pdf

Thomas, J. E., O'Connell, B., & Gaskin, C. J. (2013). Residents' perceptions and experiences of social interaction and participation in leisure activities in residential aged care. *Contemporary Nurse, 45*, 244–254. https://doi.org/10.5172/conu.2013.45.2.244

Thomas, W. H. (1996). *Life worth living: How someone you love can still enjoy life in a nursing home: The Eden alternative in action.* Vander-Wyk & Burnham.

Thomson, S. (2014). Adulterated play: An empirical discussion surrounding adults' involvement with children's play in the primary school playground. *Journal of Playworks Practice, 1*, 5–21. https://doi.org/10.1332/205316214X13944535662152

Townsend, E. A., & Polatajko, H. J. (2007). *Advancing an occupational therapy vision for health, well-being, and justice through occupation.* Canadian Association of Occupational Therapists.

Townsend, E., & Wilcock, A. (2004). Occupational justice and client-centred practice: A dialogue in progress. *Canadian Journal of Occupational Therapy, 71*, 75–87. https://doi.org/10.1177/000841740407100203

Tse, T., & Linsey, H. (2005). Adult day groups: Addressing older people's needs for activity and companionship. *Australasian Journal on Ageing, 24,* 134–140. https://doi.org/10.1111/j.1741-6612.2005.00117.x

Turner, H., Chapman, S., McSherry, A., Krishnagiri, S., & Watts, J. (2000). Leisure assessment in occupational therapy: An exploratory study. *Occupational Therapy in Health Care, 12,* 73–85. https://doi.org/10.1080/J003v12n02_05

Ville, I., Ravaud, J.-F., & Tetrafigap Group. (2001). Subjective well-being and severe motor impairments: The Tetrafigap survey on the long-term outcome of tetraplegic spinal cord injured persons. *Social Science & Medicine, 52,* 369–384. https://doi.org/10.1016/s0277-9536(00)00140-4

Vizenor, K. V. (2014). *Binary lives: Digital citizenship and disability participation in a user content created virtual world.* State University of New York at Buffalo.

Waldman-Levi, A., & Bundy, A. (2016). A glimpse into co-occupations: Parent/caregiver's support of young children's playfulness scale. *Occupational Therapy in Mental Health, 32,* 217–227. https://doi.org/10.1080/0164212X.2015.1116420

Wang, H.-X., Jin, Y., Hendrie, H. C., Liang, C., Yang, L., Cheng, Y., Unverzagt, F. W., Ma, F., Hall, K. S., Murrell, J. R., Li, P, Bian, J., Pei, J-J., Gao, S., & Kritchevsky, S. (2012). Late life leisure activities and risk of cognitive decline. *The Journals of Gerontology, 68,* 205–213. https://doi.org/10.1093/gerona/gls153

Warchol, K. (2006). Facilitating functional and quality-of-life potential: Strength-based assessment and treatment for all stages of dementia. *Topics in Geriatric Rehabilitation, 22,* 213–227. https://aging.idaho.gov/wp-content/uploads/2019/06/Habilitation_Concepts.pdf

Weigl, R., & Bundy, A. (2013). Die spielerische Herangehensweise (Playfulness) Erwachsener an ihre Freizeitaktivitäten. The Experience of Leisure Scale (TELS) mit deutsch-sprachigen Erwachsenen [The playful approach of adults to their leisure time activities with German-speaking adults]. *Ergoscience, 8,* 11–21.

White, R. W. (1959). Motivation reconsidered: The concept of competence. *Psychological Review, 66,* 297–323. https://doi.org/10.1037/h0040934

Wilcock, A. A. (2007). Active ageing: Dream or reality. *New Zealand Journal of Occupational Therapy, 54,* 15–20. https://www.otnzwna.co.nz/download/32/nzjot-archived/1212/volume-54-issue-01.pdf#page=17

Wilkes, S., Cordier, R., Bundy, A., Docking, K., & Munro, N. (2011). A play-based intervention for children with ADHD: A pilot study. *Australian Occupational Therapy Journal, 58,* 231–240. https://doi.org/10.1111/j.1440-1630.2011.00928.x

Wilkes-Gillan, S., Bundy, A., Cordier, R., & Lincoln, M. (2014a). Evaluation of a pilot parent-delivered play-based intervention for children with attention deficit hyperactivity disorder. *American Journal of Occupational Therapy, 68,* 700–709. https://doi.org/10.5014/ajot.2014.012450

Wilkes-Gillan, S., Bundy, A., Cordier, R., & Lincoln, M. (2014b). Eighteen-month follow-up of a play-based intervention to improve the social play skills of children with attention deficit hyperactivity disorder. *Australian Occupational Therapy Journal, 61,* 299–307. https://doi.org/10.1111/1440-1630.12124

Wilkes-Gillan, S., Bundy, A., Cordier, R., & Lincoln, M. (2016a). Child outcomes of a pilot parent-delivered intervention for improving the social play skills of children with ADHD and their playmates. *Developmental Neurorehabilitation, 19,* 238–245. https://doi.org/10.3109/17518423.2014.948639

Wilkes-Gillan, S., Bundy, A., Cordier, R., Lincoln, M., & Chen, Y.-W. (2016b). A randomised controlled trial of a play-based intervention to improve the social play skills of children with attention deficit hyperactivity disorder (ADHD). *PLoS One, 11*(8), 1–22. https://doi.org/10.1371/journal.pone.0160558

Wilkes-Gillan, S., Bundy, A., Cordier, R., Lincoln, M., & Hancock, N. (2015). Parents' perspectives on the appropriateness of a parent-delivered intervention for improving the social play skills of children with ADHD. *British Journal of Occupational Therapy, 78,* 644–652. https://doi.org/10.1177/0308022615573453

Wilkes-Gillan, S., Cantrill, A., Cordier, R., Barnes, G., Hancock, N., & Bundy, A. (2017). The use of video-modelling as a method for improving the social play skills of children with attention deficit hyperactivity disorder (ADHD) and their playmates. *British Journal of Occupational Therapy, 80,* 196–207. https://doi.org/10.1177/0308022617692819

Willard, H. S., & Spackman, C. S. (1963). *Occupational therapy* (3rd ed.). Lippincott Williams & Wilkins.

Willard, H. S., Spackman, C. S., Hopkins, H. L., & Smith, H. D. (1978). *Willard & Spackman's occupational therapy* (5th ed.). Lippincott Williams & Wilkins.

Willard, H. S., Spackman, C. S., Hopkins, H. L., & Smith, H. D. (1993). *Willard & Spackman's occupational therapy* (8th ed.). Lippincott Williams & Wilkins.

Wood, W., Harris, S., Snider, M., & Patchel, S. A. (2005). Activity situations on an Alzheimer's disease special care unit and resident environmental interaction, time use, and affect. *American Journal of Alzheimer's Disease and Other Dementias, 20,* 105–118. https://doi.org/10.1177/153331750502000210

Ziegler, L. H. (1924). Some observations on recreations. *Archives of Occupational Therapy, 3,* 255–265.

Ziviani, J., Poulsen, A., & Cuskelly, M. (2012). *The art and science of motivation: A therapist's guide to working with children.* Jessica Kingsley.

Sleep and Rest

Jo M. Solet

LEARNING OBJECTIVES

After reading this chapter, you will be able to:

1. Understand the elements of sleep architecture and sleep changes through the life cycle.
2. Develop an epidemiologic perspective on sleep deficiency.
3. Relate sufficient sleep to individual health outcomes, memory, cognition, and occupational performance.
4. Describe multiple factors that may influence sleep.
5. Recognize common medical and psychiatric diagnoses treated by occupational therapists in which sleep may be implicated.
6. Organize client options for sleep hygiene, including sleep habits and environments; relate these to self-care and occupational balance.
7. Describe common primary sleep disorders.
8. Provide basic client sleep education and screening assessment and anticipate need for specialized referrals and occupational therapy participation on the treatment team.

Why Learn About Sleep?

We spend one-third of our lives asleep. Once thought of as a period of simple repose enforced by limited daylight, we now know sleep is a complex, dynamic state critical to growth and development. Many common medical and psychiatric disorders treated by occupational therapists affect client sleep or carry sleep-related signs and symptoms (Zee & Turek, 2006). Disordered sleep is a major public health concern affecting both genders, all races, and socioeconomic levels (Choi et al., 2006; Hale, 2005; Kim & Young, 2005) that increases with age (Ancoli-Israel & Cooke, 2005; Basner et al., 2007; Hale, 2005; Hale & Do, 2007; Patel et al., 2004). Sleep has documented impacts on health and safety, psychological well-being, learning and memory, and cognitive and occupational performance (Classen et al., 2011; Connor et al., 2002; Dorrian et al., 2011; Drake et al., 2010; Pizza et al., 2010; Poe et al., 2010; Smith & Phillips, 2011; Van Dongen et al., 2003). Inadequate sleep has been implicated in performance deficits and can place individuals and those they are responsible for at risk. Excessive sleepiness has contributed to environmental disasters such as oil spills, air traffic–control failures, medical errors, and auto and truck accidents. Sleep medicine is a dynamic, evolving field; research is underway at multiple levels, from genetic through epidemiologic (Hobson, 2011; Shepard et al., 2005). New insights with clinical significance can be expected on a continuing basis. The 2020 "Occupational Therapy Practice Framework" (American Occupational Therapy Association, 2020) categorizes sleep and rest as occupations. This chapter provides a sleep foundation in this emerging area of practice for occupational therapists.

Now, as our technology continues to evolve, we have developed the ability to monitor sleep outside the laboratory and even to detect some disorders through our personal devices. These same devices can now also deliver personalized sleep health behavior support through artificial intelligence (AI) counseling for problems such as insomnia. Already under development are techniques for enhancing learning and memory through sleep stage, wave-specific subliminal stimulation.

The Structure of Sleep

Beginning in 1929 with the introduction of the **electroencephalogram (EEG)**, it was revealed that sleep consists of patterns of changing brain waves that present in cycles of about 90 minutes throughout the night. Within these cycles, different stages of sleep are identified by the frequency and amplitude of the brain waves. When comparing the EEG readings of waking and sleep stages, researchers and clinicians assess the frequency of the brain waves, measured in hertz (Hz), and the size, or amplitude, of the brain waves, measured in microvolts, which differ for various stages of wakefulness and sleep.

Sleep Stages and Architecture

The stages of sleep fall into two categories: **rapid eye movement sleep** or **REM sleep**, in which most dreaming occurs, and **nonrapid eye movement sleep**, called **NREM sleep** or **non-REM sleep**, which displays progressively deeper stages identified as NREM1, NREM2, and NREM3. Infants and children have higher proportions of REM sleep than adults.

Transition from wakefulness begins with light sleep, known as stage 1 (NREM1), and deepens to stage 2 sleep (NREM2). In early cycles of the night, slow brain waves with low frequency and high amplitude characteristic of stage 3 or deep sleep (NREM3) are common. As morning approaches, the proportion of time in deep sleep drops, whereas the proportion in REM sleep—characterized by higher-frequency and lower-amplitude brain waves—increases. During REM sleep, there is diminished muscle tone, preventing the sleeper from acting out dream experiences. The map of a typical adult night's sleep showing the REM and NREM stages in 90-minute cycles through the night is called a **hypnogram** (Figure 48.1).

Current sleep medicine research explores the roles of REM and NREM sleep stages in contributing to specific

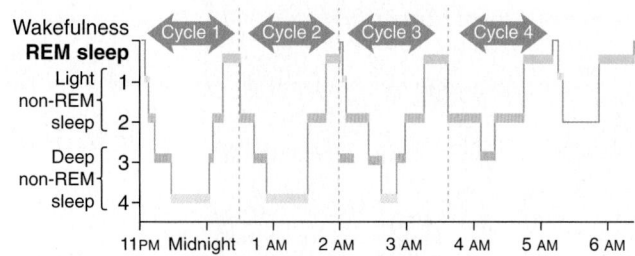

FIGURE 48.1 Sleep cycles across the night "hypnogram." REM, rapid eye movement.

functions, including emotional regulation, cognition, learning, and memory consolidation (American Academy of Sleep Medicine [AASM], 2009; Haack & Mullington, 2005; Poe et al., 2010; Stickgold, 2005; Walker & Stickgold, 2004).

Sleep Drives

Two processes interact to determine the drive for sleep: **sleep–wake homeostasis** and the circadian biological clock. The sleep–wake homeostatic drive increases with accumulated time awake. The **circadian biological clock** organizes a physiological cycle of body temperature and hormone release regulating the variability of sleepiness and wakefulness throughout the night and day. These two drives are not simply additive because with an increase in accumulated sleep debt, the circadian drive has been shown to exert greater impact on sleepiness (Figure 48.2).

The suprachiasmatic nucleus (SCN), a group of cells in the hypothalamus that respond to light and dark, controls the circadian biological clock. Signals generated by light reaching the optic nerve through the eyes travel to the SCN, carrying the message to the internal clock for wakefulness. With exposure to morning light, the SCN orchestrates

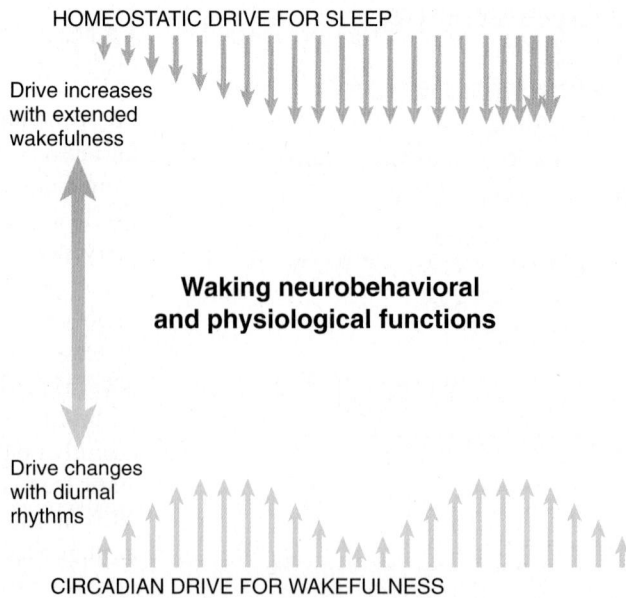

FIGURE 48.2 Sleep and wakefulness are regulated by two processes.

signals to other parts of the brain, raising body temperature and regulating certain hormone levels. Light delays the release of the hormone melatonin, which rises in the evening and stays elevated through the night, promoting sleep (Brendel et al., 2001; Edlund, 2003).

Sleep and the Life Cycle

Sleep changes through the life cycle, becoming shorter and lighter with aging (Figure 48.3). The period it takes to fall asleep,

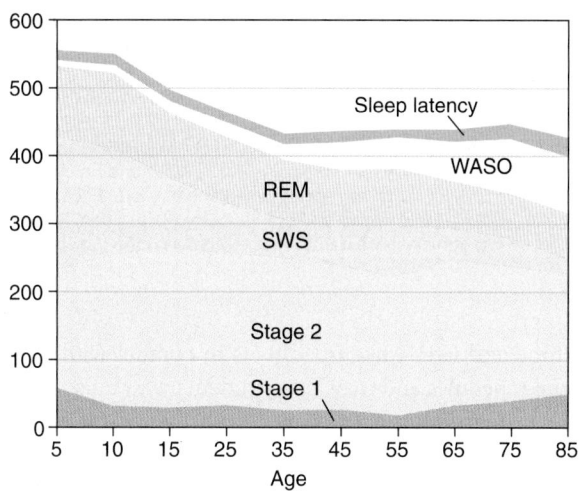

Minutes of sleep stage per night versus age

WASO: Wake after sleep onset (more with age)

REM: Rapid eye movement sleep (slightly less with age)

SWS: Non-REM, deep stages 3 and 4 combined (less with age)

FIGURE 48.3 Sleep: less and lighter with aging.

(Source: Reprinted with permission from Ohayon, N. M., Carskadon, M. A., Guilleminault, C., & Vitiello, M. V. [2004]. Meta-analysis of quantitative sleep parameters from childhood to old age in healthy individuals: Developing normative sleep values across the human lifespan. *Sleep, 27,* 1255–1273. https://doi.org/10.1093/sleep/27.7.1255)

known as **sleep latency**, changes little over the life course, but the amount of time in restorative deep sleep drops off and the time spent **awake after sleep onset (WASO)** increases. The proportion of individuals with sleep–wake impairments also increases substantially with age (Hale, 2005; Ohayon, 2002; Ohayon & Vecchierini, 2005). As the baby boomers age, disordered sleep will require substantial attention and consumption of healthcare resources (Leland et al., 2014).

Sleep and Modern Life
Epidemiology

The average sleep time for Americans has dropped over the past five decades from 8.5 to 7 hours at the same time as obesity and diabetes rates have risen (Ayas, 2010; Flier & Elmquist, 2004; Hale, 2005; Patel & Hu, 2008; Quan et al., 2010; Watanabe et al., 2010; Watson et al., 2010). Furthermore, Centers for Disease Control and Prevention (CDC) overlay maps show an alarming congruence; states, especially in the Deep South, with populations having the most limited sleep also have the highest rates of obesity and diabetes (Figure 48.4) (see CDC website). Not only does inadequate sleep increase appetite, lower satiation, and alter glucose metabolism, but as part of a dangerous cycle, obesity also increases the risk for disordered sleep. Insufficient sleep is common even among children. Parents may not be aware of child sleep requirements and or may not enforce consistent sleep schedules (Owens & Mindell, 2005). Many believe that insufficient sleep is in part responsible for the alarming rise in childhood obesity.

Individual Health Impacts

The range of negative health impacts from insufficient or disrupted sleep includes elevated stress hormones, impaired

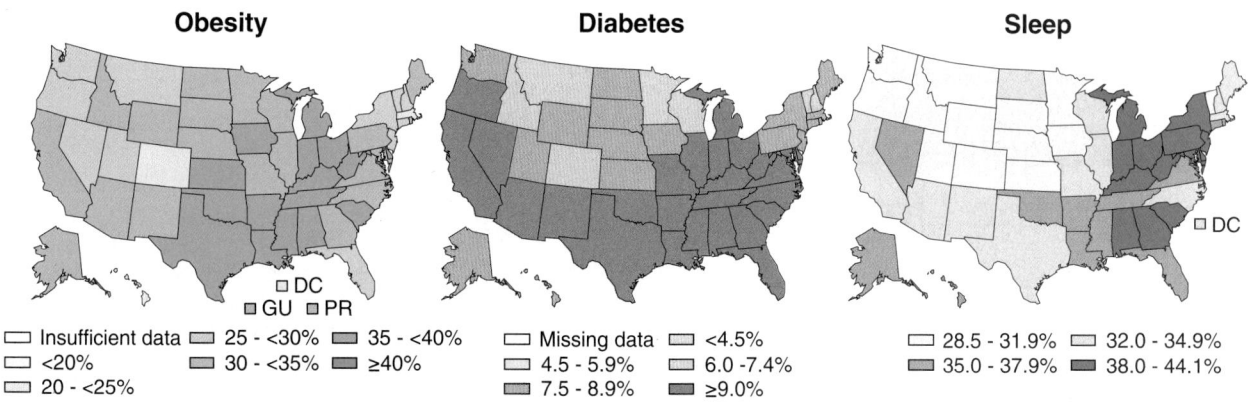

FIGURE 48.4 Intersecting epidemics.

(Sources: Data from the following sources: Obesity: Centers for Disease Control and Prevention. [2020]. *Adult obesity prevalence maps.* https://www.cdc.gov/obesity/data/prevalence-maps.html; Diabetes: Centers for Disease Control and Prevention, Division of Diabetes Translation. [2015]. *Maps of trends in diagnosed diabetes.* https://www.cdc.gov/diabetes/statistics/slides/maps_diabetes_trends.pdf; Insufficient sleep: Centers for Disease Control and Prevention, National Center for Chronic Disease Prevention and Health Promotion. [2014]. *Sleep and sleep disorders: Data and statistics.* http://www.cdc.gov/sleep/data_statistics.htm.)

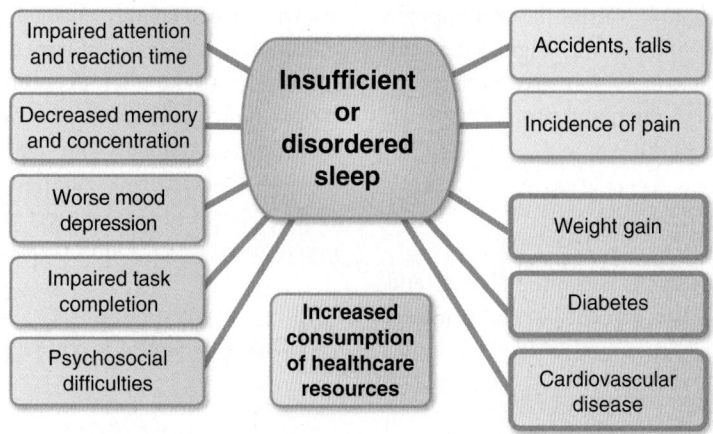

FIGURE 48.5 Insufficient or disordered sleep.

(Copyright Jo Solet, MS, EdM, PhD, OTR/L; Data from Ancoli-Israel, S., & Cooke, J. R. [2005]. Prevalence and comorbidity of insomnia and effect on functioning in elderly populations. *Journal of the American Geriatrics Society, 54*, S264–S271. https://doi.org/10.1111/j.1532-5415.2005.53392.x; Choi, S. W., Peek-Asa, C., Sprince, N. L., Rautiainen, R. H., Flamme, G. A., Whitten, P. S., & Zwerling, C. [2006]. Sleep quantity and quality as a predictor of injuries in a rural population. *American Journal of Emergency Medicine, 24*, 189–196. https://doi.org/10.1016/j.ajem.2005.09.002; and Spiegel, K., Knutson, K., Leproult, R., Tasali, E., & Van Cauter, E. [2005]. Sleep loss: A novel risk factor for insulin resistance and type 2 diabetes. *Journal of Applied Physiology, 99*, 2008–2019. https://doi.org/10.1152/japplphysiol.00660.2005; Chien, K. L., Chen, P. C., Hsu, H. C., Su, T. C., Sung, F. C., Chen, M. F., & Lee, Y. T. [2010]. Habitual sleep duration and insomnia and the risk of cardiovascular events and all-cause death: Report from a community-based cohort. *Sleep, 33*, 177–184. https://doi.org/10.1093/sleep/33.2.177)

glucose tolerance, diabetes (Zizi et al., 2011), obesity (Flier & Elmquist, 2004), cardiovascular disease, and stroke (Ayas, White, Al-Delaimy, et al., 2003; Ayas, White, Manson, et al., 2003). In addition, insufficient or disrupted sleep may be associated with **hyperalgesia** (Chhangani et al., 2009; Hamilton et al., 2007; Kristiansen et al., 2011; Roehrs et al., 2006), lowered mood, irritability, aggressiveness, and psychosocial difficulties (AASM, 2009; Owens et al., 2010). Decreased memory consolidation (Poe et al., 2010; Stickgold, 2005; Walker & Stickgold, 2004), impairments in concentration, impaired task completion, and decreased occupational performance have also been documented (Banks et al., 2010; Cohen et al., 2010; Durmer & Dinges, 2005; Ohayon & Vecchierini, 2005). Industrial, truck, and auto accidents are also associated with insufficient sleep (Classen et al., 2011; Connor et al., 2002; Drake et al., 2010; Pizza et al., 2010; Smith & Phillips, 2011; Tregear et al., 2009; Figure 48.5).

Sleep Requirements Through the Life Cycle

Whereas newborns sleep as much as 16 hours a day, by 6 months, babies typically sleep 12 hours during the night plus take two naps during the day (Figure 48.6). Well-rested preschoolers may still take an afternoon nap while sleeping 12 consolidated hours at night. Elementary school children require as much as 10 to 12 hours. Teenagers are understood as a group to experience **delayed sleep phase**—their natural sleep inclinations, based on timing release of the sleep-inducing hormone melatonin, are often toward later

bedtime and later wake up. This is in conflict with typical school schedules and may leave students who must awaken early feeling underslept and inattentive. Experiments with later high school start times showed improvements in multiple areas, including mood and academic performance as well as positive reactions from teachers (Owens et al., 2010). These findings are now driving policy initiatives supported by the American Academy of Pediatrics to delay junior and high school start times. School-based occupational therapists are in the position to bring awareness of sleep impacts to parents, teachers, and administrators.

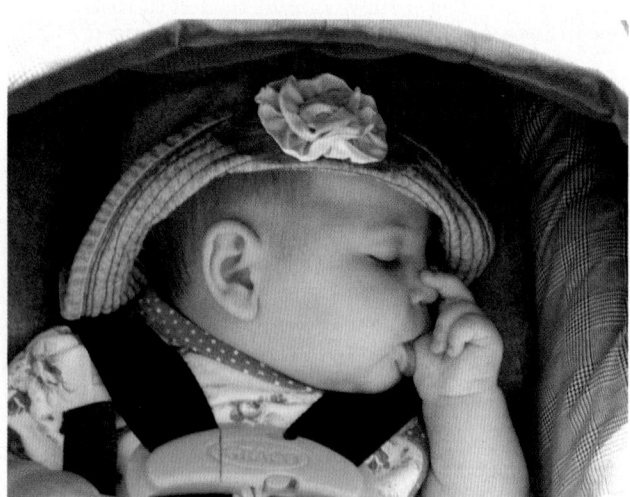

FIGURE 48.6 Infants have a faster sleep homeostasis and a greater percentage of REM sleep than older children.

(Courtesy of Jo Solet, MS, EdM, PhD, OTR/L.)

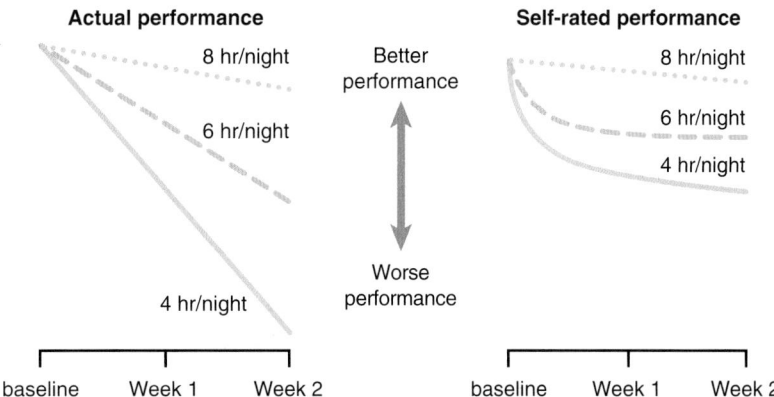

FIGURE 48.7 Restricting sleep impairs vigilance without parallel insight into increased deficits.

(Source: Reprinted with permission from Van Dongen, H. P., Maislin, G., Mullington, J. M., & Dinges, D. F. [2003]. The cumulative cost of additional wakefulness: Dose–response effects on neurobehavioral functions and sleep physiology from chronic sleep restriction and total sleep deprivation. *Sleep, 26*, 117–126. https://doi.org/10.1093/sleep/26.2.117. As redrawn by Orfeu Buxton.)

Along with changes during growth and development, there are individual differences in adult sleep requirements and schedule preferences. Ideally, individuals choose occupations that match their natural proclivities. However, it may be that many of us have become accustomed to a level of functioning that results from less-than-optimal sleep. In sleep restriction vigilance studies, subjects actually show limited insight into their deepening performance decrements over a 2-week period (Van Dongen et al., 2003; Figure 48.7). Although 7.5 hours is frequently cited as adequate for healthy adults, recent sleep extension studies with college athletes showed performance enhancements at 10 hours of time in bed (TIB; Mah et al., 2011).

Although elderly people may sleep less, in part owing to higher levels of medical disorders and pain or because they lack a consolidated night sleep period, napping on and off during the day, there is no evidence to support the common belief that elderly people actually require less sleep.

Influences on Sleep

As part of the clinical reasoning process and treatment planning, the occupational therapist is aware of multiple influences on sleep (Figure 48.8), which fall into five realms of concern: (a) common medical conditions and psychiatric disorders, (b) health habits and behaviors, (c) stress and occupational balance, (d) sleep environments, and (e) sleep disorders. The next sections of the chapter review each of these realms of concern with reference to these influences.

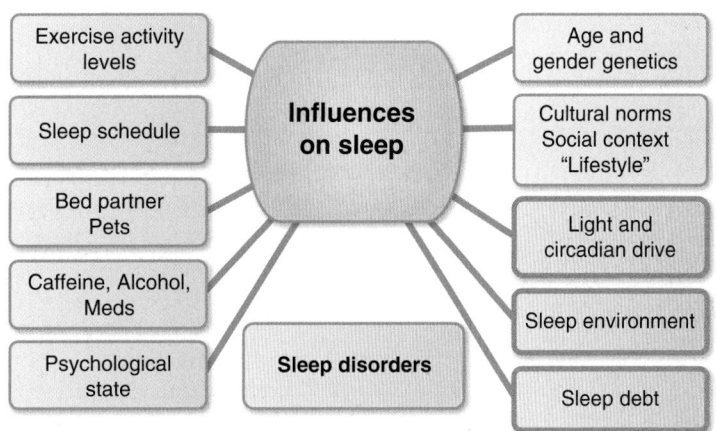

FIGURE 48.8 Influences on sleep: Many of these influences are open to modification as a part of occupational therapy collaborative treatment.

(Courtesy of Jo Solet, MS, EdM, PhD, OTR/L.)

Sleep and Common Medical Conditions and Psychiatric Disorders

The majority of conditions and disorders treated by occupational therapists (see Appendix I) may either impact client sleep, be exacerbated by insufficient or disordered sleep, or both (Stroe et al., 2010; Zee & Turek, 2006). The examples shown in Box 48.1 include possible mechanisms through which sleep may mediate functional disability.

Additional common medical conditions with sleep-disrupting symptoms include **adenotonsillar hypertrophy** (breathing difficulties, especially in childhood), ulcers and gastroesophageal reflux disease, pain, **benign prostatic hypertrophy** (**nocturia**), and **atopic dermatitis** (itching). Pregnancy, especially the last trimester (discomfort, difficulty breathing, nocturia), postpartum (infant care), and menopause (autonomic instability, hot flashes) may compromise sleep for some women. Although it is beyond the scope of this chapter to fully describe sleep issues associated with each of these disorders, the occupational therapist becomes familiar with this information for the specific diagnostic categories that present in his or her clinical practice, using chapter references and other resources. OT Story 48.1 describes a client with a sleep disorder.

OT STORY 48.1 ELVIRA

Celia is an occupational therapist called for a bedside activities of daily living (ADL) evaluation of Elvira, a 40-year-old naturalized citizen, following colostomy reversal surgery. Communicating with the help of a Spanish interpreter, Elvira complains that her pain is still "so bad" that she is having "fears and visions" about her surgical experiences and that "her legs are kicking and waking her up at night." Yet, in terms of ADL, Celia finds Elvira only requires minimal assistance.

Questions

1. How should Celia prioritize the multiple concerns that Elvira has raised?
2. Are there possible interactions between Elvira's pain report and her other complaints?
3. Which members of the clinical team should be called for consultation?
4. How might cultural competency help Celia and other team members address Elvira's complaints?

BOX 48.1 MECHANISMS THROUGH WHICH SLEEP MAY MEDIATE FUNCTIONAL DISABILITY IN COMMON CONDITIONS AND DISORDERS

Acute or Chronic Pain

- Arthritis
- Burns
- Low back pain

Central Nervous System Disease or Injury

- Alzheimer disease, dementias
- Parkinson disease
- Head injury
- Stroke/cerebrovascular disease
- Spinal cord injury
- Multiple sclerosis

Reward System, Appetite Satiation, or Metabolic Dysregulation

- Substance abuse
- Eating disorders
- Obesity
- Diabetes
- Cardiovascular disease

Respiratory Compromise, Disordered Breathing

- Chronic obstructive pulmonary disease
- Asthma
- Allergies

Perceived Lack of Safety, Insufficient Environmental Resources

- Posttraumatic stress disorder
- Anxiety disorders
- Poverty
- Homelessness

Failure of Self-Care, Isolation

- Major mental illness
- Developmental delays
- Autism

Compiled from Bondoc and Siebert (2008); Braley and Chervin (2010); Brown et al. (2011); Burton et al. (2010); Buxton and Marcelli (2010); Chandola et al. (2010); Coelho et al. (2010); Copinschi (2005); Epstein and Brown (2010); Fogelberg et al. (2012, 2016, 2017); Irwin et al. (2008); Johnson and Johnson (2010); Jozwiak et al. (2017); Luyster et al. (2011); McCall et al. (2009); Ownby et al. (2010); Parcell et al. (2008); Redline (2009); Sixel-Döring et al. (2011); Spiegel et al. (2004, 2005); Watson (2010); as well as comprehensive sleep textbook by Kryger et al. (2011).

Health Habits and Behaviors

Exercise for both adults and children is sleep enhancing (Buxton et al., 2003; Passos et al., 2010; Youngstedt & Buxton, 2003; Figure 48.9). Ideally, it is undertaken several hours before sleep. Following evening exercise, at least 2 hours are thought to be required for the body temperature to cooldown into sleep; a tepid shower may speed the process.

Caffeine—as coffee, colas, or energy drinks—is very commonly used at "wake up" and to fight fatigue and sleepiness. Caffeine can be an asset when used judiciously. Individuals develop tolerance for caffeine, needing more and more to provide the same effect. Especially when used to fight the midafternoon energy decline, caffeine may delay night sleep onset and reduce deep sleep (Roehrs & Roth, 2008). Depending on the planned sleep schedule, it is often recommended that the last caffeine be no later than early afternoon. Caffeine withdrawal can produce headache, fatigue, and drowsiness.

Although tobacco has multiple well-known negative health impacts, it remains among the chosen substances individuals use to manage mood and energy. Smokers are more likely to report problems falling asleep and staying asleep and may experience decreased REM sleep as compared with nonsmokers. Increased arousals from sleep may be reported with smoking cessation efforts (Roehrs & Roth, 2011a).

Alcohol is used by some to help bring on sleep. In healthy adults, alcohol has an initial sedative effect, but later during the night, following completed metabolism of alcohol, a rebound effect may actually interfere with sleep. In addition to effects on sleep initiation and sleep maintenance, alcohol also can also affect the proportion of the various sleep stages, including suppressing REM sleep. There is some evidence that alcohol may behave differently in insomniacs. Many questions remain, including whether insomniacs develop tolerance to alcohol's sedative effects and then increase intake (Roehrs & Roth, 2011b). A new category of beverage is one that combines caffeine and alcohol. These drinks are thought to be dangerous because caffeine can produce a perception of wakefulness and mask insight into deficits caused by alcohol.

Numerous drugs, recreational, over-the-counter, and prescription medications, including marijuana, herbs, and "nutraceuticals," can impact sleep (Albert et al., 2017; Schweitzer, 2011). Chart review and careful history taking may identify these substances; information can be brought to the attention of the treating physician for review, including analysis of drug interactions and polypharmacy, the latter being especially common in the elderly (Frazier, 2005).

Stress and Occupational Balance

The ideal sleep–wake pattern dedicates sufficient time for uninterrupted sleep, is congruent with natural circadian clock rhythms, and is regular and consistent. Yet, compelling opportunities and requirements for night activity, as well as situational stressors, at times override sleep needs. For some, these reflect lifestyle choices and leisure pursuits, with the option for easy reversal to increased TIB. For others, it is a challenge to complete work, school, family caregiving, and home responsibilities within a schedule that leaves adequate time for self-care and sleep (Berkman et al., 2010; Bibbs, 2011; Luckhaupt et al., 2010). For example, an increasing number of mothers of young children have joined the workforce and may struggle to maintain occupational balance (Anaby et al., 2010). Technologies bring work into the home setting, even well after normal work hours, demanding immediate attention. Occupations such as nursing, medicine, and air traffic controller must be accomplished around the clock, requiring night shift work (Edlund, 2003; Levine et al., 2010; Nurok et al., 2010). Daytime sleep must then be undertaken against natural circadian rhythms. Travel to other time zones can disrupt natural sleep patterns, requiring alertness and high functioning during natural circadian sleep periods. This experience is colloquially known as jet lag (Youngstedt & Buxton, 2003). Finally, situations of grief, loss, and trauma, common in client populations that OT practitioners encounter, have ripple effects that can damage sleep.

OT Story 48.2 illustrates some of the difficulties clients and occupational therapists can encounter while addressing sleep and occupational performance. The reader is urged to

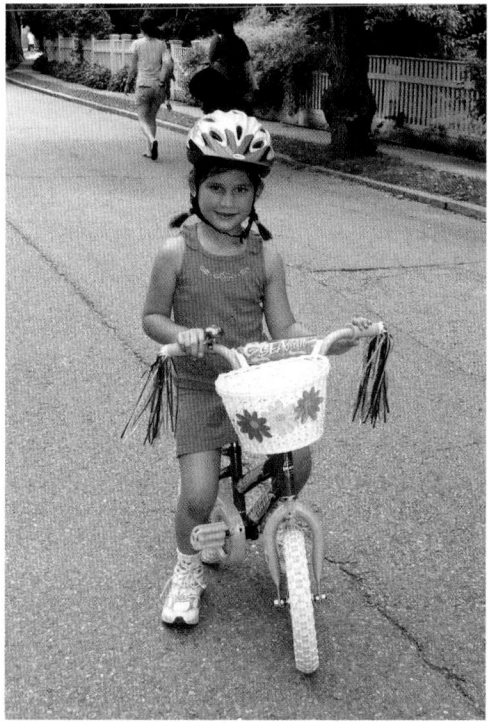

FIGURE 48.9 **Exercise enhances sleep.**

(Courtesy of Jo Solet, MS, EdM, PhD, OTR/L.)

OT STORY 48.2 MR. CHEVY

Stanley is an occupational therapist working in an outpatient facility. During evaluation of Mr. Chevy, a 58-year-old overweight truck driver with high blood pressure (partially controlled by medication), he notices the client falling asleep midmorning.

Upon questioning, Mr. Chevy admits he sometimes "feels himself falling asleep" even while driving, especially on long hauls at night. In answering some basic screening questions about his sleep schedule, sleep experience, and sleep environment, he mentions that his wife gets angry with him on nights when he sleeps at home because his snoring wakes her up repeatedly at night.

Mr. Chevy has been referred to occupational therapy by orthopedics for "energy conservation training and back school" to improve his driving comfort and lifting safety. He is afraid that any mention of sleep problems in his record could cause him to lose his job. He has just 2 years left before planned retirement. Mr. Chevy threatens to leave treatment entirely if Stanley will not agree to keep sleep problems off his record.

Questions

1. What should Stanley do in this situation?
2. What additional information should Stanley seek to help with his decision?
3. How might Stanley help educate Mr. Chevy about risks to himself and others?
4. Should Stanley reach out to Mrs. Chevy for help in supporting diagnosis or treatment?
5. Should Stanley make a referral for further assessment?

develop initial responses to the questions posed here and then to return to them after completing the chapter for discussion with colleagues.

Social Context

Eliciting the client's social context as part of the occupational profile and initial assessment can be particularly relevant with regard to sleep behaviors and occupational balance. For example, presleep stimulating computer use and video games and all-night texting are documented peer-driven sleep hazards for many young people (American College of Chest Physicians, 2010; Weaver et al., 2010). Developing and maintaining balance in an environment where this is far from the norm, such as in a college dormitory, can be difficult.

A social context of emotional isolation experienced as loneliness has been identified as an independent risk factor for sleep problems (Hawkley et al., 2010, 2011; McHugh & Lawlor, 2011). In addition, individuals who have little contact with others, owing to advanced age or disability, may have insufficient daily life structure. They may spend much of their TIB, napping on and off. Providing for daily activities and companionship, which are common goals of OT intervention, may help to consolidate and improve sleep.

Naps and Safe Management of Fatigue

Naps have historically been part of occupational balance in some cultures, especially in the heat of midday. Like exercise, planned napping can be integrated into daily routines to enhance health and well-being. Even brief naps can have restorative effects. However, misplaced or extended napping can interfere with daily activities, social integration, and night sleep (Leland et al., 2016). There are times when the OT practitioner may recommend napping to manage fatigue and to improve safety and alertness, especially in anticipation of night performance requirements, such as driving, infant care, or medical shift work.

Short naps of 20 to 30 minutes, or longer naps of a full sleep cycle, 90 minutes, are more likely to allow for awakening without significant sleep inertia (Mednick & Ehrman, 2006). The sleep stage content of the nap is thought to affect the resulting enhancements, with REM-containing naps shown to decrease negative emotional bias and amplify recognition of positive emotions (Gujar et al., 2010). When naps are required even after adequate TIB, it can be a signal that further assessment is required. Chronic illnesses such as multiple sclerosis (MS) may increase fatigue levels for extended periods (Stout & Finlayson, 2011); under these circumstances, it may be useful to schedule naps and rest periods into the daily routine. In cases of excessive daytime sleepiness, safety must be given the highest priority, including arrangements for alternative transportation rather than driving and extra attention given to fall and accident prevention.

Sleep Environments

Along with healthy sleep habits, an optimal sleep environment is a component of **sleep hygiene**. The ideal sleep environment is *quiet*, *dark*, *cool*, *comfortable*, *clean*, and *safe*. As part of a home visit or review of a long-term care facility, the occupational therapist helps to adapt and organize the sleep environment (Figure 48.10).

Numerous studies document the disruptive effects of noise on sleep (Basner et al., 2011; Buxton et al., 2012; Hume, 2011; Solet et al., 2010). Ensuring quiet includes blocking disturbances from within the room, home, or building. This may include simple solutions such as closing doors and soliciting family and partner (or roommate) commitments to limit noisy activities after an agreed on hour. Sometimes, external noise sources from the streetscape, such as truck deliveries and cycling air-handling equipment, disrupt sleep. Soothing sound and white noise machines or earplugs may be successful in blocking these disturbances. Be

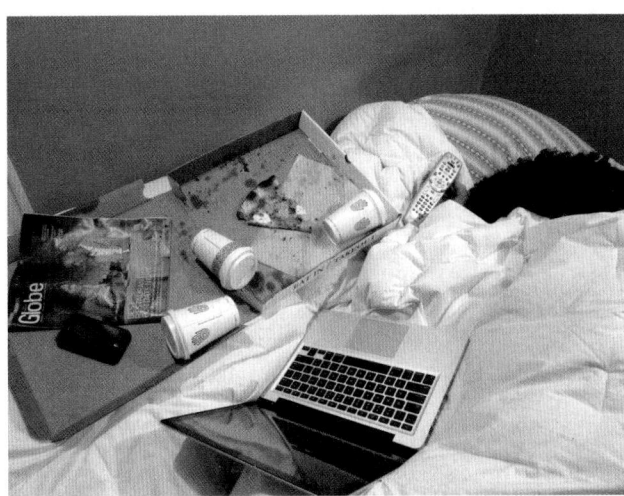

FIGURE 48.10 **Inappropriate environment for sleep.**

(Courtesy of Jo Solet, MS, EdM, PhD, OTR/L.)

sure smoke alarms, phone signals, and other emergency alerts can penetrate.

Some communities have noise ordinances that limit decibel levels, especially during night hours. Night noise, from airplane overflights and truck traffic, for example, may be quite prevalent in some communities. Many American cities have homeless populations, limited shelter beds, and people sleeping on the streets. Availability of a safe, quiet place for sleep is an occupational justice issue. According to Blakeney and Marshall (2009), occupational justice rests on two important principles: that "occupational participation is a determinant of health" and the "principle of empowerment through occupation" (p. 47). Sleep qualifies on both counts (see Chapter 10).

Ironically, some of the most difficult sleep environments are healthcare facilities, including critical care units (Busch-Vishniac et al., 2005; Dogan et al., 2005; Friese et al., 2007; Solet & Barach, 2012; Weinhouse & Schwab, 2006). Complaints of "noise around room" are among the most common in hospital quality-of-care surveys. In most states, since 2006, construction codes for new hospitals require single-bed patient rooms, preventing disturbance through roommates. Research demonstrating the sleep disruptive character of common hospital sounds has informed the most recent edition of *Design and Construction Guidelines for Healthcare Facilities*, which now includes acoustic guidelines for hospital rooms (Facility Guidelines Institute, 2010; Solet et al., 2010). Patient sleep disruption by hospital night staff led to the development of the Somerville Protocol, an evidence-based night routine solution that can be implemented by staff in healthcare settings to preserve patient sleep (Bartick et al., 2010).

Because light is naturally alerting, providing darkness in the sleep environment is also an important protector of sleep (Edlund, 2003). As the negative impacts of night lighting on sleep are being documented, community efforts to limit LED streetlights have become vigorous (Solet, 2016). Light sources within the room, such as bright digital clocks, should be dimmed or removed. The bedroom can be conditioned for sleep and sex, not meals, technology, and TV. Ideally, space allows the TV and computer to be placed elsewhere; screens including cellphones should be shut down well before sleep. This can be part of a consistent "wind-down period" with a relaxing presleep ritual, such as a bath and reading, or "story time" for children.

Night shift workers, who are at special risk because they sleep during daylight against natural circadian rhythms, are found to sleep more efficiently when true darkness is provided. Eye masks or "blackout" window shades may be useful in the effort to limit ambient light intrusion.

Body temperature drops as part of the sleep cycle. A cool bedroom is thus most conducive to sleep. Most people report the mid-to-high 60s as quite comfortable. Conflicts between bed partners over room temperature are legendary. For this and other reasons, partners sometimes do not sleep well next to each other. Mismatched sleep schedules or even specific disorders in one partner (e.g., excessive movement during sleep, use of equipment to normalize breathing) may disturb the sleep of the other. Splitting into individual beds in the same room may be sufficient to preserve sleep; separate rooms, if available, may serve to protect sleep and ultimately preserve relationships. "Visits" can be planned.

A significant percentage of Americans responding to the US census listed pets as family members. Pets are common bed partners. However, pets may have natural sleep cycles that are different from their owners', for example, becoming most active as the sun rises. Many people report that sleeping with their pets is a great comfort. This decision should be made in consideration of the degree of pet-induced sleep disruption and the individual's health status. A separate comfortable pet bed should be an option (Figure 48.11).

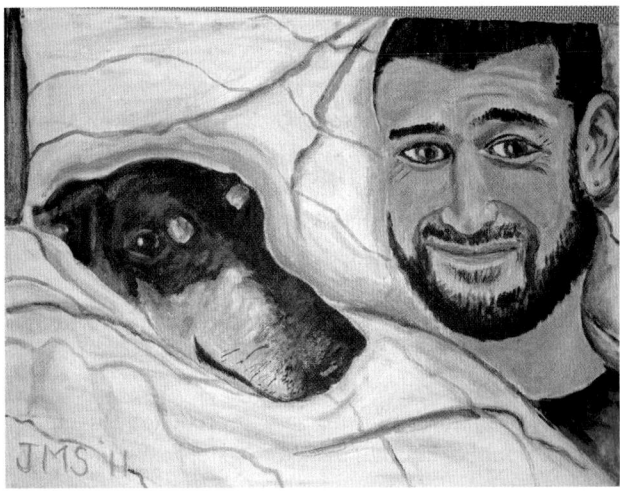

FIGURE 48.11 **Sleeping with a pet may be comforting yet at times may disrupt sleep.**

(Courtesy of Jo Solet, MS, EdM, PhD, OTR/L.)

A clean environment is especially important to those with allergies, who may experience breathing difficulties during sleep owing to accumulated allergens, such as pet hair. HEPA air-cleaning machines may be helpful. A clean environment is also safer, with clothes and other items off the floor. Any cord, equipment, or furniture that blocks the exit or the path to the bathroom should be relocated as part of fall prevention. Availability of a full set of fresh bedclothes should be ensured and a weekly room-cleaning schedule put in place.

Sleep Disorders

Patients may describe significant distress related to impairment in occupational and social functioning and yet have little insight that disordered sleep is driving their difficulties. Although making a diagnosis of a sleep disorder is outside the professional expertise of occupational therapists, it is important to be aware of the International Classification of Sleep Disorders (ICSD-2) (available for download) to have access to criteria and standards as resources and to recognize sleep disorders that are commonly diagnosed. The newest edition of the *Diagnostic and Statistical Manual of Mental Disorders* (*DSM-5*), published in 2013, offers a revised categorization of sleep disorders.

Sleep disorders can be understood through descriptions of the ways in which sleep is disturbed: inability to fall asleep, multiple awakenings, inability to fall back asleep, nonrestorative sleep, inadequate breathing during sleep (may be described as snoring and or gasping for breath), disruptive movements during sleep, nonsleep activities intruding into sleep, and mistimed or uncontrolled sleep. Although shortened sleep conveys health risks and decreases longevity, when sleep is disrupted and discontinuous, this impact is even greater.

Insomnias

The **insomnias** are defined by repeated problems of sleep initiation, duration, consolidation, or quality that occur despite adequate time and opportunity for sleep and result in some form of daytime impairment (Haynes, 2009; Passos et al., 2010; Roth et al., 2007; Vitiello et al., 2009). Using stringent criteria of sleep disturbance every night for 2 weeks or more, a consistent prevalence ranging between 9% and 17.7% of the adult population has been documented as affected (Ohayon, 2002). This translates into 30 to 40 million Americans. Historically, the insomnias have been organized into multiple subtypes with variable patterns at different phases of the life course: pediatric, pregnancy, menopause, and geriatric. Insomnia can be primary or **secondary insomnia** that is comorbid, at times related to pain, depression, posttraumatic stress disorder, and other medical conditions that should be identified and addressed in treatment planning.

Treatments may include use of the relaxation response such as meditation, progressive muscle relaxation, or biofeedback; cognitive behavioral therapy (especially addressing sleep-related anxieties and conditioning the bed for sleep only); improved sleep habits and environments; limits on caffeine and alcohol; and sometimes prescription medications.

Obstructive Sleep Apnea

Obstructive sleep apnea (OSA) is caused by partial or complete blockage of airway passages during sleep. Diagnosis typically follows from laboratory sleep testing, frequently after the individual's roommate or sleep partner has reported hearing "loud snoring" or "gasping for breath" during the night. The index of OSA severity, called the **apnea/hypopnea index (AHI)**, typically increases in untreated individuals with age and relates to the number of repeated awakenings per hour driven by decreased **oxygen saturation**. Awakenings may occur dozens or even hundreds of times a night; individuals may have no awareness, perhaps only reporting excessive daytime sleepiness. Morning headache is a common complaint (Vaughn & D'Cruz, 2011). Certain jaw, overbite, tongue and soft tissue proportions, and large neck girth as well as excessive weight are recognized as anatomic risk factors. OSA can be a serious disorder, depriving the brain of oxygen, leading to **hypertension**, metabolic changes, weight gain, diabetes, and cardiovascular disease (O'Connor et al., 2009; Peppard, 2009; Redline, 2009). Increased risks for dementia documented with OSA may be a result of retention of toxic metabolites, normally drained through increased interstitial space during adequate sleep (Xie et al., 2013). Excessive sleepiness also places these individuals, like others with serious sleep disorders, at increased risk for auto and industrial accidents (Tregear et al., 2009).

Treatments for OSA include use of a **continuous positive airway pressure (CPAP)** system that pushes air through the nose (Tomfohr et al., 2011), sleep positioning to side-lying, dental devices, corrective surgery (Verse & Hörmann, 2011), and weight loss to decrease obstructive tissue. CPAP "machines" now include technology to monitor their use. Some individuals find the masks inconvenient or uncomfortable or feel the devices negatively impact intimate relationships. The consequences of untreated chronic OSA can be severe; support for seeking a comfortable CPAP mask fit and reinforcing treatment adherence through continuous monitoring are valuable therapeutic interventions (Cooke et al., 2009).

See instructional video http://healthysleep.med.harvard.edu/sleep-apnea.

Restless Legs Syndrome and Periodic Limb Movement Disorder

Restless legs syndrome (RLS) is a sleep disorder in which there is an urge to move the legs in order to stop unpleasant leg sensations that may be described as "crawling" or "tingling." During sleep, involuntary leg movements can lead to awakenings and may occur repeatedly without being remembered (Bayard et al., 2008; Kushida, 2007). Risk factors include peripheral neuropathy, chronic kidney disease, iron deficiency, Parkinson disease, and side effects of certain medications; there is also higher prevalence among clients with a history of stroke (Coelho et al., 2010) and fibromyalgia (Viola-Saltzman et al., 2010). Genetic factors are implicated because certain families as well as populations, especially northern Europeans, show higher incidence. Some individuals experience movements without the sensations; upper extremities can also be involved. This is called **periodic limb movement disorder (PLMD).** Along with treatment of predisposing conditions, exercise, stretching, massage, and warm baths may provide some relief. In some cases, medications may be prescribed.

Parasomnias

Parasomnias are nonsleep behaviors that intrude during sleep. Sleepwalking and sleep-eating episodes can occur during deep sleep through partial awakening (Howell et al., 2009). Typically, individuals have no memory of these behaviors, which are reported to them by others or are discovered through evidence found in the morning. Sleepwalking is more common in children, who often outgrow the disorder. Organizing secure environments and alerting systems for parents or partners are practical safety measures.

Healthy REM sleep involves muscle paralysis (**atonia**). In **REM sleep behavior disorder (RBD)**, this paralysis fails and the individual moves, as if acting out a dream. Bed partners can be at risk of injury from these uncontrolled actions and may be the initiators of the search for diagnosis. Research demonstrates RBD may be a precursor to dementia or Parkinson disease (Sixel-Döring et al., 2011). When it does occur, RBD in Parkinson disease is associated with a more impaired cognitive profile and more severe and widespread neurodegeneration (Jozwiak et al., 2017).

Other parasomnias include **night terrors, rhythmic movement disorders in children, bruxism** (tooth grinding), and **confusional arousals** in adults. Secondary insomnia can result from an effort to block frightening parasomnia experiences by avoiding sleep.

Narcolepsy

Narcolepsy is characterized by an excessive uncontrollable daytime sleepiness even after adequate sleep at night. According to the National Institutes of Health, it is estimated to be as common as Parkinson disease or MS but is underdiagnosed. Experiences that affect some, but not all, narcoleptics include **cataplexy** (a sudden loss of muscle function ranging from weakness to full collapse, which may have an emotional trigger); inability to talk or move while falling asleep or waking up; and vivid, sometimes frightening, images in transition to sleep, called **hypnagogic hallucinations**. In narcolepsy, the architecture of

sleep is disturbed with REM rather than NREM occurring at sleep onset and REM experiences actually intruding into waking periods. The main treatments are lifestyle adaptations to maintain safety, central nervous system stimulants, and antidepressant or other medications that suppress REM sleep.

Additional Resources for Sleep Disorders

Readers are also encouraged to visit http://healthysleep.med.harvard.edu/healthy/getting/treatment/an-overview-of-sleep-disorders. This is a section of online resources provided by the Division of Sleep Medicine at Harvard Medical School in collaboration with the WGBH (public television) Educational Foundation.

The National Institutes of Health also offers valuable online sleep disorder information: https://www.nhlbi.nih.gov/science/sleep-science-and-sleep-disorders.

National Sleep Foundation can be found at http://www.sleepfoundation.org/articles/sleep-disorders.

Also see the comprehensive text: Kryger, M. H., Roth, T., & Dement, W. C. (Eds.). (2016). *Principles and practice of sleep medicine* (6th ed.). Elsevier Saunders.

Sleep Screening and Referral

Because the majority of medical and psychiatric disorders treated by occupational therapists may affect or be affected by sleep and because sleep disorders are so common, brief sleep screening as part of initial OT assessment is valuable (Zee & Turek, 2006). The attuned occupational therapist will be alert to a history or current report of excessive daytime sleepiness and will probe for the degree to which sleep is experienced as nonrestorative and the extent to which daytime activities may be impaired. Some clients will report functional problems without recognizing any link to their sleep difficulties. Others, despite complaints of excessive sleepiness, may have little insight even into multiple night arousals, for example, owing to OSA or RLS. Bed partners or family members of clients may be resources for supplying additional details and documentation, especially women (Umberson, 1992). As always, to protect privacy, clients' permission must be sought before these discussions.

Sleep History and Self-Reports

Standardized client self-report questionnaires, such as the Epworth Sleepiness Scale, supplement the occupational profile and may be useful for screening and for tracking effectiveness of certain treatments (Box 48.2; Johns, 1991). Many clinical settings make available preferred tools for sleep

BOX 48.2 EPWORTH SLEEPINESS SCALE

The Epworth Sleepiness Scale is used to determine the level of daytime sleepiness. A score of 10 or more is considered sleepy.

Use the following scale to choose the most appropriate number for each situation:

0 = would *never* doze or sleep
1 = *slight* chance of dozing or sleeping
2 = *moderate* chance of dozing or sleeping
3 = *high* chance of dozing or sleeping

Situations: Chance of Dozing or Sleeping

1. Sitting and reading _____
2. Watching TV _____
3. Sitting inactive in a public place _____
4. Being a passenger in a motor vehicle for an hour or more _____
5. Lying down in the afternoon _____
6. Sitting and talking to someone _____
7. Sitting quietly after lunch (no alcohol) _____
8. Stopped for a few minutes in traffic while driving _____

Total (add the scores up) _____

Johns, M. W. (1991). A new method for measuring daytime sleepiness: The Epworth Sleepiness Scale. *Sleep, 14*, 540–545. https://doi.org/10.1093/sleep/14.6.540

---

screening that have been validated for the specific treated population, such as school-aged children (Owens, Spirito, & McGuinn, 2000; Owens, Spirito, McGuinn, & Nobile, 2000).

When clients complain of *excessive daytime sleepiness*, a **sleep diary** or a wrist-worn sleep-monitoring device, showing sleep timing and perceived refreshment, can be useful in collaborating to gain a picture defining sleep patterns (Figure 48.12). **Sleep inertia** is the normal period at awakening in which full alertness is not yet achieved. Diary rating of sleep should be completed after the individual is fully awake and through this transition period.

When diary or device results confirm insufficient TIB or an erratic schedule, a critical OT sleep education and treatment goal is to evoke a cognitive shift: away from perceiving limited sleep as "no problem," "heroic," or "efficient," toward perceiving it as "a drain on well-being and performance," "an unwise health risk," or "a factor complicating recovery." Individuals suffering from certain medical, psychiatric, or sleep disorders can be doubly challenged and their health risks raised further by poor sleep habits. This cognitive shift initiates readiness for a program to include sleep as a priority. The occupational therapist helps clients develop strategies to incorporate energy conservation and fatigue management techniques to cope with the extra demands associated with these conditions.

Recent research suggests that sleep symptoms are common but are not routinely screened for in primary care settings (Haponik et al., 1996; Senthilvel et al., 2011; Sorscher, 2008). Although efforts are underway to enhance medical attention to sleep, an OT encounter could include the first sleep screening a client receives. Referral for follow-up, potentially including a home or laboratory sleep study, may be made to neurology, pulmonology, psychiatry, occupational health, or directly to sleep medicine, depending on comorbid diagnosis, potential severity, and available resources.

As part of the referral process and in follow-up team meetings, the occupational therapist takes the opportunity to make colleagues aware of his or her tools for addressing sleep problems and documents sleep interventions in care notes.

Sleep Evaluation

The technology used for sleep evaluation is evolving toward more complete home testing. **Actigraphy** is a wristband-mounted accelerometer system that records periods of motion during sleep and indicates sleep latency, arousals, and time of awakening (Sadeh, 2011; Sánchez-Ortuño et al., 2010). Actigraphy systems for personal use can now be run through downloadable apps for smartphones. Consumer/home sleep-tracking devices paired with smartphone apps can provide a more accurate picture of sleep than diary recording alone.

Polysomnography is comprehensive testing that includes three simultaneously recorded parts: the EEG, which traces brain wave activity through scalp electrodes, recording differing frequencies identified as alpha, beta, delta, and theta rhythms; **electrooculograms,** which measure eye movements through electrodes placed on the skin around the eyes; and **electromyograms,** which measure motor activity through electrodes placed on the skin over muscles. As part of sleep evaluation, sensors may be used to track breathing and oxygen saturation in the blood. Video recordings are used for monitoring client positioning and movements during sleep, especially as coordinated with other readouts. Sleep stages (REM and NREM1, NREM2, and NREM3) have specific "fingerprints" based on brain activity and coordinated muscle and eye movements. Certain sleep disorders are more likely to occur during specific stages. Furthermore, alterations in architecture of sleep, as shown in the hypnogram, can be produced by environmental or medical conditions. Standardized scoring criteria are applied to analyze these recordings to identify stages, arousals, and anomalies supporting diagnoses (Chervin, 2010).

SLEEP HEALTHCENTERS®
...better sleep. better health.

SLEEP DIARY

NAME: ____________________

WEEK OF: ____________________

Day	Duration of Naps (minutes)	Bedtime	Time to Fall Asleep (minutes)	Number of Awakenings	Duration of Awakenings (minutes)	Final Waketime	Out of Bed Time	Time Spent Asleep (hours)	Medications Taken	Next Day Alertness 1-10 (10=most alert)
Monday										
Tuesday										
Wednesday										
Thursday										
Friday										
Saturday										
Sunday										

- Please begin to complete the sleep diary on a daily basis. It will provide a subjective tracking of your sleep schedule for you and your sleep clinician to use as you work together to improve your sleep.
- Do not look at the clock to complete this form. You should complete this diary each morning with respect to your previous night of sleep. Do not complete it during the night or keep it in your bedroom.
- Use it only as a guideline and spend no more than 30 seconds filling it out in the morning.

BSM-DIRY-0002_1 Reviewed 3/05/10

FIGURE 48.12 Sleep diary.

(Source: Reprinted with permission from Sleep HealthCenters, LLC: http://www.sleephealth.com.)

Summary: Sleep and Occupational Therapy Interventions

Occupational therapy interventions to improve sleep and manage fatigue are based in client education, self-care and health habits, occupational balance, and optimal environments (see OT Story 48.3). As part of the continuum of care provided by occupational therapists, sleep-enhancing interventions may be adapted for primary prevention and health promotion, such as work-based and school wellness programs (Beebe et al., 2010; Gangwisch et al., 2005, 2010; Quan et al., 2010); may address sleep problems related to aging, injury, illness, or disability; and may contribute to treatments directed specifically at sleep disorders. School and work wellness programs focus on life cycle sleep requirements and schedules, health habits and behaviors that influence sleep, and adequate sleep environments.

Occupational therapy treatments for common medical conditions and psychiatric disorders, many of which carry comorbid sleep difficulties, may be directed toward pain, anxiety, depression, limited mobility, poor self-care, respiratory compromise, substance abuse, insufficient resources, and/or social isolation. Broad components of treatment for these clients, which may also improve comorbid sleep difficulties, include (but are not limited to) cognitive behavioral therapy, relaxation response, graded exercise, activities to increase social integration, and resources for safety (Solet, 2014). Improvement in any of these complaint areas can also be expected to improve sleep; the effects are reciprocal (Zee & Turek, 2006).

Treatment components directed specifically at sleep either as a primary problem or a comorbidity include reinforcing consistent sleep schedules, sufficient TIB, conditioning bed for sleep only, and sleep environment modifications: quiet, dark, cool, safe, and clean. Sleep interventions also target related health habits including use of caffeine, alcohol, tobacco, or other substances; exercise; and support for treatment adherence such as use of CPAP equipment and weight-loss programs (Barnes et al., 2009).

OT STORY 48.3 ALBERTA

Alberta is a 15-year-old private high school student who complains of "being so tired." Although she showed early academic ability, the high school "scene" has posed increasing problems. She is 5 ft 9 in, 170 lb, and her athletic activities are restricted owing to asthma, which she has suffered since early childhood. She recently had an experience of social network bullying, which left her isolated from and unable to trust her female classmates. Her strong interest in math and science has allowed her to forge some friendships with boys in the class. Her mother has described her as "depressed." Alberta has been referred to a group private OT practice by her long-time pediatrician for help with "fatigue, fitness, and fitting in."

Questions

1. What information should Alberta's OT seek from the pediatrician?
2. Describe components of a first OT meeting with Alberta?
3. What could be helpful in establishing rapport?
4. What screening and assessments might shed light on her fatigue?
5. Could bullying and isolation affect adolescent sleep?
6. Through what mechanisms might sleep affect fitness, mood?
7. Suggest possible components for an OT treatment program to improve adolescent self-care and sleep.

Although the primary focus of this chapter is sleep, occupational balance encompasses both patterns and cycles of activity, including periods of rest. Yoga, meditation, and other spiritual or relaxation practices, especially when undertaken consistently, may not only improve sleep by lowering autonomic arousal and bringing mindful attention to the present but also have important independent adaptive and restorative qualities (Benson & Proctor, 2010; Solet, 2014). In *The Power of Rest*, Dr. Matthew Edlund (2010) offers an accessible, comprehensive review of the benefits of rest, including through music and companionship.

Conclusion

Sleep medicine is a new frontier, an opportunity to enhance health, safety, well-being, performance, and even longevity. As occupational therapists, our unique perspective on daily living, together with the relationships we enjoy with our clients and colleagues, puts us in a unique position to contribute to this dynamic area of science and healthcare.

As part of your professional commitment, improve sleep awareness, evaluation, and treatment and sleep well!

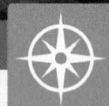

EXPANDING OUR PERSPECTIVES

Sleep Quality in the 21st Century

Clover Hutchinson

Sleep is an occupation that is often taken for granted, yet it is a biological necessity for all living creatures. Although sleep is essential, global capitalism has shattered the concept of rest and restful sleep. We are available twenty-four hours a day and seven days a week granting access at all times of the day and night, infringing on sleep. Human beings spend a third of their lifetime sleeping, making it a prerequisite to daily functioning. Getting adequate amount of rest is associated with good health and well-being. Sleep deprivation and common sleep problems have been linked to various health problems, such as obesity, diabetes, hypertension, stroke, and mortality. Additionally, it may cross other variables such as life span, culture, and gender, and needs to be further explored to gain a deeper understanding of the phenomenon of sleep.

Current research explores sleep within the lens of occupational routines. Sleep health and sleep disorders are not equitably distributed across racial and ethnic groups owing to a lack of research on additional factors such as environment, family structure, socioeconomic class, and social cohesion. Considering a person's income, education, and access to healthcare can influence their disease profile, their overall health, and risk of mortality related to sleep. Sleep impairment across various racial and ethnic groups may be challenging to interpret; however, understanding these factors is vital to understanding sleep. Sleep is a vital component of restorative sleep.

Restorative sleep influences physical, mental, and spiritual well-being. Sleep is not often given priority and is viewed as an expendable luxury. Globally, many individuals face challenges with migration, insecurities in housing, food, and work, which affect their ability to engage in the meaningful occupation of sleep. Now, with the COVID-19 pandemic and its restrictions, for example, working from home has disrupted the relationship between social and biological sleep–wake timing. Consequently, owing to work from home coupled with a possible false perception of flexibility and availability, it is not a surprise that overall sleep quality for many has been reduced. Having a solid understanding of all the factors that may affect sleep can aid healthcare practitioners, including occupational therapists, provide a holistic guide to total health and well-being.

Resources for More Information About Sleep and Rest

Websites

Centers for Disease Control and Prevention: http://www.cdc.gov/sleep/

Center for Health Design: http://www.healthdesign.org/chd/research/validating-acoustic-guidelines-healthcare-facilities

Harvard Medical School, Division of Sleep Medicine: http://healthysleep.med.harvard.edu/portal/; Section on Sleep Disorders: http://healthysleep.med.harvard.edu/healthy/getting/treatment/an-overview-of-sleep-disorders

International Network for Occupational Therapists Interested in Sleep: http://www.sleepOT.org (new resource to empower OT practitioners, students, and researchers to consider, identify, and address sleep and sleep problems)

National Institute of Alcohol Abuse and Alcoholism: http://www.niaaa.nih.gov/

National Sleep Foundation Sleep in America Polls: http://www.sleepfoundation.org/category/article-type/sleep-america-polls

National Sleep Foundation: http://www.sleepfoundation.org/articles/sleep-disorders

YMCA: http://www.ymca.net/healthy-family-home/sleep-well.html

Additional Resources

American Academy of Sleep Medicine: http://www.aasmnet.org

Journal of Clinical Sleep Medicine: http://www.aasmnet.org/JCSM

Sleep Centers: http://www.sleepcenters.org

SLEEP: http://www.journalsleep.org

Acknowledgments

I would like to thank the patients who have been my teachers for the more than 40 years I have been an occupational therapist as well as Jenny Lee Olsen, former director of Library Services at Cambridge Health Alliance, for help in the literature search, the chapter peer reviewers for their careful attention and thoughtful comments, and the editors for offering me the opportunity to contribute this chapter on sleep, an important emerging area of practice.

Lippincott® Connect *For additional resources on the subjects discussed in this chapter, visit Lippincott Connect.*

REFERENCES

Albert, S. M., Roth, T., Toscani, M., Vitiello, M. V., & Zee, P. (2017). Sleep health and appropriate use of OTC sleep aids in older adults. *The Gerontologist, 57*, 163–170. https://doi.org/10.1093/geront/gnv139

American Academy of Sleep Medicine. (2009). *Naps with rapid eye movement sleep increase receptiveness to positive emotion.* http://www.aasmnet.org/articles.aspx?id=1317

American College of Chest Physicians. (2010, November). *Electronic media taking its toll on teens.* Paper presented at the 76th CHEST Annual Meeting of American College of Chest Physicians, Vancouver, Canada. http://www.chestnet.org/accp/article/electronic-media-taking-its-toll-teens

American Occupational Therapy Association. (2020). Occupational therapy practice framework: Domain and process (4th ed.). *American Journal of Occupational Therapy, 74*(Suppl. 2), 7412410010. https://doi.org/10.5014/ajot.2020.74S2001

Anaby, D. R., Backman, C. L., & Jarus, T. (2010). Measuring occupational balance: Theoretical exploration of two approaches to occupational balance. *Canadian Journal of Occupational Therapy, 77*, 280–288. https://doi.org/10.2182/cjot.2010.77.5.4

Ancoli-Israel, S., & Cooke, J. R. (2005). Prevalence and comorbidity of insomnia and effect on functioning in elderly populations. *Journal of the American Geriatrics Society, 53*, S264–S271. https://doi.org/10.1111/j.1532-5415.2005.53392.x

Ayas, N. T. (2010). If you weigh too much, maybe you should try sleeping more. *Sleep, 33*, 143–144. https://doi.org/10.1093/sleep/33.2.143

Ayas, N. T., White, D. P., Al-Delaimy, W. K., Manson, J. E., Stampfer, M. J., Speizer, F. E., & Hu, F. B. (2003). A prospective study of self-reported sleep duration and incipient diabetes in women. *Diabetes Care, 26*, 380–384. https://doi.org/10.2337/diacare.26.2.380

Ayas, N. T., White, D. P., Manson, J. E., Stampfer, M. J., Speizer, F. E., Malhotra, A., & Hu, F. B. (2003). A prospective study of sleep duration and coronary heart disease in women. *Archives of Internal Medicine, 163*, 205–209. https://doi.org/10.1001/archinte.163.2.205

Banks, S., Van Dongen, H. P., Mailsen, G., & Dinges, D. F. (2010). Neurobehavioral dynamics following chronic sleep restriction: Dose-response effects of one night for recovery. *Sleep, 33*, 1013–1026. https://doi.org/10.1093/sleep/33.8.1013

Barnes, M., Goldsworthy, U. R., Cary, B. A., & Hill, C. J. (2009). A diet and exercise program to improve clinical outcomes on patients with obstructive sleep apnea—A feasibility study. *Journal of Clinical Sleep Medicine, 5*, 409–421. https://doi.org/10.5664/jcsm.27594

Bartick, M. C., Thai, X., Schmidt, T., Altaye, A., & Solet, J. M. (2010). Decrease in as needed sedative use by limiting nighttime sleep disruptions from hospital staff. *Journal of Hospital Medicine, 5*, E20–E24. https://doi.org/10.1002/jhm.549

Basner, M., Fomberstein, K. M., Razavi, F. M., Banks, S., William, J. H., Rosa, R. R., & Dinges, D. F. (2007). American time use survey: Sleep time and its relationship to waking activities. *Sleep, 30*, 1085–1095. https://doi.org/10.1093/sleep/30.9.1085

Basner, M., Müller, U., & Elmenhorst, E. M. (2011). Single and combined effects of air, road, and rail traffic noise on sleep and recuperation. *Sleep, 34*, 11–23. https://doi.org/10.1093/sleep/34.1.11

Bayard, M., Avonda, T., & Wadzinski, J. (2008). Restless legs syndrome. *American Family Physician, 78*, 235–240. https://doi.org/10.1177/1755738019876672

Beebe, D. W., Ris, D. M., Kramer, M. E., Long, E., & Amin, R. (2010). The association between sleep disordered breathing, academic grades, and cognitive and behavioral functioning among overweight subjects during middle to late childhood. *Sleep, 33*, 1447–1457. https://doi.org/10.1093/sleep/33.11.1447

Benson, H., & Proctor, W. (2010). *Relaxation revolution: Enhancing your personal health through the science and genetics of mind body healing.* Scribner.

Berkman, L. F., Buxton, O., Ertel, K., & Okechukwu, C. (2010). Managers' practices related to work-family balance predict employee cardiovascular risk and sleep duration in extended care settings. *Journal of Occupational Health Psychology, 15*, 316–329. https://doi.org/10.1037/a0019721

Bibbs, M. (2011). A wake up call to sleepy workers. *Sleep Diagnosis and Therapy, 6*, 14. https://www.headpaininstitute.com/lack-of-sleep-can-be-deadly/

Blakeney, A., & Marshall, A. (2009). Water quality, health, and human occupations. *American Journal of Occupational Therapy, 63*, 46–57. https://doi.org/10.5014/ajot.63.1.46

Bondoc, S., & Siebert, C. (2008). *The role of occupational therapy in chronic disease management.* American Occupational Therapy Association.

Braley, T. J., & Chervin, R. D. (2010). Fatigue in multiple sclerosis: Mechanisms, evaluation, and treatment. *Sleep, 33*, 1061–1067. https://doi.org/10.1093/sleep/33.8.1061

Brendel, D. H., Florman, J., Roberts, S., & Solet, J. M. (2001). "In sleep I almost never grope": Blindness, neuropsychiatric deficits, and a chaotic upbringing. *Harvard Review of Psychiatry, 9*, 178–188.

Brown, C. A., Berry, R., Tan, M. C., Khoshia, A., Turlapati, L., & Swedlove, F. (2011). A critique of the evidence-base for non-pharmacological sleep interventions for persons with dementia. *Dementia, 12*, 174–201. https://doi.org/10.1177/1471301211426909

Burton, A. R., Rahman, K., Kadota, Y., Lloyd, A., & Vollmer-Conna, U. (2010). Reduced heart rate variability predicts poor sleep quality in a case-control study of chronic fatigue syndrome. *Experimental Brain Research, 204*, 71–78. https://doi.org/10.1007/s00221-010-2296-1

Busch-Vishniac, I. J., West, J. E., Barnhill, C., Hunter, T., Orellana, D., & Chivukula, R. (2005). Noise levels in Johns Hopkins Hospital. *The Journal of the Acoustical Society of America, 118*, 3629–3645. https://doi.org/10.1121/1.2118327

Buxton, O. M., Ellenbogen, J. M., Wang, W., Carballeira, A., O'Connor, S., Cooper, D., Gordhandas, A.J., McKinney, S.M. & Solet, J. M. (2012). Sleep disruption due to hospital noises: A prospective evaluation. *Annals of Internal Medicine, 157*, 170–179. https://doi.org/10.7326/0003-4819-157-3-201208070-00472

Buxton, O. M., Lee, C. W., L'Hermite-Baleriaux, M., Turek, F. W., & Van Cauter, E. (2003). Exercise elicits phase shifts and acute alterations of melatonin that vary with circadian phase. *American Journal of Physiology. Regulatory, Integrative and Comparative Physiology, 284*, R714–R724. https://doi.org/10.1152/ajpregu.00355.2002

Buxton, O. M., & Marcelli, E. (2010). Short and long sleep are positively associated with obesity, diabetes, hypertension, and cardiovascular disease among adults in the United States. *Social Science and Medicine, 71*, 1027–1036. https://doi.org/10.1016/j.socscimed.2010.05.041

Chandola, T., Ferrie, J. E., Perski, A., Akbaraly, T., & Marmot, M. G. (2010). The effect of short sleep duration on coronary heart disease risk is greatest among those with sleep disturbance: A prospective study from Whitehall II cohort. *Sleep, 33*, 739–744. https://doi.org/10.1093/sleep/33.6.739

Chervin, R. D. (2010). Use of clinical tools and tests in sleep medicine. In M. H. Kryger, T. Roth, & W. C. Dement (Eds.), *Principles and practice of sleep medicine* (5th ed., pp. 666–679). Elsevier Saunders.

Chhangani, B. S., Roehrs, T. A., Harris, E. J., Hyde, M., Drake, C., Hudgel, D. W., & Roth, T. (2009). Pain sensitivity in sleepy pain-free normals. *Sleep, 32*, 1011–1017.

Choi, S. W., Peek-Asa, C., Sprince, N. L., Rautiainen, R. H., Flamme, G. A., Whitten, P. S., & Zwerling, C. (2006). Sleep quantity and quality as a predictor of injuries in a rural population. *American Journal of Emergency Medicine, 24*, 189–196. https://doi.org/10.1016/j.ajem.2005.09.002

Classen, S., Levy, C., Meyer, D. L., Bewernitz, M., Lanford, D. N., & Mann, W. C. (2011). Simulated driving performance of combat veterans with mild traumatic brain injury and posttraumatic stress disorder: A pilot study. *American Journal of Occupational Therapy, 65*, 419–427. https://doi.org/10.5014/ajot.2011.000893

Coelho, F. M., Georgsson, H., Narayansingh, M., Swartz, R. H., & Murray, B. J. (2010). Higher prevalence of periodic limb movements of sleep in patients with history of stroke. *Journal of Clinical Sleep Medicine, 6*, 428–430. https://doi.org/10.5664/jcsm.27930

Cohen, D. A., Wang, W., Wyatt, J. K., Kronauer, R. E., Dijk, D. J., Czeisler, C. A., & Klerman, E. B. (2010). Uncovering residual effects of chronic sleep loss on human performance. *Science Translational Medicine, 2*, 14ra3. https://doi.org/10.1126/scitranslmed.3000458

Connor, J., Norton, R., Ameratunga, S., Robinson, E., Civil, I., Dunn, R., Bailey, J., & Jackson, R. (2002). Driver sleepiness and risk of serious injury to car occupants: Population-based case control study. *BMJ, 324*, 1125. https://doi.org/10.1136/bmj.324.7346.1125

Cooke, J. R., Ayalon, L., Palmer, B. W., Loredo, J. S., Corey-Bloom, J., Natarajan, L., Liu, L., & Ancoli-Israel, S. (2009). Sustained use of CPAP slows deterioration of cognition, sleep, and mood in patients with Alzheimer's disease and obstructive sleep apnea: A preliminary study. *Journal of Clinical Sleep Medicine, 5*, 305–309. https://doi.org/10.5664/jcsm.27538

Copinschi, G. (2005). Metabolic and endocrine effects of sleep deprivation. *Essentials of Psychopharmacology, 6*, 341–347.

Dogan, O., Ertekin, S., & Dogan, S. (2005). Sleep quality in hospitalized patients. *Journal of Clinical Nursing, 14*, 107–113. http://dx.doi.org/10.1111/j.1365-2702.2004.01011.x

Dorrian, J., Sweeney, M., & Dawson, D. (2011). Modeling fatigue-related truck accidents: Prior sleep duration, recency and continuity. *Sleep and Biological Rhythms, 9*, 3–11. https://doi.org/10.1111/j.1479-8425.2010.00477.x

Drake, C., Roehrs, T., Breslau, N., Johnson, E., Jefferson, C., Scofield, H., & Roth, T. (2010). The 10-year risk of verified motor vehicle crashes in relation to physiologic sleepiness. *Sleep, 33*, 745–752. https://doi.org/10.1093/sleep/33.6.745

Durmer, J. S., & Dinges, D. F. (2005). Neurocognitive consequences of sleep deprivation. *Seminars in Neurology, 25*, 117–129. https://doi.org/10.1055/s-0029-1237117

Edlund, M. (2003). *The body clock advantage: Finding your best time to succeed in love, work, play, and exercise.* Adams Media.

Edlund, M. (2010). *The power of rest: Why sleep alone is not enough. A 30-day plan to reset your body.* HarperOne.

Epstein, J. E., & Brown, R. (2010). Sleep disorders in spinal cord injury. In V. W. Lin (Ed.), *Spinal cord medicine: Principles and practice* (2nd ed., pp. 230–240). Demos.

Facility Guidelines Institute. (2010). *Guidelines for design and construction of health care facilities—2010 edition.* American Hospital Association Services.

Flier, J. S., & Elmquist, J. K. (2004). A good night's sleep: Future antidote to the obesity epidemic? *Annals of Internal Medicine, 141*, 885–886. https://doi.org/10.7326/0003-4819-141-11-200412070-00014

Fogelberg, D. J., Hoffman, J. M., Dikmen, S., Temkin, N. R., & Bell, K. R. (2012). Association of sleep and co-occurring psychological conditions at 1 year after traumatic head injury. *Archives of Physical Medicine Rehabilitation, 93*, 1313–1318. https://doi.org/10.1016/j.apmr.2012.04.031

Fogelberg, D. J., Hughes, A. B., Vitiello, M. V., Hoffman, J. M., & Amtmann, D. (2016). Comparison of sleep problems in individuals with spinal cord injury and multiple sclerosis. *Journal of Clinical Sleep Medicine, 12*, 695–701. https://doi.org/10.5664/jcsm.5798

Fogelberg, D. J., Leland, N. E., Blanchard, J., Rich, T. J., & Clark, F. A. (2017). Qualitative experience of sleep in individuals with spinal cord injury. *OTJR: Occupation, Participation and Health, 37*, 89–97. https://doi.org/10.1177/1539449217691978

Frazier, S. C. (2005). Health outcomes and polypharmacy in elderly individuals: An integrated literature review. *Journal of Gerontological Nursing, 31*, 4–11. https://doi.org/10.3928/0098-9134-20050901-04

Friese, R. S., Diaz-Arrastia, R., McBride, D., Frankel, H., & Gentilello, L. M. (2007). Quantity and quality of sleep in the surgical intensive care unit: Are our patients sleeping? *The Journal of Trauma, 63*, 1210–1214. https://doi.org/10.1097/TA.0b013e31815b83d7

Gangwisch, J. E., Babiss, L. A., Malaspina, D., Turner, B., Zammit, G. K., & Posner, K. (2010). Earlier parental set bedtimes as a protective factor against depression and suicidal ideation. *Sleep, 33,* 97–106. https://doi.org/10.1093/sleep/33.1.97

Gangwisch, J. E., Malaspina, D., Boden-Albala, B., & Heymsfield, S. B. (2005). Inadequate sleep as a risk factor for obesity: Analyses of the NHANES I. *Sleep, 28,* 1289–1296. https://doi.org/10.1093/sleep/28.10.1289

Gujar, N., McDonald, S. A., Nishida, M., & Walker, M. P. (2010). A role for REM sleep in recalibrating the sensitivity of the human brain to specific emotions. *Cerebral Cortex, 21,* 115–123. https://doi.org/10.1093/cercor/bhq064

Haack, G., & Mullington, J. M. (2005). Sustained sleep restriction reduces emotional and physical well-being. *Pain, 119,* 56–64. https://doi.org/10.1016/j.pain.2005.09.011

Hale, L. (2005). Who has time to sleep? *Journal of Public Health, 27,* 205–211. https://doi.org/10.1093/pubmed/fdi004

Hale, L., & Do, D. P. (2007). Racial differences in self-reports of sleep duration in a population-based study. *Sleep, 30,* 1096–1103. https://doi.org/10.1093/sleep/30.9.1096

Hamilton, N. A., Catley, D., & Karlson, C. (2007). Sleep and affective response to stress and pain. *Health Psychology, 26,* 288–295. https://doi.org/10.1037/0278-6133.26.3.288

Haponik, E. F., Frye, A. W., Richards, B., Wymer, A., Hinds, A., Pearce, K., McCall, J., & Konen, J. (1996). Sleep history is neglected diagnostic information. Challenges for primary care physicians. *Journal of General Internal Medicine, 11,* 759–761. https://doi.org/10.1007/BF02598994

Hawkley, L. C., Cacioppo, J. T., & Preacher, K. J. (2011). As we said, loneliness (not living alone) explains individual differences in sleep quality: Reply. *Health Psychology, 30,* 136. https://doi.org/10.1037/a0022366

Hawkley, L. C., Preacher, K. J., & Cacioppo, J. T. (2010). Loneliness impairs daytime functioning but not sleep duration. *Health Psychology, 29,* 124–129. https://doi.org/10.1037/a0018646

Haynes, P. L. (2009). Is CBT-I effective for pain? *Journal of Clinical Sleep Medicine, 5,* 363–364. https://doi.org/10.5664/jcsm.27548

Hobson, J. A. (2011). *Dream life: An experimental memoir.* MIT Press.

Howell, M. J., Schenck, C. H., & Crow, S. J. (2009). A review of night-time eating disorders. *Sleep Medicine Reviews, 13,* 23–34. https://doi.org/10.1016/j.smrv.2008.07.005

Hume, K. I. (2011). Noise pollution: A ubiquitous unrecognized disruptor of sleep? *Sleep, 34,* 7–8. https://doi.org/10.1093/sleep/34.1.7

Irwin, M. R., Wang, M., Ribeiro, D., Cho, H. J., Olmstead, R., Breen, E. C., Martinez-Maza, O., & Cole, S. (2008). Sleep loss activates cellular inflammatory signaling. *Biological Psychiatry, 64,* 538–554. https://doi.org/10.1016/j.biopsych.2008.05.004

Johns, M. W. (1991). A new method for measuring daytime sleepiness: The Epworth Sleepiness Scale. *Sleep, 14,* 540–545. https://doi.org/10.1093/sleep/14.6.540

Johnson, K. G., & Johnson, C. D. (2010). Frequency of sleep apnea in stroke and TIA patients: A meta-analysis. *Journal of Clinical Sleep Medicine, 6,* 131–137. https://doi.org/10.5664/jcsm.27760

Jozwiak, N., Postuma, R. B., Montplaisir, J., Latreille, V., Panisset, M., Chouinard, S., Bourgouin, P. A., & Gagnon, J. F. (2017). REM sleep behavior disorder and cognitive impairment in Parkinson's disease. *Sleep, 40,* zsx101. https://doi.org/10.1093/sleep/zsx101

Kim, H., & Young, T. (2005). Subjective daytime sleepiness: Dimensions and correlates in the general population. *Sleep, 28,* 625–634. https://doi.org/10.1093/sleep/28.5.625

Kristiansen, J., Perrson, R., Björk, J., Albin, M., Jakobsson, K., Ostergren, P. O., & Ardö, J. (2011). Work stress, worries, and pain intersect synergistically with modeled traffic noise on cross-sectional associations with self-reported sleep problems. *International Archives of Occupational and Environmental Health, 84,* 211–224. https://doi.org/10.1007/s00420-010-0557-8

Kryger, M. H., Roth, T., & Dement, W. C. (Eds.). (2011). *Principles and practice of sleep medicine* (5th ed.). Elsevier Saunders.

Kushida, C. A. (2007). Clinical presentation, diagnosis, and quality of life issues in restless legs syndrome. *American Journal of Medicine, 120,* S4–S12. https://doi.org/10.1016/j.amjmed.2006.11.002

Leland, N. E., Fogelberg, D., Sleight, A., Mallinson, T., Vigen, C., Blanchard, J., Carlson, M., & Clark, F. (2016). Napping and nighttime sleep: Findings from an occupation-based intervention. *American Journal of Occupational Therapy, 70,* 7004270010p1–7004270010p7. https://doi.org/10.5014/ajot.2016.017657

Leland, N. E., Marcione, N., Schepens, S. L., Kelkar, K., & Fogelberg, D. (2014). What is occupational therapy's role in addressing sleep problems among older adults? *OTJR: Occupation, Participation and Health, 4,* 141–149. https://doi.org/10.3928/15394492-20140513-01

Levine, A. C., Adusumilli, J., & Landrigan, C. P. (2010). Effects of reducing or eliminating resident work shifts over 16 hours: A systematic review. *Sleep, 32,* 1043–1053. https://doi.org/10.1093/sleep/33.8.1043

Luckhaupt, S. E., Tak, S., & Calvert, G. M., (2010). The prevalence of short sleep by industry and occupation in the National Health Interview Survey. *Sleep, 33,* 149–159. https://doi.org/10.1093/sleep/33.2.149

Luyster, F. S., Chasens, E. R., Wasko, M. C., & Dunbar-Jacob, J. (2011). Sleep quality and functional disability in patients with rheumatoid arthritis. *Journal of Clinical Sleep Medicine, 7,* 49–55. https://doi.org/10.5664/jcsm.28041

Mah, C. D., Mah, K. E., Kezerian, E. J., & Dement, W. C. (2011). The effects of sleep extension on the athletic performance of collegiate basketball players. *Sleep, 34,* 943–950. https://doi.org/10.5665/SLEEP.1132

McCall, W. V., Kimball, J., Boggs, N., Lasater, B., D'Agostino, R. B., & Rosenquist, P. B. (2009). Prevalence and prediction of primary sleep disorders in a clinical trial of depressed patients with insomnia. *Journal of Clinical Sleep Medicine, 5,* 454–458. https://doi.org/10.5664/jcsm.27602

McHugh, J., & Lawlor, B. (2011). Commentary: Living alone does not account for the association between loneliness and sleep in older adults: Response to Hawkley, Preacher, and Cacioppo, 2010. *Health Psychology, 30,* 135. https://doi.org/https://doi.org/10.1037/a0022433

Mednick, S. C., & Ehrman, M. (2006). *Take a nap! Change your life.* Workman.

Nurok, M., Czeisler, C. A., & Lehmann, L. S. (2010). Sleep deprivation, elective surgical procedures, and informed consent. *The New England Journal of Medicine, 36,* 2577–2579. https://doi.org/10.1056/NEJMp1007901

O'Connor, G. T., Caffo, B., Newman, A. B., Quan, S. F., Rapoport, D. M., Redline, S., Resnick, H. E., & Shahar, E. (2009). Prospective study of sleep-disordered breathing and hypertension: The Sleep Heart Health Study. *American Journal of Respiratory Critical Care Medicine, 179,* 1159–1164. https://doi.org/10.1164/rccm.200712-1809OC

Ohayon, M. M. (2002). Epidemiology of insomnia: What we know and what we still need to learn. *Sleep Medicine Reviews, 6,* 97–111. https://doi.org/10.1053/smrv.2002.0186

Ohayon, M. M., & Vecchierini, M. F. (2005). Normative sleep data, cognitive function and daily living activities in older adults in the community. *Sleep, 28,* 981–989. http://dx.doi.org/10.1093/sleep/28.8.981

Owens, J. A., Belon, K., & Moss, P. (2010). Impact of delaying school start time on adolescent sleep, mood, and behavior. *Archives of Pediatrics and Adolescent Medicine, 164,* 608–614. https://doi.org/10.1001/archpediatrics.2010.96

Owens, J. A., & Mindell, J. A. (2005). *Take charge of your child's sleep: The all-in-one resource for solving sleep problems in kids and teens.* Marlowe & Company.

Owens, J. A., Spirito, A., & McGuinn, M. (2000). The Children's Sleep Habits Questionnaire (CSHQ): Psychometric properties of a survey instrument for school-aged children. *Sleep, 23,* 1043–1051.

Owens, J. A., Spirito, A., McGuinn, M., & Nobile, C. (2000). Sleep habits and sleep disturbance in elementary school-aged children. *Journal of Developmental and Behavioral Pediatrics, 21,* 27–36. https://doi.org/10.1097/00004703-200002000-00005

Ownby, R. L., Saeed, M., Wohlgemuth, W., Capasso, R., Acevedo, A., Peruyera, G., & Sevush, S. (2010). Caregiver reports of sleep problems in non-Hispanic white, Hispanic, and African American patients with Alzheimer dementia. *Journal of Clinical Sleep Medicine, 6*, 281–289. https://doi.org/10.5664/jcsm.27827

Parcell, D. L., Ponsford, J. L., Redman, J. R., & Rajaratnam, S. M. (2008). Poor sleep quality and changes in objectively recorded sleep after traumatic brain injury: A preliminary study. *Archives of Physical Medicine and Rehabilitation, 89*, 843–850. https://doi.org/10.1016/j.apmr.2007.09.057

Passos, G. S., Poyares, D., Santana, M. G., Garbuio, S., Tufik, S., & Mello, M. T. (2010). Effect of acute physical exercise on patients with chronic primary insomnia. *Journal of Clinical Sleep Medicine, 6*, 270–275. https://doi.org/10.5664/jcsm.27825

Patel, S. R., Ayas, N. T., Malhotra, M. R., White, D. P., Schernhammer, E. S., Speizer, F. E., Stampfer, M. J., & Hu, F. B. (2004). A prospective study of sleep duration and mortality risk in women. *Sleep, 27*, 440–444. https://doi.org/10.1093/sleep/27.3.440

Patel, S. R., & Hu, F. B. (2008). Short sleep duration and weight gain: A systematic review. *Obesity, 16*, 643–653. https://doi.org/10.1038/oby.2007.118

Peppard, P. E. (2009). Is obstructive sleep apnea a risk factor for hypertension?—Differences between the Wisconsin sleep cohort and the Sleep heart health study. *Journal of Clinical Sleep Medicine, 5*, 404–405. https://doi.org/10.5664/jcsm.27592

Pizza, F., Contardi, S., Antognini, A. B., Zagoraiou, M., Borrotti, M., Mostacci, B., Mondini, S., & Cirignotta, F. (2010). Sleep quality and motor vehicle crashes in adolescents. *Journal of Clinical Sleep Medicine, 6*, 41–45. https://doi.org/10.5664/jcsm.27708

Poe, G. R., Walsh, C. M., & Bjorness, T. E. (2010). Both duration and timing of sleep are important to memory consolidation. *Sleep, 33*, 1277–1280. https://doi.org/10.1093/sleep/33.10.1277

Quan, S. F., Parthasarathy, S., & Budhiraja, R. (2010). Healthy sleep education—a salve for obesity? *Journal of Clinical Sleep Medicine, 6*, 18–19. https://doi.org/10.5664/jcsm.27705

Redline, S. (2009). Does sleep disordered breathing increase hypertension risk? A practical perspective on interpreting the evidence. *Journal of Clinical Sleep Medicine, 5*, 406–408. https://doi.org/10.5664/jcsm.27593

Roehrs, T., Hyde, M., Blaisdell, B., Greenwald, M., & Roth, T. (2006). Sleep loss and REM sleep loss are hyperalgesic. *Sleep, 29*, 145–151. https://doi.org/10.1093/sleep/29.2.145

Roehrs, T., & Roth, T. (2008). Caffeine: Sleep and daytime sleepiness. *Sleep Medicine Reviews, 12*, 153–162. https://doi.org/10.1016/j.smrv.2007.07.004

Roehrs, T., & Roth, T. (2011a). Medication and substance abuse. In M. H. Kryger, T. Roth, W. C. Dement (Eds.), *Principles and practice of sleep medicine* (5th ed., pp. 1512–1523). Elsevier Saunders.

Roehrs, T., & Roth, T. (2011b). *Sleep, sleepiness, and alcohol use.* http://pubs.niaaa.nih.gov/publications/arh25-2/101-109.htm

Roth, T., Roehrs, T., & Pies, R. (2007). Insomnia: Pathophysiology and implications for treatment. *Sleep Medicine Reviews, 11*, 71–79. https://doi.org/10.1016/j.smrv.2006.06.002

Sadeh, A. (2011). The role and validity of actigraphy in sleep medicine: An update. *Sleep Medicine Reviews, 15*, 259–267. https://doi.org/10.1016/j.smrv.2010.10.001

Sánchez-Ortuño, M. M., Edinger, J. D., Means, M. K., & Almirall, D. (2010). Home is where the sleep is: An ecological approach to test the validity of actigraphy for the assessment of insomnia. *Journal of Clinical Sleep Medicine, 6*, 21–29. https://doi.org/10.5664/jcsm.27706

Schweitzer, P. (2011). Drugs that disturb sleep and wakefulness. In M. H. Kryger, T. Roth, & W. C. Dement (Eds.), *Principles and practice of sleep medicine* (5th ed., pp. 542–562). Elsevier Saunders.

Senthilvel, E., Auckley, D., & Dasarathy, J. (2011). Evaluation of sleep disorders in the primary care setting: History taking compared to questionnaires. *Journal of Clinical Sleep Medicine, 7*, 41–48. https://doi.org/10.5664/jcsm.28040

Shepard, J. W., Buyesse, D. J., Chesson, A. L., Dement, W. C., Goldberg, R., Guilleinault, C., Harris, C. D., Iber, C., Mignot, E., Mitler, M. M., Moore, K. E., Phillips, B. A., Quan, S. F., Rosenberg, R. S., Roth, T., Schmidt, H. S., Silber, M. H., Walsh, J. K., & White, D. P. (2005). History of the development of sleep medicine in the United States. *Journal of Clinical Sleep Medicine, 1*, 61–81. https://doi.org/10.5664/jcsm.26298

Sixel-Döring, F., Schweitzer, M., Mollenhauer, B., & Trenkwalder, C. (2011). Intraindividual variability of REM sleep behavior disorder in Parkinson's disease: A comparative assessment using a new REM Sleep Behavior Disorder Severity Scale (RBDSS) for clinical routine. *Journal of Clinical Sleep Medicine, 7*, 75–80. https://doi.org/10.5664/jcsm.28044

Smith, B., & Phillips, B. A. (2011). Truckers drive their own assessment for obstructive sleep apnea: A collaborative approach to online self-assessment for obstructive sleep apnea. *Journal of Clinical Sleep Medicine, 7*, 241–245. https://doi.org/10.5664/JCSM.1060

Solet, J. M. (2014). Optimizing personal and social adaptation. In M. V. Radomski & C. A. Trombly Latham (Eds.), *Occupational therapy for physical dysfunction* (7th ed., pp. 925–954). Lippincott Williams & Wilkins.

Solet, J. M. (2016). Translating sleep science into policy. *Sleep Health, 2*, 264–265. https://doi.org/10.1016/j.sleh.2016.09.005

Solet, J. M., & Barach, P. (2012). Managing alarm fatigue in cardiac care. *Progress in Pediatric Cardiology, 33*, 85–90. https://doi.org/10.1016/j.ppedcard.2011.12.014

Solet, J. M., Buxton, O. M., Ellenbogen, J. M., Wang, W., & Carballiera, A. (2010). Validating acoustic guidelines for healthcare facilities. Evidence-based design meets evidence-based medicine: The sound sleep study. The Center for Health Design. http://www.healthdesign.org/chd/research/validating-acoustic-guidelines-healthcare-facilities

Sorscher, A. J. (2008). How is your sleep: A neglected topic for health care screening. *Journal of the American Board of Family Medicine, 21*, 141–148. https://doi.org/10.3122/jabfm.2008.02.070167

Spiegel, K., Knutson, K., Leproult, R., Tasali, E., & Van Cauter, E. (2005). Sleep loss: A novel risk factor for insulin resistance and type 2 diabetes. *Journal of Applied Physiology, 99*, 2008–2019. https://doi.org/10.1152/japplphysiol.00660.2005

Spiegel, K., Tasali, E., Penev, P., & Van Cauter, E. (2004). Brief communication: Sleep curtailment in healthy young men is associated with decreased leptin levels, elevated ghrelin levels, and increased hunger and appetite. *Annals of Internal Medicine, 141*, 846–850. https://doi.org/10.7326/0003-4819-141-11-200412070-00008

Stickgold, R. (2005). Sleep-dependent memory consolidation. *Nature, 437*, 1272–1285. https://doi.org/10.1038/nature04286

Stout, K., & Finlayson, M. (2011). Fatigue management in chronic illness: The role of occupational therapy. *OT Practice, 16*(1), 16–19.

Stroe, A. F., Roth, T., Jefferson, C., Hudgel, D. W., Roehrs, T., Moss, K., & Drake, C. L. (2010). Comparative levels of excessive daytime sleepiness in common medical disorders. *Sleep Medicine, 11*, 890–896. https://doi.org/10.1016/j.sleep.2010.04.010

Tomfohr, L. M., Ancoli-Israel, S., Loredo, J. S., & Dimsdale, J. E. (2011). Effects of continuous positive airway pressure on fatigue and sleepiness in patients with obstructive sleep apnea: Data from a randomized controlled trial. *Sleep, 34*, 121–126. https://doi.org/10.1093/sleep/34.1.121

Tregear, S., Reston, J., Schoelles, K., & Phillips, B. (2009). Obstructive sleep apnea and risk of motor vehicle crash: A systematic review and meta-analysis. *Journal of Clinical Sleep Medicine, 5*, 573–581. https://doi.org/10.5664/jcsm.27662

Umberson, D. (1992). Gender, marital status and the social control of health behaviors. *Social Science & Medicine, 34*, 907–917. https://doi.org/10.1016/0277-9536(92)90259-S

Van Dongen, H. P., Maislin, G., Mullington, J. M., & Dinges, D. (2003). The cumulative cost of additional wakefulness: Dose-response effects on neurobehavioral functions and sleep physiology from chronic sleep restriction and total sleep deprivation. *Sleep, 26*, 117–126. https://doi.org/10.1093/sleep/26.2.117

Vaughn, B. V., & D'Cruz, O. (2011). Cardinal manifestations of sleep disorders. In M. H. Kryger, T. Roth, & W. C. Dement (Eds.), *Principles and practice of sleep medicine* (5th ed., pp. 647–657). Elsevier Saunders.

Verse, T., & Hörmann, K. (2011). The surgical treatment of sleep-related upper airway obstruction. *Deutsches Ärzteblatt International, 108*, 216–221. https://doi.org/10.3238/arztebl.2010.0216

Viola-Saltzman, M., Watson, N. F., Bogart, A., Goldberg, J., & Buchwald, D. (2010). High prevalence of restless legs syndrome among patients with fibromyalgia: A controlled cross-sectional study. *Journal of Clinical Sleep Medicine, 6*, 423–427. https://doi.org/10.5664/jcsm.27929

Vitiello, M. V., Rybarczk, B., Von Korff, M., & Stepanski, E. J. (2009). Cognitive behavioral therapy for insomnia improves sleep and decreases pain in older adults with co-morbid insomnia and osteoarthritis. *Journal of Clinical Sleep Medicine, 5*, 355–362. https://doi.org/10.5664/jcsm.27547

Walker, M. P., & Stickgold, R. (2004). Sleep-dependent learning and memory consolidation. *Neuron, 44*, 121–133. https://doi.org/10.1016/j.neuron.2004.08.031

Watanabe, M., Kikuchi, H., Katsutoshi, T., & Takahashi, M. (2010). Association of short sleep duration with weight gain and obesity at 1 year follow-up: A large-scale prospective study. *Sleep, 33*, 161–167. https://doi.org/10.1093/sleep/33.2.161

Watson, N. F. (2010). Stroke and sleep specialists: An opportunity to intervene? *Journal of Clinical Sleep Medicine, 6*, 138–139. https://doi.org/10.5664/jcsm.27761

Watson, N. F., Buchwald, D., Vitiello, M. V., Noonan, C., & Goldberg, J. (2010). A twin study of sleep duration and body mass index. *Journal of Clinical Sleep Medicine, 6*, 11–17. https://doi.org/10.5664/jcsm.27704

Weaver, E., Gradisar, M., Dohnt, H., Lovato, N., & Douglas, P. (2010). The effect of presleep video-game playing in adolescent sleep. *Journal of Clinical Sleep Medicine, 6*, 184–185. https://doi.org/10.5664/jcsm.27769

Weinhouse, G. L., & Schwab, R. J. (2006). Sleep in the critically ill patient. *Sleep, 29*, 707–716. https://doi.org/10.1093/sleep/29.5.707.

Xie, C., Kang, H., Xu, Q., Chen, M. J., Liao, Y., Thiyagarajan, M., O'Donnell, J., Christensen, D. J., Nicholson, C., Iliff, J. J., Takano, T., Deane, R., & Nedergaard, M. (2013). Sleep drives metabolite clearance from the adult brain. *Science, 342*, 373–377. doi: 10.1126/science.1241224

Youngstedt, S. D., & Buxton, O. M. (2003). Jet lag and athletic performance. *American Journal of Medicine and Sports, 5*, 219–226.

Zee, P. C., & Turek, F. W. (2006). Sleep and health: Everywhere and in both directions. *Archives of Internal Medicine, 166*, 1686–1688. https://doi.org/10.1001/archinte.166.16.1686

Zizi, F., Jean-Louis, G., Brown, C. D., Ogedegbe, G., Boutin-Foster, C., & McFarlane, S. I. (2011). Sleep duration and risk of diabetes mellitus: Epidemiologic evidence and pathophysiologic insights. *Current Diabetes Reports, 10*, 43–47. https://doi.org/10.1007/s11892-009-0082-x

Social Participation

Leanne Yinusa-Nyahkoon and Mary Alunkal Khetani

OUTLINE

LEARNING OBJECTIVES

After reading this chapter, you will be able to:

1. Describe how social participation is defined in comparison to the related concepts of performance and quality of life.
2. Evaluate the strengths and limitations of available assessments to develop participation profiles of diverse clients seeking occupational therapy services.
3. Describe ways that you might appraise a client's participation using available measures.
4. Describe ways that you can incorporate information about a client's environment to appraise a client's participation.
5. Describe ways of intervening to promote participation at the individual, group, or organizational level.

Introduction

It has been nearly two decades since the *International Classification of Functioning, Disability and Health* (ICF) and the *ICF Version for Children and Youth* (ICF-CY) were introduced. In these classification systems, disability is conceptualized as a state in which the individual experiences challenges to their health and well-being as shaped, in part, by their attempts to participate in society on an equal basis with others (World Health Organization [WHO], 2001, 2007). This definition of disability emphasizes the importance of understanding individuals' experiences of disability, acknowledges the role of systems and policies in shaping opportunities for participation in meaningful occupations, and marks a significant paradigmatic shift and opportunity for occupational therapists to contribute to interprofessional practice.

The occupational therapy (OT) profession focuses on promoting participation in everyday occupations that are meaningful and purposeful (American Occupational Therapy Association [AOTA], 2020). This chapter introduces you to contemporary thinking about social participation—how it is currently understood, assessed, and promoted—to best target it in your career.

Understanding Social Participation

The Distinction Between Performance and Social Participation

A client's social participation is complementary but separate from the skills used to perform discrete tasks of everyday life (e.g., putting on clothes, eating with hands or utensils) (Granlund, 2018). Clients with different task-related competencies can derive equal value from participating in the same occupations (Imms et al., 2015). Thus, a client with a spinal cord injury may enjoy participating in team sports with their peers, although they may navigate the court, rink, competition room, or playing field using a wheelchair. Similarly, a client with sensory processing challenges may participate in their family ritual of dining out, although they may request a modified meal, use technology to order and interact with others during mealtime, and use adaptive utensils brought from home to eat and drink. Regardless of their approach to performing these tasks, both clients have access to satisfying experiences when participating in their chosen occupation. They demonstrate their presence and interest in the occupation, and they each derive personal or social connection to the occupation (see Figure 49.1 and OT Stories 49.1 and 49.2).

The Distinction Between Social Participation and Quality of Life

A second important distinction is between the concepts of social participation and quality of life (Whiteneck,

2006). According to the WHO, **participation** is defined as a person's "involvement in life situations," whereas **quality of life** is defined as a person's overall well-being, including "perceptions of their position in life in the context of the culture and value system where they live and in relation to their goals, expectations, standards, and concerns" (Quality of Life Assessment by World Health Organization Quality of Life [WHOQOL] Group [WHO, 1998, p. 27, 2012]). Quality of life measures have often been developed without input from persons with disabilities (Hays et al., 2002) and often contain questions about independence versus quality of life (Fayed et al., 2012; Jarvis & Fink, 2021; Ow et al., 2021). However, the WHO definitions of both participation and quality of life suggest an objective quality to participation and a subjective aspect of quality of life.

From an OT perspective, a client's social participation is considered an indicator of their overall quality of life as described in the latest Occupational Therapy Practice Framework (AOTA, 2020). Practitioners gather information about the objective component of a client's social participation, such as their attendance and their level of involvement in a valued activity (Imms et al., 2015). Because participation observations may differ from the lived experience of participating in an activity, it is important to evaluate the subjective component of a client's social participation. Pairing objective and subjective inquiries reflects best practice and recognizes the perspectives of clients across the globe and life course, including those of parents and caregivers of children and youth with disabilities (Bedell et al., 2011; Khetani et al., 2013) and adults with disabilities living in different geographic regions (Hammel et al., 2008; Murchland & Parkyn, 2010; Simpson et al., 2021).

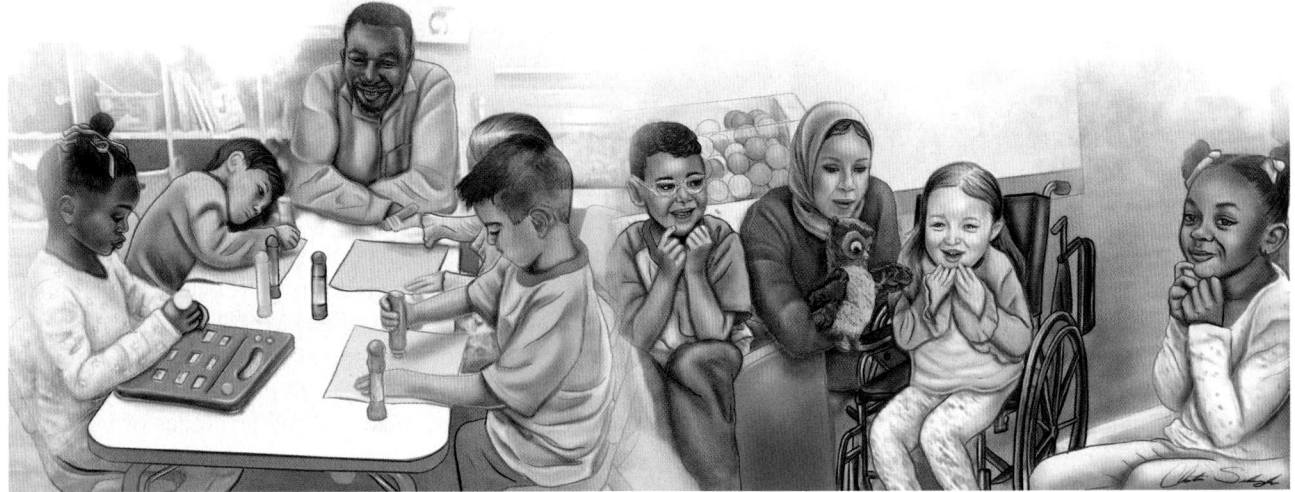

FIGURE 49.1 Clients with different task-related competencies can actively participate and derive equal value from the same occupations. (Used with permission from artist Christina Sidorowych.)

OT STORY 49.1 DIFFERENTIATING PERFORMANCE AND PARTICIPATION IN AN END-OF-LIFE CONTEXT

Leon (they, them, their) is a 79-year-old man with a complex history of neurologic anomalies and multiple C-spine surgeries, which contribute to pervasive balance deficits and frequent syncopal episodes with falls. Leon lives at home with their partner and primary caregiver, Micah, and has the local support of their three adult children and their families. Leon ambulates with a cane, refuses to transition to a walker, and requires assistance for most activities of daily living (ADLs) owing to decreased balance, strength, range of motion, and activity tolerance. Leon values religion, traditions, and family and celebrates Christmas and Kwanzaa as their most cherished time of the year. Leon takes pride in these annual celebrations but is experiencing increased difficulty decorating and hosting. In July, Leon was diagnosed with stage

4 lung cancer, has declined treatment, and has an estimated life expectancy of 6 months. Leon reports that their most important priorities are spending one more Christmas and Kwanzaa season decorating, preparing traditional recipes, celebrating the seven principles, exchanging gifts, watching classic movies like *The Preacher's Wife*, singing and storytelling with family, and dying with dignity at home.

1. How have Leon's health conditions impacted their skills to perform ADLs and celebrate?
2. What does Leon still want to participate in to achieve their end-of-life wishes?
3. What about Leon's performance and environment could support participation in occupations?

OT STORY 49.2 DIFFERENTIATING PERFORMANCE AND PARTICIPATION FOR A WORKING MOM

Elyse (she, her, hers) is an active 30-year-old single mother of young twin boys who are avid members of their school's Battle-of-the-Books team, and she co-owns a hair salon with a full client base as a senior stylist. Elyse experienced a traumatic C4–C5 spinal cord injury (SCI) in a motocross accident, resulting in functional quadriplegia and severe depression and anxiety. After a year in hospitals and SCI rehabilitation, she wants to go home so she can be present with her children and remotely maintain her salon. Elyse is dependent for ADLs, so her mother will be her primary caregiver. She maintains enough function in her left arm to hold a stylus and operate a tablet. She can bring her hand to mouth for

feeding but lacks the grip strength and coordination to manipulate standard utensils. Her priorities include maintaining her leadership role and client base at the salon and reading books with her children so they can compete in the upcoming city championship.

Questions

1. How have Elyse's injuries impacted the skills she needs to perform the key tasks related to styling hair and reading books with her children?
2. How might Elyse's environment be modified to ensure her participation in each of these valued occupations?

The Relationship Between Participation and Social Participation

Current thinking about *participation* and *social participation* is that they are interchangeable terms. The ICF and ICF-CY define participation as "involvement in life situations" (WHO, 2001, 2007) without referring to social participation as a separate concept. Similarly, the Occupational Therapy Practice Framework, 4th edition (AOTA, 2020, p. 83), defines social participation *broadly* as "interweaving of occupations to support desired engagement in community and family activities, as well as those

involving peers and friends," such as "involvement in a subset of activities that incorporate social situations with others and that support social interdependence" (Bedell, 2012; Khetani & Coster, 2019; Magasi & Hammel, 2004; Schell & Gillen, 2019; Figure 49.2). With the expanded use of technology and social media, we expand this definition to acknowledge that social participation can be synchronous or asynchronous and occurs in person or remotely using technology, such as a cell phone, computer, laptop, tablet, video game console, or other modes of virtual or video interaction.

Although the concepts of *participation* and *social participation* are considered interchangeable, there has been dialogue about identifying like terms and consistently

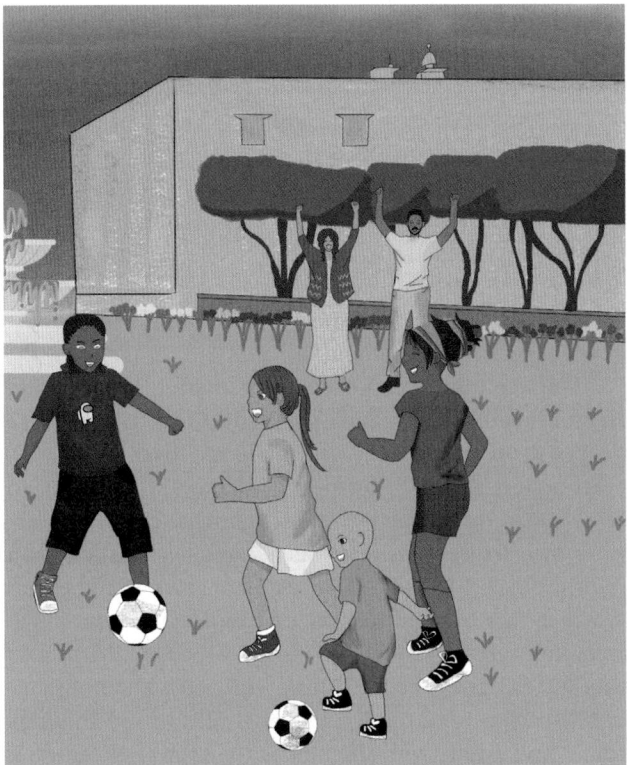

FIGURE 49.2 For children, life situations are organized sets and sequences of activities that typically involve the presence and engagement of others. These life situations may be directed toward development of skills and capacities as well as enjoyment. (Used with permission of the artist Zurisadai Salgado.)

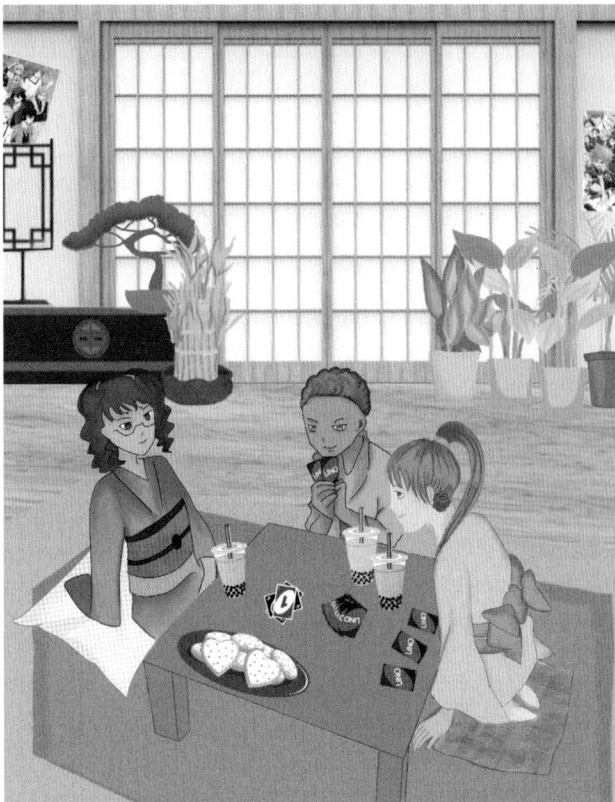

FIGURE 49.3 Social participation and participation are considered interchangeable terms. (Used with permission of the artist Zurisadai Salgado.)

defining participation in order to guide research and practice. For example, when referring to children, McConachie and colleagues (2006) classified "life situations" as sets of activities that were pursued for survival, supporting the child's development, discretionary, or educationally enriching. For children and youth, life situations typically involve the presence and engagement of others, are environment-specific, and are directed toward a personally or socially meaningful goal—like physical health, development of skills, and emotional well-being (Coster & Khetani, 2008; Khetani et al., 2013). Similarly, for adults, participation is intrinsically social and entails engagement in productivity, social, and community situations (Chang & Coster, 2014; Figure 49.3).

Across these definitions, there are two common underlying assumptions: (a) any life situation can be social and (b) social participation is best classified according to where the interaction takes place rather than whether they include a social element. Thinking about social participation along these terms will help us to consistently organize our thinking about social participation when working with clients across the life course. We can assume all important life situations for a client can have a social element, and we can expect to appraise a host of intrinsic and extrinsic

factors that influence the client's social participation in an activity. For example, we might consider the availability and adequacy of resources to play basketball at home, which may be different from resources needed to play basketball in the neighborhood, at the community center, or for the school team (Heinemann, 2010). This approach places high demand on contextual thinking because client desires and expectations may differ across activities, environments, and time even when personal factors align (Khetani et al., 2013; Tamis-Monda et al., 2007).

In the remainder of this chapter, we choose to use the term *participation* only. We discuss ways to assess and promote participation outcomes across a broad range of activities that a client might engage in with or without others and across the life course.

Evaluating Participation

As occupational therapists, one of our first tasks when working with clients is to create their occupational profile, which focuses on the client's current and desired participation in occupation (AOTA, 2020). Because participation is a *multidimensional* and *context-dependent* concept, we need to recognize that there is more than one way to ascertain whether clients are participating in the activities they need and want to do (i.e., multidimensional) and how clients' participation may differ depending on what they are doing and where the activity takes place (i.e., context-dependent). Hence, it takes significant resources to collaboratively generate a profile of how diverse clients participate across a full range of occupations in home, educational, employment, and/or community situations (O'Connor et al., 2021). Because participation is influenced by the environment in which activities take place (Anaby et al., 2013; Hammel et al., 2015), evaluating the client's participation is coupled with close consideration of the environments the client encounters in the course of their daily life.

There is no single measure of participation that is suitable for use with all clients across diverse contexts (including personal factors and environmental factors that comprise a person's life situation). In addition, measures can be more or less useful depending on whether they are being used as assessments as they were intended to be used (Bedell & Coster, 2008). In the next section, we include descriptions of assessments of participation designed to guide intervention planning for persons across diverse backgrounds and the life course.

Common Features of Participation Assessments

Assessment approaches described in this section reinforce the use of a top-down and client-centered approach to evaluating clients' participation needs. When using a top-down approach, we first focus on identifying the client's current and desired participation. We then focus on determining the contextual factors, both personal and environmental, that proximally support or hinder the client in taking part in

occupations that they need or want to do more. Finally, we select intervention approaches to address the identified capacities, competencies, and contextual factors (e.g., natural and human made environment; technology; relationships; attitudes; and systems) that are restricting their participation in a valued activity (AOTA, 2020). Assessments described in this section provide an organized way to obtain information about participation, to develop clients' occupational profiles and more sharply focus interventions toward those activities that clients most want or need to participate in but experience restriction(s).

One common approach to gathering information about a client's participation preferences is to ask them via interview or survey. This assessment approach allows OT practitioners to build therapeutic alliances with clients, to be able to partner effectively in designing and enacting services that are responsive to their identified participation priorities (see Chapter 26). Assessments vary in the extent to which they have been developed with stakeholder input, including service providers (Chang & Coster, 2014); parents and caregivers of individuals with and without disabilities (Bedell et al., 2011; Khetani et al., 2013); and children, youth, and adults with disabilities themselves (Kramer & Hammel, 2011; Majnemer et al., 2010; Shahin et al., 2022; Shikako-Thomas et al., 2009). Best practice guidelines also emphasize user engagement to culturally adapt participation assessments (Arestad et al., 2017; Tomas et al., 2021) because many assessments were developed in Western, English-speaking contexts, validated primarily on persons with social privilege and primarily used to build knowledge about disparities in participation in those contexts (Fauconnier et al., 2009; Ullenhag et al., 2012).

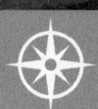

EXPANDING OUR PERSPECTIVES

A Picture Is Worth a Thousand Words

Leanne Yinusa-Nyahkoon and Mary Alunkal Khetani

A recent review of the pictures included in participation assessments across the life course caused us to pause and reflect on the status of diversity and inclusion of participation assessments commonly used within OT. The images within many of the measures that were reviewed for inclusion in this chapter seem to have historically centered around the participation norms of white, able-bodied, middle-class, cisgendered, adult individuals living in North America and who value individualism and independence. Few images of participation in valued occupations feature individuals who present as Black, Indigenous, and People of Color (BIPOC), individuals with an observable physical disability, individuals of various gender identities, or

individuals who identify with an intersection of these minoritized identities (e.g., race, ability, gender). For example, we found that, of those participation measures in this chapter that contained images, less than 3% of the images included individuals presenting as women of color, and individuals of color presenting with an observable physical disability were excluded altogether.

When images of underrepresented individuals were included, their presentation lacked cultural sensitivity. Participation cards hand drawn in black and white used shading or stripes to demonstrate darker skin tones. Drawn or photographed hair textures and styles of individuals presenting as BIPOC appeared uniform and seemed to align with acceptable North American norms and standards (e.g., straightened or moderately curly and voluminous hair). The clothing choices of featured individuals lacked diversity or uniqueness so as to reinforce dominant

Northern American cultural views on what it means to be "professional," "business casual," "gender conforming," or expected when participating in an area of occupation (e.g., work, education, play). In addition, participation images that included minoritized groups perpetuated colonial hierarchies and historical and systemic power differences. For example, images of volunteer and leisure participation consistently featured older, white adults leading activities for children of color. In the few images that included a child or adult with an observable physical disability, all similarly displayed these individuals sitting in a wheelchair. Related assessment questions and response options seemed to center around the dominant Western values of individualism and independence, minimizing the assets and values of non-Western cultures, such as community and interdependence, that are congruent with the concept of participation.

As BIPOC OT scholars who have each contributed in different ways to building capacity for participation-focused practice for more than 20 years, we are left wondering why there is not more diversity in the images within participation assessments. This messaging implies that only individuals from dominant societal groups participate in the occupations featured in participation measures. Practitioners and clients alike can experience harm when tasked to administer or complete these assessments to enact the OT process. It remains unclear how these Western norms have been challenged in cultural adaptation of participation assessments. It has been our experience that undertaking cultural adaptation of participation assessments, particularly as a BIPOC scholar, is challenging. The images from this chapter reflect this effort to upgrade one participation assessment included in this chapter.

The Occupational Therapy Practice Framework, 4th edition, recognizes the need to consider a broad range of personal factors, or unique features, that impact an individual's life and daily living (AOTA, 2020). Similarly, legislation such as the Creating a Respectful and Open World for Natural Hair (CROWN) Act reminds us that it is discriminatory to ignore the diversity of personal factors, or natural characteristics, that exist among us, and challenges unspoken normative assumptions (CROWN Act, 2021–2022). We therefore recommend that authors consider expanding the personal factors included in the development and revisions of participation assessments. We encourage all OT stakeholders to pause and reflect on the diversity and inclusion of the participation assessments they have access to and choose to use. Where do we go from here?

References

American Occupational Therapy Association. (2020). Occupational therapy practice framework: Domain and process (4th ed.). *American Journal of Occupational Therapy, 74*(Suppl. 2), 7412410010. https://doi.org/10.5014/ajot.2020.74S2001
Creating a Respectful and Open World for Natural Hair (CROWN) Act of 2022, H.R. 2116, 117th Cong. (2021–2022). https://www.congress.gov/bill/117th-congress/house-bill/2116/titles

Overview of Selected Participation Measures

For this chapter, we build on what has been covered in other chapters and review a set of measures that explicitly address participation in a broad range of activities that have some psychometric evidence to support their use in practice (Adair et al., 2018; McConachie et al., 2006; Morris et al., 2005) and have some published evidence of efforts to culturally adapt the assessment (i.e., adapt their content and administration, both of which are needed for assessment completion) to maximize their clinical utility (Pizur-Barnekow et al., 2011; Tomas et al., 2021).

The subset of measures selected for review in this chapter vary in terms of their comprehensiveness, how they are administered, how long they take to complete, the population of focus they are designed for, and the extent to which they have been culturally adapted for use across diverse clinical contexts. In this section, we describe assessments of participation that have been developed for young children, children and youth, adults, and older adults.

Table 49.1 provides a brief overview of what information each assessment can help you gather as you assess your clients. For each selected measure, we have indicated (a) whether its content addresses home, school, work, and/or community participation; (b) whether it gathers objective or subjective data or both; and (c) whether it includes an assessment of environment.

Many participation assessments are endorsed as common data elements in intervention studies involving individuals with disabilities (e.g., National Institutes of Health Common Data Elements Initiative [National Institutes of Health, 2017]). Assessment details are also summarized and routinely updated for and by practitioners (e.g., Rehabilitation Measures Database [Shirley Ryan AbilityLab, 2010]).

Selected Participation Measures for Young Children

All available instruments for young children rely on parent report but vary in their content and mode of administration (paper vs. electronic). Young children are typically in close

TABLE 49.1	Overview of Select Participation Measures for Young Children, School-Aged Youth and Young Adults, Adults, and Older Adults					
	Area(s) of Participation Addressed			**Dimensions Addressed**		**Environmental Impact Addressed**
Assessment	Home	School or Work	Community	Objective Assessment	Subjective Assessment	
Participation Measures for Young Children						
Preschool Activity Card Sort (PACS)	✔	✔	✔	Frequency Extent	Importance Satisfaction	✔
Assessment of Preschool Children's Participation (APCP)	✔		✔	Diversity Intensity Where With whom	Enjoyment Preferences	
Children's Engagement in Daily Life (CEDL)	✔		✔	Frequency	Enjoyment	
Young Children's Participation and Environment Measure (YC-PEM)	✔	✔	✔	Frequency Involvement	Desire for change	✔
Participation Measures for Children and Youth						
Children's Assessment of Participation and Enjoyment (CAPE) and Preferences for Activities (PAC)	✔		✔	Diversity Intensity Where With whom	Enjoyment Preferences	
Picture My Participation (PMP)	✔	✔	✔	Frequency Involvement	Priorities for change	
School Function Assessment (SFA)		✔		Involvement		✔
Child and Adolescent Scale of Participation (CASP)	✔	✔	✔	Degree of restriction		✔
Assessment of LIFE-Habits for Children (LIFE-H)	✔	✔	✔	Accomplishment	Satisfaction	✔
Participation and Environment Measure for Children and Youth (PEM-CY)	✔	✔	✔	Frequency Involvement	Desire for change	✔
Participation Measures for Adults and Older Adults						
Activity Card Sort (ACS)	✔		✔	% Maintained		
Craig Handicap Assessment and Reporting Technique (CHART)		✔	✔	Time spent No. of social contacts		✔
Community Integration Questionnaire (CIQ)	✔	✔		How often With whom Assistance		
The Participation Measure for Post-Acute Care (PM-PAC)			✔	Frequency Extent of limitation	Satisfaction	

contact with and guided by their caregivers to participate in home and community activities. Therefore, parent-report measures are commonly used to make inferences about the young child's participation. We describe four measures of young children's participation (Figure 49.4).

Preschool Activity Card Sort

The Preschool Activity Card Sort (PACS) (Berg & LaVesser, 2006) is a semistructured interview for use with parents of children 3 to 6 years of age. PACS contains 85 photographs of

children engaged in one of seven types of activities: self-care, community mobility, leisure, social interaction, domestic chores, and education. Parents view each of the 85 photographs and respond to the question "Does your child participate in this activity?" using one of six response options: (a) yes, child participates; (b) yes, child participates but requires adult assistance beyond that typically required of preschoolers; (c) yes, with environmental assistance (e.g., can ride a bike on some surfaces—hard, smooth surfaces but not grass); (d) no (does not participate in the activity), for

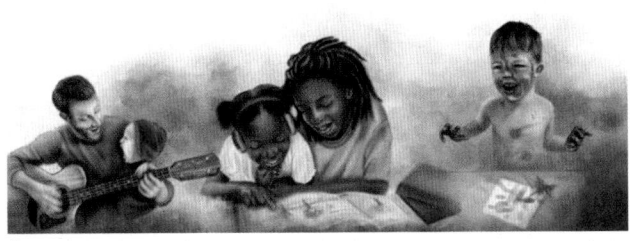
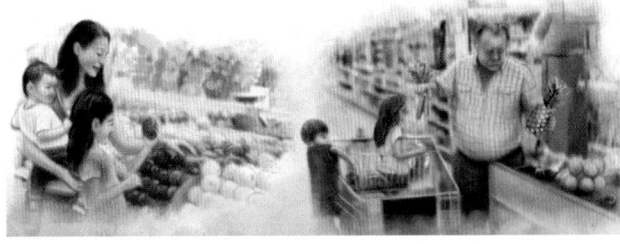

A   **B**

FIGURE 49.4 Young children are typically in close contact with and guided by their parents or caregivers to participate in **(A)** home-based and **(B)** community-based activities. Therefore, parent-report measures are commonly used to make inferences about the young child's participation. (Used with permission of artist Christina Sidorowych.)

child reasons (e.g., owing to pain, balance); (e) no, for adult reasons (e.g., financial); or (f) no, for environmental reasons (e.g., community resources unavailable, neighborhood safety). Parents are then asked to identify five activities that they would like to be the focus of intervention and rate the relative importance of each activity, the frequency with that the activity is performed, the extent of participation (from 0 = *currently not participating at all* to 10 = *fully participating*), and satisfaction with participation. There have been efforts to culturally adapt PACS for Spanish-speaking families (Stoffel & Berg, 2008), in Arabic-speaking countries (Malkawi et al., 2015, 2017), and in Japan (Igarashi et al., 2020).

Assessment of Preschool Children's Participation

The Assessment of Preschool Children's Participation (APCP) scale (Law et al., 2012) has been modeled after the Children's Assessment of Participation and Enjoyment (CAPE) and the Preferences for Activities of Children (PAC; King et al., 2004) and is designed for use with children ages 2 to 5 years and 11 months. The APCP assesses young children's participation in voluntary, day-to-day activities outside of preschool. The APCP is a parent-report, paper–pencil survey that contains 45 drawings of activities across the areas of play (9 items); skill development (15 items); active physical recreation (10 items); and social activities (11 items). Parents identify activities that their child has participated in during the past 4 months (yes/no) and, if yes, how often they did them (7-point scale). Diversity and intensity scores can be generated for each activity area. There has been effort to culturally adapt the APCP for use with Chinese and Dutch families (Bult et al., 2013; Kang et al., 2017).

Young Children's Participation and Environment Measure

The Young Children's Participation and Environment Measure (YC-PEM; Khetani, 2015; Khetani et al., 2015) is a parent-report questionnaire designed to assess the young child's current and desired participation, environmental impact on participation, and strategies used to promote participation in activities that take place in three settings: home, daycare/preschool, and community. This measure can be used with families of children aged 0 to 5 years. The YC-PEM allows parents to rate their child's frequency of participation (0 = *never* to 7 = *once or more each day*), the child's level of involvement (0 = *not very involved* to 5 = *very involved*), and the caregiver's desire for their child's participation to change (*yes/no*). If parents desire change in their child's participation in an activity, they can specify ways that they want the child's participation to change (e.g., participate more often, be more involved, and/or participate in a broader variety of activities) and describe strategies used to promote participation. Parents are also asked to evaluate the impact of a broad range of environmental features and resources, including the demands of activities, on participation in occupation. There has been effort to culturally adapt the YC-PEM, with and without language translation, for use by Hispanic and Singaporean families (Arestad et al., 2017; Lim et al., 2018) and with families in Sweden (Astrom et al., 2018) and Hong Kong (Chien et al., 2021), and carefully appraise requests for changes to its administration (e.g., not removing the color black from its aesthetic so that it better conforms to a cultural norm that privileges lighter colors) (Tomas et al., 2021).

Child Engagement in Daily Life

The Child Engagement in Daily Life measure (CEDL; Chiarello et al., 2014) is a parent-completed measure for use with young children with and without cerebral palsy between 1.5 and 5 years of age. The CEDL contains 18 items that address participation in family and recreational activities (11 items) and self-care (7 items). For each activity in the family and recreational activities section, the parent is asked to report on the child's frequency of participation (how often the child participates, from 1 = *never* to 5 = *very often*) and the child's enjoyment of participation (from 1 = *not at all* to 5 = *a great deal*). For each activity in the self-care section, the parent is asked to report on the child's degree of participation in their daily self-care activities (from 1 = *no, unable* to 5 = *yes, initiates and performs consistently*). Summary scores for each area of participation can be computed to obtain estimates of frequency of participation in family and recreational activities (sum frequency), enjoyment of participation in family and recreational activities (average enjoyment), and participation in self-care (sum participation). There is evidence of effort to culturally adapt the CEDL self-care domain (Alghamdi et al., 2021).

Selected Participation Measures for School-Aged Youth and Young Adults

We review six participation measures designed for school-aged youth and young adults.

Children's Assessment of Participation and Enjoyment

The CAPE (King et al., 2004) is a 55-item measure designed to obtain a participation profile specific to leisure and recreation activities that take place outside of the school setting (e.g., hobbies, crafts, games, organized sports, clubs, groups, arts, and entertainment). The CAPE contains activity drawings on cards and visual response forms to help enable children to complete this assessment via self-report or interview. The CAPE assesses five dimensions of participation in reference to a 4-month time frame: (a) diversity of activities (whether child participates), (b) intensity or how often the child participates, (c) with whom the child participates, (d) where the child participates, and (e) extent of enjoyment in activities. The CAPE can be completed separately from the PAC and takes 30 to 45 minutes to complete. There have been efforts to culturally adapt it for use in Spain (Longo et al., 2014), and in Dutch (Bult et al., 2013), German (Fink et al., 2016), and Norwegian (Nordtorp et al., 2013) contexts.

Picture My Participation

Picture My Participation (PMP) is a self-report measure designed as part of a structured interview using the Talking Mats approach (Arvidsson et al., 2020, 2021; Balton et al., 2022). PMP has 20 items that are converted into graphic symbols and visual scales to facilitate conversation with the child about their frequency of participation in home, school, and community activities (from never to always), three prioritized activities that they desire change, and perceived level of involvement (from minimally to very) in these three prioritized activities. PMP is valid for children and youth with intellectual disability (ID) in low-income

and middle-income settings, like South Africa, and in high-income settings, like Sweden (Arvidsson et al., 2021; Samuels et al., 2020). There have also been efforts to culturally adapt it for use in mainland China (Liao et al., 2019; Shi et al., 2021).

School Function Assessment

The School Function Assessment (SFA; Coster et al., 1998) begins with a section on participation in six different school settings: (a) classroom (regular or specialized), (b) playground or recess, (c) transportation, (d) bathroom or toileting, (e) transitions, and (f) mealtime or snack time, with one item for each section. These six items are each rated on a 6-point scale that reflects the extent to which the child participates in the tasks and activities compared to peers (from 1 = *extremely limited* to 6 = *child fully participates in all tasks and activities within each setting*). The participation subscale can be completed by the child's teacher in about 5 to 10 minutes when used separately from the larger measure and has reported evidence of test–retest reliability and internal consistency. SFA addresses the environment in separate scales that assess the use of adult assistance and/or adaptations (modifications of equipment, environment, activity, program) to complete school tasks. Efforts have been made to develop a Chinese version for cross-cultural use in Taiwan (Hwang et al., 2004).

Child and Adolescent Scale of Participation

Child and Adolescent Scale of Participation (CASP; Bedell, 2009) was developed as part of the Child and Family Follow-up Survey (CFFS) to monitor outcomes and needs of children with acquired brain injuries and subsequently has been used separately from the CFFS to assess children with other diagnoses (Bedell, 2004, 2009; Bedell & Dumas, 2004). CASP includes four subsections that address the extent to which children aged 5 years and older participate in broad types of home, school, and community activities compared to same-aged peers. All items are rated on a 4-point scale (from 1 = *unable* to 4 = *age expected*). CASP includes open-ended questions that ask about effective strategies and supports and barriers that affect participation. CASP alone takes about 10 minutes to complete and has reported evidence of test–retest reliability, internal consistency, and construct and discriminant validity (Bedell, 2004, 2009; Bedell & Dumas, 2004; Golos & Bedell, 2016). The 18-item Child and Adolescent Scale of Environment (CASE) is a separate but compatible measure that can be used with CASP to get information about environmental barriers to participation (from 1 = *no problem* to 3 = *big problem*). There is a youth self-report version of CASP (McDougall et al., 2013) and culturally adapted version for use with clients speaking traditional Chinese (Hwang et al., 2013).

Assessment of Life Habits in Children

The Assessment of Life Habits (LIFE-H; Noreau et al., 2005, 2007) was initially designed for adults but has been adapted for use as a parent-report survey for families of children aged 5 years and older. Its purpose is to identify disruptions in the accomplishment of 11 types of life habits, with 6 categories of life habits that fall into the daily activities domain (e.g., personal care, fitness) and five life habits that fall into the social roles domain (e.g., recreation, education, community life). LIFE-H has a long form (197 items, 1–2 hours to complete) and a short form (64 items, 3–45 minutes to complete). LIFE-H assesses one's (a) level of accomplishment (according to the level of difficulty and type of assistance) and (b) level of satisfaction. Level of accomplishment and satisfaction scores can be computed for items and life habit categories and globally. Efforts to culturally adapt this measure include a version for use with Turkish-identifying families (Akbas et al., 2021).

Participation and Environment Measure for Children and Youth

The Participation and Environment Measure for Children and Youth (PEM-CY; Coster et al., 2010) is a caregiver-report instrument that combines assessment of participation and environment in a single measure. The PEM-CY contains 25 participation items reflecting broad types of activities that are typically done at home, at school, or in the community. Each participation item is rated in three ways: according to (a) frequency (from 0 = *never* to 7 = *daily*), (b) involvement (from 1 = *minimally* to 5 = *very involved*), and (c) desire for change (parents are asked if they want their child's participation to change [yes/no], and if yes, the parent is asked to indicate all of the ways in which change is desired [e.g., more or less frequency, more or less involvement, and/or more variety]). For each setting, parents are asked whether features of the environment help or hinder their child's participation and whether there are available or adequate resources to support their child's participation. The online PEM-CY takes 20 to 30 minutes to complete and is reliable and valid for children and youth aged 5 to 17 years (Coster et al., 2011). A youth and young adult version is under development (Shahin et al., 2022), and efforts have been made to develop versions for use with German- (Krieger et al., 2020), Hindi- (Srinivasan et al., 2021), Korean- (Jeong et al., 2016), and Chinese-speaking users (Chien et al., 2020).

Selected Participation Measures for Adults and Older Adults

We describe four adult participation measures, some of which have been reviewed in greater detail in other chapters in this text. We chose to include measures that demonstrate

inclusivity, highlight diversity, or have begun the ongoing work of cultural adaptation.

Activity Card Sort

The Activity Card Sort (ACS; Baum & Edwards, 2008) is intended to document older adult clients' (≥60 years) participation in instrumental, leisure, and social activities. The ACS uses Q-sort methodology, which is a rank-order procedure in which the client sorts photographs into categories based on the question being posed by the person administering the assessment. There are 89 photographs of activities (20 instrumental, 35 low–physical demand leisure, 17 high–physical demand leisure, and 17 social). There are three versions of the ACS. The Community-Living Version involves community-dwelling older adults sorting photographs into five categories: never done, do now, do less, and given up. The Institutional Version is intended for use with clients receiving services in a hospital, rehabilitation, or skilled nursing facility and asks clients to sort the same 89 photographs into two groups: (a) done prior to illness or injury or (b) never done. The Recovering Version is intended for use with clients to record changes in activity patterns owing to current illness or injury. The client sorts photographs into categories: not done prior to current illness or injury, continued during current illness or injury, performed less since current illness or injury, gave up owing to illness or injury, and new activity since illness or injury. The score reflects the percentage of activities that the client maintains or retains.

Culturally adapted versions of the ACS expand beyond activities perceived to be common in the continental United States and instead reflect the occupations of older adults in specific geographic regions. The activity cards in each culturally adapted version of ACS feature select generationally and culturally relevant scenarios and settings. For example, the Activity Card Sort-Spain Version (ACS-SP) includes 79 activities, including napping, seeing sports in a stadium, and voting, whereas the Hong Kong Version (ACS-HK) has 67 activities and uniquely features food preservation (Alegre-Muelas et al., 2019). The ACS has been adapted for clients in several countries, including Australia (ACS-Aus), Brazil (ACS-Brazil), Holland (ACS-NL), Israel (ACS-Israeli version), Japan (ACS-JPN) (Uemura et al., 2019), Korea, Puerto Rico (PR-ACS), Singapore, and the United Kingdom (ACS-UK), as well as for clients worldwide who identify with Arab Heritage (A-ACS) (Hamed & Holm, 2013).

Craig Handicap Assessment and Reporting Technique

The Craig Handicap Assessment and Reporting Technique (CHART; Whiteneck et al., 1992) was originally developed as a self-report instrument for persons with SCI, but it has since been used with individuals aged 15 years and older with physical disabilities and cognitive impairments. The measure assesses participation in the years after initial onset of illness or injury, and content development was originally guided by the original International Classification of Impairments, Disabilities, and Handicaps (ICIDH). The revised version of the CHART includes 32 questions grouped into six domains: physical independence, mobility, occupation, social integration, economic self-sufficiency, and cognitive independence. Questions focus on objective and observable indicators, such as time engaged in an ADL or IADL activity (e.g., working, leisure participation) and number of individuals within a household (e.g., family members, roommates, care attendants). The 19-item short form, CHART-SF (Whiteneck, 2011), asks a subset of questions from the six domains and therefore requires less time to administer. The CHART-SF has been translated and validated for individuals in countries and communities where Persian is the native or heritage language (Golhasani-Keshtan et al., 2013).

Community Integration Questionnaire-Revised

The Community Integration Questionnaire-Revised (CIQ-R; Callaway et al., 2014, 2016; Corrigan & Deming, 1995; Sander et al., 2007; Willer et al., 1993) is an 18-item measure that assesses an individual's home integration, social integration, productivity, and electronic social networking following an acute injury (e.g., acquired brain injury) or when managing a chronic illness or degenerative condition (multiple sclerosis; Hirsh et al., 2011). The CIQ-R can be administered in person, administered over the phone, self-administered, or administered by proxy. Scores are based on the frequency of participation and level of assistance needed. The CIQ-R recognizes the expansion of cyber-participation, so the revised version assesses electronic communication as a means of social networking and integration (Stiers et al., 2012). The initial and revised versions of the questionnaire have been translated from English into other several languages (Fraga-Maia et al., 2015; Liu et al., 2014; Negahban et al., 2013; Rintala et al., 2002; Saeki et al., 2006). The CIQ-R- is available in Croatian, Italian, and Malay (Ioncoli et al., 2020; Saeki et al., 2006).

Participation Measure for Post-Acute Care

The Participation Measure for Post-Acute Care (PM-PAC; Gandek et al., 2007) examines the participation outcomes of community-dwelling adolescents and adults (≥13 years old) following rehabilitation services. The measure assesses perceived participation limitations across nine domains including mobility; role functioning; work; education; economic life; domestic life; community, social, and civic life; interpersonal relationships; and communication. The 51-item measure consider diversity-of-life situations and ask generally about participation (e.g., did your means of transportation allow you to get to all the places you wanted to go?). Most of the PM-PAC items ask respondents to rate the extent to which they are currently limited in a life situation using the response options *not at all limited, a little, somewhat, very much, extremely limited,* and *don't do/not applicable (N/A).* Other items measure duration of participation (e.g., all of the time, none of the time) or the degree of participation satisfaction (e.g., very satisfied, very dissatisfied). Efforts have been made to develop a Brazilian Portuguese version of the PM-PAC (Souza et al., 2018).

In summary, measures offer different approaches to gathering information about client participation. When selecting the best measure to gather information, it is important to first identify the assessment purpose and then identify those measures that best match that need by considering the following: (a) the characteristics of the population of focus (e.g., a 3-year-old child with developmental delay, in which case only a subset of measures that have been validated on young children would be appropriate); (b) the type of information needed (e.g., areas where a child is least satisfied with their participation in community activities, which would require gathering information about the subjective qualities of participation in a comprehensive set of activities within a specific setting); (c) whether it is important to obtain estimates of change in a client's participation; and (d) how much time is available to gather this information in the context of daily practice (Bedell & Coster, 2008).

Interventions to Promote Social Participation

The measures described in this chapter provide robust knowledge about participation that can inform the implementation of evidence-based practice, minimize disparities in participation across contexts and populations (Arakelyan et al., 2019; Benjamin et al., 2017; Kaelin et al., 2021; Shabat et al., 2021), navigate determinants of participation outcomes (Chiarello et al., 2016; Jarvis et al., 2020), and increase the emphasis on the role of strategies (Jarvis et al., 2019) and the environment in predicting participation outcomes (Anaby et al., 2013; Di Marino et al., 2018; Khetani et al., 2020; Vaughan et al., 2017). There are a growing number of studies of participation change (Imms & Adair, 2017; Khetani, 2017; Khetani et al., 2018) and efforts to systematically translate this knowledge for participation-focused practice (Anaby et al., 2021).

Participation in everyday occupation is the reason for OT (Law, 2002) and the promise of rehabilitation (Baum, 2011). Assuming that individuals are motivated to engage in meaningful activities, participation should always be considered when designing OT intervention. Participation may be incorporated into intervention in one of two ways: (a) participation as an *end goal* of intervention and (b) participation as a *component* of a multifaceted intervention.

Promoting Participation as End Goal of Intervention

When participation is the end goal, interventions are designed to empower individuals who are socially isolated owing to stigmatization, remove barriers that limit their access to desired social activities, and/or help facilitate changes in their major life roles following the onset of an acute injury or a chronic health condition. Various interventions can promote a client's participation and may be directed toward the client or the client's environment. As an example, Law and colleagues (2011) examined child-focused and context-focused intervention approaches for young children with cerebral palsy and found them to be equally effective (Figure 49.5).

Client-Centered Approaches to Promoting Participation as End Goal

Occupational therapists can intervene with individual clients to help them become participating members of a community, like linking individual clients to various resources and services and by helping them develop support and peer networks. For example, Occupational Performance Coaching (OPC) is an approach to improve participation in children and adults (Bernie et al., 2021; Chien et al., 2021; Graham et al., 2018; Kessler et al., 2017). As another example, Kramer and colleagues applied a participatory action research approach to develop and pilot test a Teens Making Environment and Activity Modifications (TEAM) intervention to help youth with disabilities identify and advocate for removal of environmental barriers that prevent them from participating in school and community life (Kramer et al., 2013, 2014). Recently, Anaby and colleagues developed and demonstrated the effectiveness of a similar type of intervention approach called Pathways and Resources for Engagement and Participation (PREP; Anaby et al., 2015, 2016, 2017, 2018, 2020; Anaby & Pozniak, 2020). As another example,

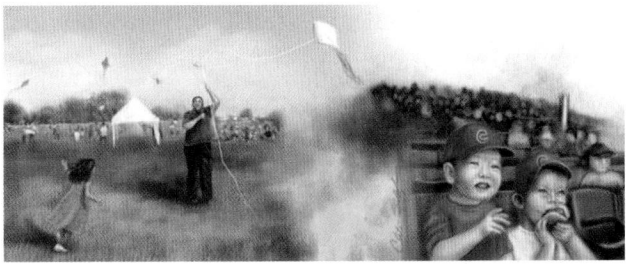

FIGURE 49.5 There is more than one valid way to develop interventions to promote a client's participation. These interventions may be directed toward the client or the client's environment. (Used with permission of artist Christina Sidorowych.)

Schelly et al. (2011) at the Center for Community Partnerships at Colorado State University are implementing a peer-mentored approach to help autistic students create strategies to navigate challenges related to college life like time management, study skills, effective communication, forming relationships, and learning to advocate for themselves in educational settings. In these examples, the methods of intervention depend on the nature of the identified barriers limiting participation. Barriers owing to lack of knowledge about available resources may be addressed through client education and guided exploration. However, barriers owing to lack of accessibility may need to be addressed through advocacy with planning, building, and policy groups.

When participation is the client's primary goal, it is important to ensure that the client's own definition of meaningful and satisfying participation guides intervention design. Individuals have different preferences for how they engage with others: some are "group" people, others may seek friendship with a few people; some enjoy conversation as a main activity, others prefer to engage in activities with others. Therefore, it is not enough to simply identify situations that offer opportunities for participation: the setting and their activities need to fit with individuals' values, interests, and preferences. The opportunity for choice is an important component to facilitating self-determination for meaningful participation, and clients may need a period of guided exploration to discover the options that offer the best fit (Angell et al., 2019).

There are increasing efforts to explore the use of familiar technology to provide guided support for client engagement by designing interventions that focus on participation as the end goal. For example, the Social Participation and Navigation (SPAN) is an app-based coaching intervention to support social participation in youth with traumatic brain injury (Bedell et al., 2016; Narad et al., 2018; Wade et al., 2018). As another example, the Participation and Environment Measure Plus (PEM+) is an app that extends the use of PEM participation assessment results for person-centered goal-setting (Bosak et al., 2019; Jarvis et al., 2019, 2020; Khetani et al., 2017). Video calling and conferencing technology is used daily by many adolescents and adults, and it is increasingly used by individuals with intellectual and physical disabilities for leisure participation and communication with preferred peers and partners (Lancioni et al., 2020). In addition, there may also be value to emerging health information technologies that personalize interventions, address known gaps in the use of artificial intelligence (Kaelin et al., 2021), and use exemplars of promising strategies, like virtual conversational agents, to drive behavior change among minoritized communities (Gardiner et al., 2021; Kramer et al., 2021).

Context-Based Interventions to Promote Participation as End Goal

Universal design principles to directly intervene on the environment have been applied by OT practitioners to promote participation (see Chapter 24). For example, ensuring that residences have a single-level entrance and 32-in-wide access to a bathroom on the main level are ways to ensure the "visitability" of a home (Maisel, 2006). As an example of this environmentally focused approach to intervention, OT researchers have provided guidance on how to consult with museums, arenas and other community agencies to increase access to and learning by visitors with neurological and developmental differences (Laskowski, 2022; Umeda et al., 2017). Technology-based approaches, like the Jooay app, were developed for use by community organizations to link youth to accessible community spaces for participation in leisure activities (Thornton et al., 2021).

Another focus of context-based intervention considers the human dimensions of environments, particularly in supported work and living situations, such as group homes or assisted living facilities. Staff in these programs may view their primary role as enabling clients to complete daily tasks, such as dressing, grooming, or eating, and may need to be educated by an occupational therapist to facilitate client participation in meaningful occupation. Studies have shown that the appropriate training of direct-care staff in group homes increases the social participation of residents with intellectual and developmental disabilities (Jones et al., 1999). Emerging approaches to audit case notes and other documents support routine implementation of participation-focused practice by staff (Graham et al., 2020; Kolehmainen et al., 2020).

Interventions to Promote Participation as a Component of a Broader Program

Some interventions address social participation to enhance the therapeutic value of the program. This key idea underlies various health promotion initiatives such as the Well Elderly Study 2 (Clark et al., 1997, 2011) as well as adult day programs (Horowitz & Chang, 2004) and programs for older adults in senior housing (Matsuka et al., 2003). This is also the underlying premise of peer support groups, where it is believed that connecting with others who experience similar challenges will decrease social isolation and provide emotional support and resources for daily health management. Examples include symptom self-management programs for people with multiple sclerosis (Finlayson et al., 2011), stroke (Lee et al., 2017; Wolf et al., 2016), and Parkinson disease (Tickle-Degnen et al., 2010). Some intervention programs may have specific goals to provide positive social experiences as a component of an overall prevention effort. For example, Bazyk and Bazyk (2009) have developed

school-based social skills groups for urban youth and anti-bullying programs that foster respect for diversity by engaging individuals from different groups in collaborative learning experiences. It is important to realize that simply incorporating social interaction into a group is insufficient to ensure meaningful participation. Just as activities need to be carefully selected to support achieving skill-based client goals, the group process and activities also need to be carefully selected to facilitate meaningful social participation. Relevant considerations include the size and makeup of group, type of leadership, decision-making processes, and member roles and responsibilities.

Conclusions and Future Directions

Participation in valued everyday occupations is a central focus of OT. Given its importance, we recommend that practitioners try to stay current with developments in the following key areas and consider ways of contributing to them while in practice: (a) development and testing of culturally relevant measures of participation; (b) routinely applying measures of participation within organizational workflows to generate occupational profiles; and (c) implementing evidence-based interventions to promote participation, including technology-based approaches to intervention with individuals, groups, and populations.

Acknowledgments

We thank Boston University and University of Illinois at Chicago pre-OT and OT students Asia Anderson, Marlene Angulo, Sophie Lieberman, and Zurisadai Salgado who have helped with updating descriptions of selected participation assessments, inserting references, and/or providing critical feedback. We also thank our colleague, Lori Sutton, MS, OTR/L, for contributing two case studies inspired by her lived and professional experiences promoting participation that guide her practice at Desert Rose Therapy Services.

Lippincott® Connect *For additional resources on the subjects discussed in this chapter, visit Lippincott Connect.*

REFERENCES

Adair, B., Ullenhag, A., Rosenbaum, P., Granlund, M., Keen, D., & Imms, C. (2018). Measures used to quantify participation in childhood disability and their alignment with the family of participation-related constructs: A systemic review. *Developmental Medicine & Child Neurology, 60*(11), 1101–1116. https://doi.org/10.1111/dmcn.13959

Akbas, N. A., Ozal, C., Cankaya, O., Seyhan Biyik, K., Unes, S., Tuncdemir, M., Arslan, U. E., Ozcebe, L. H., & Kerem Gunel, M.

(2021). Reliability and construct validity of the Turkish adaptation of the assessment of life habits for children and adolescents with cerebral palsy. *Marmara Medical Journal, 34*(2), 101–111. https://doi.org/10.5472/marumj.943118

Alegre-Muelas, C., Alegre-Ayala, J., Huertas-Hoyas, E., Martínez-Piédrola, M. R., Pérez-Corrales, J., Máximo-Bocanegra, N., Sánchez-Camarero, C., & Pérez-De-Heredia-Torres, M. (2019). Spanish transcultural adaptation of the Activity Card Sort. *Occupational Therapy International, 2019*, 4175184. https://doi.org/10.1155/2019/4175184

Alghamdi, M. S., Chiarello, L. A., Abd-Elkafy, E. M., Palisano, R. J., Orlin, M., & McCoy, S. W. (2021). Cross-cultural adaptation of the Arabic version of self-care domain of child engagement in daily life and ease of caregiving for children measures. *Research in Developmental Disabilities, 110*(October 2019), 103853. https://doi.org/10.1016/j.ridd.2021.103853

American Occupational Therapy Association. (2020). Occupational therapy practice framework: Domain and process, 4th edition. *American Journal of Occupational Therapy, 74*, 7412410010p1–7412410010p87. https://doi.irg/10.5014/ajot.2020.74S2001

Anaby, D., Hand, C., Bradley, L., DiRezze, B., Forhan, M., DiGiacomo, A., & Law, M. (2013). The effect of the environment on participation of children and youth with disabilities: A scoping review. *Disability and Rehabilitation, 35*, 1589–1598. https://doi.org/10.3109/09638288.2012.748840

Anaby, D., Khetani, M., Piskur, B., van der Holst, M., Bedell, G., Schakel, F., de Kloet, A., Simeonsson, R., & Imms, C. (2021). Towards a paradigm shift in pediatric rehabilitation: Accelerating the uptake of evidence on participation into routine clinical practice. *Disability and Rehabilitation, 44*(9), 1746–1757. https://doi.org/10.1080/09638288.2021.1903102

Anaby, D., Law, M., Majnemer, A., & Feldman, D. (2016). Improving the participation of youth with physical disabilities: The effectiveness of the Pathways and Resources for Engagement and Participation (PREP) intervention. *Developmental Medicine and Child Neurology, 58*, 41–41. https://doi.org/10.1111/dmcn.56_13224

Anaby, D., Law, M., Teplicky, R., & Turner, L. (2015). Focusing on the environment to improve youth participation: Experiences and perspectives of occupational therapists. *International Journal of Environmental Research in Public Health, 12*(10), 13388–13398. https://doi.org/10.3390/ijerph121013388

Anaby, D., Mercerat, C., & Tremblay, S. (2017). Enhancing youth participation using the PREP intervention: Parents' perspectives. *International Journal of Environmental Research in Public Health, 14*(9), 1–10. https://doi.org/10.3390/ijerph14091005

Anaby, D., & Pozniak, K. (2019). Participation-based intervention in childhood disability: A family-centred approach. *Developmental Medicine and Child Neurology, 61*(5), 502. https://doi.org/10.1111/dmcn.14156

Anaby, D., Vrotsou, K., Kroksmark, U., & Ellegård, K. (2020). Changes in participation patterns of youth with physical disabilities following the pathways and resources for engagement and participation intervention: A time-geography approach. *Scandinavian Journal of Occupational Therapy, 27*(5), 364–372. https://doi.org/10.1080/11038128.2018.1554088

Anaby, D. R., Law, M., Feldman, D., Majnemer, A., & Avery, L. (2018). The effectiveness of the Pathways and Resources for Engagement and Participation (PREP) intervention: Improving participation of adolescents with physical disabilities. *Developmental Medicine and Child Neurology, 60*(5), 513–519. https://doi.org/10.1111/dmcn.13682

Angell, A. M., Carroll, T. C., Bagatell, N., Chen, C., Kramer, J.M., Schwartz, A., Tallon, M. B., & Hammel, J. (2019). Understanding self-determination as a crucial component in promoting the distinct value of occupational therapy in post-secondary transition planning. *Journal of Occupational Therapy, Schools, & Early Intervention, 12*(1), 129–143. https://doi.org/10.1080/19411243.2018.1496870

Arakelyan, S., Maciver, D., Rush, R., O'hare, A., & Forsyth, K. (2019). Family factors associated with participation of children with disabilities: A systematic review. *Developmental Medicine and Child Neurology, 61*(5), 514–522. https://doi.org/10.1111/dmcn.14133

Arestad, K. E., MacPhee, D., Lim, C. Y., & Khetani, M. A. (2017). Cultural adaptation of a pediatric functional assessment for rehabilitation outcomes research. *BMC Health Services Research, 17*(1), 1–13. https://doi.org/10.1186/s12913-017-2592-6

Arvidsson, P., Dada, S., Granlund, M., Imms, C., Bornman, J., Elliott, C., & Huus, K. (2020). Content validity and usefulness of Picture My Participation for measuring participation in children with and without intellectual disability in South Africa and Sweden. *Scandinavian Journal of Occupational Therapy, 27*(5), 336–348. https://doi.org/10.4102/AJOD.V10I0.763

Arvidsson, P., Dada, S., Granlund, M., Imms, C., Shi, L. J., Kang, L. J., Hwang, A. W., & Huus, K. (2021). Structural validity and internal consistency of Picture My Participation: A measure for children with disability. *African Journal of Disability, 10*, 1–8. https://doi.org/10.4102/AJOD.V10I0.763

Astrom, F., Khetani, M., & Axelsson, A. (2018). Young children's participation and environment measure: Swedish cultural adaptation. *Physical & Occupational Therapy in Pediatrics, 38*(3), 329–342. https://doi.org/10.1080/01942638.2017.1318430

Balton, S., Arvidsson, P., Granlund, M., Huus, K., & Dada, S. (2022). Test-retest reliability of Picture My Participation in children with intellectual disability in South Africa. *Scandinavian Journal of Occupational Therapy, 29*(4), 315–324. https://doi.org/10.1080/11038128.2020.1856922

Baum, C., & Edwards, D. (2008). *Activity card sort* (2nd ed.). American Occupational Therapy Association.

Baum, C. M. (2011). Fulfilling the promise: Supporting participation in daily life. *Archives of Physical Medicine and Rehabilitation, 92*, 169–175. https://doi.org/10.1016/j.apmr.2010.12.010

Bazyk, S., & Bazyk, J. (2009). Meaning of occupation-based groups for low-income urban youths attending after-school care. *American Journal of Occupational Therapy, 63*, 69–80. https://doi.org/10.5014/ajot.63.1.69

Bedell, G. (2012). Measurement of social participation. In V. Anderson & M. H. Beauchamp (Eds.), *Developmental social neuroscience and childhood brain insult: Theory and practice* (pp. 185–204). The Guilford Press.

Bedell, G., & Coster, W. (2008). Measuring participation of school-aged children with traumatic brain injuries: Considerations and approaches. *Journal of Head Trauma Rehabilitation, 23*(4), 220–229. https://doi.org/10.1097/01.HTR.0000327254.61751.e7

Bedell, G. M. (2004). Developing a follow-up survey focused on participation of children and youth with acquired brain injuries after discharge from inpatient rehabilitation. *Neuro Rehabilitation, 19*, 191–205. https://doi.org/10.1080/0269905031000110517

Bedell, G. M. (2009). Further validation of the Child and Adolescent Scale of Participation (CASP). *Developmental Neurorehabilitation, 12*, 342–351. https://doi.org/10.3109/17518420903087277

Bedell, G. M., & Dumas, H. M. (2004). Social participation of children and youth with acquired brain injuries discharged from inpatient rehabilitation: A follow-up study. *Brain Injury, 18*, 65–82. https://10.1080/0269905031000110517

Bedell, G. M., Khetani, M. A., Cousins, M. A., Coster, W. J., & Law, M. C. (2011). Parent perspectives to inform development of measures of children's participation and environment. *Archives of Physical Medicine and Rehabilitation, 92*, 765–773. https://doi.org/10.1016/j.apmr.2010.12.029

Bedell, G.M., Wade, S. L., Turkstra, L. S., Haarbauer-Krupa, J., & King, J. A. (2016). Informing design of an app-based coaching intervention to promote social participation of teenagers with traumatic brain injury. *Developmental Neurorehabilitation, 2016*, 1–10. https://doi.org/10.1080/17518423.2016.1237584

Benjamin, T. E., Lucas-Thompson, R. G., Little, L. M., Davies, P. L., & Khetani, M. A. (2017). Participation in early childhood educational environments for young children with and without developmental disabilities. *Physical & Occupational Therapy in Pediatrics, 37*, 87–107. https://doi.org/10.3109/01942638.2015.1130007

Berg, C., & LaVesser, P. (2006). The preschool activity card sort. *OTJR: Occupation, Participation and Health, 26*, 143–151. https://doi.org/10.1177/153944920602600404

Bernie, C., Mitchell, M., Williams, K., & May, T. (2021). Parent-directed intervention versus controls whilst their child waits for diagnostic assessment: A systematic review protocol. *Systematic Reviews, 10*(1), 1–8. https://doi.org/10.1186/s13643-021-01615-7

Bosak, D. L., Jarvis, J. M., & Khetani, M. A. (2019). Caregiver creation of participation-focused care plans using Participation and Environment Measure Plus (PEM+), an electronic health tool for family-centred care. *Child: Care, Health and Development, 45*(6), 791–798. https://doi.org/10.1111/cch.12709

Bult, M. K., Verschuren, O., Gorter, J. W., Jongmans, M. J., Piškur, B., & Ketelaar, M. (2013). Cross-cultural validation and psychometric evaluation of the Dutch language version of the Children's Assessment of Participation and Enjoyment (CAPE) in children with and without physical disabilities. *Clinical Rehabilitation, 24*(9), 843–853. https://doi.org/10.1177/0269215510367545

Callaway, L., Winkler, D., Tippett, A., Migliorini, C., Herd, N., & Willer, B. (2014). *The Community Integration Questionnaire-Revised (CIQ-R).* Summer Foundation Ltd.

Callaway, L., Winkler, D., Tippett, A., Herd, N., Migliorini, C., & Willer, B. (2016). The Community Integration Questionnaire – Revised: Australian normative data and measurement of electronic social networking. *Australian Occupational Therapy Journal, 63*(3), 143–153. https://doi.org/10.1111/1440-1630.12284

Chang, F. H., & Coster, W. J. (2014). Conceptualizing the construct of participation in adults with disabilities. *Archives of Physical Medicine and Rehabilitation, 95*(9), 1791–1798. https://doi.org/10.1016/j.apmr.2014.05.008

Chiarello, L. A., Bartlett, D. J., Palisano, R. J., McCoy, S. W., Fiss, A. L. F., Jeffries, L., & Wilk, P. (2016). Determinants of participation in family and recreational activities of young children with cerebral palsy. *Disability and Rehabilitation, 38*(25), 2455–2468. https://doi.org/10.3109/09638288.2016.1138548

Chiarello, L. A., Palisano, R. J., McCoy, S. W., Bartlett, D. J., Wood, A., Chang, H., Kang, L. J., & Avery, L. (2014). Child engagement in daily life: A measure of participation for young children with cerebral palsy. *Disability and Rehabilitation, 36*, 1804–1816. doi:10.3109/09638288.2014.88241

Chien, C. W., Lai, Y. Y. C., Lin, C. Y., & Graham, F. (2021). Occupational performance coaching with parents to promote community participation of young children with developmental disabilities: Protocol for a feasibility and pilot randomized control trial. *Frontiers in Pediatrics, 9*, 1–12. https://doi.org/10.3389/fped.2021.720885

Chien, C. W., Li-Tsang, C. W. P., Cheung, P. P. P., Leung, K. Y., & Lin, C. Y. (2020). Development and psychometric evaluation of the Chinese version of the participation and environment measure for children and youth. *Disability and Rehabilitation, 42*(15), 2204 2214. https://doi.org/10.1080/09638288.2018.1553210

Clark, F. A., Azen, S. P., Zemke, R., Jackson, J. M., Carlson, M. E., Hay, J., Josephson, K., Cherry, B., Hessel, C., Palmer, J., & Lipson, L. (1997). Occupational therapy for independent-living older adults: A randomized controlled trial. *JAMA, 278*, 1321–1326. https://doi.org/10.1001/jama.278.16.1321

Clark, F. A., Jackson, J. M., Carlson, M. E., Chou, C. P., Cherry, B. J., Jordan-Marsh, M., Knight, B. G., Mandel, D., Blanchard, J., Granger, D. A., Wilcox, R. R., Lai, M. Y., White, B., Hay, J., Lam, C., Marterella, A.,

& Azen, S. P. (2011). Effectiveness of a lifestyle intervention in promoting the well-being of independently living older people: Results of the Well Elderly 2 Randomised Controlled Trial. *Journal of Epidemiology and Community Health, 66*, 782–790. https://doi.org/10.1136/jech.2009.099754

Corrigan, J. D., & Deming, R. (1995). Psychometric characteristics of the community integration questionnaire: Replication and extension. *The Journal of Head Trauma Rehabilitation, 10*, 41–53. https://doi.org/10.1097/00001199-199508000-00005

Coster, W. J., Bedell, G. M., Law, M., Khetani, M., Teplicky, R., Liljenquist, K., Gleason, K., & Kao, Y. (2011). Psychometric evaluation of the participation and environment measure for children and youth. *Developmental Medicine and Child Neurology, 53*, 1030–1037. https://doi.org/10.1111/j.1469-8749.2011.04094.x

Coster, W. J., Deeney, T., Haltiwanger, J., & Haley, S. M. (1998). *School function assessment.* PsychCorp.

Coster, W. J., & Khetani, M. (2008). Measuring participation of children with disabilities: Issues and challenges. *Disability and Rehabilitation, 30*, 639–648. https://doi.org/10.1080/09638280701400375

Coster, W. J., Law, M., & Bedell, G. M. (2010). *Participation and environment measure for children and youth (PEM-CY).* Boston University.

Di Marino, E., Tremblay, S., Khetani, M. A., & Anaby, D. (2018). The effect of child, family and environmental factors on the participation of young children with disabilities. *Disability and Health Journal, 11*, 36–42. https://doi.org/10.1016/j.dhjo.2017.05.005

Fauconnier, J., Dickinson, H. O., Beckung, E., Marcelli, M., McManus, V., Michelsen, S. I., Parkes, J., Parkinson, K. N., Thyen, U., Arnaud, C., & Colver, A. (2009). Participation in life situations of 8-12 year old children with cerebral palsy: Cross sectional European study. *BMJ (Online), 338*(7703), 1116–1121. https://doi.org/10.1136/bmj.b145

Fayed, N., De Camargo, O. K., Kerr, E., Rosenbaum, P., Dubey, A., Bostan, C., Faulhaber, M., Raina, P., & Cieza, A. (2012). Generic patient-reported outcomes in child health research: A review of conceptual content using World Health Organization definitions. *Developmental Medicine and Child Neurology, 54*(12), 1085–1095. https://doi.org/10.1111/j.14698749.2012.04393.x

Fink, A., Gebhard, B., Erdwiens, S., Haddenhorst, L., & Nowak, S. (2016). Reliability of the German version of the Children's Assessment of Participation and Enjoyment (CAPE) and Preferences for Activities of Children (PAC). *Child: Care, Health and Development, 42*(5), 683 691. https://doi.org/10.1111/cch.12360

Finlayson, M., Preissner, K., Cho, C., & Plow, M. (2011). Randomized trial of a teleconference-delivered fatigue management program for people with multiple sclerosis. *Multiple Sclerosis, 17*, 1130–1140. https://doi.org/10.1177/1352458511404272

Fraga-Maia, H. M. S., Werneck, G., Dourado, I., Fernandes, R. de C. P., & Brito, L. L. (2015). Translation, adaptation and validation of "community integration questionnaire." *Ciencia e Saude Coletiva, 20*(5), 1341–1352. https://doi.org/10.1590/1413-81232015205.08312014

Gandek, B., Sinclair, S. J., Jette, A. M., & Ware, J. E., Jr. (2007). Development and initial psychometric evaluation of the participation measure for post-acute care (PM-PAC). *American Journal of Physical Medicine & Rehabilitation, 86*, 57–71. https://doi.org/10.1097/01.phm.0000233200.43822.21

Gardiner, P., Bickmore, T., Yinusa-Nyahkoon, L., Reichert, M., Julce, C., Sidduri, N., Martin Howard, J., Woodhams, E., Aryan, J., Zhang, Z., Fernandez, J., Loafman, M., Srinivasan, J., Cabral, H., & Jack, B. W. (2021). Using health information technology to engage African American women on nutrition and supplement use during the preconception period. *Frontiers in Endocrinology, 11*(January), 1–11. https://doi.org/10.3389/fendo.2020.571705

Golhasani-Keshtan, F., Ebrahimzadeh, M. H., Fattahi, A. S., Soltani-Moghaddas, S. H., & Omidi-Kashani, F. (2013). Validation and cross-cultural adaptation of the Persian version of Craig Handicap Assessment and Reporting Technique (CHART) short form. *Disability and Rehabilitation, 35*(22), 1909–1914. https://doi.org/10.3109/09638288.2013.768710

Golos, A., & Bedell, G. (2016). Psychometric properties of the Child and Adolescent Scale of Participation (CASP) across a 3-year period for children and youth with traumatic brain injury. *NeuroRehabilitation, 38*, 311–319. https://doi.org/10.3233/NRE-161322

Graham, F., Boland, P., Ziviani, J., & Rodger, S. (2018). Occupational therapists' and physiotherapists' perceptions of implementing Occupational Performance Coaching. *Disability and Rehabilitation, 40*(12), 1386–1392. https://doi.org/10.1080/09638288.2017.1295474

Graham, F., Timothy, E., Williman, J., & Levack, W. (2020). Participation-focused practices in paediatric rehabilitation for children with neurodisability in New Zealand: An observational study using MAPi audit tool. *Child: Care, Health and Development, 46*(5), 552–562. https://doi.org/10.1111/cch.12789

Granlund, M. (2018). Is independence the same as participation for young people with disabilities? *Developmental Medicine and Child Neurology, 61*(2), 116–117. https://doi.org/10.1111/dmcn.14041

Hamed, R., & Holm, M. B. (2013). Psychometric properties of the Arab heritage activity card sort. *Occupational Therapy International, 20*(1), 23–34. https://doi.org/10.1002/oti.1335

Hammel, J., Magasi, S., Heinemann, A., Gray, D. B., Stark, S., Kisala, P., Carlozzi, N. E., Tulsky, D., Garcia, S. F., & Hahn, E. A. (2015). Environmental barriers and supports to everyday participation: A qualitative insider perspective from people with disabilities. *Archives of Physical Medicine and Rehabilitation, 96*(4), 578–588. https://doi.org/10.1016/j.apmr.2014.12.008

Hammel, J., Magasi, S., Heinemann, A., Whiteneck, G., Bogner, J., & Rodriguez, E. (2008). What does participation mean? An insider perspective from people with disabilities. *Disability and Rehabilitation, 30*, 1445–1460. https://doi.org/10.1080/09638280701625534

Hays, R., Hahn, H., & Marshall, G. (2002). Use of the SF-36 and other health-related quality of life measures to assess persons with disabilities. *Archives of Physical Medicine and Rehabilitation, 83*, S4–S9. https://doi.org/10.1053/apmr.2002.36837

Heinemann, A. W. (2010). Measurement of participation in rehabilitation research. *Archives of Physical Medicine and Rehabilitation, 92*, 1729–1730. https://doi.org/10.1016/j.apmr.2009.08.155

Hirsh, A. T., Braden, A. L., Craggs, J. G., & Jensen, M. P. (2011). Psychometric properties of the Community Integration Questionnaire in a heterogeneous sample of adults with physical disability. *Archives of Physical Medicine and Rehabilitation, 92*(10), 1602–1610. https://doi.org/10.1016/j.apmr.2011.05.004

Horowitz, B. P., & Chang, P. F. J. (2004). Promoting well-being and engagement in life through occupational therapy lifestyle redesign: A pilot study with adult day programs. *Topics in Geriatric Rehabilitation, 20*, 46–58. https://doi.org/10.1097/00013614-200401000-00007

Hwang, A. W., Liou, T. H., Bedell, G. M., Kang, L. J., Chen, W. C., Yen, C. F., Chang, K. H., & Liao, H. F. (2013). Psychometric properties of the Child and Adolescent Scale of Participation Traditional Chinese version. *International Journal of Rehabilitation Research, 36*(3), 211–220. https://doi.org/10.1097/MRR.0b013e32835d0b27

Hwang, J. L., Nochajski, S. M., Linn, R. T., & Wu, Y. W. B. (2004). The development of the School Function Assessment - Chinese version for cross-cultural use in Taiwan. *Occupational Therapy International, 11*(1), 26–39. https://doi.org/10.1002/oti.195

Igarashi, G., Karashima, C., & Uemura, J. I. (2020). Items selection for the Japanese version of the preschool activity card sort. *OTJR: Occupation, Participation and Health, 40*(3), 166–174. https://doi.org/10.1177/1539449220906794

Imms, C., & Adair, B. (2017). Participation trajectories: Impact of school transitions on children and adolescents with cerebral palsy. *Developmental Medicine and Child Neurology, 59*, 174–182. https://doi.org/10.1111/dmcn.13229

Imms, C., Adair, B., Keen, D., Ullenhag, A., Rosenbaum, P., & Granlund, M. (2015). "Participation": A systematic review of language, definitions, and constructs used in intervention research with children with disabilities. *Developmental Medicine and Child Neurology, 58*, 29–38. https://doi.org/10.1111/dmcn.12932

Ioncoli, M., Berardi, A., Tofani, M., Panuccio, F., Servadio, A., Valente, D., & Galeoto, G. (2020). Crosscultural validation of the community integration questionnaire-revised in an Italian population. *Occupational Therapy International, 2020*, 8916541. https://doi.org/10.1155/2020/8916541

Jarvis, J. M., Gurga, A. R., Lim, H., Cameron, J., Gorter, J. W., Choong, K., & Khetani, M. A. (2019). Caregiver strategy use to promote children's home participation after pediatric critical illness. *Archives of Physical Medicine and Rehabilitation, 100*(11), 2144–2150. https://doi.org/10.1016/j.apmr.2019.05.034

Jarvis, J. M., Fayed, N., Fink, E. L., Choong, K., & Khetani, M. A. (2020). Caregiver dissatisfaction with their child's participation in home activities after pediatric critical illness. *BMC Pediatrics, 20*(1), 415. https://doi.org/10.1186/s12887-020-02306-3

Jarvis, J. M., & Fink, E. L. (2021). More than a feeling: Understanding function and health related quality of life after pediatric neurocritical illness. *Neurocritical Care, 35*(2), 308–310. https://doi.org/10.1007/s12028-021-01270-9

Jeong, Y., Law, M., Stratford, P., DeMatteo, C., & Kim, H. (2016). Cross-cultural validation and psychometric evaluation of the Participation and Environment Measure for Children and Youth in Korea. *Disability and Rehabilitation, 38*(22), 2217–2228. https://doi.org/10.3109/09638288.2015.1123302

Jones, E., Perry, J., Lowe, K., Felce, D., Toogood, S., Dunstan, F., Allen, D., & Pagler, J. (1999). Opportunity and the promotion of activity among adults with severe intellectual disability living in community residences: The impact of training staff in active support. *Journal of Intellectual Disability Research, 43*, 164–178. https://doi.org/10.1046/j.1365-2788.1999.00177.x

Kaelin, V. C., Valizadeh, M., Salgado, Z., Parde, N., & Khetani, M. A. (2021). Artificial intelligence in rehabilitation targeting the participation of children and youth with disabilities: Scoping review. *Journal of Medical Internet Research, 23*(11), e25745. https://doi.org/10.2196/25745

Kaelin, V. C., Wallace, E. R., Werler, M. M., Collett, B. R., Rosenberg, J., & Khetani, M. A. (2021). Caregiver perspectives on school participation among students with craniofacial microsomia. *American Journal of Occupational Therapy, 75*(2), 1–10. https://doi.org/10.5014/ajot.2021.041277

Kang, L., Hwang, A., Palisano, R., King, G., Chiarello, L., & Chen, C. (2017). Validation of the Preschool Children's Participation for children with physical disabilities. *Developmental Neurorehabilitation, 20*(5), 266–273. https://doi.org/10.3109/17518423.2016.1158746

Kessler, D., Egan, M., Dubouloz, C. J., McEwen, S., & Graham, F. P. (2017). Occupational Performance Coaching for stroke survivors: A pilot randomized controlled trial. *American Journal of Occupational Therapy, 71*(3), 7103190020p1–7103190020p7. https://doi.org/10.5014/ajot.2017.024216

Khetani, M. A. (2015). Validation of environmental content in the Young Children's Participation and Environment Measure. *Archives of Physical Medicine and Rehabilitation, 96*, 317–322. https://doi.org/10.1016/j.apmr.2014.11.016

Khetani, M. A. (2017). Capturing change: Participation trajectories in cerebral palsy during life transitions. *Developmental Medicine and Child Neurology, 59*(2), 118–119. https://doi.org/10.1111/dmcn.13260

Khetani, M. A., Albrecht, E. C., Jarvis, J. M., Pogorzelski, D., Cheng, E., & Choong, K. (2018). Determinants of change in home participation among critically ill children. *Developmental Medicine and Child Neurology, 60*(8), 793–800. https://doi.org/10.1111/dmcn.13731

Khetani, M. A., Cohn, E., Orsmond, G., Law, M., & Coster, W. (2013). Parent perspectives of participation in home and community life when receiving Part C early intervention services. *Topics in Early Childhood Special Education, 32*(4), 234–245. https://doi.org/10.1177/0271121411418004

Khetani, M. A., & Coster, W. (2019). Social participation. In B. A. B. Schell & G. Gillen (Eds.), *Willard and Spackman's occupational therapy* (13th ed., pp. 847–860). Wolters Kluwer.

Khetani, M. A., Graham, J. E., Davies, P. L., Law, M. C., & Simeonsson, R. J. (2015). Psychometric properties of the Young Children's Participation and Environment Measure (YC-PEM). *Archives of Physical Medicine and Rehabilitation, 96*, 307–316. https://doi.org/10.1016/j.apmr.2014.11.016

Khetani, M. A., Lim, H., & Corden, M. (2017). Caregiver input to optimize the design of a pediatric care planning guide for rehabilitation: Descriptive study. *JMIR Rehabilitation and Assistive Technologies, 4*, e10. https://doi.org/10.2196/rehab.7566

Khetani, M. A., McManus, B. M., Albrecht, E. C., Kaelin, V. C., Dooling-Litfin, J. K., & Scully, E. A. (2020). Early intervention service intensity and young children's home participation. *BMC Pediatrics, 20*(1), 1–10. https://doi.org/10.1186/s12887-020-02182-x

King, G. A., Law, M., King, S., Hurley, P., Rosenbaum, P., Hanna, S., Kertoy, M., & Young, N. (2004). *Children's Assessment of Participation & Enjoyment (CAPE) and Preferences for Activities of Children (PAC).* PsychCorp.

Kolehmainen, N., Marshall, J., Hislop, J., Fayed, N., Kay, D., Ternent, L., & Pennington, L. (2020). Implementing participation-focused services: A study to develop the Method for using Audit and Feedback in Participation Implementation (MAPi). *Child: Care, Health and Development, 46*(1), 37–45. https://doi.org/10.1111/cch.12723

Kramer, J., Barth, Y., Curtis, K., Livingston, K., O'Neil, M., Smith, Z., Vallier, S., & Wolfe, A. (2013). Involving youth with disabilities in the development and evaluation of a new advocacy training: Project TEAM. *Disability and Rehabilitation, 35*, 614–622. https://doi.org/10.3109/09638288.2012.705218

Kramer, J., & Hammel, J. (2011). "I do lots of things": Children with cerebral palsy perceptions of competence for everyday activities. *International Journal of Disability, Development, and Education, 58*, 121–136. https://doi.org/10.1080/1034912x.2011.570496

Kramer, J. M., Roemer, K., Liljenquist, K., Shin, J., & Hart, S. (2014). Formative evaluation of project TEAM (Teens Making Environment and Activity Modifications). *Intellectual and Developmental Disabilities, 52*, 258–272. https://doi.org/10.1352/1934-9556-52.4.258

Kramer, J., Yinusa-Nyahkoon, L., Olafsson, S., Penti, B., Woodhams, E., Bickmore, T., & Jack, B. W. (2021). Black men's experiences with health care: Individuals' accounts of challenges, suggestions for change, and the potential utility of virtual agent technology to assist black men with health management. *Qualitative Health Research, 31*(10), 1772–1785. https://doi.org/10.1177/10497323211013323

Krieger, B., Schulze, C., Boyd, J., Amann, R., Piškur, B., Beurskens, A., Teplicky, R., & Moser, A. (2020). Cross-cultural adaptation of the Participation and Environment Measure for Children and Youth (PEM-CY) into German: A qualitative study in three countries. *BMC Pediatrics, 20*(1), 1–15. https://doi.org/10.1186/s12887-020-02343-y

Lancioni, G. E., Singh, N. N., O'Reilly, M. F., Sigafoos, J., Alberti, G., Perilli, V., Chiariello, V., Grillo, G., & Turi, C. (2020). A tablet-based program to enable people with intellectual and other disabilities to access leisure activities and video calls. *Disability and Rehabilitation: Assistive Technology, 15*(1), 14–20. https://doi.org/10.1080/17483107.2018.1508515

Laskowski, A. (2022). Agganis arena's new sensory room debuts. https://www.bu.edu/articles/2022/agganis-arenas-new-sensory-room-debuts/?utm_campaign=bu_today&utm_source=email_20221221_full&utm_medium=2_must_read_2&utm_content=community

Law, M. (2002). Participation in the occupations of everyday life. *American Journal of Occupational Therapy, 56*, 640–649. https://doi.org/10.5014/ajot.56.6.640

Law, M., Darrah, J., Pollock, N., Wilson, B., Russell, D., Walter, S., Rosenbaum, P., & Galuppi, B. (2011). Focus on function: A cluster, randomized controlled trial comparing child- versus context-focused intervention for young children with cerebral palsy. *Developmental Medicine and Child Neurology, 53*, 621–629. https://doi.org/10.1111/j.1469-8749.2011.03962.x

Law, M., King, G., Petrenchik, T., Kertoy, M., & Anaby, D. (2012). The assessment of preschool children's participation: Internal consistency and construct validity. *Physical & Occupational Therapy in Pediatrics, 32*, 272–287. https://doi.org/10.3109/01942638.2012.662584

Lee, D., Fischer, H., Zera, S., Robertson, R., & Hammel, J. (2017). Examining a participation-focused stroke self-management intervention in a day rehabilitation setting: A quasi-experimental pilot study. *Topics in Stroke Rehabilitation, 24*, 601–607. https://doi.org/10.1080/10749357.2017.1375222

Liao, Y. T., Hwang, A. W., Liao, H. F., Granlund, M., & Kang, L. J. (2019). Understanding the participation in home, school, and community activities reported by children with disabilities and their parents: A pilot study. *International Journal of Environmental Research and Public Health, 16*(12), 2217. https://doi.org/10.3390/ijerph16122217

Lim, C., Law, M., Khetani, M., Rosenbaum, P., & Pollock, N. (2018). Psychometric evaluation of the Young Children's Participation and Environment Measure (YC-PEM) for use in Singapore. *Physical & Occupational Therapy in Pediatrics, 38*(3), 316–328. https://doi.org/10.1080/01942638.2017.1347911

Liu, T. W., Ng, S. S. M., & Ng, G. Y. F. (2014). Translation and initial validation of the Chinese (Cantonese) version of community integration measure for use in patients with chronic stroke. *BioMed Research International, 2014*, 623836. https://doi.org/10.1155/2014/623836

Longo, E., Badia, M., Orgaz, B., & Verdugo, M. A. (2014). Cross-cultural validation of the children's assessment of participation and enjoyment (CAPE) in Spain. *Child: Care, Health and Development, 40*(2), 231–241. https://doi.org/10.1111/cch.12012

Magasi, S., & Hammel, J. (2004). Social support and social network mobilization in African American woman who have experienced strokes. *Disability Studies Quarterly, 24*(4). https://doi.org/10.18061/dsq.v24i4.878

Maisel, J. L. (2006). Toward inclusive housing and neighborhood design: A look at visitability. *Community Development, 37*, 26–34. https://doi.org/10.1080/15575330.2006.10383105

Majnemer, A., Shikako-Thomas, K., Chokron, N., Law, M., Shevell, M., Chlingaryan, G., Poulin, C., & Rosenbaum, P. (2010). Leisure activity preferences for 6- to 12-year-old children with cerebral palsy. *Developmental Medicine and Child Neurology, 52*, 167–173. https://doi.org/10.1111/j.1469-8749.2009.03393.x

Malkawi, S. H., Abu-Dahab, S. M. N., Amro, A. F., & Almasri, N. A. (2017). The psychometric properties of the Arabic preschool activity card sort. *Occupational Therapy International, 2017*, 5180382. https://doi.org/10.1155/2017/5180382

Malkawi, S. H., Hamed, R. T., Abu-Dahab, S. M. N., Alheresh, R. A., & Holm, M. B. (2015). Development of the Arabic Version of the Preschool Activity Card Sort (A-PACS). *Child: Care, Health and Development, 41*(4), 559–568. https://doi.org/10.1111/cch.12209

Matsuka, K., Giles-Heinz, A., Flinn, N., Neighbor, M., & Bass-Haugen, J. (2003). Outcomes of a pilot occupational therapy wellness program for older adults. *American Journal of Occupational Therapy, 57*, 220–224. https://doi.org/10.5014/ajot.57.2.220

McConachie, H., Colver, A., Forsyth, R., Jarvis, S., & Parkinson, K. (2006). Participation of disabled children: How should it be characterised and measured? *Disability and Rehabilitation, 28*, 1157–1164. https://doi.org/10.1080/09638280500534507

McDougall, J., Bedell, G., & Wright, V. (2013). The youth report version of the Child and Adolescent Scale of Participation (CASP): Assessment of psychometric properties and comparison with parent report.

Child: Care, Health and Development, 39(4), 512–522. https://doi .org/10.1111/cch.12050

Morris, C., Kurinczuk, J., & Fitzpatrick, R. (2005). Child or family assessed measures of activity performance and participation for children with cerebral palsy: A structured review. *Child: Care, Health and Development, 31*, 397–407. https://doi.org/10.1111/j.1365-2214.2005.00519.x

Murchland, S., & Parkyn, H. (2010). Using assistive technology for schoolwork: The experience of children with physical disabilities. *Disability and Rehabilitation: Assistive Technology, 5*(6), 438–447. https://doi.org/10.3109/17483107.2010.48177

Narad, M. E., Bedell, G., King, J. A., Johnson, J., Turkstra, L. S., Haarbauer-Krupa, J., & Wade, S. L. (2018). Social Participation and Navigation (SPAN): Description and usability of app based coaching intervention for adolescents with TBI. *Developmental Neurorehabilitation, 21*(7), 439–448. https://doi.org/10.1080/17518423.2017.1354092

National Institutes of Health. (2017). *NINDS common data elements.* https://www.commondataelements.ninds.nih.gov/#page=Default

Negahban, H., Fattahizadeh, P., Ghasemzadeh, R., Salehi, R., Majdinasab, N., & Mazaheri, M. (2013). The Persian version of community integration questionnaire in persons with multiple sclerosis: Translation, reliability, validity, and factor analysis. *Disability and Rehabilitation, 35*(17), 1453–1459. https://doi.org/10.3109/09638288.2012.741653

Nordtorp, H., Nyquist, A., Jahnsen R., Moser, T., & Liv Inger, S. (2013). Reliability of the Norwegian Version of the Children's Assessment of Participation and Enjoyment (CAPE) and Preferences for Activities of Children (PAC). *Physical & Occupational Therapy in Pediatrics, 33*(2), 199–212. https://doi.org/10.3109/01942638.2012.739269

Noreau, L., Fougeyrollas, P., Post, M., & Asano, M. (2005). Participation after spinal cord injury: The evolution of conceptualization and measurement. *Journal of Neurologic Physical Therapy, 29*, 147–156. https://doi.org/10.1097/01.npt.0000282247.15911.dc

Noreau, L., Lepage, C., Boissiere, L., Picard, R., Fougeyrollas, P., Mathieu, J., Desmarais, G., & Nadeau, L. (2007). Measuring participation in children with disabilities using the Assessment of Life Habits. *Developmental Medicine and Child Neurology, 49*, 666–671. https:// doi.org/10.1111/j.1469-8749.2007.00666.x

O'Connor, B., Kerr, C., Shields, N., Adair, B., & Imms, C. (2021). Steering towards collaborative assessment: A qualitative study of parents' experiences of evidence-based assessment practices for their child with cerebral palsy. *Disability and Rehabilitation, 43*(4), 458–467. https:// doi.org/10.1080/09638288.2019.1629652

Ow, N., Appau, A., Matout, M., & Mayo, N. E. (2021). What is QOL in children and adolescents with physical disabilities? A thematic synthesis of pediatric QOL literature. *Quality of Life Research, 30*(5), 1233–1248. https://doi.org/10.1007/s11136-021-02769-6

Pizur-Barnekow, K., Patrick, T., Rhyner, P. M., Cashin, S., & Rentmeester, A. (2011). Readability of early intervention program literature. *Topics in Early Childhood Special Education, 31*(1), 58–64. https://doi .org/10.1177/0271121410387676

Rintala, D. H., Novy, D. M., Garza, H. M., Young, M. E., High, W. M., & Chiou-Tan, F. Y. (2002). Psychometric properties of a Spanish-language version of the Community Integration Questionnaire (CIQ). *Rehabilitation Psychology, 47*(2), 144–164. https://doi .org/10.1037/0090 5550.47.2.144

Saeki, S., Okazaki, T., & Hachisuka, K. (2006). Concurrent validity of the community integration questionnaire in patients with traumatic brain injury in Japan. *Journal of Rehabilitation Medicine, 38*(5), 333–335. https://doi.org/10.1080/16501970600780245

Samuels, A., Dada, S., Van Niekerk, K., Arvidsson, P., & Huus, K. (2020). Children in South Africa with and without intellectual disabilities' rating of their frequency of participation in everyday activities. *International Journal of Environmental Research and Public Health, 17*(18), 1–12. https://doi.org/10.3390/ijerph17186702

Sander, A. M., Seel, R. T., Kreutzer, J. S., Hall, K. M., High, W. M., & Rosenthal, M. (2007). Agreement between persons with traumatic brain injury and their relatives regarding psychosocial outcome using the Community Integration Questionnaire. *Archives of Physical Medicine and Rehabilitation, 78*, 353–357. https://doi.org/10.1016/s0003-9993(97)90225-2

Schell, B. A. B., & Gillen, G. (2019). Glossary. In B. A. B. Schell & G. Gillen (Eds.), *Willard and Spackman's occupational therapy* (13th ed., pp. 1191–1215). Wolters Kluwer.

Schelly, C., Davies, P., & Spooner, C. (2011). Student perceptions of faculty implementation of universal design for learning. *Journal of Postsecondary Education and Disability, 24*, 17–28.

Shabat, T., Fogel-Grinvald., Anaby, D., & Golos, A. (2021). Perfil de participación de niños y jóvenes, de 6 a 14 años, con y sin TDAH, y el impacto de los factores ambientales. *Revista Ciencias de La Actividad Física, 18*(2), 1–16. https://www.mdpi.com/1660-4601/18/2/537

Shahin, S., DiRezze, B., Ahmed, S., & Anaby, D. (2022). Development and content validity of the youth and young-adult participation and environment measure (Y-PEM). *Disability and Rehabilitation, 45*, 1–13. https://doi.org/10.1080/09638288.2022.2030809

Shi, L., Granlund, M., Zhao, Y., Hwang, A. W., Kang, L. J., & Huus, K. (2021). Transcultural adaptation, content validity and reliability of the instrument 'Picture My Participation' for children and youth with and without intellectual disabilities in mainland China. *Scandinavian Journal of Occupational Therapy, 28*(2), 147–157. https://doi.org/10.1 080/11038128.2020.1817976

Shikako-Thomas, K., Lach, L., Majnemer, A., Nimignon, J., Cameron, K., & Shevell, M. (2009). Quality of life from the perspective of adolescents with cerebral palsy: "I just think I'm a normal kid, I just happen to have a disability." *Quality of Life Research, 18*, 825–832. https://doi .org/10.1007/s11136-009-9501-3

Shirley Ryan AbilityLab. (2010). *Rehabilitation measures database.* http://www.rehabmeasures.org/default.aspx

Simpson, K., Imms, C., & Keen, D. (2021). The experience of participation: Eliciting the views of children on the autism spectrum. *Disability and Rehabilitation, 44*, 1700–1708. https://doi.org/10.1080/09638 288.2021.1903100

Souza, M. A. P. De, Mancini, M. C., Coster, W. J., Kirkwood, R. N., Figueiredo, E. M. De, & Sampaio, R. F. (2018). Cross-cultural adaptation to Brazilian Portuguese of the Activity Measure for Post-Acute Care (AM-PAC) short forms for outpatients in rehabilitation. *Brazilian Journal of Physical Therapy, 22*(2), 135–143. https://doi .org/10.1016/j.bjpt.2017.07.003

Srinivasan, R., Kulkarni, V., Smriti, S., Teplicky, R., & Anaby, D. (2021). Cross-cultural adaptation and evaluation of the participation and environment measure for children and youth to the Indian context—A mixed-methods study. *International Journal of Environmental Research and Public Health, 18*(4), 1–16. https://doi.org/10.3390/ijerph18041514

Stiers, W., Carlozzi, N., Cernich, A., Velozo, C., Pape, T., Hart, T., Gulliver, S., Rogers, M., Villarrea, E., Gordon, S., Gordon, W., & Whiteneck, G. (2012). Measurement of social participation outcomes in rehabilitation of veterans with traumatic brain injury. *Journal of Rehabilitation Research and Development, 49*(1), 139–154. https://doi .org/10.1682/JRRD.2010.07.0131

Stoffel, A., & Berg, C. (2008). Spanish translation and validation of the Preschool Activity Card Sort. *Physical & Occupational Therapy in Pediatrics, 28*, 171–189. https://doi.org/10.1080/01942630802031859

Tamis-Monda, C. S., Way, N., Hughes, D., Yoshikawa, H., Kalman, R. K., & Niwa, E. Y. (2007). Parents' goals for children: The dynamic coexistence of individualism and collectivism in cultures and individuals. *Social Development, 17*, 183–209. https://doi .org/10.1111/j.1467-9507.2007.00419.x

Thornton, A. L., Hackett, E., Wilkie, A., Gallon, J., Grisbrook, T. L., Elliott, C. M., & Ciccarelli, M. (2021). A qualitative exploration of motivations and barriers for community leisure organisations' engagement with the Jooay™ mobile app. *Disability and Rehabilitation, 44*, 1–9. https://doi.org/10.1080/09638288.2021.1986581

Tickle-Degnen, L., Ellis, T., Saint-Hilaire, M. H., Thomas, C. A., & Wagenaar, R. (2010). Self-management rehabilitation and health-related quality of life in Parkinson's disease: A randomized controlled trial. *Movement Disorders, 25*, 194–204. https://doi.org/10.1002/mds.22940

Tomas, V., Srinivasan, R., Kulkarni, V., Teplicky, R., Anaby, D., & Khetani, M. (2021). A guiding process to culturally adapt assessments for participation-focused pediatric practice: The case of the Participation and Environment Measures (PEM). *Disability and Rehabilitation, 44*, 1–13. https://doi.org/10.1080/09638288.2021.1960645

Uemura, J. I., Tanikaga, M., Tanaka, M., Shimose, M., Hoshino, A., & Igarashi, G. (2019). Selection of activity items for development of the activity Card Sort–Japan Version. *OTJR Occupation, Participation and Health, 39*(1), 23–31. https://doi.org/10.1177/1539449218784729

Ullenhag, A., Bult, M. K., Nyquist, A., Ketelaar, M., Jahnsen, R., Krumlinde-Sundholm, L., Almqvist, L., & Granlund, M. (2012). An international comparison of patterns of participation in leisure activities for children with and without disabilities in Sweden, Norway and the Netherlands. *Developmental Neurorehabilitation, 15*(5), 369–385. https://doi.org/10.3109/17518423.2012.694915

Umeda, C. J., Fogelberg, D., Jirikowic, T., Pitonyak, J. S., Mroz, T., & Ideishi, R. (2017). Expanding the implementation of the Americans with Disabilities Act for populations with intellectual and developmental disabilities: The role of organization-level occupational therapy consultation. *American Journal of Occupational Therapy, 71*, 7104090010p1–7104090010p6. https://doi.org/10.5014/ajot.2017.714001

Vaughan, M. W., Felson, D. T., LaValley, M. P., Orsmond, G. I., Niu, J., Lewis, C. E., Segal, N. A., Nevitt, M. C., & Keysor, J. J. (2017). Perceived community environmental factors and risk of five-year participation restriction among older adults with or at risk of knee osteoarthritis. *Arthritis Care & Research (Hoboken), 69*, 952–958. https://doi.org/10.1002/acr.23085

Wade, S. L., Bedell, G., King, J. A., Jacquin, M., Turkstra, L. S., Haarbauer-Krupa, J., Johnson, J., Salloum, R., & Narad, M. E. (2018). Social participation and navigation (SPAN) program for adolescents with acquired brain injury: Pilot findings. *Rehabilitation Psychology, 63*(3), 327–337. https://doi.org/10.1037/rep0000187

Whiteneck, G. (2006). Conceptual models of disability: Past, present, and future. In M. J. Field & A. M. Jette (Eds.), *The future of disability in America* (pp. 50–64). The National Academies Press.

Whiteneck, G., Charlifue, S., Gerhart, K., Overholser, J., & Richardson, G. (1992). Quantifying handicap: A new measure of long-term rehabilitation outcomes. *Archives of Physical Medicine and Rehabilitation, 73*, 519–526. https://doi.org/10.5555/uri:pii:000399939290185Y

Whiteneck, G. G. (2011). Craig handicap assessment and reporting technique. *Encyclopedia of Clinical Neuropsychology, 2011*, 728–730. https://doi.org/10.1007/978-0-387-79948-3_1789

Willer, B., Rosenthal, M., Kreutzer, J. S., Gordon, W. A., & Rempel, R. (1993). Assessment of community integration following rehabilitation for traumatic brain injury. *The Journal of Head Trauma Rehabilitation, 8*, 75–87. https://doi.org/10.1097/00001199-199308020-00009

Wolf, T., Baum, C. M., Lee, D., & Hammel, J. (2016). The development of the Improving Participation after Stroke Self-Management Program (IPASS): An exploratory randomized clinical study. *Topics in Stroke Rehabilitation, 23*, 284–292. https://doi.org/10.1080/10749357.2016.1155278

World Health Organization. (1998). *Quality of life.* http://www.who.int/healthpromotion/about/HPR%20Glossary%201998.pdf

World Health Organization. (2001). *International classification of functioning, disability and health: ICF.* Author.

World Health Organization. (2007). *International classification of functioning, disability and health: Version for children and youth.* Author.

World Health Organization. (2012). *WHOQOL user manual.* https://www.who.int/tools/whoqol

The Role of Occupational Therapy in Health Management

The Time to Act Is Now!

Margaret Swarbrick and Laurie L. Knis-Matthews

LEARNING OBJECTIVES

After reading this chapter, you will be able to:

1. Discuss how the evolution and addition of health management in the Occupational Therapy Practice Framework (4th ed.) as the ninth occupation can advance the profession in the 21st century.
2. Define the occupation of health management and its seven subcomponents: personal care device management, nutrition management, physical activity, medication management, communication with the healthcare system, symptom and condition management, and social and emotional health promotion and maintenance.
3. Describe how expanding our understanding of health, to include a focus on wellness, social determinants of health, and health disparities, can help to support health management across the life span.
4. Examine opportunities and skills needed to effectively enhance health management for individuals, groups, and populations.

Introduction

Many challenges and opportunities lie ahead for the occupational therapy (OT) profession to meet the total needs of individuals, groups, and populations to effectively support the health of people in society across the life span. The profession has an important chance to assume a lead role using a wellness lens to address health disparities. Health management, as an occupation, can play a key role by focusing on preventable and chronic diseases, particularly in populations that have historically been marginalized by the healthcare system. Health disparities must be addressed to ensure optimal health outcomes. In the OT philosophy, this is a social justice issue. We are armed with a framework, Occupational Therapy Practice Framework: Domain and Process, 4th edition (American Occupational Therapy Association [AOTA], 2020a), that can direct care that is adaptive and holistic.

The OT profession is in an ideal position to design and deliver effective interventions and new programs to support health management. This chapter begins by defining the evolution of health management—as well as health, wellness, and social determinants of health (SDOH). Core competencies, including health literacy, a wellness promotion model, and new roles

857

will be reviewed. Implications for OT practice will be suggested. This chapter will highlight how health management, as an area of occupation, can assure the OT professional has an important powerful role in ensuring that people are able to care for themselves and self-direct their health and wellness.

The Evolution of Health Management

OT continues to respond to society's needs using occupation as both the means and the end of assisting people to health and well-being in all facets of their lives (Amini, 2021; AOTA, 2020a). We are a pragmatic profession that empowers people by facilitating their ability to adapt and organize their daily routines to prevent and minimize dysfunction; promote and develop a healthy lifestyle; and facilitate adaptation and recovery from injury, disease, or developmental challenges. The profession has long recognized the importance of wellness habits and routines that promote the adoption and maintenance of healthy behaviors that impact quality of life and life span. Practitioners help people create new health habits and routines across their life span. For example, OT practitioners can design and deliver health-promoting play activities for children to enhance physical well-being and social skills; develop and implement injury prevention programs for adult workers; and educate seniors on home and activity modifications to prevent falls and manage medications. Many of these examples relate to health management, an addition to the list of occupations for which the profession has distinct tools and techniques to assist clients.

Health management, as an occupation, is important because it outlines important areas of functioning where the profession is competent to address to ensure that people served in the 21st century can care for themselves to promote a high quality of life and longer quality of life functioning as independently as possible. **Health management** is defined as "activities related to developing, managing, and maintaining health and wellness routines, including self-management, with the goal of improving or maintaining health to support participation in other occupations" (AOTA, 2020a, p. 32). The seven health management subcomponents include personal care device management, nutrition management, physical activity, medication management, communication with the healthcare system, symptom and condition management, and social and emotional health promotion and maintenance (Figure 50.1). Table 50.1 outlines the health management subcomponents that practitioners may examine and play a role in assisting individuals, groups, and populations across one's life span.

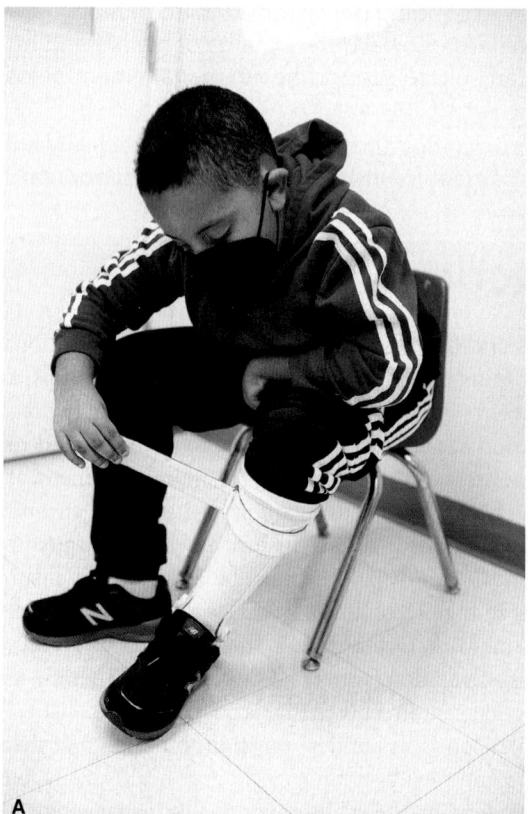
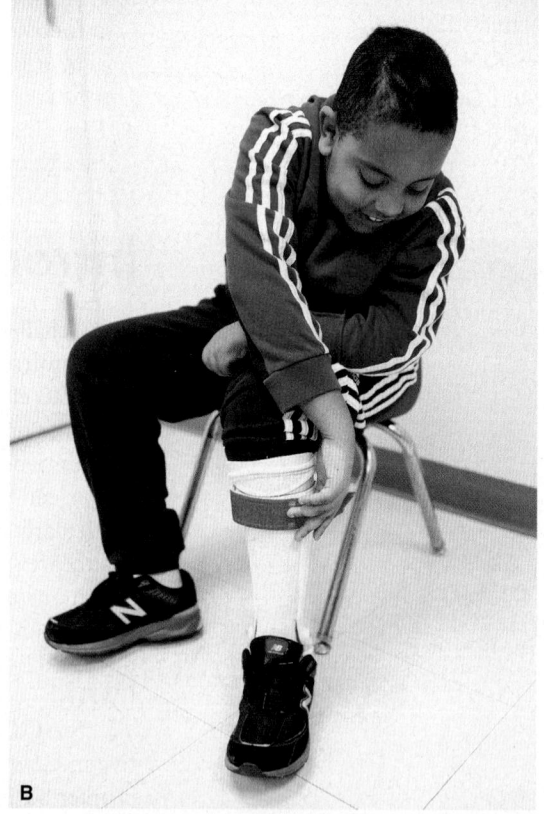

FIGURE 50.1 One of the subcomponents of health management is personal care device. Here, an OT practitioner teaches a young boy to put on his orthotics so he can go outside to play with his brother. (Picture courtesy of Brielle Hassa.)

TABLE 50.1	**Health Management Subcomponents**
Subcomponents	**Description**
1. Social and emotional health promotion and maintenance	• Identifying personal strengths and assets, managing emotions, expressing needs effectively • Seeking occupations and social engagement to support health and wellness • Developing self-identity • Making choices to improve quality of life in participation
2. Symptom and condition management	• Managing physical and mental health needs, including using coping strategies for illness, trauma history, or societal stigma; managing pain; managing chronic disease • Recognizing symptom changes and fluctuations • Developing and using strategies for managing and regulating emotions • Planning time and establishing behavioral patterns for restorative activities (e.g., meditation) • Using community and social supports; navigating and accessing the healthcare system
3. Communication with the healthcare system	• Expressing and receiving verbal, written, and digital communication with healthcare and insurance providers, including understanding and advocating for self or others
4. Medication management	• Communicating with the physician about prescriptions, filling prescriptions at the pharmacy • Interpreting medication instructions • Taking medications on a routine basis, refilling prescriptions in a timely manner
5. Physical activity	• Completing cardiovascular exercise, strength training, and balance training to improve or maintain health and decrease risk of health episodes, such as by incorporating walks into daily routine
6. Nutrition management	• Implementing and adhering to nutrition and hydration • Preparing meals to support health goals • Participating in health-promoting diet routines
7. Personal care device management	• Procuring, using, cleaning, and maintaining personal care devices, including hearing aids, contact lenses, glasses, orthotics, prosthetics, adaptive equipment, pessaries

To provide context in the fourth edition of the Occupational Therapy Practice Framework: Domain and Process (Amini, 2021; AOTA, 2020a), health management was added as a ninth occupation to the previous list of eight occupations (activities of daily living, instrumental activities of daily living, rest and sleep, education, work, play, leisure, and social participation), elevating its importance to the identity, value, and meaning for each person, group, or population served. As part of the evolutionary process of the Framework, expanded descriptions emphasize the seven subcomponents of health management.

The third edition of the Framework identified the components of nutrition, medication routines, and physical fitness. Medication management has been expanded to emphasize our explicit role in the process of ensuring that people have their medication, are safe with their medication, and can remember and physically take their medication. Practitioners can play an important role in communicating with the medical team, including the physician, if medication side effects are noted, as well as ensuring that a prescription is current and refills are available and that the pharmacy has the meds in stock. OT practitioners can help the person interpret instructions, ensure that a routine for taking medication is in place, and establish a plan for medication refills (Amini, 2021; AOTA, 2020a). Schwartz and Smith (2016) examined the effectiveness of an OT intervention for 19 adults with chronic illnesses and poor medication adherence. The adults in the OT group reported greater compliance managing their medications and demonstrated new adaptive strategies relating to such practices as advocacy, education, and use of assistive technology. Occupational therapists are well prepared to address issues of medication management and adherence (AOTA, 2017).

The fourth edition of the Framework also places a greater emphasis on nutrition management and physical activity for individuals, groups, and populations, an important facet of a person's overall health management. Physical exercise, diet, and fluid intake are essential components of a healthy lifestyle. It is necessary to understand the context for which physical activity occurs to each person, group or population served. For example, Mische-Lawson and Little (2017) examined a sensory-based swim program for 42 children diagnosed with autism spectrum disorder. Results of this study demonstrated an improvement in swim skills, interest in swimming, and increased physical activity maintenance as a part of health management.

There is a modest amount of evidence describing the value of health management research and interventions. Arbesman and Mosley (2012) present a systematic review of the literature on occupation- and activity-based health management and maintenance interventions for productive aging (see "Commentary on the Evidence" section). Brown and associates (2015) examined the Nutrition and Exercise for Wellness and Recovery (NEW-R) weight-loss intervention with participants from a community-based mental health program. Over the eight weekly NEW-R sessions, knowledge of nutrition and changes in weight outcomes were measured immediately post-intervention and at 6 months. Nutrition and physical activity knowledge increased and there were slight weight decreases. Influenced by the Well Elderly Lifestyle Redesign program (Jackson et al., 1998), a variety of interventions have been developed that address health management for a range of populations. Uyeshiro and Collins (2017) examined the efficacy of the Well Elderly Lifestyle Redesign program

for people living with chronic pain. Research is sparse on the role of OT practitioners in pain programs because prescription medication continues to dominate pain intervention plans. This is truly an important area for practice given the high rates of pain conditions and negative impacts of pain medications. Schepens and colleagues (2021) designed a lifestyle redesign intervention program for rural-dwelling late-midlife Latinos, which resulted in gains in health-related outcomes in terms of knowledge, practice, and well-being 1 year after the intervention program was completed. See OT Story 50.1.

OT STORY 50.1 HELPING JANE

Jane is a divorced woman who lives with her two small dogs in a house that she rents on the outskirts of an older city in the United States. Even though she has a college degree and a good work history, she struggled to find well-paying job after moving to a new state at 60 years of age. She was working for the 2020 Census during the COVID-19 lockdown, going out each day in the summertime heat to knock on doors and take census data. The work was hard on her physically. She is overweight; has arthritis in her hands, neck, and back; and was struggling with the high temperatures and the steps she had to climb to people's front doors. She had been feeling poorly for a few days and woke up one Sunday morning feeling even worse. Eventually, she realized something was wrong. Then, she thought she should go to the hospital, but when she went outside, she could not figure out how to open her car door, so she went to a neighbor's house. Once there, she was unable to tell the neighbor what was wrong, so he called 9-1-1. Jane was having a stroke, and it was eventually discovered that the stroke was caused by a blood clot from atrial fibrillation. After a week in the hospital, she was discharged home, and her sister came to help get her through the first few weeks.

Jane's low income and lack of health insurance qualified her for Medicaid, which the hospital enrolled her in. Through Medicaid, she was assigned a home health nurse, a speech-language pathologist, and an occupational therapist, each of whom would visit her at home.

The occupational therapist, Casey, started visiting Jane right away. Her family found Casey to be very helpful. Here are some of the suggestions from Casey that the family implemented:

- Local friends had taken in the dogs while Jane was hospitalized, and Casey suggested that the friends should keep the dogs for a few weeks until Jane's new routines were solidified.
- He suggested that the family buy Jane two large pill organizers in two different colors—one for morning pills and one for evening pills.
- He also suggested that she get a cross-body bag so that she could keep her smartphone with her at all times in case she fell.
- He surveyed Jane's house and suggested removing area rugs, installing grab bars in the bathrooms, and lowering the height of her bed.

- Casey strongly urged Jane to start walking every day, even though at that point she could only walk about half a block. Whenever he came to see her, he would take her out for a walk. He said that any walking was better than no walking, and if she walked a little every day, by the time her dogs came home, she would be able to walk them around the block.

In the beginning, Jane had trouble finding words, pronouncing words, and organizing her thoughts. All of that improved in the months after the stroke. She eventually developed her own system for taking the many medications she needed, organizing them in multiple pill boxes and using a smartphone app to remind her when to take them. Jane used the cross-body bag for a few months but eventually put it aside. She replaced her area rugs when her dogs came home because she said her floors were too slippery for the dogs. She has tripped over them many times since the stroke. Jane did not keep up with the walking program.

Two years after the stroke, Jane's health has continued to deteriorate. Since the stroke, she has had two procedures to remove kidney stones, a procedure to reduce pressure in her eyes owing to acute-angle glaucoma, and surgery to repair her L5 vertebra, which had disintegrated owing to arthritis. At 65 years of age, her mobility is very limited. She can go up steps only by holding onto railings on both sides. She is living in a rented room in a house, having lost her small house when the owners decided to sell it.

Questions

1. The seven health management subcomponents in the fourth edition of the AOTA Practice Framework include personal care device management, nutrition management, physical activity, medication management, communication with the healthcare system, symptom and condition management, and social and emotional health promotion and maintenance.
2. How would you prioritize these multiple components to assist Jane in maintaining/improving her occupational performance?
3. How can principles from the Well Elderly Study be applied to a person such as Jane who is living with multiple chronic conditions?

> **" COMMENTARY ON THE EVIDENCE**

Arbesman and Mosley (2012) present a systematic review of the literature on occupation- and activity-based health management and maintenance interventions for productive aging.

They found moderate-to-strong evidence that OT improved physical functioning and occupational performance related to health management in community-dwelling older adults as well as in adults with osteoarthritis and macular degeneration.

Health education programs were shown to reduce pain and increase physical activity and individualized health action plans were shown to improve activities of daily living function and participation in physical activities.

Programs that incorporated cognitive–behavioral principles into physical activity improved long-term participation in exercise. Although the evidence for skill-specific training in isolation is limited, effectiveness increases when skill-specific training is combined with health management programs.

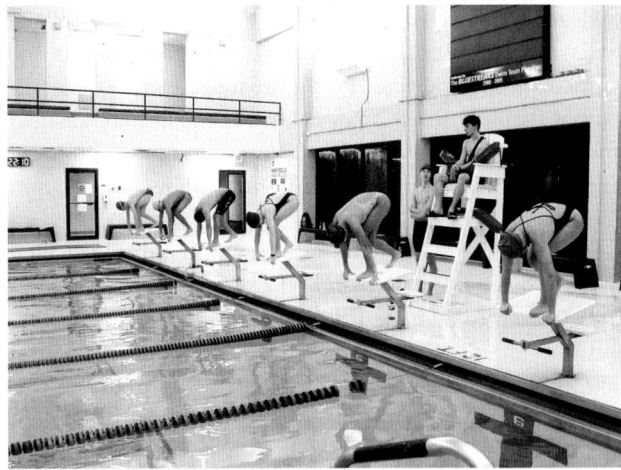

FIGURE 50.2 Swimming is a sport or recreational activity that will help individuals lead a more active lifestyle and manage stress. (Picture courtesy of Christine Gentile.)

Wellness and Social Determinants of Health

For the profession to effectively support health management as an occupation, it is important to expand our understanding of health, wellness, and the SDOH. Health is not just the absence of disease; it must be examined through the lens of wellness and the impact of SDOH that drive health disparities. As previously stated, health management includes activities related to developing, managing, and maintaining health and wellness routines, including self-management, with the goal of improving or maintaining health to support participation in other occupations. It is important to reexamine the definition of health to include the holistic focus of wellness with a clear understanding of inequities and SDOH.

Historically, health was equated with the absence of disease. This implies that health is directed at efforts to remove diseases and diminish the number of individuals impacted negatively. There has been a growing awareness that the definition of health must include recognition of a person's ability to actively participate in the many spheres of their life, including social participation, education, employment, leisure, activities of daily living, and health management. The involvement of functioning in the definition of health reflects a recognition that promotes health as a process by which the capacity of individuals to cope will be enhanced and strengthened. This is aligned with the profession's focus on strengths and function. For example, well-being and stress management can include engaging in habits and routines that involve some form of regular

physical exercise or physical activity (Figure 50.2). Risk factors such as sedentary lifestyle, smoking, poor eating habits, and insufficient application of hygienic measures, such as washing one's hands, are all factors that do impact the development of medical conditions and diseases and can impact functional performance.

Health, and creating healthy lifestyles, does not stop at efforts to remove diseases and to diminish risk factors that might lead to illness, chronic disability, and premature mortality. It involves the individuals whose health is to be promoted in an active way by addressing the values of individuals, groups, and populations to ensure that health is a priority. Values are shaped throughout life. Values are influenced by caregivers, friends, schools, the media, laws, and life experiences. Changing values—for example, to give health and wellness a higher value—is an essential task for all of those involved in shaping individuals', groups', and communities' values. OT practitioners can play an important role by helping individuals, groups, and communities to clearly define health within the context of the eight wellness dimensions (see Figure 63.2 in Chapter 63).

Wellness is a conscious, deliberate process that requires a person to become aware of and make choices for engaging in health habits (Swarbrick, 1997, 2006). A wellness lifestyle includes a "self-defined balance" of health habits and routines. The habits include adequate sleep, rest, and healthy food choices; productivity and exercise; participation in meaningful activity; and connections with supportive relationships (Swarbrick, 1997, 2006, 2012). Wellness is holistic and includes eight areas that can represent strengths and needs of an individual in terms of physical, social, emotional, intellectual, occupational, financial, spiritual, and environmental dimensions (refer to Chapter 63 for a detailed explanation). The image is like a kaleidoscope where the focus can be on one dimension while keeping all the other dimensions in mind as strengths and needs that enhance well-being. The eight-dimensional wellness model aligns well with social and emotional health promotion as the individual is empowered to be proactive in the preservation of their own well-being. The individual is encouraged and supported to assume an active role in defining and self-monitoring their own health and wellness habits and routines.

This model is different from a medical model, in which the healthcare provider defines the problem and prescribes the methods to address problems defined by professionals. In the wellness model, the OT practitioner collaborates and acts as a coach, helping to guide the person to define valued treatment goals and plans congruent with strengthen and valued life roles. Occupational therapists can use motivational interviewing (Shaw & Wilson, 2021) and wellness coaching strategies (Brice et al., 2014; Gao et al., 2021; Swarbrick et al., 2011, 2016), which have been shown to be effective in assisting people with co-occurring physical health, mental health, and substance-use challenges.

The wellness model views motivation through personal control and valuing health (in contrast to the health models that use fear to drive change and instill compliance). The focus is on people's strengths and needs in the various eight dimensions rather than on their limitations and weaknesses that create barriers to progress. Physical wellness strengths include engaging in regular walking or meditation routines to help manage stress and symptoms of depression and anxiety, with the purpose of preventing exacerbation of either mental disorders or physical health conditions. The wellness model recognizes the strengths in the eight wellness dimensions as protective factors to manage and cope with stress and adversity in many of life's crises. For example, social wellness strengths can have a powerful impact on lessening the incidence of mental and substance-use disorders and stress-related illness. OT practitioners can design and deliver services focusing on the strength-based wellness lens to address health and wellness management for people across the life span at risk and people who are living with a range of disabilities and social barriers.

Health management that considers wellness habits and routines can be effective to assist people at risk or and/or living with a chronic mental substance-use or medical condition or for those experiencing the long-term impacts of chronic stress and trauma. Managing chronic conditions also involves learning specific health management skills. Depending on the condition, skills could include regularly monitoring blood pressure, weight, blood glucose, or pain levels; planning, shopping for, and preparing meals according to specific requirements or restrictions; administering oral, injected, or inhaled medications; or creating and sustaining a regular physical activity routine. To manage chronic health conditions, it is important to help people learn or relearn skills and consistently and habitually apply the skills, so they become integrated into their existing routines. Practitioners can help people examine the barriers that prevent them from integrating health management tasks successfully into their daily routines and, if necessary, incorporate adaptations to overcome these barriers. The profession is particularly skilled in helping people manage chronic conditions in a way that fits with existing routines and patterns so changes feel less disruptive and are more likely to be consistently integrated into daily routines.

OT practitioners are skilled at understanding the emotional challenges associated with living with a chronic condition, such as anger and depression, feelings of uncertainty about the future, and changes in relationships with family and friends. Social isolation is frequently a result of illness or disability or, as we have recently experienced, a global pandemic. However, research has been clear that social participation is associated with improved physical and cognitive health, emotional well-being, and quality of life (Townsend et al., 2021). Well-being is more than controlling symptoms or managing daily tasks, so it is important to help individuals engage in activities that are meaningful to them. OT practitioners engage individuals, and sometimes their caregivers, in taking charge of their own care and sustaining the responsibilities and relationships important for them to maintain their highest level of functional independence. OT practitioners evaluate the fit between abilities and challenges imposed by those activities and the environment. Recommendations may include energy conservation, pain management, simplifying the activities, and improving safety and independent functioning in home, school, work, or community environments. Table 50.2 outlines a few examples of opportunities and roles for practitioners to focus on health and wellness management for individuals, groups, and populations. The wellness model is an important lens as we design and deliver interventions or develop programs to support health management. The wellness lens is a framework to keep in focus the health disparities and inequities among many groups and underrepresented marginalized groups and populations the profession currently serves or can and should be serving. See Lippincott Connect for recommended readings and resources for health management.

Social Determinants of Health: Zip Code Matters

Where you live (which is the focus of the environmental wellness dimension) matters in terms of your quality of life and longevity. Scientific and technological advancements affect society's health and wellness; however, the right of all citizens to resources that support wellness and quality timely affordable healthcare is not guaranteed. Although the general population is now living longer, people who are disadvantaged and disenfranchised often experience a shorter life span. Far too many live with chronic, disabling,

TABLE 50.2	Health Management Examples
Category	**Examples**
Social and emotional health promotion and maintenance	• Classes for caregivers who became parents during the pandemic; support for new parents and caregivers who are reintegrating into their communities with children during the extended quarantine and COVID-19 precautions • Emotion regulation programs • Weekend transition-to-college program created for adolescents with special needs who are interested in pursuing college after high school to experience living in a dorm, eating in a college cafeteria, observing a class of interest • School-based programs to support emotional and behavioral health and positive social participation • Adoption of best practices in trauma informed care
Symptom and condition management	• Workplace injury prevention and wellness programs • Ergonomic assessments for computer workstations to decrease repetitive motion and musculoskeletal disorders • Specialized summer camps emphasizing constraint-induced movement therapy to children diagnosed with hemiplegia • Self-management programs to enable those with chronic diseases like diabetes, rheumatoid arthritis, and cardiac conditions to optimize health through appropriate routines (modifications when necessary) and participate in meaningful occupations • Self-regulation, sensory diet, and distress tolerance strategies for individuals who experience trauma
Communication with the healthcare system	• Caregiver education to prevent injury and/or burnout • Advocacy on the behalf of an individual or caregiver for adaptative equipment or social support resources to promote functioning in least restrictive environment • Organizing a wellness fair with multiple members of the interprofessional team to answer questions
Medication management	• Teaching caregivers or clients how to create routines using technological or environment cures as reminders • Using health literacy principles to teach individuals with memory or adherence issues
Physical activity	• Community walking group for at-risk groups or helping individuals to establish a walking habit and routine • Tai chi program for individuals with Parkinson disease • Programs for drivers to accommodate their needs (e.g., limited neck mobility) through minor adaptations and adjustments to the car • Community-based fall prevention programs for seniors • School-based programs that integrate the use of physical activity to create meaningful occupational participation in children
Nutrition management	• Collaborating with a chef to create a community cooking class with people who are at risk of or living with diabetes, high blood pressure, obesity, or other health conditions requiting dietary restrictions • NEW-R program to develop knowledge and skills for healthy meal planning
Personal care device management	• Managing dentures, hearing aids, orthoses • Educate a person who is experiencing lower body paralysis how to insert tampons during menstruation

preventable medical conditions that may be directly and/or indirectly affected by unjust laws and policies, discrimination, and stigma. Across populations, health is affected by many factors including where people live (environment dimension), their income (financial dimension), educational status (intellectual and occupational dimension), and their social relationships (social dimension). These factors are known as **social determinants of health (SDOH)** and include the physical, economic, and social conditions under which people live that determine their health. These conditions include political forces, and physical, social, and economic factors (World Health Organization [WHO],

2021). SDOH have been recognized by the WHO (2021) and include income and social status; social support networks; education and literacy (including health literacy); employment and working conditions; social and physical environments; health practices and coping skills; child development; genetic factors; access to health services; gender; and culture.

In most societies, people who are considered to be in lower socioeconomic status face poverty and generally experience poorer health outcomes in terms of mortality and morbidity. People in different socioeconomic groups experience differing health outcomes. Many major diseases are determined by a network of interacting exposures that increase or decrease the risk for the disease. COVID-19 has illustrated many of these intersectional factors, as discussed below.

The SDOH framework broadens our view of health management when we consider the unequal distribution of power, income, goods, and services at global and national levels. These very real conditions—access to healthcare, schools, and education, conditions of work and leisure, residential settings, and larger communities, towns, or cities—play a role in increasing the risk of reduced quality of life and poor health outcomes. Environmental determinants of health include physical, chemical, and biologic factors external to a person and all the related factors impacting behaviors. This definition excludes behavior not related to the environment, as well as behavior related to the social and cultural environment, and genetics. For example, an increased rate of crime in a community might indirectly influence a child's frequency of physical exercise and/or exploration of active leisure interests. Concerns about unsafe neighborhood activity may influence children to remain inside their residence and play video games or have more screen time.

Contagious diseases have been experienced unequally, with higher rates of infection and mortality among the most disadvantaged communities—particularly in more socially unequal countries. The COVID-19 pandemic has placed the spotlight on SDOH and on health inequalities that have been known for decades. Emerging evidence from a variety of countries suggests that these inequalities are being mirrored today in the COVID-19 pandemic (Bambra et al., 2020). Both then and now, these inequalities have emerged through the syndemic nature of COVID-19 (i.e., a synergistic epidemic where a disease clusters in specific populations)—because it interacts with and exacerbates existing inequalities in chronic disease and the SDOH. COVID-19 has illuminated the long-standing social, economic, and political inequalities that existed even before the COVID-19 pandemic. For example, life expectancy among the poorest groups was already declining in the United Kingdom and the United States and health inequalities in some European countries have been increasing over the last decade (Bambra et al., 2020; Forster et al., 2018). The SDOH appear to have placed marginalized communities more vulnerable to infection from COVID-19—even when they have no underlying health conditions. The reader is encouraged to view local and national level data from their country where these inequities are evidenced in rising rates of chronic medical conditions, including mental and substance-use disorders, as well as increases in post-traumatic stress disorder (PTSD).

Researchers on SDOH have found that the chronic stress of material and psychological deprivation is associated with immunosuppression (Segerstrom & Miller, 2004).

Psychosocial feelings of subordination or inferiority because of occupying a low position on the social hierarchy stimulate physiologic stress responses (e.g., raised cortisol levels), which, when prolonged (chronic), have long-term adverse consequences for physical and mental health (Biondi & Zannino, 1997). Studies have found consistent associations between low job status (e.g., low control and high demands); stress-related morbidity; and various chronic conditions, including coronary heart disease, hypertension, obesity, musculoskeletal conditions, and psychological ill health. There is increasing evidence that living in disadvantaged environments may produce a sense of powerlessness and collective threat, leading to chronic stressors that, in time, damage health (Segerstrom & Miller, 2004). Adverse psychosocial experiences (Boullier & Blair, 2018) and circumstances increase susceptibility—influencing the onset, course, and outcome of infectious diseases—including respiratory diseases like COVID-19. Recent data collected have also confirmed the presence of racial and ethnic disparities affecting stress, mental health conditions, and increased substance use among adults because of the COVID-19 pandemic (McKnight-Eily et al., 2021).

COVID-19 disproportionately affected historically stigmatized minoritized underrepresented groups in the United States. Analysis of trends suggests that infection and death rates in majority-Black counties were, respectively, 3 and 6 times those in predominantly majority-White counties (Thebault, 2020). The causes of this disparity are numerous and underlying medical conditions and SDOH contributed significantly. Many of the health conditions that increase the risk for poor COVID-19 outcomes are the same conditions already seen at higher rates in underrepresented minority groups. Amid marked visibility of anti-Asian violence and macroaggression spurred by the pandemic, Asian populations in the United States experienced health-related disparities regarding morbidity, mortality, and access to care for COVID-19. In addition, low-income individuals are more likely to be essential workers and less likely to be able to work remotely, putting these individuals at increased risk. It is also worth noting that people in these communities are often subjected to higher-density living environments and experience poorer access to insurance and healthcare.

These issues are further compounded by the inherent mistrust of the medical field that exists in underrepresented minoritized communities because of racist actions and policies that exist even in healthcare. These factors have resulted in a community that is both medically vulnerable and skeptical of the medical system. Within the LGBTQ+ community, COVID-19 has exacerbated the health consequences of an already stigmatized population (Salerno et al., 2020). Relative to the COVID-19 pandemic, LGBTQ+ people face unique health challenges that put them at compounded risk (Krause, 2021). The LGBTQ+ population has greater rates of chronic disease compared to their non-LGBTQ+

counterparts (Gonzales et al., 2016; Phillips et al., 2020). Rates of diabetes, coronary artery disease, cancer, human immunodeficiency virus, and asthma have all been reported to be higher in LGBTQ+ populations. LGBTQ+ individuals experience stigmatizing experiences in healthcare settings and lack of provider knowledge on healthcare needs and elders often encounter social isolation and loneliness. Mental health is much more prevalent in LGBTQ+ populations. LGBTQ+ populations report increased risk of violence, discrimination, exclusion, loneliness, depression, anxiety, substance abuse, and suicide (Krause, 2021).

OT practitioners across practice settings should consider how SDOH impact client performance and ability to manage health conditions (Synovec & Aceituno, 2020). Hammell (2021) urges the profession to prioritize education, research, and action on systemic injustices and SDOH and occupation, aligning our commitment with the WHO standards to reduce the health inequalities by promoting health and access to quality healthcare (see Recommended Readings, "Social Determinants of Health" section, online for relevant resources). Occupational therapists need to gather and use information on SDOH to develop and deliver effective individual-, group-, and population-level health management interventions especially for underrepresented and minoritized groups. Prevention and wellness promotion models will be an important lens and tool for OT practitioners. Additionally, it is essential to strengthen our understanding of health promotion principles and health literacy as a new vital sign.

Health Promotion and Health Literacy Skills

Prevention is a process using actions designed to prevent health problems before they start. *Secondary prevention* is the recognition of problems early in development. The goal is to identify underlying causes and change contributing behaviors to halt disease development or progression. It is well known that many untimely deaths and hospitalizations are linked to largely preventable behaviors, such as tobacco use, alcohol abuse, sedentary lifestyle, and overeating. Healthy lifestyle habits and behaviors, such as eating nutritious foods, being physically active, and avoiding tobacco use, can prevent or control the devastating effects of many diseases.

Health promotion is a process of enhancing wellness through education, guidance, and support and is believed to contribute to positive behavioral change. Health promotion is a planned approach. Educational strategies are used to empower people to assume responsibility for their own individual lifestyle habits.

Health promotion models are based on the belief that individuals should be supported in their effort to exert control over SDOH and mitigate potential adverse effects

(see Chapter 40 for more information). Health promotion strategies include creating supportive organizational environments and strengthening social empowerment through community action. Prevention and health promotion models consider many of the SDOH to be population-level issues, such as inequality, poverty, and education. Health promotion and prevention efforts require that professionals shift from an orientation focused on illness to one of health and wellness. This will require some changes in terms of education and training for occupational therapists.

Health Literacy

Health literacy is an essential competency for OT practitioners assisting people with health management, especially medication management, communication with the healthcare system, and social and emotional health promotion and maintenance. **Health literacy** is the ability to find, understand, and use health information and services to make appropriate health decisions and act on health information. Examples include the ability to read and understand a prescription label, understand the healthcare professional's recommendations and intervention plans (including OT), read educational brochures provided by healthcare providers, comprehend a written consent form before a medical procedure, figure out what health benefits are available from third-party payers, and negotiate the complex healthcare delivery system. Health literacy is an important element to address with parents or caregivers of children with special needs—ensuring full understanding of the rehabilitative and educational process and being able to advocate for the best care. Health literacy is a central focus of Healthy People 2030. One of the overarching goals of the initiative demonstrates this focus: "Eliminate health disparities, achieve health equity, and attain health literacy to improve the health and well-being of all."

As OT practitioners, it is important that we understand the complex skills involved in health literacy. While basic skills are required to understand and apply health information, such as reading and listening, more complex skills are also needed. These skills include but are not limited to comprehending and evaluating health information and problem-solving and analyzing skills. Health literacy is low among people with limited education and those who live in poverty. Many have low levels of general literacy, which contributes to low health literacy. Well-educated individuals may also have low health literacy. For example, some individuals even with college graduate degrees report that health topics are so emotional that they have a hard time comprehending information shared by healthcare professionals. Many colleagues in the United States report significant health literacy issues related to healthcare insurance options, payments, and billing procedures. Improving health literacy is very important. OT practitioners should become competent in these areas so that they can help the people and communities they serve comprehend health information and access health services.

OT health literacy universal precautions can be focused on

- simplifying communication (written and verbal) and confirming comprehension to minimize miscommunication when addressing health management topics;
- adjusting the environment where services are offered;
- helping individuals navigate the complexities of the healthcare system; and
- supporting individual efforts to develop skills to improve general health, as well as manage mental and substance-use disorders, and to address other risk factors related to SDOH.

Universal precautions are needed to address health literacy because we cannot know which people served are challenged by health information and tasks at any given time. Health literacy skills are varied, complex, and evolving and are influenced by personal factors, such as individual development and personal health needs, environmental factors such as technology and available resources, and SDOH that disproportionately affect minority populations. OT practitioners should be competent to assess health literacy needs and apply effective strategies for training individuals and caregivers in finding, understanding, evaluating, and using quality health management information. Health literacy aligns with wellness and prevention. Strengthening health literacy competencies can empower the practitioner and client to engage in habits and routines that may protect their health as well as better manage those problems and unexpected situations that happen. Empowering people served through engagement and support based on individualized health literacy needs is a proactive approach to address health disparities. Helping people access quality health education and not become overwhelmed with misinformation has become an important focus we have learned from the COVID-19 pandemic (Gabarron et al., 2021).

Even people who read well and are comfortable using numbers can face health literacy issues. Some may not be familiar with medical terms; others may have difficulty interpreting statistics. Many have challenges evaluating risks and benefits that affect their health and safety. In the authors' experience for decades, we have observed that when diagnosed with a serious illness it is very common for people to feel scared and confused. In our experience, we have seen individuals become overwhelmed and depressed when health conditions require complicated self-care. These emotional factors can create additional barriers for listening to and understanding health information.

Practitioners working to address health management can take advantage of health literacy resources available to strengthen health literacy skills when

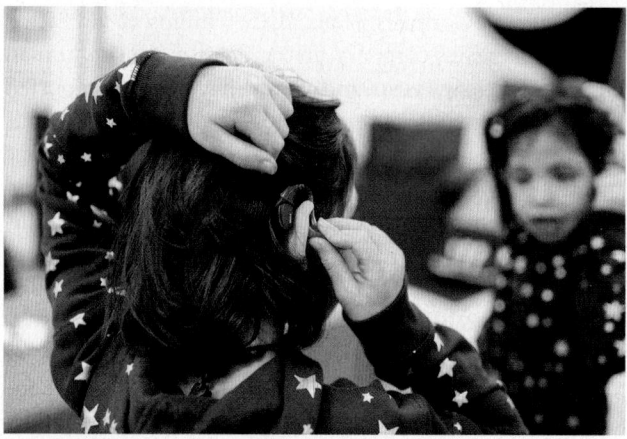

FIGURE 50.3 **This child was educated by the OT practitioner so that she could independently put on her hearing aid. (Picture courtesy of Brielle Hassa.)**

designing and implementing wellness promotion group and population-level programs as well as creating health and wellness promotion educational resources (see Recommended Readings, "Health Literacy" section, on Lippincott Connect for useful resources for occupational therapists). Practitioners may be responsible for educating others and creating or adapting health education materials for medication management, physical activity, nutrition management, symptom or condition management, or personal care device management, and they need to ensure that the information is accessible and accurate (Figure 50.3). OT practitioners armed with health literacy competencies will be better able to design and deliver information accurately and in ways that people can understand and apply that information in their own lives (See chapter 23 for more detail on Health Education).

Opportunities

Beyond helping individuals and groups served in traditional roles, OT practitioners can assume consultation roles helping organizations, such as business and health insurance companies, to create programs based on population-level data. Addressing health management as an occupation is an important role for OT in primary care settings (AOTA, 2020b). OT practitioners are well prepared to offer wellness coaching and fulfill case management roles, which includes skills to address health management (AOTA, 2018). Case management is defined as the process of managing client wellness and autonomy through advocacy, communication, education, and identification and facilitation of services (Health2 Resources, 2013). This definition is aligned with the holistic principles and philosophy of OT. OT practitioners may work directly to offer case management for individuals addressing health management and may provide supportive and educational strategies for caregivers. Work with caregivers includes education, emotional support, problem-solving, referral to helpful community resources, and training in strategies to better cope with client-related issues, such as cancer-related fatigue or maintenance of sobriety (Gitlin et al., 2015).

There is a modest amount of research describing the role of OT practitioners in addressing health management. It is expected that this paradigm shift will strengthen within our profession as practitioners engage in more research and program development applying community-based participatory action research methods (Turcotte et al., 2019) and co-production approaches that best align with stakeholder inclusion to be meet needs (see Recommended Readings, Community-Based Participatory Action Research/Co-Production Resources, on Lippincott Connect). Occupational therapists have valuable skills to contribute: they engage in research to examine the efficacy and cost-effectiveness of wellness and health promotion guidelines. For OT practitioners to implement the

use of the wellness promotion model into our professional practices, as a group we must develop practice guidelines for working with groups and communities. Our profession needs to promote the use of health and wellness principles beyond the absence of diseases and be sure to view individuals, groups, and populations using an SDOH framework.

Health management is an important occupation that leads to OT practitioners becoming expert consultants in a wellness-focused occupation paradigm shift. This will require placing close attention to SDOH as they impact individuals, groups, and populations especially around structural barriers related to intersectionality. There needs to be more emphasis on health and wellness embedded in all aspects of the OT curriculum, from introducing these constructs through to application for all persons served. Infusing these threads in the curriculum will direct students, practitioners, and academicians to engage in scholarly activities, such as research inquiry, development of updated guidelines for practice, and ways to influence needed policy changes at the professional, state, and federal levels. For one example, see "Expanding Our Perspectives" section.

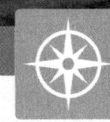

EXPANDING OUR PERSPECTIVES

Health Management Through Spoon Theory and Disability Justice

Pamela Block

Disabled people and those who experience chronic conditions have developed strategies for supporting each other in maintaining health and wellness. One such strategy is called "spoon theory" and those who use this strategy call themselves "spoonies." The story of how spoon theory came to be is compelling and best learned from the person who coined the term Christine Miserandino (n.d.) (https://butyoudontlooksick.com/articles/written-by-christine/the-spoon-theory/). Explaining to a friend what it was like to have to manage every activity knowing she had limited energy, she handed her friend a handful of spoons. Every activity for the day cost spoons and when the spoons were gone, so was the ability to do anything. Whereas someone who is not disabled or experiencing a chronic condition does not usually have to think in these terms, a spoonie knows that you must manage your spoons carefully. Sometimes, you must make choices between needed activities (shopping or showering? cooking or homework?) because once the spoons are gone, they are gone, and if you try to go beyond your limits, you might find yourself in bed or even in hospital, with days or weeks of recovery needed. Spoon theory is a useful way of helping people who are

new to the experience how to navigate life with a disability or chronic condition.

Other approaches disabled people teach each other have been articulated by disability justice activists at Sins Invalid (2015), including the 10 Principles of Disability Justice and the essays and books written by Leah Lakshmi Piepzna-Samarasinha (2018), Sins Invalid (2019), and Aimi Hamraie (2017): these focus on collective access and mutual care relationships. Instead of seeing care as a transactional commodity, where some give care and others receive it—which is a typical biomedical model understanding of care—a disability justice understanding of care is seen as something that is constituted mutually in different ways and times among individuals and groups. Similarly, collective access challenges notions of individuals requesting and receiving "accommodations" based on static rules or regulations. Instead, collective access frames access as a dynamic and fluid but imperfect process that is constantly being enacted among groups of people to ensure the most people have the most access possible amid realities fraught with access conflicts and failures. According to the disability justice activists Mia Mingus, Alice Wong, and Sandra Ho in the Disability Visibility Project: "Access is Love" (disability visibility project, n.d.). The principles of disability justice grow out of intersectional understandings of Indigenous, Black, and other People of Color, as well as people from LGBTQ+ communities, and their

(continued)

lived experiences with disability and chronic conditions alongside other forms of systemic inequality and injustice. These are the people who face the biggest health disparities owing to experiencing multiple barriers to high-quality healthcare. Given that OT services in North America are largely based on access to health insurance, providing strategies and resources for mutual support and ways to connect with disability and spoonie community are important means for occupational therapists to support people in contexts of health management, including health education and discharge planning.

References

Disability Visibility Project. (n.d.). *Access is love.* https://disabilityvisibilityproject.com/2019/02/01/access-is-love/

Hamraie, A. (2017). *Building access: Universal design and the politics of disability.* Minnesota University Press.

Miserandino, C. (n.d.). *The spoon theory.* https://butyoudontlooksick.com/articles/written-by-christine/the-spoon-theory/

Piepzna-Samarasinha, L. L. (2018). *Care work: Dreaming disability justice.* Arsenal Pulp Press.

Sins Invalid. (2015). *10 principles of disability justice.* https://www.sinsinvalid.org/blog/10-principles-of-disability-justice

Sins Invalid. (2019). *Skin, tooth, and bone: The basis of movement is our people* (2nd ed.). Primedia eLaunch LLC.

Conclusion

The time is now to focus on health and wellness. This chapter is meant to challenge OT practitioners to examine their own lifestyle and the lifestyle of persons served to fulfill a mandate of a health-oriented society. The addition of the ninth occupation provides the opportunity to assume leadership roles to help individuals, groups, and populations society to focus on health management to foster a wellness lifestyle for all. OT practitioners can expand knowledge of wellness, SDOH, and health literacy, and they can fulfill roles areas, such as case management, consultant, co-producing health management, and wellness programs for and with individuals and groups, especially those who have been underrepresented and underserved. As we have these knowledge and skills, it is time to lead our next generation of OT practitioners toward these models and embrace this paradigm shift by engaging in program development and creating research agendas that design and evaluate effective and useful health management guidelines.

Acknowledgments

We wish to acknowledge Serina Figueiras for her invaluable assistance in organizing resources for this chapter and Dr Lynne Richard for reviewing the chapter and submitting the direct practice section.

Lippincott® Connect *For additional resources on the subjects discussed in this chapter, visit Lippincott Connect.*

REFERENCES

American Occupational Therapy Association. (2017). Occupational therapy's role in medication management. *American Journal of Occupational Therapy, 71*(Suppl. 2), 7112410025. https://doi.org/10.5014/ajot.716S02

American Occupational Therapy Association. (2018). Occupational therapy's role in case management. *American Journal of Occupational Therapy, 68*(Suppl. 1), 7212410050. https://doi.org/10.5014/ajot.2018.72S206

American Occupational Therapy Association. (2020a). Occupational therapy practice framework: Domain and process (4th ed.). *American Journal of Occupational Therapy, 74*(Suppl. 2), 7412410010. https://doi.org/10.5014/ajot.2020.74S2001

American Occupational Therapy Association. (2020b). Role of occupational therapy in primary care. *American Journal of Occupational Therapy, 74*(Suppl. 3), 7413410040. https://doi.org/10.5014/ajot.2020.74S3001

Amini, D. (2021). *The OTPF-4: Continuing our professional journey through change.* American Occupational Therapy Association. https://www.aota.org/-/media/Corporate/Files/Publications/CE-Articles/CEA_February_2021.pdf

Arbesman, M., & Mosley, L. J. (2012). Systematic review of occupation and activity-based health management and maintenance interventions for community-dwelling older adults. *American Journal of Occupational Therapy, 66*(3), 277–283. https://doi.org/10.5014/ajot.2012.003327

Bambra, C., Riordan, R., Ford, J., & Matthews, F. (2020). The COVID-19 pandemic and health inequalities. *Journal of Epidemiology and Community Health, 74*(11), 964–968. https://doi.org/10.1136/jech-2020-214401

Biondi, M., & Zannino, L. G. (1997). Psychological stress, neuroimmunomodulation, and susceptibility to infectious diseases in animals and man: A review. *Psychotherapy and Psychosomatics, 66*(1), 3–26. https://doi.org/10.1159/000289101

Boullier, M., & Blair, M. (2018). Adverse childhood experiences. *Paediatrics and Child Health, 28*(3), 132–137. https://doi.org/10.1016/j.paed.2017.12.008

Brice, G. H., Swarbrick, M. A., & Gill, K. J. (2014). Promoting wellness of peer providers through coaching. *Journal of Psychosocial Nursing and Mental Health Services, 52*(1), 41–45. https://doi.org/10.3928/02793695-20130930-03

Brown, C., Read, H., Stanton, M., Zeeb, M., Jonikas, J. A., & Cook, J. A. (2015). A pilot study of nutrition and exercise for wellness and recovery (NEW-R): A weight loss program for individuals with serious mental illness. *Psychiatric Rehabilitation Journal, 38*(4), 371–373. https://doi.org/10.1037/prj0000115

Forster, T., Kentikelenis, A., & Bambra, C. (2018). *Health inequalities in Europe: Setting the stage for progressive policy action.* Foundation for European Progressive Studies. https://www.feps-europe.eu/attachments/publications/1845-6%20health%20inequalities%20inner-hr.pdf

Gabarron, E., Oyeyemi, S. O., & Wynn, R. (2021). COVID-19-related misinformation on social media: A systematic review. *Bulletin of the World Health Organization, 99*(6), 455–463A. https://doi.org/10.2471/BLT.20.276782

Gao, N., Solomon, P., Clay, Z., & Swarbrick, P. (2021). A pilot study of wellness coaching for smoking cessation among individuals with mental illnesses. *Journal of Mental Health,* 1–7. https://doi.org/10.1080/09638237.2021.1922630

Gitlin, L. N., Marx, K., Stanley, I. H., & Hodgson, N. (2015). Translating evidence-based dementia caregiving interventions into practice: State-of-the-science and next steps. *The Gerontologist, 55*(2), 210–226. https://doi.org/10.1093/geront/gnu123

Gonzales, G., Przedworski, J., & Henning-Smith, C. (2016). Comparison of health and health risk factors between lesbian, gay, and bisexual adults and heterosexual adults in the United States: Results from the national health interview survey. *JAMA Internal Medicine, 176*(9), 1344–1351. https://doi.org/10.1001/jamainternmed.2016.3432

Hammell, K. W. (2021). Social and structural determinants of health: Exploring occupational therapy's structural (in)competence. *Canadian Journal of Occupational Therapy, 88*(4), 365–374. https://doi.org/10.1177/00084174211046797

Health2 Resources. (2013). Case managers strengthen health care's weakest link: Improving care transitions. *CCMC Issue Brief, 4*(3), 1–8.

Jackson, J., Carlson, M., Mandel, D., Zemke, R., & Clark, F. (1998). Occupation in lifestyle redesign: The well elderly study occupational therapy program. *The American Journal of Occupational Therapy, 52*(5), 326–336. https://doi.org/10.5014/ajot.52.5.326

Krause, K. D. (2021). Implications of the COVID-19 pandemic on LGBTQ communities. *Journal of Public Health Management and Practice, 27*(Suppl. 1), S69–S71. https://doi.org/10.1097/PHH.0000000000001273

Mische-Lawson, L., & Little, L. M. (2017). Feasibility of a swimming intervention to improve sleep behaviors of children with autism spectrum disorder. *Therapeutic Recreation Journal, 51*(2), 97–108. https://doi.org/10.18666/trj-2017-v51-i2-7899

McKnight-Eily, L. R., Okoro, C. A., Strine, T. W., Verlenden, J., Hollis, N. D., Njai, R., Mitchell, E. W., Board, A., Puddy, R., & Thomas, C. (2021). Racial and ethnic disparities in the prevalence of stress and worry, mental health conditions, and increased substance use among adults during the COVID-19 pandemic—United States, April and May 2020. *Morbidity and Mortality Weekly Report, 70*(5), 162–166. https://doi.org/10.15585/mmwr.mm7005a3

Phillips, G., II., Felt, D., Ruprecht, M. M., Wang, X., Xu, J., Pérez-Bill, E., Bagnarol, R. M., Roth, J., Curry, C. W., & Beach, L. B. (2020). Addressing the disproportionate impacts of the COVID-19 pandemic on sexual and gender minority populations in the United States: Actions toward equity. *LGBT Health, 7*(6), 279–282. https://doi.org/10.1089/lgbt.2020.0187

Salerno, J. P., Williams, N. D., & Gattamorta, K. A. (2020). LGBTQ populations: Psychologically vulnerable communities in the COVID-19 pandemic. *Psychological Trauma, 12*(Suppl. 1), S239–S242. https://doi.org/10.1037/tra0000837

Schepens Niemiec, S. L., Vigen, C. L., Martínez, J., Blanchard, J., & Carlson, M. (2021). Long-term follow-up of a lifestyle intervention for late-midlife, rural-dwelling Latinos in primary care. *American Journal of Occupational Therapy, 75*(2), 7502205020. https://doi.org/10.5014/ajot.2021.042861

Schwartz, J. K., & Smith, R. O. (2016). Intervention promoting medication adherence: A randomized, phase I, small-N study. *American Journal of Occupational Therapy, 70*(6), 7006240010p1–7006240010p11. https://doi.org/10.5014/ajot.2016.021006

Segerstrom, S. C., & Miller, G. E. (2004). Psychological stress and the human immune system: A meta-analytic study of 30 years of inquiry. *Psychological Bulletin, 130*(4), 601–630. https://doi.org/10.1037/0033-2909.130.4.601

Shaw, D. S., & Wilson, M. N. (2021). Taking a motivational interviewing approach to prevention science: Progress and extensions. *Prevention Science, 22*(6), 826–830. https://doi.org/10.1007/s11121-021-01269-w

Swarbrick, M. (1997, March). A wellness model for clients. *Mental Health Special Interest Section Quarterly, 20,* 1–4.

Swarbrick, M. (2006). A wellness approach. *Psychiatric Rehabilitation Journal, 29*(4), 311–314. https://doi.org/10.2975/29.2006.311.314

Swarbrick, M. (2012). A wellness approach to mental health recovery. In A. Rudnick (Ed.), *Recovery of people with mental illness: Philosophical and related perspectives* (pp. 30-38). Oxford Press.

Swarbrick, M., Gill, K. J., & Pratt, C. W. (2016). Impact of peer delivered wellness coaching. *Psychiatric Rehabilitation Journal, 39*(3), 234–238. https://doi.org/10.1037/prj0000187

Swarbrick, M., Murphy, A., Zechner, M., Spagnolo, A., & Gill, K. (2011). Wellness coaching: A new role for peers. *Psychiatric Rehabilitation Journal, 34*(4), 328–331. https://doi.org/10.2975/34.4.2011.328.331

Synovec, C. E., & Aceituno, L. (2020). Social justice considerations for occupational therapy: The role of addressing social determinants of health in unstably housed populations. *Work, 65*(2), 235–246. https://doi.org/10.3233/WOR-203074

Thebault, R., Ba Tran, A., & Williams, V. (2020). The coronavirus is infecting and killing black Americans at an alarmingly high rate. *Washington Post.* https://www.washingtonpost.com/nation/2020/04/07/coronavirus-is-infecting-killing-black-americans-an-alarmingly-high-rate-post-analysis-shows/

Townsend, B. G., Chen, J. T., & Wuthrich, V. M. (2021). Barriers and facilitators to social participation in older adults: A systematic literature review. *Clinical Gerontologist, 44*(4), 359–380. https://doi.org/10.1080/07317115.2020.1863890

Turcotte, P. L., Carrier, A., & Levasseur, M. (2019). Community-based participatory research remodeling occupational therapy to foster older adults' social participation. *Canadian Journal of Occupational Therapy, 86*(4), 262–276. https://doi.org/10.1177/0008417419832334

Uyeshiro Simon, A., & Collins, C. E. (2017). Lifestyle Redesign® for chronic pain management: A retrospective clinical efficacy study. *American Journal of Occupational Therapy, 71*(4), 7104190040p1-7104190040p7. https://doi.org/10.5014/ajot.2017.025502

World Health Organization. (2021). *Social determinants of health to advance equity.* https://www.who.int/publications/m/item/social-determinants-of-health-to-advance-equity

Routines and Habits

Elizabeth A. Pyatak

LEARNING OBJECTIVES

After reading this chapter, you will be able to:

1. Articulate the relevance of habits and routines to occupational therapy (OT) interventions.
2. Describe factors that influence the formation, maintenance, and disruption of habits.
3. Explain strategies to analyze habits and routines within an OT evaluation.
4. Construct an OT goal related to performance of habits and routines.
5. Identify intervention strategies to promote habit formation and discontinuation.
6. State relevant outcomes resulting from intervening on habits and routines within an OT plan of care.

Introduction

This chapter provides an overview of evaluation, intervention, and outcomes related to habits and routines. Habits and routines are the building blocks of our lives, and they comprise much of what we do on a day-to-day basis. As defined in Chapter 13, **habits** are specific, automatic behaviors that are performed repeatedly, relatively automatically, and with little variation. **Routines** are "a type of higher-order habit involves sequencing and combining processes, steps, or occupation and provide a structure for life" (Clark, 2000, p. 128S). Thus, habits and routines can be powerful influences on health and well-being, in both positive and negative respects. Habits and routines create a structure that makes our daily lives more predictable, reducing the mental energy we have to expend on familiar, repeated activities. This allows us to conserve energy for situations that require conscious deliberation and decision-making, which is much more mentally taxing.

The disruption caused by an illness, onset of a disabling condition, or any other significant life event can create difficulty in maintaining positive habits and routines, and occupational therapy (OT) can play an important role in helping individuals and groups reestablish these habits and routines. Such disruptions can have a positive element, as well: they can be an opportune time to discontinue habits and routines that are not in line with a person's current goals and desires. Breaking habits and routines can also be the focus of OT intervention, as clients may have deeply entrenched, well-established habits and routines that are not aligned with their long-term goals, and the occupational therapist may intervene to disrupt these habits and routines and establish new ones.

Because habits and routines are so integral to the maintenance of occupations over time, they are important to consider in almost any OT intervention setting. This chapter therefore will describe intervention strategies to create, maintain, and change habits and routines. It will also outline important considerations for habits and routines in intervention planning.

Evaluation

Chapter 13 contains several examples of assessments that can be used to evaluate habits and routines. In addition to structured assessments, reviewing a typical day or weekly schedule with a client can help to illustrate overall patterns of occupation, including habits and routines. Habits can also be inferred by asking about the frequency and context in which an activity occurs. If an activity takes place repeatedly in a stable context, it is likely to be a habit. There are several dimensions to consider when evaluating a client's habits and routines, as outlined below.

Temporality

Habits and routines may operate on various time cycles. For example, a habit could be carried out many times a day (such as washing hands after using the restroom), once daily (such as some bathing or grooming activities), or once a week (such as attending a religious service or scheduled extracurricular activity). Similarly, routines may vary across different spans of time. For instance, people often have different routines on weekdays as compared to weekends, or on workdays as compared to days off. Understanding the temporality of a given habit or routine may provide valuable insights regarding intervention strategies. For example, setting reminders or alarms can sometimes be an effective strategy for people seeking to make a new habit—but, if the habitual activity is performed several times a day, the reminders may become an annoyance and hinder, rather than support, the development of a habit.

Personal Factors

Various personal factors that may influence habits and routines should be considered in the evaluation process. Cognition is an important factor to consider, as individuals with cognitive impairment may particularly benefit from having established habits and routines, to minimize the likelihood of forgetting to carry out important tasks during their day.

At the same time, they may have more difficulty in developing or breaking habits and routines and may benefit from additional supports such as environmental cues or caregiver involvement to facilitate changes in existing habits and routines.

Personality and temperament are also important considerations in relation to habits and routines. Although everyone benefits to some degree from having habits and routines that create structure in their daily life, people vary a great deal in how much they enjoy novelty versus predictability. Someone who favors a very predictable environment is likely to crave a high degree of structure and routine, and conversely, someone with a high need for novelty and new experiences may resist making their daily life more routinized than absolutely necessary.

Environmental Factors

Understanding the environmental factors that support or undermine your client's ability to create and maintain habits and routines is essential. Many individuals, groups, and populations lack sufficient control over their environment to establish and maintain consistent habits and routines. You may relate to this as an OT student, as you likely are required to attend classes on specific days and times, which may or may not align with your preferred routines. This schedule likely changes a few times a year when a new quarter or semester begins, which requires you to establish new routines on a seasonal basis. Consider that many workers, in the United States and globally, are employed in "gig" jobs that lack consistent hours—typically, to maximize efficiency at the expense of providing a predictable schedule and income to employees. Being unable to predict one's schedule more than a few days ahead is a significant barrier to establishing consistent routines.

Similarly, one's social environment can either support or undermine the establishment of routines. Consider a child living in a household where meals, bedtime, and other family routines take place at consistent times as compared to a household that carries out these activities on a less predictable basis. If the child is working with an occupational therapist learning to complete and turn in homework assignments on time, it may be easier for the first child than the second child to develop a routine for doing homework and putting it in their backpack to bring to school.

Evaluating Habits

Evaluating habits can be challenging, because, by definition, they operate outside of conscious awareness. Therefore, people often lack insight into when, how, and why they perform habitual behaviors. One signifier that a behavior is habitual is that we engage in it despite our intention to do otherwise. For example, when traveling to a new destination on the highway I take to commute home from work,

I occasionally find myself getting off at the exit that goes toward my house, rather than continuing toward my intended destination. This happens because my brain has formed a strong habit to drive home from work when on that section of highway, which overrides my intention to travel to a different destination. This can also be seen clinically when someone has difficulty making a behavior change despite their stated desire or intention to change their behavior. Clinicians sometimes make the mistake of attributing their clients' difficulty with making behavior changes to a lack of knowledge, motivation, or engagement, when in fact they are fighting with long-established habits that are difficult to change. Box 51.1 outlines how to distinguish whether a given behavior is a habit.

Evaluating Routines

Routines can often be elicited by reviewing an individual's "typical day." Routines, by definition, unfold in a predictable sequence and therefore the description of a typical day will often highlight daily routines. Keep in mind that, as noted above, routines may unfold on a less frequent basis. Reviewing an individual or family's weekly schedule is another opportunity to identify recurring events that comprise a routine, and it may also be helpful to probe for events that occur routinely but less frequently (e.g., monthly, seasonally).

A Balance Wheel (see Figure 51.1), daily or weekly schedule (see Figure 51.2), or other visual depiction of a typical day or week can be helpful in identifying aspects of a client's routine that are not aligned with their goals and interests. For example, the Balance Wheel depicted in Figure 51.1 depicts a daily routine with significant time devoted to school, work, and studying (the brown segments indicating time spent in "productivity" occupations), but very little time spent in play or leisure occupations; the client may desire to shift their routine to incorporate more time for leisure. The schedule shown in Figure 51.2 depicts an irregular eating routine, with 10 hours between breakfast and lunch on one

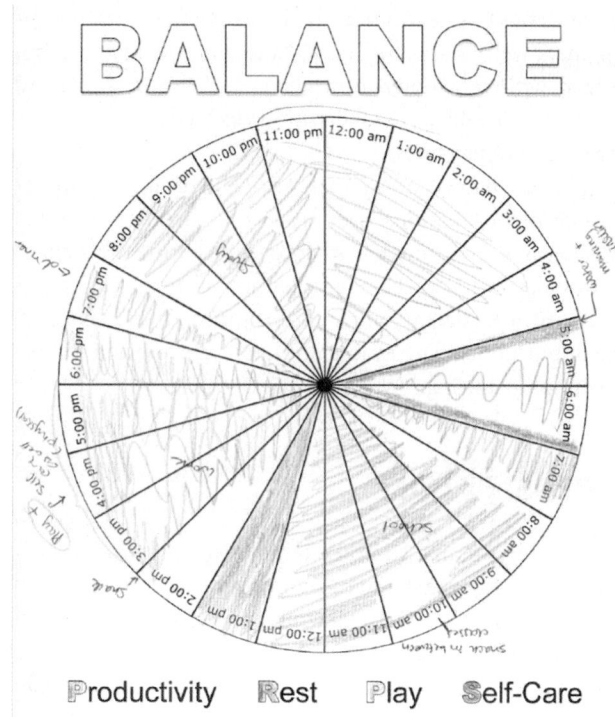

Productivity   Rest   Play   Self-Care

FIGURE 51.1 **Balance wheel.**

BOX 51.1 **IS IT A HABIT?**

What do habits look like "in the wild?" How do you know if a behavior has become a habit? Compared to behaviors that are not habits (i.e., goal-directed behaviors), someone performing a habitual behavior will be (Smith & Graybiel, 2014):

- Faster at initiating and completing the task
- More accurate while completing the task
- Less likely to be distracted during the task
- Less sensitive to negative feedback (i.e., the behavior will persist even if the outcome is not what was desired)

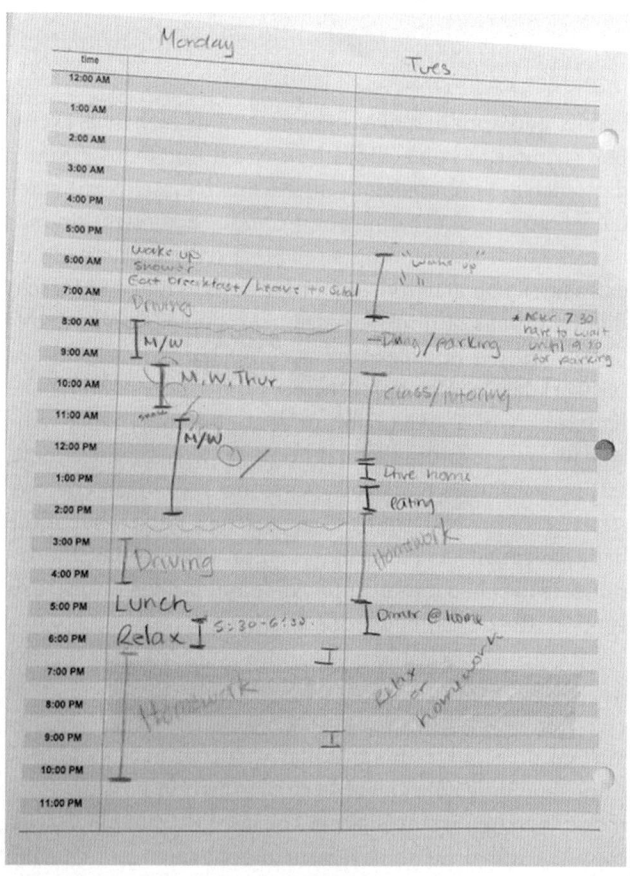

FIGURE 51.2 **Daily schedule.**

day—this large gap in mealtimes may adversely impact the client's mood, energy, and occupational performance, which could be addressed through changes to their routine.

Writing Goals for Habits and Routines

The goal of intervening on habits and routines is usually to alter the performance of the activity or activities embedded within a habit or routine. Thus, a goal may focus on the frequency, context, and/or performance quality of one or more activities within the context of a habit or routine. Some examples include:

- Mohammed will take his morning medication 5/7 days immediately after showering and dressing. [Current performance: 3/7 days]

  The goal above represents a **chaining strategy**: integrating a new activity within an existing routine to increase the likelihood of it becoming a habit. In doing so, the activity immediately before the target activity (in this case, showering and dressing) becomes the cue to trigger the new habit. If the client is already in the habit of showering once daily, and taking medication can be incorporated in this existing routine, this may promote enhanced medication adherence.

- During the next workweek, at the beginning of morning and afternoon breaks, Mariah will walk outdoors for 10 minutes and note her energy levels thereafter at 8/10 opportunities.

  Although not stated explicitly in the goal, this encompasses the three requirements to form a habit: a cue (start of breaktime at work), a targeted behavior (taking a walk), and a reward (increased energy). This goal may represent the culmination of an activity analysis session in which the occupational therapist guided the client in developing a plan to increase her physical activity. See an example in Figure 51.3.

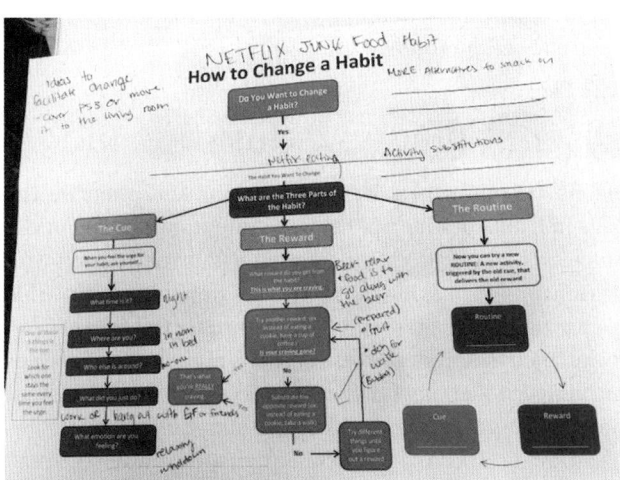

FIGURE 51.3 **Habit change worksheet.**

Intervention

Interventions to modify habits and routines have a storied history in OT, dating back to our profession's founding when habit training formed a cornerstone of Eleanor Clark Slagle's approach to OT (Reed, 2019). Although habits and routines have always been considered essential aspects of OT, our understanding of how to intervene on habits and routines has evolved rapidly in recent years. This section describes evidence-based strategies to address habit formation, habit discontinuation, and creating routines—three essential aspects of intervening on habits and routines.

Developing New Habits

New habits are created when a particular behavior is repeated over time in a stable context, followed (at least some of the time) by a reward (Wood & Neal, 2016). This repetition over time, with the expectation of a possible reward, causes the brain to create a shortcut: when exposed to that context, you automatically perform the behavior, without having to consciously think about doing it. Indeed, you may find it effortful to resist performing the habitual behavior! The basic ingredients of creating a habit, thus, are relatively simple: Identify a cue for the desired behavior, perform that behavior in response to the cue, and receive a reward. However, although this process is simple in theory, it can be quite challenging in practice. It takes trial and error to identify appropriate contextual cues and rewards for a desired behavior, and even once those are in place, it takes time for a behavior to become habitual. A commonly heard guideline is that it takes 21 days, or 3 weeks, to form a habit. Is there any science to support this claim? In short, no! The amount of time it takes to form a habit varies widely, depending on the person, task, and environmental factors. One study found that it took anywhere from 18 to 264 days for a given behavior to become a habit—on average, new habits were formed after 66 days (Lally et al., 2009). The amount of time it takes for a behavior to become a habit depends on a range of individual and contextual factors including, importantly, the "key ingredients" outlined below. Below, we outline considerations for each of the three elements necessary to create a new habit; See Table 51.1 for examples of habit formation in clinical practice.

Contextual Cues

For habits to form, some aspect of the context or environment has to serve as the trigger for the behavior to take place, as opposed to goal-directed behaviors that are triggered by an individual's intentions. Contextual cues can come from a broad array of sources, both physical and social, and both internal and external. Aspects of the sensory environment can be powerful cues. For example, when the lights dim at a theater, a hush reliably settles over the audience, and when I bake chocolate chip cookies, the smell inevitably lures my children into the kitchen looking for a snack. The social environment can also provide cues; for instance, when someone to whom you are being introduced extends their hand, you may instinctually extend yours as well for a handshake. (How many of you struggled to stop automatically shaking hands when it became frowned upon during the COVID pandemic?) Internal states can also trigger habits; for many people, boredom has become a cue to look at their smartphones for entertainment. A sequence of events can also become a contextual cue: chaining is a strategy in which you introduce a new behavior after an already established habit.

Targeted Behavior

Habitual behaviors can range from simple to highly complex, as illustrated in a typology of habit proposed by Clark et al. (2007), which describes habits ranging in complexity from simple motor tics to **habitus**, one's overarching character and disposition. The habitual behaviors most often addressed in OT interventions tend to be single, commonly performed activities, which fall in the middle of this range. Generally speaking, the more consistently the behavior can be performed, the more readily it will become a habit. Thus, performing an activity as consistently as possible will generally promote habit formation. For example, while I cook both eggs and vegetables nearly every day, I have a stronger habit for cooking eggs than for vegetables. My egg frying is highly predictable: each egg is approximately the same size and shape, is seasoned the same way, and takes the same amount of time to cook. I almost always cook eggs first thing in the morning, using a cast iron pan I have had for many years. Conversely, when I sauté vegetables, the activity varies a great deal according to the size and type of vegetables I'm using, how long I will cook them and at what temperature, and the seasonings I plan to use. This example illustrates how activities that are performed more consistently become habits more readily than activities that are more variable.

Rewards

Just as cues may be internal or external, rewards may be intrinsic to the activity (such as an endorphin "high" someone gets after exercise) or extrinsic (such as rewarding oneself for exercise with a piece of candy). Intrinsic rewards are a natural consequence of the activity itself, whereas extrinsic rewards are separate from the activity. Although intrinsic and extrinsic rewards are each effective for habit formation, they have distinct advantages and disadvantages. Intrinsic rewards are more likely to be consistently available over time, and they also increase **intrinsic motivation**, or the desire to engage in an activity for its own sake. By contrast, extrinsic rewards tend to *decrease* intrinsic motivation, and some extrinsic rewards lose their value over time (will a

piece of candy feel as rewarding after the 25th workout as it did after the first?). An additional drawback is that extrinsic rewards may not always be available, as compared to intrinsic rewards that are inherent to the activity. Yet, there are also advantages, such as the ability to customize extrinsic rewards to individual preferences (perhaps you find a peanut butter cup more rewarding than a piece of toffee?) and one can more easily provide graduated rewards if desired (e.g., one piece of toffee per 15 minutes of exercise). Lastly, when an activity is not especially intrinsically rewarding, extrinsic rewards may be the only or best option.

Whether intrinsic or extrinsic, rewards are most effective when they happen right after the behavior. Using the exercise example above, either the intrinsic "endorphin high" reward or the extrinsic chocolate reward immediately after working out will be much more effective at creating a habit than will the reward of increased strength or endurance (or a larger piece of chocolate!) weeks or months in the future. To put it simply, for our brain to perceive a reward as being associated with a behavior, it should come as soon after the behavior as possible.

Rewards are also most effective when they happen intermittently and are somewhat unpredictable. Decades of psychological research have shown that once the expectation of a reward is established, habitual behaviors will be most persistent when they are rewarded on an unpredictable basis (e.g., Bijou, 1957; Perkins & Cacioppo, 1950). This principle has been employed in various contexts, both positive and negative, to promote addictive patterns of behavior. For instance, slot machines operate on an intermittent reward schedule, which heightens the addictive potential of gambling. Although addiction is clearly an outcome to be avoided, intermittent rewards can be employed to promote the formation of health-promoting habits. For example, when I pick up prescriptions from the pharmacy each month, I receive coupons on my receipt of varying value. Occasionally, I receive a coupon for a deep discount on a product I need and use, which is an intermittent reward that reinforces my habit of filling prescriptions at this particular pharmacy each month.

Discontinuing Undesired Habits

Habits are powerful drivers of behavior, and often we engage in habits despite our desire or intention not to. For example, someone recently diagnosed with hypertension who has a habit of snacking on salted nuts or potato chips while preparing dinner may want to discontinue this behavior to lower their sodium intake. Yet, they may find themselves reaching for their habitual pre-dinner snack almost without noticing, and they find it difficult to stop this behavior.

Having a conscious desire and motivation to break a "bad habit" is not enough to produce a change, because habits happen outside of our conscious awareness. Indeed,

TABLE 51.1	Principles of Habit Formation in Action		
Key Principle	Definition	Clinical Example #1: Office Worker With Low Back Pain	Clinical Example #2: Full-inclusion Kindergarten Class
Performance in stable contexts	Context cues "trigger" habitual behaviors. Cues can include time, place, sequence, physical or emotional states, or almost any other aspect of the internal or external environment.	Standing and stretching once per hour in response to smartwatch vibration	Teacher claps in rhythm, indicating the end of free play and transition to morning meeting.
Repetition	The more often an activity is repeated, the more likely it is to become a habit.	Every workday while seated at their desk, approximately 6×/d, 5 d/wk	Once every school day, at the end of free play
Rewards (preferably varying or intermittent)	Specific rewards, either intrinsic or extrinsic, can promote habit formation - especially when receiving these rewards is unpredictable.	Decreased pain and muscle tension after stretching	Teacher provides varying verbal affirmations for listening and following directions.

people often persist in engaging in their undesired habits despite having a very strong intention to stop, which can understandably cause frustration and distress! In supporting a client through the process of habit change, it is important to provide education about the nature of habits and reassure them that setbacks are to be expected in the process. As you have learned, habits are triggered by contextual cues, and when a person with a strong habit is exposed to those cues, the habitual behavior is likely to be triggered despite their intentions otherwise. Because cues are sometimes not obvious, it may take some trial and error to identify what specifically is triggering a habit, which is something to keep in mind regardless of what strategy is used to try to break the habit.

Once habits are "hard-wired" into our brain, they can't simply be reversed. In keeping with this insight, three interventions have been demonstrated to help to break unwanted habits:

1. Making environmental modifications (which either eliminate the cue triggering the habit or make an alternative activity easier than the habitual one)
2. Using vigilant self-monitoring to disrupt the habit
3. Taking advantage of a naturally occurring disruption of the habit.

Each of these approaches is described in more detail below.

Eliminate Exposure to Cues

Because contextual cues are responsible for triggering habits, the most effective (though not always the most practical) strategy is to eliminate the cue that is triggering the unwanted habit. As noted above, sometimes the cue for a particular habit is not obvious at first, and it takes some experimentation to discern. For instance, let's return to the example above of a person who was recently diagnosed with

hypertension and wants to stop snacking on salted nuts and chips while they cook dinner, in order to reduce their sodium intake. A simple approach, if it is acceptable to the client and their household members, is to stop buying these salty snacks altogether. If they are not in the house at dinnertime when the client starts cooking, the client is unlikely to interrupt their meal preparation to procure some, no matter how much they are craving them.

As another example, many people experience distractions from their smartphones or other digital devices, which exhibit visual, auditory, or tactile cues when new information is available on the devices. These cues often prompt the response of picking up your device to see what is new, and the reward of some novel information. Typically, the device settings can be adjusted to eliminate these cues, which helps to avoid triggering the habitual behavior of picking up your device many times per day, which may disrupt participation in other valued occupations.

Enhance Availability of Alternatives

In situations where it is not possible to eliminate a cue to an undesired habit, habit change can be effected by making it harder to carry out the habitual behavior and easier to carry out an alternative activity. When substituting an alternative behavior for a habitual one, keep in mind that the substitute must also be rewarding—otherwise, the brain will keep craving the reward provided by the habitual behavior, which is counterproductive. You can see this principle in action with the smoking cessation strategy of using nicotine gum in the place of cigarettes. The gum provides a similar reward—the short-term dose of nicotine—without the other harmful effects of smoking. This alternative can make it easier to break the habit of reaching for a cigarette when a craving strikes.

In another example of using an alternate behavior, suppose a client is aiming to break their habit of hitting the snooze button on their alarm several times in the morning and instead wants to get up when the alarm goes off and go for a walk outdoors. Modifying the environment to make this alternative more likely could entail moving the alarm clock across the room and placing the client's exercise clothes on the nightstand where the alarm clock was previously. In doing so, hitting snooze on the alarm becomes more difficult than it was previously, whereas getting dressed to go for a walk becomes easier. These environmental modifications don't eliminate the cue entirely (because they are still using the alarm clock to wake up), but they make it harder to carry out the undesired habit and easier to carry out the desired alternative. With time and repetition, the cue of the alarm clock may eventually create a habitual response to get dressed for a walk, rather than to hit the snooze button for a few extra minutes of sleep. The reward, in this case, may be the increased energy and wakefulness that results from the morning walk which is an acceptable substitute for the increased energy gained from a few extra minutes of sleep.

As a final example, consider again the client with hypertension. Suppose that the client's spouse still wants to have salted nuts and potato chips in the house to eat, and objects to eliminating these from the environment altogether. The client could potentially negotiate to store the salty snacks in an inconvenient location—perhaps the top shelf of the pantry—and to keep their preferred alternative within close proximity of where they prepare dinner. In doing so, these environmental modifications create more difficulty in carrying out the habitual behavior of snacking on nuts or chips and make it easier to snack on their preferred alternative.

Vigilant Self-Monitoring

In some situations, it is not practical to change an unwanted habit by modifying the environment to eliminate exposure to cues or enhance the availability of alternatives. In these cases, another approach to habit change is to maintain a heightened awareness of situations that trigger the undesired habit, and the intention to substitute an alternate behavior. This strategy works by increasing a person's conscious control over their behavior, which competes with the automatic triggering of behaviors through habits (Wood & Ruenger, 2016). Because this strategy is very mentally taxing, it is most likely to be effective when an individual is both highly motivated to change their habits and has adequate mental resources to maintain a high level of self-control over their behavior (Lally & Gardner, 2011).

To reduce the difficulty of maintaining constant vigilance over one's behavior, it is helpful to develop an understanding of the contexts in which a habit is likely to be triggered. Identifying the cues that are likely to trigger an undesired habit allows an individual to be alert to situations where they may need to more closely monitor their behavior. For example, if you are trying to break a habit of

drinking soda, and you know that you are most likely to want a soda at the end of a long workday when you are physically and mentally fatigued, you can be better prepared to self-monitor your behavior at the end of the workday. When in a setting that may trigger an undesired habit, exerting self-control by using simple statements like "Don't do it!" can be effective in reducing the likelihood of performing an unwanted habit (Quinn et al., 2010).

Self-monitoring can also be supported by using implementation intentions, or specific statements that describe the circumstances that may trigger an undesired habit, and how to avoid engaging in the unwanted behavior. These intentions can often be framed as "if-then" or "when-then" statements (Fritz & Cutchin, 2016). For example, an individual with a habit of biting their nails when they are anxious might tell themselves, "when I feel anxious, then I will squeeze a stress ball." Implementation intentions are most effective if, as in this example, the alternative behavior is incompatible with the unwanted habit.

Making Changes During a Life Event or Transition

Major life events, such as relocating, starting a new job, or experiencing a significant medical event, often disrupt existing habits. Although this is a problem insofar as it disrupts desirable habits, it also creates an opportunity to discontinue unwanted habits. Because occupational therapists are often called upon to provide intervention during or following such life events, they present an opportune time to investigate whether there are any habits the client would like to change. For example, a client receiving inpatient rehabilitation after a stroke may be interested in discussing strategies for smoking cessation, particularly if they recognize the connection between smoking and the risk of stroke. Their smoking habit has been temporarily disrupted by the hospitalization, creating an opportunity to identify the triggers that typically cue them to smoke, and proactively creating a plan to avoid or eliminate them when they return home after the hospitalization.

An important limitation to this approach is that identifying cues for a habit and developing strategies to avoid or change one's response to them is an ongoing and sometimes lengthy process of trial and error, yet occupational therapists often see clients for only a brief amount of time following a major life event. Ideally, an occupational therapist seeing a client in an acute or subacute setting for a limited amount of time would share the client's goals related to habit change with an outpatient or home health occupational therapist to continue the process of problem-solving. When this is not possible, the occupational therapist can educate the client and family members about the process of habit change, to anticipate relapses of old habits as a normal part of the process, and to develop strategies to get back on track with changing habits.

Creating, Maintaining, and Changing Routines

When clients describe their daily lives and the accommodations that they make to sustain a routine, they are providing information with deep implications for intervention planning. (Gallimore & Lopez, 2002, p. 76S)

As illustrated by the above quote, routines are essential to consider in any OT intervention context, even those that do not seek explicitly to change a client's existing routines. Many of the underlying issues that lead people to seek OT services represent breaches of routine that have disrupted their daily lives. Consider that even taking time out of their day to attend an OT session likely represents a departure from your client's typical routine. Furthermore, an occupational therapist's recommendation to adopt, change, or stop doing a particular activity or occupation all represent potential changes in the client's routine. Examples of such changes are nearly limitless, and often taken for granted: donning and doffing compression garments to manage lymphedema, taking "brain breaks" while doing homework to support self-regulation, or doing periodic range of motion exercises to preserve joint mobility all represent changes to a client's usual routine. Thus, working with clients to identify *how* they will implement these changes to their routines is an essential aspect to supporting their performance of these activities and attaining the benefits of therapy.

In considering how to support clients to create, maintain, or change their routines, it is best to use a collaborative approach that centers the client's expertise about how their daily life is structured, what works well in their current routines, and what is amenable to change. Routines are often used to coordinate activity within a social group, as in a family routine or a classroom routine. Thus, it is also important to consider how changing a routine will impact various members of the group. There are a wide range of tools that can be used to support routines, many of which you are already likely familiar with, including visual schedules, day planners (paper or app-based), and calendars. In selecting tools to support a client's change in routines, it is important to consider what is feasible and, if possible, already embedded into a client's daily life. For example, suppose you are adapting a student's homework routine to incorporate periodic "brain breaks," and the student works on most of their homework assignments through their school's web portal. Rather than using a timer or other external means to schedule brain breaks, it may be possible to install a plugin for the web browser itself, so that the student is automatically reminded to take breaks whenever they launch the school website. For more examples of strategies to adapt routines, see OT Story 51.1 and Expanding Our Perspectives.

OT STORY 51.1 COVID IN A GROUP HOME

Refer to Chapter 13 to review the case of Rob, a 46-year-old man with Down syndrome who resides in a group home and is experiencing occupational disruption due to COVID-19. During the occupational therapist's initial evaluation, she noted that Rob and his housemates' habits and routines had been significantly disrupted by the stay-at-home order imposed by their local public health department. Rob's inability to participate in his valued work, leisure, and social occupations contributed to an increase in depressive symptoms and disengagement from activities of daily living. During the evaluation, Rob, his housemates, and the occupational therapist collaborated to set goals related to reestablishing consistent habits and routines.

Before the stay-at-home order, the housemates' mealtimes varied due to their different schedules. However, they decided that having shared morning and evening meals provided an opportunity to establish a consistent routine and socialize with one another whereas their activities outside the home were curtailed. They also developed a "buddy system" in which a housemate would check in with anyone who missed a meal unexpectedly.

Because in-person contact with other group homes was restricted, the housemates also discussed ideas to replace the routine social and leisure activities they had engaged in before COVID. They brainstormed activities that were still permitted under the public health guidelines, and they created a schedule of recurring weekly events in which housemates could elect to participate. This provided housemates with predictable opportunities to engage in social activities and a routine to help them structure and organize their time. As a group, they identified activities such as morning and afternoon walks in the neighborhood; shared daily chores such as sweeping, raking, and snow shoveling outside; and playing games after dinner.

In addition, Rob worked one-on-one with the occupational therapist to establish a new morning routine because of his struggle to get out of bed and engage in activities of daily living. He decided to place his music player at the side of his bed to play gentle music to help him go to sleep and play music from his favorite musicals to help him wake up. Together, they also created a daily breakfast menu that Rob could help cook and looked forward to eating.

Questions

1. What would be an example of a goal Rob and his occupational therapist might set to reestablish consistent habits and routines in his daily life?
2. What is an additional routine or habit you would want to establish with Rob to support his well-being?

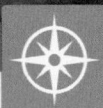

EXPANDING OUR PERSPECTIVES

Letting Go Ceremony

Debbie Bub (B.Sc. occupational therapy)

I worked in an inpatient addiction treatment facility. People whose lives had been negatively affected by all sorts of addictions came for treatment. One of the activities I designed was a Letting Go Ceremony. In fact, I did not design it alone. This was done in collaboration with the service users, but more about that later.

My thinking behind the Letting Go Ceremony was to give the community a therapeutic experience that dramatized the loss of a way of life. People facing active addiction need to make and sustain an enormous change in their daily habits and routines in order to recover. Addiction is so hijacking of people's everyday way of doing things, it takes over. Facing addiction is difficult, as so much time and energy get consumed in the service of one's addiction that is inevitably never satisfied. And so, a Letting Go Ceremony was a way of offering service users an opportunity to gain insight into what they needed to leave behind as they moved away from their addictive behaviors, as well as offering emotional support in the process of doing this.

The first part of this process was to call the whole service user community together and explain to them that we would be having a Letting Go Ceremony in a week's time. The aim of this first meeting was to discuss the idea and then to plan the form the ceremony would take. I would facilitate this discussion making sure to support the group in designing a ceremony that made sense to them. If necessary, I would give cues like suggesting there be a beginning, middle, and end to the proceedings. I also would suggest that the ceremony provide each service user an opportunity to have their turn in letting go of whatever they were struggling with (the choice was theirs) and to find a symbol that represents that. I would have paper and pen so I could take minutes of the order of proceedings, and community members would volunteer to take on different tasks. The session would end with a confirmation of the order of proceedings for clarity so that the community was well informed. After this, I would also type out the order of proceedings and distribute this to the community.

The therapeutic team would be informed of the Letting Go Ceremony and in their individual and group therapy sessions, they would support the service users' processes.

Service users tended to engage really well in this therapeutic process.

The therapeutic aim was to help individuals identify what they were letting go of and then decide how to symbolize this for the Letting Go Ceremony. This provided an opportunity to explore with service users the detail of their addictive routines that needed alteration. There was often an accompanying sense of grief that seemed to emerge in the community as service users prepared for their ceremony. This then led to a greater intensity of therapy in all aspects of the program, often allowing insight into a service user's internal motivation.

The design was always unique in all but one aspect—service users almost always chose to make a fire to burn whatever they were letting go of. Only once did a community decide to dig a grave.

And then the day for the ceremony arrived and there was always a sense of anticipation and even anxiety. The service users would gather. Sometimes someone would read something, or sing a song, or say what we were about to do. Every group had a different design. But each ceremony gave each service user their chance to be witnessed by the group as they explained their symbol and then let go of it. Some examples were a service user burning their pencil case where they had kept the syringe and needles they needed to use heroin. Another service user let go of their shoes that had walked many a street in their pursuit of drugs, and another wrote a letter that they read out, releasing a long-held secret. Someone else burnt their sim card so that using friends and dealers would no longer be able to contact them. Someone else removed a piercing as they began to change how they presented themselves to the world. The list goes on but represents how service users were able to use the Letting Go Ceremony to demonstrate changes they were beginning to make in their daily habits and routines. This event enabled service users to identify environmental cues that needed to be avoided and new habits to be practiced. And though it was different for each person, everyone was in a similar position of needing to let go of old habits while learning new ones. And so, the ceremony united everyone in this transition and held each member accountable. Once everyone had a turn, the ceremony was concluded.

Thereafter the community and staff would gather to celebrate and mingle, with treats to eat and drink.

Outcomes

Habit Change Outcomes

The outcomes of interventions to address habits and routines can be multifaceted and wide-ranging. At the level of the targeted activity, strengthening or extinguishing habits will make it more or less likely that the activity is carried out. For example, if an intervention aiming to strengthen a client's habit of taking their arthritis medication is successful, the outcome will be that the client takes the medication more consistently. A successful outcome of an intervention focused on extinguishing a client's undesired habit of smoking cigarettes would be fewer cigarettes smoked. Outcomes may also relate to the *consequences* of performing a given activity more or less frequently: for example, the client who is taking their arthritis medication more consistently may have fewer and less painful arthritis flare-ups. The client who is smoking fewer cigarettes may notice that they are coughing less, or that they no longer crave a cigarette upon waking in the morning. Finally, habit change interventions can result in improved self-efficacy, decreased illness intrusiveness (illness-related disruptions to other life activities), or other psychosocial benefits. These outcomes often result from the client's success in making a desired change in their patterns of activity, more so than the direct impact of how often they carry out a given activity.

Routine Change Outcomes

Similar to habits, interventions to change routines can have a wide range of possible outcomes. As with habit change interventions, creating routines can facilitate more consistent performance of activities that are embedded within routines, while altering routines to eliminate an undesired activity can help to reduce the performance of that activity. As noted in Chapter 13, routines create a consistent and predictable structure in our daily lives, and thus developing routines can give people a greater sense of control over their lives, which contributes to improved psychosocial well-being (Deci & Ryan, 2008). Creating stronger routines can also improve the efficiency of carrying out daily activities, an energy conservation strategy that may facilitate participation in other valued occupations and contribute to overall well-being.

Conclusion

As the building blocks of our daily lives, habits and routines have a powerful influence on our occupational engagement, participation, and quality of life. Habits and routines that are aligned with our goals, interests, and desires for how we spend our time are essential tools for maintaining our health and well-being. However, habits and routines can also undermine our health and well-being when they lead us to repeatedly engage in activities that are not aligned with our goals, interests, and desires. The strategies outlined in this chapter provide a starting point for occupational therapists to evaluate, intervene, and track outcomes related to creating, maintaining, and changing habits and routines. In doing so, occupational therapists can assist clients in structuring their daily lives in ways that best support their health, well-being, and quality of life. See OT Story 51.2 describing interventions for performance patterns related to sleep and nutrition.

Lippincott® Connect *For additional resources on the subjects discussed in this chapter, visit* Lippincott Connect.

OT STORY 51.2 KARINA

Karina (she/her/), a 51-year-old woman, was referred to OT by her primary care physician for the management of diabetes and hypertension. When the occupational therapist meets with Karina for the first time, they take a thorough occupational history, focusing particularly on Karina's habits and routines, and how they impact her ability to carry out occupations relevant to managing her chronic conditions. Please refer to Chapter 13 for details about Karina's occupational history.

During the OT evaluation, the therapist identifies occupational performance deficits in the domains of rest/sleep, health management, and instrumental activities of daily living (IADLs) that compromise Karina's overall health and well-being. Karina notes that she is interested in making lifestyle changes to improve her health, but she feels overwhelmed and doesn't know where to start. Together with Karina, the therapist identifies Karina's performance patterns related to sleep preparation and nutrition management as primary areas to address in occupational therapy.

In the area of nutrition management, the therapist and Karina focus first on the snack that Karina typically eats during her overnight shift. She habitually chooses snacks that are high in added sugars, which elevate her blood sugar and contribute to fatigue. Karina and the therapist review possible cues for Karina to choose these snacks on her overnight shift, and they identify that the hunger she feels at the start of her break is the most likely cue. They brainstorm alternative snacks that will satisfy her hunger while meeting nutritional recommendations, and they create a plan for substituting these alternatives when she is cued to snack during her shift. Karina aims to substitute a lower-sugar snack at three out of five opportunities over the coming week.

Questions

1. What would be your next step to addressing Karina's overnight snack habit, if during her next visit, she notes that she was not successful with her initial plan?
2. With respect to sleep preparation, what is important to know about Karina's bedtime routine? How might changing her bedtime routine help to promote better quality sleep?

REFERENCES

Bijou, S. W. (1957). Patterns of reinforcement and resistance to extinction in young children. *Child Development, 28*(1), 47–54. https://doi.org/10.1111/j.1467-8624.1957.tb04830.x

Clark, F. (2000). The concepts of habit and routine: A preliminary synthesis. *OTJR: Occupation, Participation and Health, 20,* 123S–137S. https://doi.org/10.1177/15394492000200S114

Clark, F., Sanders, K., Carlson, M., Blanche, E., & Jackson, J. (2007). Synthesis of habit theory. *OTJR: Occupation, Participation, and Health, 27*(Suppl), 7S–23S. https://doi.org/10.1177/15394492070270S103

Deci, E. L., & Ryan, R. M. (2008). Facilitating optimal motivation and psychological well-being across life's domains. *Canadian Psychology/Psychologie canadienne, 49*(1), 14–23. https://doi.org/10.1037/0708-5591.49.1.14

Fritz, H., & Cutchin, M. P. (2016). Integrating the science of habit: Opportunities for occupational therapy. *OTJR: Occupation, Participation and Health, 36*(2), 92–98. https://doi.org/10.1177/1539449216643307

Gallimore, R., & Lopez, E. M. (2002). Everyday routines, human agency, and ecocultural context: Construction and maintenance of individual habits. *Occupational Therapy Journal of Research, 22*(Suppl), 70S–77S. https://doi.org/10.1177/15394492020220S109

Lally, P., & Gardner, B. (2011). Promoting habit formation. *Health Psychology Review, 7*(Suppl. 1), S137–S158. https://doi.org/10.1080/17437199.2011.603640

Lally, P., van Jaarsveld, C. H. M., Potts, H. W. W., & Wardle, J. (2009). How are habits formed: Modelling habit formation in the real world. *European Journal of Social Psychology, 40*(6), 998–1009. https://doi.org/10.1002/ejsp.674

Perkins, C. C., Jr., & Cacioppo, A. J. (1950). The effect of intermittent reinforcement on the change in extinction rate following successive reconditionings. *Journal of Experimental Psychology, 40*(6), 794–801. https://doi.org/10.1037/h0054216

Quinn, J. M., Pascoe, A., Wood, W., & Neal, D. T. (2010). Can't control yourself? Monitor those bad habits. *Personality and Social Psychology Bulletin, 36*(4), 499–511. https://doi.org/10.1177/0146167209360665

Reed, K. L. (2019). The beliefs of Eleanor Clarke Slagle: Are they current or history? *Occupational Therapy in Healthcare, 33*(3), 265–285. https://doi.org/10.1080/07380577.2019.1619215

Smith, K. S., & Graybiel, A. M. (2014). Investigating habits: Strategies, technologies, and models. *Frontiers in Behavioral Neuroscience, 8,* 39. https://doi.org/10.3389/fnbeh.2014.00039

Wood, W., & Neal, D. T. (2016). Healthy through habit: Interventions for initiating & maintaining health behavior change. *Behavioral Science & Policy, 2*(1), 71–83. https://doi.org/10.1353/bsp.2016.0008

Wood, W., & Ruenger, D. (2016). Psychology of habit. *Annual Review of Psychology, 67,* 289–314. https://doi.org/10.1146/annurev-psych-122414-033417

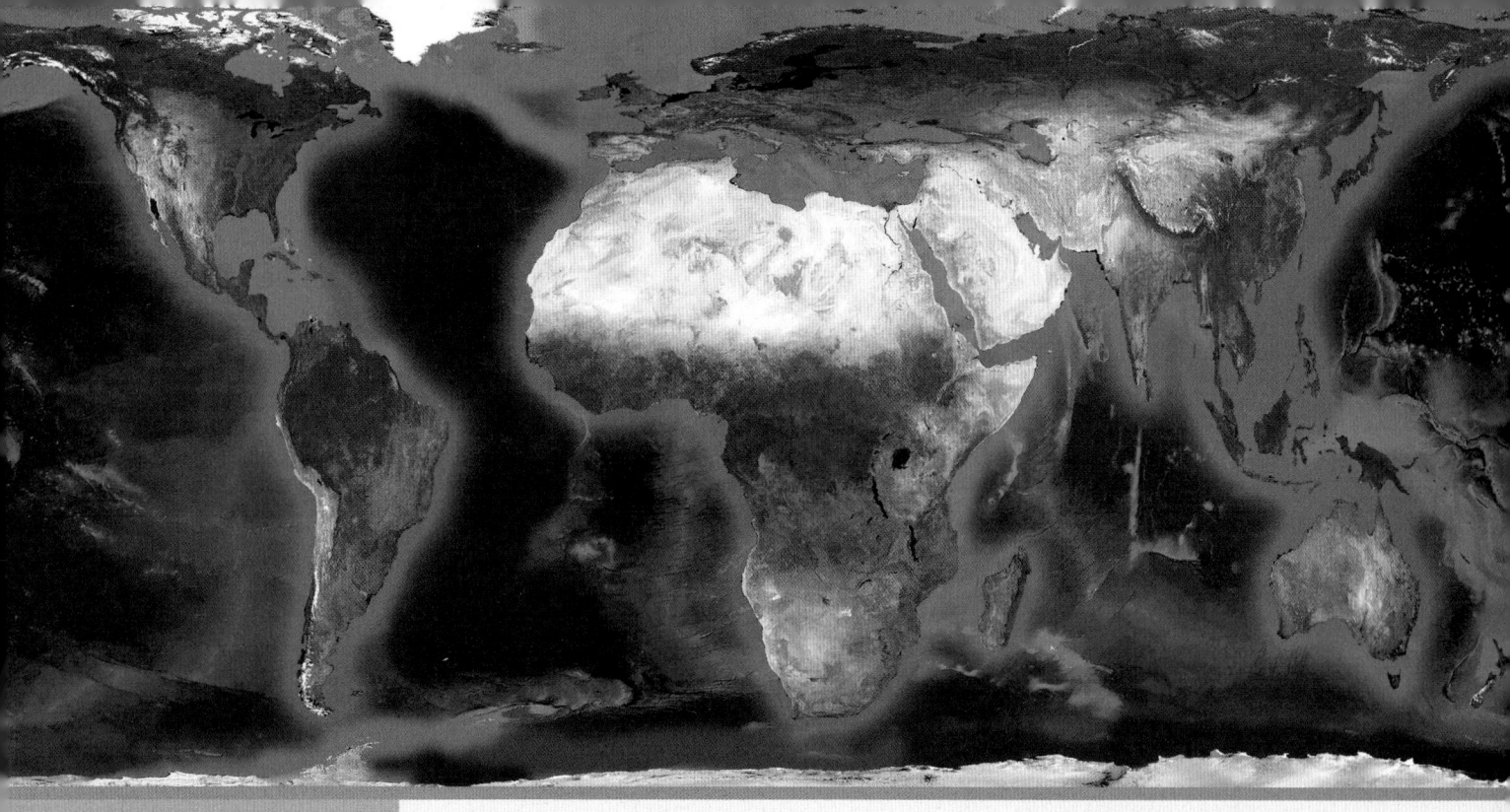

UNIT VIII

Evaluation, Interventions, and Outcomes for Performance Skills and Client Factors

Media Related to Evaluation, Intervention, and Outcomes for Performance Skills and Client Factors

Readings
- The Curious Incident of the Dog in the Night-Time: Fictional mystery novel by Mark Haddon about a 15-year-old boy who investigates the death of his neighbor's dog. According to the author, the novel is about difference, about being an outsider, and about seeing the world in a surprising and revealing way. (2003)

Movies/Television
- Special: Ryan O'Connell accounts for his life as a gay man with cerebral palsy pursing friendship, relationship, and self-sufficiency. (2019–2021)
- Still Alice: American film based on the 2007 novel by Lisa Genova. It follows a linguistics professor diagnosed with early-onset Alzheimer disease shortly after her 50th birthday. (2014)

Art
- *Lorenza Böttner's Venus de Milo:* Chilean-German transgendered artist, stood onstage, statuesque, in a Munich theater. She was covered in a fine layer of white plaster and with a cloth draped around her waist and was posed in a manner resembling the Venus de Milo. Like the ancient Greek statue, Böttner is armless, and her provocative performance invited the sorts of stares she was used to receiving. Yet she asked her viewers to bring a new awareness to their gaze. She was pointing out how impairment can seem downright romantic when it's presented as a metaphor or suggested by ruins; meanwhile, in daily life, disabled people are regularly gawked at. (1987)

Evaluating Quality of Occupational Performance: Performance Skills

Anne G. Fisher and Lou Ann Griswold

LEARNING OBJECTIVES

After reading this chapter, you will be able to:

1. Use the Transactional Model of Occupation to describe the difference between (a) performance skills and (b) body functions.
2. Implement an analysis of performance skills (performance analysis) and document a person's quality of occupational performance.
3. Describe how the results of a performance analysis are used to collaboratively establish client-centered goals and indicate change in occupational performance.

Introduction to Performance Skills

Performance skills are the smallest observable actions—units of occupational performance—that we can observe as people carry out their daily life tasks. When people are engaged in carrying out their daily life tasks, they are engaged in broad activities (e.g., activities of daily living [ADLs], social activities) or specific task performances (e.g., eating dinner, socializing with friends, reading a book). Noting the degree of performance skill that can be observed during those task performances is critical for evaluating the quality of a person's occupational performance. Consider, for example, what Karla observes as she watches Maurice perform daily life tasks (see OT Story 52.1).

In OT Story 52.1, Karla evaluated the quality of Maurice's occupational performance by observing the small goal-directed actions Maurice enacted one by one as he engaged in relevant and meaningful daily life task performances. More specifically, she observed the quality of his performance skills (Fisher, 2009; Fisher & Kielhofner, 1995; Fisher & Marterella, 2019; Kielhofner, 2008). Kielhofner (2008) referred to these observable performance skills as "discrete purposeful actions [that] can be discerned" (p. 103). Performance skills are links in a larger chain of actions, which link by link, action by action, become the whole chain—the task performance (Fisher & Marterella, 2019; Figure 52.2).

OT STORY 52.1 PERFORMANCE SKILLS—OBSERVABLE CHAINS OF GOAL-DIRECTED ACTIONS

Karla, Maurice's occupational therapist, observes him as he is engaged in preparing himself a glass of orange juice. As she observes his **motor skills**, she observes that he momentarily props (*stabilizes*) on the kitchen counter as he *walks* to the refrigerator. He then *bends* forward, *reaches* out, and grasps (*grips*) the handle on the door of the refrigerator without any evidence of clumsiness or increased physical effort. When he attempts to open the door of the refrigerator (*moves*), he does not pull hard enough (*calibrates*)—the door does not open. She then observes him as he pulls again (*moves, calibrates*) on the handle of the refrigerator door and, this time, she sees the refrigerator door open. Karla then observes that Maurice effectively *reaches* in, *grips* a container of orange juice, *lifts* it, and takes it out of the refrigerator, but that he is somewhat unstable (*stabilizes*) when he *walks* and *transports* the container of juice over to the counter where he has placed a glass. See Figure 52.1.

As Karla observes Maurice as he is engaged in preparing his breakfast, she also observes his **process skills**. For example, Karla observes that although Maurice *initiates* most task actions without a delay, he pauses momentarily before reaching for the handle of the refrigerator door. She also sees that he *continues* each action through to completion without any unnecessary pauses (e.g., continuing pulling on the refrigerator door until it is open, continuing walking until the orange juice is transported to the counter). As Maurice *initiates* pouring orange juice into the glass on the counter, he again pauses. Moreover, Karla observes that he does not *terminate* pouring the orange juice before some orange juice spills over the rim of the glass. She also observes that Maurice performs task actions in a logical order (*sequences*). For example, she observes that he opens the lid of the orange juice container and then pours juice into the glass and not vice versa. Finally, she observes Maurice as he *searches* for and *locates* the orange juice container in the refrigerator, *chooses* orange juice, *gathers* the orange juice container to the same workspace where he has placed the glass, and *organizes* his workspace effectively—not too crowded, not too spread out.

Later, as Karla observes Maurice as he is engaged in a social exchange with his care provider, Joyce—planning the weekly meals and making a shopping list—she observes Maurice's **social interaction skills**. More specifically, she observes that he readily *approaches* his social partner and *starts* a conversation. As he does so, and throughout the social exchange, Maurice *turns toward*, but frequently does not *look* at his social partner when they are talking to each other. As Maurice is talking, Karla observes that he *produces speech* that is clearly audible and that he *gesticulates* by nodding his head and smiling in a manner that is socially appropriate. She also observes that Maurice often stammers and pauses during his spoken messages (*speaks fluently*), and that he occasionally starts messages but leaves them "hanging in the air" and never finishes them (*times duration*). When Joyce asks Maurice questions (e.g., "What would you like to eat this week?"), he frequently *replies* with messages that are markedly irrelevant to the ongoing conversation (e.g., "My son called me last night."). Finally, Karla observes Maurice as he *takes turns* with his social partner, and that he frequently "talks over" and interrupts his social partner (*times response*).

Questions

1. How does conducting and using the results of a performance analysis to describe the quality of a person's occupational performance differ from other assessments you might have seen or used?
2. Based on the description of Karla's observation of Maurice pouring himself a glass of orange juice, what skills seem to be effective and what skills seem to be ineffective during his task performance?
3. What other tasks might you want to observe Maurice perform and how might you prioritize these while ensuring you retain a client-centered perspective?

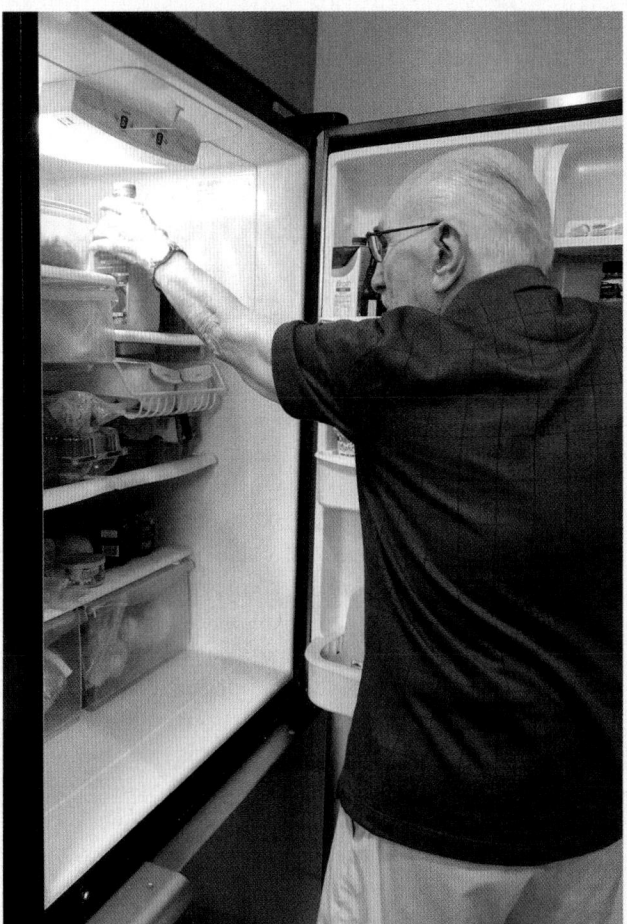

FIGURE 52.1 Maurice reaching into refrigerator to get the bottle of orange juice.

Occupational performance
A chain of small actions

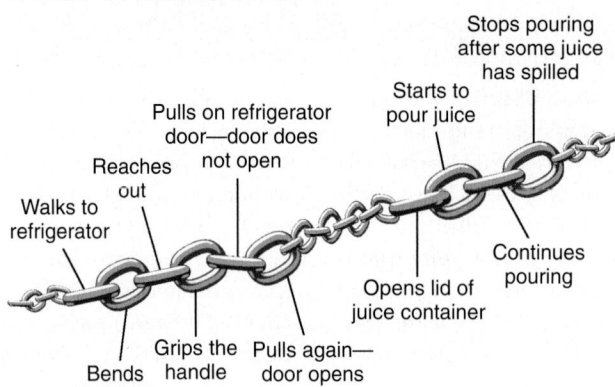

FIGURE 52.2 Performance skills: smallest observable units of occupational performance—links in a chain of ongoing actions that people perform one by one as they "construct" overall daily life task performances (e.g., preparing a glass of orange juice and a bowl of cereal).

(Adapted from Fisher, A. G., & Marterella, A. [2019]. *Powerful practice: A model for authentic occupational therapy.* Center for Innovative OT Solutions. Reprinted with permission.)

The term *performance skills* has been used to refer to the smallest observable units of occupational performance because the people we evaluate demonstrate more or less occupational skill when they complete (i.e., "construct") daily life task performances. These small units of observable actions were first conceptualized in the mid-1980s (Fisher, 2006), and they have now been incorporated into major occupational therapy (OT) models of practice, including the Model of Human Occupation (Kielhofner, 1995, 2008; Taylor, 2017), the Occupational Therapy Intervention Process Model (Fisher, 1998, 2009; Fisher & Marterella, 2019), and the Transactional Model of Occupation (Fisher & Marterella, 2019). They are also included in the *Occupational Therapy Practice Framework* (American Occupational Therapy Association [AOTA], 2020). The smallest observable actions of occupational performance have been variously referred to as *performance skills* (AOTA, 2020; Fisher, 2006; Fisher & Kielhofner, 1995), *performance units* (Hagedorn, 2000), *units* or *subunits of occupational performance* (Fisher, 2006; Polatajko et al., 2000), *occupational skill* (Kielhofner, 2008), and *actions of performance* (Fisher, 1998). Within the *International Classification of Functioning, Disability and Health* (ICF; World Health Organization [WHO], 2001), performance skills are analogous to the smaller discrete actions that are part of larger task performances defined within the "Activities" and "Participation" domains. In all of these instances, performance skills have been clearly differentiated from underlying body functions. Body functions are discussed in more detail in Chapter 53.

Using the Transactional Model of Occupation to Conceptualize the Difference Between Performance Skills and Body Functions

The Transactional Model of Occupation shown in Figure 52.3 was developed by Fisher and Marterella (2019) to capture the true complexity of occupation as recognized by a transactional perspective on occupation. This perspective on occupation was introduced into occupational science by Dickie and colleagues (Aldrich, 2008; Dickie et al., 2006).

Within the Transactional Model of Occupation, **occupation** is viewed as being comprised of three interwoven elements that mutually influence each other: occupational performance, occupational experience, and participation. More specifically, **occupational performance** pertains to the observable aspects of occupation—what one is doing. As we noted above, at the more global level of occupational performance, people engage in activities or task performances (e.g., preparing a glass of orange juice). At the more discrete level of occupational performance, we have the smallest observable units of occupation: performance skills—the links in the chain of observable action shown in Figure 52.2.

Occupational experience pertains to what the person experiences during occupational performance and can only become known to the outsider via the person's verbal or nonverbal report (e.g., experiencing occupational performance as satisfying, effortful, painful, productive, and/or pleasurable). Finally, **participation** (i.e., occupational engagement) emerges when one's doing (occupational performance) occurs in combination with the specific occupational experience of *personal value* in that doing (e.g., feeling that what you are doing is necessary or worthwhile, feeling that it is important to do what you are doing because you said you would do it or because it is your responsibility to do it, feeling that what you are doing is helpful or is making a difference, feeling that you are included or socially connected when doing with others). "Thus, when people are doing something and experiencing personal value in that doing, they are participating" (Fisher & Marterella, 2019, pp. 21–22).

Inherent to the Transactional Model of Occupation is the recognition that the interwoven elements of occupation arise from and are inextricably intertwined with all of the elements of the situational context shown in Figure 52.3 (e.g., sociocultural elements, geopolitical elements, client elements). That is, in addition to influencing each other, the three occupational elements are continually influencing the various elements of the situational context, and the elements of the situational context are simultaneously mutually influencing each other as well as the three occupational elements. The lines between all situational elements and the occupation shown in Figure 52.3 are designed to illustrate how various situational elements and occupation are inextricably intertwined and mutually shape each other. Thus, as Fisher and Marterella (2019) pointed out, we must remain "constantly aware that any change in any given situational or occupational element will occur reciprocally with changes in other elements because of the constant interplay among them" (p. 18).

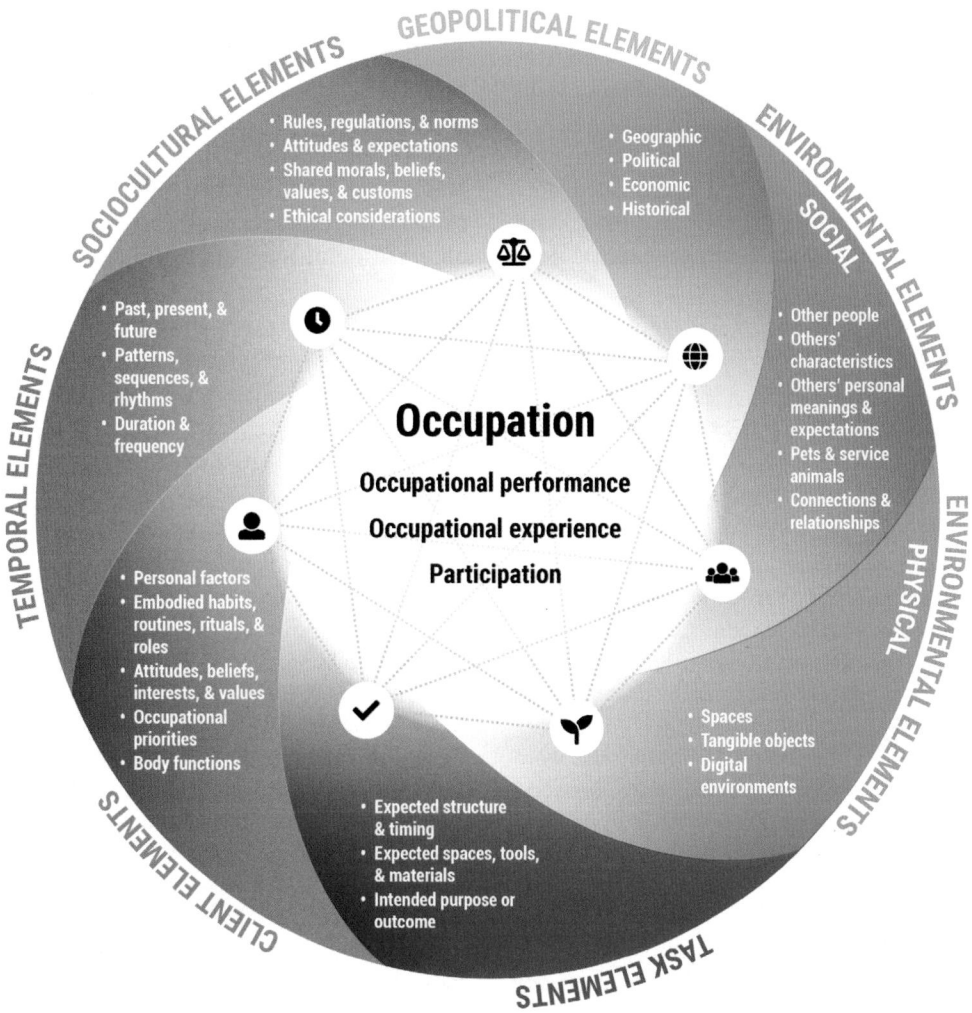

FIGURE 52.3 Graphic representation of the *Transactional Model of Occupation.*

(From Fisher, A. G., & Marterella, A. [2019]. *Powerful practice: A model for authentic occupational therapy.* Center for Innovative OT Solutions. Reprinted with permission.)

When we use the Transactional Model of Occupation to conceptualize the difference between performance skills and body functions, we can begin by recognizing that body functions are part of the situational context—a client element. Examples of body functions include memory, motor planning and praxis skill, perceptual skill, joint mobility, muscle power, fine motor coordination, and emotional regulation.

In contrast, performance skills pertain to occupational performance—*what people do* as they interact with task objects (e.g., *swing* a baseball bat and *hit* a baseball, *jump* rope, *choose* a pencil and *use* it to *write*) in the context of their engagement in activities or task performances (playing baseball with friends, jumping rope with classmates, completing a schoolwork task). When a person is engaged in occupation that includes social interaction with others, it also becomes possible to observe social interaction skills (*greet* one's friends, *laugh* at a friend's joke).

Thus, as shown in Figure 52.3, body functions (a client element) are not the same thing as performance skills (an occupational element: occupational performance). Although body functions (and all of the other situational and occupational elements) can support or hinder the quality of occupational performance, body functions and performance skills represent very different constructs. Swinging a bat and hitting a ball may be supported by the person having strength and coordination, but being strong and coordinated does not mean that the person can skillfully swing a bat and hit a ball. Moreover, people can demonstrate occupational skills

despite having impairments of their body functions (see the Commentary on the Evidence box).

In fact, a critical feature of the Transactional Model of Occupation is the recognition that the influence of body functions on occupation is neither more nor less than is the influence of the other situational elements that mutually influence and are influenced by occupation. In addition, occupation, including occupational performance, is not produced by people (or their body functions), it is produced by the transactional whole shown in Figure 52.3 (Fisher & Marterella, 2019).

In OT Story 52.1, we noted that when Karla observed Maurice as he attempted to open the refrigerator door, he did not pull hard enough and the door did not open. From the perspective of occupational performance (what Maurice did), Karla observed that Maurice did not pull with enough force to open the refrigerator door. When Karla began to speculate about reasons why Maurice might not have pulled with enough force to open the door, one possibility she considered was that he might have diminished strength in his upper limb.

In such instances, occupational therapists may think they "see" decreased strength, but in fact, they do not. Rather, they observe the person to perform some action that has an underlying demand for strength and therefore reason that diminished strength is the cause of the occupational performance problem observed. But Karla has not observed diminished strength because strength cannot be

COMMENTARY ON THE EVIDENCE

Performance Skills Cannot Be Equated With Body Functions

Many respected authors within OT incorrectly equate performance skills with body functions. That is, (a) process skills sometimes are referred to as cognitive skills and/or (b) motor planning, executive functions, and perceptual skills sometimes are considered to be performance skills. One such example is the second edition of the *Occupational Therapy Practice Framework* (AOTA, 2008). Within that earlier edition of the framework, performance skills were described as including motor and praxis skills, sensory-perceptual skills, emotional regulation skills, cognitive skills, and communication and social skills. When considered in relation to the Transactional Model of Occupation (see Figure 52.3), praxis skill (i.e., motor planning), perceptual skill, cognitive skill, and emotional regulation are viewed as client elements, specifically underlying body functions, not performance skills. In contrast, performance skills pertain to occupational performance—the smallest observable units of what a person does.

What is the evidence to support the differentiation between performance skills and these underlying body functions? One such resource comes from Rexroth and colleagues (2005) who implemented a study where they compared the level of motor and process skill between 1,939 people with right hemispheric strokes and 1,939 people with left hemispheric strokes. If we compare these two groups, people who have had right hemispheric strokes are much more likely to demonstrate visual perceptual impairments and unilateral neglect, whereas people who had left hemispheric strokes are much more likely to demonstrate aphasia and apraxia (Bartels et al., 2016). These are impairments of body functions.

If performance skills, specifically motor and process skills, are to be equated with praxis and perceptual skills, it should follow that people with right versus left hemispheric stroke will differ significantly in terms of their levels of motor and/or process skill. Yet, Rexroth et al. (2005) found that there was no significant difference between the two groups in any of the 36 motor and process skills studied. These results indicate that performance analysis, focused on performance skill (i.e., the person's observed quality of doing), is very different from assessment methods focused on underlying body functions. See Table 52.1 for a list of the 36 performance skills they compared.

TABLE 52.1   **Universal Performance Skills**

Universal Performance Skills	Description
Motor Skills	
Stabilizes	Moves through task environment and interacts with task objects without *momentary* propping or loss of balance
Aligns	Interacts with task objects without evidence of *persistent* propping or *persistent* leaning
Positions	Positions oneself an effective distance from task objects and without evidence of awkward body positions
Reaches	Effectively extends the arm and, when appropriate, bends the trunk to effectively get or place task objects that are out of reach
Bends	Flexes or rotates the trunk as appropriate when sitting down or when bending to grasp or place task objects that are out of one's reach
Grips	Effectively pinches or grasps task objects such that the objects do not slip (e.g., from between one's fingers, from between the teeth, from between one's hand and a supporting surface)
Manipulates	Uses dexterous finger movements, without evidence of fumbling, when manipulating task objects (e.g., manipulating buttons when buttoning)
Coordinates	Uses two or more body parts together to manipulate and hold task objects without evidence of fumbling task objects or task objects slipping from one's grasp
Moves	Effectively pushes or pulls task objects along a supporting surface, pulls to open or pushes to close doors and drawers, or pushes on wheels to propel a wheelchair
Lifts	Effectively raises or lifts task objects without evidence of increased effort
Walks	During the task performance, ambulates on level surfaces without shuffling the feet, becoming unstable, propping, or using assistive devices
Transports	Carries task objects from one place to another while walking or moving in a wheelchair
Calibrates	Uses movements of appropriate force, speed, or extent when interacting with task objects (e.g., not crushing task objects, pushing a door with enough force that it closes but does not bang)
Flows	Uses smooth and fluid arm and wrist movements when interacting with task objects
Endures	Persists and completes the task without *obvious* evidence of physical fatigue, pausing to rest, or stopping to catch one's breath
Paces	Maintains a consistent and effective rate or tempo of performance throughout the entire task performance
Process Skills	
Paces	Maintains a consistent and effective rate or tempo of performance throughout the entire task performance
Attends	Does not look away from what he or she is doing, interrupting the ongoing task progression
Heeds	Carries out and completes the task originally agreed upon or specified by another person
Chooses	Selects necessary and appropriate type and number of task objects for the task, including the task objects that the person was directed to use (e.g., by a teacher) or that were specified by the person
Uses	Applies task objects as they are intended (e.g., using a pencil sharpener to sharpen a pencil, but not to sharpen a crayon) and in a hygienic fashion
Handles	Supports or stabilizes task objects in an appropriate manner, protecting them from damage, slipping, moving, or falling
Inquires	(a) Seeks needed verbal or written information by asking questions or reading directions or labels and (b) does not ask for information in situations where the person had been fully oriented to the task and environment and had immediate prior awareness of the answer
Initiates	Starts or begins the next task action or task step without any hesitation
Continues	Performs single actions or steps without any interruptions, such that once an action or task step is initiated, one continues without pauses or delays until the action or step is completed
Sequences	Performs steps in an effective or logical order and with an absence of (a) randomness or lack of logic in the ordering and/or (b) inappropriate repetition of steps
Terminates	Brings to completion single actions or single steps without inappropriate persistence or premature cessation
Searches/Locates	Looks for and locates task objects in a logical manner
Gathers	Collects related task objects into the same workspace, and regathers task objects that have spilled, fallen, or been misplaced

(continued)

TABLE 52.1 **Universal Performance Skills (*continued*)**

Universal Performance Skills	Description
Organizes	Logically positions or spatially arranges task objects in an orderly fashion within a single workspace, and between multiple appropriate workspaces, such that the workspace is not too spread out or too crowded
Restores	Puts away task objects in appropriate places, and ensures that the immediate workspace is restored to its original condition
Navigates	Moves the arm, body, or wheelchair without bumping into obstacles when moving in the task environment or interacting with task objects
Notices/Responds	Responds appropriately to (a) nonverbal task-related cues (e.g., heat, movement), (b) the spatial arrangement and alignment of task objects to one another, and (c) cupboard doors or drawers that have been left open during the task performance
Adjusts	Effectively (a) goes to new workspaces; (b) moves task objects out of the current workspace; and (c) adjusts knobs, dials, switches, or water taps to overcome problems with ongoing task performance
Accommodates	Prevents ineffective performance of all other motor and process skills, and asks for assistance only when appropriate or needed
Benefits	Prevents ineffective performance of all other motor and process skills from recurring or persisting
Social Interaction Skills	
Approaches/Starts	Approaches or initiates interaction with the social partner in a manner that is socially appropriate
Concludes/ Disengages	Effectively terminates the conversation or social interaction, brings to closure the topic under discussion, and disengages or says goodbye
Produces speech	Produces spoken, signed, or augmentative (i.e., computer generated) messages that are audible and clearly articulated
Gesticulates	Uses socially appropriate gestures to communicate or support a message
Speaks fluently	Speaks in a fluent and continuous manner, with an even pace (not too fast, not too slow), and without pauses or delays during the message being sent
Turns toward	Actively positions or turns the body and the face toward the social partner or the person who is speaking
Looks	Makes eye contact with the social partner
Places self	Positions oneself at an appropriate distance from the social partner during the social interaction
Touches	Responds to and uses touch or bodily contact with the social partner in a manner that is socially appropriate
Regulates	Does not demonstrate irrelevant, repetitive, or impulsive behaviors that are not part of social interaction
Questions	Requests relevant facts and information and asks questions that support the intended purpose of the social interaction
Replies	Keeps conversation going by replying appropriately to suggestions, opinions, questions, and comments
Discloses	Reveals opinions, feelings, and private information about oneself or others in a manner that is socially appropriate
Expresses emotion	Displays affect and emotions in a way that is socially appropriate
Disagrees	Expresses differences of opinion in a socially appropriate manner
Thanks	Uses appropriate words and gestures to acknowledge receipt of services, gifts, or compliments
Transitions	Handles transitions in the conversation or changes the topic without disrupting the ongoing conversation
Times response	Replies to social messages without delay or hesitation and without interrupting the social partner
Times duration	Speaks for reasonable length of time given the complexity of the message sent
Takes turns	Takes one's turn and gives social partners the freedom to take their turn
Matches language	Uses a tone of voice, dialect, and level of language that is socially appropriate and matched to the social partner's abilities and level of understanding
Clarifies	Responds to gestures or verbal messages from the social partner signaling that the social partner does not comprehend or understand a message, and ensures that the social partner is "following" the conversation
Acknowledges/ Encourages	Acknowledges receipt of messages, encourages the social partner to continue interaction, and encourages all social partners to participate in social interaction

| TABLE 52.1 | Universal Performance Skills (*continued*) |

Universal Performance Skills	Description
Empathizes	Expresses a supportive attitude toward the social partner by agreeing with, empathizing with, or expressing understanding of the social partner's feelings and experiences
Heeds	Uses goal-directed social interactions that are focused toward carrying out and completing the intended purpose of the social interaction
Accommodates	Prevents ineffective or socially inappropriate social interaction
Benefits	Prevents problems with ineffective or socially inappropriate social interaction from recurring or persisting

From Fisher, A. G., & Marterella, A. (2019). *Powerful practice: A model for authentic occupational therapy.* Center for Innovative OT Solutions. Reprinted with permission.

directly observed, nor was diminished strength necessarily the reason Maurice did not open the refrigerator door.

When Karla reasoned as to why did Maurice not open the door on his first attempt, she actually considered many possibilities besides diminished upper limb strength, such as "Is the seal on the refrigerator door unusually tight?" "Is he unfamiliar with this particular refrigerator and more familiar with one that opens more easily?" "Had Joyce criticized him for being unsafe when getting things from the refrigerator?" She could not determine the answer based solely on what she had observed. She needed to use her professional reasoning skills to speculate about possible reasons why Maurice did not open the door on his first attempt. Thus, Karla considered all occupational or situational elements in her speculation. Karla knew that while people engage in occupation and perform tasks, people do not produce occupation. Again, occupation arises from the inextricably intertwined whole shown in Figure 52.3 (Fisher & Marterella, 2019).

Universal Versus Task-Specific Performance Skills

Universal Performance Skills

Performance skills can be viewed as being *universal* or more *task specific*. The brief definitions of universal motor, process, and social interaction performance skills included in Table 52.1 are based on the operational definitions of each skill within three standardized tests of performance skill: the Assessment of Motor and Process Skills (AMPS; Fisher & Jones, 2012, 2014), the School Version of the Assessment of Motor and Process Skills (School AMPS; Fisher et al., 2007), and the Evaluation of Social Interaction (ESI; Fisher & Griswold, 2018). They are considered to be universal because they can be observed in virtually any daily life task

performance and, in the case of social interaction skills, virtually any daily life task performance involving social interaction. As we will discuss next, these universal performance skills can be complemented by an endless number of task-specific performance skills.

Using the AMPS as an example, Figure 52.4 helps to clarify the concept of *universal skills*. Because the AMPS is a test of a person's ability to perform personal activities of daily living (PADL) tasks and instrumental activities of daily living (IADL) tasks (collectively, activities of daily living [ADL]), the motor and process performance skills included in the AMPS are referred to as ADL skills. There are more than 120 standardized ADL tasks in the current edition of the AMPS (Fisher & Jones, 2014). No matter which of these ADL tasks a person is observed performing, the occupational therapist can observe the person's degree of performance skill as the person *lifts* tasks objects, *moves* objects, *walks* within the task environment, *chooses* needed tools and materials, *initiates* task actions, and so on. Moreover, when performing ADL tasks, easier performance skills (e.g., *endures, lifts, uses, chooses*) are likely to be easier actions to perform in a skilled manner no matter which ADL task the person performs. Which ADL motor and ADL process skills are harder or easier, and the extent to which the challenge of an ADL task can affect the degree of observed performance skill has been based on a many-facet Rasch analysis of more than 148,000 people who were included in the international standardization sample of the AMPS (Fisher & Jones, 2012). These same principles also apply to the school motor and school process skills included in the School AMPS and the social interaction skills included in the ESI.

Task-Specific Performance Skills

Although the occupational therapist can use the existing taxonomies of universal motor, process, and social interaction skills listed in Table 52.1 in either a standardized or a nonstandardized manner, the occupational therapist is never restricted to these taxonomies. Rather, the occupational therapist may observe and evaluate the quality of any

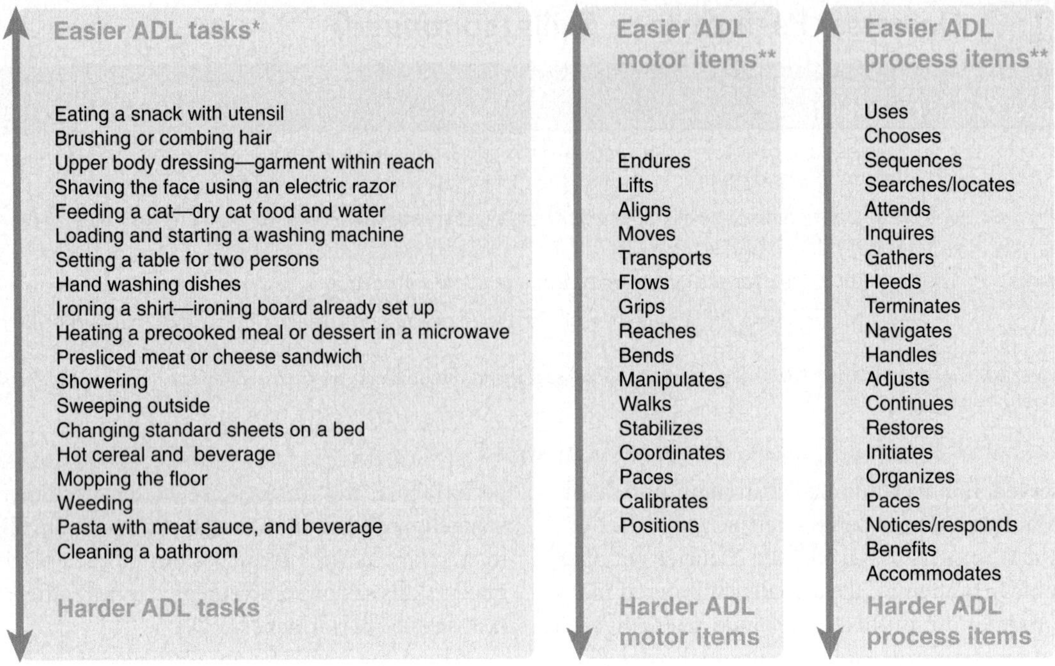

Easier ADL tasks*	Easier ADL motor items**	Easier ADL process items**
Eating a snack with utensil		Uses
Brushing or combing hair		Chooses
Upper body dressing—garment within reach	Endures	Sequences
Shaving the face using an electric razor	Lifts	Searches/locates
Feeding a cat—dry cat food and water	Aligns	Attends
Loading and starting a washing machine	Moves	Inquires
Setting a table for two persons	Transports	Gathers
Hand washing dishes	Flows	Heeds
Ironing a shirt—ironing board already set up	Grips	Terminates
Heating a precooked meal or dessert in a microwave	Reaches	Navigates
Presliced meat or cheese sandwich	Bends	Handles
Showering	Manipulates	Adjusts
Sweeping outside	Walks	Continues
Changing standard sheets on a bed	Stabilizes	Restores
Hot cereal and beverage	Coordinates	Initiates
Mopping the floor	Paces	Organizes
Weeding	Calibrates	Paces
Pasta with meat sauce, and beverage	Positions	Notices/responds
Cleaning a bathroom		Benefits
		Accommodates
Harder ADL tasks	Harder ADL motor items	Harder ADL process items

*   Each person evaluated using the AMPS chooses to perform, from among over 120 ADL tasks included in the AMPS manual, two ADL tasks that are meaningful, perceived as presenting a challenge, and prioritized for intervention.

** The 16 ADL motor and 20 ADL process items (universal performance skills) that can be observed during any ADL task performance and are scored based on the person's quality of performance of each of the two chosen ADL tasks.

FIGURE 52.4 Selected standardized tasks included in the *Assessment of Motor and Process Skills* (AMPS) and each of the activities of daily living (ADL) motor and ADL process items (task actions, performance skills) that are scored based on the person's quality of performance of each ADL task action (degree of skill as indicated by lack of observable clumsiness or physical effort, inefficiency, safety risk, and/or need for assistance).

motor, process, or social action that is part of the observed occupational performance (i.e., the observable links in the chain of task actions). Moreover, many daily life task performances involve the performance of motor, process, and social actions that are more unique to the particular task performed. For example, when Michaela watches José as he is playing baseball, she observes him *throw* the ball to the first baseman, and she observes the first baseman *catch* the ball. Later, when José is up to bat, she observes him *swing* the bat, *drop* the bat, *run*, and *slide* into first base. Finally, she observes José's mother *smile* and the audience *cheer*.

A Rationale for Implementing Performance Analyses

There are several interrelated advantages of implementing a **performance analysis**, either standardized or nonstandardized. The first is that by implementing performance analyses, we, as occupational therapists, focus our evaluations on the quality of occupational performance, not body functions or other aspects of the situational context that may be reasons for a person's ineffective occupational performance (see Figure 52.3). The second advantage is that we make explicit which performance skills the person performed effectively and which were performed ineffectively (i.e., errors of occupational performance). The result is that we become better able to describe to others (i.e., the client, team members, and third-party payers) using "everyday language," the person's observed problems of occupational performance. The final two advantages may be the ones that are most important. That is, if we use "everyday language" in describing the quality of occupational performance, the result will be that we more readily (a) work collaboratively with our clients to establish occupation-focused goals, and plan and implement occupation-based interventions and (b) use "occupation-first" language in our documentation and in our communication with others. The advantage is that people will better understand that occupation is the primary focus of our profession.

Advantages and Disadvantages of Standardized and Nonstandardized Performance Analyses

Although standardized performance analyses such as the AMPS, School AMPS, and ESI have several advantages, they also have a number of disadvantages. One major advantage is that the use of standardized performance analyses allows the trained occupational therapist to generate an objective linearized measure (Bond & Fox, 2015) of the person's quality of occupational performance that can be used to document outcomes and implement evidence-based practice. The second advantage is that evaluation practices become more consistent, which promotes the ability to compare results across world regions, occupational therapists, clients, and settings (e.g., hospital vs. community). Another important advantage is that the person's linear performance measure can be compared to established criterion measures and normative values that enable the interpretation of the person's results from a criterion-referenced and a norm-referenced perspective. The final advantage is that formal training in standardized performance analysis methods facilitates the occupational therapist's ability to perform nonstandardized performance analyses and avoid common misperceptions that performance skills can be likened to body functions.

An important disadvantage of existing standardized performance analyses is that formal training and rater calibration often are required. Another disadvantage is that standardized assessments sometimes lack the flexibility needed to observe virtually any daily life task performance. For example, the AMPS is a test of ADL, and the School AMPS is a test of schoolwork task performance (e.g., cutting, writing, drawing, computing). Neither can be used to assess the quality of task performance in the areas of work or play.

Obviously, the major advantage of nonstandardized performance analyses is their flexibility. That is, the occupational therapist can implement an informal evaluation of performance skills based on the observation of performance of any daily life task. The only requirements are that the occupational therapist and the people observed must have a clear idea of what each person plans to do, or, if directed by another, what each person has been directed to do. For example, if the occupational therapist plans to observe a child in a classroom setting, the occupational therapist must know what the teacher has asked the students to do and what objects they are expected to use to complete the task. Then, after observing the person's performance, the occupational therapist must systematically rate each universal or

task-specific motor skill, process skill, and (when relevant) social interaction skill observed. For example, the occupational therapist can subjectively judge whether the observed actions were skilled, and if not, if the actions (i.e., performance skills) were mildly, moderately, or markedly ineffective. The occupational therapist can also note the frequency or duration of any observed occupational performance errors. More detailed directions for implementing nonstandardized performance analyses, including more detailed rating criteria, are provided by Fisher and Marterella (2019).

Differentiating Performance Analyses from Task, Activity, and Occupational Analyses

Performance analysis should not be confused with **task analysis** or **activity analysis**, which are intended for the purposes of identifying (a) the contextual factors (e.g., body functions, environmental factors) that might be the underlying reasons for the person's observed problems with occupational performance or (b) how to best adapt, grade, or modify various situational elements to design an effective intervention (Hagedorn, 1995; Llorens, 1993; Mosey, 1981, 1986; Piersol, 2014; Watson, 1997). See Table 52.2 for a comparison of performance analysis, task analysis, and activity analysis. An example of a standardized *task analysis* is the Neurobehavioral (NB) scale of the ADL-focused Occupation-based Neurobehavioral Evaluation (A-ONE; Árnadóttir, 1990, 2016; Árnadóttir et al., 2009). The NB scale of the A-ONE was designed to be used to evaluate the underlying neurobehavioral impairments that are speculated to cause diminished ADL task performance based on direct observation within the natural context of those ADL task performances. More specifically, scoring of the A-ONE requires that the trained occupational therapist use the operational definitions of the NB items, combined with his or her professional reasoning skills and knowledge of neurology and neuropsychology, to formulate hypotheses related to interpreting the observed errors of ADL task performance. The goal is to identify what underlying neurobehavioral impairments are speculated to be the cause of the person's diminished occupational performance (Árnadóttir, 2016; Árnadóttir et al., 2009, 2010).

Standardized task analyses such as the NB scale of the A-ONE; Kitchen Task Assessment (KTA, Baum & Edwards, 1993); Children's Kitchen Task Assessment (CKTA; Rocke et al., 2008); Executive Function Performance Test (EFPT; Baum & Wolf, 2013); the Perceive, Recall, Plan, and Perform (PRPP) System of Task Analysis (Aubin et al., 2009;

| TABLE 52.2 | Comparison among Different Types of Occupational Analyses: Performance Analyses, Task Analyses, and Activity Analyses |

Occupational Analyses		
Performance Analysis—Analysis of What We Observe	**Task Analysis** ("Explanatory Analysis")—Analysis of Why We Observed What We Have Observed	**Activity Analysis** ("Solution Analysis")—Analysis of How Could We Minimize the Person's Problem
• **Occupation-focused**: Focus is on quality of occupational performance skills	• **Not occupation-focused**: Focus is on how body functions and other contextual factors impact occupational performance	• **Not occupation-focused**: Focus is on how to make changes to various situational elements to design therapeutic occupation
• **Occupation-based**: The occupational therapist must always observe the person performing a task	• **Occupation-based**: The occupational therapist must always observe the person performing a task	• **Not occupation-based**: The occupational therapist does *not* observe the person performing a task; sometimes done as a decontextualized "academic exercise"
• The occupational therapist asks, "During the observation, what do *I know*, what did I actually see?"	• The occupational therapist asks, "Now that I have observed, what do *I hypothesize* might be the reasons I saw what I did?"	• The occupational therapist asks, "What do *I think* might be some good possibilities for intervention?"

Adapted from Fisher, A. G. (2009). *Occupational Therapy Intervention Process Model: A model for planning and implementing top–down, client-centered, and occupation-based interventions.* Three Star Press. Reprinted with permission.

Nott et al., 2009); and the visual motor, fine motor, and gross motor scales of the Miller Function and Participation Scales (M-FUN; Miller, 2006) were all designed to fulfill an important need within OT for more ecologically relevant assessments of underlying body functions (e.g., cognition, including executive functions and information processing; gross and fine motor coordination; motor planning; visual motor skills) based on professional reasoning to speculate about the reasons for observed occupational performance errors. They also fulfill, however, an important need that is very different from the one that is filled by standardized or nonstandardized performance analyses. Performance analyses are used at the stages of the OT intervention process where the occupational therapist (a) observes a person's quality of occupational performance as they perform prioritized daily life tasks and then (b) rates their observed quality of occupational performance (i.e., performance skills performed effectively or ineffectively). In contrast, task analyses are used to help the occupational therapist proceed to the point of finalizing the results of an evaluation and speculating about the reasons for the person's occupational challenges (Figure 52.5).

Performance analyses also should not be confused with the terms activity analysis or **occupational analysis** as described in Chapter 43. As noted in Table 52.2, activity analyses are decontextualized "academic exercises." In contrast, an occupational analysis includes steps in the OT intervention process that precede as well as follow the actual performance analysis, including task analyses (e.g., evaluation of body functions and structures, the evaluation of the physical and social environments) and activity analyses. Thus, a performance analysis can be viewed as one part of a more global occupational analysis.

Implementing Performance Analyses: Evaluations of Occupational Performance Skill

With this background information related to performance skills and performance analysis, we will turn to discussing in more detail how an occupational therapist implements a performance analysis. Our focus, and the case example, will be on implementing nonstandardized performance analyses.

When an occupational therapist implements a performance analysis, the evaluation always occurs within the context of observing one or more people as they are engaged in the performance of a prioritized task. That is, each task performance observed should be one that each person has identified as a concern and prioritized as a potential target for intervention. Which tasks to observe are typically determined based on a thorough OT interview where the occupational therapist gathers information needed to understand the complex relationship between the person's occupations and the situational contexts of those occupations (see Figure 52.5).

Once the person and the occupational therapist have collaboratively determined which occupational performances to prioritize, the occupational therapist introduces the idea of observing the person perform prioritized tasks and initiates one or more performance analyses. Each

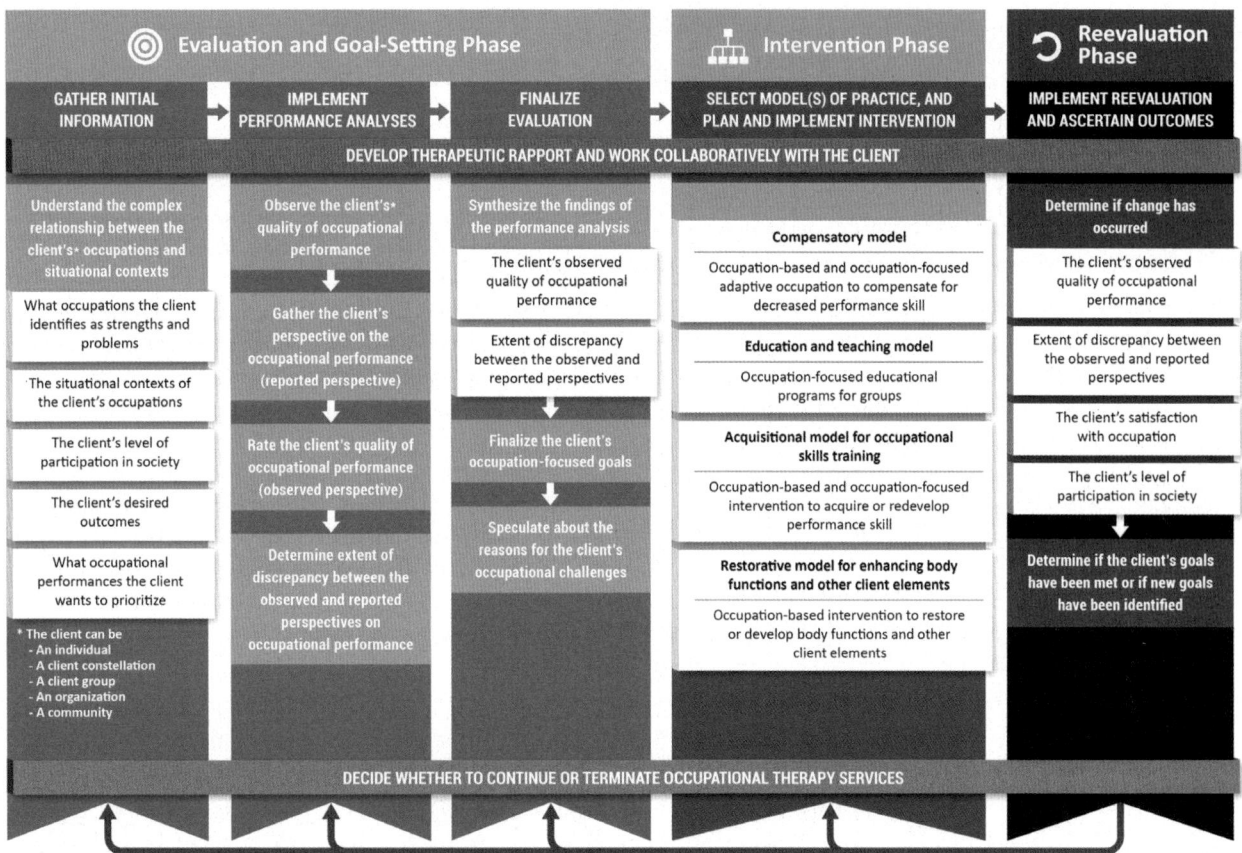

FIGURE 52.5 **Graphic representation of the phases of the true top-down and occupation-centered reasoning process defined in the *Occupational Therapy Intervention Process Model*.**

(From Fisher, A. G., & Marterella, A. [2019]. *Powerful practice: A model for authentic occupational therapy.* Center for Innovative OT Solutions. Reprinted with permission.)

performance analysis progresses over three steps shown in Figure 52.5:

- **Step 1:** Observe people's quality of occupational performance as they perform chosen and prioritized daily life tasks in their usual manner and take observational notes of observed occupational performance errors.
- **Step 2:** Rate each person's quality of occupational performance. Either the universal performance motor, process, and social interaction skills shown in Table 52.1 or more task-specific motor, process, and social interaction skills can be evaluated. Each performance skill is rated in terms of ease (physical effort and/or clumsiness), efficiency (time and space organization), safety (risk of harm to person or damage to task objects), independence, or, in the case of social interaction skills, social appropriateness. The occupational therapist can use (a) standardized scoring criteria outlined in the respective test manual or (b) a nonstandardized qualitative scale (e.g., no problem, mild problem, moderate problem, or severe problem) to rate the observed quality of each performance skill. More detailed nonstandardized rating criteria are provided by Fisher and Marterella (2019).

- **Step 3:** Synthesize the findings of the performance analysis by
  - Making a list of all the ineffective performance skills observed and select up to 10 motor and process skills and/or 10 social interaction skills that best capture the person's diminished quality of occupational performance. In a similar manner, the motor, process, and/or social interaction skills that best capture the person's strengths of occupational performance also should be identified.
  - Creating clusters of interrelated performance skills and write summary statements that can be used to document the person's quality of occupational performance.

Figure 52.5 also includes steps beyond the scope of this chapter where the occupational therapist gathers people's perspectives on their occupational performances. This information may include gathering information about their occupational experiences during the observed occupational performances (e.g., their levels of satisfaction), or their perspectives on their quality of occupational performance (e.g., how effortful or safe their task performances were; Fisher & Marterella, 2019).

EXPANDING OUR PERSPECTIVES

Implementing Performance
Analyses to Promote Authentic
Occupational Therapy in a Rural
Argentinian Community

Fernanda M. Suppicich

I have been an occupational therapist for 11 years. I grew up in a rural town 110 km from the City of Buenos Aires where I studied occupational therapy. My first job was at an outpatient clinic in the city. Occupational therapy at this clinic was well known for their focus on everyday functioning of clients with neurological conditions. My supervisor encouraged me to implement performance analyses as part of my occupation-based and occupation-focused services.

Later, I moved back to my hometown. Together with a colleague, we began working at a residence for older adults. Suddenly, I experienced challenges I had not experienced in the city. Although my colleague and I were well received by the doctors and nurses, they also became our first and primary barrier. They viewed occupational therapists as the people who were there to "entertain" the residents by "keeping them busy."

My colleague and I quickly realized that we needed to work together, not only to support each other but also to be able to respond to the needs of the 63 residents. Rather than just keep them busy, we chose to implement authentic occupational therapy. It took us 2 months to assess all 63 residents. To gather the information needed to understand each resident and their occupational concerns, we first reviewed their medical records and interviewed each resident and/or their assistants. We then implemented informal performance analyses, observing each resident perform two tasks that were relevant and significant to them (e.g., eating, playing cards, drinking mate, weaving).

Yes, it was 2 months of intensive occupation- and client-centered evaluations! But in the end, our performance analyses of each resident enabled us to better understand the occupational strengths and problems of each resident. Thus, we were able to present a report to the head of the institution. In our report, we recommended a variety of individual and group activities not only appropriate to the facility but also centered on the residents' occupational interests, goals, and levels of occupational performance: gardening, cooking, card playing, library/reading, handicrafts, among others.

To this day, we continue to focus on the residents' engagement in occupation, no matter their ages, conditions, or limitations. We are clear that our role is to enable them to remain engaged in occupation and promote their sense of well-being and participation. This means that we regularly use performance analyses to identify how to best "keep their performance skills going." Our evaluations, which include performance analyses, rarely take more than 45 minutes and we have found the performance analyses to be critical to implementing client-centered services focused on occupation.

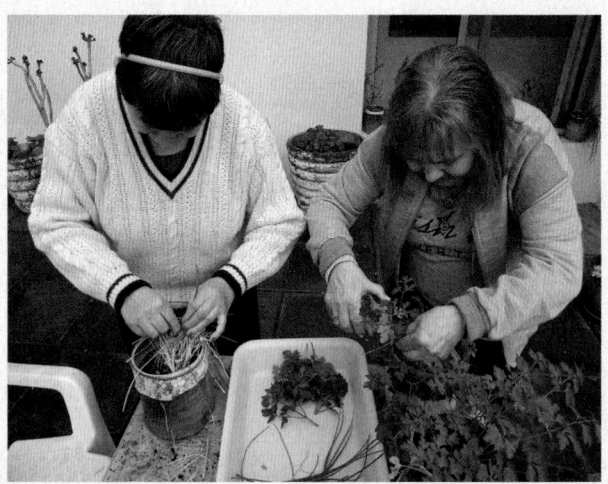

During their chosen gardening group activity, two residents *position* themselves an effective distance from task objects, *reach* for and use two hands (*coordinate*) as they *pinch*, *grip*, *manipulate*, and *cut* chives and parsley.

OT STORY 52.2 IMPLEMENTING NONSTANDARDIZED PERFORMANCE ANALYSES

Background: Referral and Occupational Therapy Interview

Maurice is 78 years of age and lives in his own home. Until recently, Maurice was considered a healthy aging adult, but over the past 6 months, he has fallen on several occasions and was hospitalized for observation and treatment of severe lacerations on the back of his head. These falls and hospitalizations have taken their toll; Maurice has become increasingly frail. His doctor has spoken to Maurice and his family, and he has recommended that they consider some form of alternative housing for Maurice, somewhere where he would have 24-hour supervision.

Maurice, however, is determined to continue living at home. He already pays for a woman, Joyce, to come in each day and help him with his daily chores. Because his family wants to support Maurice's wishes, they have requested an OT evaluation to ensure Maurice's safety, particularly during the time that Joyce is not with him. When they contacted Karla, the occupational therapist, they mentioned not only Maurice's recent falls but also that he often seems to be "a bit confused." They feel that his confusion, combined with moderate hearing loss, has led to increasing challenges when they are trying to communicate with him. They expressed concern that Maurice and Joyce may also be having similar problems when discussing his desires and needs.

With this background information gathered during the referral process, Karla contacted Maurice and made arrangements for a visit. Karla began her OT interview by introducing herself and telling Maurice that she was an occupational therapist and that her role was to help him do the things that he wanted to do, such as dressing, doing activities around the house, going out in the community, and engaging in leisure activities. She then transitioned to asking Maurice to tell her about what he currently does during a typical day, what he would like to do, and what are his concerns and priorities.

During this OT interview, Karla also gathered information needed to understand the situational contexts of his occupations, his level of participation in society, and his desired outcomes. She learned that Maurice is satisfied overall with his current living situation. He has a supportive family with whom he has daily telephone contact and biweekly visits. He explained that Joyce comes in 4 to 5 hours a day, 6 days a week to prepare his lunch and dinner, clean, take him on errands, and spend time with him. Maurice has daily routines that include getting dressed, preparing his breakfast, and reading the newspaper, all of which he performs before Joyce comes for the day. He also showers twice each week before Joyce arrives. During the day, he watches television, uses his computer, talks to family on the phone, and reads. He likes to go to town two or three times a week to go to the bank, post office, and grocery store. Joyce drives him to town and accompanies him, but Maurice takes care of his own errands. He has had his bathroom adapted to include grab bars, a raised toilet seat, and a shower bench, which, according to Maurice, enable him to remain independent in personal activities of daily living (PADL).

As the interview progressed, Karla guided the discussion to learn about tasks that Maurice currently does that are challenging for him and to hear about other tasks that Maurice does not currently do but might want to do. Her aim was to find out from Maurice what occupational performances he wanted to prioritize for further evaluation and possible intervention. Maurice stated that he is satisfied with most of the tasks he is doing and does not have others

that he wants to do at this time. He said that he is having difficulty putting on his shoes and socks. He also said that preparing his breakfast (orange juice and cold cereal) has gradually become more difficult and that he wants to be able to keep doing that for himself each morning. When she focused on other aspects of dressing and showering, tasks Karla reasoned also were likely to be challenging, Maurice denied any problems.

Desiring to maintain a client-centered focus and to ensure that Maurice is safe in doing the two tasks that he identified as more challenging and important to him, Karla and Maurice decided that she would observe him perform these. She told Maurice that after she observed his performance, she would be able to make suggestions to help him do these tasks more easily. As Maurice had also acknowledged that he does not always "follow conversations" when he is interacting with others, he also agreed that Karla could observe him when he and Joyce would be deciding on meals for the week and writing a shopping list for the grocery store.

Implementing a Performance Analysis: Step 1—Observe the Person Perform Chosen Daily Life Tasks

When Karla observed Maurice perform the two activities of daily living (ADL) tasks and the social interaction with Joyce, she ensured that he performed each task in his usual manner and she remained an unobtrusive observer. During each of his task performances, she took notes of any occupational performance errors that reflected diminished quality of Maurice's occupational performance.

Implementing a Performance Analysis: Step 2—Rating the Person's Quality of Performance

After Karla had observed Maurice perform the two ADL tasks and engage in social interaction with Joyce, she proceeded to rate Maurice's quality of performance in relation to each of the motor, process, and social interaction skills shown in Table 52.1. When she did her rating, she used a four-category qualitative scale: no problem, mild problem, moderate problem, and marked problem.

Synthesizing the Findings of the Performance Analysis: Step 3a—Defining the Actions of Performance That Were Effective Versus Ineffective

After rating both of the observed ADL tasks and the social exchange, Karla transitioned to making a list of all of the motor and process skills and all of the social interaction skills that she had observed to be ineffective. When she did this, she first listed each performance skill and then she made note of what behavior she had observed that led to her rating. Finally, Karla put a check mark (✓) on those performance

(continued)

OT STORY 52.2 IMPLEMENTING NONSTANDARDIZED PERFORMANCE ANALYSES (*continued*)

skills that she reasoned best captured Maurice's diminished quality of occupational performance (Tables 52.3 and 52.4 show Karla's lists for *Putting on socks and shoes* and *Planning the weekly meals and making a shopping list*). As she also wanted to capture Maurice's relative strengths, she made similar lists of the motor, process, and social interaction skills that most supported his occupational performance.

Synthesizing the Findings of the Performance Analysis: Step 3b—Identifying Clusters of Interrelated Skills and Writing Summary Statements for Use in Documentation

Karla's next step was to create clusters of performance skills that she judged to be interrelated. Once she created each cluster, she wrote a summary statement that she used to document Maurice's baseline level of occupational performance. For example, she created three clusters of motor and process skills related to the task of *Putting on shoes and socks* and four clusters related to social interaction skills. Those clusters and her summary statements were as follows:

Putting on Socks and Shoes

- **Stabilizes, Reaches, Bends, Lifts:** *Marked fall risk when standing and bending to reach down and lift his shoes up from the floor.*
- **Reaches, Bends, Moves, Endures:** *Moderate increase in effort and audible shortness of breath when reaching forward to pull his leg up over his opposite knee and when pulling up his socks.*
- **Accommodates, Benefits:** *Did not anticipate and prevent problems from occurring; his problems persisted throughout the task performance.*

Planning Weekly Meals and Making a Shopping List Together With Care Provider

- **Looks, Regulates:** *Frequently looked down and away from social partner; occasionally "fidgeted" with task objects (e.g., pencil and notepad).*
- **Speaks Fluently, Times Duration:** *Frequently paused "mid-message." On two occasions, these pauses were*

TABLE 52.3	Maurice's Motor and Process Skills That Most Reflected His Diminished Quality of Activity of Daily Living Task Performance— Putting on His Socks and Shoes

ADL Motor Skills	Behavior Observed	Rating
✓ Stabilizes	• Risk of a fall—standing and bending down to get shoes	• Marked
✓ Reaches	• Increased effort and risk for fall—reaching down to get shoes • Increased effort and audible shortness of breath—reaching forward to pull leg up over opposite knee	• Marked • Moderate
✓ Bends	• Increased effort and risk of a fall—bending down to get shoes • Increased effort and audible shortness of breath—bending forward to pull leg up over opposite knee	• Marked • Moderate
Grips	• Grip slips from socks when pulling them up	• Mild
Manipulates	• Fumbles shoelaces	• Mild
✓ Moves	• Increased effort and audible shortness of breath—pulling leg up over opposite knee and pulling up socks	• Moderate
✓ Lifts	• Increased effort and risk of a fall—lifting shoes from the floor	• Marked
Walks	• Walks using a walker	• Mild
✓ Endures	• Audible shortness of breath	• Moderate
ADL Process Skills	Behavior Observed	Rating
Initiates	• Occasional short pauses before initiating task steps	• Mild
Continues	• Starts to pull up sock, pauses, returns to pulling up sock	• Mild
✓ Accommodates	• Demonstrates risk of a fall (*reaches, bends, lifts*); he did not prevent his problems	• Marked
✓ Benefits	• Audible shortness of breath persisted (*reaches, bends, moves, endures*)	• Moderate

ADL, activity of daily living.

OT STORY 52.2 IMPLEMENTING NONSTANDARDIZED PERFORMANCE ANALYSES (*continued*)

TABLE 52.4	**Maurice's Social Interaction Skills That Most Reflected His Ineffective Quality of Social Interaction—Planning Weekly Meals and Making a Shopping List Together with Joyce**

Social Interaction Skills	Behavior Observed	Rating
✓ *Concludes/Disengages*	• J starts to bring discussion to a close, but M continues to talk about what he will eat	• Mild
Speaks fluently	• Speaks in a hesitant manner, with short pauses and stammering, "I think w-we . . . should . . . buy some apples" • On two occasions, M pauses 3–4 seconds in the middle of a message	• Mild • Moderate
✓ *Looks*	• Frequently looks down and away from J	• Mild
✓ *Regulates*	• Occasionally fidgets with pencil and notepad used for shopping list	• Mild
✓ *Replies*	• Replies with markedly irrelevant responses (e.g., when asked what he wants to eat, he replies, "My son called")	• Marked
✓ *Transitions*	• Transitions to a markedly irrelevant topic (e.g., abruptly changes topic to getting a phone call from his son)	• Marked
✓ *Times response*	• M interrupts J as she is speaking; occasionally delays before replying to J's questions	• Moderate
✓ *Times duration*	• Starts messages, but leaves two messages "hanging in the air"	• Moderate
✓ *Clarifies*	• J asks M to clarify what he meant, "Let's buy some scrapple"; he does not clarify; his reply is markedly irrelevant, "I need to make a doctor's appointment"	• Marked
✓ *Heeds*	• When engaged in a social interaction with an intended purpose of making a shopping list, M begins to discuss his son and a doctor's appointment	• Moderate
✓ *Accommodates*	• Demonstrated markedly inappropriate Replies, Transitions, and Clarifies skill; he did not prevent his problems	• Marked
✓ *Benefits*	• Several of M's moderately inappropriate social interaction skill deficits persisted	• Moderate

J, Joyce; M, Maurice.

3 to 4 seconds in length, and on two additional occasions, he began but never finished sending his messages.
- **Replies, Transitions, Clarifies, Heeds:** On two occasions, his replies were markedly irrelevant to the intended purpose of the social exchange.
- **Accommodates, Benefits:** Did not modify his social interactions to prevent problems from occurring; his problems often reoccurred during the ongoing social exchange.

When Karla actually documented Maurice's baseline level of occupational performance, she wanted to place her summary statements in the context of her overall observation. Therefore, she began with an introductory phrase to clarify what it was that Maurice had done (e.g., put on his socks and shoes) and incorporated into that a global baseline statement that would document his overall quality of ADL task performance. Then, she added her summary statements to document his specific baseline. For example, her final documentation for *Putting on socks and shoes* was as follows:

While Maurice was independent when putting on his shoes and socks, he demonstrated marked safety risk and moderate increase in physical effort. More specifically, Maurice demonstrated marked fall risk when

standing and bending to reach down and lift his shoes up from the floor. He also demonstrated moderate increase in effort and audible shortness of breath when reaching forward to pull his leg up over his opposite knee and when pulling up his socks. Maurice did not anticipate and prevent problems from occurring, and his problems persisted throughout the task performance.

Progressing From Synthesizing the Findings of the Performance Analysis to Finalizing the Client's Occupation-Focused Goals

When Karla documented his baseline level of occupational performance, she also discussed with Maurice her observations and engaged him in a discussion of how he felt about his performance and what might be his desired outcomes of OT services. For example, she pointed out to Maurice that even though he was holding onto his rollator, he almost fell when he bent down and picked up his shoes from the floor. Maurice acknowledged that falling has been a major issue and is one of the reasons his doctor does not want him living at home anymore. Maurice indicated that he wanted to be able to perform tasks without fall risk.

(continued)

OT STORY 52.2 IMPLEMENTING NONSTANDARDIZED PERFORMANCE ANALYSES (*continued*)

Karla, therefore, discussed with him his baseline statement related to putting on socks and shoes—*marked fall risk when standing and bending to reach down and lift his shoes up from the floor*—and engaged Maurice in determining what was his desired goal. As Maurice specified that he did not want to have a fall risk, Karla and Maurice decided that his goal would be *no fall risk when putting on socks and shoes.* Karla did not refer to Maurice's standing, bending down, or lifting his shoes because she wanted to leave open the option for introducing compensatory strategies that would enable Maurice to avoid fall risk. Karla engaged Maurice in similar collaborative discussions related to his obviously increased physical effort and shortness of breath when putting on his socks and shoes as well as the challenges he faced with preparing his breakfast and engaging in social interaction with his care provider. After implementing the intervention, Karla planned to reevaluate Maurice's occupational performance quality by carrying out another performance analysis. This would enable her to ascertain the outcomes of intervention and determine if Maurice's goals have been met (see Figure 52.5).

Questions

1. Given that Maurice likely has problems with balance, would you have been inclined to use a different assessment approach than was described in this chapter?
2. How might Maurice's goals have changed had Karla focused on evaluating body functions rather than analyzing performance skills observed during desired task performances?
3. What was the benefit of Karla's separately describing the quality of each of Maurice's task performances, based on her analysis of his observed level of performance skill, when she wrote her documentation?
4. How does conducting a performance analysis support a collaborative process between the occupational therapist and client?
5. Three visits from OT are not many. Karla decided to use one visit for evaluation, leaving her with only two more visits. Discuss the benefit of spending time doing a performance analysis for Maurice.
6. How does conducting a performance analysis contribute to the role of OT in an interprofessional team?

Once the occupational therapist has completed the performance analysis and determined which performance skills most reflect and best describe the person's quality of occupational performance, the occupational therapist has progressed to the phase in the OT intervention process where the occupational therapist and the person work collaboratively to finalize and document the person's occupation-focused goals (see Figure 52.5). The summary statements developed in step 3 of the performance analysis represent the person's baseline level of occupational performance. They provide the foundation for collaboratively developing observable and measurable client-centered and occupation-focused goals.

Finally, the occupational therapist speculates about the reasons for the person's occupational challenges, including diminished quality of occupational performance (see Figure 52.5). The various factors that may be contributing to and influencing the quality of the person's occupational performance include all of the occupational and situational elements shown in Figure 52.3. Fisher and Marterella (2019) recommend using the Transactional Model of Occupation to reason about possible factors supporting or hindering the person's quality of occupational performance. The process of implementing a performance analysis is preceded by gathering thorough information needed to understand the complex relationship between the person's occupations and the situational contexts of those occupations; and, followed by finalizing the person's occupation-focused goals, as illustrated in OT Story 52.2.

Lippincott® Connect *For additional resources on the subjects discussed in this chapter, visit Lippincott Connect.*

REFERENCES

Aldrich, R. M. (2008). From complexity theory to transactionalism: Moving occupational science forward in theorizing the complexities of behavior. *Journal of Occupational Science, 15,* 147–156. https://doi.org/10.1080/14427591.2008.9686624

American Occupational Therapy Association. (2008). Occupational therapy practice framework: Domain and process, 2nd edition. *American Journal of Occupational Therapy, 62,* 625–683. https://doi.org/10.5014/ajot.62.6.625

American Occupational Therapy Association. (2020). Occupational therapy practice framework: Domain and process, fourth edition. *American Journal of Occupational Therapy, 74*(Suppl. 2), 7412410010. https://doi.org/10.5014/ajot.2020.74S2001

Árnadóttir, G. (1990). *The brain and behavior: Assessing cortical dysfunction through activities of daily living.* Mosby.

Árnadóttir, G. (2016). Impact of neurobehavioral deficits on activities of daily living. In G. Gillen (Ed.), *Stroke rehabilitation: A function-based approach* (4th ed., pp. 573–609). Mosby.

Árnadóttir, G., Fisher, A. G., & Löfgren, B. (2009). Dimensionality of nonmotor neurobehavioral impairments when observed in the natural contexts of ADL task performance. *Neurorehabilitation & Neural Repair, 23,* 579–586. https://doi.org/10.1177/1545968308324223

Árnadóttir, G., Löfgren, B., & Fisher, A. G. (2010). Difference in impact of neurobehavioural dysfunction on activities of daily living performance between right and left hemispheric stroke. *Journal of Rehabilitation Medicine, 42*, 903–907. https://doi.org/10.2340/16501977-0621

Aubin, G., Chapparo, C., Gélinas, I., Stip, E., & Rainville, C. (2009). Use of the Perceive, Recall, Plan, and Perform System of Task Analysis for persons with schizophrenia: A preliminary study. *Australian Occupational Therapy Journal, 56*, 189–199. https://doi.org/10.1111/j.1440-1630.2007.00725.x

Bartels, M. N., Duffy, C. A., & Beland, H. E. (2016). Pathophysiology, medical management, and acute rehabilitation of stroke survivors. In G. Gillen (Ed.), *Stroke rehabilitation: A function-based approach* (4th ed., pp. 2–45). Mosby.

Baum, C. M., & Edwards, D. F. (1993). Cognitive performance in senile dementia of the Alzheimer's type: The Kitchen Task Assessment. *American Journal of Occupational Therapy, 47*, 431–436. https://doi.org/10.5014/ajot.47.5.431

Baum, C. M., & Wolf, T. J. (2013). *Executive Function Performance Test (EFPT) manual.* Program in Occupational Therapy. Washington University School of Medicine. http://www.ot.wustl.edu/about/resources/executive-function-performance-test-efpt-308

Bond, T. G., & Fox, C. M. (2015). *Applying the Rasch model: Fundamental measurement in the human sciences* (3rd ed.). Routledge.

Dickie, V., Cutchin, M. P., & Humphry, R. (2006). Occupation as transactional experience: A critique of individualism in occupational science. *Journal of Occupational Science, 13*, 83–93. https://doi.org/10.1080/14427591.2006.9686573

Fisher, A. G. (1998). Uniting practice and theory in an occupational framework: 1998 Eleanor Clarke Slagle lecture. *American Journal of Occupational Therapy, 52*, 509–521. https://doi.org/10.5014/ajot.52.7.509

Fisher, A. G. (2006). Overview of performance skills and client factors. In H. M. Pendleton & W. Schultz-Krohn (Eds.), *Pedretti's occupational therapy: Practice skills for physical dysfunction* (6th ed., pp. 372–402). Mosby.

Fisher, A. G. (2009). *Occupational Therapy Intervention Process Model: A model for planning and implementing top–down, client-centered, and occupation-based interventions.* Three Star Press.

Fisher, A. G., Bryze, K., Hume, V., & Griswold, L. A. (2007). *School AMPS: School Version of the Assessment of Motor and Process Skills* (2nd ed.). Three Star Press.

Fisher, A. G., & Griswold, L. A. (2018). *Evaluation of Social Interaction* (4th ed.). Three Star Press.

Fisher, A. G., & Jones, K. B. (2012). *Assessment of Motor and Process Skills: Development, standardization, and administration manual* (7th ed., Rev. ed.). Three Star Press.

Fisher, A. G., & Jones, K. B. (2014). *Assessment of Motor and Process Skills: User manual* (8th ed.). Three Star Press.

Fisher, A. G., & Kielhofner, G. (1995). Skill in occupational performance. In G. Kielhofner (Ed.), *A model of human occupation: Theory and application* (2nd ed., pp. 113–137). Williams & Wilkins.

Fisher, A. G., & Marterella, A. (2019). *Powerful practice: A model for authentic occupational therapy.* Center for Innovative OT Solutions.

Hagedorn, R. (1995). *Occupational therapy: Perspectives and processes.* Churchill Livingstone.

Hagedorn, R. (2000). *Tools for practice in occupational therapy: A structured approach to core skills and processes.* Churchill Livingstone.

Kielhofner, G. (1995). *A model of human occupation: Theory and application* (2nd ed.). Williams & Wilkins.

Kielhofner, G. (2008). *Model of Human Occupation: Theory and application* (4th ed.). Lippincott Williams & Wilkins.

Llorens, L. A. (1993). Activity analysis: Agreement between participants and observers on perceived factors in occupation components. *Occupational Therapy Journal of Research, 13*, 198–211. https://doi.org/10.1177/153944929301300304

Miller, L. J. (2006). *Miller Function and Participation Scales.* PsychCorp.

Mosey, A. C. (1981). *Occupational therapy: Configuration of a profession.* Raven Press.

Mosey, A. C. (1986). *Psychosocial components of occupational therapy.* Raven Press.

Nott, M. T., Chapparo, C., & Heard, R. (2009). Reliability of the Perceive, Recall, Plan and Perform System of Task Analysis: A criterion-referenced assessment. *Australian Occupational Therapy Journal, 56*, 307–314. https://doi.org/10.1111/j.1440-1630.2008.00763.x

Piersol, C. V. (2014). Occupation as therapy: Selection, gradation, analysis, and adaptation. In M. V. Radomski & C. A. Trombly Latham (Eds.), *Occupational therapy for physical dysfunction* (7th ed., pp. 360–393). Lippincott Williams & Wilkins.

Polatajko, H. J., Mandich, A., & Martini, R. (2000). Dynamic performance analysis: A framework for understanding occupational performance. *American Journal of Occupational Therapy, 54*, 65–72. https://doi.org/10.5014/ajot.54.1.65

Rexroth, P., Fisher, A. G., Merritt, B. K., & Gliner, J. (2005). Ability differences in persons with unilateral hemispheric stroke. *Canadian Journal of Occupational Therapy, 72*, 212–221. https://doi.org/10.1177/000841740507200403

Rocke, K., Hays, P., Edwards, D., & Berg, C. (2008). Development of a performance assessment of executive function: The Children's Kitchen Task Assessment. *American Journal of Occupational Therapy, 62*, 528–537. https://doi.org/10.5014/ajot.62.5.528

Taylor, R. R. (2017). *Kielhofner's Model of Human Occupation: Theory and application* (5th ed.). Wolters Kluwer.

Watson, D. E. (1997). *Task analysis: An occupational performance approach.* American Occupational Therapy Association.

World Health Organization. (2001). *International classification of functioning, disability and health (ICF).* Author.

Individual Variance

Body Structures and Functions

Glen Gillen and Barbara A. Boyt Schell

LEARNING OBJECTIVES

After reading this chapter, you will be able to:

1. Consider how personal characteristics and factors are related to occupations and occupational performance.
2. Discuss how knowledge of personal factors is used in occupational therapy (OT) evaluation and intervention.
3. Identify examples of body functions and structures that are considered in OT process.

Introduction

Throughout this text, there is recognition that occupation is a function of the individual performing within a specific context. How that occupational performance occurs, then, is a reflection of all the unique characteristics of the person doing the acting as well as the specific context in which the action occurs. In this unit, we examine the personal factors that may influence occupational performance.

This chapter provides an overview of the various personal characteristics and factors that affect occupational performance. **Personal factors** is a broad term used here to encompass several aspects of the human condition. Different professional groups, such as the American Occupational Therapy Association (AOTA, 2020) and the World Health Organization (WHO, 2001), organize these descriptors of individuals in different ways. The AOTA Practice Framework uses the term *client factors* (AOTA, 2020, p. 15) to encompass many aspects of the person, the WHO uses the term *body structures and body functions* (WHO, 2001, p. 10), and other international models may use the term *performance components* or *occupational performance components* (Chapparo et al., 2017) to refer to many aspects of personal factors.

Regardless of the specific terminology used, occupational therapy (OT) requires close attention to the many ways that individuals are unique. Examples include basic information such as the person's age, gender identity, and ethnicity. People also vary in body structures, or anatomical parts, such as bones and organs and body functions, or physiological processes of the body, including psychological function (WHO, 2001). For instance, people may vary physically in terms of height, weight, and bodily strength; they may vary in their responses to different sensory experiences such as a preference for spicy food or cold drinks, and they may vary in their emotional responses to specific situations. Furthermore, these differences may or may not impact the person's occupational performance, depending on the demands and challenges the individual experiences in life. ***It is important to note that client factors and performance skills are different*** (see Chapter 52). While client factors are specific capacities, characteristics, or beliefs, performance skills are observable goal-directed actions (AOTA, 2020).

See OT Story 53.1 as an illustration of the many personal factors affecting individual occupational performance. Later in the chapter are tables listing many of the personal factors that may be considered by occupational therapists.

The Whole Is Greater Than the Sum of the Parts

Personal factors do not operate in isolation. Anyone who has tried to maneuver in unfamiliar space in the dark (such as finding the bathroom in a dark hotel room in the middle of the night) can attest to the importance of vision to movement. All bodily factors work synergistically, which is why it is difficult to generate a definitive list of factors to which practitioners should attend. That is the case in this chapter as well, and the selected lists of factors and descriptions are presented to prompt your thinking. The categorizations that are presented here are not, nor can they be, a complete list of

OT STORY 53.1 CYNDE: PERSONAL FACTORS REQUIRED TO BE A NATURALIST ON A WHALE-WATCHING BOAT

Cynde is a naturalist on a whale-watching boat. In this description, some of the personal factors affecting her performance are noted. Refer to Tables 53.1 to 53.3 (presented later in the chapter) to see if you can pinpoint the specific terms. Additionally, try to match other terms that connect to the many personal factors affecting her performance.

Cynde has been passionate about whales for as long as she can remember, and she is deeply committed to preserving the ocean habitat to ensure their survival (values and beliefs). Her job requires that she orient tourists to the whaleboat safety rules, educate tourists about whales, and help them understand what they are seeing when they observe whale surface behavior. Because of her commitment to sustainability, she also tries to explain how personal actions in daily life can impact marine life many miles away from home.

Cynde starts each trip by standing on the dock, going over boat safety rules, and also explaining a bit about whales (Figure 53.1). Note that she has to hold (body function—musculoskeletal) the microphone with one hand (body structure—nervous system, movement-related structures) while demonstrating with another. She had to memorize (body function—long-term memory) what she needs to say (body function—language expression and working memory) and deliver her talk in a certain amount of time (body function—organization, planning, self-monitoring) while the boat is being readied for departure. She demonstrates enthusiasm and humor (body function—range of emotion, appropriate level of excitement) during her presentation. Once on the boat, she has to climb a steep ladder to get to the captain's area, where she will again use the microphone to call attention to the whales and their behavior. She works with the boat captain to detect whales at a long distance, using her visual skills. When she gets closer, she recognizes the distinctive patterns on the whale tails (called flukes), as

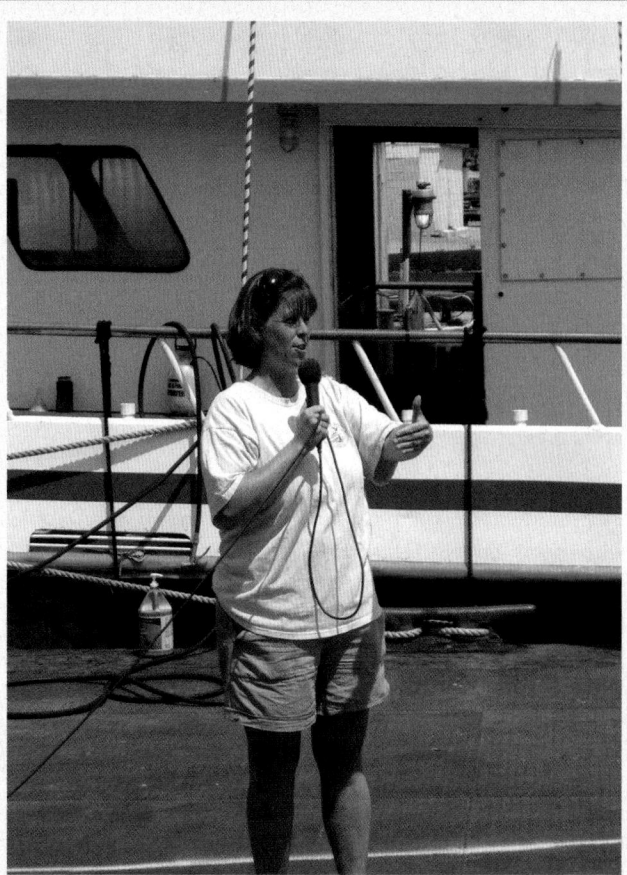

FIGURE 53.1 **Cynde is going over boat safety rules and also explaining a bit about whales.**

this is important to track individual whales. While she is providing commentary, she is also photographing whales and supervising science interns as they collect scientific data about whale sightings and surface behavior.

all the factors that affect human behavior. They are, at best, suggestions of factors to consider in analyzing occupational performance.

Practitioners can consider all of these factors from an objective standpoint or as subjectively experienced by the client. When considering personal factors objectively, therapists typically start by carefully observing occupational performance. If more information is needed to understand why the person is acting in a particular way, the therapist may evaluate body functions and structures using standardized approaches that other observers can replicate. Examples include muscle testing, sensory testing, and cognitive testing in relation to occupational performance. Chapters 19 and 20 address the use of objective assessments and the importance of using reliable and valid measures to obtain objective data. Although objective approaches are undeniably useful for informing professional reasoning, the client's subjective experience is also important. For example, objective measurement may indicate impairment; however, the person may not consider this limitation problematic in terms of daily life. Consequently, there may not be a need for intervention. Alternatively, comparison of objective and subjective findings may show that a client is unaware of safety concerns that are observed by the therapist. Therefore, skilled practitioners consider both the client's perspective and the objective information during the OT process. Box 53.1 provides some examples of objective and subjective reports related to body functions and structures.

BOX 53.1 OBJECTIVE AND SUBJECTIVE REPORTS OF BODY FUNCTIONS AND STRUCTURES

"I Didn't Have a Clue"

In a study seeking to understand the subjective experience of regaining self-care skills after a stroke or spinal cord injury, Guidetti et al. (2007) reported numerous examples of what it felt like for the study participants to attempt familiar tasks with various impairments. For instance, one participant who was recovering from a stroke appears to have had what objectively might be documented as a sensory loss, along with neglect of the affected upper extremity. She described her experience this way: "I didn't have a clue where it [her hand] was, it was behind my back and like this, so the first night it could have been anybody's hand" (Guidetti et al., 2007, p. 306).

"When You're Sitting There by Yourself, You're Just Eating"

In a study examining supported socialization for people with mental illness, Davidson and colleagues (2004) argued that people with persistent mental illness are lonely and isolated, not by choice (or objective impairments) but because of lack of opportunity and encouragement. When viewed solely from an objective perspective, people with persistent mental illness have been described as having impairments in volition, self-awareness, or coping (affective and cognitive impairments) and are thought to no longer desire human connection, with a preference for being alone. In a randomized control trial of supported socialization intervention, Davidson and colleagues (2001) found that people with mental illness desire friendships. One participant in the study commented that eating with her friend was better than eating alone at Burger King: "I'm alone. I sit down at the table, I eat a hamburger. But when I go with somebody else, and I'm sitting there at the table and eating it, she'll say 'Oh, is your hamburger good?' Then it becomes, the hamburger becomes noticeable, and then your mind starts to think about the taste. But when you're sitting there by yourself, you're just eating" (Davidson et al., 2001, p. 380).

This woman's description of eating with a friend illustrates the importance of considering clients' subjective experience. Without consideration of the subjective experience, intervention may not address aspects of occupational performance that were meaningful to this woman.

"I Didn't Understand the 'Meaning' of the Part Surrounded by the Outline of the Object"

Kikuko Yamada is a medical doctor in Japan who struggled with impaired perceptive and cognitive dysfunctions after having three cerebral hemorrhages and one cerebral infarction with moyamoya disease as the underlying disease. According to her autobiography (Yamada, 2004), she had difficulties with ADL due to "visual agnosia" and "spatial relations dysfunction" due to damage to the parietal lobe, primarily in the right hemisphere. For example, during a meal, she put the plate which she was holding in the soup and messed up the dinner tray (in Japan, the main dish and side dishes are served in separate plates and bowls, so many plates and bowls were placed on the tray), and she plunged her feet into a Japanese-style toilet bowl. She described her situation as follows: "… I often got thoughtful in front of the serving tray with lots of tableware … Whenever I tried to put the plate back on the tray, I made a mistake. Well, where should I put the plate? … A similar thing happened in the Japanese-style toilet. For the time being, I put my foot on the place where I felt that it seemed to be the most stable. But it was a flat puddle in the toilet bowl … I was in a world with few irregularities including the surrounding scenery, and if I look closely, it seemed that only the contour lines barely showed the boundary between objects …. Even dishes on the tray, only the outline of each dish looked like a flat cartoon drawn by an amateur, there is no information on height or distance, the dish is bounded by the boundary of different colors, and I think I could not recognize the existence of it … I didn't understand the 'meaning' of the part surrounded by the outline of the object."

Our job as OT practitioners is twofold. First, we must carefully observe occupational performance so as to understand which personal factors support occupational engagement and which ones are limiting engagement. Additionally, we must go beyond the generic labeling and understanding of diagnostic conditions to a deeper and more personal understanding of how clients perceive and experience their specific situations.

Reasoning About Personal Factors: Occupational Therapy as a Bridge

OT practitioners like to say that they treat the whole person. Whereas other professions (such as nursing) legitimately make a similar claim, OT is unique in its focus on how daily occupations are the synergistic product of the personal factors within the individual and factors that are external to the person in the larger context.

Another way to think about OT and how we consider the factors under discussion is to contrast OT with other professions. Think of OT as a bridge between the medical world and the lifeworld. In the medical world, there are many professions that focus on particular sets of body structures and functions. The field of medicine has obvious examples, with specialties in dermatology, endocrinology, gynecology, psychiatry, ophthalmology, and the list goes on and on. But other professions can also be examples. For instance, nutritionists focus on the digestive system, physical therapists focus on the neuromuscular and musculoskeletal systems, and speech-language pathologists focus primarily on the cognitive and oral-motor systems as they relate to communication. Although all of these professionals are interested in improving an individual's function, their contribution is very specific, and their knowledge about body functions and structures within their specific scope is typically quite extensive.

In contrast, other professions organize themselves around major roles or tasks of life. For instance, vocational evaluators and rehabilitation counselors focus on work-related concerns, educators focus on helping people learn to become productive citizens, recreation professionals focus on play and leisure, and social workers focus on family and community life. These professionals may attend to the impact of personal factors. So, for example, vocational rehabilitation practitioners know a great deal about job demands, employer requirements, and government standards related to work. Special education teachers are particularly aware of the impact of cognitive abilities and limitations for students in the classroom. Similarly, recreation therapists are quite knowledgeable about recreational spaces and places, the value of leisure in life, and the kinds of equipment that individuals might use to pursue leisure interests. However, for the most part, these professionals are very different from those in the medically oriented fields in that they typically have little or no background related to anatomy, physiology, and the specific impact of different health conditions on performance. Additionally, these professions typically are less likely to attend to the full array of social and psychological factors affecting performance. Rather, they have broad working knowledge about the skills and social demands that are required for their area of interest.

Occupational therapists have the education and ability to understand and address the impact of body structures and functions on life roles and tasks. This is done with full appreciation of the interconnected nature of occupations as well as how occupations are learned and change over the life course. In addition, OT practitioners recognize the transactions among personal factors and the environments in which the person must function (AOTA, 2020). As a result, OT as a profession provides information that bridges the clients' personal factors with the roles and task competencies required in daily life.

Complexity: An Asset and a Challenge

OT is unique as a profession in its willingness to consider all the client's personal factors along with all contextual factors as they shape engagement in the daily activities and routines of life. It is this appreciation of the transactional nature of occupational performance that makes OT so customized and effective for helping to solve complex problems of daily life. This uniqueness is a tremendous asset. However, for new practitioners and even some experienced ones, it can be challenging not to get absorbed in one aspect and thus lose sight of the larger picture. Practitioners who focus on one area of function may refer to themselves as hand therapists, cognitive therapists, or vision therapists and lose sight of the totality of our work as occupational therapists. Depth of knowledge about the personal factors is very important to expert practice; however, clients are best served when these factors are viewed in relation to the use of occupation as a means for intervention. Further, occupational engagement is the desired outcome regardless of how individual differences affect the ways in which this outcome is achieved. For example, as opposed to "doing hand therapy," our focus should be stated as "improving occupational performance after a hand injury." All of the practitioners in Unit IX indicate a deep understanding of body functions and structures that are relevant to their clients, but they view these factors in relation to occupational performance. Furthermore, OT practitioners grade their use of interventions in a way that is mindful of each person's individual characteristics, development, impairments, potential for recovery, and/or need for adaptive approaches. Practitioners also are very cognizant of how social and cultural contexts influence their clients' lives (see Expanding Our Perspectives). ***Thus, OT practitioners specialize not in body parts or body functions but in achieving health, well-being, and participation in life through engagement in occupation*** (AOTA, 2020).

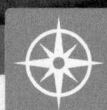

EXPANDING OUR PERSPECTIVES

Individual Variance From an East Asian Perspective

Asako Matsubara

Occupations and their meanings often vary depending on the person who performs them and the contexts in which they are performed. For example, when considering "eating," various eating utensils are used depending on location and culture. In Japan, as in other Asian countries, a lot of people use *hashi* (chopsticks). Despite the commonality of this utensil, the length and material of chopsticks can vary according to country and local customs. Moreover, some people shun the use of utensils altogether, using their hands instead when eating. Clearly, we can appreciate cultural customs and influences on the occupations of eating.

Different eating utensils require different body functions. For example, chopsticks are comprised of two separate parts (sticks), requiring higher hand dexterity and spatial relation functions than when using singular utensils. Therefore, occupational therapists need to be mindful of the impact and value of such habits and cultural differences on occupation.

When choosing to engage in a particular occupation, it is important to know that personal factors and the meaning and value of those occupations for the client are greatly influenced by culture. Iwama (2006) pointed out that "Depending on others, in Japanese cultural contexts, constitutes a very important basis to their occupations." In the context of a collectivist society where interdependence is a tacitly accepted social norm, Iwama noted that "… Japanese might prefer 'ningen kankei' (human relation) or Lebra's (1976) derivative, 'belonging,' as the ethos to their existence," as a primary driver to their occupational behavior.

Based on these unique cultural patterns, practitioners may observe such situations as follows; our clients might choose to participate in community (interdependent) activities that make them feel valued to their group rather than solitary self-care skills that aim toward the goal of independence. In Japan, families can often be observed helping their family members with self-care activities even though they are actually capable of performing these activities independently. The ethos of belonging is set strongly enough in Japanese society to drive other occupational behaviors; many Japanese people will often feel the need to engage and participate in certain activities simply because people around them are doing them, regardless of any intrinsic or personal value of the activity. As much as it matters in the Western world, an occupational therapist's thorough understanding of the meaning and value of their client's occupations of their will inform local practitioners to provide effective interventions that are culturally congruent and safe.

Japanese poet Misuzu Kaneko wrote in her poem "Me and the Little Bird and the Bell": "The bell, the little bird, and I, everyone is different, everyone is good." Interpreted through an occupational therapy perspective, the lyric suggests that the lives and personal factors of our clients are appreciated as being different, and uniquely formed. On this premise, that "everyone is different," the practitioner is challenged to carry out evaluation and intervention processes that are integrated to effectively capture the complexities of the client's daily life realities, as well as their aspirations.

Intertwining Knowledge and Theories

For OT practitioners to work effectively with people who have impairments or developmental conditions that affect their performance, practitioners must intertwine knowledge about occupation with knowledge about the client's particular health problems. As noted earlier, this chapter provides only a topical overview of the many person factors that practitioners may consider. Knowing what to do requires an in-depth appreciation of relevant theories and research in order to assure effective intervention. Units VI and VII provide the reader with examples of how theories guide practice to improve occupational performance in the focused areas of motor control, cognition and perception, sensory processing, emotional regulation, and communication/social interaction. Readers are encouraged to look at those chapters for examples of how to integrate theories about body functions and structures into an OT intervention.

Personal Factors That Are Commonly Considered

In this section, we provide several tables that readers might find helpful to prompt consideration of one or more personal factors (Tables 53.1–53.4). Readers will likely find the language useful in communicating about personal factors. As was discussed earlier, there is no practical way to make a comprehensive list, so we make no claim that the tables are all inclusive. Information for these tables was drawn primarily from the *International Classification of Functioning, Disability and Health* (WHO, 2001), the Occupational Therapy Practice Framework (AOTA, 2020), and topical areas that are addressed in this unit.

TABLE 53.1	Examples of Personal Factors (Excluding Body Functions and Structures) That Are Considered in Occupational Therapy
Factor	**Common Categories or Descriptors**
Age	Historical cohort (e.g., people who lived through the Vietnam War and how that experience affects their worldview) Internalization of societal expectations regarding development and achieving a particular developmental milestone at a given time in the life course Personal expectations about age-related behavior
Gender	Personally adopted social/cultural norms and roles regarding gender
Values	Meanings associated with physical and social spaces Importance of family Standards of conduct Qualities considered desirable Principles considered worthwhile
Beliefs	Knowledge that is held to be truth Beliefs about causes and interventions related to illness Perceived locus of control Cognitive content held as truth
Spirituality	Beliefs about the meaning of life Quest to understand ultimate life questions Religious and sacred beliefs
Family and significant others	Internalized family experiences that shape worldview Internalized expectations about relationships
Socioeconomic status	Financial status Work status Educational attainment
Ethnicity	Internal beliefs about membership in groups of common descent; can include race, culture, language, religion, and politics
Sexual orientation	An individual's sexuality, usually related to an individual's romantic, emotional, and/or sexual attraction to persons of a particular gender

TABLE 53.2	Examples of Body Structures Considered in Occupational Therapy
Structure	**Common Categories or Descriptors**
Nervous system	Brain (cortical, subcortical including brain stem) Spinal cord Spinal nerves Sympathetic and parasympathetic systems
Eye and ear	Eye (retina, cornea, lens) External ocular muscles Ear (inner, middle, outer)
Voice and speech	Mouth (lips, cheek, tongue, teeth, palate) Nose Pharynx (nasal and oral) Larynx (vocal cords)
Cardiovascular, immunological, respiratory	Heart Veins Arteries Lungs Trachea Bronchial tubes Muscles of respiration Lymphatic system
Digestive, metabolic, endocrine	Esophagus Stomach Intestine Many glands

TABLE 53.2	Examples of Body Structures Considered in Occupational Therapy (*continued*)
Structure	**Common Categories or Descriptors**
Genitourinary, reproductive	Bladder, ureters, urethra Reproductive structures
Movement-related structures (head/neck, upper and lower extremities, trunk, pelvic region)	Bones Joints Muscles Tendons Ligaments Fascia
Skin and related structures	Skin layers Skin glands Hair Sensing organs in skin

Sources: American Occupational Therapy Association. (2020). Occupational therapy practice framework: Domain and process, 4th edition. *American Journal of Occupational Therapy, 74*(Supp. 2), 74124110010; and World Health Organization. (2001). *International classification of functioning, disability and health (ICF)*. Author.

TABLE 53.3	Examples of Body Functions Considered by Occupational Therapists
Category	**Examples**
ICF: Global mental functions (affective, cognitive, perceptual)	
Consciousness	Alertness Arousal level Continuity of wakeful state
Orientation	Person Place Time Self Others Past Present
Intellectual functions	Understanding Integration of cognitive functions
Psychosocial functions	Interpersonal skills Social interactions
Temperament/personality	Emotional stability Disposition Confidence
Energy and drive	Energy level Motivation Impulse control Appetite
Sleep functions	Amount and onset of sleep Quality Sleep cycle functions
ICF: Specific mental functions (affective, cognitive, perceptual)	
Attention	Selectivity Sustainability Shifting Divided
Memory	Short term Long term Working

TABLE 53.3	Examples of Body Functions Considered by Occupational Therapists (*continued*)
Category	**Examples**
Perception	Auditory Visual Olfactory Gustatory Tactile Visuospatial
Sensory processing	Reception Organization Assimilation Integration
Thought	Ideation Pace of thought Content
Higher level cognitive functions	Volition Organization/planning Purposeful action Self-awareness Self-monitoring Decision making Problem solving Judgment Time management Coping
Emotional	Behavioral regulation Range of emotion
Psychomotor functions	Appropriate affect Response time Level of excitement/agitation Speed of behavior
Mental functions of language	Reception of language (spoken, written, and sign) Expression of language (spoken, written, and sign)
Mental functions of sequencing complex movement	Praxis
ICF: Sensation and pain	
Taste	Quality Intensity
Smell	Quality Intensity
Touch	Light Deep pressure
Temperature	Hot Cold
Pain	Sharp Stabbing Aching Burning
Proprioception	Quick Sustained
Vestibular	Linear Angular
Visual	Acuity Intensity Contrast
Interoception	Detection of changes in one's internal organs
Auditory	Acuity Intensity Contrast Rhythm

(continued)

TABLE 53.3 **Examples of Body Functions Considered by Occupational Therapists (*continued*)**

Category	Examples
ICF: Neuromuscular and movement	
Joint mobility	Passive ROM Active ROM
Muscle strength	Pinch Grip Force
Muscle tone	Quality
Voluntary motor control	Coordination (dexterity, gross motor, bilateral integration) Motor execution (mobility)
Involuntary motor control	Reflexes Unconscious movement
Posture	Alignment Orientation Stability Control Balance Adaptation
ICF: Cardiovascular, immunological, respiratory	
Heart rate	Beats per minute
Blood pressure	Range of pressure exerted on arteries
Respiration	Rhythm Depth Rate

ICF, International Classification of Functioning, Disability and Health; ROM, range of motion.

From American Occupational Therapy Association. (2014). Occupational therapy practice framework: Domain and process, 3rd edition. *American Journal of Occupational Therapy, 68*, S1–S48; Dunn, W. (2011). *Best practice occupational therapy: In community service with children and families* (2nd ed.). SLACK; and World Health Organization. (2001). *International classification of functioning, disability and health (ICF)*. Author.

TABLE 53.4 **Examples of Impaired Body Functions and Potential Impact on Occupational Performance**

Impairment of Body Function	Potential Difficulty With Daily Life Occupations
Impaired visuospatial processing	Inability to orient clothing to self Misjudging distance when reaching for a utensil Inability to align car in parking space Spilling juice when pouring from carton into glass Difficulty finding the way in new environments and fear of getting lost results in self-imposed participation restrictions (Árnadóttir, 2021)
Decreased shoulder range of motion	Inability to manage hair care Unable to tuck shirt into back of pants Inability to retrieve book from high shelves at the library Inability to change a light bulb Difficulty holding and playing with one's children or grandchildren Role strain from inability to perform job responsibilities and inability to fulfill the role of primary financial provider
Poor emotional regulation	Poor performance at job interview Inability to cope during finals week at college, resulting in poor test performance Social isolation due to inappropriate affect Difficulty initiating, developing, and maintaining interpersonal relationships Inability to make decisions due to overwhelming anxiety

TABLE 53.4	Examples of Impaired Body Functions and Potential Impact on Occupational Performance (*continued*)
Impairment of Body Function	**Potential Difficulty With Daily Life Occupations**
Sensory loss in feet	Increased incidence of falls during community outings Inability to walk on rough terrains (beach, hiking trails, etc.) Inability to drive a car Decreased participation in social/leisure activities due to fear of falling
Decreased attention	Difficulty attending to one conversation at a time at a dinner party Unable to attend school lectures/lessons Inability to cook toast and tea at the same time Difficulty following verbal and written instructions on the job Experiences of relationship strain as a partner may perceive a lack of interest due to easy distractibility (Gillen, 2009)
Memory deficits	Inability to remember whether one has eaten, difficult thinking about what was eaten Inability to complete normal errands Going to the store and coming back home without buying what was needed Inability to go to the hospital on the day of appointment see a doctor Difficulty remembering people one has met before Inability to remember whether one took required medications

Clues to personal factors that could be affecting performance are gained from at least three sources:

- **Reason for referral.** Referral information may contain a medical, psychological, or educational diagnosis and sometimes precautions to consider during intervention. Even when precautions, symptoms, or other descriptors are not included, knowledge about typical body structures and functions that are affected by the condition can guide practitioners regarding factors to consider.

   Example: Diagnosis—rotator cuff tear. Knowledge of the body structure will lead practitioners to evaluate for the *impact* that pain, weakness, and limited shoulder range of motion may have on identified limitations in occupational performance. Limitations may include inability to perform self-care (e.g., shampooing hair), inability to fulfill a homemaker role (e.g., putting groceries away, washing windows), inability to engage in leisure activities (e.g., fly fishing), inability to perform job responsibilities (e.g., writing on a blackboard), and/or inability to fulfill child-care responsibilities (e.g., lifting a toddler into a high chair).

   Example: Diagnosis—head trauma, scapula fracture, bilateral radius fracture, pelvic fracture, and so on. *Precautions to consider during intervention*: The client jumped from the 5th floor of a condominium and was injured. She had previously been seen by a physician at a psychiatric hospital. She may injure herself with sharps and might experience flashbacks of this accident, especially when situated at heights. Knowledge of the body structure, body function, and illness will lead OT practitioners to evaluate for the *impact* that pain, limited range of motion, muscle weakness, impaired perception and cognition, and mental status

may have on identified limitations in occupational performance. Limitations may include the inability to perform self-care (e.g., grooming, dressing), inability to fulfill a homemaker role (e.g., cooking with a knife, drying laundry on the balcony), inability to fulfill child-care responsibilities (e.g., taking a child to a private-tutoring school) and the inability to drive a car.

- **Client self-report.** Clients themselves, their families, and other key people in their social environments (e.g., teachers, employers, caregivers) often give practitioners information about factors that they believe are affecting client performance.

   Example: A third-grade teacher reports to the occupational therapist that Alicia is highly distractible in class, requires multiple prompts and cues to stay on task, and is falling behind her classmates in reaching educational objectives. Alicia expresses a desire to play with other girls during recess but doesn't quite know how to join the group.

   Example: After the onset of subarachnoid hemorrhage, a woman came to the hospital for outpatient rehabilitation care after discharge. She said, "My shoulder on the paralyzed side is not painful like before. I can take a bath using adaptive equipment. I can hold vegetables with my paralyzed hand and cut them now."

- **Observation of client.** Observations of the client engaging in occupations often prompt practitioners to consider one or more factors that are affecting performance.

   Example: During an evaluation of meal preparation skills, the OT practitioner notes that Mr. Brown is unable to independently complete a task as he did before his recent decline in cognitive function. He now requires step-by-step cues to sequence and organize the process of making a soup and salad.

Example: Coleman attends a residential school for adolescents with traumatic brain injury. Since his accident, Coleman becomes fatigued, withdrawn, and apathetic by mid-afternoon. Every week, six teenage boys plan a Thursday evening community outing to relax and have fun together. The occupational therapist observes that Coleman does not offer suggestions for outings and rarely interacts with his peers during the outing. To accommodate for Coleman's personal factors and engage during a time of day when his performance is optimal, the practitioner plans to change the community outings to Saturday morning.

Example: During a driving evaluation using a driving simulator, the attending OT practitioner found that the client did not notice a road sign on his left side. The practitioner plans to show a video that was recorded in the driving simulator to the client to assess his perception—particularly to his left side—and to facilitate his ability to pay attention to the left side.

Skillful intervention requires that practitioners respond to these cues and then use credible resources to obtain needed objective information. This information, combined with the subjective data provided by the client, is then synthesized to develop interventions that enable the client's occupational performance. It is important to remember that the "presence or absence of specific body functions and body structures do not necessarily ensure a client's success or difficulty with daily life occupations" (AOTA, 2020, p. 15). A person with memory loss may be able to fully participate in most aspects of life using compensatory strategies such as memory notebooks/diaries, electronic paging systems, written reminder lists posted in the environment, and/or smartphone alarm reminders. Optical aids, text-to-speech translators, and the use of guide dogs can provide a person with vision loss with the ability to live life fully and independently.

Conclusion

OT practitioners routinely consider body functions, structures, and other personal factors during intervention.

By integrating knowledge and theories about these personal factors with theories that relate to occupation and occupational contexts, practitioners provide a unique contribution to society and to the clients they serve.

Acknowledgments

The authors would like to acknowledge the contributions of Marjorie E. Scaffa and Ellen S. Cohn to earlier editions of this chapter.

Lippincott® Connect *For additional resources on the subjects discussed in this chapter, visit* Lippincott Connect.

REFERENCES

American Occupational Therapy Association. (2020). Occupational therapy practice framework: Domain and process, 4th edition. *American Journal of Occupational Therapy, 74*(Suppl. 2), 74124110010. https://doi.org/10.5014/ajot.2020.74S2001

Árnadóttir, G. (2021). Impact of neurobehavioral deficits on activities of daily living. In G. Gillen & D. M. Nilsen (Eds.), *Stroke rehabilitation: A function-based approach* (5th ed., pp. 556–592). Elsevier.

Chapparo, C., Ranka, J., & Nott, M. (2017). The Occupational Performance Model (Australia): A description of constructs, structure and propositions. In M. Curtin, M. Egan, & J. Adams (Eds.), *Occupational therapy for people experiences illness, injury or impairment* (7th ed., 134–147). Elsevier.

Davidson, L., Shahar, G., Stayner, D. A., Chiman, M. J., Rakfeldt, J., & Tebes, J. K. (2004). Supported socialization for people with psychiatric disabilities: Lessons from a randomized control trial. *Journal of Community Psychology, 32*, 453–477. https://doi.org/10.1002/jcop.20013

Davidson, L., Stayner, D. A., Nickou, C., Styron, T. H., Rowe, M., & Chinman, M. L. (2001). "Simply to be let in": Inclusion as a basis for recovery. *Psychiatric Rehabilitation Journal, 24*, 375–388. https://doi.org/10.1037/h0095067

Gillen, G. (2009). *Cognitive and perceptual rehabilitation: Optimizing function.* Elsevier/Mosby.

Guidetti, S., Asaba, E., & Tham, K. (2007). The lived experience of recapturing self-care. *American Journal of Occupational Therapy, 61*, 303–310. https://doi.org/10.5014/ajot.61.3.303

Iwama, M. K. (2006). *The Kawa model: Culturally relevant occupational therapy.* Elsevier/Churchill Livingstone.

Lebra, T. S. (1976). *Japanese patterns of behavior.* The University Press of Hawaii.

World Health Organization. (2001). *International classification of functioning, disability and health (ICF).* Author.

Yamada, K. (2004). *Kowareta Nou Seizonsuru Chi.* Tankobon Hardcover.

CHAPTER 54

Motor Function and Occupational Performance

Dawn M. Nilsen and Glen Gillen

LEARNING OBJECTIVES

After reading this chapter, you will be able to:

1. Understand how motor function supports occupational performance throughout the life course.
2. Explain how impairments related to motor function limit occupational performance across the life course.
3. Compare and contrast the approaches that are used to guide the occupational therapy process related to improving occupational performance for those with motor impairments.
4. Become familiar with assessments that are used to measure motor function across the life course.
5. Begin to construct evidence-based intervention plans that improve occupational performance for those living with motor impairments.

Introduction: Motor Function and Everyday Living

This morning, you may have rolled over in bed, reached over to your nightstand to turn off the alarm, and transitioned to a seated position on your bed, followed by a transition to a standing posture before walking to the bathroom. On your way to the bathroom, you might step into your slippers by shifting your weight from one foot to the other. Your **postural control** system combined with your trunk and limb function worked together to support your functional mobility and activities of daily living (ADLs).

Kamal is taking care of his child. As he lifts his child from the crib, he must generate enough force in his upper limbs to move his child, calibrate this force as to not harm his child with too much pressure in his hands, maintain his balance as he lifts his child toward him, and coordinate/plan his movements so that his hand supports his child's head as he lifts. Kamal's parenting role is being supported by various motor functions.

Danielle is going ice-skating for the first time today at the age of 4 years. To be successful, she will need to learn to maintain her center of gravity, use various postural reflexes (e.g., righting and equilibrium responses) to maintain an upright position, learn that she can integrate her upper limbs to maintain her balance, and coordinate her limbs to glide over the ice. In addition, she requires enough strength and endurance to complete the task. Danielle's ability to engage in play is supported by multiple systems and structures related to motor function. To be successful, Danielle must also process and adapt to incoming information from her sensory systems (e.g., vestibular, proprioception, vision; see Chapter 56 for more details).

Most of the day (and night albeit to a much lesser extent) is spent engaging in occupations that require motor functions to support performance. Occupational therapy (OT) practitioners treat various conditions that result in limited motor function and loss of motor control. As you can infer from the examples earlier, any change in motor function has a tremendous impact on our ability to engage in meaningful occupations. The following two cases illustrate these points.

Approaches That Guide Therapy

Various approaches may be used when working with clients with motor deficits. Many times, approaches are combined and/or the therapist may switch from one to another based on the client's response or preference (see Chapter 21).

Biomechanical Approach

The **biomechanical approach** is considered a remediation approach. It is focused at the level of the client factor/impairment when these impairments are limiting occupational performance. Examples of impairments that are addressed by this approach include weakness, limitations

in joint **range of motion**, edema, pain, low endurance, sensory changes, joint instability, poor coordination, and so on. Clients living with cardiopulmonary diseases, various forms of arthritis, burns, cumulative trauma disorders/repetitive strain injuries, tendon tears or lacerations, fractures, and so on, may be appropriate for interventions based on the biomechanical approach.

More recently, components of this approach (e.g., resistance training) have been applied to those living with acquired brain injuries such as a stroke. Data suggests that resistance training may be beneficial in improving muscle force, motor function, health-related quality of life (HRQoL), independence, and reintegration (Veldema & Jansen, 2020).

This approach is based on several assumptions:

- The underlying impairment is amenable to remediation.
- Engagement in occupation and various other therapeutic activities has the potential to remediate the underlying impairment(s).
- This remediation will result in improved occupational performance.

See OT Story 54.1 for a demonstration of the biomechanical approach.

The key to successfully using this approach is linking the underlying impairment to the occupational performance deficit. This linking must occur in both the intervention planning process and goal writing. For example:

- ***Incorrect goal focused on impairment:*** Client will demonstrate a 20° increase in shoulder external rotation.
- ***Correct goal focused on change in performance:*** Client will demonstrate a 20° increase in shoulder external rotation in order to comb the back of her hair with minimal assistance.

OT STORY 54.1 KAMAL: LIMITED OCCUPATIONAL PERFORMANCE DUE TO A MUSCULOSKELETAL INJURY

Kamal (as discussed in the opening paragraphs) fell while jogging. He landed on his dominant right shoulder and returned home complaining of weakness and excruciating pain. Kamal's orthopedist diagnosed him with a full-thickness tear of his rotator cuff. Surgery was scheduled, and the tear was repaired. Postoperatively, Kamal was referred for OT. The occupational therapist performed evaluations focused on Kamal's impairments and activity limitations related to areas of occupation. Various standardized measures were used. A Visual Analogue Scale documented that his pain was rated as 8 on a 0 to 10 scale. His **active range of motion** and strength, as tested by a

manual muscle test, were intact with the exception of his right shoulder. These tests were deferred for his injured shoulder because the medical orders allowed only passive motion until the repair site began to heal. **Passive range of motion** of his involved shoulder was limited by pain as expected. Kamal reported and demonstrated difficulty with both basic and instrumental activities of daily living (ADLs), stating, "I am very right dominant." The occupational therapist administered the Disabilities of the Arm, Shoulder, and Hand (DASH) Outcome Measure including the work module because Kamal was employed as a grocery store manager. The DASH is a 30-item, self-report questionnaire

OT STORY 54.1 KAMAL: LIMITED OCCUPATIONAL PERFORMANCE DUE TO A MUSCULOSKELETAL INJURY (*continued*)

designed to measure physical function and symptoms in people with any of several musculoskeletal disorders of the upper limb. The DASH provided the occupational therapist with specific information regarding how Kamal's shoulder injury was impacting his daily functioning. Kamal's long-term goals were defined as (a) independent in all basic ADL, (b) independent in child care, and (c) return to work part time.

The occupational therapist used various interventions that were graded as Kamal's tendons healed over time. The interventions were based on both rehabilitative and biomechanical approaches. These included the following:

- ADL retraining using one-handed techniques and assistive devices. This was an early focus because Kamal was not allowed to actively move his right shoulder for several weeks. Although he lived with his wife, he did not want to be a burden as she was taking care of their newborn. Therefore, he was highly motivated to be as independent as possible. These techniques were only employed temporarily.
- Physical agent modalities such as **cryotherapy** (ice) for pain control

- Education related to sleep postures
- Progressive mobilization of Kamal's shoulder (passive range of motion, active assisted range of motion, active range of motion, and strengthening)
- Physical agent modalities such as therapeutic heat to increase flexibility before therapy
- Engaging Kamal's right arm to support performance of occupations that were graded over time. The occupational therapist began with low-height activities such as reaching into cabinets under the sink, followed by medium-height activities (e.g., applying deodorant), and followed by overhead reach activities such as hanging up clothing and putting groceries away on high shelves.
- Resumption of bilateral ADL
- Simulated work activities

Using the aforementioned approaches and interventions, Kamal was able to meet his goals and soon after resumed full-time duties at work.

Questions

1. What is the priority of Kamal's intervention plan?
2. What are some assistive devices that Kamal can use to perform ADLs?

For the correct version of the goal, it is assumed that a self-care evaluation has been documented to demonstrate the impact of the loss of range of motion on basic ADL.

Standard assessments and evaluations associated with the biomechanical approach include:

- Standardized objective tests of occupational performance (see Unit VIII)
- Self-report measures of how impairments limit occupational performance (e.g., DASH, Manual Ability Measure)
- Goniometry: active and passive range of motion
- Manual muscle tests
- Dynamometry (grip and pinch strength testing)
- Sensory testing (e.g., Semmes Weinstein Monofilament Examination, 2-point discrimination)
- Coordination testing
- Provocative tests (tests used to provoke underlying symptoms)
- Circumferential or volumetric measures to quantify edema
- Pain scales
- Examination of skin integrity/wounds
- Borg Rating of Perceived Exertion Scale (endurance)
- Ergonomic evaluations

Interventions commonly used in the biomechanical approach include:

- ADL retraining
- Work hardening
- Active, active assistive, passive range of motion exercises
- High-load brief stretch
- Low-load prolonged stretch
- Orthoses (static and dynamic) (see Figures 54.1 and 54.2)
- Strengthening
- Endurance training
- Joint protection techniques
- Physical agent modalities (e.g., superficial heat, deep heat, cold/cryotherapy, electrical modalities)
- Therapeutic exercise (e.g., passive, isotonic, active assistive, resistive, isometric, and isokinetic exercises)
- Edema control techniques (e.g., massage and mobilization, positional elevation, wrapping techniques)
- Desensitization for hypersensitivity
- Sensory retraining
- Scar management
- Joint mobilization
- Tendon and nerve gliding

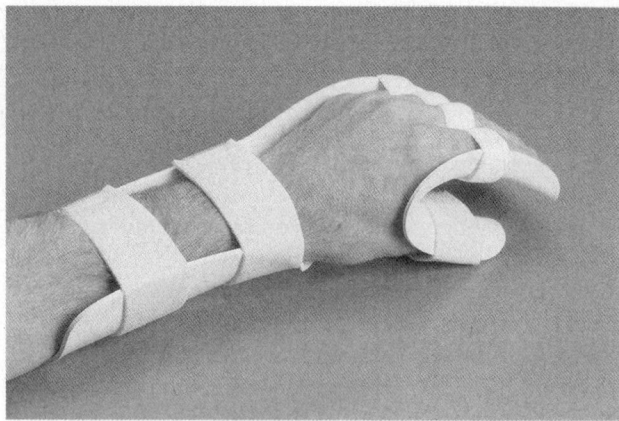

FIGURE 54.1 One common static orthoses is the resting orthosis, which is used for clients with rheumatoid arthritis, traumatic injuries, burns, tendon injuries, stroke, spinal cord injury, infections, and post-op Dupuytren's.

(Photo courtesy of the Rehabilitation Division of Smith & Nephew, Germantown, WI.)

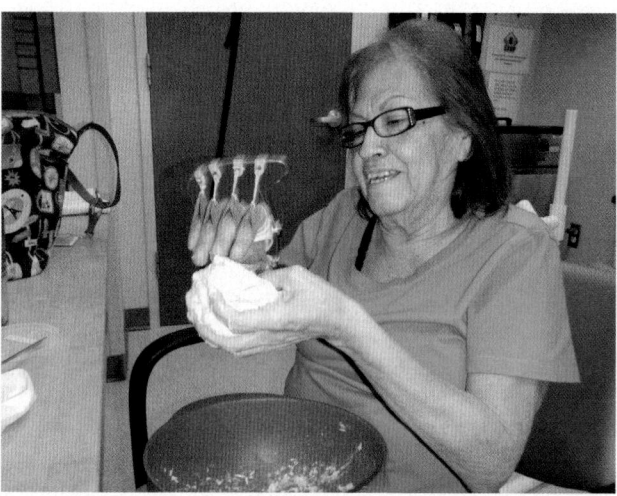

FIGURE 54.2 Using a dynamic orthosis to support engagement in occupation.

(Photo courtesy of Lauro A. Munoz, OTR, MOT.)

See Table 54.1 for examples of evidence that supports interventions used in the biomechanical approach.

Rehabilitative Approach

The **rehabilitative approach** includes the concepts of adaptation, compensation, and environmental modifications (see Chapter 21 for more details). It may be used in conjunction with other approaches or in isolation. This approach places an emphasis on the client's strengths as opposed to their limitations. The ultimate goal is to maximize independence despite the presence of persistent impairments. This approach may be most appropriate for clients who are living with impairments that are permanent, including both static and progressive impairments. This approach may also be useful when an underlying impairment is potentially amenable to remediation but the client is not motivated to participate in the sometimes long and difficult process of remediation. Contextual factors such as limited therapy visits may also lead therapists to adopt this approach because some may argue that functional independence is achieved quicker.

Clients living with the following disorders may be candidates for the rehabilitative approach in isolation or in conjunction with the other approaches discussed: multiple sclerosis, amyotrophic lateral sclerosis, severe stroke, advanced arthritis, advancing Parkinson disease, spinal cord injuries, and so on. Readers should note that the rehabilitative approach is used for various impairments beyond motor deficits.

In many cases, the occupational therapist takes on the role of "teacher" when using this approach and must consider the following questions:

1. What is the client's potential to learn?
2. Is the client motivated to learn?
3. What is the client's optimal learning style?

Motor learning principles to promote skill acquisition will be discussed later in this chapter. Assessments and evaluations used for the rehabilitative approach as it relates to motor deficits include:

- Standardized objective tests of occupational performance
- Self-report measures of occupational performance
- Ergonomic evaluations
- Evaluations to determine client's strengths
  - ◆ Cognitive evaluations (to evaluate learning potential)
  - ◆ Range of motion and strength testing of nonaffected limbs
  - ◆ Balance testing
- Evaluations of environmental and social contexts to determine supports and limitations

Sample interventions commonly associated with the rehabilitative approach include:

- Energy conservation
- Work simplification
- Recommending and training with assistive devices to support occupational performance
- Recommending and training with durable medical equipment
- Recommending and training with assistive technology
- Home modifications
- Work modifications
- Wheeled mobility and seating recommendations
- Fabrication of orthoses that support function

See OT Story 54.2 for a demonstration of the rehabilitation approach and Table 54.2 for evidence that supports using a rehabilitative approach.

TABLE 54.1	Sample Evidence That Supports Interventions Used When Adopting the Biomechanical Approach	
Author/Year	**Objective**	**Conclusion**
Egan and Brousseau (2007)	To review the evidence regarding the effectiveness of splinting for carpometacarpal osteoarthritis	Research to date indicates that splinting may help relieve pain in persons with carpometacarpal osteoarthritis.
M. J. Page, Massy-Westropp, et al. (2012)	To compare the effectiveness of splinting for carpal tunnel syndrome (CTS) with no treatment, placebo, or another nonsurgical intervention	Overall, limited evidence that a splint worn at night is more effective than no treatment, but insufficient evidence regarding safety/effectiveness of one type of splint or wearing schedules over others, and of splinting over other nonsurgical interventions.
Veldema and Jansen (2020)	Systematic review and meta-analysis investigating the effects of resistance training in supporting recovery in stroke patients	There is evidence that resistance training can improve muscle force and motor function of the upper and lower limbs and HRQoL.
Hurkmans et al. (2009)	To assess the effectiveness and safety of short-term and long-term dynamic exercise therapy programs (aerobic capacity and/or muscle strength training) for people with rheumatoid arthritis (RA)	Based on the evidence, aerobic capacity training combined with muscle strength training is recommended as routine practice in patients with RA.
Saunders et al. (2016)	To determine whether fitness training after stroke reduces death, dependence, and disability and to assess the effects of training regarding adverse events, risk factors, physical fitness, mobility, physical function, quality of life, mood, and cognitive function	Cardiorespiratory training and, to a lesser extent, mixed training reduce disability during or after usual stroke care. Sufficient evidence to incorporate cardiorespiratory and mixed training, involving walking, within poststroke rehabilitation programs. Insufficient evidence to support the use of resistance training. The effects of training on death and dependence are unclear. Impact on cognitive function is under investigated.
Werner et al. (2005)	To determine whether night splinting of workers identified through active surveillance with symptoms consistent with CTS would improve symptoms and median nerve function as well as impact medical care	The results suggest that a short course of nocturnal splinting may reduce wrist, hand, and/or finger discomfort among active workers with symptoms consistent with CTS.

HRQoL, health-related quality of life.

OT STORY 54.2 SIMONE: LIMITED OCCUPATIONAL PERFORMANCE DUE TO MULTIPLE FRACTURES

Simone was admitted to the local hospital's acute care unit after falling off her motorcycle. She had recently lost her job due to the COVID-19 pandemic and is uninsured. She presented with multiple rib fractures, a left shoulder fracture, and a right wrist/thumb fracture. In addition, she presented with a small bleed in her left temporal lobe (language is unaffected and there is no evidence of apraxia). Simone lives in a first-floor apartment with her girlfriend Stacey. The team believes that she will be in the hospital for 4 days before being discharged home with Stacey.

Simone's OT practitioner realizes that she will only be able to offer three to four therapy sessions. Postdischarge will not include any rehabilitation services due to Simone's lack of insurance. A rehabilitation approach was chosen to guide intervention. Interventions included:

- Inviting Stacey to OT sessions to train her how to help Simone with bed mobility, transfers, and ADL. Simone requires minimal assistance due to pain and her multiple fractures.
- Providing adaptive equipment (rocker knife, button hook, and cutting board) to help Simone participate in ADL.
- Giving Stacey suggestions on how to modify the bathroom to ensure safety (remove bathmats, add suction bottom rubber mats in the shower). Simone can walk but is slow and unsteady due to pain.
- Teaching a simple exercise program to maintain mobility in Simone's unaffected joints.

Questions

1. What precautions would you teach Stacey to use when assisting Simone during ADLs?
2. What community resources would you recommend for Stacey and Simone to maximize her recovery?

TABLE 54.2	Sample Evidence That Supports Interventions Used When Adopting the Rehabilitation Approach	
Author/Year	**Objective**	**Conclusion**
Ashfaq et al. (2019)	To find the effectiveness of adaptive devices on functionality and quality of life of patients with multiple conditions	Marked improvement according to the results of FIM scoring and WHQOL showed the importance of adaptive devices and their great role in person's independence level. Use of adaptive devices is very important to provide independent life as the main goal of Occupational Therapy treatment and to improve the functionality and quality of life as well.
Mann et al. (1999)	To evaluate a system of assistive technology and environmental interventions provision designed to promote independence and reduce health care costs for physically frail elderly persons	Results indicate rate of functional decline can be slowed, and institutional and certain in-home personnel costs reduced through a systematic approach to providing these interventions.
Yachnin et al. (2017)	To investigate whether technology-assisted toilets improve toileting independence, quality of life, and whether technology-assisted toilets can provide sufficient toileting hygiene in stroke rehabilitation	Technology-assisted toilets improved stroke patients' psychosocial outcomes compared to standard toileting and completely cleaned participants in the majority of cases.

FIM, functional independence measure; WHOQOL, World Health Organization Quality of Life.

Task-Oriented Approaches

Task-oriented approaches—also described as task-specific training, repetitive task practice, goal-directed training, and functional task practice—are considered the most current approach related to impaired motor function and motor control for those living with brain damage. The assumptions of the OT task-oriented approach are based on the following systems model of motor behavior:

- Functional tasks help organize behavior.
- Personal and environmental systems, including the central nervous system, are heterarchically organized.
- Occupational performance emerges from the interaction between persons and their environment.
- Experimentation with various strategies leads to optimal solutions to motor problems.
- Recovery is variable because patient factors and environmental contexts are unique.
- Behavioral changes reflect attempts to compensate and to achieve task performance.

Timmermans et al. (2010) describe the components of task-oriented training. In this approach, movement emerges as an interaction between many systems in the brain and is organized around a goal and constrained by the environment (Shumway-Cook & Woollacott, 2017). Rensink et al. (2009) describe task-oriented training as including a wide range of interventions such as walking training on the ground, bicycling programs, endurance training and circuit training, sit-to-stand exercises, and reaching tasks for improving balance. A major focus of task-oriented training is on arm training using functional tasks, such as grasping objects, and constraint-induced movement therapy (CI therapy; Wolf et al., 2006). This approach is task focused and client focused and not therapist focused (Rensink et al., 2009). See Table 54.3 for examples of evidence that support the use of a task-oriented approach.

Training components of the task-oriented approach have been described (adapted from Timmermans et al., 2010).

1. **Functional movements:** A movement involving task execution that is not directed toward a clear ADL goal.
2. **Clear functional goal:** A goal that is set during everyday life activities and/or hobbies (e.g., washing dishes, grooming activity, dressing oneself, playing golf).
3. **Client-centered patient goal:** Therapy goals that are set through the involvement of the patient himself or herself in the therapy goal decision process. The goals respect patients' values, preferences, and expressed needs and recognize the clients' experience and knowledge.
4. **Overload:** Overload is determined by the total time spent on therapeutic activity, the number of repetitions, the difficulty of the activity in terms of coordination, muscle activity type and resistance load, and the intensity, that is, number of repetitions per time unit.
5. **Real-life object manipulation:** Manipulation that makes use of objects that are handled in normal everyday life activities (e.g., cutlery, hairbrush).
6. **Context-specific environment:** A training environment (supporting surface, objects, people, room, etc.) that equals or mimics the natural environment for a specific task execution in order to include task characteristic sensory/perceptual information, task-specific context characteristics, and cognitive processes involved.
7. **Exercise progression:** Exercises with an increasing difficulty level that is in line with the increasing abilities of the patient in order to keep the demands of the exercises and challenges optimal for motor learning.

TABLE 54.3 — Sample Evidence That Supports Interventions Used When Adopting the Task-Oriented Approach

Author/Year	Objective	Conclusion
Almhdawi et al. (2016)	To evaluate the functional and the impairment effects of the Occupational Therapy Task-Oriented Approach on upper limb function via a randomized clinical trial using a crossover design	The results supported the approach as indicated by significant and clinically meaningful changes in the Canadian Occupational Performance Measure, the Motor Activity Log, and the time scale of the Wolf Motor Function Test. The author concluded that the approach is an effective upper extremity (UE) poststroke rehabilitation approach in improving the UE functional abilities.
Chisari et al. (2017)	The aim was to test the impact of an intensive task-oriented training intervention on motor function and quality of life in patients with MS.	The intensive task-oriented rehabilitation protocol was effective in improving motor function and had a positive impact on quality of life in MS patients with moderate disability.
Corbetta et al. (2015)	To determine the efficacy of CIMT, modified CIMT (mCIMT), or forced use (FU) for arm management in people with hemiparesis after stroke	CIMT was effective at reducing impairments and improving arm motor function, but these benefits did not reduce disability.
French et al. (2016)	To determine if RTT improves upper limb function/reach and lower limb function/balance in adults after stroke	Low to moderate quality evidence that RTT improves upper and lower limb function with improvements sustained up to 6 months poststroke.
Nilsen et al. (2015)	To determine the effectiveness of interventions to improve occupational performance in people with motor impairments after stroke	Evidence suggests that repetitive task practice, constraint-induced or modified constraint-induced movement therapy can improve upper extremity function, balance and mobility, and/or activity and participation. Commonalities among several of the effective interventions include the use of goal-directed, individualized tasks that promote frequent repetitions of task-related or task-specific movements.
Soke et al. (2021)	To examine the effects of task-oriented circuit training combined with aerobic training (TOCT-AT) on gait, balance, functional mobility, disease severity and quality of life in patients with PD	Results suggest TOCT-AT improves balance, gait performance, functional mobility, and quality of life in patients with PD.
Wolf et al. (2010)	To compare functional improvements between stroke participants randomized to receive constraint-induced movement therapy (CI therapy) within 3–9 mo (early group) to participants randomized on recruitment to receive the identical intervention 15–21 mo after stroke (delayed group)	CI therapy can be delivered to eligible patients 3–9 mo or 15–21 mo after stroke. Both groups achieved approximately the same level of significant arm motor function 24 mo after enrollment.

CIMT, constraint-induced movement therapy; MS, multiple sclerosis; PD, parkinson disease; RTT, repetitive task training.

8. *Exercise variety*: Various exercises are offered to support motor skill learning of a certain task because of the person experiencing different movement and context characteristics (within task variety) and problem-solving strategies.
9. *Feedback*: Specific information on the patient's motor performance that enhances motor learning and positively influences patient motivation.
10. *Multiple movement planes*: Movement that uses more than one degree of freedom of a joint, therefore occurring around multiple joint axes.
11. *Patient-customized training load*: A training load that suits the individualized treatment targets (e.g., endurance, coordination, or strength training) as well as the patient's capabilities.
12. *Total skill practice*: The skill is practiced in total, with or without preceding skill component training (e.g., via chaining).
13. *Random practice*: In each practice session, the tasks are randomly ordered.
14. *Distributed practice*: A practice schedule with relatively long rest periods.
15. *Bimanual practice*: Tasks where both arms and hands are involved.

See OT Story 54.3 for a demonstration of the Task-Oriented Approach.

Occupational Therapy Task-Oriented Approach

In the early 1990s, Mathiowetz and Bass-Haugen (1994) argued for a shift away from the traditional neurophysiologic approaches that were being used in OT. They proposed the occupational therapy task-oriented approach (OT-TOT) that continues to develop (Mathiowetz, 2016; Mathiowetz & Bass-Haugen, 2008). The approach is based on current

OT STORY 54.3 JACOB: LIMITED OCCUPATIONAL PERFORMANCE DUE TO HEMIPARESIS

Jacob is an 8-year-old boy with a hemiparetic right upper limb secondary to cerebral palsy. Jacob's parents are frustrated because he has minimal movement in his arm and hand. They report constantly "nagging" Jacob to use his arm when he is outside of a structured therapy session. They also describe that his arm appears "useless" when he is at school or play. Both Jacob and his parents are getting frustrated with therapy. Specifically, his parents would like to see "carryover" from his present therapy. Jacob's occupational therapist informed the parents that there was a local therapeutic camp held during school holidays. Jacob was enrolled in this camp that incorporated an intervention called constraint-induced movement therapy (CI therapy).

The occupational therapist at the camp evaluated Jacob via observing his arm use during unstructured play in addition to two standardized assessments of motor function (the speed and dexterity subtest of the Bruininks–Oseretsky Test and the Jebsen–Taylor Test of Hand Function). Jacob's goals were established as (a) Jacob will use his right hand to drink without cues, (b) Jacob will be able to apply paste to his toothbrush using his right hand, and (c) Jacob will swing a bat using both hands.

The CI therapy intervention consisted of the following components (Gordon et al., 2005; Morris et al., 2006):

- Restraint of Jacob's less involved extremity (left) using a sling.

- Encouraging the involved side to be active via engaging Jacob in unimanual activities with the involved extremity (right) 6 hours a day for 10 days (60 hours).
- Repetitive practice embedded in play and functional activities. Examples of activities include arts and crafts, board games, card games, puzzles, cleaning a table after a meal, and so on.
- The technique of shaping was used. Shaping involves approaching a behavioral objective (task) in small steps by successive approximation. As Jacob's performance improved, the task was made more challenging, taking into consideration his abilities. The occupational therapist graded the tasks accordingly to target movements he wanted Jacob to achieve.
- Adherence-enhancing behavioral strategies ("the transfer package") such as a caregiver contract, home diary, home practice, and so on.

Following the therapy, Jacob's parents reported that he was using his involved arm more spontaneously and automatically. Jacob was able to meet his goals.

Questions

1. What are some examples of play activities that can be used to promote repetitive practice?
2. How can you assist Jacob and his family with adhering to the CIMT protocol?

understandings of motor control, recovery, and development as well as contemporary motor learning principles. Almhdawi et al. (2016) found the OT-TOT approach was effective at improving upper extremity function in stroke patients in the subacute to chronic phases of recovery.

The evaluation framework for OT-TOT includes five main areas of assessment:

1. Role performance (social participation)
2. Occupational performance tasks (areas of occupation)
3. Task selection and analysis
4. Person (client factors; performance skills and patterns)
5. Environment (context and activity demands)

Intervention principles for OT-TOT include:

- Interventions are occupation based and client focused.
- Keep clients active during treatment.
- Use natural objects and environments.
- Help patients adjust to role and task performance limitations.
- Create an environment that uses the common challenges of everyday life.

- Practice functional tasks or close simulations to find effective and efficient strategies for performance.
- Provide opportunities for practice outside of therapy time.
- Structure practice of the task to promote motor learning.
- Minimize ineffective and inefficient movement patterns.
- Remediate a client factor (impairment) if it is the critical control parameter.
- Adapt the environment, modify the task, use assistive technology, and/or reduce the effects of gravity.
- For persons with poor control of movement, constrain the degrees of freedom.
- For persons who do not use returned function in their involved extremities, use constraint-induced movement therapy (CI therapy).

Motor Relearning Program

The Motor Relearning Program (MRP; Carr & Shepherd, 1987, 2003) is specific to the rehabilitation of patients following stroke. The program is based on four factors that are thought to be essential for the learning of motor skills and assumed to be essential for the relearning of motor control: (a) elimination of unnecessary muscle activity, (b) feedback, (c) practice, and (d) the interrelationship of postural adjustment and movement. In this program, treatment is directed toward relearning of control rather than to activities incorporating exercise or to facilitation or inhibition techniques. Treatment is directed toward enhancing motor performance, and the emphasis is on the practice of specific tasks, the training of controllable muscle action, and control over the movement components of these tasks. The major assumptions about motor control underlying this approach include the following:

- In regaining motor control, learning is required. This learning follows the same principles and factors as those incurred in normal learning. Therefore, practice, receiving feedback, and understanding the goal are essential for treatment.
- Motor control is exercised in both anticipatory and ongoing modes.
- Sensory input is related to motor output and helps to modulate action.
- Control of a specific task can be effectively regained by practice of that specific motor task in various contexts.
- Conscious practice of tasks builds up awareness of the ability to elicit motor control activity.
- Progression of practice is from conscious awareness to practice at a more automatic level in order to ensure that a skill is learned.
- Cognitive function is emphasized. If the client is to learn, then the environment must encourage the learning process.

- When clients can perform a task effectively and efficiently without thinking about it in a variety of contexts, learning has occurred.
- Contemporary theories of motor control emphasize distributed control rather than a top-down or bottom-up approach. Therefore, in the Motor Relearning Program, recovery is directed to relearning control through many systems.
- The client is defined as an active participant in the treatment process. The major goal in rehabilitation is to relearn effective strategies for performing functional activities.
- The role of the therapist is to prevent the use of inefficient strategies by the client.
- The program addresses seven categories of functional daily activities: upper limb function, orofacial function, sitting up over the side of the bed, balanced sitting, standing up and sitting down, balanced standing, and walking.

A four-step sequence is followed for skill acquisition (Carr & Shepherd, 1987):

1. Analysis of the task, including observation
2. Practice of missing components, including goal identification, instruction, practice, and feedback with some manual guidance
3. Practice of the task with the addition of reevaluation and encouraging of task flexibility
4. Targets transfer of training

Randomized controlled trials comparing the MRP to the Bobath approach found that the MRP was more effective at improving ADL and ambulation (Bhalerao et al., 2013) and preventing poststroke apathy (Chen et al., 2019) in patients with acute stroke undergoing rehabilitation.

EXPANDING OUR PERSPECTIVES

Motor Function and Occupational Performance From an Asian Perspective

Asako Matsubara

There are many meaningful occupations in daily life, and motor functions are essential to perform them. Even when performing similar occupations such as ADLs, our clients use their individual abilities and instruments in different ways, in different environments. The motor functions required for such activity are greatly affected by the environment. Among common occupations, the performance of ADLs may differ little between individuals. In other occupations including IADL, work, and leisure activities, our clients may use different tools, in different ways, in different environments, with the required motor functions differing

between individuals. Occupational therapists need to be familiar with the client's environment in which the occupation is performed, as well as how the occupation is performed. The occupational therapist evaluates in detail the motor functions involved and provides the appropriate intervention.

When considering our Japanese clients' daily lives in the community after discharge, it is important to consider their residence and the environment around it. In Asian countries, especially in Japan, traditional Japanese style houses are known to have special features. For example, the "agarikamachi" is a piece of wood regularly seen at front edge of entranceway floor, and the boundaries between rooms. The floors are covered with "tatami," on to which futons are placed for sleeping. These straw-woven mats are conducive to a more traditional lifestyle in which

(continued)

⊕ **EXPANDING OUR PERSPECTIVES** (*continued*)

many ADL and body functions are performed on or close to the floor. In addition, the "Japanese Style" toilets in such traditional abodes differ from their Western counterparts, and some houses even have special toilets designed for men. The motor functions of the clients who live in such traditional places and lifestyles may differ markedly from others who abide in more modern places and lifestyles. Rather than performing common activities in a standing or upright position, the client in a traditional style home would likely perform a lot of standing-up movements from the floor, requiring specific motor functions for that purpose.

After suffering a neurological disorder such as stroke, it may become difficult for the client to live in the same (traditional) lifestyle. If so, it may be necessary to make home modifications, changing the lifestyle from Japanese style to Western style. For example, the client may have to use a bed instead of a futon. And the traditional style tatami mats may need to be replaced by Western style flooring, and steps/stairs may have to be eliminated. Furthermore, if cognitive impairments are also present, it may be difficult for the client to learn adaptive movements in a new, unfamiliar environment. However, it may be easier to perform such new tasks when they are performed in a familiar environment and by using familiar tools. Therefore, the occupational therapist needs to know the environment in detail and how their clients had performed these activities in the past. Practicing with familiar tools in the client's actual or similar environment will likely enhance the person's ability to return to and live in the community.

Motor Control and Motor Learning

Motor control is "the ability to regulate or direct the mechanisms essential to movement" (Shumway-Cook & Woollacott, 2017, p. 3), and motor control theories "describe viewpoints regarding how movement is controlled" (Shumway-Cook & Woollacott, 2017, p. 7). In contrast, **motor learning** is defined as "a set of processes associated with practice or experience leading to relatively permanent changes in the capability for skilled movement" (Schmidt & Lee, 2011, p. 327). Thus, motor learning theories describe the processes involved in motor skill acquisition, retention, and generalization. Motor learning is a key component of many of the earlier described intervention approaches. Over the years, various *motor control* and *motor learning* theories have been proposed, each with its own merit. These theories are summarized in Table 54.4.

TABLE 54.4   Summary of Motor Control and Motor Learning Theories*

Theory	Key Components of Theory
Motor Control Theories	
Reflex theory	• Stimulus-response view of motor control • Complex patterns of movement are the result of combining individual reflexes.
Hierarchical theory	• Top-down organizational control of movement with higher levels always exerting full control over lower levels
Motor programming theory	• *Central motor program* contains the "rules" for generating an action. • Program can be activated by sensory input or by central processes.
System theory	• Describes the body as a *mechanical system* that is subject to both external (e.g., gravity) and internal forces (e.g., inertial forces) • *Self-organization:* movement emerges from an interaction of multiple systems—no need for "higher centers" or "central motor program." • *Nonlinearity:* motor output is not proportional to input—variability expected and needed in the system. • *Control parameters:* a variable that regulates a change in behavior (e.g., velocity may be considered the control parameter that shifts the action of walking to running). • *Attractor states:* preferred patterns of movements that are highly stable • *Attractor wells:* the degree of flexibility to change an attractor state: *shallow well*—unstable pattern that is easy to change; *deep well*—stable pattern that is difficult to change.

TABLE 54.4	**Summary of Motor Control and Motor Learning Theories (*continued*)**
Theory	**Key Components of Theory**
Motor Control Theories	
Ecological theory	• Motor control evolved so that animals can cope with their environment: *perception–action coupling* • Gibson's theory of affordances—perception of environmental factors that are critical to the task
Motor Learning Theories	
Schmidt's schema theory	• Draws heavily on *motor programming theory* of motor control. • Emphasis on open loop control processes and the development of the *generalized motor program* (GMP), which contains the "*rules*" for creating the pattern of muscle activity needed to perform the movement. • After a movement is made there are four elements available for short-term memory storage: (a) initial movement conditions; (b) parameters used in the GMP; (c) outcome of the movement (knowledge of results); (d) sensory consequences of the movement (knowledge of performance). This information is stored as two schemas: *Recall schema* (motor) and *Recognition Schema* (sensory). • *Recall schema* is used to select a specific set of responses and the *Response schema* is used to evaluate the responses. • *Learning* occurs as a result of the updating of the two schemas each time a movement is attempted, and it is augmented by the amount of practice and variability of practice.
Ecological theory	• Draws heavily on *systems* and *ecological theories* of motor control. • During practice there is a search for *optimal strategy* to solve the task problem—search for most salient perceptual cues and optimal motor response. • *Learning* occurs as a performer searches for the optimal solution; this process strengthens perception–action coupling, and is augmented by helping the learner understand the nature of the perceptual/motor workspace, identifying the natural search strategies employed by the learner, and using augmented feedback to aid the search for the optimal solution.
Fitts and Posner three-stage model	• *Cognitive stage:* learner is figuring out what is to be done; determining appropriate strategies to complete the task. Effective strategies are maintained and ineffective ones are discarded. Performance is variable, but improvements are large. High cognitive demands are placed on the learner. The therapist uses instructions, models, feedback, etc., to assist in learning the task at hand. • *Associative stage:* learner as determined the best strategy for the task and is now refining it. Performance is less variable and improvements are slower. Cognitive demands decrease. • *Autonomous stage:* skill is performed automatically requiring little attention.
Bernstien's three-stage model	• Draws heavily on the *systems theory* of motor control and solving the *degrees of freedom* problem. • *Stage 1:* reduction in the number of degrees of freedom that must be controlled—learner will constrain the degrees of freedom and develop an *effective strategy* for task performance, but the *strategy is not energy efficient or flexible.* • *Stage 2:* release of additional degrees of freedom and muscle synergies are used across multiple joints resulting in *well-coordinated movement* that is more efficient and flexible. • *Stage 3:* release of all the degrees of freedom needed for task performance; performer has *learned to exploit external and internal forces* acting on the system to produce the most coordinated and efficient movement pattern.

(continued)

TABLE 54.4	Summary of Motor Control and Motor Learning Theories (*continued*)
Theory	**Key Components of Theory**
Motor Learning Theories	
Gentile's two-stage model	• *Initial Stage:* learner develops an understanding of the task and generates a movement pattern that enables some degree of success; key element of this stage is learning to discriminating between *regulatory features* (characteristic of environment that determine movement requirements) and *non-regulatory features* in the environment; high cognitive load. • *Later Stage:* (aka: *fixation/diversification*) learner is refining the movement so that it can be performed to meet the demands of any situation, and so that it is performed consistently and efficiently. • *Closed tasks:* environmental conditions are stable and little variability is needed—*fixation*. • *Open tasks:* environmental conditions are changing requiring multiple movement patterns—*diversification*.
OPTIMAL (Optimizing Performance Through Intrinsic Motivation and Attention for Learning) theory	• Goal-action coupling: learning is associated with structural brain changes and task-specific neural connections across brain regions (functional connectivity). • Evidence demonstrates strong motivational and attentional focus influences on motor performance and learning—enhances goal-action coupling • Key motivational variables include: enhanced expectancies for future performance (need high expectancies of success) and learner autonomy (choices and a sense of control) • External focus of attention (concentration on task goal) is critical during practice.

*No single theory accounts for all of the experimental evidence to date.

Source: Table 34-1 in Nilsen, D. M., & Gillen, G. (2020). Motor learning and task-oriented approaches. In D. Powers Dirette & S. A. Gutman (Eds.), *Occupational therapy for physical dysfunction* (8th ed., pp. 699–716). Wolters Kluwer, Lippincott, Williams, & Wilkins.

See Table 54.5 for a summary of motor learning principles that have evolved from these theories and Table 54.6 for examples of evidence that support the use of motor learning principles in clinical populations.

As our clients are learning or relearning skills, they must first acquire the skill (acquisition phase). This occurs during initial instruction on and practice of a skill or task. This usually occurs in the initial OT sessions. Following acquisition, the client must retain the skill (retention phase); this refers to *persistence of performance*. This occurs after the initial practice period, and the client is asked to demonstrate how he or she performs the newly acquired skill. Clients must then be able to transfer their performance (transfer phase). *Transfer of learning* refers to the gain in capability for performance in one task as a result of practice on another task. The individual can use the skill in a new context. Our clients can generalize the strategies learned in the therapy setting and use them in real-life situations (Sabari, 2016; Schmidt et al., 2019; Figure 54.3).

Sabari (2016) summarized the literature about skill acquisition and therapeutic interventions that promote generalization of learning. These concepts can be categorized into three major groups: type of feedback, development of underlying strategies, and practice conditions (Figure 54.4).

An Overview of Motor Development

Motor development is a process during which a person acquires skills and movement patterns. Malina (2004) has described motor development as a continuous process of modification that involves the interaction of several factors:

1. Neuromuscular maturation;
2. The physical growth and behavioral characteristics of the child;
3. The tempo of physical growth, biological maturation, and behavioral development;
4. The residual effects of prior movement experiences;
5. The new movement experiences. (p. 50)

Although many consider motor development a process specific to children, it is in fact a lifelong process

TABLE 54.5   Summary of Motor Learning Principles

Principles/Consideration	Example
Stage of the Learner: How Practice is Structured is Dependent on the Stage of the Learner	
• Early stages of learning: focus is on understanding the action goal in a functionally relevant context, identifying key regulatory features in the environment, and attempting to generate a movement strategy that leads to goal attainment. • Later stages of learning: focus is on developing skill; cognitive demands are lower; the general movement strategy is refined through practice so that there is consistency in goal attainment and efficiency in the movement.	• During retraining of drinking from a cup, the therapist uses a cup filled with a desired beverage and makes sure the patient is aware of the task goal (i.e., drinking a cup of coffee using their right hand); prior to initiating an attempt to drink from the cup the therapist asks the patient to describe the size, shape, and weight of the cup, as well as its location on the table surface. The therapist then models the performance of the activity for the patient and asks to patient to perform the task. Feedback is provided (see below) and task attempts are repeated. • During retraining of drinking from a cup, the therapist now uses multiple types of cups that are placed in various locations on the table surface and the patient is encouraged to practice drinking from the various cups. Feedback is provided as needed (see below).
Task Specificity: Learning is Contingent on the Type of Task Being Learned	
• Discrete tasks: tasks with a recognizable beginning and end. • Continuous tasks: tasks without a recognizable beginning or end; the task is performed until arbitrarily stopped • Serial tasks: tasks that contain a series of movements linked together to make a "whole" • Closed tasks: performed in predictable and stable environments; movements can be planned in advance. • Open tasks: performed in constantly changing environments that may be unpredictable. • Variable motionless tasks: involve interacting with a stable and predictable environment, but specific features of the environment are likely to vary between performance trials. • Consistent motion tasks: involve interacting with environmental features that are in motion, but the motion is consistent and predictable between trials	• Kicking a ball, pushing a button, standing up from a chair, writing your name • Walking, swimming, driving • Playing an instrument, dressing, making a sandwich, lighting a fire • Oral care, signing a check, bowling • Driving in traffic, walking down a busy street, playing a game of soccer. • Performing ADLs outside of the home environment • Stepping onto an escalator, assembly line work, retrieving luggage from an airport carousel
Feedback: Information Learners Receive About Their Attempts to Learn a Skill Can Enhance Learning	
• Inherent (intrinsic) feedback: information that is normally received during performance of a task. • Augmented (extrinsic) feedback: information about task or motor performance that is fed back to the patient by artificial means; supplements intrinsic feedback (can be verbal or non-verbal) • Concurrent feedback: information that is provided during task performance. • Terminal feedback: information that is provided after task performance. • Immediate feedback: information that is provided immediately after performance. • Delayed feedback: information provided is delayed by some amount of time. • Accumulated feedback: information that represents an accumulation of past performance. • Distinct feedback: information that represents each performance separately. • Knowledge of results: information about the outcome of the task performance. • Knowledge of performance: information about the nature of the task performance.	• Seeing and feeling water spill from a cup as you are attempting to drink. • Therapist provides verbal information to a patient: "you need to lock your wheelchair breaks before standing up" or non-verbal information (e.g., using a mirror to show the patient their sitting posture). • While the patient is reaching for the toothpaste the therapist says, "Don't hike your shoulder." • After the patient reaches for the cup the therapist says, "You didn't open your hand wide enough." • Right after the patient attempts a tub transfer the therapist says, "That was perfect." • At the end of the day the therapist says to the patient, "Your transfers were better today, keep checking your wheelchair brakes." • The therapist says, "Your feet were placed perfectly during 3 out of 5 of your transfers today." • The therapist says, "Your feet were placed perfectly during that transfer." • The therapist says, "Your shirt is on backwards." or "You dropped the cup." • The therapist says, "Next time dress your right arm first." or "Your elbow was bent."

(continued)

TABLE 54.5	**Summary of Motor Learning Principles** (*continued*)	

Principles/Consideration	Example
Practice Variables: Learning is Contingent on the Amount and Type of Practice Provided	
<ul><li>External focus of attention: learner's attention is directed outside the body to an object or environmental goal.</li><li>Internal focus of attention: learner's attention is direct inward toward body movements.</li><li>Massed practice: practice time is greater than rest time.</li><li>Distributed practice: practice time is equal to or less than rest time.</li><li>Blocked practice: repetitive practice of the same task, uninterrupted by practice of other tasks.</li><li>Random practice: tasks being practiced are ordered randomly; attempt multiple tasks or variations of a task before mastering any one of the tasks.</li><li>Whole practice: task is practiced in its entirety and not broken into parts.</li><li>Part practice: task is broken down into its parts for separate practice.</li><li>Motivational influences:<ul><li>Enhancing learner's expectancy of success; practice conditions that enhance self-efficacy or confidence enhance learning.</li><li>Autonomy: giving the learner control over certain aspects of practice conditions enhances learning.</li></ul></li></ul>	<ul><li>Therapist instructs the patient to focus on keeping their cup straight prior to practicing the task of drinking.</li><li>Therapist instructs the patient focus on their wrist position prior to practicing the task of drinking.</li><li>Patient practices the task of typing on a computer for 15 minutes, takes a brief rest for 2 minutes, and then practices typing again for 15 minutes.</li><li>Patient practices transferring to and from a commode for 10 minutes, takes a rest for 10 minutes and then practices transferring again for 10 minutes.</li><li>Patient practices moving from sit to stand multiple times in a row. Practice sequence of tasks "A," "B," and "C": AAAAABBBBBBBCCCCC.</li><li>Patient practices transferring to multiple surfaces (couch, toilet, bench, chair, stool, car) in one occupational therapy session. Practice sequence of tasks "A," "B," and "C": ACBACABCCBACABCACABBACCACB.</li><li>Practicing dressing</li><li>Don/doff shirt.</li><li>Therapist sets up a just-right-challenge task, highlights the learnability of the task and provides information that helps reduce the perceived difficulty of the task.</li><li>Therapist provides the patient with choices over tasks to be practiced, when feedback is provided, or choices over irrelevant aspects of the task (e.g., color of a cup).</li></ul>

Source: Table 34-2 in: Nilsen, D. M., & Gillen, G. (2020). Motor learning and task-oriented approaches. In D. Powers Dirette & S. A. Gutman (Eds.), *Occupational therapy for physical dysfunction* (8th ed., pp. 699–716). Wolters Kluwer, Lippincott, Williams, & Wilkins.

TABLE 54.6	**Sample Evidence That Supports Motor Learning–Based Interventions**	

Author/Year	Objective	Conclusion
Bhalerao et al. (2013)	To compare the effectiveness of MRP versus Bobath approach on activities of daily living (ADLs) and ambulation at every in acute stroke rehabilitation	MRP is significantly more effective than Bobath approach in early enhancement of ADL and ambulation after stroke.
Bar-Haim et al. (2010)	To evaluate effectiveness of motor learning coaching on retention and transfer of gross motor function in children with cerebral palsy	In higher functioning children with cerebral palsy, the motor learning coaching treatment resulted in significantly greater retention of gross motor function and transfer of mobility performance to unstructured environments than neurodevelopmental treatment.
Chen et al. (2019)	To compare the MRP to Bobath concept on preventing the onset of poststroke apathy	Motor Relearning program was significantly more effective in preventing new onset of apathy following stroke compared with Bobath approach.
Sidaway et al. (2016)	To examine the effects of blocked versus random practice conditions on the learning of a fine motor control task (peg sequencing) in individuals with PD	Overall, the results showed that the random practice schedule lead to enhance retention and transfer of the peg sequencing task.
Subramanian et al. (2010)	To determine if the provision of extrinsic feedback results in improved motor learning in the upper limb poststroke	The author's systematic review "found strong evidence supporting the provision of explicit feedback for implicit motor learning in the upper limb of stroke survivors." The results suggest that "stroke survivors are able to use explicit feedback and preserve motor learning abilities despite having underlying upper limb motor control deficits. An important consideration is that the ability to use explicit feedback applies to both the less- and more-affected sides" (p. 121).

MRP, Motor Relearning Program; PD, parkinson disease.

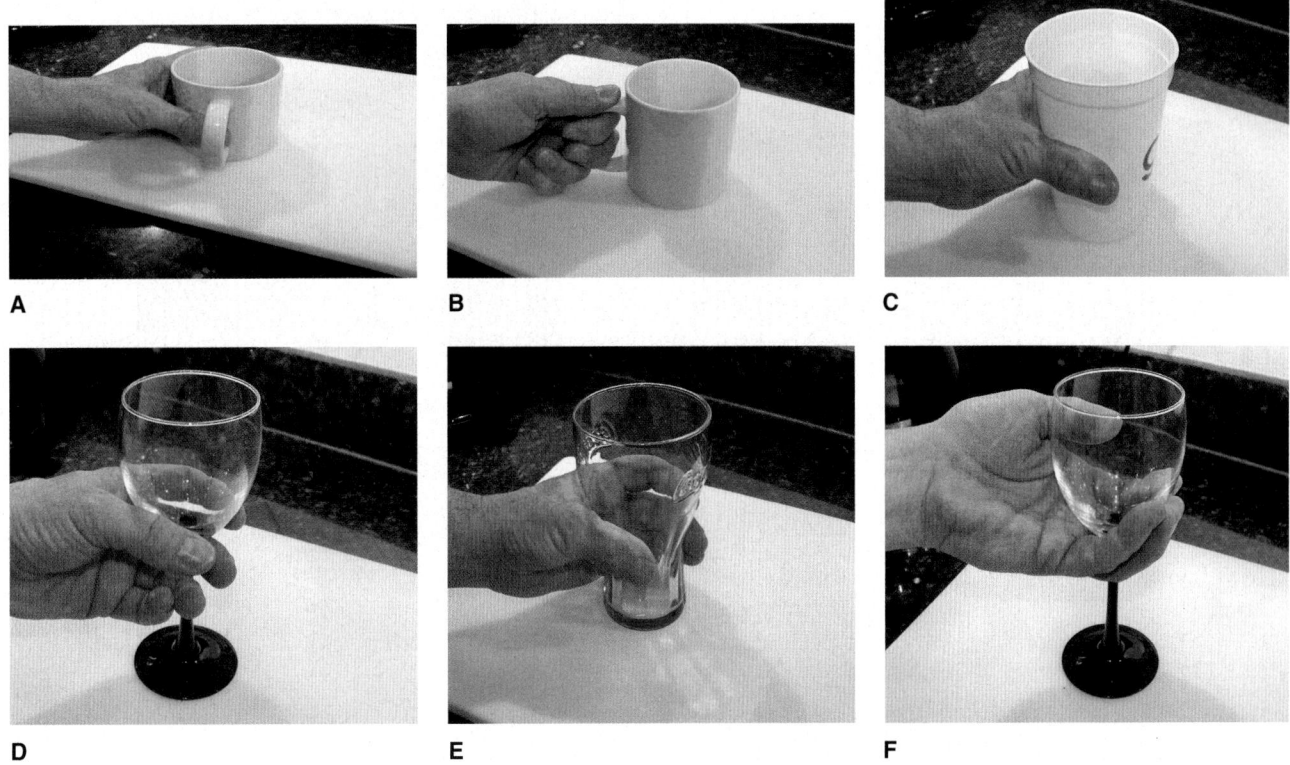

FIGURE 54.3 Variability in practice promotes both generalization and learning.

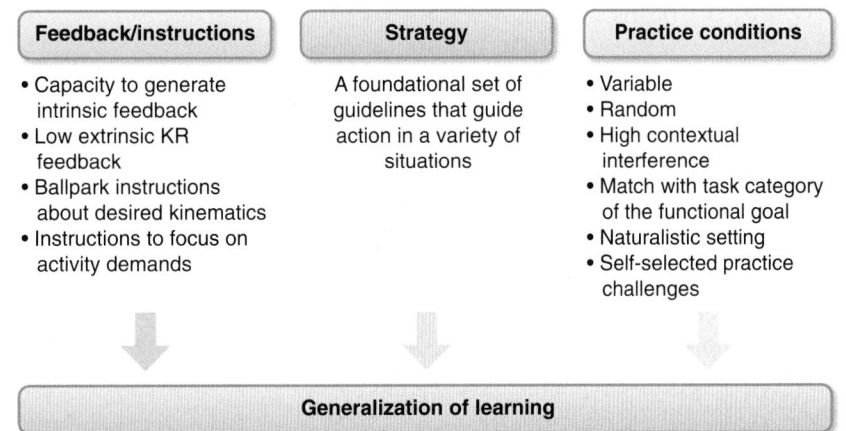

FIGURE 54.4 Factors that contribute to generalization of learning. *KR,* knowledge of results.

(Reprinted with permission from Sabari, J. [2016]. Activity-based interventions in stroke rehabilitation. In G. Gillen [Ed.], *Stroke rehabilitation a function-based approach* [3rd ed., p. 8099]. Mosby.)

that should be considered from a life course perspective. Typical developmental changes that occur in infancy and childhood are considered positive when milestones are met and new skills are acquired (Figure 54.5). Maximum performance may be reached in adolescence and adulthood. As the aging process continues, there comes a decline in performance with loss of speed, accuracy, and precision of movement. That being said, "a progression

to regression" of skills description of motor development may not be completely accurate. Older adults have the potential to acquire quite intricate new motor skills as well. Think of older adults in your life who have mastered new leisure activities such as knitting, paddle boarding, or ballroom dancing.

Although neurodevelopment follows a predictable course, it is important to understand that intrinsic and

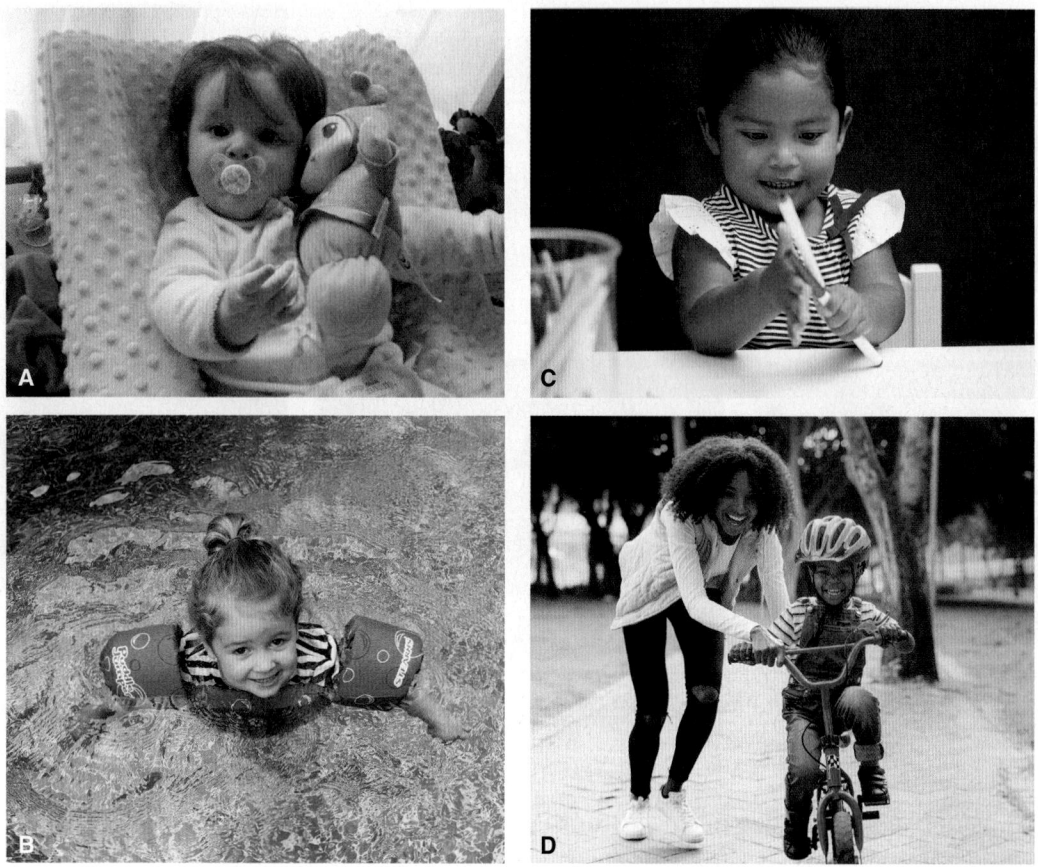

FIGURE 54.5 **Development of motor control.**

extrinsic forces produce individual variation, making each child's developmental path unique. Intrinsic influences include genetically determined attributes (e.g., physical characteristics, temperament) as well as the child's overall state of wellness. Extrinsic influences during infancy and childhood originate primarily from the family. Parent and sibling personalities, the nurturing methods used by caregivers, the cultural environment, and the family's socioeconomic status with its effect on resources of time and money all play a role in the development of children. Developmental theory has, itself, developed as clinicians have

tried to grapple with which influence is more predominant (Gerber et al., 2010, p. 267).

Although there is a typical order of motor development that is commonly discussed and described (Table 54.7), it is important to remember that individuals may achieve their developmental milestones in various orders, may skip a milestone step, may achieve them within different time periods (Figure 54.6), and so on. For example, Gerber et al. (2010) note that crawling is not a prerequisite to walking; pulling to stand is the skill infants must develop before they take their first steps.

TABLE 54.7 **Examples of Developmental Motor Milestones**

Age	Gross Motor	Fine Motor
1 mo	Chin up in prone position Turns head in supine position	Keeps hands fisted near face
2 mo	Can hold head up and begins to push up when lying prone Makes smoother movements with arms and legs	Hands not fisted 50% of the time Retains rattle if placed in hand Holds hands together
4 mo	Holds head steady, unsupported Pushes down on legs when feet are on a hard surface May be able to roll over from prone to supine Brings hands to mouth. When lying on stomach, pushes up to elbows	Hands held predominately open Clutches at clothes Reaches persistently Can hold a toy and shake it and swing at dangling toys

TABLE 54.7	Examples of Developmental Motor Milestones (*continued*)	
Age	**Gross Motor**	**Fine Motor**
6 mo	Rolls from tummy to back Pushes up with straight arms when on tummy When sitting, leans on hand for support	
9 mo	Can get into sitting position Sits without support Crawls	Transfers hand to hand Rakes food
1 yr	Pulls up to stand Walks holding on to furniture ("cruising")	• Drinks from a cup without a lid, as you hold it • Picks things up between thumb and pointer finger, like small bits of food
18 mo	Walks alone • Climbs on and off a couch or chair without help	Drinks from a cup without lid (may spill) Tries to eat with a spoon Finger feeds Scribbles
2 yrs	• Kicks a ball • Runs • Walks (not climbs) up a few stairs with or without help	Eats with a spoon
3 yrs	• Puts on some clothes by himself, like loose pants or a jacket	Strings large items Uses a fork
4 yrs	• Catches a large ball most of the time • Serves himself food or pours water, with adult supervision	• Unbuttons some buttons • Holds crayon or pencil between fingers and thumb (not a fist)
5 yrs	Hops on one foot	Buttons some buttons

Data from Centers for Disease Control and Prevention. (2022). *Learn the signs. Act early.* https://www.cdc.gov/ncbddd/actearly/index.html; and Zubler, J. M., Wiggins, L. D., Macias, M. M., Whitaker, T. M., Shaw, J. S., Squires, J. K., Pajek, J. A., Wolf, R. B., Slaughter, K.S., Broughton, A. S., Gerndt, K. L., Mlodoch, B. J., & Lipkin, P. H. (2022). Evidence-informed milestones for developmental surveillance tools. *Pediatrics, 149*(3), e2021052138. https://doi.org/10.1542/peds.2021-052138

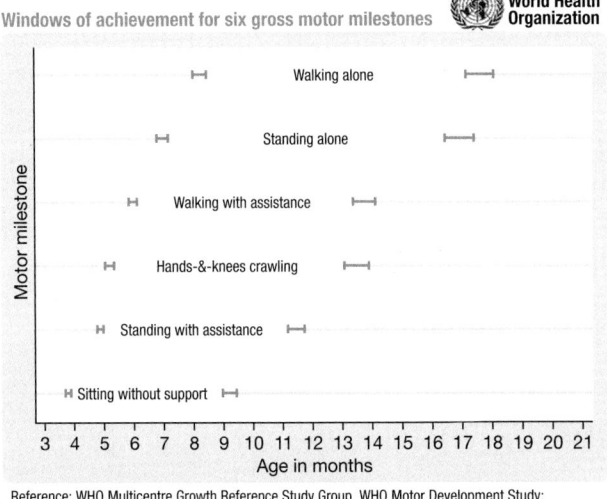

FIGURE 54.6 **Windows of achievement for six gross motor milestones.**

It is of critical importance that therapists and parents are aware of the warning signs that indicate delays in motor development. Gerber et al. (2010) discuss three key "red flags":

1. Lack of steady head control at 4 months while sitting
2. Inability to sit by 9 months
3. Inability to walk by 18 months

As will be discussed next, there are various standardized tools that occupational therapists can use to monitor motor development.

Evaluation and Assessment of Motor Function

Many tools and procedures are available to document our client's level of motor function. These include developmental assessments, neurological screening methods, self-report measures, assessments of postural control, assessments of limb function, and assessments performed in natural contexts. The following paragraphs and Table 54.8 give examples of each.

Developmental Assessments

These tools are used to assess the development and capability of functional skills in children. The assessments in this category consist of screening instruments, criterion-referenced

TABLE 54.8 **Standardized Assessments of Motor Function**

Assessment	Areas of Occupation			Client Factors		
	Activity	Participation	Quality of Life	Body Structures and Functions	Values, Beliefs, and Spirituality	Performance Skills
ABILHAND Questionnaire and ABILHAND-Kids	X					
Action Research Arm Test				X		X
Activities-Specific Balance Confidence (ABC) Scale	X					
Arm Motor Ability Test	X					
Ashworth Scale				X		
Assessment of Motor and Process Skills	X	X				X
Assisting Hand Assessment	X					X
Bayley Scales of Infant Development, Second Edition				X		X
Bennett Hand-Tool Dexterity Test	X					X
Berg Balance Scale (adult and pediatric versions)	X			X		X
Box and Block Test				X		X
Bruininks-Oseretsky Test of Motor Proficiency, Second Edition	X			X		
Chedoke Arm and Hand Activity Inventory	X					
Clinical Observations of Motor and Postural Skills-Second Edition				X		
Complete Minnesota Dexterity Test				X		X
Crawford Small Parts Dexterity Test				X		X
Disabilities of the Arm, Shoulder, and Hand (DASH)	X	X				
Dynamometry				X		
Erhardt Developmental Prehension Assessment	X					X
Evaluation Tool of Children's Handwriting	X					X
FirstSTEp: Screening Test for Evaluating Preschoolers	X			X		
Frenchay Arm Test	X					X
Functional Upper Extremity Levels (FUEL)	X					X
Fugl-Meyer Sensorimotor Assessment				X		
Functional Reach Test and Multi-Directional Functional Reach Test						X
Goniometry				X		
Grooved Pegboard Test				X		
Gross Motor Function Measure	X					
Infant Neurological International Battery (INFANIB)				X		

| TABLE 54.8 | **Standardized Assessments of Motor Function (*continued*)** |

Assessment	Areas of Occupation		Client Factors			
	Activity	Participation	Quality of Life	Body Structures and Functions	Values, Beliefs, and Spirituality	Performance Skills
Jebsen-Taylor Test of Hand Function	X					
Manual Ability Measure	X					
Manual Muscle Testing				X		
Melbourne Assessment of Unilateral Upper Limb Function	X					X
Miller Assessment for Preschoolers	X			X		
Miller Function and Participation Scales	X	X		X		
Minnesota Rate of Manipulation Test				X		
Modified Ashworth Scale				X		
Motor Activity Log (adult and pediatric versions)	X					
Motor Assessment Scale	X			X		X
Motricity Index			X			X
Movement Assessment Battery for Children (Movement ABC)				X		X
National Institutes of Health (NIH) Pain Scales				X		
Nine-Hole Peg Test				X		
O'Connor Dexterity Tests				X		X
Peabody Developmental Motor Scales, Second Edition				X		X
Pediatric Evaluation of Disability Inventory	X	X				
Postural Assessment Scale for Stroke Patients	X					
Purdue Pegboard Test				X		
Quick Neurological Screening Test (QNST)				X		
Reflex Testing				X		
Rivermead Motor Assessment	X			X		
Sensory Organization Test				X		
School Assessment of Motor and Process Skills	X	X				X
School Function Assessment	X	X				
Tardieu Scale				X		
Tinetti Balance and Gait Evaluation	X			X		
Timed Up and Go Test	X					
Trunk Control Test	X					
Upper Extremity Performance Test for the Elderly or *Test d'Evaluation des Membres Supérieurs de Personnes Agées* (TEMPA)	X					
Wolf Motor Function Test	X					X

See Appendix II for more details related to these tools.

measures, rating scales, and norm-referenced measures, some of which can be completed by a teacher or caregiver or through direct interaction with the child being assessed.

The Pediatric Evaluation of Disability Inventory (PEDI) examines three categories: self-care, mobility, and social function. This test is designed for use with children, ages 6 months to 7 years, who have various disabilities that result in functional problems. The PEDI is standardized on a normative sample; therefore, one can calculate both standard and scaled performance scores. The PEDI provides resources to assess a child on three different measurement scales. The first, Functional Skills, establishes the ability of the child to complete discrete functional skills. The Caregiver Assessment scale determines the amount of assistance that the child is provided with during complex functional skills. And finally, the Modification Skills scale assesses what types of modifications the child requires to complete and support his or her function. The scales can be used concurrently or independently of one another depending on the domain of interest for each individual child (Haley et al., 1992).

The Peabody Gross Motor Scale (2nd edition) compares fine and gross motor skills to normally developing children ages 0 to 5 years. There are 170 activities that are assessed regarding reflexes, stationary skills, locomotion, object manipulation, grasping, and visual motor integration. Results from these subtests are used to generate the three composite scores: Gross Motor Quotient, Fine Motor Quotient, and Total Motor Quotient. Scores are presented as percentiles, standard scores, and age equivalents. Norms, based on a nationally representative sample of more than 2,000 children, are stratified by age (Folio & Fewell, 2000).

The Erhardt Developmental Prehension Assessment was designed to measure components of arm and hand development in children of all ages and cognitive levels who have cerebral palsy, multiple disabilities, and developmental delays. It can be used to identify intervention needs, modify programs with ongoing assessment, and provide accountability with retesting. Three hundred forty-one items are divided into three sections: (a) positional-reflexive: involuntary arm–hand patterns; (b) cognitively directed: voluntary movements of approach, grasp, manipulation, and release; and (c) prewriting skills: pencil grasp and drawing (Erhardt, 1994).

Neurological Screening Methods

Various procedures are used to document the presence of atypical motor performance and movements associated with neurological damage. These screening procedures related to motor function are outlined in Table 54.9.

TABLE 54.9 **Neurological Damage, Typical Clinical Signs, and Associated Assessments**

Category	Description	Test
Lower Motor Neuron Dysfunction		
Weakness and eventual muscle atrophy (wasting)	• Weakness of individual muscles; atrophy can be observed during visual inspection.	Assessed by asking patient to perform voluntary movements; Manual muscle testing and visual inspection/palpation
Fibrillations or fasciculation	• Spontaneous twitches due to involuntary contractions of one motor unit (fibrillation) or groups of motor units (fasciculation)	Visual inspection can be used to note the presence of fasciculation (observed as a flicker of movement under the skin.
Hypotonia	• Decreased involuntary resistance of a muscle to passive stretch	Assessed by passively moving the limb (e.g., to assess the muscle tone of the biceps the elbow would be passively extended)
Hyporeflexia or areflexia	• Weak (hypo) or absent (areflexia) deep tendon reflexes	Assessed by eliciting deep tendon reflexes by properly positioning the patient, palpating a muscle tendon, and tapping the muscle tendon briskly with a reflex hammer
Upper Motor Neuron Dysfunction		
Weakness (paresis) or paralysis (plegia)	Weakness or paralysis of groups of muscles. • Mono (paresis/plegia): impacts one limb • Hemi (paresis/plegia): impacts one side of the body • Para (paresis/plegia): impacts lower limbs • Tetra/Quad: impacts all four limbs	Assessed by asking patient to perform voluntary movements; Manual muscle testing and visual inspection/palpation.
Hypertonia/Spasticity	• Hypertonia: increased involuntary resistance of a muscle to passive stretch • Spasticity is a velocity-dependent increase in the stretch reflex coupled with an exaggeration of deep tendon reflexes.	Assessed by passively moving the limb (e.g., to assess the muscle tone of the biceps the elbow would be passively extended); MASS

TABLE 54.9	**Neurological Damage, Typical Clinical Signs, and Associated Assessments** (*continued*)	

Category	Description	Test
Hyperreflexia	• Overactive deep tendon reflexes	Assessed by eliciting deep tendon reflexes by properly positioning the patient, palpating a muscle tendon, and tapping the muscle tendon briskly with a reflex hammer
Babinski sign	• Dorsiflexion of the great toe and outward fanning of the rest of the toes in response to firm stroking along the lateral aspect of the foot's sole	Assessed by placing patient in a supine or long sitting position. Therapist supports the patient's foot in neutral and applies stimulation to the plantar aspect of the foot, typically moving lateral to medial from the heel to the metatarsals, with the blunt end of a reflex hammer.
Cerebellar Dysfunction		
Intention tremor	• Occurs during voluntary movement, is less apparent or absent during rest, and intensifies at the termination of the movement • Evident in multiple sclerosis.	• Finger-to-finger test, finger-to-nose test • May have trouble performing tasks that require accuracy and precision of limb placement (e.g., drinking from a cup or inserting a key in a lock)
Essential familial tremor	• Inherited as an autosomal-dominant trait, visible when client is carrying out a fine precision and accuracy task	• Have the person reach for an item. Positive if tremors are present during the reach.
Dysdiadochokinesia	• Decreased ability to perform rapid alternating movements smoothly	• Supinate/pronate, flex/extend elbow, grasp/release hand, alternating bilateral tasks. Number of alternations within a time period and the differences between extremities are noted.
Dysmetria	• Inability to control muscle length results in overshooting when pointing to target objects. • Inability to estimate range of motion necessary to reach a target. Two types include hypermetria (overshoot) and hypometria (undershoot).	• Finger-to-finger or finger-to-nose tests
Dyssynergia	• Movements are broken up into their component parts and appear jerky. Jerky movements are due to lack of synergy between agonist/antagonist. • Can cause problems in articulation and phonation	• Alternating movement, finger-to-nose, finger-to-finger tests
Ataxia	• Delayed initiation of movement responses, errors in range and force of movement, errors in rate and regularity of movement. Poor agonist/antagonist coordination, results in jerky, poorly controlled movements, poor postural stability	• When reaching for object, shortest distance between the client and object is not a straight line.
Ataxic gait	• Unsteady, wide-based gait, tendency to veer or fall toward side of lesion • Staggering, wide-based gait with reduced or no arm swing, uneven step length and tendency to fall	• Observation of walking, turning quickly, walking toe to heel along straight line
Rebound phenomenon of Holmes	• Lack of a check reflex • Inability to stop a motion quickly to avoid striking something	• Therapist releases resistance to client's elbow flexion unexpectedly; client's hand hits his or her own chest if unable to check motion.
Hypotonia	• Decreased muscle tone, decreased resistance to passive movement	• Can observe clinically and perform a quick stretch
Nystagmus	• Involuntary (oscillating) movement of eyes. Interferes with head control and balance. Can occur as result of vestibular system, brainstem, or cerebellar lesions	• Can observe by having the person look at a fixed object. Is positive if the eyes make small rapid oscillations (tremor-like movements)

(continued)

TABLE 54.9	Neurological Damage, Typical Clinical Signs, and Associated Assessments (*continued*)	
Category	**Description**	**Test**
Dysarthria	• Explosive or slurred speech caused by incoordination of the speech mechanism • Speech may vary in pitch, seem nasal or tremulous.	• Can observe if ability to articulate words due to the oral-motor and/or larynx musculature. This is a motor problem, not due to aphasia.
Posterior Column Dysfunction		
Ataxia	• Wide-based gait results from loss of proprioception, but client can self-correct using vision by watching their feet (compare with cerebellar dysfunction).	• Can observe in any part of the body. Is characterized by "large" tremors
Romberg sign	• Inability to maintain standing balance with feet together and eyes closed	• The test is the same as the definition.
Basal Ganglia Dysfunction		
Athetoid movements	• Continuous, slow, wormlike, arrhythmic movements that primarily affect the distal portions of the extremities. Occur in the same patterns in the same subject, not present during sleep. Co-occurrence with athetosis = choreoathetosis	• Therapist should note proximal or distal involvement extremities involved, pattern of motions, and which stimuli increase/decrease abnormal movements. Its occurrence can be documented through observation.
Dystonia	• A form of athetosis that causes twisting movements of the trunk and proximal muscles of the extremities, distorted postures, and torsion spasms. • Persistent posturing of the extremities (e.g., hyperextension or hyperflexion of the wrist and fingers) often with concurrent torsion of the spine and twisting of the trunk Movements are often continuous and seen in conjunction with spasticity. Subtypes included segmental, generalized, focal, and multifocal.	• Its occurrence can be documented through observation.
Chorea	• Irregular, purposeless, involuntary, coarse, quick, jerky, and dysrhythmic movements of variable distribution. May occur in sleep	• Its occurrence can be documented through observation.
Ballism	• A rare symptom produced by continuous, abrupt contraction of axial and proximal musculature of the extremity. Causes the limb to fly out suddenly. Occurs on one side (hemiballism) and is caused by lesions of the opposite subthalamic nucleus	• Its occurrence can be documented through observation.
Resting tremors	• Stop at the initiation of voluntary movement, resume during holding phase of motor task (e.g., pill rolling tremor of Parkinsonism). • Occurs at rest and subsides when voluntary movement is attempted. Seen in Parkinson's disease	• Have the person reach for an item. Positive if tremors are present before initiation of the reach but stop when the reach begins.
Bradykinesia	• Movement is very slow or even nonexistent (akinesia), with accompanying rigidity.	• Ask the person to move; on attempting to move, the person's motions are extremely slow, if at all. Tone appears to be high.

MASS, modified ashworth spasticity scale.

Sources: Data from Giuffrida, C. G., & Rice, M. S. (2008). Motor skills and occupational performance: Assessments and interventions. In E. B. Crepeau, E. S. Cohn, & B. A. B. Schell (Eds.), *Willard & Spackman's occupational therapy* (11th ed., pp. 658–680). Lippincott Williams & Wilkins; and Nilsen, D. M., & Gillen, G. (2020). Motor control assessment. In D. Powers Dirette & S. A. Gutman (Eds.), *Occupational therapy for physical dysfunction* (8th ed., pp. 290–310). Wolters Kluwer, Lippincott, Williams, & Wilkins.

Self-Report Measures

Several measures are available that allow clients to report their level of motor function. The Disabilities of the Arm, Shoulder, and Hand (DASH), as described in OT Story 54.1, is an example of this level of measurement that is typically used by therapists. The Motor Activity Log is also a self-report questionnaire (report by patient or family) related to actual use of the involved upper extremity outside of structured therapy time. It uses a semistructured interview format. Quality of movement ("How well" scale) and amount of use ("How much" scale) are graded on a 6-point scale. At present, there are 30-, 28-, and 14-item versions of the tool. Sample items include hold book, use a towel, pick up a glass, write/type, steady myself, and so on (Uswatte et al., 2005). The Pediatric Motor Activity Log is a structured interview intended to examine how often and how well a child uses his or her involved upper extremity in his or her natural environment outside the therapeutic setting. The child's primary caregiver is asked standardized questions about the amount of use of the child's involved arm and the quality of the child's movement during the functional activities specified in the instrument (e.g., point to a picture, turn pages in a book; Uswatte et al., 2012; Wallen et al., 2009).

The 36-item Manual Ability Measure (MAM-36) is a Rasch-developed, self-report disability outcome measure. It contains 36 gender-neutral, commonly performed everyday hand tasks. The patient is asked to report the ease or difficulty of performing such items. It uses a 4-point rating scale, with 1 indicating *unable* ("I am unable to do the task all by myself"), 2 indicating *very hard* ("It is very hard for me to do the task and I usually ask others to do it for me unless no one is around"), 3 indicating *a little hard* ("I usually do the task myself, although it takes longer or more effort now than before"), and 4 indicating *easy* ("I can do the task without any problem"). Item examples include zip a jacket, turn a key, and take things/cards out of a wallet. The MAM-36 can be accessed (Chen et al., 2007). A lookup table from raw scores to converted 0 to 100 Rasch measures is available (Chen & Bode, 2009).

The ABILHAND questionnaire asks clients to use a 3-point scale (0 = *impossible*, 1 = *difficult*, 2 = *easy*) to rate how difficult it would be to complete 23 bimanual activities (e.g., hammering a nail, wrapping a gift, thread a needle, file nails, cut meat, peel onions, open jar; Penta et al., 2001). The ABILHAND-Kids is comprised of 21 mainly bimanual daily activities. The difficulty experienced by the child to perform the required tasks is scored on a 3-point ordinal scale (Arnould et al., 2004).

Assessments of Postural Control

Various postural control measures are available based on client status. Examples follow. The Trunk Control Test examines four functional movements: roll from supine to the weak side, roll from supine to the strong side, sitting up from supine, and sitting on the edge of the bed for 30 seconds (feet off the ground). Each task is scored as follows: 0, unable to perform with assistance; 12, able to perform but in an abnormal manner; and 25, able to complete movement normally. The range of scores is 0 to 100 (Collin & Wade, 1990).

The Postural Assessment Scale for Stroke Patients contains 12 four-point items graded from 0 to 3 (Benaim et al., 1999). Higher scores indicate better performance. Items include sitting without support, standing with and without support, standing on the nonparetic leg, standing on the paretic leg, supine to affected side, supine to unaffected side, supine to sit, sit to supine, sit to stand, stand to sit, and standing and picking up a pencil from the floor.

The Berg Balance Scale (BBS) was developed to measure balance among older people with impairment in balance function by assessing the performance of functional tasks. It is a valid instrument used for evaluation of the effectiveness of interventions and for quantitative descriptions of function in clinical practice and research. It includes 14 items such as sit to stand, transfers, and retrieving an object from the floor (Berg et al., 1989).

Assessments of Limb Function

Assessments of limb function are usually composed of items that are best described as simulated ADL or movements that mimic those required to engage in daily activities. The Fugl-Meyer Upper Extremity subscale (FM-UE; Fugl-Meyer et al., 1975) has been used to reliably measure change in the upper extremity in a variety of stroke motor intervention trials (Bushnell et al., 2015). It assesses movement of the upper extremity via the performance of 33 tasks. Performance of each task is rated on a 3-point ordinal scale from 0 (cannot perform) to 2 (performs fully). Velozo and Woodbury (2011) developed a key form recovery map for use with the FM-UE. Recording patient responses to the standardized items on the form allows the therapist to quickly see what items the patient is struggling with. This information can then be used to tailor upper extremity training to the specific needs of the patient. In addition, minimally clinically important differences (MCID) have been established for the FM-UE for people with stroke across various stages of recovery (Arya et al., 2011; S. J. Page, Fulk, & Boyne, 2012; Shelton et al., 2001).

The Arm Motor Ability Test has been used to determine the effectiveness of interventions and includes 13 unilateral and bilateral tasks. Sample items include tying a shoe, opening a jar, wiping up spilled water, using a light switch, using utensils, and drinking. The therapist times task performance and rates movement quality on a 6-point scale. The test is appropriate for evaluating motor skills in high-level clients with active wrist and finger extension (Kopp et al., 1997).

The Wolf Motor Function Test has been used to document the outcomes related to CI therapy and other interventions and includes various tasks such as basic reaching tasks (e.g., lifting arm from lap to table, extending elbow with and without a weight attached) as well as more functional activities that involve fine motor control (e.g., picking up a pencil, turning a key in a lock). All tasks but one are unilateral and appropriate for both the dominant and nondominant arms. Because many tasks do not require distal control, it is appropriate for people with a more involved upper extremity. The therapist times task performance and qualitatively grades movement (Wolf et al., 2001).

The Jebsen-Taylor Test of Hand Function includes the performance of seven test activities: writing a short sentence, turning over index cards, picking up small objects and placing them in a container, stacking checkers, simulating eating, moving empty large cans, and moving weighted large cans during timed trials. The original paper is based on data collected from 360 normal subjects and patients, including patients with hemiparesis resulting from a stroke. The mean times and standard deviations for normal subjects (with their dominant and nondominant hand) are published in the paper. The test is standardized and reliable and does not have a practice effect. Therapists must be aware that some of the tasks are simulated activities, and some tasks cannot be considered ADL tasks (Jebsen et al., 1969).

The Melbourne Assessment of Unilateral Upper Limb Function measures quality of unilateral upper limb movement in children with neurological conditions aged 5 to 15 years. The assessment is designed to provide general information about levels of ability/disability rather than specific diagnostic information. The tool consists of 16 items that involve reach, grasp, release, and manipulation. A child's performance is recorded on videotape for subsequent scoring. Each test item has an individual scoring system so that various aspects of the movement can be considered such as range of movement, accuracy of reach and placement, fluency of reach and release, and developmental level of grasp. The test items and scoring system aim to be representative of the most important components of upper limb function (Randall et al., 1999).

The Assisting Hand Assessment (Krumlinde-Sundholm & Eliasson, 2003) examines how effectively a child actually uses a hemiplegic hand in bimanual activities. The spontaneous use is evaluated during a semistructured play session with toys requiring bimanual handling. The items that are scored include general use, arm use, grasp and release, fine motor adjustments, and coordination and pace. All items are scored from 0 (*does not do*) to 4 (*effective use*).

Assessments Performed in Natural Contexts

There are a limited number of tools that measure motor skills in a naturalistic context. The Assessment of Motor and

Process Skills (AMPS) and School AMPS are two examples. The therapist evaluates motor and process skills within the context of basic ADL and instrumental ADL. The quality of the person's ADL performance is assessed by rating the effort, efficiency, safety, and independence of 16 ADL motor and 20 ADL process skill items while the person is doing chosen, familiar, and life-relevant ADL tasks. There are more than 100 tasks to choose from, thus promoting a client-centered approach to assessment. Evaluated motor skills include skills related to body position (stabilizes, aligns, positions), obtaining and holding objects (reaches, bends, grips, manipulates, coordinates), moving self and objects (moves, lifts, walks, transports, calibrates, flows), and sustaining performance (endures, paces) (Fisher & Jones, 2014). See Chapter 52 for more details.

The School AMPS is a naturalistic, observation-based assessment that is administered in the natural classroom setting while the student performs schoolwork tasks assigned by the teacher. No disruption of the normal classroom routine occurs during its administration. The School AMPS helps an occupational therapist answer the following questions:

- What is the quality of this student's schoolwork task performance?
- How does the quality of this student's task performance compare with that of his or her same-age peers?
- Which school motor and/or school process skills are most impacting this student's occupational performance in the classroom?
- What intervention strategies will have the most impact on this student's performance in the classroom?
- Was there a change in this student's quality of schoolwork task performance since the last School AMPS evaluation?

The School AMPS examines the transaction between a student, a schoolwork task, and a classroom environment and evaluates the quality of the student's schoolwork task performance, measured at the level of complex activity and participation, not body functions (Fingerhut et al., 2002; Fisher et al., 2000, 2007).

Examples of Evidence-Based Interventions

Since the last edition of this book, there has been a substantial increase and focus on testing interventions for those with limitations in motor function. When using evidence to guide practice, it is important to reflect on the type of outcome measures used as described previously. One should consider the following questions when interpreting evidence:

1. Is the population that was tested similar to my client?
2. Has the intervention been shown to be effectively related to measures of activity and participation (areas of occupation) in addition to impairment measures (measurement of client factors)?

Although interventions have been discussed throughout this chapter (orthoses, strengthening, physical agent modalities, task-oriented training, motor learning techniques such as mental practice, etc.), the following paragraphs provide the reader with further examples of contemporary evidence-based interventions.

Task-Oriented Training Interventions

Constraint-Induced Movement Therapy

The term *learned nonuse* was coined by Taub et al. (1993). The learned nonuse phenomenon originally was identified in animal studies and later applied to chronic stroke survivors and others. Taub et al. hypothesized that the nonuse or limited use of an affected upper extremity in human beings after a neurologic event results from a phenomenon of learned suppression. CI therapy is an intervention developed to reverse the effects of learned nonuse. This intervention has become the gold standard to improve daily use of neurologically impaired upper extremities in both the adult population (stroke) and children with cerebral palsy who meet the motor inclusion criteria. Refer back to OT Story 54.3 for a description of pediatric applications. Box 54.1 provides more details related to how to implement this intervention.

Repetitive Task Practice/ Task-Specific Training

Repetitive Task Practice (French et al., 2016) and Task-Specific Training (Waddell et al., 2014) are terms used to describe training approaches that include the performance of goal-directed activities that require high-intensity repetition of task-related or task-specific movements.

BOX 54.1 CONSTRAINT-INDUCED MOVEMENT THERAPY PROTOCOLS

Traditional Protocol

The EXCITE trial defined the intervention as: "Participants in the intervention group were taught to apply an instrumented protective safety mitt and encouraged to wear it on their less-impaired upper extremity for a goal of 90% of their waking hours over a 2-week period, including 2 weekends, for a total of 14 days. On each weekday, participants received shaping (adaptive task practice) and standard task training of the paretic limb for up to 6 hours per day. The former is based on the principles of behavioral training that can also be described in terms of motor learning derived from adaptive or part-task practice. Standard task practice is less structured (i.e., repetition of tasks is not conducted as individual trials of discrete movements); it involves functional activities performed continuously for a period of 15 to 20 minutes (e.g., eating, writing)" (Wolf et al., 2006).

Modified Protocols

Page et al. (2008) described the following protocol consisting of two components. "The first component consisted of half-hour, one-on-one sessions of more affected arm therapy occurring 3 days per week during a 10-week period. This component included shaping in which operant conditioning was applied in such a way that subjects received positive verbal encouragement to more fully perform selected motor skills with their more affected arm. Shaping was applied with 2 or 3 upper limb activities (e.g., writing, using a fork) chosen by the subjects with help from their therapist. In the second component of the mCIT intervention, during the same 10-week period, subjects' less affected arms were restrained every weekday for 5 hours identified as a time of frequent arm use, as identified by the subjects with assistance from the therapist. Their arms were restrained using a cotton hemi-sling, while their hands were placed in mesh, polystyrene-filled mitts with Velcro straps around the wrist."

Lin et al. (2009) defined their protocol as "restraint of the less affected limb combined with intensive training of the affected limb for 2 hours daily 5 days per week for 3 weeks and restraint of the less affected hand for 5 hours outside of the rehabilitation training."

Sterr and colleagues (2002) defined their protocol as 14 consecutive days; constraint of unaffected hand for a target of 90% of waking hours, with 3 hours of shaping training with the affected hand per day. To note, they concluded that: "The 3-hour CIMT training schedule significantly improved motor function in chronic hemiparesis, but it was less effective than the 6-hour training schedule."

CIMT, constraint-induced movement therapy; EXCITE, extremity constraint-induced therapy evaluation; mCIT, modified constraint-induced movement therapy.

They are frequently used to remediate upper and lower limb dysfunction in persons who have sustained neurological injuries, such as stroke (French et al., 2016).

Bilateral Arm Training/Bimanual Training

Bilateral arm training has emerged as a promising intervention to improve arm function after stroke. Stoykov et al. (2009) summarized the technique:

- Has been shown to be efficacious not only with stroke survivors who are only mildly impaired but also those with moderate and severe motor impairments
- Protocols reported in the literature are diverse and can be categorized as categories: repetitive reaching with and fixed, isolated muscle repetitive training, and whole arm functioning
- May be combined with rhythmic auditory cueing and is coupled with repetitive reaching with hand-fixed activities

Examples of treatment activities include opening and closing two identical drawers, wiping a table with both arms using both arms symmetrically, bilateral reaching and placing objects, and so on. Stoykov et al. (2009) compare the effectiveness of bilateral training with unilateral training for individuals with moderate upper limb hemiparesis. They concluded that both bilateral and unilateral training are efficacious for moderately impaired chronic stroke survivors and that bilateral training may be more advantageous for proximal arm function.

Gordon et al. (2007) developed a bimanual intervention, Hand-Arm Bimanual Intensive Therapy (HABIT), which is specifically aimed at upper extremity impairments in congenital hemiplegia. The authors describe HABIT as

- A form of functional training
- Focusing on intensive practice
- Focused on improving coordination of the two hands using structured task practice embedded in bimanual play and functional activities
- Using principles of motor learning (practice specificity, types of practice, feedback)
- Using principles of neuroplasticity (practice-induced brain changes arising from repetition, increasing movement complexity, motivation, and reward)

The authors conducted a randomized trial to examine the effectiveness of this intervention. Children were engaged in play and functional activities that provided structured bimanual practice 6 hours per day for 10 days. They concluded that for this carefully selected subgroup of children with hemiplegic cerebral palsy, HABIT appears to be efficacious in improving bimanual hand use.

Of note is that Gordon et al. (2011) conducted a randomized trial comparing CI therapy and HABIT that maintains the intensity of practice associated with CI therapy but where children are engaged in functional bimanual tasks. The children received 90 hours of CI therapy or HABIT. They concluded that both CI therapy and bimanual training lead to similar improvements in hand function. They note that a potential benefit of bimanual training is that participants may improve more on self-determined goals.

Use of Cognitive Strategies to Improve Performance

The use of cognitive strategies is emerging as an effective intervention for children with developmental coordination disorder (DCD). This term is used to describe children with motor skill impairment who experience problems with the performance of various motor-based tasks, such as catching/throwing a ball, playing in a jungle gym, dressing, feeding, riding a bicycle, and handwriting.

Hyland and Polatajko (2012) describe the Cognitive Orientation to daily Occupational Performance (CO-OP) approach as a multifaceted top-down approach that combines elements from various disciplines such as behavioral and cognitive psychology, health, and human movement science. They further describe it as a verbally based individualized approach that focuses on teaching children to use self-talk and problem-solving strategies to solve their motor-based performance problems. The children choose their own goals, and problem-solving strategies are used to identify and address performance issues.

The CO-OP therapist guides the child in the learning of a global problem-solving strategy and the discovery of domain-specific cognitive strategies that improve motor performance. The global cognitive strategy is a problem-solving strategy taken from the work of Meichenbaum (1977), which provides a structure within which the child can learn to talk through occupational performance problems. Domain-specific strategies (DSS) are used in specific tasks or situations to help achieve specific occupational performance goals (Sangster et al., 2005, p. 70).

Sangster et al. (2005) argue that their research supports the use of a cognitively-based approach such as CO-OP in assisting children with DCD in developing cognitive strategies when solving occupational performance problems. They state that the CO-OP approach has two hypotheses: (a) that children with DCD do not independently generate effective cognitive strategies to solve performance problems and (b) that cognitive strategy use changes with the CO-OP intervention. Examples of strategies that are employed include verbal guidance, feeling the movement, attention to doing, practice, and so on. Indeed, the authors' pilot work has supported the use of a cognitively based approach such as

CO-OP in assisting children with DCD in developing cognitive strategies when solving occupational performance problems.

Cognitive strategies have also been used to enhance motor skill acquisition poststroke. McEwen et al. (2009) examined the literature and concluded that

- Research investigating cognitive strategies to improve motor skill acquisition in people with stroke is emerging in the peer-reviewed literature.
- The cognitive strategies studied included three general strategies (those that are applicable in many different situations) and four task-specific strategies: motor imagery (MI) (also known as *mental practice*); Feldenkrais Attention to Movement; goal setting with assigned, high, specific goals; and preparatory arousal.
- None of the strategies have been studied exhaustively.
- There is strong evidence that general strategy training combined with MI during practice improves and maintains performance in both trained and untrained ADL compared to traditional functional training in people in the early rehabilitation phase after a stroke.
- There is strong evidence that general strategy training improves performance in untrained ADL compared to traditional OT in people with apraxia as a result of stroke (see Chapter 55 for more information on apraxia).

Wolf et al. (2016) examined the impact of combining CO-OP with task-specific training on cognition and upper extremity function in subacute stroke survivors. They found that the group receiving CO-OP had measurable improvements over usual care on all of the included outcome measures related to arm function, cognition, and participation.

Additionally, combining repetitive task practice with cognitive strategies such as mirror therapy (MT) and action observation (AO) have also been shown to be effective at improving upper extremity function in adults poststroke (Borges et al., 2018; Nilsen et al., 2015; Thieme et al., 2018) and children with cerebral palsy (Buccino et al., 2012; Park et al., 2016; Sgandurra et al., 2013). Likewise, there is emerging evidence that MT and AO may produce beneficial effects for persons with PD. For example, Bonassi et al. (2016) found that MT improves the speed of hand movement in the more affected hand of persons with PD, and AO has been shown to improve functional mobility, ADL performance, and quality of life in persons with PD (Buccino et al., 2011; Di Iorio et al., 2018).

Postural Control/Balance Interventions

Adding purpose to daily occupations has been shown to improve standing balance (Hsieh et al., 1996) in those with hemiplegia. Hsieh et al. (1996) examined three types of standing balance interventions. They hypothesized that the two added-purpose occupations would elicit more exercise repetitions than a rote exercise. They examined a dynamic standing balance exercise that involved bending down, reaching, standing up, and extending the arm. One condition of added purpose involved the use of materials (small balls and target); a second added-purpose condition involved the subjects' imagination of the small balls. The third condition was the rote exercise without added purpose. The subjects did significantly more exercise repetitions in the added-materials condition and in the imagery-based condition than in the rote exercise condition. The authors concluded that this study demonstrates how added purpose can enhance motor performance in persons with hemiplegia. They demonstrated that purpose may be effectively added to an exercise through the use of materials or imagery.

The concept of using reaching activities has also been shown to be effective in retraining seated postural control (Dean & Shepherd, 1997). As technology continued to be more and more commonplace, games such as the Wii are being used in rehabilitation settings to address multiple impairments including improving balance (Gil-Gómez et al., 2011).

Electrical Stimulation

Electrical stimulation and electromyography (EMG)-triggered electrical stimulation are being used for those with impaired motor function. Electrical stimulation has been used in poststroke upper extremity rehabilitation for many years. Potential uses have included reduction of shoulder subluxation, reduction of pain, improved motor control, and increasing use of the involved extremity. In general, the effects of electrical stimulation have been the most consistent at improving limb impairments such as range of motion and reducing pain. The effects on function and ADL have received less attention and have been inconsistent. Electrical stimulation can be triggered by voluntary movement or nontriggered. The EMG-triggered stimulation detects underlying muscle activity when it reaches a threshold level before providing the stimulation. The stroke survivor must voluntarily activate the correct muscles before the stimulation facilitating the motor response. This type of stimulation assures that the intervention is not passive in nature. Triggered electrical stimulation may be more effective than nontriggered electrical stimulation in facilitating upper extremity motor recovery following stroke (de Kroon et al., 2005). This intervention has been shown to be effective at improving wrist extension, a key movement to be considered a candidate for some task-oriented approaches such as CI therapy. Findings from systematic reviews and meta-analyses have been inconsistent. However,

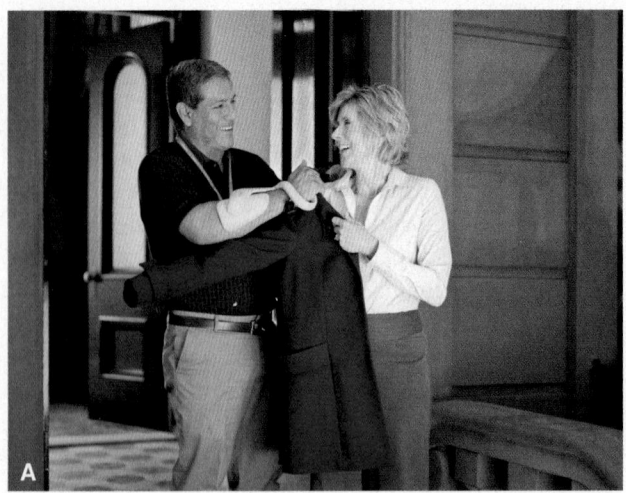
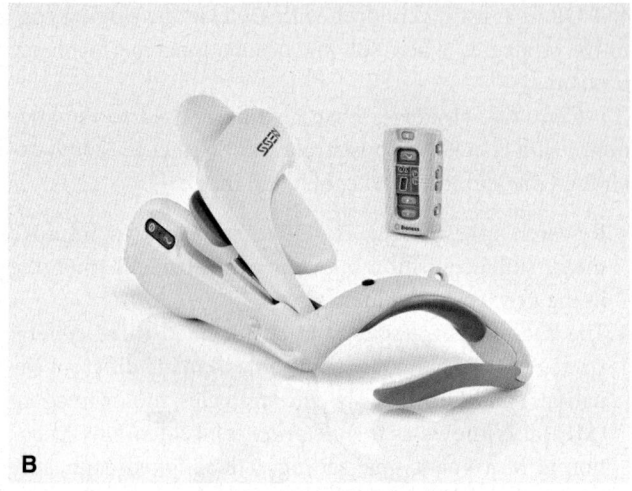

FIGURE 54.7 A neuroprosthesis (H200 Wireless) used to support occupational performance. This device combines a wrist/hand orthosis (to provide stabilization) with integrated surface electrodes to activate muscles of a paralyzed forearm and hand.

(Photo courtesy of Bioness, Inc., Valencia, California.)

there is enough evidence to continue to integrate these modalities with other task-oriented training activities. Further investigation is warranted (see Figure 54.7).

Conclusion

Motor function and control is a multifaceted concept that relies on multiple body structures and functions, performance skills, and so on. Successful rehabilitation is based on the adoption of a clear therapeutic approach or approaches; the interpretation of standardized, valid, and reliable assessments; and the adoption of evidence-based interventions. Remember, the goal of motor-based interventions is to improve overall occupational performance and *not* only reduce motor impairment.

Lippincott® Connect *For additional resources on the subjects discussed in this chapter, visit Lippincott Connect. See* **Appendix I, Table of Interventions** *for a comprehensive list of interventions, and* **Appendix II, Table of Assessments** *for a comprehensive list of assessments.*

REFERENCES

Almhdawi, K. A., Mathiowetz, V. G., White, M., & delMas, R. C. (2016). Efficacy of occupational therapy task-oriented approach in upper extremity post-stroke rehabilitation. *Occupational Therapy International, 23*(4), 444–456. https://doi.org/10.1002/oti.1447

Arnould, C., Penta, M., Renders, A., & Thonnard, J. L. (2004). ABILHAND-Kids: A measure of manual ability in children with cerebral palsy. *Neurology, 63*, 1045–1052. doi:10.1212/01.wnl.0000138423.77640.37

Arya, K. N., Verma, R., & Garg, R. K. (2011). Estimating the minimal clinically important difference of an upper extremity recovery measure in subacute stroke patients. *Topics in Stroke Rehabilitation, 18*(Suppl. 1), 599–610. https://doi.org/10.1310/tsr18s01-599

Ashfaq, F., Soomro, N., Zubia, S., Bushra, E., & Sagar, P. (2019). Efficacy of adaptive devices for improving ADL's and quality of life in patients with multiple conditions. *International Journal of Research and Innovation in Social Science (IJRISS), III*(X) 405–408. https://www.rsisinternational.org/virtual-library/papers/efficacy-of-adaptive-devices-for-improving-adls-and-quality-of-life-in-patients-with-multiple-conditions/.

Bar-Haim, S., Harries, N., Nammourah, I., Oraibi, S., Malhees, W., Loeppky, J., Perkins, N. J., Belokopytov, M., Kaplanski, J., & Lahat, E.; MER Project. (2010). Effectiveness of motor learning coaching in children with cerebral palsy: A randomized controlled trial. *Clinical Rehabilitation, 24*, 1009–1020. https://doi.org/10.1177/0269215510371428

Benaim, C., Pérennou, D. A., Villy, J., Rousseaux, M., & Pelissier, J. Y. (1999). Validation of a standardized assessment of postural control in stroke patients: The Postural Assessment Scale for Stroke Patients (PASS). *Stroke, 30*, 1862–1868. https://doi.org/10.1161/01.str.30.9.1862

Berg, K., Wood-Dauphinee, S., Williams, J. I., & Gayton, D. (1989). Measuring balance in the elderly: Preliminary development of an instrument. *Physiotherapy Canada, 41*, 304–311. https://doi.org/10.3138/ptc.41.6.304

Bhalerao, G., Kulkarani, V., Doshi, C., Rairikar, S., & Sancheti, P. (2013). Comparison of motor relearning program versus Bobath approach at every two weeks interval for improving activities of daily living and ambulation in acute stroke rehabilitation. *International Journal of Basic and Applied Medical Sciences, 3*(3), 70–77. http://www.cibtech.org/jms.htm

Bonassi, G., Pelosin, E., Ogliastro, C., Cerulli, C., Abbruzzese, G., & Avanzino, L. (2016). Mirror visual feedback to improve bradykinesia in Parkinson's disease. *Neural Plasticity, 2016*, 8764238. https://doi.org/10.1155/2016/8764238

Borges, L. R., Fernandes, A. B., Melo, L. P., Guerra, R. O., & Campos, T. F. (2018). Action observation for upper limb rehabilitation after stroke. *The Cochrane Database of Systematic Reviews, 8*, CD011887. https://doi.org/10.1002/14651858.CD011887.pub3

Buccino, G., Arisi, D., Gough, P., Aprile, D., Ferri, C., Serotti, L., Tiberti, A., & Fazzi, E. (2012). Improving upper limb motor functions through action observation treatment: A pilot study in children with cerebral palsy. *Developmental Medicine and Child Neurology, 54*, 822–828. https://doi.org/10.1111/j.1469-8749.2012.04334.x

Buccino, G. R., Giusti, M. C., Negrotti, A., Rossi, A., Calzetti, S., & Cappa, S. F. (2011). Action observation treatment improves autonomy in daily activities in Parkinson's disease patients: Results of a pilot study. *Movement Disorders, 26*(10), 1963–1964. https://doi.org/10.1002/mds.23745

Bushnell, C., Bettger, J. P., Cockroft, K. M., Cramer, S. C., Edelen, M. O., Hanley, D., Katzan, I. L., Mattke, S., Nilsen, D. M., Piquado, T., Skidmore, E. R., Wing, K., & Yenokyan, G. (2015). Chronic stroke outcome measures for motor function intervention trials: Expert panel recommendations. *Circulation: Cardiovascular Quality and Outcomes, 8*, S163–S169. https://doi.org/10.1161/CIRCOUTCOMES.115.002098

Carr, J. H., & Shepherd, R. B. (1987). *A motor relearning program for stroke* (2nd ed.). Aspen.

Carr, J. H., & Shepherd, R. B. (2003). *Stroke rehabilitation: Guidelines for exercise and training to optimize motor skill.* Butterworth-Heinemann.

Chen, C. C., & Bode, R. K. (2009, April). *MAM-36: Psychometric properties and differential item functioning in neurologic and orthopedic patients.* Paper presented at the AOTA 88th annual conference, Long Beach, CA.

Chen, C. C., Kasven, N., Karpatkin, H. I., & Sylvester, A. (2007). Hand strength and perceived manual ability among patients with multiple sclerosis. *Archives of Physical Medicine and Rehabilitation, 88*, 794–797. https://doi.org/10.1016/j.apmr.2007.03.010

Chen, L., Xiong, S., Liu, Y., Lin, M., Zhu, L., Zhong, R., Zhao, J., Liu, W., Wang, J., & Shang, X. (2019). Comparison of motor relearning program versus Bobath approach for prevention of poststroke apathy: A randomized controlled trial. *Journal of Stroke and Cerebrovascular Diseases: The Official Journal of National Stroke Association, 28*(3), 655–664. https://doi.org/10.1016/j.jstrokecerebrovasdis.2018.11.011

Chisari, C., Venturi, M., Bertolucci, F., Fanciullacci, C., & Rossi, B. (2017). Benefits of an intensive task-oriented circuit training in multiple sclerosis patients with mild disability. *Neurorehabilitation, 35*(3), 509–518. https://doi.org/10.3233/NRE-141144

Collin, C., & Wade, D. (1990). Assessing motor impairment after stroke: A pilot reliability study. *Journal of Neurology, Neurosurgery, and Psychiatry, 53*, 576–579. https://doi.org/10.1136/jnnp.53.7.576

Corbetta, D., Sirtori, V., Castellini, G., Moja, L., & Gatti, R. (2015). Constraint-induced movement therapy for upper extremities in people with stroke. *The Cochrane Database of Systematic Reviews, 2015*(10), CD004433. https://doi.org/10.1002/14651858.CD004433.pub

Dean, C. M., & Shepherd, R. B. (1997). Task-related training improves performance of seated reaching tasks after stroke. A randomized controlled trial. *Stroke, 28*, 722–728. https://doi.org/10.1161/01.str.28.4.722

de Kroon, J., Ijzerman, M., Chae, J., Lankhorst, G., & Zilvold, G. (2005). Relation between stimulation characteristics and clinical outcome in studies using electrical stimulation to improve motor control of the upper extremity in stroke. *Journal of Rehabilitation Medicine, 37*, 65–74. https://doi.org/10.1080/16501970410024190

Di Iorio, W., Ciarimboli, A., Ferriero, G., Feleppa, M., Baratto, L., Matarazzo, G., Gentile, G., Masiero, S., & Sale, P. (2018). Action observation in people with Parkinson's disease. A motor-cognitive combined approach for motor rehabilitation. A preliminary report. *Diseases (Basel, Switzerland), 6*(3), 58. https://doi.org/10.3390/diseases6030058

Egan, M. Y., & Brousseau, L. (2007). Splinting for osteoarthritis of the carpometacarpal joint: A review of the evidence. *American Journal of Occupational Therapy, 61*, 70–78. https://doi.org/10.5014/ajot.61.1.70

Erhardt, R. (1994). *Developmental hand dysfunction: Theory, assessment, and treatment* (2nd ed.). Pro-Ed.

Fingerhut, P., Madill, H., Darrah, J., Hodge, M., & Warren, S. (2002). Classroom-based assessment: Validation for the school AMPS. *American Journal of Occupational Therapy, 56*, 210–213. https://doi.org/10.5014/ajot.56.2.210

Fisher, A. G., Bryze, K., & Atchison, B. T. (2000). Naturalistic assessment of functional performance in school settings: Reliability and validity of the School AMPS scales. *Journal of Outcome Measurement, 4*, 504–522. https://pubmed.ncbi.nlm.nih.gov/11272598/

Fisher, A. G., Bryze, K., Hume, V., & Griswold, L. A. (2007). *School AMPS: School version of the assessment of motor and process skills* (2nd ed.). Three Star Press.

Fisher, A. G., & Jones, K. B. (2014). *Assessment of motor and process skills: User manual* (8th ed.). Three Star Press.

Folio, M. R., & Fewell, R. R. (2000). *Peabody developmental motor scales: Examiner's manual* (2nd ed.). Pro-ED.

French, B., Thomas, L. H., Coupe, J., McMahon, N. E., Connell, L., Harrison, J., Sutton, C. J., Tishkovskaya, S., & Watkins, C. L. (2016). Repetitive task training for improving functional ability after stroke. *The Cochrane Database of Systematic Reviews, 11*(11), CD006073. https://doi.org/10.1002/14651858.CD006073.pub3

Fugl-Meyer, A. R., Jääskö, L., Leyman, I., Olsson, S., & Steglind, S. (1975). The post-stroke hemiplegic patient. 1. A method for evaluation of physical performance. *Scandinavian Journal of Rehabilitation Medicine, 7*, 13–31. https://pubmed.ncbi.nlm.nih.gov/1135616/

Gerber, R. J., Wilks, T., & Erdie-Lalena, C. (2010). Developmental milestones: Motor development. *Pediatrics in Review, 31*, 267–277. https://doi.org/10.1542/pir.31-7-267

Gil-Gómez, J. A., Lloréns, R., Alcañiz, M., & Colomer, C. (2011). Effectiveness of a Wii balance board-based system (eBaViR) for balance rehabilitation: A pilot randomized clinical trial in patients with acquired brain injury. *Journal of Neuroengineering and Rehabilitation, 8*, 30. https://doi.org/10.1186/1743-0003-8-30

Gordon, A. M., Charles, J., & Wolf, S. L. (2005). Methods of constraint-induced movement therapy for children with hemiplegic cerebral palsy: Development of a child-friendly intervention for improving upper-extremity function. *Archives of Physical Medicine and Rehabilitation, 86*, 837–844. https://doi.org/10.1016/j.apmr.2004.10.008

Gordon, A. M., Hung, Y. C., Brandao, M., Ferre, C. L., Kuo, H. C., Friel, K., Petra, E., Chinnan, A., & Charles, J. R. (2011). Bimanual training and constraint-induced movement therapy in children with hemiplegic cerebral palsy: A randomized trial. *Neurorehabilitation and Neural Repair, 25*, 692–702. https://doi.org/10.1177/1545968311402508

Gordon, A. M., Schneider, J. A., Chinnan, A., & Charles, J. R. (2007). Efficacy of hand-arm bimanual intensive therapy (HABIT) for children with hemiplegic cerebral palsy: A randomized control trial. *Developmental Medicine and Child Neurology, 49*, 830–838. https://doi.org/10.1111/j.1469-8749.2007.00830.x

Haley, S., Coster, W., Ludlow, L., Haltiwanger, J., & Andrellos, J. (1992). *Pediatric evaluation of disability inventory (PEDI).* Trustees of Boston University.

Hsieh, C. L., Nelson, D. L., Smith, D. A., & Peterson, C. Q. (1996). A comparison of performance in added-purpose occupations and rote exercise for dynamic standing balance in persons with hemiplegia. *American Journal of Occupational Therapy, 50*, 10–16. https://doi.org/10.5014/ajot.50.1.10

Hurkmans, E., van der Giesen, F. J., Vliet Vlieland, T. P., Schoones, J., & Van den Ende, E. C. (2009). Dynamic exercise programs (aerobic capacity and/or muscle strength training) in patients with rheumatoid arthritis. *The Cochrane Database of Systematic Reviews, 2009*(4), CD006853. https://doi.org/10.1002/14651858.CD006853.pub2

Hyland, M., & Polatajko, H. J. (2012). Enabling children with developmental coordination disorder to self-regulate through the use of dynamic performance analysis: Evidence from the CO-OP approach. *Human Movement Science, 31*, 987–998. https://doi.org/10.1016/j.humov.2011.09.003

Jebsen, R. H., Taylor, N., Trieschmann, R. B., Trotter, M. J., & Howard, L. A. (1969). An objective and standardized test of hand function. *Archives of Physical Medicine and Rehabilitation, 50*, 311–319. https://pubmed.ncbi.nlm.nih.gov/5788487/

Kopp, B., Kunkel, A., Flor, H., Platz, T., Rose, U., Mauritz, K. H., Gresser, K., McCulloch, K. L., & Taub, E. (1997). The Arm Motor Ability Test: Reliability, validity, and sensitivity to change of an instrument for assessing disabilities in activities of daily living. *Archives of Physical Medicine and Rehabilitation, 78*, 615–620. https://doi.org/10.1016/s0003-9993(97)90427-5

Krumlinde-Sundholm, L., & Eliasson, A. C. (2003). Development of the Assisting Hand Assessment, a rash-built measure intended for children with unilateral upper limb impairments. *Scandinavian Journal of Occupational Therapy, 10,* 16–26. https://doi.org/10.1080/11038120310004529

Lin, K. C., Wu, C. Y., Liu, J. S., Chen, Y. T., & Hsu, C. J. (2009). Constraint-induced therapy versus dose-matched control intervention to improve motor ability, basic/extended daily functions, and quality of life in stroke. *Neurorehabilitation and Neural Repair, 23,* 160–165. https://doi.org/10.1177/1545968308320642

Malina, R. (2004). Motor development during infancy and early childhood: Overview and suggested directions for research. *International Journal of Sport and Health Science, 2,* 50–66. https://doi.org/10.5432/ijshs.2.50

Mann, W. C., Ottenbacher, K. J., Fraas, L., Tomita, M., & Granger, C. V. (1999). Effectiveness of assistive technology and environmental interventions in maintaining independence and reducing home care costs for the frail elderly. A randomized controlled trial. *Archives of Family Medicine, 8,* 210–217. https://doi.org/10.1001/archfami.8.3.210

Mathiowetz, V. (2016). Task-oriented approach to stroke rehabilitation. In G. Gillen (Ed.), *Stroke rehabilitation a function-based approach* (4th ed., pp. 59–78). Elsevier.

Mathiowetz, V., & Bass-Haugen, J. (1994). Motor behavior research: Implications for therapeutic approaches to central nervous system dysfunction. *American Journal of Occupational Therapy, 48,* 733–745. https://doi.org/10.5014/ajot.48.8.733

Mathiowetz, V., & Bass-Haugen, J. (2008). Assessing abilities and capacities: Motor behavior. In M. V. Radomski & C. A. Trombly-Latham (Eds.), *Occupational therapy for physical dysfunction* (6th ed., pp. 186–211). Lippincott Williams & Wilkins.

McEwen, S. E., Huijbregts, M. P., Ryan, J. D., & Polatajko, H. J. (2009). Cognitive strategy use to enhance motor skill acquisition post-stroke: A critical review. *Brain Injury, 23,* 263–277. https://doi.org/10.1080/02699050902788493

Meichenbaum, D. (1977). *Cognitive-behaviour modification: An integrative approach.* Plenum Press.

Morris, D. M., Taub, E., & Mark, V. W. (2006). Constraint-induced movement therapy: Characterizing the intervention protocol. *Europa Medicophysica, 42*(3), 257–268. https://pubmed.ncbi.nlm.nih.gov/17039224/

Nilsen, D. M., Gillen, G., Geller, D., Hreha, K., Osei, E., & Saleem, G. T. (2015). Effectiveness of interventions to improve occupational performance of people with motor impairments after stroke: An evidence-based review. *American Journal of Occupational Therapy, 69,* 6901180030p1. https://doi.org/10.5014/ajot.2015.011965

Page, M. J., Massy-Westropp, N., O'Connor, D., & Pitt, V. (2012). Splinting for carpal tunnel syndrome. *The Cochrane Database of Systematic Reviews, 2012*(7), CD010003. https://doi.org/10.1002/14651858.CD010003

Page, S. J., Fulk, G. D., & Boyne, P. (2012). Clinically important differences for the upper-extremity Fugl-Meyer scale in people with minimal to moderate impairment due to chronic stroke. *Physical Therapy, 92,* 791–798. https://doi.org/10.2522/ptj.20110009

Page, S. J., Levine, P., Leonard, A., Szaflarski, J. P., & Kissela, B. M. (2008). Modified constraint-induced therapy in chronic stroke: Results of a single-blinded randomized controlled trial. *Physical Therapy, 88,* 333–340. https://doi.org/10.2522/ptj.20060029

Park, E., Baek, S., & Park, S. (2016). Systematic review of the effects of mirror therapy in children with cerebral palsy. *Journal of Physical Therapy Science, 28,* 3227–3231. https://doi.org/10.1589/jpts.28.3227

Penta, M., Tesio, L., Arnould, C., Zancan, A., & Thonnard, J. L. (2001). The ABILHAND questionnaire as a measure of manual ability in chronic stroke patients: Rasch-based validation and relationship to upper limb impairment. *Stroke, 32,* 1627–1634. https://doi.org/10.1161/01.str.32.7.1627

Randall, M., Johnson, L., & Reddihough, D. (1999). *The Melbourne assessment of unilateral upper limb function: Test administration manual.* Royal Children's Hospital.

Rensink, M., Schuurmans, M., Lindeman, E., & Hafsteinsdóttir, T. (2009). Task-oriented training in rehabilitation after stroke: Systematic review. *Journal of Advanced Nursing, 65,* 737–754. https://doi.org/10.1111/j.1365-2648.2008.04925.x

Sabari, J. (2016). Activity-based interventions in stroke rehabilitation. In G. Gillen (Ed.), *Stroke rehabilitation: A function-based approach* (4th ed., pp. 79–95). Elsevier.

Sangster, C. A., Beninger, C., Polatajko, H. J., & Mandich, A. (2005). Cognitive strategy generation in children with developmental coordination disorder. *Canadian Journal of Occupational Therapy, 72,* 67–77. https://doi.org/10.1177/000841740507200201

Saunders, D. H., Sanderson, M., Hayes, S., Kilrane, M., Greig, C. A., Brazzelli, M., & Mead, G. E. (2016). Physical fitness training for stroke patients. *The Cochrane Database of Systematic Reviews, 2016,* CD003316. https://doi.org/10.1002/14651858.CD003316.pub6

Schmidt, R. A., & Lee, T. D. (2011). *Motor control and learning: A behavioral emphasis* (5th ed.). Human Kinetics.

Schmidt, R. A., Lee, T. D., Winstein, C. J., Wulf, G., & Zelaznik, H. N. (2019). *Motor control and learning a behavioral emphasis* (6th ed.). Human Kinetics.

Sgandurra, G., Ferrari, A., Cossu, G., Guzzetta, A., Fogassi, L., & Cioni, G. (2013). Randomized trial of observation and execution of upper extremity actions versus action alone in children with unilateral cerebral palsy. *Neurorehabilitation and Neural Repair, 27,* 808–815. https://doi.org/10.1177/1545968313497101

Shelton, F., Volpe, B. T., & Reding, M. (2001). Motor impairment as a predictor of functional recovery and guide to rehabilitation treatment after stroke. *Neurorehabilitation and Neural Repair, 15,* 229–237. https://doi.org/10.1177/154596830101500311

Shumway-Cook, A., & Woollacott, M. (2017). *Motor control: Translating research into clinical practice* (5th ed.). Lippincott Williams & Wilkins.

Sidaway, B., Ala, B., Baughman, K., Glidden, J., Cowie, S., Peabody, A., Roundy, D., Spaulding, J., Stephens, R., & Wright, D. L. (2016). Contextual interference can facilitate motor learning in older adults and in individuals with Parkinson's disease. *Journal of Motor Behavior, 48*(6), 509–518. https://doi.org/10.1080/00222895.2016.1152221

Soke, F., Guclu-Gunduz, A., Kocer, B., Fidan, I., & Keskinoglu, P. (2021). Task-oriented circuit training combined with aerobic training improves motor performance and balance in people with Parkinson's disease. *Acta Neurologica Belgica, 121,* 535–543. https://doi.org/10.1007/s13760-019-01247-8

Sterr, A., Elbert, T., Berthold, I., Kölbel, S., Rockstroh, B., & Taub, E. (2002). Longer versus shorter daily constraint-induced movement therapy of chronic hemiparesis: An exploratory study. *Archives of Physical Medicine and Rehabilitation, 83,* 1374–1377. https://doi.org/10.1053/apmr.2002.35108

Stoykov, M. E., Lewis, G. N., & Corcos, D. M. (2009). Comparison of bilateral and unilateral training for upper extremity hemiparesis in stroke. *Neurorehabilitation and Neural Repair, 23,* 945–953. https://doi.org/10.1177/1545968309338190

Subramanian, S. K., Massie, C. L., Malcolm, M. P., & Levin, M. F. (2010). Does provision of extrinsic feedback result in improved motor learning in the upper limb poststroke? A systematic review of the evidence. *Neurorehabilitation and Neural Repair, 24,* 113–124. https://doi.org/10.1177/1545968309349941

Taub, E., Miller, N. E., Novack, T. A., Cook, E. W., III, Fleming, W. C., Nepomuceno, C. S., Connell, J. S., & Crago, J. E. (1993). Technique to improve chronic motor deficit after stroke. *Archives of Physical Medicine and Rehabilitation, 74,* 347–354. https://pubmed.ncbi.nlm.nih.gov/8466415/

Thieme, H., Morkisch, N., Mehrholz, J., Pohl, M., Behrens, J., Borgetto, B., & Dohle, C. (2018). Mirror therapy for improving motor function after stroke. *The Cochrane Database of Systematic Reviews, 7*(7), CD008449. https://doi.org/10.1002/14651858.CD008449.pub3

Timmermans, A. A. A., Spooren, A. I. F., Kingma, H., & Seelen, H. A. M. (2010). Influence of task-oriented training content on skilled arm-hand performance in stroke: A systematic review. *Neurorehabilitation and Neural Repair, 24*, 858–870. https://doi.org/10.1177/1545968310368963

Uswatte, G., Taub, E., Griffin, M. A., Vogtle, L., Rowe, J., & Barman, J. (2012). The pediatric motor activity log-revised: Assessing real-world arm use in children with cerebral palsy. *Rehabilitation Psychology, 57*, 149–158. https://doi.org/10.1037/a0028516

Uswatte, G., Taub, E., Morris, D., Vignolo, M., & McCulloch, K. (2005). Reliability and validity of the upper-extremity Motor Activity Log-14 for measuring real-world arm use. *Stroke, 36*, 2493. https://doi.org/10.1161/01.STR.0000185928.90848.2e

Veldema, J., & Jansen, P. (2020). Resistance training in stroke rehabilitation: systematic review and meta-analysis. *Clinical Rehabilitation, 34*(9), 1173–1197. https://doi.org/10.1177/0269215520932964

Velozo, G. A., & Woodbury, M. L. (2011). Translating measurement findings into rehabilitation practice: An example using Fugl-Meyer Assessment-Upper Extremity with patients following stroke. *Journal of Rehabilitation Research and Development, 48*, 1211–1222. https://doi.org/10.1682/JRRD.2010.10.0203

Waddell, K. J., Birkenmeier, R. L., Moore, J. L., Hornby, T. G., & Lang, C. E. (2014). Feasibility of high-repetition, task-specific training for individuals with upper-extremity paresis. *American Journal of Occupational Therapy, 68*, 444–453. https://doi.org/10.5014/ajot.2014.011619

Wallen, M., Bundy, A., Pont, K., & Ziviani, J. (2009). Psychometric properties of the Pediatric Motor Activity Log used for children with cerebral palsy. *Developmental Medicine and Child Neurology, 51*, 200–208. https://doi.org/10.1111/j.1469-8749.2008.03157.x

Werner, R. A., Franzblau, A., & Gell, N. (2005). Randomized controlled trial of nocturnal splinting for active workers with symptoms of carpal tunnel syndrome. *Archives of Physical Medicine and Rehabilitation, 86*, 1–7. https://doi.org/10.1016/j.apmr.2004.05.013

Wolf, S. L., Catlin, P. A., Ellis, M., Archer, A. L., Morgan, B., & Piacentino, A. (2001). Assessing Wolf Motor Function Test as outcome measure for research in patients after stroke. *Stroke, 32*, 1635–1639. https://doi.org/10.1161/01.str.32.7.1635

Wolf, S. L., Thompson, P. A., Winstein, C. J., Miller, J. P., Blanton, S. R., Nichols-Larsen, D. S., Morris, D. M., Uswatte, G., Taub, E., Light, K. E., & Sawaki, L. (2010). The EXCITE stroke trial: Comparing early and delayed constraint-induced movement therapy. *Stroke, 41*, 2309–2315. https://doi.org/10.1161/STROKEAHA.110.588723

Wolf, S. L., Winstein, C. J., Miller, J. P., Taub, E., Uswatte, G., Morris, D., Giuliani, C., Light, K. E., & Nichols-Larsen, D.; EXCITE Investigators. (2006). Effect of constraint-induced movement therapy on upper extremity function 3 to 9 months after stroke: The EXCITE randomized clinical trial. *JAMA, 296*, 2095–2104. https://doi.org/10.1001/jama.296.17.2095

Wolf, T. J., Polatajko, H., Baum, C., Rios, J., Cirone, D., Doherty, M., & McEwen, S. (2016). Combined cognitive-strategy and task-specific training affects cognition and upper-extremity function in subacute stroke: An exploratory randomized controlled trial. *American Journal of Occupational Therapy, 70*, 7002290010p10. https://doi.org/10.5014/ajot.2016.017293

Yachnin, D., Gharib, G., Jutai, J., & Finestone, H. (2017). Technology-assisted toilets: Improving independence and hygiene in stroke rehabilitation. *Journal of Rehabilitation and Assistive Technologies Engineering, 4*, 1–8. https://doi.org/10.1177/2055668317725686

Cognition, Perception, and Occupational Performance

Joan Pascale Toglia and Yael Goverover

LEARNING OBJECTIVES

After reading this chapter, you will be able to:

1. Define functional cognition and describe how cognitive impairments can limit the performance of activities and decrease participation in meaningful occupations.
2. Discuss the role of occupational therapy practitioners in cognitive interventions.
3. Describe the key characteristics and process of a comprehensive approach to evaluate functional cognition across the life span.
4. Compare and contrast different models and approaches for cognitive interventions.
5. Discuss the factors that need to be considered when choosing evaluation and intervention approaches, including the evidence that supports decisions.
6. Describe specific areas of cognition and perception; their assessment and approaches for intervention.

Introduction

Cognition can be described as the mental processes involved in perceiving, understanding, organizing, assimilating, and processing information. It encompasses a broad range of skills involved in learning, and everyday life such as attention, visual-spatial perception, memory, executive functions, and metacognition. The term **functional cognition** involves the integration of cognitive skills with motor skills and/or the demands of the activity and environment during the performance of everyday activities. Functional cognition describes how cognition is applied in everyday life and interacts dynamically with the task and environment during the performance (Giles et al., 2020).

Functional cognitive impairments can significantly limit an individual's daily life activities (e.g., self-care, household activities, financial management, driving), restrict participation in meaningful occupations, or contribute to high-risk behaviors related to substance abuse, obesity, gambling, and inability to maintain a job. Additionally, functional cognitive impairments can significantly affect an individual's ability to recognize potential hazards, anticipate consequences of actions and behaviors, follow safety precautions, and respond to emergencies. Mild difficulties in cognition can compromise health and well-being by limiting the ability to adhere to dietary and exercise recommendations, manage medications and appointments, and seek information from health providers (Katz, 2018). Functional cognition limitations can also diminish a person's sense of competence, self-efficacy, and self-esteem, further compounding difficulties in adapting to the demands of everyday living and adopting to the new "self" postinjury (Nalder et al., 2019).

Who Could Benefit From Cognitive Intervention?

Traditionally, **cognitive rehabilitation** was recommended for people following traumatic brain injury (TBI) or stroke (Cicerone et al., 2019). In the past 15 years, researchers have begun applying cognitive rehabilitation interventions to chronic illnesses to prevent or delay disease progression and functional decline. In fact, research has shown that interventions that address cognition can be effective for a wide range of persons across the life span. For example, cognitive rehabilitation can be effective for children with various diagnoses including but not limited to attention-deficit disorders (Ziabakhsh et al., 2020), spina bifida (Stubberud et al., 2021), and autism (Dhamodharan et al., 2020). It can also be effective for people with chronic diseases such as cancer (Fernandes et al., 2019; Wolf et al., 2016), chronic pulmonary disease (Park et al., 2021), multiple sclerosis (Ferry, 2021), Parkinson's disease (Foster et al., 2018; Sanchez-Luengos et al., 2021), schizophrenia (Vizzotto et al., 2021), and addiction (Anderson et al., 2021). Recently, cognitive rehabilitation principles have been applied to occupational therapy (OT) for an individual with long COVID-19 (Wilcox & Frank, 2021). In addition, cognitive rehabilitation methods have been used to both promote cognitive health in healthy older adults as well as to provide early intervention for at-risk populations (Glenthøj et al., 2020; Toglia & Katz, 2018).

Since cognitive rehabilitation has broadened in scope and is no longer limited to traditional rehabilitation settings, we use the term **cognitive interventions** to reflect this shift in practice. The aim of OT intervention for people with functional cognitive limitations is to improve engagement and participation in everyday activities and help individuals gain the abilities they need to take control over their lives and develop healthy and satisfying ways of living.

In this chapter, the process of cognitive intervention will be discussed, starting with evaluation, moving to treatment approaches, and followed by a discussion of specific cognitive perceptual problems encountered in clinical practice across the life span. OT assessment and treatment of confusional states, self-awareness, executive functions, spatial neglect, visual perception, and motor planning deficits will each be reviewed along with OT assessment, treatment, and examples of how deficits in these areas affect engagement in everyday activities.

Evaluation

Occupational therapists screen individuals for functional cognitive deficits and provide comprehensive information on the effect of **cognitive impairments** on basic and instrumental activities of daily living (BADL; IADL), education, work, play, leisure, social participation, and role competence. Evaluation requires consideration of other factors such as language impairments, pain, fatigue, low motivation, depression, anxiety, or psychological distress that may impact and mask the person's performance and true cognitive abilities (Lier et al., 2021). This section provides detailed information about the cognitive evaluation process that occupational therapists need to consider when choosing and conducting assessments.

The Cognition Evaluation Process

Occupational therapists approach the evaluation process with the goal of identifying functional cognitive challenges that influence accomplishment of everyday activities and participation in life roles (Giles et al., 2017). There are two main reasons to perform a cognitive evaluation. First, evaluations provide evidence and information about the presence of impairments and performance competencies. Such information can be used to establish baselines, estimate functional cognitive abilities, plan discharge, and measure intervention effectiveness (e.g., rehabilitation outcomes). Second, evaluations are used to gather information for intervention planning.

The *Cognitive–Functional Evaluation (C-FE) Process* (Bar-Haim Erez & Katz, 2018; Rotenberg & Maeir, 2019) and the *international classification of health model* (ICF; World Health Organization, 2001) can guide the evaluation process. Both the C-FE and ICF guide therapists to select evaluations that provide information about a client's[1] cognitive capabilities, activity, and participation. The goal of the C-FE and the ICF is to help therapists gather information

---

[1]According to the American Occupational Therapy Association (AOTA, 2020a, p. S75), the term *client* refers to *persons* (including those involved in care of a client), *groups* (a collection of individuals having shared characteristics or common or shared purpose, e.g., family members, workers, students, and those with similar interests or occupational challenges), and *populations* (aggregates of people with common attributes such as contexts, characteristics or concerns, including health risks. However, in countries other than the United States, the term *client* often refers to persons who are paying for their care directly. In most countries, *patient* is used to describe persons who are in hospital or rehabilitation. *Service user* and *person* are terms in general use that describe those in need of OT services. For this chapter, we are using *client* without implying the source of payment for services.

on factors involved in the interaction between cognition and everyday functioning and participation and thus provide a comprehensive understanding of cognition in context. The C-FE suggests assessment of five major domains that are listed below (Rotenberg & Maeir, 2019).

1. Clients' perspective of functional cognitive limitations and behaviors; interviews and ratings of everyday participation.
2. Cognitive profile: Domain-specific tests to describe cognitive impairments and capacities.
3. Functional assessments of cognition: performance-based testing.
4. Self-awareness regarding cognitive deficits and functional cognition
5. Assessment of environmental and contextual factors

Initial interviews or questionnaires along with cognitive screenings may be followed by domain-specific assessments and functional cognitive assessments. When combined, the data from the C-FE process provides the therapist with a comprehensive perspective of the potential interaction of the influence of cognitive symptoms on performance within the context of the environment. Whenever feasible, standardized evaluation tools or questionnaires with established psychometric properties such as validity, reliability, and sensitivity to change in occupational performance should be used to establish an objective baseline of performance and allow for measurement of progress. Tables 55.1 and 55.2 outline a variety of assessment tools for different aspects of client evaluation. It should be kept in mind that formal assessments should also be combined with observations of performance and client perspectives as described below.

TABLE 55.1 **Examples of Cognitive Perceptual Assessments for Children**

Note: *Sources for all assessments can be found online at* Lippincott Connect

Interviews, Questionnaires, and Rating Scales—Perspective of Child and Others

Occupational Profile	**Ratings of Everyday Cognitive Symptoms**
Children's Assessment of Participation and Enjoyment (CAPE) (ages 6–21 yr)	Behavior Rating Inventory of Executive Function (BRIEF 2) (5–18 yr) and Preschool Version BRIEF-P (2–5.11 yr)
Child Occupational Self-Assessment 2.2. (COSA) (7–17 yr)	Children Visual Behavior checklist (7–12.11 yr)
Pediatric Activity Card Sort (PACS) (6–12 yr)	Developmental Coordination Disorder DCDQ-R questionnaire (5–14.6 yr)
Short Child Occupational Profile (SCOPE), v. 2.2, (birth–21 yr)	Executive Function and Occupational Routines Scale (EFORTS) (3–10 yr)
Functional/Cognitive IADL Activities	Multidimensional everyday memory ratings for youth (MEMRY) (ages 5–21)
Pediatric Evaluation of Disability Inventory Computer Adaptive Test PEDI-CAT (birth–20 yr)	**Awareness Questionnaires or Rating Scales**
The Roll Evaluation of Activities of Life (REAL) (2–18.11 yr)	Pediatric Awareness Questionnaire (PAQ) (8–16)
School Function Assessment (SFA) (K–6th grade)	**Diagnostic-Specific Rating Scales**
	Childhood (4–12) and Teenage (13–19) Executive Function Inventory (CHEXI and TEXI) (ADHD)

Cognitive Screening Instruments

Delirium Screening	**Comprehensive Cognitive Screening**
Preschool Confusion Assessment Method for the ICU (psCAM-ICU) < 5 yr	Dynamic Occupational Therapy Cognitive Assessment for Children (DOTCA-Ch) (6–12 yr)
Pediatric Confusion Assessment Method for the Intensive Care Unit (pCAM-ICU) ≥ 5	

Performance-Based Tests of Functional Cognition

Level of Cues or Assistance Needed	**Types of Performance Errors**
Children's Kitchen Task Assessment (8–12 yr)	Children's Cooking Task (CCT) (8–18 yr)
Preschool Executive Task Assessment (PETA) (3–5 yr)	Weekly Calendar Planning Activity (WCPA) (above age 11)
Skills Interfering With Performance	
Do-Eat (EF rating) (5–8 yr)	
School AMPS (3–15 yr)	

Domain-Specific Cognitive Perceptual Tests

Executive Function and Memory	**Visual Perception**
Behavioural Assessment of the Dysexecutive Syndrome for Children (BADS-C). (8–16 yrs)	Beery-Buktenica Developmental Test of Visual-Motor Integration, 6th ed. (BEERY VMI) (age 2 and up)
Contextual Memory Test (CMT-2)—Children	Developmental Test of Visual Perception—3rd ed. (DTVP-3) (4–12.11 yr)
Motor Planning	Motor-Free Visual Perception Test-4 (MVPT-4) (4–80 yr)
Motor Planning Maze Assessment (MPMA) (3–teens)	Test of Visual-Perceptual Skills—4th ed. (TVPS-4) (5–21 yr)
Movement Assessment Battery (M-ABC-2)	
Test of Ideational Praxis (TIP) (3–8 yr)	
Spatial Neglect	
Letter Cancellation Test (9 yr and above)	
Teddy Bear Cancellation Test (TBCT) (3–8 yr)	

TABLE 55.2   Examples of Cognitive Perceptual Assessment for Adults

Note: *Sources for all assessments can be found online at Lippincott Connect*

Interviews, Questionnaires, and Rating Scales—Perspective of Client and Others

Occupational Profile
Activity Card Sort (ACS), 2nd ed.
Canadian Occupational Performance Measure 5th ed. (COPM)
Functional Activities/Cognitive IADL
Activity Measure for Post-Acute Care (AM-PAC®) Applied
  Cognitive Scale
Daily Living Questionnaire (DLQ)
Nottingham Extended Activities of Daily Living Scale (NEADL)
Occupational Self-Assessment – Short-Form (OSA-SF)
  version 2.2
Ratings of Everyday Cognitive Symptoms
Behavior Rating Inventory of Executive Function-Adult Version
  (BRIEF-A)
Brief Assessment of Prospective Memory (BAPM)
Moss Attentional Rating Scale (MARS)

Diagnostic-Specific Rating Scales
Functional Assessment of Cancer Therapy—Cognition
  (FACT-Cog)
Subjective Scale to Investigate Cognition in Schizophrenia
  (SSTICS)
Awareness Questionnaires or Rating Scales
Abridged Anosognosia Questionnaire (dementia) Awareness
  Questionnaire (AQ)
Self-Awareness of Deficits Interview (SADI)
Self-Awareness Multilevel Assessment Scale
Scale to Assess Unawareness in Mental Disorder in
  schizophrenia (SUMD)

Cognitive Screening Instruments

Mental Status Exams
Mini-Mental State Exam (MMSE)
Montreal Cognitive Assessment (MoCA)
Medi-Cog—R

Comprehensive Cognitive Screenings
Dynamic Loewenstein Occupational Therapy Cognitive
  Assessment (DLOTCA)
Geriatric version available: (LOTCA-G)

Performance-Based Tests of Functional Cognition

Accuracy
Kohlman Evaluation of Living Skills (KELS) 4th ed.
Safe at Home
Test of Grocery Shopping Skills (TOGSS)
Texas Functional Living Scale (TFLS)
University of California, San Diego Performance-Based Skills
  Assessment-Brief (UPSA-Brief)
Level of Cognitive Functioning
Allen Cognitive Level Screen (ACLS-5) and large version
  (LACLS)
Cognitive Performance Test (CPT)
Routine Task Inventory (RTI)

Level of Cues or Assistance Needed
Kettle Test
Executive Function Performance Test (EFPT) and enhanced
  version. EFPT-e
Performance Assessment of Self-Care Skills, Version 4.0
Skills Interfering with Performance
ADL-Focused Occupation-Based Neurobehavioral Evaluation
  (A-ONE)
Actual Reality Task
Assessment of Motor and Process Skills (AMPS)
Types of Performance Errors
Multiple Errands Test–Revised (MET)
Perceive, recall, plan and perform (PRPP)
Weekly Calendar Planning Activity (WCPA)

Domain-Specific Cognitive Perceptual Tests

Memory
Contextual Memory Test (Online version:CMT-2)
Rivermead Behavioural Memory Test |Third Edition (RBMT-3)
  (16–96)
Motor Planning
Diagnostic Instrument for Limb Apraxia-Short Version (DILA-S)

Spatial Neglect
Bell's Cancellation Test
Kessler Foundation Neglect Assessment Process (KF-NAP™)
The Baking Tray Test (BTT)
Visual Perception
Motor-Free Visual Perception (MVPT-4)
Brain Injury Visual Assessment Battery for Adults (biVABA)

Clients' Perspective of Functional Cognitive Limitations and Behaviors

Occupational therapists typically begin the evaluation process with a structured or semistructured interview of the client or informant that inquires about the client's typical routines and meaningful occupations. Such information helps occupational therapists to develop an **occupational profile** of the client's past functioning and goals for the future (AOTA, 2020b). The client or informant is usually asked to identify everyday activities that they are most concerned about or would like to be able to do with greater ease (see Tables 55.1 and 55.2).

Interviews can be supplemented by structured questionnaires or rating scales to provide information on the client's perceived functioning as well as the perceptions of others (clinicians, significant others, parents, or teachers). There are different types of questionnaires or rating scales. Some questionnaires assess general level of function or participation while others have been specifically developed to assess perceived functioning in cognitively demanding activities (cognitive IADL scales). In addition, there are several questionnaires or rating scales that examine the frequency of reported general or diagnostic-specific cognitive symptoms occurring within the context of everyday life. For example, the Behavior Rating Inventory of Executive Function

(BRIEF; Baron, 2000) assesses executive function behaviors from preschool to adults, within the school or home, and was designed to be used across a wide range of diagnostic groups. Other questionnaires are tailored toward cognitive symptoms occurring within daily life for specific diagnostic groups such as people with attention-deficit/hyperactivity disorder (ADHD), concussion, mild cognitive impairment (MCI), schizophrenia, stroke, or cancer. In some cases, there may be questions about the extent that the person's self-report reflects actual function due to limitations in **self-awareness** or an inability to recognize functional cognitive problems. Nonetheless, the person's perspectives and lived experiences are important to understand and respect, regardless of whether they match observations. Self-awareness and specific methods for assessment are described later in this chapter.

There is evidence that self or informant reports of cognitive functioning assess different underlying constructs than performance-based measures that directly observe function (Muzzatti et al., 2020; Spreij et al., 2021). Reports by clients and informants are based on subjective perceptions and experiences across time within the context of everyday life and add a unique perspective that should be validated and highly valued. Performance-based tests (i.e., objective tests) involve direct task observation and are based on one point in time. However, they provide the opportunity to gain in-depth information on the process of how a person goes about the task. Both subjective reports and performance-based measures provide important and complementary information. This highlights the need to administer both subjective and objective performance-based assessments whenever feasible (Schmitter-Edgecombe et al., 2020).

Explore Cognitive Profile/Factors

Cognitive Screening. Cognitive screening tools identify cognitive changes that can significantly impact functional independence or discharge recommendations as well as cognitive areas that may need further attention and assessment. Most brief cognitive screenings assess mental status and provide global ratings of the client's orientation, attention, and memory. Some screening tools include short assessments of language, visuospatial abilities, and executive functions. Cognitive screening tools provide an overall score or diagnostic cutoff score that differentiates "normal" from suspect or impaired cognitive functioning. In choosing a screening, the published sensitivity (i.e., persons correctly identified as having cognitive impairment) and specificity (i.e., correct identification of persons without cognitive impairment) need to be considered within the population that is being tested. Typically, cognitive screening exams are short, standardized assessments that require minimal equipment (e.g., paper and pencil and computerized versions) making them convenient for bedside and office testing. In addition, many of these tests are in the public domain or freely available on the Internet. Screening tools such as the popular Montreal Cognitive

Assessment (MoCA; Nasreddine et al., 2005) have been used and validated in various populations and languages and have been found to be predictive of functional outcomes (Jaywant, Toglia, et al., 2020; Lim et al., 2018; Zietemann et al., 2018). For more information see https://www.mocatest.org/.

Cognitive screening tests are particularly useful within acute care settings where there are time constraints or the client may be unaware of limitations and specialized cognitive assessment is not available (Wolf, 2019). In inpatient settings, cognitive screening is particularly important because mild cognitive deficits can be easily missed by health professionals and families (Goverover, Chiaravalloti, & DeLuca, 2019; Wolf, 2019). Also, in the early stages of an illness or injury, the presence of obvious physical deficits often receives greater attention than cognitive deficits.

Cognitive screening tests have several disadvantages. They rely heavily on verbal skills, are culturally biased, and have substantial false-negative rates (i.e., missing possible cognitive impairments). A recent cognitive screening tool, the Medi-Cog combines recall of three words and a clock drawing task with a functional cognitive task that requires placing pills into a pillbox according to instructions (Marks et al., 2020). This brief screening measure has been shown to be useful in detecting possible functional cognitive deficits in community-dwelling older adults and addresses some of the limitations of traditional measures.

In general, cognitive screening assessments may miss more subtle impairments that are displayed by clients with mild impairments. For example, Toglia and colleagues (2017) found that one-third of people with stroke who did not show impairment on the MoCA at admission to an acute inpatient rehabilitation unit exhibited IADL deficits on discharge. Therefore, administration of a functional cognitive performance-based IADL test for those that score within normal ranges on a cognitive screening test is recommended (Toglia et al., 2017). In these situations, complex performance-based measures as described below should be used in an inpatient setting or the person should be referred to outpatient OT for further assessment and follow-up. Screening is the first stage of the evaluation process that should be followed with tests of functional cognition and cognitive tests for specific domains if needed.

Domain-Specific Cognitive Assessments. When the client's performance in either cognitive screening or functional cognitive measures indicates the potential for cognitive impairments, occupational therapists may administer more specific standardized cognitive assessments (see Table 55.1) or if available, refer the person for neuropsychological testing to better understand their cognitive strengths and weaknesses and quantify the level of impairment. Neuropsychological assessments have strong psychometric properties and can provide valuable insights into specific cognitive abilities, compared to a normative sample. Neuropsychological and standardized cognitive assessments, however, focus on isolated cognitive skills and are administered in quiet structured environments whereas functional performance requires the integration and interleaving of cognitive abilities and the ability to function in a variety of environments (Toglia & Foster, 2021). The relationship between standardized cognitive tests and functional cognitive tests has been found to be weak-moderate indicating that although they share commonalities, each type of test provides unique information (Goverover, Toglia, & DeLuca, 2019; Weber, Goverover, & DeLuca, 2019). Therefore, standardized cognitive or neuropsychological tests are not a substitute for functional cognitive tests or direct observation of functional performance. OT is therefore uniquely positioned to observe and document functional cognitive performance and outcome using performance-based assessment tools described in the next section because neuropsychological or standardized cognitive assessments alone do not provide a full picture of the person's function.

Performance-Based Testing of Functional Cognition

Functional cognitive *performance-based tests* are designed to assess how an individual responds to the cognitive demands of everyday situations. They include observation of performance of everyday activities (real or simulated). Since IADL have greater cognitive demands and rely more heavily on executive functions, most performance-based tests use IADL tasks. Performance-based tests can be categorized according to the methods used to observe and rate functional performance. These include (a) breaking a task into key task subcomponents and rating accuracy or competency; (b) level of assistance/cues needed to successfully complete each task component or to support executive function skills; (c) characterizing cognitive levels; (d) rating underlying process skills or impairments interfering with successful performance; and (e) identifying types of performance errors (no cues) (Toglia & Foster, 2021). Some tools use a combination of methods; however, each performance-based method provides different types of information that should be considered in selecting an assessment. For example, if information is needed on the level and type of support the client needs, a performance-based assessment that uses progressive cues or assesses cognitive level should be considered. While there are several standardized tools available, performance-based methods can also be used with any task that is relevant to the client by adopting a systematic method of analyzing and rating performance of task components (Toglia & Foster, 2021; Velikonja et al., 2017)

There are numerous performance-based measures available for use listed in Tables 55.1 and 55.2. Descriptions of a few performance-based tests are provided below to illustrate differences in methods as well as applications across ages and populations.

The Test of Grocery Skills Shopping (TOGSS; Harris et al., 2021) is performed in a supermarket or real-world environment. Although it was designed for persons with schizophrenia, it can be used with other populations. The test measures the ability to locate 10 items in a grocery store according to specific rules. Scores reflect accuracy and efficiency in completing the grocery shopping task and are correlated with measures of executive function. While the TOGGS focuses on accuracy, The Executive Function Performance Test (EFPT; Baum et al., 2008, 2017) examines how much assistance and what type of cues a person needs to successfully accomplish daily life tasks. The EFPT is based on performance of four IADL tasks: cooking, making a phone call, taking medication, and paying a bill), and it has four alternate tasks (Hahn et al., 2014) as well as two Internet tasks (online bill paying and telephone use). An enhanced version, EFPT-e, includes more complex tasks than the original EFPT (see Table 55.2). The EFPT has been used with varied populations including older adults, those with neurological, disorders, mental health disorders, and chronic diseases (Baum et al., 2017, 2019). In addition, the EFPT has been used as a basis for development of two performance-based measures for children, the Preschool Executive Task Assessment (PETA), and the Children's Kitchen Task Assessment (CKTA), which involve following a recipe to make play dough for ages 8 to 12. Another functional cognitive assessment, The Weekly Calendar Planning Assessment (WCPA; Toglia, 2015), involves entering a list of appointments into a weekly schedule while adhering to multiple rules and managing conflicts without cues or assistance. Similar to the TOGSS, both accuracy and efficiency in completing the task are scored. The WCPA, however, also rates the number and type of strategies used, analyzes error types, and examines the person's awareness of strategies used as a way to characterize and interpret performance. In addition, normative data is available from ages 12 to 94. The WCPA has been used with at-risk youth, healthy older adults, and across a variety of mental health and neurological disorders (Goverover, Toglia, & DeLuca, 2019; Lussier et al., 2019; Zlotnik & Toglia, 2018).

It is important to acknowledge that performance-based tests that simulate performance in a treatment setting may not be predictive of performance in natural contexts in which the person must establish goals, plan, initiate, problem-solve, and manage both subtle and complex environmental cues.

The Environment and Contextual Factors

The environment where cognitive tasks are performed may either support or hinder a client's occupational performance. Situations that require higher-level cognitive perceptual skills are difficult to create in structured treatment environments. Some environmental assessments were designed for specific cognitively impaired populations, such as Home Environmental Assessment Protocol (HEAP; Gitlin et al.,

2002) which was developed for individuals with dementia and their caregivers (Struckmeyer et al., 2020).

Assessment for Clients With Severe Cognitive Impairments

A client who presents with significant confusion, agitation, or language and object recognition impairments will most likely be unable to follow the instructions of a standardized assessment. Observational rating scales such as the Moss Attentional Rating Scale (MARS; see Table 55.2) can be used to systematically characterize abilities in those with severe cognitive or language impairments. Simple functional performance-based tasks such as brushing teeth, washing hands, or buttering a slice of bread should be used when is feasible. Such tasks can be broken down into small subcomponents or steps for systematic assessment. Accurate completion of each task component with or without cues can be rated to provide an objective measure of task performance (e.g., the E-ADL assessment; Luttenberger et al., 2012). Appropriate selection and use of objects within the context of a simplified functional task can be assessed by including irrelevant objects or distractors, as described by Toglia (2011). Note that once the client can attend for at least 10 minutes and reliably follow directions, the therapist may engage in more formal evaluation of the client's cognitive perceptual skills.

Overview of Cognitive Intervention Models and Approaches

Cognitive intervention approaches reflect different perspectives on learning and the ability to apply or generalize information to daily life. Each approach differs in the areas targeted for change or emphasized in intervention. For example, some approaches emphasize change in the task or environment (e.g., functional approaches), whereas others emphasize change in the person's skills (e.g., remedial). Evaluation and treatment guidelines reflect these different areas of focus.

This section describes different cognitive intervention approaches as well as factors that are critical in the selection and application of the treatment approaches. There are five main approaches: (a) functional, (b) remedial, (c) cognitive strategy, (d) combined approaches, and (e) health promotion and prevention. Each of these approaches is described below.

Functional Approaches

Functional approaches emphasize the ability to successfully perform everyday tasks and routines by building on the person's assets and/or residual skills. Activity limitations

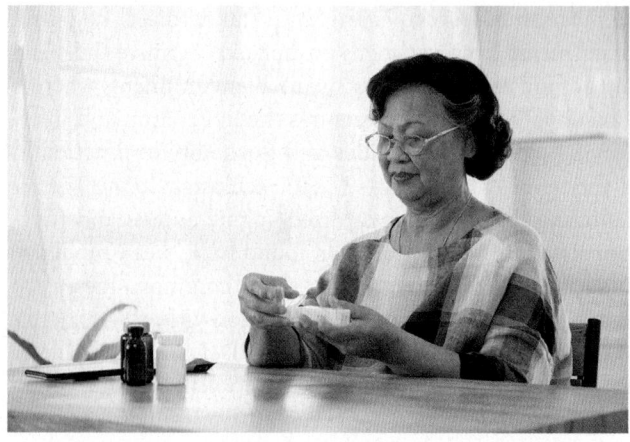

FIGURE 55.1 A pillbox organizer can be an important contextual cue to help those with memory impairments to safely self-administer medications.

and participation restrictions are reduced by changing the task and environment or enhancing specific task performance rather than remediating or restoring impaired skills (Figure 55.1). Common methods used within the functional approach include the following:

- Adaptation or modification of tasks or the environment
- Matching or prescribing activities appropriate to the person's level (Allen, 1985)
- Compensatory methods, strategies, or technologies such as smart phones, smart homes, and digital assistants (Gentry, 2018)
- Caregiver education, training, collaboration, or coaching (Döpp et al., 2015; Gitlin et al., 2016)
- Task-specific methods include errorless learning (i.e., the person is prevented from making incorrect or inappropriate responses during the learning process), vanishing cues, and spaced retrieval (Ferry, 2021; Giles, 2018)

It is important to acknowledge that functional methods can require different levels of learning, environmental support, and awareness. For example, adaptations, task modifications, and/or technologies may be set up, implemented, and monitored by others or practiced repeatedly to encourage automatic learning. On the other hand, individuals can be taught compensatory methods to modify or adapt activities themselves. This latter approach requires self-awareness and higher levels of learning

Task or Environmental Adaptations

Adaptations, such as alarms or restructuring of the environment (e.g., eliminating distractors, providing bright light) may be used to compensate for cognitive impairments. The assumption of this approach is that errors in daily tasks may be reduced by simplifying the relationship between the environment and the required response (Kessler et al., 2015). Such adaptations to the environment require implementation and support by others, and therefore, adaptive methods go hand in hand with caregiver training. Involvement of a caregiver in treatment is crucial for successful outcomes.

The Cognitive Disability Model. Allen (1985) developed the Cognitive Disability Model (CDM), which provides guidelines for matching and adapting the individual's functional cognitive capacities with activity demands and contexts. In this model, function is organized into six ordinal levels of global functional cognitive capacities, ranging from normal (Level 6) to profoundly disabled (Level 1). Modes of performance within each level further qualify behavior variations and allow for more sensitive measurement of the person's global functional capacity. The CDM has been most frequently applied to persons with mental health conditions, hospitalized and community-dwelling older adults, and those with dementia. It has provided a strong foundation for the development of other interventions described below (e.g., Cognitive Adaptation Training [CAT], Tailored Activity Program [TAP], and the Care of Older Persons in their Environment [COPE]) that share similarities in principles with a focus on task and environmental modifications or supports and caregiver training to optimize functional cognition. To obtain a comprehensive description of the CDM and Allen Cognitive Levels, refer to Allen (1985), McCraith and Earhart (2018), and Levy (2018). Please refer to this website for resources and more details: https://allencognitive.com/.

Programs Involving Adaptation for Persons With Mental Health Conditions: Cognitive Adaptation Training. CAT is an evidence-based strategy to improve functional performance by integrating environmental supports into routines, home, or work contexts (Velligan, 2018; Velligan et al., 2015). **Environmental supports** include signs, reminders, checklists, and organizing the environment. Velligan et al. (2009) collaborated with occupational therapists to create a systematic approach for the use of environmental supports and compensatory strategies for persons with schizophrenia to improve their functional behaviors (Velligan et al., 2009, 2015). Persons with different cognitive behaviors (e.g., decreased initiation vs. disinhibition) were found to benefit from different types of adaptations (Velligan et al., 2009). Adaptations and environmental supports should address the problems and needs identified by the client and/or family/caregivers as well as be appropriate to the client's culture and cognitive capacities. This adaptation program is supported by evidence from randomized controlled trials that have resulted in reduced levels of symptomatology, lower relapse rates, decreased caregiver burden, increased levels of adaptive functioning and attainment of goals, improved quality of life, and improved medication adherence

(Allott et al., 2017; Kidd et al., 2018; Stiekema et al., 2020). Further information on the CAT program can be found on the following website: https://div12.org/treatment/cognitive-adaptation-training-cat-for-schizophrenia.

Programs Involving Adaptation for Persons With Dementia: Tailored Activity Program and the Care of Older Persons in Their Environment. TAP is an individually designed, client-centered program implemented by occupational therapists that involves identifying the interests and abilities of those with dementia and closely collaborating with caregivers to use tailored activities as part of everyday routines (Gitlin et al., 2016, 2021). The TAP was influenced by the CDM and includes a system of matching task and environmental demands with the individual's capabilities. TAP can be delivered in home, hospital, residential, or adult day services settings (Marx et al., 2019). Studies have found that TAP reduces the frequency of behavioral symptoms, caregiver upset, and the need for assistance from others; in addition, it improves caregiver skills, efficacy, and mood and decreases healthcare costs (Gitlin et al., 2016, 2021; Oliveira et al., 2019). A certification course is available for occupational therapists to implement this evidence-based program. Similarly, the COPE program is a dyad evidence-based intervention that includes both the caregiver and the person with dementia within the home environment. The COPE focus is on reducing environmental stressors and enhancing knowledge and skills of the caregiver. Compared to controls, persons with dementia receiving COPE experienced less functional decline and more activity engagement, while care partners reported improved well-being and greater ability to keep family members at home (Clemson et al., 2021; Fortinsky et al., 2020). For more information on COPE, visit https://drexel.edu/cnhp/research/centers/agewell/Research-Studies/COPE/.

Adaptations for Children. Occupational therapists can collaborate with parents and teachers to adapt tasks at home or school to enhance ADL, and academic performance, or support child participation. Adaptations may include color-coding locations for materials, posting cue signs, pictures, or large checklists for multiple-step activities such as cleaning a room or packing a backpack. It can also include establishing fixed routines, breaking down directions or assignments into small components, and reorganizing or creating organizational systems for rooms, lockers, binders, backpacks, or desk draws to enhance organization (Waldman-Levi & Steinmann Obermeyer, 2018).

Formal parent coaching programs such as the Occupational Performance Coaching Program include guiding parents in identifying possible ways that they can modify tasks to facilitate occupational performance (e.g., changing the sequence of tasks in the bedtime routine or seating arrangement during homework activities; Chien et al., 2020, 2021).

Functional Task Training: The Neurofunctional Approach and Errorless Learning

The neurofunctional approach (NFA) emphasizes the use of **task-specific training** or rote repetition of specific tasks or routines within natural contexts to develop habits or functional behavioral routines. Repetitive practice reduces the demands on cognitive resources needed for task performance and increases automaticity of performance. Emphasis is on the mastery of functional task performance through the practice of "doing" meaningful activities. Intervention involves systematically breaking down a functional task into essential subcomponents for the person (Clark-Wilson et al., 2014; Giles et al., 2019). Practice using errorless learning methods facilitates learning and performance for those with significant memory deficits. Key techniques such as goal setting, task analysis, repetition, practice, cue experimentation, chaining, feedback, and reinforcement methods (Giles, 2018) may be used to promote skill acquisition.

The NFA was initially designed for persons with chronic or severe cognitive impairments as a result of TBI (Clark-Wilson et al., 2014; Giles, 2018). Similar approaches have been applied to persons with a history of cerebrovascular accidents (CVA; Rotenberg-Shpigelman et al., 2012), and individuals with TBI in acute rehabilitation (Trevena-Peters et al., 2018). Please see case example using the NFA approach and an evidence commentary in the online material.

Functional task training using errorless learning capitalizes on procedural or implicit memory of "how-to" do something rather than verbal memory for facts and events. Electronic devices, including tablets and smartphones, can be used to provide pictures or videos of task steps as prompts to facilitate errorless learning of habits and routines during task-specific training. Errorless learning methods have been demonstrated to be effective in people with dementia (Voigt-Radloff et al., 2017), autism (Leaf et al., 2020), Korsakoff syndrome (Rensen et al., 2019), and schizophrenia (Kern et al., 2018). For example, work outcomes were significantly improved following treatment with errorless learning in people with serious mental illness (Kern et al., 2018).

Compensation

Compensation bypasses or minimizes the effects of impairment by teaching the person to use methods that capitalize on their strengths and reduce demands on areas of weakness. For example, the client is taught to modify tasks and environments themselves or use compensatory strategies such as a checklist, smartphone reminder app, or an internal strategy such as self-talk to overcome a limitation presented by their cognitive impairment or the environment.

Task-specific strategies are taught within targeted tasks and environments and combined with errorless learning and adaptive methods. For example, in learning to use a new microwave oven the person can be taught a verbal rehearsal strategy of stating the steps out loud. Through repetition and practice of operating the microwave, initiation of the verbal rehearsal strategy can become automatic and may facilitate performance. Teaching to use a task-specific strategy is for the sole goal of enabling the client to perform the specific task they need to perform. The use of compensatory strategies beyond a specific task or context requires self-awareness and generalization of learning. **Compensatory strategies** can be provided by the therapist and taught directly or they can be integrated within metacognitive strategy approaches (described later in this section) that promote strategy generation and use through guided learning methods.

Summary of Evidence for Functional Approaches

The effectiveness of the functional approach has been demonstrated in persons with schizophrenia (Kessler et al., 2015; Velligan, 2018), brain injury (Clark-Wilson et al., 2014), dementia (Ferry, 2021; Gitlin et al., 2021, p. 202), and children with various conditions (Caprì et al., 2021).

In general, modification or adaptation of tasks, environments, and social contexts including collaboration or coaching with caregivers has wide evidence support across the life span for improving quality of life, decreasing behavioral problems, maintaining function, or enhancing participation in productive activities. Similarly, functional task training can produce significant changes in performance of ADL and vocational tasks in people with severe or long-term cognitive impairments. The NFA has been evaluated in several single-case, small group, and a large randomized controlled study, supporting robust changes in daily living skills for people with acquired brain injury (ABI; Giles, 2018). Functional approaches require continued consistency and support from others. Challenges in implementation can include poor carryover by others or an overwhelmed caregiver who is stressed and unable to consistently follow through with adaptations or systems of prompts required for errorless learning. In these situations, full analysis of the context and potential obstacles for implementation together with support for both the caregiver and the client may be needed. In some settings, reimbursement for services to caregivers for a person with chronic, progressive, or severe cognitive deficits may be an obstacle. In these situations, it is important to advocate for services by presenting a rationale, supported by evidence-based research.

Compensatory methods are widely used in clinical practice by occupational therapists and supported by evidence for people with psychosis (Allott et al., 2020) and TBI (Cicerone et al., 2019), and for children (Resch et al., 2018) and older adults (Tomaszewski Farias et al., 2018).

Remedial Approaches

Remedial approaches place an emphasis on evaluating and restoring impaired cognitive perceptual skills. They focus on identifying and targeting the person's underlying deficits or skills rather than manipulating the activity demands or context (Kim et al., 2018). This approach assumes that repetitive training on impaired tasks stimulates neuroplasticity and allows the brain to reorganize its structural and functional connections (Sala & Gobet, 2019).

In traditional remedial approaches, cognitive skills are divided into a hierarchy of discrete subskills, such as attention, discrimination, memory, sequencing, categorization, concept formation, and problem-solving. The lower-level skills such as attention provide the foundation for more complex skills and behaviors such as problem-solving (Toglia, 2018). Nonetheless, improvement in underlying cognitive or perceptual deficits is thought to promote recovery or reorganization of the impaired skill. Information on functional reorganization and adult brain plasticity support this view (Goverover, 2018).

Targeted and intense training of discrete skills that complies with the principles of neuroplasticity (direct stimulation of a cognitive domain, ongoing adaptive adjustment of task difficulty, and immediate objective feedback on task performance) has better remedial benefits than the use of repetitive memory drills or general cognitive stimulation activities (Cicerone et al., 2019). Thus, the adaptive capabilities of newer technologies that adjust the level of challenge to the person's abilities is a critical ingredient to improve cognitive function (Pedullà et al., 2016). Populations with the most positive responses (and most research studies) include healthy older adults (Nguyen et al., 2019), people with MS (Goverover, Chiaravalloti, O'Brien, & DeLuca, 2018), and those with schizophrenia (Harvey et al., 2018). However, in general, there is insufficient evidence that demonstrates the impact of such intervention on everyday functioning (Goverover, 2018).

Many commercial computerized programs are available for use. They are easy to administer and adaptive but evidence is inadequate to support isolated use in practice. Additional information regarding these programs is available in a review (Shah et al., 2017) that describes the characteristics of such training programs, and assesses the number and quality of studies evaluating the empirical evidence related to commercial programs, with inclusive results.

In sum, remedial interventions have been criticized because a person can show changes in specific cognitive exercises without changes in everyday function or cognitive skills that were not trained (Bharadwaj et al., 2022; Sala & Gobet, 2019; Simons et al., 2016). Remedial interventions are more effective when combined with coaching, goal setting, peer support (Goverover, 2018), self-monitoring techniques, and strategy training (Cicerone et al., 2019). Therefore, it is recommended that remedial activities be combined with other intervention approaches if used.

Metacognitive Cognitive Strategy Approaches

Metacognition includes knowledge or awareness of one's thinking and strengths or weaknesses as well as control or moment-to-moment self-monitoring including ability to recognize potential obstacles, adjust and use strategies effectively, and self-assess performance in comparison to goals or outcomes. **Metacognitive strategy approaches** within OT represent a broad group of interventions that use structured metacognitive processes within the context of occupational performance and focus on cognitive strategies rather than discrete cognitive skills. Effective strategy use requires metacognitive skills such as the ability to assess task demands or recognize when a strategy is needed, monitor performance, detect errors, make adjustments, and self-evaluate performance (Toglia & Foster, 2021). Some metacognitive strategy approaches place a greater emphasis on self-awareness or self-monitoring skills while others focus on goal management or problem-solving methods; however, all such approaches focus on methods to enhance strategy use, learning, and performance within everyday activities.

Within metacognitive strategy approaches, strategies are viewed from a broad perspective and are considered to be an inherent and normal part of occupational performance. Strategies extend beyond compensation and are described as methods, tools, or procedures that are used to improve information processing, learning, and/or performance. They help a person acquire new information or skills and cope with cognitive challenges. Cognitive strategies can be *internal* and include self-talk, self-cues, or use of mental practice, or they can be *external* and include the use of a checklist. Healthy people use multiple strategies in everyday life (Toglia et al., 2012).

Metacognitive strategy approaches have been used with both children and adults across various conditions including ADHD (Levanon-Erez et al., 2019), schizophrenia (Ishikawa et al., 2020; Vizzotto et al., 2021), TBI (Radomski et al., 2018, 2020), healthy older adults (Coe et al., 2019) and a wide range of other developmental, mental health and neurological diagnostic groups. OT treatment approaches that use a metacognitive strategy approach include the following: multicontext approach (Toglia, 2018; Toglia & Foster, 2021), the Cognitive Orientation to Occupational Performance (CO-OP) approach (McEwen et al., 2018; Polatajko et al., 2012); and the Cog-Fun approach (for more information see https://medicine.ekmd.huji.ac.il/en/occupationalTherapy/research/cogfun/Pages/default.aspx).

The Multicontext Approach

The multicontext approach is based on the Dynamic Interactional Model (DIM) of Cognition. The DIM explains how the interaction between personal factors with activity and environmental demands influences occupational performance (Toglia, 2018; Toglia & Foster, 2021). There are six treatment components of the multicontext approach:

1. Focus on use of cognitive strategies
2. Activities structured to promote transfer and generalization
3. Metacognitive framework
4. Therapeutic support focused on enhancing self-efficacy
5. Treatment activities that are functionally relevant and at an optimal level of challenge
6. Goal setting and revision

The first three components are specific to this approach while the latter three present generic therapeutic methods. However, all components are used simultaneously in treatment. The multicontext approach uses a metacognitive framework that focuses on assisting clients in anticipating challenges, monitoring performance, generating strategies, and evaluating performance themselves through the use of mediated learning techniques and guided questions. The metacognitive framework is embedded within activities that are structured to promote transfer and generalization. For example, the person practices recognizing application of a strategy such as the use of a checklist, mental rehearsal, or self-cues across purposeful and occupation-based activities that systematically differ in appearance yet remain at a similar level of difficulty. Such practice of strategies places gradual demands on the ability to transfer learning because the more two situations or activities are physically similar, the easier it is to transfer strategies learned in one situation to another (Toglia & Foster, 2021). Table 55.3 shows an example of intervention activities presented along the transfer continuum. Activity demands are not graded in difficulty until evidence of spontaneous strategy use along the entire transfer continuum is observed.

Assessments used in the multicontext approach determine how external variables such as activity demands, alterations in the environment, and mediation from others influence a person's strategy use and self-awareness during task performance (Toglia, 2018; Toglia & Foster, 2021).

The multicontext approach was originally developed for use with adults with TBI (Toglia, 2018); however, it has been applied to children and adolescents (Cermak & Toglia, 2018; Josman & Rosenblum, 2018; Waldman-Levi & Steinmann Obermeyer, 2018), Persons with schizophrenia (Josman & Rosenblum, 2018; Kaizerman-Dinerman et al.,

2018), adults with lupus (Harrison et al., 2005), and most recently an individual with cognitive deficits post COVID (Wilcox & Frank, 2021). There is now evidence to support this treatment approach for persons with ABI (Goverover et al., 2007b), TBI (Toglia et al., 2010), MS (Goverover, Chiaravalloti, Genova, & DeLuca, 2018), Parkinson disease (Foster et al., 2018), and stroke (Jaywant, Steinberg, et al., 2020; Nagelkop et al., 2021; Toglia & Chen, 2020). Comprehensive guidelines for this approach are detailed by Toglia and Foster (2021) and additional information can be found on the multicontext website: www.multicontext.net.

The Cognitive Orientation to Occupational Performance Approach

The CO-OP approach emphasizes the use of cognitive strategies in the development and acquisition of motor skills and daily living skills. It draws on dynamic systems theory as well as literature in motor performance, educational or cognitive psychology, and OT (McEwen et al., 2018).

The key components of the CO-OP approach include:

- Client-centered goals
- Dynamic performance analysis
- Cognitive strategy use
- Guided discovery
- Principles that include methods for promoting client engagement and learning
- Parent or significant other involvement
- A structured intervention format (i.e., preparation phase, acquisition phase, and check verification phase)

The CO-OP approach uses a combination of a global strategy "Goal, Plan, Do, Check" and domain-specific strategies to acquire skills that will support the person's daily functioning (McEwen et al., 2018). The global strategy is used as an overall problem-solving framework throughout intervention. Domain-specific strategies such as visual charts, lists, walking away, counting to 10, and punching a bag when feeling angry to manage specific tasks or situations are facilitated using guided discovery and enabling principles. In one case, children created and wrote their own goals and plans, reward charts, and time logs, and were encouraged to discover their own solutions using coaching, modeling, and feedback (Rodger & Vishram, 2010).

TABLE 55.3   The Transfer Continuum

Strategy Emphasized in All Activities: Use a Checklist to Gather and Keep Track of Items to:							
Very Similar		Somewhat Similar			Different		Very Different
Make vegetable salad (6–8 items)	Make fruit salad (6–8 items)	Set a table for dinner (for 6–8)	Pack 6–8 items in a lunchbox	Pack 6–8 items in a bag for an overnight stay	Put a list of 6–8 appointments in a calendar	Use a list to complete 6–8 party invitations	Use a list to complete 6–8 errands

The CO-OP approach was originally developed to enhance skill acquisition in children with developmental coordination disorder (DCD; McEwen et al., 2018) and subsequently applied to children with autism (Rodger & Vishram, 2010; Wilson, 2014), cerebral palsy (Gimeno et al., 2021), brain injury (Jackman et al., 2018), and pervasive developmental disorder (Phelan et al., 2009), as well as adults with stroke (Polatajko et al., 2012; Skidmore et al., 2015), brain injury (Dawson et al., 2009), older adults with MCI (Dawson et al., 2014), and women with chemotherapy-induced cognitive impairment (Wolf et al., 2016). More information can be found at https://icancoop.org/.

Summary of Metacognative Approaches

There is strong evidence supporting metacognitive strategy approaches across ages and diagnostic groups (Cicerone et al., 2019); however, this type of intervention requires the ability to learn from mistakes and respond to guidance from others. Therefore, it is not appropriate for a person with global or severe cognitive deficits, limited communication or language comprehension skills, or someone who completely denies any functional or cognitive difficulties and concerns.

Metacognitive strategy interventions can present challenges in implementation because therapists have to switch from jumping in to assist or providing direct cues and instruction whenever the client has difficulty, to asking guided questions. This requires a therapist to learn to reframe how they speak, prompt, and interact with clients during treatment. Training courses as well as practice, role-playing, and feedback support for therapists are needed to attain the skills necessary for proper implementation (Chui et al., 2020; Toglia & Foster, 2021).

Combined Approaches

Different treatment approaches might also be used at different points along the recovery trajectory or to address different problem areas or goals. An approach that includes components from both functional and remedial methods has been described within an OT cognitive rehabilitation framework by Schwartz and Sagiv (2018). Simultaneous combination of treatment methods requires further study and investigation and is usually delivered depending on the clients' abilities, stage of recovery, or disability.

Several studies have begun to examine combinations of cognitive treatment approaches. For example, Williams et al. (2020) describe a feasibility study exploring the integration of cognitive adaptation and remedial intervention for early psychosis and encourage future research in this area. In addition, there are several studies exploring feasibility and use of metacognitive strategy methods with computerized remedial programs in children (Resch et al.,

2021) and healthy older adults (Rosi et al., 2019), and in people with schizophrenia (Reeder et al., 2017) and cancer (Maeir et al., 2021).

Addressing Cognition Within Health Promotion and Prevention

Cognitive interventions with a focus on health promotion and prevention in healthy populations and in people with non-neurological conditions are emerging. These interventions use a broad, holistic approach that combines, cognitive adaptation and supports, compensatory cognitive strategies, or metacognitive strategies, with exercise, lifestyle modifications, self-management, or behavioral interventions. There is evidence that individual differences in cognitive abilities such as executive functions in healthy populations and those with non-neurological conditions have an impact on health, well-being, and participation. At the same time, stress, poor sleep, nutrition, or negative health behaviors further diminish cognitive abilities and illustrate a reciprocal relationship between cognition and health (Toglia & Katz, 2018).

Programs that include supporting, optimizing, or strengthening cognitive skills for establishment and management of healthy routines have emerged in the area of obesity (Eichen et al., 2021; Hayes et al., 2018) and substance abuse (Anderson et al., 2021; Mistler et al., 2021). Similarly, those who have a chronic disease are often burdened with increased cognitive demands needed for health management tasks while also being vulnerable to lower cognitive skills due to factors described above. This creates a negative cycle that leads to functional decline (Toglia & Foster, 2021). Greater attention and provider training are needed to recognize these issues and provide cognitive interventions, particularly in rural and lower socioeconomic areas.

For people in the early stages of chronic disease, optimization of cognitive skills such as executive functions through modifications, cognitive supports, or strategies has potential to lessen health disparities and the negative spiral of cognitive and functional decline and increase ability to manage complex health-related tasks. For example, cognitive skills can be supported through preprogrammed text reminders to help a person recall foods that need to be avoided, medication management organizational systems, or problem-solving strategies to adjust ingredients and amounts in recipes or plan the steps needed to implement a new exercise routine.

In addition, programs that optimize cognitive health in older adults involve supporting and maximizing participation in meaningful and cognitively challenging activities or occupations such as learning a new skill (taking or editing photos on an iPad; Chan et al., 2016; Dawson et al., 2014). These programs often combine cognitive challenges with physical and social activities as a means of fostering healthy cognitive aging.

Selecting Intervention Approaches

Five main approaches that are used across ages and diagnostic categories were presented in this section. Each of these approaches alone and in combination could be used to optimize functional cognition. The process of selecting an intervention is multifaceted and requires integration of information from different sources. Given the wide range of severity, symptoms, ages, populations, and performance challenges that characterize individuals with cognitive perceptual dysfunction, there is not one model or approach that will fit all clients.

In planning intervention, the clinician uses clinical reasoning and considers various variables such as the client's goals, severity of the cognitive and functional deficits, practice setting, the evidence supporting the approach, the context including external supports, significant others, and resources; the trajectory of the client's neurological condition and age. For a person who is completely unaware of their own difficulties, is unresponsive to cues, has severe global deficits, and does not show potential for change within the intervention time frame, a treatment approach that focuses on teaching others to change the environment or activity (e.g., TAP; CDM), may result in greater functional outcomes. The NFA, which uses repetitive practice to change performance on a specific task, might also be indicated to increase functional performance. However, a treatment approach that targets changes in strategy use such as the multicontext approach or CO-OP approach, might not be appropriate. Alternatively, a client who shows awareness or partial awareness of task error patterns that affect performance across situations, and/or decreased use of strategies, might benefit from a metacognitive strategy approach. This process is reflected in the scenarios described in OT Story 55.1.

Treatment Delivery Format

Traditionally, interventions for cognitive dysfunction are performed in person; however, such practice cannot always be maintained. For example, during the COVID-19 pandemic, restrictive measures were hampering their implementation. Therefore, everyday technology, virtual reality, and emerging technologies (augmented reality) are used to deliver cognitive interventions across different approaches to either support, optimize, or improve cognitive function (Gentry, 2018; Maggio et al., 2020). Remote communication technologies are now regarded as potential effective options to maintain and deliver cognitive interventions. Efficacy studies are growing in number with promising results (Burton & O'Connell, 2018; Hewitt et al., 2020). Note that each delivery format has its own limitations and clients' context, preferences, learning style, and resources should be taken into consideration when choosing treatment delivery method (see Chapter 67 for more information).

Importance of Context, Environment, and Culture When Tailoring Intervention to Improve Functional Cognition

Interventions to improve functional cognition should emphasize specific goals and related knowledge, beliefs, and values of the clients. The context of the person's life needs to be considered in planning and choosing intervention activities (Bjørkedal et al., 2020). This includes the person's occupations, personality, interests, premorbid level of functioning, culture, values, external supports, and resources. Interventions that address cognitive limitations need to be blended

---

OT STORY 55.1 USING A METACOGNITIVE APPROACH FOR A PATIENT WITH LONG COVID-19

Rhonda is a 52-year-old female who lives with her 22-year-old daughter. She worked full time as a senior project manager and event coordinator, a job that required a high level of organization, planning, and attention to detail. Rhonda was diagnosed with a mild case of COVID-19 and did not require hospitalization. She attempted to return to work after 5 weeks but was overwhelmed, fatigued, and unable to keep track of things. She then began to develop additional symptoms including vertigo, shortness of breath, low endurance, anxiety, "brain fog" and inability to concentrate. After 5 months, she has still not been able to return to work. Her physical capacity, endurance, and vertigo have greatly improved but "brain fog" and anxiety continue to create obstacles for return to her

former roles. She stated, "I lose track of things I am supposed to do all the time. My day slips away and I don't get things done. I feel disorganized and out of control."

The occupational therapist integrated a metacognitive strategy approach across a wide range of higher-level cognitively challenging functional activities in preparation for return to work. All activities were related to work (e.g., creating a work schedule, choosing a restaurant based on multiple criteria). These activities involved the ability to integrate information from different sources. During activities, there was a focus on guiding Rhonda to anticipate and identify challenges, recognize triggers or early warning signs of anxiety and mental fatigue, and generate her own solutions or

OT STORY 55.1 USING A METACOGNITIVE APPROACH FOR A PATIENT WITH LONG COVID-19 (*continued*)

strategies. During activity experiences, she realized "I don't think of taking breaks until my brain shuts down." She began to identify and anticipate the task conditions that negatively impacted performance and generated strategies. For example, she recognized that when she was involved in two consecutive cognitively challenging tasks, she was more vulnerable to cognitive overload and mental exhaustion. She learned to plan ahead to arrange tasks with mental load in mind or balance the day by alternating tasks that required low and high mental energy. She also set a timer as a reminder for mental and visual rest breaks, and she learned to break down and simplify tasks that appeared overwhelming. As confidence and self-efficacy in managing cognitively challenging tasks increased, she was able to return to work on a part-time schedule with the plan to gradually increase her hours.

Questions

1. Why was the metacognitive strategy approach chosen to treat Rhonda?

2. What would be a secondary approach you would choose to alleviate some of her symptoms?

Commentary on Related Evidence

The use of metacognitive strategy intervention for executive function deficits is evidence-based for people with stroke or TBI and executive function deficits. This led Wilcox et al. to apply and describe the multicontext approach to OT functional cognitive treatment for a case with long COVID (Wilcox & Frank, 2021). In this case report, Wilcox et al. provide a description of how assessment and intervention helped to improve a person's cognitive performance in work-related activities. This case illustrates that there are instances when there is a lack of evidence for a particular condition, yet evidence for similar symptoms can be taken into account along with consideration of client characteristics and goals and applied in practice.

---

with those that address interpersonal skills; social participation; and everyday activities, routines, and roles (Jamieson et al., 2020). In addition, interventions should also target factors that may affect functional cognition capacities such as noise, sleep, screen time, nutrition, and physical activity.

Cognitive Perceptual Capacities and Their Impact on Activities and Participation

This section describes and explains the main constructs involve in cognition, including their definitions, evaluation, and treatment. These constructs are as follows:

- *Confusional state: Orientation, delirium, and dementia:* Confusional state is prevalent in acute care, global or diffuse brain injuries, or in long-term care settings.
- *Self-awareness and metacognition:* Prevalent across diagnosis and across the life span.
- *Executive function and cognitive control:* Impairments in executive functions are prevalent across the life span, diagnostic groups, and stages of care (e.g., could be observed in children who live in the community and clients in subacute mental health units).
- *Memory:* Memory concerns may be observed in aging, as well as in people with neurological and mental health conditions across the life span.

- *Spatial neglect:* Most commonly observed in adults with stroke or a right hemisphere brain lesions but also observed in children with neurological conditions.
- *Visual processing and visual motor:* Impairments are observed in people with developmental, neurological, or psychiatric conditions across the life span.
- *Motor planning:* DCD is observed in children and adults; apraxia is common after stroke with left hemisphere lesions but can also be observed in other acquired neurological or neurodegenerative conditions.

Although each of these areas is discussed separately for the purposes of description, it is important to recognize that cognitive problems are interrelated and rarely occur in isolation. Similarly, examples of intervention approaches applied to specific cognitive perceptual domains are discussed; however, in clinical practice, various intervention methods are used in combination with each other.

Confusional States Across the Life Span

Confusional states, such as delirium, involve disturbances in orientation, fluctuating periods of consciousness, and reduced ability to focus or sustain attention, remember, or think. The person may not know where they are or what day it is, and they may not be able to remember personal details about themselves such as their address or names of family members. Individuals may call out or ramble on without making sense and be unable to focus on a conversation or a simple task such as combing one's hair or self-feeding.

Some people in a confusional state may experience hallucinations and become restless or agitated or aggressive (hyperactive delirium), while others appear lethargic and apathetic (hypoactive delirium) (Greenberg et al., 2020).

Acute confusional states are known as delirium and often occur without any structural abnormalities in the brain. Delirium is most commonly observed in an intensive care unit or acute care settings and develops within a short period of time following surgery, trauma, or critical illness, and it can be seen not only in older adults but also in children (Thom et al., 2019). For example, children with developmental disabilities are at high risk for developing delirium when critically ill (Kaur et al., 2020). Older adults over age 65 are at risk of developing delirium following surgery. In general children and adults who sustain moderate to severe TBI often experience a transitory state of impaired consciousness and confusion called posttraumatic confusional state (Sherer et al., 2020). Delirium may also be observed due to many other medical conditions such as very low blood sugar, severe infections, carbon monoxide poisoning, or substance withdrawal. Older adults with moderate to severe dementia also experience confusional states; however, unlike delirium, the onset develops slowly over many years and is irreversible (Greenberg et al., 2020).

Delirium can be missed or misinterpreted as behavioral problems, particularly in critically ill children. For both children and adults who survive a critical illness, the presence and duration of delirium in the early stages of an illness is a strong predictor of long-term subtle cognitive deficits that can significantly impact participation and quality of life years after the illness (C. M. Kim, van der Heide, et al., 2021; Mattison, 2020). Therefore, the detection, prevention, and treatment of delirium have become a priority in healthcare.

Evaluation

Confusion and disorientation are indicative of significant impairments in attention and memory and global disruption in cognition (Bodien et al., 2020). Assessments need to be brief and under 5 minutes. In the acute care environment, the gold standard for assessing delirium for both children and adults is the Confusion Assessment Method (Shi et al., 2013; see Tables 55.1 and 55.2). This brief assessment of orientation and attention is often carried out by interdisciplinary team members to assist in monitoring the patient's status. When feasible, other assessments such as the Abbreviated Mental Test Score (Pendlebury et al., 2015) or Orientation Log (Penna & Novack, 2007) can also be used to track a person's confusional state across different times within a day as well as across days. Fluctuations in orientation during the day should be noted because patients might experience **sundowning**, a syndrome in which confusion or neuropsychiatric symptoms become worse in the late afternoon or evening (Canevelli et al., 2016).

Although a standardized functional assessment cannot be easily administered at this stage, it is important to assess and carefully observe patients performing familiar, simple, and repetitive BADL that they used to do before hospitalization such as brushing their hair, washing their face with a washcloth, or buttering bread using systematic observational methods. Observations during functional performance include the ability to stay on task, initiate, select and use objects appropriately, switch from one step to the next, detect hazards, and notice important details.

Intervention

Delirium Prevention. In the acute environment, there has been an increasing emphasis on strategies to reduce the incidence and duration of delirium. Delirium prevention programs involve a multidisciplinary, nonpharmacological approach including early mobilization, reorientation, sleep enhancement programs, environmental adaptation (lighting control, noise reduction), education of family and staff, minimization of psychoactive medication, and adequate pain relief (Bannon et al., 2019; Thomas et al., 2021). A key aspect of improving outcomes for those at risk for delirium is creating a context for the engagement and participation of family members or caregivers by helping them to understand the signs and symptoms of delirium and the importance of cognitive stimulation and activity engagement (McKenzie & Joy, 2020). A randomized pilot study demonstrated that OT intervention that was provided twice a day was effective in lowering the duration and incidence of delirium and improving functional outcomes compared to controls. The OT treatment included a combination of cognitive stimulation and basic functional activities on top of standard care for individuals above the age of 60, who were in the ICU but not on mechanical ventilation (Álvarez et al., 2017).

An OT practitioner could guide family members and rehabilitation staff on brief frequent activities that could be used to provide general cognitive stimulation including meaningful conversations, listening to music, word or card games, looking through family photos, or engaging in simple self-care activities.

Management of Delirium and Confusional States. Interventions to address confusion should focus on adaptations of the task or focus on creation of a familiar environment and orientation information. Adaptations that decrease stimulation (noise, visual clutter), and increase the saliency of key environmental cues can be used to help a person feel less confused and more attentive (Pozzi et al., 2020). Note that when creating such adaptations, the amount of visual information presented at one time must match the person's processing abilities. Some examples of tools to increase orientation include:

- Large orientation board that includes key facts about the person, place, and time.
- Large calendar posted in an accessible place
- Electronic devices preset to automatically announce the day and time on an hourly basis

- Talking picture frame that contains pictures of family members
- Music or personal objects (e.g., favorite pillow) that are familiar
- Audio or video recording of family members

When feasible, it is best to ask the patient to locate orientation tools in their environment. For example, if they want to know what day it is, it is better to ask the patient where they should look rather than telling them the answer. A "get to know me card" that has key facts about the patient (hobbies, music interests, cultural background, occupations, family members) can be placed in the room so that everyone who walks in the room can initiate conversations about topics relevant to the patient.

The principles of adaptation can be used to promote engagement in simple functional tasks. Tasks that are predictable, repetitive, and familiar should be introduced first with adaptations, prompts, or manual guidance as needed. In the task of brushing teeth, for example, unnecessary items should be removed from the sink, and the items that are required for use can be made prominent with contrasting colors to aid discrimination or introduced one item at a time. To initiate the task, the therapist may need to place the toothbrush in the patient's hand or complete the initial steps while they complete the rest. Gradually, the patient takes over more of the activity themselves. Functional approaches such as the CDM or TAP can be used to match activities to the appropriate cognitive level of the person and train staff or caregivers. Additionally, task-specific training techniques used within the NFA (e.g., errorless learning) can also be used to improve performance on specific functional tasks or learn new skills such as a wheelchair or use of a mobility device.

Self-Awareness and Metacognition

Impaired self-awareness includes a person's lack of knowledge about their own cognitive perceptual limitations and/or their functional implications as well as deficiencies in metacognitive skills (e.g., the ability to anticipate difficulties, recognize errors, and/or monitor performance within the context of an activity; Toglia & Kirk, 2000). From a developmental perspective, self-awareness gradually develops during childhood, starting with awareness of concrete, attributes of behavior or physical characteristics, and graduating into more abstract attributes (Lloyd et al., 2015; Toglia & Maeir, 2018). The process of becoming self-aware starts by experiencing various everyday life tasks while receiving reflections, personal feedback, and social feedback. Such guidance is an essential element of this development process (Rasheed et al., 2019). Among clinical populations, decreased self-awareness is observed across a wide range of developmental, neurological, and mental health conditions.

For example, such impairments are observed in conditions such as TBI (Engel et al., 2019); MS (Chen & Goverover, 2021); schizophrenia (S.-J. Kim, Jung, et al., 2021), and children and adolescents with ADHD (Levanon-Erez et al., 2019; Steward et al., 2017). Limitations in self-awareness can result in diminished motivation and compliance, decreased self-advocacy, lack of sustained effort, unrealistic expectations, incongruence between goals of the client and family, impaired judgment and safety, inability to adopt the use of compensatory strategies, and increased caregiver burden (Kelleher et al., 2016; Toglia & Maeir, 2018). In addition, children with ADHD with impaired self-awareness had worse social and academic performance (Steward et al., 2017). Creative approaches are needed to engage clients in treatment and structure experiences in a way that helps them discover their abilities as described in the intervention section (p. 23).

A traditional way to conceptualize awareness is by the hierarchical pyramid model of awareness (Crosson et al., 1989), which distinguishes between intellectual awareness, emergent awareness, and anticipatory awareness. Clients with *intellectual awareness* verbally describe limitations in functioning, whereas clients with *emergent awareness* recognize a problem only when it is actually happening. Clients with *anticipatory awareness* are able to anticipate that an impairment will likely cause a challenge before performing a given activity (Crosson et al., 1989). The Dynamic Comprehensive Model of Awareness (DCMA; Toglia & Kirk, 2000) expanded upon the pyramid model of awareness. It describes awareness as nonhierarchical and proposes that levels of awareness vary across different tasks and contexts within the same domain. It implies that awareness needs to be assessed both outside and inside the context of an activity. In addition, the model describes how a person can further develop and improve their self-awareness. The model implies that self-knowledge or beliefs about abilities that exist before an activity (i.e., intellectual awareness) and "online" awareness that is activated within the context of performing an activity (which includes self-monitoring and self-regulatory processes) improve specific self-awareness which in turn could improve general self-awareness. In addition, it suggests that awareness involves both an interplay between neurological mechanisms as well as the task, context, and personal factors such as personality, coping mechanisms, and culture (Toglia & Goverover, 2022).

Lack of awareness can be a result of psychological sources, such as denial. Denial is a psychological defense mechanism that is related to premorbid personality traits and is characterized by over-rationalization, hostility, resistance to feedback, and an unwillingness to confront problems (Prigatano & Sherer, 2020). For example, it is known that persons with addiction disorder do not report that addiction is a problem, and this is a form of denial that may hold a significant barrier to intervention (Rogers et al., 2019). A person who has a history of denying inadequacies and resisting help from others and a strong desire to be "in control" is more likely to use denial as a coping strategy. In many cases, neurological and psychological sources of unawareness coexist and cannot be easily differentiated. If denial is the predominant source of unawareness, methods of awareness training might not be effective (Toglia & Maeir, 2018). However, other methods that provide opportunities for choice, autonomy, and success within a supportive context may minimize defensive reactions (Toglia & Foster, 2021).

Evaluation

Evaluation of self-awareness should be done for clients across the life span and with any diagnosis. The need for assessment of self-awareness in children and adolescents with ADHD and epilepsy has been identified, even though impaired self-awareness is not recognized as a primary symptom of these conditions (Fisher et al., 2022; Zlotnik & Toglia, 2018).

Intellectual self-awareness can be assessed by two different methods: The first involves clinician rating of responses to semistructured interviews; the second compares the person's self-report of their functioning to the report of a caregiver or clinician (Toglia & Maeir, 2018). In both methods, it is assessed outside the context of an activity. Online awareness of performance is assessed within the context of a specific activity and involves recording error detection or correction as well as quantification of the person's assessment of their performance before and immediately after task performance (Toglia & Goverover, 2022). In general, questionnaires and discrepancy scores are not sufficient to assess awareness, because there can be a disassociation between knowledge of limitations and the ability to use that knowledge to recognize and monitor errors during actual performance (Krasny-Pacini et al., 2015).

A comprehensive evaluation of awareness plays a key role in guiding and selecting methods of intervention. For example, if awareness is severely impaired both during an interview and within an activity, intervention methods that do not require awareness, such as functional skill training, errorless learning, and adaptation of the environment, may be most appropriate in facilitating occupational performance. If a lack of understanding of strengths and limitations prevents a person from choosing goals that are realistic and attainable, the therapist should assist the client in focusing on skills or tasks that are needed for the "here and now." On the other hand, if a person generally recognizes errors within the context of an activity, (online awareness) treatment can focus on further enhancing awareness of performance during functional activities (regardless of responses during an interview).

Intervention

Metacognitive strategy approaches are recommended for addressing limitations in self-awareness because they enhance the person's understanding of their own strengths and limitations and focus on self-monitoring of performance. These approaches stress the importance of helping a person discover his or her own errors and generate his or her own solutions.

Toglia and Kirk (2000) emphasize that directly pointing out errors or telling clients that they have problems is the least effective in increasing awareness, as this approach tends to elicit defensive reactions. They recommend a therapeutically supportive context, and use of familiar activities at the "just right challenge level," within a metacognitive framework to enhance the emergence of awareness. Recently, a systematic review by Engel et al. (2019) found support for use of multiple awareness intervention techniques including metacognitive strategy intervention, guided discussion, external feedback, and multimodal feedback within the context functional task practice to produce positive outcomes at an activity and participation level. This supports the need to focus on online awareness of performance within the context of functional activities as advocated by several authors with both children and adults (Krasny-Pacini et al., 2014; Toglia & Goverover, 2022). Group metacognitive strategy intervention, has been applied to adults with schizophrenia (Kaizerman-Dinerman et al., 2018) and ABI (Toglia & Foster, 2021). The group's intervention focused on increasing use of self-monitoring strategies, self-questioning, and self-assessment skills within the context of group activities such as planning a supermarket trip or bake sale (Figure 55.2; Kaizerman-Dinerman et al., 2018; Toglia & Foster, 2021).

Clearly, awareness interventions are critical to improving function when warranted. Following are descriptions of

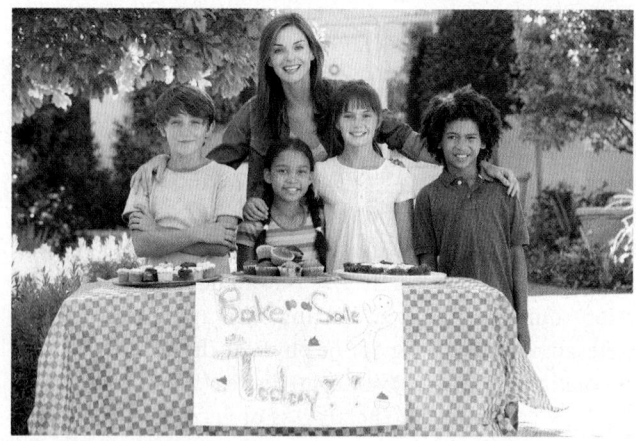

FIGURE 55.2 Planning and carrying out a bake sale is an appropriate group activity for those with metacognitive and executive function impairments.

specific techniques that can be used in a wide range of activities to enhance awareness (see also Table 55.4). These techniques are often used in combination with one other, can be blended with strategy training, and may be incorporated into all treatment sessions. The multicontext approach provides additional guidelines for simultaneously addressing awareness and strategy use (Toglia & Foster, 2021). Note, that awareness intervention is not appropriate for clients with depression, denial, or dementia.

Executive Functions and Cognitive Control

Executive function and **self-regulation** skills are the mental processes that enable us to plan, focus attention, remember instructions, and juggle multiple tasks successfully. In addition, executive functions are crucial for enabling persons to adapt to new situations and cope with unfamiliar activities and environments. Persons with good executive function skills can filter distractions, prioritize tasks, set and achieve goals, and control impulses (McCoy, 2019). Executive function is composed of a set of interrelated core skills including working memory, inhibition and flexibility, and

initiation. These skills are involved in every activity a person does across their life span (Toglia & Foster, 2021) and when integrated create cognitive control. **Cognitive control** is the ability to actively guide performance of a task including choosing strategies, coordinate and regulating responses. Cognitive control is associated with a wide range of processes and is not restricted to a particular cognitive domain. For example, a person in a busy grocery store looking for nongluten bread in the bread section needs to keep the goal and criteria in mind while searching, switch between aisles, and inhibit distractions. A child who is playing with a ball during recess needs to demonstrate restraint and inhibition if another child suddenly grabs the ball from him. Instead of responding by hitting or fighting, the child with inhibitory control is able to complain to the teacher. For more examples see Table 55.5. In addition, impaired executive function in developmental, neurological, psychiatric, or chronic conditions can affect the ability to benefit from treatment and is a strong indicator of functional outcome and participation (Goverover et al., 2013; Kim et al., 2020; Sandry et al., 2016).

Vulnerabilities in executive functions are related to various personal factors such as stress, sleep deprivation, and anxiety as well as individual disease processes. Individual differences in executive functions within healthy

TABLE 55.4 Summary of Techniques to Improve Self-Awareness

Specific Awareness Techniques	Description	Treatment Method
Self-Prediction (Goverover et al., 2007a; Toglia & Maeir, 2018).	Anticipation of difficulties or prediction of performance on a task. Client rates activity difficulty or identifies challenges that might be encountered before an activity.	Immediately following performance, actual results are compared with predicted results, and any discrepancies are discussed.
Specific Goal Ratings (Toglia & Foster, 2021).	Daily or weekly self-ratings of defined goals, behaviors, or strategies. Self-ratings of goals can be charted or graphed over time and tracked to improve awareness.	Client self-ratings of goal attainment are compared with therapist ratings or significant others, and discrepancies are discussed.
Videotape Feedback (Doig et al., 2020; Engel et al., 2019)	Video review of oneself during activity performance. Videotape feedback allows clients to reexperience their performance and self-evaluate difficulties as they are occurring rather than discussing them after the fact.	Video replays are paused and the client is encouraged to reflect on performance, recognize errors and generate strategies for future performance.
Self-Evaluation (Miyahara et al., 2018; Nagelkop et al., 2021)	Client self-evaluates their performance after a task. Structured systems (e.g., set of questions, a checklist) or a self-rating system may be used to guide self-assessment.	Client is asked to identify challenges or use a self-evaluation checklist, e.g., "Have I attended to all the necessary information?" "Did I check over my work?"
Self-Questioning and Experience With the Task (Toglia & Maeir, 2018)	Self-questions designed to cue the client to monitor their behavior during activity performance are identified and written on an index card or memorized.	At specific time intervals during a task, the client stops and answers the same two or three questions, such as "Am I sure that I am looking all the way to the left?" "Am I paying attention to the details?" or "Am I going too quickly?"
Journaling (Goverover et al., 2007a; Toglia & Foster, 2021).	Client records activity experiences and performance results in a journal immediately after task performance. Client is encouraged to think about what they have learned about themselves and summarize strengths and weaknesses.	Journal is reviewed at the end of the session and beginning of the following session. Client reflects on and interprets activity experiences during discussion of journal entries.

TABLE 55.5	Core Executive Functions Skills	
Executive Function Components	**Functional Examples**	**Prevalence**
Working memory (Ramos et al., 2020): Holding information in mind	Keeping track of what has already been done in a multistep cooking task and remembering which medication or pill was just taken. At school, children may have difficulty remembering their teachers' instructions, recalling the rules to a game, and paying attention.	ADHD brain injury, mental illness
Cognitive flexibility (Uddin, 2021): Set shifting, mental flexibility or shifting of attention	The ability to shift between adding and subtracting when balancing a checkbook; answering the telephone; going back to typing, or baking a cake while following a written recipe; view information from different perspectives, generate alternative solutions.	Autism, TBI, and addiction
Inhibition (Toglia & Katz, 2018): Inhibitory control of actions or thoughts	Resisting distractions when finding specific items in a closet, resisting food when you are on a diet, restraining impulsive responses, and staying within a fixed budget when shopping.	Older adults, MCI, ADHD, obesity, drug and alcohol abuse
Initiation (Toglia & Katz, 2018): Independently start a task, including generating ideas	Completes the final step of one job and moves on to the next job; ability to brainstorm and initiate ideas; understands when to ask for help and when to keep trying to solve a problem independently.	ADHD, Parkinson disease, schizophrenia

populations can affect mental and physical health, school readiness and success, social competence, resilience, success at work, and cognitive, social, and psychological development (Diamond, 2013; Mousavi et al., 2022). In fact, the wide distribution of executive function networks across different areas of the brain makes executive functions highly sensitive to risk factors (e.g., growing up in a chaotic and stressful environment) and disruptions caused by disease processes, biochemical, and molecular changes.

Impairments in executive function are reflected by neuroscientific findings within distributed networks involving several subcortical and cortical areas (including the prefrontal regions) rather than isolated regions (Peskin et al., 2020). Executive function impairments are found to be prevalent in almost every condition that affects information processing, learning, and brain function. For example, lower executive function skills have been identified in people with autism and/or ADHD; chronic health conditions such as kidney disease, COPD, cancer, or poorly controlled diabetes; neurological disorders such as TBI, stroke, or MS; mental health issues including bipolar disease, OCD, substance abuse, and eating disorders, schizophrenia; and in older adults. Weaknesses in executive function may have significant effect on health behavior and self-management of the disease and symptoms that accompany it (Toglia & Katz, 2018). For example, a person with a chronic condition who needs to change their eating habits (to manage diabetes or lose weight) may have problems in inhibitory control or mindset shift that are required to adapt to a new diet.

Executive function starts to develop in infancy and continues through adulthood. For example, an infant starts to understand object consistency in the first year of life. Initial understanding of cause and effect can also be observed in the first year of life. Later during the toddler years,

inhibitory control over initial responses is learned. In general, working memory develops from preschool through adolescence with a gradual increase in the number of items that can be remembered simultaneously through the years. Inhibitory control and cognitive flexibility develop rapidly during preschool years (Cermak & Toglia, 2018).

Evaluation

Executive function impairments represent a distinct challenge because they can be masked within familiar ADL or routines but are most apparent when the client is required to function in situations that are less structured, require multitasking, or managing novel and unexpected situations (Redick et al., 2016). Therefore, executive functions can be best observed in adults and children while performing a multistep activity such as cooking, following instructions for an art and crafts project, or online shopping and purchasing (Toglia & Foster, 2021). Most standardized cognitive assessments are structured and do not adequately examine the area of executive functions (Baum et al., 2019; Goverover, Toglia, & DeLuca, 2019). Newer ecologically valid functional cognitive evaluations for executive function have been designed such as the Multiple Errands Test (Morrison et al., 2013), its home version (Burns & Neville, 2017), WCPA (Toglia, 2015), EFPT (Baum et al., 2008), CKTA (Berg et al., 2012), and Do-Eat assessment for children (Josman et al., 2010; see Tables 55.1 and 55.2).

Intervention

Functional Approach: Adaptations of Task or Environment and Task-Specific Training. Adaptations that minimize demands on executive functions include collaborating with teachers, parents, or caregivers to reduce the number of items or choices presented to the client at one time, decrease distractions such as clutter or interruptions, and preorganize an activity or activity materials. For example, instead of working in groups of five kids in a classroom, work in groups of two to three kids; prearrange grooming items on the sink in the correct sequence; or if a student is easily distracted, provide them with the option of sitting at a desk closer to the board or provide visual cues to help them to remain goal focused (see Figure 55.3). Table 55.6 provides additional examples of adaptations.

Executive function demands can also be reduced through establishment of routines and repetitive task practice. As tasks become more habitual and automatic, the need for top-down executive function control decreases (Waldman-Levi & Steinmann Obermeyer, 2018). Organizational systems can be provided, directly taught, and practiced to enhance school success and participation. For example, children can be directly taught compensatory strategies such as using checklists for organizing school materials and managing homework responsibilities (Langberg et al., 2018).

Metacognitive Strategy-Based Approach. A variety of strategies that maximize executive functioning have been described in the literature For example, a group of

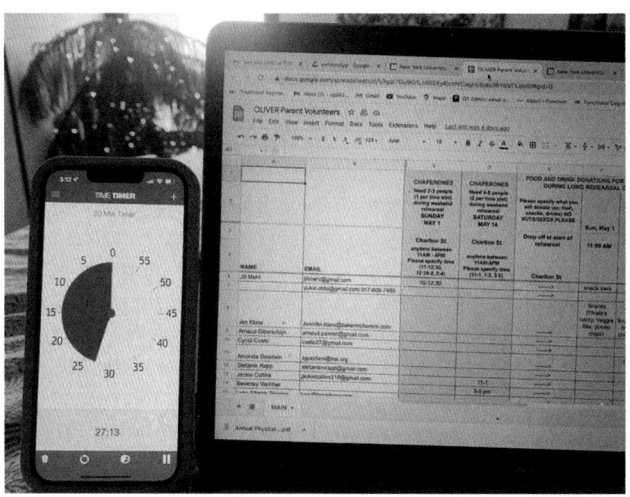

FIGURE 55.3 **Use of a visual timer app to maintain goal focus, resist distractions while completing a scheduling task.**

activity management strategies provide structured frameworks to help a person manage multistep activities, remain focused on the goals, and cope with obstacles or problems that arise during activity performance (Toglia & Foster, 2021, p. 97). One such strategy is stop, think, organize, and plan (STOP). Another goal management strategy is to (a) "stop" and define what I am going to do, (b) "define" the main task, (c) "list" the steps, (d) "learn" the steps and *do* it, and (e) "check" if am I doing what I planned to do (Hypher et al., 2019; Krasny-Pacini et al., 2014). Both provide a top-down structured system for approaching activities, thereby replacing the impulsive, disorganized, or unsystematic approach often observed in people with executive dysfunction. These strategies also help the person maintain the focus of goals and intentions and are frequently reinforced by metacognitive strategy approaches that use self-questioning techniques and emphasize monitoring and evaluating effectiveness of strategy use (Toglia & Foster, 2021).

The multicontext approach (Toglia et al., 2010) emphasizes application and practice of strategies across a wide variety of activities. For example, activity management strategies can be practiced when planning a weekly schedule, organizing a backpack or school binder, planning social get-togethers, organizing medications according to a schedule, planning an overnight trip and packing a suitcase, or obtaining and organizing a list of local business phone numbers. The use of a checklist strategy combined with self-awareness training and practiced across multiple tasks has also been shown to improve occupational performance of clients with executive function impairments as a result of brain injury (Jaywant, Steinberg, et al., 2020) or Parkinson disease (Foster et al., 2018). Intervention incorporates practice in identifying the situations or activities in which the use of a checklist could be helpful, for example, in managing finances (Grant et al., 2012; Toglia et al., 2010). The multicontext approach can be applied across the life span. For example, children who have problems with schoolwork such as keeping track of homework assignments and their schedule could be asked guided questions that help them anticipate the need to plan out their week or use a calendar. A child could be encouraged to create reminder strategies such as placing a cue sign in their room or setting an alarm

TABLE 55.6	Examples of Adaptations to the Environment or the Task
Problem	**Adaptation**
Difficulty with getting started with tasks, moving from step to step, or performing steps in the correct order	Provide structure such as a checklist, video or audio instructions that cue the client to initiate an activity and perform each step at a time in its proper sequence.
Difficulty in answering open-ended questions on a test or in daily life (e.g., what would you like to eat for lunch?)	Questions should provide a limited number of choices whenever feasible (e.g., would you like a pasta or rice?).
Problems initiating and following a daily routine	Predictable and structured daily routine (e.g., daily schedule is written on a board)

message to check the calendar. This differs from a direct strategy instruction approach because treatment focuses on helping the child understand when and how the strategy should be applied and assess its usefulness (Toglia & Foster, 2021; Waldman-Levi & Steinmann Obermeyer, 2018).

Metacognitive strategy attention training programs for children with brain injury have been reported by several studies (Luton et al., 2011; Séguin et al., 2018). For example, Luton et al. (2011) taught children (ages 6–15) with various neurological deficits key phrases or "magic words" to help alert and prepare themselves for focusing. They were also taught to restate task directions in their own words and write down or draw visual cues to remind them what to do. The strategy program was associated with improvement in several aspects of parent-reported attention and children's performance on tasks requiring organization, and problem-solving.

Another example of intervention directed at enhancing strategy use is provided by pilot studies that examined the applicability of the CO-OP approach for use with adults

executive dysfunction arising from brain injury (Dawson et al., 2009) and Cancer (Maeir et al., 2021) and children with executive function impairments (Lebrault et al., 2021).

Metacognitive Strategy-Based Approach for Children With Attention-Deficit/Hyperactivity Disorder. Recently, evidence-based interventions for young children with impairments in executive function and ADHD have been developed. The Parental Occupation Executive Training (POET) is a parent-training program that promotes the use of cognitive strategies to support daily functioning of children with ADHD from the ages of 4 to 7 years. In this program, parents learn about the nature of executive function and its implications for everyday functioning, as well as about strategies to support daily functioning (Frisch et al., 2020). In addition, the Cog-Fun approach is a strategy-based treatment designed to specifically address executive functions in school-age children with ADHD (Kim et al., 2020). See OT Story 55.2.

OT STORY 55.2 USING COG-FUN FOR A STUDENT WITH ADHD

Harlan is an 11-year-old school student diagnosed with ADHD. She attends school regularly, however, as school work progressed with each grade, she is expected to learn and remember more information, and she finds it difficult to recall the material she has learned in class. Having always been an excellent student, Harlan felt frustrated with her inability to keep up. She puts extra effort into studying but still gets poor grades. She expressed her frustration to the occupational therapist who treats her regularly and exclaimed: I can hear and read the information, but I feel it doesn't "stick" in my brain, studying doesn't help, I'm just not smart, school is too hard. Harlan is facing a difficulty that will grow and be more prominent in the future if she is not able to take care of it sooner rather than later. The therapist introduced Harlan to the Cog-Fun approach. The treatment goals were to help her maintain and improve her academic performance by promoting executive strategy acquisition.

Cog-Fun is composed of four main components that were incorporated into Harlan's cognitive treatment. First was developing self-awareness about her strengths and limitations. The therapist worked with Harlan on discovering her strengths within the academic context and understanding the challenges caused by ADHD and their effect on learning. The second component of the treatment is strategy acquisition in a functional context. Harlan learned to use an internal strategy of "stop and test herself on the information learned." During treatment, Harlan discovered that if she takes breaks in between learning trials, information is retained better than just repeating the information over and over again. During treatment sessions, the therapist

and Harlan constantly monitored her performance at home and school using these strategies and started to think and discover more ways to promote information organization to enable better learning. Importantly, her parents were asked to supervise and support Harlan at home while she does homework. Her teachers were also notified about the strategies she uses and some environmental modifications were noted. Integration of caretakers and teachers is the third component of the Cog-Fun. The fourth component of the treatment is related to promoting transfer and generalization of treatment gains. Harlan presented what she learned during treatment to her parents and her school adviser. During this process, she learned to self-advocate and express what would help her to be a better learner.

Questions

1. What are Harlan's main cognitive and functional limitations?
2. How can utilization of the Cog-Fun approach help address Harlen's problem areas?

Commentary on Evidence

The Cog-Fun was first described in 2011. Research on the Cog-Fun approach over the past 11 years has accumulated enough high-quality evidence to indicate its effectiveness. For example, two randomized controlled trials tested the efficacy of the Cog-Fun intervention for children with ADHD with very positive results, providing strong evidence (Hahn-Markowitz et al., 2017, 2020). This was further supported by a recent systematic review that classified the Cog-Fun approach as an effective approach with enough evidence to be applied in practice (Novak & Honan, 2019). The Cog-Fun has also been investigated with adolescents with ADHD using the Teen Cog-Fun (Levanon-Erez et al.,

2019) and with adults with ADHD (Kastner et al., 2022). These studies also provided promising results. However, they were done as feasibility or pilot studies, and therefore, more evidence is needed to support this approach with adults and adolescents.

Remedial Training. Recently, several commercial, computer-based, working memory training programs have been developed. From those, Endeavor RXTM was approved for use by the Food and Drug Administration (FDA) for children with ADHD ages 8 to 12 years (see https://www.cnn.com/2020/06/16/health/ADHD-fda-game-intl-scli-wellness/index.html). Endeavor RXTM is a videogame-delivered cognitive training treatment designed to improve cognitive impairments associated with ADHD such as attention and working memory (Evans et al., 2021). Another example is CogMed, which is widely used in schools and clinics. This program is based on eight different exercises involving both visuospatial and verbal working memory tasks, in which the difficulty level varies adaptively during training. The effectiveness of these programs has been mostly measured by neuropsychological tests. Evidence for generalization to function has not been adequately assessed. Generalization in such programs is challenging because computerized exercises or games do not include as many demands as clients may have while performing activities in complex environments required for daily functions (e.g., school and work; Evans et al., 2021).

Memory

Memory gives individuals the ability to draw on past experiences and learn new information (Dudai et al., 2015). This provides us with a sense of continuity in the environment and frees us from dependency in here-and-now situations. Memory is dependent on other cognitive skills such as executive functions and attention and can be described as a

process that includes three stages described in Table 55.7 (Goverover et al., 2013; Guo et al., 2019). Once information is in long-term memory it can be classified into declarative and nondeclarative memory. *Declarative memory* is explicit and is consciously remembered. There are two types of declarative memory: semantic and episodic. *Semantic memory* refers to knowledge about the world (e.g., when you see a red traffic light you need to stop your car). *Episodic memory* refers to the memory of personal experiences such as your children's birthdays. *Prospective memory* is also a type of explicit episodic memory that involves the ability to remember intentions or activities that will be required in the future (Toglia & Foster, 2021). Prospective memory is dependent on good executive functions (Weber, Chiaravalloti, et al., 2019). *Nondeclarative memory* is considered an implicit memory and refers to knowledge that is not consciously accessed. Thus, *implicit memory* refers to how learning influences behavior, even if the individual is not aware of those influences. *Procedural memory* is part of implicit memory and is memory that involves the ability to remember how to perform an activity or procedure without conscious awareness. The ability to crawl, walk, and run are procedures, and adults have no conscious memory of how or when they learned them (Hicks et al., 2018). Importantly, implicit and explicit memory work in parallel to model our behavior (Squire & Dede, 2015).

Evaluation

It is important to distinguish whether everyday memory problems are due to failures to keep track of a conversation or what was just said (e.g., working memory), recall of past

TABLE 55.7 Three Stages of the Memory Process

Memory Stages	Example
1. Encoding (registration): How memories are formed	Create a mental image of a story you need to remember or think about what would be the consequences if you forget to pay the bill at the end of the month.
2. Retention and storage: How memories are retained	Remembering a phone number for 60 s would be an example of short-term memory, while remembering a phone number for a long time of years is a long-term memory.
3. Retrieval: Remembering and recalling the information or events that were previously encoded and stored	**Free recall:** Try to remember where you put your watch. **Cued:** Ask yourself questions such where was the last time you wore your watch? **Recognition:** Three places you might have put the watch, and recall the location.

events or conversations from the day before (e.g., episodic, event-based memory), or failures in carrying out future activities (e.g., prospective memory). A comprehensive evaluation of memory examines the different types of memory and methods of retrieval (see Tables 55.1 and 55.2). Assessments must consider factors such as the modality in which the information is presented (auditory, verbal, or visual), the type of instructions (general or specific), the number of stimuli presented, the familiarity and meaningfulness of the information, the presence of contextual cues during recall phases, the type of information to be remembered (factual or skill related), and the length of retention. Dynamic assessment of memory such as Toglia's (1993) Contextual Memory Test (CMT) evaluates awareness of memory capabilities and use of strategies.

Intervention

Memory impairments are closely related to other cognitive impairments, particularly executive function and processing speed. Some investigators have suggested that an indirect approach that addresses other cognitive skills such as executive functions, attention, organization, and processing speed rather than memory may be effective to improve learning and memory (Duckworth et al., 2019). In addition, some researchers found that in order to benefit from memory treatment and use of strategies, clients need to present with good working memory and cognitive control (i.e., executive functions; Goverover et al., 2013; Guo et al., 2019).

Interventions for memory impairments can be organized as internal compensatory strategies, external compensatory aids, and rehearsal-based strategies (Chudoba et al., 2020; Lambez & Vakil, 2021). In addition, adaptations and use of technology to compensate for memory problems are gaining more attention (Goodall et al., 2021). Importantly, a recent systematic review concluded that a combination of cognitive interventions that include internal and external cognitive strategies seems to have the most positive effect on cognitive memory symptomology (Henry, 2021; Lambez & Vakil, 2021).

Functional Approach
Adaptations of Task or Environment. Demands on memory can be reduced through adaptations or modifications of tasks or environments such as:

- Using cue cards or signs in key places (e.g., a sign on door where it will be seen before leaving: "Take keys and . . .")
- Labeling the outside of drawers or closets to minimize the need to recall the location of items
- Providing step-by-step directions to reduce memory demands
- Providing checklists to assist in keeping track of task steps
- Using technology including smart homes technologies to facilitate performance of everyday activities (Chen, Bodine, & Lew, 2021)

Significant others can be trained to use methods that increase the likelihood that the client will remember material, such as asking them to repeat instructions or important information in their own words, encouraging the client to ask questions, and presenting material in small groups, clusters, or categories.

Task-Specific Training. Task-specific methods such as errorless learning or spaced retrieval (i.e., learning trials are spaced), can be used to teach a person with moderate-severe memory impairments to use an external memory aide or device (e.g., reminder app on a smartphone or smartwatch). In the initial stages of intervention, the client might be expected to use the aid or device only when it is initiated by another person. Gradually, the client can be trained to initiate the use of the aid independently. Usually, clients with high motivation, high intelligence, excellent organizational skills, and who were young at the time of amnesia-onset and have good social support would probably be more successful in implementing external strategies (Halder et al., 2021).

Compensatory Strategies. External strategies utilize aids to organize and retrieve information. The use of external strategies or aids may decrease the burden on executive control and memory processes (Chudoba & Schmitter-Edgecombe, 2020; Lanzi & Bourgeois, 2020). Devices and aids that can support memory function include the following: timers, voice recorders, alarm messages on smart devices, electronic devices such as pillbox organizers, lists, daily planners, notebooks or digital diaries, smart watches, and commercially available applications (i.e., apps) for mobile/smart phones, tablets, and computers. Studies have documented the effectiveness of technology and aids to support those with memory impairments in both children and adults (Lanzi & Bourgeois, 2020; Resch et al., 2018). Intervention is most effective when the client is motivated, involved in identifying the memory problem, and has good executive functions (Pizzonia & Suhr, 2022). In addition, interventions can use a combination of external aids and strategies with awareness training to improve prospective memory device use (Lanzi & Bourgeois, 2020).

The successful use of a new device or memory aid may require structured training and may not fit every client who presents with memory problems. Several evidence-based programs have been developed to train use of memory aids and digital memory notebooks systematically (Chudoba & Schmitter-Edgecombe, 2020; Dewar et al., 2018; Lanzi et al., 2022). For example, the Structured External Memory Aid Treatment (SEMAT; Lanzi et al., 2022) uses a three-step training program based on previous work by Sohlberg and Mateer (1989). Using this program, participants had to: (a) explore several examples of external strategies, (b) role-play using the strategy in everyday situations, and then (c) use the strategies in their home environment. Participants were encouraged to choose an external strategy or aid that was most relevant for them. Increased use of external memory strategies and aids during everyday activities was observed immediately and 18 months post-treatment (Lanzi et al., 2022).

When choosing external memory aids, it is important to remember that such aids are focused on supporting the users' abilities rather than strengthening them. The person's needs and lifestyle should be considered when selecting devices or memory aids (Dewar et al., 2018; Lanzi & Bourgeois, 2020). Devices that were previously used by clients may tap into procedural memory and be more easily accepted and applied to support memory. In any case, training to use memory aids or devices needs to take place in the context of various everyday activities.

Some of the current trends in the use of technology in rehabilitation include the following:

- Digital voice assistants and "smart-home" technologies can be used as reminders or monitoring systems to enhance safety. For example, sensors placed in the home can assist in physiologic monitoring and alert systems for medication reminders. Remote video monitoring and automated door locks and openers can be used to facilitate entry, safety, and security (Chen, Bodine, & Lew, 2021, p. 202).
- Reminder apps for smartphones and tablets can send text reminders or alarms to remind individuals to complete tasks (Gentry, 2018).
- Wearable devices, such as smart glasses, watches, or cameras such as SenseCam (Silva et al., 2018), and visual lifelogging (van Teijlingen et al., 2021) allow for continuous recording of everyday life in the real world over an extended period of time.
- Apps for IADL tasks such as grocery shopping (Figure 55.4) can help clients categorize and arrange items in a logical manner. Other apps may help the individual correctly sequence a task through video/photo modeling and/or voice instructions (Ramirez-Hernandez et al., 2021), and even public transportation assistance that uses GPS and handheld devices (Alsaqer, 2021).

Strategy Training: Internal Strategies. Training in internal memory strategies is most appropriate for people with mild memory deficits and those in whom other areas of cognition are intact (Cicerone et al., 2019). Internal compensatory strategies rely on mnemonic techniques to organize and learn new information. Internal compensatory strategies cannot be used to learn large quantities of information that may need to be remembered on a daily basis (Chudoba et al., 2020).

Internal memory strategies may be directed primarily at registration and retention stages (i.e., encoding operations, getting information in) or the retrieval stage of memory (i.e., getting information out). Some examples of such strategies include:

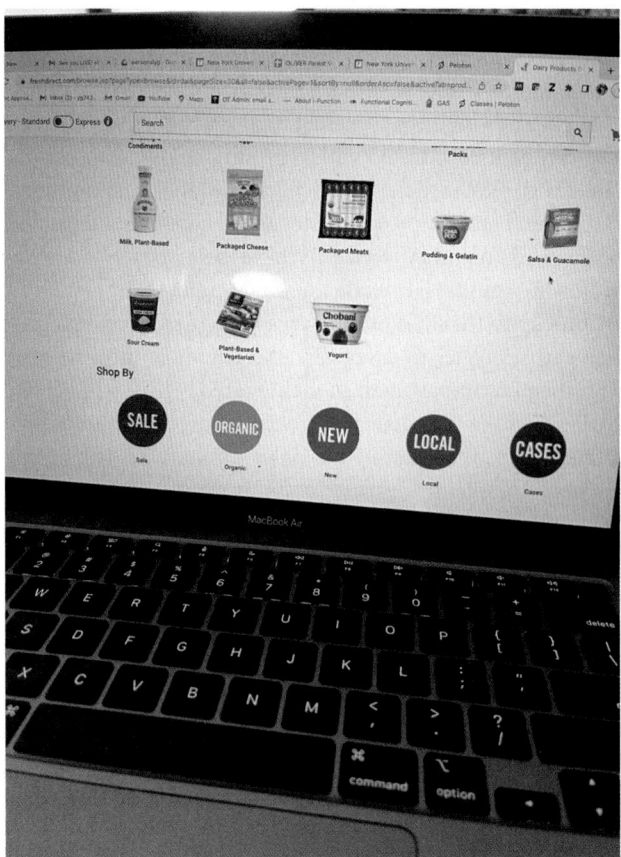

FIGURE 55.4 **Use of a computer to aid organizing groceries for clients with memory and executive function impairments.**

- ***Mnemonics:*** Useful when we need to remember a large quantity of information, such as certain facts. Chunking is an example of a mnemonic
- ***Association:*** Connect items we need to remember with a visual or another word. For example, if a client needs to remember to buy milk today, they may associate it with the coffee they would like to drink in the morning, and imagine the consequences of not having milk for the morning coffee.

The modified Story Memory Technique (mSMT) is an example of an internal strategy in which clients are asked to learn words, embed the words in a story, and then visualize that story (Chiaravalloti et al., 2016, 2020; DeLuca et al., 2020). This treatment is manualized and ready to use by practitioners; for more information, visit https://www.kflearn.org/courses/kf-msmt. Internal strategies help the learned information to become associated with something more accessible or meaningful, which, in turn, provides better retention of the information. The benefits of using internal strategies are potentially greater when combined with other strategies such as association or visualization (Henry, 2021). Internal memory strategies may be taught directly as described above or integrated into metacognitive strategy approaches.

Group Interventions. Individual memory interventions seem to be the most frequently used, but the use of group memory interventions is also recommended (Leśniak et al., 2018). Cognitive rehabilitation principles and strategies can be incorporated within group programs and combined with psychosocial or psychoeducational interventions.

Several group programs to assist caregivers or older adults with memory concerns have been described with promising results. For example, the Memory Strategy Education Group (MSEG) program was designed to provide advice and strategies to caregivers and clients on how to deal with memory impairment in their everyday lives (Coe et al., 2019). Another example is an occupation-based metacognitive group intervention for older adults with subjective memory complaints designed to improve occupational goal attainment and metamemory (Rotenberg & Maeir, 2018). In this program, participants met as a book club group, and within the book club format, internal and external memory strategies were introduced using a metacognitive framework.

Spatial Neglect

Spatial neglect (SN) (also referred to as visuospatial neglect or unilateral neglect), is a failure to orient to, respond to, or report stimuli presented on one side of the environment or body. The neglected space is contralateral to the side of the brain lesion (Heilman et al., 2012). SN is most common with right hemispheric lesions in adults and affects the left side of space; however, right-sided neglect following left hemisphere lesions can also be observed, although it is typically less severe and less chronic (Esposito et al., 2021). SN has been reported in 30% to 50% of clients with right hemispheric stroke (Barrett, 2021). SN can also occur after TBI,

or brain tumor at any age (Purpura et al., 2022). In children, SN occurs with the equal frequency following right or left hemisphere lesions; however, left hemisphere lesions to produce a greater degree of bilateral inattention (Thareja et al., 2012). It occurs in children following perinatal, neonatal, or childhood stroke and is observed in unilateral spastic cerebral palsy (Adamos et al., 2022; Ickx et al., 2018).

SN can involve one or more modalities (e.g., tactile, visual, and auditory), and can vary with activity demands including the number, salience, or complexity of the stimuli (Nijboer & Van Der Stigchel, 2019). Several main SN subtypes have been described (Rode et al., 2017):

- *Extrapersonal neglect:* Demonstrate neglect symptoms in large spaces, such as a room
- *Personal neglect:* Have impaired awareness of their body
- *Peripersonal neglect:* Difficulty with paper and pencil tasks
- *Representational neglect:* Internal mental images
- *Motor neglect:* Decreased movement into or toward the contralesional space.
- *Sensory neglect:* Decreased ability to perceive sensory stimuli in contralesional space.

People with SN behave as though one-half of the world does not exist. They often begin scanning on the right side and fail to explore most of the stimuli on the left, missing key information in their environment (see Figure 55.5). This can lead to accidents or falls and compromise the ability to safely cross the street, drive, or navigate in the community. SN results in difficulties completing everyday life tasks (see Box 55.1).

SN occurs as a result of disturbed visual-spatial attentional and perceptual processes and is not caused by primary sensory deficits such as a visual field cut or decreased sensation on one side (Heilman et al., 2012). The term *neglect* connotes a volitional component to the disorder, but

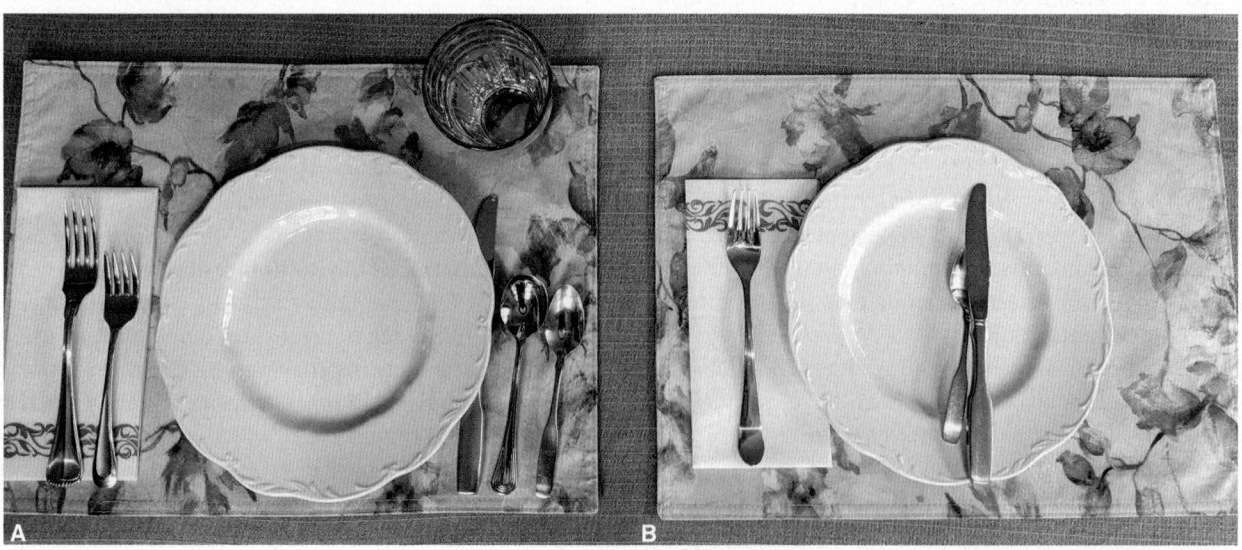

FIGURE 55.5 **A:** Place setting activity a person with left spatial neglect was asked to copy during OT treatment. **B:** The client omitted right-sided items or deviated items toward the left.

BOX 55.1 FUNCTIONAL SIGNS AND SYMPTOMS OF SPATIAL NEGLECT

- Misses objects or people on the one side of space (see Figure 55.5)
- Bumps into walls or doorways on one side
- Collides with people or obstacles on one side when walking or navigating a wheelchair
- Washes one-half of face
- Dresses one-half of their body
- Food is missed on one side of the plate
- Draws only one side of a figure
- Writing is crowded on the one side of paper
- One side of words or sentences may be missed
- Misreads the first letter of a particular word
- Fails to attend to all information while copying from a blackboard

this is a misnomer. The person with SN is unaware of the incompleteness of their perception and responses to the environment. They perceive the world as complete and are often surprised or shocked to learn that they have missed information (Chen & Toglia, 2019). The conflicting perceptions that confront those with SN can cause stress, anxiety, frustration, and a wide range of emotional and social challenges (Klinke et al., 2015). Both clients and their families need support and assistance to fully understand and interpret their experiences. The consequences of SN can be far-reaching and affect all aspects of everyday function. There are negative impacts on independence in ADL, mobility, functional recovery, caregiver burden, participation, and quality of life (Bosma et al., 2020). Individuals with SN have more difficulty resuming life activities including self-care, household tasks, driving, social activities, community mobility, and work. There is also slower recovery, longer hospital stays, increased risk for falls or accidents, and higher disability and dependence levels compared to those without neglect (Chen et al., 2015; Tarvonen-Schröder et al., 2020). In addition, neglect is a predictor of upper arm use during ADL and is associated with UE motor recovery (Doron & Rand, 2019; Vanbellingen et al., 2017).

SN is sometimes confused with hemianopsia or a visual field cut. It is important to recognize that while a visual field cut or hemianopsia can occur with SN, the two are separate disorders and one does not cause the other. People with visual field cuts typically have awareness of their visual field loss and make compensatory eye and head movements toward the affected side while SN is characterized by decreased awareness of the contralesional side of space. Visual scanning toward the neglected space is frequently limited or nonexistent. SN also varies with attentional demands or task complexity and can be observed across sensory modalities, whereas a visual field cut is limited to the visual modality and unlike SN, symptoms do not fluctuate with task demands or context (Chen & Toglia, 2019).

Evaluation

Given the variety and type of SN symptoms, it is generally recommended that a set of assessment tools or tasks that are sensitive to different SN symptoms, be used to evaluate it (Klinke et al., 2018).

Traditional Paper and Pencil Assessments. The most common method of assessing SN involves use of cancellation tasks that require detection of target stimuli such as letters, symbols, or shapes, distributed on both sides of space (see Table 55.2). Tasks with a scattered arrangement, greater number of stimuli, more density, and less discriminability are more sensitive to mild cases of SN. The percentage of targets detected are compared on the right and left side. SN is indicated by a greater percentage of missed targets on the contralesional side of space. Examples of cancellation tasks for adults and children are listed in Tables 55.1 and 55.2. Other traditional paper and pencil tasks used to assess SN include copying figures, bisecting a line in the middle, or drawing a house, person, or clock.

Traditional SN assessments suffer from two main limitations. First, some of the most commonly used tests, such as the cancellation task, do not provide information regarding different forms of neglect. The cancellation test provides information on spatial biases in attention in peripersonal space but not on personal neglect or neglect in extrapersonal space. Second, the traditional paper and pencil tests may be insensitive to mild forms of neglect. Therefore, it is important not to rely completely on traditional assessments in identifying SN (Pitteri et al., 2018).

Contemporary Assessment of Spatial Neglect. The Kessler Foundation Neglect Assessment Process (KF-NAP; https://www.kflearn.org/courses/KF-NAP), a 10-item behavioral assessment that involves rating neglect in everyday tasks (Chen & Hreha, 2015) was found to be more sensitive in detecting functional impairment related to SN, compared to conventional tests (Gillen et al., 2021; Pitteri et al., 2018). The KF-NAP has not been used with children; however, the items are applicable. Although SN has been reported during ADL in children, studies of SN in children have not reported use of formal functional assessments. In addition to observations of ADL, bimanual tasks such as stringing beads, locating and picking up toys spread in the environment, dealing or placing cards on both sides of the environment, kicking small items located while walking, and age-appropriate reading, writing, or drawing tasks have been reported in the literature (Hart et al., 2021). The different behavioral manifestations and subtypes of neglect need to be considered during observation of performance (Evald et al., 2021; Rode et al., 2017). The need to further refine neglect assessment and focus on differentiating between neglect subtypes has been recognized in the literature as it could allow for more individualized and targeted treatment strategies.

Intervention

Different treatment methods for SN have been described, with a focus on adults with right hemisphere lesions. Studies investigating treatment of SN for children have used the same intervention approaches reported for adults; however, research in children is limited (Hart et al., 2021). No single treatment approach for SN has been demonstrated to be more effective than others (Longley et al. 2021). Despite this, there are a variety of therapeutic options that are supported by clinical experience and research, thereby providing a basis for practice guidelines and recommendations forming intervention of SN.

Task or Environmental Adaptations and Functional Skill Training. Adaptation of the task or environment is commonly used to enhance functional performance, for clients with SN. Collaboration with caregivers and family members to minimize the effects of SN within everyday environments is crucial. Such collaboration involves educating clients and families throughout the entire course of recovery (Chen et al., 2018). This involves identifying activities that are impacted by SN symptoms and discussing potential solutions such as those listed below.

- Increasing the saliency of items on the left side, such as placing red tape on the client's wheelchair brakes, edges of doorways, and furniture.
- Rearranging the position or placement of items, for example, placing brightly colored objects such as a napkin or cup on the left side of a plate.
- Using electronic devices with vibrating, auditory, or visual cues placed within the environment or in left pockets, clipped on the left side of a belt, or placed on a wrist to encourage attention to the left side of the body (Fong et al., 2011).

Metacognitive Strategy Intervention. Strategy use in people with neglect has been observed to be related to awareness (Tham et al., 2001). This underscores the importance of deeply embedding awareness training techniques, and metacognitive strategy methods such as those described earlier, into all intervention activities. For example, before performance, the client can be asked to identify challenges and methods they could use to ensure they would see items on both sides of space.

Strategies can include guiding the client in locating external cues that serve as an "anchor" or spatial point of reference that lets them know when they have attended to the left. This includes highlighting the left margin of a page or placing colored tape, a bright object, or their arm on the left border of a place setting. The same strategy is practiced across different activities and situations (Toglia & Foster, 2021). Toglia and Chen (2020) presented a study examining the multicontext treatment approach for spatial exploration strategy training in clients with stroke and SN. The therapist provided supportive feedback and semistructured guidance to promote strategy learning and self-discovery of errors. The treatment decreased neglect symptoms and improved online self-awareness.

Other intervention strategies for SN include tactile search and use of mental imagery. *Tactile search* includes teaching the client to feel the left side of space with eyes closed or to feel the left edges of objects before visual search (Toglia & Chen, 2020). *Mental imagery* teaches imagining and describing familiar scenes or routes and using mental images during movement of limbs or visual scanning (Welfringer et al., 2011). Reduction in neglect symptoms and increased performance on functional tasks were reported after a mental imagery program that involved teaching people with neglect to imagine their eyes as sweeping beams of a lighthouse from left to right across the visual field (McCarthy et al., 2002; Niemeier et al., 2001).

Strategies for SN can be practiced within a wide variety of everyday activities including setting a large table for six people; reading a newspaper, dealing a deck of cards to four people, filling multiple bowls with salad, placing cookie dough on a baking sheet, arranging photographs in a picture album, or copying a place setting (Toglia & Foster, 2021). Intervention should include practice in identifying situations in which SN symptoms are most likely and least likely to occur. Because SN symptoms vary with activity demands (e.g., size of space, amount, complexity), activity characteristics needed to be matched with neglect symptoms.

Remedial Training. A variety of interventions have been used to remediate disorders of SN, including visual scanning training (VST), prism adaptation (PA), eye patching, limb activation (Cicerone et al., 2019), mirror therapy (Zhang et al., 2022), neck vibration on the affected side (Ceyte et al., 2019; Kamada et al., 2011), general alertness or sustained attentional training (Van Vleet & DeGutis, 2013) noninvasive brain stimulation (Kashiwagi et al., 2018), virtual reality (Azouvi et al., 2017; Choi et al., 2021; Gillen et al., 2015; Ogourtsova et al., 2017), and music- assisted rehabilitation (Tramontano et al., 2021). Many of these techniques can be used within the context of functional activities.

Several systematic reviews have found the strongest level of evidence for VST or eye pursuit training in reducing neglect symptoms (Azouvi et al., 2017; Cicerone et al., 2019; Gillen et al., 2015). VST typically involves searching and locating stimuli in space with a focus on eye pursuits to the affected side. The amount and complexity of visual information presented is gradually increased. A systematic review concluded that there is Level I evidence to support VST and recommended it as a practice standard for individuals with visual neglect after a right hemisphere stroke (Cicerone et al., 2019). Although VST is the most widely used treatment for neglect, it should be kept in mind that VST selectively focuses on visual neglect, but SN symptoms often extend beyond the visual system (e.g., motor neglect, representational neglect; Kerkhoff et al., 2021). The application of VST combined with other evidence-based treatment techniques was illustrated in a case description of OT treatment for a person with a stroke and SN (Nilsen et al., 2015). The case illustrated how methods such as VST and videotape feedback could be integrated into occupation-based activities.

Active left-limb movement in the left side of space has been shown to improve visual scanning and leftward attention for some clients with SN. During limb activation, the person is asked to make limb movements with their contralesional arm while performing spatial or functional tasks. Similarly, forced use of the affected UE through restraint or CMIT during functional tasks or play activities has been observed to increase attention and awareness of the neglected side in both children and adults (Bollea et al., 2007; Chen et al., 2018).

The combination of forced limb activation or movements of the left arm or hand on the left side of space in conjunction with visual scanning has shown positive results and is recommended as a practice guideline (Cicerone et al., 2019).

More recently, there is accumulating evidence to support the combination of visual scanning and mirror therapy (MT) as well as MT alone. MT involves attempting to move the paretic upper extremity to mimic movements of the nonparetic limb reflected in a mirror on the side of the paretic limb. A review of five randomized controlled studies demonstrated that MT effectively improved neglect and daily living activities in adults with SN after stroke (Zhang et al., 2022).

The combination of limb activation or MT with VST suggests that a combination of treatment techniques that address different symptoms of SN may be more effective than one technique alone (Cicerone et al., 2019). Limb activation and MT address may address personal neglect or motor neglect whereas VST affects visual search and attention.

Prism adaptation (PA) has also been shown to alleviate the symptoms of SN and has been a popular area of research in adults with stroke. It has also been piloted in children with unilateral brain lesions. Prisms cause an optical deviation of the visual field to the right so that objects appear to be moved farther to the right than they actually are. A pilot study with children ages 6 to 11 found that PA used with games produced short-term improvements in SN after treatment and appears promising (Riquelme et al., 2015).

A systematic review of the impact of PA treatment on daily life activities in adults found evidence suggesting that PA improves daily functioning, particularly in the area of reading and writing (Champod et al., 2018; Chen, Diaz-Segarra, et al., 2021). Others, however, have argued that PA improves neglect symptoms for SN poststroke in the short term, but its long-term effects and impact on daily activities are inconclusive and still need further research (Li et al., 2021). Different neglect subtypes may respond differentially to PA treatment. There is initial evidence that better response to PA treatment is associated with those with frontal lesions and motor neglect or direction-specific motor abnormalities (Goedert et al., 2020).

Summary of Evidence. Given the heterogeneity of the neglect syndrome, it is unlikely that one intervention method would be suitable for all people with SN. Experts that were asked how to treat adults with SN identified visual scanning, active limb activation, sustained attention training, and PA as the top-five selections indicating that all are used frequently (Chen et al., 2018). Different treatment methods target different types of symptoms. Although one particular treatment has not been demonstrated to be superior over others, it is clear that interventions for SN are effective in helping to reduce neglect symptoms and improve functional recovery in some clients (Matano et al., 2015). It is recommended that intervention be tailored to the types of neglect symptoms that the person exhibits and that combination of intervention methods be utilized (Spaccavento et al., 2017). OT practitioners are encouraged to use clinical reasoning to determine the combination of treatment approaches that might be most beneficial for their clients.

Visual Perception

Visual perception is a broad term that refers to the ability to process, integrate, represent or interpret what is seen. We notice visual details, identify the context of the environment, interpret scenes with multiple interacting objects and people, search and locate visual information, recognize similarities, differences, or patterns between visual stimuli, and learn how things are related through our visual perceptual system. Visual perceptual dysfunction can affect the ability of children and adults to successfully engage in daily occupations. For example, visual perceptual deficits have been associated with difficulties in self-care skills (Chi & Lin, 2021; Chiu et al., 2019), mathematics (Critten et al., 2018), reading comprehension, handwriting legibility (Lee, 2021), social participation and difficulties in navigation within the environment (Rivest et al., 2018). Visual perception interacts with and affects numerous aspects of development, including neuromotor, cognitive, language, and emotional development (Ben Itzhak et al., 2021).

The term *cerebral visual impairment* (CVI) is used to describe a heterogeneous group of visual disorders in children (including visual perceptual deficits) that cannot be attributed to ocular impairments. CVI refers to damage to the cerebral visual pathways often known as the dorsal and ventral pathways, and associated structures (Ben Itzhak et al., 2021). CVI is observed in children with neurodevelopmental disorders such as cerebral palsy, spina bifida, autism, nonverbal learning disability, and DCD.

In adults, neurological disorders such as stroke (Chiu et al., 2019), TBI (Berger et al., 2016), and neurodegenerative diseases (Pelak, 2022) can result in visual perceptual deficits, depending on the areas of the brain involved in the injury or illness. In addition, deficits in visual perceptual skills, particularly, perceptual organization have been identified in adults with schizophrenia (Kurylo et al., 2018).

Visual perception can be viewed on an information-processing continuum involving reception, organization, and assimilation of visual information. On one end of the continuum, basic visual processing skills develop early in toddlers and occur automatically or with minimal effort in adults. Basic visual processing skills include:

- Discriminating between objects, pictures of objects, and basic shapes
- Detecting gross differences in size, position, direction, angles, distance, and rotations
- Searching and locating single visual targets in space
- Detecting simple part-whole relationships in objects or basic shapes

On the other end of the continuum, complex or higher-order visual tasks include unfamiliar or ambiguous stimuli or subtle discriminations within visually crowded arrays. These complex visual skills have been reported to be fully developed in adolescence (Dekker et al., 2011; Ebaid & Crewther, 2019). Across ages, visual perceptual performance varies depending on interactions between the person, activity demands (e.g., number of items, spacing, organization of visual stimuli), and the context (e.g., meaningfulness, familiarity) (Toglia, 2011).

Perceptual development generally progresses from being based on parts or piecemeal to being based on wholes (Pereira & Smith, 2009). During development, children learn to switch between local and global features of objects. Children with developmental delays may tend to over-focus on pieces of a shape, object, or figure, resulting in visual recognition errors (Guy et al., 2019). The ability to recognize objects or tools from unusual views is developed by age 10 with higher-order higher perceptual skills fully developed in early adolescence (Dekker et al., 2011). Young children with delays may struggle to match socks or utensils, especially when the differences are subtle. They might not notice differences between similar letters or numbers and may struggle to find information on a busy blackboard.

In adults, failure to recognize an object is labeled *visual agnosia*. The term *simultaneous agnosia* is described as an inability to simultaneously perceive multiple elements or objects and interpret the meaning of a basic visual scene, despite being able to perceive the discrete elements of the scene (Mazza, 2017). The person may have difficulty in familiar and routine activities and may easily misinterpret or misidentify objects. There are many different underlying reasons for visual agnosia. For example, a person might fail to attend to the critical feature of an object or the part of the object that identifies what it is (e.g., prongs of a fork). Attention might be captured by salient but irrelevant aspects of the object (e.g., the utensil's decorative handle) or scene (Toglia, 1989). Similar to observations of visual perceptual errors in children, an adult with neurological injury might be unable to process the overall shape and the details simultaneously. They might miss important details or over-focus on pieces of an object or scene, resulting in misinterpretations (Mazza, 2017). A child or adult might also have difficulty recognizing and interpreting facial expressions, recognizing social cues, or making sense of ambiguous, incomplete, fragmented, or distorted visual stimuli.

Evaluation

Evaluation of visual perceptual impairments involves examining visual foundation skills and visual perceptual abilities with and without a motor response. Any disruption of foundational skills can affect interpretations of higher-level visual processing assessments (Warren, 1993).

Visual Foundation Skills. The Brain Injury Visual Assessment Battery for Adults (biVABA; Warren, 1998, 2005) is an example of an evaluation that includes screening of visual foundation skills. It includes visual acuity; ocular alignment; visual pursuits, smooth tracking of moving objects; and saccades, or quick eye movements to place an object of interest in view (Aravich & Troxell, 2021). Visual fields should also be evaluated before a visual processing evaluation to screen out visual problems that will interfere with the accuracy of perceptual testing (Cate & Richards, 2000; Hanna et al., 2017). If a screening indicates possible difficulties in visual acuity, binocular coordination, or visual foundation skills, close collaboration with an optometrist is indicated (Aravich & Troxell, 2021).

Several clinical observations during functional tasks can alert occupational therapists to the need for a formal visual assessment, such as compensatory head movements and tilting, squinting, shutting off one eye, or a tendency to lose one's place while reading. To understand a client's visual perceptual abilities and the effects of impairments on functioning, therapists are encouraged to analyze the types of errors, as well as the activity conditions (complexity, amount, familiarity, and predictability) and context under which they occur (Toglia, 1989; 2011). Functional tasks that require visual-spatial skills such as locating or finding items in a room, desk, shelves, draws, or closets, reading and interpreting maps, diagrams, graphs, or charts; setting a table, fitting and positioning items within containers or discriminating between similar letters or objects can be directly observed and analyzed. The person's ability to recognize and correct visual perceptual errors should be investigated across functional tasks. For example, some clients do not recognize visual-spatial errors even when attention is directed to the problem area, whereas other clients recognize errors but are unable to correct them. The inability to correct visual perceptual errors that are recognized may suggest difficulties in visual motor integration.

Visual Perceptual Abilities. Standardized nonmotor assessments of visual perception (see Tables 55.1 and 55.2) generally involve identifying differences or similarities among visual figures. These tests categorize visual perception into specific components or subskills such as figure-ground (distinguishing a figure or object from the background or irrelevant visual information), form constancy (recognizing a shape or object despite variations in size, angle, position, or context visual closure (recognize an object, shape or picture based on partial information), and position in space or spatial relations (understanding and interpreting distance, direction, position or relationships between objects, oneself or other people) (Brown & Peres, 2018a, 2018b).

There is little evidence to support the existence of discrete areas of visual perception as represented by standardized tests. Most children and adults with visual perceptual difficulties score low across multiple subtests (Brown & Peres, 2018b; Sullivan et al., 2018). This is because individuals with visual perceptual impairments may have difficulty performing different types of visual processing tasks for similar reasons. For example, the terms "figure-ground" or position in space describe the type of task rather than the underlying difficulties. In addition, the connection between the results obtained in standardized tests of visual perception and functional performance is not always clear. For example, more than half of a sample that was identified as having significant difficulty with functional visual perceptual skills was not identified as having significant difficulty by a standardized visual perceptual test (Sullivan et al., 2018). Standardized visual perceptual tests are often required in clinical practice to provide objective evidence of the need for services. Such assessments, however, need to be combined with direct observation and performance analysis of functional visual perceptual tasks and/or parent/teacher questionnaires that assess functional visual perceptual skills. An example of a standardized ADL assessment that identifies the effect of visual-spatial impairments on self-care tasks such as grooming, feeding, and dressing is

the A-ONE (Gillen, 2009). Visual perceptual assessment should examine responses to activities with and without a motor response to examine performance differences under varied conditions.

Assessments for children include Parent Questionnaires such as the Cerebral Vision Impairment Inventory (CVI-I; Gorrie et al., 2019), and the Higher Visual Function Question Inventory (HVFQI-51; Chandna et al., 2021) screens functional difficulties that children with CVI might experience such as finding items in environmental clutter, and bumping into things when walking. Additionally, the Children's Visual Behaviour Checklist (CVBC) includes visual perceptual difficulties that can be observed in self-care, play/leisure, or school including reading, math, and writing (Sullivan et al., 2018).

Visual Motor Integration. *Visual motor integration* (i.e., perceptual-motor integration) is a broad term that is described as the ability to perceive and process visual information and coordinate a motor response. It includes eye-hand coordination, praxis, visual perceptual skills, gross or fine motor coordination that may be affected by developmental or neurological disorders (Carsone et al., 2021). Visual motor tasks encompass both graphomotor tasks such as writing, copying, and drawing tasks (e.g., drawing a map, copying shapes or a design), and constructional tasks that involve assembling pieces into a whole (e.g., assembling a coffeepot or a toy).

Children with difficulties in visual motor integration may have difficulty using scissors, opening a combination lock, tying shoelaces, or handwriting. Activities such as drawing, mazes, puzzles, and block-building activities are often avoided. Gross motor activities involving eye-hand coordination such as throwing or catching a ball, playing baseball or basketball may also present challenges. The child may bump into people or objects due to poor spatial awareness and have difficulty negotiating obstacle courses. These difficulties may also be observed in DCD as described below. In adults, the term *constructional apraxia* is used to refer to difficulty withdrawing or assembly tasks that cannot be attributed to primary motor or sensory impairment, visual processing deficits, ideomotor apraxia, or general cognitive impairments (Trojano, 2020). Constructional abilities are closely related to ADL performance. Clients may have difficulty dressing (dressing apraxia,) orienting clothes correctly on a hanger, or assembling a coffee pot.

Assessment of Visual Motor Skills. Assessment of visual motor skills typically involves copying geometric designs or shapes that vary in complexity or constructional tasks such as block designs or puzzles. Performance on these types of tasks can be difficult to relate to function. Observation of performance on functional tasks that require visual motor skills such as assembling a toy, completing an arts and crafts project, copying a graph, diagram, or poster layout, packing a lunchbox, assembling a thermos, folding clothes, or wrapping a package is recommended. These types of tasks are multifaceted and difficulties in assembly or graphomotor tasks can occur for many different reasons including deficits in executive functions, attention, visual scanning, motor planning, impaired discrimination of size and angle, poor ability to locate, align, position, or rotate items accurately. Analysis of the qualitative types of errors observed (omission of pieces or details versus spatial disorganization of the pieces without the overall gestalt as well) as the activity demands, and context can provide important insights into performance difficulties

Intervention

Adaptations of Task or Environment.
Adaptations of the task and environment to minimize the effects of visual perceptual difficulties are frequently used in practice (Yoo et al., 2020). Key principles include (a) reduce the amount of visual information presented simultaneously, minimize clutter and eliminate visual distractions, (b) keep visual information well organized, and (c) make the distinctive features of objects or figures more salient with color cues or use high contrast.

In a school setting, this may involve reorganizing worksheets to simplify the structure, reducing the amount of information presented on a page, or organizing visual information into quadrants or color-coded sections. Items in the classroom or home environment can be reorganized using color coding, written labels, high contrast, and large spacing between items when feasible. Pictures of what a desk, cubby, backpack, or room should look like can be provided to keep it organized. Adaptations for schoolwork may also include highlighting aspects of a geometric figure, line graph, or symbol in math, or placing a dark placemat under a worksheet or on top of a desk to increase contrast. Bolded or raised lines on a page, can help a child use lines and support writing efficiency. Enlarged print for worksheets or books, modifications to lighting, and a reading guide to help keep one's place also enhance reading. Consistent locations for objects (e.g., in the classroom, refrigerator, closet, drawer, or a countertop) increase predictability and provide contextual cues for recognition. Cues such as colored marks or tape at spatial landmarks (e.g., label of a shirt, key, or combination lock) reduce spatial demands and make it easier to orient and align parts of an item. Colored tape on buttons to operate appliances or salient color cues on objects make them easier to locate and discriminate (e.g., bright pink tape on a medication bottle). Significant others should be instructed to introduce only a small amount of visual information at one time and to decrease visual distractions in rooms and within tasks by limiting designs and patterns or by using solid colors with high contrast. Patterns, designs, and decorations make it harder to select and recognize critical features of an object. Task-specific training using errorless learning methods has also been reported to improve performance on visual-spatial functional tasks such as setting a table (Bier et al., 2019), or using a navigation app successfully (Rivest et al., 2018).

Metacognitive Strategy Approach.
Metacognitive strategy approaches such as the multicontext approach focus on helping the person learn to anticipate and understand the types of activity conditions that present greater risk for visual perceptual errors. Treatment includes anticipating challenges and generating strategies to prevent or manage visual processing errors. Strategies that maximize the client's ability to process visual information can include getting a sense of the whole before looking at the parts (Chen et al., 2012); teaching the person to partition space before localizing details; using one's finger to scan, trace visual stimuli, or focus on details; covering or blocking visual stimuli when too much information is presented at once; verbalizing salient visual features or subtle differences; and mentally visualizing a particular item before looking for it (Toglia, 1989, 2011). These strategies can be practiced across a variety of everyday activities such as choosing among objects that are similar in shape and size (e.g., matching socks, sorting teaspoons and soup spoons); locating information within calendars, schedules, pictures of scenes, or playing spot the difference games, arranging information within grids; copying patterns in arts and craft activities; or finding information in crowded spaces. Intervention involves careful manipulation of activity parameters related to visual perception while using strategies to promote task performance as listed in Box 55.2.

BOX 55.2 STRATEGIES FOR MANIPULATING ACTIVITY PARAMETERS

Activity parameters that require ...	
LESS attention, effort, and visual analysis	**MORE attention, effort, and visual analysis**
Features are distinct	Features are blended
Few details	A lot of details
Solid colors	Mixed colors and patterns
Solid backgrounds	Patterned backgrounds
Contrasting colors	Similar colors
Items in usual positions	Items in unusual positions
Familiar items	Unfamiliar items
Small number of items	A lot of items

Strategy use promoted within a multicontext paradigm, structures a wide range of activities horizontally (e.g., similar visual processing demands), so that carryover and generalization of strategy use are repeatedly practiced. This is different than a compensational paradigm that trains a visual perceptual strategy within a specific task or context (without generalization).

Remedial Exercises. Remedial exercises may be recommended for individuals with oculomotor or visual field deficits. For example, range of motion eye exercises to the involved muscle has been advocated for individuals with eye muscle paresis. Occlusion of the intact visual field with eye patching has been employed to force use of the impaired visual field (Warren, 1993), and VST has been used to increase saccadic eye movements or rapid visual search for both children and adults with visual field deficits (Hazelton et al., 2019; Ivanov et al., 2018) with preliminary evidence of effectiveness (Berger et al., 2016; Kerkhoff et al., 2021). These treatments involve repetitions of graded scanning activities. Visual perceptual exercises have also been used across various populations including children (Harpster et al., 2022), and adults with schizophrenia (Silverstein et al., 2020) or brain injury, but there is limited evidence of generalization to function when exercises are used in isolation (Berger et al., 2016). Visual scanning skills can also be directly integrated into play, school, or functional activities such as locating or searching for items on a shelf, hallway, or within one's environment.

Motor Planning

Motor planning, or praxis, is the ability to organize and execute skilled and purposeful movements. Difficulties in motor planning can be observed in children (developmental dyspraxia or developmental coordination) or adults (apraxia) and are not attributable to lower-level sensory or motor impairment, comprehension, inattention, or perceptual deficits (Worthington, 2016). Apraxia is defined as a disorder of intentional and *learned* movement following neurological conditions in adults (Foundas & Duncan, 2019). Unlike apraxia, developmental dyspraxia or DCD represents difficulties in the early *acquisition* of new motor skills (rather than learned skills). These latter conditions can persist through adolescence and adulthood (Costini et al., 2017). Since apraxia and DCD are distinct, these two disorders will be described separately in children and adults, along with clinical assessment and treatment.

Developmental Coordination Disorder/ Developmental Dyspraxia

DCD is common in school-aged children and is defined as impairment in the acquisition and execution of coordinated age-appropriate motor skills and skill learning that has a significant and persistent impact on daily living activities or academic achievement. The motor skill deficits are not explained by intellectual, developmental, or neurological disorders or visual impairments (Yu et al., 2018). The term *developmental dyspraxia* is commonly used synonymously with DCD in the literature; however, DCD has also been described as an umbrella term that includes developmental dyspraxia. In this context, developmental dyspraxia relates to the ability to learn, plan and perform skilled motor actions or motor sequences, and the ability to use tools (Costini et al., 2017). In this section, we will use the general term DCD as synonymous with developmental dyspraxia. Children who are born preterm are at higher risk of developing DCD (Spittle et al., 2021). DCD is typically diagnosed around the ages of 6 to 7; however, subtle signs and symptoms may be present earlier. Children with DCD are often described as clumsy, awkward, with slower or less accurate gross and fine motor skills compared to peers. Problems in sensory skills, visuospatial processing, or executive functions often accompany motor planning difficulties, although they do not fully explain the observed symptoms.

The motor skill problems in DCD can have a wide and pervasive impact on performance in everyday activities and participation. For example, the child or adolescent may have difficulty in tasks varying from self-care activities such as tying shoes or managing a zipper to leisure tasks such as riding bikes and engaging in sports activities or physical games. Activities such as physical education or sports are frequently avoided due to struggles, repeated failures, and low self-esteem. Children may be hesitant to play in the playground and are often socially isolated (Araújo et al., 2019). Adolescents with DCD may have difficulty learning to drive, causing embarrassment among teenage peers (Gentle et al., 2021). The functional consequences of DCD often persist and extend into adulthood, impacting physical and mental health as well as social participation and quality of life (Yu et al., 2018). For example, reduced physical activity participation and lower fitness increase the risk of obesity and cardiovascular disease. Many individuals with DCD have co-occurring problems including ADHD, autism, behavioral issues, and experience social isolation, anxiety, depression, and lower self-efficacy. Greater severity of DCD is associated with more comorbid issues and poorer outcomes (Smits-Engelsman et al., 2018). In general, adults who continue to exhibit DCD symptoms report lower quality of life.

Assessment. The most commonly used standardized test for identification of DCD in children is the Movement Assessment Battery for Children-Test (M-ABC-2 Test; Wuang et al., 2012). Specific handwriting assessments are also commonly utilized since the legibility of writing is frequently affected. In addition to motor skills, assessment should identify the types of activities the child avoids or finds difficult and observe and analyze its performance.

The Do-Eat is a performance-based assessment that has been validated for children with DCD (Josman et al., 2010). It involves making a sandwich, making chocolate milk, and writing a certificate. Performance accuracy as well as sensory-motor and executive control factors are examined. Additionally, dynamic performance analysis (DPA), described in the CO-OP approach provides a framework for an observation-based process of identifying performance problems or performance breakdown in activities that are meaningful to the child (McEwen et al., 2018).

Questionnaires provide important perspectives from parents or teachers on the functional impact of DCD symptoms in everyday activities. Some examples include the DCD-Questionnaire (DCDQ-R; Wilson et al., 2009) and the DCD Daily-Q, which is a parental questionnaire that focuses on acquisition and participation in ADL activities (van der Linde et al., 2014). An adult checklist of DCD symptoms for those who continue to struggle into adulthood is also available (Kirby et al., 2010).

Intervention. Treatment for DCD often includes a combination of treatment methods. The MATCH strategy, for example, is a combined approach (Modify the task, Alter expectations, Teach strategies, Change the environment, Help by understanding) to optimize learning in the classroom setting (Missiuna et al., 2004). A systematic review and meta-analysis of interventions for DCD found that activity-oriented approaches that focus on task-specific skills showed consistent improvements in both activity-based outcomes and client factors. This reinforces the importance of using meaningful tasks that are relevant to the child's everyday life (Smits-Engelsman et al., 2018). In addition, the importance of holistic treatment approaches including promotion of an active lifestyle and nutrition to minimize the risk of long-term health problems associated with DCD such as obesity, physical inactivity, and cardiovascular problems is advocated (Smits-Engelsman et al., 2018; Yu et al., 2018).

Functional Approach and Adaptations. Children and adolescents often need accommodations in school and at home to reduce motor demands and increase the ease of daily activities. For example,

- Dressing can be facilitated by selecting clothing or shoes that are easy to get on and off or that use Velcro closures rather than laces, buttons or snaps, or zippers (Missiuna et al., 2004).
- Extra time may be needed to complete writing assignments, gather and organize belongings, or for dressing (e.g., changing clothes for gym or recess).
- Handwriting or tool use can be facilitated with adaptations such as pencil grips, slant board for writing, thick-handled utensils or tools, and spring-loaded scissors.

- Writing demands can be reduced by photocopies of notes, voice recognition software, oral reports or oral test-taking, and worksheets with minimal writing such as fill in the blanks or matching.

Education of teachers and caregivers about the impact of DCD on children's ability to complete home and academic tasks is important in creating an environment that supports performance. This should include collaboration, coaching, or guidance in the identification and use of adaptations that can be employed to promote successful performance (Blank et al., 2019). In addition to adaptations, repetitive practice of specific tasks has also been shown to improve performance in children with DCD.

Metacognitive Strategy. The CO-OP approach has been shown to be effective in improving activity performance and participation in children with DCD and has been recommended for practice around the world (Blank et al., 2019). The CO-OP approach has been applied successfully to both individual and group interventions (Krajenbrink et al., 2022). In addition to a focus on meaningful everyday tasks and goals, the CO-OP approach helps the child problem-solve motor challenges encountered within tasks and recognize monitor, and correct problems during performance (Krajenbrink et al., 2022; Schwartz et al., 2020; Thornton et al., 2016). It has been argued that children with DCD need to learn to monitor, cope and manage motor challenges (Schoemaker & Smits-Engelsman, 2015), therefore, task practice should be combined with a metacognitive approach (Missiuna et al., 2012).

Remedial Interventions. Several interventions focus on directly improving motor abilities through practice in complex motor planning activities such as negotiating obstacle courses, use of exergames, virtual reality, perceptual-motor activities, or use of methods such as balance, strength training, oculomotor training, kinesthetic training, and sensory integration. Sensory integration methods focus on integrating sensory processing (e.g., tactile, proprioceptive, kinesthetic, or vestibular input) with activities requiring motor sequences, bilateral integration, or crossing the midline to reduce the interference of reflexes and promote higher-level motor planning skills. It is recommended that these interventions be combined with play or functional tasks to promote generalization (Smits-Engelsman et al., 2018); however, there is a lack of research studying the long-term effects of these interventions on everyday function (Yu et al., 2018). Refer to Chapter 56, Sensory Processing in Everyday Life, for more information.

Apraxia

Apraxia occurs most commonly after stroke; however, it can also be seen in persons with dementia, MS, Parkinson disease, and movement disorders such as Huntington disease

(Buchmann, Dangel, et al., 2020; Foundas & Duncan, 2019). Apraxia may be seen after lesions in either hemisphere, although it is more frequently encountered in clients who have sustained a left hemisphere lesion. Aphasia is often associated with apraxia because the left hemisphere is also dominant for language (Foundas & Duncan, 2019).

Apraxia can have a negative impact on ADL, functional outcomes, quality of communicative gestures, and the ability to engage in meaningful activities (Cosar et al., 2020; Pazzaglia & Galli, 2019). People with apraxia may have difficulty performing routine activities such as getting dressed, brushing teeth, and using utensils for eating or preparing food. As a result, apraxia can increase caregiver burden (Lindsten-McQueen et al., 2014) as well as increase anxiety, depression, and social isolation (Alashram et al., 2021). Apraxia can persist over time, and individuals can continue to have significant functional limitations in both the learning of new motor tasks, such as one-handed shoe tying and in the efficiency and accuracy of actions to verbal command or demonstration (Poole, 2000).

Four traditional forms of upper limb apraxia have been identified (Heilman, 2021):

1. *Ideomotor apraxia* involves the execution of an action plan. The greatest difficulty is observed when the client is asked to pretend to use a tool or object or to perform limb gestures. Some improvement may be seen when the client is asked to imitate the motion or perform the motion with the actual object, but the movement is still imprecise. These clients know what they want to do, but actions are carried out in an awkward, inefficient, or clumsy manner. Spatial-temporal errors or errors of preservation, timing, spatial orientation or position, or inefficiencies (e.g., extra joint movements or excessive co-contraction) may be observed.

2. *Limb-kinetic apraxia* is characterized by unilateral clumsy distal movements that affect the production of hand and finger sequences. The person has difficulty with buttoning or manipulating coins that cannot be explained by sensory loss, ataxia, weakness, or impaired muscle tone.

3. *Conceptual apraxia* involves the loss of knowledge about the functional properties of an object, the object action or knowledge about the needed tool to perform an action, and knowledge about alternative tools. Some individuals demonstrate a tool selection deficit. They understand what needs to be done but cannot recognize the object or tool needed to perform the action. Others demonstrate a tool-action-association deficit and are unable to retrieve the type of action that is associated with specific objects or tools. For example, a person might be able to accurately name and identify a toothbrush and hairbrush but might try to brush his or her hair with a toothbrush. Although object recognition is intact, the person is unable to associate the object with its corrective action plan.

4. *Ideational apraxia* is a loss of knowledge of action sequences and involves difficulty in carrying out sequences of objects in the correct order. For example, in attempting to brush one's teeth the person may brush teeth without putting toothpaste on the toothbrush and then puts toothpaste in one's mouth. Ideational apraxia is sometimes included under conceptual apraxia because the person has lost the concept of an action sequence or the knowledge of the correct order of steps even though the individual elements may be intact.

Both ideomotor and limb-kinetic apraxia are thought to reflect problems in the praxis production system that controls execution of learned motor plans whereas ideational and conceptual apraxia reflect problems in the praxis conceptual system that involves the knowledge of object-related action plans (Foundas & Duncan, 2019).

In addition to the traditional forms of limb apraxia, the term action disorganization syndrome (ADS), has been used to describe omission and substitution errors in tool use or steps during tasks that involve multiple objects, sequencing, and multistep actions. For example, the person may have preserved single object use but when making toast and coffee, they may pick up a spoon instead of a knife to spread butter on the toast (Morady & Humphreys, 2011). ADS explains difficulties in multistep tasks as a combination of poor retrieval of stored knowledge about the task steps as well as decreased executive control of attention or poor error monitoring (Nakajima et al., 2020). Unlike traditional views of apraxia, ADS highlights how action errors can be influenced by cognitive demands of activities.

Dressing apraxia and *constructional apraxia* are additional subtypes of apraxia, previously described in the section on visual motor integration. Traditional labels of apraxia are narrow in scope and do not account for the wide range of skills that underlie motor planning and constructional abilities.

Evaluation. Motor planning and action sequencing involve an integration of multiple skills including visual-spatial, executive functions, language, and somatosensory skills as well as knowledge and understanding of object properties and sequences. OT practitioners are encouraged to analyze error patterns and the underlying factors contributing to difficulties in performance rather than attempting to classify clients within traditional categories. If aphasia and apraxia coexist, information on the client's language skills should be obtained from a speech-language pathologist or be screened for by testing for "yes" or "no" comprehension and ability to follow one-step commands.

In evaluating apraxia, the clinician typically observes the client's performance of different types of functional movements and tasks, noting the method of evocation (e.g., command, imitation, or object use), quality of movement, type of errors made, and the influence of familiarity and context (Haaland, 1993). Tasks that involve both single object use as well as multiple objects and steps should be examined. For example, a subtest of the Diagnostic Instrument of Limb Apraxia -short version (DILA-S) involves observing the person prepare a breakfast including a toasted slice of bread with butter and jam as well as a cup of tea with sugar. The number of steps accurately completed as well as the number and type of errors are scored (Buchmann, Dangel, et al., 2020).

Apraxia is also assessed in the A-ONE evaluation through observation of self-care activities and ratings on a neurobehavioral scale (Árnadóttir, 2016). A dynamic assessment approach for adults with aphasia and apraxia that analyzes the response to different types of cues across functional tasks with increasing number of steps has also been described (Toglia, 2011).

Intervention. In general familiar tasks that are performed in context are easier for people with motor planning disorders because the context provides cues that facilitate the desired action. Interventions can be graded by gradually increasing the number of tools and distractors, increasing the degrees of freedom (Gillen, 2009), or introducing activities and environments that have less stability and predictability, such as negotiating around obstacles in a crowded store.

Adaptations of Task or Environment. Simple adaptations to objects that draw attention to the critical features of the object or activity can facilitate action and motor planning (e.g., colored tape on the knife handle or toothbrush handle). Patterns and designs on utensils or clothing might draw attention to the wrong detail and result in an inappropriate motor response. Tool use should be minimized (Poole, 2000), and adaptive equipment should be selected with caution for clients with apraxia. For example, some adaptations such as a button hook, one-handed shoe tying, or a one-arm drive wheelchair might be confusing for clients with apraxia and place greater demands on motor planning abilities. Other adaptations, such as adaptive clothing closures, may simplify the task or motor pattern required to manipulate or hold objects, reduce the number of steps, and facilitate function in the client with apraxia.

Training caregivers to modify instructions so that the activity is broken into one command at a time and to use simple whole commands (e.g., "Get up") can put the activity on an automatic level and effectively enhance motor planning (Zoltan, 2007).

Task-specific training using errorless learning principles and immediate feedback has been found to be effective in training specific functional tasks (Buchmann, Dangel, et al., 2020; Goldenberg & Hagmann, 1998). Task-specific strategies such as rehearsal of a verbal script of action sequences for a particular task have also been demonstrated to increase specific task performance. For example, naturalistic

action therapy trains object selection and task execution with an errorless learning approach during functional activities. Verbal and visual supports (e.g., photos, demonstration, imitation) and if necessary physical guidance is provided to facilitate motor patterns or manipulation of objects within tasks such as pouring water into a glass, preparing a letter, or filling a pill organizer box (Buchmann, Finkel, et al., 2020). As performance improves, cues are withdrawn. This method of treatment is similar to the NFA, which emphasizes mastery of functional task performance through practice (Giles, 2018).

Recently technology has also been used to provide immediate feedback within task-specific training. The system Cogwatch uses sensors embedded in household objects connected to a display and central processor that provides errorless feedback and can be used to guide a person through simple tasks. A randomized controlled trial that focused on tea-making training reduced time required and errors compared to a control group (Howe et al., 2022). No generalization, however, was observed in a complex tea preparation task (making two different cups of tea simultaneously) reflecting the specificity of the training.

Metacognitive Strategy Intervention. Clients can be encouraged to generate or use verbal or visual, internal or external strategies to enhance movement while performing everyday activities (Pazzaglia & Galli, 2019). For example, before performing an activity, the client can mentally practice or imagine task performance (e.g., making tea or brushing teeth), or imagine how an object such as a toothbrush should look in his or her hand before picking it up. Audiotapes or verbal scripts can be used to guide mental practice (Wu et al., 2011). Incorrect patterns of movement, such as holding an object in the wrong way, can also be visualized with an emphasis on having the client solve the problem and mentally practice correct the movement.

Visual external strategies include pictorial cues or encouraging creation and use of step-by-step written lists or photo sequences across activities (Moinuddin et al., 2022). Object pointing strategies before use, help a person focus on object features that are critical to various actions. Self-verbalization strategies (talk aloud or internal self-talk) describe individual actions or steps either before or as they are carried out and can increase awareness of actions and prevent action errors across situations. For example, Nakajima et al. (2020) used metacognitive techniques that included asking a client to report the details of any action slips that had occurred during daily activities. The client was then asked to analyze the context in which each slip occurred and generate strategies for preventing future occurrences. This type of self-reflection also heightens awareness and self-monitoring skills and prevents action errors.

Several studies have reported improvements in everyday activities as a result of strategy interventions (Alashram et al., 2021; Geusgens et al., 2006; Moinuddin et al., 2022). Systematic reviews of apraxia interventions consistently indicate that strategy training is one of the most promising interventions for improving everyday function (Alashram et al., 2021; Worthington, 2016). Strategy-based treatment has therefore been recommended as a practice standard (Cicerone et al., 2019).

Remedial Training. Remedial or restorative approaches to apraxia include gestural training, action observation, mirror box therapy, and virtual or augmented reality. Several studies and reviews have supported the use of gesture training in apraxia when used in combination with functional or strategy approaches; however, additional research is needed (Aguilar-Ferrándiz et al., 2022; Alashram et al., 2021). Gesture training includes gesture-production and recognition exercises such as pantomime, imitation, or producing gestures involving manipulation of objects, which are gradually increased in difficulty level. The use of action observation or modified mirror box therapy has been suggested in the treatment of apraxia and is an emerging area of interest (Romano et al., 2021). The use of immersive virtual reality and augmented reality for the treatment of ideomotor apraxia in adults with stroke is another area of promising research. Augmented reality offers a way to provide and manipulate salience of objects and contextual features that may induce automatic motor responses (Park et al., 2021; Rohrbach et al., 2021).

Occupational Therapy Role Within the Interprofessional Team

A strong interdisciplinary approach is needed to address the complex issues that arise from cognitive perceptual problems. Team goals should be identified as well as specific discipline goals. The family, client, and caregivers, when appropriate, are also members of the team; they should be involved in team discussions and provide input into the overall intervention plan.

Once goals and targeted behaviors for intervention have been clearly identified, the OT practitioner and OTA collaborate to identify various activities that can be used to reinforce the desired behaviors. The practice setting may determine the depth of the OT practitioner's involvement because of the nature of that setting and the client's length of stay.

An interdisciplinary intervention program should emphasize the same major goals during treatment rather than working on separate skills. For example, a speech-language pathologist might address working memory problems within the context of language material such as listening to and keeping track of conversations; a neuropsychologist might use remedial working memory exercises; a physical therapist might reinforce working memory by asking the person to keep track of things in the environment as they are ambulating; and an OT practitioner might address the ability to keep track of information within the context of IADL, leisure, community, and/or work activities. An integrated approach that assists the person in seeing patterns of behaviors across different activities is strongly advocated rather than a fragmented approach.

Conclusion

It is clear from the content in this chapter that cognitive impairments can significantly disrupt everyday life across multiple groups of clients and ages. It is also clear that functional cognitive intervention is crucial for clients across the life span for various reasons, from prevention of decline in ADL to maintenance, support, or promotion of cognitive or daily life skills.

OT has made substantial gains in our ability to assess and manage functional cognition by developing performance-based measures and by developing and fostering various cognitive intervention approaches that take into account client and environmental factors. These performance-based assessments (e.g., EFPT, WCPA) represent substantial advances over impairment-based assessments or conventional ADL scales that were used in practice (i.e., FIM). In addition, an evidence-based cognitive intervention that focuses on improving and maintaining daily life performance has shown significant improvement in the life of clients who received such treatment.

As occupational therapists, we are equipped with the tools to understand (a) how cognition is linked with engagement in everyday occupations; (b) how context and environment affect people's functional capacity, and (c) how activity can facilitate and stimulate various cognitive processes. We should embrace this understanding and knowledge and use it in our practice, education, and research. It is time to think out of the box, expand perspectives and focus OT treatment on promoting health behaviors, preventing functional decline, and optimizing function, participation, and well-being using cognitive intervention approaches described in this chapter (see Expanding Our Perspectives).

Furthermore, the changing perspectives on cognition and executive functioning and the significant impact of subtle cognitive deficits on participation and quality of life expand opportunities for occupational therapists in new and emerging areas. As reviewed in this chapter, cognitive interventions can also be applied to nontraditional or at-risk populations. For example, negative early childhood experiences, impoverished environments, or prolonged stress can have adverse effects on brain development and cognitive skills that place children and adolescents at risk for weaknesses or vulnerabilities in executive function skills. Individual differences in executive functioning abilities have been related to behavioral problems, risky behaviors academics, and achievement throughout life. Earlier intervention may be able prevent the secondary mental health challenges of children and even young adults with DCD, perceptual impairments or mild visual motor or executive function delays.

Another example is clients with chronic conditions such as obesity, kidney failure, cancer, or chronic fatigue syndrome who may be experiencing subtle changes in cognition and are at risk for negative health outcomes. In this group of clients, functional cognitive interventions that support or optimize executive functions for successful management of health-related tasks could be beneficial in preventing hospital readmissions and functional decline. Note, however, that significant access barriers still exist among people from lower socioeconomic status. Additionally, OTs need to articulate our scope of practice to eliminate confusion with other allied health professions such as speech therapy in cognitive rehabilitation

In conclusion, this chapter describes substantial progress in our recognition of the impact of functional cognitive intervention on daily life and the acknowledgment that it is engagement in meaningful activities and roles that is most important to the clients impacted. As OTs continue to focus efforts on implementing functional cognitive interventions, it is essential that we continue to recognize the importance of optimizing cognition within the context of a person's life including their goals, routines, valued activities, and life roles.

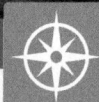

EXPANDING OUR PERSPECTIVES

Advocacy With Cognitive Rehabilitation in Rural Health

Maggie M. Heyman Hotch, MOT, OTR/L

My own discovery of OT at the age of ten was when my father suffered a severe CVA at age thirty-six, resulting in right hemiparesis and severe expressive aphasia. Seeing his usual optimistic spirit finally return following an OT session several months into his intensive hospital-based rehabilitation, I realized that would be a very fun and powerful job. Twenty-five years later, when I began practicing year-round in rural Alaska, one of my first referrals was a former AP Journalist who had broken the West Virginia Coal Mining story just before a CVA very similar to my father's three years prior at age 44. Having attended intensive rehabilitation for the first year and a half following his stroke, he had been referred through our relationship with Division of Vocational Rehabilitation, planning to reinvent himself as a farmer. The opportunity for placement was at a farm 18 miles out of town with no local public transportation. Had I done driver rehabilitation before? No! Was I a little nervous about the endeavor? Yes! Was there anyone else that was going to step up to help him? Likely not. Before being referred, while still holding a valid West Virginia driver's license, he followed the correct procedure and took the written test with his wife arranging accommodations to read the questions aloud to him at the local DMV (department of motor vehicles). He passed. The state trooper in the nearby office had observed him walk into the DMV with his cane, overheard the written test being read aloud, and presumed as I had frustratingly witnessed so many people do of my father over the years of my youth, that aphasia indicates incompetence. Following evaluation of visual motor skills, visual perception, and functional cognition, while feeling frustrated at how many cognitive assessments cannot be administered to those who have expressive aphasia, I determined it would be safe to begin driver rehabilitation. We began using a small cart converted with left-footed gas pedal on the quiet back roads of his neighborhood first and progressing in stages. We then learned of the trooper's ableist action of having his license revoked which limited our ability to continue temporarily. When the letter came from West Virginia DMV revoking his license, I countered with a letter containing assessment scores and, more importantly, clinical observation of his functional cognition. This was enough to reinstate the license, but another barrier presented in obtaining the paperwork for a DMV road test from primary care. His provider stated "needs evaluation" on many of the items that I had already evaluated and reported back in the plan of care, rather than approving. After many phone calls with the RN (I was never given

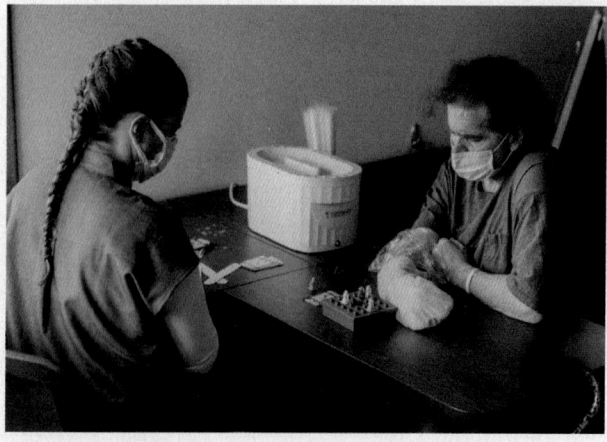

Courtesy of Katlyn Hickman, Haines, Alaska.

EXPANDING OUR PERSPECTIVES (continued)

access to the Dr directly to share my experience of being in the vehicle with my client), we were strung along for several months with the local clinic telling me the paperwork was sent, and DMV telling me it had not been received. I began planting myself in the clinic once a week asking after the paperwork. Eventually, the client switched primary care providers, and once allowed a road test he passed easily. While he did not plan to ever drive in a city or area other than our rural small town and the surrounding areas, having the driver's license allowed him to maintain his role as a parent by shuffling his middle school age children around to their activities. His license

also enabled him to perform all household management and IADL tasks such as grocery shopping, cooking, and household errands in the community so that his wife could continue working full time. He generalized this to farm his own property with peonies and vegetables with a small tractor outfitted with a left-foot gas pedal and steering knob. He continues six years later to run a small business farming and mowing lawns in our community as well as maintaining a booth at the weekly local farmer's market, interacting with community members, and changing perceptions about the relationship between functional cognition and spoken language.

Lippincott® Connect *For additional resources on the subjects discussed in this chapter, visit Lippincott Connect.*

REFERENCES

Adamos, T., Chukoskie, L., Townsend, J., & Trauner, D. (2022). Spatial attention in children with perinatal stroke. *Behavioural Brain Research, 417,* 113614. https://doi.org/10.1016/j.bbr.2021.113614

Aguilar-Ferrándiz, M. E., Toledano-Moreno, S., García-Ríos, M. C., Tapia-Haro, R. M., Barrero-Hernández, F. J., Casas-Barragán, A., & Pérez-Mármol, J. M. (2022). Effectiveness of a functional rehabilitation program for upper limb apraxia in poststroke patients: A randomized controlled trial. *Archives of Physical Medicine and Rehabilitation.* https://doi.org/10.1016/j.apmr.2022.02.002

Alashram, A. R., Annino, G., Aldajah, S., Raju, M., & Padua, E. (2021). Rehabilitation of limb apraxia in patients following stroke: A systematic review. *Applied Neuropsychology. Adult, 29*(6), 1658–1668. https://doi.org/10.1080/23279095.2021.1900188

Allen, C. K. (1985). *Occupational therapy for psychiatric diseases: Measurement and management of cognitive disabilities* (1st ed.). Little Brown & Co.

Allott, K. A., Killackey, E., Sun, P., Brewer, W. J., & Velligan, D. I. (2017). Improving vocational outcomes in first-episode psychosis by addressing cognitive impairments using Cognitive Adaptation Training. *Work, 56*(4), 581–589. https://doi.org/10.3233/WOR-172517

Allott, K. A., van-der-EL, K., Bryce, S., Parrish, E. M., McGurk, S. R., Hetrick, S., Bowie, C. R., Kidd, S., Hamilton, M., Killackey, E., & Velligan, D. (2020). Compensatory interventions for cognitive impairments in psychosis: A systematic review and meta-analysis. *Schizophrenia Bulletin, 46*(4), 869–883. https://doi.org/10.1093/schbul/sbz134

Alsaqer, M. (2021). Aging and technology: Understanding the issues and creating a base for technology designers. *Journal of Medical Engineering & Technology, 45*(4), 258–283. https://doi.org/10.1080/03091902.2021.1891313

Álvarez, E. A., Garrido, M. A., Tobar, E. A., Prieto, S. A., Vergara, S. O., Briceño, C. D., & González, F. J. (2017). Occupational therapy for delirium management in elderly patients without mechanical ventilation in an intensive care unit: A pilot randomized clinical trial. *Journal of Critical Care, 37,* 85–90. https://doi.org/10.1016/j.jcrc.2016.09.002

American Occupational Therapy Association. (2020a). Occupational therapy practice framework: Domain and process, 4th edition. *American Journal of Occupational Therapy, 74*(Suppl. 2), 7412410010. https://doi.org/10.5014/ajot.2020.74S2001

American Occupational Therapy Association. (2020b). *AOTA's occupational profile template for documentation.* https://www.aota.org/practice/practice-essentials/documentation/improve-your-documentation-with-aotas-updated-occupational-profile-template

Anderson, A. C., Youssef, G. J., Robinson, A. H., Lubman, D. I., & Verdejo-Garcia, A. (2021). Cognitive boosting interventions for impulsivity in addiction: A systematic review and meta-analysis of cognitive training, remediation and pharmacological enhancement. *Addiction, 116*(12), 3304–3319. https://doi.org/10.1111/add.15469

Araújo, C. R. S., Cardoso, A. A., & Magalhães, L. de C. (2019). Efficacy of the cognitive orientation to daily occupational performance with Brazilian children with developmental coordination disorder. *Scandinavian Journal of Occupational Therapy, 26*(1), 46–54. https://doi.org/10.1080/11038128.2017.1417476

Aravich, D., & Troxell, L. (2021). Clinical practice guidelines for occupational therapists in the evaluation and treatment of oculomotor impairment following traumatic brain injury. *Current Physical Medicine and Rehabilitation Reports, 9*(3), 93–99. https://doi.org/10.1007/s40141-021-00310-x

Árnadóttir, G. (2016). Impact of neurobehavioral deficits on activities of daily living. In G. Gillen (Ed.), *Stroke rehabilitation: A function-based approach* (4th ed., pp. 573–611). Elsevier. https://doi.org/10.1016/B978-0-323-17281-3.00026-5

Azouvi, P., Jacquin-Courtois, S., & Luauté, J. (2017). Rehabilitation of unilateral neglect: Evidence-based medicine. *Annals of Physical and Rehabilitation Medicine, 60*(3), 191–197. https://doi.org/10.1016/j.rehab.2016.10.006

Bannon, L., McGaughey, J., Verghis, R., Clarke, M., McAuley, D. F., & Blackwood, B. (2019). The effectiveness of non-pharmacological interventions in reducing the incidence and duration of delirium in critically ill patients: A systematic review and meta-analysis. *Intensive Care Medicine, 45*(1), 1–12. https://doi.org/10.1007/s00134-018-5452-x

Bar-Haim Erez, S. A., & Katz, N. (2018). Cognitive functional evaluation. In N. Katz & J. Toglia (Eds.), *Cognition, occupation, and participation across the life span: Neuroscience, neurorehabilitation, and models of intervention in occupational therapy* (4th ed., pp. 69–86). AOTA Press.

Baron, I. S. (2000). Behavior rating inventory of executive function. *Child Neuropsychology, 6*(3), 235–238. https://doi.org/10.1076/chin.6.3.235.3152

Barrett, A. M. (2021). Spatial neglect and anosognosia after right brain stroke. *Continuum (Minneapolis, Minn.), 27*(6), 1624–1645. https://doi.org/10.1212/CON.0000000000001076

Baum, C. M., Connor, L. T., Morrison, T., Hahn, M., Dromerick, A. W., & Edwards, D. F. (2008). Reliability, validity, and clinical utility of the executive function performance test: A measure of executive function in a sample of people with stroke. *The American Journal of Occupational Therapy, 62*(4), 446–455. https://doi.org/10.5014/ajot.62.4.446

Baum, C. M., Edwards, D. F., Al-Heizan, M., & Giles, G. M. (2019). The executive function performance test. In T. Wolf, D. F. Edwards, & G. M. Giles (Eds.), *Functional cognition and occupational therapy: A practical approach to treating individuals with cognitive loss* (pp. 67–73). AOTA Press.

Baum, C. M., Wolf, T. J., Wong, A. W. K., Chen, C. H., Walker, K., Young, A. C., Carlozzi, N. E., Tulsky, D. S., Heaton, R. K., & Heinemann, A. W. (2017). Validation and clinical utility of the executive function performance test in persons with traumatic brain injury. *Neuropsychological Rehabilitation, 27*(5), 603–617. https://doi.org/10.1080/09602011.2016.1176934

Ben Itzhak, N., Kooiker, M. J. G., van der Steen, J., Pel, J. J. M., Wagemans, J., & Ortibus, E. (2021). The relation between visual orienting functions, daily visual behaviour and visuoperceptual performance in children with (suspected) cerebral visual impairment. *Research in Developmental Disabilities, 119,* 104092. https://doi.org/10.1016/j.ridd.2021.104092

Berg, C., Edwards, D. F., & King, A. (2012). Executive function performance on the children's kitchen task assessment with children with sickle cell disease and matched controls. *Child Neuropsychology: A Journal on Normal and Abnormal Development in Childhood and Adolescence, 18*(5), 432–448. https://doi.org/10.1080/09297049.2011.613813

Berger, S., Kaldenberg, J., Selmane, R., & Carlo, S. (2016). Effectiveness of interventions to address visual and visual-perceptual impairments to improve occupational performance in adults with traumatic brain injury: A systematic review. *The American Journal of Occupational Therapy, 70*(3), 7003180010p1–7003180010p7. https://doi.org/10.5014/ajot.2016.020875

Bharadwaj, S. V., Yeatts, P., & Headley, J. (2022). Efficacy of cogmed working memory training program in improving working memory in school-age children with and without neurological insults or disorders: A meta-analysis. *Applied Neuropsychology. Child, 11*(4), 891–903. https://doi.org/10.1080/21622965.2021.1920943

Bier, N., El-Samra, A., Bottari, C., Vallet, G. T., Carignan, M., Paquette, G., Brambati, S., Demers, L., Génier-Marchand, D., & Rouleau, I. (2019). Posterior cortical atrophy: Impact on daily living activities and exploration of a cognitive rehabilitation approach. *Cogent Psychology, 6*(1), 1634911. https://doi.org/10.1080/23311908.2019.1634911

Bjørkedal, S. T. B., Bejerholm, U., Eplov, L. F., & Møller, T. (2020). Meaningful Activities and Recovery (MA&R): The effect of a novel rehabilitation intervention among persons with psychiatric disabilities on activity engagement—Study protocol for a randomized controlled trial. *Trials, 21*(1), 789. https://doi.org/10.1186/s13063-020-04722-3

Blank, R., Barnett, A. L., Cairney, J., Green, D., Kirby, A., Polatajko, H., Rosenblum, S., Smits-Engelsman, B., Sugden, D., Wilson, P., & Vinçon, S. (2019). International clinical practice recommendations on the definition, diagnosis, assessment, intervention, and psychosocial aspects of developmental coordination disorder. *Developmental Medicine and Child Neurology, 61*(3), 242–285. https://doi.org/10.1111/dmcn.14132

Bodien, Y. G., Martens, G., Ostrow, J., Sheau, K., & Giacino, J. T. (2020). Cognitive impairment, clinical symptoms and functional disability in patients emerging from the minimally conscious state. *NeuroRehabilitation, 46*(1), 65–74. https://doi.org/10.3233/NRE-192860

Bollea, L., Rosa, G. D., Gisondi, A., Guidi, P., Petrarca, M., Giannarelli, P., & Castelli, E. (2007). Recovery from hemiparesis and unilateral spatial neglect after neonatal stroke. Case report and rehabilitation of an infant. *Brain Injury, 21*(1), 81–91. https://doi.org/10.1080/02699050601148882

Bosma, M. S., Nijboer, T. C. W., Caljouw, M. A. A., & Achterberg, W. P. (2020). Impact of visuospatial neglect post-stroke on daily activities, participation and informal caregiver burden: A systematic review.

Annals of Physical and Rehabilitation Medicine, 63(4), 344–358. https://doi.org/10.1016/j.rehab.2019.05.006

Brown, T., & Peres, L. (2018a). A critical review of the Motor-Free Visual Perception Test—fourth edition (MVPT-4). *Journal of Occupational Therapy, Schools, & Early Intervention, 11*(2), 229–244. https://doi.org/10.1080/19411243.2018.1432441

Brown, T., & Peres, L. (2018b). An overview and critique of the Test of Visual Perception Skills—fourth edition (TVPS-4). *Hong Kong Journal of Occupational Therapy, 31*(2), 59–68. https://doi.org/10.1177/1569186118793847

Buchmann, I., Dangel, M., Finkel, L., Jung, R., Makhkamova, I., Binder, A., Dettmers, C., Herrmann, L., Liepert, J., Möller, J. C., Richter, G., Vogler, T., Wolf, C., & Randerath, J. (2020). Limb apraxia profiles in different clinical samples. *The Clinical Neuropsychologist, 34*(1), 217–242. https://doi.org/10.1080/13854046.2019.1585575

Buchmann, I., Finkel, L., Dangel, M., Erz, D., Maren Harscher, K., Kaupp-Merkle, M., Liepert, J., Rockstroh, B., & Randerath, J. (2020). A combined therapy for limb apraxia and related anosognosia. *Neuropsychological Rehabilitation, 30*(10), 2016–2034. https://doi.org/10.1080/09602011.2019.1628075

Burns, S., & Neville, M. (2017). Assessing the impact of real-life cognitive functioning in the home: Development and psychometric study of the Multiple Errands Test–Home. *The American Journal of Occupational Therapy, 71*(4_Suppl._1), 7111500030p1. https://doi.org/10.5014/ajot.2017.71S1-PO2138

Burton, R. L., & O'Connell, M. E. (2018). Telehealth rehabilitation for cognitive impairment: Randomized controlled feasibility trial. *JMIR Research Protocols, 7*(2), e9420. https://doi.org/10.2196/resprot.9420

Canevelli, M., Valletta, M., Trebbastoni, A., Sarli, G., D'Antonio, F., Tariciotti, L., de Lena, C., & Bruno, G. (2016). Sundowning in dementia: Clinical relevance, pathophysiological determinants, and therapeutic approaches. *Frontiers in Medicine, 3.* https://www.frontiersin.org/article/10.3389/fmed.2016.00073

Caprì, T., Nucita, A., Iannizzotto, G., Stasolla, F., Romano, A., Semino, M., Giannatiempo, S., Canegallo, V., & Fabio, R. A. (2021). Telerehabilitation for improving adaptive skills of children and young adults with multiple disabilities: A systematic review. *Review Journal of Autism and Developmental Disorders, 8*(2), 244–252. https://doi.org/10.1007/s40489-020-00214-x

Carsone, B., Green, K., Torrence, W., & Henry, B. (2021). Systematic review of visual motor integration in children with developmental disabilities. *Occupational Therapy International, 2021,* e1801196. https://doi.org/10.1155/2021/1801196

Cate, Y., & Richards, L. (2000). Relationship between performance on tests of basic visual functions and visual-perceptual processing in persons after brain injury. *The American Journal of Occupational Therapy, 54*(3), 326–334. https://doi.org/10.5014/ajot.54.3.326

Cermak, S. A., & Toglia, J. (2018). Cognitive development across the lifespan: Development of cognition and executive functioning in children and adolescents. In N. Katz & J. Toglia (Eds.), *Cognition, occupation, and participation across the life span: Neuroscience, neurorehabilitation, and models of intervention in occupational therapy* (4th ed., pp. 9–28). AOTA Press.

Ceyte, H., Beis, J.-M., Simon, M., Rémy, A., Anxionnat, R., Paysant, J., & Caudron, S. (2019). Lasting improvements in left spatial neglect following a protocol combining neck-muscle vibration and voluntary arm movements: A case-study. *Disability and Rehabilitation, 41*(12), 1475–1483. https://doi.org/10.1080/09638288.2018.1430178

Champod, A. S., Frank, R. C., Taylor, K., & Eskes, G. A. (2018). The effects of prism adaptation on daily life activities in patients with visuospatial neglect: A systematic review. *Neuropsychological Rehabilitation, 28*(4), 491–514. https://doi.org/10.1080/09602011.2016.1182032

Chan, M. Y., Haber, S., Drew, L. M., & Park, D. C. (2016). Training older adults to use tablet computers: Does it enhance cognitive function? *The Gerontologist, 56*(3), 475–484. https://doi.org/10.1093/geront/gnu057

Chandna, A., Ghahghaei, S., Foster, S., & Kumar, R. (2021). Higher Visual Function Deficits in Children With Cerebral Visual Impairment and Good Visual Acuity. *Frontiers in human neuroscience, 15,* 711873. https://doi.org/10.3389/fnhum.2021.711873

Chen, M. H., & Goverover, Y. (2021). Self-awareness in multiple sclerosis: Relationships with executive functions and affect. *European Journal of Neurology, 28*(5), 1627–1635. https://doi.org/10.1111/ene.14762

Chen, P., Diaz-Segarra, N., Hreha, K., Kaplan, E., & Barrett, A. M. (2021). Prism adaptation treatment improves inpatient rehabilitation outcome in individuals with spatial neglect: A retrospective matched control study. *Archives of Rehabilitation Research and Clinical Translation, 3*(3), 100130. https://doi.org/10.1016/j.arrct.2021.100130

Chen, P., Hartman, A. J., Priscilla Galarza, C., & DeLuca, J. (2012). Global processing training to improve visuospatial memory deficits after right-brain stroke. *Archives of Clinical Neuropsychology, 27*(8), 891–905. https://doi.org/10.1093/arclin/acs089

Chen, P., & Hreha, K. (2015). KF-NAP 2015 manual. Kessler Foundation.

Chen, P., Hreha, K., Kong, Y., & Barrett, A. M. (2015). Impact of spatial neglect on stroke rehabilitation: Evidence from the setting of an inpatient rehabilitation facility. *Archives of Physical Medicine and Rehabilitation, 96*(8), 1458–1466. https://doi.org/10.1016/j.apmr.2015.03.019

Chen, P., Pitteri, M., Gillen, G., & Ayyala, H. (2018). Ask the experts how to treat individuals with spatial neglect: A survey study. *Disability and Rehabilitation, 40*(22), 2677–2691. https://doi.org/10.1080/09638288.2017.1347720

Chen, P., & Toglia, J. (2019). Online and offline awareness deficits: Anosognosia for spatial neglect. *Rehabilitation Psychology, 64*(1), 50–64. https://doi.org/10.1037/rep0000207

Chen, S.-C., Bodine, C., & Lew, H. L. (2021). Assistive technology and environmental control devices. In D. X. Cifu (Ed.), *Braddom's physical medicine and rehabilitation* (6th ed., pp. 374–388.e1). Elsevier. https://doi.org/10.1016/B978-0-323-62539-5.00019-9

Chi, I.-J., & Lin, L.-Y. (2021). Relationship between the performance of self-care and visual perception among young children with autism spectrum disorder and typical developing children. *Autism Research, 14*(2), 315–323. https://doi.org/10.1002/aur.2367

Chiaravalloti, N. D., Moore, N. B., & DeLuca, J. (2020). The efficacy of the modified Story Memory Technique in progressive MS. *Multiple Sclerosis Journal, 26*(3), 354–362. https://doi.org/10.1177/1352458519826463

Chiaravalloti, N. D., Sandry, J., Moore, N. B., & DeLuca, J. (2016). An RCT to treat learning impairment in traumatic brain injury: The TBI-MEM trial. *Neurorehabilitation and Neural Repair, 30*(6), 539–550. https://doi.org/10.1177/1545968315604395

Chien, C.-W., Lai, Y. Y. C., Lin, C.-Y., & Graham, F. (2020). Occupational performance coaching with parents to promote community participation and quality of life of young children with developmental disabilities: A feasibility evaluation in Hong Kong. *International Journal of Environmental Research and Public Health, 17*(21), 7993. https://doi.org/10.3390/ijerph17217993

Chien, C.-W., Lai, Y. Y. C., Lin, C.-Y., & Graham, F. (2021). Occupational performance coaching with parents to promote community participation of young children with developmental disabilities: Protocol for a feasibility and pilot randomized control trial. *Frontiers in Pediatrics, 9,* 1290. https://doi.org/10.3389/fped.2021.720885

Chiu, E.-C., Yu, M.-Y., Wu, W.-C., Chou, C.-X., Hung, J.-W., & Chen, P.-C. (2019). Validation of the Test of Visual Perceptual Skills-Third Edition in patients with stroke. *Disability and Rehabilitation, 41*(1), 104–109. https://doi.org/10.1080/09638288.2017.1378389

Choi, H.-S., Shin, W.-S., & Bang, D.-H. (2021). Application of digital practice to improve head movement, visual perception and activities of daily living for subacute stroke patients with unilateral spatial neglect: Preliminary results of a single-blinded, randomized controlled trial. *Medicine, 100*(6), e24637. https://doi.org/10.1097/MD.0000000000024637

Chudoba, L. A., Church, A. S., Dahmen, J. B., Brown, K. D., & Schmitter-Edgecombe, M. (2020). The development of a manual-based digital memory notebook intervention with case study illustrations. *Neuropsychological Rehabilitation, 30*(9), 1829–1851. https://doi.org/10.1080/09602011.2019.1611606

Chudoba, L. A., & Schmitter-Edgecombe, M. (2020). Insight into memory and functional abilities in individuals with amnestic mild cognitive impairment. *Journal of Clinical and Experimental Neuropsychology, 42*(8), 822–833. https://doi.org/10.1080/13803395.2020.1817338

Chui, A., Mazzitti, D., Nalder, E., Cameron, D., Polatajko, H. J., & Dawson, D. R. (2020). Therapists' experience of the cognitive orientation to daily occupational performance (CO-OP) approach: Shifting from conventional practice. *Scandinavian Journal of Occupational Therapy, 27*(2), 133–141. https://doi.org/10.1080/11038128.2018.1483424

Cicerone, K. D., Goldin, Y., Ganci, K., Rosenbaum, A., Wethe, J. V., Langenbahn, D. M., Malec, J. F., Bergquist, T. F., Kingsley, K., & Nagele, D. (2019). Evidence-based cognitive rehabilitation: Systematic review of the literature from 2009 through 2014. *Archives of Physical Medicine and Rehabilitation, 100*(8), 1515–1533.

Clark-Wilson, J., Giles, G. M., & Baxter, D. M. (2014). Revisiting the neurofunctional approach: Conceptualizing the core components for the rehabilitation of everyday living skills. *Brain Injury, 28*(13–14), 1646–1656. https://doi.org/10.3109/02699052.2014.946449

Clemson, L., Laver, K., Rahja, M., Culph, J., Scanlan, J. N., Day, S., Comans, T., Jeon, Y.-H., Low, L.-F., Crotty, M., Kurrle, S., Cations, M., Piersol, C. V., & Gitlin, L. N. (2021). Implementing a reablement intervention, "Care of People With Dementia in Their Environments (COPE)": A hybrid implementation-effectiveness study. *The Gerontologist, 61*(6), 965–976. https://doi.org/10.1093/geront/gnaa105

Coe, Á., Martin, M., & Stapleton, T. (2019). Effects of an occupational therapy memory strategy education group intervention on Irish older adults' self-management of everyday memory difficulties. *Occupational Therapy in Health Care, 33*(1), 37–63. https://doi.org/10.1080/07380577.2018.1543911

Cosar, S. N. S., Ozen, S., Selcuk, S. T., & Yemisci, U. (2020). Does the presence of ideomotor apraxia in stroke patients adversely affect rehabilitation outcomes? A prospective study. *Neurology Asia, 25*(4), 459–465. http://neurology-asia.org/articles/neuroasia-2020-25(4)-459.pdf

Costini, O., Roy, A., Remigereau, C., Faure, S., Fossoud, C., & Le Gall, D. (2017). Nature and specificity of gestural disorder in children with developmental coordination disorder: A multiple case study. *Frontiers in Psychology, 8.* https://www.frontiersin.org/article/10.3389/fpsyg.2017.00995

Critten, V., Campbell, E., Farran, E., & Messer, D. (2018). Visual perception, visual-spatial cognition and mathematics: Associations and predictions in children with cerebral palsy. *Research in Developmental Disabilities, 80,* 180–191. https://doi.org/10.1016/j.ridd.2018.06.007

Crosson, B., Barco, P. P., Velozo, C. A., Bolesta, M. M., Cooper, P. V., Werts, D., & Brobeck, T. C. (1989). Awareness and compensation in postacute head injury rehabilitation. *The Journal of Head Trauma Rehabilitation, 4*(3), 46–54. https://doi.org/10.1097/00001199-198909000-00008

Dawson, D. R., Gaya, A., Hunt, A., Levine, B., Lemsky, C., & Polatajko, H. J. (2009). Using the cognitive orientation to occupational performance (CO-OP) with adults with executive dysfunction following traumatic brain injury. *Canadian Journal of Occupational Therapy, 76*(2), 115–127. https://doi.org/10.1177/000841740907600209

Dawson, D. R., Richardson, J., Troyer, A., Binns, M., Clark, A., Polatajko, H., Winocur, G., Hunt, A., & Bar, Y. (2014). An occupation-based strategy training approach to managing age-related executive changes: A pilot randomized controlled trial. *Clinical Rehabilitation, 28*(2), 118–127. https://doi.org/10.1177/0269215513492541

Dekker, T., Mareschal, D., Sereno, M. I., & Johnson, M. H. (2011). Dorsal and ventral stream activation and object recognition performance in school-age children. *NeuroImage, 57*(3), 659–670. https://doi .org/10.1016/j.neuroimage.2010.11.005

DeLuca, J., Chiaravalloti, N. D., & Sandroff, B. M. (2020). Treatment and management of cognitive dysfunction in patients with multiple sclerosis. *Nature Reviews Neurology, 16*(6), 319–332. https://doi .org/10.1038/s41582-020-0355-1

Dewar, B.-K., Kapur, N., & Kopelman, M. (2018). Do memory aids help everyday memory? A controlled trial of a Memory Aids Service. *Neuropsychological Rehabilitation, 28*(4), 614–632. https://doi.org/10 .1080/09602011.2016.1189342

Dhamodharan, T., Thomas, M., Ramdoss, S., JothiKumar, K., SaravanaSundharam, S., Muthuramalingam, B., Hussainalikhan, N., Ravichandran, S., Vadivel, V., Suresh, P., Buddhan, S., & Madhusudanan, A. (2020). Cognitive rehabilitation for autism children mental status observation using virtual reality based interactive environment. In T. Ahram, W. Karwowski, A. Vergnano, F. Leali, & R. Taiar (Eds.), *Intelligent human systems integration 2020* (pp. 1213–1218). Springer International Publishing. https://doi.org/10.1007/978-3-030-39512-4_185

Diamond, A. (2013). Executive functions. *Annual Review of Psychology, 64*(1), 135–168. https://doi.org/10.1146/annurev-psych-113011-143750

Doig, E. J., Fleming, J., & Ownsworth, T. (2020). Evaluation of an occupation-based metacognitive intervention targeting awareness, executive function and goal-related outcomes after traumatic brain injury using single-case experimental design methodology. *Neuropsychological Rehabilitation, 31*(10), 1527–1556. https://doi.org/10.1 080/09602011.2020.1786410

Döpp, C. M. E., Graff, M. J. L., Teerenstra, S., Olde Rikkert, M. G. M., Nijhuis-van der Sanden, M. W. G., & Vernooij-Dassen, M. J. F. J. (2015). Effectiveness of a training package for implementing a community-based occupational therapy program in dementia: A cluster randomized controlled trial. *Clinical Rehabilitation, 29*(10), 974–986. https://doi.org/10.1177/0269215514564699

Doron, N., & Rand, D. (2019). Is unilateral spatial neglect associated with motor recovery of the affected upper extremity poststroke? A systematic review. *Neurorehabilitation and Neural Repair, 33*(3), 179–187. https://doi.org/10.1177/1545968319832606

Duckworth, A. L., Taxer, J. L., Eskreis-Winkler, L., Galla, B. M., & Gross, J. J. (2019). Self-control and academic achievement. *Annual Review of Psychology, 70*(1), 373–399. https://doi.org/10.1146/ annurev-psych-010418-103230

Dudai, Y., Karni, A., & Born, J. (2015). The consolidation and transformation of memory. *Neuron, 88*(1), 20–32. https://doi.org/10.1016/j .neuron.2015.09.004

Ebaid, D., & Crewther, S. G. (2019). Visual information processing in young and older adults. *Frontiers in Aging Neuroscience, 11*. https:// www.frontiersin.org/article/10.3389/fnagi.2019.00116

Eichen, D. M., Pasquale, E. K., Twamley, E. W., & Boutelle, K. N. (2021). Targeting executive function for weight loss in adults with overweight or obesity. *Physiology & Behavior, 240*, 113540. https://doi .org/10.1016/j.physbeh.2021.113540

Engel, L., Chui, A., Goverover, Y., & Dawson, D. R. (2019). Optimising activity and participation outcomes for people with self-awareness impairments related to acquired brain injury: An interventions systematic review. *Neuropsychological Rehabilitation, 29*(2), 163–198. https://doi.org/10.1080/09602011.2017.1292923

Esposito, E., Shekhtman, G., & Chen, P. (2021). Prevalence of spatial neglect post-stroke: A systematic review. *Annals of Physical and Rehabilitation Medicine, 64*(5), 101459. https://doi.org/10.1016/j .rehab.2020.10.010

Evald, L., Wilms, I., & Nordfang, M. (2021). Assessment of spatial neglect in clinical practice: A nationwide survey. *Neuropsychological Rehabilitation, 31*(9), 1374–1389. https://doi.org/10.1080/09602011 .2020.1778490

Evans, S. W., Beauchaine, T. P., Chronis-Tuscano, A., Becker, S. P., Chacko, A., Gallagher, R., Hartung, C. M., Kofler, M. J., Schultz, B. K., Tamm, L., & Youngstrom, E. A. (2021). The efficacy of cognitive videogame training for ADHD and what FDA clearance means for clinicians. *Evidence-Based Practice in Child and Adolescent Mental Health, 6*(1), 116–130. https://doi.org/10.1080/23794925.2020.1859960

Fernandes, H. A., Richard, N. M., & Edelstein, K. (2019). Cognitive rehabilitation for cancer-related cognitive dysfunction: A systematic review. *Supportive Care in Cancer, 27*(9), 3253–3279. https://doi .org/10.1007/s00520-019-04866-2

Ferry, K. (2021). *Exploring the effectiveness of errorless learning and use of memory aids for people with dementia and mild cognitive impairment* [DClinPsy]. University of Glasgow. https://theses.gla.ac.uk/ 82488/

Fisher, O., Berger, I., Grossman, E. S., & Maeir, A. (2022). Online and intellectual awareness of executive functioning in daily life among adolescents with and without ADHD. *Journal of Attention Disorders, 26*(6), 870–880. https://doi.org/10.1177/10870547211031982

Fong, K. N., Lo, P. C., Yu, Y. S., Cheuk, C. K., Tsang, T. H., Po, A. S., & Chan, C. C. (2011). Effects of sensory cueing on voluntary arm use for patients with chronic stroke: A preliminary study. *Archives of Physical Medicine and Rehabilitation, 92*(1), 15–23. https://doi.org/10 .1016/j.apmr.2010.09.014

Fortinsky, R. H., Gitlin, L. N., Pizzi, L. T., Piersol, C. V., Grady, J., Robison, J. T., Molony, S., & Wakefield, D. (2020). Effectiveness of the care of persons with dementia in their environments intervention when embedded in a publicly funded home- and community-based service program. *Innovation in Aging, 4*(6), igaa053. https://doi.org/10 .1093/geroni/igaa053

Foster, E. R., Spence, D., & Toglia, J. (2018). Feasibility of a cognitive strategy training intervention for people with Parkinson's disease. *Disability and Rehabilitation, 40*(10), 1127–1134. https://doi.org/10 .1080/09638288.2017.1288275

Foundas, A. L., & Duncan, E. S. (2019). Limb apraxia: A disorder of learned skilled movement. *Current Neurology and Neuroscience Reports, 19*(10), 82. https://doi.org/10.1007/s11910-019-0989-9

Frisch, C., Tirosh, E., & Rosenblum, S. (2020). Parental Occupation Executive Training (POET): An efficient innovative intervention for young children with attention deficit hyperactive disorder. *Physical & Occupational Therapy in Pediatrics, 40*(1), 47–61. https://doi.org/10 .1080/01942638.2019.1640336

Gentle, J., Brady, D., Woodger, N., Croston, S., & Leonard, H. C. (2021). Driving skills of individuals with and without developmental coordination disorder (DCD/Dyspraxia). *Frontiers in Human Neuroscience, 15*. https://www.frontiersin.org/article/10.3389/fnhum.2021.635649

Gentry, T. (2018). Consumer technologies as cognitive aids. In N. Katz & J. Toglia (Eds.), *Cognition, occupation, and participation across the life span: Neuroscience, neurorehabilitation, and models of intervention in occupational therapy* (4th ed., pp. 219–230). AOTA Press.

Geusgens, C., van Heugten, C., Donkervoort, M., van den Ende, E., Jolles, J., & van den Heuvel, W. (2006). Transfer of training effects in stroke patients with apraxia: An exploratory study. *Neuropsychological Rehabilitation, 16*(2), 213–229. https://doi.org/10.1080/ 09602010500172350

Giles, G. M. (2018). Neurofunctional approach to rehabilitation after brain injury. In N. Katz & J. Toglia (Eds.), *Cognition, occupation, and participation across the life span: Neuroscience, neurorehabilitation, and models of intervention in occupational therapy* (4th ed., pp. 419–442). AOTA Press.

Giles, G. M., Clark-Wilson, J., Baxter, D. M., Tasker, R., Holloway, M., & Seymour, S. (2019). The interrelationship of functional skills in individuals living in the community, following moderate to severe traumatic brain injury. *Brain Injury, 33*(2), 129–136. https://doi.org/ 10.1080/02699052.2018.1539762

Giles, G. M., Edwards, D. F., Baum, C., Furniss, J., Skidmore, E., Wolf, T., & Leland, N. E. (2020). Making functional cognition a professional priority. *The American Journal of Occupational Therapy, 74*(1), 7401090010p1–7401090010p6. https://doi.org/10.5014/ajot.2020.741002

Giles, G. M., Edwards, D. F., Morrison, M. T., Baum, C., & Wolf, T. J. (2017). Screening for functional cognition in postacute care and the Improving Medicare Post-Acute Care Transformation (IMPACT) Act of 2014. *The American Journal of Occupational Therapy, 71*(5), 7105090010p1–7105090010p6. https://doi.org/10.5014/ajot.2017.715001

Gillen, G. (2009). *Cognitive and perceptual rehabilitation: Optimizing function* (1st ed.). Mosby.

Gillen, G., Nilsen, D. M., Attridge, J., Banakos, E., Morgan, M., Winterbottom, L., & York, W. (2015). Effectiveness of interventions to improve occupational performance of people with cognitive impairments after stroke: An evidence-based review. *The American Journal of Occupational Therapy, 69*(1), 6901180040p1–6901180040p9. https://doi.org/10.5014/ajot.2015.012138

Gillen, R. W., Fusco-Gessick, B., & Harmon, E. Y. (2021). How we assess spatial neglect matters: Prevalence of spatial neglect as measured by the Catherine Bergego Scale and impact on rehabilitation outcomes. *American Journal of Physical Medicine & Rehabilitation, 100*(5), 443–449. https://doi.org/10.1097/PHM.0000000000001710

Gimeno, H., Jackman, M., & Novak, I. (2021). Cognitive orientation to daily occupational performance (CO-OP) intervention for people with cerebral palsy: A systematic review with meta-analysis. *Journal of Pediatrics, Perinatology and Child Health, 5*(3), 177–193. https://doi.org/10.26502/jppch.74050077

Gitlin, L. N., Marx, K., Piersol, C. V., Hodgson, N. A., Huang, J., Roth, D. L., & Lyketsos, C. (2021). Effects of the tailored activity program (TAP) on dementia-related symptoms, health events and caregiver wellbeing: A randomized controlled trial. *BMC Geriatrics, 21*(1), 1–14. https://doi.org/10.1186/s12877-021-02511-4

Gitlin, L. N., Piersol, C. V., Hodgson, N., Marx, K., Roth, D. L., Johnston, D., Samus, Q., Pizzi, L., Jutkowitz, E., & Lyketsos, C. G. (2016). Reducing neuropsychiatric symptoms in persons with dementia and associated burden in family caregivers using tailored activities: Design and methods of a randomized clinical trial. *Contemporary Clinical Trials, 49*, 92–102. https://doi.org/10.1016/j.cct.2016.06.006

Gitlin, L. N., Schinfeld, S., Winter, L., Corcoran, M., Boyce, A. A., & Hauck, W. (2002). Evaluating home environments of persons with dementia: Interrater reliability and validity of the Home Environmental Assessment Protocol (HEAP). *Disability and Rehabilitation, 24*(1–3), 59–71. https://doi.org/10.1080/09638280110066325

Glenthøj, L. B., Mariegaard, L. S., Fagerlund, B., Jepsen, J. R. M., Kristensen, T. D., Wenneberg, C., Krakauer, K., Medalia, A., Roberts, D. L., Hjorthøj, C., & Nordentoft, M. (2020). Cognitive remediation plus standard treatment versus standard treatment alone for individuals at ultra-high risk of developing psychosis: Results of the FOCUS randomised clinical trial. *Schizophrenia Research, 224*, 151–158. https://doi.org/10.1016/j.schres.2020.08.016

Goedert, K. M., Chen, P., Foundas, A. L., & Barrett, A. M. (2020). Frontal lesions predict response to prism adaptation treatment in spatial neglect: A randomised controlled study. *Neuropsychological Rehabilitation, 30*(1), 32–53. https://doi.org/10.1080/09602011.2018.1448287

Goldenberg, G., & Hagmann, S. (1998). Therapy of activities of daily living in patients with apraxia. *Neuropsychological Rehabilitation, 8*(2), 123–141. https://doi.org/10.1080/713755559

Goodall, G., Taraldsen, K., & Serrano, J. A. (2021). The use of technology in creating individualized, meaningful activities for people living with dementia: A systematic review. *Dementia, 20*(4), 1442–1469. https://doi.org/10.1177/1471301220928168

Gorrie, F., Goodall, K., Rush, R., & Ravenscroft, J. (2019). Towards population screening for cerebral visual impairment: Validity of the five questions and the CVI questionnaire. *PLoS One, 14*(3), e0214290. https://doi.org/10.1371/journal.pone.0214290

Goverover, Y. (2018). Cognitive rehabilitation: Evidence-based interventions. In N. Katz & J. Toglia (Eds.), *Cognition, occupation, and participation across the life span: Neuroscience, neurorehabilitation, and models of intervention in occupational therapy* (4th ed., pp. 51–68). AOTA Press.

Goverover, Y., Chiaravalloti, N. D., O'Brien, A. R., & DeLuca, J. (2018). Evidenced-based cognitive rehabilitation for persons with multiple sclerosis: An updated review of the literature from 2007 to 2016. *Archives of Physical Medicine and Rehabilitation, 99*(2), 390–407. https://doi.org/10.1016/j.apmr.2017.07.021

Goverover, Y., Chiaravalloti, N., & DeLuca, J. (2013). The influence of executive functions and memory on self-generation benefit in persons with multiple sclerosis. *Journal of Clinical and Experimental Neuropsychology, 35*(7), 775–783. https://doi.org/10.1080/13803395.2013.824553

Goverover, Y., Chiaravalloti, N., & DeLuca, J. (2019). Money management in multiple sclerosis: The role of cognitive, motor, and affective factors. *Frontiers in Neurology, 10*, 1128. https://doi.org/10.3389/fneur.2019.01128

Goverover, Y., Chiaravalloti, N., Genova, H., & DeLuca, J. (2018). A randomized controlled trial to treat impaired learning and memory in multiple sclerosis: The self-GEN trial. *Multiple Sclerosis Journal, 24*(8), 1096–1104. https://doi.org/10.1177/1352458517709955

Goverover, Y., Johnston, M. V., Toglia, J., & Deluca, J. (2007a). *Treatment to improve self-awareness and functional independence for persons with TBI: A pilot randomized trial.* Paper presented at the Neuropsychological Society 35th annual meeting, Portland, OR.

Goverover, Y., Johnston, M. V., Toglia, J., & Deluca, J. (2007b). Treatment to improve self-awareness in persons with acquired brain injury. *Brain Injury, 21*(9), 913–923. https://doi.org/10.1080/02699050701553205

Goverover, Y., Toglia, J., & DeLuca, J. (2019). The weekly calendar planning activity in multiple sclerosis: A top-down assessment of executive functions. *Neuropsychological Rehabilitation, 30*(7), 1372–1387. https://doi.org/10.1080/09602011.2019.1584573

Grant, M., Ponsford, J., & Bennett, P. C. (2012). The application of goal management training to aspects of financial management in individuals with traumatic brain injury. *Neuropsychological Rehabilitation, 22*(6), 852–873. https://doi.org/10.1080/09602011.2012.693455

Greenberg, D., Aminoff, M., & Simon, R. (2020). *Lange clinical neurology* (11th ed.). McGraw Hill/Medical.

Guo, J. Y., Ragland, J. D., & Carter, C. S. (2019). Memory and cognition in schizophrenia. *Molecular Psychiatry, 24*(5), 633–642. https://doi.org/10.1038/s41380-018-0231-1

Guy, J., Mottron, L., Berthiaume, C., & Bertone, A. (2019). A developmental perspective of global and local visual perception in Autism Spectrum Disorder. *Journal of Autism and Developmental Disorders, 49*(7), 2706–2720. https://doi.org/10.1007/s10803-016-2834-1

Haaland, K. Y. (1993). *Assessment of limb apraxia.* AOTA Neuroscience Institute Treating Adults with Apraxia.

Hahn, B., Baum, C., Moore, J., Ehrlich-Jones, L., Spoeri, S., Doherty, M., & Wolf, T. J. (2014). Development of additional tasks for the executive function performance test. *The American Journal of Occupational Therapy: Official Publication of the American Occupational Therapy Association, 68*(6), e241–e246. https://doi.org/10.5014/ajot.2014.008565

Hahn-Markowitz, J., Berger, I., Manor, I., & Maeir, A. (2017). Impact of the Cognitive–Functional (Cog-Fun) intervention on executive functions and participation among children with attention deficit hyperactivity disorder: A randomized controlled trial. *The American Journal of Occupational Therapy, 71*(5), 7105220010p1–7105220010p9. https://doi.org/10.5014/ajot.2017.022053

Hahn-Markowitz, J., Berger, I., Manor, I., & Maeir, A. (2020). Efficacy of Cognitive–Functional (Cog-Fun) occupational therapy intervention among children with ADHD: An RCT. *Journal of Attention Disorders*, *24*(5), 655–666. https://doi.org/10.1177/1087054716666955

Halder, T., Schenk, T., Wlasich, E., Vollmar, C., Uttner, I., & Danek, A. (2021). Living with global amnesia: Self-established compensation strategies of a patient with severe memory impairment—a narrative report. *Neurocase*, *27*(3), 287–296. https://doi.org/10.1080/13554794.2021.1938134

Hanna, K. L., Hepworth, L. R., & Rowe, F. (2017). Screening methods for post-stroke visual impairment: A systematic review. *Disability and Rehabilitation*, *39*(25), 2531–2543. https://doi.org/10.1080/09638288.2016.1231846

Harpster, K., Weckherlin, N., Engsberg, J. R., Powell, S. K., Barnard, H., Kadis, D., Dodd, J. N., Garrett, M. L., Mangano, F. T., Limbrick, D. D., Altaye, M., & Yuan, W. (2022). An iPad-based intervention to improve visual-motor, visual-attention, and visual-perceptual skills in children with surgically treated hydrocephalus: A pilot study. *Child's Nervous System*, *38*(2), 303–310. https://doi.org/10.1007/s00381-021-05379-2

Harris, M., Blanco, E. A., & Rempfer, M. (2021). Cognition and daily life functioning among persons with serious mental illness: A cluster analytic examination of heterogeneity on the Test of Grocery Shopping Skills. *Neuropsychology*, *35*(1), 57–68. https://doi.org/10.1037/neu0000700

Harrison, M. J., Morris, K. A., Horton, R., Toglia, J., Barsky, J., Chait, S., Ravdin, L., & Robbins, L. (2005). Results of intervention for lupus patients with self-perceived cognitive difficulties. *Neurology*, *65*(8), 1325–1327. https://doi.org/10.1212/01.wnl.0000180938.69146.5e

Hart, E., Grattan, E., Woodbury, M., Herbert, T. L., Coker-Bolt, P., & Bonilha, H. (2021). Pediatric unilateral spatial neglect: A systematic review. *Journal of Pediatric Rehabilitation Medicine*, *14*(3), 345–359. https://doi.org/10.3233/PRM-200779

Harvey, P. D., McGurk, S. R., Mahncke, H., & Wykes, T. (2018). Controversies in computerized cognitive training. *Biological Psychiatry: Cognitive Neuroscience and Neuroimaging*, *3*(11), 907–915. https://doi.org/10.1016/j.bpsc.2018.06.008

Hayes, J. F., Eichen, D. M., Barch, D. M., & Wilfley, D. E. (2018). Executive function in childhood obesity: Promising intervention strategies to optimize treatment outcomes. *Appetite*, *124*, 10–23. https://doi.org/10.1016/j.appet.2017.05.040

Hazelton, C., Pollock, A., Walsh, G., & Brady, M. C. (2019). Scanning training for rehabilitation of visual field loss due to stroke: Identifying and exploring training tools in use. *British Journal of Occupational Therapy*, *82*(8), 502–511. https://doi.org/10.1177/0308022618809900

Heilman, K. M. (2021). Upper limb apraxia. *Continuum (Minneapolis, Minn.)*, *27*(6), 1602–1623. https://doi.org/10.1212/CON.0000000000001014

Heilman, K. M., Watson, R. T., & Valenstein, E. (2012). Neglect and related disorders. In K. M. Heilman & E. Valenstein (Eds.), *Clinical neuropsychology* (5th ed., Vol. 20, pp. 296–348). Oxford University.

Henry, J. D. (2021). Prospective memory impairment in neurological disorders: Implications and management. *Nature Reviews Neurology*, *17*(5), 297–307. https://doi.org/10.1038/s41582-021-00472-1

Hewitt, K. C., Rodgin, S., Loring, D. W., Pritchard, A. E., & Jacobson, L. A. (2020). Transitioning to telehealth neuropsychology service: Considerations across adult and pediatric care settings. *The Clinical Neuropsychologist*, *34*(7–8), 1335–1351. https://doi.org/10.1080/13854046.2020.1811891

Hicks, R., Alexander, V., & Bahr, M. (2018). Explicit and implicit memory loss in aging. *International Journal of Psychological Studies*, *10*(3), 40. https://doi.org/10.5539/ijps.v10n3p40

Howe, J., Chua, W., Sumner, E., Drozdowska, B., Laverick, R., Bevins, R. L., Jean-Baptiste, E., Russell, M., Rotshtein, P., & Wing, A. M. (2022). The efficacy of a task model approach to ADL rehabilitation in stroke apraxia and action disorganisation syndrome: A randomised controlled trial. *PLoS One*, *17*(3), e0264678. https://doi.org/10.1371/journal.pone.0264678

Hypher, R. E., Brandt, A. E., Risnes, K., Rø, T. B., Skovlund, E., Andersson, S., Finnanger, T. G., & Stubberud, J. (2019). Paediatric goal management training in patients with acquired brain injury: Study protocol for a randomised controlled trial. *BMJ Open*, *9*(8), e029273. https://doi.org/10.1136/bmjopen-2019-029273

Ickx, G., Hatem, S. M., Riquelme, I., Friel, K. M., Henne, C., Araneda, R., Gordon, A. M., & Bleyenheuft, Y. (2018). Impairments of visuospatial attention in children with unilateral spastic cerebral palsy. *Neural Plasticity*, *2018*, 1435808. https://doi.org/10.1155/2018/1435808

Ishikawa, R., Ishigaki, T., Shimada, T., Tanoue, H., Yoshinaga, N., Oribe, N., Morimoto, T., Matsumoto, T., & Hosono, M. (2020). The efficacy of extended metacognitive training for psychosis: A randomized controlled trial. *Schizophrenia Research*, *215*, 399–407. https://doi.org/10.1016/j.schres.2019.08.006

Ivanov, I. V., Kuester, S., MacKeben, M., Krumm, A., Haaga, M., Staudt, M., Cordey, A., Gehrlich, C., Martus, P., & Trauzettel-Klosinski, S. (2018). Effects of visual search training in children with hemianopia. *PLoS One*, *13*(7), e0197285. https://doi.org/10.1371/journal.pone.0197285

Jackman, M., Novak, I., Lannin, N. A., Galea, C., & Froude, E. (2018). The cognitive orientation to daily occupational performance (CO-OP) approach: Best responders in children with cerebral palsy and brain injury. *Research in Developmental Disabilities*, *78*, 103–113. https://doi.org/10.1016/j.ridd.2018.04.019

Jamieson, M., Jack, R., O'Neill, B., Cullen, B., Lennon, M., Brewster, S., & Evans, J. (2020). Technology to encourage meaningful activities following brain injury. *Disability and Rehabilitation: Assistive Technology*, *15*(4), 453–466. https://doi.org/10.1080/17483107.2019.1594402

Jaywant, A., Steinberg, C., Lee, A., & Toglia, J. (2020). Feasibility and acceptability of the multicontext approach for individuals with acquired brain injury in acute inpatient rehabilitation: A single case series. *Neuropsychological Rehabilitation*, *32*(2), 211–230. https://doi.org/10.1080/09602011.2020.1810710

Jaywant, A., Toglia, J., Gunning, F. M., & O'Dell, M. W. (2020). Subgroups defined by the Montreal Cognitive Assessment differ in functional gain during acute inpatient stroke rehabilitation. *Archives of Physical Medicine and Rehabilitation*, *101*(2), 220–226. https://doi.org/10.1016/j.apmr.2019.08.474

Josman, N., Goffer, A., & Rosenblum, S. (2010). Development and standardization of a "do-eat" activity of daily living performance test for children. *The American Journal of Occupational Therapy*, *64*(1), 47–58. https://doi.org/10.5014/ajot.64.1.47

Josman, N., & Rosenblum, S. (2018). A metacognitive model for children with neurodevelopmental disabilities. In N. Katz & J. Toglia (Eds.), *Cognition, occupation, and participation across the life span: Neuroscience, neurorehabilitation, and models of intervention in occupational therapy* (4th ed., pp. 273–294). AOTA Press.

Kaizerman-Dinerman, A., Roe, D., & Josman, N. (2018). An efficacy study of a metacognitive group intervention for people with schizophrenia. *Psychiatry Research*, *270*, 1150–1156. https://doi.org/10.1016/j.psychres.2018.10.037

Kamada, K., Shimodozono, M., Hamada, H., & Kawahira, K. (2011). Effects of 5 minutes of neck-muscle vibration immediately before occupational therapy on unilateral spatial neglect. *Disability and Rehabilitation*, *33*(23–24), 2322–2328. https://doi.org/10.3109/09638288.2011.570411

Kashiwagi, F. T., Dib, R. E., Gomaa, H., Gawish, N., Suzumura, E. A., da Silva, T. R., Winckler, F. C., de Souza, J. T., Conforto, A. B., Luvizutto, G. J., & Bazan, R. (2018). Noninvasive brain stimulations for unilateral spatial neglect after stroke: A systematic review and meta-analysis of randomized and nonrandomized controlled trials. *Neural Plasticity*, *2018*. https://doi.org/10.1155/2018/1638763

Kastner, L., Velder-Shukrun, Y., Bonne, O., Bar-Ilan, R. T., & Maeir, A. (2022). Pilot study of the Cognitive–Functional Intervention for Adults (Cog-Fun A): A metacognitive–functional tool for adults with attention deficit hyperactivity disorder. *The American Journal of Occupational Therapy, 76*(2), 7602205070. https://doi.org/10.5014/ajot.2022.046417

Katz, N. (2018). Introduction to cognition and participation. In N. Katz & J. Toglia (Eds.), *Cognition, occupation, and participation across the life span: Neuroscience, neurorehabilitation, and models of intervention in occupational therapy* (4th ed., pp. 3–8). AOTA Press.

Kaur, S., Silver, G., Samuels, S., Rosen, A. H., Weiss, M., Mauer, E. A., Gerber, L. M., Greenwald, B. M., & Traube, C. (2020). Delirium and developmental disability: Improving specificity of a pediatric delirium screen. *Pediatric Critical Care Medicine, 21*(5), 409–414. https://doi.org/10.1097/PCC.0000000000002248

Kelleher, M., Tolea, M. I., & Galvin, J. E. (2016). Anosognosia increases caregiver burden in mild cognitive impairment. *International Journal of Geriatric Psychiatry, 31*(7), 799–808. https://doi.org/10.1002/gps.4394

Kerkhoff, G., Rode, G., & Clarke, S. (2021). Treating neurovisual deficits and spatial neglect. In T. Platz (Ed.), *Clinical pathways in stroke rehabilitation: Evidence-based clinical practice recommendations* (pp. 191–217). Springer International Publishing. https://doi.org/10.1007/978-3-030-58505-1_11

Kern, R. S., Zarate, R., Glynn, S. M., Turner, L. R., Smith, K. M., Mitchell, S. S., Sugar, C. A., Bell, M. D., Liberman, R. P., Kopelowicz, A., & Green, M. F. (2018). Improving work outcome in supported employment for serious mental illness: Results from 2 independent studies of errorless learning. *Schizophrenia Bulletin, 44*(1), 38–45. https://doi.org/10.1093/schbul/sbx100

Kessler, R. K., Rhodes, E., & Giovannetti, T. (2015). Environmental adaptations improve everyday action in schizophrenia. *Journal of the International Neuropsychological Society, 21*(5), 319–329. https://doi.org/10.1017/S1355617715000260

Kidd, S. A., Kerman, N., Ernest, D., Maples, N., Arthur, C., de Souza, S., Kath, J., Herman, Y., Virdee, G., Collins, A., & Velligan, D. (2018). A pilot study of a family cognitive adaptation training guide for individuals with schizophrenia. *Psychiatric Rehabilitation Journal, 41*(2), 109–117. https://doi.org/10.1037/prj0000204

Kim, C. M., van der Heide, E. M., van Rompay, T. J. L., Verkerke, G. J., & Ludden, G. D. S. (2021). Overview and strategy analysis of technology-based nonpharmacological interventions for in-hospital delirium prevention and reduction: Systematic scoping review. *Journal of Medical Internet Research, 23*(8), e26079. https://doi.org/10.2196/26079

Kim, E. J., Bahk, Y.-C., Oh, H., Lee, W.-H., Lee, J.-S., & Choi, K.-H. (2018). Current status of cognitive remediation for psychiatric disorders: A review. *Frontiers in Psychiatry, 9*, 461. https://doi.org/10.3389/fpsyt.2018.00461

Kim, M. J., Park, H. Y., Yoo, E.-Y., & Kim, J.-R. (2020). Effects of a cognitive–functional intervention method on improving executive function and self-directed learning in school-aged children with attention deficit hyperactivity disorder: A single-subject design study. *Occupational Therapy International, 2020*, 1250801. https://doi.org/10.1155/2020/1250801

Kim, S.-J., Jung, D.-U., Moon, J.-J., Jeon, D.-W., Seo, Y.-S., Jung, S.-S., Lee, Y.-C., Kim, J.-E., & Kim, Y.-S. (2021). Relationship between disability self-awareness and cognitive and daily living function in schizophrenia. *Schizophrenia Research: Cognition, 23*, 100192. https://doi.org/10.1016/j.scog.2020.100192

Kirby, A., Edwards, L., Sugden, D., & Rosenblum, S. (2010). The development and standardization of the adult developmental co-ordination disorders/dyspraxia checklist (ADC). *Research in Developmental Disabilities, 31*(1), 131–139. https://doi.org/10.1016/j.ridd.2009.08.010

Klinke, M. E., Hjaltason, H., Tryggvadóttir, G. B., & Jónsdóttir, H. (2018). Hemispatial neglect following right hemisphere stroke: Clinical course and sensitivity of diagnostic tasks. *Topics in Stroke Rehabilitation, 25*(2), 120–130. https://doi.org/10.1080/10749357.2017.1394632

Klinke, M. E., Zahavi, D., Hjaltason, H., Thorsteinsson, B., & Jónsdóttir, H. (2015). "Getting the left right": The experience of hemispatial neglect after stroke. *Qualitative Health Research, 25*(12), 1623–1636. https://doi.org/10.1177/1049732314566328

Krajenbrink, H., Lust, J., van Heeswijk, J., Aarts, P., & Steenbergen, B. (2022). Benefits of an intensive individual CO-OP intervention in a group setting for children with DCD. *Occupational Therapy International, 2022*, e8209128. https://doi.org/10.1155/2022/8209128

Krasny-Pacini, A., Chevignard, M., & Evans, J. (2014). Goal management training for rehabilitation of executive functions: A systematic review of effectiveness in patients with acquired brain injury. *Disability and Rehabilitation, 36*(2), 105–116. https://doi.org/10.3109/09638288.2013.777807

Krasny-Pacini, A., Limond, J., Evans, J., Hiebel, J., Bendjelida, K., & Chevignard, M. (2015). Self-awareness assessment during cognitive rehabilitation in children with acquired brain injury: A feasibility study and proposed model of child anosognosia. *Disability and Rehabilitation, 37*(22), 2092–2106. https://doi.org/10.3109/09638288.2014.998783

Kurylo, D. D., Waxman, R., Silverstein, S. M., Weinstein, B., Kader, J., & Michalopoulos, I. (2018). Remediation of perceptual organisation in schizophrenia. *Cognitive Neuropsychiatry, 23*(5), 267–283. https://doi.org/10.1080/13546805.2018.1493986

Lambez, B., & Vakil, E. (2021). The effectiveness of memory remediation strategies after traumatic brain injury: Systematic review and meta-analysis. *Annals of Physical and Rehabilitation Medicine, 64*(5), 101530. https://doi.org/10.1016/j.rehab.2021.101530

Langberg, J. M., Dvorsky, M. R., Molitor, S. J., Bourchtein, E., Eddy, L. D., Smith, Z. R., Oddo, L. E., & Eadeh, H.-M. (2018). Overcoming the research-to-practice gap: A randomized trial with two brief homework and organization interventions for students with ADHD as implemented by school mental health providers. *Journal of Consulting and Clinical Psychology, 86*(1), 39–55. https://doi.org/10.1037/ccp0000265

Lanzi, A. M., & Bourgeois, M. S. (2020). Structured external memory aid treatment for mild cognitive impairment. *American Journal of Speech-Language Pathology, 29*(1S), 474–484. https://doi.org/10.1044/2019_AJSLP-CAC48-18-0209

Lanzi, A. M., Wallace, S. E., Cohen, M. L., & Bourgeois, M. S. (2022). Structured external memory aid treatment (SEMAT) for older adults with mild cognitive impairment: Long-term adherence and acceptability of treatment. *Aphasiology, 36*(2), 234–250. https://doi.org/10.1080/02687038.2020.1868395

Leaf, J. B., Cihon, J. H., Ferguson, J. L., Milne, C. M., Leaf, R., & McEachin, J. (2020). Comparing error correction to errorless learning: A randomized clinical trial. *The Analysis of Verbal Behavior, 36*(1), 1–20. https://doi.org/10.1007/s40616-019-00124-y

Lebrault, H., Chavanne, C., Abada, G., Latinovic, B., Varillon, S., Bertrand, A.-F., Oudjedi, E., Krasny-Pacini, A., & Chevignard, M. (2021). Exploring the use of the cognitive orientation to daily occupational performance approach (CO-OP) with children with executive functions deficits after severe acquired brain injury: A single case experimental design study. *Annals of Physical and Rehabilitation Medicine, 64*(5), 101535. https://doi.org/10.1016/j.rehab.2021.101535

Lee, S. C. (2021). Visual perceptual skills as predictors of handwriting skills of children grades 1-3. *Journal of Occupational Therapy, Schools, & Early Intervention, 15*(3), 265–273. https://doi.org/10.1080/19411243.2021.1959484

Leśniak, M. M., Mazurkiewicz, P., Iwański, S., Szutkowska-Hoser, J., & Seniów, J. (2018). Effects of group versus individual therapy for patients with memory disorder after an acquired brain injury: A randomized, controlled study. *Journal of Clinical and Experimental Neuropsychology, 40*(9), 853–864. https://doi.org/10.1080/13803395.2018.1441379

Levanon-Erez, N., Kampf-Sherf, O., & Maeir, A. (2019). Occupational therapy metacognitive intervention for adolescents with ADHD: Teen Cognitive–Functional (Cog-Fun) feasibility study. *British Journal of Occupational Therapy, 82*(10), 618–629. https://doi.org/10.1177/0308022619860978

Levy, L. (2018). Neurocognition and function: Intervention in dementia based on the cognitive disabilities model. In N. Katz & J. Toglia (Eds.), *Cognition, occupation, and participation across the life span: Neuroscience, neurorehabilitation, and models of intervention in occupational therapy* (4th ed., pp. 499–522). AOTA Press.

Li, J., Li, L., Yang, Y., & Chen, S. (2021). Effects of prism adaptation for unilateral spatial neglect after stroke: A systematic review and meta-analysis. *American Journal of Physical Medicine & Rehabilitation, 100*(6), 584–591. https://doi.org/10.1097/PHM.0000000000001598

Lier, E. J., Rijn, C. M. van, Vries, M. de, Goor, H. van, & Oosterman, J. M. (2021). The interaction between pain and cognition: On the roles of task complexity and pain intensity. *Scandinavian Journal of Pain.* https://doi.org/10.1515/sjpain-2021-0119

Lim, K.-B., Kim, J., Lee, H.-J., Yoo, J., You, E.-C., & Kang, J. (2018). Correlation between montreal cognitive assessment and functional outcome in subacute stroke patients with cognitive dysfunction. *Annals of Rehabilitation Medicine, 42*(1), 26–34. https://doi.org/10.5535/arm.2018.42.1.26

Lindsten-McQueen, K., Weiner, N. W., Wang, H.-Y., Josman, N., & Connor, L. T. (2014). Systematic review of apraxia treatments to improve occupational performance outcomes. *OTJR: Occupation, Participation and Health, 34*(4), 183–192. https://doi.org/10.3928/15394492-20141006-02

Lloyd, O., Ownsworth, T., Fleming, J., & Zimmer-Gembeck, M. J. (2015). Awareness deficits in children and adolescents after traumatic brain injury: A systematic review. *The Journal of Head Trauma Rehabilitation, 30*(5), 311–323. https://doi.org/10.1097/HTR.0000000000000113

Longley, V., Hazelton, C., Heal, C., Pollock, A., Woodward-Nutt, K., Mitchell, C., Pobric, G., Vail, A., & Bowen, A. (2021). Interventions for spatial neglect after stroke or nonprogressive brain injury: A Cochrane systematic review. *Stroke, 52*(9), e548–e549. https://doi.org/10.1161/STROKEAHA.121.036590

Lussier, A., Doherty, M., & Toglia, J. (2019). Weekly calendar planning activity. In T. Wolf, D. Edwards, & G. Giles (Eds.), *Functional cognition and occupational therapy: A practical approach to treating individuals with cognitive loss* (pp. 75–89). AOTA Press.

Luton, L. M., Reed-Knight, B., Loiselle, K., O'Toole, K., & Blount, R. (2011). A pilot study evaluating an abbreviated version of the cognitive remediation programme for youth with neurocognitive deficits. *Brain Injury, 25*(4), 409–415. https://doi.org/10.3109/02699052.2011.558044

Luttenberger, K., Schmiedeberg, A., & Gräßel, E. (2012). Activities of daily living in dementia: Revalidation of the E-ADL test and suggestions for further development. *BMC Psychiatry, 12*(1), 208. https://doi.org/10.1186/1471-244X-12-208

Maeir, T., Nahum, M., Makranz, C., Hoba, A., Peretz, T., Nagary, S. N., Silberman, N., & Gilboa, Y. (2021). The feasibility of a combined model of online interventions for adults with cancer-related cognitive impairment. *British Journal of Occupational Therapy, 84*(7), 430–440. https://doi.org/10.1177/0308022620950993

Maggio, M. G., De Luca, R., Manuli, A., & Calabrò, R. S. (2020). The five "W" of cognitive telerehabilitation in the COVID-19 era. *Expert Review of Medical Devices, 17*(6), 473–475. https://doi.org/10.1080/17434440.2020.1776607

Marks, T. S., Giles, G. M., Al-Heizan, M. O., & Edwards, D. F. (2020). Can brief cognitive or medication management tasks identify the potential for dependence in instrumental activities of daily living? *Frontiers in Aging Neuroscience, 12*, 33. https://doi.org/10.3389/fnagi.2020.00033

Marx, K. A., Scott, J. B., Piersol, C. V., & Gitlin, L. N. (2019). Tailored activities to reduce neuropsychiatric behaviors in persons with dementia: Case report. *The American Journal of Occupational Therapy, 73*(2), 7302205160p1–7302205160p9. https://doi.org/10.5014/ajot.2019.029546

Matano, A., Iosa, M., Guariglia, C., Pizzamiglio, L., & Paolucci, S. (2015). Does outcome of neuropsychological treatment in patients with unilateral spatial neglect after stroke affect functional outcome? *European Journal of Physical and Rehabilitation Medicine, 51*(6), 737–743. PMID: 25739509

Mattison, M. L. P. (2020). Delirium. *Annals of Internal Medicine, 173*(7), ITC49–ITC64. https://doi.org/10.7326/AITC202010060

Mazza, V. (2017). Simultanagnosia and object individuation. *Cognitive Neuropsychology, 34*(7–8), 430–439. https://doi.org/10.1080/02643294.2017.1331212

McCarthy, M., Beaumont, J. G., Thompson, R., & Pringle, H. (2002). The role of imagery in the rehabilitation of neglect in severely disabled brain-injured adults. *Archives of Clinical Neuropsychology, 17*(5), 407–422. https://doi.org/10.1093/arclin/17.5.407

McCoy, D. C. (2019). Measuring young children's executive function and self-regulation in classrooms and other real-world settings. *Clinical Child and Family Psychology Review, 22*(1), 63–74. https://doi.org/10.1007/s10567-019-00285-1

McCraith, D., & Earhart, C. (2018). Cognitive disabilities model: Creating a fit between functional cognitive abilities and activity demands for best ability to function. In N. Katz & J. Toglia (Eds.), *Cognition, occupation, and participation across the life span: Neuroscience, neurorehabilitation, and models of intervention in occupational therapy* (4th ed., pp. 469–497). AOTA Press.

McEwen, S., Mandich, A., & Polatajko, H. (2018). CO-OP Approach™: A cognitive-based intervention for children and adults. In N. Katz & J. Toglia (Eds.), *Cognition, occupation, and participation across the life span: Neuroscience, neurorehabilitation, and models of intervention in occupational therapy* (4th ed., pp. 315–334). AOTA Press.

McKenzie, J., & Joy, A. (2020). Family intervention improves outcomes for patients with delirium: Systematic review and meta-analysis. *Australasian Journal on Ageing, 39*(1), 21–30. https://doi.org/10.1111/ajag.12688

Missiuna, C. A., Pollock, N. A., Levac, D. E., Campbell, W. N., Whalen, S. D. S., Bennett, S. M., Hecimovich, C. A., Gaines, B. R., Cairney, J., & Russell, D. J. (2012). Partnering for change: An innovative school-based occupational therapy service delivery model for children with developmental coordination disorder. *Canadian Journal of Occupational Therapy, 79*(1), 41–50. https://doi.org/10.2182/cjot.2012.79.1.6

Missiuna, C. A., Rivard, L., & Pollock, N. (2004). They're bright but can't write: Developmental coordination disorder in school aged children. *Teaching Exceptional Children Plus, 1*(1). https://eric.ed.gov/?id=EJ966505

Mistler, C. B., Shrestha, R., Gunstad, J., Sanborn, V., & Copenhaver, M. M. (2021). Adapting behavioural interventions to compensate for cognitive dysfunction in persons with opioid use disorder. *General Psychiatry, 34*(4), e100412. https://doi.org/10.1136/gpsych-2020-100412

Miyahara, T., Shimizu, H., Yamane, S., & Hanaoka, H. (2018). Occupation-based intervention to improve self-awareness in persons with acquired brain injury: A single-case experimental design. *Asian Journal of Occupational Therapy, 14*(1), 33–41. https://doi.org/10.11596/asiajot.14.33

Moinuddin, A., Faridi, K., Sethi, Y., & Goel, A. (2022). A systematic review on strategy training: A novel standardized occupational therapy program for apraxia patients to perform activities of daily living. *Cureus*, *14*(3). https://doi.org/10.7759/cureus.23547

Morady, K., & Humphreys, G. (2011). Multiple task demands in action disorganization syndrome. *Neurocase*, *17*(5), 461–472. https://doi.org/10.1080/13554794.2010.532144

Morrison, M. T., Giles, G. M., Ryan, J. D., Baum, C. M., Dromerick, A. W., Polatajko, H. J., & Edwards, D. F. (2013). Multiple Errands Test-Revised (MET-R): A performance-based measure of executive function in people with mild cerebrovascular accident. *The American Journal of Occupational Therapy*, *67*(4), 460–468. https://doi.org/10.5014/ajot.2013.007880

Mousavi, E., Akbarfahimi, N., Moein, S., & Vahedi, M. (2022). A Study of the relationship between executive function and school function in children with Cerebral Palsy. *Journal of Occupational Therapy, Schools, & Early Intervention*. https://doi.org/10.1080/19411243.2022.2027840

Muzzatti, B., Cattaruzza, N., Piccinin, M., Flaiban, C., Agostinelli, G., Berretta, M., & Annunziata, M. A. (2020). Cognitive function in long-term lymphoma survivors: Relationship between subjective reports and objective assessments and with quality of life. *Psychology, Health & Medicine*, *26*(8), 968–979. https://doi.org/10.1080/13548506.2020.1770815

Nagelkop, N. D., Rosselló, M., Aranguren, I., Lado, V., Ron, M., & Toglia, J. (2021). Using multicontext approach to improve instrumental activities of daily living performance after a stroke: A case report. *Occupational Therapy in Health Care*, *35*(3), 249–267. https://doi.org/10.1080/07380577.2021.1919954

Nakajima, A., Funayama, M., & Nakamura, T. (2020). Scooping rice into a glass and putting a cell phone in the refrigerator: Action slips in an individual with a diffuse axonal injury. *Cognitive and Behavioral Neurology*, *33*(4), 259–265. https://doi.org/10.1097/WNN.0000000000000246

Nalder, E., Hartman, L., Hunt, A., & King, G. (2019). Traumatic brain injury resiliency model: A conceptual model to guide rehabilitation research and practice. *Disability and Rehabilitation*, *41*(22), 2708–2717. https://doi.org/10.1080/09638288.2018.1474495

Nasreddine, Z. S., Phillips, N. A., Bédirian, V., Charbonneau, S., Whitehead, V., Collin, I., Cummings, J. L., & Chertkow, H. (2005). The Montreal Cognitive Assessment, MoCA: A brief screening tool for mild cognitive impairment. *Journal of the American Geriatrics Society*, *53*(4), 695–699. https://doi.org/10.1111/j.1532-5415.2005.53221.x

Nguyen, L., Murphy, K., & Andrews, G. (2019). Immediate and long-term efficacy of executive functions cognitive training in older adults: A systematic review and meta-analysis. *Psychological Bulletin*, *145*(7), 698–733. https://doi.org/10.1037/bul0000196

Niemeier, J. P., Cifu, D. X., & Kishore, R. (2001). The lighthouse strategy: Improving the functional status of patients with unilateral neglect after stroke and brain injury using a visual imagery intervention. *Topics in Stroke Rehabilitation*, *8*(2), 10–18. https://doi.org/10.1310/7UKK-HJ0F-GDWF-HHM8

Nijboer, T. C. W., & Van Der Stigchel, S. (2019). Visuospatial neglect is more severe when stimulus density is large. *Journal of Clinical and Experimental Neuropsychology*, *41*(4), 399–410. https://doi.org/10.1080/13803395.2019.1566444

Nilsen, D., Gillen, G., Arbesman, M., & Lieberman, D. (2015). Occupational therapy interventions for adults with stroke. *The American Journal of Occupational Therapy*, *69*(5), 6905395010p1–6905395010p3. https://doi.org/10.5014/ajot.2015.695002

Novak, I., & Honan, I. (2019). Effectiveness of paediatric occupational therapy for children with disabilities: A systematic review. *Australian Occupational Therapy Journal*, *66*(3), 258–273. https://doi.org/10.1111/1440-1630.12573

Ogourtsova, T., Souza Silva, W., Archambault, P. S., & Lamontagne, A. (2017). Virtual reality treatment and assessments for post-stroke unilateral spatial neglect: A systematic literature review. *Neuropsychological Rehabilitation*, *27*(3), 409–454. https://doi.org/10.1080/09602011.2015.1113187

Oliveira, A. M. de, Radanovic, M., Mello, P. C. H. de, Buchain, P. C., Vizzotto, A. D., Harder, J., Stella, F., Piersol, C. V., Gitlin, L. N., & Forlenza, O. V. (2019). An intervention to reduce neuropsychiatric symptoms and caregiver burden in dementia: Preliminary results from a randomized trial of the tailored activity program–outpatient version. *International Journal of Geriatric Psychiatry*, *34*(9), 1301–1307. https://doi.org/10.1002/gps.4958

Park, W., Kim, J., & Kim, M. (2021). Efficacy of virtual reality therapy in ideomotor apraxia rehabilitation: A case report. *Medicine*, *100*(28), e26657. https://doi.org/10.1097/MD.0000000000026657

Pazzaglia, M., & Galli, G. (2019). Action observation for neurorehabilitation in apraxia. *Frontiers in Neurology*, *10*. https://www.frontiersin.org/article/10.3389/fneur.2019.00309

Pedullà, L., Brichetto, G., Tacchino, A., Vassallo, C., Zaratin, P., Battaglia, M. A., Bonzano, L., & Bove, M. (2016). Adaptive vs. non-adaptive cognitive training by means of a personalized App: A randomized trial in people with multiple sclerosis. *Journal of NeuroEngineering and Rehabilitation*, *13*(1), 88. https://doi.org/10.1186/s12984-016-0193-y

Pelak, V. S. (2022). The clinical approach to the identification of higher-order visual dysfunction in neurodegenerative disease. *Current Neurology and Neuroscience Reports*, *22*(4), 229–242. https://doi.org/10.1007/s11910-022-01186-7

Pendlebury, S. T., Klaus, S. P., Mather, M., de Brito, M., & Wharton, R. M. (2015). Routine cognitive screening in older patients admitted to acute medicine: Abbreviated mental test score (AMTS) and subjective memory complaint versus Montreal Cognitive Assessment and IQCODE. *Age and Ageing*, *44*(6), 1000–1005. https://doi.org/10.1093/ageing/afv134

Penna, S., & Novack, T. A. (2007). Further validation of the orientation and cognitive logs: Their relationship to the mini-mental state examination. *Archives of Physical Medicine and Rehabilitation*, *88*(10), 1360–1361. https://doi.org/10.1016/j.apmr.2007.07.005

Pereira, A. F., & Smith, L. B. (2009). Developmental changes in visual object recognition between 18 and 24 months of age. *Developmental Science*, *12*(1), 67–80. https://doi.org/10.1111/j.1467-7687.2008.00747.x

Peskin, N., Koren, D., & Gabay, S. (2020). Subcortical neural tracks play an important role in executive function in schizophrenia: An experimental study among patients with schizophrenia and healthy comparisons. *Schizophrenia Research: Cognition*, *22*, 100185. https://doi.org/10.1016/j.scog.2020.100185

Phelan, S., Steinke, L., & Mandich, A. (2009). Exploring a cognitive intervention for children with pervasive developmental disorder. *Canadian Journal of Occupational Therapy*, *76*(1), 23–28. https://doi.org/10.1177/000841740907600107

Pitteri, M., Chen, P., Passarini, L., Albanese, S., Meneghello, F., & Barrett, A. M. (2018). Conventional and functional assessment of spatial neglect: Clinical practice suggestions. *Neuropsychology*, *32*(7), 835–842. https://doi.org/10.1037/neu0000469

Pizzonia, K. L., & Suhr, J. A. (2022). Systematic review of correlates of internal and external memory strategy use in older adults. *Journal of Applied Gerontology*, 7334648211065427. https://doi.org/10.1177/07334648211065427

Polatajko, H. J., McEwen, S. E., Ryan, J. D., & Baum, C. M. (2012). Pilot randomized controlled trial investigating cognitive strategy use to improve goal performance after stroke. *The American Journal of Occupational Therapy*, *66*(1), 104–109. https://doi.org/10.5014/ajot.2012.001784

Poole, J. L. (2000). A comparison of limb praxis abilities of persons with developmental dyspraxia and adult onset apraxia. *The Occupational Therapy Journal of Research*, *20*(2), 106–120. https://doi.org/10.1177/153944920002000202

Pozzi, C., Tatzer, V. C., Álvarez, E. A., Lanzoni, A., & Graff, M. J. L. (2020). The applicability and feasibility of occupational therapy in delirium care. *European Geriatric Medicine, 11*(2), 209–216. https://doi.org/10.1007/s41999-020-00308-z

Prigatano, G. P., & Sherer, M. (2020). Impaired self-awareness and denial during the postacute phases after moderate to severe traumatic brain injury. *Frontiers in Psychology, 11.* https://www.frontiersin.org/article/10.3389/fpsyg.2020.01569

Purpura, G., Guzzetta, A., & Tinelli, F. (2022). Visual neglect: Does it exist in children with unilateral brain lesion? A systematic review. *Neuropsychological Rehabilitation.* https://doi.org/10.1080/09602011.2022.2032762

Radomski, M. V., Giles, G., Finkelstein, M., Owens, J., Showers, M., & Zola, J. (2018). Implementation intentions for self-selected occupational therapy goals: Two case reports. *The American Journal of Occupational Therapy, 72*(3), 7203345030p1–7203345030p6. https://doi.org/10.5014/ajot.2018.023135

Radomski, M. V., Giles, G. M., Owens, J., Showers, M., Rabusch, S., Kreiger, R., Zola, J., & Kath, K. (2020). Can service members with mild traumatic brain injury learn to develop implementation intentions for self-identified goals? *Disability and Rehabilitation, 44*(12), 2640–2647. https://doi.org/10.1080/09638288.2020.1841309

Ramirez-Hernandez, D., Stolwyk, R. J., Ownsworth, T., & Wong, D. (2021). A comparison of systematic instruction, error-based learning and trial and error to train the use of smartphone memory apps after acquired brain injury: A three-armed phase II randomised controlled trial study protocol. *Brain Impairment, 22*(2), 217–232. https://doi.org/10.1017/BrImp.2020.10

Ramos, A. A., Hamdan, A. C., & Machado, L. (2020). A meta-analysis on verbal working memory in children and adolescents with ADHD. *The Clinical Neuropsychologist, 34*(5), 873–898. https://doi.org/10.1080/13854046.2019.1604998

Rasheed, S. P., Younas, A., & Sundus, A. (2019). Self-awareness in nursing: A scoping review. *Journal of Clinical Nursing, 28*(5–6), 762–774. https://doi.org/10.1111/jocn.14708

Redick, T. S., Shipstead, Z., Meier, M. E., Montroy, J. J., Hicks, K. L., Unsworth, N., Kane, M. J., Hambrick, D. Z., & Engle, R. W. (2016). Cognitive predictors of a common multitasking ability: Contributions from working memory, attention control, and fluid intelligence. *Journal of Experimental Psychology. General, 145*(11), 1473–1492. https://doi.org/10.1037/xge0000219

Reeder, C., Huddy, V., Cella, M., Taylor, R., Greenwood, K., Landau, S., & Wykes, T. (2017). A new generation computerised metacognitive cognitive remediation programme for schizophrenia (CIRCuiTS): A randomised controlled trial. *Psychological Medicine, 47*(15), 2720–2730. https://doi.org/10.1017/S0033291717001234

Rensen, Y. C. M., Egger, J. I. M., Westhoff, J., Walvoort, S. J. W., & Kessels, R. P. C. (2019). The effect of errorless learning on psychotic and affective symptoms, as well as aggression and apathy in patients with Korsakoff's syndrome in long-term care facilities. *International Psychogeriatrics, 31*(1), 39–47. https://doi.org/10.1017/S1041610218000492

Resch, C., Hurks, P., de Kloet, A., & van Heugten, C. (2021). Rationale and description of BrainLevel: Computerized repeated practice with strategy use instruction for children with acquired brain injury. *Clinical Rehabilitation, 35*(6), 787–800. https://doi.org/10.1177/0269215521989652

Resch, C., Rosema, S., Hurks, P., de Kloet, A., & van Heugten, C. (2018). Searching for effective components of cognitive rehabilitation for children and adolescents with acquired brain injury: A systematic review. *Brain Injury, 32*(6), 679–692. https://doi.org/10.1080/02699052.2018.1458335

Riquelme, I., Henne, C., Flament, B., Legrain, V., Bleyenheuft, Y., & Hatem, S. M. (2015). Use of prism adaptation in children with unilateral brain lesion: Is it feasible? *Research in Developmental Disabilities, 43–44*, 61–71. https://doi.org/10.1016/j.ridd.2015.06.009

Rivest, J., Svoboda, E., McCarthy, J., & Moscovitch, M. (2018). A case study of topographical disorientation: Behavioural intervention for achieving independent navigation. *Neuropsychological Rehabilitation, 28*(5), 797–817. https://doi.org/10.1080/09602011.2016.1160833

Rode, G., Pagliari, C., Huchon, L., Rossetti, Y., & Pisella, L. (2017). Semiology of neglect: An update. *Annals of Physical and Rehabilitation Medicine, 60*(3), 177–185. https://doi.org/10.1016/j.rehab.2016.03.003

Rodger, S., & Vishram, A. (2010). Mastering social and organization goals: Strategy use by two children with Asperger syndrome during cognitive orientation to daily occupational performance. *Physical & Occupational Therapy in Pediatrics, 30*(4), 264–276. https://doi.org/10.3109/01942638.2010.500893

Rogers, S. M., Pinedo, M., Villatoro, A. P., & Zemore, S. E. (2019). "I don't feel like I have a problem because I can still go to work and function": Problem recognition among persons with substance use disorders. *Substance Use & Misuse, 54*(13), 2108–2116. https://doi.org/10.1080/10826084.2019.1630441

Rohrbach, N., Krewer, C., Löhnert, L., Thierfelder, A., Randerath, J., Jahn, K., & Hermsdörfer, J. (2021). Improvement of apraxia with augmented reality: Influencing pantomime of tool use via holographic cues. *Frontiers in Neurology, 12*, 711900. https://doi.org/10.3389/fneur.2021.711900

Romano, D., Tosi, G., Gobbetto, V., Pizzagalli, P., Avesani, R., Moro, V., & Maravita, A. (2021). Back in control of intentional action: Improvement of ideomotor apraxia by mirror box treatment. *Neuropsychologia, 160*, 107964. https://doi.org/10.1016/j.neuropsychologia.2021.107964

Rosi, A., Vecchi, T., & Cavallini, E. (2019). Metacognitive-strategy training promotes decision-making ability in older adults. *Open Psychology, 1*(1), 200–214.

Rotenberg, S., & Maeir, A. (2018). Occupation-based metacognitive group intervention for older adults experiencing memory problems: Feasibility study. *British Journal of Occupational Therapy, 81*(10), 582–590. https://doi.org/10.1177/0308022618760787

Rotenberg, S., & Maeir, A. (2019). The cognitive–functional evaluation framework. In T. J. Wolf, D. F. Edwards, & G. M. Giles (Eds.), *Functional cognition and occupational therapy: A practical approach to treating individuals with cognitive loss* (pp. 39–46). AOTA Press.

Rotenberg-Shpigelman, S., Erez, A. B.-H., Nahaloni, I., & Maeir, A. (2012). Neurofunctional treatment targeting participation among chronic stroke survivors: A pilot randomised controlled study. *Neuropsychological Rehabilitation, 22*(4), 532–549. https://doi.org/10.1080/09602011.2012.665610

Sala, G., & Gobet, F. (2019). Cognitive training does not enhance general cognition. *Trends in Cognitive Sciences, 23*(1), 9–20. https://doi.org/10.1016/j.tics.2018.10.004

Sanchez-Luengos, I., Balboa-Bandeira, Y., Lucas-Jiménez, O., Ojeda, N., Peña, J., & Ibarretxe-Bilbao, N. (2021). Effectiveness of cognitive rehabilitation in Parkinson's disease: A systematic review and meta-analysis. *Journal of Personalized Medicine, 11*(5), 429. https://doi.org/10.3390/jpm11050429

Sandry, J., Chiou, K. S., DeLuca, J., & Chiaravalloti, N. D. (2016). Individual differences in working memory capacity predicts responsiveness to memory rehabilitation after traumatic brain injury. *Archives of Physical Medicine and Rehabilitation, 97*(6), 1026–1029.e1. https://doi.org/10.1016/j.apmr.2015.10.109

Schmitter-Edgecombe, M., Sumida, C., & Cook, D. J. (2020). Bridging the gap between performance-based assessment and self-reported everyday functioning: An ecological momentary assessment approach. *The Clinical Neuropsychologist, 34*(4), 678–699. https://doi.org/10.1080/13854046.2020.1733097

Schoemaker, M. M., & Smits-Engelsman, B. C. M. (2015). Is treating motor problems in DCD just a matter of practice and more practice? *Current Developmental Disorders Reports, 2*(2), 150–156. https://doi.org/10.1007/s40474-015-0045-7

Schwartz, S. P., Northrup, S. R. K., Izadi-Najafabadi, S., & Zwicker, J. G. (2020). CO-OP for children with dcd: Goals addressed and strategies used. *Canadian Journal of Occupational Therapy*, 87(4), 278–286. https://doi.org/10.1177/0008417420941980

Schwartz, Y., & Sagiv, A. (2018). Cognitive rehabilitation: A retraining model for clients with neurological disabilities. In N. Katz & J. Toglia (Eds.), *Cognition, occupation, and participation across the life span: Neuroscience, neurorehabilitation, and models of intervention in occupational therapy* (4th ed., pp. 405–418). AOTA Press.

Séguin, M., Lahaie, A., Matte-Gagné, C., & Beauchamp, M. H. (2018). Ready! Set? Let's Train!: Feasibility of an intensive attention training program and its beneficial effect after childhood traumatic brain injury. *Annals of Physical and Rehabilitation Medicine*, 61(4), 189–196. https://doi.org/10.1016/j.rehab.2017.05.001

Shah, T. M., Weinborn, M., Verdile, G., Sohrabi, H. R., & Martins, R. N. (2017). Enhancing cognitive functioning in healthy older adults: A systematic review of the clinical significance of commercially available computerized cognitive training in preventing cognitive decline. *Neuropsychology Review*, 27(1), 62–80. https://doi.org/10.1007/s11065-016-9338-9

Sherer, M., Katz, D. I., Bodien, Y. G., Arciniegas, D. B., Block, C., Blum, S., Doiron, M., Frey, K., Giacino, J. T., Graf, M. J. P., Greenwald, B., Hammond, F. M., Kalmar, K., Kean, J., Kraus, M. F., Nakase-Richardson, R., Pavawalla, S., Rosenbaum, A., Stuss, D. T., & Yablon, S. A. (2020). Post-traumatic confusional state: A case definition and diagnostic criteria. *Archives of Physical Medicine and Rehabilitation*, 101(11), 2041–2050. https://doi.org/10.1016/j.apmr.2020.06.021

Shi, Q., Warren, L., Saposnik, G., & Macdermid, J. C. (2013). Confusion assessment method: A systematic review and meta-analysis of diagnostic accuracy. *Neuropsychiatric Disease and Treatment*, 9, 1359–1370. https://doi.org/10.2147/NDT.S49520

Silva, A. R., Pinho, M. S., Macedo, L., & Moulin, C. J. A. (2018). A critical review of the effects of wearable cameras on memory. *Neuropsychological Rehabilitation*, 28(1), 117–141. https://doi.org/10.1080/09602011.2015.1128450

Silverstein, S. M., Seitz, A. R., Ahmed, A. O., Thompson, J. L., Zemon, V., Gara, M., & Butler, P. D. (2020). Development and evaluation of a visual remediation intervention for people with schizophrenia. *Journal of Psychiatry and Brain Science*, 5, e200017. https://doi.org/10.20900/jpbs.20200017

Simons, D. J., Boot, W. R., Charness, N., Gathercole, S. E., Chabris, C. F., Hambrick, D. Z., & Stine-Morrow, E. A. L. (2016). Do "Brain-Training" programs work? *Psychological Science in the Public Interest*, 17(3), 103–186. https://doi.org/10.1177/1529100616661983

Skidmore, E. R., Dawson, D. R., Butters, M. A., Grattan, E. S., Juengst, S. B., Whyte, E. M., Begley, A., Holm, M. B., & Becker, J. T. (2015). Strategy training shows promise for addressing disability in the first 6 months after stroke. *Neurorehabilitation and Neural Repair*, 29(7), 668–676. https://doi.org/10.1177/1545968314562113

Smits-Engelsman, B., Vinçon, S., Blank, R., Quadrado, V. H., Polatajko, H., & Wilson, P. H. (2018). Evaluating the evidence for motor-based interventions in developmental coordination disorder: A systematic review and meta-analysis. *Research in Developmental Disabilities*, 74, 72–102. https://doi.org/10.1016/j.ridd.2018.01.002

Sohlberg, M., & Mateer, C. (1989). *Introduction to cognitive rehabilitation: Theory and practice*. Guilford Press.

Spaccavento, S., Cellamare, F., Falcone, R., Loverre, A., & Nardulli, R. (2017). Effect of subtypes of neglect on functional outcome in stroke patients. *Annals of Physical and Rehabilitation Medicine*, 60(6), 376–381. https://doi.org/10.1016/j.rehab.2017.07.245

Spittle, A. J., Dewey, D., Nguyen, T.-N.-N., Ellis, R., Burnett, A., Kwong, A., Lee, K., Cheong, J. L. Y., Doyle, L. W., & Anderson, P. J. (2021). Rates of developmental coordination disorder in children born very preterm. *The Journal of Pediatrics*, 231, 61–67.e2. https://doi.org/10.1016/j.jpeds.2020.12.022

Spreij, L. A., Sluiter, D., Gosselt, I. K., Visser-Meily, J. M. A., & Nijboer, T. C. W. (2021). CoCo—Participation: The development and clinical use of a novel inventory measuring cognitive complaints in daily life. *Neuropsychological Rehabilitation*, 31(2), 255–277. https://doi.org/10.1080/09602011.2019.1691017

Squire, L. R., & Dede, A. J. O. (2015). Conscious and unconscious memory systems. *Cold Spring Harbor Perspectives in Biology*, 7(3), a021667. https://doi.org/10.1101/cshperspect.a021667

Steward, K. A., Tan, A., Delgaty, L., Gonzales, M. M., & Bunner, M. (2017). Self-awareness of executive functioning deficits in adolescents with ADHD. *Journal of Attention Disorders*, 21(4), 316–322. https://doi.org/10.1177/1087054714530782

Stiekema, A. P. M., van Dam, M. T., Bruggeman, R., Redmeijer, J. E., Swart, M., Dethmers, M., Rietberg, K., Wekking, E. M., Velligan, D. I., Timmerman, M. E., Aleman, A., Castelein, S., van Weeghel, J., Pijnenborg, G. M. H., & van der Meer, L. (2020). Facilitating recovery of daily functioning in people with a severe mental illness who need longer-term intensive psychiatric services: Results from a cluster randomized controlled trial on cognitive adaptation training delivered by nurses. *Schizophrenia Bulletin*, 46(5), 1259–1268. https://doi.org/10.1093/schbul/sbz135

Struckmeyer, L. R., Pickens, N., Brown, D., & Mitchell, K. (2020). Home environmental assessment protocol–revised initial psychometrics: A pilot study. *OTJR: Occupation, Participation and Health*, 40(3), 175–182. https://doi.org/10.1177/1539449220912186

Stubberud, J., Holthe, I. L., Løvstad, M., Schanke, A.-K., Brandt, A., & Finnanger, T. (2021). The feasibility and acceptability of goal management training of executive functions in children with spina bifida and acquired brain injury. *Neuropsychological Rehabilitation*, 31(4), 601–620. https://doi.org/10.1080/09602011.2020.1723649

Sullivan, C., Lynch, H., & Kirby, A. (2018). Does visual perceptual testing correlate with caregiver and teacher reported functional visual skill difficulties in school-aged children? Considerations for practice. *Irish Journal of Occupational Therapy*, 46(2), 89–105. https://doi.org/10.1108/IJOT-03-2018-0005

Tarvonen-Schröder, S., Niemi, T., & Koivisto, M. (2020). Clinical and functional differences between right and left stroke with and without contralateral spatial neglect. *Journal of Rehabilitation Medicine*, 52(6), jrm00072. https://doi.org/10.2340/16501977-2699

Tham, K., Ginsburg, E., Fisher, A. G., & Tegnér, R. (2001). Training to improve awareness of disabilities in clients with unilateral neglect. *The American Journal of Occupational Therapy*, 55(1), 46–54. https://doi.org/10.5014/ajot.55.1.46

Thareja, T., Ballantyne, A., & Trauner, D. (2012). Spatial analysis after perinatal stroke: Patterns of neglect and exploration in extra-personal space. *Brain and Cognition*, 79(2), 107–116. https://doi.org/10.1016/j.bandc.2012.02.009

Thom, R. P., Levy-Carrick, N. C., Bui, M., & Silbersweig, D. (2019). Delirium. *The American Journal of Psychiatry*, 176(10), 785–793. https://doi.org/10.1176/appi.ajp.2018.18070893

Thomas, C., Spank, J., Weller, S., & Eschweiler, G. W. (2021). Nonpharmaceutical concepts for prevention and treatment of delirium. *Zeitschrift Fur Gerontologie Und Geriatrie*, 54(8), 759–767. https://doi.org/10.1007/s00391-021-01988-3

Thornton, A., Licari, M., Reid, S., Armstrong, J., Fallows, R., & Elliott, C. (2016). Cognitive orientation to (daily) occupational performance intervention leads to improvements in impairments, activity and participation in children with developmental coordination disorder. *Disability and Rehabilitation*, 38(10), 979–986. https://doi.org/10.3109/09638288.2015.1070298

Toglia, J. (1989). Visual perception of objects: An approach to assessment and intervention. *The American Journal of Occupational Therapy*, 43(9), 587–595. https://doi.org/10.5014/ajot.43.9.587

Toglia, J. (1993). *The contextual memory test*. Therapy Skill Builders.

Toglia, J. (2011). The dynamic interactional model of cognition in cognitive rehabilitation. In N. Katz (Ed.), *Cognition, occupation, and participation across the life span: Neuroscience, neurorehabilitation, and models of intervention in occupational therapy* (3rd ed., pp. 161–201). AOTA Press.

Toglia, J. (2015). *Weekly calendar planning activity.* AOTA Press. https://myaota.aota.org/shop_aota/product/900369

Toglia, J. (2018). The dynamic interactional model and the multicontext approach. In N. Katz & J. Toglia (Eds.), *Cognition, occupation, and participation across the life span: Neuroscience, neurorehabilitation, and models of intervention in occupational therapy* (4th ed., pp. 355–385). AOTA Press.

Toglia, J., Askin, G., Gerber, L. M., Taub, M. C., Mastrogiovanni, A. R., & O'Dell, M. W. (2017). Association between 2 measures of cognitive instrumental activities of daily living and their relation to the montreal cognitive assessment in persons with stroke. *Archives of Physical Medicine and Rehabilitation, 98*(11), 2280–2287. https://doi.org/10.1016/j.apmr.2017.04.007

Toglia, J., & Chen, P. (2020). Spatial exploration strategy training for spatial neglect: A pilot study. *Neuropsychological Rehabilitation, 32*(5), 792–813. https://doi.org/10.1080/09602011.2020.1790394

Toglia, J., & Foster, E. R. (2021). *The multicontext approach to cognitive rehabilitation: A metacognitive strategy intervention to optimize functional cognition.* Gatekeeper Press.

Toglia, J., & Goverover, Y. (2022). Revisiting the dynamic comprehensive model of self-awareness: A scoping review and thematic analysis of its impact 20 years later. *Neuropsychological Rehabilitation, 32*(8), 1676–1725. https://doi.org/10.1080/09602011.2022.2075017

Toglia, J., Johnston, M. V., Goverover, Y., & Dain, B. (2010). A multicontext approach to promoting transfer of strategy use and self regulation after brain injury: An exploratory study. *Brain Injury, 24*(4), 664–677. https://doi.org/10.3109/02699051003610474

Toglia, J., & Katz, N. (2018). Executive function: Prevention and health promotion for at-risk populations and those with chronic disease. In N. Katz & J. Toglia (Eds.), *Cognition, occupation, and participation across the life span: Neuroscience, neurorehabilitation, and models of intervention in occupational therapy* (4th ed., pp. 129–142). AOTA Press.

Toglia, J., & Kirk, U. (2000). Understanding awareness deficits following brain injury. *NeuroRehabilitation, 15*(1), 57–70. https://doi.org/10.3233/NRE-2000-15104

Toglia, J., & Maeir, A. (2018). Self-awareness and metacognition: Effect on occupational performance and outcome across the lifespan. In N. Katz & J. Toglia (Eds.), *Cognition, occupation, and participation across the life span: Neuroscience, neurorehabilitation, and models of intervention in occupational therapy* (4th ed., pp. 143–163). AOTA Press.

Toglia, J., Rodger, S., & Polatajko, H. (2012). Anatomy of cognitive strategies: A therapist's primer for enabling occupational performance. *Canadian Journal of Occupational Therapy, 79*(4), 225–236. https://doi.org/10.2182/cjot.2012.79.4.4

Tomaszewski Farias, S., Schmitter-Edgecombe, M., Weakley, A., Harvey, D., Denny, K. G., Barba, C., Gravano, J. T., Giovannetti, T., & Willis, S. (2018). Compensation strategies in older adults: Association with cognition and everyday function. *American Journal of Alzheimer's Disease & Other Dementias®, 33*(3), 184–191. https://doi.org/10.1177/1533317517753361

Tramontano, M., De Angelis, S., Mastrogiacomo, S., Princi, A. A., Ciancarelli, I., Frizziero, A., Iosa, M., Paolucci, S., & Morone, G. (2021). Music-based techniques and related devices in neurorehabilitation: A scoping review. *Expert Review of Medical Devices, 18*(8), 733–749. https://doi.org/10.1080/17434440.2021.1947793

Trevena-Peters, J., McKay, A., Spitz, G., Suda, R., Renison, B., & Ponsford, J. (2018). Efficacy of activities of daily living retraining during posttraumatic amnesia: A randomized controlled trial. *Archives of Physical Medicine and Rehabilitation, 99*(2), 329–337. https://doi.org/10.1016/j.apmr.2017.08.486

Trojano, L. (2020). Constructional apraxia from the roots up: Kleist, Strauss, and their contemporaries. *Neurological Sciences, 41*(4), 981–988. https://doi.org/10.1007/s10072-019-04186-7

Uddin, L. Q. (2021). Cognitive and behavioural flexibility: Neural mechanisms and clinical considerations. *Nature Reviews Neuroscience, 22*(3), 167–179. https://doi.org/10.1038/s41583-021-00428-w

Vanbellingen, T., Ottiger, B., Maaijwee, N., Pflugshaupt, T., Bohlhalter, S., Müri, R. M., Nef, T., Cazzoli, D., & Nyffeler, T. (2017). Spatial neglect predicts upper limb use in the activities of daily living. *Cerebrovascular Diseases (Basel, Switzerland), 44*(3–4), 122–127. https://doi.org/10.1159/000477500

van der Linde, B. W., van Netten, J. J., Otten, B. E., Postema, K., Geuze, R. H., & Schoemaker, M. M. (2014). Psychometric properties of the DCDDaily-Q: A new parental questionnaire on children's performance in activities of daily living. *Research in Developmental Disabilities, 35*(7), 1711–1719. https://doi.org/10.1016/j.ridd.2014.03.008

van Teijlingen, T., Oudman, E., & Postma, A. (2021). Lifelogging as a rehabilitation tool in patients with amnesia: A narrative literature review on the effect of lifelogging on memory loss. *Neuropsychological Rehabilitation, 32*(10), 2646–2672. https://doi.org/10.1080/09602011.2021.1974891

Van Vleet, T. M., & DeGutis, J. M. (2013). The nonspatial side of spatial neglect and related approaches to treatment. *Progress in Brain Research, 207*, 327–349. https://doi.org/10.1016/B978-0-444-63327-9.00012-6

Velikonja, D., Oakes, J., Brum, C., & Sachdeva, M. (2017). Assessing the validity of task analysis as a quantitative tool to measure the efficacy of rehabilitation in brain injury. *Brain Injury, 31*(1), 68–74. https://doi.org/10.1080/02699052.2016.1212090

Velligan, D. I. (2018). The implementation of cognitive adaptation training (CAT) across countries. *Schizophrenia Bulletin, 44*(Suppl 1), S30–S31. https://doi.org/10.1093/schbul/sby014.074

Velligan, D. I., Diamond, P., Mueller, J., Li, X., Maples, N., Wang, M., & Miller, A. L. (2009). The short term impact of generic versus individualized environmental supports on functional outcomes and target behaviors in schizophrenia. *Psychiatry Research, 168*(2), 94–101. https://doi.org/10.1016/j.psychres.2008.03.016

Velligan, D. I., Roberts, D., Mintz, J., Maples, N., Li, X., Medellin, E., & Brown, M. (2015). A randomized pilot study of MOtiVation and Enhancement (MOVE) Training for negative symptoms in schizophrenia. *Schizophrenia Research, 165*(2–3), 175–180. https://doi.org/10.1016/j.schres.2015.04.008

Vizzotto, A., Celestino, D., Buchain, P., Oliveira, A., Oliveira, G., Di Sarno, E., Napolitano, I., & Elkis, H. (2021). Occupational goal intervention method for the management of executive dysfunction in people with treatment-resistant schizophrenia: A randomized controlled trial. *The American Journal of Occupational Therapy, 75*(3), 7503180050. https://doi.org/10.5014/ajot.2021.043257

Voigt-Radloff, S., de Werd, M. M. E., Leonhart, R., Boelen, D. H. E., Olde Rikkert, M. G. M., Fliessbach, K., Klöppel, S., Heimbach, B., Fellgiebel, A., Dodel, R., Eschweiler, G. W., Hausner, L., Kessels, R. P. C., & Hüll, M. (2017). Structured relearning of activities of daily living in dementia: The randomized controlled REDALI-DEM trial on errorless learning. *Alzheimer's Research & Therapy, 9*(1), 22. https://doi.org/10.1186/s13195-017-0247-9

Waldman-Levi, A., & Steinmann Obermeyer, I. (2018). Addressing executive functions in schools. In N. Katz & J. Toglia (Eds.), *Cognition, occupation, and participation across the life span: Neuroscience, neurorehabilitation, and models of intervention in occupational therapy* (4th ed., pp. 259–272). AOTA Press.

Warren, M. (1993). Visuospatial skills: Assessment and intervention strategies. In C. B. Royeen (Ed.), *AOTA self-study series: Cognitive rehabilitation* (pp. 6–76). AOTA Press.

Warren, M. (1998). *The brain injury visual assessment battery for adults.* VisABILITIES Rehab Services.

Warren, M. (2005). *Brain injury visual assessment battery for adults* (4th ed.). visAbilities Rehab Services. https://www.visabilities.com/pdf/9_18- biVABA%20Brochure.pdf

Weber, E., Chiaravalloti, N. D., DeLuca, J., & Goverover, Y. (2019). Time-based prospective memory is associated with functional performance in persons with MS. *Journal of the International Neuropsychological Society, 25*(10), 1035–1043. https://doi.org/10.1017/S135561771900095X

Weber, E., Goverover, Y., & DeLuca, J. (2019). Beyond cognitive dysfunction: Relevance of ecological validity of neuropsychological tests in multiple sclerosis. *Multiple Sclerosis Journal, 25*(10), 1412–1419. https://doi.org/10.1177/1352458519860318

Welfringer, A., Leifert-Fiebach, G., Babinsky, R., & Brandt, T. (2011). Visuomotor imagery as a new tool in the rehabilitation of neglect: A randomised controlled study of feasibility and efficacy. *Disability and Rehabilitation, 33*(21–22), 2033–2043. https://doi.org/10.3109/09638288.2011.556208

Wilcox, J., & Frank, E. (2021). Occupational therapy for the long haul of post-COVID syndrome: A case report. *The American Journal of Occupational Therapy, 75*(Suppl._1), 7511210060p1–7511210060p7. https://doi.org/10.5014/ajot.2021.049223

Williams, R. S., Virdee, G. K., Bowie, C. R., Velligan, D. I., Maples, N. J., Herman, Y., & Kidd, S. A. (2020). Development and feasibility exploration of a combined compensatory and restorative approach to addressing cognitive challenges in early intervention psychosis. *Cognitive and Behavioral Practice, 27*(4), 454–469. https://doi.org/10.1016/j.cbpra.2020.02.004

Wilson, B. N., Crawford, S. G., Green, D., Roberts, G., Aylott, A., & Kaplan, B. J. (2009). Psychometric properties of the revised Developmental Coordination Disorder Questionnaire. *Physical & Occupational Therapy in Pediatrics, 29*(2), 182–202. https://doi.org/10.1080/01942630902784761

Wilson, J. (2014). *Concept mapping and the cognitive orientation to daily occupational performance (CO-OP) approach as an intervention framework for adolescents with autism spectrum disorder (ASD)* [Electronic Thesis and Dissertation Repository]. https://ir.lib.uwo.ca/etd/2379

Wolf, T. J. (2019). Occupational profile: The anchor of functional–cognitive assessment. In T. J. Wolf, D. F. Edwards, & G. M. Giles (Eds.), *Functional cognition and occupational therapy: A practical approach to treating individuals with cognitive loss* (pp. 47–52). AOTA Press.

Wolf, T. J., Doherty, M., Kallogjeri, D., Coalson, R. S., Nicklaus, J., Ma, C. X., Schlaggar, B. L., & Piccirillo, J. (2016). The feasibility of using metacognitive strategy training to improve cognitive performance and neural connectivity in women with chemotherapy-induced cognitive impairment. *Oncology, 91*(3), 143–152. https://doi.org/10.1159/000447744

World Health Organization. (2001). International classification of functioning, disability and health: ICF. Author.

Worthington, A. (2016). Treatments and technologies in the rehabilitation of apraxia and action disorganisation syndrome: A review. *NeuroRehabilitation, 39*(1), 163–174. https://doi.org/10.3233/NRE-161348

Wu, A. J., Radel, J., & Hanna-Pladdy, B. (2011). Improved function after combined physical and mental practice after stroke: A case of hemiparesis and apraxia. *The American Journal of Occupational Therapy, 65*(2), 161–168. https://doi.org/10.5014/ajot.2011.000786

Wuang, Y.-P., Su, J.-H., & Su, C.-Y. (2012). Reliability and responsiveness of the Movement Assessment Battery for Children-Second Edition Test in children with developmental coordination disorder. *Developmental Medicine and Child Neurology, 54*(2), 160–165. https://doi.org/10.1111/j.1469-8749.2011.04177.x

Yoo, P. Y., Scott, K., Myszak, F., Mamann, S., Labelle, A., Holmes, M., Guindon, A., & Bussieres, A. E. (2020). Interventions addressing vision, visual-perceptual impairments following acquired brain injury: A cross-sectional survey. *Canadian Journal of Occupational Therapy, 87*(2), 117–126. https://doi.org/10.1177/0008417419892393

Yu, J. J., Burnett, A. F., & Sit, C. H. (2018). Motor skill interventions in children with developmental coordination disorder: A systematic review and meta-analysis. *Archives of Physical Medicine and Rehabilitation, 99*(10), 2076–2099. https://doi.org/10.1016/j.apmr.2017.12.009

Zhang, Y., Xing, Y., Li, C., Hua, Y., Hu, J., Wang, Y., Ya, R., Meng, Q., & Bai, Y. (2022). Mirror therapy for unilateral neglect after stroke: A systematic review. *European Journal of Neurology, 29*(1), 358–371. https://doi.org/10.1111/ene.15122

Ziabakhsh, M., Sharifi, M., Fath Abad, J., & Nejati, V. (2020). Comparison of the effectiveness of cognitive rehabilitation method with neurofeedback method in students with attention deficit disorder. *Journal of Psychological Achievements, 27*(1), 167–192. https://doi.org/10.22055/psy.2020.31763.2452

Zietemann, V., Georgakis, M. K., Dondaine, T., Müller, C., Mendyk, A.-M., Kopczak, A., Hénon, H., Bombois, S., Wollenweber, F. A., Bordet, R., & Dichgans, M. (2018). Early MoCA predicts long-term cognitive and functional outcome and mortality after stroke. *Neurology, 91*(20), e1838–e1850. https://doi.org/10.1212/WNL.0000000000006506

Zlotnik, S., & Toglia, J. (2018). Measuring adolescent self-awareness and accuracy using a performance-based assessment and parental report. *Frontiers in Public Health, 6*. https://www.frontiersin.org/article/10.3389/fpubh.2018.00015

Zoltan, B. (2007). *Vision, perception, and cognition: A manual for the evaluation and treatment of the adult with acquired brain injury* (4th ed.). Slack Incorporated.

Sensory Processing in Everyday Life

Evan E. Dean, Lauren M. Little, Anna Wallisch, Spencer Hunley, and Winnie Dunn

LEARNING OBJECTIVES

After reading this chapter, you will be able to:

1. Examine the history that has led to occupational therapy becoming a leader in applying sensory processing ideas to daily life.
2. Explain the core concepts of sensory processing using Dunn's Sensory Processing Framework.
3. Apply sensory processing concepts to the daily life routines and adaptations of the general population, using the Ecology of Human Performance (EHP) as a conceptual basis.
4. Assess the current evidence about sensory processing concepts and its application to people's everyday lives.
5. Assess the current evidence related to intervention and explain how adjusting routines and contexts can support sensory processing patterns.
6. Design ways to discuss sensory processing intervention options with families, individuals, and other colleagues.

Introduction

Individuals experience the world through their senses. The ways in which we structure our days, coordinate routines, and engage in social activities are all influenced by how we prefer sensory experiences. **Sensory processing** is a key factor that occupational therapists assess to understand the participation of clients they serve. When occupational therapy (OT) practitioners understand how an individual's sensory processing patterns influence participation, they can design intervention approaches to meet the individual's needs.

There have been decades of research about sensory processing in the OT literature, and ideas continue to develop. This chapter discusses the history of sensory processing theory as it has evolved from Dr. Jean Ayres's original ideas. It explains Dunn's Sensory Processing Framework and outlines how different behaviors fit within each sensory processing pattern (i.e., registration, seeking, sensitivity, and avoidance). In addition, this chapter examines current evidence about how sensory processing influences everyday activities among a variety of populations. Using the Ecological Model of Human Performance (Dean et al., 2018; Dunn et al., 1994), sensory processing concepts are applied to different intervention approaches (e.g., Establish/Restore, Alter, Adapt/Modify, Prevent). This chapter also identifies how specific methods of assessing sensory processing, including observation, interview, and self-report, may be combined with direct measures of participation. Finally, it synthesizes evidence related to interventions focused on supporting participation in everyday life using a sensory processing approach.

History of Sensory Processing in Occupational Therapy

From the 1950s to 1970s, Dr. Jean Ayres was unsettled about some of the children she encountered in her work as an occupational therapist. Dr. Ayres dared to ask questions that others had not considered; in doing so, she opened the floodgates of what is possible to know about sensory processing and its impact on everyday life. It is important to remember the context of Dr. Ayres's work. During this time period, children with disabilities were segregated in care centers or special schools outside of public education. Prior to the passage of the Education of All Handicapped Children Act of 1975, some children were not allowed in school at all. Dr. Ayres noticed certain children who had characteristics that did not receive attention because the focus at the time was on serving children with more frank disorders such as cerebral palsy and intellectual disabilities. As a further reflection of the time, people started using the term "minimal brain dysfunction" to describe these children's conditions.

As Dr. Ayres worked, she observed details about how children with less noticeable conditions and subtle differences responded to sensory stimuli in their play and other routines (Ayres, 1972). Based on her work with these children, she identified the possible relationship between children's responses to sensory events and subsequent behaviors. Being one of the few occupational therapists with a background in research at the time, Dr. Ayres began to examine what she observed in practice. She designed a standardized test to document and measure her observations about sensory processing, the Southern California Sensory Integration Tests (SCSIT; Ayres, 1980). Dr. Ayres used the data from the SCSIT to create a model of sensory integration (SI) that linked the findings to her background in neuroscience. Basically, the model incorporated sensory input, integration of sensory inputs, and behavioral outputs into a cohesive set of ideas. She hypothesized that when sensory input works differently than expected, the integration and outputs are affected as well; in this way, she linked sensory input to behavioral output. She provided a model that invited professionals to think about the process that led to observed behavior. Her model removed the judgment about behaviors being "bad"

and illustrated how an integrated conceptual model created a new understanding about children's behavior and therefore opened new paths for intervention. These ideas were revolutionary for the time. They had great appeal and spread quickly, especially within the OT community.

After the passage of the Education of All Handicapped Children Act of 1975 in the United States (which later became the Individuals with Disabilities Education Act [IDEA], 1990), there were many more possibilities for serving all children. Dr. Ayres's ideas about the impact of sensory processing on children's behavior became tools for therapists and teachers working with school-aged children in public education. Implementation of Dr. Ayres's ideas and the passage of Education of All Handicapped Children Act of 1975 occurred at a time when all children were given the opportunity to obtain services, which would have been impossible to consider before this point. Although the Education of All Handicapped Children Act of 1975 explicitly stated that children were to be served in the "least restrictive environment," "clinical" settings continued to exist within public schools. In creating these separate spaces for children and removing them from natural environments, the approach to serving children reflected a medical model (i.e., fix what is wrong with the child).

Over time, therapists began to recognize opportunities for applying OT knowledge in a more integrated way in school routines and settings. For example, tools from traditional SI clinical settings started to be used in preschools (e.g., scooter boards). Therapists began to embrace their role as *related service* professionals at school, which compelled them to examine how they contributed to educational outcomes. This cultural shift in service delivery, specifically how to deliver OT using sensory processing theory, reflected how ideas evolve when contexts and environmental opportunities change.

The professional culture also changed over the next two decades. There were strong calls for professionals to test their ideas systematically and create convincing methods of applying such ideas (i.e., evidence-based practices). OT practitioners started going to graduate school to learn about research. People designed systematic ways to evaluate children; standardized tests became more available, and therapists used them more often in practice. Over time, data accumulated from studies, leading the way for both practical application and research. (These research trends are reviewed in a later section of this chapter.)

The history of OT and the cultural shifts that impact service delivery affect our ability to understand the evolution of ideas and subsequent application of such ideas. A significant benchmark in the development of the OT profession is Dr. Ayres's explication of the impact of sensory processing on behavior and therapists' ability to interpret behavior. Many researchers have followed her to provide further research about this topic, and their contributions build on the strong scaffolding Dr. Ayres created.

Today, work in sensory processing looks very different from Dr. Ayres's original ideas and work. We draw from her innovative thinking for her time; however, because contexts change and scientific methods and approaches evolve, new ways have been developed to study sensory processing and apply its concepts in practice.

Application of Sensory Processing to the General Population

It is important to note that this chapter places sensory processing concepts and research within the context of the general population, or all people. OT practitioners recognize that all sensory processing occurs on a continuum and that individuals have distinct sensory preferences and aversions. Sensory processing can be defined as how an individual detects sensory information from the environment and regulates behavioral responses associated with such sensory information (Dunn, 2014). To describe how people process sensory information and behave in accordance, researchers and clinicians have used various terms. Terminology can become confusing because individuals from different fields (e.g., OT vs. neuroscience) often use different words to describe similar behaviors (Baranek et al., 2014; Cascio et al., 2016; Schaaf & Lane, 2015). Although there is a significant body of research concerning children with autism spectrum disorder (ASD) and other childhood conditions (because children in these groups have different ways of responding to sensory events in everyday life), sensory processing is actually about everyone. The terms "sensory processing differences" and "sensory features" are used to describe all people's sensory experiences. Certainly, research shows that some groups (e.g., children with ASD and attention-deficit/hyperactivity disorder [ADHD]) demonstrate distinct sensory processing preferences and aversions; however, such differences should not be considered as dysfunction, abnormalities, or deficits. In the book *Saving Normal: An Insider's Look at What Caused the Epidemic of Mental Illness and How to Cure It*, Frances (2013) argues against pathologizing people's experiences by stating the following:

> This brings us to the question of the moment—can we use statistics in some simple and precise way to define mental normality? Can the bell curve provide a scientific guide in deciding who is mentally normal and who is not? Conceptually, the answer is "why not," but practically the answer is "hell no". . . . There are just too many statistical, contextual, and value judgments that perplex a simple statistical solution. (p. 7)

Just as other person characteristics (e.g., cognition, emotion) occur on a bell curve, sensory processing characteristics

present on a bell curve. Most people display responses to sensory stimuli in a similar range, but there will always be people who demonstrate responses outside of that range who can still participate successfully in their daily lives. Consider yourself or any other individual. You may be in the top 5% on height but still appear in the middle of the bell curve because you have brown eyes, which are more common across the globe. In sensory processing, you might be in the "just like others" range for seeking and respond "much more than others" in sensitivity. Perhaps your motor coordination is in the bottom 20% compared with others. This places your characteristics all over the bell curve, so you cannot be classified as "normal" or "not normal" as a person. Individuals can adapt to their situations no matter where their characteristics might be on the bell curve, so the difference cannot be used to identify dysfunction. Frances (2013) continues:

> We must reconcile to there not being any simple standard to decide the question of how many of us are abnormal. The normal curve tells us a great deal about the distribution of everything from quarks to koalas, but it doesn't dictate to us where normal ends and abnormal begins. . . . Human difference was never meant to be reducible to an exhaustive list of diagnoses . . . it takes all types to make a successful tribe and a full palette of emotions to make a fully lived life. We shouldn't medicalize difference and attempt to treat it away. . . . (p. 8)

Again, sensory processing is a characteristic that applies to everyone; it is not associated with abnormality. Although some people use the term "sensory processing disorder," it is not an official term in diagnostic manuals such as the *Diagnostic and Statistical Manual of Mental Disorders*, 5th edition (*DSM-5*) (American Psychiatric Association, 2013). The American Academy of Pediatrics (Zimmer et al., 2012) issued a statement on *sensory processing disorder* for pediatricians, which suggests that the term should not be used. Rather, the American Academy of Pediatrics emphasizes that services should focus on daily life, which supports OT's core tenets.

Because of the diligent work of many OT practitioners and other researchers, sensory processing concepts have permeated people's work and lives. Many people recognize that sensory processing differences, just as other human differences, are reflective of how people prefer to live. Words such as "sensory seeker" and "sensory avoider" have become everyday language to describe an individual's responses to sensory events. People's sensory preferences influence the ways in which they prefer to contribute to work and relationships. For example, Seekers create new ideas, Avoiders create structure, and Bystanders are easy-going in challenging situations. In summary, a core assumption in this chapter is that everyone has particular sensory processing patterns that affect their lives. OT practitioners can contribute by helping individuals gain insight into their own patterns so they can mindfully plan how to create a satisfying life (see OT Story 56.1, for an example).

OT STORY 56.1 WHAT DO WE RISK BY PATHOLOGIZING SENSORY PREFERENCES?

What may be a painful, miserable sensitivity to sound for one person may be the catalyst behind another's exceptional linguistic aptitude, acting talent, musical ability, or engineering expertise.

Take Sloan, for example; as a child, their parents found that they were uninterested in the visuals on the television screen but were incredibly sensitive to its sound. Loud, chaotic action scenes with explosions and startling sounds were overwhelming; but symphonies, opera singers, orchestras, and other similar sounds were captivating and soothing for Sloan. Sloan's parents encouraged Sloan to explore music—learning about different instruments, how they produced sound, how it's composed, and more; their auditory senses were so attuned that Sloan could pick out and name what instruments were being played in any piece by their 15th birthday.

As Sloan grew into adulthood, they not only found other audiophiles, but also a multitude of careers that embraced their interest: sound engineering, writing and composing music, sound editing and production, and even being a musician. Sloan still wears noise-canceling headphones to avoid unwanted auditory stims, but finds them unnecessary in their home studio, where they can close their eyes and absorb every note of a song as they optimize and edit their clients' music.

Questions

1. For younger people, how can you support the person to identify activities, groups, or environments that match their sensory preferences?
2. How can you work with families to recognize their child's sensory preferences and identify or create activities and environments that match those sensory preferences?
3. Sloan was fortunate to come from a family that had the resources and access for music lessons. How would you support a child with Sloan's interests and sensory preferences who did not have Sloan's resources and access?
4. How can you work with people to identify career interests based on their sensory preferences?
5. Based on this OT Story, do you believe Sloan is disabled? Why, or why not?

Dunn's Sensory Processing Framework

This section describes a commonly used model of sensory processing, Dunn's Sensory Processing Framework (Dunn, 2014); explains the terminology and concepts used in this model; and provides examples of behaviors within each sensory processing pattern. Additionally, it describes the ways in which researchers in OT have organized sensory processing knowledge by grouping individuals according to their particular sensory patterns.

In a recent scoping review of how sensory factors impact children's everyday lives and occupations (Dunn, Little, et al., 2016), evidence showed that the most commonly used model to investigate sensory features is Dunn's Sensory Processing Framework. In 1997, Dunn proposed a model of sensory processing describing the interaction of individual sensory detection thresholds (i.e., how quickly one detects a sensation) and self-regulation strategies (i.e., one's behavioral responses to the sensation) (Dunn, 1997). Since then, the model has been updated and is now referred to as Dunn's Sensory Processing Framework (Dunn, 2014). In this model, detection thresholds range from high (i.e., slow to notice or perceive a sensation) to low (i.e., quick to notice or perceive a sensation). Self-regulation ranges from passive to active. These two continua interact to create four sensory processing patterns (Figure 56.1):

1. **Registration:** high threshold and passive self-regulation
2. **Seeking:** high threshold and active self-regulation
3. **Sensitivity:** low threshold and passive self-regulation
4. **Avoiding:** low threshold and active self-regulation

Sensory processing patterns occur across systems (e.g., tactile, auditory, olfactory) and reflect behaviors affected by neurologic thresholds and self-regulation strategies. Individuals can exhibit specific behaviors that align with each sensory processing pattern, referred to as bystanders, seekers, avoiders, and sensors.

- *Bystanders* are individuals who have difficulty with registration and may take longer to notice sensory information or need sensory events to be more intense to notice. Examples of behaviors that bystanders may show include lack of response to one's name or not noticing when someone new enters a room.
- *Sensory seekers* are individuals who crave intense sensory experiences. Sensory seeking behaviors include active involvement in activities or actions that provide intense sensory input (e.g., a lot of movement), preferring

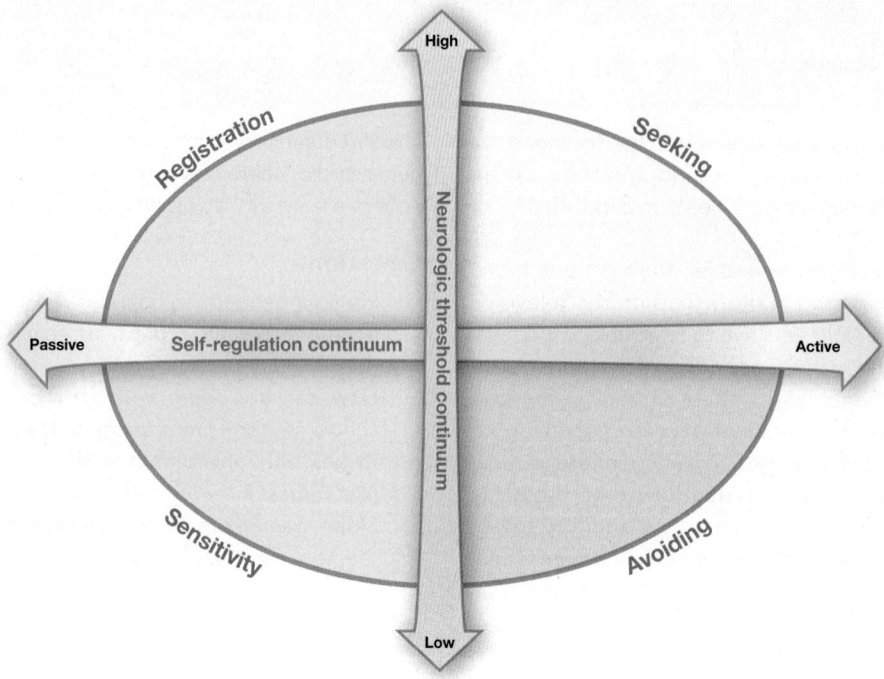

FIGURE 56.1 **Dunn's sensory processing framework.**

environments that are colorful or bright, and needing busy or loud environments (see Figure 56.2).

- *Avoiders* are individuals who detect sensory stimuli very quickly and exhibit active behavior responses in an attempt to disengage from such stimuli Avoidance behaviors include covering one's ears to block noise, not attending an event or place that is known to be loud or bright, and not being willing to try a novel food (see Figure 56.3).
- *Sensors* are individuals who detect sensory information quickly but do not use active strategies to disengage. Sensors may prefer specific brands of foods or clothing and

may have distinct preferences about what restaurants or stores are acceptable.

Sensory Processing Classifications

As you read descriptions of behaviors that fall within each sensory processing pattern, you may wonder about the senses themselves. You may think, "I am a seeker with movement, but I am very sensitive to smells." OT researchers have been interested in this topic and have therefore studied the

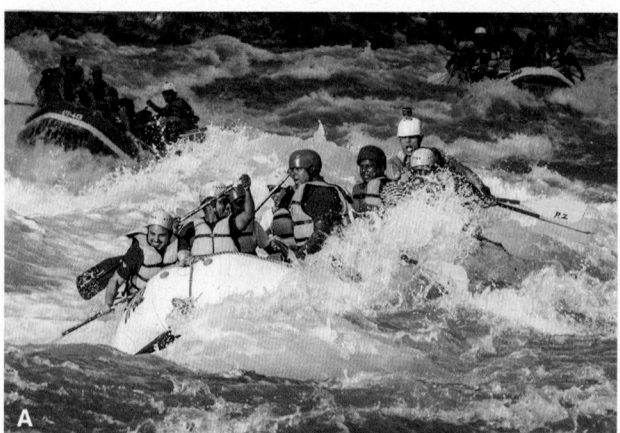
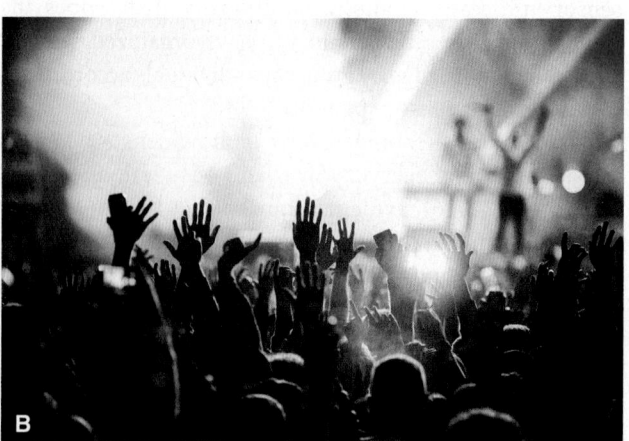

FIGURE 56.2 **Sensory seekers are individuals who crave intense sensory experiences. A:** These river rafters may be seeking intense, multi-sensory experiences, including movement, proprioception, touch, and sound. **B:** These concert goers may be seeking an intense experience with sound, movement, and touch.

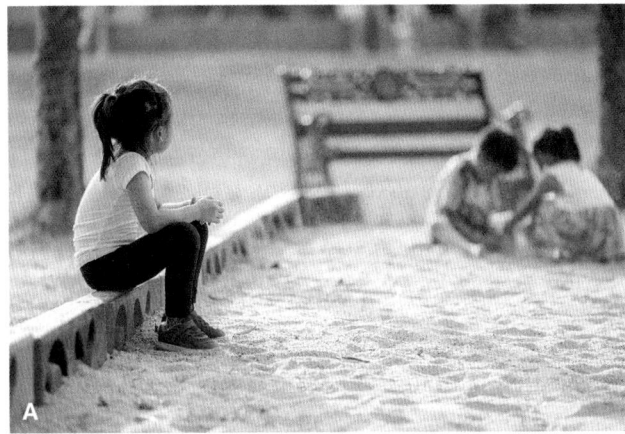
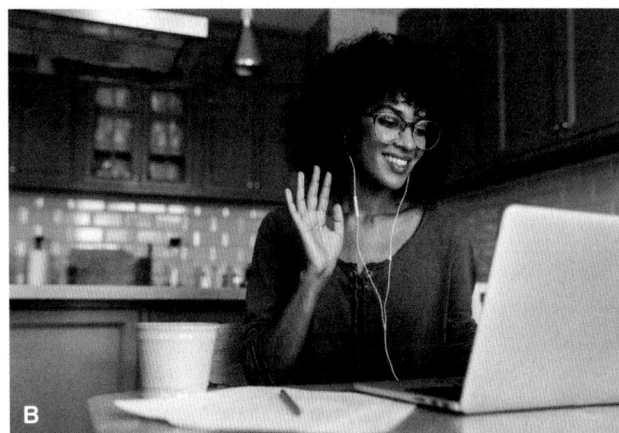

FIGURE 56.3 Avoiders seek less sensory input. **A:** This child may be avoiding the sand, her classmates, or both. **B:** Some adults who are sensory avoiders prefer working at home.

different combinations of sensory features among individuals with typical development as well as those with conditions. Evidence shows that individuals can show unique combinations of sensory patterns based on activity contexts and task demands (Baranek et al., 2014; Little et al., 2015). That is, individuals' behavior is affected by a combination of the sensory aspects of contexts, task factors, and their own sensory preferences. For example, a bright, loud sporting stadium may expose a person's sensitivity, but a dark movie theater may not activate such sensitivity. Additionally, a child may show aversion to playing with play dough because of the sticky texture; however, the same child may play at a water table without hesitation.

When an individual shows different sensory responses across different tasks and environments, therapists may need to use a variety of strategies to increase adaptation. One study, using the Sensory Profile (Dunn, 1999), showed that parents and teachers rated children's sensory processing differently (Brown & Dunn, 2010). This suggests that children may show varying sensory-related behaviors based on contextual characteristics. For example, children may be more avoidant at school or engage in more sensory seeking because of the noise in the environment and number of other children. First-hand accounts from individuals with ASD (Grandin, 1986) suggest that busy, multisensory, and social environments may become overstimulating. Such overstimulation results in some individuals becoming withdrawn or unable to select the most relevant sensory stimuli.

Previous research has focused on how sensory patterns can be grouped to characterize people into "sensory subtypes." Many of these studies have focused on children with ASD because they have high rates of sensory features. A few studies have identified four groups that characterize children with ASD. Lane and colleagues (2014) used the *Short Sensory Profile* (McIntosh et al., 1999) to examine sensory

subtypes of children with ASD and found four subtypes: (a) sensory adaptive, (b) taste–smell sensitive, (c) postural inattentive, and (d) generalized sensory difference. Another group of researchers used the *Sensory Experiences Questionnaire* (Baranek, 2009) and also found four sensory subtypes of children with ASD: (a) mild, (b) sensitive-distressed, (c) attenuated–preoccupied, and (d) extreme-mixed (Ausderau et al., 2014). These studies suggest that four subtypes describe the combinations of sensory responses among children with ASD. Subtypes were characterized by overall intensity of sensory features and the different presentation of sensory responses. Specifically:

- The mild group was similar to the sensory adaptive group; these children with ASD showed very few sensory processing differences.
- Children in the sensitive–distressed group were somewhat similar to the taste–smell sensitive subtype and showed high rates of sensory sensitivities, particularly in taste and olfactory processing.
- Children in the attenuated–preoccupied group were similar to the postural inattentive group, showing high rates of sensory seeking and registration.
- The extreme–mixed group was similar to the generalized sensory difference group; these children showed high rates of sensory processing differences across all sensory processing patterns.

The abovementioned studies showed that children with ASD may be grouped according to their sensory responses. However, all individuals have sensory preferences and aversions; sensory processing patterns occur across the general population, including among children with and without conditions (Dunn, Tomchek, et al., 2016). Therefore, Little and colleagues (2017) examined sensory subtypes among a general population of children with and without conditions using the *Sensory Profile-2* (Dunn,

2014). Five groups characterized all children and included the following:

1. *Balanced:* characterized by evenly distributed and low frequency of sensory behaviors
2. *Interested:* increased sensory seeking behaviors with other sensory patterns in the expected range
3. *Intense:* high frequencies of all sensory patterns; that is, they concurrently show high avoidance, sensitivities, registration, and seeking
4. *Mellow until . . . :* increased scores in avoidance and registration (i.e., misses more cues). Children in this profile may not notice sensory stimuli (low registration) as quickly as other children. However, when a stimulus becomes salient enough for the child to notice, the stimuli may quickly become aversive (avoiding).
5. *Vigilant:* increased sensitivity and avoidance. This group of children likely avoid sensory experiences and show aversion to different types of sensory stimuli.

All five subtypes included children with and without conditions such as ASD, ADHD, learning disabilities, and typical development. The findings suggest that all individuals, regardless of condition, demonstrate different combinations of sensory preferences and aversions.

As individuals show distinct sensory preferences and aversions, some researchers have studied whether individuals' sensory processing patterns are consistent across time.

For example, if someone is a bystander as a child, can they develop into an avoider? Studies suggest that individuals' sensory processing patterns remain relatively stable over time. For example, one study showed that toddlers with sensory sensitivity and avoidance show similar sensory processing patterns over 2 years (Green et al., 2012), and another study showed that preschool children with ASD exhibit stability in their sensory processing patterns until they are school aged (Perez Repetto et al., 2017). McCormick et al. (2016) also showed that children with ASD and a developmental disability (DD) showed stability in sensory processing patterns from early childhood to school age. The one sensory processing pattern that may significantly change is sensory seeking. Toddlers and early childhood aged children may show increased sensory seeking, and as children enter school age, sensory seeking has been shown to decline among all children (e.g., Baranek et al., 2019; Dunn, 2014). What this tells us is that sensory processing can be considered a person characteristic that likely does not significantly change over the course of development, and that behaviors associated with sensory seeking can be considered as developmentally appropriate through early childhood.

OT Story 56.2 is an example of how using a strengths-based approach can support a family member to reframe sensory preferences and create opportunities to partner with an OT and teacher to identify effective ways of altering a classroom environment for her son.

EXPANDING OUR PERSPECTIVES

From a Self-Advocate: Thinking Bigger Than Classifications

Spencer Hunley

Isn't it interesting that the behaviors most associated with autism are things autistic people do when we're distressed?

In much of the modern world, there is a supposition that autistics are few and far between; that most people believe they don't know anyone autistic—and if they do, they're either children or childlike adults who either work menial jobs or just live with their parents for nearly their entire lives. It's a stereotype that refuses to be fully extinguished, despite the fact that at some point in your own life, you were next to—or even interacted with—an autistic person.

For autistics and other neurodivergent individuals, modern environments that serve communities of people can be hotbeds of sensory nightmares: harsh, burning lights; eardrum-breaking noise echoing off of hard surfaces; an olfactory assault of heavy, caustic scents; being forced to hug or touch hands when greeting someone; and more. It shouldn't come as a surprise when an

autistic child has a meltdown while having to endure such nerve-wracking sensory overload; yet very little is done with respect to prevention and preparation.

A major autistic "coming of age" milestone is the realization that we are forced to adapt to a society that demands a high sensory threshold from everyone. Part of that adaptation is communicating with other neurodivergent individuals, finding out how they cope with that demand. Whether it be using noise-canceling headphones, hats/glasses, earplugs, nose plugs, timing outings to avoid crowds, and so on—as well as first-person suggestions for sensory assistance regulation, alleviation, and even comfort.

Parents and professionals focus so much on deficits, distress, and low sensory thresholds that they miss out on the intrinsic elements of being autistic. Despite the best of intentions, they may unwittingly cause the very circumstances leading to a response they're trying to prevent, such as meltdowns. An autistic child who enjoys the feel of a shoelace, and uses it to stim, would find it much more difficult to tolerate hostile sensory environments if the shoelace was prohibited in favor of more "socially acceptable" methods.

OT STORY 56.2 GETTING JEFFREY READY FOR KINDERGARTEN

A mother named Rachel reached out to you about her son Jeffery. Jeffery is a 5-year-old boy diagnosed with ASD who is getting ready to transition to kindergarten. Although Rachel reports many concerns, her primary concern is getting Jeffery's "sensory issues" under control prior to starting kindergarten. She further explains that Jeffery used to see an outpatient OT practitioner who said Jeffery may have sensory processing disorder (SPD). Because of a recent move, Rachel reports they never received the diagnosis. Rachel has indicated communication with Jeffery's school is especially difficult, and she fears the new classroom environment may need to make certain accommodations for Jeffery's "sensory issues." Without an SPD diagnosis, she worries the school will not accommodate Jeffery. Rachel requests help with receiving the SPD diagnosis to ease Jeffery's transition into a new classroom.

As a new OT practitioner with this family, you want to support them and build rapport; however, you find yourself in a dilemma. That is, a dilemma between the controversial evidence on SPD and supporting Rachel's request for an SPD diagnosis. You have read the policy statement from the American Academy of Pediatrics recommending not using the SPD diagnosis because it is difficult to distinguish whether SPD is an actual disorder of our sensory systems or if it is characteristic of other diagnoses (Zimmer et al., 2012). You also know that with Jeffery's ASD diagnosis, the school should accommodate his sensory preferences, especially if this is written into his Individualized Education Plan (IEP).

You've studied the evidence indicating the therapeutic benefit of using a strengths-based perspective to focus planning on the child's strengths and interests while offering support when needed. You would like to talk with Rachel about reframing Jeffery's "sensory issues" as sensory preferences while still honoring Rachel's experiences. You expand the conversation about "sensory issues" by saying "we all have preferences on which environments are too loud, too

bright, or just right. When we find environments with sensory features that match our preferences, we participate and feel more comfortable. However, when environments do not match our preferences, we can develop strategies to help us. For example, some individuals with certain sensory patterns may be very detail oriented; however, this may mean certain environments are very distracting. For instance, sitting at the front of a classroom may help to avoid visual distractions, whereas sitting at the back of the classroom may create too many distractions." This begins a conversation with Rachel about ways she supports Jeffery to incorporate his participation by pairing his preferences and sensory features within the environment. This conversation helps the therapist and kindergarten teacher think of strategies to support Jeffery's participation in the classroom.

From this perspective, we think about a child's preferences and finding sensory features within environments that support participation.

Questions

1. When presented only with information about "problems," it can be difficult to support family members or other supporters to see the humanity and strengths of their child. When parents report only problem behaviors or things they are struggling with, how would you reframe the conversation to learn more about the child?

2. OT practitioners are always hearing about the latest evidence-based practices that will solve all of the problems of their clients. Many of these practices actually have little evidence of effectiveness, and the developers (and sellers) of the interventions often overstate the evidence or only provide testimony from a few clients. How will you determine the evidence base of interventions you learn about?

The Ecology of Human Performance: A Framework to Understand Sensory Processing

As explained above, a person's response to sensory stimuli is a result of the person's sensory preferences as well as the demands of the context and task. Given this relationship, the Ecology of Human Performance (EHP) provides a guiding framework for understanding aspects of sensory

processing and identifying an appropriate intervention focus (Dean et al., 2018; Dunn et al., 1994). Four primary factors guide EHP: person, task, context, and performance. Five therapeutic intervention approaches (i.e., Establish/Restore, Adapt/Modify, Alter, Prevent, and Create) address the dynamic relationship among the four constructs.

Similarly, the underlying assumptions of Dunn's Sensory Processing Framework also focus on the importance of matching an individual's characteristics with contextual factors and task demands to increase participation and performance in meaningful activities. The theoretical underpinnings of EHP provide a structure for considering one's sensory processing patterns in light of the demands of everyday life. The following section outlines the four primary factors of EHP, which guide an understanding of evidence related to how sensory features impact everyday life. EHP is covered in more depth in Chapter 35, although the model is briefly described here because the chapter uses EHP to structure the discussions of research related to sensory processing.

Ecology of Human Performance Factors

According to EHP, *person factors* include the combination of sensorimotor and psychosocial abilities as well as a person's interests, values, and experiences (Dean et al., 2018; Dunn et al., 2003). Applied to sensory processing, person factors may also include sensory preferences and patterns (i.e., sensors, avoiders, seekers, or bystanders).

Each *task* or activity requires specific behaviors and performance ranges to reach the end goal and therefore places different demands on a person for successful engagement. In the context of sensory processing, each task involves different sensory features (e.g., kneading pizza dough compared to washing dishes) and may either match or not match a person's preferences.

The *performance* construct refers to how an individual engages in tasks. Each person has a performance range based on the interaction of person and context factors (Dunn et al., 2003). Specifically, individuals may perform best in contexts with certain sensory features.

Lastly, *context*, or the environment, is key to the EHP framework and refers to the physical, social, temporal, and cultural environments surrounding a person (Dunn et al., 2003). Each context has inherent sensory features (e.g., sounds in an auditorium). By understanding contextual features, one may better understand how sensory preferences (i.e., person factors) fit best within certain contexts and tasks.

A key assumption of EHP is that the four factors dynamically interact with one another. Particularly, it is not possible from an EHP perspective to truly understand person factors or a person's performance range without understanding the context for performance (Dunn et al., 1994). Contexts may facilitate performance of tasks or serve as a barrier to performance in any given task. For instance, someone who lives far from the ocean who is interested in surfing may not have the same opportunities to learn surfing as someone living on a coast who is also interested in surfing; therefore, the context creates a barrier to surfing for one individual (i.e., the person living far from the ocean) while facilitating performance for another (i.e., individual living on the coast). One's sensory preferences and patterns are an important feature of person factors; consequently, certain sensory patterns may make certain activities or contexts more appealing, whereas other sensory patterns might make people feel more apprehensive.

Ecology of Human Performance Intervention Approaches

Sensory processing patterns impact many areas of occupation and shape the ways in which individuals experience the world. As sensory processing patterns impact people's participation, researchers have tried to understand how to best design intervention approaches that incorporate knowledge of or directly address sensory features. This section places sensory processing concepts within the EHP framework, showing how the five intervention approaches of EHP address the dynamic interactions among the four factors (i.e., person, task, performance, context). Table 56.1 provides examples of how each intervention approach can be used with Dunn's Sensory Processing Framework.

TABLE 56.1 Strategies That Exemplify Ecology of Human Performance Interventions by Sensory Processing Pattern

Intervention Approach	Sensory Processing Pattern			
	Seeker	Avoider	Sensor	Bystander
Establish/Restore (learn something new every day)	Teach individual to recognize what his or her body needs and acceptable ways to get the input.	Teach individual to recognize situations in which he or she might get overloaded and develop strategies to manage input.	Develop strategies to manage input so individual can successfully participate in desired settings.	Develop strategies to create awareness of missed sensory input (e.g., to help you remember to take your bag to work, put car keys in the bag so you can't drive off without the bag).
Adapt/Modify (make it easier to do)	Insert ways to move during a computer work task.	Wear ear plugs when in noisy environment.	Use a mixer instead of hands to mix dough.	Gather all ingredients on a tray before starting to follow a recipe.

TABLE 56.1	Strategies That Exemplify Ecology of Human Performance Interventions by Sensory Processing Pattern (*continued*)			
Intervention Approach	**Sensory Processing Pattern**			
	Seeker	Avoider	Sensor	Bystander
Alter (find a better place)	Choose concert venues that encourage standing, with clear exit and enter points.	Allow students to work in a library when the classroom is noisy.	Divide classroom into small groups to limit input.	Find a grocery store with clear overhead signs and aisle markers.
Prevent (think ahead)	Provide magazines and fidget toys in a waiting room.	Make quiet rooms available at a noisy building.	Arrive at class or appointment early to avoid crowds.	Make numerous navigation signs that are easy to see in a building.
Create (make it work for everyone)	Serve on the community park board to construct playgrounds that meet diverse sensory needs.	Work with the museum to create "get away" spaces within exhibits.	Consult with designers to find the most "accessible" fabrics for a convention center seating.	Collaborate with the shopping mall to design signage that is easy to see.

Establish/Restore: Learn Something New Every Day

The Establish/Restore approach to intervention focuses on improving person factors by establishing new skills or restoring a person's performance in a task. For instance, the weather during the summer time (i.e., physical context) is more conducive to swimming (i.e., task); however, at the beginning of the summer, the individual may need to focus on restoring swimming skills (i.e., person) and potentially establishing new skills (e.g., backstroke, free style).

Adapt/Modify: Make It Easier to Do

The Adapt/Modify approach focuses on both the context and task demands to best facilitate performance (Dean et al., 2018; Dunn et al., 1994). With sensory processing, a therapist can facilitate an individual's performance by adjusting the task features to match their sensory preferences or by making the context of the task best match the person's sensory preferences. For example, the sound of a lawn mower may be too loud for sensors and avoiders. To make the task a better match for their sensory preferences, they may wear noise-canceling headphones or use a battery-operated lawn mower; both adaptations result in less noise.

Alter: Find a Better Place

The Alter method of intervention focuses on changing contextual factors to support a person's current strengths and abilities as a way to facilitate task performance (Dunn, 2007). This approach aligns with sensory processing in that many people select the places where they engage in activities based on their sensory preferences. For instance, when attending a class, an individual may select a seat based on their social context (i.e., friends) or based on their sensory preferences. A seat in the front row provides fewer visual distractions for a sensor, whereas a seat in the middle may match the preferences of a seeker.

Prevent: Think Ahead

The Prevent intervention method addresses all factors (i.e., person, task, context, performance) to identify and address potential barriers to performance, thus preventing negative events from occurring. When applied to sensory processing, parents may think ahead and address potential contexts that may not be best suited for them or their children. For instance, a music concert may provide a context where seekers may thrive, but it may also provide a context too overwhelming for an avoider or a sensor. Therefore, one may think ahead and prevent the contextual features from impacting engagement in attending a music concert by bringing ear plugs, carefully selecting a seating location, and establishing an exit plan ahead of time.

Create: Make It Work for Everyone

The Create intervention approach focuses on creating strategies to support the performance of a community or population (Dean et al., 2018). Similar to the Prevent approach, the Create approach may focus on all four factors to develop an intervention strategy (Dunn et al., 2003). In fact, many Create intervention approaches begin as Alter approaches but result in a solution that benefits the population as a whole (Dean et al., 2018). For instance, by having grocery stores of varying sizes, with varying foods and options within a community, people may find a store that best matches their preferences. Specifically, the contextual factors of a small grocery store with more limited options may provide the best match for a sensor or avoider (e.g., less noisy, easier to navigate, less visually stimulating). A larger store, with many options and taste testings may provide a better match for a seeker or bystander (e.g., noisier, more people to talk to, stimulating for

OT STORY 56.3 ALTERING THE WORKPLACE TO SUPPORT PARTICIPATION

Rowan is 20 years old and working as a dishwasher at a restaurant. This work requires standing for long periods of time and involves little interaction with other people. The restaurant owner considers Rowan a valuable employee who shows up on time and is fun to work with. However, recently, the owner has voiced concerns about Rowan's productivity.

The owner reports that Rowan frequently walks away from his dishwashing station and visits with other workers in the dining room. Rowan's coworkers also express that Rowan is sometimes rude when they offer help. Rowan expresses he is unhappy with his job. Rowan likes working in the restaurant, and the owner wants to find a way for Rowan to increase his productivity so he can keep his job. Rowan's father, who also serves as his legal guardian, contacted vocational rehabilitation (VR) to find out how they could support Rowan. Rowan and his father completed an application to gain access to VR supports.

An OT practitioner who contracted with a VR provider came to the restaurant to assess Rowan's strengths and preferences related to work. The OT practitioner administered the Adolescent/Adult Sensory Profile (AASP; Brown & Dunn, 2002), talked with Rowan and his boss, and observed Rowan at work. Rowan stated that he loved working at the restaurant, but sometimes became bored with dishwashing because "he did the same thing over and over and didn't have anyone to talk to." He also stated that his goal was to work in the dining room "because they move fast and get tips." During the observation, the OT practitioner noticed that Rowan stayed on task at his dishwashing station for about 5 minutes before he walked around to either go to the restroom or visit with other employees. The practitioner also noticed that when the kitchen was busy and noisy (which is where the dishwashing station was located), Rowan would become irritable and sometimes respond rudely when another employee or the owner asked him a question or directed him back to his task.

The AASP indicated that Rowan scored in the "more than others" range on the "high threshold" quadrants (seeking and registration). Based on this result, along with observations and information from the restaurant owner,

the OT practitioner concluded that Rowan was most successful when doing tasks that allowed him to move around frequently and minimized auditory cues (e.g., verbal instructions). She hypothesized that altering Rowan's workplace tasks based on his sensory preferences may make him more successful at work—and could better align with Rowan's goals.

The practitioner talked with Rowan and Rowan's job coach from VR about approaching the owner about assigning new work tasks for Rowan for a trial period. During the trial period, Rowan's job included seating customers, wiping down tables, and taking dishes to the kitchen. Rowan enjoyed the fast pace of the restaurant. He recognized when he needed to clear a table because he could see that the customers had left, and their plates were still on the table. Additionally, Rowan had brief social interactions with customers, which he and the customers enjoyed.

In this example, the context of the restaurant provided many options for productive work so that Rowan could remain a loyal employee there. The OT practitioner recognized the sensory characteristics of the restaurant context and, with strong activity analysis skills, found the combination of tasks that would match Rowan's sensory patterns throughout his shift. The restaurant did not have to make adjustments to their routines or environment to accommodate Rowan; partnering with the OT practitioner, they found a situation that already existed and matched Rowan with these work tasks. From an EHP perspective, this would be an "Alter" intervention, finding a better match without changing the person's characteristics or the context.

Questions

1. How would you work with people to align their goals with their sensory processing preferences?
2. If the restaurant owner was hesitant to let Rowan try working in the dining room, how could you set up the dishwashing environment to match Rowan's sensory processing preference so that he could convince the owner he could work in the dining room?

tastes and smells). OT Story 56.3 shows an example of how altering a workplace environment based on sensory processing patterns can support a person with employment.

Measurement

The first step to successful intervention is to administer an appropriate, validated measure to help understand the sensory processing patterns of an individual and how they affect participation in daily life. A variety of assessment tools

measure sensory processing through direct observation of behavior or questionnaires completed by family members, caregivers, teachers, and/or self-report.

Measures are designed to reflect differing theoretical foundations (e.g., sensory processing or SI), and therefore, utility and supporting evidence varies by measure. Additionally, the theoretical foundations guide whether a measure is developed with a top-down (i.e., measuring and focusing on the person as a whole or participation-focused) versus a bottom-up approach (i.e., focusing on details first or skill-focused) framework. Because measures guide intervention development, it is important for OT practitioners to understand the theoretical assumptions of a measure as well as the specific type of information gathered. Although sensory processing assessments provide information about sensory features in everyday life contexts, it is helpful to use additional measures that directly assess participation; participation-based assessments can help practitioners further understand how sensory patterns impact participation and how to develop intervention approaches to best suit the needs of an individual. Table 56.2 presents various measures related to sensory processing, SI, and participation. It is not intended to be an exhaustive list of measures of participation; rather, it provides examples that may be helpful for OT practitioners to administer in conjunction with an assessment of sensory features.

TABLE 56.2 **Assessment Measures Related to Sensory Processing, Sensory Integration, and Participation**

Measure	Category	Population	Type	Description	Approach
Measures of Sensory Processing and Sensory Integration					
Participation and Sensory Environment Questionnaire-Teacher Version (Piller & Pfeiffer, 2016) and Community Version (Pfeiffer et al., 2019)	SP	3–5 yrs old	Questionnaire	Deigned to measure the environmental sensory influences on preschool children's participation	Top-down
Sensory Profile-2 (Dunn, 2014) Short Sensory Profile-2 (Dunn, 2014) Adolescent/Adult Sensory Profile (Brown & Dunn, 2002)	SP	Across the life course	Questionnaire	Caregiver questionnaire designed to measure sensory preferences in four quadrants: Low Registration, Sensory Seeking, Sensory Sensitivity, and Sensory Avoiding. A short form and adolescent/adult self-report form are also available.	Top-down
Sensory Experiences Questionnaire Version 3.0 (Baranek, 2009)	SP	2–12 yrs	Questionnaire	Caregiver-report questionnaire designed to measure behaviors associated with everyday sensory experiences. Measures the frequency of behaviors associated with four sensory response patterns: hyporesponsiveness, hyperresponsiveness, sensory seeking, and enhanced perception	Top-down
Sensory Processing Measure (Parham & Ecker, 2007) Sensory Processing Measure-Preschool (SPM-P) (Miller Kuhaneck et al., 2010; Parham & Ecker, 2007)	SI	5–12 yrs; 2–5 yrs	Questionnaire	Parent or teacher questionnaire for assessing SP challenges at school and at home. Detects problem behaviors in sensory processing, praxis, and social participation. The SPM-P provides information on social participation; praxis; and the visual, auditory, tactile, proprioceptive, and vestibular sensory systems.	Bottom-up
The Sensory Perception Quotient (Tavassoli et al., 2014)	SP	Adults	Questionnaire	Self-report questionnaire that assesses sensory perception in adults. Assesses basic hypersensitivity and hyposensitivity across five modalities (touch, hearing, vision, smell, taste). A short form is also available.	Top-down

(continued)

TABLE 56.2	Assessment Measures Related to Sensory Processing, Sensory Integration, and Participation (*continued*)				
Measures of Participation					
Activity Card Sort (Baum & Edwards, 2001)		18–65+ yrs	Questionnaire	Individuals sort activity cards (i.e., instrumental, social, and leisure). Examines individual's engagement in the activity and if he or she discontinues an activity	Top-down
Pediatric Activity Card Sort (Mandich et al., 2004)		5–14 yrs	Questionnaire	Children sort activity cards in four domains: personal care, school, hobbies/social, and sports. Examines a child's engagement in the activity and if he or she discontinues an activity	Top-down
Assessment of Preschool Activity Participation (King et al., 2006)		2–5 yrs	Questionnaire	Caregiver-report scale that characterizes children's engagement in activities in four categories: play, skill development, active physical recreation, and social activities	Top-down
Child and Adolescent Scale of Participation (Bedell, 2009)		3–22 yrs	Questionnaire	Caregiver-report scale that measures child participation in home, school, and community activities in four subdomains: home participation, community participation, school participation, and home and community living participation	Top-down
Participation and Environment Measure for Children and Youth (Coster et al., 2010)		5–17 yrs	Questionnaire	Parent-report measure for participation at home, school, and the community, including environmental features	Top-down
The Young Children's Participation and Environment Measure (Khetani et al., 2013)		0–5 yrs	Questionnaire	Parent-report measure of participation at home, preschool/day care, and the community	Top-down

SP, sensory processing; SI, sensory integration; SPM-P, Sensory Processing Measure-Preschool.

Evidence on Sensory Processing and Everyday Life

As described above, senses can enhance an individual's enjoyment of a place or activity, but sensory experiences can also make daily life challenging. For example, a person may love to cook at home because the smells of their family recipes remind them of childhood, and the repetitive movement of chopping or mixing is relaxing. However, creating the same recipe when multiple children are running around the kitchen may not be so pleasant. The addition of extra noise, touching, and a crowded work environment changes the experience of cooking the same recipe. This section describes the research on how sensory processing contributes to daily life, with an emphasis on how sensory aspects of the person, task, and context interaction relate to performance. Family and person narratives are also a source of evidence, as you will see in our example.

School and Learning

For all children, success in school is in part dependent on how well the child can attend to instruction and self-regulate behavior to match classroom expectations, the demands of specific learning activities, and teachers' teaching styles. Research has investigated how sensory processing impacts learning and school performance among typically developing children as well as those with conditions. In preschoolers, how quickly children identify and focus on changing stimuli is related to reading and spelling performance (Boets et al., 2008). Children with a learning disability may struggle to integrate auditory and visual input, which can impact their learning (Boliek et al., 2010). Additionally, children with dyslexia may have more difficulty filtering noise when people are speaking, indicating that a quiet classroom may support learning for these students (Geiger et al., 2008). One study (Jirikowic et al., 2008) reported that children with fetal alcohol spectrum disorder (FASD) have differences in sensory processing that affect academic and behavioral performance. Children with ASD may also need more support to be successful in some learning environments. For instance, Ashburner et al. (2008) reported that academic performance for students with ASD may be affected by a mismatch between the classroom context (e.g., background noise in the classroom) and the students' sensory processing preferences (e.g., toleration of auditory or touch stimuli). This mismatch can lead to difficulties with attention, hyperactivity, and oppositional behaviors. As more children access educational content in different contexts (e.g., remote learning), another area for possible research and practice could be related to understand the effects of different learning environment for children who have different sensory processing preferences.

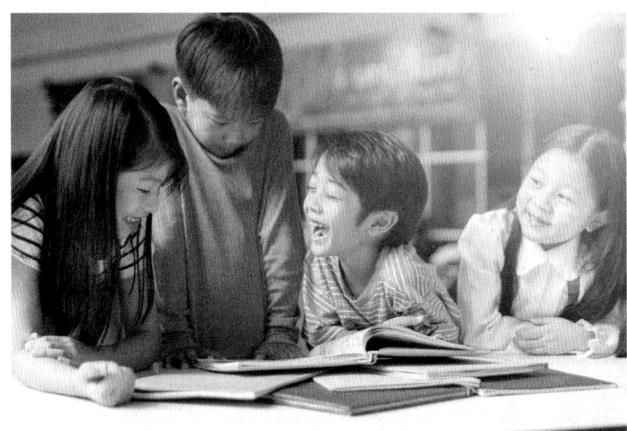

FIGURE 56.4 **Sensory processing demands of schools can be different from those at home, indicating the importance of considering sensory processing patterns in the specific context in which the therapist is working with a child.**

As shown in Figure 56.4, it is important to note that the sensory processing demands of schools can be different from those at home, indicating the importance of considering sensory processing patterns in the specific context in which the OT practitioner is working with the child (Brown & Dunn, 2010). OT Story 56.4 is an example of how adapting a classroom environment based on sensory processing patterns can support classroom participation. See Chapter 45, for details related to the role of OT in educational settings.

OT STORY 56.4 ADAPTING CLASSROOM EXPECTATIONS TO SUPPORT PARTICIPATION

Jonel is a 7-year-old boy who attends a first-grade classroom. He loves his teacher and says that he "has lots of friends" in the class. He says his favorite subject is "recess," but he also likes math but "not too much"—meaning he doesn't like to do math for too long at one time. Jonel also says that he gets frustrated because he gets in trouble a lot but can't seem to "do what I'm supposed to."

Jonel's teacher contacted the school's OT practitioner because she felt that his classroom behavior was preventing him from reaching academic potential. The teacher explained that Jonel was a "sweet kid" but would disrupt the class (especially during quiet, seated work) by walking or running around the classroom, talking to the teacher at her desk, or fidgeting at his desk. Jonel frequently did not complete assignments and would often claim he did not hear the teacher's instructions about completing the assignment.

The teacher had tried providing rewards and consequences for completing assignments and staying in his seat, but these interventions frustrated Jonel because he could not seem to meet the teacher's expectation to get the reward or avoid the punishment.

At home, Jonel's mother claimed that she did not have trouble with Jonel being disruptive and stated he spent most of his time riding his bike outside or playing with his four brothers. She did note, however, that Jonel had difficulty following directions, but she didn't think he was being defiant. She stated, "I just don't think he hears me all of the time."

The OT practitioner administered the *Sensory Profile School Companion 2* (SPSC2; Dunn, 2014) and observed Jonel in the classroom and on the playground. The practitioner noticed that Jonel could sit still for about 5 minutes but then

(continued)

OT STORY 56.4 ADAPTING CLASSROOM EXPECTATIONS TO SUPPORT PARTICIPATION (continued)

would start shaking his leg. When he came to school in the morning, he was friendly with his classmates, but as the day went on, he would get up from his seat and poke or kick classmates as he walked around the classroom. On the playground, Jonel would play soccer or tag the entire recess and cooperated with classmates.

The SPSC2 indicated that Jonel scored in the "more than others" range on the "high threshold" quadrants (seeking and registration). Based on this result, along with classroom and playground observations and information from his teacher, the OT practitioner concluded that Jonel was most successful when doing tasks that allowed him to move around frequently and minimized auditory cues (e.g., verbal instructions). She hypothesized that adapting classroom expectations would support Jonel's academic performance.

The OT practitioner worked with Jonel's teacher to develop teaching strategies to provide more opportunities for movement and also limit verbal instructions. The teacher said that she would find "errands" for Jonel to run before long periods of sitting time and also experiment with dynamic seating options, such as ball seats for more sensory input. Finally, the teacher said she would ask the class to write down their homework assignments before they finished the lesson and ensure that Jonel wrote down the assignments. Jonel loved the ball seat, and his teacher noted that Jonel stayed in his seat longer when using it. He still got fidgety and needed to walk around but usually only once an hour rather than every 10 minutes. The teacher designated Jonel as the "assignment collector," which allowed him to walk around the classroom and collect the assignments. On days when Jonel needed extra movement, the class would time him to see how fast he could do the job. When Jonel wrote down his homework assignments, he increased his assignment completion from "almost never" to "about half the time." The teacher resolved to talk with his family about organizational strategies that would enable Jonel to complete his homework more often.

In this example, the classroom environment was not a good match for Jonel's sensory preferences. Through observation and collaboration with the teacher, the OT practitioner identified classroom modifications that would better match Jonel's sensory input needs. From an EHP perspective, this "Adapt" intervention supported Jonel's academic participation by modifying the classroom to meet Jonel's sensory preferences.

Questions

1. What was different between the home and school environments that may explain why Jonel's behavior at school was different from his behavior at home?
2. What are ways OT practitioners can ensure they understand a person's behavior (and the environmental features that support or inhibit participation) in multiple environments?
3. What suggestions or scheduling changes could you suggest to the teacher/school that might benefit all children?

Adaptive Behavior

Evidence shows that individuals' adaptive behavior (i.e., how they function in social communication and daily living skills) is impacted by their sensory processing patterns. Among individuals with ASD, the overall degree of sensory features (e.g., how loud, bright, or crowded a room is or how much movement is required in a task [Rogers et al., 2003]) as well as specific sensory response patterns (Ashburner et al., 2008) may be related to adaptive behavior difficulties. Specifically, sensory seeking and registration patterns have been found to contribute to such difficulties among individuals with ASD (Adams et al., 2011; Baker et al., 2008; Reynolds et al., 2011). Studies have found similar findings among individuals with FASD and ADHD (Mattard-Labrecque et al., 2013).

With regard to self-care, a few studies (Stein et al., 2011, 2013) reported that children with ASD struggle with dental care because of the sensory challenges associated with the task; the authors proposed modifications to reduce the sensory input in dental care environments.

Overall, the relationship between adaptive behavior and sensory features is complex. There are many behavioral domains associated with adaptive behavior (e.g., social communication, self-care, community skills), all of which may be differentially impacted by a person's sensory processing characteristics as well as task and contextual demands. In OT, more investigations are needed to unravel the complexities of how specific sensory features support and interfere with adaptive behavior.

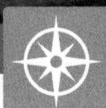

EXPANDING OUR PERSPECTIVES

The Value of Stimming

Spencer Hunley

Stimming is the most recognizable autistic trait, although the type of stim may vary from person to person. The word "stim" is shorthand for "self-stimulation," which is a wide range of actions that are repeated again and again, sometimes with specific interval or rhythm. In this process, autistic individuals are using their own senses to calm and regulate themselves. Stimming can be done with external objects or with the autistic's own body incorporating visual, auditory, olfactory, tactile, vestibular, and even proprioceptive senses. Stims are as unique and plentiful as the number of autistic persons across the globe; the list would be inexhaustible. Below are some examples of stims organized by sensory system:

Visual:

- Looking through a kaleidoscope
- Holding a fidget spinner close to one's face to watch it flicker
- Spinning or playing with an object that has flashing or changing light patterns

Auditory:

- Playing the same song over and over (or a specific part)
- Nonspeaking vocalizations (humming, moaning, grunting)
- Rubbing a finger on the edge of the glass to produce a sound

Olfactory:

- Putting one's face close to a book to smell the paper
- Holding a washed blanket close to one's nose
- Making coffee or baking cookies to fill the room with a specific scent

Tactile:

- Holding and/or rubbing a piece of fabric or string (like a shoelace) between one's fingers
- Rubbing one's hands on a smooth or rough wall
- Twisting and/or rubbing one's hair

Vestibular:

- Shifting balance from one foot to another
- Spinning in an office chair, while standing, or on a swing
- Doing cartwheels, somersaults, or hanging upside down

Proprioceptive:

- Rocking back and forth
- Bouncing on a trampoline or bed
- Pulling on a rubber band

Stimming is a natural and healthy response, and it serves many vital purposes. Some stims and sensory needs can actually lead into lifelong pursuits as a hobby or a career. For example, a young adult who stims using doughlike textures and items may find a career in pottery or masonry later in life; another with high sensitivity for sound might possibly decide to study sound engineering or another audio career; even a child who has a low sensory threshold for intolerably bright lighting may pursue astronomy or another field with low-light conditions.

What may be a painful, miserable sensitivity to sound for one person may be the catalyst behind another's exceptional linguistic aptitude, acting talent, musical ability, or engineering expertise.

Yet, if stims and sensory needs are contravened through the desire to "fix" them, such endeavors may never be realized. This misstep can be avoided by heeding these fundamental principles of the neurodiversity paradigm:

- Neurodiversity is a natural and valuable form of human diversity.
- Presuming that there is one "normal" or "healthy" type of brain—or one "right" style of neurocognitive functioning—is a culturally constructed fiction, just as invalid as the assumption that there is one "normal" or "right" ethnicity, gender, or culture.

The second principle is one of the most important—and it should be a critical guiding principle when working with neurodivergent individuals. By adopting it, appreciating sensory differences, and embracing stims, you will build a more substantial understanding—and provide a much more beneficial practice.

Activity and Social Participation

Individuals are likely to choose activities that match their sensory preferences and aversions. Overall, studies suggest that sensory avoidance and sensitivities negatively impact the amount of activity participation among individuals with ASD (Hochhauser & Engel-Yeger, 2010; Jasmin et al., 2009; Lane et al., 2010; Marquenie et al., 2011) and ADHD

(Engel-Yeger et al., 2011). Parents have reported that home activities are more manageable for children with ASD because of the unpredictability of sensory features in community contexts (Bagby et al., 2012). Findings are mixed with regard to the roles that cognition and attention play in how sensory features impact activity participation. Some findings suggest that difficulties are more related to cognition and attention (Zingerevich, 2009), whereas other findings suggest that sensory processing contributes to difficulties in activity participation regardless of cognition (Little et al., 2015).

Although most research has focused on sensory barriers to participation, there are likely sensory features that support children's activity participation. Little et al. (2015) found that enhanced perception (i.e., sensory hyperacuity and attention to details) was associated with increased activity participation among individuals with ASD, and children with increased sensory seeking scores participated in more adult/ child play time in the home. Additionally, Dean, Little, et al. (2018) studied children in the general population and found that the Avoiding and Seeking patterns can affect resiliency and the Avoiding pattern also affects adaptability. The authors concluded that people who notice sensory responses quickly and actively respond to the stimuli (e.g., try to get away or reduce the input) may need more support to overcome obstacles or adjust to changes in routine. Higher frequencies of seeking behaviors, on the other hand, may make children more resilient. For an example of how sensory seeking behaviors can support participation, refer to Expanding Our Perspectives above on the vital purposes that stimming serves.

Sensory processing is also related to how individuals participate in social situations. Researchers have begun to gain insight about effective approaches to supporting people's sensory preferences based on the perspective of autistic people (Stump, 2017), who tend to consider their sensory features as part of who they are and consider self-regulation strategies and accommodating environments as critical to social participation (Robison, 2008; Shore, 2003; Zaks, 2006). Grandin and Barron (2005) noted that until sensory aspects of the environment "are addressed and alleviated, forget trying to teach more advanced aspects of behavior and sociability" (p. 181).

This quote highlights the need to consider sensory processing preferences when supporting participation. Research with children suggests a similar relationship between sensory processing patterns and preferences for social environments. Children with avoidance and sensory sensitivities get more enjoyment out of socializing with family or a few close friends than a larger group of peers (Cosbey et al., 2010). Also, typically developing children and children with ASD who demonstrate higher frequency of sensory processing behaviors also demonstrate more needs for support with social interactions (Hilton et al., 2007; Matsushima & Kato, 2013). Individuals' sensory characteristics contribute to and detract from activity participation. When OT practitioners understand the interface between people's sensory characteristics and the features of the context or task, they can best support activity participation.

Eating and Mealtime

Eating is an important daily activity that has intense sensory qualities; in fact, the sensory features of food are what can make eating enjoyable for many people. The sights, smells, and tastes of our favorite foods can make eating a central aspect of many social, cultural, and family activities. When children show sensory sensitivities and avoidances, however, eating and mealtime can become challenging.

Overall, children with ADHD, ASD, and gastrointestinal (GI) conditions tend to show increased taste and smell sensitivities (Davis et al., 2013; Ghanizadeh, 2013; Zobel-Lachiusa et al., 2015). Children with ASD who show sensory sensitivities also demonstrate more challenges with mealtime, including the number of foods eaten, amount and variety of foods eaten, ability to sit at the table with others, and ability to stay seated at mealtime (Nadon et al., 2011).

Among individuals with typical development, sensory processing is related to how people approach novel foods. Research suggests that when trying new food, children are more attracted to foods that are visually similar to familiar foods, whereas adults are more likely to use touch to decide whether they will try a new food (Dovey et al., 2012). Children with taste and smell sensitivities may also be more likely to reject fruits and vegetables than other children (Coulthard & Blissett, 2009). Knowing these issues related to sensory processing and mealtime, OT practitioners can work with families to create mealtime routines that match the sensory processing patterns of all people in the family and honor cultural and family preferences (Figure 56.5).

Play

Play is a central occupation for children, and children's sensory processing patterns can inform practitioners about the types of play activities that are likely to be more enjoyable for different children. When typically developing children show more sensory processing differences, they engage in less mature and less socially based play than peers (Cosbey et al., 2010). Additionally, typically developing children with increased sensitivities are less likely to change their body positions during play (Mische Lawson & Dunn, 2008).

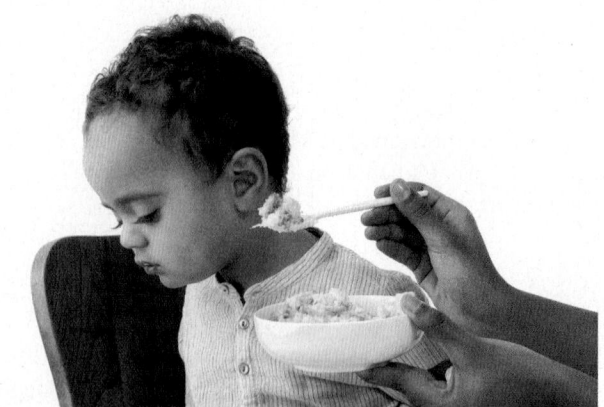

FIGURE 56.5 When children show sensory sensitivities and avoidances, eating and mealtime can become challenging.

The play opportunities of children are likely influenced by their parents' sensory preferences. One study showed that child and parent sensory avoiding and sensitivity scores are significantly related, which contributes to parents offering nonseeking play activities (Welters-Davis & Mische Lawson, 2011). For children with ASD, researchers have shown relationships between sensory processing and social play; specifically, the overall sensory processing scores relate to how children create play opportunities with others (Kuhaneck & Britner, 2013).

When addressing play with children and their families, it is important for OT practitioners to understand the sensory preferences of the child and the sensory experiences that particular activities afford. For example, a child who has a low threshold for movement may not enjoy playing organized sports but may enjoy the predictability of swinging on a swing set. When the preference of the child matches the sensory characteristics of the activity, the child is more likely to be successful. See Chapter 47, for more information on OT and play.

Sleep

A child's sleep routines can have a significant impact on a family's quality of life. The relationship between sensory processing and sleep has not been studied extensively; however, research is beginning to focus on these issues, specifically among children with conditions. Children with FASD, who are more sensitive to sensory input, may not sleep as long and may take longer to go to sleep (Wengel et al., 2011). Similarly, children who seek more sensory input tend to stay awake longer and sleep less. Children with ASD who show increased sensory sensitivities have also been shown to have sleep difficulties (Mazurek & Petroski, 2015; Reynolds et al., 2012). Researchers suggest that when children arouse to more stimuli, it is harder to fall asleep again because they detect more sensory events. They also hypothesize that these sensory and sleep patterns could be associated with anxiety.

When OT practitioners work with individuals on sleep and bedtime routines, it is important to consider the sensory characteristics of the person as well as how the sensory features of the environment and family preferences (e.g., co-sleeping) may be impacting overall sleep (Figure 56.6). See Chapter 48, for more information related to OT and sleep.

Evidence Related to Intervention

Interventions designed to address sensory processing vary by what aspect of occupational performance they emphasize and therefore differently align with EHP intervention

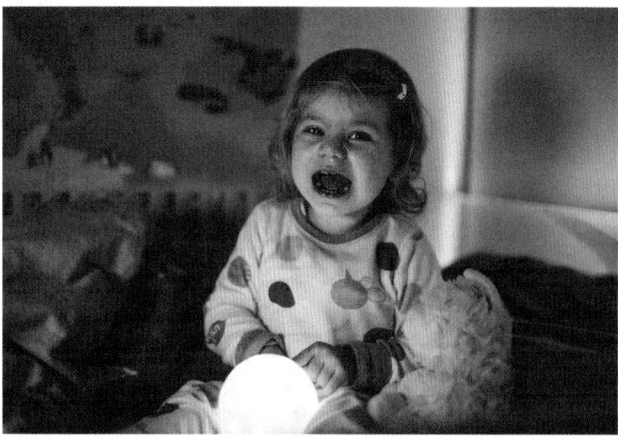

FIGURE 56.6 A child's sleep routines can have a significant impact on a family's quality of life.

approaches. Similar to sensory measures, sensory-focused interventions use differing theoretical bases (e.g., sensory processing vs. SI) as well as the conceptualization of the mechanism of change (i.e., the process or specific way in which participation increases). This section discusses the evidence related to a number of interventions, including environmental modifications, occupation-based coaching, targeted parent education, and SI, and explains how each intervention fits within an EHP intervention approach (i.e., Establish/Restore, Alter, Adapt/Modify, Prevent, Create). (Refer to Table 56.1, for examples of how specific strategies match each sensory pattern and EHP intervention approach.)

When deciding which intervention approach to use, it is critical for OT practitioners to determine the approach that best meets the needs of the families and individuals they serve. The following questions can help OT practitioners think through this decision:

- Does the intervention use materials and tools readily available in the family's home?
- Does the intervention reflect everyday life?
- Can underserved and marginalized populations afford or access the intervention?
- Can the intervention be used as part of the individual's or family's authentic activities and routines?
- Does the intervention focus on family and individual interests and priorities?
- Does the intervention take time away from other childhood experiences (e.g., camps, school, time with family)?
- Would other children be doing activities associated with the intervention with the same frequency?

OT Story 56.5 is an example of how an OT practitioner might discuss the evidence base of different sensory approaches.

OT STORY 56.5 UNDERSTANDING THE EVIDENCE RELATED TO INTERVENTION

A parent named Keith is interested in understanding more about what he can do to support his daughter, Veronica, with sensory-related activities. He reports he completed many Internet searches and learned OT practitioners are often certified in these activities. He wants to learn more about how these interventions will help Veronica's sensory challenges. He hands you a list of interventions, including Auditory Integration Training and the Wilbarger Brushing Protocol.

You know that parents taking responsibility to research information is especially important; however, you also know the evidence for these methods is lacking. Although you want to continue to support Keith, you also have a responsibility to report accurate evidence on the interventions he found during his search.

You first talk with Keith about sensory preferences and explain that understanding Veronica's sensory preferences may help us target activities that are the most supportive to Veronica's needs. You normalize sensory preferences by telling Keith that we all have sensory preferences; and over time, we learn strategies to help us when activities do not match our preferences. By understanding Veronica's sensory processing patterns, we can develop strategies to support her.

You then encourage Keith by affirming that the Internet research he completed is very important, and that you are encouraged that he took the time to learn and understand Veronica this way. You then share evidence on the two methods he read about. You explain that the studies showed different findings with these two methods, and certain studies were stronger than others as well. This makes it especially confusing to sift through the evidence. You explain that the idea behind Auditory Integration Training is that listening to specialized auditory input will fix Veronica's central nervous system. However, to date, studies are showing no benefits to Auditory Integration Training for child behavior (Case-Smith et al., 2015). You then explain that the Wilbarger Protocol is very similar; however, instead of auditory input, you use a small brush to apply pressure to different joints of the body to change the sensory systems of Veronica (Wilbarger & Wilbarger, 1991). However, like Auditory Integration Training, there is little to no evidence indicating the Wilbarger Brushing Protocol will help child behavior.

You go on to offer alternative strategies that can support Veronica while also highlighting how her sensory preferences can make her life richer. You explain that her sensory preferences are part of how she understands the world; her discerning auditory system can be distracting in noisy places, but this might also mean she hears details in songs that you and I would miss. Her touch sensitivity makes it hard to get dressed, but we can find the right fabrics and textures for her wardrobe so she can fully participate without her clothing bothering her. So we can take advantage of understanding her preferences by planning activities that match her needs and by thinking ahead about activities that might be more challenging.

Questions

1. What are essential considerations you will use to determine which interventions to recommend to families (this section can help identify essential considerations)?
2. OT practitioners are always hearing about the latest practices that claim to be "evidence-based practices." Many of these practices actually have little evidence of effectiveness, and the developers (and sellers) of the interventions often overstate the evidence or provide testimony from only a few clients. How will you determine the evidence base of new interventions?

Environmental Modifications

Most public environments were created for people who fit within the majority of others on the bell curve, which can create challenges for people who process sensory input differently. Environmental modifications can be used to address specific elements of contexts that elicit aversive responses from individuals. Such modifications can be made to match children's sensory preferences. For example, classrooms are bright and loud for many children with sensory differences, and a few studies have investigated the effects of modifying the classroom environment. One study found positive effects on student engagement when classroom lighting and sound were altered for children with ASD (Kinnealey et al., 2012). Specifically, the students in this study expressed that the halogen lighting and sound-absorbing walls helped them focus and feel more comfortable in the classroom. Another study (Bagatell et al., 2010) found that young children with ASD benefited from using therapy ball chairs in the classroom, particularly if they had frequent seeking behaviors. The therapy balls were not helpful, however, for children with poor postural stability, as they were less engaged.

Visual schedules have been shown to be a very effective environmental modification intervention among children with ASD, likely because of strengths in visual processing (Case-Smith & Arbesman, 2008). Research shows that when using visual schedules, children show decreased problem behavior and increased engagement; the visual schedules seem to offer the children control because they have pictures to sequentially depict activities (for a review, see Lequia et al., 2012).

Research findings about environmental modifications show that OT practitioners should consider the individual sensory preferences of each child when designing these types of interventions. Children with differing levels of sensory seeking, registration, sensitivities, and avoidance may respond differently to varying types of modifications. For example, a bright light or strong scent may be activating for some children with registration difficulties; however, if a child shows sensory avoidance, the bright light or strong scent may lead to more problem behaviors.

In the context of EHP intervention approaches, environmental modifications may be considered to be an Alter intervention. When we alter the sensory elements of contexts, individuals may be better able to participate. For example, dimming fluorescent lighting and soundproofing walls may help students with sensory sensitivities focus in the classroom. These interventions may also support many other students to focus as well.

Although we think about changing the environment to meet the needs of specific individuals with sensory processing challenges and distinct preferences, such environmental modifications may also result in a Create intervention. Interventions that use the Create approach are designed to support optimal performance for all persons and populations. There are few examples in the literature of using the create strategy to support sensory processing, but environmental modifications are being increasingly used to create environments acceptable for various people. For example, therapy balls provide seating for individuals who seek movement; however, some research suggests that therapy ball chairs may help other children maintain focus in a classroom (Fedewa & Erwin, 2011; Schilling et al., 2003). Other examples include businesses that understand the potential of matching customers' sensory preferences with sensory-friendly environments. Some movie theaters offer "sensory-friendly" times in which the sound is down and the lights are up, which are appealing to a wide variety of people. Some museums offer tactile, visual, and movement opportunities to interact with displays.

OT practitioners can use their knowledge of sensory processing to play key roles in supporting businesses to create sensory-friendly environments for all people.

Occupation-Based Coaching

Occupation-based coaching (OBC) directly engages caregivers in identifying their own goals for their children and working with an OT practitioner to understand how to embed sensory-based, communication, and play strategies into everyday activities. In OBC, OT practitioners work with caregivers to gain a deeper understanding of the caregivers' own knowledge and the impact of their strategies on their children's behavior (Rush & Shelden, 2020). The role of the OT practitioner is to support caregivers to generate their own solutions to challenges in everyday life through the use of reflective questions and comments so that caregivers have opportunities to evaluate their own strategies and daily routines. Differences in sensory preferences among family members often play a role in family life, and parents must understand their children's particular sensory patterns to best provide them with learning opportunities that match their needs.

A number of studies suggest that OBC is an effective intervention method. Among families of children with ASD, a 12-week OBC intervention resulted in positive effects related to parent self-efficacy and child participation (Dunn et al., 2012). At the end of intervention, families of children with ASD reached goals such as going to the grocery store and having their child engage in a bath time routine. One study implemented OBC via telehealth and found a significant increase in parent self-efficacy and child participation (Little et al., 2018). A recent study using a shorter timeline (4 weeks) for three parents of children with ASD aged 3 to 5 years showed improvements in child behavior (Bulkeley et al., 2016).

The American Academy of Pediatrics identified coaching as a best practice method in early intervention (Baio, 2014) and is a recommended practice from the Division of Early Childhood (DEC, 2014; see http://www.dec-sped.org/dec-recommended-practices, for more information). Through coaching, parents become empowered to support their child's everyday routines. OT practitioners are in a unique position to use the principles of coaching in combination with their knowledge of how children's sensory processing influences participation in everyday routines and activities. More information on coaching can be found at http://www.coachinginearly-childhood.org/.

Targeted Parent Education Models

Another intervention that has shown promise is structured parent education that incorporates sensory processing knowledge. After participating in a 6-week intervention, parents showed a significant increase in self-confidence about their children's particular characteristics as well as a significant decrease in anxiety (Farmer & Reupert, 2013). Other studies have found that the parents were empowered when they understood how to implement sensory strategies at home and take control over their child's therapy (Dunstan & Griffiths, 2008). Gibbs and Toth-Cohen (2011) used structured parent education and sensory diets (activities spread throughout the day that match the person's sensory preferences) for four families of children with ASD and found a decrease in self-stimulatory behaviors and an increase in fine motor skills.

In the context of EHP intervention approaches, parent-led models may be considered as an Adapt/Modify intervention and/or a Prevent intervention. When parents adapt and modify task features to match children's sensory preferences, children may be able to better participate in occupations. For example, if a child needs to attend a siblings' school concert in a crowded and noisy auditorium, an OT practitioner can coach a family to think through strategies to make the event tolerable for the child. On the other hand, when parents engage in parent-led interventions with OT practitioners, they can better understand how to set up environments and tasks for their children in a way that will mitigate negative responses before they occur. For example, a parent may know that a child with taste and smell sensitivity will not eat dinner with the family if ketchup is on anyone's plate. The parent would then simply not use ketchup; by removing something from the task or environment, the parent is preventing a negative reaction to mealtime.

Sensory Integration

Although we have described a contextual approach to supporting participation, another approach that targets changing people's sensory processing patterns is sensory integration or sensory integration therapy (SIT), which is a time-intensive, clinic-based, play-focused intervention that uses sensory-enhanced interactions to elicit child adaptive responses (Case-Smith et al., 2015). SIT uses controlled sensory stimulation and provides children with structured opportunities in sensory-focused activities that are designed to elicit adaptive behavioral responses from children. In other words, gross motor activities activate somatosensory, vestibular, and proprioceptive systems and are believed to help the child integrate environmental sensory information. The hypothesis of SI is that the "integration" that occurs in the clinic will translate to the child's organization of communication and adaptive behavior across everyday contexts. In terms of EHP intervention approaches, SIT is an Establish/Restore approach. The underlying assumption of SI is that by targeting changes in the person's central nervous system, outcomes may be seen related to the child's ability to respond differently to demands. The focus of these interventions is on changing the child's ability to integrate sensory information as opposed to focusing on the environment to meet the needs of the child or changing the task to match a child's preferences.

It is important to note that research on SIT is mixed, and studies that compare SIT with other treatment approaches vary in their findings. As compared with Applied Behavior Analysis (Devlin et al., 2011), sensorimotor (Dunbar et al., 2012), social skills (Iwanaga et al., 2014), and fine motor interventions (Pfeiffer et al., 2011), SIT showed similar, and not significantly different, results in supporting the outcome of interest (i.e., challenging behaviors, play,

cognition/social skills, fine motor goal attainment). However, a few studies suggest that SIT may be efficacious compared with usual treatment (e.g., other services received by participants, such as behavioral or pharmacologic services) (Miller et al., 2007; Schaaf et al., 2014); yet, it is important to recognize that children in SIT received many more hours of therapy than children who received therapy in typical community settings. This means it is difficult to disentangle findings associated with SIT from findings associated with increased hours, or attention, in therapy. Overall, OT practitioners considering using SIT in their practice must consider the child behavior that the therapy is intended to impact. If sensory factors are impacting a child's play or self-care skills, the OT practitioner may instead use an occupation-based intervention to directly address such play or self-care skills. In order to provide best practice and serve families in an efficient, efficacious manner, OT practitioners must talk with families about how and why interventions work and the evidence related to the interventions. Further, OT practitioners must ensure the intervention approaches and intended outcomes match the goals of the family, child, and educators want to see.

Lippincott® Connect *For additional resources on the subjects discussed in this chapter, visit Lippincott Connect.*

REFERENCES

Adams, J. B., Audhya, T., McDonough-Means, S., Rubin, R. A., Quig, D., Geis, E., Gehn, E., Loresto, M., Atwood, S., Barnhouse, S., & Lee, W. (2011). Nutritional and metabolic status of children with autism vs. neurotypical children, and the association with autism severity. *Nutrition & Metabolism, 8*(1), 34. https://doi.org/10.1186/1743-7075-8-34

American Psychiatric Association. (2013). *Diagnostic and statistical manual of mental disorders* (5th ed.). Author.

Ashburner, J., Ziviani, J., & Rodger, S. (2008). Sensory processing and classroom emotional, behavioral, and educational outcomes in children with autism spectrum disorder. *American Journal of Occupational Therapy, 62*, 564–573. https://doi.org/10.5014/ajot.62.5.564

Ausderau, K. K., Furlong, M., Sideris, J., Bulluck, J., Little, L. M., Watson, L. R., Boyd, B. A., Belger, A., Dickie, V. A., & Baranek, G. T. (2014). Sensory subtypes in children with autism spectrum disorder: Latent profile transition analysis using a national survey of sensory features. *Journal of Child Psychology and Psychiatry, and Allied Disciplines, 55*(8), 935–944. https://doi.org/10.1111/jcpp.12219

Ayres, A. J. (1972). *Sensory integration and learning disorders.* Western Psychological Services.

Ayres, A. J. (1980). *Southern California Sensory Integration Tests Manual.* Western Psychological Services.

Bagatell, N., Mirigliani, G., Patterson, C., Reyes, Y., & Test, L. (2010). Effectiveness of therapy ball chairs on classroom participation in children with autism spectrum disorders. *American Journal of Occupational Therapy, 64*, 895–903. https://doi.org/10.5014/ajot.2010.09149

Bagby, M. S., Dickie, V. A., & Baranek, G. T. (2012). How sensory experiences of children with and without autism affect family occupations. *American Journal of Occupational Therapy, 66*, 78–86. https://doi.org/10.5014/ajot.2012.000604

Baio, J. (2014). Prevalence of autism spectrum disorder among children aged 8 years—Autism and developmental disabilities monitoring network, 11 sites, United States, 2010. *Surveillance Summaries, 63,* 1–21. https://doi.org/10.15585/mmwr.ss6706a1

Baker, A. E., Lane, A., Angley, M. T., & Young, R. L. (2008). The relationship between sensory processing patterns and behavioural responsiveness in autistic disorder: A pilot study. *Journal of Autism and Developmental Disorders, 38,* 867–875. https://doi.org/10.1007/s10803-007-0459-0

Baranek, G. T. (2009). Sensory *experiences questionnaire versi*on 3.0 [Unpublished manuscript]. University of North Carolina at Chapel Hill, North Carolina.

Baranek, G. T., Carlson, M., Sideris, J., Kirby, A. V., Watson, L. R., Williams, K. L., & Bulluck, J. (2019). Longitudinal assessment of stability of sensory features in children with autism spectrum disorder or other developmental disabilities. *Autism Research, 12*(1), 100–111. https://doi.org/10.1002/aur.2008

Baranek, G. T., Little, L. M., Parham, L., Ausderau, K. K., & Sabatos-DeVito, M. G. (2014). Sensory features in autism spectrum disorders. In F. R. Volkmar, S. J. Rogers, R. Paul, & K. Pelphrey (Eds.), *Handbook of autism and pervasive developmental disorders* (4th ed., Vol. 1, pp. 378–408). Wiley.

Baum, C. M., & Edwards, D. (2001). *ACS: Activity card sort.* Washington University School of Medicine.

Bedell, G. (2009). Further validation of the Child and Adolescent Scale of Participation (CASP). *Developmental Neurorehabilitation, 12,* 342–351. https://doi.org/10.3109/17518420903087277

Boets, B., Wouters, J., van Wieringen, A., De Smedt, B., & Ghesquiére, P. (2008). Modelling relations between sensory processing, speech perception, orthographic and phonological ability, and literacy achievement. *Brain and Language, 106,* 29–40. https://doi.org/10.1016/j.bandl.2007.12.004

Boliek, C., Keintz, C., Norrix, L., & Obrzut, J. (2010). Auditory-visual perception of speech in children with learning disabilities: The McGurk effect. *Canadian Journal of Speech-Language Pathology and Audiology, 34,* 124–131.

Brown, C., & Dunn, W. (2002). *Adolescent/adult sensory profile: User's manual.* Therapy Skill Builders.

Brown, N. B., & Dunn, W. (2010). Relationship between context and sensory processing in children with autism. *American Journal of Occupational Therapy, 64,* 474–483. https://doi.org/10.5014/ajot.2010.09077

Bulkeley, K., Bundy, A., Roberts, J., & Einfeld, S. (2016). Family-centered management of sensory challenges of children with autism: Single-case experimental design. *American Journal of Occupational Therapy, 70,* 7005220040p1–7005220040p8. https://doi.org/10.5014/ajot.2016.017822

Cascio, C. J., Woynaroski, T., Baranek, G. T., & Wallace, M. T. (2016). Toward an interdisciplinary approach to understanding sensory function in autism spectrum disorder. *Autism Research, 9,* 920–925. https://doi.org/10.1002/aur.1612

Case-Smith, J., & Arbesman, M. (2008). Evidence-based review of interventions for autism used in or of relevance to occupational therapy. *American Journal of Occupational Therapy, 62,* 416–429. https://doi.org/10.5014/ajot.62.4.416

Case-Smith, J., Weaver, L. L., & Fristad, M. A. (2015). A systematic review of sensory processing interventions for children with autism spectrum disorders. *Autism, 19,* 133–148. https://doi.org/10.1177/1362361313517762

Cosbey, J., Johnston, S. S., & Dunn, M. L. (2010). Sensory processing disorders and social participation. *American Journal of Occupational Therapy, 64,* 462–473. https://doi.org/10.5014/ajot.2010.09076

Coster, W., Law, M., Bedell, G., & Teplicky, R. (2010). *Participation and environment measure for children and youth (PEM-CY).* Trustees of Boston University.

Coulthard, H., & Blissett, J. (2009). Fruit and vegetable consumption in children and their mothers. Moderating effects of child

sensory sensitivity. *Appetite, 52,* 410–415. https://doi.org/10.1016/j.appet.2008.11.015

Davis, A. M., Bruce, A. S., Khasawneh, R., Schulz, T., Fox, C., & Dunn, W. (2013). Sensory processing issues in young children presenting to an outpatient feeding clinic. *Journal of Pediatric Gastroenterology and Nutrition, 56,* 156–160. https://doi.org/10.1097/MPG.0b013e3182736e19

Dean, E. E., Little, L., Tomchek, S., & Dunn, W. (2018). Sensory processing in the general population: Adaptability, resiliency, and challenging behavior. *American Journal of Occupational Therapy, 72,* 7201195060p1–7201195060p8. https://doi.org/10.5014/ajot.2018.019919

Dean, E. E., Wallisch, A., & Dunn, W. (2018). Adaptation as a transaction with the environment: Perspectives from an ecological model of OT. In L. C. Grajo & A. Boisselle (Eds.), *Occupation and adaptation: Multidimensional perspectives.* SLACK.

Devlin, S., Healy, O., Leader, G., & Hughes, B. M. (2011). Comparison of behavioral intervention and sensory-integration therapy in the treatment of challenging behavior. *Journal of Autism and Developmental Disorders, 41,* 1303–1320. https://doi.org/10.1007/s10803-011-1303-0

Division for Early Childhood. (2014). *DEC recommended practices in early intervention/early childhood special education 2014.* http://www.dec-sped.org/dec-recommendedpractices

Dovey, T. M., Aldridge, V. K., Dignan, W., Staples, P. A., Gibson, E. L., & Halford, J. C. (2012). Developmental differences in sensory decision making involved in deciding to try a novel fruit. *British Journal of Health Psychology, 17,* 258–272. https://doi.org/10.1111/j.2044-8287.2011.02036.x

Dunbar, S. B., Carr-Hertel, J., Lieberman, H. A., Perez, B., & Ricks, K. (2012). A pilot study comparison of sensory integration treatment and integrated preschool activities for children with autism. *Internet Journal of Allied Health Sciences and Practice, 10,* 6. https://doi.org/10.46743/1540-580X/2012.1407

Dunn, W. (1997). The impact of sensory processing abilities on the daily lives of young children and their families: A conceptual model. *Infants and Young Children, 9,* 23–35. https://doi.org/10.1097/00001163-199704000-00005

Dunn, W. (1999). *The Sensory Profile manual.* The Psychological Corporation.

Dunn, W. (2007). Ecology of Human Performance model. In S. Dunbar (Ed.), *Occupational therapy models for intervention with children and families* (pp. 127–156). SLACK.

Dunn, W. (2014). *Sensory Profile-2.* Pearson.

Dunn, W., Brown, C., & McGuigan, A. (1994). The ecology of human performance: A framework for considering the effect of context. *American Journal of Occupational Therapy, 48,* 595–607. https://doi.org/10.5014/ajot.48.7.595

Dunn, W., Brown, C., Youngstrom, M. J., Kramer, P., Hinojosa, J., & Royeen, C. (2003). Ecological model of occupation. In P. Kramer, J. Hinojosa, & C. B. Royeen (Eds.), *Perspectives in human occupation: Participation in life* (pp. 222–263). Lippincott Williams & Wilkins.

Dunn, W., Cox, J., Foster, L., Mische-Lawson, L., & Tanquary, J. (2012). Impact of a contextual intervention on child participation and parent competence among children with autism spectrum disorders: A pretest-posttest repeated-measures design. *American Journal of Occupational Therapy, 66,* 520–528. https://doi.org/10.5014/ajot.2012.004119

Dunn, W., Little, L., Dean, E., Robertson, S., & Evans, B. (2016). The state of the science on sensory factors and their impact on daily life for children: A scoping review. *OTJR: Occupation, Participation and Health, 36*(Suppl.), 3S–26S. https://doi.org/10.1177/1539449215617923

Dunn, W., Tomchek, S., Little, L., & Dean, E. (2016). Prevalence of sensory characteristics in the general population: A person-centered approach. *American Journal of Occupational Therapy, 70,* 7011500001p1. https://doi.org/10.5014/ajot.2016.70S1-RP202A

Dunstan, E., & Griffiths, S. (2008). Sensory strategies: Practical support to empower families. *New Zealand Journal of Occupational Therapy, 55*, 5. https://doi.org/10.3316/informit.194572153682279

Education of All Handicapped Children Act of 1975, Pub. L. No. 94-142, 89 Stat. 773, *codified as amended at* title 20 U.S.C. §1401 (1975).

Engel-Yeger, B., Hardal-Nasser, R., & Gal, E. (2011). Sensory processing dysfunctions as expressed among children with different severities of intellectual developmental disabilities. *Research in Developmental Disabilities, 32*, 1770–1775. https://doi.org/10.1016/j.ridd.2011.03.005

Farmer, J., & Reupert, A. (2013). Understanding autism and understanding my child with autism: An evaluation of a group parent education program in rural Australia. *The Australian Journal of Rural Health, 21*, 20–27. https://doi.org/10.1111/ajr.12004

Fedewa, A. L., & Erwin, H. E. (2011). Stability balls and students with attention and hyperactivity concerns: Implications for on-task and in-seat behavior. *American Journal of Occupational Therapy, 65*, 393–399. https://doi.org/10.5014/ajot.2011.000554

Frances, A. (2013). *Saving normal: An insider's look at what caused the epidemic of mental illness and how to cure it.* William Morrow.

Geiger, G., Cattaneo, C., Galli, R., Pozzoli, U., Lorusso, M. L., Facoetti, A., & Molteni, M. (2008). Wide and diffuse perceptual modes characterize dyslexics in vision and audition. *Perception, 37*, 1745–1764. https://doi.org/10.1068/p6036

Ghanizadeh, A. (2013). Parents reported oral sensory sensitivity processing and food preference in ADHD. *Journal of Psychiatric and Mental Health Nursing, 20*, 426–432. https://doi.org/10.1111/j.1365-2850.2011.01830.x

Gibbs, V., & Toth-Cohen, S. (2011). Family-centered occupational therapy and telerehabilitation for children with autism spectrum disorders. *Occupational Therapy in Health Care, 25*, 298–314. https://doi.org/10.3109/07380577.2011.606460

Grandin, T. (1986). *Emergence: Labeled autistic.* Arena Press.

Grandin, T., & Barron, S. (2005). *Unwritten rules of social relationships: Decoding social mysteries through the unique perspectives of autism.* Future Horizons.

Green, S. A., Ben-Sasson, A., Soto, T. W., & Carter, A. S. (2012). Anxiety and sensory over-responsivity in toddlers with autism spectrum disorders: Bidirectional effects across time. *Journal of Autism and Developmental Disorders, 42*(6), 1112–1119. https://doi.org/10.1007/s10803-011-1361-3

Hilton, C., Graver, K., & LaVesser, P. (2007). Relationship between social competence and sensory processing in children with high functioning autism spectrum disorders. *Research in Autism Spectrum Disorders, 1*, 164–173. https://doi.org/10.1016/j.dcn.2017.04.010

Hochhauser, M., & Engel-Yeger, B. (2010). Sensory processing abilities and their relation to participation in leisure activities among children with high-functioning autism spectrum disorder (HFASD). *Research in Autism Spectrum Disorders, 4*, 746–754. https://doi.org/https://doi.org/10.1016/j.rasd.2010.01.015

Individuals with Disabilities Education Act, Pub. L. No. 101-476, 104 Stat. 1142, *codified as amended at* title 20 U.S.C. §1400 (1990).

Iwanaga, R., Honda, S., Nakane, H., Tanaka, K., Toeda, H., & Tanaka, G. (2014). Pilot study: Efficacy of sensory integration therapy for Japanese children with high-functioning autism spectrum disorder. *Occupational Therapy International, 21*, 4–11. https://doi.org/10.1002/oti.1357

Jasmin, E., Couture, M., McKinley, P., Reid, G., Fombonne, E., & Gisel, E. (2009). Sensorimotor and daily living skills of preschool children with autism spectrum disorders. *Journal of Autism and Developmental Disorders, 39*, 231–241. https://doi.org/10.1007/s10803-008-0617-z

Jirikowic, T., Olson, H. C., & Kartin, D. (2008). Sensory processing, school performance, and adaptive behavior of young school-age children with fetal alcohol spectrum disorders. *Physical & Occupational Therapy in Pediatrics, 28*, 117–136. https://doi.org/10.1080/01942630802031800

Khetani, M., Coster, W., Law, M., & Bedell, G. (2013). *Young children's participation and environment measure (YC-PEM).* Colorado State University.

King, G., Law, M., Petrenchik, T., & Kertoy, M. (2006). *Assessment of preschool children's participation (APCP).* CanChild Centre for Childhood Disability Research, McMaster University.

Kinnealey, M., Pfeiffer, B., Miller, J., Roan, C., Shoener, R., & Ellner, M. L. (2012). Effect of classroom modification on attention and engagement of students with autism or dyspraxia. *American Journal of Occupational Therapy, 66*, 511–519. https://doi.org/10.5014/ajot.2012.004010

Kuhaneck, H. M., & Britner, P. A. (2013). A preliminary investigation of the relationship between sensory processing and social play in autism spectrum disorder. *OTJR: Occupation, Participation and Health, 33*, 159–167. https://doi.org/10.3928/15394492-20130614-04

Lane, A. E., Molloy, C. A., & Bishop, S. L. (2014). Classification of children with autism spectrum disorder by sensory subtype: A case for sensory-based phenotypes. *Autism Research, 7*, 322–333. https://doi.org/10.1002/aur.1368

Lane, A. E., Young, R. L., Baker, A. E., & Angley, M. T. (2010). Sensory processing subtypes in autism: Association with adaptive behavior. *Journal of Autism and Developmental Disorders, 40*, 112–122. https://doi.org/10.1007/s10803-009-0840-2

Lequia, J., Machalicek, W., & Rispoli, M. J. (2012). Effects of activity schedules on challenging behavior exhibited in children with autism spectrum disorders: A systematic review. *Research in Autism Spectrum Disorders, 6*, 480–492. https://doi.org/10.1016/j.rasd.2011.07.008

Little, L. M., Ausderau, K., Sideris, J., & Baranek, G. T. (2015). Activity participation and sensory features among children with autism spectrum disorders. *Journal of Autism and Developmental Disorders, 45*, 2981–2990. https://doi.org/10.1007/s10803-015-2460-3

Little, L. M., Dean, E., Tomchek, S. D., & Dunn, W. (2017). Classifying sensory profiles of children in the general population. *Child: Care, Health and Development, 43*, 81–88. https://doi.org/10.1111/cch.12391

Little, L. M., Pope, E., Wallisch, A., & Dunn, W. (2018). Occupation-based coaching by means of telehealth for families of young children with autism spectrum disorder. *American Journal of Occupational Therapy, 72*, 7202205020. https://doi.org/10.5014/ajot.2018.024786

Mandich, A., Polatajko, H., Miller, L., & Baum, C. (2004). *Paediatric activity card sort (PACS).* Canadian Association of Occupational Therapists.

Marquenie, K., Rodger, S., Mangohig, K., & Cronin, A. (2011). Dinnertime and bedtime routines and rituals in families with a young child with an autism spectrum disorder. *Australian Occupational Therapy Journal, 58*, 145–154. https://doi.org/10.1111/j.1440-1630.2010.00896.x

Matsushima, K., & Kato, T. (2013). Social interaction and atypical sensory processing in children with autism spectrum disorders. *Hong Kong Journal of Occupational Therapy, 23*, 89–96. https://doi.org/10.1016/j.hkjot.2013.11.003

Mattard-Labrecque, C., Ben Amor, L., & Couture, M. M. (2013). Children with autism and attention difficulties: A pilot study of the association between sensory, motor, and adaptive behaviors. *Journal of the Canadian Academy of Child and Adolescent Psychiatry, 22*, 139–146.

Mazurek, M. O., & Petroski, G. F. (2015). Sleep problems in children with autism spectrum disorder: Examining the contributions of sensory over-responsivity and anxiety. *Sleep Medicine, 16*, 270–279. https://doi.org/10.1016/j.sleep.2014.11.006

McCormick, C., Hepburn, S., Young, G. S., & Rogers, S. J. (2016). Sensory symptoms in children with autism spectrum disorder, other developmental disorders and typical development: A longitudinal study. *Autism, 20*(5), 572–579. https://doi.org/10.1177/1362361315599755

McIntosh, D. N., Miller, L. J., Shyu, V., & Dunn, W. (1999). Overview of the short sensory profile (SSP). In W. Dunn (Ed.), *The sensory profile: Examiner's manual* (pp. 59–73). The Psychological Corporation.

Miller, L. J., Coll, J. R., & Schoen, S. A. (2007). A randomized controlled pilot study of the effectiveness of occupational therapy for children with sensory modulation disorder. *American Journal of Occupational Therapy, 61*, 228–238. https://doi.org/10.5014/ajot.61.2.228

Miller Kuhaneck, H., Ecker, C., Parham, L., Henry, D., & Glennon, T. (2010). *Sensory processing measure-preschool (SPM-P): Manual.* Western Psychological Services.

Mische Lawson, L., & Dunn, W. (2008). Children's sensory processing patterns and play preferences. *Annual in Therapeutic Recreation, 16*, 1–14.

Nadon, G., Feldman, D. E., Dunn, W., & Gisel, E. (2011). Association of sensory processing and eating problems in children with autism spectrum disorders. *Autism Research and Treatment, 2011*, 541926. https://doi.org/10.1155/2011/541926

Parham, L. D., & Ecker, C. (2007). *Sensory processing measure (SPM).* Western Psychological Services.

Perez Repetto, L., Jasmin, E., Fombonne, E., Gisel, E., & Couture, M. (2017). Longitudinal study of sensory features in children with autism spectrum disorder. *Autism Research and Treatment, 2017*, 1–8. https://doi.org/10.1155/2017/1934701

Pfeiffer, B. A., Koenig, K., Kinnealey, M., Sheppard, M., & Henderson, L. (2011). Effectiveness of sensory integration interventions in children with autism spectrum disorders: A pilot study. *The American Journal of Occupational Therapy, 65*(1), 76–85. https://doi.org/10.5014/ajot.2011.09205

Reynolds, S., Bendixen, R. M., Lawrence, T., & Lane, S. J. (2011). A pilot study examining activity participation, sensory responsiveness, and competence in children with high functioning autism spectrum disorder. *Journal of Autism and Developmental Disorders, 41*, 1496–1506. https://doi.org/ 10.1007/s10803-010-1173-x

Reynolds, S., Lane, S. J., & Thacker, L. (2012). Sensory processing, physiological stress, and sleep behaviors in children with and without autism spectrum disorders. *OTJR: Occupation, Participation and Health, 32*, 246–257. https://doi.org/10.3928/15394492-20110513-02

Robison, J. E. (2008). *Look me in the eye: My life with Asperger's.* Random House.

Rogers, S. J., Hepburn, S., & Wehner, E. (2003). Parent reports of sensory symptoms in toddlers with autism and those with other developmental disorders. *Journal of Autism and Developmental Disorders, 33*, 631–642. https://doi.org/10.1023/b:jadd.0000006000.38991.a7

Rush, D. D., & Shelden, M. L. L. (2020). *The early childhood coaching handbook.* Brookes.

Schaaf, R. C., Benevides, T., Mailloux, Z., Faller, P., Hunt, J., van Hooydonk, E., Freeman, R., Leiby, B., Sendecki, J., & Kelly, D. (2014). An intervention for sensory difficulties in children with autism: A randomized trial. *Journal of Autism and Developmental Disorders, 44*, 1493–1506. https://10.1007/s10803-013-1983-8

Schaaf, R. C., & Lane, A. E. (2015). Toward a best-practice protocol for assessment of sensory features in ASD. *Journal of Autism and Developmental Disorders, 45*, 1380–1395. https://doi.org/10.1007/s10803-014-2299-z

Schilling, D. L., Washington, K., Billingsley, F. F., & Deitz, J. (2003). Classroom seating for children with attention deficit hyperactivity disorder: Therapy balls versus chairs. *American Journal of Occupational Therapy, 57*, 534–541. https://doi.org/10.5014/ajot.57.5.534

Shore, S. M. (2003). *Beyond the wall: Personal experiences with autism and Asperger syndrome.* Autism Asperger Publishing Company.

Stein, L. I., Polido, J. C., & Cermak, S. A. (2013). Oral care and sensory over-responsivity in children with autism spectrum disorders. *Pediatric Dentistry, 35*, 230–235.

Stein, L. I., Polido, J. C., Mailloux, Z., Coleman, G. G., & Cermak, S. A. (2011). Oral care and sensory sensitivities in children with autism spectrum disorders. *Special Care in Dentistry, 31*, 102–110. https://doi.org/10.1111/j.1754-4505.2011.00187.x

Stump, K. (2017). *Children with autism wearing action cameras: Changing parent/child interactions using point-of-view video modeling* [Doctoral dissertation]. https://kuscholarworks.ku.edu

Tavassoli, T., Hoekstra, R. A., & Baron-Cohen, S. (2014). The Sensory Perception Quotient (SPQ): Development and validation of a new sensory questionnaire for adults with and without autism. *Molecular Autism, 5*, 29. https://doi.org/10.1186/2040-2392-5-29

Welters-Davis, M., & Mische Lawson, L. (2011). The relationship between sensory processing and parent–child play preferences. *Journal of Occupational Therapy, Schools, and Early Intervention, 4*, 108–120. https://doi.org/10.1080/19411243.2011.595300

Wengel, T., Hanlon-Dearman, A. C., & Fjeldsted, B. (2011). Sleep and sensory characteristics in young children with fetal alcohol spectrum disorder. *Journal of Developmental and Behavioral Pediatrics, 32*, 384–392. https://doi.org/10.1097/DBP.0b013e3182199694

Wilbarger, P., & Wilbarger, J. L. (1991). *Sensory defensiveness in children aged 2–12: An intervention guide for parents and other caretakers.* Therapro.

Zaks, Z. (2006). *Life and love: Positive strategies for autistic adults.* Autism Asperger Publishing Company.

Zimmer, M., Desch, L., Rosen, L. D., Bailey, M. L., Becker, D., Culbert, T. P., McClafferty, H., Sahler, Z., Vohra, S., & Liptak, G. S. (2012). Sensory integration therapies for children with developmental and behavioral disorders. *Pediatrics, 129*(6), 1186–1189. https://doi.org/10.1542/peds.2012-0876

Zingerevich, C. (2009). The contribution of executive functions to participation in school activities of children with high functioning autism spectrum disorder. *Research in Autism Spectrum Disorders, 3*, 429–437. https://doi.org/10.1016/j.rasd.2008.09.002

Zobel-Lachiusa, J., Andrianopoulos, M. V., Mailloux, Z., & Cermak, S. A. (2015). Sensory differences and mealtime behavior in children with autism. *American Journal of Occupational Therapy, 69*, 6905185050p1–6905185050p8. https://doi.org/10.5014/ajot.2015.016790

Emotion Regulation

Jami E. Flick and Marjorie E. Scaffa

LEARNING OBJECTIVES

After reading this chapter, you will be able to:

1. Describe the neurophysiologic and developmental aspects of emotion regulation.
2. Discuss the relationship between emotion regulation and trauma.
3. Understand how emotion regulation supports or limits occupational performance.
4. Identify assessments that are used to measure emotion regulation.
5. Develop intervention plans that address the needs of persons with emotion dysregulation and improve occupational performance.
6. Discuss a strength-based approach to emotion regulation.

Introduction

Emotions are an essential component of being human. It is impossible to be alive and not experience emotions. According to Mahoney (2005), "emotional processes are among the most powerful and primitive of human self-organizing processes" (p. 747). Although the term emotion is difficult to define, there is consensus that emotions are evaluative mental states that occur in the present moment and consist of neurobiologic arousal, perceptual-cognitive processes, subjective experience, and affective expression (Izard, 2010). Emotions arise when a situation appears that has relevance to one's goals. Situations that are likely to enhance goal attainment elicit pleasurable emotions, whereas situations that are likely to inhibit goal attainment elicit negative or unpleasant feelings. Emotions provide us with qualitative information on which to make decisions that result in adaptive responses in our everyday lives. Emotions serve various functions including "motivating and focusing individual endeavors, social interactions, and the development of adaptive and maladaptive behavior" (Izard, 2010, p. 368).

Some emotions are ubiquitous and experienced by all human beings, for example, love, anger, grief/sadness, fear, joy, and disgust. Other emotions are often melds of these primary emotions. For example, surprise could be conceived of as a melding or combination of joy and fear, whereas contempt is a melding of anger and disgust. Emotions

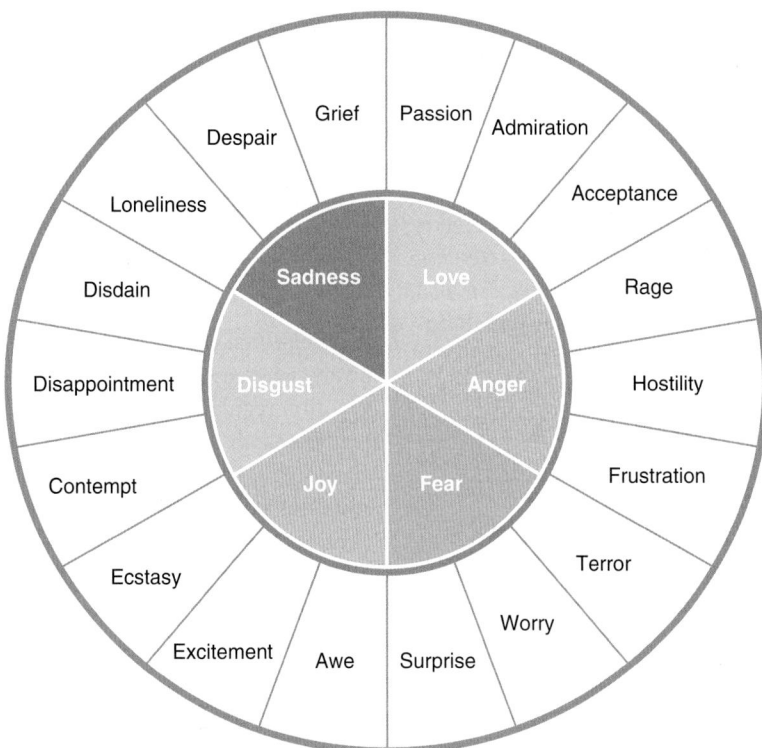

FIGURE 57.1 **Emotions wheel.**

vary in intensity. For example, hostility, frustration, and rage are varying intensities of anger, whereas anticipation, happiness, and ecstasy are varying intensities of joy (Nussbaum, 2001). One way to illustrate the variety and intensities of emotion is through an emotions wheel (Figure 57.1).

Emotions can affect health directly and indirectly, and that impact can be either positive or negative. Emotions can influence health directly through their impact on the immune, endocrine, cardiovascular, and nervous systems. Emotions affect health indirectly through adherence to medical regimens and participation in healthy or unhealthy behaviors (Kiecolt-Glaser et al., 2002). For example, health habits among couples are "contagious," meaning a companion with unhealthy behaviors increases the likelihood that their partner will share negative habits and health consequences, but if one partner improves their health behavior then the other partner likely will follow suit (Kiecolt-Glaser & Wilson, 2017; Sbarra et al., 2015).

An Overview of Emotion Regulation

Emotions are rarely obligatory or automatic and are therefore subject to self-regulation and response modulation. Eisenberg and Spinrad (2004) define *emotion-related self-regulation* as

the process of initiating, avoiding, inhibiting, maintaining, or modulating the occurrence, form, intensity, or duration of internal feeling states, emotion-related physiological, attentional processes, motivational states, and/or the behavioral concomitants of emotion in the service of accomplishing affect-related biological or social adaptation or achieving individual goals. (p. 338)

More simply, *emotion regulation processes* are those behaviors, skills, and strategies that monitor, evaluate, modulate, modify, inhibit, or enhance emotional experiences in the pursuit of one's goals. Emotion dysregulation occurs when despite a person's best efforts, they are unable to "change in a desired way their emotional cues, experiences, actions, verbal responses, and/or nonverbal expressions under normal conditions" (Neacsiu et al., 2014, p. 493). Emotion dysregulation can interfere with goal-directed pursuits, interpersonal relationships, or healthy adaptation (Schore, 2003).

Individuals who are referred for occupational therapy (OT) services with diagnoses of traumatic brain injury (TBI), cerebrovascular accident (CVA), autism spectrum disorders (ASD), dementia, diabetes, cancer, chronic obstructive pulmonary disease (COPD), heart disease, progressive neurologic disorders, attention deficit disorder, eating disorders, addictions of all types, depression, bipolar disorder, posttraumatic stress disorder (PTSD), and other psychiatric diagnoses often present with emotion dysregulation problems that interfere with their occupational performance and participation.

Emotion regulation may be intrinsic or extrinsic. *Intrinsic* refers to factors within the person that contribute to emotion regulation, for example, temperament, cognitive processes, and neurologic and physiologic functions. *Extrinsic* refers to social and contextual influences that affect emotion regulation, for example, interactions with caregivers, sibling and peer relationships, and cultural context (Fox & Calkins, 2003). Although typically focused on reducing negative or painful emotions, emotion regulation can also involve heightening positive emotions (Eisenberg & Spinrad, 2004).

The modal model of emotion consists of five components: the situation, attention to the situation, appraisal of the situation, the emotional and behavioral response to the situation based on the appraisal, and feedback on the effects of the response. Emotions can be regulated before (antecedent focused), during, and after (response focused) they occur. Although these regulatory mechanisms are described separately, they are often employed in combination. Antecedent-focused emotion regulation involves selecting and modifying situations that typically give rise to emotional response tendencies. Situation selection involves taking actions that increase or decrease the likelihood that one will end up in a situation that evokes desirable or undesirable emotional reactions. Examples include avoiding a negative classmate or arranging an outing after an exam to decompress. Situation modifying involves consciously altering external environmental conditions to reduce or enhance the emotional impact of the situation (Gross, 2014). For example, playing upbeat music at a party to set a fun mood or meeting someone at a neutral location to discuss something difficult.

Regulating emotions in the midst of experiencing them may take the form of attentional deployment or cognitive change. *Attentional deployment* refers to individuals "directing their attention within a given situation to influence one's emotions" and includes distraction, or focusing attention away from the situation, and concentration, or focusing on the emotional aspects of the situation to gain control over them (Gross, 2014, p. 10). *Cognitive change*, sometimes referred to as cognitive reappraisal, involves changing one's evaluation of a situation, its consequences, or one's ability to manage the consequences to alter its emotional significance or modify its impact.

Response-focused emotion regulation, also called response modulation, involves modifying the physiologic effects, the experiential aspects, and/or the behavioral expression of emotion. Emotional responses are not adaptive or maladaptive in and of themselves but rather are adaptive or maladaptive depending on the context. For example, crying may be adaptive in one situation and maladaptive in another. Cultural values also determine emotional response modulation and the interpretation of what is socially appropriate, desirable, and adaptive (Gross, 2014).

Neurophysiologic Aspects of Emotion Regulation

Emotion regulation occurs along a continuum from fully automatic and subconscious to conscious and voluntary. Deliberate and effortful attempts to manage emotional reactions are referred to as *intentional emotion regulation*, whereas unintentional and effortless responses are referred to as *incidental emotion regulation*. The neural mechanisms of intentional emotion regulation have been studied extensively, whereas there is much less research on incidental emotion regulation (Berkman & Lieberman, 2009).

Research has demonstrated that the areas of the brain most involved in emotion regulation are the sensory thalamus, amygdala, the hippocampus, and several areas of the prefrontal cortex (PFC) (Davidson et al., 2007; Johnstone & Walter, 2014; Ochsner & Gross, 2014). The amygdala is the primary brain structure involved in the generation of normal and pathologic emotional behavior and is responsible for directing attention to salient stimuli and determining whether further processing is needed. The PFC is often considered the locus of cognitive control, but it also has a role in affective processing. The PFC develops and stores goals and the means to their achievement. Therefore, the PFC appraises the situation to determine whether it is a facilitator or threat to one's goals. In stressful situations, threat stimuli are registered in the sensory thalamus and are almost instantaneously relayed to the amygdala, which is the emotional center responsible for fight-or-flight responses. From there, the message travels to the hippocampus and PFC. The hippocampus applies context to the threat situation and regulates the amygdala, whereas the cortex incorporates memory (Davidson et al., 2007; Johnstone & Walter, 2014; Ochsner & Gross, 2014).

Research on populations with focal brain damage has yielded the following insights regarding emotional processing and emotion regulation:

- Lesions in the lateral frontal lobes are linked to blunted emotional responses or the absence of expected emotions.
- Right orbital frontal lobe damage is associated with increased anger and depression and inability to maximize positive emotion.
- Lesions in the caudate produce inappropriate laughing or crying.
- Regulation of aversive emotions may not require awareness or memory as evidenced by damage to the temporal lobes (Beer & Lombardo, 2007).

Trauma exposure compromises neurologic function particularly in the hippocampus, which is responsible for learning and memory, and in the frontal limbic systems, which are responsible for emotion regulation (Karl et al., 2006). There is evidence to suggest that at least half of psychiatric disorders are characterized by emotion dysregulation, possibly because of dysfunction of the prefrontal-amygdala pathway (Mennin et al., 2005; Ochsner & Gross, 2014; Price & Drevets, 2012; Suveg & Zeman, 2004). As a result, OT practitioners should be particularly alert to the presence of emotion dysregulation in children, adolescents, adults, and older adults who have experienced trauma.

Developmental Aspects of Emotion Regulation

The biologic foundations for emotion regulation develop prenatally. For example, maternal stress during pregnancy has been associated with emotional and self-regulatory difficulties among offspring, such as hyperactivity, limited attention, and maladaptive social behaviors (Calkins & Hill, 2007; Korja et al., 2017). The ability to self-regulate emotional states begins to develop in infancy. Research on infant temperament has demonstrated biologically based tendencies toward the experience and expression of particular emotions. *Temperament* refers to the speed and intensity of emotional reactivity and the ability to modify or self-regulate the intensity and duration of the emotional experience (Rothbart, 2011). Babies and toddlers self-regulate using strategies such as gaze aversion, self-sucking, and seeking proximity to their caregiver (Cole et al., 2004).

Young children learn to self-regulate through their attachment relationships with their primary caregivers (Figure 57.2). Parents influence their child's emotional states by interpreting the infant's emotional signals, modulating the baby's level of physiologic arousal, and reinforcing the child's efforts at self-regulation. For example, when an infant cries, the caregiver often tries to calm and soothe the

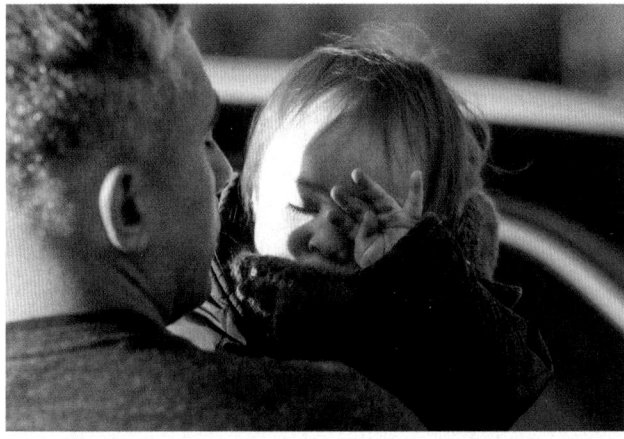

FIGURE 57.2 **Learning emotion regulation through relationships with caregivers.**

child through gentle, rhythmic rocking. Cole et al. (2004) postulate that the "quality of these emotional exchanges . . . is an important precursor of the developing child's ability to regulate his or her own emotions" (p. 324).

During the first year of life, infants develop these attachment relationships to parental figures based on the child's expectation of the caregiver's behavior. These expectations are based on repeated daily interactions with the parent. According to Bowlby (1978), infants who experience consistent, supportive responses to their emotional signals develop secure attachments. An insecure attachment is developed if the child experiences inconsistent, or selective attention to their emotional signals. Insecure attachment has two subtypes, avoidant and anxious. Avoidant attachment is characterized by compulsive self-reliance and distrust in the intentions of others. Anxious attachment is characterized by worries that others will be unresponsive to their emotional needs and compulsive-seeking affirmation, love, and support from others.

Attachment style can have significant implications for later emotion regulation in childhood and adulthood. Individuals with secure attachments tend to be more optimistic about life, more confident in their ability to deal with challenges, and utilize more productive and effective emotion regulation strategies. Individuals with insecure attachments tend to deny or suppress emotions associated with real or imagined abandonment (avoidant attachment), or to exaggerate or overemphasize their feelings of vulnerability and helplessness in order to elicit attention and care from others (anxious attachment). Both insecure attachment styles result in ineffective emotion regulation strategies. Attachment-related differences in emotion regulation are evident in the brain. On functional magnetic resonance imaging (MRI), persons with insecure attachment demonstrate heightened activity in the amygdala in contrast to persons with secure attachment in response to stressful stimuli (Mikulincer & Shaver, 2019).

Toddlers and preschoolers learn to incorporate these caregiver-directed strategies into their behavioral repertoires for self-regulation of emotion. Children at this age typically demonstrate a decrease in self-soothing strategies and an increase in more complex emotion regulation approaches using objects and interpersonal interactions (Cole et al., 2004). These emotion regulation skills can then be applied across various situations in both deliberate and automatic ways. Failure to develop these early emotion self-regulatory skills may constrain the development of more complex emotional skills later and can lead to poor school adjustment and a low level of social competence (Calkins & Hill, 2007; Eisenberg et al., 2014).

For older children, "learning to tolerate distress; correctly label uncomfortable situations, internal feelings, and emotions; and develop appropriate ways to respond to emotions are central to healthy development" (Giroux et al., 2019, p. 388). This is accomplished through the development of effortful control. Effortful control refers to a volitional ability to shift attention, inhibit the tendency to enact a dominant response, and/or activate an alternative response as needed (Rothbart & Bates, 2006). Other factors that impact the development of adaptive emotion regulation are the maturation of language skills that enable the labeling and expression of emotions, observation of the expression of emotions by others in various contexts, and cultural values and mores (Gross, 2014). Neurophysiologic processes continue to mature during adolescence, enabling teenagers to develop self and other awareness, empathy, impulse control, mastery over the environment, and self-regulation of emotion.

Among healthy adults, emotional experience and emotion regulation are well maintained into late adulthood and typically do not deteriorate with aging. However, the frequency of use of different modes of regulation may change. In middle adulthood, suppression of emotion may be used more frequently to succeed in higher education and work, whereas in older adulthood, there appears to be more of a tendency to use cognitive reappraisal to lessen unpleasant emotional experiences and heighten positive emotional states (Benson et al., 2019; Gross, 2014). Older adults perceive daily stressors as less threatening and therefore report less negativity as a result when compared to their younger counterparts (Benson et al., 2019; Birditt et al., 2005).

Relationship between Emotion Regulation and Trauma

Many children and adults have been impacted by trauma. The effects of exposure to trauma are dependent, in part, on the developmental stage of the individual when the trauma occurs. Exposure to trauma during childhood is referred to as **adverse childhood experiences (ACEs)** and often take the form of physical, emotional and sexual abuse, household mental health disorders or substance abuse, or parental incarceration. ACEs can result in negative health outcomes, such as depression, heart disease, lung disease, high risk behaviors, violence victimization, homelessness, criminal activity, and poverty (Merrick et al., 2018). Nearly 60% of adults in the United States have experienced at least one ACE, and 21% have experienced three or more ACEs during childhood (Giano et al., 2020). Trauma early in life has a negative effect on a child's ability to establish and maintain healthy interpersonal attachments and their capacity for emotional self-regulation (Hughes, 2004). Disrupted attachment relationships between children and their caregivers are a significant predictor of risk for child emotional or behavioral problems (Choi et al., 2020). These emotional or behavior problems manifest as poorly moderated affect and impulse control; distrust of others and problems with intimacy; and the lack of a stable, predictable sense of self (van der Kolk, 2003).

Children and adolescents exposed to trauma, in the form of neglect and child abuse in all its forms, as well as witnessing domestic violence, war, and violent crime, have difficulty identifying and describing internal arousal states, labeling, and expressing emotions, and making their needs and wants known. Childhood trauma increases the risk of major depressive disorder later in life often with earlier onset and longer duration. The consistent presence of a competent, emotionally supportive caregiver can mitigate these effects. There appear to be three critical factors in a caregiver's response to their child's trauma experience that facilitate adaptive emotional functioning. These are believing and validating the child's experience, accepting, and understanding the child's affect, and managing the caregiver's own emotional reactions (Cook et al., 2005).

Even mentally healthy, competent adults demonstrate significant declines in cognitive and emotional functioning when traumatized. Adults with PTSD experience persistent arousal (e.g., sleep difficulties, concentration problems, irritability, and exaggerated startle responses) and continue to reexperience the traumatic event after it is over through flashbacks, nightmares, and intrusive thoughts, which produce emotional distress. In their attempts to regulate these distressing emotions, persons exposed to trauma may exhibit externalizing and/or internalizing behaviors (Box 57.1). Internalizing behaviors are often associated with fearful emotions, whereas externalizing behaviors are typically the result of irritable and angry emotions.

BOX 57.1 EXTERNALIZING AND INTERNALIZING BEHAVIORS

Acting Out—Externalizing Behaviors

- Anger
- Violence toward others
- Truancy
- Criminal acts

Acting In—Internalizing Behaviors

- Denial, repression
- Substance abuse (self-medicating)
- Eating disorders
- Self-injury
- Dissociation

Impact of Emotional Dysregulation on Occupational Performance

Poorly regulated emotions can impair occupational functioning and are therefore important considerations in OT evaluation and intervention. In the fourth edition of the "Occupational Therapy Practice Framework (OTPF)" (American Occupational Therapy Association [AOTA], 2020), emotions are categorized as a specific mental function that includes regulation of emotions; expressing a range of emotions (i.e., love, anger, tension, and anxiety); and appropriate use of emotions. According to the OTPF, expressing emotion is a performance skill that entails conveying appropriate affect and emotion for the social situation. The fourth edition of the OTPF does not contain an explicit description of emotional regulation skills, but Gratz and Roemer (2004) suggest that emotion regulation skills include the ability to:

- Accept unpleasant, negative emotional experiences as an inevitable aspect of living
- Redirect and focus one's attention during the presence of intense emotion
- Soothe oneself in response to emotion-related physiologic arousal
- Inhibit inappropriate behaviors related to intense emotional experiences
- Initiate, organize, and persist in goal-directed activity regardless of mood state

Emotional regulation skills are critical elements to social and emotional health promotion and maintenance that is found under the new category of health management as an occupation (AOTA, 2020). Social and emotional health promotion and maintenance consists of:

- Identifying personal strengths and assets
- Managing emotions
- Expressing needs effectively
- Seeking occupations and social engagement to support health and wellness
- Developing self-identity
- Making choices to improve quality of life in participation

Under healthy conditions, these skills are acquired as part of the normal developmental process. However, some children demonstrate impairment in self-regulation secondary to emotional hyperreactivity and a poorly organized stress response system. This reflects an excessive reaction of the autonomic nervous system to relatively low levels of stress that results in intense reactions to emotional stimuli and a slow return to baseline or homeostasis. Linehan (1993a) believes that emotion dysregulation results when a child with high emotional vulnerability is exposed to an invalidating, neglectful, or abusive environment. These children demonstrate affective instability, impulsiveness, irritability, and distractibility all of which interfere with school performance, play, and family and peer relationships. Box 57.2 presents a day in the life of Henry, a child with emotional dysregulation.

In adults, affective instability and the accompanying behavior patterns interfere with the development and maintenance of healthy habits and routines and the

BOX 57.2 THE DYNAMICS OF DYSREGULATION: A DAY IN THE LIFE OF A CHILD WITH EMOTION DYSREGULATION

Henry is a 7-year-old child who experiences emotional dysregulation. Although he has not been formally diagnosed, his parents and teachers agree that many things in life are more difficult for Henry than for his siblings and his peers.

Morning mayhem: *Activities of daily living (ADLs)*	Henry has little trouble awakening in the morning, although he is somewhat grouchy. The first thing Henry must do as part of his morning routine is discreetly throw away his "pull-up," being careful not to let any of his siblings see, even though he knows that they know. At 7 years old, Henry is not fully potty trained, and bedwetting continues to be a problem despite his parent's efforts. Henry feels embarrassed every morning because his 2-year-old brother wears regular underwear to sleep. "What is wrong with me?" He worries and he wonders.
Bad luck on the bus: *Work*	Henry's dad is responsible for making sure that he gets to the bus stop on time. His father makes sure that the morning routine is kept structured to reduce anxiety for Henry and assist with the family's busy morning routine. But today, when Henry climbs on to the bus and attempts to sit down in his assigned seat, a new child is sitting where he is supposed to sit. The bus driver asks Henry to please be seated so that she can continue. Henry's eyes well up with tears because he doesn't know how to explain that someone is sitting in his seat. One of the older boys on the bus sees Henry crying and says tauntingly, "Cry baby!"

(continued)

BOX 57.2 THE DYNAMICS OF DYSREGULATION: A DAY IN THE LIFE OF A CHILD WITH EMOTION DYSREGULATION (*continued*)

Suffering through school: *Education*	At school, Henry's teacher is working with the children on writing paragraphs from a prompt. The class has formed paragraphs together for weeks, and today, the teacher will give the students a prompt and ask the students to write a paragraph on their own. The teacher notes that Henry participates verbally when the class works together but notices that it takes Henry longer to copy the class paragraph from the board to his paper. Today, the teacher notes that as the other children are attempting to write their paragraph, Henry is off-task, playing in his desk. She quietly asks him to please get started, and he appears to be compliant. But when she collects the paragraphs, Henry has only written three sentences, whereas the other children have produced more than double the amount of sentences.
Cafeteria crisis: *Social participation*	Henry has several close friends; most of them are people he has known for a long time because they attended the same preschool as he did. One of the boys is in Henry's class. Henry usually sits next to his friend at the lunch table. But today, his friend is absent from school. Henry sits at the same table but eats his lunch in solitude because he is too shy to talk to any of the other children.
"It's not fair." *Play and leisure*	Henry has three siblings. He usually makes good choices when it comes to following the rules of games. But he gets overly angry when other people do not follow the rules. Often, he storms out in the middle of games with both siblings and peers if he thinks something is "unfair." His peers have difficulty with this pattern of behavior, which often results in them not wanting to include Henry in play.
Homework hostility: *Work*	One of Henry's parents' most difficult tasks is helping Henry complete his homework. They report that Henry has a difficult time focusing, often becomes distracted, and must have a quiet environment with no disruptions to complete even simple assignments. In a busy household, this is seldom possible. Henry also often cries if he cannot quickly figure out new material, and he is sensitive about even gentle corrections from his parents.
Medication complication: "I can't sleep." *Rest and sleep*	Recently, the pediatrician has recommended medication for Henry to help alleviate some of his noted anxiety and to improve his level of concentration. Henry's mother feels uncertain but decides to agree with her husband and try the medication. At times, the medication seems to be helping. But at night, Henry cannot sleep. This side effect bothers his parents, and they feel that this sleep disruption may erase any benefit of the medication.

ability to perform occupational roles effectively. Persons with emotion regulation deficits typically have occupational performance problems in work, instrumental activities of daily living, leisure, and social participation (Figure 57.3) (Scheinholz, 2011).

The way people regulate their emotions affects their social participation, interactions, and relationships. In one study of college students, emotion regulation ability was positively correlated with several social interaction quality indicators. These were "self-reports and peer nominations of interpersonal sensitivity, reciprocal friendship nominations, and the proportion of positive versus negative peer nominations" (Lopes et al., 2005, p. 115). In addition, poor emotional regulation can produce both internalizing and externalizing behaviors, which have a negative impact on social functioning (Eisenberg et al., 2000). Box 57.3 presents a day in the life of Rebecca, an adult with emotional dysregulation.

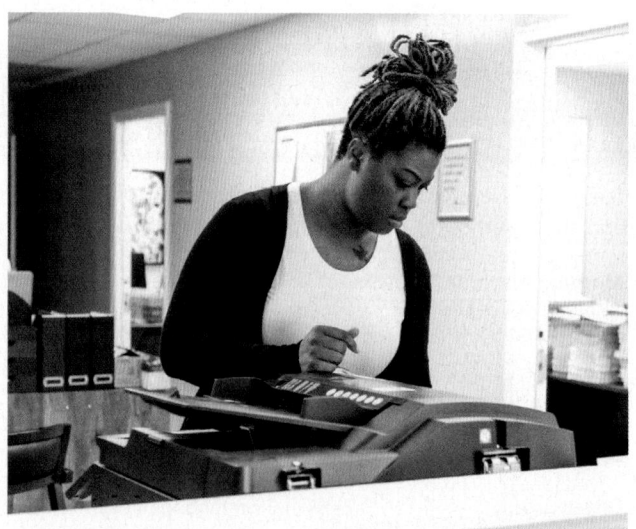

FIGURE 57.3 The workplace can be very stressful and challenge one's ability to self-regulate emotions.

BOX 57.3 THE DYNAMICS OF DYSREGULATION: A DAY IN THE LIFE OF AN ADULT WITH EMOTION DYSREGULATION

Rebecca is a 36-year-old adult who experiences emotional dysregulation. Rebecca is married and has one child. She works as a legal secretary in a large law practice. Rebecca reports her mother was abusive and abandoned the family when she was 14 years old. Rebecca was expected to take over the often overwhelming role of helping to raise her siblings after her mother left.

Mad already and it's only morning: *Rest and sleep*	The alarm goes off every day at 5:30 AM, and every day, Rebecca hits the snooze button because she dreads getting out of bed. Today, she doesn't have the opportunity to hit the snooze button; she has forgotten to set her alarm the night before. Instead, she awakens to her husband who says, "Rebecca, the alarm didn't go off, hurry up, get up, we've overslept." As is frequently the case, her misdirected anger causes her to snap at both her husband and her daughter repeatedly before leaving for work. Her husband, fed up with this treatment, looks at her and says, "It's only morning, and you are already mad. I'm starting to wonder if you wake up this way?"
Breakfast on the run; life on the run: *Activities of daily living (ADLs)*	Even though Rebecca considers herself an organized person, she often rushes through tasks because she has so many responsibilities. Most of her life, she has been expected to complete more than the reasonable amount of activities. She has come to believe that if she doesn't get it all done, she will not be valued. She also has difficulty saying "no" when people ask her for help. She feels that her self-worth is dependent on task completion. Throughout her life, her ADL and personal care have taken a backseat to other people's needs. This morning is no different. In her hurry, after oversleeping, Rebecca skips breakfast and hurries out the door, forgetting also the lunch in the refrigerator her husband had packed for her.
"Never mind, I will do it myself." *The world of work*	At work, the firm has hired an additional legal secretary because of expansion. Rebecca feels threatened by the new legal secretary because she is younger and performs many tasks more quickly than Rebecca. Rebecca knows that she should ask the new secretary to share some of her workload, and today, she decides to ask for help because she is running late. After greeting the new coworker, she asks if she can complete the morning summaries for her while Rebecca moves on to the next item. Morning summaries are an area that the new secretary has not done before, and so she agrees to do the work but says she will need to ask a few questions. Before her new colleague can ask the first question, Rebecca snatches the papers from her hand and says, "Never mind, I will just do it myself." Her coworker comments later to their mutual supervisor that, "Rebecca seems a bit passive–aggressive to me." She follows with details of their earlier interaction.
Stop the stress: *Health promotion and maintenance*	Rebecca's job is busy and stressful. A trip to her doctor earlier that month confirmed that Rebecca has extremely high blood pressure, placing her at risk of various illnesses. He had insisted that she begin taking blood pressure medication but also told her that she must find other ways to reduce her stress and anxiety.
Finding friends, no time for play: *Social participation/play and leisure*	Rebecca has difficulty trusting other people and therefore feels that she has little peer support. She went to counseling during adulthood to try to cope with the rejection, loneliness, fear of abandonment, and depression that she has experienced since her mother left. Because she had to help raise her siblings and even now takes on more than a reasonable share of responsibility at home and work, Rebecca has little opportunity to pursue hobbies. Also, she has few opportunities for social participation.
Taking care of everything and everyone: *Instrumental activities of daily living (IADL) overload*	Rebecca is still taking care of her siblings in addition to her responsibilities to her spouse and child. As a result, she manages several households and supplements her siblings financially as well. This causes marital stress because Rebecca is unable to say no to her siblings, and her spouse and child suffer as a result. When her spouse and/or child express their concerns or displeasure, Rebecca either retreats into isolation or becomes angry and verbally abusive toward them.
"I can't rest, I can't relax, and I can't SLEEP!" Turning off the emotionally dysregulated brain: *Rest and sleep*	Most nights, Rebecca lays in her bed, and she cannot stop thinking about how many things that she didn't finish that day, worried about how she will finish the next day's responsibilities, and feels that she cannot quiet her brain or her emotions. Rebecca sometimes uses alcohol to "quiet her mind." Her husband worries because this is a pattern that seems to be happening more frequently.

Evaluation and Assessment of Emotion Regulation

There are several validated assessments to measure emotional regulation skills, and the impact on overall health and well-being; however, none is specific to OT. The social history interview and occupation-based interview assessment tools are useful in identifying occupational performance issues related to emotion dysregulation. However, naturalistic observation of emotion regulation skills in various contexts may be the most informative.

Developed for adults, the Difficulties in Emotion Regulation Scale (DERS) is a comprehensive assessment that has demonstrated "high internal consistency, good test–retest reliability, and adequate construct and predictive validity" (Gratz & Roemer, 2004, p. 41). The DERS has undergone translation and validation among multiple countries, including Argentina, Brazil, Chile, China, Ecuador, Iran, Italy, Mexico, Portugal, Spain, and Turkey (Cremades et al., 2021; Giromini et al., 2012; Guzmán-González et al., 2014; Li et al., 2018; Machado et al., 2020; Mazaheri, 2015; Navarro Carrascal et al., 2021; Reivan-Ortiz et al., 2020; Veloso et al., 2011; Yigit & Guzey, 2019). Several short versions of the form are available and the DERS is frequently used in research studies.

The DERS was designed to measure the following dimensions of emotion regulation:

- Awareness and acceptance of emotions
- Ability to persist in goal-directed behavior when experiencing negative emotions
- Access to emotion regulation strategies that are perceived to be efficacious

The DERS consists of 36 items that make up the following six subscales with higher scores indicating deficits in emotion regulation:

1. Acceptance of emotional responses
2. Engagement in goal-directed behavior
3. Impulse control
4. Emotional awareness
5. Access to emotion regulation strategies
6. Emotional clarity

One assessment, although not directly measuring emotion regulation, that may be useful to measure affective states is the Positive and Negative Affect Schedule (PANAS). The PANAS is a 20-item assessment that measures positive and negative affective dispositions. High negative affect scores indicate the presence of subjective distress and unpleasant engagement, whereas low negative affect scores represent the absence of these feeling states. High positive affect scores indicate enthusiasm and pleasurable engagement with the environment, whereas low positive affect scores represent a lack of pleasurable engagement and lethargy. Using a large sample of the general adult population, the PANAS demonstrated adequate to good reliability and validity (Crawford & Henry, 2004). Like the DERS, the PANAS has also been translated and validated among diverse populations and found to be effective in clinical and community contexts (Lim et al., 2010; Merz et al., 2013).

Another assessment that might provide an insight on emotional regulation is the Mayer-Salovey-Caruso Emotional Intelligence Test, Version 2.0 (MSCEIT V2.0). This tool is designed as a performance-based assessment of the ability to reason using emotional information, including the capacity to access, perceive, and understand emotions; to use emotional knowledge; and to regulate emotions. It can be administered individually or in groups and presents individuals with eight tasks that require emotional problem-solving. The test has norms based on data from over 5,000 participants in various countries, has demonstrated acceptable reliability and validity, and has been frequently utilized in research (Mayer et al., 2003).

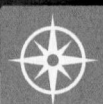

EXPANDING OUR PERSPECTIVES

The Effect of the Cultural Lens of the Therapist

Lisa Mahaffey

In the early 1990s, I worked for an organization providing consultation to long-term care facilities that housed people with significant mental disabilities. Most of the people I consulted for came from black and brown cultural groups. My experiences as a white, cisgendered female, who until then spent my time in primarily white communities, was very different from what I was experiencing in this position. Initially I interpreted actions I observed around emotional regulation, communication, and interpersonal relationships from my perspective and bias. This inevitably translated into assessment, documentation, and consultation that was out of sync with the people I was supposed to be helping. I am grateful to the few people I worked with who were comfortable enough to call me out and engage me in more culturally sensitive discourse. The range and acceptance of personal expression is as much part of diversity as lived experiences, language, and other measures of culture. Although the authors of this chapter speak to a wide application of emotional regulation, the end goal is finding strategies

EXPANDING OUR PERSPECTIVES (*continued*)

and learning skills to manage emotion in pursuit of goal attainment. As with any therapeutic process, the cultural lens of the therapist influences the outcomes of therapy, and as such, the parameters for a "well-regulated" emotion.

I argue that a requirement for emotional regulation has the potential to be a microaggression if bias is unchecked. According to Wing Sue et al. (2007), one of the primary microaggressions is when cultural values and communication styles are pathologized, leading to "the notion that the values and communication styles of the dominant/White culture are ideal" (p. 276). Normal, or ideal, cannot be established without the social construction of that which is abnormal, or not ideal. The potential for our personal bias, established through dominant cultural social construction, is always built in. These "norms" are often expressed through our cliches, for example different sensitivities to social situations might be called out by saying "you have a chip on your shoulder," or more recently, "liberal snowflake." According to Wing Sue et al. (2007), when black and brown people experience a microaggression, they face a double-edged sword. The choice to regulate or suppress their emotional response allows everyone to avoid the negative consequences, or even danger, that can happen when emotions are high. However, research shows that people who suppress emotion in complex interpersonal situations face negative psychologic and physical outcomes (Wing Sue et al., 2007).

Far too often our interventions for those with disabilities are centered around what our society and teachings establish as normal or ideal. Increasingly, the disability community is pushing back on the expectation to work hard to fit in. Although no one would argue with an approach that supports resilience, the expected outcomes for people with disability too often center around

behavior shaping, establishing social interaction skills and tolerance of sensory or social situations. The Neurodiversity Affirming Model (RDs for Neurodiversity, n.d.) states that people who identify as neurodivergent are not sick, or abnormal but part of the variation of humanity. This form of affective justice is respectful of body and emotional autonomy, considers the biases of abelism and sanism, and recognizes the impact of the trauma experienced by people with these identities. A trauma that often includes uncomfortable, sometimes painful therapy that comes with trying to fix people, and a message that acceptance is based on overcoming something that may be an integral part of who they are. McArthur and Gill (2021) remind us that decisions in therapy are ethical decisions. They advocate for incorporating disability ethics, and disability voice in our discourse around JEDI because it will enable us to appreciate the diversity of all human experience, including the variability of emotional expression.

References

McArthur, A. R., & Gill, C. J. (2021). The issue is—Building bridges: Integrating disability ethics into occupational therapy practice. *American Journal of Occupational Therapy, 75*, 7504347010. https//doi.org/10.5014/ajot.2021.044164

Ramzan, N., & Amjad, N. (2017). Cross cultural variation in emotional regulation: A systematic review. *Annals of King Edward Medical University, 23*, 77–90. https://doi.org/10.21649/akemu.v23i1.1512

RDs for Neurodiversity. (n.d.). *The neurodiversity affirming model (NAM).* https://www.rdsforneurodiversity.com/neurodiversity-affirming-model

Wing Sue, D., Capodilupo, C. M., Torino, G. C., Bucceri, J. M., Holder, A. M. B., Nadal, K. L., & Eaquilin, M. (2007). Racial Microaggressions in everyday life: Implications for clinical practice. *American Psychology Association, 62*, 271–286. https://doi.org/10.10370003-066X.62.4.271.

Interventions to Enhance Emotion Regulation

Dialectical Behavior Therapy

Dialectical behavior therapy (DBT) is based on cognitive behavioral principles. Cognitive behavioral intervention approaches are based on evidence that suggests that cognitive processes influence emotional states. These cognitive processes occur when people use situational cues, judgment, and memory to identify the source of their physiologic arousal, to recognize other people's emotions, and to

interpret and respond effectively to emotionally charged situations (Nussbaum, 2001). The term dialectic in this context refers to the tension between acceptance and change (Swales & Dunkley, 2020).

Developed by Linehan (1993a, 1993b), the focus of DBT from the beginning was to "build a life worth living" (Linehan & Wilks, 2015, p. 98). Originally, DBT was designed as an outpatient psychotherapy protocol to treat persons with suicidality and borderline personality disorder (BPD). BPD is considered a pervasive emotional regulation disorder primarily involving the brain's limbic system (amygdala), insula, and PFC (Martin & Ochsner, 2016).

Over time, DBT has been adapted for use with a variety of populations, including persons with eating disorders

(Lenz et al., 2014; Linardon et al., 2017), PTSD (Görg et al., 2017; Meyers et al., 2017), and substance use disorders (Stotts & Northrup, 2015). Although originally developed for use with adults, there is some preliminary evidence that DBT, with age-appropriate modifications, can be effective with children (Perepletchikova et al., 2011).

The DBT philosophy is based on the following principles and assumptions, which are critical to the effectiveness of the approach:

- The individual wants to change and is trying but may not always appear so.
- The individual's emotional responses and behaviors are best understood in the context of personal history and present circumstances.
- The individual is not to blame for their current situation but is responsible for making changes in their life.
- Blaming and labeling the individual as manipulative, deceptive, etc. will not enhance the therapeutic intervention.
- An individual does not fail at DBT, it is the intervention that is not working and needs to be modified (Linehan, 1993a).

DBT combines individual psychotherapy with group-based skills training. Although OT practitioners are not qualified to provide traditional psychotherapy, they are adequately prepared to implement aspects of the DBT skills training component. Moro (2007) describes the use of DBT by OT practitioners in the treatment of persons who engage in non-suicidal self-injury in response to emotion dysregulation.

DBT skills are divided into *acceptance skills* including mindfulness and distress tolerance, and *change skills* including interpersonal effectiveness and emotion regulation (Linehan & Wilks, 2015). Mindfulness training facilitates the awareness of emotional states without judgment and thereby decreases the arousal associated with negative mood states. Mindfulness also encourages living in the moment, observing, interpreting, and experiencing emotions in productive ways to satisfy one's own needs and to meet the demands of the environment. Distress tolerance training facilitates the ability to cope with stressful events, self-soothe, and persist in tasks despite frustration. This requires the capacity to accept the current reality, experience negative emotions without judgment, and thoughtfully determine a course of action. There are four stages of DBT intervention with corresponding goals:

Stage 1: Stabilization and behavioral control
Stage 2: Experience a full range of emotions
Stage 3: Reduce ordinary problems in living
Stage 4: Increase a sense of completeness and find joy in living

Interpersonal effectiveness training facilitates the development of effective communication skills, conflict management, and interpersonal problem-solving. Participants learn how to meet their needs in interpersonal encounters without damaging their relationships with their significant others. Emotion regulation training is designed to help individuals understand their emotions, reduce emotional suffering, and increase emotional resilience. Skills taught include identifying emotions, expressing emotions appropriately, managing difficult emotions, and responding to the feelings of others. Skills develop through acquisition, strengthening, and generalization. Acquisition is learning the basics of the skill; strengthening occurs through repetition, successive approximations and feedback; and generalization is the ability to apply the skill in a variety of contexts (Swales & Dunkley, 2020).

Woods-Jaeger and colleagues (2018) tested an intervention, Dialectical Behavior Therapy Skills Training for Parents (DBT4P), designed to prevent the intergenerational cycle of toxic stress and ACEs. Parents were taught mindfulness and emotion regulation skills to improve their capacity to respond effectively to their children's emotional, behavioral, and developmental needs. The mixed methods study indicated, although there were many barriers to parental participation, that those who completed the training described several benefits, including an increase in confidence in parenting skills, decreased anxiety, and improved interactions and relationships with their children. In addition, participants' scores on measures of depression, parental distress, and difficulties in emotion regulation significantly decreased from pre to post intervention ($P < .05$).

Maffei and colleagues (2018) evaluated the effects of an intensive 3-month DBT skills training program on duration of abstinence and changes in emotion regulation with alcohol-dependent individuals. The initial sample consisted of 244 subjects, 61% male, 39% female, between the ages of 21 and 71. The 157 participants who completed the program demonstrated statistically significant ($P < .001$) improvements in consecutive days of abstinence from alcohol, and in emotion regulation. These results were independent of initial levels of alcohol addiction severity.

The effectiveness of DBT for improving emotion regulation has been validated through research for a variety of populations. OT practitioners who wish to infuse their practice with DBT principles and strategies should participate in continuing education in order to gain knowledge and skills regarding the science and practice of DBT. See OT Story 57.1 for an example.

Emotional Intelligence Interventions

The concept of emotional intelligence (EI) was first introduced into the popular media by Goleman (1995). The Four-Branch Model of Emotional Intelligence posits that a person's emotional quotient (EQ) consists of four skill sets:

OT STORY 57.1 JASON: COPING WITH EMOTION DYSREGULATION ASSOCIATED WITH PTSD

Jason is a 29-year-old veteran of Operation Enduring Freedom (OEF) and Operation Iraqi Freedom (OIF), who presented for treatment nearly a year after his honorable discharge from the Army.

Background

Jason (he/him) was born the youngest of three boys in a small, rural town. He reported "my father was an abusive alcoholic who deserted the family when I was 6 years old." His mother was 24 years old when Jason was born, and she was diagnosed with bipolar disorder when she was 32. He described two significant traumatic events that occurred during his adolescence. When Jason was 12 years old, his mother died by suicide. After his mother's death, he went to live with his maternal grandfather on the family farm. When he was 16 years old, his oldest brother died in a motorcycle crash while intoxicated. Jason admitted to using cannabis daily and binge drinking during high school. Immediately after high school graduation, he enlisted in the military in order to get away from his small hometown and his family.

Jason was deployed three times, once to Afghanistan and twice to Iraq, and served as an Army medic for 10 years. During his deployments, he experienced a number of traumatic incidents. He witnessed convoys being hit by improvised explosive devices (IEDs), and fellow soldiers killed and injured. Some of the wounded he tended to could not be saved. However, Jason reports the most distressing event he witnessed was a small boy who was playing in the street being run over by a tank. When he returned home, he never told anyone about this experience.

Jason mentioned that prior to his deployment, he was proud of being a soldier and protecting his country from terrorism. He indicated that the structure and discipline of basic training was beneficial for him, and he valued the sense of family that developed with his fellow soldiers. Jason met and married his wife between his first and second deployment. She was working as a respiratory therapist in a Veterans Administration hospital where he had gone to visit a friend who was recuperating from surgery. Between his second and third deployment, his son was born. Since his discharge and return home, Jason has been experiencing insomnia, mood swings, hypervigilance, and flashbacks. He was diagnosed with PTSD and is receiving treatment at Veterans Recovery Resources, a nonprofit, community-based intensive outpatient program.

Occupational Therapy Evaluation

Jason arrived 30 minutes early to his first scheduled OT visit. He appeared agitated, uncomfortable, and restless, repositioning himself and getting up and down out of the chair frequently. At one point, he got up and moved to another chair so that he could face the door.

Jason completed the DERS with subscale scores indicating deficits in impulse control, emotional awareness, and access to emotion regulation strategies. The Canadian Occupational Performance Measure (COPM) was used to identify his occupational performance challenges and goals. Jason indicated low levels of performance and satisfaction in sleep, health maintenance, driving, employment seeking, and social participation. In addition, the OT practitioner observed Jason in a group activity using the Comprehensive Occupational Therapy Evaluation (COTE). The COTE indicated strengths in reality orientation, following directions, cooperation, and interest in accomplishments. Deficits were noted in frustration tolerance, problem-solving, and organization.

Goals

Jason indicated his desire to improve his ability to identify, manage, and express his personal thoughts and feelings with his wife. In addition, he wants to work on finding a job, developing new habits, roles, and routines; and finding meaning and purpose in life.

Intervention

As a component of his intensive outpatient treatment program, Jason participated in an OT intervention based on Lifestyle Redesign® principles and DBT. He attended eight OT group sessions, and five individual sessions.

Questions

1. Describe the elements of emotional dysregulation that are illustrated in this case.
2. How has developmental exposure to trauma (adverse childhood experiences) impacted the individual's emotional self-management abilities?
3. Describe the OT theoretical approach(es) that you would use to support your emotional regulation intervention.
4. What principles and assumptions of the DBT philosophy apply to this case?
5. Identify Jason's strengths and discuss how you might incorporate these in the intervention process.
6. Describe specific intervention strategies you would use to address Jason's goals.
7. What discharge recommendations would you make for this individual?

(a) perceiving emotions in self and others, (b) understanding emotional information, (c) incorporating emotions into one's thought processes, and (d) managing or regulating one's emotions (Mayer et al., 2016). Emotion management or regulation (i.e., Branch 4) in this model consists of the ability to:

- Be open to both pleasant and unpleasant emotional feelings
- Monitor and reflect on the reasonability of emotional states
- Engage with emotions if helpful and if not, then disengage
- Maintain, reduce, or increase an emotional response
- Manage one's own emotions
- Respond to the emotions of others (Mayer et al., 2016)

Other aspects of EI are Branches a to c that include:

- Knowledge that an individual possesses regarding how and when emotions can be regulated
- Knowledge of strategies for emotion regulation and when to deploy them
- Ability to implement emotion regulation strategies
- Ability to identify and describe one's emotional experience
- Ability to express one's feelings in words or some other symbolic expression

Many studies have linked EI to overall health and well-being, academic and occupational success, quality of life, and resilience. Over the last 10 years, there has been increased attention to the development of interventions that enhance EQ, but research is still needed in this area. One experimental study consisting of 37 participants (19 in the intervention group and 18 in the control group) evaluated the effectiveness of a psychoeducational approach based on the Four-Branch Model of Emotional Intelligence. The intervention consisted of four weekly sessions of 2.5 hours each. The sessions consisted of mini-lectures, role-play, group discussions, readings, and homework. Results indicated positive changes in trait EI, emotion identification, and emotion management for the intervention group but not for the control group, and the changes were sustained at the 6-month follow-up (Nelis et al., 2009). More recently, videogame-based interventions with adolescents have been conducted to determine impact on EI. Cejudo et al. (2019) found a brief intervention with the Spock videogame statistically improved EI scores on the MSCEIT with 92 adolescents aged 17 to 19. A randomized control trial was performed with 119 adolescents 11 to 15 years old using *emoTIC*, a game-based social–emotional program designed in accordance with Mayer, Caruso, and Salovey's model of EI (de la Barrera et al., 2021). The participants exhibited improvements in self-esteem and balancing affect, as well as managing emotional symptoms, behavioral problems, and hyperactivity. Participants with low to medium anxiety reported improved self-esteem after the intervention; however, no improvements in self-esteem were noted for those with high anxiety.

Social and Emotional Learning

Social and emotional learning (SEL) is a strategy to teach children, adolescents, and adults the skills needed for self-management and the establishment of healthy relationships. These skills include, but are not limited to, identifying and managing one's emotions, initiating and maintaining interpersonal relationships, handling challenges effectively, and making responsible decisions. The overall goal of SEL is to reduce risk factors and enhance resiliency factors for positive adjustment. The five core competencies in SEL are the following:

1. self-awareness
2. self-management
3. social awareness
4. relationship skills
5. responsible decision-making (Collaborative for Academic, Social, and Emotional Learning [CASEL], 2021).

A large-scale meta-analysis indicated that SEL programs are effective for racially and ethnically diverse students at the elementary, middle, and high school levels and can be implemented successfully in both school and after-school settings. The outcomes identified by this study included higher achievement test scores and improved social–emotional skills, prosocial behavior, and attitudes toward self, others, and school for students who participated in SEL. In addition, a reduction in conduct problems and emotional distress was noted (Durlak et al., 2011). A 2021 systematic review found that young people's social and emotional skills were enhanced and symptoms of depression and anxiety reduced by universal SEL interventions (Clarke et al., 2021). The SEL interventions were more effective than mindfulness or positive youth development interventions (Clarke et al., 2021).

The most effective SEL programs incorporated four best practices. These programs were sequenced (S), active (A), focused (F), and explicit (E). This has become known as the SAFE approach to SEL. The interaction of these practices produces greater results than any single factor alone. *Sequenced* means breaking down complex skills into smaller steps and mastering them sequentially within a developmental perspective. *Active learning* involves incorporating opportunities to experiment and practice the skills being taught in various contexts, for example, through role-play and behavioral rehearsal. *Focused* means that sufficient time and attention are allotted for the development of specific skills, and *explicit* refers to the importance of specific, rather than general, learning objectives (Durlak et al., 2011).

Taylor et al. (2017) discovered that SEL approaches are consistently effective across diverse demographic groups in the United States and in international settings. When the focus is on social and emotional assets (i.e., strengths-focused), this helps to support positive social–emotional development among diverse families and geographical context. All SEL interventions must be culturally and contextually relevant to maximize on the benefits of SEL. Wigelsworth et al. (2016) found that the largest effect size for SEL interventions are the ones that keep context and culture at the forefront of the design. A one-size-fits-all approach is not recommended for SEL approaches. Quality SEL programming should arise from authentic and equitable school–family–community partnerships (CASEL, 2021).

Sensory-Based Approaches

Sensory-based approaches to intervention are based on the biologic aspects of emotion regulation and are neuroregulatory in nature. The underlying concept, although not well researched, is that it is possible to regulate emotional states by managing and/or controlling physiologic responses. Sensory integration as a therapeutic approach is designed to help children develop the ability to self-regulate. Self-regulation involves various processes such as sensory modulation and emotion regulation. Sensory integration theory posits that some developmental problems in children are due in part to hyposensitivity or hypersensitivity to sensory stimuli. This undersensitivity or oversensitivity results in emotional hypoarousal or hyperarousal, respectively. Hypoarousal may manifest as flat affect, detachment, withdrawal, depression, and passive–aggressive behavior. Hyperarousal may appear in the form of emotional tantrums, hypervigilance, anxiety, fear, and overreaction to perceived threats (Champagne, 2011). Sensory modulation is the ability to comfort, calm, or alert oneself and to regulate responses to sensory stimuli in order to engage in goal-directed behavior. Self-soothing is an important skill to reduce sensory and emotional arousal when it becomes uncomfortable and distressing. Sensory-based interventions include therapeutic sensorimotor groups, sensory activities, sensory diet, and environmental enhancements such as multisensory rooms (Champagne et al., 2010).

Champagne (2006) describes the use of multisensory rooms as an intervention that addresses the emotion regulation needs of adults with psychiatric disorders. Multisensory rooms are designed to reduce an individual's exposure to chaotic, sensory overload and thereby elicit a relaxation response. This is typically accomplished through the use of muted, soft paint colors; a variety of comfortable seating options; soothing music; and visually appealing imagery. For more information about sensory integration evaluation and intervention, see Chapter 56.

Use of the arts in OT also improves sensory processing. Art making is a sensory activity that is naturally self-soothing. Because emotion regulation is a mind–body phenomenon, embodied multisensory experiences, such as the arts and mindfulness practices, may prove useful in therapy. One study of adults with a variety of mental health challenges, using a multiple case study design, demonstrated the efficacy of an art-based self-soothing kit. An art-based self-soothing kit was defined as "a container, such as a box, bag, or a bin, that contains multi-sensory and multimodal materials that a person uses to engage in meaningful creative and contemplative activities" (Sokmen & Watters, 2016, p. 350). Each participant created their own personalized self-soothing kit. The items chosen to be included in order of frequency were music, gratitude journaling, scented candles, audio meditations, painting, jewelry-making supplies, doodling/coloring, modeling materials, and gardening. During the first 4 weeks, use of the kits varied from every other day to multiple times a day. The length of these self-directed sessions ranged from 15 minutes to 3 hours. The results indicated that making and regularly using the kits fostered self-awareness, interrupted intrusive thoughts and flashbacks, decreased impulsive negative coping behaviors, and improved emotion regulation. An unexpected finding was that the participants used their self-soothing kits as a means of improving social connections and facilitating social participation (Sokmen & Watters, 2016).

❝ COMMENTARY ON THE EVIDENCE

Bailliard and Whigham (2017) conducted a scoping review on the relationship between sensory processing and mental health disorders in order to identify areas in need of further research. Neuroscientific research has identified a link between atypical neurosensory activity and mental health conditions using functional MRIs and electroencephalography. The OT literature primarily focused on sensory rooms in inpatient settings and studies linking occupational participation challenges with sensory processing deficits were limited. Bailliard and Whigham (2017) recommended that more research should be conducted on the efficacy of sensory-based interventions and how it impacts occupational participation for individuals with mental health disorders and atypical sensory

processing. Sensory-based interventions need further research that is replicable and robust.

Although research in this area is limited, there are indications of the effectiveness of various approaches including sensory-based interventions, DBT, emotional intelligence (EI) interventions, social–emotional learning, and strengths-based approaches. Occupational therapy (OT) practitioners and researchers are in a unique position to develop and evaluate occupation-based assessment tools and interventions related to emotion regulation and EI. Future research should focus on the impact of emotional regulation on social and emotional health promotion and maintenance, and how OT can support individuals, groups, and populations in this area of occupation.

Future Directions

Most research in emotion regulation focuses on decreasing and/or managing negative, distressing emotions and behaviors. An alternative approach is to focus on enhancing positive emotions, strengths, and resilience. The health benefits of positive emotion are being documented in the literature. For example, greater optimism predicted better health outcomes among persons with heart disease (Scheier et al., 1999). The mechanisms through which positive emotion impacts health are not yet clear but are likely to involve endocrine and immune system functions (Kiecolt-Glaser et al., 2002).

The ability to access positive emotion is an important aspect of coping. Coping can be described as "conscious, volitional efforts to regulate emotion, cognition, behavior, physiology, and the environment in response to stressful events or circumstances" (Compas et al., 2001, p. 89). Eliciting positive emotions reduces stressful reactions and returns the body to a more balanced state. For example, prompting positive emotions such as gratitude and joy in response to stressful situations resulted in reduced heart rate, blood pressure, and vasoconstriction (Fredrickson & Levenson, 1998).

Cumming et al. (2022) adapted a strengths-based approach used primarily in sport for performance enhancement for youth experiencing homelessness. The psychoeducational intervention, based on mental skills training, offered an opportunity for participants to recognize, develop, apply, refine, and transfer intrapersonal and interpersonal strengths into a variety of contexts to maximize their ability to cope and adapt to stressful situations. Mental skills are the capabilities that enable athletes to effectively manage their thoughts, feelings, and behaviors and ultimately improve their performance. This approach has also been successfully applied in medicine, law enforcement, and the military. Outcomes of the intervention included increased strengths and intentional self-regulation, reduction in risk behaviors, and enhanced self-worth, resilience, and well-being.

Fredrickson's (2001) Broaden and Build Model provides a framework for enhancing positive emotions and resilience. She asserts that negative, distressing emotions narrow an individual's attention and focus to the problem or source of dissatisfaction, whereas positive emotion broadens the field of attention. The broader field of attention facilitates creative problem-solving that builds personal resources and resilience (Fredrickson, 2001). As a result, *broadening* a person's range of attention, cognition, and action and *building* their physical, intellectual, emotional, and social resources can enhance resilience and improve physical and mental health. Positive affect, especially curiosity, also encourages exploration and mastery (Peterson & Seligman, 2004).

Conclusion

Effective OT interventions focus on helping individuals participate in meaningful occupations. For some individuals, emotional dysregulation impairs occupational performance and limits participation. In addition, adults with emotion regulation difficulties report more physical and cognitive fatigue, less overall satisfaction with life, and less satisfaction with performance of daily activities (Hebert, 2017).

It is for this reason that OT practitioners must attend to and attempt to enhance the emotional regulation and EI of the people they serve. However, emotion regulation skills cannot be considered in isolation. They must be addressed in the context of the individual's desired and meaningful occupations; their habits, roles, and routines; and their values and beliefs. In addition, emotion regulation is a complex phenomenon that requires attention to be paid to the physiologic, cognitive, affective, behavioral, and motivational aspects of the individual. Our unique role as OT clinicians is to help people find successful strategies to support emotional regulation within the context of occupational performance and identify the appropriate contextual supports that are needed to enhance emotion regulation and thereby facilitate occupational participation.

Lippincott® Connect *For additional resources on the subjects discussed in this chapter, visit Lippincott Connect.*

REFERENCES

American Occupational Therapy Association. (2020). Occupational therapy practice framework: Domain and process (4th edition). *American Journal of Occupational Therapy*, 74(Suppl. 2), S1–S87. https://doi.org/10.5014/ajot.2020.74S2001

Bailliard, A. L., & Whigham, S. C. (2017). Linking neuroscience, function, and intervention: A scoping review of sensory processing and mental illness. *American Journal of Occupational Therapy*, 71(5), 1–18. https://doi.org/10.5014/ajot.2017.024497

Beer, J. S., & Lombardo, M. V. (2007). Insights into emotion regulation from neuropsychology. In J. J. Gross (Ed.), *Handbook of emotion regulation* (pp. 69–86). Guilford Press.

Benson, L., English, T., Conroy, D. E., Pincus, A. L., Gerstorf, D., & Ram, N. (2019). Age differences in emotion regulation strategy use, variability, and flexibility: An experience sampling approach. *Developmental Psychology*, 55(9), 1951–1964. https://doi.org/10.1037/dev0000727

Berkman, E. T., & Lieberman, M. D. (2009). Using neuroscience to broaden emotion regulation: Theoretical and methodological considerations. *Social and Personality Psychology Compass*, 3, 475–493. https://doi.org/10.1111/j.1751-9004.2009.00186.x

Birditt, K. S., Fingerman, K. L., & Almeida, D. M. (2005). Age differences in exposure and reactions to interpersonal tensions: A daily diary study. *Psychology and Aging*, 20, 330–340. https://doi.org/10.1037/0882-7974.20.2.330

Bowlby, J. (1978). Attachment theory and its therapeutic implications. *Adolescent Psychiatry*, 6, 5–33.

Calkins, S. D., & Hill, A. (2007). Caregiver influences on emerging emotion regulation: Biological and environmental transactions in early development. In J. J. Gross (Ed.), *Handbook of emotion regulation* (pp. 229–248). Guilford Press.

Cejudo, J., López-Delgado, M. L., & Losada, L. (2019). Effectiveness of the videogame "Spock" for the improvement of the emotional intelligence on psychosocial adjustment in adolescents. *Computers in Human Behavior, 101*, 380–386. https://doi.org/10.1016/j.chb.2018.09.028

Champagne, T. (2006). Creating sensory rooms: Environmental enhancements for acute inpatient mental health settings. *Mental Health Special Interest Section Quarterly, 29*(4), 1–4.

Champagne, T. (2011). *Sensory modulation & environment: Essential elements of occupation* (3rd ed.). Pearson.

Champagne, T., Koomar, J., & Olson, L. (2010). Sensory processing evaluation and intervention in mental health. *OT Practice, 15*(5), CE1–CE7.

Choi, K. R., Stewart, T., Fein, E., McCreary, M., Kenan, K. N., Davies, J. D., Naureckas, S., & Zima, B. T. (2020). The impact of attachment-disrupting adverse childhood experiences on child behavioral health. *The Journal of Pediatrics, 221*, 224–229. https://doi.org/10.1016/j.jpeds.2020.03.006

Clarke, A., Sorgenfrei, M., Mulcahy, J., Davie, P., Friedrich, C., & McBride, T. (2021). *Adolescent mental health: A systematic review on the effectiveness of school-based interventions.* Early Intervention Foundation.

Cole, P. M., Martin, S. E., & Dennis, R. A. (2004). Emotion regulation as a scientific construct: Methodological challenges and directions for child development research. *Child Development, 75*, 317–333. https://doi.org/10.1111/j.1467-8624.2004.00673.x

Collaborative for Academic, Social, and Emotional Learning. (2021). *What is the CASEL framework?* Retrieved December 30, 2021, from https://casel.org/fundamentals-of-sel/what-is-the-casel-framework/

Compas, B. E., Connor, J. K., Saltzman, H., Thomsen, A. H., & Wadsworth, M. E. (2001). Coping with stress during childhood and adolescence: Problems, progress, and potential in theory and research. *Psychological Bulletin, 127*, 87–127. https://psycnet.apa.org/doi/10.1037/0033-2909.127.1.87

Cook, A., Spinazzola, J., Ford, J., Lanktree, C., Blaustein, M., Cloitre, M., DeRosa, R., Hubbard, R., Kagan, R., Liautaud, J., Mallah, K., Olafson, E., & van der Kolk, B. (2005). Complex trauma in children and adolescents. *Psychiatric Annals, 35*, 390–398. https://doi.org/10.3928/00485713-20050501-05

Crawford, J. R., & Henry, J. D. (2004). The Positive and Negative Affect Schedule (PANAS): Construct validity, measurement properties and normative data in a large non-clinical sample. *British Journal of Clinical Psychology, 43*, 245–265. https://doi.org/10.1348/0144665031752934

Cremades, C. F., Garay, C. J., Etchevers, M. J., Muiños, R., Peker, G. M., & Gómez Penedo, J. M. (2021, November 9). Difficulties in Emotion Regulation Scale (DERS): Adaptation and validation for its use in adults in the Metropolitan Area of Buenos Aires (Argentina) [Escala de Dificultades en la Regulación Emocional (Difficulties in Emotion Regulation Scale [DERS]): Adaptación y validación para su uso en adultos en el Área Metropolitana de Buenos Aires (Argentina)]. *PsyArXiv.* https://doi.org/10.31234/osf.io/5fsu7

Cumming, J., Whiting, R., Parry, B. J., Clarke, F. J., Holland, M. J., Cooley, S. J., & Quinton, M. L. (2022). The My Strengths Training for Life program: Rationale, logic model, and description of a strengths-based intervention for young people experiencing homelessness. *Evaluation and Program Planning, 91*, 102045. https://doi.org/10.1016/j.evalprogplan.2021.102045

Davidson, R. J., Fox, A., & Kalin, N. H. (2007). Neural bases of emotion regulation in nonhuman primates and humans. In J. J. Gross (Ed.), *Handbook of emotion regulation* (pp. 47–68). Guilford Press.

de la Barrera, U., Mónaco, E., PostigoZegarra, S., Gil-Gómez, J-A., & Montoya-Castilla, I. (2021). EmoTIC: Impact of a game-based social-emotional programme on adolescents. *PLoS One, 16*(4), e0250384. https://doi.org/10.1371/journal.pone.0250384

Durlak, J. A., Weissberg, R. P., Dymnicki, A. B., Taylor, R. D., & Schellinger, K. B. (2011). The impact of enhancing students' social and emotional learning: A meta-analysis of school-based universal interventions. *Child Development, 82*, 405–432. https://doi.org/10.1111/j.1467-8624.2010.01564.x

Eisenberg, N., Fabes, R. A., Guthrie, I. K., & Reiser, M. (2000). Dispositional emotionality and regulation: Their role in predicting quality of social functioning. *Journal of Personality and Social Psychology, 78*, 136–157. https://doi.org/10.1037//0022-3514.78.1.136

Eisenberg, N., Hofer, C., Sulik, M. J., & Spinrad, T. L. (2014). Self-regulation, effortful control, and their socioemotional correlates. In J. J. Gross (Ed.), *Handbook of emotion regulation* (pp. 157–172). Guilford Press.

Eisenberg, N., & Spinrad, T. L. (2004). Emotion-related regulation: Sharpening the definition. *Child Development, 75*, 334–339. https://doi.org/10.1111/j.1467-8624.2004.00674.x

Fox, N. A., & Calkins, S. D. (2003). The development of self-control of emotion: Intrinsic and extrinsic influences. *Motivation and Emotion, 27*, 7–26. https://doi.org/10.1023/A:1023622324898

Fredrickson, B. L. (2001). The role of positive emotions in positive psychology. The broaden-and-build theory of positive emotions. *The American Psychologist, 56*(3), 218–226. https://doi.org/10.1037//0003-066x.56.3.218

Fredrickson, B. L., & Levenson, R. W. (1998). Positive emotions speed recovery from the cardiovascular sequelae of negative emotions. *Cognition & Emotion, 12*(2), 191–220. https://doi.org/10.1080/026999398379718

Giano, Z., Wheeler, D. L., & Hubach, R. D. (2020). The frequencies and disparities of adverse childhood experiences in the U.S. *BMC Public Health, 20*, 1327–1339. https://doi.org/10.1186/s12889-020-09411-z

Giromini, L., Velotti, P., de Campora, G., Bonalume, L., & Cesare Zavattini, G. (2012). Cultural adaptation of the difficulties in emotion regulation scale: reliability and validity of an Italian version. *Journal of Clinical Psychology, 68*(9), 989–1007. https://doi.org/10.1002/jclp.21876

Giroux, J. L., McLaughlin, R., & Scheinholz, M. (2019). Emotion. In C. Brown, V. C. Stoffel, & J. P. Muñoz (Eds.), *Occupational therapy in mental health: A vision for participation.* F. A. Davis.

Goleman, D. (1995). *Emotional intelligence: Why it can matter more than IQ.* Bantam Books.

Görg, N., Priebe, K., Böhnke, J. R., Steil, R., Dyer, A. S., & Kleindienst, N, (2017). Trauma-related emotions and radical acceptance in dialectical behavior therapy for posttraumatic stress disorder after childhood sexual abuse. *Borderline Personality Disorder and Emotion Dysregulation, 4*, 1–12. https://doi.org/10.1186/s40479-017-0065-5

Gratz, K. L., & Roemer, L. (2004). Multidimensional assessment of emotion regulation and dysregulation: Development, factor structure, and initial validation of the Difficulties in Emotion Regulation Scale. *Journal of Psychopathology and Behavioral Assessment, 26*, 41–54. https://doi.org/10.1023/B:JOBA.0000007455.08539.94

Gross, J. J. (2014). Emotion regulation: Conceptual and empirical foundations. In J. J. Gross (Ed.), *Handbook of emotion regulation* (pp. 3–20). Guilford Press.

Guzmán-González, M., Trabucco, C., Urzúa, M. A., Garrido, L., & Leiva, J. (2014). Validez y Confiabilidad de la Version Adaptada al Español de la Escala de Dificultades de Regulación Emocional (DERS-E) en Población Chilena [Validity and reliability of the Adapted Spanish Version of the Difficulties in Emotion Regulation Scale in Chilean population]. *Terapia Psicológica, 32*(1), 19–29. https://doi.org/10.4067/S0718-48082014000100002

Hebert, K. (2017). The relationship between emotion regulation and quality of life in healthy adults: Implications for occupational therapy. *American Journal of Occupational Therapy, 71*(4_Suppl. 1), 7111505138p1. https://doi.org/10.5014/ajot.2017.71S1-PO5107

Hughes, D. (2004). An attachment-based treatment of maltreated children and young people. *Attachment & Human Development, 6*(3), 263–278. https://doi.org/10.1080/14616730412331281539

Izard, C. E. (2010). The many meanings/aspects of emotion: Definitions, functions, activation, and regulation. *Emotion Review, 2,* 363–370. https://doi.org/10.1177/1754073910374661

Johnstone, T., & Walter, H. (2014). The neural basis of emotional dysregulation. In J. J. Gross (Ed.), *Handbook of emotion regulation* (pp. 58–71). Guilford Press.

Karl, A., Schaefer, M., Malta, L. S., Dörfel, D., Rohleder, N., & Werner, A. (2006). A meta-analysis of structural brain abnormalities in PTSD. *Neuroscience and Biobehavioral Reviews, 30,* 1004–1031. https://doi.org/10.1016/j.neubiorev.2006.03.004

Kiecolt-Glaser, J. K., McGuire, L., Robles, T., & Glaser, R. (2002). Emotions, morbidity, and mortality: New perspectives from psychoneuroimmunology. *Annual Reviews of Psychology, 53,* 83–107. https://doi.org/10.1146/annurev.psych.53.100901.135217

Kiecolt-Glaser, J. K., & Wilson, S. J. (2017). Lovesick: How couples' relationships influence health. *Annual Reviews of Clinical Psychology, 13*(1), 421–443. https://doi.org/10.1146/annurev-clinpsy-032816-045111

Korja, R., Nolvi, S., Grant, K. A., & McMahon, C. (2017). The relations between maternal prenatal anxiety or stress and child's early negative reactivity or self-regulation: A systematic review. *Child Psychiatry & Human Development, 48,* 851–869. https://doi.org/10.1007/s10578-017-0709-0

Lenz, A. S., Taylor, R., Fleming, M., & Serman, N. (2014). Effectiveness of dialectical behavior therapy for treating eating disorders. *Journal of Counseling and Development, 92*(1), 26–35. https://doi.org/10.1002/j.1556-6676.2014.00127.x

Li, J., Han, Z. R., Gao, M. M., Sun, X., & Ahemaitijiang, N. (2018). Psychometric properties of the Chinese version of the Difficulties in Emotion Regulation Scale (DERS): Factor structure, reliability, and validity. *Psychological Assessment, 30*(5), e1–e9. https://doi.org/10.1037/pas0000582

Lim, Y. J., Yu, B. H., Kim, D. K., & Kim, J. H. (2010). The positive and negative affect schedule: Psychometric properties of the Korean version. *Psychiatry Investigation, 7*(3), 163–169. https://doi.org/10.4306/pi.2010.7.3.163

Linardon, J., Fairburn, C. G., Fitzsimmons-Craft, E. E., Wilfley, D. E., & Brennan, L. (2017). The empirical status of the third wave behaviour therapies for the treatment of eating disorders: A systematic review. *Clinical Psychology Review, 58,* 125–140. https://doi.org/10.1016/j.cpr.2017.10.005

Linehan, M. M. (1993a). *Cognitive-behavioral treatment of borderline personality disorder.* Guilford Press.

Linehan, M. M. (1993b). *Skills training manual for treating borderline personality disorder.* Guilford Press.

Linehan, M. M., & Wilks, C. R. (2015). The course and evolution of dialectical behavior therapy. *American Journal of Psychotherapy, 69*(2), 97–110. https://doi.org/10.1176/appi.psychotherapy.2015.69.2.97

Lopes, P. N., Salovey, P., Coté, S., & Beers, M. (2005). Emotion regulation abilities and the quality of social interaction. *Emotion, 5*(1), 113–118. https://doi.org/10.1037/1528-3542.5.1.113

Machado, B. M., Gurgel, L. G., Boeckel, M. G., & Reppold, C. T. (2020). Evidences of validity of the Difficulties in Emotion Regulation Scale —DERS. *Paidéia (Ribeirão Preto) [online], 30,* e3017. https://doi.org/10.1590/1982-4327e3017

Maffei, C., Cavicchioli, M., Movalli, M., Cavallaro, R., & Fossati, A. (2018). Dialectical behavior therapy skills training in alcohol dependence treatment: Findings based on an open trial. *Substance Use & Misuse, 53*(14), 2368–2385. https://doi.org/10.1080/10826084.2018.1480035

Mahoney, M. J. (2005). Constructivism and positive psychology. In C. R. Snyder & S. J. Lopez (Eds.), *Handbook of positive psychology* (pp. 745–750). Oxford University Press.

Martin, R. E. & Ochsner, K. N. (2016). The neuroscience of emotion regulation development: Implications for education. *Current Opinion in Behavioral Sciences, 10,* 142–148. https://doi.org/10.1016/j.cobeha.2016.06.006

Mayer, J., Caruso, D., & Salovey, P. (2016). The ability model of emotional intelligence: Principles and updates. *Emotion Review, 8*(4), 290–300. https://doi.org/10.1177/1754073916639667

Mayer, J., Salovey, P., Caruso, D., & Sitarenios, G. (2003). Measuring emotional intelligence with the MSCEIT V2.0. *Emotion, 3*(1), 97–105. https://doi.org/10.1037/1528-3542.3.1.97

Mazaheri, M. (2015). Psychometric properties of the Persian version of the Difficulties in Emotion Regulation Scale DERS-6 & DERS-5-revised (in an Iranian clinical sample). *Iranian Journal of Psychiatry, 10*(2), 115–122.

Mennin, D. S., Heimberg, R. G., Turk, C. L., & Fresco, D. M. (2005). Preliminary evidence for an emotion dysregulation model of generalized anxiety disorder. *Behaviour Research and Therapy, 43*(10), 1281–1310. https://doi.org/10.1016/j.brat.2004.08.008

Merrick, M. T., Ford, D. C., Ports, K. A., & Guinn, A. S. (2018). Prevalence of adverse childhood experiences from the 2011–2014 Behavioral Risk Factor Surveillance System in 23 States. *JAMA Pediatrics, 172,* 1038–1044. doi:10.1001/jamapediatrics.2018.2537

Merz, E. L., Malcarne, V. L., Roesch, S. C., Ko, C. M., Emerson, M., Roma, V. G., & Sadler, G. R. (2013). Psychometric properties of Positive and Negative Affect Schedule (PANAS) original and short forms in an African American community sample. *Journal of Affective Disorders, 151*(3), 942–949. https://doi.org/10.1016/j.jad.2013.08.011

Meyers, L., Voller, E. K., McCallum, E. B., Thuras, P., Shallcross, S., Velasquez, T., & Meis, L. (2017). Treating veterans with PTSD and borderline personality symptoms in a 21-week intensive outpatient setting: Findings from a pilot program. *Journal of Traumatic Stress, 30*(2), 178–181. https://doi.org/10.1002/jts.22174

Mikulincer, M., & Shaver, P. R. (2019). Attachment orientations and emotion regulation. *Current Opinion in Psychology, 25,* 6–10. https://doi.org/10.1016/j.copsyc.2018.02.006

Moro, C. D. (2007). A comprehensive literature review defining self-mutilation and occupational therapy intervention approaches: Dialectical behavior therapy and sensory integration. *Occupational Therapy in Mental Health, 23*(1), 55–67. https://doi.org/10.1300/J004v23n01_04

Navarro Carrascal, O., Restrepo Ochoa, D. A., Rommel, D., Ghalaret, J.-M., & Fleury-Bahi, G. (2021). Validation of a brief version of the Difficulties in Emotion Regulation Scale with a Spanish speaking population (DERS-S SF). *CES Psicología, 14*(2), 71–88. https://doi.org/10.21615/cesp.5360

Neacsiu, A. D., Bohus, M., & Linehan, M. M. (2014). Dialectical behavior therapy: An intervention for emotion dysregulation. In J. J. Gross (Ed.), *Handbook of emotion regulation* (pp. 491–507). Guilford Press.

Nelis, D., Quoidbach, J., Mikolajczak, M., & Hansenne, M. (2009). Increasing emotional intelligence: (How) is it possible? *Personality and Individual Differences, 47*(1), 36–41. https://doi.org/10.1016/j.paid.2009.01.046

Nussbaum, M. C. (2001). *Upheavals of thought: The intelligence of emotions.* Cambridge University Press.

Ochsner, K. N., & Gross, J. J. (2014, this volume). The neural bases of emotion and emotion regulation: A valuation perspective. In J. J. Gross (Ed.), *Handbook of emotion regulation* (3rd ed., pp. 23–42). Guilford Press.

Perepletchikova, F., Axelrod, S. R., Kaufman, J., Rounsaville, B. J., Douglas-Palumberi, H., & Miller, A. L. (2011). Adapting dialectical behavior therapy for children: Towards a new research agenda for pediatric suicidal and non-suicidal self-injurious behaviors. *Child and Adolescent Mental Health, 16*(2), 116–121. https://doi.org/10.1111/j.1475-3588.2010.00583.x

Price, J. L., & Drevets, W. C. (2012). Neural circuits underlying the pathophysiology of mood disorders. *Trends in Cognitive Sciences, 16*(1), 61–71. https://doi.org/10.1016/j.tics.2011.12.011

Peterson, C., & Seligman, M. E. P. (2004). *Character strengths and virtues: A handbook and classification.* Oxford University Press.

Reivan-Ortiz, G. G., Ortiz Rodas, P. E., & Reivan Ortiz, P. N. (2020). A Brief Version of the Difficulties in Emotion Regulation Scale (DERS): Validity evidence in Ecuadorian population. *International Journal of Psychological Research, 13*(2), 14–24. https://doi.org/10.21500/20112084.4325

Rothbart, M. K. (2011). *Becoming who we are: Temperament and personality in development.* Guilford Press.

Rothbart, M. K., & Bates, J. E. (2006). Temperament. In W. Damon & N. Eisenberg (Eds.), *Handbook of child psychology: Vol. 3. Social, emotional, and personality development* (6th ed., pp. 99–166). Wiley.

Sbarra, D. A., Hasselmo, K., & Bourassa, K. J. (2015). Divorce and health: Beyond individual differences. *Current Directions in Psychological Science, 24*(2), 109–113. https://doi.org/10.1177/0963721414559125

Scheier, M. F., Matthews, K. A., Owens, J. F., Schulz, R., Bridges, M. W., Magovern, G. J., & Carver, C. S. (1999). Optimism and rehospitalization after coronary artery bypass graft surgery. *Archives of Internal Medicine, 159*(8), 829–835. https://doi.org/10.1001/archinte.159.8.829

Scheinholz, M. (2011). Emotion Regulation. In C. Brown & V. C. Stoffel, (Eds.), *Occupational Therapy in Mental Health* (pp. 350-351). F.A. Davis Company.

Schore, A. (2003). *Affect dysregulation and disorders of the self.* Norton.

Sokmen, Y. C., & Watters, A. (2016). Emotion regulation with mindful arts activities using a personalized self-soothing kit. *Occupational Therapy in Mental Health, 32*(4), 345–369. https://doi.org/10.1080/0164212X.2016.1165642

Stotts, A. L., & Northrup, T. F. (2015). The promise of third-wave behavioral therapies in the treatment of substance use disorders. *Current Opinion in Psychology, 2,* 75–81. https://doi.org/10.1016/j.copsyc.2014.12.028

Suveg, C., & Zeman, J. (2004). Emotion regulation in children with anxiety disorders. *Journal of Clinical Child and Adolescent Psychology, 33*(4), 750–759. https://doi.org/10.1207/s15374424jccp3304_10

Swales, M., & Dunkley, C. (2020). Principles of skills assessment in dialectical behavior therapy. *Cognitive and Behavioral Practice, 27*(1), 18–29. https://doi.org/10.1016/j.cbpra.2019.05.001

Taylor, R. D., Oberle, E., Durlak, J. A., & Weissberg, R. P. (2017), Promoting positive youth development through school-based social and emotional learning interventions: A meta-analysis of follow-up effects. *Child Development, 88,* 1156–1171. https://doi.org/10.1111/cdev.12864

van der Kolk, B. A. (2003). The neurobiology of childhood trauma and abuse. *Child and Adolescent Psychiatric Clinics of North America, 12*(2), 293–317. https://doi.org/10.1016/S1056-4993(03)00003-8

Veloso, M., Pinto-Gouveia, J., & Dinis, A. (2011). Estudos de validação com a versão portuguesa da Escala de Dificuldades na Regulação Emocional (EDRE). *Psychologica, 54,* 87–110. https://doi.org/10.36315/2019inpact060

Wigelsworth, M., Lendrum, A., Oldfield, J., Scott, A., ten Bokkel, I., Tate, K., & Emery, C. (2016). The impact of trial stage, developer involvement and international transferability on universal social and emotional learning programme outcomes: A meta-analysis. *Cambridge Journal of Education, 46*(3), 347–376. https://doi.org/10.1080/0305764X.2016.1195791

Woods-Jaeger, B. A., Sexton, C. C., Gardner, B., Siedlik, E., Slagel, L., Tezza, V., & O'Malley, D. (2018). Development, feasibility, and refinement of a toxic stress prevention research program. *Journal of Child and Family Studies, 27*(11), 3531–3543. https://doi.org/10.1007/s10826-018-1178-1

Yigit, I., & Guzey, M. (2019). Psychometric properties of Turkish version of Difficulties in Emotion Regulation Scale-Brief Form (DERS-16). *Current Psychology, 38,* 1503–1511. https://doi.org/10.1007/s12144-017-9712-7

Social Interaction and Occupational Performance

Lou Ann Griswold and C. Douglas Simmons

LEARNING OBJECTIVES

After reading this chapter, you will be able to:

1. Discuss the importance of addressing social interaction skills as critical for engagement in all areas of occupation.
2. Compare assessment approaches evaluating social interaction.
3. Identify factors that influence the quality of social interaction.
4. Evaluate intervention approaches to support social interaction skills.
5. Discuss how to support the quality of social interaction during a person's occupational engagement.

Introduction

People are social beings, and many occupations in which people engage involve social interaction with others. Social participation is one of nine occupations identified within the Occupational Therapy Practice Framework (OTPF-4) (American Occupational Therapy Association [AOTA], 2020). The AOTA describes social participation as "activities that involve social interaction with others" (p. 34), such as participation in the community and engaging with family and friends. Such engagement supports other areas of occupation, including work, leisure, play, education, and instrumental activities of daily living (IADLs), which require social interaction. For example, children interact with one another as they play together, do school projects, and share information about their day with their families. Teens spend a large amount of their time interacting with their peers inside and outside of school as they participate in music groups, theater, team sports, volunteering, after-school programming at a Boys or Girls Club, or casually discussing events of the day. Adults interact with others when they participate in a variety of tasks at work, at home, and in the community. Depending on the circumstances, personal activities of daily living (ADLs) and rest and sleep might also involve social interaction with others. Like other areas of occupation, social participation supports engagement in other occupations along with being a distinct area of occupation.

Depending on the occupational context, interacting with others requires a variety of intended purposes of social interaction including decision-making, collaborating, sharing information, gathering information, and conversing socially. For example, friends may prepare a meal together, which is an IADL. In doing so, they may decide who will make different dishes of the meal or who will chop the ingredients and who will do the mixing. Thus, they are *making decisions*. They then may *collaborate* to share the needed tools and cooking space. One person might *share information* regarding the recipe. All social exchanges, regardless of the intended purpose, require similar skills to support interaction (see social interaction skills discussed in Chapter 52). People initiate interaction or respond to another person's greeting to begin a social interaction. They communicate using words (i.e., speech, augmentative device, or sign language) and gestures. Furthermore, they ask questions, respond to a social partner, and take turns to support the ongoing interaction. A person also responds to messages sent by a social partner, clarifying, encouraging the other person to sustain the interaction, and empathizing as relevant. Specific expectations and demands for skills may vary with the context of the social exchange and social partners, yet each of these skills is observable during an in-person social interaction. In a virtual interaction, some social interaction skills are not possible to evaluate, for example considering how close or far a person positions themselves to a social partner. However, other skills may be particularly critical to sustain an interaction, such as providing adequate detail when responding to another person or asking questions to encourage ongoing interaction.

Because most occupations require social interaction, having difficulty interacting with others potentially influences all areas of occupation, significantly limiting full occupational participation. In fact, difficulty with social interaction skills may be *the* limiting factor for full participation in work, leisure, or IADLs. For example, the friends who are preparing a meal together may demonstrate the motor and process skills to do their tasks in meal preparation, but one person may demonstrate challenges when interacting with the others in the group. That person may not ask questions, or not respond to another person's question, or not clarify when necessary, or the person may use a judgmental tone when responding that could result in a negative experience for the persons engaged in the cooking task. As a result, the cooking experience may not be satisfying to all persons participating. Observing and noting the quality of each social interaction skill provides a way to describe the difficulty a person may be demonstrating when interacting with others, leading to decreased occupational engagement.

Social interaction skills are critical to one's success in occupations of work, education, play, and leisure and social participation in the community (Byom et al., 2020; Dillon et al., 2021; Hendricks & Wehman, 2009; Morgan & Schultz, 2012; Mulder & Cashin, 2014). In a longitudinal study, Jones et al. (2015) found social skills in children were associated with later success as adults regardless of other predictors. Lexén and Bejerholm (2016) found a correlation between social interaction skills and the number of hours worked in competitive employment and greater income for people with mental illness. Although practitioners are aware of the importance of social interaction skills for people of all ages and with various conditions, much of the research has focused on children and those with autism spectrum disorder (ASD; Verhoeven et al., 2013). However, researchers within occupational therapy (OT) have examined the influence of social interaction for people with mental health diagnoses (Søndergaard & Fisher, 2012; Williams & Chard, 2016), acquired or traumatic brain injury (Byom et al., 2020; Simmons & Griswold, 2010), and people with intellectual/developmental disabilities (Fisher et al., 2017). Collectively, the research in OT supports the importance of evaluating the quality of social interaction, and providing intervention to improve social interaction skills is relevant when working with a wide range of populations. Supporting persons' quality of social interaction during their desired occupations in natural contexts in which they spend time with others would influence their success in enhanced participation.

Assessment of Social Interaction

Because of the importance of social interaction, professionals from other disciplines evaluate and provide intervention to enhance this area of skills. Assessments of social interaction have primarily taken two forms: report by the person or others (e.g., parents or teachers) and observation (Dillon et al., 2021; Norbury, 2014). Assessments based on report are frequently in the form of checklists. Report by others allows for assessment of social communication and interaction in context in which the reporter is familiar. Dillon and colleagues (2021) identified limitations in relying on a report by others, including the quality of the relationship between informant and person, the socioeconomic status and educational level of the informant, and person's behaviors. It is important to note that adult persons may provide a self-report that may not provide the perspective of others (Byom et al., 2020). Furthermore, informants, whether the person or someone else, usually lack training to identify specific social interaction skills that may be limiting overall quality of social interaction (Dillon et al., 2021).

Observation of structured interactions provide a more objective measure of social interaction. Such observations may be contrived or "set up" to elicit certain behaviors or may be conducted in a natural context. Because the role-play situations are predetermined, they allow for a standardized observation. Assessments based on role-play reflect contrived situations based on social situations that are believed to be important to many people, but these may not be relevant situations to all persons. Assessments using role-play are common in mental health settings. An example of such an assessment was developed by Tsang and Pearson (2000) to evaluate social skills and to prepare persons with mental illness for work. Their evaluation included two work-related role-play situations: a job interview and requesting time off from work. Tsang and Pearson's assessment also included a self-report. Bellack et al. (2006) believed that assessments based on role-play provide information on a person's "behavioral capacity" rather than "real life performance" (p. 350). Although observing structured interactions allows for reliability and opportunity to evaluate change over time, the situation lacks cultural and contextual information and often the evaluator is unfamiliar to the person being observed,

influencing the person's performance (Dillon et al., 2021; Norbury, 2014). Using standardized narratives is another observational approach, often used by speech and language pathologists, for example having a child tell a story from a picture book or having a child tell a story after being prompted by a beginning story line. While providing a standardized measure, this approach does not provide understanding of how the child interacts in a natural context when interacting with usual social partners (Norbury, 2014). The need for an observation of social interaction in a natural context by an evaluator who is trained to observe specific skills and performance is evident. For more on culturally responsive interaction, see Expanding Our Perspectives.

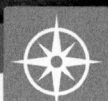

EXPANDING OUR PERSPECTIVES
Culturally Responsive Interaction

Rebecca Lord and Jaime Phillip Muñoz

Evaluation requires social interaction. Practitioners rely on the person they are assessing to make decisions, collaborate, and share information. For my doctoral capstone project, I (R.L.) explored occupational profiles of middle-school-aged refugee youth. My goal was to understand their needs and inform program development. Most of the displaced children I worked with spent their early childhood living in refugee camps. These youth often spoke three or more languages, but most were not proficient in any of these.

Communication and cultural barriers were significant. Having an interpreter present didn't guarantee effective communication. It was clear I needed to build trust, attend to the emotional needs of these children, and create a space for interaction that was grounded in respect and reciprocity. Reflecting on my early attempts, I identified several situations when I failed to create such a space. For example, when using the Child Occupational Self-Assessment, I noticed that many children would repeat the same answer for multiple questions in a row, despite an interpreter being present.

I began offering games for the children to choose from. We would engage in this activity until the child seemed comfortable interacting, then I presented a structured assessment. I implemented sensory breaks offering a choice of modulation strategies depending on the child's state of arousal. Sessions always ended with another activity chosen by the child. Play activities created opportunities to explore social participation. I learned that in many situations their efforts to interact in English were disparaged by teachers and peers. As a result, many avoided speaking at all, which only exacerbated social isolation and occupational deprivation. I learned key phrases in the first

languages of these children and clumsily tried to use these during sessions. This always created laughter and opportunities for them to teach me pronunciation and grammar. Communicating unconditional acceptance of their language abilities and playfully modeling my own difficulties with language created a shift in our social interactions. Many children became more confident using English and relied less on interpreters.

Incorporating assessments with nonverbal communication elements offered the children new options for interaction. The KAWA, which integrates drawing in the assessment process resonated with the children. Giving children space to creatively express themselves and using probes specific to their drawings created breakthroughs in our interactions. Children shared experiences and initiated storytelling with me, and also with family and friends. These stories generated opportunities for reframing and celebrating strengths each child had exhibited throughout their resettlement journeys. Encouraging them to label their strengths became a springboard for problem-solving how to overcome current challenges limiting participation. Other strategies included incorporating humor, particularly when a child started to struggle with attention or became frustrated. Incorporating child-selected music and dancing served as a sensory regulation strategy and provided opportunities for the child to share elements of their culture with me. Involving interpreters, siblings, and caregivers when possible allowed for increased communication among all parties. Participating in family rituals such as greetings or the sharing of meals increased trust with the family unit and supported carryover from sessions to everyday life. This experience was a lesson in cultural humility for me. It reinforced the critical need to purposely engage in supportive, intentional interactions with others, particularly persons with diverse cultural identities.

Occupational Therapy Assessment of Social Interaction

Two assessment tools have been developed by occupational therapists to evaluate social interaction skills: the *Assessment of Communication and Interaction Skills* (ACIS; Forsyth et al., 1998) and the *Evaluation of Social Interaction* (ESI; Fisher & Griswold, 2009, 2018). For both assessments, therapists rate the social interaction skills using a 4-point criterion-referenced scale indicating the person's level of competence for each skill.

When administering the ACIS, the OT practitioner observes the person during two or more social situations. Options for situations include interacting during (a) one-on-one conversations with another person to discuss a topic, (b) parallel tasks in which people work individually on tasks but near others, (c) cooperative groups in which several people interact to complete a task or play a game, and (d) open interactions without a preplanned agenda or limited number of persons (e.g., a break room or party) (Forsyth et al., 1998). Activities to be observed are to be determined by the person and the occupational therapist, based on what is meaningful to the person's daily life (Haglund & Thorell, 2004). Using the ACIS, the person can be observed during either naturalistic situations or in simulated situations in which the occupational therapist might become the social partner. The ACIS evaluates 20 skills in categories of (a) physicality, (b) information exchange, and (c) relations (Forsyth et al., 1998).

The psychometric properties of the ACIS were determined primarily with persons with psychiatric diagnoses (81 of the 117 subjects; Forsyth et al., 1999, p. 72). Subsequent studies using the ACIS have also primarily included that same client population (Bonsaksen et al., 2011; Fan et al., 2020; Haglund & Thorell, 2004; Hsu et al., 2008). Studies using the ACIS have also included persons with learning disabilities and neurologic disorders (Kjellberg et al., 2003).

Occupational therapists using the ESI observe the person during at least two social interactions in natural contexts with typical social partners (Fisher & Griswold, 2018). The person and occupational therapist determine what social interactions the occupational therapist will observe by discussing social interactions that are relevant to the person's daily life. The social exchanges are categorized by their intended purpose: gathering information, sharing information, problem-solving/decision-making, collaborating/producing, acquiring goods and services, providing/serving goods and services, and conversing socially/small talk. The ESI evaluates 27 skills related to (a) initiating and terminating social interaction, (b) producing social interaction, (c) physically supporting social interaction, (d) shaping content of social interaction, (e) maintaining flow of social interaction, (f) verbally supporting social interaction, and (g) adapting social interaction (Fisher & Griswold, 2018).

The latest edition of the ESI is standardized based on a sample of nearly 15,000 persons of all ages without a diagnosis and with those with various diagnostic conditions (Fisher & Griswold, 2018). Studies support using the ESI with specific populations including children with autism, learning disabilities, and anxiety disorders (Griswold & Townsend, 2012); adults with traumatic brain injury (TBI; Simmons & Griswold, 2010); adults with psychiatric disorders or neurologic disorders (Søndergaard & Fisher, 2012); and adults with intellectual disabilities (Fisher et al., 2017).

Evaluating the quality of social interaction at the level of skills, using the ACIS or ESI, enables the OT practitioner to identify the specific skills that are hindering the person's social interaction with others during desired occupations. The occupational therapist and person can then use the evaluation results to determine an intervention plan. The OT Story 58.1 of Bethany illustrates the evaluation and intervention process.

OT STORY 58.1 BETHANY

Evaluating Quality of Social Interaction
Background: Referral and Occupational Therapy Interview

Bethany is 31 years old and a survivor of two TBIs. She currently lives in an apartment associated with an independent living organization and attends a community-based program for adults with acquired brain injury (ABI). It was in this setting that Bethany sought the services of OT. The occupational therapist, Steve, met with Bethany, at which point he gathered information about Bethany as a person and learned about her goals, conducting an occupational profile (Figure 58.1). (See Chapter 18, for more information about occupational profiles.)

Bethany told Steve about herself and the accidents that resulted in two TBIs. Bethany identified herself as an artist since childhood. She loved painting and had been studying fine arts in college in a large urban area, with plans to become a studio artist and continue living in the city with her friends. On her way to class, she was crossing a busy intersection and was struck by a car and a driver who was texting and not aware of people in the crosswalk. Bethany was thrown 20 ft down the road and sustained a TBI as well as orthopedic injuries. After 10 weeks of rehabilitation, Bethany was discharged to her parents' home where she lived for 1 year and then moved back to the city to pursue an art degree. Bethany reported that she continued to have minimal issues with balance and

(continued)

OT STORY 58.1 BETHANY (continued)

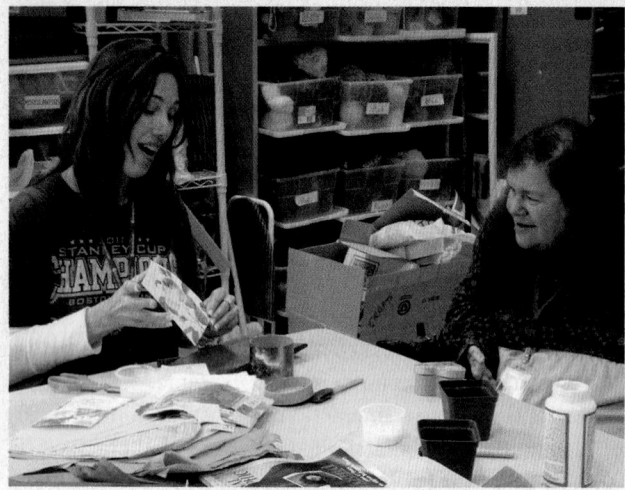

FIGURE 58.1 Bethany practicing social skills in an occupational therapy group.

after a night of clubbing returned to her apartment alone. She was on the second flight of stairs up to her third floor apartment when she had a dizzy spell and fell down a flight and a half of stairs, sustaining a second head injury. She was again discharged to her parents' home post rehabilitation. After living with her parents for about a year and a half, she moved into her apartment associated with an independent living organization in the city where her parents live.

At the time of her discharge from rehabilitation services, Bethany had no identified options for employment and had few friends with whom she had contact. She had difficulty speaking and was given an augmentative and alternative communication (AAC) device, which she did not use regularly. She felt isolated. When she learned about a community-based program for adults with ABI, she eagerly attended in hopes of meeting people and finding meaningful activities. In the program, Bethany began exploring new art media and had joined a cake decorating group, which she said she enjoyed. However, she stated that while she enjoyed the activities, she really missed having a strong social network. She recognized that her brain injuries had resulted in difficulty interacting with others.

Bethany stated her goals were to establish social networks and to use her art talents in some way to supplement her income. Steve and Bethany discussed that improved social interaction skills would be essential in supporting both of Bethany's goals. Bethany said that when she was engaged in an activity with another program member, she usually did not interact a great deal and they usually worked side by side, not working together or talking. She knew this type of experience was important for her to practice using her AAC in a productive manner and to become more social again, but she did not know how to begin working in this direction.

Steve suggested using the ESI to evaluate Bethany's social interaction skills to identify specific social skill deficits and plan intervention to address those identified. Bethany agreed, and together they identified two possible social exchanges that naturally occurred in the community program that Bethany reported were relevant and challenging for her. Bethany agreed to have Steve observe her as she (a) created a bulletin board with another program member and (b) decorated a cake with a different program member.

Evaluation Results

Steve followed the steps of implementing a standardized performance analysis using the ESI (refer to Chapter 52, for details of performance analysis and the definition of the 27 ESI items). Steve quietly observed Bethany as she engaged in the two tasks that involved social interaction. He took notes on Bethany's quality of social interaction and scored her performance using the standardized ESI scoring criteria. Bethany's score form for the cake decorating task is shown in Figure 58.2.

Steve entered Bethany's raw ESI scores into his copy of the ESI computer-scoring software to generate a linear measure of the quality of social interaction. Bethany's quality of social interaction measure is reported on the computer-generated ESI graphic report (Figure 58.3).

Bethany's ESI measures can be interpreted from a criterion-based interpretation and norm-based perspective. The arrow to the left of the scale indicates the location of Bethany's ESI measure along the scale at −0.52 logit. At this level, well below the criterion-referenced cutoff point of competent performance (at 1.0 logit, indicated by a heavy black line on the ESI scale), in the range reflecting persons who demonstrate *moderately to markedly ineffective social interaction skills*. When making a norm-referenced interpretation, Steve compared the location of Bethany's ESI measure to the bar to the left of the scale that indicates the range (±2 *SD*) of quality of social interaction of typical adults between the ages of 22 and 59 years. The black dot in the middle of the bar indicates the mean quality of social interaction for typical adults in that age group.

Using the steps of implementing a performance analysis (refer to Chapter 52), Steve began his documentation with a global baseline statement reflecting Bethany's overall quality of social interaction:

> When Bethany was engaged in two social interactions, one with a program member to create a bulletin board for the program's hallway and another interaction with a different member to decorate a cake, the quality of her social interaction was moderately to markedly ineffective for both tasks. Bethany chose not to use her augmentative communication device and she did not collaborate with her social partners during either task.

OT STORY 58.1 BETHANY (continued)

EVALUATION OF SOCIAL INTERACTION SCORE FORM (Page 1)

Name: Bethany

Occupational therapist: Steve

Gender: ___ Male   X Female

Date of evaluation: _____

Date of birth: _____ Age: 31

Major diagnosis: Traumatic brain injury

Secondary diagnosis: _____

Observation number: ___ 1 X 2 ___ 3 ___ 4

Intended purpose of social interaction:
___ Gathering information (GI)
___ Sharing information (SI)
___ Problem solving/Decision making (PD)
X Collaborating/Producing (CP)
___ Acquiring goods and services (AG)
___ Conversing socially/Small talk (CS)

Social interaction code: CP-1

Detailed task description: Decorating a cake
_____

Time of day:
___ Morning X Afternoon ___ Evening

Familiarity of the physical environment:
X Familiar
___ Somewhat familiar
___ Unfamiliar

Degree of expected structure:
___ High structure
X Relaxed structure
___ "Free" structure

Noise level:
___ Quiet
X Moderate noise
___ Extreme noise

Number of social partners: 1

Primary social partner: KL

Familiarity of primary the social partner:
X Familiar
___ Somewhat familiar
___ Unknown

Status of pri___
___ Expe___
___ Rec___
X Frien___
___ Fam___
___ Othe___

Age of prima___
___ Chil___
___ Adol___
X Adul___
___ Olde___

Social partn___
___ App___
___ Que___
___ Mini___
X Mod___
___ Mar___

Overall com___
___ Gen___
___ Que___
___ Unc___
X Very___

Person's ov___
___ App___
___ Que___
___ Mini___
___ Mod___
X Mar___

EVALUATION OF SOCIAL INTERACTION SCORE FORM (Page 2)

ITEM RAW SCORES

Initiating and Terminating Social Interaction

1. Approaches/Starts   4 3 2 ①
   Did not respond to partner's greeting
2. Concludes/Disengages   4 3 ② 1
   Ended somewhat abruptly

Producing Social Interaction

3. Produces Speech   4 3 2 ①
   Produced very little intelligible speech
4. Gesticulates   4 3 2 ①
   Minimal gestures to support interaction
5. Speaks Fluently   4 3 2 ①
   Very little intelligible speech

Physically Supporting Social Interaction

6. Turns Toward   4 3 ② 1
   Did not turn face toward partner
7. Looks   4 3 ② 1
   Looked at partner out of corner of eye
8. Places Self   4 3 ② 1
   Placed self far away from partner
9. Touches   ④ 3 2 1
10. Regulates   ④ 3 2 1

Shaping Content of Social Interaction

11. Questions   4 3 2 ①
    Did not ask partner questions
12. Replies   4 3 2 ①
    Did not reply to questions and comments
13. Discloses   ④ 3 2 1
14. Expresses Emotion   4 3 2 ①
    Did not express emotion matching partner's messages
15. Disagrees   4 3 2 ①
    Did not respond to partner's suggestions
16. Thanks   4 3 ② 1
    Did not thank partner for frosting tip

Maintaining Flow of Social Interaction

17. Transitions   ④ 3 2 1
18. Times Response   4 3 2 ①
    Long delay to respond and no response
19. Times Duration   4 3 2 ①
    Spoke briefly -- partner needed clarification
20. Takes Turns   4 3 2 ①
    Did not take social turn

Verbally Supporting Social Interaction

21. Matches Language   4 3 2 ①
    Said very little and used simple language
22. Clarifies   4 3 2 ①
    Did not clarify when partner questioned
23. Acknowledges/Encourages   4 3 2 ①
    Did not encourage partner to engage
24. Empathizes   4 3 2 ①
    No support when partner was frustrated

Adapting Social Interaction

25. Heeds   4 3 2 ①
    Did not heed intended purpose: collaborate
26. Accommodates   4 3 2 ①
    Did not prevent problems from occurring
27. Benefits   4 3 2 ①
    Social interaction problems persisted

Additional comments:

FIGURE 58.2 Bethany's Evaluation of Social Interaction (ESI) score form for her social interaction supporting decorating a cake with another person.

(From Fisher, A. G., & Griswold, L. A. [2018]. *The evaluation of social interaction* [4th ed.]. Three Star Press. Reprinted with permission.)

(continued)

OT STORY 58.1 BETHANY (continued)

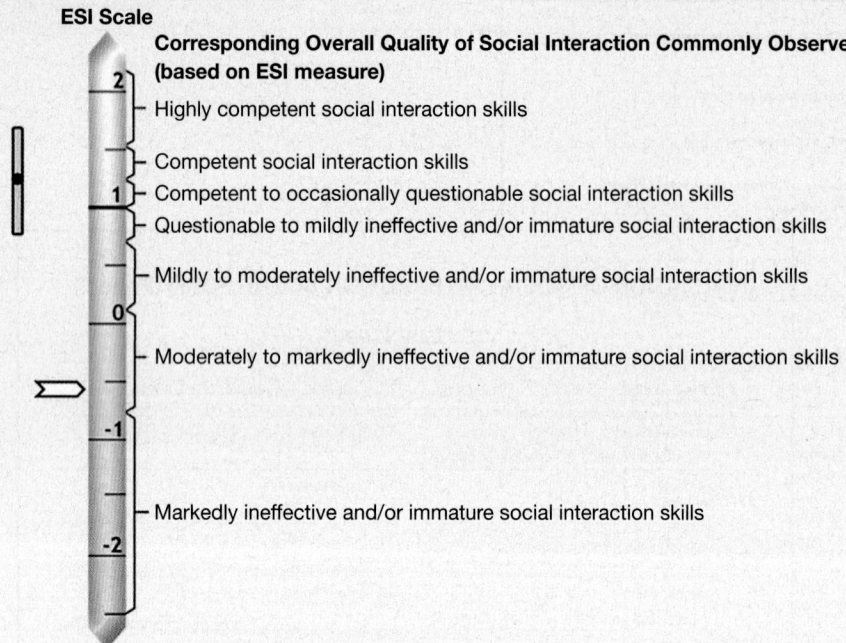

ESI Scale

Corresponding Overall Quality of Social Interaction Commonly Observed (based on ESI measure)

2 — Highly competent social interaction skills

— Competent social interaction skills

1 — Competent to occasionally questionable social interaction skills

— Questionable to mildly ineffective and/or immature social interaction skills

— Mildly to moderately ineffective and/or immature social interaction skills

0

— Moderately to markedly ineffective and/or immature social interaction skills

-1

— Markedly ineffective and/or immature social interaction skills

-2

FIGURE 58.3 The Evaluation of Social Interaction (ESI) scale illustrating Bethany's ESI measure, indicated by the arrow to the left.

(From Fisher, A. G., & Griswold, L. A. [2018]. *The evaluation of social interaction* [4th ed.]. Three Star Press. Reprinted with permission.)

Steve used the social interaction skills that had most limited Bethany's overall quality of social interaction in the two tasks he had observed and clustered the interrelated social interaction skills. He then wrote the following summary statements to document Bethany's social interaction and support her baseline statement (refer to Chapter 52 for details on clustering interrelated skills). Because Bethany's observed social interaction skills were similar in both social exchanges, creating a bulletin board and decorating a cake, Steve described them together.

- *Produces Speech, Speaks Fluently, and Matches Language:* Bethany spoke very little (two to three words per social exchange), and when she did, her speech was almost always unintelligible, with frequent pauses between words.
- *Times Response, Times Duration, Takes Turns, and Clarifies:* Bethany did not respond to most of her social partners' questions or comments, and when she did, she gave one-word responses, resulting in her partners asking for clarification, to which Bethany did not respond.
- *Expresses Emotion and Empathizes:* Bethany demonstrated little emotion throughout the two social exchanges and did not empathize with her partners' feelings when they were jovial or frustrated when they could not understand what Bethany was saying.
- *Questions, Acknowledges/Encourages, and Heeds:* Bethany did not ask her social partners any questions during either task and did not acknowledge when the

social partners made comments or encourage her social partners to continue the social interaction. The result was that Bethany did not collaborate with her partners when they were to work together to make the bulletin board and decorate the cake.

Steve shared the results of his observations with Bethany so that they could use the information to refine Bethany's goal of improving her interaction with others. Steve's documentation clearly identified skills that Bethany might work on as a means to reaching her overarching goal.

Because Bethany had difficulty with many social interaction skills, Steve and Bethany had to determine which of these to address first. Steve knew that they had two approaches to use: (a) reflect on the skills that seemed to most interfere with Bethany's overall quality of social interaction or (b) address the skills that are relatively easier. The ESI manual (Fisher & Griswold, 2018) includes a hierarchy of the relative difficulty of all ESI skills, based on Rasch analysis of all evaluations for the ESI standardization sample. Working collaboratively, Steve and Bethany used a combination of these two approaches and decided to focus first on skills of *Clarifies, Questions, and Replies.* Steve reasoned that whereas *Replies* was a relatively more difficult skill on the ESI skill hierarchy, Bethany's lack of responding to her social partners had a very large impact on her overall quality of social interaction. Steve also reasoned that if Bethany improved her ability to reply to her social partner even somewhat, her overall social interaction would be enhanced.

Bethany and Steve wrote the following goals:

1. In a collaborative task (e.g., cooking, art project), Bethany will consistently answer her social partner's questions using five or more words.
2. In a collaborative task (e.g., cooking, art project), Bethany will clarify what she had said when prompted by her social partner, responding with five or more words.
3. In a collaborative task (e.g., cooking, art project), Bethany will ask her social partner at least two questions to seek his or her perspective on the task and/or how to proceed.

The measurable goals allow Bethany to know what she is working toward and provide her with objective benchmarks against which to measure progress. Most importantly, Bethany set her own goals with Steve, using the results from her observed performance.

Questions

1. What is the value of evaluating social interaction in natural contexts?
2. How does evaluating the quality of social interaction at the level of performance skills influence intervention?
3. Why would skills be clustered when documenting a person's quality of social interaction, rather than listing the skills separately?

Intervention to Enhance Social Interaction Skills

Research on Intervention Strategies

Intervention strategies to support social interaction skills found in the literature differ based on the age and diagnostic condition (Deckers et al., 2016). Research typically has focused on one age group and one diagnosis at a time. See "Commentary on the Evidence" box, for further details. When the results of the studies are considered collectively, it appears that clear and concise assessment data allows for intervention focused on social interaction and leads to improvement in overall quality of social interaction, supporting a person's ability to participate in desired occupations.

Intervention Planning

After setting goals, together, the occupational therapist and person plan intervention. The occupational therapist brings professional reasoning, experience, theory, and evidence from research to the discussion, and the person contributes suggestions related to activities, strategies, and locations in which intervention might occur naturally. Having evaluation results based on observation in a natural context enables the occupational therapist and person to logically plan a well-targeted intervention to promote social interaction during occupational performance that is relevant and meaningful.

Several intervention models have been proposed to describe approaches to enhance social interaction (AOTA, 2020; Fisher & Marterella, 2019; Odom et al., 1999). The models promote using a *compensatory approach*, adapting the environment or demands of the social exchange, and using an *acquisitional approach*, teaching social skills and providing opportunity to practice the skills relevant during naturally occurring social exchanges. These two approaches have been supported by a number of intervention studies to support social interaction with pre- and post-test measures using the ESI or ACIS.

Simmons and Griswold (2010) conducted an early study using the ESI to evaluate the effectiveness of intervention to support the quality of social interaction for a group of 10 survivors of TBI. Williams and Chard (2016) similarly examined the effectiveness of intervention of social interaction with six males in a low secure forensic unit using the ESI. And in another study in 2019, Williams and Chard provided intervention to 12 adult mothers who had mental health challenges leading to difficulty with the occupations related to their mothering role because of diminished social interaction skills. Ávila-Álvarez and colleagues (2020) explored the effect of animal-assisted intervention (AAI) to facilitate social skills for 19 boys, 30 to 66 months of age, on the autism spectrum; they evaluated social interaction skills using the ASIC. In all four studies, the researchers provided intervention using compensatory and acquisitional approaches in naturalistic settings and reported improved social interaction for many of the study participants. Collectively, the cited research illustrates assessment based on observing persons during social interactions to guide developing goals that are relevant for the persons and lead to intervention to support social interaction in desired occupations.

Intervention Guided by Theory

Occupational therapists use theory in their professional reasoning to guide the planning of intervention. The Occupational Therapy Intervention Process Model (OTIPM; Fisher, 1998, 2009; Fisher & Marterella, 2019) guides the evaluation and intervention process in a true top-down model by first understanding the client as a person, the person's performance context, and occupations that are meaningful for the person, followed by observing the person perform meaningful tasks and conducting performance analyses. As discussed in detail in Chapter 52, performance analyses involve determining what specific goal-directed actions are effective and ineffective. This process was illustrated earlier with Bethany. The problems identified in the performance analysis provide the basis for goals and the focus of intervention.

Based on the OTIPM, after conducting a performance analysis in which the occupational therapist determines which actions (e.g., produces speech) most limit the person's social interaction, the occupational therapist considers the factors potentially leading to challenges in occupational performance (Fisher, 2009; Fisher & Marterella, 2019). Considering the factors that might contribute to performance difficulty after implementing a performance analysis is the hallmark of true top-down reasoning. Using a top-down reasoning process also keeps the occupational therapist focused on occupations that are important to the person, reflecting person-centered and occupation-based practice (Fisher, 2009; Fisher & Marterella, 2019; see Chapter 52).

Conceptual Model of Social Interaction and Factors That Impact Quality of Social Interaction. Fisher and Griswold (2018) proposed a conceptual model of social interaction and identified factors that are believed to influence a person's quality of social interaction (Figure 58.4). Factors that support or hinder a person's quality of social interaction include societal

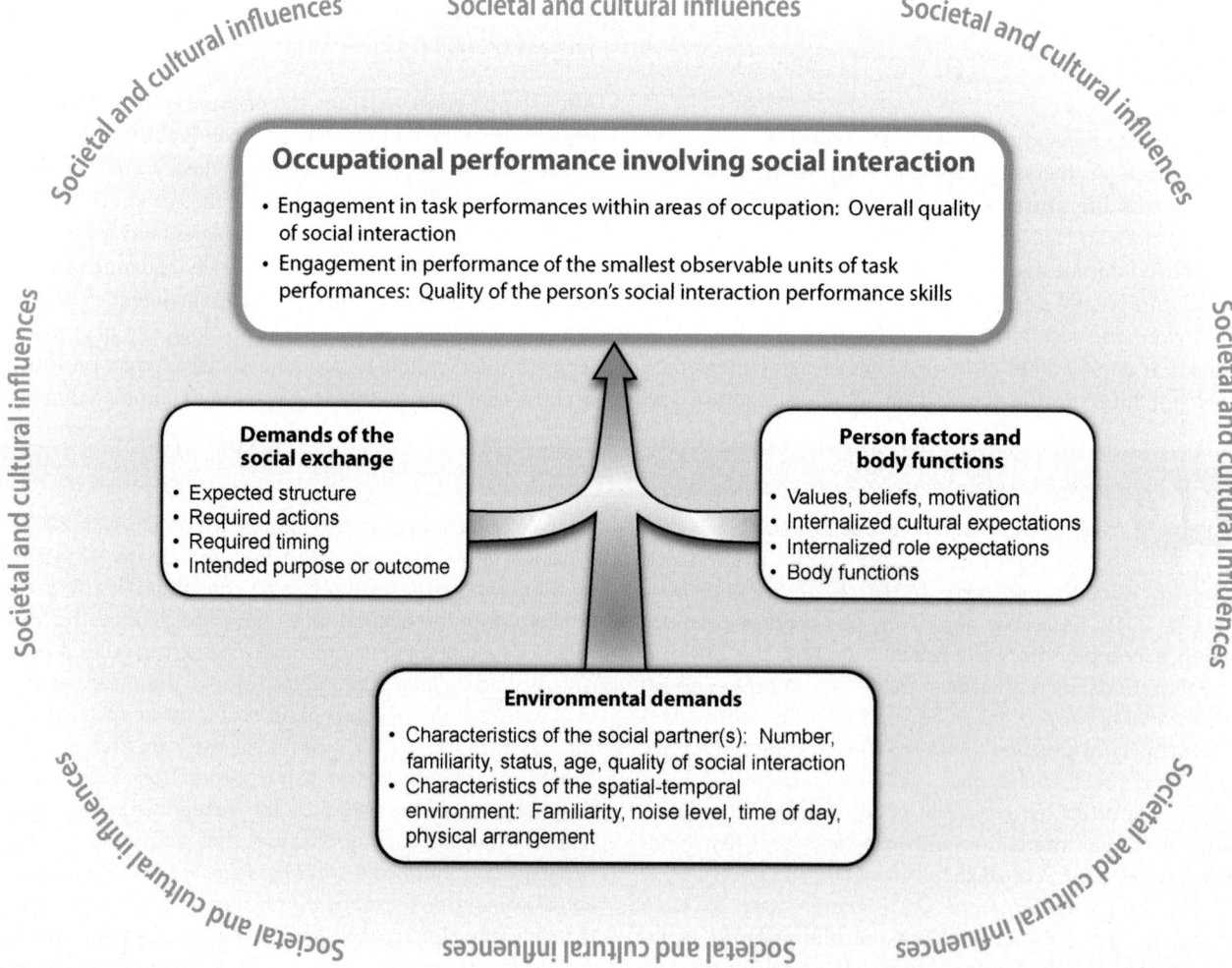

FIGURE 58.4 Schematic representation of the quality of social interaction influenced by transaction among societal and cultural influences, demands of the social exchange, environmental demands, and person factors and body functions.

(Adapted from Fisher, A. G., & Griswold, L. A. [2018]. *The evaluation of social interaction* [4th ed.]. Three Star Press. Reprinted with permission.)

and cultural influences, demands of the social exchange (e.g., the intended purpose, expected structure of the social exchange, familiarity of the setting, noise level, and time of day), social partner characteristics (e.g., number of social partners, their familiarity, their age and status, and their quality of social interaction), and influences of person factors (e.g., motivation, internalized cultural expectations, and body functions). Because each of the identified factors can impact a person's quality of social interaction, they can also contribute to the "cause" of the person's problems with social interaction. The many factors that influence the quality of one's social interaction can also provide the occupational therapist with options to consider when planning interventions to promote or support a person's quality of social interaction. A more dynamic analysis of factors that contribute to a person's occupational performance is the Transactional Model of Occupation (Fisher & Marterella, 2019), presented in Chapter 52.

Models for Intervention. Once the occupational therapist and the person have considered factors that limit the person's quality of social interaction, they need to select an intervention approach to address the identified concerns and work toward the person's goals. According to the OTIPM (Fisher & Marterella, 2019), there are four models for intervention: the *compensatory model*, using adapted methods such as adaptive equipment, assistive technology, or modifications of the environment or task demands to support performance; *acquisitional model* for occupational skills training, using occupations to promote the person to develop or reacquire skills; *restorative model*, using occupations to facilitate restoring person factors and/or body functions; and *education and teaching model*, providing education to share information on strategies to address problems. The occupational therapist uses the identified speculated reasons for decreased quality of social interaction to determine the most appropriate intervention model. The OT Story 58.2 illustrates Steve's reasoning process in planning intervention for Bethany.

OT STORY 58.2 BETHANY

Planning Intervention to Support Social Interaction

Steve considered how demands of the social exchange contributed to Bethany's quality of social interaction. Specifically, he thought that the challenge of the intended purpose of collaborating with another person was challenging for Bethany. Steve was aware that collaborating with another person requires many social interaction skills. Steve also recognized that both social exchanges did not offer much structure. Steve was aware that both interactions had occurred in the natural environments of the hallway (for the bulletin board task) and the kitchen, where other members were passing through or also engaged in tasks. He wondered about how the noise from the other people hindered Bethany's quality of social interaction. Steve also considered Bethany's social partners' characteristics for the two social exchanges. Bethany had two different social partners from the community program, both of whom also had difficulty with social interaction. Steve wondered how much of the partners' lack of social skill influenced Bethany's quality of social interaction. Finally, Steve then considered person factors and body functions. Bethany was motivated to engage with other people and to engage in both tasks. Discussion with Bethany about how well she thought she had interacted with her partners led Steve to reason that Bethany had internalized the expectations, based on her report that she knew her partners had asked questions and made comments, but she had chosen not to respond because it was "too hard." When Bethany did speak, her speech was slow, slurred, and not well articulated, making her speech

unintelligible—all factors of body functions. Steve recalled that Bethany reported that she did not use her AAC because she thought it had not been programmed to include phrases that she commonly needed, so she did not find it helpful. Steve concluded that there were many factors contributing to Bethany's ineffective quality of social interaction. Although limitation in body function was evident, Steve knew that Bethany was not likely to improve her ability to articulate her words more clearly, at least not very quickly.

As Steve and Bethany discussed the causes of Bethany's difficulty in social interaction, they began considering ways to address many of these factors. Steve considered the first three intervention models from OTIPM. Together, Steve and Bethany determined that restoring body function around oral motor control was not going to be fruitful because Bethany had already received a great deal of speech therapy with little to no improvement. They decided that using the AAC would enable other people to better understand Bethany, provided the right phrases and words were programmed into the device. Steve agreed to program Bethany's AAC with phrases that Bethany thought she would need. For example, including the question, "Do you know what I mean?" would help Bethany ensure that her social partners where understanding her and allow her to clarify as needed. Bethany suggested that adding the question, "What do you think?" would promote her to encourage her partners in interactions that were collaborative. These strategies reflected the compensatory model of intervention.

Bethany was eager to reacquire skills around social interaction using her AAC, using the acquisitional model for

(continued)

OT STORY 58.2 BETHANY (continued)

intervention. However, Bethany stated that she needed assistance to identify when she might use her augmentative device to engage in interaction more successfully. Steve and Bethany discussed the use of a subtle cuing system in which Steve could prompt Bethany to ask questions or respond to her social partner. They practiced the cuing system briefly and then tried it later that day when Bethany engaged in casual conversation with other program members during lunch. Steve explained that he could support Bethany as she acquired skills through practice in the natural opportunities while she attended the community program.

Bethany and Steve concluded that a combination of using two models for intervention would provide the basis to enhance Bethany's social interaction skills: compensatory model, using her AAC; and acquisitional model, to acquire social interaction skills.

The natural context of the community-based program included many opportunities for Bethany to practice the skills she wanted to acquire. Bethany knew that Steve would not be with her throughout the day and suggested that a few of the other staff also be shown the subtle cues to prompt her as needed. Steve knew that many of the program members wanted to work on social interaction to support their desired occupational participation. Therefore, Steve decided to offer an in-service training session to all staff using another model of intervention—*education and training model* (Fisher & Marterella, 2019). During the training session, Steve shared the conceptual model for social interaction and led the staff in a discussion of natural strategies for the program to better support social interaction by modifying the environment and structure of frequent program activities. Specifically,

the staff and Steve discussed promoting more face-to-face opportunities for members to socially interact with one another, monitoring noise in areas in which social interactions frequently occurred, and pairing members so that they were better suited to support one another's social interaction. Steve suggested strategies to provide more structure to the activities with clear social interaction demands. For example, when cooking together, members might be organized into small groups of three persons with each person having a defined role for interacting, such as one person reading directions and the other two sharing the actual cooking task. Last, Steve introduced a simple universal system of cuing to prompt members on skills that many wanted to acquire. The in-service training session resulted in support of natural opportunities to acquire and practice social interaction skills throughout the day for all program members.

Questions

1. What social interaction skills seem more critical to support a positive social exchange that would be important to address in intervention, not specific to Bethany?
2. Consider the strategies that Steve suggested to program staff to promote improved quality of social interaction for Bethany and other program members and determine which intervention model the strategies use: compensatory, acquisitional, or restorative.
3. Consider the models for intervention proposed, which ones seem more logical to implement for a person with Bethany's profile? How would your intervention differ from what Steve provided?

Effectiveness of Intervention

After intervention, it is essential that the OT practitioner reevaluates the person to determine if OT was effective. Again, using observation in natural context provides information that is relevant to the person's daily needs. A reevaluation might

indicate that the person has made significant changes and no longer needs OT. Reevaluation might also reveal new areas of concern, in which case the occupational therapist and person would use the same top-down reasoning process to consider other naturally occurring social contexts that the person is reporting as challenging. Observation in natural context could reveal additional social interaction skills to address in OT to enhance the quality of social interaction. See OT Story 58.3.

OT STORY 58.3 BETHANY

Determining Effectiveness of Occupational Therapy Intervention

After 8 weeks of working on improving her social interaction skills in the program, Bethany thought that she was meeting her goals. She requested that Steve see how she was doing by observing her again. Bethany and Steve determined two social exchanges for Steve to observe and score using the

ESI. For this evaluation, Bethany taught another member how to use a digital camera that the program had recently purchased and then how to enhance the pictures using a computer. Steve observed the two interactions, scored them, and entered Bethany's scores into the ESI computer software program. The results revealed that Bethany's overall quality of social interaction was now at 0.6 logits.

OT STORY 58.3 BETHANY (continued)

Criterion-referenced interpretation indicated that her overall quality of social interaction was *mildly to moderately ineffective*, a significant improvement from the first evaluation. Steve verified the change by comparing Bethany's ESI measures for both evaluations, finding that the difference in the two measures was greater than the sum of the mean standard error of measurement for each assessment, according to the ESI manual (Fisher & Griswold, 2018). The ESI progress report, obtained from the computer-scoring software, includes the ESI scale indicating Bethany's ESI measure for the first and second assessments, marked with a number 1 and 2 for each respective assessment (Figure 58.5). Using a standardized assessment such as the ESI enabled

Steve to confirm that Bethany had indeed made significant progress in the quality of her social interaction skill. The ESI scale in the ESI progress report provided an understandable visual aid. Bethany was eager to further improve her social interaction skills and set new goals based on the last evaluation results.

Questions

1. Steve evaluated Bethany's progress using the ESI. What other methods might he have considered?
2. What is an advantage of using a standardized assessment, such as the ESI, for reevaluation over other available options possible?

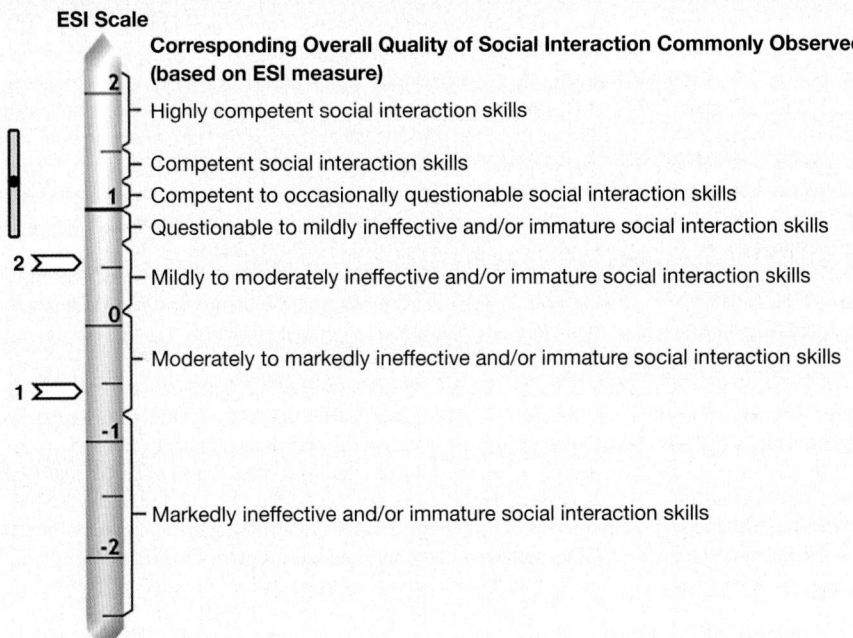

FIGURE 58.5 **The Evaluation of Social Interaction (ESI) scale illustrating Bethany's ESI measure for her first and second evaluation, indicated by arrows to the left.**

(From Fisher, A. G., & Griswold, L. A. [2018]. *The evaluation of social interaction* [4th ed.]. Three Star Press. Reprinted with permission.)

Conclusion

The OT Story illustrated how the occupational therapist listened to the person as she expressed a desire to interact with others. Occupational therapists working in any area of practice may support persons who experience challenges in social interaction that decrease their participation in desired occupations. Steve used a standardized assessment to evaluate Bethany's quality of social interaction; in doing so, he was able to document improvement in Bethany's social interaction performance. Steve could have also completed a nonstandardized performance analysis to identify social interaction skills that were challenging for Bethany and plan intervention. Using either assessment approach would result in providing intervention to enhance her social interaction using one or more of the models for

intervention. Most importantly, in either situation, evaluating in natural context during a real occupation leads to occupation-focused intervention, ultimately to support a person's social participation.

Lippincott® Connect *For additional resources on the subjects discussed in this chapter, visit* Lippincott Connect.

REFERENCES

American Occupational Therapy Association. (2020). Occupational therapy practice framework: Domain and process (4th ed.). *American Journal of Occupational Therapy, 74*(Suppl. 2), 7412410010. https://doi.org/10.5014/ajot.2020.74S2001

Ávila-Álvarez, A., Alonso-Bidegain, M., De-Rosende-Celeiro, I., Vizcaíno-Cela, M., Larrañeta-Alcalde, L., & Torres-Tobío, G. (2020). Improving social participation of children with autism spectrum disorder: Pilot testing of an early animal-assisted intervention in Spain.

Health and Social Care in the Community, 28, 1220–1229. https://doi .org/10.1111/hsc.12955

Bellack, A. S., Brown, C. H., & Thomas-Lohrman, S. (2006). Psychometric characteristics of role-play assessments of social skill in schizophrenia. *Behavior Therapy, 37,* 339–352. https://doi.org/10.1016/j.beth .2006.01.005

Bonsaksen, T., Myraunet, I., Celo, C., Granå, K. E., & Ellingham, B. (2011). Experiences of occupational therapists and occupational therapy students in using the assessment of communication and interaction skills in mental health settings in Norway. *British Journal of Occupational Therapy, 74,* 332–338. https://doi.org/10.4276/0308022 11X13099513661117

Byom, L., O'Neil-Pirozzi, T. M., Lemoncello, R., MadDoonald, S., Meulenbroek, P., Ness, B., & Sohlberg, M. M. (2020). Social communication following adult traumatic brain injury: A scoping review of theoretical models. *American Journal of Speech-Language Pathology, 29,* 1735–1748. https://doi.org/10.1044/2020_AJSLP-19-00020

Deckers, A., Muris, P., Roelofs, J., & Arntz, A. (2016). A group-administered social skills training for 8- to 12-year-old, high-functioning children with autism spectrum disorders: An evaluation of its effectiveness in a naturalistic outpatient treatment setting. *Journal of Autism and Developmental Disorders, 46,* 3493–3504. https://doi.org/10.1007/ s10803-016-2887-1

Dillon, E., Holingue, C., Herman, D., & Landa, R. J. (2021). Psychometrics of the pragmatic rating scale for school-age children with a range of linguistic and social communication skills. *Journal of Speech, Language, and Hearing Research, 64,* 3477–3488. https://doi .org/10.1044/2021_JSLHR-20-00753

Fan, C. W., Keponen, R., Piiki, S., Tsang, H. W. H., Popova, E. S., & Taylor, R. (2020). Psychometric evaluation of the Finnish translation of the assessment of communication and interaction skills (ACIS-FI). *Scandinavian Journal of Occupational Therapy, 27,* 112–121. https:// doi.org/10.1080/11038128.2018.1483425

Fisher, A. G. (1998). Uniting practice and theory in an occupational framework. 1998 Eleanor Clarke Slagle Lecture. *American Journal of Occupational Therapy, 52,* 509–521. https://doi.org/10.5014/ ajot.52.7.509

Fisher, A. G. (2009). *Occupational therapy intervention process model: A model for planning and implementing top-down, client-centered, and occupation-based occupational therapy interventions.* Three Star Press.

Fisher, A. G., & Griswold, L. A. (2009). *Evaluation of social interaction.* Three Star Press.

Fisher, A. G., & Griswold, L. A. (2018). *The evaluation of social interaction* (4th ed.). Three Star Press.

Fisher, A. G., Griswold, L. A., Munkholm, M., & Kottorp, A. (2017). Evaluating domains of everyday functioning in people with developmental disabilities. *Scandinavian Journal of Occupational Therapy, 24,* 1–9. https://doi.org/10.3109/11038128.2016.1160147

Fisher, A. G., & Marterella, A. (2019). *Powerful practice: A model for authentic occupational therapy.* Center for Innovative OT Solutions.

Forsyth, K., Lai, J., & Kielhofner, G. (1999). The assessment of communication and interaction skills (ACIS): Measurement properties. *British Journal of Occupational Therapy, 62,* 69–74. https://doi .org/10.1177/030802269906200208

Forsyth, K., Salamy, M., Simon, S., & Kielhofner, G. (1998). *The assessment of communication and interaction skills (ACIS).* Model of Human Occupation Clearinghouse, University of Illinois.

Griswold, L. A., & Townsend, S. (2012). Assessing the sensitivity of the evaluation of social interaction: Comparing social skills for children with and without disabilities. *American Journal of Occupational Therapy, 66,* 709–717. https://doi.org/10.5014/ajot.2012.004051

Haglund, L., & Thorell, L. (2004). Clinical perspective on the Swedish version of the assessment of communication and interaction skills: Stability of assessments. *Scandinavian Journal of Caring Sciences, 18,* 417–423. https://doi.org/10.1111/j.1471-6712.2004.00295.x

Hendricks, D. R., & Wehman, P. (2009). Transition from school to adulthood for youth with autism spectrum disorders. *Focus on Autism and Other Developmental Disabilities, 24,* 77–88. https://doi .org/10.1177/1088357608329827

Hsu, W., Pan, A., & Chen, T. (2008). A psychometric study of the Chinese version of the assessment of communication and interaction skills. *Occupational Therapy in Health Care, 22,* 177–185. https://doi.org/ 10.1080/07380570801991818

Jones, D. E., Greenberg, M., & Croweley, M. (2015). Early social-emotional functioning and public health: The relationship between kindergarten social competence and future wellness. *American Journal of Public Health, 105,* 2283–2290. https://doi.org/10.2105/AJPH.2015.302630

Kjellberg, A., Haglund, L., Forsyth, K., & Kielhofner, G. (2003). The measurement properties of the Swedish version of the assessment of communication and interaction skills. *Scandinavian Journal of Caring Science, 17,* 271–277. https://doi.org/10.1046/j.1471-6712.2003.00225.x

Lexén, A., & Bejerholm, U. (2016). Exploring communication and interaction skills at work among participants in individual placement and support. *Scandinavian Journal of Occupational Therapy, 23,* 314–319. https://doi.org/10.3109/11038128.2015.1105294

Morgan, R. L., & Schultz, J. C. (2012). Towards and ecological, multi-modal approach to increase employment for young adults with autism spectrum disorder. *Journal of Applied Rehabilitation Counseling, 43,* 27–35. https://doi.org/10.1891/0047-2220.43.1.27

Mulder, A. M., & Cashin, A. (2014). The need to support students with autism at university. *Issues in Mental Health Nursing, 35,* 664–671. https://doi.org/10.3109/01612840.2014.894158

Norbury, C. (2014). Practitioner review: Social (pragmatic) communication disorder conceptualization, evidence, and clinical implications. *Journal of Child Psychology and Psychiatry, 55,* 204–216. https:// doi.org/10.1111/jcpp.12154

Odom, S., McConnell, S. R., McEvoy, M. A., Peterson, C., Ostrosky, M., Chandler, L. K., Spicuzza, R., Skellenger, A., Creighton, M., & Favazza, P. C. (1999). Relative effects of interventions supporting the social competence of young children with disabilities. *Topics in Early Childhood Education, 19,* 75–91. https://doi.org/10.1177/027112149901900202

Simmons, C. D., & Griswold, L. A. (2010). Using the evaluation of social interaction in a community-based program for persons with traumatic brain injury. *Scandinavian Journal of Occupational Therapy, 17,* 49–56. https://doi.org/10.3109/11038120903350303

Søndergaard, M., & Fisher, A. G. (2012). Sensitivity of the evaluation of social interaction measures among people with and without neurologic or psychiatric disorders. *American Journal of Occupational Therapy, 66,* 356–362. https://doi.org/10.5014/ajot.2012.003582

Tsang, H., & Pearson, V. (2000). Reliability and validity of a simple measure for assessing the social skills of people with schizophrenia necessary for seeking and securing a job. *Canadian Journal of Occupational Therapy, 67,* 250–259. https://doi.org/10.1177/000841740006700407

Verhoeven, E. W. M., Smeekens, I., & Didden, R. (2013). Brief report: Suitability of the social skills performance assessment (SSPA) for the assessment of social skills in adults with autism spectrum disorders. *Journal of Autism and Developmental Disorders, 43,* 2990–2996. https://doi.org/10.1007/s10803-013-1843-6

Williams, B., & Chard, G. (2016). Using the evaluation of social interaction (ESI) with men in low secure forensic unit. *British Journal of Occupational Therapy, 79,* 206–211. https://doi.org/10.1177/ 0308022615615890

Williams, B., & Chard, G. (2019). The usefulness of the evaluation of social interaction in a mother and baby mental health unit. *British Journal of Occupational Therapy, 82,* 582–587. https://doi .org/10.1177/0308022619835399

Personal Values, Beliefs, and Spirituality

Christy Billock

> Spirituality looks like folding the towels in a sweet way and talking kindly to the people in the family even though you've had a long day.
>
> —SYLVIA BOORSTEIN (2016)

LEARNING OBJECTIVES

After reading this chapter, you will be able to:

1. Develop an understanding of the meaning of personal values, beliefs, and spirituality as related to occupational therapy (OT) practice, including definition, related themes, and distinction from religion.
2. Recognize the relationship between spirituality, occupation, health, and well-being.
3. Understand the relevance of individual experiences of spirituality through occupation by examining important factors, such as context, reflection, intention, and mindfulness.
4. Describe strategies to integrate personal values, beliefs, and spirituality into OT practice.
5. Explore how personal values, beliefs, spirituality, and occupation might intersect in your own life experiences.

Introduction

With principles of holism at the center of the occupational therapy's (OT's) founding philosophy, the profession embraces the idea that what we *do* every day matters—to body, mind, and spirit. Occupational participation provides the vehicle for experiencing meaning in life for persons, groups, and populations. Understanding the rich interconnections of personal values, beliefs, and spirituality as experienced through occupation provides OT practitioners the opportunity of enhancing the profession's unique heritage of a holistic approach to health and well-being as well as help clients to experience meaning in life. This chapter serves as an introductory resource for understanding personal values, beliefs, and spirituality in OT practice. The exploration begins by looking at the interconnections of values, beliefs, and spirituality as important facets of occupation. Second, this chapter discusses the multiple ways in which spirituality is experienced through occupation. Third, it provides strategies for integrating values, beliefs, and spirituality into OT practice.

Framing Personal Values, Beliefs, and Spirituality From an Occupational Therapy Perspective

A holistic context of care helps OT thrive where "in pursuing occupation, humans express the totality of their being, a mind-body-spirit union" (Hooper & Wood, 2014, p. 38). The transactions of mind, body, and spirit through occupational engagement help answer the question—what do you live for? At the heart of those answers is a person's values, beliefs, and spirituality. Values can be understood as "acquired beliefs and commitments, derived from culture, about what is good, right, and important to do" (American Occupational Therapy Association [AOTA], 2020, p. S84). The notion of beliefs closely relates to values and can be defined as "something that is accepted, considered to be true, or held as an opinion" (AOTA, 2020, p. S75). Both values and beliefs often influence subjective experiences of occupation because of the qualities of meaning and centrality in the person's life. Although these definitions emphasize thinking from an individualistic lens, values and beliefs often are inherently socially constructed and reliant on communal experiences and perspectives. Values and beliefs can derive from multiple sources including personal experience, friends and acquaintances, family, culture, religion, and politics, among others. The mattering inherent in daily occupation extends to how we connect with others and create shared meaning in groups and communities.

The multidimensional and complex nature of spirituality defies simple definition and a consideration of how the concept relates to occupation further complicates the pursuit. The Occupational Therapy Practice Framework (AOTA, 2020) uses Billock's (2005) definition of spirituality as "a deep experience of meaning brought about by engaging in occupations that involve the enacting of personal values and beliefs, reflection, and intention within a supportive contextual environment" (p. 887). For example, a person might experience spirituality through the occupation of walking their dog through a neighborhood park while reflecting on the love they experience together and the relationship functions as a vital and meaningful part of their life.

As a central tenet of the profession, OT practitioners believe that meaning matters for persons, communities, and populations. Experiencing meaning in life relies on the facets of *significance* of contributions and how those matter in the world, *coherence* and making sense of one's life in the world, and *purpose* where actions orient toward goals (Costin & Vignoles, 2020). Meaning-making, in its essence, can be understood as a spiritual process that seeks expression through occupation (Peloquin, 1997). Meaning

is often co-constructed with others through relationships, within communities, or among larger groups of people with shared experiences or beliefs. Wilcock and Townsend (2014) put forth meaning-making, experiencing meaning, and self-expression as the "activist element of human existence" (p. 542). The South African philosophy of Ubuntu provides a helpful concept for understanding how this activist element moves beyond just an individualistic perspective (Ramugondo & Kronenberg, 2015). The interactive ethic of Ubuntu implies that our humanity relies upon interactions with others. People and groups often experience spirituality through engagement in everyday activities; consequently, occupation creates meaning and purpose in life and helps to answer larger existential questions of the meaning of life (Christiansen, 1997; Frankl, 1959). Spirituality thrives on actual experiences of occupations that provide the opportunity to bring values and beliefs to life individually and collectively.

People oftentimes equate religion and spirituality; however, although religious participation and spiritual experience can occur together, the two are not synonymous. Religion can be defined as a set of shared beliefs and attendant practices used to relate to the sacred. As individual and communal practices, religion permeates many daily experiences of spirituality through participation in rituals and occupations such as prayer, meditation, reading theological books, and attending religious services. Not only do religions provide followers with practices directly relating to theological beliefs, but religious beliefs often ascribe spiritual meaning to daily occupations such as food preparation, work, and intimacy, especially if "understood as commanded by God" (Frank et al., 1997, p. 201). Although many people use religion as a tool for framing spirituality in their lives, spiritual experience does not depend on religious affiliation or practice.

Spirituality, health, and well-being can interconnect through occupation and lifestyle in a variety of ways. For those with mental illness, practicing religion and spirituality can serve as a powerful resource for some and impede treatment for others depending upon diagnosis and individual experience (Koenig et al., 2020). For many, spiritual experience positively influences mental health and well-being leading to increased coping and stress resilience. Evidence suggests that practicing spirituality and religion can positively influence health through the physiologic processes of the immune, neuroendocrine, and cardiovascular systems (Aldwin et al., 2014; Seeman et al., 2003). Spiritual health takes on many definitions but generally connotes being able to experience meaning, fulfillment, and connection with self, others, and a higher power or larger reality (Hawks et al., 1995). Experiences of occupational alienation (Townsend & Wilcock, 2004), that is, an inability to create meaning and express one's spirit through occupation, demonstrates a lack of spiritual health or well-being for a person (Simó-Algado et al., 2002).

At the heart of OT beats a strong reminder that people and communities need something to live for—purpose in life, meaning, connection, coping, resilience, and hope for the future. OT practitioners seek to understand which occupations will spark motivation to maximize engagement and participation in life and facilitate health and well-being. Figuring out such occupations and facilitating participation in them essentially provides a glimpse into the spirit of people and groups, thereby representing some of the best benefits OT can uniquely offer.

Experiencing Spirituality Through Occupation

Engaging in occupations can bring personal values, beliefs, and spirituality to life. Although spirituality can be experienced outside of occupation, participating in occupation is the most common and effective mechanism for making spirituality a real, tangible reality in daily life. Peloquin (1997) refers to occupation as an act of making that represents an extension and animation of the human spirit:

> To see such radical making in the acts that we commonly name *doing* purposeful activities, *performing* life roles and tasks, *adapting* to the environment, *adjusting* to disability, and *achieving* skills or mastery, is to discern the spiritual depth of occupation. (p. 167)

Linking occupation and spirituality together with the notion of "making" implies a fluid and active approach to the phenomenon. In making, a person expresses tangibly the intangible yet vital realities of life. These internal representations of values and beliefs about the meaning of reality and the world drive people to orchestrate occupations to express those meanings (Kroeker, 1997). Therein lies the importance of finding occupations that make people's faces light up and motivate them to get out of bed in the morning.

Occupations stemming from religious practice have been traditionally viewed as a path to spiritual experience. From an international perspective, the reported importance of religion in a person's life and religious service attendance varies widely based on region. Africa, the Middle East, South Asia, and Latin America tend to have high rates of people reporting religion to be important in their lives, and Europe, North America, East Asia, and Australia reflect significantly lower levels of religious importance and attendance (Pew Research Center, 2018). Dramatic shifts in the religious landscape have changed practices in recent years with a wide array of factors influencing people's occupational and ideological relationship to religion. Within the United States, membership in churches, synagogues, or mosques fell to 47% in 2020, down from 70% in 1999 (Jones, 2021). Around the world, young adults tend to report lower rates of religious affiliation and practice (Pew Research Center,

2018). Other identified trends point toward a greater number of people creating a personal construction of practices for the foundation of spiritual life and to experience purpose (Wuthnow, 1998, 2010). Although many more people identify as nonreligious, limited research exists about how meaning is cultivated in secular contexts (Baker & Smith, 2015). McColl (2002) contends that given the erosion of meaning in work from industrialization and the prevalence of secular pluralism in modern society, occupation "may be the most effective medium available through which individuals can affirm their connection with the self, with others, with the cosmos, and with the divine" (p. 352). Orchestration of and engagement in everyday occupation holds the potential of helping people to meet the fundamental need for spiritual expression. For example, the busy executive attending a yoga class, receiving a massage, or taking a hike might serve the vitally important role of facilitating their experiences of spirituality because of the deeply meaningful nature of such occupations (Figure 59.1).

Contextual Factors

Spiritual experiences through occupation depend on and are vulnerable to transactions with several environmental and contextual factors, including physical and social worlds (Billock, 2005). The physical world can serve to potentially facilitate or block spiritual experiences (Jackson, 1996). Some experience spirituality through occupations in nature such as hiking in the mountains, fly fishing in a stream, or walking along the beach. Built spaces such as churches, houses, and other structures serve to refine and make more vivid human feeling, perception, and comprehension of reality (Tuan, 1977). Out of experiencing those spaces and the objects within them, a person draws a sense of place that is "an organized world of meaning" (Tuan, 1977, p. 179). For example, a home filled with memories of family gatherings

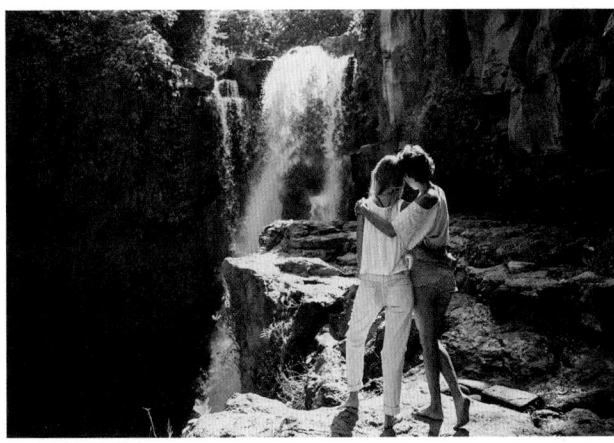

FIGURE 59.1 Taking a hike might serve the vitally important role of facilitating experiences of spirituality.

and decorated with special pieces of art and pictures of loved ones can provide support for experiencing spirituality through occupational participation. Gathering around a table appointed with grandmother's linens and pottery made by friends, then lighting candles when friends come to share a meal, mark the event as one with special meaning, personal value, and spiritual import (Figure 59.2). Whereas home can support one person's experiences of spirituality, for another, home might be a place of strained memories and relationships. For a person physically abused by their partner in the privacy of their home, experiences of occupation within the home may show less potential for spiritual experience.

Social contexts can significantly influence spiritual experience because meaning is both personally and socially constructed (Hasselkus, 2011). Attempts to understand spiritual experience involve looking at the doer of the occupation and the social and cultural worlds of engagement. Engaging in occupations with others, co-occupation (Zemke & Clark, 1996), or collective occupations (Ramugondo & Kronenberg, 2015) can potentiate or negate the likelihood of a spiritual experience. As a growing public health concern in many countries, loneliness and lack of social connection can increase mortality and a range of disease morbidities and points to the necessity for helping people find ways to connect with others (Fried et al., 2020; Holt-Lundstadt et al., 2017). Religions recognize the importance of believers practicing their faith with others as a means of mutual support and affirmation of belief and provide the context for many shared occupations and ways for parishioners to connect (Howard & Howard, 1997). Beyond religious occupations, communal occupations such as attending sporting events, concerts, or political protests as well as celebrations such as weddings, graduations, or parties can be rich environments for spiritual experience, the enacting of personal values and beliefs, and the fundamental human need for connection (Figure 59.3).

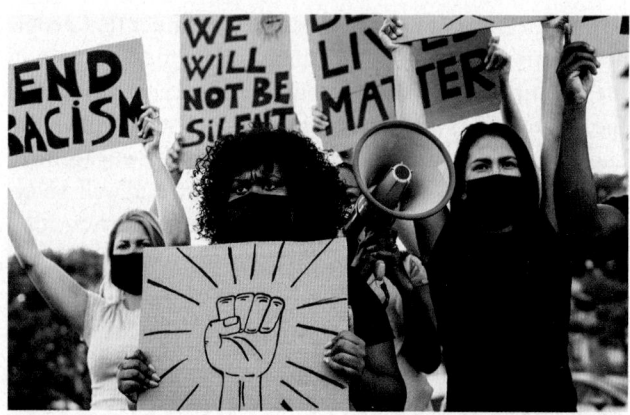

FIGURE 59.3 In the summer of 2020, many people participated in Black Lives Matter protests through the world.

Reflection, Intention, and Mindfulness

Reflection, intention, and mindfulness can enhance spiritual experience (Billock, 2005). All three of these supporting factors involve a focused, attentive engagement of the mind. *Reflection* refers to the exploration of one's inner world and necessarily involves recognition of feelings, emotions, and motivations to act. Although an internal experience, self-reflection intimately connects to the outside world and others as well. Reflection can become a tool of interpretation that can lead to a setting apart of spiritual experiences as different from everyday life, something special or transcendent (Bell, 1997). *Intention* involves using a value, belief, or ideology to guide one's occupational engagement, thereby changing the meaning of the experience.

In recent years, an awareness has grown about the value of mindfulness for supporting well-being and health. Mindful awareness is a way to mitigate the stress of everyday life and counter mindless and distracted modes of living. *Mindfulness* can be understood as a "flexible state of mind where we are actively engaged in the present, noticing new things and sensitive to context" (Langer, 2000, p. 220). Mindfulness can be both a cognitive trait and a meditative practice (Elliot, 2011). Some people use mindfulness activities such as meditation or yoga as an intentional part of their spiritual life. Mindful awareness, reflection, and intention can be active while participating in a wide array of varied occupations from hiking to drinking a cup of tea, thereby potentiating experiences of spirituality.

Occupations engaging a person's creativity offer the opportunity for deep levels of reflection, intention, mindful awareness, and ultimately spiritual experience. Kidd (1996), speaking of creativity and spirituality, says, "My creative life is my greatest prayer" (p. 123). In her classic work, *The Artist's Way: A Spiritual*

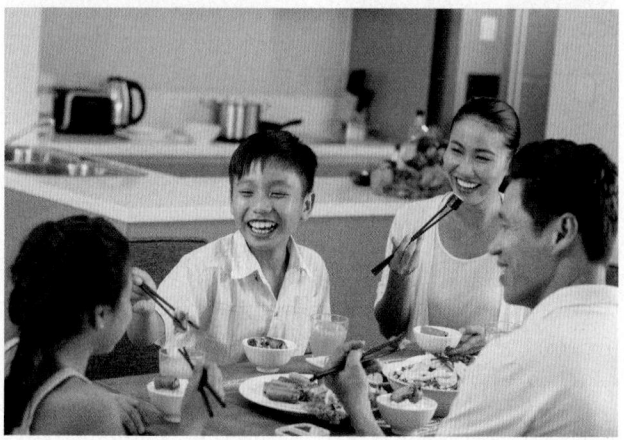

FIGURE 59.2 Gathering to share a meal can be an occupation with spiritual potential.

Path to Higher Creativity, Cameron (1992) shared a similar view of the intertwining of spirituality and creativity:

> Creativity is an experience—to my eye, a spiritual experience. It does not matter which way you think of it: creativity leading to spirituality or spirituality leading to creativity. In fact, I do not make a distinction between the two. (p. 2)

Infusing occupation with creativity allows for expression of internal states innately spiritual in nature and can translate into enhanced modes of coping (Corry et al., 2014; Simó-Algado et al., 2002). Whereas artistic occupations such as painting, making pottery, or writing poetry show high potential for spiritual experience, other everyday occupations can be filled with creativity as well (Hasselkus, 2011). Occupations such as cooking, conversing with others, playing an instrument, or planning a party, along with countless others, can be occupations in which creativity is expressed (Figure 59.4).

Occupational Participation

Not all occupations are experienced as spiritual, but all occupations hold the potential to be spiritual. Although people often name occupations stemming from religious traditions as spiritual, the lived experience might feel rote or disconnected to self and community and might not necessarily be spiritual for the person at that point in time. Everyday occupations such as work, walking the dog, or gardening might be experienced as spiritual but might not be named as religious (Howard & Howard, 1997; Unruh, 1997). Occupations that are deeply meaningful to the person, imbued with personal reflection and intention, and carried out within a supportive contextual environment offer the

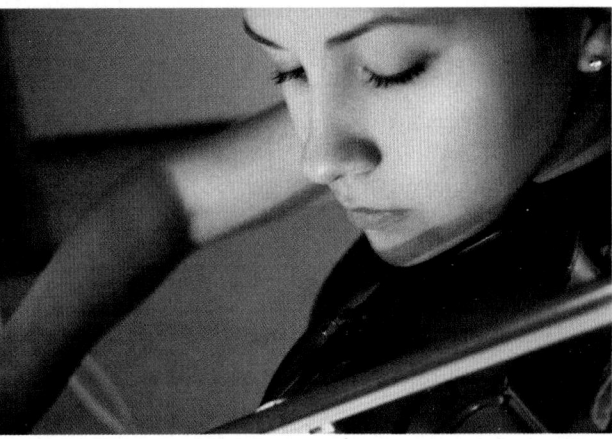

FIGURE 59.4 **An occupation that engages creativity can offer the opportunity for a spiritual experience.**

highest potential for spiritual experience (Billock, 2005). Kidd (1996) stated, "In a way all sacred experience and all journeys of soul lead us to the smallest moment of the most ordinary day" (p. 221). The line between secular and sacred becomes blurry with thoughtful examination of lived experiences of occupation. For the immigrant who left behind a homeland with limited resources, even the quotidian act of brushing her teeth with a toothbrush, toothpaste, and clean running water can spark a deep experience of meaning and gratitude. For an example of spirituality experienced through occupation, see Expanding Our Perspectives.

People frequently experience rituals as spiritual and can be used to reinforce values and beliefs (AOTA, 2020). Rituals

EXPANDING OUR PERSPECTIVES

Spirituality Through Occupation in Argentina

Mariel Pellegrini

For more than 5 years I worked in a municipal rehabilitation center for children with developmental challenges. This center was located in a poor neighborhood with limited economic resources in Buenos Aires. The children attended the different rehabilitation services once a week, accompanied by their mothers. The mothers waited in a room of the center while their children had treatments with the various professionals. The center asked me as a community occupational therapist to work with the mothers.

Seeing the mothers weekly, I observed how they really spent that time as a time of waiting, as a "between parentheses" of their daily lives. They passed the hours almost without speaking to each other. They had the possibility of

using the kitchen to have a coffee or an Argentine maté, but they did not move from their seats. They did not ask for anything; they did not exchange conversations with each other.

I had recently written a book chapter on spirituality and occupations in which I described the two dimensions of occupations, the visible and the invisible (Pellegrini, 2007). The first includes the observable, the form, the palpable of occupational doing. The second includes what accompanies doing, that which cannot be touched, but can be described as that which accompanies the human being when performing occupations, which transcends the visible, that is, spirituality.

Spirituality is connected with meaningful occupations; it manifests itself in the expression of people when they enjoy watching a sunset, listening to music, reading a book, or smelling an aroma, for example. Explain why one

(continued)

EXPANDING OUR PERSPECTIVES (*continued*)

person likes mountainous landscapes and others the sea; why some prefer the spring and others the autumn. It is that component that makes us unique (Pellegrini, 2007). Therefore, it connects us with a deep and intimate dimension that accompanies everyday life. Being something so unique to each person, it is not possible to identify what occupations facilitate their development, nor what behaviors characterize it. What can be identified is how it develops in the life of each individual and how significant occupations facilitate their development.

So I wondered where spirituality was in this space and how I could facilitate that connection in this time and space. With such a complex reality, where basic needs are not met and poverty is a cruel reality, where was the romanticism that accompanied the writings on spirituality? But I would learn from these women with their daily strength.

The beginning of the experience was to modify the environment, which I consider the unconditional ally of OT. After moving furniture to use the table as a meeting space, we were no longer sitting around the perimeter of the room. Instead, we were in a space of greater intimacy, of closeness, sharing coffee or Argentine matés.

Then I proposed an activity to repair games, toys, and cushions in the waiting room. This activity was designed to develop from their role as mothers and housewives. These were occupational roles that gave them

identity and strength, an intimate place of security and self-knowledge. In this proposal, the magic of occupation began to appear between threads, seams, glue, wool, patchworks, and toys that recovered eyes, buttons, and hair. The worktable facilitated sharing and participation. Where the mothers' gazes had another to see, their hands were used to repair, build, and collaborate. Thus, without thinking about it, spirituality began to flow, and the magic of the occupation flowed in the space with laughter, stories, recipes, advice, and daily talks.

The "between parentheses" and silence of the waiting room was transformed into a space where the occupation was the bridge of connection with that deep and intimate dimension that accompanies daily life. At that time, with those women, I learned that spirituality can occur in spaces of meditation, specific settings where romance and beauty are present, but that it can also flow when occupations connect us with the simplest things in life. Spirituality occurs when we feel intimately sure of our doing, when we share activities that facilitate those spaces of intimacy with oneself and/or with other beings with whom we feel safe and validated, and we can show ourselves as we are.

Reference

Pellegrini, M. (2007). *Fundamentos del Paradigma de Ciencia de la Ocupación. en: Terapeutas Ocupacionales, Servicio Andaluz de Salud* (Vol. I., p. 411). Editorial MAD, Sevilla.

---

can be understood as "symbolic actions with spiritual, cultural, or social meaning" (AOTA, 2020, p. S13). Common to understandings of ritual are the notions of repetition, fixedness, and predictability and are often embedded in the doing of religion (Hasselkus, 2011). Outside of religion, any occupation can take on ritualistic characteristics of formalism, tradition, invariance, sacral symbolization, and performance. It is these characteristics that differentiate sacred experience from the more mundane aspects of life (Bell, 1997). Depending on an individual's engagement, an occupation such as taking a bath could be experienced as spiritual owing to ritualized characteristics. Bell (1997) recognized the importance of ritual-like performances because they "communicate on multiple sensory levels, usually involving highly visual imagery, dramatic sounds, and sometimes even tactile, olfactory, and gustatory stimulation" (p. 160). For example, engagement in the occupations of a holiday celebration with its attendant ritual practices involving food and particular actions offers the possibility of spiritual experience in bringing together personal, familial, social, religious, and cultural aspects of life (Luboshitzky & Gaber, 2001; Figure 59.5).

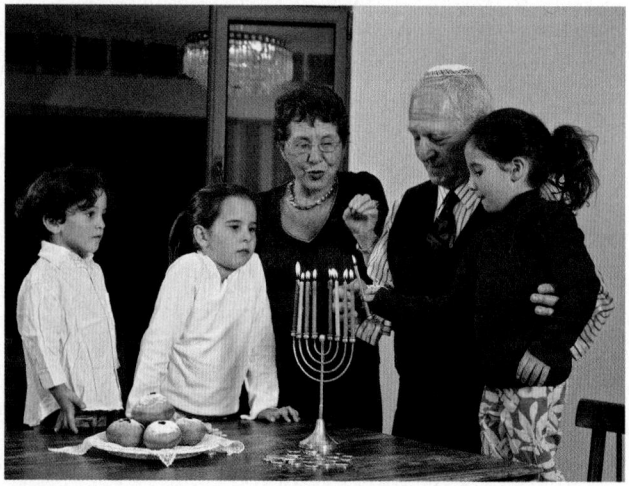

FIGURE 59.5 Engagement in the occupations of a holiday celebration with its attendant ritual practices offers the possibility of spiritual experience in bringing together personal, familial, social, religious, and cultural aspects of life.

Integrating Personal Beliefs, Values, and Spirituality Into Occupational Therapy Practice

As a profession rooted in holistic values and a person-centered approach to care, OT holds a unique opportunity to help clients experience meaning in their lives, a vitally important and essentially spiritual task. Although most OT practitioners recognize spirituality as an important aspect of life, integrating a client's personal beliefs, values, and spirituality into OT practice proves problematic because of breadth of definitions, large diversity of practitioners' understanding of the notions, and need for more extensive or further education (Enquist et al., 1997; Johnston & Mayers, 2005; Morris et al., 2014). These challenges can lead to role ambiguity and a lack of confidence in addressing spirituality in practice in spite of a recognized need for its inclusion (Belcham, 2004). As Howard and Howard (1997) indicate, "occupational therapists need not look beyond the tools, theories, and values of the profession to provide a context for acknowledging the spiritual in the clinic" (p. 185). If spirituality is a deep experience of meaning effectively experienced through occupational engagement, then OT intervention strategies that uphold holism through occupation-based and person-centered techniques will likely promote spiritual health and well-being.

Recognizing the difficulty of integrating spirituality into practice, Egan and Swedersky (2003) identified several strategies used by occupational therapists who successfully achieve this integration. Two strategies include addressing clients' religious concerns and assisting clients in dealing with suffering. Addressing clients' religious concerns can include talking about the accessibility of the clients' place of worship, practicing transfers to the type of seating in the religious setting, which might also involve kneeling down on a bench or the floor. Working with a Muslim client could involve practicing floor-to-stand transfers to be able to assume the traditional prayer posture or discussing adaptations for completing the five times daily occupation. Understanding various religious beliefs in relation to illness and suffering also proves important. For example, in the Buddhist tradition, pain and suffering are viewed as tools for spiritual insight or enlightenment. Often, OT practitioners work with clients and families dealing with a major life event or transition that demands coping and being able to find meaning and purpose to move forward—an important role that spirituality can play (Jones et al., 2016; Maley et al., 2016). See OT Story 59.1, for an example. Spiritual beliefs and personal

OT STORY 59.1 A WOMAN WITH A SPINAL CORD INJURY

You are an OT practitioner working in an inpatient rehabilitation unit with a 34-year-old woman named Sarah who sustained a T2 complete spinal cord injury in a car crash 2 weeks ago. Sarah and her husband, Uri, are active in their Orthodox Jewish synagogue and community. Sarah is the primary caregiver to her three young children aged 2, 4, and 7 years. Although she said that she is motivated to work on being able to care for herself and family, Sarah shared that she is feeling "discouraged and sad" and finds it hard to do therapy at times.

Questions
- How might Sarah's faith inform her goals for activities of daily living (ADL) and instrumental activities of daily living (IADL) participation?
- What questions would you ask to provide more information so you can address her coping skills?
- What would you want to know about Sarah's participation in her religious community?

values can inform the type of coping intervention and could include occupations such as prayer, meditation, or writing a note of gratitude to a friend. Also, leisure occupations such as gardening can be experienced as spiritual and support living and coping with stressful life events and can promote resilience (Unruh & Hutchinson, 2011).

Integrating spirituality into practice necessarily involves a reflective process of the OT practitioner (Townsend et al., 1999). Practitioners must consider their own understanding of spirituality and how their spirituality plays out in their occupations and experiences. Additionally, this self-reflective process may lead to the recognition of personal biases, values, or beliefs that could interfere with the crucially needed openness to clients' diverse beliefs and experiences. Self-reflection also aids in the ethically important need for therapeutic interventions to be consistent with the client's spiritual life or community's values and beliefs, not the therapist's (Rosenfeld, 2001). Those who practice therapeutic use of self through active listening, empathy, tolerance, unconditional acceptance, and flexibility toward the client's desires and needs demonstrate a spiritual approach to therapeutic interaction. A spiritual perspective within OT can lead practitioners to view their work as deeply meaningful and transformative (Egan & Swedersky, 2003).

Several approaches and tools can assist in the integration of spirituality for all the phases of the OT process. Many recipients of OT services experience disruptions to and loss of the occupations through which they experience spirituality and meaning. By honoring the subjective experiences of those in the evaluation, goal setting, and intervention planning processes, the practitioner moves toward integrating spirituality into practice and will likely increase the person's motivation (Townsend et al., 1999). Tools such as the Canadian Occupational Performance Measure allow for a person-centered and occupation-based approach that can address spiritual needs through actively integrating the individual into the phases of evaluation and intervention (Law et al., 2014). Conducting an occupational profile gathers relevant information about important and meaningful occupations and builds a person-centered foundation for intervention (AOTA, 2020).

Multiple healthcare professions use spiritual assessment tools as a practical method for including spirituality in practice (Koenig, 2007; Puchalski & Romer, 2000). OT practitioners have found spiritual assessments FICA and HOPE as practical and convenient for gathering vital information about their clients' spiritual lives (Anandarajah & Hight, 2001; Bouthot et al., 2011). However, these tools do not uniquely focus on OT concerns. The OT-QUEST (Schulz, 2008) is an OT spiritual assessment with a combination of Likert scale and open-ended questions.

Another spiritual assessment specifically tailored to OT is the Occupational Therapy Spiritual Assessment (OTSA; Box 59.1). The OTSA consists of guiding qualitative narrative interview questions designed to better understand a client's lived experiences of spirituality to help enable integration of holistic spiritual care in OT. The tool's design strives to facilitate a meaningful conversation between OT practitioner and client about areas of deep meaning relating to occupational participation and is meant to be flexible according to client needs. The five core categories of personal values and beliefs, coping, community, connection, and referral all have a primary question with other optional exploratory questions. Questions can be skipped, reordered, or modified as needed. Facilitation takes between five and ten minutes and can be used with adult clients, family members, or caregivers.

BOX 59.1 OCCUPATIONAL THERAPY SPIRITUAL ASSESSMENT

Personal Values and Beliefs

What activities do you do to express your personal values or beliefs?

Other ways to explore the question:

- Tell me about a time when you did an activity that made you feel connected to your personal values or beliefs.
- What do you most look forward to doing each day or week?
- What activities are you most passionate about participating in?
- What do you notice about yourself when you are connected to passions in your life?
- What activities make you feel most like yourself?
- Tell me about any beliefs that might influence your wellness, medical care, and/or recovery process.

Coping

Tell me about how you cope with difficulties in life.

Other ways to explore the question:

- Tell me about a time when you successfully managed a hardship in your life.
- What gives you hope for the future?
- When times are tough, what gets you through the day?
- What helps you feel peaceful?
- Who do you turn to when you need help?

Community

Tell me about your participation with a spiritual, religious, or other group.

Other ways to explore the question:

- Tell me about a memorable experience spending time with a spiritual, religious, or other group.
- Do you have a group that you spend time with regularly?
- What do you like to do with your spiritual/religious community or other group?
- Tell me about your connections within your spiritual/religious community or group.
- If you attend services in a spiritual or religious setting now or in the past, how do you participate?
- Tell me about any fears or concerns about participating with your group.

Connection

How do you experience connection in your life?

Other ways to explore the question:

- Tell me about a time where you did an activity that made you feel connected to other people, the world, yourself, or a higher power.
- What do you do to connect with other people, the world, yourself, or a higher power?
- How do you feel when you are doing things you love?
- Who do you love most and who loves you?
- How do you experience love and connection?

BOX 59.1 OCCUPATIONAL THERAPY SPIRITUAL ASSESSMENT (*continued*)

Referral

Would you like to talk with someone about any spiritual or religious concerns?

Other ways to explore the question:

- Tell me about a time when someone was able to help you through a difficult time.
- Who do you speak with about your spiritual or religious concerns?
- Who do you talk with when life gets hard?
- Tell me how your present concerns might be shared.
- Would you like to talk with a chaplain?
- Would you like to talk with your clergyperson?

Satisfaction

How satisfied are you with the activities and experiences that support your spirit?

1. Not satisfied
2. Slightly satisfied
3. Moderately satisfied
4. Very satisfied
5. Extremely satisfied

© 2022 Christy Billock, PhD, OTR/L, DipACLM.

After spiritual assessment, bringing spirituality into intervention proves important. A person-centered OT approach that draws spirituality into practice requires close attention to the culture, personal values, and beliefs (Simó-Algado et al., 2002). Practitioners sometimes feel uncomfortable integrating clients' religious occupations into practice. If an individual names these occupations as important in daily life, religious occupations such as prayer or reading sacred texts can be integrated into intervention sessions as deeply meaningful occupations. Addressing culture might call for learning more about rituals and religious traditions different from the practitioner's own religious experience or exposure. Clergy from the client's religion as well as family members can serve as resources for the practitioner to increase cultural and religious competence (Rosenfeld, 2001). For clients dealing with emotional trauma, occupations encouraging reflection and expression of internal states, such as artistic pursuits and storytelling, can provide opportunity for spiritual insight and coping (Simó-Algado et al., 2002). Last, engaging in mindful awareness practices may facilitate a sense of connection and open the door to spiritual experience (see Box 59.2).

Conclusion

The rich concepts of personal beliefs, values, and spirituality provide OT practitioners with valuable tools for understanding the deep meaning of engaging in occupation. Future growth in integrating spirituality into practice include strengthening education both in the preparation of and continuing education for practitioners, understanding the role of spirituality and occupation for communities and populations, gaining a deeper understanding about children's experience of spirituality (Harrison & Cox, 2017), and

BOX 59.2 NARRATIVE AS A KEY TO UNDERSTANDING: *JOURNEY TO LADAKH*

Beth Long shares her heartfelt story of finding meaning and rebuilding her life after a stroke in Appendix III, Chapter F, *Journey to Ladakh*. She illuminates the spiritual power of others providing love, support, and compassion, which transcends religious beliefs or cultural practices. Her experience of staying present in the moment for whatever life brings and recognizing the fullness of values and beliefs in the everyday can remind us of the potential for spiritual experience as fuel for coping with challenges and loss.

exploring the intersections of disability and spiritual experience to name a few. Important to clients' health and well-being, integrating spirituality into OT practice proves relevant to the profession's goal of providing person-centered care now and into the future.

Lippincott® Connect *For additional resources on the subjects discussed in this chapter, visit Lippincott Connect.*

REFERENCES

Aldwin, C. M., Park, C. L., Jeong, Y., & Nath, R. (2014). Differing pathways between religiousness, spirituality, and health: A self-regulation perspective. *Psychology of Religion and Spirituality, 6*, 9–21. https://doi.org/10.1037/a0034416

American Occupational Therapy Association. (2020). Occupational therapy practice framework: Domain and process, 4th edition. *American Journal of Occupational Therapy, 74*(2), 74124110010. https://doi.org/10.5014/ajot.2020.74S2001

Anandarajah, G., & Hight, E. (2001). Spirituality and medical practice: Using the HOPE questions as a practical tool for spiritual assessment.

American Family Physician, 63, 81–89. https://doi.org/10.1016/s1443-8461(01)80044-7

Baker, J. O., & Smith, B. G. (2015). *American secularism: Cultural contours of nonreligious belief systems.* NYU Press.

Belcham, C. (2004). Spirituality in occupational therapy: Theory in practice? *British Journal of Occupational Therapy, 67,* 39–46. https://doi.org/10.1177/030802260406700106

Bell, C. (1997). *Ritual: Perspectives and dimensions.* Oxford University Press.

Billock, C. (2005). *Delving into the center: Women's lived experience of spirituality through occupation* [Doctoral dissertation]. ProQuest Dissertations and Theses Database (Accession Order No. AAT 3219812).

Bouthot, J., Wells, T., & Black, R. (2011). Spirituality in practice: Using the FICA spiritual history assessment. *OT Practice, 18*(3), 13–16.

Cameron, J. (1992). *The artist's way: A spiritual path to higher creativity.* Penguin Putnam.

Christiansen, C. (1997). Nationally speaking: Acknowledging a spiritual dimension in occupational therapy practice. *American Journal of Occupational Therapy, 51,* 169–172. https://doi.org/10.5014/ajot.51.3.169

Corry, D. A. S., Lewis, C. A., & Mallett, J. (2014). Harnessing the mental health benefits of the creativity-spirituality construct: Introducing the theory of transformative coping. *Journal of Spirituality in Mental Health, 16,* 89–110. https://doi.org/10.1080/19349637.2014.896854

Costin, V, & Vignoles, V. L. (2020). Meaning is about mattering: Evaluating coherence, purpose, and existential mattering as precursors of meaning in life judgments. *Journal of Personality and Social Psychology, 118*(4), 864–884. https://doi.org/10.1037/pspp0000225

Egan, M., & Swedersky, J. (2003). Spirituality as experienced by occupational therapists in practice. *American Journal of Occupational Therapy, 57,* 525–533. https://doi.org/10.5014/ajot.57.5.525

Elliot, M. L. (2011). Being mindful about mindfulness: An invitation to extend occupational engagement into the growing mindfulness discourse. *Journal of Occupational Science, 18,* 366–376. https://doi.org/10.1080/14427591.2011.610777

Enquist, D. E., Short-DeGraff, M., Gliner, J., & Oltjenbruns, K. (1997). Occupational theorists' beliefs and practices with regard to spirituality and therapy. *American Journal of Occupational Therapy, 51,* 173–180. https://doi.org/10.5014/AJOT.51.3.173

Frank, G., Bernardo, C. S., Tropper, S., Noguchi, F., Lipman, C., Maulhardt, B., & Weitze, L. (1997). Jewish spirituality through actions in time: Daily occupations of young Orthodox Jewish couples in Los Angeles. *American Journal of Occupational Therapy, 51,* 199–206. https://doi.org/10.5014/ajot.51.3.199

Frankl, V. (1959). *Man's search for meaning.* Washington Square Press.

Fried, L., Prohaska, T., Burholt, V., Burns, A., Golden, J., Hawkley, L., Lawlor, B., Leavey, G., Lubben, J., O'Sullivan, R., Perissinotto, C., van Tilburg, T., Tully, M., & Victor, C. (2020). A unified approach to loneliness. *Lancet, 395*(10218), 114. https://doi.org/10.1016/S0140-6736(19)32533-4

Harrison, L., & Cox, D. (2017). Myth or reality? How do occupational therapists address the spirituality of children with disabilities? *British Journal of Occupational Therapy, 80,* 40–41. http://insight.cumbria.ac.uk/id/eprint/3240/

Hasselkus, B. R. (2011). *The meaning of everyday occupation* (2nd ed.). SLACK.

Hawks, S. R., Hull, M. L., Thalman, R. L., & Richins, P. M. (1995). Review of spiritual health: Definition, role and intervention strategies in health promotion. *American Journal of Health Promotion, 9,* 371–378. https://doi.org/10.4278/0890-1171-9.5.371

Holt-Lundstadt, J., Robles, T. F., & Sbarra, D. A. (2017). Advancing social connection as a public health priority in the United States. *American Psychologist, 72,* 517–530. https://doi.org/10.1037/amp0000103

Hooper, B., & Wood, W. (2014). The philosophy of occupational therapy: A framework for practice. In B. A. B. Schell, G. Gillen, & M. Scaffa

(Eds.), *Willard & Spackman's occupational therapy* (12th ed., pp. 35–46). Lippincott Williams & Wilkins.

Howard, B. S., & Howard, J. R. (1997). Occupation as spiritual activity. *American Journal of Occupational Therapy, 51,* 181–185. https://doi.org/10.5014/ajot.51.3.181

Jackson, J. M. (1996). Living a meaningful existence in old age. In R. Zemke & F. Clark (Eds.), *Occupational science: The evolving discipline* (pp. 339–361). F. A. Davis.

Johnston, D., & Mayers, C. (2005). Spirituality: A review of how occupational therapists acknowledge, assess, and meet spiritual needs. *British Journal of Occupational Therapy, 68*(9), 386–392. https://doi.org/10.1177/030802260506800902

Jones, J. (2021). U.S. church membership falls below majority for first time. *Gallup.* https://news.gallup.com/poll/341963/church-membership-falls-below-majority-first-time.aspx

Jones, J., Topping, A., Wattis, J., & Smith, J. (2016). A concept analysis of spirituality in occupational therapy practice. *Journal for the Study of Spirituality, 6,* 38–57. https://doi.org/10.1080/20440243.2016.1158455

Kidd, S. M. (1996). *Dance of the dissident daughter: A woman's journey from Christian tradition to the sacred feminine.* HarperCollins.

Koenig, H. G. (2007). *Spirituality in patient care: Why, how, when, and what* (2nd ed.). Templeton Press.

Koenig, H. G., Al-Zaben, F., & VanderWeele, T. J. (2020). Religion and psychiatry: Recent developments in research. *British Journal of Psychiatry Advances, 26*(5), 262–272. https://doi.org/10.1192/bja.2019.81

Kroeker, T. (1997). Spirituality and occupational therapy in a secular culture. *Canadian Journal of Occupational Therapy, 64,* 122–126. https://doi.org/10.1177/000841749706400109

Langer, E. (2000). Mindful learning. *Current Directions in Psychological Science, 9,* 220–223. https://doi.org/10.1111/1467-8721.00099

Law, M., Baptiste, S., Carswell, A., McColl, M. A., Polatajko, H., & Pollock, N. (2014). *Canadian occupational performance measure* (5th ed.). Canadian Association of Occupational Therapists.

Luboshitzky, D., & Gaber, L. B. (2001). Holidays and celebrations as a spiritual occupation. *Australian Occupational Therapy Journal, 48,* 66–74. https://doi.org/10.1046/j.1440-1630.2001.00251.x

Maley, C. M., Pagana, N. K., Valenger, C. A., & Humbert, T. K. (2016). Dealing with major life events and transitions: A systematic literature review on and occupational analysis of spirituality. *American Journal of Occupational Therapy, 70,* 7004260010p1–7004260010p6. https://doi.org/10.5014/ajot.2016.015537

McColl, M. A. (2002). Occupation in stressful times. *American Journal of Occupational Therapy, 56,* 350–353. https://doi.org/10.5014/ajot.56.3.350

Morris, D. N., Stecher, J., Briggs-Peppler, K. M., Chittenden, C. M., Rubira, J., & Wismer, L. K. (2014). Spirituality in occupational therapy: Do we practice what we teach? *Journal of Religion and Health, 53,* 27–36. https://doi.org/10.1007/s10943-012-9584-y

Peloquin, S. M. (1997). Nationally speaking: The spiritual depth of occupation: Making worlds and making lives. *American Journal of Occupational Therapy, 51,* 167–168. https://doi.org/10.5014/ajot.51.3.167

Pew Research Center. (2018). *The age gap in religion around the world.* https://www.pewforum.org/2018/06/13/how-religious-commitment-varies-by-country-among-people-of-all-ages/

Puchalski, C., & Romer, A. (2000). Taking a spiritual history allows clinicians to understand patients more fully. *Journal of Palliative Medicine, 3,* 129–137. https://doi.org/10.1089/jpm.2000.3.129

Ramugondo, E. L. & Kronenberg, F. (2015). Explaining collective occupations from a human relations perspective: Bridging the individual-collective dichotomy. *Journal of Occupational Science, 22*(1), 3–16. https://doi.org/10.1080/14427591.2013.781920

Rosenfeld, M. S. (2001). Exploring a spiritual context for care. *OT Practice, 6*(11), 18–26.

Schulz, E. (2008). OT-QUEST assessment. In B. J. Hemphill-Pearson (Ed.), *Occupational therapy assessment in mental health* (2nd ed., pp. 263–289). SLACK.

Seeman, T. E., Dubin, L. F., & Seeman, M. (2003). Religiosity/spirituality and health: A critical review of the evidence for biological pathways. *American Psychologist, 58*, 53–63. https://doi.org/10.1037/0003-066x.58.1.53

Simó-Algado, S., Mehta, N., Kronenberg, F., Cockburn, L., & Kirsh, B. (2002). Occupational therapy intervention with children survivors of war. *Canadian Journal of Occupational Therapy, 69*, 205–215. https://doi.org/10.1177/000841740206900405

Townsend, E., DeLaat, D., Egan, M., Thibeault, R., & Wright, W. A. (1999). *Spirituality in enabling occupation: A learner-centered workbook*. Canadian Association of Occupational Therapists.

Townsend, E., & Wilcock, A. (2004). Occupational justice and client-centered practice: A dialogue in practice. *Canadian Journal of Occupational Therapy, 71*, 75–87. https://doi.org/10.1177/000841740407100203

Tuan, Y. (1977). *Space and place: The perspective of experience*. University of Minnesota Press.

Unruh, A. M. (1997). Spirituality and occupation: Garden musings and the Himalayan blue poppy. *Canadian Journal of Occupational Therapy, 64*, 156–160. https://doi.org/10.1177/000841749706400112

Unruh, A. M., & Hutchinson, S. (2011). Embedded spirituality: Gardening in daily life and stressful life experiences. *Scandinavian Journal of Caring Sciences, 25*, 567–574. https://doi.org/10.1111/j.1471-6712.2010.00865.x

Wilcock, A. A., & Townsend, E. A. (2014). Occupational justice. In B. A. B. Schell, G. Gillen, & M. Scaffa (Eds.), *Willard & Spackman's occupational therapy* (12th ed., pp. 541–552). Lippincott Williams & Wilkins.

Wuthnow, R. (1998). *After heaven: Spirituality in America since the 1950's*. University of California Press.

Wuthnow, R. (2010). *After the baby-boomers: How twenty- and thirty-somethings are shaping the future of American religion*. Princeton University Press.

Zemke, R., & Clark, F. (1996). Section V: Co-occupations of mothers and children: Introduction. In R. Zemke & F. Clark (Eds.), *Occupational science: The evolving discipline* (pp. 213–215). F. A. Davis.

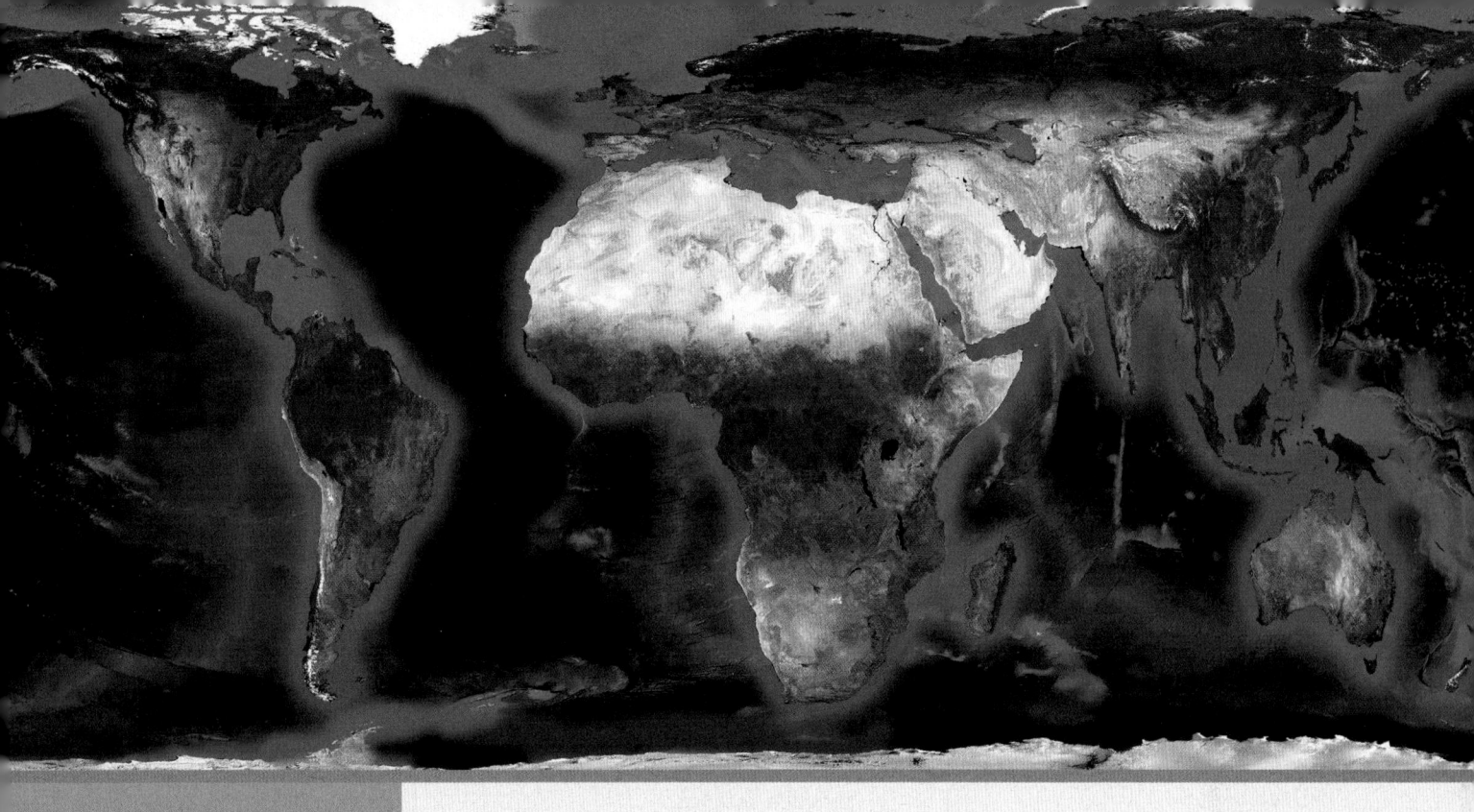

UNIT IX

The Practice Context: Therapists in Action

Media Related to The Practice Context: Therapists in Action

Readings
- *Hidden Valley Road:* Robert Kolker's book about a family with six of twelve children diagnosed with schizophrenia. (2020)

Movies
- *The Diving Bell and the Butterfly:* The story of Jean-Dominique Bauby, who experienced locked-in syndrome after a cerebral vascular seizure. Eventually he and his speech therapist were able to create a means by which he could communicate and write his story. (2007)
- *Million Dollar Baby:* A movie with a controversial ending about a woman who becomes a quadriplegic after a boxing incident and decides to end her life. (2005)

TV Shows
- *Atypical:* A comedy about an autistic high schooler. (2018–2021)
- *The Great Depresh:* Part stand-up and part documentary about Gary Gulman's experiences with severe depression. (2019)

Music and Theater
- *Freak Flag:* From *Shrek the Musical*, a song about embracing what makes you special even if it is what also makes you different. (2008)
- *TDF Autism Friendly Performances:* This organization presents Broadway musicals and plays in a friendly, supportive environment for people with ASD and other sensitivity issues. Since 2011, they have presented more than 18 autism friendly shows on Broadway.

Practice Settings for Occupational Therapy

Pamela S. Roberts and Mary E. Evenson

LEARNING OBJECTIVES

After reading this chapter, you will be able to:

1. Describe occupational therapy's typical roles in physical disability, mental health, pediatric, older adult, and work/employment practice settings.
2. Value the importance of client-centered care through the collaborative goal-setting process to guide the professional reasoning process and influence intervention planning across practice settings.
3. Recognize how client factors and contexts featured in the case studies influence discharge recommendations and disposition through an individualized path of receiving occupational therapy services across the continuum of care.
4. Be aware of key healthcare system regulations that affect a client's eligibility for services and length of stay in various practice settings.
5. Acknowledge the opportunities for population-based practice areas to meet the needs of populations with varying access to healthcare.

Introduction

This chapter provides an overview of settings in which occupational therapy (OT) practitioners practice in the areas of physical disability, mental health, pediatrics, older adults, and work/employment. Population-based services are also discussed. Case studies are featured as examples to illustrate how different services and settings can meet an individual client's needs and goals, depending on the level of care and the client's personal factors and occupational performance. These settings sometimes fall on a continuum of care that might include a variety of services spanning emergency/acute care, inpatient and outpatient rehabilitation, skilled nursing and/or extended care, partial hospital or day programs, community-based services, home care, and/or hospice. Table 60.1 provides an organizing structure to help understand the different settings This chapter is a preface to the following chapters in this unit that more comprehensively address selected populations and occupational therapist's role to support optimal function and participation.

TABLE 60.1	**Practice Settings**			
Setting	Requirements for Admission to Setting	Typical Setting	Typical Services	Role of Occupational Therapy Service
Physical Disability/Illness Practice Settings				
Acute medical/ surgical care	• Need for medical or surgical diagnosis or intervention • Admitted from emergency room, direct admission, or transfer from another facility	• Private hospital • Community hospital • Academic hospital • Veterans Administration hospital • Specialty hospital	• Trauma services • ICU • Monitored unit • Medical services • Surgical services • Consultations by allied healthcare providers	• Positioning, range of motion, splinting/casting, early mobilization, and ADL. • Safety assessment; assessment of client's abilities, roles, habits, and routines, and functional skills, such as eating/dysphagia, grooming, dressing, bathing, and toileting • Recommendations for continued services at next level of care • Discharge planning
Inpatient rehabilitation	• Transfer from a hospital, nursing home, or home • Must be able to tolerate intensive therapy • Able to engage in ongoing intervention of multiple therapies and benefit from intensive therapy • Patient is medically stable at the time of admission. • Supervision by a rehabilitation physician	• Freestanding rehabilitation center • Unit within hospital • Veterans Administration rehabilitation unit	• Rehabilitation physician • Rehabilitation nursing • PT • (OT) • Speech–language pathology • Recreational therapy • Neuropsychology or psychology • Social services • Respiratory therapy • Dietary • Pharmacy • Other services by consultation • Services usually 3 hours of therapy per day at least 5 out of 7 days	• Comprehensive evaluation • ADL and IADL assessment • Self-care skills • Functional mobility • Functional communication • Social cognition • IADL • Community reintegration • Discharge planning • Recommendations for continued services (e.g., driving evaluation) at the next level of care
Skilled nursing/ transitional care	• Require 24-h care for either a short or extended period of time • Bridge the gap with another level of care • Admitted from acute care hospital • Skilled intervention, such as intravenous medication, wound care, and so forth • Disability with new functional deficit	• Unit in a hospital • Freestanding nursing home	• Physician • Nursing • Social services • Activity therapy • PT • OT • Speech–language pathology • Other services by consultation	• Self-care skills, such as eating/dysphagia, grooming, upper and lower body dressing, bathing, and toileting • Mobility skills during ADL, such as bed, chair, and wheelchair transfers; toilet and tub/shower transfers; and locomotion activities • IADL and community skills, such as car transfers, homemaking activities, public dining, care of pets, and so forth
Outpatient rehabilitation	• Medical/surgical diagnosis with functional limitation that interferes with abilities to participate in activities and roles • Admitted from a variety of places, including institutional care or home	• Part of a freestanding rehabilitation center • Within a hospital • Within the Veterans Administration hospital • Satellite clinic (affiliated with a healthcare institution, such as hand therapy clinic) • Independent, privately owned clinic	• Rehabilitation physician • Psychology Services • PT • Speech–language pathology • OT	• Self-care skills, such as eating/dysphagia, grooming, upper and lower body dressing, bathing, and toileting • Mobility skills during ADL, such as bed, chair, and wheelchair transfers; toilet and tub/shower transfers; and locomotion activities • IADL skills • Social participation, such as student, worker, and caregiver roles

(continued)

TABLE 60.1	**Practice Settings** (*continued*)			
Setting	**Requirements for Admission to Setting**	**Typical Setting**	**Typical Services**	**Role of Occupational Therapy Service**
Long-term care	• Require 24-h care for an indefinite period of time • When functional recovery may not be possible • Lack of resources to be safe at home • Transfer from a hospital, nursing home, or home • Bridge gap between inpatient setting and home vs. determine need for permanent placement	• Freestanding hospital • Private hospital • State hospital • Veterans Administration hospital • Freestanding nursing home • Private nursing home • Custodial care, such as eating/dysphagia, grooming, and bathing	• Physician/psychiatrists • Nursing • Mental health workers • Therapy consultation as indicated for safety, assessment, self-care skills and routines, positioning, functional mobility during ADL, adaptations, and caregiver training	• Individual assessment and interventions as indicated • Consultant to program for ADL, environmental adaptations, and behavior management
Hospice, palliative care	• Eligible for Medicare Part A • Physician and hospice medical director certify terminal illness, and the patient has 6 mo or less to live if illness runs normal course • Sign statement choosing hospice care instead of other Medicare-covered benefits to treatment of terminal illness • Care from Medicare-approved hospice program	• Short-term inpatient care • Short-term respite care • Home	• Physician • Nursing • Counselors • Social services • OT • PT • Speech–language pathology • Hospice aides • Homemakers • Volunteers • Dietitian • Grief and loss counseling	• Assessment (living skills, work, leisure) • Home visits, environmental changes • Provision of aids and adaptations • Training in the use of equipment • Work simplification • Energy conservation, time management • Group activities • Group therapy (touch, role-play, psychodrama) • Education in coping with change (patient and family) • Relaxation and stress management • Therapeutic activities (arts, crafts, poetry, music) • Reminiscence therapy
Mental Health/Behavioral Health Practice Settings				
Inpatient psychiatry or substance misuse	• Require 24-h care for either a short or extended period of time • Need for psychiatric diagnosis or intervention • Admitted from the emergency room • Direct admit • Transfer from another facility • Person requires 24-h monitoring for safety • May be court ordered as in the case of forensic cases in which clients require secured (locked) units owing to safety risk to self or others	• Freestanding hospital • Private hospital • Unit within hospital • State hospital • Veterans Administration hospital	• Psychiatry • Psychology • Nursing • Mental health workers • Social services • OT • Recreational therapy • Art therapy • Expressive or music therapy • Behavior management • Other services by consultation	• Assessment of client's abilities, roles, habits, and routines • Safety assessment • Recommendations for continued services at next level of care • Discharge planning • Individual and/or group treatment • Functional skills, such as self-care, home, and community function • Reinforce behavioral or therapeutic plan

TABLE 60.1   Practice Settings (*continued*)

Setting	Requirements for Admission to Setting	Typical Setting	Typical Services	Role of Occupational Therapy Service
Partial hospitalization	• Require episodic focused psychiatric or substance misuse intervention • Transition from inpatient or as an alternative to acute psychiatric hospitalization • Structured program	• Freestanding hospital • Private hospital • Unit within hospital • State hospital • Veterans Administration hospital	• Psychiatry • Psychology • Nursing • Mental health workers • Social services • OT • Recreational therapy	• Assessment of client's abilities, roles, habits, and routines • Continuity of care for self-management goals with emphasis on productive living for home, community, and work • Individual and/or group treatment • Recommendations for continued services at next level of care
Community mental health center	• Provide ongoing support and structure to people who have mental health diagnoses to live in the community by promoting daily routine and sense of belonging to the program community and community at large • Participants may come and go based on program interests.	• Freestanding • Community health facility	• Psychiatric services • Case management • Peer support • Psychological services • May include housing and employment services • Leisure activities and groups • OT	• Establish or restore performance skills or work, self-care, and leisure, including coping strategies, interpersonal skills, time management, and decision-making • Strategies to support participants' behavior and ability to cope with challenges in social environments and adapt tasks for participant success
Group homes	• Adults with serious mental or medical illness, cognitive dysfunction, or developmental disabilities who require 24-h residential care • Foster development of social networks	• Residential facilities designed to create support, structure, and stability in a home-like setting	• Support for everyday living • Medication management • Recreational and leisure activities • OT	• Behavioral management techniques • Development of social and recreational programs at home • Facilitate independence in ADL and IADL by establishing performance patterns or modifying environment or activity demands • Evaluation to identify skills and develop behavioral plans and involvement in social, recreational, and work-related injuries
Supported housing	• Adults with serious mental illness needing support for independent community living	• Apartment complexes in the community	• Financial assistance with rent • Residential setting with intermittent support that might include assistance with money management, home management, etc.	• Assessment of home environment and living skills • Living skills training, environmental support, leisure activities
Sober living, halfway house, substance recovery center, transitional centers, re-entry centers, community-based residential facilities	• People in substance use recover leaving inpatient setting and not actively using substances or people leaving prison or jail needing support before returning to independent living in the community	• A residential facility where people live in a group environment typically with a strict set of rules and requirements before transition into independent living	• Medical, psychological, and social services to assist with reentry to community living • In some settings, residents are required to work during the day.	• Living skills training • Therapeutic activities • Assistance with transition to work and independent living

(*continued*)

TABLE 60.1   Practice Settings (*continued*)

Setting	Requirements for Admission to Setting	Typical Setting	Typical Services	Role of Occupational Therapy Service
Homeless shelters/domestic violence shelters	• People in need of emergency housing	• Freestanding buildings, locations for domestic violence shelters are confidential.	• Provide short-term relief for homelessness. Typically offer meals, shelter and supportive services. • Domestic violence shelters provide refuge and safety as well as housing, meals, and support.	• Living skills training • Assistance with transition to permanent housing • Coping/trauma-informed care
Forensic settings	• Involvement with justice system	• Prisons, jails, psychiatric hospital	• Counseling • Education • Job training • Community reentry	• Creative and therapeutic media • Emotion regulation, coping, trauma-informed care • Social skills training • Community reentry
Practice Settings Serving Children				
Early intervention	• Developmental delay in one or more area of development or has diagnosis likely to result in developmental delay • Identified disability or condition or at risk for developing a disability • Demonstrate atypical behaviors • Circumstances that place child and/or parent at risk for developmental delay • Each state has its own specific eligibility criteria.	• Home • Hospital • Clinic • Child care	• Physician • OT • Focus on family-centered model for service delivery	• Services to promote development • Promotion of parent–child interaction, ADL, especially feeding and play skills • Sensorimotor development • Gross motor skills • Fine motor skills • Self-help skills • Social–emotional development
Preschool	• Children who are 3 yr and older (until entry into elementary school) • Fit one of the categories under IDEA	• Public school setting • Childcare • Preschool setting	• OT • Preschool teacher	• Carrying out or suggesting activities that promote the child's overall development and ability to fully participate in preschool activities • Sensorimotor development • Gross motor skills • Fine motor skills • Social–emotional development
School	• Identified disability that fits one of the categories under IDEA • All eligibility and service decisions are made by a student's individual educational program.	• Public school • Private school	• OT • School teacher	• Supports student's education program and ability to fully participate in school activities, including recess • Organizing the student's daily schedule and materials • Negotiating in the cafeteria • During transition out of the school system, focus broadens to include independent living and community participation

TABLE 60.1   **Practice Settings (*continued*)**

Setting	Requirements for Admission to Setting	Typical Setting	Typical Services	Role of Occupational Therapy Service
Private practice	• Children of all ages • Decreased performance in daily tasks or desired activities	• Private clinic	• OT	• Addressing the child's needs that may not be met at school • Focus on body functions, such as sensory processing, motor planning, and visual perception, that provide foundational skills needed in school, ADL, and play
Practice Settings Serving Older Adults				
Adult day services (social, medical, dementia)	• Provide social/medical programming to increase the quality of life and health status of participants • Social: day programs to provide social/recreational activities, meals, and some health supports • Medical: provides rehabilitation and medical services to provide sufficient supports to forestall nursing home placement • Dementia: programs designed to focus on providing programming with cognitive support that improve the quality of life	• Freestanding • Associated with other community programs or health agencies, such as senior centers, mental health centers, rehabilitation centers, nursing homes, or hospitals	• Personnel from adult day services • OT • PT • Speech–language pathology	• Assistance with modifying and adapting activity programming for social, medical, and dementia programs • Assessment of ADL, IADL, safety, cognition, and so forth • Educational services to staff and family members regarding ADL, IADL, safety, fall prevention, and so forth
Assisted living	• Residential care for older adults who can no longer live independently but do not require medical services of a nursing home • Provides supportive care that enhances autonomy and choice • Provides supervision and support for ADL, IADL, safety, and so forth caused by dementia, neurologic impairment, or other medical problems • Provides activity programming to foster social engagement and participation	• Assisted living facilities	• Personnel from assisted living • OT • PT • Speech–language pathology	• Consultation to ensure that program engages residents in occupations of their choice and assist facility personnel to modify the physical/social environment to promote safety and independence • Direct services including evaluation and intervention to increase independence in ADL and IADL, prevent falls, and enhance participation in social activities • Education or direct service regarding issues related to aging, occupation, and health promotion

(continued)

TABLE 60.1	Practice Settings (*continued*)			
Setting	Requirements for Admission to Setting	Typical Setting	Typical Services	Role of Occupational Therapy Service
Work/Employment Practice Settings				
Sheltered workshops and prevocational training	• Individuals with disabilities (often developmental disabilities) that could benefit from a protective and highly supervised work environment.	• Freestanding facility	• Highly supervised work environment where individuals perform work tasks, such as parts assembly, sorting, and packing • Typically receive pay based on amount of work completed	• Evaluate workers' performance skills to match the activity demands of various possible jobs • Consultants to others to modify the work environment or activity demands for more efficient performance • Establish performance patterns and new performance skills • Maintain performance skills that workers have acquired
Supported employment	• Provide supported employment for people with serious mental illness, developmental disabilities, traumatic brain injury, etc., who desire to work in competitive employment and would benefit from supportive services to do so.	• Existing community work settings	• Rehabilitation counselors • Employment specialists • Occupational therapy	• Consultation with worksites to ensure integration of the employee and to provide education regarding adaptation to worksite environment and activity demands • Job coach to assist the employee to adapt to the worksite and to function effectively by learning job skills and interacting appropriately with other employees at worksite • Involved in matching prospective worker to potential worksites
Social firms, affirmative businesses, creative economies	• People with disabilities who desire employment in a community setting and want to work alongside other people with disabilities in a supportive setting	• Freestanding businesses, like restaurants, cafes, or industry that produces goods created to employ people with disabilities	• Employment opportunities • Workers are paid at market rates	• Environmental adaptation • Matching workers to job tasks • Skills training
Return-to-work programs	• Serve people with acquired disability who require rehabilitation to return to workforce either on job or new one.	• Freestanding • Part of other facilities, such as hospital, rehabilitation center, or community program	• Employment specialists • OT • PT • Certified vocational evaluation	• Provide rehabilitation services to enable the client to return to work • Evaluation of work tolerance • Development of work-related skills primarily using purposeful activities, such as work simulation and preparatory methods, such as work conditioning, work hardening, and exercise programs • Modification of job demands when necessary and possible to better match the current skills

ADL, activities of daily living; IADL, instrumental activities of daily living; IDEA, Individuals with Disabilities Education Act; OT, occupational therapy; PT, physical therapy.

OT practitioners work in facilities that provide a range of services to address the occupational performance needs and concerns of children and adults across the life course (Roberts & Evenson, 2009). Individuals seek OT evaluation and interventions often a result of a diagnosis/condition that requires medical, surgical, psychiatric, habilitation, or rehabilitative intervention. As a consequence, individuals experience difficulty performing daily life habits and activities and participating in social roles within their homes and communities (World Health Organization, 2001).

As part of the OT process, practitioners collaborate with clients and their caregivers to identify goals that will influence the intervention plan and subsequent delivery of services to support the individual's optimal functioning, recovery, and desired outcomes (see Chapters 18, 19, and 28). In addition to the client's goals, an occupational profile should be included in the evaluation process and ideally encompasses a biopsychosocial perspective, addressing safety, client factors, occupational performance, social support, and environmental contexts. In doing so, analysis of client functioning for areas of occupation, activities of daily living (ADL), instrumental activities of daily living (IADL), education, work, play and leisure, rest and sleep, and social participation is assessed throughout the various settings (American Occupational Therapy Association [AOTA], 2020) (see Unit XIII).

Types of Settings Providing Occupational Therapy to Individuals

One of the distinctive characteristics of OT practice is the diversity of settings in which we practice. Hospitals are one of the largest employers of occupational therapists with various levels of care; however, occupational therapists also practice in a variety of outpatient and community-based settings and in settings that are not healthcare based, such as schools and work sites. This section will describe major practice settings, but it is far from inclusive.

OT is practiced around the world and can be translated into practice in many different cultures and environments. OT programs and services for children and adults are increasing worldwide, with over 500,000 OT practitioners globally (Pattison, 2018). Hospitals employ over 130,000 occupational therapists in the United States (Bureau of Labor Statistics, 2020). Various levels of care may be available at an individual hospital, including acute care, long-term acute care, inpatient rehabilitation, and outpatient rehabilitation. Administratively, facilities may be for-profit, not-for-profit, or governmental. Hospital-based healthcare is a labor-intensive industry operating on a 24-hour-per-day, 7-day-per-week basis, facing complex issues related to finances, workforce, and information technology (American Hospital Association, 2017a, 2017b).

Schools and long-term care/skilled nursing facilities also provide a substantial percentage of job opportunities within the field (AOTA, 2019). Employment for occupational therapists in the United States is projected to increase by 17% from 2020 to 2030 (Bureau of Labor Statistics, 2020).

Once a person in need of services is medically stable (or when inpatient medical services are not needed or indicated), OT practitioners may work with them in freestanding outpatient/ambulatory care services, community

agencies, private practices, and home-based services, such as early intervention and home healthcare. Community-based settings often afford practitioners the opportunity to work in the client's[2] natural environment, such as home or school, and to focus on authentic occupation, in comparison to the focus on medical stabilization as the priority for inpatient settings.

Depending on the client's needs, an individual may receive OT services in different types of settings within the continuum of care. Determining the delivery of OT services in the various settings must be meaningful and within the scope of the individual's person-centered individualized treatment plan. Services may be face-to-face or through telehealth services. The use of telehealth has been accelerated to increase access during the pandemic health emergency. Including a method of live online service delivery through video software, by telephone, or by other means of electronic communications needs to be considered in the delivery options throughout the continuum of care (see Chapter 67 for more information on providing OT services via telehealth).

Balancing clients' needs, resources, personal factors, and occupational performance in consideration of their future goals also involves review and use of the best available evidence. This complex decision-making process requires practitioners to use their professional reasoning to make appropriate and meaningful recommendations to support and facilitate a client's progression through the continuum of care (see Chapter 25). Individual personal factors and levels of occupational performance, along with the contexts and environments in which one participates, greatly influence the options for discharge both between the levels of care and toward a final discharge disposition, ultimately enabling the client to be in a residential or home context.

Evidence Supporting Occupational Therapy in Selected Practice Settings

Health policy evidence has found OT to be the only spending category where additional spending has statistically significant association with lower readmission rates for

[2]According to the AOTA (2020, p. S75), the term *client* refers to *persons* (including those involved in care of a client), *groups* (a collection of individuals having shared characteristics or common or shared purpose, e.g., family members, workers, students, and those with similar interests or occupational challenges), and *populations* (aggregates of people with common attributes, such as contexts, characteristics, or concerns, including health risks). However, in countries other than the United States, the term *client* often refers to persons who are paying for their care directly. In most countries, *patient* is used to describe persons who are in hospital or rehabilitation. *Service user* and *person* are terms in general use that describe those in need of OT services. For this chapter, we are using *client* without implying the source of payment for services.

heart failure, pneumonia, and acute myocardial infarction (Rogers et al., 2016). Spending resources on OT has been shown to place a unique focus on patients' functional and social needs, which are important indicators to address. It was noted that this spending category (OT) affects both the clinical and social determinants of health and that investment in OT in the acute care setting has the potential to improve quality of care without significantly increasing overall hospital spending (Rogers et al., 2016). In another study involving OT in the community, it was found that a structured Community Aging in Place, Advancing Better Living for Elders (CAPABLE) program was associated with improved physical functioning, including improving from four to two difficulties with ADL, could enable the person to continue living at home instead of having to move to assisted living or institution (Szanton et al., 2016). These client dimensions of care intersect with legislative and funding/payment parameters to determine a client's eligibility for the frequency and duration of receiving OT services (see Table 60.1).

The goal of healthcare globally is to expand access and services, improve quality of life and work with available resources. This has led government agencies to develop and implement initiatives to improve the delivery of healthcare for increased quality, safety, and efficiency of care. An example would be the expansion of telehealth practice and payment options during the COVID-19 public health emergency. In examining international healthcare systems, it is important to consider the provision of OT services. This involves knowledge of each country's unique set of economic and social factors that influence the payment of OT services (refer Chapter 76).

Occupational Therapy Stories in Selected Practice Settings

To better understand the scope of OT services, the OT stories illustrate examples of practice areas. Each OT Story includes an occupational profile, performance, needs, goals, and practice context. Refer Table 60.1 for additional specifics on each area of practice featured in this chapter. See OT stories 60.1 to 60.5.

OT STORY 60.1 PHYSICAL ILLNESS: ADULT WITH CEREBRAL VASCULAR ACCIDENT

Jack is a man in his mid-70s who had a sudden onset of right-sided weakness as well as aphasia at 10 PM. Jack's wife immediately drove him to the local hospital, which had a certified stroke center. Within an hour of the onset of symptoms, he was assessed by the triage nurse and emergency department physician who consulted the neurologist on call. Jack was taken to imaging for a computed tomography (CT) scan, which showed no evidence of hemorrhage and a left middle cerebral artery infarct. The neurologist determined that Jack was a candidate for tissue plasminogen activator (tPA). Tissue plasminogen activator, if provided within an established time frame, can significantly reduce the effects of stroke and permanent disability. Jack was transferred to the neurointensive care unit where he was continuously monitored.

OT was consulted in the neurointensive care unit. The occupational therapist performed an evaluation using an occupational profile to learn of Jack's active lifestyle prior to admission to the hospital. Jack lived with his wife in a one-story home with five steps to enter. Jack is a retired lawyer. He is active with guest lecturing at a local law school and in volunteering at the animal shelter in his community. Jack loves to cook for his wife, two children, and four grandchildren. Additionally, Jack enjoyed driving, going to the theater, and dining at restaurants at least two times per week. Jack's goals are to be able to return to his previous active lifestyle, especially being able to cook for his family.

Jack's past medical history is significant for coronary artery disease, osteoarthritis, and borderline renal insufficiency. The OT assessment revealed right hemiparesis and expressive aphasia, resulting in activity limitations in daily activities requiring maximum assistance for eating, grooming, dressing, bathing, toileting, and mobility. Jack is dependent on others to perform IADL. OT started in the intensive care unit and continued on the acute stroke floor, with the focus on improving Jack's participation in daily activities and functional mobility. It was determined that Jack met admission criteria for inpatient rehabilitation (see Table 60.1) based on the diagnosis of stroke and functional limitations. Jack required intervention from multiple therapies, including physical therapy (PT), OT, and speech–language pathology (SLP). During his acute care hospitalization, Jack was actively participating in therapies (PT, OT, and SLP). After 4 days in the acute hospital, Jack was admitted to the inpatient rehabilitation hospital with a focus on restoration of function for eventual home with his wife.

The OT practitioner performed a standardized evaluation to assess ADL, mobility, safety, and the Canadian Occupational

OT STORY 60.1 PHYSICAL ILLNESS: ADULT WITH CEREBRAL VASCULAR ACCIDENT (*continued*)

Performance Measure (COPM) (Law et al., 2014), which revealed that Jack's goals were to be independent in self-care and cooking and, eventually, to return to his community activities. Within the first week, the interprofessional team had a conference that included Jack and his wife, discussing Jack's functional status, barriers, and goals. This collaboration provided the foundation for the interprofessional treatment plan with focus on Jack's goals to increase his independence for self-care, functional mobility, and IADL. Jack demonstrated significant improvement throughout his inpatient stay and was able to perform his daily activities with minimal assistance and cook simple meals with moderate assistance. He was able to eat a regular diet; however, he required assistance with cutting his food. Discharge planning included an evaluation of the home environment, ordering of durable medical equipment, and provision of referrals for community resources

and support groups. After discharge, Jack plans to continue his therapy at home with home health services until he is no longer homebound, when he will then plan to transition to outpatient rehabilitation to support his goals of increased independence for home and community reintegration, including eventual return to driving. See Figures 60.1 and 60.2.

Questions

1. How would Jack's cultural and social background influence the OT plan of care?
2. Taking into consideration from the OT profile and the responses on the COPM, what would be the priorities of care for Jack in this practice area?
3. Returning to driving is one of Jack's long-term goals, how can you learn more about OT's role in driving assessment and safety?

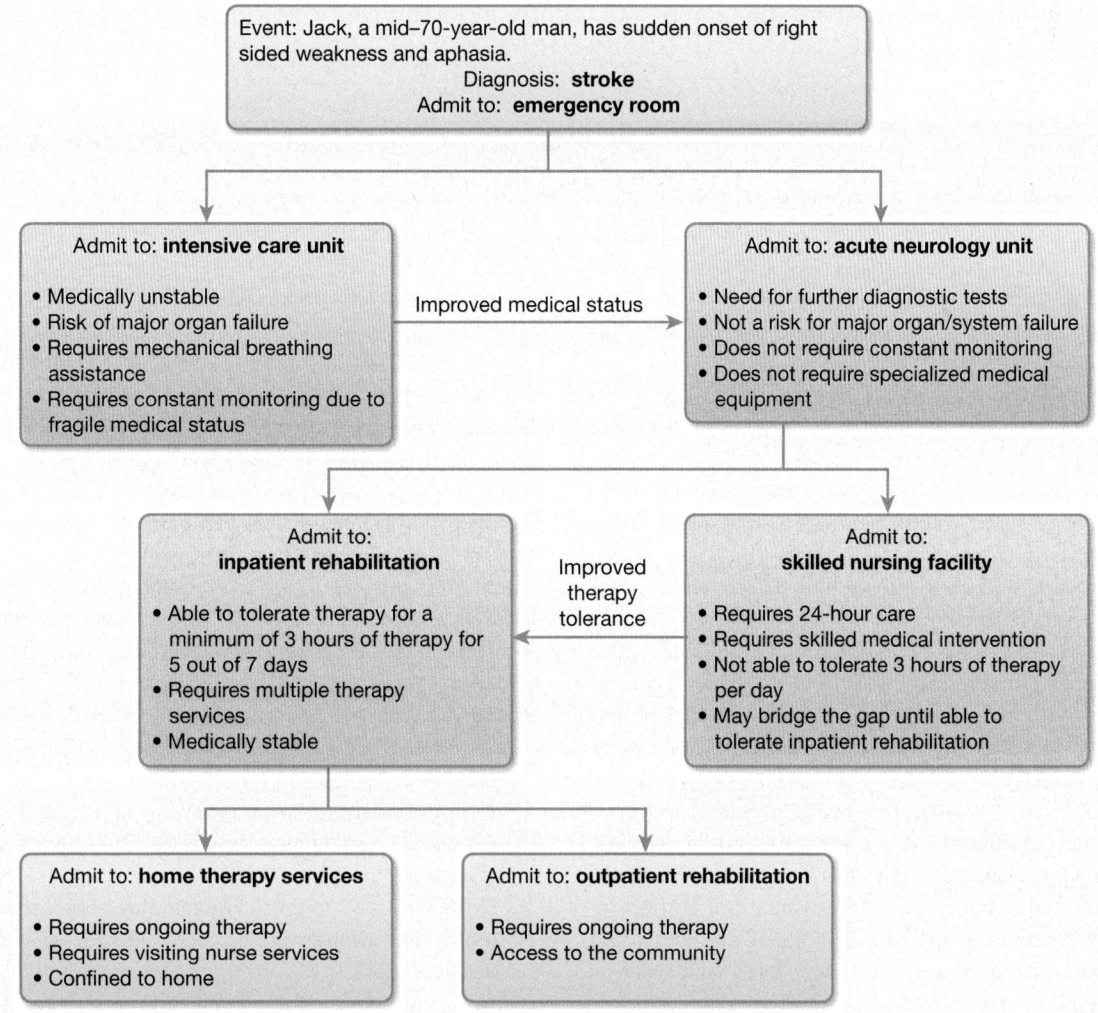

FIGURE 60.1 Example of transitioning through the continuum of care.

(continued)

OT STORY 60.1 PHYSICAL ILLNESS: ADULT WITH CEREBRAL VASCULAR ACCIDENT (continued)

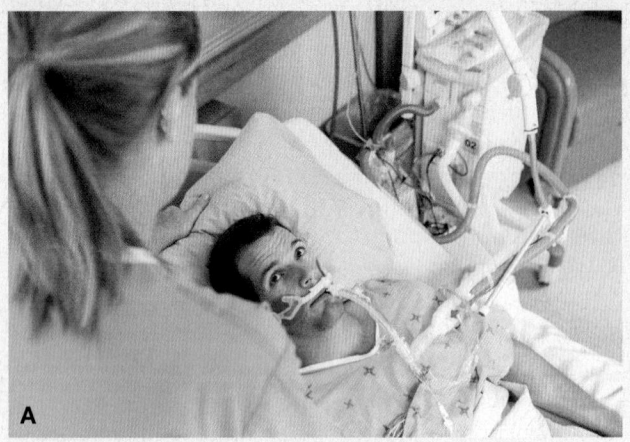
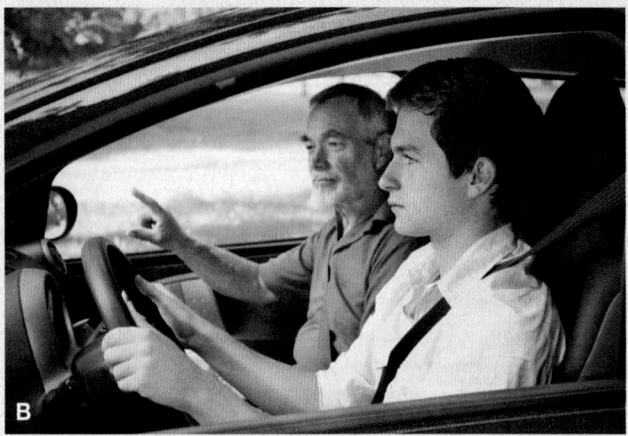

FIGURE 60.2 Occupational therapy practitioners work with clients throughout the continuum. **A:** In severe cases, we may first start to interact as part of early mobilization intensive care unit teams. **B:** Our role may continue all the way through community reentry including return to driving.

OT STORY 60.2 PHYSICAL DISABILITY: ADULT WITH TOTAL HIP REPLACEMENT

Episodes of care may occur within multiple facilities to meet the individual patient needs. Eligibility for services may vary in the amount and location of services provided. This applies to Marion, a female in her early 90s who has severe osteoarthritis. Prior to hospitalization, Marion was having increasing pain in her right hip, which was limiting her ability to perform her daily activities, including walking. She had an elective right total hip arthroplasty. The orthopedic surgeon ordered post-surgery precautions with toe-touch weight bearing on the right lower extremity. Marion's past medical history was significant for hypertension and congestive heart failure, which were controlled with medications. Prior to admission, Marion lived alone in an assisted living community. She was active within this community, participating in the daily social activities and leading flower-arranging activities. Marion has three sons who are grown and have their own families and do not live locally.

One day after surgery, the acute care occupational therapist was consulted. The occupational profile revealed that Marion's goal was to eventually return to her assisted living residential community. Upon evaluation, Marion required maximum assistance for functional mobility using a walker and maximum assist for lower body ADL. Marion also had pain and intermittent confusion since surgery, which limited her ability to engage in therapy. It was determined that Marion would continue her rehabilitation at the local skilled nursing facility because she required skilled intervention but did not require an intensive therapy program of 3 hours daily.

The OT practitioner performed the facility's initial evaluation, including the ADL, mobility, safety, and the COPM (Law et al., 2014). The COPM revealed Marion's desire to be independent in self-care and to return to her assisted living community. Intervention at the skilled nursing facility focused on self-care and functional mobility retraining. Within 20 days, Marion was independent in self-care except for minimal assistance for seated bathing in the shower and functional mobility using a front-wheeled walker. The OT practitioner provided caregiver training to the hired personal care attendant, ordered appropriate equipment for bathroom adaptations, and arranged for continued therapy in Marion's assisted living community to support her optimal recovery.

Questions

1. With the goal of Marion returning to her assisted living residential community, how does OT facilitate safe discharge planning?
2. How can OT create meaningful interventions related to flower-arranging activities to facilitate goal achievement?
3. Upon discharge, Marion will require assistance from a hired personal care giver. What key factors can OT address to decrease care giver burden and assist Marion in her recovery toward independence?

OT STORY 60.3 MENTAL HEALTH: ADULT WITH DEPRESSION AND ANXIETY

Sarah is a female in her early 30s who has experienced a history of minor depression and anxiety beginning when she was in college. Initially, her symptoms were most noticeable at the end of the semester, stemming from the pressures of final examinations and erratic study habits, resulting in irregular sleep patterns. Typically, Sarah managed her symptoms through social drinking of alcohol and partying with friends, sometimes binge drinking. On a few occasions, Sarah sought out behavioral health counseling services offered by the university when she faced trouble focusing her attention or feeling panicky. With her parents living abroad, Sarah has relied heavily on classmates and coworkers for her social support. After college graduation, she met her spouse at an after-work social gathering featuring alcoholic drinks and dancing.

Soon after, they were married and immediately started to try to build a family. However, after 2 years of having difficulty getting pregnant, Sarah sought infertility treatments while struggling with feelings of failure and emotional insecurity about the lack of control. Increasing stress and distractions about her infertility treatments started to affect Sarah's job performance. Ultimately, she was laid off when her company was downsizing personnel, and she found herself increasingly distressed, ruminating on her feelings of failure, both personally and professionally. Although she subsequently became pregnant several times, she experienced multiple miscarriages. Consequently, Sarah's emotional condition escalated, and she was hospitalized to treat major depression. This hospitalization was precipitated by Sarah experiencing many of the following symptoms nearly every day for at least 2 weeks: feeling sad or empty most of the day (depressed mood), significant loss of interest or pleasure in activities that used to be enjoyable, significant weight gain, fatigue, poor concentration and slowing down of thoughts, sleeping too much, and feelings of worthlessness and guilt that are related to thoughts about death or suicide. After a few days in the hospital and a new medication regimen, Sarah was discharged home. She felt isolated and alone, while her spouse was at work and she started to drink alcohol during the day, with her spouse often finding her still in her pajamas and intoxicated when he got home from work. Her alcohol abuse further compromised her ability to cope with her feelings of depression and anxiety, impacting her ability to consistently perform basic self-care and home management activities. Frustrated with Sarah's debilitating symptoms, her marital relationship became significantly strained and her spouse moved out of their apartment, asking for a separation and possibly a divorce.

Struggling to manage her symptoms, this change in her marital relationship triggered Sarah's contemplation of suicide. Consequently, Sarah sought voluntary readmission to an inpatient psychiatric hospital unit to treat her dual diagnosis of major depression and alcohol abuse. This hospitalization addressed adjustment of her medications, along with Sarah's participation in an OT evaluation, such as the Occupational Self-Assessment (OSA) (Kielhofner et al., 2009) and group interventions focusing on the use of cognitive behavioral therapy coping strategies (Ellis, 1992) (see Chapters 19 and 29). Sarah's goals are to be able to more effectively cope with and manage her symptoms; to regain her ability to productively engage in basic self-care, home management, and exploration of job search opportunities; and to work on her marital relationship. After a week, Sarah was discharged from the hospital and referred to a partial hospital program to participate in a structured program to support her continued work toward meeting her goals.

Partial hospital programs extend care and serve as a transition from inpatient hospitalization. This level of care enables occupational therapists to support clients' goals for IADL, work, and social participation. Sarah was a candidate to participate in this type of program based on her motivation to gain coping skills to manage her symptoms and to reengage in her daily routine, including explorations of marital reconciliation and potential to work. Initially, Sarah participated in the program for 5 days each week for a month, then tapered to 3 days a week. She took initiative to explore community resources to build a support network and to begin to volunteer in order to transition into a workplace context, taking steps toward her longer-term goal of paid employment. Identifying vocational skills necessary to reenter the workforce became a focus of Sarah's rehabilitation program and volunteer experience. This skill set capitalized on her work experience and included practicing communication skills to foster effective peer and supervisory relationships, sustaining concentration and using problem-solving skills, and regaining confidence and self-reliance for beginning a job search.

Questions

1. How would Sarah's sexual orientation/gender identity influence the OT plan of care?
2. Given that returning to work is one of Sarah's long-term goals, how can you learn more about OT's role in return to work?
3. What are key factors that could be integrated into Sarah's treatment plan that focus on roles, habits, and routines to promote coping and self-management?

OT STORY 60.4 PEDIATRICS: CHILD WITH TRAUMATIC BRAIN INJURY, ORTHOPEDIC FRACTURE, AND AMPUTATION

Joshua is a sixth-grade male who experienced a traumatic brain injury along with multiple fractures and a severe crush injury as a result of being hit by a truck when riding his bike home after a soccer game. Unconscious at the scene of the accident, emergency medical personnel transported Joshua to the nearest Children's Hospital Emergency Services via medic flight. Joshua underwent extensive orthopedic surgery to stabilize his left humeral fracture with an open reduction internal fixation (ORIF) and to perform a below-the-knee (BKA) amputation of his right lower extremity owing to the severe nature of his ankle and foot crush injury. Following surgery, Joshua was treated in the hospital's pediatric intensive care unit (PICU) to closely monitor his status while in a comatose state for 5 days. In the PICU, the occupational therapist performed an initial evaluation and found that Joshua responded to localized stimuli before he eventually emerged from the coma. At first signs of consciousness, Joshua was sluggish and complained of feeling tired. He was disoriented, not knowing where he was or what had happened—common symptoms of posttraumatic amnesia.

After a week, Joshua became emotionally agitated, trying to get out of the hospital bed and repeatedly yelling, "It hurts . . . I want to go home!" After a few days, Joshua's confusion and agitation started to subside, and he began to more cooperatively participate in all of his nursing care and therapy sessions. This medical stabilization enabled transfer from the PICU to the hospital's pediatric unit and, eventually, to the inpatient rehabilitation unit. Once in rehabilitation, the OT practitioner worked closely with his mother and the nursing staff to engage Joshua in participating in his basic self-care, such as eating, brushing his teeth, and dressing his upper and lower body. Nursing, OT, and PT provided collaborative interventions to assist Joshua with his functional mobility in getting in and out of bed, building up his sitting tolerance, and toileting and bathing with adaptive equipment and assistance. Joshua tended to be impulsive and impatient with the extra time and effort required for getting from one place to another, requiring step-by-step verbal cueing and moderate physical assistance to support his safety. Joshua used a wheelchair and practiced standing pivot functional transfers using his left leg for weight bearing. Therapy involved teaching Joshua and his mother important safety precautions to prevent falls and to adhere to his orthopedic precautions. Another aspect of care that was addressed during inpatient rehabilitation was coordination with Joshua's school. The interprofessional team obtained Joshua's school records, and they were able to address skills necessary for eventual return to school. These skills included improving attention and concentration as well as other executive functioning activities. After 2 weeks in inpatient rehabilitation, Joshua was discharged home, having progressed to needing only minimal assistance from his mother or nursing staff for his basic self-care and functional transfers. The left distal humerus ORIF was still healing, and he was using a wheelchair for functional mobility until his right lower extremity prosthetic training progressed.

Initially, Joshua received home care OT and PT to ensure a safe transition to home. However, once the left upper extremity ORIF was fully healed, Joshua started outpatient OT and PT 3 days a week with his mother driving him to the hospital. Joshua's goals focused on "being able to do what I did before," requiring the support of the healthcare team and his mother to help him accept that he will need to find some new ways to do things after his accident. Because his accident was in the summer, Joshua will be returning to his middle school. Joshua's mother is very concerned about him going back to school and being frustrated with the challenges that he will face, especially ambulating with his new prosthesis and crutches while using a backpack. Although the neuropsychological testing in the hospital revealed Joshua's performance to be at the low end of normal for his age, it is unknown to what extent his cognitive deficits, as a result of his traumatic brain injury, might pose to his academic performance in returning to school. Therefore, Joshua's outpatient rehabilitation program focused on transition to school-based OT (see Chapter 45). The school-based therapists (PT, OT, SLP, and neuropsychology) collaborated with the outpatient rehabilitation therapists to determine the skills and adaptations that would be necessary in order to have a smooth transition back to school in the fall. The individualized learning plan (IEP) identifies aspects of continued care in the school system for participation in adaptive physical education and other identified strategies for taking notes and test taking since Joshua's brain injury. Coping and adaptation to disability within the educational setting is another transitional aspect that will need to be addressed through individual therapy and/or participation in a support group.

Questions

1. Taken into consideration Joshua's behavior and early responses, what would be OT's role to modify the environment and integrate the care team and family to facilitate engagement in meaningful occupation?
2. Given that returning to school is one of Joshua's goals, how can you learn more about OT's role in return to school?
3. What are key factors that could be integrated into Joshua's treatment plan that focus on roles, habits, and routines to promote coping, adjustment, and return to daily activities?

Population-Based Practice

Some specific examples of OT's contributions in population-based practice involve consultation (see Chapter 74), program development, health promotion education, and grant-funded demonstration projects. Considerations across the life span may vary according to individual country and government regulations influencing access to OT services. An important guiding rationale for population-based practice has been identified as "the successful promotion of participation in occupations among individuals, groups, or communities through the development of OT services to underserved or unserved clients" (Holmes & Scaffa, 2009, p. 196). However, a common barrier for population-based practice is the lack of resources or payment for populations of all ages, including, but not limited to, children and adults with chronic disabilities, those who are homeless, and at-risk older adults. Opportunities for population-based OT practice are evolving in day programs, transitional housing and employment programs, and specialized services such as low vision and ergonomics and community-based practices.

Once young adults reach the age of 21 or 22 years, most are no longer eligible for school-based special education services. For this population, parents and guardians are responsible to assume a full-time caregiving role. Group homes provide residential options for young adults with disabilities to transition from living with parents/guardians into the community. Centers for independent living provide consumer services and resources to promote independent living skills. Occupational therapists can influence the quality of life for this population by offering consultation services to group homes or centers for independent living. Such services may address making recommendations for activity adaptations and environmental modifications and training clients in self-advocacy and support staff in approaches to provide quality care.

For adults with chronic conditions such as HIV/AIDS, fibromyalgia, arthritis, chronic fatigue syndrome, multiple sclerosis, and so forth, performance of desired occupations is often experienced in conjunction with pain and/or fatigue. For these populations, occupational therapists have collaborated and partnered with professional organizations that provide consumer services, resources, and support. Development of educational self-management programs that outline strategies to control and cope with symptoms and to simplify daily activities has been enhanced by OT's unique perspective. Fall prevention programs have been developed targeting at-risk older populations with interventions to promote wellness through active lifestyles and healthy habits for exercise as well as to assess home safety risks and to offer assistance with home modifications. The following case study describes an example of OT—emerging practice in the area of low vision.

EXPANDING OUR PERSPECTIVES

Applying a Community-Centered Practice Approach to the COVID Vaccine Rollout in Australia

Nerida Hyett

In May 2021, I was granted leave from my academic position at the university to work on the COVID vaccine rollout in a regional planning and coordination position funded by the Australian Government.

In Australia, at this time, we had had some of the lowest COVID case numbers in the world, but this came with major occupational disruption caused by extended lockdowns. Public health experts recommended that high vaccination rates were needed to end lockdowns and to return to a life that resembled what we remembered as normal. As an occupational therapist with knowledge and previous experiences of working at the community level, I accepted this employment role because I wanted to apply my occupational lens and community-centered practice approach to this complex population health challenge.

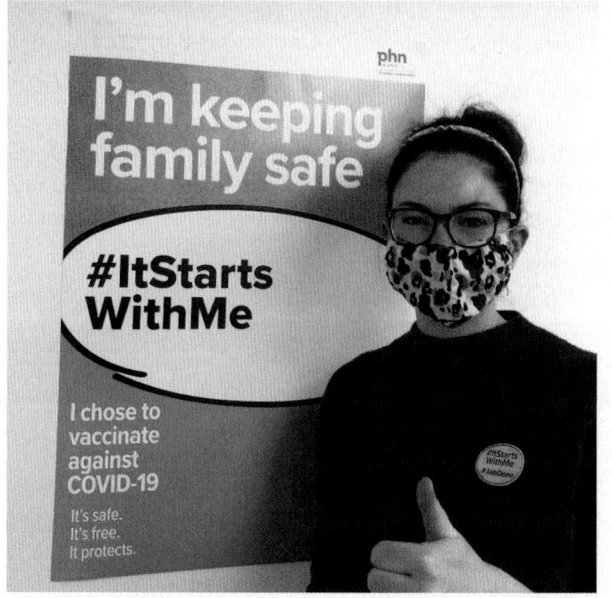

(continued)

EXPANDING OUR PERSPECTIVES (*continued*)

Understanding Community Identities and Limits and Limitations of My Own

In this role, it was important to have an in-depth understanding of the rural communities that I was working with, including histories, cultures, political and economic contexts, social networks, and institutions and businesses. I had grown up and worked my entire career in this rural region, enabling me to draw on my own lived experiences. However, as a white, middle-class, able-bodied woman, I needed to be conscious of the limits and limitations of my lived experiences and worldview. This involved critical reflection and proactively seeking out and learning from people with different perspectives to my own. I did this by developing partnerships with disability services across the region and facilitating a regular cross-region meeting for COVID vaccination planning and strategy. My team also developed a funding strategy with Aboriginal Community Controlled Health Organisations, enabling the design and implementation of culturally safe vaccination services for First Nation communities.

Practice Built on a Foundation of Strong Community Relationships

My role involved collaborating with primary healthcare providers, government officials, and various community leaders across Northern Victoria. It was critical to make time to identify key contacts, build relationships, and grow my networks. Relationships with local community leaders built on reciprocity, accountability, trust, and honesty; provided me with valuable insights into communities; and created new opportunities for community engagement.

Strengths-Based Approach Utilizing Community Assets and Resources to Overcome Barriers

All communities across the region had different strengths, assets, and resources to draw upon for implementing vaccination programs. An important part of my role involved collecting information and data to develop community profiles and to identify strengths and resources that could be used to address unmet needs or service gaps creating systemic and environmental barriers to vaccination.

For example, I provided funding and clinical guidance to primary healthcare providers enabling the design and implementation of pop-up vaccination clinics in familiar and accessible community spaces, which included a shopping mall, a car park drive-through clinic for families with children, a church hall, and neighborhood parks.

An equity lens was applied to all aspects of this work to address inequities in vaccination uptake within communities caused by existing socioeconomic disadvantages, including stigma, marginalization, and exclusion caused by poverty, racism, and discrimination.

Enabling Community Participation in Occupation Is the End Result

Work at the community level requires a client-centered approach informed by comprehensive understandings of clinical guidelines and evidence-based practice. This involved ongoing reflection and learning, identifying my knowledge gaps, seeking out evidence and resources, and learning from colleagues and communities. I needed a comprehensive understanding of the COVID vaccines and best practice in vaccination programs to ensure I could develop evidence-based plans and provide timely and accurate information to primary healthcare providers and community leaders. I drew upon my OT knowledge to provide specialist advice on vaccine hesitancy, environmental accessibility, and social and cultural inclusion.

Occupation was used as a means to achieving community vaccination in some programs; for example, vaccine clinics were delivered in parks while providing food and activities. In all communities, occupation was the motivating factor and the goal or end result of the vaccination program. Achieving high vaccination rates in communities aimed to reduce occupational disruption and increase participation, and this was promoted in advertisements and social media campaigns and legislated through vaccination mandates for specific employment groups.

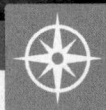

EXPANDING OUR PERSPECTIVES

No Need to Dress Up, Just Turn Up!

Ellen Adomako

The CHIPS system is an existing approach at the community level used by the public health services in Ghana. My week is structured such that I have days I spend at the clinic, but I spend other days at the Community-Based Health Implementation and Planning Services (CHIPS) compounds. The CHIPS zones, which are all located within the community, are closer to people's home, which reduces the cost of traveling and the need, especially for the mothers or caregivers and, for the children to feel that they need to dress up to "travel" to access services. The CHIPS compounds are community health centers that have resident staff. The CHIPS zones on the other hand can be any place from church buildings, mosques,

EXPANDING OUR PERSPECTIVES (*continued*)

community centers, in front of the chief's palace, people's houses, or simply under a tree with a shade. Items and personnel required to set up at the CHIP zones are usually transported from nearby health centers, clinics, and the CHIP compounds. This way of offering services has significantly increased birth registration, access to child welfare clinics for child growth monitoring, and vaccination of children both within the rural and urban communities in Ghana. What was missing in the CHIPS team was the involvement of allied health professionals, such as occupational therapists, who could assist with screening for developmental delays.

Below is a summary of the conversation I had with Daniella,[2] a practicing occupational therapist leading the only community-based OT service in Ghana—The Shai Osudoku Community-Based Occupational Therapy Centre.

OT in Ghana is in its early stages with practice settings in hospitals within the national capital (Accra). This is a significant progress from what was prevailing in 2012, where there were no Ghanaian practicing occupational therapist or services within any of the government physical health settings. Taking a population-based approach has always been at the core of the education of OT students in Ghana, with two courses in the accredited BSc program focusing on health promotion and community therapy services.

When Daniella assumed her post in 2017, she was tasked to help set up the new OT service within the district hospital. We completed a need assessment that helped identify that within the team that she would be working, there was an opportunity to develop OT service at the population level. Using a public health approach, the service was uniquely placed for staff to go out to the community to carry out OT assessments and interventions and to make the necessary referrals to appropriate secondary and tertiary services. Working with the team that ran the CHIP compound, Daniella is able to assess babies and children, screen for any developmental delay, make the appropriate referrals, and follow up with the assessment and the interventions for those who will directly benefit from OT services. Through health education and OT awareness programs within the community, people now understand the role of OT and the services that we offer to children with special needs. This has helped increased the number of people accessing the services.

As part of information gathered on home visits, the community team identifies older adults and persons with disability within households that they visit. This data have facilitated the set up of three activity-based groups within the communities for the older people, with a focus on promoting engagement in meaningful occupation. With the number of qualified occupational therapists in the country growing, it is assumed that this community-level involvement of occupational therapists will be expanded to other areas in the country.

---

2 Daniella Korletey is the occupational therapist at post implementing the community occupational therapy services.

OT STORY 60.5 OLDER ADULTS: COMMUNITY-BASED ADULT WITH LOW VISION

Mr. Gonzales is a Spanish-speaking male in his late 70s who immigrated from Mexico more than 40 years ago with his wife and brother. When his wife died, he relocated to a subsidized housing development for older individuals where he has been living for the past 10 years. Mr. Gonzales has a history of diabetes mellitus with associated visual impairment as a result of glaucoma. He does not seek regular medical care and has not had a recent ophthalmologic examination. He is aware that some of his neighbors have taken advantage of free vision screenings that are offered through a grant-funded mobile van service. Mr. Gonzales has told some of his neighbors that his glasses do not work as well as they used to, and his neighbors have encouraged him to go to the mobile van for a vision screening the next time that it comes to the housing development.

Mr. Gonzales voluntarily participated in a low-vision screening that was administered by an occupational therapist with specialty certification in low-vision rehabilitation. Besides recommending and referring him to an

ophthalmologist, the therapist suggested that she could also virtually visit his apartment and help adapt the environment for safety and improved vision via telemedicine. Mr. Gonzales agreed with encouragement from his daughter who agreed to coordinate the cell phone video technology for the virtual home visit. The therapist conducted a telehealth home safety assessment to identify risks and to recommend environmental adaptations, such as installing an overhead light in both his kitchen and his bathroom.

Questions

1. How would Mr. Gonzales' cultural, language, and social background influence the OT plan of care?

2. How can you learn more about OT's role in low-vision screening and treatment interventions for individuals and populations?

3. How would you understand options for OT service delivery through the use of technology to address Mr. Gonzales' goals?

Conclusion

Today's different areas of practice are ever changing and complex (Porter, 2010; Porter & Teisberg, 2006). OT practice focuses on the client based on where they are receiving services across different practice settings. Other factors that may affect the client's transition and ultimate outcome are the severity of the disability as well as the client's social, cultural, and financial support systems. Quality care requires interprofessional teamwork, which can be informal and/or formal. Occupational therapists have the opportunity to advocate for the client by identifying necessary transitions and resources based on service delivery and systems of care. This goal can be accomplished by collaborating with and exchanging information between providers to ensure that the client's needs and preferences for care are understood and provided. It is important for practitioners to keep in mind the client's priorities as related to satisfaction and participation in life roles. Regardless of practice setting, the role of OT is to support our clients' successful participation and engagement in daily activities.

Lippincott® Connect *For additional resources on the subjects discussed in this chapter, visit* Lippincott Connect.

REFERENCES

American Hospital Association. (2017a). *AHA fast facts on U.S. hospitals.* http://www.aha.org/research/rc/stat-studies/fast-facts.shtml

American Hospital Association. (2017b). *AHA hospital statistics, 2017 edition.* https://ams.aha.org/eweb/DynamicPage.aspx?WebCode=ProdDetailAdd&ivd_prc_prd_key=886dfb06-826f-4258-b843-77ae9416b895

American Occupational Therapy Association. (2019). *Occupational therapy compensation and workforce study.* https://www.aota.org/career/state-of-the-profession/how-much-can-i-earn/2019-salary-workforce-survey

American Occupational Therapy Association. (2020). Occupational therapy practice framework: Domain and process, 4th edition. *American Journal of Occupational Therapy, 74*(Supplement 2), 7412410010p.1–7412410010p87. https://doi.org/10.5014/ajot.2020.74S2001

Bureau of Labor Statistics. (2020). *Occupational outlook handbook.* Author. https://www.bls.gov/ooh/healthcare/occupational-therapists.htm

Ellis, A. (1992). Group rational-emotive and cognitive-behavioral therapy. *International Journal of Group Psychotherapy, 42*, 63–80. https://doi.org/10.1080/00207284.1992.11732580

Holmes, W. M., & Scaffa, M. E. (2009). The nature of emerging practice in occupational therapy: A pilot study. *Occupational Therapy in Health Care, 23*, 189–206. https://doi.org/10.1080/07380570902976759

Kielhofner, G., Forsyth, K., Kramer, J., & Iyenger, A. (2009). Developing the occupational self assessment: The use of Rasch analysis to assure internal validity, sensitivity, and reliability. *British Journal of Occupational Therapy, 72*(3), 94–104. https://doi.org/10.1177/030802260907200302

Law, M., Baptiste, S., Carswell, A., McColl, M., Polatajko, H., & Pollock, N. (2014). *Canadian occupational performance measure* (5th ed.). Canadian Association of Occupational Therapists.

Pattison, M. (2018). Message from the president: Global health policy. *World Federation of Occupational Therapists Bulletin, 74*(1), 3–7. https://doi.org/10.1080/14473828.2018.1432472

Porter, M. E. (2010). What is value in health care? *The New England Journal of Medicine, 363*, 2477–2481. https://doi.org/10.1056/nejmp1011024

Porter, M. E., & Teisberg, E. O. (2006). *Redefining health care.* Harvard Business School.

Roberts, P., & Evenson, M. E. (2009). Occupational therapy resource summaries: Practice settings. In E. B. Crepeau, E. S. Cohn, & B. A. B. Schell (Eds.), *Willard & Spackman's occupational therapy* (11th ed., pp. 1070–1083). Lippincott Williams & Wilkins.

Rogers, A. T., Bai, G., Lavin, R. A., & Anderson, G. F. (2016). Higher hospital spending on occupational therapy is associated with lower readmission rates. *Medical Care Research and Review, 74*, 668–686. https://doi.org/10.1177/1077558716666981

Szanton, S. L., Leff, B., Wolff, J. L., Roberts, L., & Gitlin, L. N. (2016). Home-based care program reduces disability and promotes aging in place. *Health Affairs, 35*, 1558–1563. https://doi.org/10.1377/hlthaff.2016.0140

World Health Organization. (2001). *International classification of functioning, disability, and health (ICF).* Author.

Providing Occupational Therapy for Autistic Individuals

Panagiotis (Panos) A. Rekoutis

LEARNING OBJECTIVES

After reading this chapter, you will be able to:

1. Gain a broader understanding of the different levels and forms of disparity and inequality associated with autistic people and their families.
2. Explain the daily challenges that autistic individuals face and how those can shape different life trajectories.
3. Differentiate autism spectrum disorder across different life stages.
4. Outline the scope of occupational therapy (OT) practice as it relates to autistics and their families with different needs of support from childhood through adulthood.
5. Describe the role of OT evaluation and intervention as part of multidisciplinary team approaches in the field of autism.

Introduction

> By the time Katie was 18 months, the more manifest sign was no sounds were coming in. We were supposed to have a three-session evaluation with this notable speech therapist. Right before we went over to see her, I got a book on autism. It was like a slow death for me reading that book. Because of all the signs: the crying, the lining up of all the toys, the speech delays with her; the non-relatedness when you called her name. There was no babbling. The only thing Katie would relate to was music, and she would light up with music and maybe "Ring around the Rosy." Very few things would interest her. The worst was when you would call her name, and she would be completely unresponsive. (Rekoutis, 2013, p. 144)

The number of parents in this country who find themselves in the same position as Katie's mother has kept rising steadily in the last 20 years. According to the Centers for Disease Control and Prevention (CDC, 2020) and the epidemiologic data from the 11 sites participating in the Autism and Developmental Disabilities Monitoring (ADDM) Network, in the United States, 1 in 54 children aged 8 years were diagnosed with an **autism spectrum diagnosis (ASD)** in 2016 (Maenner et al., 2020). This rate of occurrence translates into more than 1.85% of the general population being diagnosed with ASD.

Before delving further into the realm of autism and the role of occupational therapy (OT) practice, two important elements need to be acknowledged and discussed because of their inextricable connection to the topic of autism: first is the ongoing debate regarding the use of person-first language versus identity-first language and second is the multilayered and ongoing disparity and inequality in the identification of, diagnosis of, and intervention in autism.

Autistic Versus Person With Autism

The issue of preferred identifying language has been ongoing within the larger community of ASD (affected individuals, parents, families and health professionals) during the last 15 years or so. Proponents of using person-first language (PFL) (e.g., person with autism) feel that these terms respect the person's humanity and individuality primarily while acknowledging their condition as a secondary attribute (Shakes & Cashin, 2020). Although PFL has been adopted by the health and human services community, identity-first language (IFL) (e.g., autistic individual) is the preferred use among autistic adults (Dunn & Andrews, 2015; Kenny et al., 2016). The perspective here is not that of honoring humanity; rather it is that of respecting diversity. It is not about seeing individuals past their disorder; it is more about acknowledging and celebrating their difference. The issue of identification language is about reconceptualizing "autistics" as a minority group within a society of "neurotypicals." Using IFL allows us to reframe autism as a society-induced disability construct. Through this lens, the onus is then on how society can change to accommodate, include, and integrate autistics. At the same time, the collective mindset can shift toward a strength-based approach, which can further transform our diagnostic, assessment, and intervention efforts (Koenig & Williams, 2017; Urbanowicz et al., 2019). Through this guiding principle, IFL will be used throughout this chapter.

The Disparities of Autism

The phenomenon of ASDs is characterized by its multilayered disparities. At the forefront is the disparity of the diagnostic process between the past and the present: during various periods of time in the past 120 years or so, the origin of autism, the identification and interpretation of autistic features, and behaviors related to autism have been strongly influenced by the psychosocial trends of each period. At the beginning of the 20th century, the word *autism* was used by Bleuler (Tomchek & Koenig, 2016) to describe socially withdrawn mental health patients. In the 1940s through 1960s, the focus shifted to "infantile autism" with Kanner's (1943) description of "extreme autistic aloneness" and Bettelheim's (1967) "refrigerator mothers" reflecting the predominant trend of Freudian psychoanalysis during that period. It was not until 1980 that autism was recognized as a developmental disorder in the *Diagnostic and Statistical Manual of Mental Disorders* (DSM-III; American Psychiatric Association [APA], 1980). Over the next 33 years in the *DSM-IV* (APA, 2000) and *DSM-5* (APA, 2013), the APA refined the diagnostic processes, models, and autism-related manifestations. These changes were informed by the progression of educational and societal changes regarding the integration and inclusion of students with special needs. Today, autism disorders are regarded as a spectrum described by a confluence of challenges in verbal and nonverbal communication and restricted and repetitive behaviors (*DSM-5* (R); APA, 2015). Such challenges appear very early in life and are present with differing levels of severity among individuals with ASD (Tanner & Dounavi, 2021). Within the current classification system, three distinct severity levels are identified. Each level reflects the need for varying levels and types of support across the life course of an autistic individual as seen in Table 61.1.

The diagnostic disparities through time are important to acknowledge as they do inform the next disparity—that of autism prevalence. In the time of DSM-III, 1 in 5,000 were diagnosed as autistic. Today, this rate has multiplied by a hundredfold (1 in 54 children) (CDC, 2020). Contributing factors for this epidemiologic explosion can be explained by modern social trends, changes in medical practices, and environmental

| **TABLE 61.1** | Selected Diagnostic Criteria for Autism Spectrum Disorder | |

Severity	Deficits in Social Communication and Interaction	Restricted, Repetitive Patterns
Level 1 (requiring support)	• Decreased interest to interact with others • Challenges with initiating and responding to typical back-and-forth conversations (e.g., difficulty making friends)	• Challenges with demonstrating flexibility in different contexts • Daily performance is affected by difficulties with executive function skills.
Level 2 (requiring substantial support)	• Observable challenges with both verbal and non-verbal communication • Limited ability to engage in communicative exchanges (i.e., poor eye contact, use of short sentences, tendency to only talk about personal special interests)	• Inflexible adherence to routines and insistence on sameness paired with restricted/repetitive behaviors that disrupt daily function • Becoming distressed or having obvious challenges when needing to shift focus between different actions or activities
Level 3 (requiring very substantial support)	• Very limited verbal and nonverbal communication (possibly nonverbal or having few intelligible words) • Social interaction is limited to responding to direct social approaches initiated by others.	• High frequency of repetitive behaviors/motor movements • Ritualized patterns or use of objects • Change or unpredictable events can cause extreme distress and coping difficulties.

Adapted from American Psychiatric Association. (2015). *Diagnostic and statistical manual of mental disorders* (5th ed.). Author.

exposures (Russell, 2021). Embedded in the prevalence issue is yet another disparity: that of socioeconomic status and its impact on frequency and age of diagnosis.

For example, more urbanized states in the United States appear to have a higher rate of diagnosis compared to more rural states (1.7% in Wisconsin vs. 3.1% in New Jersey; CDC, 2020). Hispanic children are identified with autism at lower rates than Black or White children. That discrepancy increases for non-English-speaking families (McManus et al., 2020). In addition, data indicate that Hispanic children receive evaluations at older ages than white children (Durkin et al., 2017). Even within states, disparities exist in age at diagnosis between urban/suburban and rural areas. In a study conducted by Hall-Lande et al. (2021), Somali children in metropolitan areas of Minnesota were diagnosed earlier than same ethnic background children in more rural areas of that state.

This type of socioeconomic disparity is a global phenomenon. For example, Koller et al. (2021) identified prevalence and age of diagnosis disparities among secular and modern religious Jews, ultra-Orthodox Jews, and Arabs in Jerusalem. Comparable concerns were raised in a study by Alotaibi et al. (2021) about the diagnostic procedures in Saudi Arabia. In Austria, differences were identified between children with migrant and nonmigrant background (Garcia Primo et al., 2020). Discrepancies in diagnostic procedures result in lack or delayed service provision (McManus et al., 2020; Salomone et al., 2016). Such challenges continue beyond elementary and secondary education (Sarrett, 2018). Autistic individuals face an uphill road with college enrollment, successful attendance, and graduation.

When entering the workforce, the opportunities for employment are rather bleak. A recent study estimated that roughly 70,000 to 110,000 autistic teens become adults each year in the United States—thereby losing school-based autism services (Shattuck et al., 2020). Of those adults, approximately 80% are unemployed. In neighboring Canada, employment rate for adults with autism is estimated at only 14.3% for individuals over 15 years of age (Nicholas, 2020). A similar study in Australia reported that people on the autism spectrum have lower employment rates (42%) than people with other types of disabilities (53%) (Hatfield et al., 2018). These trends are disheartening, especially because a large percentage of autistic individuals have well above average IQs (Clouse et al., 2020). The rates of employment become even more dismal for autistic adults who also have an intellectual impairment (Taylor & Seltzer, 2011). For many of them, the only available option is sheltered workshops or day activity centers. And even then, of the nearly 18,000 people with autism who used state-funded vocational rehabilitation programs in 2014, only 60% left the program with a job and only 2,160 worked at a job that paid above the poverty level (Anderson et al., 2021).

The role and contributions of OT practice for autistic children changes along the continuum of a child's life from early childhood through adulthood. The OT stories at the end of this chapter provide meaning and context regarding the scope of OT for autistic individuals. Jonathan and Brandon had different starting points and trajectories from early childhood through late adolescence. Their journeys will shed a guiding light on the challenging, but highly rewarding and fascinating, practice of OT in the field of autism. For other perspectives, see Box 61.1 and Expanding Our Perspectives.

BOX 61.1 THERAPIST NARRATIVE—INSIGHTS TO A CLINICIAN'S APPROACH

Across the years, many different elements shape and change one's approach to treatment. The unwavering constants in my work with individuals with ASD and their families have been the following three aspects: work with the family and not just the child, know what you do and why you do it, and be part of a village. The common thread and most essential part is effective communication. What may take therapists one step closer is to be direct, yet gentle and sensitive, and optimistic, yet realistic (Rekoutis, 2013).

Challenges in the ability to communicate are the defining criterion for ASDs. Combined with the complexity of other symptoms and a plethora of different therapists involved in the intervention process, the impact on family life can be very stressful, and the need for effective communication can be overwhelming. That aspect constantly ebbs and flows among parents and their children, parents and the therapists, among members of the therapeutic team, and between different agents of the multilayered healthcare and educational

systems. Across all ages, symptoms, and severity, we are working in tandem with the families. Parents value communicative exchanges by their outcome. If deemed successful or effective, they lead to broader shared experiences and promote extended exchanges. On the contrary, when deemed as less effective or not helpful, the underlying message is discarded, the experience devalued, and future exchanges can be met with skepticism and disbelief.

As an occupational therapist, I see myself as uniquely educated and equipped to aid individuals with ASD in making useful sense of their bodies and their environment on their way to living a meaningful and happy life. Children lost within their own bodies, or uncomfortable and threatened by their surroundings, do not know how to regulate, or modulate, or achieve homeostasis for long periods of time. The goal (early on) is to help open up a window to teach skills and strategies so that they can then better negotiate their environment and increase their function. A powerful tool in that direction is

(continued)

BOX 61.1 THERAPIST NARRATIVE—INSIGHTS TO A CLINICIAN'S APPROACH (continued)

finding their hidden interests and turning them into motivating strengths. As a therapist, you need to be good enough, creative enough, quick on your feet enough, and imaginative and resourceful enough to go with the child's flow and embed learning in what the child wants to do. In that regard, occupational therapists can be the ones to help them start connecting their brain to the rest of their body and begin to make sense of the world around them. That leads to being less anxious and better able to maintain socially acceptable behaviors.

Our daily interactions with individuals with ASD do not happen in isolation. More often than not, occupational therapists are parts of distinct teams (in home care, school and clinical settings, vocational and assisted living facilities). They need to be able to navigate the dynamics of those teams, clearly explain their role, and help set appropriate expectations. When successfully doing so, they can become effective advocates for the individuals they work with and their families.

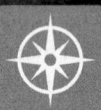

EXPANDING OUR PERSPECTIVES

I Am a Cliché

Sarah Selvaggi Hernandez, MOT, OTR/L

Identity-first language: Autistic, Deaf

Pronouns: She/They

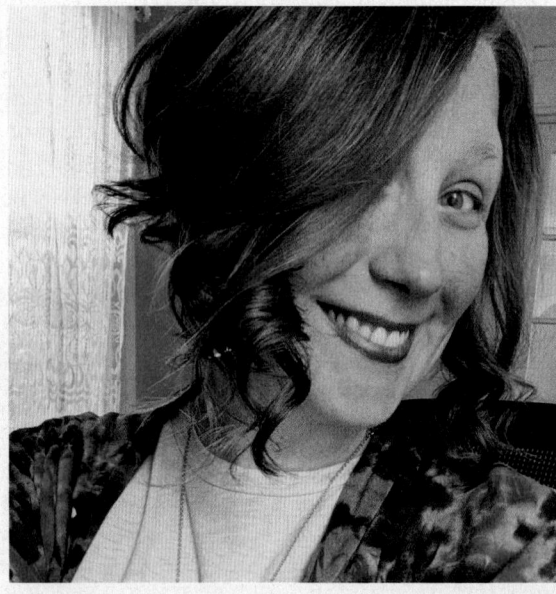

I am a cliché: a white woman, in her 30s, finding her autism diagnosis after her son was identified as being autistic. This is a familiar story for so many autistic adults—a teacher/therapist suggests our child may be on the autism spectrum and we respond, "No way—they're just like me!" Indeed, they are.

I clearly remember being in Dr Lori Vaughn's class and looking at the results of my Adult/Adolescent Sensory Profile. It was the first time I was validated that I experienced sensory information differently than other people in a significant way. I always knew it, but society had expectations of compliance for me.

I was to be ladylike and quiet, studious and productive. This meant masking my reactions to uncomfortable sensory stimuli. It meant practicing conversations in the mirror for hours before an interaction, only to come home and perseverate on the many ways I could be perceived as socially inept. Masking means internalizing dysregulation to appear more feminine.

This shattered my sense of self. I cannot underscore enough the decades of work I have before me to untangle the trauma of living an inauthentic, neuronormative life.

This is what happened because I worked to "appear indistinguishable from my peers." The harm of placing neuronormative expectations on autistic neurology and autistic bodies means I have autoimmune disorders, mental illness, reduced quality of life, and an increased risk for premature death. At 42 years, I am already an older adult in my community. In fact, I have passed the life expectancy of autistic people, which is 41 years.

To be clear, it never had to be this way. Society explicitly and implicitly created a damaging context for my autistic development. People, organizations, and systems groomed me for compliance to the detriment of my health and well-being.

But, I am a white woman with privilege. The potential for harm is even greater for additional intersections with autism that include black, indigenous, and people of color (BIPOC), the queer community, and multiply disabled autistic people. We do not fully understand the needs of the whole autistic community because of misdiagnosis, missed diagnosis, and other barriers to receiving diagnosis and support.

I believe the science and practice of occupation can change this damaging trajectory. I believe occupational practitioners are uniquely suited to do the extraordinary work of shifting the paradigm of abuse. I believe in the reciprocal relationship between occupation and health.

Help us to identify autistic occupations and create a better understanding of what autistic health means. We need to eradicate the barriers to diagnosis. With autistic stakeholders, create autistic development scales, autistic contexts, and autistic environments. Advocate for us. Protect our authenticity.

I know, with your help, we can create an inclusive world that provides equity in access for all.

Providing Occupational Therapy for Young Autistic Children

Working With the Families

Autistic toddlers and preschoolers can demonstrate differences across all domains of daily performance. Before discussing them in more detailed terms, it is imperative to consider the children's parents and caregivers at this particular junction. Receiving the diagnosis of autism can be an earth-shattering moment in any parent's life (Rekoutis, 2013). Parents may feel relief because for the first time, they have a framework that can begin to explain some of their child's unique features and behaviors. In these early stages, parents try to come to terms with the still-prevalent societal perception of a "disorder" that cannot be cured. They are suddenly forced to reconcile their life dreams about their child while paving the path toward acceptance. Supporting and empowering them to reframe their dreams and expectations through a strengths-based perspective can become a positive road map toward navigating services and intervention approaches. In the early stages of recruiting health providers and building the child's support team, parents have to advocate for and navigate through uncharted waters. They need to become knowledgeable about different treatments and approaches, negotiate mandates, secure funding, and deal with the scheduling puzzle. Parents are required to be and become—almost overnight—effective and efficient team managers, planners, facilitators, communicators, and decision-makers about things they probably have very little prior exposure to or knowledge of (see Box 61.2).

Parents and caregivers of autistic children often lean on the service providers for technical knowledge and expertise, guidance, and support. That need for support morphs, ebbs, and flows through the years, but caregivers always rely on service providers. They tend to identify the following attributes as critical qualities of the therapists who interact with their children: professional knowledge, respectfulness, consistency, openness, and willingness to collaborate (Grindle et al., 2009; MacKean et al., 2005; Rekoutis, 2013). At the very least, parents expect therapists to be "direct, yet gentle and sensitive; and optimistic, yet realistic" (Rekoutis, 2013, p. 270).

Working With the Children

Children's ability to explore and understand the world around them is influenced by sensory processing differences (Ben-Sasson et al., 2013; Schaaf, Benevides, et al., 2015; Wigham et al., 2015). Autistic children can demonstrate intense interests and focus, guardedness around others, avoidance of eye contact, and idiosyncratic movements. These are accompanied by preoccupation with specific interests, lack of flexibility, ritualistic types of behavior, and insistence on sameness. More specifically, young children with ASD may demonstrate differences with how they process tactile (Cascio et al., 2016; Puts et al., 2014; Tavassoli et al., 2016), visual (Sabatos-DeVito et al., 2016), auditory (Brandwein et al., 2015; Chang et al., 2012), and proprioceptive and vestibular input (Ament et al., 2015; Hazen et al., 2014).

Autistic children may demonstrate distinct sensory patterns or combinations of sensory behaviors depending on the environments they find themselves in or the demands that are placed on them. Children may be sensory over responsive (SOR) to sensory input (Baranek et al., 2007), which is associated with increased sensitivity (defensiveness), described as "a tendency to react negatively or with alarm to sensory input that is generally considered harmless or nonirritating" (Wilbarger & Wilbarger, 1991, p. 3). Surrounding environments and conditions are perceived as dangerous, and children can be fearful and anxiety ridden (Ben-Sasson et al., 2013). Some children appear to be sensory under responsive (SUR). Often, those children appear to have challenges related to muscle tone and their responses to sensory input are usually slower or "sluggish." For example, they may demonstrate decreased awareness of temperature or pain (Ausderau et al., 2014). Finally, children with autism may also be described as "sensory seeking" when they present with prolonged and repetitive engagement (e.g., twirling objects, observing lights, looking from the corner of their eyes) that can be interpreted as attempts toward self-initiated soothing, grounding, or coping with

BOX 61.2 NARRATIVE PERSPECTIVE: *WHO IS DRIVING THE BUS*

In this online chapter, a mother (Laura), father (Craig), and son (Will, who was diagnosed with Asperger syndrome at 3 years of age) describe Will's early years, diagnosis, therapy, and the challenges of school. Sections are written by each member of the family from birth through 18 years of age. "Who's driving the bus" is a metaphor that Laura uses to describe the journey the family took with doctors, therapists, teachers, school counselors, etc., with Laura at the wheel, acting as the driver.

See the full story, see Appendix III, Chapter B, at Lippincott Connect.

stressful situations. See Chapter 56 for more information on sensory processing.

Further differences can be observed with motor co-ordination and motor planning (Green et al., 2009; Jasmin et al., 2009; Liu, 2012). Autistic children may often have challenges with the development of self-care skills, play skills, and meaningful engagement in age-appropriate occupations (Liu & Breslin, 2013; Lloyd et al., 2013; Tomchek et al., 2015). For these young children and their families, such issues often translate into frequent behavioral and emotional overreactions, difficulties with eating, and disturbed sleeping patterns that can place significant strains on the entire family's life and routines.

Based on the child's age and needs, services can vary in nature and intensity. Home-based and private practice/clinic instruction programs are usually organized with a primary focus on facilitating skill development across domains. Center-based programs can provide the same focus in addition to exposing children to social participation and integration opportunities (Koegel et al., 2012; Stahmer & Ingersoll, 2004). Occupational therapists find themselves working hand in hand with speech–language pathologists, special education teachers, mainstream teachers, day care teachers, psychologists, behavior therapists, and, to a lesser degree, physical therapists and social workers. Depending on the nature of the program and the composition of the team, interventions that occupational therapists may directly or indirectly utilize can include the following: Picture Exchange Communication System (PECS™) or Prompts for Restructuring Oral Muscular Phonetic Targets (PROMPT©) systems to improve communication; classroom protocols such as Treatment and Education of Autistic and Related Communication Handicapped Children (TEACCH); play-based relationship-based therapy (Developmental Individual-

difference Relationship-based model [DIR®] Floortime) (Brunner & Seung, 2009); applied behavior analysis (ABA); sensory integration approaches; sensorimotor activities and developmental interventions; strengths-based approaches (Braun et al., 2017; Dunst et al., 2012; Steiner, 2011; Tomchek & Koenig, 2016); and parent-mediated interventions (PACT; Tanner et al., 2015). See Box 61.3 for examples of commonly used interventions, and see Chapter 56 for more information on sensorybased approaches.

Providing Occupational Therapy for Individuals for Autistic Individuals During School Years

By the time autistic children reach elementary school age, support services become primarily school-based and focused, although children often continue to receive services in a clinical setting or at home (Bilaver et al., 2016) to either complement the school program or to add further layers of necessary intensity. Based on the child's needs, classroom placements can range from inclusion in classrooms with typically developing peers to much more restricted special education settings with highly increased ratios between adults/instructors and students (1:1 or 2:1). Occupational therapists who function within these environments may continue to focus their efforts to help students develop age-appropriate skills in academics, social participation, and play/leisure-related occupations. For students without intellectual impairment, therapy often focuses on strengthening executive

---

BOX 61.3 EXAMPLES OF COMMONLY USED INTERVENTIONS

- **Strength-based approaches:** The practitioner focuses on identifying and building on the students' abilities versus focusing on their limitations or disabilities.
- **Picture Exchange Communication System (PECS™):** This intervention allows people with little or no communication abilities to communicate using pictures. People using PECS™ are taught to approach another person and give them a picture of a desired item in exchange for that item. By doing so, the person is able to initiate communication. A child or adult with autism can use PECS™ to communicate a request, a thought, or anything that can reasonably be displayed or symbolized on a picture card.
- **Prompts for Restructuring Oral Muscular Phonetic Targets (PROMPT©):** The technique is a tactile-kinesthetic approach that uses touch cues to a patient's articulators (jaw, tongue, lips) to manually guide them through a

targeted word, phrase, or sentence. The technique develops motor control and the development of proper oral muscular movements while eliminating unnecessary muscle movements.
- **Developmental Individual-difference Relationship-based model (DIR®) Floortime:** This is a specific technique to both follow the child's natural emotional interests and at the same time challenge the child toward greater and greater mastery of the social, emotional, and intellectual capacities. With young children, these playful interactions may occur on the floor but go on to include conversations and interactions in other places.
- **Applied behavior analysis (ABA):** It is the process of systematically applying interventions based on the principles of learning theory to improve socially significant behaviors to a meaningful degree.

OT STORY 61.1 JONATHAN (JOHNNIE)

Initial Evaluation and Findings

Johnnie was diagnosed at the age of 18 months with ASD. He received his diagnosis from an early intervention state-funded agency. Using today's diagnostic criteria, he would have been classified as Level 3, "requiring very substantial support." At the time of the evaluation, Johnnie presented as a nonverbal toddler, showing no interest in his surrounding, with a tendency to produce only repetitive sounds and movements when excited. Johnnie would start crying and become emotionally overwhelmed when his parents attempted to take away some of the objects he enjoyed holding in his hands. He also demonstrated fearful reactions to different sounds and noises, types of foods, and textures. He was particularly fearful of large spaces and encounters with groups of people. At the time of his initial evaluation, Johnnie had just started walking independently and demonstrated significant low tone in both large and small muscles. Based on the team's diagnosis and recommendations, he received home-based special education instruction, speech–language pathology, and physical therapy at the time but no OT.

Progress Through the Years

The Preschool Years

At age 3 years 6 months: Johnnie demonstrated minimal progress in communication skills. He was still nonverbal and demonstrated minimal eye contact with peers or adults. Overall sensory processing was challenged, and Johnnie presented with fleeting joint attention and poor frustration tolerance. Repetitive behaviors were frequent and intensified when he was frustrated. His parents were frustrated with the lack of progress and enrolled Johnnie at a private special education school that provided an intense ABA program paired with speech–language therapy and OT.

At age 4 years 2 months: By the end of his first school year, Johnnie was starting to verbalize more and was actively communicating his desire during games by saying "go," using "more" to initiate or continue with a motor task (i.e., swinging or jumping on the trampoline), or using "ball" when he wanted a ball thrown at him. Johnnie would almost always stand up at the sight of the occupational therapist stepping into his classroom and would verbalize "jump—jump." His oral motor skills also improved because Johnnie was now able to blow bubbles and different types of whistles independently on request. Johnnie's overall tactile sensitivity had decreased, and he could tolerate handling a variety of textures (play dough, finger paint, and lotion). However, he still was not demonstrating any self-driven interest to engage with these materials. Johnnie required physical prompting and/or verbal cues to redirect him during tasks that were

repetitive in nature (i.e., climb to reach for an object and bring it to a specified area in the room). In that first year of school, Johnnie also made improvements in his gross motor skills and overall strength, which seemed to help increase his overall alertness and endurance. However, he still had significant issues with sensory processing and tactile defensiveness. Haircutting was an impossible task for his parents who either had to hold him down or tried to snip his hair while he was asleep. The same applied to nail clipping. For his second year at school, these goals were identified as high priority and became the focus of his OT sessions. An incremental and simplified process of desensitization was initiated. We paired a simple token rewards system with the different steps involved in a haircut (allowing his hair to be combed, wearing a bib, allowing his hair to be wet, becoming used to the presence of scissors around him) to increase Johnnie's engagement. Several of those components were carried over in the classroom during direct instruction time with his ABA teacher (Figure 61.1).

At age 5 years 3 months: At the end of the second school year, Johnnie had demonstrated measurable improvement across all areas and programs. Although more words were becoming part of his everyday speech, his communicative interactions were still quite limited to sentences of two to three words. His verbalizations were almost exclusively about satisfying basic needs. Johnnie had also started using PECS and visual schedules successfully. Sensory processing difficulties continued to persist despite gains. For example, although Johnnie had successfully participated in a Therapeutic Listening© auditory integration protocol, he was still immensely scared of the noise during birthday parties. However, he had successfully overcome

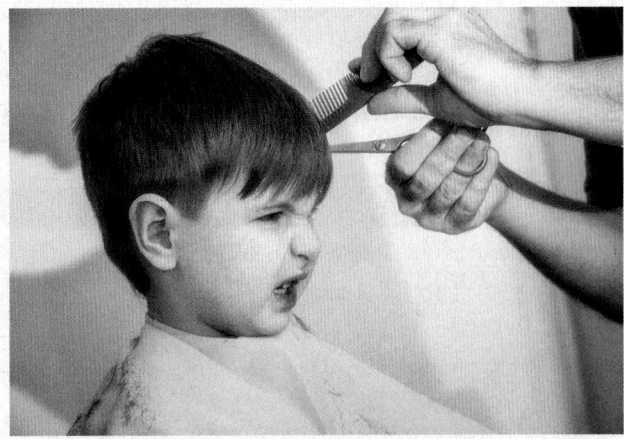

FIGURE 61.1 Johnnie had significant issues with sensory processing and tactile defensiveness. Haircutting became an impossible task.

(continued)

OT STORY 61.1 JONATHAN (JOHNNIE) (continued)

difficulties that had to do with waking up in the middle of the night from the sound of sirens and not being able to go back to sleep. While going through the first cycle with the protocol, Johnnie also stopped being annoyed by the ringing of the phone at home. His mother, actually, asked to have him start back on the protocol after about 4 weeks since they had found that Johnnie would participate nicely during dinner at the table when he was listening to the modified music. In the weeks that ensued, Johnnie started becoming more restless again during dinner time. However, by the end of the second cycle, those gains became solidified.

Beyond these gains, Johnnie's engagement in tabletop activities and fine motor tasks led to small improvements that were measurable enough to be identified in his Peabody Developmental Motor Scales, Second Edition (PDMS-2) scoring between the beginning and end of the school year as demonstrated in Table 61.2.

The School Years

Johnnie's progress through the years across all domains and occupations continued at a slow pace. Each victory and milestone was a big cause of celebration for his family and his team. New skills would come in after targeting them for a number of years and after a lot of plateaus. Often, we would make one step forward, followed by a regression of shorts. Johnnie did not sleep in his own bed until he was 9 years old. Until that point, he was sharing the same bed with his mother and father at home. It took him 5 years before he could tolerate having a haircut with a barber at a hair salon. The day he came back with his first haircut, we threw a big party for him at the school. By that time, he had learned to enjoy parties and other school gatherings. A little time later, he tolerated having an orthodontic retainer placed in his mouth by the dentist with no overreactions. Talking to his mother, at the time, she mentioned that getting to that point really made all the efforts we had put in through the years worthwhile and worth waiting for. Johnnie spent several years learning how to write his name but was quite proficient with learning to type. Once introduced to computers and electronic tablets, he demonstrated an affinity for scanning the keyboard for the correct letters in order to find his favorite video clips on the Internet. He enjoyed typing up e-mails and telling his mother how his day was going at school. Within this, functional format typing instruction became one of his preferred school tasks. His overall motor skills, motor planning, and coordination continued to be delayed despite concerted efforts to help him in those domains. Table 61.3 demonstrates his performance and overall change in scores when tested with the Bruininks–Oseretsky Test of Motor Proficiency, Second Edition (BOT-2). In all this time, all the areas of needs were addressed collectively by all the team members through sharing of expertise, cross-training, and daily collaboration (Figure 61.2).

TABLE 61.2   Johnnie's Occupational Therapy Evaluation Scores During His First Year at School

Subtest	Beginning of School Year (Age Equivalent in Months)	End of School Year (Age Equivalent in Months)
Stationary	28	35
Locomotion	22	29
Object manipulation	32	32
Grasping	11	28
Visual–motor integration	30	30

TABLE 61.3   Johnnie's Occupational Therapy Evaluation Bruininks–Oseretsky Test of Motor Proficiency, Second Edition Scores

	11 Years, 3 Months	12 Years, 3 Months	Progress Made
Fine motor precision	4:0–4:1	5:0–5:1	+12 months
Fine motor integration	4:10–4:11	5:6–5:7	+8 months
Manual dexterity	5:2–5:3	5:6–5:7	+4 months
Upper-limb coordination	7:3–7:5	7:6–7:8	+3 months
Bilateral coordination	7:3–7:5	8:9–8:11	+18 months
Balance	5:2–5:3	5:4–5:6	+2 months
Running speed and agility	4:2–4:3	4:2–4:3	No change
Strength	4:8–4:9	5:6–5:7	+10 months

OT STORY 61.1 JONATHAN (JOHNNIE) (*continued*)

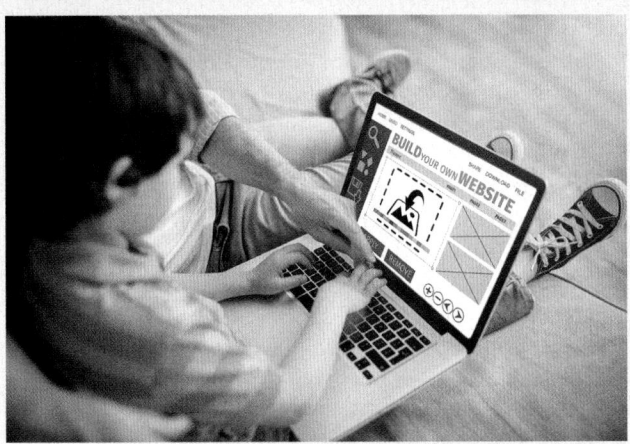

FIGURE 61.2 Johnnie developed an affinity for computers and electronic tablets. Computer skills became one of his strengths and resulted in improved school performance.

Jonathan's verbal skills also improved through the years. Johnnie grew apparently tired of being called "Johnnie" because around the time of his ninth birthday, he announced that his name was Jonathan. The entire school staff never called him Johnnie after that day. At the age of 10 years, Jonathan was the master of ceremonies (emcee) during a school event announcing the different skits in front of a crowd of more than 100 people. He was wearing a blazer and stood behind a microphone, reading his script and smiling. All of us who experienced his journey up to that point were crying tears of joy. Jonathan also revealed an affinity for pranks. His favorite task during his school day was to practice his navigational skills and follow multistep directions in delivering mail and different forms to staff. It was his opportunity to come and place plastic bugs at our work stations or give us a handshake and jolt us with a little contraption between his fingers. Our surprised expressions would always crack him up.

By the time Jonathan was 11 years, he had already started participating in different types of prevocational activities that aimed at further developing his organizational skills and also focused on professional behaviors. He learned very quickly how to distribute mail to different staff members. He was also able to file worksheets in alphabetic order. During one of our sessions, he was asked to look at a picture of a kitchen at a fast-food restaurant. I asked him to pretend that he was working there and tell me what he would cook. He quickly replied, "Hamburgers." I then showed him a picture of the same kitchen with a big fire on top of the grill. When I asked him what he would do if there was a big fire, his response was "I will cook a Big Burger." On another occasion, when I asked him what he would do if there was a fire at the restaurant that he was eating as a customer, he responded that he would leave and go to a different restaurant.

During his school day, Jonathan continued to participate in training programs that targeted aspects of safety awareness in different contexts (home, school, community) whether it was on an individual basis or part of his classroom group curriculum. Occupational therapists, speech–language pathologists, and classroom teachers all contributed their respective roles. Social skills from an early stage involved learning how to go through a meal at a restaurant, tolerating and eventually enjoying trips to entertainment venues (the zoo, movie theaters, and amusement parks). Jonathan's OT sessions involved meal planning and meal preparation as he started getting older. In the area of health and wellness, Jonathan—while at his school—learned how to use a gym membership and practiced arriving, checking in, changing into his gym outfit in the locker rooms, using the treadmills there, changing back to his clothes, and returning to school. Beyond the memberships, we were able to develop a collaboration between the school and that particular neighborhood gym, where Jonathan and other students would go and clean up the equipment during low "foot-traffic periods" as part of their vocational training with the occupational therapist being the most knowledgeable team member to act as the liaison.

Latest Update

Jonathan graduated school at the age of 21 years, and he was hired part time at a small business that manufactures T-shirts. Jonathan started at the company as an unpaid intern and really enjoyed the environment. Jonathan will continue living with his family for the foreseeable future, especially now that his job is within walking distance from their apartment.

Questions

1. What modifications would you recommend allowing Jonathan to feel more comfortable in his home and school environment when he was younger?
2. Provide a list of strengths that you were able to identify from the narrative about Jonathan.
3. What kind of assistive technology applications would you recommend for Jonathan that would improve his overall independence?

OT STORY 61.2 BRANDON

Initial Evaluation and Findings

Brandon was initially evaluated by a multidisciplinary team at the age of 2 years. The diagnostic center where he was evaluated included a developmental pediatrician, psychologist, speech–language pathologist, and an occupational therapist. His parents were concerned about his delay in meeting several milestones, his limited use of language, and diminished eye contact. In addition, his parents felt that Brandon was not interested in other people and was shying away from interactions with his parents and infant brother. During parental interviewing, his mother mentioned characteristically that Brandon "was there, but was practically absent" while the family celebrated his second birthday.

Brandon was seen separately by each clinician but demonstrated consistent behaviors across testing administrations. He had had observable difficulty following verbal directions and tended to simply repeat everything he heard while requiring visual and gestural prompts to perform simple tasks. At times, he showed signs of hyper-responsiveness to sound, covering his ears and/or would sing to himself, in an attempt to disengage from the process. Brandon was particularly drawn to visual stimulation, evidenced by his enjoyment and prolonged looking at spinning and shiny objects. Furthermore, he demonstrated difficulty transitioning from preferred activities (such as playing with train toys) to adult-directed tasks. As a result, he was not able to complete the corresponding standardized expressive and receptive language assessment as well as an intelligence scale. During his evaluation, Brandon appeared very distracted while inside a large sensory gym. He had marked difficulty with visual–vestibular processing, showing signs of gravitational insecurity (a fear of having his feet off the ground) and fear of imposed movement. He further appeared to lack depth perception, necessary for safe navigation around his environment, very frequently tripping over objects. Brandon avoided touching certain textures and walked primarily on his toes, presenting signs of tactile defensiveness. In addition, his mother reported that Brandon almost always resisted having his teeth brushed and frequently refused to try new foods. Brandon presented with low to average muscle tone, normal to slightly increased range of motion (joint laxity), and poor strength and stability throughout his body. Righting, equilibrium, and protective reactions were slow to emerge, causing him to seek out stationary, familiar activities and to resist imposed and novel movements in all planes of motion. Brandon was observed drooling when physical demands were placed on him, demonstrating difficulty with motor planning and dissociation of major muscle groups. Brandon demonstrated similar difficulties with fine motor tasks and age-appropriate self-care tasks, such as taking

off his socks and shoes on his own. As was the case with the other assessments, it was not possible to engage Brandon in all the necessary tasks as part of his PDMS-2, and thus, he was not able to receive scores for any of the five subtests.

Brandon received the diagnosis of pervasive developmental disorder not otherwise specified (PDD-NOS) from the DSM-IV (APA, 2000). The recommendation to his parent was that he received an intensive early intervention program that included one-to-one special education instruction, relationship-based home intervention, speech therapy, physical therapy, and OT. His early programming amounted to almost 30 hours of weekly intervention time that took place at a private clinic and at home. Brandon's parents were able to fund his program by combining compensation through private pay, their health insurance plans, and early intervention services funded by Individuals with Disabilities Education Act (IDEA) part C.

OT services were provided in a sensory clinic with additional home consultations to help adapt his environment and teach parents strategies to promote self-care skills. Specific interventions were put in place to address sensory processing difficulties and gross, fine, and visual–motor, cognitive, and self-care skill deficits.

Progress Through the Years
The Preschool Years

At age 3 years 11 months: Brandon had demonstrated impressive gains in expressive language and was able to form short sentences. Repetitive answers and stereotypical speech were still frequent, but they were considerably reduced since the onset of services. At this point, Brandon had been enrolled in a small preschool class with typically developing peers and a "shadow" teacher in a part-time program. Brandon continued to have a very hard time regulating his behavior and was becoming distracted and disengaged when his environment was too stimulating or expectations were overwhelming. Brandon's ability to process auditory information remained a relative weakness but following multiple-step verbal directions had improved. The focus of intervention was to further improve response times and ability to remain focused on the task at hand. Walking on tiptoes diminished with the use of the Wilbarger Brushing protocol. Through direct intervention following the sequential oral sensory (SOS) approach to feeding, his food repertoire and willingness to try new foods in different environments improved 10-fold. New foods were added in practically every food category. Brandon's mother attributed a lot of the gains to the trusting bond that he had developed with his therapist. At the same time, defensiveness and avoidance behaviors with toothbrushing, blowing horns, blowing bubbles, and blowing candles were successfully

OT STORY 61.2 BRANDON (continued)

addressed and resolved through gradual exposure and pairing with tangible rewards. Although Brandon demonstrated improvements in tolerating vestibular input and improved balancing and protective reactions, his sensory system was still becoming overwhelmed by the vestibular input that he received. Although still not using a mature running pattern, Brandon could walk up and down stairs alternating feet without the need to hold onto a hand rail. He was also jumping forward, jumping down from a height, and jumping over obstacles by taking off and landing with both feet. However, overall gross motor coordination performance was still well below age-level expectancy. Brandon continued to be disinterested in catching and throwing ball games. At that point in time, Brandon was much more efficient with fine motor skills and dressing skills. Brandon, nevertheless, was showing a keen interest in all the suspended equipment available to him during his OT sessions. He enjoyed participating in imaginary journeys to faraway places, where he had to overcome ominous creatures and obstacles to reach his destination while navigating the different parts of elaborate obstacle courses. With the passing of time, he started adding comments and parts to the narrative and enjoyed building his own obstacle courses.

At age 5 years 3 months: Brandon continued to make impressive gains across all domains of communication, social interactions, and sensory processing. However, he started demonstrating anxiety-related issues and was placed on medication. Some of his improvements and overall functioning in gross and fine motor skills are presented in Table 61.4. The team and his parents made the decision—at that point—to prolong his preschool stay for another year, although he would typically be eligible for kindergarten.

Throughout this time, Brandon enjoyed participating in OT sessions and continued to excitedly engage in "jungle gym" type of obstacle courses (Figure 61.3). He was able to show a creative side in organizing his environment and was demonstrating a bubbly personality. His interest in the jungle gym "stories" translated in more elaborate drawings and became a spark for his early forays with letter formation and writing using the vocabulary from his "journeys."

The School Years

At age 7 years 3 months: After Brandon remained in preschool for a second year, he was then placed at a kindergarten classroom with typically developing peers and a shadow teacher. However, at the end of that year, and because of his increasing anxiety, the decision was made to place him at a school for students with learning difficulties. At that point, Brandon started receiving OT sessions at home instead of the sensory gym environment. Sessions focused on age-appropriate leisure skills, such as learning how to ride his bike and play different types of interactive video games (Wii Sports). Brandon's relationship with his therapist evolved to that of him having an older brother after working together for almost 6 years. Brandon would confide about his problems at school, and we would try to look for solutions together. At the same time, his improvements in communication and social skills did land him in "hot water." For example, Brandon texted one of his home tutors, pretending to be his mother and attempted to cancel his session. More seriously, he managed to also use his parents' credit card information to order a series of religious books (religion becoming one of his special interests at the time). Facilitating his interest in matters of

TABLE 61.4	Brandon's Occupational Therapy Evaluation Scores at Age 5 Years and 3 Months			
Brandon's PDMS-2 Scores at 41 Months and 63 Months				
Subtest	Age Equivalent Months 41 Months	Age Equivalent Months 63 Months	Percentile Rank (%) at 63 Months	Progress Made
Stationary	43	58	37	15 months
Locomotion	39	57	37	18 months
Object manipulation	37	41	9	4 months
Grasping	40	40	5	No change
Visual–motor integration	51	62	50	11 months
Beery–Buktenica Developmental Test of Visual–Motor Integration (6th Edition) (VMI)				
	VMI	Visual	Motor	
Percentile Rank	50%	63%	12%	
Age Equivalence	5 years, 2 months	5 years, 6 months	4 years, 6 months	

PDMS-2, Peabody Developmental Motor Scales, Second Edition.

(continued)

OT STORY 61.2 BRANDON (*continued*)

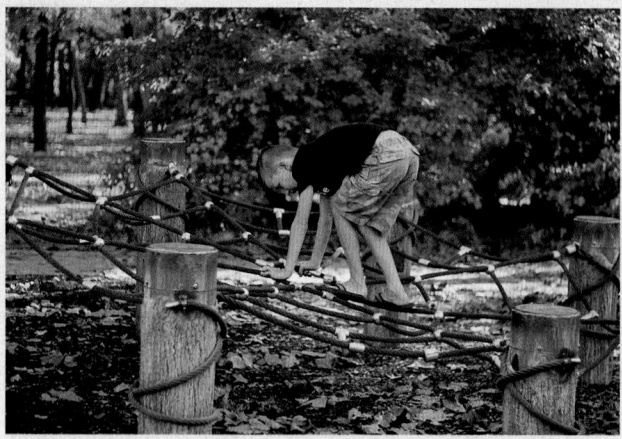

FIGURE 61.3 Brandon enjoyed participating in OT sessions and continued to excitedly engage in "jungle gym" types of obstacle courses.

religion allowed Brandon to gain increased social opportunities with other children attending rites and ceremonies. It helped further increase his ability to attend long events with sustained attention and better body control. Brandon was very motivated and decided to participate in the chorus of his church.

At age 8 years 11 months: Brandon demonstrated a resolute ability and motivation to overcome difficulties and excelled with his learning at his school. Parent and teacher reports indicated that he was well organized and able to follow classroom instruction. At the same time, Brandon could manage frustration very effectively and would easily follow the "voice of reason." Brandon developed a keen sense of humor, which, combined with strong verbal skills, made him a very affable young boy with strong and well-argued opinions who was a pleasure to interact with. In his OT sessions, Brandon was working on developing organizational strategies and strengthening his executive functioning to guide him in following specific steps toward completing the task at hand. Progressively, these strategies would translate into habits and routines associated with how he prepares, works through, and completes academic projects and performs during school testing procedures. Furthermore, he continued to explore new movement and exercise strategies that helped him remain regulated. Brandon excelled in learning how to jump rope and used an app to practice yoga and meditation.

A couple of months before his ninth birthday, Brandon managed to wander off outside his weekend home in a wooded area and got lost for a few hours. Police and rescue parties were notified. He was found about half a mile from his home because he decided to stay in place and wait until somebody would call him for dinner. During one of our sessions—while addressing safety awareness—I asked him what he would do if he woke up at night and smelled fire. He responded that he would run out of the house. When I asked him, if he would alert anybody else in case they were still asleep, he responded, "No, because my life is too precious to lose." Empathy was still a skill that required further development, apparently. In late spring of that school year, we decided to discharge Brandon. He was getting ready to go to a sleepaway camp in the summer, and he felt that he was ready after 7 years of working together.

About 6 months later, I received an e-mail from his mother. She shared with me what another girl at Brandon's class wrote in an essay at school (sent to Brandon's mother by the girl's mother):

> My friends named Brandon and J. made school a fun place to be because they taught me how to do new things I never did. Some things my friends taught me were how to play box ball, how to jump rope while the rope is spinning, how to use the spinny thing, how to do forward rolls and how to play the fire drill game.

Latest Update

Brandon decided to cut down on commuting time between school and home and has been living in the residential part of his school for the past 2 years. This is the third consecutive year that he has campaigned successfully to be the class president. His latest aspirations include studying political science in college.

Questions

1. When working in an elementary school, which of the following areas would be more appropriate to focus on while working with Brandon: self-care skills, leisure occupations, academic function, handwriting, movement?

2. What roles could an occupational therapist have while working at Brandon's middle school that is part of a residential program?

3. What kind of assessments would be used to promote self-determination when interacting with Brandon at his residential placement (e.g., COSA)?

functioning skills (Zingerevich & Patricia, 2009). During the middle school years, students who continue to require support engage in OT interventions that address independence across the range of self-care skills, activities of daily living, aspects of self-efficacy, and wellness (Rekoutis & Dimitropoulou, 2018; Tomchek et al., 2017). Those interventions expand at some point to include prevocational and vocational training (Dunn et al., 2015). See OT Stories 61. and 61.2.

Providing Occupational Therapy for Autistic Adolescents and Adults

For older autistic students in mainstream secondary education, occupational therapists may assist with their transition toward college by supporting them in exploring studies and college programs of interest, creating a study path, and helping with the application process. At the same time, both the students and their families may need support while preparing for life away from home. Furthermore, students may need guidance and scaffolding in the area of work skills, including such tasks as learning how to perform job searches, creating resumes, and preparing for job interviews (Seaman & Cannella-Malone, 2016). These can prove essential catalysts in the pursuit of employment because many large corporations already acknowledge the unique skillset of autistic individuals and the need to integrate them in the workforce (Clouse et al., 2020). Many autistic individuals can possess valuable work-related qualities and skills, including attention to detail, strong sense of morality, mathematical abilities, creative talents, good memory, cognitive and technical skills, trustworthiness, and loyalty (De Schipper et al., 2016; Lee et al., 2020; Lei & Russell, 2021). In addition to addressing work for adolescents with ASD, OT services can address continuing needs for independent daily living, functional limitations with self-care skills, community mobility, work-related practices, and leisure activities.

Conclusion

OT practice can play a vital and dynamic role in supporting autistic individuals and their families. The two case studies illustrate the strong bonds that therapists can develop with autistic children, adolescents, and adults and their families. Our strength-based perspective in developing and implementing interventions places us firmly in the forefront of the service provision system. The role of OT continues to be increasingly acknowledged as an integral part of the intensive and comprehensive intervention programming (Bilaver et al., 2016; Christon et al., 2015; Shattuck et al., 2011; Turcotte et al., 2016). As part of a multidisciplinary team approach, occupational therapists assume distinct parts in both the assessment and intervention processes. Qualified occupational therapists are being sought after across many clinical and educational settings. Accordingly, interest in OT research in autism has become a focused topic, and opportunities for associated funded projects are expanding in frequency and scope (American Occupational Therapy Association, 2017; Case-Smith et al., 2014; Schaaf, Schoen, et al., 2015; Tomlin & Swinth, 2015). As occupational therapists, we possess a unique lens for understanding the needs of autistic individuals and their families.

Lippincott® Connect *For additional resources on the subjects discussed in this chapter, visit Lippincott Connect.*

REFERENCES

Alotaibi, A. M., Craig, K. A., Alshareef, T. M., AlQathmi, E. S., Aman, S. M., Aldhalaan, H. M., & Oandasan, C. L. (2021). Sociodemographic, clinical characteristics, and service utilization of young children diagnosed with autism spectrum disorder at a research center in Saudi Arabia: The road to autism spectrum disorder diagnosis. *Saudi Medical Journal, 42*(8), 878–885. https://doi.org/10.15537/smj.2021.42.8.20210297

Ament, K., Mejia, A., Buhlman, R., Erklin, S., Caffo, B., Mostofsky, S., & Wodka, E. (2015). Evidence for specificity of motor impairments in catching and balance in children with autism. *Journal of Autism and Developmental Disorders, 45,* 742–751. https://doi.org/10.1007/s10803-014-2229-0

American Occupational Therapy Association. (2017). Research opportunities in the area of people with autism spectrum disorder. *American Journal of Occupational Therapy, 71,* 7102400010p1–7102400010p2. https://doi.org/10.5014/ajot.2017.712002

American Psychiatric Association. (1980). *Diagnostic and statistical manual of mental disorders (DSM-III)* (3rd ed.). Author.

American Psychiatric Association. (2000). *Diagnostic and statistical manual of mental disorders (DSM-IV)* (4th ed., rev. ed.). Author.

American Psychiatric Association (2013). *Diagnostic and statistical manual of mental disorders (DSM-5)* (5th ed.). Author.

American Psychiatric Association. (2015). *Diagnostic and statistical manual of mental disorders (DSM-5 (R))* (5th ed., revised). Author.

Anderson, C., Butt, C., & Sarsony, C. (2021). Young adults on the autism spectrum and early employment-related experiences: Aspirations and obstacles. *Journal of Autism and Developmental Disorders, 51*(1), 88–105. https://doi.org/10.1007/s10803-020-04513-4

Ausderau, K. K., Furlong, M., Sideris, J., Bulluck, J., Little, L. M., Watson, L. R., Boyd, B. A., Belger, A., Dickie, V. A., & Baranek, G. T. (2014). Sensory subtypes in children with autism spectrum disorder: Latent profile transition analysis using a national survey of sensory features. *Journal of Child Psychology and Psychiatry, and Allied Disciplines, 55,* 935–944. https://doi.org/10.1111/jcpp.12219

Baranek, G. T., Boyd, B. A., Poe, M. D., David, F. J., & Watson, L. R. (2007). Hyperresponsive sensory patterns in young children with autism, developmental delay, and typical development. *American Journal on Mental Retardation, 112,* 233–245. https://doi.org/10.1352/0895-8017(2007)112[233:HSPIYC]2.0.CO;2

Ben-Sasson, A., Soto, T. W., Martínez-Pedraza, F., & Carter, A. S. (2013). Early sensory over-responsivity in toddlers with autism spectrum disorders as a predictor of family impairment and parenting stress. *Journal of Child Psychology and Psychiatry, and Allied Disciplines, 54,* 846–853. https://doi.org/10.1111/jcpp.12035

Bettelheim, B. (1967). *The empty fortress: infantile autism and the birth of self.* Free Press.

Bilaver, L., Cushing, L., & Cutler, A. (2016). Prevalence and correlates of educational intervention utilization among children with autism spectrum disorder. *Journal of Autism and Developmental Disorders, 46,* 561–571. https://doi.org/10.1007/s10803-015-2598-z

Brandwein, A., Foxe, J., Butler, J., Frey, H., Bates, J., Shulman, L., & Molholm, S. (2015). Neurophysiological indices of atypical auditory processing and multisensory integration are associated with symptom severity in autism. *Journal of Autism and Developmental Disorders, 45,* 230–244. https://doi.org/10.1007/s10803-014-2212-9

Braun, M. J., Dunn, W., & Tomchek, S. D. (2017). A pilot study on professional documentation: Do we write from a strengths perspective? *American Journal of Speech-Language Pathology, 26,* 972–981. https://doi.org/10.1044/2017_AJSLP-16-0117

Brunner, D. L., & Seung, H. (2009). Evaluation of the efficacy of communication-based treatments for autism spectrum disorders: A literature review. *Communication Disorders Quarterly, 31,* 15–41. https://doi.org/10.1177/1525740108324097

Cascio, C., Lorenzi, J., & Baranek, G. (2016). Self-reported pleasantness ratings and examiner-coded defensiveness in response to touch in children with ASD: Effects of stimulus material and bodily location. *Journal of Autism and Developmental Disorders, 46,* 1528–1537. https://doi.org/10.1007/s10803-013-1961-1

Case-Smith, J., Weaver, L. L., & Fristad, M. A. (2014). A systematic review of sensory processing interventions for children with autism spectrum disorders. *Autism, 19,* 133–148. https://doi.org/10.1177/1362361313517762

Centers for Disease Control and Prevention. (2020). *Autism prevalence rises in communities monitored by CDC.* https://www.cdc.gov/media/releases/2020/p0326-autism-prevalence-rises.html

Chang, M. C., Parham, L. D., Blanche, E. I., Schell, A., Chou, C.-P., Dawson, M., & Clark, F. (2012). Autonomic and behavioral responses of children with autism to auditory stimuli. *American Journal of Occupational Therapy, 66,* 567–576. https://doi.org/10.5014/ajot.2012.004242

Christon, L. M., Arnold, C. C., & Myers, B. J. (2015). Professionals' reported provision and recommendation of psychosocial interventions for youth with autism spectrum disorder. *Behavior Therapy, 46,* 68–82. https://doi.org/10.1016/j.beth.2014.02.002

Clouse, J. R., Wood-Nartker, J., & Rice, F. A. (2020). Designing beyond the Americans With Disabilities Act (ADA): Creating an autism-friendly vocational center. *Herd-Health Environments Research & Design Journal, 13*(3), 215–229. https://doi.org/10.1177/1937586719888502

De Schipper, E., Mahdi, S., de Vries, P., Granlund, M., Holtmann, M., Karande, S., Almodayfer, O., Shulman, C., Tonge, B., Wong, V. V. C. N., Zwaigenbaum, L., & Bölte, S. (2016). Functioning and disability in autism spectrum disorder: A worldwide survey of experts. *Autism Research, 9*(9), 959– 969. https://doi.org/10.1002/aur.1592

Dunn, D. S., & Andrews, E. E. (2015). Person-first and identity-first language: Developing psychologists' cultural competence using disability language. *American Psychologist, 70*(3), 255–264. https://doi.org/10.1037/a0038636

Dunn, L., Diener, M., Wright, C., Wright, S., & Narumanchi, A. (2015). Vocational exploration in an extracurricular technology program for youth with autism. *Work, 52,* 457–468. https://doi.org/10.3233/WOR-152160

Dunst, C. J., Trivette, C. M., & Hamby, D. W. (2012). Meta-analysis of studies incorporating the interests of young children with autism spectrum disorders into early intervention practices. *Autism Research and Treatment, 2012,* 462531. https://doi.org/10.1155/2012/462531

Durkin, M. S., Maenner, M. J., Baio, J., Christensen, D., Daniels, J., Fitzgerald, R., Imm, P., Li-Ching Lee, Schieve, L. A., Van Naarden Braun, K., Wingate, M. S., & Yeargin-Allsopp, M. (2017). Autism spectrum disorder among US children (2002-2010): Socioeconomic, racial, and ethnic disparities. *American Journal of Public Health, 107*(11), 1818–1826. https://doi.org/10.2105/AJPH.2017.304032

Garcia Primo, P., Weber, C. Posada de la Paz, P., Fellinger, J., Dirmhirn, A. & Holzinger, D. (2020). Explaining age at autism spectrum diagnosis in children with migrant and non-migrant background in Austria. *Brain Sciences, 10*(448), 448. https://doi.org/10.3390/brainsci10070448

Green, D., Charman, T., Pickles, A., Chandler, S., Loucas, T., Simonoff, E., & Baird, G. (2009). Impairments in movement skills of children with autistic spectrum disorders. *Developmental Medicine and Child Neurology, 51,* 311–316. https://doi.org/10.1111/j.1469-8749.2008.03242.x

Grindle, C. F., Kovshoff, H., Hastings, R. P., & Remington, B. (2009). Parent's experiences of home-based applied behavior analysis programs for young children with autism. *Journal of Autism and Developmental Disorders, 39,* 42–56. https://doi.org/10.1007/s10803-008-0597-z

Hall-Lande, J., Esler, A. N., Hewitt, A., & Gunty, A. L. (2021). Age of initial identification of autism spectrum disorder in a diverse urban sample. *Journal of Autism & Developmental Disorders, 51*(3), 798–803. https://doi.org/10.1007/s10803-018-3763-y

Hatfield, M., Ciccarelli, M., Falkmer, T., & Falkmer, M. (2018). Factors related to successful transition planning for adolescents on the autism spectrum. *Journal of Research in Special Educational Needs, 18*(1), 3–14. https://doi.org/10.1111/1471-3802.12388

Hazen, E. P., Stornelli, J. L., O'Rourke, J. A., Koesterer, K., & McDougle, C. J. (2014). Sensory symptoms in autism spectrum disorders. *Harvard Review of Psychiatry, 22,* 112–124. https://doi.org/10.1097/01.hrp.0000445143.08773.58

Jasmin, E., Couture, M., McKinley, P., Reid, G., Fombonne, E., & Gisel, E. (2009). Sensori-motor and daily living skills of preschool children with autism spectrum disorders. *Journal of Autism and Developmental Disorders, 39,* 231–241. https://doi.org/10.1007/s10803-008-0617-z

Kanner, L. (1943). Autistic disturbances of affective contact. *Nervous Child, 2,* 217–250. http://neurodiversity.com/library_kanner_1943.pdf

Kenny, L., Hattersley, C., Molins, B., Buckley, C., Povey, C., & Pellicano, E. (2016). Which terms should be used to describe autism? Perspectives from the UK autism community. *Autism, 20*(4), 442–462. https://doi.org/10.1177/1362361315588200

Koegel, L., Matos-Freden, R., Lang, R., & Koegel, R. (2012). Interventions for children with autism spectrum disorders in inclusive school settings. *Cognitive and Behavioral Practice, 19,* 401–412. https://doi.org/10.1016/j.cbpra.2010.11.003

Koenig, K. P., & Williams, L. H. (2017). Characterization and utilization of preferred interests: A survey of adults on the autism spectrum. *Occupational Therapy in Mental Health, 33,* 129–140. https://doi.org/10.1080/0164212X.2016.1248877

Koller, J., Shalev, R., Schallamach, C., Gumpel, T. P., & Begin, M. (2021). The role of demographics in the age of autism diagnosis in Jerusalem. *Journal of Autism & Developmental Disorders, 51*(3), 769–777. https://doi.org/10.1007/s10803-019-04107-9

Lee, E. A. L., Black, M. H., Falkmer, M., Tan, T., Sheehy, L., Bölte, S., & Girdler, S. (2020). "We can see a bright future": Parents' perceptions of the outcomes of participating in a strengths-based program for adolescents with autism spectrum disorder. *Journal of Autism & Developmental Disorders, 50*(9), 3179–3194. https://doi.org/10.1007/s10803-020-04411-9

Lei, J., & Russell, A. (2021). Understanding the role of self-determination in shaping university experiences for autistic and typically developing students in the United Kingdom. *Autism: The International Journal of Research & Practice, 25*(5), 1262–1278. https://doi.org/10.1177/1362361320984897

Liu, T. (2012). Motor milestone development in young children with autism spectrum disorders: An exploratory study. *Educational Psychology in Practice, 28,* 315–326. https://doi.org/10.1080/02667363.2012.684340

Liu, T., & Breslin, C. M. (2013). Fine and gross motor performance of the MABC-2 by children with autism spectrum disorder and typically developing children. *Research in Autism Spectrum Disorders, 7,* 1244–1249. https://doi.org/10.1016/j.rasd.2013.07.002

Lloyd, M., MacDonald, M., & Lord, C. (2013). Motor skills of toddlers with autism spectrum disorder. *Autism, 17,* 133–146. https://doi.org/10.1177/1362361311402230

MacKean, G. L., Thurston, W. E., & Scott, C. M. (2005). Bridging the divide between families and health professionals' perspectives on family-centered care. *Health Expectations, 8,* 74–85. https://doi.org/10.1111/j.1369-7625.2005.00319.x

Maenner, M. J., Shaw, K. A., Baio, J., Washington, A., Patrick, M., DiRienzo, M., Christensen, D. L., Wiggins, L. D., Pettygrove, S., Andrews, J. G., Lopez, M., Hudson, A., Baroud, T., Schwenk, Y., White, T., Rosenberg, C. R., Lee, L., Harrington, R. A., Huston, M., . . . Dietz,

P. M. (2020). Prevalence of autism spectrum disorder among children aged 8 years—Autism and developmental disabilities monitoring network, 11 sites, United States, 2016. *MMWR Surveillance Summaries*, *69*(No. SS-4), 1–12. http://doi.org/10.15585/mmwr.ss6904a1

McManus, B.M., Richardson, Z., Schenkman, M., Murphy, N.J., Everhart, R.M., Hambidge, S., & Morrato, E. (2020). Child characteristics and early intervention referral and receipt of services: A retrospective cohort study. *BMC Pediatrics*, *20*(84), 1–10. https://doi.org/10.1186/s12887-020-1965-x

Nicholas, D. B. (2020). Employment in autism: Reflections on the literature and steps for moving forward. *Autism & Developmental Disorders*, *18*(3), 5–11. https://doi.org/10.17759/autdd.2020180301

Puts, N. A., Wodka, E. L., Tommerdahl, M., Mostofsky, S. H., & Edden, R. A. (2014). Impaired tactile processing in children with autism spectrum disorder. *Journal of Neurophysiology, 111*, 1803–1811. https://doi.org/10.1152/jn.00890.2013

Rekoutis, P. A. (2013). *Parents of children with autism: Their perceptions and experiences with occupational therapy*. LAP Lambert Academic Publishing AG & Co. KG.

Rekoutis, P. A., & Dimitropoulou, K. A. (2018, April). *Individual movement-based protocols to reduce stereotypies and increase academic participation in school-age children with ASD* [Poster session]. 2018 AOTA annual conference & expo, Salt Lake City, UT.

Russell. G. (2021). *The rise of autism: Risk and resistance in the age of diagnosis*. Routledge.

Sabatos-DeVito, M., Schipul, S., Bulluck, J., Belger, A., & Baranek, G. (2016). Eye tracking reveals impaired attentional disengagement associated with sensory response patterns in children with autism. *Journal of Autism and Developmental Disorders, 46*, 1319–1333. https://doi.org/10.1007/s10803-015-2681-5

Salomone, E., Beranová, Š., Bonnet-Brilhault, F., Briciet Lauritsen, M., Budisteanu, M., Buitelaar, J., Canal-Bedia, R., Felhosi, G., Fletcher-Watson, S., Freitag, C., Fuentes, J., Gallagher, L., Garcia Primo, P., Gliga, F., Gomot, M., Green, J., Heimann, M., Jónsdóttir, S. L., Kaale, A., . . . Charman, T. (2016). Use of early intervention for young children with autism spectrum disorder across Europe. *Autism: The International Journal of Research and Practice, 20*(2), 233–249. https://doi.org/10.1177/1362361315577218

Sarrett, J. C. (2018). Autism and accommodations in higher education: Insights from the autism community. *Journal of Autism and Developmental Disorders, 48*(3), 679–693. https://doi.org/10.1007/s10803-017-3353-4

Schaaf, R. C., Benevides, T., Leiby, B., & Sendecki, J. (2015). Autonomic dysregulation during sensory stimulation in children with autism spectrum disorder. *Journal of Autism and Developmental Disorders, 45*, 461–472. https://doi.org/10.1007/s10803-013-1924-6

Schaaf, R. C., Schoen, S. A., May-Benson, T. A., Parham, L. D., Lane, S. J., Roley, S. S., & Mailloux, Z. (2015). State of the science: A road map for research in sensory integration. *American Journal of Occupational Therapy, 69*, 6906360010p1–6906360010p7. https://doi.org/10.5014/ajot.2015.019539

Seaman, R., & Cannella-Malone, H. (2016). Vocational skills interventions for adults with autism spectrum disorder: A review of the literature. *Journal of Developmental and Physical Disabilities, 28*, 479–494. https://doi.org/10.1007/s10882-016-9479-z

Shakes, P., & Cashin, A. (2020). An analysis of twitter discourse regarding identifying language for people on the autism spectrum. *Issues in Mental Health Nursing, 41*(3), 221–228. https://doi.org/10.1080/01612840.2019.1648617

Shattuck, P. T., Garfield, T., Roux, A. M., Rast, J. E., Anderson, K., Hassrick, E. M., & Kuo, A. (2020). Services for adults with autism spectrum disorder: A systems perspective. *Current Psychiatry Reports*, *22*(3), 1–12. https://doi.org/10.1007/s11920-020-1136-7

Shattuck, P. T., Wagner, M., Narendorf, S., Sterzing, P., & Hensley, M. (2011). Post-high school service use among young adults with an autism spectrum disorder. *Archives of Pediatrics and Adolescent Medicine, 165*, 141–146. https://doi.org/10.1001/archpediatrics.2010.279

Stahmer, A. C., & Ingersoll, B. (2004). Inclusive programming for toddlers with autism spectrum disorders: Outcomes from the children's toddler school. *Journal of Positive Behavior Interventions, 6*, 67–82. https://doi.org/10.1177/10983007040060020201

Steiner, A. M. (2011). A strength-based approach to parent education for children with autism. *Journal of Positive Behavior Interventions, 13*, 178–190. https://doi.org/10.1177/1098300710384134

Tanner, A., & Dounavi, K. (2021). The emergence of autism symptoms prior to 18 months of age: A systematic literature review. *Journal of Autism & Developmental Disorders, 51*(3), 973–993. https://doi.org/10.1007/s10803-020-04618-w

Tanner, K., Hand, B. N., O'Toole, G., & Lane, A. E. (2015). Effectiveness of interventions to improve social participation, play, leisure, and restricted and repetitive behaviors in people with autism spectrum disorder: A systematic review. *American Journal of Occupational Therapy, 69*, 6905180010p1–6905180010p12. https://doi.org/10.5014/ajot.2015.017806

Tavassoli, T., Belleshein, K., Tommerdahl, M., Holden, J. M., Kolevzon, A., & Buxbaum, J. D. (2016). Altered tactile processing in children with autism spectrum disorder. *Autism Research, 9*, 616. https://doi.org/10.1002/aur.1563

Taylor, J. J., & Seltzer, M. (2011). Employment and post-secondary educational activities for young adults with autism spectrum disorders during the transition to adulthood. *Journal of Autism and Developmental Disorders, 41*, 566–574. https://doi.org/10.1007/s10803-010-1070-3

Tomchek, S., & Koenig, K. P. (2016). *Occupational therapy practice guidelines for individuals with autism spectrum disorder*. AOTA Press.

Tomchek, S., Koenig, K. P., Arbesman, M., & Lieberman, D. (2017). Evidence connection—Occupational therapy interventions for adolescents with autism spectrum disorder. *American Journal of Occupational Therapy, 71*, 7101395010. https://doi.org/10.5014/ajot.2017.711003

Tomchek, S. D., Little, L. M., & Dunn, W. (2015). Sensory pattern contributions to developmental performance in children with autism spectrum disorder. *American Journal of Occupational Therapy, 69*, 6905185040p1. https://doi.org/10.5014/ajot.2015.018044

Tomlin, G. S., & Swinth, Y. (2015). Contribution of qualitative research to evidence in practice for people with autism spectrum disorder. *American Journal of Occupational Therapy, 69*, 6905360010p1–6905360010p4. https://doi.org/10.5014/ajot.2015.017988

Turcotte, P., Mathew, M., Shea, L., Brusilovskiy, E., & Nonnemacher, S. (2016). Service needs across the lifespan for individuals with autism. *Journal of Autism and Developmental Disorders, 46*, 2480. https://doi.org/10.1007/s10803-016-2787-4

Urbanowicz, A., Nicolaidis, C., den Houting, J., Shore, S. M., Gaudion, K., Girdler, S., & Savarese, R. J. (2019). An expert discussion on strengths-based approaches in autism. *Autism in Adulthood, 1*(2), 82–89. https://doi.org/10.1089/aut.2019.29002.aju

Wigham, S., Rodgers, J., South, M., McConachie, H., & Freeston, M. (2015). The interplay between sensory processing abnormalities, intolerance of uncertainty, anxiety and restricted and repetitive behaviours in autism spectrum disorder. *Journal of Autism and Developmental Disorders, 45*, 943–952. https://doi.org/10.1007/s10803-014-2248-x

Wilbarger, P., & Wilbarger, J. (1991). *Sensory defensiveness in children aged 2–12: An intervention guide for parents and other caretakers*. Avanti Educational Programs.

Zingerevich, C., & Patricia, D., L. (2009). The contribution of executive functions to participation in school activities of children with high functioning autism spectrum disorder. *Research in Autism Spectrum Disorders, 3*, 429–437. https://doi.org/10.1016/j.rasd.2008.09.002

Providing Occupational Therapy for Individuals With Traumatic Brain Injury

Intensive Care to Community Reentry

Steven D. Wheeler, Amanda Acord-Vira, and Diana Davis

LEARNING OBJECTIVES

After reading this chapter, you will be able to:

1. Identify the role of occupational therapy throughout the full spectrum of traumatic brain injury (TBI) recovery.
2. Appreciate the manner in which impairments, activity limitations, personal factors, and environmental barriers interact to impact successful and meaningful occupational performance following TBI.
3. Understand the importance of therapeutic relationship building and occupation-based practice in facilitating optimal community reentry following TBI.

Introduction

Few conditions challenge the diverse knowledge base and skill set of occupational therapy (OT) practitioners like traumatic brain injury (TBI). TBI is a complex condition characterized by varying degrees of cognitive, physical, psychological, behavioral, and emotional impairment. Although successful **community integration,** which involves attaining the personal, social, and vocational competency to successfully participate in the community (CARF International, 2022), represents the ultimate goal of the TBI recovery process, for most individuals, the road from initial assessment and intake to community reentry is a long and arduous one. Each patient's presentation after TBI depends on the extent and location of damage to the brain mixed with that person's cultural background, personality, and life experiences. As a result, no two individuals presenting to the OT practitioner are exactly alike, necessitating a true client-centered approach to assessment and treatment (see Box 62.1 and Chapter 28).

Persons with TBI can receive medical care and/or rehabilitation in a variety of settings. These areas might be categorized as follows:

Acute care phase:

- Intensive care unit (ICU)/acute care

Acute rehabilitation phase:

- Structured, ongoing therapy in acute care hospital or separate rehabilitation hospital

Post-acute rehabilitation phase:

- Outpatient rehabilitation
- Home therapy services
- Skilled long-term care
- Skilled residential care
- Transitional living/work
- Educational/school settings

There are many factors that influence the continuum of care following TBI. These are summarized in Figure 62.2 and discussed in Box 62.2. Regardless of the path following injury, OT is likely to play an important role. See also Commentary on the Evidence.

BOX 62.1 NARRATIVE AS A KEY TO UNDERSTANDING: THE IMPORTANCE OF THERAPEUTIC RELATIONSHIP BUILDING IN TBI REHABILITATION

Unsuccessful efforts to return to "normal" after TBI can be damaging to one's self-esteem and, subsequently, one's willingness to take chances and risk failure. This can pose a considerable challenge to OT practitioners responsible for encouraging clients to try new tasks necessary for the attainment of meaningful goals. Working within a client's comfort zone (i.e., doing activities that they're already competent at) can make a treatment session manageable but may not be moving toward those meaningful occupations identified by the client and family in the early stages of therapy. Additionally, always keeping things "safe" prevents the client from learning about their impairments, an important component in the development of self-awareness. Impaired self-awareness, which is associated with executive dysfunction (Pettemeridou et al., 2020), can negatively impact a person's perceived need for rehabilitation along with motivation for behavior change and a more productive daily routine (Trudel et al., 1998).

The development of an unconditional, therapeutic relationship is central to building a climate of trust. Clients who believe that their therapist will remain supportive regardless of whether they succeed or fail at an activity are more likely to take those risks necessary to experience meaningful accomplishments and enhance self-esteem. Rapport building with many clients takes time and may even require the therapist to "prove" his or her commitment to the relationship by staying supportive with the client during periods of acting out, defiance, and other acts. Therapists who discharge or transfer clients to other therapists because of difficult behavior or "noncompliance" may be missing an opportunity to establish the therapeutic relationship needed to encourage clients risk-taking and the attainment of major life accomplishments.

The personal narrative of Mary Feldhaus Weber and her 16-year journey following severe TBI highlights the individualized nature of TBI and depicts why effective "listening" and client-centered OT is so critical to the rehabilitation process (see Figure 62.1). To read her full story, see Appendix III, Chapter H, at Lippincott Connect.

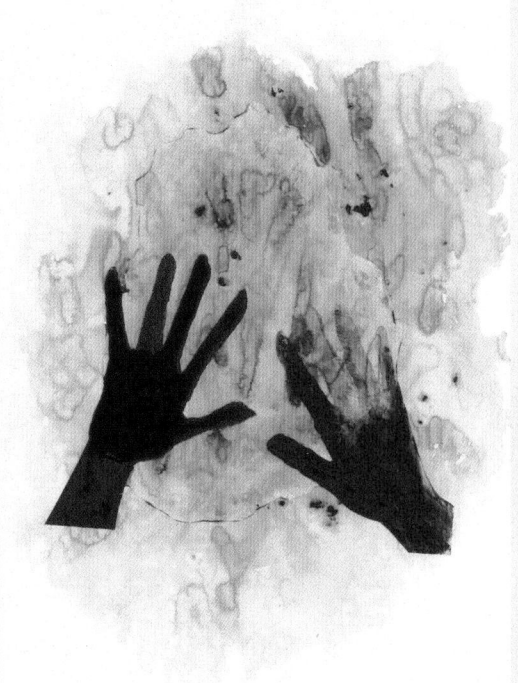

FIGURE 62.1 Mary Feldhaus Weber's painting "Blue Seizure."

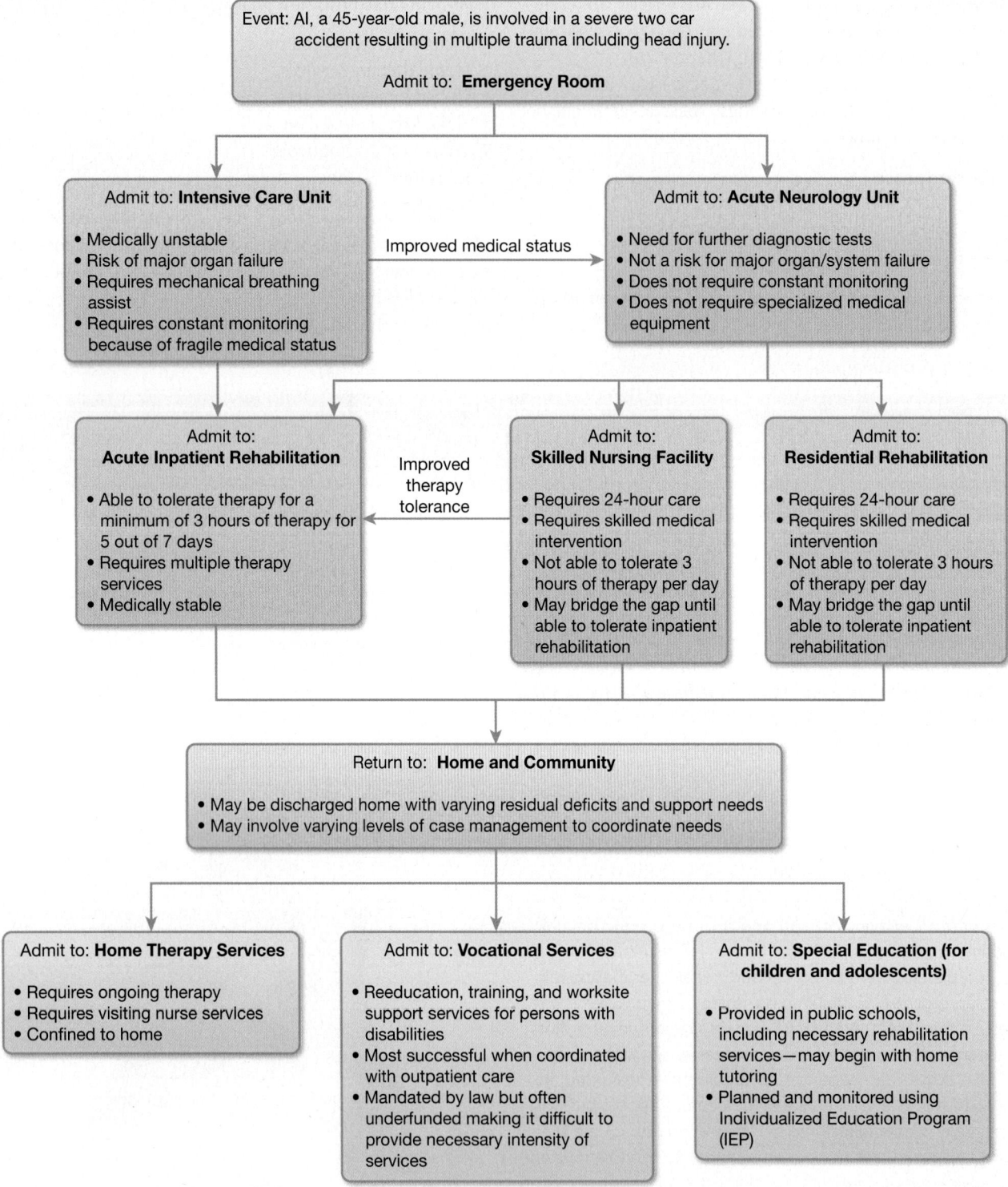

FIGURE 62.2 Potential continuum of care after traumatic brain injury.

BOX 62.2 MARKETPLACE REALITIES AFFECTING THE TBI CONTINUUM OF CARE

The need to shift from the medical model of traumatic brain injury (TBI) rehabilitation to a more client-centered philosophy as an individual becomes medically stable is commonly cited in the literature (Lash, 2009). Unfortunately, the realities of the US marketplace present considerable challenges to providing rehabilitation care for many in need (Ullmann, 2015). Health insurance coverage for rehabilitation becomes incrementally more difficult across the continuum of care outlined in Figure 62.2—from inpatient to outpatient to residential and community services. For many, funding shifts from private to public sources such as Medicaid or Medicare for long-term care. The adequacy of public funding varies between states as some have developed Medicaid waivers to provide long-term home and community services that would otherwise be covered in institutional settings such as a nursing home (Katz et al., 2007). Understanding the complexities of reimbursement and sources of alternative funding such as vocational rehabilitation and/or Center for Independent Living Programs is a challenging but essential element for clinicians, especially those providing services at the community level.

COMMENTARY ON THE EVIDENCE

Interventions to Improve Psychosocial and Emotional Impairments After Brain Injury

The high prevalence of psychological impairments among individuals with TBI supports continued efforts to identify appropriate and empirically based interventions. Depression, anxiety, suicidal ideation, posttraumatic stress disorder, substance abuse, and sleep disorders are among the conditions commonly cited across the continuum of recovery. Psychological issues are commonly cited among unmet rehabilitation needs following TBI (Mahoney et al., 2021), and these directly fall within OT's scope of practice. There is strong evidence to support the use of cognitive-behavioral approaches to improve symptoms of depression, anxiety, and emotional distress (Wheeler et al., 2016). Cognitive-behavioral therapy techniques emphasize challenging and altering cognitive distortions and behaviors to facilitate more effective coping strategies and improved functioning (Potter et al., 2016). The approach can be linked to specific OT individual and group interventions to support occupational performance outcomes. Evidence also supports the use of goal-directed interventions to increase life satisfaction, psychosocial reintegration (Doig et al., 2011), and emotional control (Tornås et al., 2016). Additional evidence-based interventions to improve various aspects of psychosocial functioning include peer mentoring (Hanks et al., 2012), education and skills training (Vuletic et al., 2016), physical exercise (Rzezak et al., 2015), mindfulness-based programs (Combs et al., 2018), and yoga (Donnelly et al., 2017).

There is tremendous heterogeneity of symptoms and severity across the population of TBI survivors. To effectively implement the evidence to improve psychosocial functioning, it is essential that OT practitioners consider severity of injury, physical and cognitive capacity, demographic characteristics, and environmental factors. A client-centered approach is essential to selecting an intervention and delivery method best suited to the needs of the individual and family.

Occupational Therapy in Action: Miles's Journey From the ICU to College Graduation

The case of Miles characterizes the complexity of TBI rehabilitation and the important impact of OT throughout the recovery spectrum. His experience following severe TBI also demonstrates the barriers to full community participation from the standpoint of both the individual and society.

Background Information

At the age of 22, Miles sustained a severe TBI in a motor vehicle crash while performing his job as a laborer with a local homebuilder. At the time of the injury, Miles was living with his mother, girlfriend, and infant daughter. He was a high school graduate who enjoyed sports, computers, and social events. He remained in a coma for approximately 3 months, with computed tomography (CT) scan showing extensive brainstem damage and multiple contusions throughout his brain. OT at this stage focuses on both managing impairments resulting from the injury and preventing secondary impairments that can occur over periods of unconsciousness.

The evidence supports a team-coordinated multimodal approach with close observation of the client designed to improve alertness and arousal (Li et al., 2020). This approach typically involves using familiar and meaningful sensory stimulation of the visual, auditory, olfactory, gustatory, cutaneous, and/or kinesthetic system tailored to both client tolerance and premorbid preferences. Additionally, interventions such as passive range of motion (PROM), motor training, splinting, casting, and positioning are among the interventions to support occupations are used to either restore motor function or prevent secondary complications such as joint and muscle contractures during coma (Leung et al., 2019).

Miles had numerous medical complications during his acute care admission, including a lower-extremity deep vein thrombosis (DVT), pneumonia, atelectasis, bradycardia, and questionable seizure activity. When his medical status stabilized, he was transferred to a skilled nursing facility where he continued the coma recovery program as described earlier. He remained in this setting until he emerged from coma and became progressively more alert. At that point he was assessed at a level III (localized response) on the Rancho Los Amigos Levels of Cognitive Functioning Scale (RLAS; Hagen, 1998) and was transferred to a rehabilitation hospital for intensive interdisciplinary rehabilitation—approximately 6 months after the date of his injury. OT at this stage employs remedial and compensatory approaches to address sensorimotor and self-care skill impairments, functional cognitive remediation, and environmental modifications, along with caregiver education and training (Mortera, 2015). Depending on the client's level of agitation, structured, basic self-care tasks can be initiated along with structured simple activities requiring physical movements and/or cognitive skills. Bogner and colleagues (2019) found that increasing contextualized interventions (e.g., self-care, real-life activities) during inpatient rehabilitation improved community participation 1 year later. New learning at this stage is generally limited because of posttraumatic amnesia, agitation, overstimulation, and confusion (Wheeler & Acord-Vira, 2016). After 5 weeks of intensive, inpatient interdisciplinary rehabilitation, Miles was assessed at a level V (confused, inappropriate) on the RLAS (Hagen, 1998). Miles's progress was considered to have reached a plateau and he was subsequently transferred back to the skilled nursing facility because of his current level of functioning as he continued to require assistance will all basic activities of daily living (ADL). He had a percutaneous endoscopic gastrostomy (PEG) tube in place, was on a pureed diet with moderately thickened liquids, and was nonambulatory, dependent on others for wheelchair mobility. His verbal expression was described as "profoundly impaired," and he communicated via a communication board.

Referral

Approximately 2 months into his second admission to the skilled nursing facility, Miles's specialized care was extended by referring him to a TBI post-acute, residential rehabilitation program. This program would provide opportunities for Miles to improve his independence and community living (Rosenbaum et al., 2018). As part of the community reentry rehabilitation team, I had the opportunity to complete a comprehensive assessment with Miles followed by an intensive rehabilitation program.

Evaluation

Initial Impressions

Given the severity of Miles's injury, I was very aware of the challenges that were to lie ahead for him, and how that could affect my treatment planning. Schutz and Schutz (2010) noted that for injuries where coma is less than 1 day, most survivors regain independence and perform adequately in a competitive job. However, for more severe injuries, as was the case for Miles, even the most intense therapy may not restore full functioning in productive tasks, social outings and community participation years post-injury (Malone et al., 2019; Schutz & Schutz, 2010). While reviewing Miles's medical record, I was able to gain an appreciation of recent positive changes in his level of alertness, initiation, and desire to participate in intensive rehabilitation.

Community-Based Occupational Therapy Assessment—Considerations

Helping people to be productive and satisfied in their least restrictive environment is central to OT regardless of treatment setting or medical diagnosis. McColl and colleagues (2001) categorized meaningful aspects of community integration to include the following:

1. Activities to fill one's time
2. Independence in one's living situation
3. Relationships with other people

Additionally, I've found the constructs of the International Classification of Functioning, Disability, and Health (ICF; World Health Organization, 2001) to be helpful in organizing my approach to both assessment and treatment. Both perspectives consider the interaction of person and environment and its impact on participation in meaningful occupations.

Assessment Priority No. 1— Therapeutic Relationship Building

If I were to name one thing that was essential to a positive outcome when working with persons with severe brain injury, it would be the establishment of a strong therapeutic relationship. That process begins with the very first interaction with the client. Standardized interview tools such as the Occupational Performance History Interview II (Kielhofner et al., 2004) and the Canadian Occupational Performance Measure (COPM; Law et al., 2005) are excellent for collecting important information and establishing client-centered goals. However, care should be taken to ensure that the interview isn't so structured that it hinders rapport building (refer back to Box 62.1). For persons with a low frustration tolerance, moderate-to-severe cognitive impairments, and/or difficulty regulating environmental stimulation, adaptations to the interview duration, wording of questions, and interview setting may be required in order to collect meaningful data. When initial rapport is established, clients are more likely to participate in home and community assessment tasks likely to be both challenging and frustrating for them.

Assessment Results

Selected assessments were implemented to complete Miles's occupational profile, a summary of his "history and experiences, patterns of daily living, interests, values, and needs" (American Occupational Therapy Association [AOTA], 2020, p. S21). Miles's initial assessment was completed over a period of approximately 1 week, a time frame that is longer than in many settings but necessary for community-based rehabilitation given the need to observe performance in home and community settings. The assessments used with Miles are outlined in Table 62.1.

During our initial interview, Miles presented as extremely motivated and eager to participate in assessment tasks. After collecting some background information, Miles was asked to identify long-term goals and areas of life that were most important to him. They included the following:

1. Getting reunited with his girlfriend and infant daughter who had relocated to her parents' home more than 1,000 miles away
2. Being able to move more effectively and walk—"getting out of this wheelchair"
3. Being able to complete morning dressing, grooming, self-feeding, and toileting tasks without assistance

TABLE 62.1 Community-Based Assessment Data Collection to Complete an Occupational Profile

Assessment Method	Rationale	Interpretation
Initial interview	Rapport building, establish client goals and meaningful occupations, screen cognitive impairments, and orientation	Positive transition from skilled nursing; patient concerned about girlfriend and daughter relocating and not available to visit. Therapeutic relationship initiated with OT practitioners.
Canadian Occupational Performance Measure (COPM; Law et al., 2005)	Capture a client's self-perception of performance and satisfaction with occupational performance	Scores range from 1 to 10, with higher scores indicating greater perception of performance and satisfaction. Average change in scores for performance was 2.0 and satisfaction was –1.6.
Self-Care and Mobility Section GG Items (AOTA, 2018)	Self-Care and Mobility Sections of the GG items. Provides performance levels and can be used in any adult care setting.	Partial/moderate (less than half the effort) to substantial/maximal (more than half the effort) assist required for all aspects of basic self-care and functional transfers to bed and chair from wheelchair. Total assistance was required for transfer into a standard bathtub.
Community Integration Questionnaire (CIQ; Willer et al., 1994)	Brain injury–specific measure to address actual participation in categories related to community integration 1. Integration into a homelike setting 2. Social integration 3. Integration into productive activities	A total CIQ score can range from 0 to 29, with higher scores indicating greater community integration. Miles's score reflects virtually no current participation in activities inside or outside home.
Satisfaction with Life Scale (SWLS; Diener et al., 1985)	Measure of general life satisfaction, a factor of subjective well-being; quick administration, well-established validity, and reliability	Scores on the SWLS range from 5 (very dissatisfied) to 35 (highly satisfied). Miles's score of 24 represented "mild satisfaction."

(continued)

TABLE 62.1	Community-Based Assessment Data Collection to Complete an Occupational Profile (*continued*)

Assessment Method	Rationale	Interpretation	
Neurobehavioral Functioning Inventory (Kreutzer et al., 1999)	Completing patient form in concert with family caregiver form allows assessment of awareness of impairments, an important aspect of executive cognitive functioning and an area considered important to rehabilitation program compliance	*Miles*　　*Caregiver* Depression 45　　51 Somatic complaints 45　　74 Memory 46　　51 Communication 58　　54 Aggression 39　　44 Motor impairments 51　　60	Comparison of patient and caregiver raw scores suggests possibility of deficit of self-awareness based on Miles reporting less severity of symptoms in all areas except communication.

from others—"taking care of myself and having some privacy"

4. Being able to communicate more effectively—"talking better without drooling so much"
5. Going back to school—wanted to attend college prior to injury
6. Being able to play sports—expressed a particular interest in basketball and running

Having Miles identify these areas was important as client-centered goal setting using occupation-based interventions in a relevant environmental context can improve occupational performance (Powell et al., 2016) and motivation for working on their goals (Evans & Krasny-Pacini, 2017). Given the gap between Miles's current and desired level of functioning, his full commitment to the program was especially essential.

Further testing was carried out to determine which impairments limited occupational performance. Sensorimotor testing revealed severe ataxia affecting his ability to coordinate movements throughout the muscles of his extremities and trunk. Functional transfers from wheelchair to bed and toilet were poor. Generalized weakness and decreased endurance were also noted. Grip strength, evaluated by dynamometer, was 20 lb on the dominant right side and 34 lb on the left. Range of motion was within normal limits, with the exception of right shoulder abduction and flexion, which were both limited to approximately 30° actively and 90° passively. Miles had sustained a severe fracture to his right forearm in his accident, resulting in prolonged immobilization of his right arm. He did not report discomfort with movement of his right upper extremity and no exercise restrictions were noted. Sensation was grossly intact.

In addition to the assessments listed in Table 62.1, Miles and I completed a community living skills assessment (Angle

& Buxton, 1991) that demonstrated moderate-to-severe difficulty with all home and community tasks except money management and telephone use, which were mildly impaired. Although it appeared that physical impairments were the primary contributor to these functional difficulties, cognitive deficits such as impulsivity and reduced awareness of impairments were also evident during observations. Such executive cognitive dysfunctions are commonly associated with damage to the brain's frontal lobes. These executive dysfunctions significantly impact other higher-order cognitive skills such as decision-making, goal setting, self-evaluation, and, ultimately, successful performance of the majority of life roles. Short-term memory impairments were also evident but appeared influenced by time of day and nature of the content to be remembered. Vision was tested prior to his admission and was determined to be consistent with pre-injury acuity. Miles demonstrated functional vision during reading, computer keyboard access, and other evaluation activities.

Treatment Planning: Mapping Out Strategies to Turn Assessment Findings Into Performance Outcomes

Assessment findings revealed a large performance discrepancy between Miles's current functioning and his stated goals. Assisting clients in overcoming the factors contributing to reduced community participation following TBI is generally much more challenging for OT practitioners

BOX 62.3 INCLUDING FAMILY TO MAXIMIZE THE EFFECTIVENESS OF TBI REHABILITATION

The occurrence of a significant brain injury is life altering for both the individual and their family. Bogner and colleagues (2019) found that individuals with TBI whose families attended therapy at least 10% of the time during inpatient rehabilitation were more active in the communities after discharge. Of particular concern is the effect of brain injury on the functioning and effectiveness of supportive relationships. Occurrence of relationship dysfunction, stress, and failure following a TBI is prevalent. Evidence supports direct, couple-based, face-to-face intervention addressing communication, empathy, positive behavioral support, and coping to improve relationship functioning and satisfaction. Ensuring ongoing success of a support relationship can be key in improving the outcomes for individuals who have experienced a TBI (Backhaus et al., 2019; Kreutzer et al., 2020).

than identifying them. My treatment plan with Miles was heavily influenced by the client-centered philosophy and the person–environment models of OT (see Chapters 28 and 35). To me, this model represents the "ideal" scenario for a community reentry OT plan because it integrates the client-centered, occupation-based focus of OT with what we've learned about through the course of brain injury recovery. Unfortunately, the ability to fully implement the approach in most healthcare settings and systems is difficult, but clinicians should do all that is possible within the settings that they work. Working in Miles's favor was the fact that his health insurance (Workers Compensation) and case manager appeared supportive of intensive, long-term rehabilitation. Providing early onset and more intensive rehabilitation following Miles's TBI could improve his outcomes with functional tasks (Königs et al., 2018). However, the chronic, complex, and evolving nature of TBI makes it very difficult to determine the optimal and most cost-effective amount of intervention for any particular individual (Wheeler & Acord-Vira, 2016).

Given the gap between Miles's current functional level and his desired goals, regular communication with him regarding his progress was essential so that he could see how small incremental goals were related to his long-term goals. Success experiences are essential to building self-esteem and self-confidence as well as fueling motivation. Encouragement and support from outside his treatment program would be negatively affected by the fact that his girlfriend and child relocated with her parents after his accident and were more than 1,000 miles away (see Box 62.3). Additionally, although his mother expressed a strong interest in helping Miles recover, both she and Miles acknowledged a turbulent and unstable family history that included little contact with his father. Miles's community-based rehabilitation program included a multidisciplinary treatment team that comprised myself, a certified occupational therapy assistant (COTA), a psychologist, speech-language pathologist, physical therapist, nurse, and social worker. Key target areas of the interdisciplinary treatment program are described in Table 62.2.

TABLE 62.2 Selected Target Areas of the Interdisciplinary Treatment Program

Occupational Therapy	Speech Therapy	Psychology	Physical Therapy
Basic ADL performance/functional transfers	Speech clarity	Counseling for adjustment to disability	Functional ambulation using walker
Fine motor skills (e.g., handwriting) to facilitate day planner/memory notebook use	Swallowing/oral motor skills	Memory training and compensation	Strengthening exercises with home exercise program
Meal preparation/home management	Memory—recall of sentences and paragraphs	Family counseling	Balance training
Leisure and social community outings	Augmentative communication	Attention training	Transfers and bed/mat mobility
Prevocational preparation including computer access	Respiratory exercises	Comprehensive neuropsychological assessment	Family/caregiver training related to ambulation and exercises

ADL, activities of daily living.

Implementing the Treatment Plan

Miles's treatment program tested our therapeutic relationship from the onset. His severe ataxia contributed to poor motor coordination and frequent frustration during our sessions. Despite his high drive to participate in tasks with me and the COTA, functional gains were slow, accompanied by growing self-awareness of the fact that getting physically stronger was not going to resolve his severe ataxic movements. Miles was less interested in compensatory strategies than being the person he was prior to his injury, and that contributed to resistance when it came to trying adaptive equipment and compensatory techniques.

OT treatment sessions used both home and community settings. In the home, ADL training and home management activities were in an actual bedroom, bathroom, kitchen, living room, and office area. Whenever possible, we practiced tasks at normal times—dressing, grooming, transfers, meal preparation, using the computer, handwriting in his memory notebook, planning and participating in community outings, doing household chores, and doing leisure activities. Repetition during activities was used to strengthen muscles and improve performance in conjunction with daily upper-extremity strengthening exercises. Although often considered an adjunct to occupation, Miles's upper-extremity strengthening program was additionally important as exercise was a meaningful occupation pre-injury.

With repeated struggles, Miles appeared more accepting of adaptive equipment to improve his independence in activities that were particularly important to him. For example, weighted feeding utensils with built-up handles, dishes with higher lips, and cups with a top were effective at improving motor function to improve his ability to feed himself and drink more efficiently without excessive spillage. Building up handles on writing and grooming utensils also improved quality of performance, although to a lesser degree. We attempted to use weighted wrist cuffs to improve movement efficiency during computer keyboard use. However, Miles insisted on a one-handed typing technique that involved stabilizing his wrist using the opposite hand (Figure 62.3).

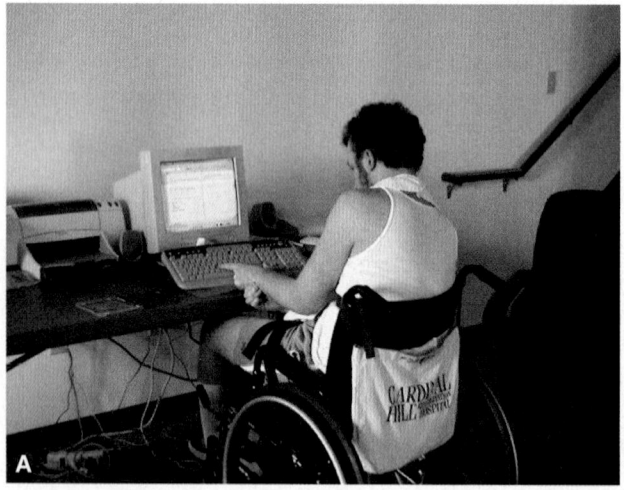

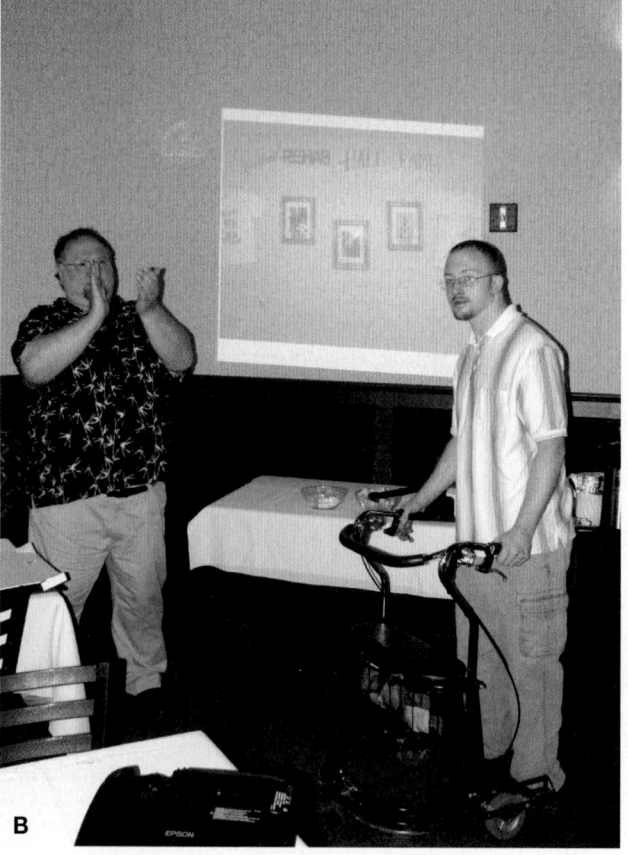

FIGURE 62.3 Miles's educational program progressed from **(A)** basic computer keyboard access to **(B)** speaking to other survivors of brain injury.

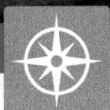

EXPANDING OUR PERSPECTIVES

Importance of Treating the Client, Not the Diagnosis

Kaitlin Bristol

In the spring of my third year of college, I experienced a mild traumatic brain injury (mTBI). Following a workup and observation in the emergency room (ER), I was discharged with instructions for two weeks of rest. They told me to pace myself when returning to sports and that I would be able to return to classes immediately following rest. Overlooked as insignificant in my patient history were four prior mTBIs spanning from childhood through adolescence, increasing the likelihood for complications. However, with reassurance from my care team that it was "just a concussion," and having previously fully recovered from mTBIs, I expected to return to baseline quickly.

When this injury proved itself to be different, I was unequipped to handle it. For months, I experienced fatigue, headache, and sensory and cognitive changes. Suddenly, names of acquaintances became difficult to remember, so I self-isolated. My chosen tool of self-expression, writing, became impossible because of difficulty with word-finding, so I stopped. Lectures were hard to follow and I grew self-conscious of frequently asking professors to repeat themselves, so I grew silent. Despite recognizing that I was struggling, I held onto the well-meaning insistence of my care team that I would be fine, paralyzed by a fear of being dismissed as faking if I questioned them. My grades slipped and I grew depressed.

That summer, I was seen by a neurologist and given accommodations. They were approved by my college's Disability Student Support (DSS) center, but I avoided the intake meeting. However, when that semester began as the last had ended, I began to accept that this injury was unique despite being the same in name as those prior and set up a meeting with a counselor. We determined that my resistance to accepting help was multifaceted. Minimal

education combined with little reevaluation of the treatment plan left me vulnerable to expectations of normalcy. A lack of progressive return to academics meant the inability to monitor my cognitive exertion to avoid provocation of symptoms. The loss of valued occupations and increased self-doubt meant that while my skull may not have fractured, my spirit did.

The turning point for me was a statement she made; "Accommodations are not meant to enable someone to get ahead of their peers but to level the playing field." This forced me to confront my belief that my injury wasn't severe enough to have accommodations. With the help of the DSS, I learned strategies to manage my symptoms and slowly used my accommodations. Most importantly, they taught me how to advocate for myself in order to navigate both obstacles in accessibility and negative viewpoints in the educational and post-professional world. Although I continued to experience headaches and auditory processing deficits, with the proper supports in place, I accomplished my goal of becoming an occupational therapist.

It is easy to make the mistake of seeing a diagnosis and not the individual. As occupational therapists, we must remember that each individual's presentation is unique to them because of their distinct occupational profile. Although the diagnosis bears the name "mild," the impact of the injury on my life was severe and it was vital to my recovery that it wasn't minimized. My counselor recognized this and validated my feelings, which led to building trust. Though not an OT, she was able to consider my lived experiences, values, and occupations and make recommendations that wouldn't feel obtrusive. When making recommendations for our clients, we must be thoughtful and consider the intersection of all client factors to find the best fit for them and not what seems best on paper. When we are able to do this, our practice becomes truly client-centered.

Miles had his first session in the community approximately 3 weeks into his program—a trip to a department store to purchase clothing. From that point on, sessions in the community were a regular aspect of his program, occurring approximately two to three times a week. Community outings included visits to restaurants, visiting his mother at her home, and attending sporting events, including a wheelchair basketball game. During outings, OT focused on evaluating skills such as money management, functional mobility, planning, initiative, problem-solving, and decision-making in relation to his degree of independence for each task.

Although functional gains were positive, the rate of progress was inconsistent. Success was complicated by medical factors such as frequent medication changes attempting to manage upper-extremity tremors and severe esophageal reflux, which negatively impacted self-feeding and nutritional intake. His status 3 months after the onset of his post-acute, residential program and 8 months from the date of his injury is summarized in Table 62.3. Despite his functional gains, Miles reported less satisfaction with life, frustration with his current situation, more frequent periods of agitation, and depressed mood. Additionally, he demonstrated increased self-awareness based on statements

TABLE 62.3	Selected Test Scores From 90-Day Evaluation		
Evaluation	Baseline	90-Day Reassessment	Interpretation
CIQ	Home integration, 0	Home integration, 3	Significant progress in home management and initiation and participation in social activities
	Social integration, 2	Social integration, 5	
	Productive activity, 0	Productive activity, 0	
COPM	Self-care tasks I=9, P=5, S=6	Self-care tasks P=8, S=5	Significant progress in perception of performance and perceived satisfaction decreased with top 5 rated areas of importance.
	School I=9, P=1, S=3	School P=3, S=2	
	Basketball I=7, P=2, S=4	Basketball P=5, S=2	
	Meal preparation I=8, P=2, S=4	Meal preparation P=5, S=3	
	Socialization I=7, P=5, S=6	Socialization P=4, S=3	
Self-Care and Mobility Section GG Tasks	Eating, 2	Eating, 4	Notable functional gains in ADL independence. Assistance required for tasks requiring balance and fine motor coordination because of continued ataxia
	UB dressing, 3	UB dressing, 5	
	LB dressing, 2	LB dressing, 4	
	Shoes, 1	Shoes, 4	
	Oral hygiene, 2	Oral hygiene, 4	
	Shower/bath, 2	Shower/bath self, 4	
	Toilet hygiene, 2	Toilet hygiene, 4	
	Transfers (bed to chair), 2	Transfers (bed to chair), 4	
SWLS	24	12	Despite progress, significant reduction in self-reported life satisfaction

ADL, activities of daily living; COPM, Canadian Occupational Performance Measure; LB, lower body; SWLS, Satisfaction with Life Scale; UB, upper body.

regarding the severity of his impairments and similarities between his and staff responses on the Neurobehavioral Functioning Inventory (Kreutzer et al., 1999).

Revising the Treatment Plan: Expanding Occupations

With it becoming increasingly clear that Miles would have lifelong physical impairments, especially ataxia, aspects of Miles's program were modified to expand his occupations by putting greater emphasis on productivity and leisure goals. Up to this point in his treatment program, the occupations occupying Miles's typical day were almost entirely centered on self-care. The effort required for basic ADL and home management left little time and energy for other activities. That, combined with an increasing level of awareness of impairments, negatively affected life satisfaction. Aspects of leisure and productivity, so central to Miles pre-injury daily routine, were very limited and impacted his psychological well-being. It was hoped by balancing self-care and home management goals with productive activity and leisure, Miles would develop a greater sense

of accomplishment and gain a more positive outlook in the face of residual disability. The plan to increase Miles's productive occupations included two primary objectives identified by Miles: (1) taking college courses to eventually obtain a degree and (2) taking greater responsibility of his finances to demonstrate capacity to become his own legal guardian. Additionally, OT continued working on self-care skills, home management, and community participation to help Miles and the clinical team make decisions on his least restrictive living environment after his discharge from the residential treatment program.

Planning was initiated to look at options for community living. During family sessions, it became increasingly clear that Miles would not be residing with his parents, and his girlfriend had expressed an intention to break off their relationship. The therapeutic relationships established with many clinical team members served as a critical source of support during this period of social isolation and an uncertain future. Although supportive of Miles during his struggles, adherence to professional boundaries by the OT team and all staff was essential at all times. Haddad and colleagues (2018) describe strategies to express genuine care for clients and building positive relationships based on respect while maintaining some distance. Given Miles's emotional vulnerability, it would be understandable for him to misinterpret the nature of his relationships with health-care providers (e.g., social friendships, intimacy). Strategies used by the treatment team to maintain professional boundaries included:

- Having Miles participate in team meetings where issues about his progress were discussed
- Dividing outings and activities between team members
- Limiting visits/interactions to work hours
- Working with Miles to expand his relationships beyond the rehabilitation setting
- Selectively sharing with Miles's personal incidents from everyday life

The stages of Miles's education, independent living, and leisure goals are detailed in Figure 62.4. Each phase is characterized by significant clinical progress and incorporation of meaningful occupations into his daily routine. Each was also characterized by significant struggle and testing of the therapist–client relationship. On occasion, Miles would appear to sabotage his progress, acting out or refusing to

participate in tasks that had been weeks, and sometimes months, in planning. The roles of the OT team changed throughout the phases, moving from predominantly teaching direct skills to advocacy and working with landlords, builders, and school personnel (e.g., office of accessibility services, professors) to help Miles face environmental barriers in terms of accessibility and prejudice.

It took 8 years for Miles to receive his Bachelor of Arts in Psychology (Figure 62.5). At the time of graduation, he was living in the community with homemaker support, and he gained legal authority to manage his own finances. His outcomes defy the expected for persons with severe TBI. But despite these accomplishments, he also faces an uncertain future. Without secured employment, an absence of leisure activities, few friends, and residual motor impairments present continuing challenges. It is likely that he will continue to require various rehabilitative and social services, but with his perseverance and services, Miles may continue to defy expectations.

Lippincott® Connect *For additional resources on the subjects discussed in this chapter, visit* Lippincott Connect.

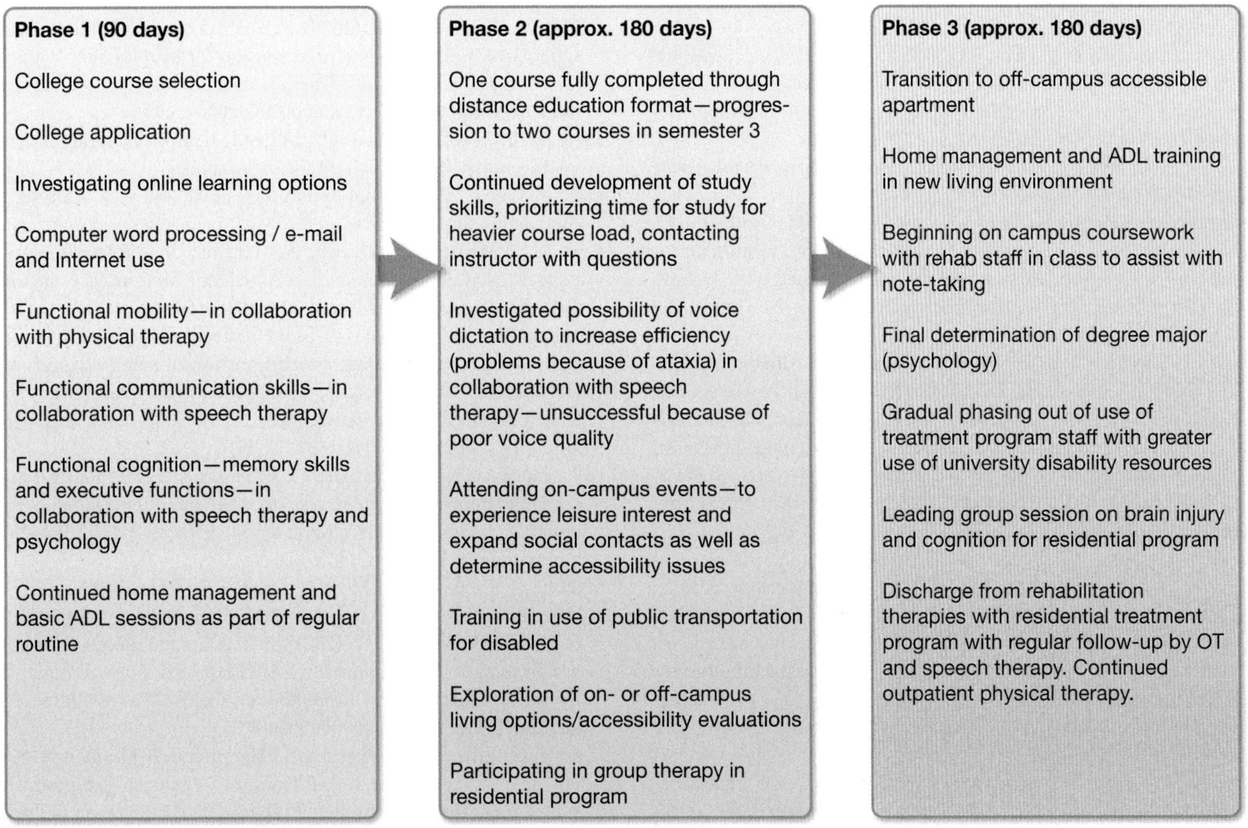

Phase 1 (90 days)

College course selection

College application

Investigating online learning options

Computer word processing / e-mail and Internet use

Functional mobility—in collaboration with physical therapy

Functional communication skills—in collaboration with speech therapy

Functional cognition—memory skills and executive functions—in collaboration with speech therapy and psychology

Continued home management and basic ADL sessions as part of regular routine

Phase 2 (approx. 180 days)

One course fully completed through distance education format—progression to two courses in semester 3

Continued development of study skills, prioritizing time for study for heavier course load, contacting instructor with questions

Investigated possibility of voice dictation to increase efficiency (problems because of ataxia) in collaboration with speech therapy—unsuccessful because of poor voice quality

Attending on-campus events—to experience leisure interest and expand social contacts as well as determine accessibility issues

Training in use of public transportation for disabled

Exploration of on- or off-campus living options/accessibility evaluations

Participating in group therapy in residential program

Phase 3 (approx. 180 days)

Transition to off-campus accessible apartment

Home management and ADL training in new living environment

Beginning on campus coursework with rehab staff in class to assist with note-taking

Final determination of degree major (psychology)

Gradual phasing out of use of treatment program staff with greater use of university disability resources

Leading group session on brain injury and cognition for residential program

Discharge from rehabilitation therapies with residential treatment program with regular follow-up by OT and speech therapy. Continued outpatient physical therapy.

FIGURE 62.4 Stages of Miles's school/independent living progression with occupational therapy (OT) focus areas. ADL, activities of daily living.

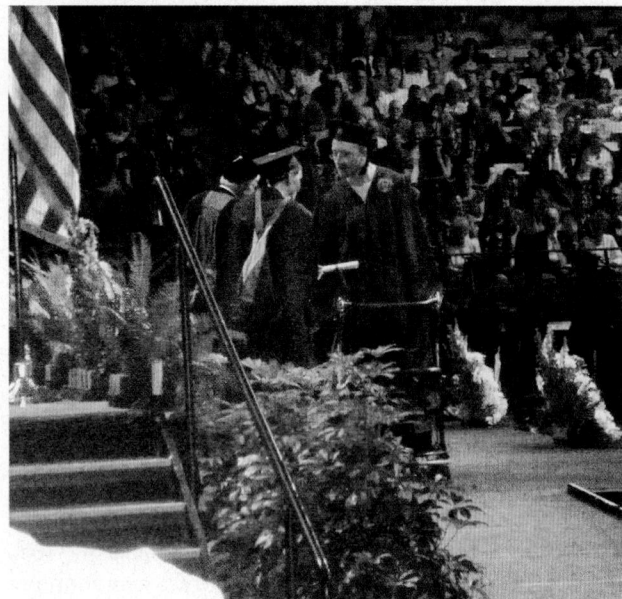

FIGURE 62.5 An intensive, occupation-based rehabilitation program helped Miles accomplish his goal of college graduation.

REFERENCES

American Occupational Therapy Association. (2018). *Self-care and mobility section GG items.* https://www.aota.org/-/media/Corporate/Files/Practice/Manage/Documentation/Self-Care-Mobility-Section-GG-Items-Assessment-Template.pdf

American Occupational Therapy Association. (2020). Occupational therapy practice framework: Domain and process, 4th edition. *American Journal of Occupational Therapy, 74*(S2), 1–87. https://doi.org/10.5014/ajot.2020.74S2001

Angle, D., & Buxton, J. (1991). *Community living skills workbook for the head injured adult.* Aspen.

Backhaus, S., Neumann, D., Parrott, D., Hammond, F. M., Brownson, C., & Malec, J. (2019). Investigation of a new couples intervention for individuals with brain injury: A randomized controlled trial. *Archives of Physical Medicine and Rehabilitation, 100*(2), 195–204. https://doi.org/10.1016/j.apmr.2018.08.174

Bogner, J., Dijkers, M., Hade, E. M., Beaulieu, C., Montgomery, E., Giuffrida, C., Timpson, M., Peng, J., Gilchrist, K., Lash, A., Hammond, F. M., Horn, S. D., & Corrigan, J. D. (2019). Contextualized treatment in traumatic brain injury inpatient rehabilitation: Effects on outcomes during the first year after discharge. *Archives of Physical Medicine and Rehabilitation, 100*(10), 1810–1817. https://doi.org/10.1016/j.apmr.2018.12.037

CARF International. (2022, January 29). *Community integration.* Programs. http://www.carf.org/Programs/ProgramDescriptions/ECS-Community-Integration/

Combs, M. A., Critchfield, E. A., & Soble, J. R. (2018). Relax while you rehabilitate: A pilot study integrating a novel, yoga-based mindfulness group intervention into a residential military brain injury rehabilitation program. *Rehabilitation Psychology, 63*(2), 182–193. https://doi.org/10.1037/rep0000179

Diener, E., Emmons, R. A., Larsen, R. J., & Griffin, S. (1985). The satisfaction with life scale. *Journal of Personality Assessment, 49*, 71–75. https://doi.org/10.1207/s15327752jpa4901_13

Doig, E., Fleming, J., Kuipers, P., Cornwell, P., & Khan, A. (2011). Goal-directed outpatient rehabilitation following TBI: A pilot study of programme effectiveness and comparison of outcomes in home and day hospital settings. *Brain Injury, 25*(11), 1114–1125. https://doi.org/10.3109/02699052.2011.607788

Donnelly, K. Z., Linnea, K., Grant, D. A., & Lichtenstein, J. (2017). The feasibility and impact of a yoga pilot programme on the quality-of-life of adults with acquired brain injury. *Brain Injury, 31*(2), 208–214. https://doi.org/10.1080/02699052.2016.1225988

Evans, J. J., & Krasny-Pacini, A. (2017). Goal setting in rehabilitation. In B. A. Wilson, J. Winegardner, C. M. van Heugten, & T. Ownsworth (Eds.), *Neuropsychological rehabilitation* (pp. 49–58). Taylor & Francis.

Haddad, A., Doherty, R., & Purtilo, R. (2018). *Health professional and patient interaction* (9th ed.). Elsevier.

Hagen, C. (1998). *The Ranchos Los Amigos levels of cognitive functioning: The revised levels* (3rd ed.). Ranchos Los Amigos.

Hanks, R. A., Rapport, L. J., Wertheimer, J., & Koviak, C. (2012). Randomized controlled trial of peer mentoring for individuals with traumatic brain injury and their significant others. *Archives of Physical Medicine and Rehabilitation, 93*(8), 1297–1304. https://doi.org/10.1016/j.apmr.2012.04.027

Katz, D., Zasler, N., & Zafonte, R. (2007). Clinical continuum of care and natural history. In N. Zasler, D. Katz, & R. Zafonte (Eds.), *Perspectives on rehabilitation care and research.* Demos.

Kielhofner, G., Mallinson, T., Crawford, C., Nowak, M., Rigby, M., Henry, A., & Walens, D. (2004). *Occupational performance history interview—II (version 2.1).* MOHO Clearinghouse.

Königs, M., Beurskens, E. A., Snoep, L., Scherder, E. J., & Oosterlaan, J. (2018). Effects of timing and intensity of neurorehabilitation on functional outcome after traumatic brain injury: A systematic review and meta-analysis. *Archives of Physical Medicine and Rehabilitation, 99*(6), 1149–1159. https://doi.org/10.1016/j.apmr.2018.01.013

Kreutzer, J. S., Marwitz, J. H., Sima, A. P., Graham, K. M., Hsu, N. H., Mills, A., & Lukow, H. R. (2020). Evaluation of a brief, skill-building, supportive, and educational intervention for couples after brain injury. *The Journal of Head Trauma Rehabilitation, 35*(3), 175–186. https://doi.org/10.1097/HTR.0000000000000519

Kreutzer, J. S., Seel, R., & Marwitz, J. (1999). Neurobehavioral functioning inventory. The Psychological Corporation.

Lash, M. (2009). *The essential brain injury guide* (4th ed.). Brain Injury Association of America.

Law, M., Baptiste, S., Carswell, A., McColl, M., Polatajko, H., & Pollock, N. (2005). *Canadian occupational performance measure.* Canadian Association of Occupational Therapists.

Leung, J., King, C., & Fereday, S. (2019). Effectiveness of a programme comprising serial casting, botulinum toxin, splinting and motor training for contracture management: A randomized controlled trial. *Clinical Rehabilitation, 33*(6), 1035–1044. https://doi.org/10.1177/0269215519831337

Li, J., Cheng, Q., Liu, F. K., Huang, Z., & Feng, S. S. (2020). Sensory stimulation to improve arousal in comatose patients after traumatic brain injury: A systematic review. *Neurological Sciences, 41*(9), 2367–2376. https://doi.org/10.1007/s10072-020-04410-9

Mahoney, E. J., Silva, M. A., Reljic, T., Dams-O'Connor, K., Hammond, F. M., Monden, K. R., Chung, J. S., Dillahunt-Aspillaga, C., & Nakase-Richardson, R. (2021). Rehabilitation needs at 5 years post-traumatic brain injury: A VA TBI model systems study. *The Journal of Head Trauma Rehabilitation, 36*(3), 175–185. https://doi.org/10.1097/HTR.0000000000000629

Malone, C., Erler, K. S., Giacino, J. T., Hammond, F. M., Juengst, S. B., Locascio, J. J., Nakase-Richardson, R., Verduzco-Gutierrez, M., Whyte, J., Zasler, N., & Bodien, Y. G. (2019). Participation following inpatient rehabilitation for traumatic disorders of consciousness: A TBI model systems study. *Frontiers in Neurology, 10*, 1314. https://doi.org/10.3389/fneur.2019.01314

McColl, M., Davies, D., Carlson, P., Johnston, J., & Minnes, P. (2001). The community integration measure: Development and preliminary validation. *Archives of Physical Medicine and Rehabilitation, 82*, 429–434. https://doi.org/10.1053/apmr.2001.22195

Mortera, M. (2015). The acute, inpatient, and subacute rehabilitation phases of recovery. In K. Golisz & M. V. Radomski (Eds.), *Traumatic brain injury (TBI): Interventions to support occupational performance* (pp. 175–229). American Occupational Therapy Association.

Pettemeridou, E., Kennedy, M. R. T., & Constantinidou, F. (2020). Executive functions, self-awareness and quality of life in chronic moderate-to-severe TBI. *Neurorehabilitation, 46*(1), 109–118. https://doi.org/10.3233/NRE-192963

Potter, S. D. S., Brown, R. G., & Fleminger, S. (2016). Randomised, waiting list controlled trial of cognitive behavioural therapy for persistent postconcussional symptoms after predominantly mild-moderate traumatic brain injury. *Journal of Neurology, Neurosurgery and Psychiatry, 87*(10), 1075–1083. https://doi.org/10.1136/jnnp-2015-312838

Powell, J. M., Rich, T. J., & Wise, E. K. (2016). Effectiveness of occupation-and activity-based interventions to improve everyday activities and social participation for people with traumatic brain injury: A systematic review. *American Journal of Occupational Therapy, 70*(3), 7003180040p1–7003180040p9. https://doi.org/10.5014/ajot.2016.020909

Rosenbaum, A., Gordon, W., Joannou, A., & Berman, B. (2018). Functional outcomes following post-acute rehabilitation for moderate-to-severe traumatic brain injury. *Brain Injury, 32*(7), 907–914. https://doi.org/10.1080/02699052.2018.1469040

Rzezak, P., Caxa, L., Santolia, P., Antunes, H. K., Suriano, I., Tufik, S., & de Mello, M. T. (2015). Affective responses after different intensities of exercise in patients with traumatic brain injury. *Frontiers in Psychology, 6*, 839–839. https://doi.org/10.3389/fpsyg.2015.00839

Schutz, L., & Schutz, M. (2010). *Head injury recovery in real life.* Plural.

Tornås, S., Løvstad, M., Solbakk, A. K., Schanke, A. K., & Stubberud, J. (2016). Goal management training combined with external cuing as a means to improve emotional regulation, psychological functioning, and quality of life in patients with acquired brain injury: A randomized controlled trial. *Archives of Physical Medicine and Rehabilitation, 97*(11), 1841–1852. https://doi.org/10.1016/j.apmr.2016.06.014

Trudel, T., Tryon, W., & Purdum, C. (1998). Awareness of disability and long-term outcome after traumatic brain injury. *Rehabilitation Psychology, 43*, 267–281. https://doi.org/10.1037/0090-5550.43.4.267

Ullmann, S. G. (2015). Access to rehabilitation services in the affordable care era. *AMA Journal of Ethics, 17*(6), 553–557. https://doi.org/10.1001/journalofethics.2015.17.6.pfor1-1506

Vuletic, S., Bell, K. R., Jain, S., Bush, N., Temkin, N., Fann, J. R., Stanfill, K. E., Dikmen, S., Brockway, J. A., He, F., Ernstrom, K., Raman, R., Grant, G., Stein, M. B., Gahm, G. A., & CONTACT Investigators. (2016). Telephone problem-solving treatment improves sleep quality in service members with combat-related mild traumatic brain injury: Results from a randomized clinical trial. *The Journal of Head Trauma Rehabilitation, 31*(2), 147–157. https://doi.org/10.1097/HTR.0000000000000221

Wheeler, S., & Acord-Vira, A. (2016). *Occupational therapy practice guidelines for adults with traumatic brain injury.* American Occupational Therapy Association.

Wheeler, S., Acord-Vira, A., & Davis, D. (2016). Effectiveness of interventions to improve occupational performance for people with psychosocial, behavioral, and emotional impairments after brain injury: A systematic review. *The American Journal of Occupational Therapy, 70*(3), 1–9. https://doi.org/10.5014/ajot.115.020677

Willer, B., Ottenbacher, K., & Coad, M. (1994). The community integration questionnaire. A comparative examination. *American Journal of Physical Medicine & Rehabilitation, 73*, 103–111. https://doi.org/10.1097/00002060-199404000-00006

World Health Organization. (2001). *International classification of functioning, disability, and health.* Author.

Providing Wellness-Oriented Occupational Therapy Services for Persons With Mental Health Challenges

Margaret Swarbrick

LEARNING OBJECTIVES

After reading this chapter, you will be able to:

1. Define mental health, mental illness, and co-occurrence of mental and substance use disorders.
2. Discuss concepts of recovery and wellness as they relate to people with mental illness and substance use concerns.
3. Identify areas of occupation that present challenges for people with mental illness.
4. Describe emerging and evidence-based occupational therapy practice models.

Introduction

Mental health is more than just the absence of a mental or substance use disorder. Good mental health has long been associated with the sense that individuals are able to cope with the normal stresses of life, work or complete school tasks productively, and participate socially in school, home, work, or community contexts (World Health Organization, n.d.). What we think, what we do, and how we feel may be observed and categorized, and this is how we report our mental health. Good mental health sometimes is observed by how well people are prepared to manage stress and the inevitable challenges of life. Mental health is so important for participation in all valued occupations. Promoting mental health and preventing and treating mental illness have become important concerns for individuals, communities, and societies throughout the world, especially since the advent of COVID-19. Mental health problems are prevalent in society and have been so throughout history. Mental health practice is also historically at the core of the development of occupational therapy (OT). There are many opportunities for occupational therapists to contribute to preventing the onset of mental illness, treating those with mental health challenges, and supporting wellness for people across the life span. It is essential for the profession of OT to continue to place emphasis on mental health treatment for children, adults, people who are aging, the healthcare workforce, and people living with and at risk for mental illness and substance use challenges. For an alternative way of looking at mental illness, see Expanding Our Perspectives.

According to the Substance Abuse and Mental Health Services Administration (SAMHSA, 2020), nearly one in five US adults lives with a mental illness (51.5 million in 2019). There are two broad categories used to describe mental

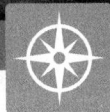

EXPANDING OUR PERSPECTIVES

Mad Perspectives on Mental Health and Treatment

Aster (né Elizabeth) Harrison

Author Pronouns: They/Them

When I was diagnosed with mental illness as a teenager, I was taught that it was a chemical imbalance in my brain, an impairment that I should treat to minimize its symptoms. Years later, I came into contact with the consumer/survivor/ex-patient (c/s/x) movement, the Mad Pride movement, and Mad Studies, which offered me alternative ways of looking at my mental illness.

As used in the Mad Pride movement and Mad Studies, the word "mad" comes from the British word for "crazy," versus the American usage of "angry." "Mad" is a reclaimed slur (similar to the words "queer" or "crip") that is proudly used by some people with mental illness to indicate a community and political affiliation with the mad movement. People in the Mad Pride movement believe that mental difference can be a point of pride. Some speak about special insights or skills related to their mental differences. They celebrate their identities and their community and may connect with others in groups that respect and affirm their differences, such as peer support groups offered by the Hearing Voices Network or the Fireweed Collective. In many cultures, experiences such as hearing voices or seeing visions may be acknowledged as spiritual experiences rather than medical issues.

The c/s/x movement consists of psychiatric consumers, people who identify as survivors of the harm of the psychiatric system, and ex-patients of the psychiatric system. Mad Studies is an academic discipline that critiques the mainstream mental health system. The c/s/x movement and Mad Studies also offer new perspectives on mental illness. They bring attention to the injustices built into the psychiatric system, such as when someone is incarcerated in a mental institution, subjected to shock treatments, or medicated against their will. Such traumatic experiences can worsen mental distress and increase symptoms. OT is sometimes part of this psychiatric system that the c/s/x movement criticizes. C/s/x activists and Mad Studies scholars urge healthcare providers to always allow self-determination of people who are mentally ill—allowing patients to choose what happens to them even when their behavior is unusual or extreme. They also emphasize the importance of peer support from other people

with experience navigating the psychiatric system or living with mental distress. A few Mad Studies books that helped me learn include *Talking Back to Psychiatry* (Morrison, 2005), *Searching for a Rose Garden* (Russo & Sweeney, 2016), *Mad Matters* (LeFrançois et al., 2013), and *Alternatives Beyond Psychiatry* (Stastny & Lehmann, 2007).

Especially in recent years, mad and disability justice activists have made connections with the Black Lives Matter movement and other movements against mass incarceration and police brutality. This is especially important given that approximately 22% of people killed by police have a mental illness (The Washington Post, 2022), and Black people with mental illnesses are disproportionately impacted by this violence. Organizations such as Project LETS build alternatives to calling the police during mental health crises (Project LETS, 2021). Activists highlight involuntary institutionalization in nursing homes and mental hospitals as a form of incarceration and fight for the right for mad and disabled people to live in the community.

Mad activists and scholars offer alternatives to involuntary treatment, including voluntary supportive housing arrangements. The Soteria model offers one voluntary housing alternative to acute psychiatric hospitalization (Calton et al., 2008). Another important tool is safety planning (see, e.g., Fukui, n.d.), which allows a mad person to identify the supports that work best for them in a time of crisis. For example, I made a document for my partner about things that help me and people she can contact for support if I am in crisis. Such plans can equip the loved ones of people with mental illness with tools to prevent reliance on police or involuntary treatment. In addition to safety planning, people can also complete psychiatric living wills that identify the kinds of medications and treatments that they consent to, so that healthcare providers can follow their wishes in times of crisis.

The most important impact of the c/s/x movement and Mad Studies on my life has been in highlighting the role of *sanism*. Sanism refers to the oppression of mad people, people considered "insane," or people labeled with psychiatric diagnoses. Sanism can manifest in discrimination against and bias toward people with mental illnesses. Learning about sanism put a powerful word to something that I saw all around me. I encountered sanism when I sat in a class in OT school about my diagnosis and heard my classmates worry about working with people with "severe mental illness" because they believed them to be dangerous and difficult. I encountered sanism when my fieldwork

(continued)

EXPANDING OUR PERSPECTIVES (*continued*)

supervisor called my university behind my back after receiving my letter of accommodation, telling them that they only wanted the "best students" and not students with disabilities. I encountered sanism when I was asked about my disability status before being allowed to be licensed as an OT—especially since I knew other people with mental illnesses whose licensure was contested or delayed if they disclosed a psychiatric diagnosis.

Discrimination and bias can intensify physical and mental health problems. Some disability justice, healing justice, and mad organizations offer approaches to treatment of mental illness that consider the role of societal oppression (including sanism, but also other intersecting forms of oppression). For example, the Fireweed Collective has created a useful "Madness and Oppression" guide (Fireweed Collective, 2015).

Some mad people identify as ex-patients or survivors of the psychiatric system and choose to have nothing to do with formal mental healthcare because of the harms that they suffered at the hands of mental health providers. Some people, like me, remain consumers within the psychiatric system—although we also push the system to be better. Although they are not right for everyone and should never be forced on anyone, medication and therapy have been helpful tools for me in managing mental distress. Identifying as mad and being in community with other mad people has also been healing for me. I see myself as part of a minority group of mad people—a group with its own culture, history, and struggle for human rights.

As a mad occupational therapist, I take a critical approach to mental illness. I recognize that people can understand their mental differences in a wide variety of ways—and not all of these will be negative. I believe deeply in peer support and acknowledge the role of

oppression in worsening mental distress or physical health problems. I trust clients as the experts of their lived experience and practice *radical client centeredness*—promoting client self-determination even when clients disagree with me or other healthcare providers. This includes fighting for someone's right to live at home when others believe they should be institutionalized.

In order to improve the health and wellness of mad people in the long term, societal change is needed. OT practitioners should have a role in combating sanism wherever we encounter it—especially within our own profession.

References

Calton, T., Ferriter, M., Huband, N., & Spandler, H. (2008). A systematic review of the Soteria paradigm for the treatment of people diagnosed with schizophrenia. *Schizophrenia Bulletin, 34*(1), 181–192. https://doi.org/10.1093/schbul/sbm047

Fireweed Collective (formerly known as The Icarus Project). (2015). *Madness and oppression: Paths to personal transformation and collective liberation.* https://fireweedcollective.org/publication/madness-oppression-paths-to-personal-transformation-and-collective-liberation/

Fukui, E. (n.d.). *Mad survival tools: Stay mad, stay together.* https://madqueer.org/madsurvival

LeFrançois, B. A., Menzies, R., & Reaume, G. (Eds.). (2013). *Mad matters: A critical reader in Canadian mad studies.* Canadian Scholars' Press.

Morrison, L. J. (2005). *Talking back to psychiatry: The psychiatric consumer/survivor/ex-patient movement* (1st ed.). Routledge.

Project LETS. (2021). *Vision and primary goals.* https://projectlets.org/about

Russo, J., & Sweeney, A. (Eds.). (2016). *Searching for a rose garden: Challenging psychiatry, fostering mad studies.* PCCS Books.

Stastny, P., & Lehmann, P. (2007). *Alternatives beyond psychiatry.* Peter Lehmann.

The Washington Post. (2022). *Fatal force database.* https://www.washingtonpost.com/graphics/investigations/police-shootings-database

health: Any Mental Illness (AMI), which encompasses all recognized mental illnesses, and Serious Mental Illness (SMI). SMI includes diagnoses such as schizophrenia, bipolar disorder, and major depression when these illnesses have a significant impact on the person's ability to function (SAMHSA, 2022). The prevalence of AMIs and SMIs in the United States can be found on the SAMHSA website at https://www.nimh.nih.gov/health/statistics/mental-illness

Occupational therapists work with people with a variety of mental health and substance use conditions (schizophrenia, bipolar disorder, major depression, anxiety disorder, personality disorder, etc.) across the life span. Occupational therapists will encounter people with mental illness in many settings, not only in mental health settings. For example, there is growing recognition that traumatic experiences can result in an increased risk for mental and physical health conditions (Grummitt et al., 2021). Many people affected by trauma report distress, including new

or worsening symptoms of depression, anxiety, and insomnia. Some people who experienced trauma develop chronic symptoms severe enough to meet criteria for posttraumatic stress disorder (PTSD) or major depressive disorder. People with such conditions may also develop physical conditions such as stroke, cardiac disease, or spinal cord injury that will require OT services in a hospital or rehabilitation facility.

Mental Illness and Physical Health

Researchers have documented for over two decades that adults with serious forms of mental illness die earlier than the general population, and this mortality gap is growing, with the lost years of life increasing to as much as 28 years (Kim et al., 2017; Lee et al., 2018; Reininghaus et al., 2015). Over the past few decades, there has been a greater recognition of growing rates of comorbid mental disorders, substance use disorders, and chronic medical conditions, which appear to be impacted by issues of poverty, chronic stressors, and socioeconomic status (Walker & Druss, 2017). Recent data have also confirmed the presence of racial and ethnic disparities affecting stress, mental health conditions, and increased substance use among adults as a result of the COVID-19 pandemic (McKnight-Eily et al., 2021). Among adults with SMI, 50% to 90% also have a co-occurring chronic medical condition. Worldwide studies found significant disparities in treatment and screening for cardiovascular disease and cancer for people with mental illness (Solmi et al., 2020, 2021). A study examining factors that contribute to excess mortality found that most of the disparity could be attributed to poverty, lifestyle behaviors, and poor quality of medical care (Druss et al., 2011). This intersection of risk factors leads to higher rates of chronic disease and medical conditions (see Figure 63.1).

Experiences of violence, poverty, and homelessness impact mental and physical health and make it challenging to continue or resume valued life roles, such as living independently, working, or going to school. Mental illness, substance use, and physical illness can impact sleep and rest, social participation, health management, work/school obligations, activities of daily living (ADL), and instrumental activities of daily living (IADL). For an example, see Box 63.1.

In April of 2021, Joshua Gordan, the director of the National Institute of Mental Health, provided an important overview of the impact of COVID-19 on mental health. It has impacted the mental health of many in society,

BOX 63.1 NARRATIVE PERSPECTIVE: HOMELESS AND RESILIENCE: PAUL CABELL'S STORY

Paul Cabell grew up in a chaotic home, which he left as a teenager. He experienced depression, homelessness, and violence through most of his life. He has lived in Alabama, Puerto Rico, Kansas, California, Illinois, Indiana, and Germany (when he was in the Army), Iowa, Nevada, New York, Utah, and Wyoming. He has worked as a day laborer, in restaurants, as a comedian and actor, and in the Army. He was eventually diagnosed with depression and substance use disorder. The Veteran's Administration and the Mormon Church helped Paul recover.

To read the full story, see Appendix III, Chapter C, at Lippincott Connect.

including those already living with mental and physical health conditions, healthcare workers, the people who have had COVID-19, and so many others as a result of being isolated or quarantined (Wu et al., 2021). Surveys, including those collected by the Centers for Disease Control and Prevention (CDC), have shown substantial increases in self-reported mental health and substance use symptoms during the pandemic.

According to a CDC report by Czeisler and colleagues (2020), which surveyed adults across the United States in late June of 2020, 31% of respondents reported symptoms

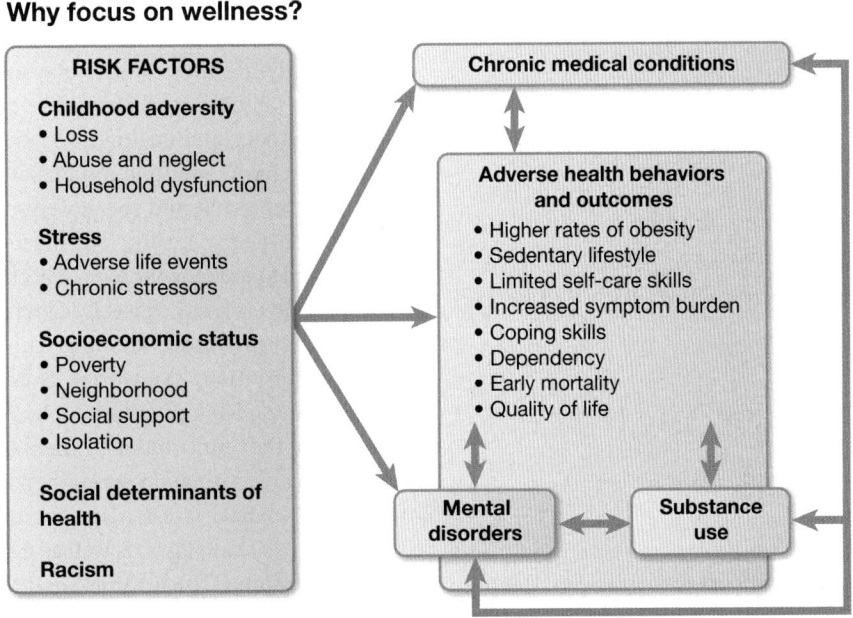

FIGURE 63.1 Model of the interaction between mental illness and medical illness.

Source: Adapted from Druss, B. G., & Walker, E. R. (2011). Mental disorders and medical comorbidity. The Synthesis project. Research Synthesis Report, (21), 1–26.

BOX 63.2 RECOVERY AND WELLNESS

Recovery has been defined as a process of change through which individuals improve their health and wellness, live a self-directed life, and strive to reach their full potential (SAMHSA, 2011, para. 3). *Wellness* is defined as a conscious, deliberate process that requires a person to become aware of and make choices for a more satisfying lifestyle. A wellness lifestyle includes a balance of health habits, including adequate sleep and rest, good nutrition, productivity, exercise, participation in meaningful activity, and connections with supportive relationships (Swarbrick, 1997). Wellness views a person holistically and includes physical, intellectual, emotional, social, environmental, occupational, financial, and spiritual dimensions (Swarbrick, 2012).

of anxiety or depression, 13% reported having started or increased substance use, 26% reported stress-related symptoms, and 11% reported having serious thoughts of suicide in the past 30 days. Risk factors for reporting anxiety symptoms or suicidal ideation included food insufficiency, financial concerns, and loneliness (Nagata et al., 2021). Black and Hispanic persons were more likely to report not having enough food, and harassment and discrimination contributed to chronic stress among these groups (McKnight-Eily et al., 2021). Emerging data indicate that people with schizophrenia and other SMIs have been disproportionately impacted by COVID-19. Individuals with schizophrenia, for instance, are nearly 10 times more likely to contract COVID-19 and are nearly three times more likely to die from it if they do fall ill, compared with individuals who do not have a mental illness. Deaths because of opioid overdose have increased substantially during the pandemic (Alter et al., 2020). The mental health impacts of COVID-19 continue. Occupational therapists can play an important role by applying evidence-based strategies to support mental health needs of people across the life span in a variety of settings. Occupational therapists can assume an important role in promoting recovery and wellness (Box 63.2).

Wellness Approach to Mental Illness

Wellness is an important framework for managing and preventing mental illness. Wellness is a conscious, deliberate process that requires a person to become aware of and make choices each day for a self-defined lifestyle. Healthy lifestyle behaviors include getting adequate sleep and rest, balancing habits and routines, engaging in purposeful and

meaningful work, and making time for play and educational activities (Swarbrick, 1997, 2006, 2012). Wellness habits are self-defined, and social support is an important factor in helping people create and sustain health lifestyles (Swarbrick, 1997, 2006, 2012). The concept of the 8 Dimensions of Wellness (Swarbrick, 2006, 2012; Swarbrick & Nemec, 2016) has been embraced in recent years by the behavioral healthcare field. Developed as an OT program model (Swarbrick, 1997) to address disparities in physical health for people with mental illness, the model has become more widely used and accepted by people with the lived experiences of trauma, substance use, and mental health challenges.

Wellness is multidimensional and includes emotional, intellectual, physical, social, occupational, environmental, financial, and spiritual dimensions, all of which are reflected in the 8 Dimensions of Wellness model (Figure 63.2). This model focuses on the strengths and potential of individuals with mental and substance use conditions across these eight dimensions, building resilience for people to survive and thrive.

For decades, the wellness model has been used by occupational therapists to help people manage trauma and mental and substance use challenges. The model outlines ways for people living with or at risk of mental health trauma and substance use challenges to create wellness habits (Swarbrick, 1997, 2012). The 8 Dimensions of Wellness model shows how each of the dimensions overlaps and how all dimensions are connected and impact one another. An important focus of this approach congruent with OT tenets is the emphasis on strengths. The model helps therapists provide interventions that focus on building or recreating daily habits and routines important for balance and well-being. Occupational therapists can help people identify key activities they do each day and develop a plan for enhancing wellness in that area. For example, sleep, regular physical activity, and healthy food choices that are affordable help support multiple dimensions, including physical, emotional, financial, and social wellness.

For short-term health, long-term health, and recovery, many people benefit from regularly checking in to consider what they do each day or week across each of the 8 wellness dimensions, providing an opportunity to build healthy habits and routines (Swarbrick & Nemec, 2016). Occupational therapists can help people identify what they are doing now that contributes to their wellness and consider how they can continue to strengthen these daily habits and routines to manage stress, manage symptoms of mental and substance use challenges, as well as deal with the long-term effects of trauma. The occupational therapist can help the person consider important habits that promote balance. Addiction, trauma, and stress can impact wellness; however, wellness habits help maintain balance and well-being (Swarbrick, 2012).

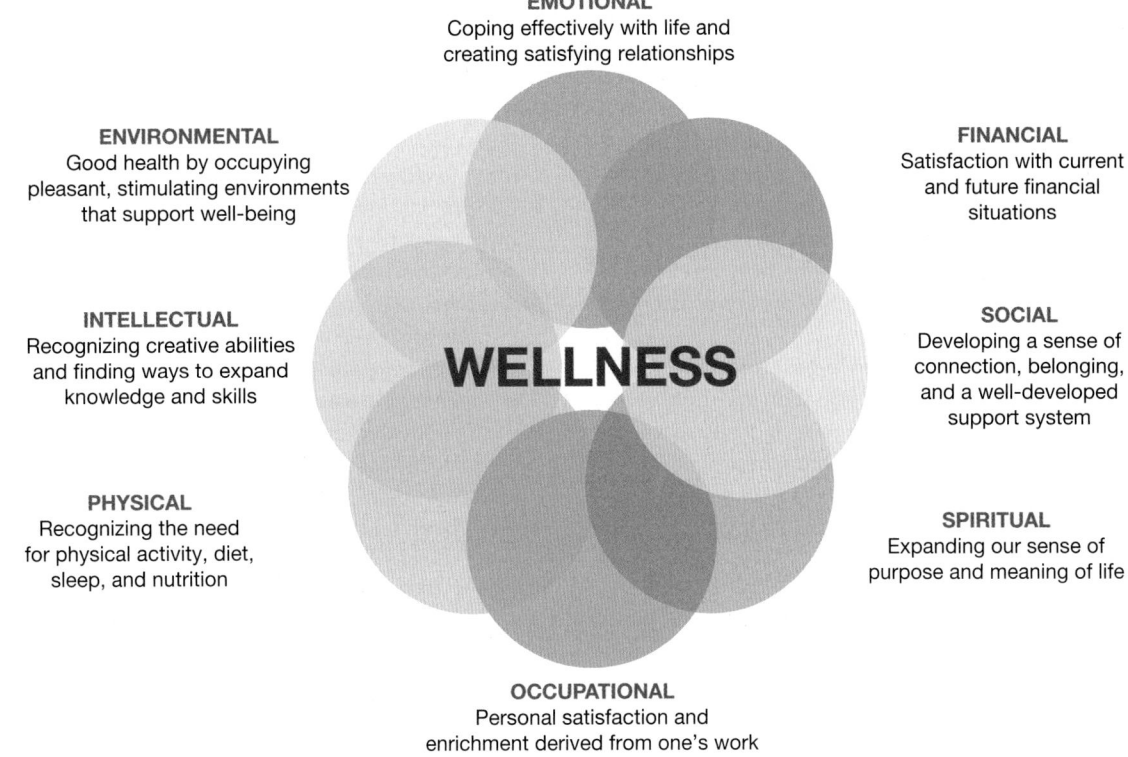

FIGURE 63.2 The 8 Dimensions of Wellness model.

Adapted from Swarbrick, M. (2006). A wellness approach. *Psychiatric Rehabilitation Journal, 29*(4), 311–314.

OT practice is based on a person-centered, holistic approach that fits well with wellness and recovery. Occupational therapists have a strong skill set to bring to serving persons with a mental and/or substance use disorder. Because occupational therapists have educational grounding in psychology, therapeutic use of self, task analysis, neuroscience, and the teaching of self-care skills, they can be effective members of interprofessional teams. Occupational therapists can be found in a wide array of settings and programs, such as acute or longer-term inpatient units, partial hospitalization programs, intensive outpatient programs, and community settings serving people who experience homelessness. Occupational therapists are beginning to work on integrated primary care teams and in certified community behavioral health clinics (CCBHCs). Occupational therapists are also assuming important roles as service providers in early psychosis programs designed to promote recovery and independence among young people with a goal of preventing or reducing long-term disability. Occupational therapists assume many roles in various capacities, from direct service provider to consultant, program coordinator, or director. Occupational therapists can serve as case managers and often facilitate groups that address sleep and rest, social participation, work and education, health management, and ADL.

In all capacities, occupational therapists contribute their unique expertise to increase the individual's occupational participation and quality of life. Box 63.3 outlines the added value of occupational therapists working with interprofessional behavioral healthcare teams.

Occupations Impacted by Mental Illness

The following section outlines occupations that are impacted by major mental illness where occupational therapists can assist people with recovery and wellness.

Sleep

Sleep is very important for people to manage symptoms of mental and substance use disorders. Additionally, sleep and rest are important for long-term recovery and both physical and emotional well-being. In the author's 35-year experience, creating and sustaining a good sleep-and-wake cycle has been essential for many people living with acute and chronic mental and substance use disorders. The wellness benefits of sleep and rest are profound. Gardner and colleagues (2017) revealed that sleep was one of the most frequently cited occupations where individuals with mental disorders had difficulty. Another study by Gardner et al. (2021) explored the habits and routines connected to the occupation of sleep preparation and participation in individuals with mental and/or substance use disorders. Participants ($N = 52$) attended community wellness centers in New Jersey where they completed the Pittsburgh Sleep Quality Index (PSQI) and discovered how habits and routines affect their sleep. Most (78.6%) participants initially reported poor sleep. After participating in the program,

BOX 63.3 ADDED VALUE OF OCCUPATIONAL THERAPISTS ON INTERPROFESSIONAL BEHAVIORAL HEALTHCARE TEAMS

- Occupational therapy (OT) is a deeply person-centered approach, and OT practitioners are trained to assess cognitive and functional impairments.
- OT practitioners help determine the likelihood that an individual will engage in services, effectively participate in treatment, and change their behaviors as necessary to sustain recovery.
- OT practitioners use performance-based testing, which provides information about participation in everyday activities. These assessments also have high potential to engage clients in a relatively brief amount of time.
- Cognitive function testing helps a team to engage individuals in planning the treatment and recovery support that is right for them (i.e., self-care, household management, childcare, and workplace tasks).
- OT practitioners assess each client's ability to perform tasks to determine how or whether the client initiates a real-world task; avoids and/or corrects errors, sequences, and executes task steps; and demonstrates intrapersonal skill and good time management.
- OT practitioners can help calibrate interventions (group or individual) based on sensory needs and cognitive capacity, develop health promotion plans, and support chronic disease management (i.e., habits and routines related to medication physical activity, occupational engagement, and sleep).

participants reported that the strategies they used to get a better night's sleep included turning off lights, listening to music, and taking a bath/shower, whereas barriers to better sleep included taking a nap, smoking, and using the phone closer to bedtime. There is a need for further research by occupational therapists on sleep interventions for a variety of populations because sleep problems are associated with so many mental health, substance use, and medical conditions and associated symptoms. OT assessment and intervention for sleep is an emerging area for research and development. See Chapter 48 for more information.

Employment

Mental and substance use disorders impact people's ability to perform worker roles and achieve employment goals and dreams. This can be quite devastating for individuals and their families. Supported employment is one approach to vocational rehabilitation that helps people with mental illness attain and succeed in their desired jobs. The Individual Placement and Support (IPS) model of supported employment has a strong evidence base that reinforces its value in vocational rehabilitation for people with major mental disorders. The program has defined training procedures, a fidelity scale, and a clear procedural manual (Swanson & Becker, 2013), and its effectiveness has been supported by numerous randomized control trials (Carmona et al., 2017; Kinoshita et al., 2013). Recent research is examining the effectiveness of using compensatory cognitive enhancement strategies to enhance employment success (McGuirk et al., 2015), which indicates a key role for OT practitioners within the IPS model. IPS is a team-based model that is often integrated with one or more interprofessional teams (e.g., assertive community treatment, intensive case management, case management, supportive housing). In the area of employment supports, occupational therapists can use their knowledge and skills in task analysis, grading of tasks, and modifying work environments to help clients achieve success and provide direct services as job coaches. Occupational therapists can also assist with assessing, planning, developing, acquiring, mastering, retaining, and changing jobs.

Education

Like employment, education is an important occupation. Education also offers an important avenue to better paying and more fulfilling jobs. Often mental and substance use disorders impact an individual's ability to perform in a student role and achieve educational goals. In recent years, supported education has evolved as a best practice to help individuals with major mental disorders succeed in higher education. Educational advancement boosts earning power, preventing people from being stuck in low-wage jobs and poverty. Supported education funding often emphasizes employment-related educational goals rather than just general educational achievement. Occupational therapists assist prospective students to identify educational skills and interests, enter the educational setting, and access needed resources such as financial aid and tutoring (Schindler & Kientz, 2013; Schindler & Sauerwald, 2013). Occupational therapists can be effective in helping students of all ages overcome barriers to school attendance, including self-esteem issues, challenges in social relationships, and managing personal and family issues. Occupational therapists have many relevant areas of expertise, such as strategies for stress and symptom management and improving memory, retention, concentration, and problem-solving. Occupational therapists can play an important role in helping people achieve college success, avoid unemployment, secure economic self-sufficiency, and improve their quality of life.

Health Management

Health management is defined as "activities related to developing, managing, and maintaining health and wellness routines, including self-management, with the goal of improving or maintaining health to support participation in other occupations" (American Occupational Therapy Association, 2020, p. 32). The subcomponents of health management include personal care device management, nutrition management, physical activity, medication management, communication with the healthcare system, symptom and condition management, and social and emotional health promotion and maintenance. Chapter 50 outlines some specific examples for people with mental health, substance use, and trauma-related challenges.

To address physical activity and nutrition management, Catana Brown and collaborators created and revised a weight-loss program, now called *Nutrition and Exercise for Weight Loss and Recovery* (NEW-R; Brown et al., 2015). The NEW-R curriculum provides both a leader manual and a participant manual to guide each session over the 2 months of the program, using a 90-minute session format individualized to each participant's needs, personal situation, strengths, and interests. The written curriculum is supplemented by free videos for the exercise segments of the program. Designed by occupational therapists, the videos feature OT students and people in recovery dancing, doing yoga, building upper and lower body strength, and performing other exercises. The NEW-R can be taught in mental health or social service agencies, peer-run programs, community health clinics, or in a private space in the community.

Emerging and Evidence-Based Treatment Models

Treatment models developed by occupational therapists are increasingly recognized as effective based on research evidence demonstrating positive outcomes. Five programs are described here.

Action Over Inertia

Action over Inertia is a manualized intervention that uses a strengths-based approach to help individuals with SMI increase their participation in daily activities and the community (Krupa et al., 2022) with a view to enabling health, well-being, and informed choice. The intervention approach is one of "supporting doing." It engages individuals in making small but quick changes in activity and participation

as an opening to longer-term changes. Information about the factors that can derail meaningful activity and participation is shared, and these factors are considered in ongoing planning and support. In addition, there is a focus on creating opportunities for activities and participation that bring meaning and social inclusion. A range of worksheets, resources, vignettes, and other tools are provided to support this practice. In addition to interventions directed to individuals, the approach engages occupational therapists and other service providers, in considering how the services they work within can be designed to facilitate practice oriented to activity and participation.

A randomized controlled design of the first version of Action over Inertia (Krupa et al., 2010) offered to individuals receiving services from assertive community treatment teams demonstrated positive changes in the balance of activity patterns with less time spent in sleep and incidental naps and more time distributed across self-care, leisure, and productivity. Qualitative evaluation of the experiences of clinicians and intervention recipients identified positive experiences with the approach and offered suggestions for improvement (Edgelow & Krupa, 2011). A study conducted in Germany demonstrated positive change with an increase in time directed to self-care (Höhl et al., 2017). In the second version of the intervention, the intervention approach has been adapted to more clearly align with evidence-informed conceptual frameworks that link activity and participation to health and well-being (e.g., the Do-Live-Well Framework; Moll et al., 2014) to provide a more robust description of the intervention approaches and to specifically outline key competencies and critical components.

International dissemination of Action over Inertia has seen the adaptation and evaluation of the approach to meet a broad range of needs within local contexts. For example, an Australian qualitative study in community residential services examined the experiences of individuals receiving Action over Inertia in a group format and highlighted positive impacts on daily routines, the importance of addressing inertia, the nature of challenges experienced and helpful intervention processes, including the benefits and drawbacks of using groups to implement the approach (Rees et al., 2021). In Israel, an open group intervention called "Occupational Connections" (OC) was designed to address the activity and participation needs of individuals with SMI in inpatient settings (Lipskaya-Velikovwsky et al., 2016). Evaluation of OC using an experimental, single-blind, pre-post design and control group using convenience sampling with sequential group allocation demonstrated that the intervention positively impacted intentions with respect to activities and participation and the participants' impressions of the service as being recovery-oriented. The study suggested that OC was associated with improvements in functional capacity, several cognitive abilities, and symptoms of schizophrenia.

Let's Get Organized

Let's Get Organized (LGO) was developed to support individuals with co-occurring mental and substance use disorders to improve their organization and time management skills so they can perform occupations such as work, social participation, and health management. Success in these occupations supports continued sobriety. The original program demonstrated improvements in the participants' time management skills, which are critical to successful reentry into the community (White, 2007). Over time, the program has been translated into nine languages, and it has demonstrated benefits for participant's time management (Holmefur et al., 2021; White et al., 2013; Wingren et al., 2021).

The LGO program focuses on time management skills, including an awareness that time can be managed effectively through the active use of skills, strategies, and tools. The focus of the program is to help participants create and maintain an electronic calendar or appointment book. The program helps the individual to create and maintain a flexible routine while exercising emotional control. Occupational therapists using this approach employ learning principles, task analysis, task sequencing, trial-and-error learning strategies, and behavioral strategies.

The program structure helps participants to integrate and generalize new learning and establish/form new habits (White, 2007). Each group session has a different theme, and the following six stages that are common to all sessions:

- **Stage 1:** Participants sign the attendance sheets and indicate the time of their arrival. They identify and record their current emotional state and choose a sensory tool to use during the session.
- **Stage 2:** Appointment books are distributed if the participants do not have their own. Participants review and enter new information in their calendar, share ways to personalize their calendars, and discuss habit-building experiences.
- **Stage 3:** The theme of the day is presented, and participants are given activity worksheets relating to time management and organization from Precin's *Living Skills for Recovery Workbook* (2015). Sensory and cognitive strategies are used to facilitate learning.
- **Stage 4:** Participants discuss the completed worksheet. They are encouraged to recognize their own learning styles, to notice the learning styles of others in the group, and to use new strategies learned in the group.
- **Stage 5:** Participants are given homework that requires them to use their calendars daily and to integrate the strategies they have learned in the sessions.
- **Stage 6:** Participants are informed of the next group topic. Sessions end with a joint expression of thanks.

As part of LGO, an outcome measure, the Assessment of Time Management Skills (ATMS), was developed. The ATMS was normed on the US general public and in Sweden on their general population and recipients of care. A Rasch analysis of the ATMS identified three subscales within the assessment: time management, organization and planning, and regulation of emotions (Janeslätt et al., 2018; White et al., 2013). The results created the ATMS 2.0 and ATMS-S titled "Activity in time with structure—*self-estimation instrument for time management and organizational skills.*" The ATMS 2.0 includes 27 items and is reliable and practical; this sample's average score of 75.6 out of a possible "best" score of 108 indicates that many people do not regularly use the most efficient time management practices. The ATMS-S is used in adult habilitation and outpatient psychiatry groups including individuals with a variety of diagnoses, such as intellectual disability, cerebral palsy, spina bifida, and autism. Both ATMS versions measure functional skills and executive function needed for daily time management (Regev & Josman, 2020).

In 2019, a multicenter randomized controlled trial (RCT) was begun to evaluate the Swedish version of the Let's Get Organized Intervention, the LGO-S, using translations of all of the ATMS and LGO materials. A pilot study, a quality review at 3 months, and a 1-year post-intervention informed the RCT. A pilot study with 55 participants (Holmefur et al., 2019) showed that participants significantly improved their time management capabilities measured by ATMS-S after participating in Keep Track (LGO-S). The improvement lasted after 3 months. The results also showed that participants significantly increased their performance of, and their satisfaction with, daily activities measured by the Instrument Satisfaction with Daily Occupations (SDO; Eklund et al., 2014).

LGO appears to help participants to develop practical skills needed in everyday life to create consistent routines, keep track of time and appointments, become more organized, and follow through with responsibilities A few studies have looked at the benefits of the LGO-S intervention. Participants were able to manage time better and accomplish more tasks in daily life. Participants reported improved sense of control, self-esteem, and ability to manage stress (Lidström-Holmqvist et al., 2020). Another study demonstrated long-term maintenance of time management skills following intervention (Wingren et al., 2021).

Early Psychosis Programs

Early psychosis programs are meant to address individuals who are at a clinically high risk for developing a psychotic disorder. This means that individuals experiencing their first episode of schizophrenia or in the prodrome period when early signs of psychosis appear but before a diagnosis can be made are targeted for intervention. Research indicates that early intervention helps maintain individuals in meaningful roles such as student or worker, prevents hospitalization, and reduces psychopathology (Kane et al., 2016).

Most early psychosis programs emphasize individualized plans of care that are developed and implemented with an interprofessional behavioral healthcare team. Team members often include occupational therapists, psychiatrists, family supporters or therapists, social workers, supported education and employment specialists, peer supporters, and psychologists. The occupational therapist focuses on designing interventions, which promote skill development and mastery in meaningful activities in areas of education, vocation, and socialization. Depending on each young person's needs and goals, the occupational therapist may provide skill-based assessments, occupational-based interventions, and/or caregiver education. Psychoeducational group interventions for individuals with psychosis and their families also have been beneficial (Calvo et al., 2015). Adam's story in OT Story 63.1 illustrates the role of occupational therapists as members of first-episode teams.

OT STORY 63.1 ADAM

Ruth Ramsey

Adam, age 19 years, likes to paint and draw, is gifted musically, and plays guitar and drums. As a child he did well in school. In his first year of college, he began to have difficulties, which included inability to attend classes and complete assignments, lack of attention to personal self-care, disturbed sleeping, trouble concentrating, hearing voices, and social withdrawal. He started drinking alcohol and smoking marijuana heavily. He was found singing loudly in the halls of his dorm several times at 3 AM. A friend called his parents, who came to the school and suggested Adam be seen by a physician. By this time, he was sleep-deprived and became angry and agitated when his parents told him their intention to have him hospitalized as a "danger to self." The police were called, and Adam was escorted to the emergency department of a local community hospital, where he was involuntarily committed. He was able to reestablish normal sleeping and eating patterns while in the hospital and, together with his team, make plans for future treatment.

The psychiatrist diagnosed Adam as having schizophrenia and referred him to an early psychosis program. Team members included an occupational therapist, psychiatrist, peer support specialist, a supported education and employment specialist, and family support specialist. The family support specialist met with Adam's family to help them understand the implications of his new diagnosis and how they could support him in his recovery. Adam meets with a psychiatrist to evaluate his response to medications and confer with the staff about his progress. The occupational therapist, Rita, met with Adam for an initial OT evaluation to help him identify personally meaningful treatment goals. Adam reported that he decided he would return to live with his parents, who converted their garage into a studio apartment for him. He feels this will allow him space to practice his music and art. He reported he will be able to fix himself a sandwich in his mini kitchen.

Rita met with Adam to develop a daily grooming schedule and agreed to review it with him daily before morning meeting. They also made plans to meet individually twice weekly so he could learn some mindfulness approaches. Adam appeared very motivated to go back to school. He adjusted well to the antipsychotic medication with few side effects and started sleeping better. He said that the mindfulness meditation helped him learn to relax, focus, and ignore the voices he was hearing. Rita and Adam discussed his plans to create a structured routine that would include a balance of sleep, physical activity, and participation in meaningful activity, and Adam planned to live with his parents while he continued his recovery. He continued to meet with his psychiatrist to ensure that the medications were helping to control his symptoms. The supported education and employment specialist helped Adam find a part-time job at a local art supply store and register for one class at a local community college. The peer support specialist provided Adam information about a young adult wellness program for individuals experiencing mental health challenges. Over time, Rita, the occupational therapist, helped Adam with time management and activity engagement, whereas the peer support specialist helped him become more comfortable and empowered to socialize with other young people, use the computers at the college computer lab, attend outings, and take additional classes on topics such as computer graphics and tai chi.

Questions

1. Consider how LGO or other time management strategies can be used to help Adam with his OT treatment goals.
2. Discuss how supported education/employment programs can help Adam pursue academic or employment goals. Consider the value using the Physical Wellness for Work booklet to guide a session, https://www.center4healthandsdc.org/physical-wellness-for-work.html.
3. Identify the importance of sleep and strategies to assist Adam to get better quality sleep for managing mental illness and pursuing educational goals. Research sleep resources, including apps, that are evidence-based and can be useful for Adam based on his needs.
4. Discuss how Adam's arrest and involuntary hospitalization may have interrupted his occupational roles. Are there alternative options for Adam at this point in his trajectory?

Sensory Rooms

Occupational therapists have been involved in the design, development, and therapeutic application of *sensory rooms.* These are rooms that include calming elements (such as weighted blankets for deep pressure, rocking chairs, soothing music, and relaxing oils such as lavender or vanilla) and stimulating elements (such as exercise equipment, peppermint or citrus oils, art materials, and energetic music). Interventions designed to calm or stimulate sensory systems are a humane alternative to the severe interventions psychiatric facilities have sometimes instituted, such as seclusion and restraint (Champagne, 2006; Champagne & Stromberg, 2004). These multisensory activities have been used to good effect in inpatient and community-based residential facilities.

Occupational therapists conducted a study of adults living with mental illness in the community ($n = 55$) to explore sensory preferences using the Adolescent/Adult Sensory Profile (AASP) (Brown & Dunn, 2002). The participants scored significantly higher in the quadrants of low registration ($P = .042$), sensory sensitivity ($P = .039$), and sensation avoiding ($P = .010$). Individuals diagnosed with bipolar disorder scored significantly higher in the quadrants of sensory sensitivity ($P = .039$) and sensation avoiding ($P = .021$). Occupational therapists are in an ideal position to offer sensory processing approaches that impact occupational performance. Knowledge of these sensory preferences would help OT practitioners to create more individualized treatment. In addition, the awareness

of sensory preferences among the mental health population would also aid in successful sensory integration and management of mental and behavioral facets of life through promotion of self-organization (Champagne & Stromberg, 2004).

Housing Transition Program

The Housing Transition Program (Gutman et al., 2016) was designed to support adults experiencing homelessness, major mental disorders, and substance use challenges. This 3-week intervention was offered at a homeless shelter using instructional videos, graphics, and opportunities for hands-on practice of functional skills in a simulated apartment setting. Participants in a pilot study indicated that the program was engaging and helped them better understand the housing transition process.

Occupational therapists are playing an important role helping people who experience homelessness to take care of themselves. Paul's story (Box 63.1 and Appendix III, Chapter C) illustrates his journey and the people and supports he needed to enhance resilience. He shares how he learned how to manage his finances and apartment and take care of himself through the support of occupational therapists at a day program. Another occupational therapist helped him engage with peers to share his knowledge.

OT Story 63.2 illustrates the needs of one man, Joseph, and provides examples of roles for occupational therapists in wellness and recovery.

OT STORY 63.2 JOSEPH

Joseph is a 55-year-old man who has received services from the public mental health system for over 30 years. He has been hospitalized many times and received numerous mental health diagnoses. He was first diagnosed with schizophrenia at age 21 years but is currently diagnosed with bipolar disorder and co-occurring alcohol dependence. Joseph is the second of seven siblings. At age 9 years, he experienced a traumatic incident (sexual abuse by a relative). He recently was enrolled in a certified community behavioral health clinic (CCBHC) where Julie, an occupational therapist, is a member of the interprofessional team. Julie met with Joseph to complete an Occupational Profile and Activity Engagement measure (Krupa et al., 2010), reviewing his strengths, needs, and goals and to develop a strengths-based wellness plan.

Joseph recently was diagnosed with fibromyalgia and reports intense pain and bouts of sleeplessness. He reported that he seems to feel better physically, emotionally, and socially when he follows a regular sleep-and-wake schedule. However, he has significant difficulty adhering to a regular routine and was unable to pinpoint and describe the many factors that contribute to this. Joseph is currently prescribed

bimonthly medications that make him feel tired, and he believes they have caused his significant weight gain. He states that he realizes he needs to take medication to maintain stability, although he has major concerns regarding side effects (short- and long term), especially how the medication slows him down and contributes to weight gain. He has been smoking for more than 30 years and is planning to quit smoking sometime soon.

Joseph is a high school graduate. He hopes to find volunteer or paid work opportunities to use his talents and skills so he can improve his sense of purpose and meaning. He periodically walks a neighbor's dogs, which he finds quite rewarding. He feels very disheartened because family and professionals often discourage him from working, which they believe would be too stressful for him. He believes that he can get and keep a job. He is interested in learning new information, particularly in the areas of the environment, and recently was able to purchase a computer. He likes to share what he learns. Joseph reports that he frequently feels lonely. He is currently living on a very limited budget and receives a housing subsidy to offset the costs for living in a studio apartment. He can manage money effectively. Joseph takes pride in his appearance and apartment. He has determined a budget so he can do his laundry and purchase healthy food and household supplies. He wants a part-time job so he can eat out once in a while, purchase new clothing, and eventually plan to save for the future. He reported that walking the dogs provides purpose and a reason to get up in the morning, which helps him prioritize going to bed early on a consistent basis so he can wake up in time to walk the dogs. Julie, the occupational therapist working on the CCBHC team, will help Joseph with the following wellness goals that he identified to help him develop an increased sense of purpose and self-sufficiency.

- Maintain a daily healthy routine: Wake up and go to sleep at set times and create a daily routine for balance and emotional equilibrium.

- Secure a part-time job at least three to four times a week (3–5 hours per day).
- Increase physical activity to prevent further weight gain and risks of sedentary lifestyle.

Questions

1. Discuss how to plan an LGO session for Joseph and outline possible benefits and outcomes.
2. Review the modules in NEW-R and outline how the OT can implement this manual to assist Joseph in terms of health management goals, https://www.center-4healthandsdc.org/new-r.html.
3. Explore sleep hygiene strategies that can be beneficial for Joseph. Discuss the benefits of offering the intervention in a group compared to an individual session.

Conclusion

Major mental and substance use disorders continue to impact people in society at increasing rates. It is inevitable that occupational therapists will encounter individuals with major mental disorders, regardless of their chosen practice setting. Given the aftermath of COVID-19 worldwide, these encounters seem even more likely. Because OT is a profession that focuses on occupational engagement and the links to health and well-being, occupational therapists are becoming more valued in new practice arenas and assisting people in the areas of employment, education, sleep, health management, and ADL. Occupational therapists have an important role as a member of interprofessional team collaborating with people served to help increase their involvement in meaningful occupation, providing functional skills assessment, planning, and implementing wellness-focused interventions. An emerging evidence base supports several structured interventions, with time-use interventions and activity engagement tools being examples of strategies that can enhance mental health and recovery outcomes. Occupational therapists can make meaningful contributions to improving the lives of people with major mental disorders, especially in the areas of managing comorbid conditions and promoting wellness.

Lippincott® Connect *For additional resources on the subjects discussed in this chapter, visit Lippincott Connect.*

REFERENCES

Alter, A., Yeager, C., & Analyst, O. (2020). *COVID-19 impact on US national overdose crisis.* http://odmap.org/Content/docs/news/2020/ODMAP-Report-May-2020.pdf

American Occupational Therapy Association. (2020). Occupational therapy practice framework: Domain and process (4th ed.). *American Journal of Occupational Therapy, 74*(Suppl. 2), 7412410010p1–7412410010p87. https://doi.org/10.5014/ajot.2020.74S2001

Brown, C., & Dunn, W. (2002). *The adult/adolescent sensory profile user's manual.* Pearson.

Brown, C., Read, H., Stanton, M., Zeeb, M., Jonikas, J., & Cook, J. (2015). A pilot study of the nutrition and exercise for weight loss and recovery (NEW-R): A weight loss program for individuals with serious mental illness. *Psychiatric Rehabilitation Journal, 38,* 371–373. https://doi.org/10.1037/prj0000115

Calvo, A., Moreno, M., Ruiz-Sancho, A., Rapado-Castro, M., Moreno, C., Sanchez-Gutierrez, T., Arango, C., & Mayoral, M. (2015). Psychoeducational group intervention for adolescents with psychosis and their families: A two-year follow-up. *Journal of the American Academy of Child and Adolescent Psychiatry, 54,* 984–990. https://doi.org/10.1016/j.jaac.2015.09.018

Carmona, V. R., Gómez-Benito, J., Huedo-Medina, T. B., & Rojo, J. E. (2017). Employment outcomes for people with schizophrenia spectrum disorder: A meta-analysis of randomized controlled trials. *International Journal of Occupational Medicine and Environmental Health, 30*(3), 345–366. https://doi.org/10.13075/ijomeh.1896.01074

Champagne, T. (2006). *Sensory modulation and environment: Essential elements for occupation. General handbook and references* (2nd ed.). Champagne Conferences and Consultation.

Champagne, T., & Stromberg, N. (2004). Sensory approaches in inpatient psychiatric settings: Innovative alternatives to seclusion & restraint. *Journal of Psychological Nursing, 42*(9), 1–8. https://doi.org/10.3928/02793695-20040901-06

Czeisler, M. É., Lane, R. I., Petrosky, E., Wiley, J. F., Christensen, A., Njai, R., Weaver, M. D., Robbins, R., Facer-Childs, E. R., Barger, L. K., Czeisler, C. A., Howard, M. E., & Rajaratnam, S. M. W. (2020). Mental health, substance use, and suicidal ideation during the COVID-19 pandemic - United States, June 24-30, 2020. *MMWR. Morbidity and Mortality Weekly Report, 69*(32), 1049–1057. https://doi.org/10.15585/mmwr.mm6932a1

Druss, B. G., Zhao, L., Von Esenwein, S., Morrato, E. H., & Marcus, S. C. (2011). Understanding excess mortality in persons with mental illness: 17-year follow up of a nationally representative US survey. *Medical Care, 49,* 599–604. https://doi.org/10.1097/MLR.0b013e31820bf86e

Edgelow, M., & Krupa, T. (2011). Randomized controlled pilot study of an occupational time-use intervention for people with serious mental illness. *American Journal of Occupational Therapy, 65,* 267–276. https://doi.org/10.5014/ajot.2011.001313

Eklund, M., Bäckström, M., & Eakman, A. (2014) Psychometric properties and factor structure of the 13-item satisfaction with daily occupations scale when used with people with mental health problems. *Health Quality of Life Outcomes, 24*(12), 191. https://doi.org/10.1186/s12955-014-0191-3

Gardner, J., Swarbrick, M., Ackerman, A., Church, T., Rios, V., Valente, L., & Rutledge, J. (2017). Effects of physical limitations on daily activities among adults with mental health disorders: Opportunities for nursing and occupational therapy interventions. *Journal of Psychosocial Nursing Mental Health Services, 55*(10), 45–51. https://doi.org/10.3928/02793695-20170818-05

Gardner, G., Swarbrick, M., Dennis, S., Franklin, M., Pricken, M., & Palmer, K. (2021). Sleep habits and routines of individuals diagnosed with mental and/or substance-use disorders. *Occupational Therapy in Mental Health, 37*(2), 158–177. https://doi.org/10.1080/0164212X.2021.1877592

Gordan, J. A. (2021). *One year in: COVID-19 and mental health.* https://www.nimh.nih.gov/about/director/messages/2021/one-year-in-covid-19-and-mental-health

Grummitt, L. R., Kreski, N. T., Kim, S. G., Platt, J., Keyes, K. M., & McLaughlin, K. A. (2021). Association of childhood adversity with morbidity and mortality in US adults: A systematic review. *JAMA Pediatrics, 175*(12), 1269–1278. https://doi.org/10.1001/jamapediatrics.2021.2320

Gutman, S. A., Raphael-Greenfield, E. I., & Simon, P. M. (2016). Feasibility and acceptability of a pilot housing transition program for homeless adults with mental illness and substance use. *Occupational Therapy in Health Care, 30,* 124–138. https://doi.org/10.3109/07380577.2015.1060660

Höhl, W., Moll, S., & Pfeiffer, A. (2017). Occupational therapy interventions in the treatment of people with severe mental illness. *Current Opinion in Psychiatry, 30*(4), 300–305. https://doi.org/10.1097/yco.0000000000000339

Holmefur, M., Roshanay, A., Lidström-Holmqvist, K., Arvidsson, P., White, S., & Janeslätt, G. (2019). Pilot study of the "Let's Get Organized": A group intervention for improving time management. *American Journal of Occupational Therapy, 73,* 7305205020p1–7305205020p10. https://doi.org/10.5014/ajot.2019.032631

Holmefur, M., Roshanany, A., White, S., Janeslätt, G., Vimefall, E., & Lidström-Holmqvist, K. (2021). Evaluation of the "Let's Get Organized" group intervention to improve time management: Protocol for a multi-centre randomised controlled trial. *Trials, 22,* 640. https://doi.org/10.1186/s13063-021-05578-x

Janeslätt, G. K., Holmqvist, K. L., White, S., & Holmefur, M. (2018). Assessment of time management skills: Psychometric properties of the Swedish version. *Scandinavian Journal of Occupational Therapy, 25*(3), 153–161. https://doi.org/10.1080/11038128.2017.1375009

Kane, J. M., Robinson, D. G., Schooler, N. R., Mueser, K. T., Penn, D. L., Rosenheck, R. A., Addington, J., Brunette, M. F., Correll, C. U., Estroff, S. E., Marcy, P., Robinson, J., Meyer-Kalos, P. S., Gottlieb, J. D., Glynn, S. M., Lynde, D. W., Pipes, R., Kurian, B. T., Miller, A. L., . . . Heinssen, R. K. (2016). Comprehensive vs. usual care for first-episode psychosis: 2-year outcomes from the NIMH RAISE early treatment program. *American Journal of Psychiatry, 173,* 362–272. https://doi.org/10.1176/appi.ajp.2015.15050632

Kim, W., Jang, S. Y., Chun, S. Y., Lee, T. H., Han, K. T., & Park, E. C. (2017). Mortality in schizophrenia and other psychoses: Data from the South Korea National Health Insurance Cohort, 2002–2013. *Journal of Korean Medical Science, 32*(5), 835–842. https://doi.org/10.3346/jkms.2017.32.5.835

Kinoshita, Y., Furukawa, T. A., Kinoshita, K., Honyashiki, M., Omori, I. M., Marshall, M., Bond, G. R., Huxley, P., Amano, N., & Kingdon, D. (2013). Supported employment for adults with severe mental illness. *The Cochrane Database of Systematic Reviews, 2013*(9), CD008297. https://doi.org/10.1002/14651858.CD008297.pub2

Krupa, T., Edgelow, M., Chen, S. P., Mieras, C., Almas, A., Perry, A., Radloff-Gabriel, D., Jackson, J., & Bransfield, M. (2010). *Action over inertia: Addressing the activity-health needs of individuals with serious mental illness.* CAOT.

Krupa, T., Edgelow, M., Mieras, C., & Chen, S. P. (2022). *Promoting activity and participation in individuals with serious mental illness the action over inertia approach.* Routledge.

Lee, E. E., Liu, J., Tu, X., Palmer, B. W., Eyler, L. T., & Jeste, D. V. (2018). A widening longevity gap between people with schizophrenia and general population: A literature review and call for action. *Schizophrenia Research, 196,* 9–13. https://doi.org/10.1016/j.schres.2017.09.005

Lidström-Holmqvist, K., Tollén, A., & Holmefur, M. (2020). Toward control over time: Participants' experiences of attending the group intervention Let's Get Organized (LGO). *American Journal of Occupational Therapy, 74*(4), 7411515440p1. https://doi.org/10.5014/ajot.2020.74S1-PO7510

Lipskaya-Velikovsky, L., Kotler, M., & Krupa, T. (2016). Description of and preliminary findings for occupational connections, an intervention for inpatient psychiatry settings. *American Journal of Occupational Therapy, 70*(6), 1–5. https://doi.org/10.5014/ajot.2016.014688

McGuirk, S., Mueser, K., Xie, H., Welsh, J., Kaiser, J., Drake, R., Becker, D. R., Bailey, E., Fraser, G., Wolfe, R., & McHugo, G. (2015). Cognitive enhancement treatment for people with a mental illness who do not respond to supported employment: A randomized control trial. *American Journal of Psychiatry, 172,* 852–861. https://doi.org/10.1176/appi.ajp.2015.14030374

McKnight-Eily, L. R., Okoro, C. A., Strine, T. W., Verlenden, J., Hollis, N. D., Njai, R., Mitchell, E. W., Board, A., Puddy, R., & Thomas, C. (2021). Racial and ethnic disparities in the prevalence of stress and worry. Mental health conditions, and increased substance use among adults during the COVID-19 pandemic - United States, April and May 2020. MMWR. *Morbidity and Mortality Weekly Report, 70*(5), 162–166. https://doi.org/10.15585/mmwr.mm7005a3

Nagata, J. M., Ganson, K. T., Whittle, H. J., Chu, J., Harris, O. O., Tsai, A. C., & Weiser, S. D. (2021). Food insufficiency and mental health in the U.S. during the COVID-19 pandemic. *American Journal of Preventive Medicine, 60,* 453–461. https://doi.org/10.1016/j.amepre.2020.12.004

Moll, S. E., Gewurtz, R. E., Krupa, T. M., Law, M. C., Lariviere, N., & Levasseur, M. (2014). Do-live-well: A Canadian framework for promoting occupation, health, and well-being. *Canadian Journal of Occupational Therapy, 82,* 9–23. https://doi.org/10.1177/0008417414545981

Precin, P. (2015). *Living skills recovery workbook.* Echo Point Books and Media.

Rees, E. F., Ennals, P., & Fossey, E. (2021). Implementing an action over inertia group program in community residential rehabilitation services: Group participant and facilitator perspectives. *Frontiers in Psychiatry, 12,* 624803. https://doi.org/10.3389/fpsyt.2021.624803

Regev, S., & Josman, N. (2020). Evaluation of executive functions and everyday life for people with severe mental illness: A systematic review. *Schizophrenia Research: Cognition, 21,* 100178. https://doi.org/10.1016/j.scog.2020.100178

Reininghaus, U., Dutta, R., Dazzan, P., Doody, G. A., Fearon, P., Lappin, J., Heslin, M., Onyejiaka, A., Donoghue, K., Lomas, B., Kirkbride, J. B., Murray, R. M., Croudace, T., Morgan, C., & Jones, P. B. (2015). Mortality in schizophrenia and other psychoses: A 10-year follow-up of the ÆSOP first-episode cohort. *Schizophrenia Bulletin, 41*(3), 664–673. https://doi.org/10.1093/schbul/sbu138

Schindler, V., & Kientz, M. (2013). Supports and barriers to higher education and employment for individuals diagnosed with mental illness. *The Journal of Vocational Rehabilitation, 39,* 39–41. https://doi.org/10.3233/JVR-130640

Schindler, V., & Sauerwald, C. (2013). Outcomes of a 4-year program with higher education and employment goals for individuals diagnosed with mental illness. *Work, 4,* 325–336. https://doi.org/10.3233/WOR-121548

Solmi, M., Fiedorowicz, J., Poddighe, L., Delogu, M., Miola, A., Høye, A., Heiberg, I. H., Stubbs, B., Smith, L., Larsson, H., Attar, R., Nielsen, R. E., Cortese, S., Shin, J. I., Fusar-Poli, P., Firth, J., Yatham, L. N., Carvalho, A. F., Castle, D. J., . . . Correll, C. U. (2021). Disparities in screening and treatment of cardiovascular diseases in patients with mental disorders across the world: Systematic review and meta-analysis of 47 observational studies. *The American Journal of Psychiatry, 178*(9), 793–803. https://doi.org/10.1176/appi.ajp.2021.21010031

Solmi, M., Firth, J., Miola, A., Fornaro, M., Frison, E., Fusar-Poli, P., Dragioti, E., Shin, J. I., Carvalho, A. F., Stubbs, B., Koyanagi, A., Kisely, S., & Correll, C. U. (2020). Disparities in cancer screening in people with mental illness across the world versus the general population: Prevalence and comparative meta-analysis including 4 717 839 people. *The Lancet. Psychiatry, 7*(1), 52–63. https://doi.org/10.1016/S2215-0366(19)30414-6

Substance Abuse and Mental Health Services Administration. (2011). *SAMHSA news release: SAMHSA announces a working definition of "recovery" from mental disorders and substance use disorders.* http://www.samhsa.gov/newsroom/advisories/1112223420.aspx

Substance Abuse and Mental Health Services Administration. (2020). *Key substance use and mental health indicators in the United States: Results from the 2019 National Survey on Drug Use and Health (HHS Publication No. PEP20-07-01-001).* Center for Behavioral Health Statistics and Quality, Substance Abuse and Mental Health Services Administration. https://www.samhsa.gov/data/sites/default/files/reports/rpt29393/2019NSDUHFFRPDFWHTML/2019NSDUHFFR1PDFW090120.pdf

Substance Abuse and Mental Health Services Administration. (2022). *Living well with serious mental illness.* https://www.samhsa.gov/serious-mental-illness

Swanson, S. J., & Becker, D. R. (2013). *Individual placement and support (IPS) supported employment: A practical guide.* Dartmouth Psychiatric Research Center.

Swarbrick, M. (1997). A wellness model for clients. *Mental Health Special Interest Section Newsletter, 20,* 1–4.

Swarbrick, M. (2006). A wellness approach. *Psychiatric Rehabilitation Journal, 29*(4), 311–314. https://doi.org/10.2975/29.2006.311.314

Swarbrick, M. (2012). A wellness approach to mental health recovery. In A. Rudnick (Ed.), *Recovery of people with mental illness: Philosophical and related perspectives* (pp. 30–38). Oxford University Press.

Swarbrick, M., & Nemec, P. B. (2016). Supporting the health and wellness of individuals with psychiatric disabilities. *Rehabilitation Research, Policy, and Education, 30*(3), 321–333. https://doi.org/10.1891/2168-6653.30.3.321

Walker, E. R., & Druss, B. G. (2017). Cumulative burden of comorbid mental disorders, substance use disorders, chronic medical conditions, and poverty on health among adults in the U.S.A. *Psychological Health Medicine, 22*(6), 727–735. https://doi.org/10.1080/13548506.2016.1227855

White, S. M. (2007). Let's Get Organized: An intervention for persons with co-occurring disorders. *Psychiatric Services, 58,* 713. https://doi.org/10.1176/ps.2007.58.5.713

White, S. M., Riley, A. W., & Flom, P. (2013). Assessment of time management skills (ATMS): A practice-based outcome questionnaire. *Occupational Therapy in Mental Health, 29,* 1–17. https://doi.org/10.1080/0164212X.2013.819481

Wingren, M., Lidström-Holmqvist, K., Roshanai, A. H., Arvidsson, P., Janeslätt, G., White, S., & Holmefur, M. (2021). One-year follow-up after the time management group intervention Let's Get Organized. *Scandinavian Journal of Occupational Therapy, 29*(4), 305–314. https://doi.org/10.1080/11038128.2021.1954687

World Health Organization (n.d.). *Mental health.* https://www.who.int/data/gho/data/themes/theme-details/GHO/mental-health

Wu, T., Jia, X., Shi, H., Niu, J., Yin, X., Xie, J., & Wang, X. (2021). Prevalence of mental health problems during the COVID-19 pandemic: A systematic review and meta-analysis. *Journal of affective disorders, 281,* 91–98. https://doi.org/10.1016/j.jad.2020.11.117

CHAPTER 64

Providing Occupational Therapy for an Individual With a Hand Injury

Marci L. Baptista and Maryam Farzad

LEARNING OBJECTIVES

After reading this chapter, you will be able to:

1. Identify assessments for pain, functional ability, and sensation.
2. Understand the importance of incorporating the biopsychosocial model in hand therapy.
3. Increase awareness of orthotic fabrication and considerations for the client.
4. Cite benefits of using occupations with hand therapy interventions.
5. Develop an appreciation of cultural diversity when treating clients in hand therapy.

Introduction

The World Federation of Occupational Therapists (WFOT) defines *occupational therapy* (OT) as a person-centered profession that promotes health and well-being through occupation (WFOT, 2010). The primary goal of OT interventions is to enable individuals to participate in activities of daily living (ADL) that they want, need, or are expected to do in their social and cultural context (WFOT, 2010).

Hand therapy, a specialty practice area of OT, aims to optimize the functional use of the hand and arm, using a person-centered approach to identify the participation needs of the individual; maintain their ability to engage in desired roles within their family and the community; and, most importantly, experience quality of life as they define it (American Occupational Therapy Association [AOTA], 2017). The Hand Therapy Certification Committee (2009) describes hand therapy as follows:

> Using specialized skills in assessment, planning and treatment, hand therapists provide therapeutic interventions to prevent dysfunction, restore function and/or reverse the progression of pathology of the upper limb in order to enhance an individual's ability to execute tasks and to participate fully in life situations.

The occupational therapist must balance interventions for the hand carefully considering the medical, temporal, physiologic, and occupational components of the healing structures while considering the individual's intrinsic motivation to optimize compliance and outcomes.

The Process of Hand Therapy

Through use of our hands, we interact with our environment, participate in occupations, and influence our world. Injuries of the hand can greatly impact occupation and self-image. Specialized knowledge of this intricate part of our anatomy is required to diagnose, treat, and rehabilitate injuries of the upper extremity (UE). The OT practitioner specializing in hand therapy will typically see conditions that include trauma and postoperative conditions, such as fractures of the hand, wrist, or elbow, tendon and nerve lacerations, amputations, burns, and reattachment of amputated fingers (replants). Acquired conditions such as tendonitis, tendinosis, carpal tunnel syndrome, and arthritic conditions are also treated by OT practitioners specializing in hand rehabilitation.

When treating UE injuries such as fractures the therapist must follow a protocol congruent with the temporal aspect of healing structures. Understanding the physical and biomechanical demands of muscle, tendon, ligament, and bone tissue with healing structures is vital for successful functional outcomes. The appropriate activities and exercises must be carefully chosen by the therapist to safely increase range of motion (ROM), stability, and strength in order to successfully guide the rehabilitation and, thus, restore meaningful occupation. Evidence indicates that individuals view themselves in relation to their occupational abilities and roles. Injuries and conditions that interfere with life roles, habits, time use, activity patterns, occupational experiences, and full participation will create a sense of dysfunction and yearning for normalcy (Custer et al., 2015). Occupation-based interventions (OBIs) should consider the individual's goals, values, beliefs, well-being, and occupational needs. Task analysis becomes a primary component of the therapist's critical thinking in order to incorporate meaningful occupations safely and therapeutically.

Evaluation

The OT evaluation includes interviews, observation, and assessments to determine impairments and measure function. This includes the occupational profile and the analysis of occupational performance, which are synthesized to inform the intervention plan (Hinojosa et al., 2014). Active and passive ROM, strength, sensibility, endurance, edema, coordination, and dexterity are assessed to ascertain how these components influence occupations. Subsequently, treatment intervention and goals are formulated and determined based on the client's occupational roles, occupational performance, and occupational performance skills.

Objective and subjective assessments are used to establish a baseline at the initial visit. Impairment of effect of

injury or trauma to the hand can be evaluated with different objective evaluations. Depending on diagnosis and contraindications, common tools for objective assessment of hand function include a dynamometer to determine gross grip strength; a pinch gauge to determine finger and thumb strength including lateral pinch, palmar pinch, and pincer pinch; and a goniometer to measure active and passive ROM. Assessment of sensation may include the Semmes–Weinstein monofilament test and 2-point discrimination tests. Edema is typically assessed using a volumeter (measuring displacement of water when the hand is placed inside a plastic container) or circumferential measurements that are taken with a measuring tape. Wounds are assessed and documented by appearance, if healing routinely, or if infection is suspected.

Subjective assessments include different patient-reported outcome measures. Occupational therapists should incorporate outcome measures that capture patients' perspectives for outcome evaluation. Considering an occupational perspective in assessment should be a flow-through initial evaluation, interventions, and the outcomes (Hocking, 2010). Subjective assessment may include the client's report of pain, sensation, functional tolerance, volunteer and work occupations, home and family responsibilities, and leisure occupations. Hand therapists administer outcome measures that consider patients' occupations and perspectives, using these results to create person-centered occupational goals and interventions (Weinstock-Zlotnick & Bear-Lehman, 2015). The patient-reported outcome measures (PROs) are either general for evaluating all types of hand and upper limb injuries or disease specific to evaluate the impact of specified injury or disease on a patient's hand function.

The Disability of the Arm, Shoulder, and Hand (DASH) questionnaire is a 30-item general questionnaire developed to evaluate a patient's ability to perform certain hand UE activities. Thus, the final score will show the level of ability/disability in all types of hand and upper limb–injury patients. In contrast, there are different disease-specified PROs, such as Patient-Rated Wrist Evaluation—which is a 15-item questionnaire designed to measure wrist pain and disability in ADL—and the Boston Carpal Tunnel Questionnaire (BCTQ)—which is widely used for assessing function and/or symptoms in patients with carpal tunnel syndrome.

As part of the evaluation, it is important for the hand therapist to assess functional ability and dexterity for ADL, leisure, and work tasks. Valid functional assessments assist the hand therapist to determine baseline function, an intervention plan, and goals. Some examples of functional assessments are the Minnesota Haptic Functional test, the Box and Block test, the Nine Hole Peg test, and the Functional Dexterity Test (Table 64.1). Functional assessments allow the therapist not only to collect objective outcome data but

TABLE 64.1   Evaluation of Body Structure and Function for the Upper Extremity

Body Structure and Function	Objective Test	Subjective Test	Functional Test
Range of motion	Goniometer (active and passive ROM)		
Pain	Algometer	• Visual analogue scale • Numeric rating scale • Verbal Rating Scale (VRS) • Shultz UE Pain Assessment (SUEPA)	
Edema	• Volumetric water displacement • Circumferential measurement (figure-of-8) • Gulick Anthropometric Tape		
Sensation	• Semmes–Weinstein Monofilament • Weinstein Enhanced Sensory • Test (WEST-Hand) • Vibrating test • Ten test • Two-point discrimination (moving and static)		• Tactile gnosis • Moberg • Dellon
Muscle testing	• Manual muscle testing • Muscle tightening		
Grip and pinch strength	• Dynamometer • Pinch gauge	The patient's outcome of surgery hand/arm (POS-Hand arm)	The Toronto Rehabilitation Institute Hand Function Test (TRI-HFT)
Vascularity of the hand	• Allen test		
Threshold tests	• Phalen test		
Burn scar	Vancouver Burn Scar Assessment		
Functional Evaluation (patient's true capabilities in performing specific tasks that extend beyond standard measures of motion, strength, or sensation)			
Dexterity			• Minnesota Rate of Manipulation Test (MRMT) • Box and Block Test (BBT) • Purdue Pegboard Test (PP) • Grooved Pegboard Test • Nine Hole Peg Test (NHP) • O'Connor Finger Dexterity Test • Functional Dexterity Test (FDT)
Activity of daily living		Hand Assessment Tool (HAT)	• Sequential Occupational Therapy Dexterity Assessment (SODA) • Chedoke Arm and Hand Activity Inventory (CAHAI)
Performance		Canadian Occupational Performance Measure (COPM)	• Wolf Motor Function Test (WMFT)
Hand function			• Suitcase Packing Activity (SPA) • Jebsen Taylor Hand Function Test (JHFT)
Work performance			• Valpar Component Work Samples (VCWS)
Evaluation of disability (activity limitation and participation restriction)		• Disability of the Arm, Shoulder, and Hand (DASH) • Patient Related Wrist [and Hand] Evaluation (PRWE/PRWHE) • Michigan Hand Outcomes Questionnaire (MHQ) • ABILHAND	

ROM, range of motion; UE, upper extremity.

also to observe patterns of grasp, pinch, reaction time, and speed, as well as compensatory movements to complete a functional task. For example, if the client demonstrates difficulty retrieving coins and placing them in a slot, the occupational therapist could write a goal that the client will be independent retrieving 10 coins from a change purse to buy an item. The therapist could introduce therapeutic activities such as picking up and placing small pieces of cotton or foam from a table using the index finger and thumb while holding the objects in their hand with the ulnar digits (in-hand translation). This activity could easily be graded up or down, depending on the type of object being picked up, the surface, the number of coins, and the rate.

Recent research has illumined the relevance of evaluating and assessing social deprivation or marginalization and socioeconomic conditions affecting outcomes in hand therapy (Stonner et al., 2022). In this study, the Area Deprivation Index (ADI) was utilized to assess social factors that would affect access to care and compliance with therapy visits and home program. It concluded that socially deprived patients attended fewer therapy sessions and obtained poorer active range of motion (AROM) and outcomes after flexor tendon repair.

Intervention

The surgeon in the following OT Story prescribes a dorsal blocking splint and an early passive motion protocol. Orthotics are an essential part of the treatment plan for many UE conditions and can be used to protect repairing structures, mobilize stiff joints, or provide function in the presence of impairments. Delay in implementation of the orthoses sometimes results in chronic stiffness, pain syndromes, and resultant atrophy. Therapists integrate their creative abilities with their knowledge of anatomy, biomechanics, physiology, and healing stages related to injury to specific tissues to fabricate an orthosis.

In order to select an appropriate orthosis for a patient, hand therapists need to develop the process of decision-making and problem-solving based on each patient's needs (see Box 64.1). One of the critical steps in orthotic interventions is monitoring patients regularly and collaborating with patients to modify the orthoses based on the healing phase. In acute patients with edema subtraction, the orthoses should be checked for any additional changes or refitting. Therapists should check the pressure points and any unnecessary restriction in joints. For example, a patient with median nerve surgery at the wrist level needs a dorsal blocking orthosis to immobilize the wrist in 30 degrees of flexion for the first 3 weeks after surgery. The position of the wrist should be changed to neutral after this time.

Orthotic intervention for occupational therapists goes beyond addressing impairments. The holistic view of OT does not limit the ability to overcome physical and anatomic issues; instead, it considers the whole picture of a patient, including lifestyle and environmental and contextual components of their occupational lives. However, much of the hand therapy literature addresses body functions and structures, with less emphasis on activities, participation, and environmental factors (Rose et al., 2011).

Many individuals in hand therapy do not adhere to splint wear recommendations. To improve the adherence to orthotic usage and enable patients' functioning, occupational therapists should consider the Client-Centered, Bio-occupational Framework for Orthotic Intervention and individualize the orthosis, considering the individual's unique biological and occupational goals, personal attributes, and environmental contexts. Occupational therapists use orthoses to minimize the effect of impairment and improve activity and participation. If a waiter has arthritis in her thumb, wearing a splint may not be appropriate because she must grasp and wash her hands frequently. In this case, incorporating a taping method might be a better choice as a "splint" to support the joint yet allow the client to be able to safely carry out job functions without compromise. An occupational therapist should consider the interaction of the environmental and personal factors with the patients' functional level to improve occupational performance. The intervention process for Josephina is described in OT Story 64.2.

The evaluation of Josephina, an individual with a hand injury, is outlined in OT Story 64.1.

BOX 64.1 FACTORS TO BE CONSIDERED FOR ORTHOTIC FABRICATION

- Consider patients' characteristics (age, job, occupational profile, occupational goal, psychological factors, acceptance).
- Identify and address the injury: biological need and anatomic parts that should be included in the orthoses.
- Consider the usability of the orthoses before deciding about the type of orthoses.
- Select the best materials and design based on all the aforementioned prerequisites.
- Be aware of bony prominences when fabricating a splint.
- Consider the arches of the hand at rest and with use when molding the splint.
- Should the splint be static or dynamic, enabling motion?
- How often should the splint be worn and for what duration.

OT STORY 64.1 JOSEPHINA: INJURY AND EVALUATION

Josephina, aged 37 years, and her husband immigrated to the United States from Guatemala 2 years ago. Her husband has only been able to work odd construction jobs without benefits. They had applied for Medicaid last year and were able to enter the County Health System. Josephina worked as a bookkeeper in Guatemala, but she is working part time cleaning homes in the United States because her English was limited. She was taking English classes to become fluent in English so that she could resume her professional occupation and attend college to complete her degree in accounting.

While preparing dinner for her family on February 8, Josephina was cutting tomatoes with a new knife when, suddenly, her cat jumped up onto the counter, startled her, and caused her to lose control of the knife. She subsequently cut her left ring finger. She was unable to stop the bleeding, and she could not move her finger actively. Her husband drove her to the emergency room at a nearby hospital, worried about the consequences of such an injury. She was immediately attended to and ushered into a room where a nurse was waiting to see her. After 15 minutes, a doctor came into the room. Dr Aziz examined Josephina's finger and after doing an x-ray and examination, the doctor determined that Josephina had a near complete laceration of left ring finger (RF), flexor digitorum superficialis (FDS), flexor digitorum profundus (FDP), ulnar digital nerve, and ulnar digital artery and that she required immediate surgery.

Early mobilization or true active flexion is considered a preferable method for flexor tendon rehabilitation for patients after flexor tendon repair (Neiduski & Powell, 2019). However, early active mobilization required strong repairs to withstand the tension of active motion in the first week after repair (Savage, 2014). There are different surgical procedures to repair flexor tendons in zone 2. Over the past three decades, significant efforts have been devoted to updating the repair techniques by increasing the number of suture strands across the repair sites, from two stands to multiple strands.

For example, in a normal hand function, the FDP tendon transmits 1 to 35 N during active finger motion, so the repaired tendon should be strong enough to withstand a force of at least 40 N during early active finger flexion without any risk of gap or rupture. All these changes were done to avoid repair gapping and failure of the repair. A stronger repair has less risk of adhesion formation and rupture. Several recent outcomes have been achieved using multi-strand core suture, pulley-venting, and early active rehabilitation techniques for flexor tendon repair in zone 2.

As the two-strand core sutures are not adequate to ensure consistently good clinical results, Dr Aziz decided to repair Josephina's lacerated tendons by using a four-strand suture, which is rather strong. The condition of the tendon was very good, and the repair went well. Dr Aziz was confident that the client would have full functional restoration of her hand if Josephina chooses to follow the therapy program. Dr Aziz placed a referral for OT twice a week, with orders to fabricate a dorsal blocking splint and to use an early passive motion protocol.

One week later, Josephina, her husband, and her son went to her initial hand therapy evaluation appointment together. The therapist, Sasha, introduced herself to the family and asked them to follow her into the hand clinic. She then explained the goals of hand therapy after flexor tendon repair, which are restoring function and returning to the previous level of function through different hand therapy techniques. She described this outcome can be achieved by preventing tendon rupture, promoting tendon healing, encouraging tendon gliding, preventing flexion contractures, restoring ROM of involved joints, and maintaining ROM of uninvolved joints. All three followed the therapist into the clinic where they were all offered chairs with Josephina seated at a hand therapy table. Her hand was in a half cast wrapped with Kerlix, a thick gauze wrap. The surgical wounds were covered with Xeroform, a thin yellow gauze strip with antibiotic ointment. Josephina saw the surgeon once since the surgery when she changed the bandages for her 2 days prior.

Sasha immediately noticed that Josephina's electronic medical record indicated that Spanish was her language of preference. She read the doctor's referral indicating the diagnosis and the preferred protocol that Dr Aziz wished the therapist to follow. There are various protocols for tendon repairs—including early active, early passive, delayed active, delayed passive motion, and place and hold techniques—depending on the physician, the surgery, the type of suture used to repair the tendon, and the condition of the tissues pre- and post-repair. Sasha brought over the interpreter videophone asking them to wait a moment while she dialed in for a Spanish interpreter. All health plans in the United States and Canada must provide a qualified interpreter either in-person, via telephone, or a video-conference platform. When the interpreter came on, she gave her ID number so that Sasha could record it in her notes. The interpreter explained first in English, then in Spanish, that the

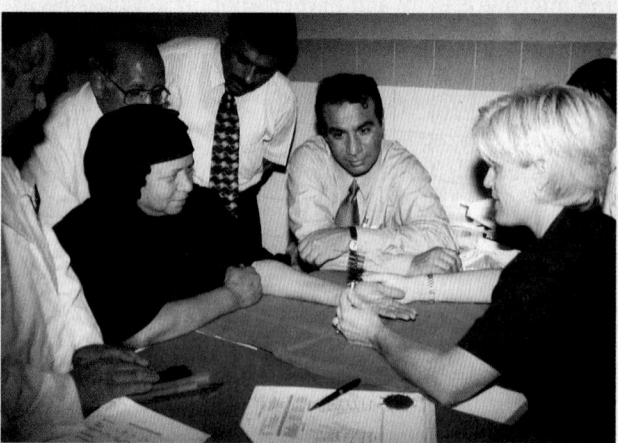

OT STORY 64.1 JOSEPHINA: INJURY AND EVALUATION (*continued*)

therapist and client are to speak to each other, not to the interpreter, and to speak slowly and clearly.

Following introductions, Sasha explained what she would be doing today for the first visit. She would interview Josephina for the subjective part of the evaluation, covering the following: how the trauma occurred, her pain levels and sensation, whether she is working and what her work tasks are, if she lives with her family, her daily and work responsibilities, and her goals. Sasha used an anatomy book to explain to Josephina what tissues were affected by her injury and how they connect to movement of the hand. The importance of following the specific exercises every 2 hours was clearly discussed to prevent tendon rupture, achieve optimal gliding of structures, and minimize adhesions that could disrupt tendon gliding and movement. Sasha spoke in short phrases so that the interpreter could interpret clearly and accurately what was spoken.

Sasha stated the precautions to the patient and instructed her to keep her wrist straight and her fingers relaxed without actively moving them. Sasha then applied her medical gloves using a sterile technique and proceeded to remove the cast and the Kerlix gauze with a bandage scissor. The Xeroform (antibiotic gauze) was slightly adherent to the wound, so it was gently removed so as not to disrupt the healing tissue. The wound appeared to be healing well. Sasha proceeded to clean the wound with wound wash and sterile gauze. After allowing the skin to air dry for a few minutes, Sasha performed passive range of motion (PROM) on each finger to assess

the condition and end feel of the finger joints. She used a finger goniometer to measure the PROM of each finger of her affected hand. Owing to repair of the nerve and Josephina's report of numbness in her RF, the Semmes–Weinstein monofilament test (an assessment for mapping out sensory loss) was administered. The wound was then redressed with a non-adherent dressing and light gauze, being careful to allow movement for exercise. Sasha asked Josephina how she was feeling to be sure she was not feeling faint as some clients are when they begin exercising after surgery. Josephina assured Sasha she was fine but her pain was a 5/10 in the RF.

Questions

1. Josephina reports she is having pain in her affected hand with strengthening exercises at 9 weeks' post-operative. What other activities, occupations, and exercises, including modalities, could Sasha incorporate into Josephina's clinic and home program for strengthening?
2. At 12 weeks' post-operative, Josephina reports difficulty with cooking tasks, including food preparation and washing dishes. She feels a lack of coordination and dexterity and occasional tingling in her affected hand. What therapeutic interventions would facilitate improved hand function for this occupation?
3. How could you encourage the client's compliance with splint wear, precautions, and home program? Discuss physical and psychosocial components.

OT STORY 64.2 JOSEPHINA'S HOME PROGRAM AND INTERVENTIONS

Sasha explained the purpose of the splint and that it is to be worn 24 hours a day during the initial 3 weeks' post-operative. She explained that the splint material will be placed in hot water, cut out, and then molded on Josephina's hand and wrist. Once it hardens, Sasha will place straps on the splint. The dorsal blocking splint (DBS) was fabricated positioning the wrist in neutral, metacarpal phalangeal (MCP) joints in 60 to 70 degrees of flexion, and the interphalangeal joints (IP) in extension (Albright et al., 2020). A perforated material to allow air circulation was used because Josephina would need to wear the splint 24 hours a day for the initial 3 weeks. A removable splint cap with a Dacron string attached allows Josephina to passively flex the affected finger because there should not be any active flexion of the finger until 3 weeks post-operative (Figure 64.1).

Now, Sasha was ready to teach Josephina the initial home exercise program. She explained that the home program should be followed exactly as described, and she demonstrated each exercise that was to be followed carefully to avoid tendon rupture and enable safe gliding of the affected

structures. Sasha explained that the exercise program would change as the tendon, nerve, and artery healed. With a nerve and artery repair, the home program is slightly delayed compared to a tendon-only repair because those structures heal more slowly. The client was told to perform 10 repetitions every 2 hours of the following: passively flex and actively extend the digit to the roof of the DBS, first just the MCP joint, then just the proximal interphalangeal (PIP) joint, then just the distal interphalangeal (DIP) joint, then the PIP and DIP joints (hook position), and finally composite flexion of all joints as close to the palm as possible. She also performed tenodesis (moving the wrist forward in flexion and backward in extension while keeping the fingers completely relaxed) from flexion to neutral wrist outside of the splint.

While explaining the home program and demonstrating each exercise, Sasha spoke clearly and slowly, allowing time for the interpreter to speak to Josephina and for Josephina to ask questions. Josephina demonstrated each exercise she was taught to ensure it was well understood. Handouts were

(*continued*)

OT STORY 64.2 JOSEPHINA'S HOME PROGRAM AND INTERVENTIONS (*continued*)

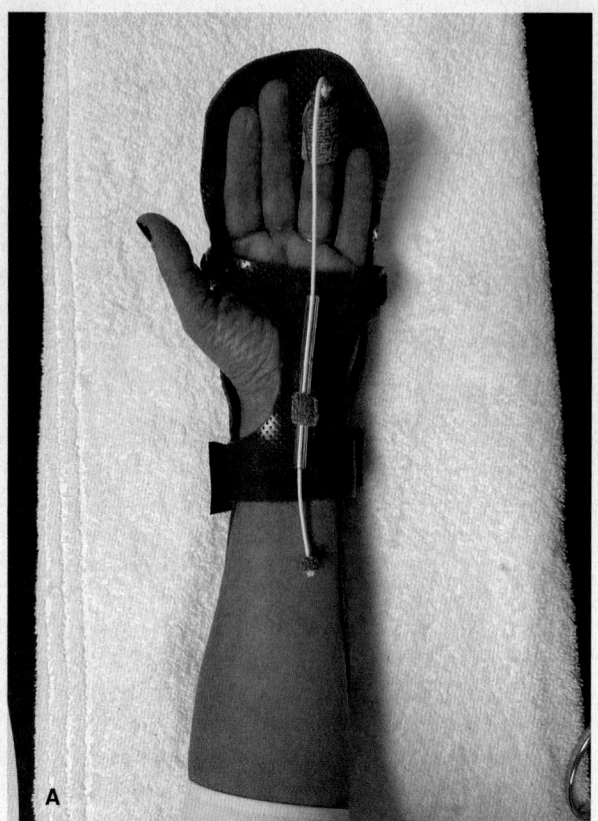 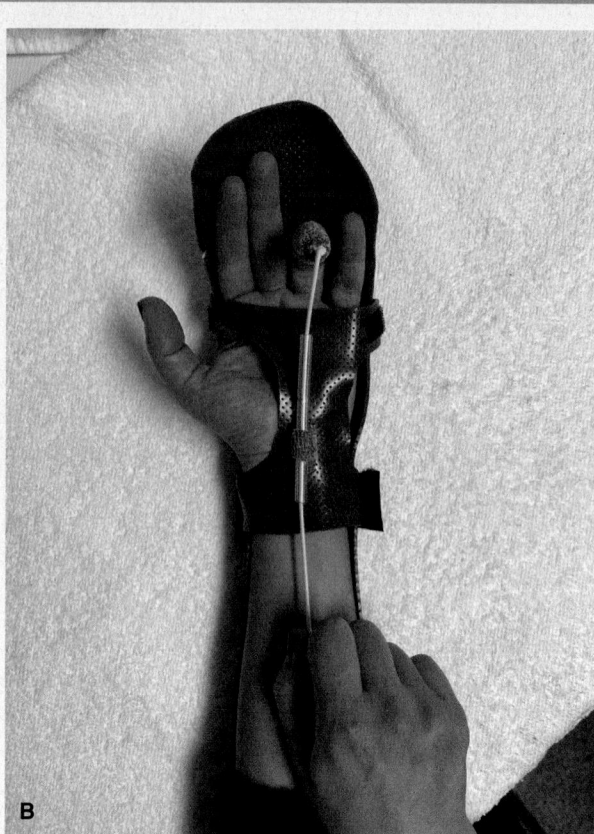

FIGURE 64.1 Dorsal blocking splint (**A**) with dynamic component (**B**).

provided in her native language of Spanish. Sasha asked Josephina to don and doff the splint before she left the clinic to be sure she was comfortable doing this. Josephina was instructed to leave the splint on 24/7, unless she is washing her hand, changing dressings, or performing the tenodesis exercise. Supplies including non-adherent dressing, sterile gauze, paper tape, and extra strapping materials were given to Josephina to take home. Her husband asked when she would need to return. Because he worked and could not bring her over on certain days, he had to be sure to schedule follow-up appointments when he or another family member was available to drive her. While the interpreter was still with us, the scheduler was asked to come over to schedule the next several appointments.

Josephina returned 2 days later for the therapist to recheck her splint and her wound and review her home program. This time, only her husband came with her. Once the Spanish interpreter was on the videophone, Josephina stated that her hand felt much better but she noticed some bloody discharge when she exercised. Sasha assured her that minimal bloody discharge is normal early on. The therapist took off the dressings and asked the client to wash her hand. New dressings were then applied to the hand. Sasha put on her gloves and began to passively move each joint and to check the PIP joint to ensure the contracture was lessening, which

it was. When asked if she was doing her home program as instructed, Josephina stated she was and sometimes she lost track of time and might have done them every hour. She thought the more she did, the better her hand would be. Sasha explained that more is not necessarily better and that if she does too much, she risks increasing inflammation or straining the stitches. Sasha verified that Josephina understood to follow the protocol exactly, not to do more or less than prescribed. Josephina appeared to understand.

Subsequent visits over the next 3 to 6 weeks included active finger exercises and decreased splint wear, along with careful and safe functional use of the hand, such as picking up pieces of cotton and cut up foam pieces for prehension, placing coins into a piggy bank, and folding clean clothes for bilateral integration. Because Josephina enjoyed knitting, she was asked to bring her knitting needles and yarn to the clinic. Utilizing task analysis, activities incorporated into interventions included picking up and manipulating the knitting needles, tying knots in yarn, cutting, and finger dexterity exercises with coins and Baoding balls (two small metal balls that can be held in one hand). Josephina also enjoyed gardening activities, so at 8 weeks she was asked to bring to the clinic a small pot, soil, and a flowering plant so that she could carry out the activity of replanting and potting a plant that she could later place in her garden at home. Her confidence grew using her affected hand more and her strength and motion improved. By 12 weeks post-operative, she was using her hand normally and continued strengthening exercises with TheraPutty and TheraBand to strengthen her upper extremities so that she could return to work without restrictions. On her last visit to the clinic, Josephina and her husband brought the therapist a bowl of pepian, a traditional chicken stew from Guatemala, to show their appreciation.

Questions

1. Josephina is recovering from her tendon injury well at 10 weeks post-op. However, she is having difficulty opening her water bottle. Considering her occupational profile, what functional interventions could you use to address this challenge now that she is able to use her hand functionally?
2. What could Sasha do if Josephina stated that the exercises hurt so she was not doing them?

The Benefits and Barriers of Using Occupation in Hand Therapy

The hand therapy approaches in evaluating and treating patients are mainly based on the medical model and biomechanical frame of reference. A core premise of OT is the intimate and inseparable connection of person and occupation, yet some occupational therapists struggle with maintaining an occupation-based focus in the field of hand therapy (Fitzpatrick & Presnell, 2004; Henrichon & Toth-Cohen, 2022; Poulsen & Hansen, 2018). Owing to the domination of the medical model in hand therapy, the methods of evaluation focus on the objective measurement of impairments (ROM, pain, muscle power, sensation). The medical model commonly uses the biomechanical frame of reference and bottom-up approaches (Hocking, 2010) to address functional deficits by treating body structure and function (James, 2003). The focus of the biomechanical frame of reference is the musculoskeletal capacity to create movement (ROM), strength, and endurance in order to carry out meaningful occupations. Movement, strength, and endurance should then be assessed within the context of a person completing their occupations (McMillan, 2016).

Creating a balance between the biomedical approach inherent within a medical model with the occupation-based philosophy and general concepts of OT is needed to move toward an occupational-based practice (OBP). There are various interpretations regarding the definition of OBI in literature, from embedding purpose and meaning to interventions to enabling performance or engagement in an occupation that a client wants to, needs to, or is expected to do. Considering all those definitions, occupational therapists can use occupation as means (OAM) and occupation as end (OAE) to reflect the OBI in hand therapy practice (Henrichon & Toth-Cohen, 2022).

However, therapists should consider the methods and risks of using "occupation as means" in intervention when

patients must follow medical precautions after surgeries (Colaianni et al., 2015). Moreover, occupational therapists have reported other barriers to OBIs, such as including logistic issues, reimbursement issues, limitations imposed by the client's medical condition, the treatment protocol, and credibility of OBIs (Colaianni & Provident, 2010).

In the early acute phase of hand injuries and the first two phases of healing, the anatomic structures should be maintained and the therapist should avoid overloading healing tissues. Therapists should modify or limit the use of occupational interventions that compromise recovery and outcomes in the early stages of healing, but they need not eliminate them. For example, it would not be appropriate to ask the client to open a bottle of water 2 weeks following a tendon repair of the FDS in zone 2 owing to lack of tensile strength of the healing tendon, but it would be appropriate to ask the client to use the affected finger(s) to gently pick up a piece of cotton and place in an open container.

Although it is important to protect healing structures in the early phases of injury, therapists must avoid neglecting the unique occupational needs of each individual by fixating on specific anatomic structures and failing to acknowledge clients as occupational beings (Robinson et al., 2016). As occupational therapists, we should maintain in our practice as a core concept of our profession that occupations are central to a client's (persons, groups, or populations) health, identity, and sense of competence and have particular meaning and value to that client (AOTA, 2020).

The focus of treatment in OT and hand therapy is to enable patients to be independent in their activities and increase their level of participation. Thus, integrating the biopsychosocial model into hand therapy is inevitable. The World Health Organization (WHO) introduced the biopsychosocial model of health as The International Classification of Function (ICF). Because using the ICF language in hand therapy evidence is not common, it has been recommended to use the ICF frame of reference to demonstrate the societal and personal impact of an impairment on a patient's life with a language understood and appreciated by many healthcare users, policymakers, and third-party payers.

Conclusion

OBI should be implemented in hand therapy by the occupational therapists to return to the OT profession's roots. However, few studies examine hand therapy's effectiveness as a purposeful or occupation-based intervention. Besides, the lack of evidence and understanding of occupational therapists regarding the method of implementing OBI is considered a barrier to integrating OBI in the practice of hand therapy (Valdes et al., 2021). In a study by Colaianni and colleagues (2015), it was found that participants demonstrated higher motivation when engaging in OBI rather than biomechanical intervention. An occupational therapist should consider the benefits of using OBIs in hand therapy.

REFERENCES

Albright, M., Alexy, C., Barteau, W., Beal, B., Bodnyk, S., Tuason Bolin, E., & Sala, J. (2020). *Diagnosis and treatment manual for physicians and therapists* (5th ed.). Indiana Hand to Shoulder Center.

American Occupational Therapy Association. (2017). *The unique role of OT in rehab of the hand.* https://www.aota.org/About-Occupational-Therapy/Professionals/RDP/hand-therapy.aspx

American Occupational Therapy Association. (2020). Occupational therapy practice framework: Domain and process—Fourth edition. *The American Journal of Occupational Therapy, 74*(Supplement_2), 7412410010p1–7412410010p87. https://doi.org/10.5014/ajot.2020.74S2001

Colaianni, D., & Provident, I. (2010). The benefits of and challenges to the use of occupation in hand therapy. *Occupational Therapy in Health Care, 24*(2), 130–146. https://doi.org/10.3109/07380570903349378

Colaianni, D., Provident, I., DiBartola, L. M., & Wheeler, S. (2015). A phenomenology of occupation-based hand therapy. *Australian Occupational Therapy Journal, 26,* 177–186. https://doi.org/10.1111/1440-1630.12192

Custer, M., Huebner, R., & Howell, D. (2015). Factors predicting client satisfaction in occupational therapy and rehabilitation. *American Journal of Occupational Therapy, 69*(1), 6901290040p1–6901290040p10. https://doi.org/10.5014/ajot.2015.013094

Fitzpatrick, N., & Presnell, S. (2004). Can occupational therapists be hand therapists? *British Journal of Occupational Therapy, 67*(11), 508–510. https://doi.org/10.1177/030802260406701107

Hand Therapy Certification Committee. (2009). *Definition of hand therapy.* htcc.org/about-htcc/definition-of-hand-therapy-and-scope-of-practice#headingOne

Henrichon, K. A., & Toth-Cohen, S. E. (2022). Perspectives and influences on occupation-based hand therapy. *Canadian Journal of Occupational Therapy, 89,* 294–306. https://doi.org/10.1177/00084174221102720

Hinojosa, J., Kramer, P., & Crist, P. (2014). Evaluation: Where do we begin? In J. Hinojosa & P. Kramer (Eds.), *Evaluation in occupational therapy: Obtaining and interpreting data* (4th ed., pp. 1–18). AOTA Press.

Hocking, C. (2010). The challenge of occupation: Describing the things people do. *Journal of Occupational Science, 16*(3), 140–150. https://doi.org/10.1080/14427591.2009.9686655

James, A. B. (2003). Biomechanical frame of reference. In E. B. Crepeau, E. S. Cohn, & B. A. B. Schell (Eds.), *Willard and Spackman's occupational therapy* (10th ed., pp. 240–242). Lippincott Williams & Wilkins.

McMillan, I. R. (2016). *The biomechanical frame of reference in occupational therapy.* Retrieved December 12, 2021, from https://musculoskeletalkey.com/the-biomechanical-frame-of-reference-in-occupational-therapy/

Neiduski, R. L., & Powell, R. K. (2019). Flexor tendon rehabilitation in the 21st century: A systematic review. *Journal of Hand Therapy, 32*(2), 165–174. https://doi.org/10.1016/j.jht.2018.06.001

Poulsen, H. S., & Hansen, A. Ø. (2018). Occupational performance problems identified by 507 patients: An insight that can guide occupation-based hand therapy. *Hand Therapy, 23*(4), 121–129. https://doi.org/10.1177/1758998318784316

Robinson, L. S., Brown, T., & O'Brien, L. (2016). Embracing an occupational perspective: Occupation-based interventions in hand therapy practice. *Australian Occupational Therapy Journal, 63*(4), 293–296. https://doi.org/10.1111/1440-1630.12268

Rose, B. W., Kasch, M, C., Aaron, D. H., & Stegink-Jansen, C. W. (2011). Does hand therapy literature incorporate the holistic view of health and function promoted by the World Health Organization? *Journal of Hand Therapy, 24*(2), 84–88. https://doi.org/10.1016/j.jht.2010.12.003

Savage, R. (2014). The search for the ideal tendon repair in zone 2: Strand number, anchor points and suture thickness. *Journal of Hand Surgery, 39*(1), 20–29. https://doi.org/10.1177/1753193413508699

Stonner, M., Keane, G., Berlet, L., Goldfarb, C., & Pet, M. (2022). The impact of social deprivation and hand therapy attendance on range of motion after flexor tendon repair. *The Journal of Hand Surgery, 47*(7), 655–661. https://doi.org/10.1016/j.jhsa.2022.03.018

Valdes, K., Naughton, N., Téllez, R. C., & Szekeres, M. (2021). The use of occupation-based interventions and assessments in hand therapy: A cross-sectional survey. *Journal of Hand Therapy.* https://doi.org/10.1016/j.jht.2021.10.008

Weinstock-Zlotnick, G., & Bear-Lehman, J. (2015). How therapists specializing in hand therapy evaluate the ability of patients to participate in their daily lives: An exploratory study. *Journal of Hand Therapy, 28*(3). 261-267. https://doi.org/10.1016/j.jt.2014.010.

World Federation of Occupational Therapists. (2010). *What is occupational therapy?* Retrieved from October 12, 2021, from http://www.wfot.org/information.asp

CHAPTER 65

Providing Occupational Therapy for Older Adults With Changing Needs

Bette R. Bonder

LEARNING OBJECTIVES

After reading this chapter, you will be able to:

1. Discuss normal age-related changes that affect occupational performance.
2. Describe health conditions and trajectories in later life as these affect occupational performance.
3. Describe environmental factors that influence the experience of growing older.
4. Discuss unique considerations in evaluating and intervening to support successful aging and minimize dysfunction in later life.
5. Describe characteristics of healthcare systems that serve older adults.
6. Describe social factors that support or impede successful aging.
7. Discuss unique considerations in providing occupational therapy services to older adults throughout late life development.
8. Analyze common ethical issues in providing occupational therapy services for older adults.
9. Discuss the ways in which the COVID-19 pandemic has altered service delivery and treatment goals for older adults and what these changes might mean for future care of older adults.

Introduction: Understanding the Life Course in Later Life

Older adults are the fastest growing segment of the population in the United States (Roberts et al., 2018). This demographic development is similar in many countries in the western world. As of 2016, there were an estimated 49.2 million older adults in the United States (Federal Interagency Forum on Aging Related Statistics, 2016). By 2050, older adults will comprise 21.4% of the US population. At present the older population is roughly 75% white, the proportion of older adults from other groups is increasing, with implications for healthcare. These demographic realities have significant implications for every aspect of life—workforce, education, economic development, and, of course, healthcare.

In 2018, life expectancy in the United States ranged from a high of 81 years in Hawaii to a low of 74.4 in West Virginia (Arias et al., 2021).

Factors that affect life expectancy, including sex, education, race, and ethnicity, were highlighted during the COVID-19 pandemic (Andrasfay & Goldman, 2021), which has reduced average life expectancy by a full year in 2020.

Although opinions vary about the impact of an aging population on the healthcare system, preventing health problems is both possible and desirable from an individual and a societal perspective. Researchers have focused on strategies to ensure **positive aging**, maintaining positive quality of life as normal age-related physical and cognitive changes occur (Wahl et al., 2016). Rowe and Kahn (1998) theorized that successful aging is based on avoiding disease and disability, maintaining mental and physical function, and maintaining active engagement with life. This early conceptualization has been broadened to consider well-being, life satisfaction, and positive aging as different, and in some cases more complex, understandings of what it means to age well (Bartholomaeus et al., 2019).

Individuals of all ages can take actions to avoid disease and disability; however, to some extent, this is not within personal control. Societal realities can impede well-being and function, which are not subject to individual control. It is also possible to take steps, within the constraints of the environment, to maintain mental and physical function, although again, these do not guarantee that decline will not occur. It is also the case that some older individuals are dealing with the combined impact of life-long health or functional issues compounded by the effects of normal aging. Every individual will experience some degree of functional decline later in life (National Institutes of Health [NIH], 2013). Maintaining active engagement with life is largely within individual control and is the central emphasis of occupational therapy (see Box 65.1; American Occupational Therapy Association [AOTA], 2020).

Occupational Therapy in Action: Mrs. Ramirez's Path Through Later Life

In general, there has been a reduction in disabling health conditions in late life in the United States (NIH, 2013),

although 40% of those over 65 have at least one disabling condition (Centers for Disease Control, 2020). Some of these conditions may reflect health and/or functional issues present in earlier life on which age-related change is superimposed. A common experience in later life is a gradual decline in aspects of body function and performance skills. Vision almost universally deteriorates. Hearing often worsens. Muscle mass decreases. These and other body function changes can affect motor and sensory-perceptual skills. Decline is often gradual for long periods of time, punctuated by acute health problems that can accelerate functional loss. A bout of pneumonia may severely reduce cardiovascular endurance, a situation compounded by the fact that older adults also take longer to recover and may never return to their pre-illness baseline (Bray & Bonder, 2018).

Further, development of chronic health conditions such as arthritis, osteoporosis, and dementia have profound consequences for function and quality of life. Issues requiring special attention in later life include the following:

- Health conditions may have more benign (some cancers) or severe (pneumonia, influenza, COVID-19) consequences in late life.
- Decrements in sensory systems, cardiovascular and musculoskeletal function, and cognition are universal, although variable in degree.
- Multiple, sometimes conflicting, health conditions can complicate treatment choices (e.g., osteoporosis and arthritis).
- Social, economic, and environmental factors profoundly influence aging.

Background Information

Mrs. Estelle Ramirez is a 78-year-old widow when she first receives OT services. She lives alone in a third-floor walk-up apartment in Brooklyn, New York—the apartment in which she raised her three daughters, now ages 56, 53, and 51 years. She and her husband remained there after the girls left home for college. Mrs. Ramirez and her husband moved to New York from Puerto Rico when Mr. Ramirez took a job in a factory 50 years earlier. Mrs. Ramirez began

BOX 65.1 THERAPIST NARRATIVE

Early in my career I served as a research assistant on a study of older adults in a low-income residential facility in an urban inner city. One question asked participants to rate how happy they were. The researchers expected a low level of happiness due to participants' economic disadvantage. They were surprised to learn that most reported being very happy with their current lives because they had the freedom to do what interested them, often after many years earning

a living at needed but unfulfilling work. My interactions with older adults over the years have further demonstrated to me that once basic needs for shelter and food are met, it is what one does and not what one has that makes for happiness in later life. Occupational therapists are central to promoting the ability of elders to do what matters most to them.

—Bette R. Bonder

working as an accountant when her girls were in high school. She retired at age 66 to take care of her husband who was then in the late stages of Alzheimer's disease (AD). He died 4 years later. Mrs. Ramirez has Social Security, a small additional pension, and Medicare (public health insurance in the United States for those age 65 and older).

Mrs. Ramirez believes herself to be in good health. She is of normal weight, and although she has joint pain that she characterizes as *artritis* (arthritis), it does not interfere very much with her function. She wears glasses, now trifocals, but sees reasonably well with them. She reports recent difficulty seeing at night so no longer drives after sunset. She has always preferred, like many New Yorkers, to use public transportation, but does not feel safe doing so after dark. This has limited her evening activities, which causes her some distress. She has also begun to complain to her daughters about her memory. They note that she tends to repeat herself when speaking with them and that she sometimes forgets appointments.

Puerto Rican culture has a strong emphasis on *familismo*, a belief in the importance of strong family ties. Her daughters are very supportive but worry about whether Mrs. Ramirez should be living by herself. There is growing tension regarding possible alternate arrangements. One daughter believes Mrs. Ramirez should stay in her home with the three girls providing supportive care, one believes her mother should come live with her, and one favors moving Mrs. Ramirez to an assisted living facility.

Since her husband's death, Mrs. Ramirez volunteers at the local elementary school. She sees her daughters frequently and takes great pleasure in spending time with her nine grandchildren and her first great-grandchild; she particularly likes cooking traditional Puerto Rican meals with them and telling them about their heritage. She spends time at the local Hispanic Senior Center. She misses her husband and regrets that she had to stop working earlier than she would have liked, but she is reasonably satisfied with her current life and enjoys her apartment and neighbors.

First Encounter

Mrs. Ramirez heard a consulting occupational therapist at the senior center make a presentation about home safety including a checklist for the participants so that they could assess their environments. As the therapist knows, falls are common among older populations and can have dire consequences (Kramarow et al., 2015), including significant disability or death. Mrs. Ramirez was very particularly pleased to hear that her Medicare would cover a cursory evaluation as part of an annual wellness assessment (Medicare.gov, n.d.). Medicare is the main healthcare payor in the United States, while other countries have other, and different, systems. In the United States, occupational therapists must be aware of what services are covered. For those needs

that Medicare does not address, therapists must identify alternative resources and/or find ways to address them in the context of what is covered as discussed below.

Reimbursement Issues and Ethical Dilemmas in Working With Older Adults

Mrs. Ramirez has typical healthcare insurance as structured in the United States. Although in the United States, individuals older than age 65 years benefit from being eligible for Medicare, a nearly universal form of health insurance for elders, Medicare has numerous—and frequently changing—limitations and regulations (Richman, 2018). Medical services associated with preventive care (e.g., vaccinations, mammography, diabetes care) are covered, but preventive OT services are not. This is unfortunate because there is strong research evidence that early intervention focused on lifestyle issues can maintain health and reduce costs (Clark et al., 2012; Lood et al., 2015).

Even when some OT services are covered, numerous regulations limit the specific treatment goals. This creates one of the many ethical dilemmas that confront occupational therapists working with older adults. How can one ensure that vital services are made available in a reimbursement environment that regulates the goals that will be covered while also limiting providers' ability to impose charges for services not covered? Creativity in selecting activities that address multiple goals is an essential component of an effective intervention plan. For example, a conversation about leisure occupations may be helpful in supporting a well-rounded occupational profile but may need to take place while the patient is working on covered services like self-care and instrumental activities.

The involvement of family can also create ethical challenges for therapists. It is not unusual for family members to have divergent views regarding the best interests of the older adult. The occupational therapist must recognize that the older adult is the client and remain focused on what is best for that individual in spite of any lobbying by family. Mrs. Ramirez's family is supportive, but it is evident that they have different views about what is best for her.

Wellness and Prevention

Evaluation

As described previously, funding for wellness and prevention in the United States can be challenging. Most often, occupational therapists provide such services by consulting with organizations rather than caring for individual clients (Bass, 2018). In such cases, the client may be a *population*

(AOTA, 2020). The process by which this occurs mirrors individual evaluation and intervention but requires focus on the needs and interests of aggregates of individuals as defined in the Occupational Therapy Practice Framework (OTPF) as well as epidemiological data that suggest what kinds of problems are most common and what health indicators can identify need and measure progress (Morrow & Johnson, 2014). Poor diet, physical inactivity, and smoking cause significant disability and premature morbidity around the world (Lisko et al., 2020). Such information is useful in framing goals of senior center activities, educational programs, and health screenings. Furthermore, data demonstrate that cognitive decline and falls are among the most common and, particularly in the case of falls, preventable health problems in later life.

Interventions to Support Positive Aging

In wellness and prevention services for older adults, the occupational therapist's most typical role is to assist in understanding the needs of clients and designing programs to be delivered by activity therapists, aides, and volunteers (Bass, 2018). Based on the information from participants and a review of literature about common health problems, the therapist generates a list of program goals and explores best practices about effective programming. Some of the interventions designed might involve populations as well as individuals (AOTA, 2020).

In the case of the Hispanic Senior Center that Mrs. Ramirez attends, one of the activities that participants most enjoy is the lunch, which includes typical Puerto Rican foods. They also enjoy listening to Hispanic music on the radio and watching Spanish-language soap operas. It is typical that senior centers establish culturally relevant programming since half of all these facilities serve minority populations (Lendon et al., 2020).

Thus, the therapist suggests a focus on culturally relevant activities encouraging physical activity through meaningful and enjoyable activities such as dancing, gardening, and nature hikes; maintaining supportive social interaction and cognitive wellness through interactive, challenging activities such as book and movie clubs, lectures, creative writing, scrapbooking; encouraging positive health promotion through nutrition and cooking demonstrations, safety awareness activities, and group discussion; and providing opportunities for altruistic activities such as reading to neighborhood children, food drives, and care for program participants who become ill.

The occupational therapist attends team meetings during which the activity therapist, part-time nurse, nutritionist, and consulting physician discuss the needs of the center's participants. Along with occupation-based programming, a series of wellness events is designed and implemented. These include blood pressure, vision, and hearing screening; quarterly visits by a dentist; and an invitation to a physical therapist to plan an appropriate exercise program for participants. These activities are relevant to Mrs. Ramirez's situation because she has not had regular screenings for common health problems and has become increasingly sedentary.

During the pandemic, the senior center had to suspend in-person operations and focus on maintaining well-being of their participants using strategies that included meal and grocery delivery, ensuring internet access for each participant with accompanying online social and educational opportunities, and regular phone check-in to ascertain the status of each participant. For an example from Sweden, see Expanding Our Perspectives.

EXPANDING OUR PERSPECTIVES

Digital Technology-Mediated Occupations

Ingeborg Nilsson

Occupational therapists are experts in enabling occupational engagement through bridging gaps between the person's needs and wishes and the demands from the environment and the occupation (Law et al., 1996). We have a responsibility to use this expertise, not only to support seniors with limitations but to promote health for all (Hammell, 2008).

I want to introduce to you Susanna, a newly retired woman in Sweden. She had been employed at the same company for decades and had been longing for retirement for the past several years. While employed she found it difficult to keep up with the rapid changes in technology development. Continuously new technical platforms for meetings and administrative routines challenged her. She thought she was good at meeting with the clients she was set to guide but more and more job tasks were carried out through digital technology which she found difficult and stressful. The contact with clients that she really enjoyed could not compensate for the stress she felt being unable to manage the digital technology.

When I as an occupational therapist met Susanna at a meeting place for seniors, she had been retired almost one year. She came to get information about ongoing activities and services available through the senior center. When we talked, she also described that she felt great emptiness. With no immediate family, an extended family spread out around Sweden, and no working colleagues to meet regularly she felt excluded and without social

EXPANDING OUR PERSPECTIVES *(continued)*

contact. Her commitment to work had reduced all other occupational arenas and she had problems to even describe what she now actually enjoyed doing. When I asked, she agreed to experiencing loneliness.

Loneliness is an experience indicating a dissatisfaction with social life (Perlman & Peplau, 1981). Loneliness is a growing concern and is identified as a public health issue (Gerst-Emerson & Jayawardhana, 2015). Reported prevalence of loneliness among older adults in Sweden varies between 25% (Lennartsson et al., 2020) and more than 50% (Nyqvist et al., 2017; Socialstyrelsen, 2020). Research indicates that loneliness is associated with severe health problems including morbidity, for example, cardiovascular diseases, dementia (Kuiper et al., 2015; Valtorta et al., 2016) as well as mortality (Holt-Lunstad et al., 2015; Rico-Uribe et al., 2018). Loneliness is a complex issue that reduces health and well-being in many ways. Conversely being socially engaged is a significant protective factor for good health (Douglas et al., 2017; Levasseur et al., 2009; Minagawa & Saito, 2015). Occupational therapists are in a good position to support social engagement (Turcotte et al., 2018).

Susanna had realized that digital technology was a necessary part of everyday life even as a retiree. Her challenges with digital technology gave consequences, she felt alienated as she for example was not active on Facebook or Instagram where updates on social events were posted. Her extended family was communicating through Messenger or FaceTime which she did not feel comfortable with. She received dinner invitations during the pandemic that she had to decline because they were meeting online through Zoom. Susanna felt restricted both in instrumental activities of daily living such as banking and healthcare as well as leisure activities like socializing, entertainment, or exercise hobbies.

During our conversation, Susanna acknowledged a need to develop her digital competence so she could participate in valued occupations. Through the principle of learning-by-doing, we started to practice relevant online occupations. As a guide for myself, I used a scheme about implementing support in online occupations (Fischl et al., 2020) which gives me a structure when applying individualized support to Susanna. The collaborative process begins by identifying areas of interests and then moves to tailoring the online occupation based on the individual's needs. In the process, emphasis is also put on identifying available support around the individual to encourage continued engagement. I found it therefore relevant to suggest Susanna to attend a group that met weekly at the city library. With supervision of a librarian, the group at the city library would practice and discuss for them relevant online platforms. I encouraged Susanna

to attend the group as it could furthermore develop her digital competence but also make her involved in a social context where she could exchange experiences. These initiatives served as a start for Susanna to get access to online occupations and get an opportunity to feel included in the digital world.

Digitalization offers many opportunities for our clients; however, they need to have sufficient digital competence to take advantage of these tools. As occupational therapists we need engagement in the area of digital occupations but also models for how to introduce, support, and adapt online activities for seniors. Since we can now do almost everything through a smartphone or tablet, this is a remarkable resource for occupational therapists in our work to support occupation and participation.

References

Douglas, H., Georgiou, A., & Westbrook, J. (2017). Social participation as an indicator of successful aging: An overview of concepts and their associations with health. *Australian Health Review, 41*(4), 455–462. https://doi.org/10.1071/AH16038

Fischl, C., Blusi, M., Lindgren, H., & Nilsson, I. (2020). Tailoring to support digital technology-mediated occupational engagement for older adults—A multiple case study. *Scandinavian Journal of Occupational Therapy, 27*(8), 577–590. https://doi.org/10.1080/11038128.2020.1760347

Gerst-Emerson, K., & Jayawardhana, J. (2015). Loneliness as a public health issue: The impact of loneliness on health care utilization among older adults. *American Journal of Public Health, 105*(5), 1013–1019. https://doi.org/10.2105/AJPH.2014.302427

Hammell, K. W. (2008). Reflections on...well-being and occupational rights. *Canadian Journal of Occupational Therapy, 75*, 61–64. https://doi.org/10.2182/cjot.07.007

Holt-Lunstad, J., Smith, T. B., Baker, M., Harris, T., & Stephenson, D. (2015). Loneliness and social isolation as risk factors for mortality: A meta-analytic review. *Perspectives on Psychological Science, 10*(2), 227–237. https://doi.org/10.1177/1745691614568352

Kuiper, J. S., Zuidersma, M., Coshaar, R. C. O., Zuidersma, S. U., van den Heuvel, E. R., Stolk, R. P., & Smidt, N. (2015). Social relationships and risk of dementia: A systematic review and meta-analysis of longitudinal cohort studies. *Ageing Research Reviews, 22*, 39–57. https://doi.org/10.1016/j.arr.2015.04.006

Law, M., Cooper, B., Strong, S., Steward, D., Rigby, P., & Letts, L. (1996). The person-environment-occupation model: A transactive approach to occupational performance. *Canadian Journal of Occupational Therapy, 63*, 9–23. https://doi.org/10.1177/000841749606300103

Lennartsson, C., Rehnberg, J., McKee, K. J., & Dahlberg, L. (2020). *Förekomst och riskfaktorer för ensamhet bland äldre personer i Norden.* Nordic Council of Ministers.

Levasseur, M., St-Cyr Tribble, D., & Desrosiers, J. (2009). Meaning of quality in life for older adults: Importance of human functioning components. *Archives in Gerontology and Geriatrics, 49*(2), e91–e100. https://doi.org/10.1016/j.archger.2008.08.013

Minagawa, Y., & Saito, Y. (2015). Active social participation and mortality risk among older people in Japan: Results from a nationally representative sample. *Research on Aging, 37*(5), 481–499. https://doi.org/10.1177/0164027514545238

(continued)

EXPANDING OUR PERSPECTIVES (continued)

Nyqvist, F., Cattan, M., Conradsson, M., Näsman, M., & Gustafsson, Y. (2017). Prevalence of loneliness over ten years among the oldest old. *Scandinavian Journal of Public Health, 45*(4), 411–418. https://doi.org/10.1177/14034948176 97511

Perlman, D., & Peplau, L. A. (1981). Toward a social psychology of loneliness. In R. Gilmour & S. Duck (Eds.), *Personal relationships: 3 Relationships in disorder* (pp. 31–56). Academic Press.

Rico-Uribe, L. A., Caballero, F. F., Martin-Maria, N., Cabello, M., Mayuso-Mateos, J. L., & Miret, M. (2018). Association of loneliness with all-cause mortality: A meta-analysis. *PLoS One, 13*(1), e0190033. https://doi.org/10.1371/journal.pone.0190033

Socialstyrelsen. (2020). In Socialstyrelsen (Ed.), Vad tycker de äldre om äldreomsorg. https://www.socialstyrelsen.se/globalassets/sharepoint-dokument/artikelkatalog/ovrigt/2020-9-6901.pdf.

Turcotte, P.-L., Carrier, A., Roy, V., & Levasseur, M. (2018). Occupational therapists' contributions to fostering older adults' social participation: A scoping review. *British Journal of Occupational Therapy, 81*, 427–449. https://doi.org/10.1177/0308022617752067

Valtorta, N. K., Kanaan, M., Gilbody, S., Ronzi, S., & Hanratty, B. (2016). Loneliness and social isolation as risk factors for coronary heart disease and stroke: Systematic review and meta-analysis of longitudinal observational studies. *Heart, 102*(13), 1009–1016. https://doi.org/10.1136/heartjnl-2015-308790

Naturally Occurring Retirement Communities

Mrs. Ramirez's apartment building is now populated almost exclusively by individuals older than 65 because young people moved out while Mrs. Ramirez and her age cohorts remained in place. The building now constitutes a **naturally occurring retirement community** (NORC) (Ivery, 2014). The emergence of NORCs reflects the wish of many older adults to **age in place**, that is, to remain in their current homes as they grow older. Advantages to doing so include the familiarity of the surroundings, social support from long-time neighbors, and access to family and healthcare professionals who know their histories and needs.

Recognizing the opportunity offered by NORCs to support positive aging, government and social agencies have begun to provide various wellness and health promotion services in these facilities. In 2008, the Administration on Aging (Parniak et al., 2022) established a funding initiative designed to

- Enhance the ability of older adults living in a residential community to continue living independently;
- Increase healthy aging behaviors through exercise, recreation, socialization, education, and culturally appropriate activities; and
- Identify needs of at-risk residents, facilitate access to existing community/government resources, and create gap-filling supportive services.

This initiative and its goals offer significant opportunities for occupational therapists to serve community-residing, well-older adults. Offering evidence-based services such as lifestyle redesign (Clark et al., 2012) can promote the goals of the AoA NORC program. Based on Mrs. Ramirez's current status, transportation services would be of particular value, as would evening activities in her building to reduce her sense of loss of evening social opportunities. Further, the NORC allowed for provision of a variety of supports during the COVID-19 pandemic as isolation was reduced by seeing friends from a distance and sharing resources like grocery delivery.

Primary Care

Occupational therapists' involvement with traditional primary care for older adults has evolved over the past few decades. Their role emphasizes assessment and management of function related to activities of daily living (ADL) that patients identify as important in their lives (Trembath et al., 2019). Interventions might emphasize pain management, community mobility, environmental redesign, health management, and other strategies for supporting and maximizing occupational engagement. As briefly noted above, this is one of the practice areas in which it may be necessary for the therapist to find strategies such as referral to community services to meet needs not explicitly covered by Medicare.

Inpatient Care

Several months after her first encounter with the occupational therapist, Mrs. Ramirez misses a week at the senior center. A concerned staff member calls her home and, when they cannot reach her, they call her oldest daughter, and discover to their dismay that Mrs. Ramirez recently fell on the steps leading to her apartment and sustained a fracture of the femur.

Evaluation

Surgery to stabilize the femur fracture was performed to insert a metal plate with several screws. The outcome is uncertain given the osteoporotic condition of her bones. The occupational therapist is involved immediately, both to help minimize any hospital-induced cognitive loss and to help Mrs. Ramirez prepare for rehabilitation.

The occupational therapist spends some time talking with Mrs. Ramirez to get to know about her interests and her life before the accident. The AOTA Practice Framework

(AOTA, 2020) encourages the completion of an occupational profile as a starting point for evaluation. The therapist is pleased when two of Mrs. Ramirez's daughters stop by to visit while she is in the room so that she can meet them and get a sense of the kind of support Mrs. Ramirez may have on her eventual return home. The therapist also administers the Montreal Cognitive Assessment (Edwards et al., 2019), a quick screening instrument for cognitive impairment, and the Functional Independence Measure (FIM) (Heinemann et al., 1994) to evaluate Mrs. Ramirez's current physical capacity. The occupational therapist finds that Mrs. Ramirez has some memory loss but her physician indicates this does not meet the standard for dementia. In addition, Mrs. Ramirez is now struggling with basic self-care such as dressing, getting herself to and from the bed to a chair or wheelchair, and moving from the wheelchair to the toilet safely.

Interventions to Minimize Dysfunction

Mrs. Ramirez will be transferred very soon to a skilled nursing facility where she can receive rehabilitation services. The therapist and Mrs. Ramirez agree that the focus of intervention will be on planning for a smooth discharge to the rehabilitation setting. For the brief time that they are together, they work on safe transfers from bed to chair and from wheelchair to toilet. They also focus on dressing because Mrs. Ramirez expresses unhappiness that she looks disheveled.

The therapist makes a point of seeing Mrs. Ramirez several times a day and encourages some of the hospital volunteers to do likewise. The daughters have expressed concern that Mrs. Ramirez seems more confused than usual. For an older adult who already has memory problems, hospital stays can lead to rapid deterioration (Ehlenbach et al., 2015). Thus, the treatment plan includes strategies to provide stimulation and orientation to time and place: providing Mrs. Ramirez a newspaper each day; discussing current events; talking about events happening in her own day ("What did you have for breakfast?" or "Have you had company today?"); and conversing about the Spanish-language soap opera that Mrs. Ramirez likes to watch.

During the COVID-19 pandemic, visitation was limited, so interaction with the family was done via phone and other electronic media. This is an example of an increase in telemedicine and other electronic service delivery by OT providers (Sarsak, 2020), a trend that may continue and improve service in otherwise underserved areas even as the pandemic abates.

Skilled Nursing

Three days after her surgery, Mrs. Ramirez is transferred to a skilled nursing facility. She expresses relief at being out of the hospital but is concerned about whether she will be able to go home. She is adamant this is what she wants and expresses this wish to every staff member she meets as well as to her daughters.

Evaluation

Skilled nursing facilities are among the most highly regulated healthcare institutions with both federal and state guidelines about the nature of services, expectations for improvement, requirements about length of stay, and outcome reporting (Centers for Medicare & Medicaid Services, 2020a; DeJong, 2016). Mrs. Ramirez will receive care from a comprehensive team while she shows improvement. If her condition does not stabilize before she can safely go home, it will be time for other arrangements. Mrs. Ramirez is highly motivated and the occupational therapist is involved early based on evidence that intensive OT is associated with shorter stay and better functional outcomes (Cimarolli & Jung, 2016).

According to Medicare guidelines, OT evaluation and interventions must focus on Mrs. Ramirez's ADL and instrumental activities of daily living (IADL). The occupational therapist reviews the report from the inpatient facility and participates with others on the team in completing the Minimum Data Set (MDS) (Centers for Medicare & Medicaid Services, 2020c). The FIM is repeated, and interviews with Mrs. Ramirez and, with her permission, her daughters, help frame goals and intervention strategies.

Intervention

Mrs. Ramirez wants to regain independence in self-care and resume her usual activities. The therapist helps her practice fundamental skills like dressing, bathing, toileting, and grooming. One goal of their sessions is to identify ways to simplify these activities, using, where appropriate, modified clothing (especially for lower extremity dressing), assistive devices (reachers, bath seat), and task modification to reduce energy expenditure.

During these treatment sessions, the therapist inquires about Mrs. Ramirez's typical patterns at home and about the environment to which she wants to return. The therapist talks with the physical therapist about the challenges of a third-floor apartment, and both agree this may be quite difficult for Mrs. Ramirez. They suggest to the social worker that she explores the possibility of moving Mrs. Ramirez to a first-floor apartment in the same building, realizing that this may not be acceptable to Mrs. Ramirez or feasible in New York's tight housing market.

It becomes apparent that Mrs. Ramirez's cognitive difficulties are interfering with her ability to master the changes in occupational patterns required by her new physical status. The therapist requests an evaluation by the psychologist who indicates that Mrs. Ramirez has mild cognitive impairment (MCI) (Parikh et al., 2016). Unlike dementia, MCI is characterized by modest forgetfulness and poor short-term memory. Well-learned functions tend to remain intact so that individuals with MCI can manage their daily activities in their accustomed environments. Function becomes much more challenging when the individual is in a new setting or when physical changes require new patterns. Mrs. Ramirez's fall and subsequent course of care have increased her confusion. Her retention from session to session is poor so the occupational therapist adds a focus on low-tech memory aids (lists, labeling, mnemonic strategies).

As with other kinds of inpatient care, much of the family's involvement would be virtual during the height of the COVID-19 pandemic. And here, too, lessons can be learned to improve care in underserved areas once the pandemic is under better control.

Transition to Home Care

Reimbursement rules from Medicare limit the amount of time that an individual can remain in skilled nursing. Very early in Mrs. Ramirez's stay, the social worker and the treatment team begin conversations with her and, with her permission, her daughters regarding a plan for her discharge. Although only one daughter supports her wish, Mrs. Ramirez remains determined to return to her home. Ultimately, one daughter agrees to stay with her for several weeks to help her readjust to the apartment. However, everyone is concerned about her ability to manage the stairs.

A week before her scheduled departure, the social worker contacts a home health agency. Given Mrs. Ramirez's continued physical limitations and the fact that she has had inpatient care, she is eligible for home health services paid for by Medicare. All agree that these services will be very helpful, and the social worker arranges for the intake nurse from the home health agency to visit Mrs. Ramirez on her first full day at home.

Home Care

As with rehabilitation, Medicare coverage of home health care is based on specific rules about services that can be provided (Centers for Medicare & Medicaid Services, 2020b; Commonwealth Fund, 2020). Occupational therapy is a covered service, as is supportive care provided by a home health aide in concert with rehabilitation. A challenge for OT is that the guidelines specify that services must focus on ADLs and IADLs, not on activities addressing quality of life. This may create an ethical dilemma for the therapist who perceives an obligation to provide comprehensive services to meet client needs. Providing intervention that can generalize to multiple activities is one helpful strategy, perhaps salsa dancing to improve balance, or calling the senior center as a way to practice using the phone for emergencies.

There is a lack of clarity about the impact the COVID-19 pandemic had on delivery of home health services (Commonwealth Fund, 2020). Such services are vital for older adults who were quarantined during the height of mandated lockdowns, and more data are needed about how to ensure adequate service at such times.

Evaluation

Home health reimbursement guidelines require that there should be an initial intake assessment, The Outcomes and Assessment Information Set (OASIS) (Centers for Medicare & Medicaid Services, 2020d) is typically completed by a nurse. The intake worker then determines what other services should be provided. These may include OT, physical therapy (PT), speech-language therapy, home aide services (but only in conjunction with therapeutic services), and nursing care. In Mrs. Ramirez's case, it is evident that OT is important to a positive outcome.

Occupational therapy evaluation in the client's own environment is often the most meaningful in terms of occupational performance. Familiarity with the environment and the psychological comfort of being at home can enhance a client's function. For Mrs. Ramirez, whose cognitive status has affected her performance, this is particularly true. On her first visit, the occupational therapist asks Mrs. Ramirez to demonstrate her daily routine: getting out of bed, toileting, grooming, bathing, and dressing. Mrs. Ramirez is able to dress independently, sitting in a chair as she was shown during her rehabilitation. However, she struggles with bathing and is unsafe getting on and off the toilet. The therapist completes a home safety evaluation (Horowitz et al., 2013), looking for unstable area rugs, inadequate lighting, and clutter.

In addition to ADL, Mrs. Ramirez will need to be able to manage some IADLs for herself. Her daughters are willing to stop by to help with laundry, grocery shopping, and light cleaning, but Mrs. Ramirez will need to fix some meals for herself and read and respond to mail, including bills. The therapist asks her to demonstrate these activities.

Intervention

If Mrs. Ramirez is to be able to manage in her home, there is much to do. The therapist orders appropriate durable medical equipment (bath seat, grab bars, raised toilet seat) to assist with safety and function. She and Mrs. Ramirez reorganize the kitchen so that frequently used items are within easy reach (Figure 65.1). With Mrs. Ramirez's approval, the therapist helps her daughters remove safety hazards from the home. They continue to work on self-care skills, bathing in particular, that are giving Mrs. Ramirez difficulty.

As a way to address leisure and social activities, the therapist structures conversation while they work on self-care so that Mrs. Ramirez can problem-solve about

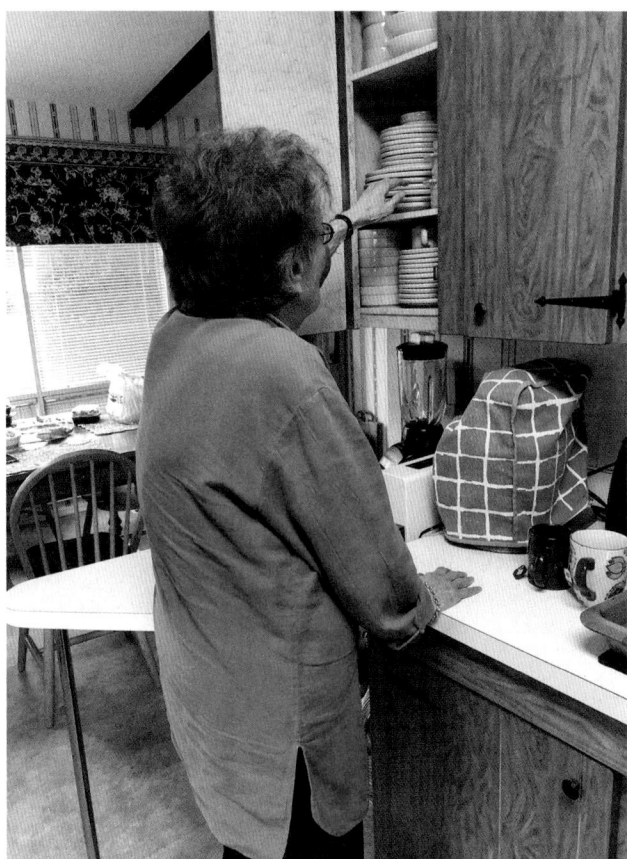

FIGURE 65.1 **An occupational therapist may work with a client to organize a kitchen for safety and ease of use.**

resuming the activities she most wants to do. She is eager to return to the Hispanic Senior Center as soon as possible, and the therapist helps her make the phone call that will arrange transportation. The therapist incorporates elements of these tasks to promote problem-solving and endurance in support of ADLs and IADLs.

Throughout their time together, the therapist notes that Mrs. Ramirez's increasing cognitive deficits create problems for her independent function. They work on organizing her space to help her find commonly used items, to lay out her grooming supplies in the bathroom, to label cabinets, and to use reminder lists, but the lists are frequently mislaid or forgotten. Mrs. Ramirez continues to be unsteady on her feet and is unable to remember the precautions that the therapist showed her regarding standing from a seated position, using her cane effectively to move around the apartment, and using the grab bars that have been installed in the bathroom.

Assisted Living

Although Mrs. Ramirez is very motivated to live on her own, ultimately, the challenges of her environment are simply too much. There are two daunting difficulties. One is

the three steep flights of stairs leading to the apartment. Although Mrs. Ramirez is increasingly functional at home, leaving and returning are painful and exhausting. Using the stairs does not fall strictly within the goals for home health services (which are intended for individuals who are homebound, not to assist such individuals with return to their community activities), the therapist feels comfortable having Mrs. Ramirez practice as a way to regain strength and endurance. However, her progress is slow and she feels increasingly isolated and depressed.

The second dilemma is Mrs. Ramirez's failing memory, which causes concern for the therapist and for Mrs. Ramirez's daughters. The therapist arranges a visit from the social worker to discuss the options. There are several very intense sessions during which the therapist, with Mrs. Ramirez's permission, reviews her skills and abilities. Ultimately, they agree that an assisted living facility is the best solution.

Evaluation

Occupational therapists typically serve as consultants for assisted living facilities, advising on programming, environmental considerations, and staff training. Residents of assisted living facilities may be referred for outpatient OT as needed, but assisted living is not designed to provide such services within the facility. Their purpose is to provide a supportive environment where meals, housekeeping, and activities are provided and healthcare can be accessed easily. Thus, Mrs. Ramirez will not be formally evaluated by an occupational therapist at the assisted living facility.

Intervention

A variety of OT interventions are helpful in assisted living facilities, including such efforts as occupational coaching (Lamarre et al., 2020). The occupational therapist encourages an array of activities that support wellness (physical activity and socialization at mealtime to encourage adequate nutrition) and quality of life (culturally appropriate, creative, spiritual, altruistic, and other meaningful and enjoyable occupations). In addition, the occupational therapist works with staff to assist in creating strategies for monitoring Mrs. Ramirez's well-being and for interacting with and supporting the family. Effective intervention and monitoring in assisted living can provide support for residents and families to prolong high-quality and meaningful life.

Conclusion

Creative occupations have been shown to have particular value in enhancing the quality of life for elders (National Endowment for the Arts, 2015). A holistic approach

TABLE 65.1	Typical Areas of Emphasis in Prevention, Inpatient Care, Skilled Nursing, Home Health, and Assisted Living			
Prevention	**Inpatient Care**	**Skilled Nursing**	**Home Health**	**Assisted Living**
Consult on design of programs to support meaningful activity	Evaluate ADL in preparation for discharge/ transition planning.	Evaluate ADL/IADL.	Evaluate ADL/IADL.	Design wellness programs.
Consult on design of physical activities	Provide stimulation to prevent cognitive loss.	As feasible, explore meaningful occupations.	As feasible, explore meaningful occupations.	Design leisure programs with an emphasis on function and meaning.
Train staff	As appropriate, discuss needs with family/other informal caregivers.	Provide interventions to increase functional ability in ADL/IADL, increase physical capacity.	Provide interventions to increase functional ability in ADL/IADL.	Consider development of day care programming.
Advise on physical design of facilities	Low vision services	Provide assistive devices as appropriate and provide training in their use.	Provide interventions to promote wellness.	Train staff.
			Complete safety assessment	Advise on physical design of facilities.
			Support environmental modifications to enhance safety and function.	
			Provide assistive devices as appropriate and provide training in their use.	
			Low vision services	
			Fall prevention	

ADL, activities of daily living; IADL, instrumental activities of daily living.

incorporating creative occupations enhances wellness and quality of life. In concert with other environmental and programmatic efforts, creative occupations can offer benefits to the individual, the family, and the community

However, as shown in Table 65.1, OT goals remain the same:

1. Prevent functional decline.
2. Maximize our client's performance in areas of occupation.
3. Decrease participation restrictions and maximize quality of life.

Acknowledgments

We would like to acknowledge the contributions of Glenn David Goodman to earlier editions of this chapter.

Lippincott® Connect *For additional resources on the subjects discussed in this chapter, visit Lippincott Connect.*

REFERENCES

Parniak, S., DePaul, V.G., Grymire, C., DePaul. S., & Donnelly, C. (2022). Naturally occurring retirement communities: Scoping Review. *Journal of Medical Internet Research, 14*(5), e34577. https://doi .org/10.2196/34577.

American Occupational Therapy Association. (2020). Occupational therapy practice framework (4th ed.). *American Journal of Occupational Therapy, 74*(Suppl. 2), 7412410010p1–7412410010p87. https:// doi.org/10.5014/ajot.2020.74S2001

Andrasfay, T., & Goldman, N. (2021). Reductions in 2020 US life expectancy due to COVID-19 and the disproportionate impact on the Black and Latino populations. *Proceedings of the National Academy of Sciences, 118*(5), e2014746118 https://doi.org/10.1073/ pnas.2014746118

Arias, E., Bastian, B., Xu, J., & Tejada-Vera, B. (2021). U.S. state life tables, 2018. *National Vital Statistics Reports, 70*(1). https://www.cdc.gov/ nchs/products/index.htm

Bartholomaeus, J. E. M., Van Agteren, M. P., Iasiello, A. J., & Kellya, D. (2019). Positive aging: The impact of a community wellbeing and resilience program. *Clinical Gerontologist, 42*(4), 377–386. https://doi .org/10.1080/7317115.2018.1561582

Bass, J. D. (2018). Health and wellness. In B. R. Bonder & V. Dal Bello-Haas (Eds.), *Functional performance in older adults* (4th ed., pp. 421–436). F. A. Davis.

Bray, P., & Bonder, B. (2018). Considerations for medical care of older adults. In B. R. Bonder & V. Dal Bello-Haas (Eds.), *Functional performance in older adults* (4th ed., pp. 263–276). F. A. Davis.

Centers for Disease Control. (2020). *Disability and health promotion.* https://www.cdc.gov/ncbddd/disabilityandhealth/infographic-disability-impacts-all.html

Centers for Medicare & Medicaid Services. (2020a). *Functional reporting.* https://www.cms.gov/Medicare/Billing/TherapyServices/Functional-Reporting

Centers for Medicare & Medicaid Services. (2020b). *Home health PPS.* https://www.cms.gov/Medicare/Medicare-Fee-for-Service-Payment/HomeHealthPPS

Centers for Medicare & Medicaid Services. (2020c). *Minimum data set (MDS) 3.0 for nursing homes and swing bed providers.* https://www.cms.gov/Medicare/Quality-Initiatives-Patient-Assessment-Instruments/NursingHomeQualityInits/NHQIMDS30

Centers for Medicare & Medicaid Services. (2020d). *OASIS user manuals.* https://www.cms.gov/Medicare/Quality-Initiatives-Patient-Assessment-Instruments/HomeHealthQualityInits/HHQIOASISUserManual

Cimarolli, V. R., & Jung, S. (2016). Intensity of occupational therapy utilization in nursing home residents: The role of sensory impairments. *Journal of the American Medical Directors Association, 17,* 939–942. https://doi.org/10.1016/j.jamda.2016.06.023

Clark, F., Jackson, J., Carlson, M., Chou, C., Cherry, B. J., Jordan-Marsh, M., Knight, B. G., Mandel, D., Blanchard, J., Granger, D. A., Wilcox, R. R., Lai, M. Y., White, B., Hay, J., Lam, C., Marterella, A., & Azen, S. (2012). Effectiveness of a lifestyle intervention in promoting the well-being of independently living older people: Results of the Well Elderly 2 Randomised Controlled Trial. *Journal of Epidemiology and Community Health, 66,* 782–790. https://doi.org/10.1136/jech.2009.099754

Commonwealth Fund. (2020). *Medicare and home health: Taking stock in the COVID-19 era.* https://www.commonwealthfund.org/publications/issue-briefs/2020/oct/medicare-home-health-taking-stock-covid-19-era

DeJong, G. (2016). Coming to terms with the IMPACT Act of 2014. *American Journal of Occupational Therapy, 70,* 7003090010p1–7003090010p6. https://doi.org/10.5014/ajot.2016.703003

Edwards, D. F., Wolf, T. J., Marks, T., Alter, S., Larkin, V., Padesky, B. L., Spiers, M., Al-Heizan, M. O., & Giles, G. M. (2019). Reliability and validity of a functional cognition screening tool to identify the need for occupational therapy. *American Journal of Occupational Therapy, 73*(2), 1–10. https://doi.org/10.5014/ajot.2019.028753

Ehlenbach, W. J., Larson, E. B., Curtis, J. R., & Hough, C. L. (2015). Physical function and disability after acute care and critical illness hospitalizations in a prospective cohort of older adults. *Journal of the American Geriatrics Society, 63,* 2061–2069. https://doi.org/10.1111/jgs.13663

Federal Interagency Forum on Aging Related Statistics. (2016). *Older Americans 2016: Key indicators of well-being.* Federal Interagency Forum on Aging Related Statistics. U.S. Government Printing Office. https://agingstats.gov/docs/LatestReport/Older-Americans-2016-Key-Indicators-of-WellBeing.pdf

Heinemann, A. W., Linacre, J. M., Wright, B. D., Hamilton, B. B., & Granger, C. (1994). Prediction of rehabilitation outcomes with disability measures. *Archives of Physical Medicine and Rehabilitation, 75,* 133–143. https://doi.org/10.1016/0003-9993(94)90385-9

Horowitz, B. P., Nochajski, S. M., & Schweitzer, J. A. (2013). Occupational therapy community practice and home assessments: Use of the home safety self-assessment tool (HSSAT) to support aging in place. *Occupational Therapy in Health Care, 27,* 216–227. https://doi.org/10.1309/07380577.2013.807450

Ivery, J. M. (2014). The NORC supportive services model: The role of social capital in community aging initiatives. *Journal of Community Practice, 22,* 451–471. https://doi.org/10.1080/10705422.2014.958635

Kramarow, E., Chen, L., Hedegaard, H., & Warner, M. (2015). *Deaths from unintentional injury among adults aged 65 and over: United States, 2000–2013* (NCHS Data Brief, 199). https://www.cdc.gov/nchs/data/databriefs/db199.pdf

Lamarre, J., Egan, M., Kessler, D., & Sauve-Schenk, K. (2020). Occupational performance coaching in assisted living. *Physical & Occupational Therapy in Geriatrics, 38*(1), 1–17. https://doi.org/10.1080/02703181.2019.1659466

Lendon, J. P., Rome, V., & Sengupta, M. (2020). Variations between adult day services centers in the United States by the racial and ethnic case-mix of center participants. *Journal of Applied Gerontology, 40,* 1029–1038. https://doi.org/10.1177/0733464820934996

Lisko, I., Kulmala, J., Annetorp, M., Ngandu, T., Mangialasche, F., & Kivipelto, M. (2020). How can dementia and disability be prevented in older adults: Where are we today and where are we going? *Journal of Internal Medicine, 289,* 807–830. https://doi.org/10.1111/joim.13227

Lood, Q., Häggblom-Kronlöf, G., & Dahlin-Ivanoff, S. (2015). Health promotion programme design and efficacy in relation to ageing persons with culturally and linguistically diverse backgrounds: A systematic literature review and meta-analysis. *BMC Health Services Research, 15,* 560. https://doi.org/10.1186/s12913-015-1222-4

Medicare.gov. (n.d.). *Yearly "Wellness" visits.* https://www.medicare.gov/coverage/yearly-wellness-visits

Morrow, C. B., & Johnson, J. A. (2014). Public health administration and practice framework. In L. Shi & J. A. Johnson (Eds.), *Novick & Morrow's public health administration: Principles for population-based management* (3rd ed., pp. 53–78). Jones & Bartlett Learning.

National Endowment for the Arts (2015). Accessibility: Creativity & Aging. https://www.arts.gov/impact/accessibility/creativity-and-aging

National Institutes of Health. (2013). *Disability in older adults.* https://report.nih.gov/nihfactsheets/ViewFactSheet.aspx?csid=37

Parikh, P. K., Troyer, A. K., Maione, A. M., & Murphy, K. J. (2016). The impact of memory change on daily life in normal aging and mild cognitive impairment. *The Gerontologist, 56,* 877–885. https://doi.org/10.1093/geront/gnv030

Richman, N. Z. (2018). Public policy and advocacy in North America. In B. R. Bonder & V. Dal Bello-Haas (Eds.), *Functional performance in older adults* (4th ed., pp. 33–44). F. A. Davis.

Roberts, A. W., Ogunwole, S. U., Blakeslee, L., & Rabel, M. A. (2018). *The population 65 years and older in the United States: 2016.* U.S. Department of Commerce. https://www.census.gov/content/dam/Census/library/publications/2018/acs/ACS-38.pdf

Rowe, J. W., & Kahn, R. L. (1998). *Successful aging.* Dell.

Sarsak, H. I. (2020). Telerehabilitation services: A successful paradigm for occupational therapy clinical services. *International Physical Medicine & Rehabilitation Journal, 5*(2), 93–98. https://doi.org/10.15406/ipmrj.2020.05.00237

Trembath, F., Dahl-Popolizio, S., Vanwinkle, M., & Milligan, L. (2019). Retrospective analysis: Most common diagnoses seen in a primary care clinic and corresponding occupational therapy interventions. *The Open Journal of Occupational Therapy, 7*(2). https://doi.org/10.15453/2168-6408.1539

Wahl, H., Deeg, D., & Litwin, H. (2016). Successful ageing as a persistent priority in ageing research. *European Journal of Ageing, 13,* 1–3. https://doi.org/10.1007/s10433-016-0364-5

CHAPTER 66

Forced Migration and the Role of Occupational Therapy

Mansha Mirza, Concettina Trimboli, Rawan AlHeresh,
Md. Ariful Islam Arman, Mary Black, Theo Bogeas,
Roshan Galvaan, Mohammad Monjurul Habib, and Yda J. Smith

LEARNING OBJECTIVES

After reading this chapter, you will be able to:

1. Explain the phenomenon of forced migration and define related terms.
2. Recognize how forced migration affects the occupational lives of forced migrants.
3. Articulate occupational therapy's role and scope of practice with forced migrants.
4. Identify a wide range of practice settings, programs, and guiding frameworks that characterize occupational therapy with forced migrants.
5. Appreciate opportunities for emerging practice, student engagement, and professional networking to address the occupational needs of those affected by forced migration.

Introduction

Worldwide, forced migration has reached crisis proportions with a record high of more than 100 million individuals, one in every 78 people, forcibly displaced from their homes and communities due to persecution, war, generalized violence, and widespread rights violations (United Nations High Commissioner for Refugees [UNHCR], 2022). This large-scale human displacement is driven by ongoing conflicts in countries including Yemen, Syria, Nigeria, Sudan, South Sudan, and the Democratic Republic of Congo. At the same time, new conflicts have erupted such as Russia's invasion of Ukraine, civil war in the Tigray region of Ethiopia, and political turbulence in Afghanistan after US withdrawal, and the Taliban's takeover of Kabul (UNHCR, 2022). Forcibly displaced individuals, also known as **forced migrants**, include those displaced internally within their country of origin as well as those who cross international borders to seek sanctuary in neighboring countries. Once application for international protection is submitted to the local authorities, individuals are considered asylum seekers, while their claim for refugee status and request for international protection are under review in the specific country where they are seeking sanctuary (Migration Data Portal, 2022). Depending on the context and conditions surrounding flight, some forced migrants who cross international borders are legally recognized as prima facie refugees under guidelines of the UNHCR. This means that their refugee status is accepted

BOX 66.1 COMMON TERMS ASSOCIATED WITH FORCED MIGRATION

Asylee: A person granted asylum and therefore allowed to legally stay in a country other than their country of origin (also used interchangeably with "refugee"; see definition below).

Asylum seeker: A person who claims refugee status, has applied for legal protection in another country, and whose application is yet to be processed (Migration Data Portal, 2022). Many countries have their own system in place to verify and review individuals' claims for asylum.

Asylum center: A residential facility, also referred to as a transit/reception center, that offers temporary accommodation, food, and other basic services to asylum seekers and refugees. These are mostly found in Europe.

Forced displacement/Forced migration: When people are dislocated from their homes and communities due to persecution, conflict, generalized violence or human rights violations (UNHCR, 2022).

Global North/South: Terms used by development organizations and development scholars to categorize high-income countries in one group, the Global North, and low and lower middle-income countries in a second group, the Global South. These categories are sometimes criticized for not being geographically consistent and for obscuring differences between countries within the same category.

Refugee: A person who is recognized under the 1951 UN Convention relating to the Status of Refugees, its 1967 Protocol, the 1969 Organization of African Unity (OAU) Convention Governing the Specific Aspects of Refugee Problems in Africa as being "outside their country of origin for reasons of feared persecution, conflict, generalized violence, or other circumstances that have seriously disturbed public order and, as a result, require[ing] international protection" (United Nations General Assembly, 1951).

Refugee camp: A temporary settlement established to provide safe accommodation for persons displaced from their homes and communities. Basic services such as food and household essentials, water, shelter, primary healthcare, and occasionally, educational opportunities are provided by the UNHCR and NGOs. In protracted refugee situations, people live in camps for years or decades. Twenty-two percent of the refugee populations lives in camps, which are typically located in countries of the Global South (USA for UNHCR, n.d.).

Resettlement: A formal process overseen by the UNHCR for transferring refugees from the country where they first sought protection in (typically a country adjacent to their country of origin) to another country that has agreed to admit them and ultimately grant them permanent residence. Only a small percentage (<3%) of refugees in urgent need of resettlement become resettled (USA for UNHCR, 2021).

United Nations High Commissioner for Refugees (UNHCR): The United Nations agency in charge of aiding and protecting displaced and stateless people. The UNHCR typically works in collaboration with other UN agencies such as the World Food Program and national and international nongovernmental organizations (NGOs/INGOs).

at first impression and without further evaluation. Henceforth in this chapter, the term *forced migrants* will be used interchangeably with *refugees* and *asylum seekers*. These and related terms are further explained in Box 66.1.

Three-fourths of the world's refugees seek immediate protection in a neighboring country, typically a developing country in the Global South (UNHCR, 2022) where they live in temporary settlements or refugee camps. Conditions in these temporary accommodations are often difficult and perilous, while safe return to their country or origin is precluded by ongoing persecution or continued conflict. Under such conditions, refugees can seek help from the UNHCR to resettle or relocate to another country willing to admit them (USA for UNHCR, 2021). Although the displacement trajectory and ultimate destination vary for refugees and asylum seekers, many share a history of physical and mental trauma having survived violence, uncertainty, and turbulent migratory journeys. According to one comprehensive review of the literature on this topic, one in six refugees have a significant physical health problem, and two-thirds experience mental health problems (Khan & Amatya, 2017). The precariousness of displacement combined with unfavorable postdisplacement social and political contexts places forced migrants at high risk of occupational injustices (see Chapter 10). The World Federation of Occupational Therapists' position statement on Human Displacement (WFOT, 2014) advocates for capacity building within the profession of occupational therapy (OT) to work with this population. This chapter discusses the various ways in which OT practitioners can address the needs of forced migrants at different stages in their displacement journeys.

Forced Migration and Occupational Lives of Refugees and Asylum Seekers

Over the years, occupational scientists and OT scholars have generated a substantial body of literature documenting how forced migration affects the occupational lives of refugees and asylum seekers. Overwhelmingly, this literature indicates that forced migrants are at risk of **occupational disruption** (Whiteford, 2000) whereby their ability to participate in meaningful occupations of choice is precluded by factors outside their control (Suleman & Whiteford, 2013). When this disruption becomes prolonged, it can lead to **occupational deprivation** (Whiteford, 2000). See Table 66.1 for OT terms associated with forced migration.

In Refugee Camps and Asylum Centers

Extraneous factors that engender occupational disruption and deprivation for forced migrants include asylum policies

that constrain freedom of choice and movement and unfavorable physical and social environments associated with refugee and asylum accommodations. These structural factors when combined with individual experiences of trauma and discrimination overshadow forced migrants' right to meaningful occupational engagement (Crawford et al., 2016). Forced migrants awaiting resettlement and asylum tend to be hosted in institutionalized, collective accommodations in countries where they first seek protection. These mass accommodations typically take the form of refugee camps in the Global South and asylum centers in the Global North (Kreichauf, 2018). Although asylum centers are more common in Europe and Australia, the practice of holding asylum seekers in surveilled detention centers is growing in the United States (Bonfiglio et al., 2020). Forced migration

TABLE 66.1 OT Terminology Associated With Forced Migration

	Definition	Example
Adaptive occupations	When an individual engages in beneficial occupations as a means of adapting to changing life circumstances or environmental demands	Spiritual activities, cooking, exercise, helping fellow refugees
Adaptive repertoire	An individual's ability to make adaptive transitions by applying past occupational experiences to new or evolving circumstances	Ability to constructively reflect on the past, ability to plan occupational engagement in the future, ability to identify and cope with trauma triggers
Downward occupational drift	When changes in occupation, specifically income-generating occupation, result in the individual's shift to a lower socioeconomic class	A forced migrant with a degree in nursing from their country of origin is unable to get a practice license in their country of asylum/resettlement and is compelled to work as a taxi driver to make ends meet.
Maladaptive occupations	When an individual engages in potentially risky or harmful occupations as a means of adapting to changing life circumstances or environmental demands	Illegal activities, recreational drug use, binge drinking
Occupational adaptation	The process of adapting to transition and the resultant new or modified occupations	Refugees learning new cultural and social norms after resettlement, learning the local language, becoming acquainted with the daily rhythms of the adopted country, meeting normative expectations related to occupational roles, and learning how to access public services
Occupational alienation	When an individual is engaging in occupations that are far removed from personal motivation, skills, aptitude, and meaning	Being unable to work in the country of resettlement due to work visa restrictions, and thus needing to subsist on welfare support
Occupational deprivation	Prolonged restriction from participation in necessary or meaningful activities due to circumstances outside the individual's control	Inability to practice familiar activities from the country of origin, such as attending a mosque, as one does not exist where the refugee is located
Occupational disruption	When the ability to participate in meaningful occupations of choice is precluded by disturbances caused by factors outside the individual's control	Forced migrants living in asylum centers being unable to participate in social outings due to institutional restrictions on entry and exit from the center
Occupational imbalance	A lack of balance when engaging in daily activities such that the individual's life satisfaction is diminished	When a person works more than one job and does not have time to participate in occupations/activities that they want to participate in (e.g., leisure, social activities)
Occupational orchestration (challenges with)	When the rhythmic routines of everyday life that allow individuals to enact occupations in ways that are responsive to personal needs and environmental expectations are disrupted	A teenager with a physical disability who needs support with daily self-care activities getting separated from her primary caregiver during displacement
Social capital	The networks of relationships an individual cultivates in a particular society that support the individual to function effectively and pursue life goals	A pregnant refugee woman joining a peer support group for new mothers living in a refugee camp

scholars argue that both refugee camps and asylum centers share a similar sociospatial configuration characterized by large numbers of people inhabiting an enclosed space with substandard and unsafe living conditions, restricted social routines, and lack of freedom of mobility (Kreichauf, 2018; Mirza, 2014). Forced migrants' ability to enter and leave these accommodations is heavily regulated with security personnel often deployed at points of entry and exit. Use of communal spaces and equipment such as kitchens and recreation centers, where available, is also restricted and contingent on rules established by nongovernmental organizations (NGOs) or private companies in charge of facility management. Most importantly, refugee camps and asylum centers represent a state of "legal exception" whereby inhabitants are included under immigration and asylum laws of host countries while being simultaneously excluded from the rights and protection available to citizens of those countries (Mirza, 2014).

Thus, exclusionary citizenship and asylum policies and the harsh realities of refugee and asylum accommodations compromise choice, personal decision-making, and engagement in daily occupations (Crawford et al., 2016; Menéndez Álvarez et al., 2021; Steindl et al., 2008). Faced with precarious living conditions, resource constraints, and institutional restrictions, survival occupations such as gathering food and fuel and caring for dependents take precedence over occupations undertaken for self-enhancement and personal fulfillment resulting in **occupational imbalance** (Alve et al., in press; Burchett & Matheson, 2011). The more marginalized among forced migrants such as frail older adults, survivors of abuse or trauma, and people with disabilities struggle to engage even in basic survival and daily life occupations. For example, forced migrants with complex trauma from preflight torture, abuse, or sexual violence can experience depleted motivation and personal capacity to engage in basic activities of daily living (ADLs) and endure difficult living conditions in refugee camps (Alve et al., in press; Whiteford, 2005). Similarly, inaccessibility of asylum centers and refugee camp facilities can be a significant barrier for occupational engagement of persons with physical and sensory disabilities. After protracted living in camps and detention centers, even previously healthy and nondisabled forced migrants can experience a decrease in ADL ability and activity levels associated with worsening of self-rated health, pain, and depression (Morville, Amris, et al., 2015; Morville, Erlandsson, et al., 2015).

Life in displacement thus challenges **occupational orchestration** (Schell et al., 2019) by disrupting the rhythmic routines of everyday life that allow individuals to enact occupations in ways that are responsive to personal needs and environmental expectations. Under these conditions, refugees and asylum seekers are compelled to adapt through occupational changes that are imposed by their extenuating circumstances and reluctantly accepted (Huot et al., 2016). Such occupational changes can be both maladaptive and

adaptive. For example, survival needs and resource constraints can provoke **maladaptive occupations** such as engaging in exploitative occupations including illicit jobs in the informal economy or sex work (Alve et al., in press; Hart, 2019). Many refugees and asylum seekers are able to cultivate more **adaptive occupations** drawing upon past experiences. Spiritual activities, cooking, exercise, and helping fellow refugees are some examples of adaptive occupations although they tend to be used as a short-term coping strategy or a way of filling the abundance of unstructured time when living in refugee camps and asylum centers rather than as a means for deriving long-term personal relevance and developing skills and aptitudes (Alve et al., in press; Ingvarsson et al., 2016; Morville & Erlandsson, 2013).

Overall, forced migrants' **adaptive repertoire** is compromised by the displacement experience. Adaptive repertoire refers to an individual's ability to make adaptive transitions by applying past occupational experiences to new or evolving circumstances (Spencer et al., 1996). A key component of adaptive repertoire is an individual's capacity for hindsight and foresight (Kielhofner, 1977). For many refugees and asylum seekers, hindsight is blurred by traumatic experiences and further obscured by the discrepancy between prearrival expectations of a safer and more stable life and the harsh realities of refugee camps and asylum detention (Mayne et al., 2016). On the other hand, foresight is marred by material uncertainties of day-to-day life and not knowing whether asylum will be granted or whether resettlement will be offered. Consequently, their adaptive repertoire is diminished and their capacity for future occupational planning is hindered (Huot et al., 2016; Mayne et al., 2016; H. C. Smith, 2015).

During and After Resettlement

Resettlement and approval of asylum alleviate some of the uncertainties faced by refugees and asylum seekers. However, occupational challenges persist and are exacerbated by various factors. Although resettlement resources and supports vary by destination country, the demand for **occupational adaptation** is a common theme (Suleman & Whiteford, 2013). Refugees and asylees need to adapt to yet another transition in their lives, albeit one ultimately more hopeful. This entails understanding new cultural and social norms, learning the local language, becoming acquainted with the daily rhythms of their adopted country, meeting normative expectations related to occupational roles, and learning how to access public services (Blankvoort, Arslan, et al., 2018). These challenges are intensified for those with complex support needs such as refugees and asylum seekers with disabilities[*] and chronic health conditions. Navigating

[*] Throughout this chapter we use the phrases "disabled persons" and "persons with disabilities" interchangeably out of respect for varying phrasing preferences in different parts of the word.

service systems becomes a necessary occupation for these individuals as they try to make sense of medical insurance regulations for the first time while also figuring out how disability rehabilitation, and other social services are organized in their adopted country (Mirza & Heinemann, 2012; Mirza et al., 2013).

Another challenge faced by newly resettled refugees and asylees is diminished **social capital**, an important precondition for occupational outlets that promotes community participation and social integration (H. C. Smith, 2015). Preresettlement social networks are often disrupted by displacement. Friends and family become separated during flight and tend to be scattered across different refugee camps and asylum countries (Y. J. Smith, 2013; Whiteford, 2005). At the same time, new networks are hard to establish after resettlement and asylum due to language and cultural barriers (Y. J. Smith, 2013).

Resettlement and asylum policies of many Global North countries emphasize social integration through economic participation rather than civic and social participation (Mirza, 2012; Morville & Jessen-Winge, 2019). The pressure for economic participation combined with limited proficiency in the dominant local language and lack of locally relevant work experience compels many refugees and asylees to take on low-paying, meaningless, and unstable jobs (Blankvoort, Arslan, et al., 2018; Gupta & Sullivan, 2008). Opportunities for economic participation can be further constrained by societal racism and negative public discourse and media representation of refugees and asylum seekers (Mayne et al., 2016). Those with professional backgrounds experience a **downward occupational drift** as credentials earned in their home country are not recognized in their country of resettlement and asylum (Blankvoort, Arslan, et al., 2018; Gupta & Sullivan, 2008). Those with agrarian or artisan backgrounds experience difficulty with transferring their skills and marketing their products in their new economic context (Y. J. Smith, 2017; Stephenson et al., 2013).

Those with disabilities are channeled toward welfare programs without regard for their aptitudes and personal

OT STORY 66.1 TEDROS MARKOS TEKLE: "WANT TO GROW AND BE PRODUCTIVE"

Tedros, who is blind, was born in Eritrea, a small country located in the Horn of Africa region. A former Italian, and later British colony, Eritrea was federated to its much larger and more powerful neighbor, Ethiopia, after World War II. After a protracted armed conflict, Eritreans declared independence from Ethiopia in 1993. Ever since the country has been under the control of an authoritarian regime with a history of political repression and human rights abuses against political activists and dissenters.

Despite the political conditions in Eritrea, Tedros was fortunate to get a good education. He earned a bachelor's degree in English and began working as a broadcast journalist. Unfortunately, his job placed him at risk of running afoul of his country's totalitarian leadership. Perceiving a significant threat to his life and well-being, Tedros fled Eritrea and sought asylum in neighboring Ethiopia with his family.

After living in Ethiopia for a few years, Tedros applied for resettlement in the United States. He was 38 years old and without much social support when he was first resettled. Although he had some friends and extended family in the United States, his immediate family was still in Ethiopia. He was mostly independent other than needing occasional help with community mobility. Over time he learned to use the many public transportation options available in the large urban metropolis he was resettled in. A refugee resettlement agency helped him access public benefits including temporary medical insurance and referred him to the Division of Rehabilitation Services. It was then that he encountered OT

services under the auspices of a program focusing on employment supports for disabled refugees. Tedros expressed keen interest in pursuing higher education with a career goal of becoming an assistive technology specialist.

The OT assisted Tedros in achieving his goals by:

- Completing vocational and occupational assessments to help him figure out educational and work options that aligned with his occupational interests
- Connecting him with a local university and helping him apply for a master's degree in rehabilitation counseling
- Referring him to the local Mayor's Office for People with Disabilities for benefits counseling
- Referring him to a local nonprofit organization to seek assistive technology supports

To read more about Tedros' journey, see Expanding Our Perspectives.

Questions

1. What occupational adaptations did Tedros need to make in the early days after resettlement in the United States?
2. What long-term occupational adaptations were important for Tedros?
3. What resources did the occupational therapist use to help Tedros build social capital after resettlement?
4. What else could be done to help Tedros build social capital?

EXPANDING OUR PERSPECTIVES

Tedros' Thoughts on Occupational Therapy for Refugees and Asylees

Tedros Markos Tekle

I landed at O'Hare International Airport on the afternoon of December 19, 2017, jet-lagged from the 23-hour flight. After four years and eight months of protracted security screening and taxing life in exile, I was eventually resettled to the United States.

It was supposedly the beginning of a promising future for someone like me, who was officially resettled to the United States, while at the same time, I was lost in the dark about where to begin. Resettlement agencies make no exception for refugees with disabilities when it comes to educational and employment pathways. In fact, they don't even know how to help refugees with disabilities network with the right resources save the Social Security Administration and the supplemental nutrition assistance program (SNAP) program. Besides being a blind refugee, my work experience and educational background have been of little avail in my quest for gainful employment.

I was introduced to a program—Partners of Refugees in Illinois Disability Employment (PRIDE)—and joined in the final quarter of 2018. PRIDE did its best to familiarize participants with federal and state resources, as well as the rights and responsibilities of employees with disabilities, thereby identifying career and educational pathways for refugees like me. Connections made through PRIDE led me to complete the Leadership Education in Neurodevelopmental and Related Disabilities (LEND) fellowship program in Illinois, and I am now enrolled in the Master's in Rehabilitation Counseling at Northeastern Illinois University.

As an active participant and peer mentor at PRIDE, I was involved in the translation and editing of training materials, mentoring, as well as supervision. I have been participating in various academic and disability-related international conferences, thanks to PRIDE. Trainers at PRIDE were well aware of the fact that a number of refugees immigrated armed with a dependable educational background and employment history. Despite being a well-researched pilot project, where the program fell short was that it was not inherently designed to network participants with employers. Many participants struggled to transition from training to gainful employment. In the future, programs such as PRIDE, and the occupational therapists working in them, should make stronger efforts to connect refugees with disabilities to viable employment opportunities.

goals (Mirza, 2012). Engaging in occupations that are far removed from personal motivation, skills, aptitude, and meaning can lead to prolonged **occupational alienation**. In addition, being unable to meet expectations of economic productivity or having to subsist on welfare support can contribute to social exclusion and perceived stigma (Burchett & Matheson, 2011; Mirza, 2012). Some refugees also experience acculturation challenges that involve negotiation of identities between their culture of origin and that of the adopted country (Jorgenson & Nilsson, 2021). Cumulatively, these experiences negatively affect the personal identity, self-efficacy, and well-being of refugees and asylees (Huot et al., 2016).

Role of Occupational Therapy With Refugees and Asylum Seekers

Working with refugees and asylum seekers is an emerging area of practice in OT. A cross-sectional survey of OT practitioners who have worked with refugees and asylum seekers in Global North countries revealed that most had been working in this practice area for 3 years or less. Many survey respondents shared potential OT interventions that could be useful for refugee and asylee clients but were not implemented likely due to a limited evidence base and established professional guidelines (Trimboli & Halliwell, 2018). Therefore, there is a need to develop and define the role of OT with refugees and asylum seekers. This section offers some suggestions drawn from existing literature in the field.

In Refugee Camps and Asylum Centers

The role of occupational therapists is likely to vary based on temporal and environmental contexts of each individual's displacement trajectory as conditions in refugee camp and asylum centers can vary based on the local and national context. Therefore, it is important for practitioners to begin with a contextual analysis of barriers and opportunities at all three levels of person–environment–occupation. In the preresettlement and preasylum period, when forced migrants are dealing with daily uncertainties, the literature recommends focusing on occupations that promote resilience and build adaptive repertoire for dealing with future transitions (De Koker et al., 2019).

During this time, OT practitioners can provide trauma-informed and creative occupational outlets to promote healing from individual and collective trauma. Occupations such as narrative storytelling, drawing, photography, videography (Moore, 2017), and community theater (Horghagen, & Josephsson, 2010) have been used with migrant youth and adults to facilitate mutual trust, reciprocal empathy, and adaptive occupational patterns. Practitioners can also create opportunities to participate in group-based art projects and team sports to break the tedium of survival occupations, restore occupational balance, and reduce migrants' social isolation (Huot et al., 2016).

The literature also recommends opportunities for altruistic occupations such as mentoring children and youth, caring for fellow refugees and asylum seekers, and volunteering as interpreters or office staff with NGOs managing the camp or asylum center. Occupations that involved "doing for others" offer forced migrants a sense of purpose, social interaction, simulation of work, and an opportunity to practice preemployment skills (Hart, 2019; Ingvarsson et al., 2016; Morville & Erlandsson, 2013; H. C. Smith, 2015). In refugee camps, where physical rehabilitation needs could be significant due to acquired injuries and illnesses (Mirza, 2011), OT might involve more standard interventions such as prescribing and fabricating low-tech adaptive aids, activity adaptations, and environmental modifications combined with biomechanical approaches for remediating limitations in occupational performance. International NGOs such as Humanity & Inclusion, Christian Blind Mission, and the International Rescue Committee have a history of hiring occupational therapists to provide direct rehabilitation services in refugee camps in the Global South (CBM et al., 2021; Handicap International, 2009; Karanja, 2009). Some low-income countries with significant refugee populations have a serious shortage of locally trained rehabilitation professionals. In such a scenario, occupational therapists based in more resourceful areas can offer telerehabilitation services or use a "train the trainer" model to support paraprofessionals or community-based rehabilitation workers to meet the rehabilitation needs in refugee camps (Mitchell-Gillespie et al., 2020). See Figure 66.1 for an example of the "train the trainer" model in practice.

During and After Resettlement

Occupational Therapists as Translators, Matchmakers, and Connectors

Occupational therapists can have instrumental roles in helping refugees and asylees build their new lives in their adopted country once they are granted resettlement or asylum. Blankvoort, Arslan, et al. (2018) suggest three roles for OT practitioners during this critical phase of adjustment. As *translators*, OT practitioners can support refugees and asylees to develop life skills that are building blocks for

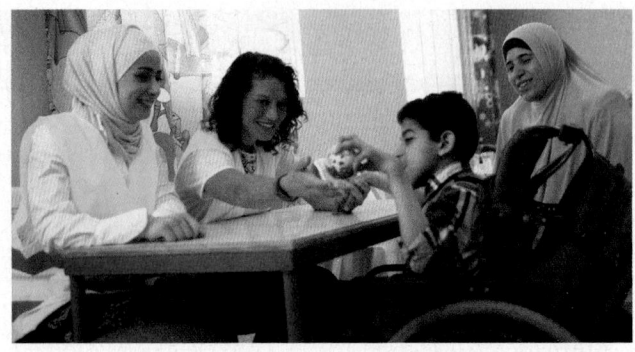

FIGURE 66.1 Occupational therapist and community worker with refugee child in Al Baqa'a refugee camp in Jordan.

occupational adaptations to the host culture and society (Blankvoort, Arslan, et al., 2018). Some occupational therapists (Crandall & Smith, 2015; Gupta & Sullivan, 2008) have developed curricula to help newly resettled refugees practice activities such as becoming familiar with local transportation options, managing time according to local expectations, using unfamiliar home appliances, identifying and safely using household chemicals, shopping in local grocery stores, safely preparing meals by learning to read food labels, and understanding expiry dates. By supporting refugees and asylees with these practical skills, occupational therapists can scaffold their adaptive repertoire for positive occupational transitions (Suleman & Whiteford, 2013).

Occupational therapists can also serve as cultural conduits between refugee families and public services such as schools, libraries, and disability-related social services. Teaching refugees and asylees to navigate these services is a critical precondition for future civic and social participation (Blankvoort, Arslan, et al., 2018; Mirza, 2012; Mirza & Heinemann, 2012). Occupational therapists can also play the role of *matchmaker* by connecting refugees and asylees with educational, vocational, volunteer, and entrepreneurial opportunities that match their prior skills, competencies, and interests and can forge a pathway for future employment (Blankvoort, Arslan, et al., 2018; Gupta & Sullivan, 2008). The matchmaking role also entails orienting refugees and asylees to workplace expectations, training them in résumé writing and interviewing skills customized to their work interests and career goals, and learning proper ergonomics and injury prevention in the workplace (Gupta & Sullivan, 2008). Occupational therapists practicing in school settings can match refugee children and youth to appropriate classroom placements, language training, educational supports, and career counseling based on a comprehensive assessment of their occupational performance related to the student role, their classroom readiness, and family expectations (Copley et al., 2011; Driver & Beltran, 1998).

A third role for occupational therapists in the post-resettlement period is that of *connector* (Blankvoort, Arslan, et al., 2018). As connectors, practitioners can connect refugees and asylees with appropriate local organizations, support groups, and other members of their ethnic community. For example, connecting disabled refugees and asylees with the local disability rights community can serve as a source of empowerment and a gateway to becoming familiar with disability laws and services in their adopted country (Mirza, 2012; Mirza & Heinemann, 2012). Similarly, fostering in-group connections among refugee and asylee communities through culturally cherished co-occupations such as traditional arts and crafts helps them build social networks, sustain cultural identity, and maintain connectivity with their past, all of which can better equip them to handle changing environments and occupational demands (Y. J. Smith et al., 2014; Stephenson et al., 2013).

Advocating for Occupational Justice

The role of OT in forced migration is not confined to direct services and community development. To address the occupational injustices faced by refugees and asylum seekers, the onus is on us as practitioners to "integrate justice with practice" (Sakellariou & Pollard, 2016). Solidarity with refugees and asylees in advocating for justice is a collaborative process. Suggestions for community advocacy include liaising with civil society organizations to promote migrants' rights and more humane asylum practices, reaching out to local politicians such as city mayors and municipal officers and sharing ideas for building inclusive and welcoming communities, and educating the general public about forced migration and occupational injustice through newsletters and podcasts (Trimboli, 2017). At the international level, organizations such as Women's Refugee Commission and Humanity and Inclusion engage in ongoing advocacy efforts to influence global policy frameworks and promote inclusive humanitarian action for displaced populations. Interested practitioners can contact these organizations to inquire how they can support their advocacy work. There is also a need for professional advocacy within the field. Practitioners can appeal to professional organizations of their respective countries to publish a clear statement and practice guidelines on the role of OT with forced migrants. Such a statement would not only support practitioners in their work but also empower them to contribute to policy discussions in their respective countries (Blankvoort, Moore, et al., 2018). Professional organizations can also be petitioned to create special interest groups and communities of practice to foster mutual support and evidence-based practice among occupational therapists working with forced migrants (Blankvoort, Moore, et al., 2018). We also need professional organizations in the field to develop accreditation standards and expanded competencies for working with forced migrants so that future generations of OT practitioners are well prepared to work in this area.

COMMENTARY ON THE EVIDENCE

Over the past two decades, the field has witnessed a growing body of research output on the occupational experiences of forced migrants. Most of this research is observational and exploratory in nature using qualitative research designs such as phenomenology and ethnography. These methodologies have allowed OT scholars to understand the complex experiences of forced migrants while also illuminating the immediate and broader contexts that shape their experiences (Huot & Laliberte Rudman, 2015). An important theme that has emerged across research studies is that refugees and asylum seekers are high-risk population for occupational deprivation and other manifestations of occupational injustice. This research has been critical in informing the role of OT with forced migrants and laying the foundation for OT interventions. However, a few gaps remain in our collective knowledge base indicating important directions for future research.

First, most of the contemporary literature on this topic has been generated by OT scholars for OT audiences (Blankvoort, Arslan, et al., 2018). Therefore, there is a need for more research using participatory and empowerment approaches, with more meaningful involvement of forced migrants and other stakeholders such as ethnic community leaders and providers of resettlement or humanitarian services (Blankvoort, Moore, et al., 2018; Huot & Laliberte Rudman, 2015). Methods such as community-mapping exercises, photovoice, community advisory boards, and nominal group techniques can be particularly useful in identifying community-specific issues and priorities for action.

Second, existing literature on this topic has been largely produced by OT scholars and scientists located in industrialized countries of the Global North. This literature has also mostly focused on refugees, asylees, and asylum seekers who have migrated to Australia, North America, or Western Europe. The field is missing diverse scholarly voices and a better understanding of the occupational experiences of forced migrants living in refugee camps and urban settlements in developing countries in the Global South.

Finally, the field is ready to move onward from exploratory research toward intervention development and

(continued)

> **COMMENTARY ON THE EVIDENCE** (*continued*)

testing. Although a few interventions programs have been developed for forced migrants resettled or granted asylum in Global North countries, these programs have only been evaluated for initial feasibility and acceptability. Therefore, an important direction for future research on this topic is testing occupation-focused interventions for efficacy on outcomes related to occupational performance, social participation, well-being, and quality of life. It is also important to investigate the effectiveness of occupational therapist-led mental health interventions with refugees and asylum seekers (Trimboli & Halliwell, 2018). Longitudinal studies that track sustained effects of occupation-focused interventions, and the role of related environmental factors,

in the long-term integration of forced migrants would also be helpful. Consolidating the OT evidence base in this area is important for informing future practice. It is also important that emerging efficacy research be disseminated both inside and outside the field via diverse channels including peer-reviewed journals, social media, news media, infographics, and podcasts. Disseminating our evidence-based interventions widely is critical for proving the unique contribution of occupational therapy in this area (Trimboli et al., 2019).

Table 66.2 provides an overview of the available research studies on this topic and their most relevant findings.

TABLE 66.2 | **Summary of the Evidence for Occupational Therapy and Forced Migration**

Citation	Study Aims	Target Population/Study Sample	Study Design	Main/Relevant Findings
Alve (in press)	To understand how refugees experience and make meaning of participation in everyday occupations while living in refugee camps	Rohingya refugees Country of resettlement/asylum: Bangladesh Country of origin: Myanmar	Qualitative, observational, phenomenology In-depth interviews and participant observations with 15 participants	Adverse environmental conditions and mental stressors inhibited performance of daily occupations, disrupted family relationships, and restricted occupational engagement and social roles. Both occupational adaptations (forming new relationships, spiritual activities, helping others) and maladaptations (engaging in unlawful and precarious occupations for survival) were noted.
Bishop and Purcell (2013)	To explore how participation in a horticultural allotment group affects feelings of health, well-being, and social inclusion for refugees and asylum seekers	Working age refugees and asylum seekers Country of resettlement/asylum: United Kingdom Countries of origin: not specified	Qualitative, observational, ethnography Semi-structured interviews, photo-elicited interviews and participant observations with five participants	Horticulture was deemed a meaningful occupation that facilitated social cohesion with other refugees and asylum seekers. Attending the horticultural group mitigated negative effects of everyday uncertainties on well-being.
Burchett and Matheson (2011)	To explore the effects of UK government restrictions on paid employment for asylum seekers	An asylum seeker who had transitioned to refugee status Country of resettlement/asylum: United Kingdom Country of origin: not specified	Qualitative, observational, grounded theory In-depth unstructured and semi-structured interviews with one participant	Government restrictions on employment led to sense of lacking control and compelled the participant to relinquish career goals. Motivation for occupational endeavors moved from self-enhancement to survival and providing for her family. Joining a refugee group brought a sense of shared experiences and relatability. However, being categorized as a refugee also brought social exclusion and perceived stigma.

TABLE 66.2	Summary of the Evidence for Occupational Therapy and Forced Migration (*continued*)			
Citation	**Study Aims**	**Target Population/ Study Sample**	**Study Design**	**Main/Relevant Findings**
Copley et al. (2011)	To develop and evaluate an occupational therapy program with high school students from refugee backgrounds	High school refugee students Country of resettlement/ asylum: Australia Country of origin: not specified	Qualitative, program development and evaluation, action research In-depth interviews with four occupational therapists, seven school staff members and two school principals Review of meeting minutes	School staff found the program to be beneficial and noted improvements in the behavior and classroom readiness of students. In response to student needs, teacher concerns, and school culture, the program evolved in focus from mastery of classroom-based tasks to development of skills to support classroom participation. The service team consulted with teachers to distinguish professional occupational therapy services from volunteer support.
Crawford et al. (2016)	To explore whether and how citizenship structures and policies contribute to occupational deprivation for asylum seekers	Asylum seekers who had previously lived in detention centers Country of resettlement/ asylum: Australia Country of origin: not specified	Qualitative, observational, constructivist grounded theory Participant observations, formal interviews with seven asylum seekers, informal interviews with three key informants, online survey with 34 service providers and document analysis of four policy documents	Study findings lend credence to the theory of Structural–Personal Interaction. Asylum policies shape the living conditions of asylum seekers. Policies and social structures that constrain the freedom of choice and movement of asylum seekers interact with personal experiences of trauma, discrimination, and stigma and contribute to asylum seekers' occupational deprivation.
Driver and Beltran (1998)	To explore refugee children's experience of traumatic events and how these experiences affect their occupational role as school students	Recently resettled refugee children (6–12 years) with past experience of trauma Country of resettlement/ asylum: Australia Country of origin: Bosnia, El Salvador, Iraq, Lebanon	Qualitative, observational, unspecified Participant observations and semi-structured interviews with five children, seven teachers, and four parents	Children demonstrated difficulty with performing tasks associated with the student role such as handwriting, reading, and homework. These difficulties were associated with limitations in performance components such as fine motor coordination, concentration, and social interaction. The home and school environment and expectations of parents and teachers affected children's adaptive response. Children were able to adapt better when their family was stable and received emotional, practical and financial support after arrival to Australia.
Hart (2019)	To explore the meaning of occupation for refugees and asylum seekers	Refugees and asylum seekers Country of resettlement/ asylum: United Kingdom Countries of origin: not specified (in the Middle East & Africa)	Qualitative, observational, phenomenology Up to three conversational interviews with 10 participants	Participants had limited opportunities for meaningful everyday occupation due to restrictions and uncertainties in the asylum process. Paid work and altruistic activities (volunteering, mentoring) were highly valued. Being busy with meaningful work provided structure and a sense of well-being. On occasion, exploitative occupations such as illicit jobs or sex work were undertaken for survival.

(continued)

TABLE 66.2	Summary of the Evidence for Occupational Therapy and Forced Migration (*continued*)			
Citation	**Study Aims**	**Target Population/ Study Sample**	**Study Design**	**Main/Relevant Findings**
Horghagen and Josephsson (2010)	To understand how theater as an occupation can promote asylum seekers' participation in other spheres of life	Asylum seekers living in a reception center Country of resettlement/ asylum: Norway Countries of origin: not specified (in Asia & Africa)	Qualitative, observational, ethnography Participant observations with 11 participants	The theatre project allowed participants to occupy a space outside the reception center, to develop their capacities, to identify shared resources, and change destructive occupational patterns. The project also facilitated mutual trust and respect and provided opportunities for asylum seekers to share their experiences with local Norwegians.
Huot et al. (2016)	To synthesize available knowledge related to the occupational experiences of forcibly displaced individuals	Refugees, asylees, and asylum seekers Countries of resettlement/ asylum: Australia, Austria, Denmark, Norway, Sweden, United Kingdom, United States Countries of origin: Afghanistan, Bhutan, Chile, Cambodia, Iran, Kosovo, Myanmar, Somalia, Thailand, Uganda	Scoping Review 24 studies	There is a dynamic interplay between occupational experiences and sense of identity among forcibly displaced individuals. Institutional limitations and resource constraints in host countries create conditions of occupational deprivation and occupational imbalance. Individuals adapt through occupational change, sometimes imposed, and sometimes welcomed. Future uncertainty can create a sense of hopelessness and daily instability especially for asylum seekers.
Ingvarsson et al. (2016)	To understand lived experiences of asylum seekers in Iceland	Asylum seekers Country of resettlement/ asylum: Iceland Countries origin: Afghanistan, Iraq, Iran	Qualitative, observational, grounded theory Semi-structured interviews with seven asylum seekers/asylees and two advocates	Participants had limited opportunities to engage in meaningful occupations dues to long processing time of their asylum applications, difficult living conditions, and legal restrictions on employment. Being dependent on social service assistance and being deprived of social integration negatively affected self-esteem and well-being. Volunteer opportunities offered purpose, social interaction, and simulation of work.
Mayne et al. (2016)	To explore existing literature on how Australian discursive climate affects the occupational experiences of refugees and asylum seekers	Refugees and asylum seekers Country of resettlement/ asylum: Australia Countries of origin: not specified	Narrative review 42 articles	Prearrival perceptions of potential occupational opportunities in Australia are countered by the reality of indefinite mandatory detention policies. Establishment and restructuring of occupational routines and habits are important during the immediate transition period postarrival. It requires adaptation to a wide range of new information. Opportunities and support for occupational engagement are linked with public discourse and media representation of refugees and asylum seekers.

TABLE 66.2	**Summary of the Evidence for Occupational Therapy and Forced Migration (*continued*)**			
Citation	**Study Aims**	**Target Population/ Study Sample**	**Study Design**	**Main/Relevant Findings**
Mirza (2012)	To explore how resettlement policies and practices in the United States support or restrict the occupational participation of disabled refugees	Refugees with disabilities resettled in the United States Country of resettlement/ asylum: United States Countries of origin: Cambodia, Somalia	Qualitative, observational, ethnography In-depth interviews with 15 disabled refugees Semi-structured interviews with 10 key experts Documentary analysis and observations	The US refugee resettlement program emphasizes economic self-sufficiency and paid work as a rite of passage for resettled refugees. This places disabled refugees often perceived as "nonemployable" at risk of occupational deprivation and limits their opportunities for social and civic participation.
Mirza and Heinemann (2012)	To examine how health and social service systems address the needs of refugees with disabilities			Disability and refugee service systems operate within their respective silos. Refugee service providers have a limited understanding of disability whereas disability service providers have a limited ability to respond to refugees' cross-cultural needs. These factors, along with resource limitations within service agencies, contribute to unmet needs among refugees with disabilities.
Mirza et al. (2013)	To identify healthcare access barriers affecting disabled and chronically ill refugees	Refugees with disabilities and chronic conditions resettled in the United States Country of resettlement/ asylum: United States Countries origin: Iraq, Myanmar, Bhutan	Qualitative, observational, (unspecified) using a CBPR approach Semi-structured interviews with 18 participants including refugee service providers and refugee community leaders	Barriers were identified at the individual, provider, and systems levels. These barriers included inadequate health insurance, unmet language and communication needs during healthcare encounters, and difficulty navigating complex health and social services systems. Newly resettled refugees with complex health conditions need support with the occupation of "navigating healthcare."
Morville and Erlandsson (2013)	To explore how asylum seekers living in an asylum center experience occupational deprivation, and how their past experiences affect value and choice of occupations	Asylum seeking men living in asylum centers run by the Danish Red Cross Country of resettlement/ asylum: Denmark Countries of origin: Afghanistan, Iran	Qualitative, observational, unspecified In-depth interviews and observations with three asylum seekers	Participants experienced occupational deprivation due to restricted living conditions in the asylum center. They were able to engage in some occupations that were based on past experiences. However, engaging in these occupations was more of a coping strategy than a sustainable means of deriving personal relevance and expressing competence.

(continued)

| TABLE 66.2 | Summary of the Evidence for Occupational Therapy and Forced Migration (*continued*) | | | |

Citation	Study Aims	Target Population/ Study Sample	Study Design	Main/Relevant Findings
Morville, Erlandsson, et al. (2015)	To describe asylum seekers' satisfaction with daily occupations and activity levels and to investigate whether these are associated with self-rated health, exposure to torture, and ADL skills	Asylum seekers living in a reception center run by the Danish Red Cross Country of resettlement/ asylum: Denmark Countries of origin: Afghanistan, Syria, Iran	Quantitative, observational, correlational Self-report questionnaires and observation-based ADL assessment completed with 43 asylum seekers at baseline and repeated with 17 asylum seekers after 10 months	Asylum seekers experienced low levels of satisfaction with daily occupations at both baseline and follow-up. There was a decrease in ADL ability, self-rated health, and an increase in depression and pain over the 10-month study period. At baseline, associations were noted between ADL ability and satisfaction with daily occupations and activity levels. Pain intensity and education were also associated with activity levels. At follow-up, associations were found between self-rated well-being and satisfaction with daily occupations. Well-being and depression were also found to be associated with activity levels.
Morville, Amris, et al. (2015)	To assess change in ADL ability of asylum seekers over a 10-month period, and to determine whether this change was associated with self-reported health and exposure to torture			ADL motor and process ability scores declined significantly over time while self-reported pain and depression increased. A significant association was found between change in ADL motor ability and exposure to physical torture, and between change in ADL process ability and change in pain. Pain and prior torture could be prognostic indicators of ADL impairment and some asylum seekers might need assistance with community living.
Morville and Jessen-Winge (2019)	To understand ideas for, and problems with, social inclusion from the perspective of an asylum seeker	An asylum seeker living in a reception center run by the Danish Red Cross Country of resettlement/ asylum: Denmark Country of origin: not specified	Qualitative, observational, phenomenology Open-ended interviews with one asylum seeker Analysis of articles and letters written by the participant	Social inclusion was hindered by living conditions in the reception center (e.g., lack of access to information, lack of daily structure) and subjective reactions (e.g., mistrust of authorities, unfamiliarity with local cultural norms). Social inclusion could be facilitated by building social networks among asylum seekers and Danes, forming a representative residents' council at the center, and creating opportunities for asylum seekers to develop vocational skills while waiting for asylum.
Schisler and Polatajko (2002)	To explore changes in the daily occupations of refugees and asylum seekers after they relocate to a new environment	English-speaking adult refugees and asylum seekers in Canada Country of resettlement/ asylum: Canada Country of origin: Burundi	Qualitative, observational, ethnography Participant observations and in-depth interviews with eight participants	Relocating to a new country instigates significant occupational changes. Although these changes are triggered by environmental factors, they are mediated by individuals themselves as they make occupational choices based on their personal values, preferences, cultural practices, and expectations, opportunities, and constraints of their new society.

TABLE 66.2	Summary of the Evidence for Occupational Therapy and Forced Migration (*continued*)			
Citation	**Study Aims**	**Target Population/ Study Sample**	**Study Design**	**Main/Relevant Findings**
Y. J. Smith (2013)	To understand the social networks of Somali Bantu refugees	Somali Bantu refugees Country of resettlement/ asylum: United States Country of origin: Somalia	Qualitative, observational, grounded theory Semi-structured interviews and participant observations with 11 participants	Social network patterns influenced participants' occupational engagement and adaptation. Participants strove to sustain traditionally strong social support systems which were disrupted by displacement and resettlement. Social connections beyond the refugee community were important to advance skills and enriching occupational engagement.
H. C. Smith (2015)	To explore individuals' experience and meaning-making of occupation during their forced displacement journeys	Refugees, asylees, and asylum seekers in the United Kingdom Country of resettlement/ asylum: United Kingdom Countries of origin: a range of nations in Africa and the Middle East	Qualitative, observational, phenomenology In-depth interviews with 10 participants	Productive and meaningful daily routines were disrupted or restricted by displacement and the asylum process. This affected participants' self-worth, physical and mental health. Societal racism, cultural adaptations, language barriers, and lack of social capital played a role in day-to-day material survival and future planning.
Y. J. Smith (2017)	To understand why refugee youth choose to participate in a traditional dance activity	Refugee youth of Karen ethnicity Country of resettlement/ asylum: United States Country of origin: Burma/Myanmar	Qualitative, observational, grounded theory Coconstructed interviews and participant observations with eight youth dancers and two adult organizers	Participation in the dance activity fostered inner strength and confidence. The dance group also served as a means for constructing and maintaining cultural identity, which was deemed important for in-group and external social inclusion.
Steindl et al. (2008)	To explore women's experience of engaging in daily occupations while living in a refugee camp in Austria	Women living in a refugee camp Countries of resettlement/ asylum: Austria Countries of origin: Georgia, Russia, Azerbaijan	Qualitative, observational, ethnography Open-ended interviews and observations with seven refugee women Review of camp rules and regulations	Institutional rules compromised choice, personal decision-making, and engagement in meaningful occupations. Daily occupations were influenced by past habits and values and seen as a conduit toward a better future.
Stephenson et al. (2013)	To explore the meaning of traditional weaving as an occupation for refugee women from Burma/ Myanmar	Refugee women of Karen ethnicity Country of resettlement/ asylum: United States Country of origin: Burma/Myanmar	Qualitative, observational, ethnography One focus group and in-depth, semi-structured interviews with eight participants	Traditional weaving was an avenue to sustain cultural identity, build social support and pursue entrepreneurship. Participants were able to integrate their traditions with their new culture by adapting woven products to US consumer preferences. Language barriers and limited financial literacy hindered participants' ability to market and sell products.

(continued)

| TABLE 66.2 | Summary of the Evidence for Occupational Therapy and Forced Migration (continued) | | | |

Citation	Study Aims	Target Population/ Study Sample	Study Design	Main/Relevant Findings
Trimboli and Halliwell (2018)	To identify interventions used by occupational therapy practitioners with refugees and asylum seekers	OT practitioners working with refugees and asylum seekers Countries represented: Australia, Canada, Germany, Netherlands, United Kingdom, United States	Quantitative, observational, descriptive Cross-sectional survey with 29 respondents	Majority of respondents had been working in this practice area for three years or less. Respondents spent most time on the following interventions during a typical week: writing/documentation; education; and leisure integration. Interventions deemed useful but not implemented frequently included: addressing sexuality, forming support groups, driving assessment and practice, home visits, and self-care
Trimboli et al. (2021)	To identify and summarize psychosocial interventions for middle childhood and to determine their effectiveness	6- to 12-year-old children who have been forcibly displaced Countries represented: United Kingdom, Turkey, Canada, Bosnia-Herzegovina, United States, Sri Lanka, Thailand, Sierra Leone, Uganda, Ethiopia, Sweden, and Germany	Systematic Review and Meta-Analysis 19 studies	None of the interventions identified were grounded in or informed by occupational therapy. Some promising interventions such as child-centered play and creative activities could fall under the domain of OT practice. Outcomes evaluated by studies focused on alleviation of symptoms of psychological distress and behavioral difficulties. Outcomes related to overall well-being and occupational participation/ performance were not addressed.
Whiteford (2005)	To understand occupational deprivation from the perspective of a refugee's lived experience	Australian citizen with prior refugee status Country of resettlement/ asylum: Australia Country of origin: Kosovo	Qualitative, observational, case study In-depth interview with one participant	Occupational deprivation occurred throughout the participant's displacement journey and was augmented by the legal and political context of displacement, asylum, and resettlement. Trauma and dislocation hindered engagement in basic survival occupations and had a lasting impact on personal and social stability. Occupational engagement in communities of interest was a source of comfort.

Examples of Occupational Therapy Programs With Forced Migrants

Occupational Therapy as Part of Integrated Services in a Refugee Camp

Occupational therapists like Ariful Islam Arman and Mohammad Monjurul Habib have played an important role in the rehabilitation of disabled refugees sheltering in camps in southeastern Bangladesh after fleeing escalating brutality in Rakhine State along the western coast of Myanmar. Practitioners work at health centers or as part of multidisciplinary home-based rehabilitation teams and are involved in conducting initial and discharge evaluations, training therapy assistants, assessing and fitting clients for appropriate assistive devices. Therapy sessions in this context often involve low-cost, homemade solutions, for example, bottle caps being used to practice fine motor skills. Training caregivers in hands-on home exercises, practicing transfers, and so on, is also an integral part of OT services considering high needs and inadequate number of trained professionals.

In addition, occupational therapists are responsible for assessing the accessibility of shelters and community spaces such as pathways, and shared water, sanitation, and hygiene facilities. Working with engineers and humanitarian professionals, occupational therapists offer innovative accessibility solutions and adaptations to facilitate participation of camp residents with disabilities. See Figure 66.2 for an example of promoting community accessibility in a refugee camp. Occupational therapists are also involved in conducting awareness-raising sessions on disability prevention and disability etiquette for caregivers and community members and also building the capacity of therapy assistants and community mobilizers. Additional roles for occupational therapists in this setting include project design and management and working as inclusion officers. In this capacity, occupational therapists conduct trainings and provide onsite technical support on disability inclusion in various areas of humanitarian intervention including health, water supply, sanitation, hygiene, and protection. Topographical barriers and humanitarian challenges in this setting compel occupational therapists to be more adaptive, think critically, and more resourceful when providing services in the context of limited resources and complex emergencies.

Occupational Therapy Programs in Asylum Centers

De Koker et al. (2019) describe the unique role of OT as part of a multidisciplinary team at a Belgian asylum center. The OT program is targeted at 6- to 12-year-old children living at the center who are unable to enroll in local schools due to restrictive policies. Drawing upon the Occupational Performance Process Model, and informed by feedback from parents, children, and staff, the program focuses on preparing children for future school placement and classroom participation. OT students work with children and families to cultivate several preparatory skills and behaviors. For example, children are engaged in structured activities with a high likelihood of success to promote self-esteem and a sense of security. Nonverbal creative activities such as shadow puppets, painting, drawing, and building models are used to foster emotional expression and communicate future hopes. Group play using developmentally appropriate toys and games is used to foster social interaction skills and a healthy relationship with toys, which many children had to leave behind during flight. Timely attendance, clean-up, and respectful communication are encouraged to help children develop classroom-appropriate behaviors. Activity sessions also incorporate writing and arithmetic practice and homework assignments to prepare children for formal education (De Koker et al., 2019). See Figure 66.3 for an example of art-based group activity with refugee children.

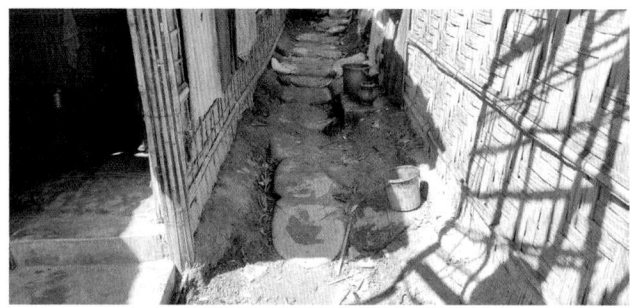

A

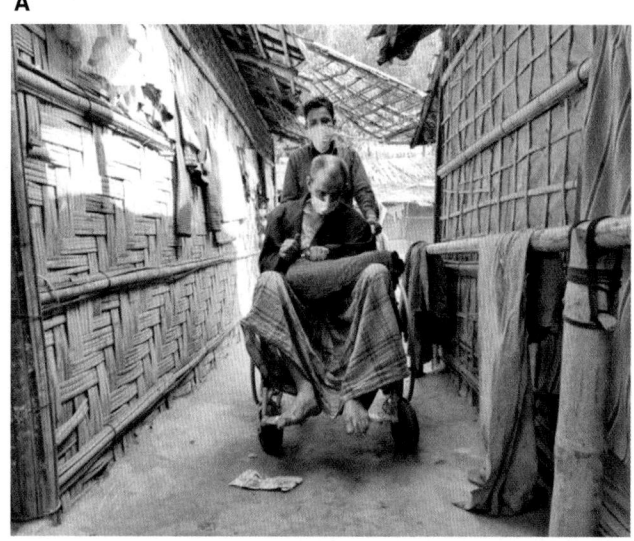

B

FIGURE 66.2 Pathway in refugee camp in Bangladesh. Before (**A**) and after (**B**) modifications.

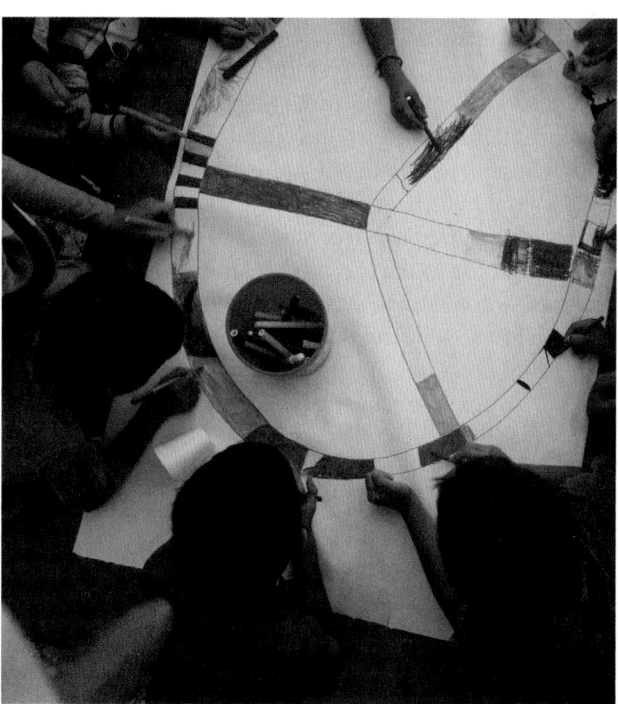

FIGURE 66.3 Designing a peace symbol with children in a refugee camp in Greece.

Occupational therapist Temple Moore (2017) has developed and implemented a strengths-based narrative storytelling program for unaccompanied refugee minors living in a shelter in Greece. The program used an OT approach informed by principles of trauma-informed recovery to promote healing and healthy identity development among teenage boys. The story-telling curriculum was designed to scaffold the boys' ability to explore their strengths and attributes while reflecting on their origins, their displacement journeys, and their hopes for the future. The program began by creating a safe space for the boys to share their stories that are audio recorded. These recordings were used to guide written accounts, illustrations, and photographs depicting each participant's story. The boys then participated in workshops where they are trained in digital photography and video editing. The final product was an audio slideshow that could be shared online with friends or family. The program was well received and garnered positive feedback. It provided participants with a safe structure and space for connecting with their past and envisioning a future while also learning new skills such as using sophisticated camera equipment and video editing software (Moore, 2017).

Community-Based Occupational Therapy Programs to Support Resettlement and Integration in a New Country

Multiple programs have been developed by OT practitioners working in Global North countries that offer resettlement and asylum to forced migrants. These programs demonstrate how occupational therapists can play the role of translators, matchmakers, and connectors (Blankvoort, Arslan, et al., 2018) to support community participation and social integration of forced migrants in a new country.

Jennifer Crandall's (Crandall & Smith, 2015) "Life Skills Program" is an effective example of the translator role. The program has been offered since 2014 under the auspices of a faith-based nonprofit organization in the southwestern US state of Arizona. The program is offered in conjunction with weekly English as second language lessons and gives participants an opportunity to practice their English skills while adapting to occupations of daily living in their new context. For example, one session involves a group outing to a local grocery store with instructions and guidance to complete specific tasks such as scouring the store brochure to identify items on sale, selecting needed items and determining their price, asking for assistance with locating items, and making the final purchase. Thus, participants learn English words for common grocery items while practicing all the steps involved in grocery shopping. Other sessions in the program focus on activities to improve general health and well-being, safe cooking with new ingredients and unfamiliar kitchen appliances, safe use of cleaning equipment and chemicals, and becoming familiar with local vegetation and wildlife (Crandall & Smith, 2015).

The matchmaker role of occupational therapists is aptly exemplified by Breakout Café, an innovative nonprofit coffee shop in Berlin that provides vocational training opportunities for vulnerable youth, mainly refugees and asylees. The café project was launched with the help of local government funding by an interdisciplinary group of professional volunteers. Berlin-based occupational therapist Sarah Novak played an important role in developing the café's occupation-focused model based on the recognition that young refugees and asylees have few opportunities to engage in meaningful income-generating occupations and develop preparatory work skills and behaviors (Blankvoort, Moore, et al., 2018). The café provides a 6-month employment and vocational training stint in the food industry and restaurant business. Professional volunteers also support employees' career goals by connecting them with further educational and job opportunities aligned with their respective interests (Blankvoort, Moore, et al., 2018). An additional goal of the café is to connect refugees and asylees with their neighborhood and its people by encouraging participation in neighborhood events such as holiday markets, art exhibitions, and musical shows (Scheer et al., 2020).

There are multiple practice examples of occupational therapists working with forced migrants that demonstrate the connector role of OT. OT practitioner and educator, Yda Smith, has worked with students at the University of Utah to develop programs that restore traditional occupations and facilitate connectedness among refugees resettled in the United States. For example, a traditional weaving group was established for women of the Karen ethnic group from Myanmar as a culturally rooted creative outlet and as an activity for income generation (Y. J. Smith et al., 2013). Dr. Smith and her students have also supported community garden projects by connecting former refugees who had a farming background to gardening programs, teaching them how to procure needed supplies, access the garden through public transportation, cultivate familiar vegetables, and sell their produce to generate supplemental income for their family and decrease potential food insecurity. Both programs offered participating refugees a social network, a sense of accomplishment, and gave them the opportunity to restore a highly valued aspect of their cultural identity (Stephenson et al., 2013).

Another example of the connector role comes from the work of occupational therapist Mary Black, at the Heartland Alliance Marjorie Kovler Center, a community-based treatment program in the US Midwest that works with survivors of state-sponsored torture (Black, 2010). The majority of Kovler clients are asylum seekers who live

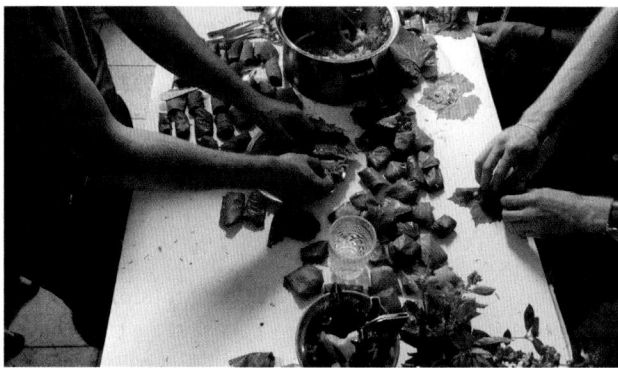

FIGURE 66.4 International cooking group at the Kovler Center.

in the community but have very limited access to public benefits and long waits for work authorization, often "doubled up" in housing or homeless shelters. The Kovler Center uses a trauma-informed approach to healing based on Judith Herman's model of trauma and recovery (Herman, 2015). Services focus on promoting safety, reconnection, and reconstruction to counter the risks of isolation caused by trauma (Gorman, 2001). OT is an integral part of the healing model focused on reclaiming voice, rebuilding community, and maximizing clients' strengths skills and interests (Fabri, 2001). In addition to one-on-one OT services, community-based groups include an international cooking group, community gardening, photovoice, and excursions to a rural organic farm, all with the goals of fostering safety, social connections, and respite from intrusive traumatic memories through engagement in meaningful self-identified occupations. The international cooking group, initiated 15 years ago, is a striking example of nurturing social connection through the universal and unifying tradition of preparing a communal meal (see Figure 66.4). Participants take turns preparing cuisine from their home countries with selected ingredients of their choice. Groups comprising adults, children, and guests all help with the meal preparation while buoyant music streams, often inspiring spontaneous dance and song. The ritual of making and sharing global cuisines not only provides welcome nutrition but also encourages pride, rekindles positive memories, and creates new community connections, purpose, and belonging.

Occupational Therapy's Role in Promoting Community Development, Systemic Change, and Human Rights

The occupation-based community development (ObCD) framework (Galvaan & Peters, 2017a) offers a useful guide for conceptualizing practice promoting occupational justice and social inclusion among marginalized communities including refugees, asylum seekers, and other migrants. Drawing on interdisciplinary theories, including occupational science, the ObCD framework focuses on collaboratively identifying possible points of leverage for change through shared understandings with marginalized groups of the limitations on occupational engagement (Galvaan, 2021). Participatory processes of change are facilitated in iterative phases of Initiating, Design, Implementing, Monitoring, Reflection, and Evaluation. Through partnerships with refugees, asylees, and key stakeholders, actions are taken to mitigate systemic, environmental, and individual factors limiting participation and social inclusion (Galvaan & Peters, 2017b). This could, for example, include addressing prejudices and xenophobic attitudes toward refugees and asylum seekers.

OT practitioners have also played a role in promoting systemic change so that refugees and asylees are better supported in countries of resettlement and asylum. The Partners of Refugees in Illinois Disability Employment (PRIDE) project based in the US state of Illinois is a pertinent example. This 3-year project was funded by the US federal government to support working-age refugees with disabilities to navigate employment resources and services and find meaningful pathways to employment using culturally and linguistically appropriate approaches (Hasnain et al., 2020). Although the overall project was interdisciplinary, bridging the fields of OT and disability studies, occupational therapists contributed significantly to its leadership, development, and implementation. Further, PRIDE's many goals and activities were jointly informed by the Social Ecological Model of Human Development (Bronfenbrenner, 1977) and the Participatory Occupational Justice Framework (Whiteford & Townsend, 2011). Multiple systemic issues that constrain disabled refugees' participation in income-generating occupations were identified and addressed by the PRIDE project. For example, partnerships were established with local disability service providers such as the Mayor's Office for People with Disabilities and the Division of Rehabilitation Services, a state agency that sponsors vocational rehabilitation programs related to employment, education, and independent living opportunities for people with disabilities. Through these partnerships, the PRIDE team strove to sensitize disability service providers to the plight of disabled refugees and helped them identify strategies to better meet refugees' cultural and language needs. To address limited disability awareness among refugee service providers, online training modules were developed focusing on disability rights and local disability services. These modules were disseminated among staff at refugee resettlement agencies to build their capacity for serving disabled refugees and to facilitate referrals to mainstream disability support services.

An information technology application was also developed to improve communication between disability and refugee service providers and to facilitate referral and tracking of refugee participants to employment supports and services (Mirza et al., 2020). Efforts were also made to raise consciousness of the broader community by creating and disseminating video testimonials of disabled refugees and service providers who participated in the PRIDE program.

The work of Theo Bogeas in Greece is an inspiring example of how OT practitioners can engage in human rights and occupational rights advocacy for forced migrants. Theo is a former manager at Human Rights 360, a nonprofit organization focused on protecting and empowering vulnerable populations, including forced migrants. The organization's many efforts include legal representation and consultation for victims of racist violence, monitoring and publishing reports on human rights violations in border areas, writing letters to and filing reports with the National Commission for Human Rights in Greece and similar European bodies, and media campaigns to counter negative stereotypes and dispel misinformation about forced migrants. Through his work in refugee camps, community centers, and NGOs, Theo discovered that by being the local, the professional, and the native speaker, he had important assets that he could incorporate in supporting the human rights of forced migrants: from escorting a refugee to a public service in order to issue a document to becoming the witness of a discriminatory behavior or mal-implementation of regulations that was reported to the local Citizen's Ombudsman. Reflexivity is one of the most valuable tools in this work that helped Theo understand the impact of societal and institutional barriers on the social inclusion and integration of forced migrants.

Opportunities for Student Engagement

Placement of OT students in forced migration settings appears to be a growing trend in the field (Trimboli & Halliwell, 2018). Such placements offer mutually beneficial opportunities where students can provide much needed community- and occupation-based programming to forced migrants under the supervision of seasoned practitioners while also building skills such as flexibility, person-centered practice, trauma-informed care, and community advocacy. Competencies needed for working with refugees and asylum seekers are outlined in Box 66.2.

Since 2004, OT students at the University of Utah have been providing life skill training for newly arrived refugees in collaboration with a local refugee resettlement agency in Salt Lake City, in the western United States. In this community-based setting, students are assigned adult individuals or couples to work with but often find that they end up working with the entire family. Common areas addressed include budgeting, bill paying, keeping track of appointments, public transportation use, home maintenance, medication management, and health system navigation. Students are also called on to help clients learn how to manage health issues such as diabetes and high blood pressure. At times, they work with children who have sensory processing disorders or developmental delays or with adults who have cognitive or orthopedic impairments as a result of traumatic injuries.

Activity analysis, development of creative intervention strategies, therapeutic-use-of-self, and culturally responsive care are utilized extensively in this learning environment (Y. J. Smith et al., 2014). Students gain an understanding of

---

BOX 66.2 COMPETENCIES FOR WORKING WITH REFUGEES AND ASYLUM SEEKERS

- Conceptual knowledge of structural racism and occupational justice (Blankvoort, Moore, et al., 2018)
- Up-to-date information about contemporary conflict situations resulting in mass human displacement
- Understanding of the global humanitarian regime including the role of the United Nations High Commissioner for Refugees and international NGOs
- Familiarity with country-level resettlement and asylum policies including systemic exclusionary practices (Blankvoort, Moore, et al., 2018)
- Awareness of how forced migration diminishes occupational roles, personal choice, and decision-making, followed by a willingness to challenge personal biases and normative assumptions about occupational roles and personal volition (Blankvoort, Arslan, et al., 2018)

- Exposure to cross-cultural practice and working with language interpreters (Blankvoort, Moore, et al., 2018)
- Proficiency in trauma-informed care including ability to recognize vicarious trauma, compassion fatigue, and burnout for service providers (Moore, 2017)
- Adaptability, flexibility, and resourcefulness toward developing ad hoc interventions at short notice as opportunities become available (De Koker et al., 2019)
- An enterprising spirit and strong networking skills for building relationships with a variety of stakeholders including governmental agencies, civic officials, NGOs, and local businesses (De Koker et al., 2019)
- Acceptance of multidisciplinary contributions to this practice area and readiness for interdisciplinary teamwork (Blankvoort, Moore, et al., 2018)

world conflicts that create refugees, local community resources, and see firsthand the occupational injustices that so many of their clients are dealing with. OT students inevitably end up experiencing what it is to be an advocate, teaching refugees how to communicate their needs to landlords, their children's schoolteachers, and many others in the systems they must engage with.

Similar to the program in Utah, Toward an All-Inclusive Jordan is an educational program that offers students in rehabilitation disciplines, including OT, opportunities for year-round placement in pro bono clinics in refugee camps in Jordan. This program, initiated in 2017, is built on an academic-community-based rehabilitation partnership model, where the community partner (United Nations Relief and Works Agency for Palestinian Refugees in the Near East) identifies annual priorities, and the academic team executes those priorities accordingly (AlHeresh & Cahn, 2020). This program focuses on grassroots community engagement. Community health workers and caregivers of children with disabilities are trained on conducting simple rehabilitation interventions themselves (such as adapting to the home environment, stretching, and strengthening through play activities), in the absence of structured services in refugee camps. OT students are paired with Jordanian OT volunteers and community workers and engage as trainers in elective coursework and doctorate capstone projects. Training themes have included topics such as inclusive education, unpacking autism, and milestones of normal child development through 330 one-on-one training sessions, 10 community workshops, and engagement of 40 US-based students and professionals in Jordan.

Networking and Communities of Practice

Creating and engaging in communities of practice is important in any area of OT practice, but perhaps even more so in role-emerging areas. Occupational therapists and OT students already involved in areas of forced migration have identified that while this area of practice is interesting and rewarding, there are various challenges. These challenges include being the sole occupational therapists, working in systems that can be unpredictable due to policy and resourcing constraints, lack of evidence to guide best practice, and often working with people who have experienced or witnessed trauma, thus being susceptible to vicarious trauma and burnout (Trimboli & Halliwell, 2018). Communities of practice are one way that occupational therapists and OT students working or interested in the area of forced migration can connect, network, and discuss particular topics; share information, tips, and best practice; and provide collegial support.

One such community of practice is "forcedmigration4OT" a Facebook page with over 500 members and four administrator volunteers from three countries. The mission behind "forcedmigration4OT" is to provide a safe space for OT practitioners to share knowledge and resources, ask questions, and disseminate relevant products, presentations, and publications on the topic of forced migration and OT. Additional country-specific communities of practice and networking opportunities are listed in Box 66.3.

BOX 66.3 NETWORKING OPPORTUNITIES AND COMMUNITIES OF PRACTICE

- **Australia:** OT Australia Special Interest Group
    https://otaus.com.au/member-resources/interest-groups/refugee-settlement
- **Canada:** Occupational Justice for Newcomers Network
    https://www.caot.ca/site/pd/otn/nn?nav=sidebar
- **Cyprus:** Bridging Occupational Gaps with Refugees and Asylum Seekers: Occupational Therapy with Refugees and Asylum Seekers as part of Clinical Practice of the Occupational Therapy Programme, European University Cyprus
    https://www.facebook.com/OccupationalTherapyWithRefugeesAndAsylumSeekers/
- **Council of Occupational Therapists for European Countries (COTEC):** Occupational Therapy with Displaced Persons Interest Group
    https://www.coteceurope.eu/ot-europe/ot-europe-interest-group-on-occupational-therapy-with-displaced-persons-in-europe/
- **Germany:** DVE Arbeitsgruppe Gemeinwesenorientierte Ergotherapie
    https://dve.info/ergotherapie/fachbereiche/gemeinwesenorientierte-ergotherapie
- **Jordon:** Toward an All-Inclusive Jordan
    https://www.facebook.com/TowardsanallinclusiveJordan/
- **International:** Forcedmigration4OT
    https://www.facebook.com/groups/1801393130103531

Conclusion

The total number of forced migrants nearly doubled during the decade between 2010 and 2020 (Migration Data Portal, 2022). In 2020 alone, 40.5 million new internal displacements were recorded across 149 countries. Although it is sometimes difficult to distinguish triggering events, new displacements are mostly attributed to conflict and violence or natural disasters (Migration Data Portal, 2022). With rising political extremism and looming climate change, forced migration is likely to increase exponentially even in countries with a history of economic and political stability. Consequently, OT practitioners across geographical and practice settings will increasingly encounter clients with a history of forced migration. OT has an important role in supporting forced migrants to rebuild their lives and deal with the many occupational disruptions caused by displacement. Investing in the further development of this role will help prepare the profession for anticipated future needs.

Lippincott® Connect *For additional resources on the subjects discussed in this chapter, visit Lippincott Connect.*

REFERENCES

AlHeresh, R., & Cahn, P. (2020). Expanding rehabilitation services through international academic-community partnerships. *Annals of Global Health, 86*(1), 71. https://doi.org/10.5334/aogh.2876

Alve, Y. A., Islam, A., Hatlestad, B., Mirza, M. (in press). Participation in everyday occupations among Rohingya refugees in Bangladeshi refugee camps. *American Journal of Occupational Therapy.*

Bishop, R., & Purcell, E. (2013). The value of an allotment group for refugees. *British Journal of Occupational Therapy, 76,* 264–269. https://doi.org/10.4276/030802213X13706169932824

Black, M. (2010). From kites to kitchens: Collaborative community based occupational therapy with refugee survivors of torture. In F. Kronenberg, N. Pollard, & D. Sakellariu (Eds.), *Occupational therapies without borders, Volume 2: Towards an ecology of occupation-based practice* (pp. 217–225). Elsevier.

Blankvoort, N., Arslan, M., Tonoyan, A., Damour, A. Q., & Mpabanzi, L. (2018). A new you: A collaborative exploration of occupational therapy's role with refugees. *World Federation of Occupational Therapists Bulletin, 74*(2), 92–98. https://doi.org/10.1080/14473828.2018.1526560

Blankvoort, N., Moore, T., Roos, K., & Schiller, S. (2018). *Report on occupational therapy with displaced persons.* Occupational Therapy Europe Interest Group Displaced Persons. http://www.oteurope.eu/wp-content/uploads/2019/01/OT-Europe-Interest-Group-Displaced-Persons-Report-on-OT-with-Displaced-Persons.pdf

Bonfiglio, G., Rosal, K., Henao-Martínez, A., Franco-Paredes, C., Poeschla, E. M., Moo-Young, J., Seefeldt, T., Dunlevy, H., Haas, M., & Young, J. (2020). The long journey inside immigration detention centres in the USA. *Journal of Travel Medicine, 27*(7), taaa083. https://doi.org/10.1093/jtm/taaa083

Bronfenbrenner, U. (1977). Toward an experimental ecology of human development. *American Psychologist, 32*(7), 513–531. https://doi.org/10.1037/0003-066X.32.7.513

Burchett, N., & Matheson, R. (2011). The need for belonging: The impact of restrictions on working on the wellbeing of an asylum seeker. *Journal of Occupational Science, 17*(2), 85–91. https://doi.org/10.1080/14427591.2010.9686679

CBM Global Disability Inclusion, CBM International and Centre for Disability in Development. (2021). *Integrated health and rehabilitation services in mass displacement. A model for inclusive healthcare from the Rohingya response in Bangladesh.* https://www.cbm.org/fileadmin/user_upload/CBM-CDD_Integrated_Health_and_Rehabilitation_Services_in_Mass_Displacement.pdf

Copley, J., Turpin, M., Gordon, S., & McLaren, C. (2011). Development and evaluation of an occupational therapy program for refugee high school students. *Australian Occupational Therapy Journal, 58*(4), 310–316. https://doi.org/10.1111/j.1440-1630.2011.0093.x

Crandall, J., & Smith, Y. J. (2015). The life skills program: Occupational therapy among resettled refugees in an urban context. *Occupational Therapy Practice, 20*(22), 18–20.

Crawford, E., Turpin, M., Nayar, S., Steel, E., & Durand, J. L. (2016). The structural-personal interaction: Occupational deprivation and asylum seekers in Australia. *Journal of Occupational Science, 23*(3), 321–338. https://doi.org/10.1080/14427591.2016.1153510

De Koker, R., Lambers, S., & Vercruysse, L. (2019). Occupational therapy at "Klein Kasteeltje" in Brussels for children of asylum seekers who cannot participate in the Belgian schooling system. *World Federation of Occupational Therapists Bulletin, 75*(1), 34–43. https://doi.org/10.1080/14473828.2019.1570703

Driver, C., & Beltran, R. (1998). Impact of refugee trauma on children's occupational role as school students. *Australian Occupational Therapy Journal, 45*(1), 23–38. https://doi.org/10.1111/j.1440-1630.1998.tb00779.x

Fabri, M. R. (2001). Reconstructing safety: Adjustments to the therapeutic frame in the treatment of survivors of political torture. *Professional Psychology: Research and Practice, 32*(5), 452–457. https://doi.org/10.1037/0735-7028.32.5.452

Galvaan, R. (2021). Generative disruption through occupational science: Enacting possibilities for deep human connection. *Journal of Occupational Science, 28*(1), 6–18. https://doi.org/10.1080/14427591.2020.1818276

Galvaan, R., & Peters, L. (2017a). Occupation-based community development: A critical approach to occupational therapy. In S. Dsouza, R. Galvaan, & E. Ramugondo (Eds.), *Concepts in occupational therapy: Understanding southern perspectives* (pp. 172–187). Manipal University Press.

Galvaan, R., & Peters, L. (2017b). Occupation-based community development: Confronting the politics of occupation In D. Sakellariou & N. Pollard (Eds.), *Occupational therapies without borders: Integrating justice with practice* (pp. 283–291). Elsevier Press.

Gorman, W. (2001). Refugee survivors of torture: Trauma and treatment. *Professional Psychology: Research and Practice, 32*(5), 443–451. https://doi.org/10.1037/0735-7028.32.5.443

Gupta, J., & Sullivan, C. (2008). Enabling immigrants to overcome participation challenges. *Occupational Therapy Practice, 13*(5), 25–32.

Hart, H. C. (2019). "Keeping busy with purpose": How meaningful occupation can shape the experience of forced migration. *Migration Studies, 38,* 1–21. https://doi.org/10.1093/migration/mnz046

Handicap International. (2009). *Dealing with disability in the Dadaab refugee camps.* Author.

Hasnain, R., Mirza, M., Gharib, A., & Tekle, T. M. (2020, December 7–8). *Empowering Illinois-based refugees/asylees with disabilities in their educational, service, and employment pursuits* [Oral Presentation]. Annual conference of the American University Centers on Disability, virtual event.

Herman, J. L. (2015). *Trauma and recovery.* Basic Books.

Horghagen, S., & Josephsson, S. (2010). Theatre as liberation, collaboration and relationship for asylum seekers. *Journal of Occupational Science, 17*(3), 168–176. https://doi.org/10.1080/14427591.2010.9686691

Huot, S., Kelly, E., & Park, S. J. (2016). Occupational experiences of forced migrants: A scoping review. *Australian Occupational Therapy Journal, 63*(3), 186–205. https://doi.org/10.1111/1440-1630.12261

Huot, S., & Laliberte Rudman, D. (2015). Extending beyond qualitative interviewing to illuminate the tacit nature of everyday occupation: Occupational mapping and participatory occupation methods. *OTJR: Occupation, Participation and Health, 35*(3), 142–150. https://doi.org/10.1177/1539449215576488

Ingvarsson, L., Egilson, S. T., & Skaptadottir, U. D. (2016). "I want a normal life like everyone else": Daily life of asylum seekers in Iceland. *Scandinavian Journal of Occupational Therapy, 23*(6), 416–424. https://doi.org/10.3109/11038128.2016.1144787

Jorgenson, K. C., & Nilsson, J. E. (2021). The relationship among trauma, acculturation, and mental health symptoms in Somali refugees. *The Counseling Psychologist, 49*, 196–232. https://doi.org/10.1177/0011000020968548

Karanja, M. (2009). Disability in contexts of displacement. *Disability Studies Quarterly, 29*(4). http://www.dsq-sds.org/article/view/969/1177

Khan, F., & Amatya, B. (2017). Refugee health and rehabilitation: Challenges and response. *Journal of Rehabilitation Medicine, 49*(5), 378–384. https://doi.org/10.2340/16501977-2223

Kielhofner, G. (1977). Temporal adaptation: A conceptual framework for occupational therapy. *American Journal of Occupational Therapy, 31*(4), 235–242.

Kreichauf, R. (2018). From forced migration to forced arrival: The campization of refugee accommodation in European cities. *Comparative Migration Studies, 6*(1), 7. https://doi.org/10.1186/s40878-017-0069-8

Mayne, J., Lowrie, D., & Wilson, J. (2016). Occupational experiences of refugees and asylum seekers resettling in Australia: A narrative review. *OTJR: Occupation, Participation and Health, 36*(4), 204–215. https://doi.org/10.1177/1539449216668648

Menéndez Álvarez, N., Diez, E., & Jimenez, E. (2021). Analysis of daily occupations and engagement in Sahrawi refugee camps. *Journal of Occupational Science, 28*, 173–184. https://doi.org/10.1080/14427591.2021.1897964

Migration Data Portal. (2022, May 27). *Types of migration: Forced migration or displacement.* https://www.migrationdataportal.org/themes/forced-migration-or-displacement

Mirza, M. (2011). *Unmet needs and diminished opportunities: Disability, displacement and humanitarian healthcare* (New Issues in Refugee Research Working Paper Series). UNHCR, Policy Development and Evaluation Service. https://www.unhcr.org/en-us/research/working/4e0dbdb29/unmet-needs-diminished-opportunities-disability-displacement-humanitarian.html

Mirza, M. (2012). Occupational upheaval during resettlement and migration: Findings of global ethnography with refugees with disabilities. *OTJR: Occupation, Participation and Health, 32*(1), S6–S14. https://doi.org/10.3928/15394492-20110906-04

Mirza, M. (2014). Refugee camps, asylum detention, and the geopolitics of transnational migration: Disability and its intersections with humanitarian confinement. In L. Ben-Moshe, C. Chapman, & A. Carey (Eds.), *Disability incarcerated: Imprisonment and disability in the United States and Canada* (pp. 217–236). Palgrave MacMillan.

Mirza, M., Black, M., Kwekel, H., & Ram, V. (2020, October 1-31). *Community collaborations to meet the occupational needs of refugees.* In Illinois Occupational Therapy Association, virtual event.

Mirza, M., & Heinemann, A. W. (2012). Service needs and service gaps among refugees with disabilities resettled in the United States. *Disability and Rehabilitation, 34*(7), 542–552. https://doi.org/10.3109/09638288.2011.611211

Mirza, M., Luna, R., Mathews, B., Hasnain, R., Hebert, E., Niebauer, A., & Mishra, U. D. (2013). Barriers to healthcare access among refugees with disabilities and chronic health conditions resettled in the US Midwest. *Journal of Immigrant and Minority Health, 16*(4), 733–742. https://doi.org/10.1007/s10903-013-9906-5

Mitchell-Gillespie, B., Hashim, H., Griffin, M., & AlHeresh, R. (2020). Sustainable support solutions for community-based rehabilitation workers in refugee camps: Piloting telehealth acceptability and implementation. *Globalization and Health, 16*(1), 82. https://doi.org/10.1186/s12992-020-00614-y

Moore, T. (2017). Strengths-based narrative storytelling as therapeutic intervention for refugees in Greece. *World Federation of Occupational Therapists Bulletin, 73*(1), 45–51. https://doi.org/10.1080/14473828.2017.1298557

Morville, A. L., Amris, K., Eklund, M., Danneskiold-Samsøe, B., & Erlandsson, L. K. (2015). A longitudinal study of changes in asylum seekers ability regarding activities of daily living during their stay in the asylum center. *Journal of Immigrant and Minority Health, 17*(3), 852–859. https://doi.org/10.1007/s10903-014-0004-0

Morville, A.-L., & Erlandsson, L.-K. (2013). The experience of occupational deprivation in an asylum centre: The narratives of three men. *Journal of Occupational Science, 20*(3), 212–223. https://doi.org/10.1080/14427591.2013.808976

Morville, A. L., Erlandsson, L. K., Danneskiold-Samsøe, B., Amris, K., & Eklund, M. (2015). Satisfaction with daily occupations amongst asylum seekers in Denmark. *Scandinavian Journal of Occupational Therapy, 22*(3), 207–215. https://doi.org/10.3109/11038128.2014.982702

Morville, A.-L., & Jessen-Winge, C. (2019). Creating a bridge: An asylum seeker's ideas for social inclusion. *Journal of Occupational Science, 26*(1), 53–64. https://doi.org/10.1080/14427591.2018.1500933

Sakellariou, D., & Pollard, N. (Eds.). (2016). *Occupational therapies without borders: Integrating justice with practice* (2nd ed.). Elsevier/Churchill Livingstone.

Scheer, S., Adamopoulou, E., Asaba, E., Grützner, R., Guerrero, M., Simó, S., & Mondaca, M. (2020). *Interdisciplinary cooperation in psychosocial interventions: A case study on refugees. Handbook for practitioners.* Interact 2020 - Erasmus+ http://interact-erasmus.eu/

Schell, B. A., Gillen, G., Crepeau, E. B., & Scaffa, M. E. (2019). Analyzing occupations and activity. In B. A. B. Schell & G. Gillen (Eds.), *Willard & Spackman's occupational therapy* (13th ed., pp. 320–334). Wolters Kluwer.

Schisler, A. M. C., & Polatajko, H. J. (2002). The individual as mediator of the person-occupation-environment interaction: Learning from the experience of refugees. *Journal of Occupational Science, 9*(2), 82–92. https://doi.org/10.1080/14427591.2002.9686496

Smith, H. C. (2015). An exploration of the meaning of occupation to people who seek asylum in the United Kingdom. *British Journal of Occupational Therapy, 78*(10), 614–621. https://doi.org/10.1177/0308022615591174

Smith, Y. J. (2013). We all Bantu—We have each other: Preservation of social capital strengths during forced migration. *Journal of Occupational Science, 20*(2), 173–184. https://doi.org/10.1080/14427591.2013.786647

Smith, Y. J. (2017). Occupational justice and advocacy: Working with former refugees and asylum seekers at personal and community levels. In D. Sakellarious & N. Pollard (Eds.), *Occupational therapies without borders: Integrating justice with practice* (pp. 433–440). Elsevier.

Smith, Y. J., Cornella, E., & Williams, N. (2014). Working with populations from a refugee background: An opportunity to enhance the occupational therapy educational experience. *Australian Occupational Therapy Journal, 61*(1), 20–27. https://doi.org/10.1111/1440-1630.12037

Smith, Y. J., Stephenson, S., & Gibson-Satterthwaite, M. (2013). The meaning and value of traditional occupational practice: A Karen woman's story of weaving in the United States. *WORK: A Journal of Prevention, Assessment and Rehabilitation, 45*(1), 25–30. https://doi.org/10.3233/WOR-131600

Spencer, J. C., Davidson, H. A., & White, V. K. (1996). Continuity and change: Past experience as adaptive repertoire in occupational adaptation. *American Journal of occupational Therapy, 50*(7), 526–534. https://doi.org/10.5014/ajot.50.7.526

Steindl, C., Winding, K., & Runge, U. (2008). Occupation and participation in everyday life: Women's experiences of an Austrian refugee camp. *Journal of Occupational Science, 15*(1), 36–42. https://doi.org/10.1080/14427591.2008.9686605

Stephenson, S. M., Smith, Y. J., Gibson, M., & Watson, V. (2013). Traditional weaving as an occupation of Karen refugee women. *Journal of Occupational Science, 20*(3), 224–235. https://doi.org/10.3233/WOR-131600

Suleman, A., & Whiteford, G. (2013). Understanding occupational transitions in forced migration: The importance of life skills in early refugee resettlement. *Journal of Occupational Science, 20*(2), 201–210. https://doi.org/10.1080/14427591.2012.755908

Trimboli, C. (2017). Occupational justice for asylum seeker and refugee children: Issues, effects, and action. In D. Sakellariou & N. Pollard (Eds.), *Occupational therapies without borders: Integrating justice with practice* (pp. 460–467). Oxford.

Trimboli, C., & Halliwell, V. (2018). A survey to explore the interventions used by occupational therapists and occupational therapy students with refugees and asylum seekers. *World Federation of Occupational Therapists Bulletin, 74*(2), 106–113. https://doi.org/10.1080/14473828.2018.1535562

Trimboli, C., Parsons, L., Fleay, C., Parsons, D., & Buchanan, A. (2021). A systematic review and meta-analysis of psychosocial interventions for 6–12-year-old children who have been forcibly displaced. *SSM-Mental Health, 1*, 100028. https://doi.org/10.1016/j.ssmmh.2021.100028

Trimboli, C., Rivas-Quarneti, N., Blankvoort, N., Roosen, I., Simó Algado, S., & Whiteford, G. (2019). The current and future contribution of occupational therapy and occupational science to transforming the situation of forced migrants: Critical perspectives from a think tank. *Journal of Occupational Science, 26*(2), 323–328. https://doi.org/10.1080/14427591.2019.1604408

United Nations General Assembly. (1951). *Convention relating to the status of refugees.* https://www.unhcr.org/protection/basic/3b66c2aa10/convention-protocol-relating-status-refugees.html

United Nations High Commissioner for Refugees. (2022). *Global trends: Forced displacement in 2022.* https://www.unhcr.org/flagship-reports/globaltrends/

USA for UNHCR. (n.d.). *What is a refugee camp?* https://www.unrefugees.org/refugee-facts/camps/

USA for UNHCR (2021, October 20). *The U.S. refugee resettlement program explained.* https://www.unrefugees.org/news/the-u-s-refugee-resettlement-program-explained/

Whiteford, G. (2000). Occupational deprivation: Global challenge in the new millennium. *British Journal of Occupational Therapy, 63*(5), 200–204. https://doi.org/10.1177/030802260006300503

Whiteford, G. (2005). Understanding the occupational deprivation of refugees: A case study from Kosovo. *Canadian Journal of Occupational Therapy, 72*(2), 78–88. https://doi.org/10.1177/000841740507200202

Whiteford, G., & Townsend, E. (2011). Participatory occupational justice framework (POJF 2010): Enabling occupational participation and inclusion. In F. Kronenberg, N. Pollard, & D. Sakellariou (Eds.), *Occupational therapies without borders – Volume 2: Towards an ecology of occupation-based practices* (pp. 65–84). Elsevier.

World Federation of Occupational Therapists. (2014). *Position statement: Human displacement (revised).* https://www.wfot.org/resources/human-displacement

Providing Occupational Therapy Services Through Telehealth

Jana Cason and Ellen R. Cohn

LEARNING OBJECTIVES

After reading this chapter, you will be able to:

1. Compare and contrast synchronous, asynchronous, and hybrid telehealth service delivery models.
2. Describe hardware, software, and videoconferencing platform features commonly used in occupational therapy (OT) telehealth sessions.
3. Identify office design and room setup considerations for effective telehealth sessions.
4. List the American Occupational Therapy Association's (AOTA's) ethics resources and competencies that promote ethical use of telehealth in OT.
5. Identify OT assessments with evidence that supports their delivery through telehealth.
6. Explain similarities and differences in documentation for OT services provided in person and through telehealth.

Introduction

Telehealth is the use of technology to deliver occupational therapy (OT) services when the practitioner and client[1] are in different physical locations at the time-of-service delivery.

Telehealth use in OT dates back more than two decades and dramatically expanded in response to the COVID-19 pandemic (American Occupational Therapy Association [AOTA], 2005; Dreyer et al., 2001; Guilfoyle

---

[1] According to the AOTA (2020c, p. S75), the term *client* refers to *persons* (including those involved in care of a client), *groups* (a collection of individuals having shared characteristics or common or shared purpose, e.g., family members, workers, students, and those with similar interests or occupational challenges), and *populations* (aggregates of people with common attributes such as contexts, characteristics, or concerns, including health risks). However, in countries other than the United States, the term *client* often refers to persons who are paying for their care directly. In most countries, *patient* is used to describe persons who are in hospital or rehabilitation. *Service user* and *person* are terms in general use that describe those in need of OT services. For this chapter, we are using *client* without implying the source of payment for services.

et al., 2003; Hoel et al., 2021; Liu, 2000; Miyazaki & Liu, 2002; Sanford et al., 2004; Sing-Fai et al., 2003).

Both the World Federation of Occupational Therapists (WFOT, 2021) and the AOTA (2018b) endorse telehealth as an appropriate and effective service delivery model for OT services. The WFOT (2021) defines telehealth as "the use of information and communication technologies to deliver health-related services when the provider and client are in different physical locations" (p. 1). Similarly, AOTA (2018b) describes telehealth as "the application of evaluative, consultative, preventative, and therapeutic services delivered through information and communication technology" (p. 1).

Telehealth technology enables OT practitioners to provide care to clients in authentic contexts (e.g., home, community, work). This chapter introduces readers to many of the fundamentals of telehealth. For an example of OT telehealth during COVID-19, see Expanding Our Perspectives.

Telehealth Delivery Models

Synchronous, Asynchronous, and Hybrid Telehealth

Three important terms describe time and place aspects of the telehealth service delivery model.

Synchronous telehealth occurs in real time with the distantly located practitioner and client having interactive, simultaneous communication. Synchronous telehealth may use phone, videoconferencing, or other technologies that enable live interaction. Examples of synchronous telehealth may include, but are not limited to, an OT practitioner using videoconferencing to coach a client on scar management techniques, recommend home modifications to a client's caregiver, or engage a

---

EXPANDING OUR PERSPECTIVES

Cooking Workshop in Pandemic Times

Mariel Pellegrini

A workshop for cooking was developed for people with mental health problems who receive OT services in their homes. Health management problems that were identified in relation to food included obesity, a lack of healthy routine, difficulty cooking food, lack of a balanced diet, among others. The objectives of this cooking workshop were to:

- Improve eating habits
- Provide resources for the identification in daily life of healthy eating habits
- Promote autonomy in the kitchen and the use of assistive technologies
- Develop social interaction skills among participants
- Create virtual support networks among the participants

This cooking workshop was originally conducted in person, but the global COVID-19 pandemic threatened its continuity. So the workshop was moved to a telehealth platform with fixed hours and days for telehealth group work. At the suggestion of the clients, a WhatsApp group was opened to share recipes and images of their dinner meals. This format of telehealth accompanied by an occupational therapist was the

beginning of many achievements, not only in food, but also in socialization and group meals (each one at home, no longer eating alone while watching television). Currently, it already works autonomously among the group's participants; once a month they have a telehealth meeting with the institution's nutritionist. The occupational therapist facilitates organization, shopping, and other operational issues for nutrition management. The WhatsApp group highly exceeded expectations. In my experience as an occupational therapist, many telehealth experiences that necessarily began in times of COVID-19 as plan B, are currently plan A for the clients of our services. Telehealth is a mode of OT without borders.

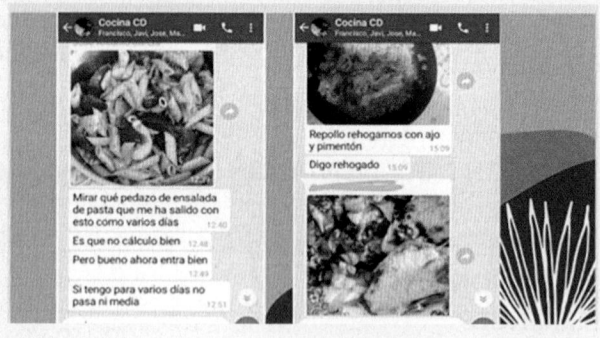

client in therapeutic activities and therapeutic exercise. Using technology to monitor real-time performance data from an online program/game or from wireless sensors while working with a client who is in a different physical location also constitutes synchronous telehealth. Similarly, phone (voice only) may be used to address specific concerns or problems, instruct a client in new therapeutic strategies such as energy conservation, or modify a home program. It is important to note, however, that payment for OT services provided through telehealth varies by payer source, and some technology exclusions may apply.

Asynchronous telehealth involves electronically shared data (e.g., video, digital images, performance data recorded from an online program, recorded data from wearable devices/sensors, text messaging, email, and other forms of communication) between the practitioner and client that occurs at a distance and does not include real-time interaction. Asynchronous telehealth is referred to as "store-and-forward" telehealth because data are stored and then forwarded between the practitioner and the client. Examples of asynchronous telehealth may include, but are not limited to, a client completing an online questionnaire-based assessment through a secure portal. Digital images and recordings may also be used within an asynchronous telehealth model. For example, an OT practitioner may view digital images of a client's home environment and provide recommendations to support transition from in-patient care to home. Or, an OT practitioner may review a digital recording sent by a client to provide a visual update on progress or to request feedback on implementation of a recommended therapeutic strategy. OT practitioners should consult their organization's policies and procedures related to use of digital images and video, secure storage, and process for integration into a client's medical or educational record.

Hybrid telehealth primarily describes a combination of in-person and telehealth services. However, it may also refer to a combination of both synchronous and asynchronous telehealth. For some clients, telehealth may be used exclusively to provide OT services, whereas for other clients, a hybrid or in-person service delivery model may be selected. For example, a client in an orthopedic setting may receive OT interventions through videoconferencing (e.g., therapeutic exercise, therapeutic activity, patient education), with some in-person OT visits to have a splint fabricated and adjusted during the course of treatment. Clinical reasoning and client preferences should guide the selection of the OT service delivery model (AOTA, 2018b).

Additional telehealth resources, including decision guides, are available at www.aota.org/telehealth.

Models of Service

Telehealth may be used for evaluation, intervention, consultation, supervision, and monitoring (AOTA, 2018b). Payer sources have established terminology and definitions aligned with models of service; these have evolved and changed over time. For example, in the United States, the Center for Medicare and Medicaid Services (CMS, 2021) defines **e-visits**, a form of consultation, as "non-face-to-face patient-initiated communications through an online patient portal" (p. 5). CMS expanded eligibility for OT practitioners to provide e-visits and other OT services through telehealth to Medicare beneficiaries during the COVID-19 pandemic (AOTA, 2020b).

Monitoring can be conceptualized broadly as monitoring clients' safety and fall risk in the home environment, progress toward outcomes, and adherence to home programs. **Remote patient monitoring** refers specifically to the use of telehealth technologies to collect physiologic health data, either synchronously or asynchronously, within a medical model (CMS, 2021).

OT practitioners should consult relevant laws, regulations, and payer guidance regarding definitions, delivery and payment of OT services, and supervision of OT students and occupational therapy assistants (OTA) when using telehealth technologies.

Ethical Considerations

Fundamentals of Ethics

Ethical conduct is central to clinical practice. It is required of all OT personnel who engage in telehealth. The AOTA (2020a) defines OT personnel as inclusive of:

> occupational therapist and occupational therapy assistant practitioners and professionals (e.g., direct service, consultation, administration); educators; students in occupational therapy and occupational therapy assistant professional programs; researchers; entrepreneurs; business owners; and those in elected, appointed, or other professional volunteer service. (p. 1)

This expansive definition of OT personnel is especially applicable to telehealth because it may require the services and support of a variety of stakeholders.

Many professional associations have their own Codes of Ethics. However, the OT profession is uniquely grounded in each of seven core values: altruism, equality, freedom, justice, dignity, truth, and prudence (AOTA, 1993, 2020a). Although these longstanding values predate the recent expansion of telehealth, each can offer guidance for evolving OT practice.

As one example, there is the ethical imperative to uphold the client's dignity. This is actualized when the tele-practitioner is knowledgeable about a client's culture and exercises cultural competence and cultural humility.

The *Principle of Beneficence*, the taking of action to benefit others, is also central to the ethical delivery of telehealth. The AOTA's Code of Ethics (2020a) provides examples of beneficence that apply to telehealth delivery. These include:

> protecting and defending the rights of others, preventing harm from occurring to others, removing conditions that will cause harm to others, offering services that benefit persons with disabilities, and acting to protect and remove persons from dangerous situations. (p. 3)

Thus, OT services provided through telehealth should benefit clients and should be conducted in a manner that ensures their safety. Telehealth requires that the practitioner recognizes when the environment is unsafe, so that the client does not suffer an accident or physical harm. The practitioner at a distance must know how to contact local emergency services associated with the client's physical location.

Additionally, both the telehealth environment and technology must ensure client confidentiality. Failure to safeguard privacy could violate the *Principle of Nonmaleficence*, which indicates that "occupational therapy personnel must refrain from causing harm, injury, or wrongdoing to recipients of service" (AOTA, 2020a, p. 3).

Central to most professional codes of ethics is that the practitioner must practice in a lawful manner. In the United States, this includes abiding by the requirements for state licensure and not engaging in price-fixing or other violations to federal antitrust law (Federal Trade Commission, n.d.).

In closing, the principles expressed in the AOTA's Code of Ethics provide guidance for clinical practice. Readers of this section might consider how each of the seven principles apply to telehealth: altruism, equality, freedom, justice, dignity, truth, and prudence, and how each might be violated. See OT Story 67.1, for an example of an ethical dilemma.

AOTA Ethics Resources

The AOTA offers rich resources on the topic of ethics. As mentioned above, the AOTA's (2020a) Code of Ethics can serve as a guide to ethical practice in OT. The AOTA's Code of Ethics outlines core values, ethical principles, and standards of conduct for OT practitioners and is applicable regardless of the service delivery model (i.e., in person, telehealth, or hybrid).

The AOTA's companion telehealth advisory opinion provides additional guidance for ethical OT practice using telehealth (AOTA, 2017). This resource addresses ethical considerations related to client comfort, practitioner competence, consent to treat, privacy and confidentiality, quality of care, and adherence to ethical standards. The AOTA's telehealth position paper also includes a section on ethical considerations when using telehealth (AOTA, 2018b).

OT STORY 67.1 MS. SMITH: ETHICAL DILEMMAS ABOUND

Ms. Smith is a school-based occupational therapist in the United States with two years of practice experience. She is licensed to practice in one state: Ohio. Ms. Smith is interested in providing telehealth during the summer months to supplement her income. She uses word-of-mouth to let parents of her students and other referral sources know that she will be accepting clients for OT telehealth services. Ms. Smith has not had any experience with telehealth, but she feels confident in her abilities because she uses videoconferencing in her personal life. Ms. Smith soon receives referrals for clients in Ohio, Kentucky, and West Virginia.

Questions
1. What ethical dilemmas are present in this scenario?
2. What actions should Ms. Smith take to ensure ethical practice using telehealth?

In addition, AOTA published a continuing education article, *Ethical Telehealth Practice,* with conceptual definitions and terminology, a brief history of telehealth, ethical principles and standards related to telehealth, and strategies for managing ethical dilemmas (Radley & Rumery, 2021).

Telehealth Technologies

Telehealth Hardware

Telehealth technologies variously employ hardware and software. **Telehealth hardware** may include computers (desktop/laptop), electronic tablets, telephones/smartphones, wearable devices such as smart watches and sensors, and peripheral devices (e.g., headsets, external microphones, document cameras).

The type of hardware that will be needed for the session will depend on the service being provided. When selecting hardware, it is important to consider whether the OT practitioner or the client will need to demonstrate motor skills requiring movement and space within the environment. A desktop computer may work well for some interventions. However, for tabletop activities requiring the practitioner to see multiviews of the client, a built-in camera on a desktop or laptop computer will not provide the necessary viewing angles. A mobile camera (e.g., tablet, smartphone, external camera) may be needed to provide viewing angles not captured by a built-in camera on a desktop or laptop computer. A document camera can provide augmented visualization of tabletop activities.

Document cameras are available commercially; however, a mobile device or an external computer camera can function similar to a document camera to provide alternate viewing angles for the practitioner or client (see Figure 67.1). Tutorials are available online describing how to make a document camera using the search terms "DIY document camera" or "homemade document camera." When using a mobile device (electronic tablet or smartphone) as a second camera, it is important that the audio is connected through only one device or one device is muted and the speaker is silenced in order to prevent audio feedback.

For seated activities, the camera should be positioned at eye level to facilitate the appearance of eye contact with the client. If the camera is too high, the practitioner will appear to be looking downward rather than at the client. Similarly, room configuration and hardware used by clients should facilitate optimal viewing of performance-based activities.

Telehealth hardware (e.g., computer, tablet, smartphone) should be plugged into an outlet during telehealth sessions to avoid loss of connection because of low battery. If possible, computers should be directly connected to the Internet using an Ethernet connection (vs. Wi-Fi connection). Wi-Fi connections are less secure and may be disrupted if multiple devices are connected to the Wi-Fi network simultaneously.

Telehealth Software

Telehealth software is operating information, programs, and data on devices that enable telehealth. Telehealth software provides access to client/patient portals, videoconferencing platforms, and applications (apps). Many healthcare organizations have secure online portals available to clients to access electronic health records and other health information. These portals may also have features for telehealth, including videoconferencing capabilities and secure messaging.

Videoconferencing platforms facilitate synchronous telehealth with both video and audio components. In the United States, OT practitioners should use videoconferencing platforms that are compliant with the Health Insurance Portability and Accountability Act of 1996 (HIPAA). Videoconferencing platforms that are HIPAA-compliant provide a **Business Associate Agreement** (BAA) to the healthcare practitioner (CMS, 2021). The BAA assures that the vendor will adhere to the same confidentiality, privacy, and security requirements as the practitioner in order to safeguard clients' health information.

Videoconferencing Platform Features

OT practitioners often use videoconferencing when providing OT services through telehealth. There are a variety of videoconferencing platform features that facilitate engaging and effective therapy sessions. These features include, but are not limited to, screen sharing, chat feature, whiteboard, and annotation tools. Web links and files can be shared with and accessed by clients using the videoconferencing chat feature. White board and annotation tools can be combined with screen sharing to enable clients to interact with online activities and worksheets shared by the practitioner. For online activities with a timing component, it is helpful to have clients access the activity on their device and then share their screen with the OT practitioner to avoid a lag in the timing that may impact performance.

Apps

Many OT practitioners use apps during in-person therapy sessions. Apps can be integrated into OT telehealth evaluations (e.g., goniometric apps, home assessment apps) and synchronous therapy sessions or recommended to clients as a component of their home therapy program. OT recommended apps are easily located by searching the Internet, with many apps grouped by population, practice setting, and skill area.

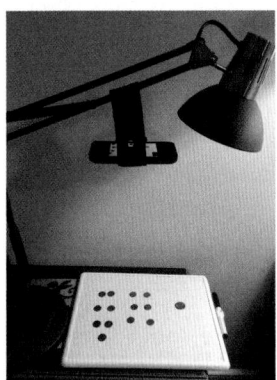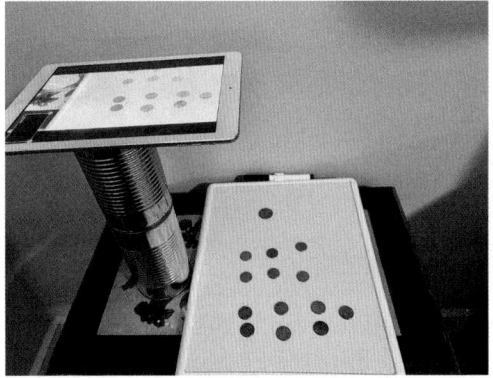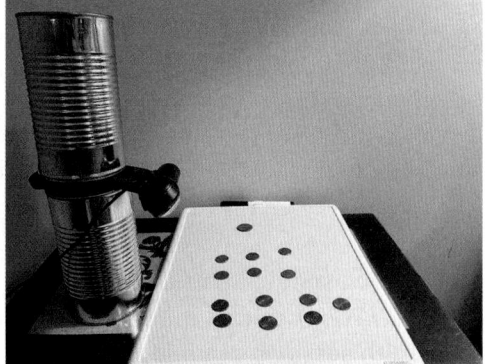

FIGURE 67.1 **A second camera provides alternate viewing angles. As shown in the photos from left to right, a mobile device, electronic tablet, and external web camera can be positioned to view a table top activity.**

Telehealth Physical Environment

Room Configuration

Office design and room setup can impact the quality of telehealth sessions. Practitioners engaged in telehealth should assure the room location and size, placement of equipment and furniture, acoustics, wall color, and background visuals are conducive to telehealth. Rooms used for telehealth should not be in "high traffic areas" where there are environmental noises and other people present. There should be a door that can be closed during telehealth sessions to protect client privacy. The room should be of sufficient size to accommodate the therapy services to be provided (i.e., seated vs. movement-based therapy, or a combination). If there will be movement-based activities demonstrated, there should be sufficient space for the OT practitioner to safely demonstrate these movements.

Lighting and Sound

When evaluating room configuration, lighting and mitigation of environmental noises should be considered. Diffused light that comes from multiple sources and includes a combination of direct and indirect lighting is optimal for telehealth sessions (California Telehealth Resource Center, 2021). Both lighting and wall color can impact image quality. Neutral wall colors, especially light blue/gray, have been shown to be optimal for telehealth sessions (California Telehealth Resource Center, 2021).

It is also important to view the space that will be used for the telehealth session through the camera as it will appear on screen for the client. Evaluate what is in the camera's view. Assure that walls are not visually cluttered with pictures, objects, and other distractions. A screen or room divider can be used to modify the background view if the room where telehealth sessions occur is a multipurpose space (e.g., bedroom; see Figure 67.2). Some videoconferencing platforms have green screen options that allow practitioners to change the view of their background. However, use of digital backgrounds can affect image quality and be distracting for some clients.

OT practitioners should minimize noise that may disrupt telehealth sessions or distract clients (e.g., a squeaky fan, rattling air conditioner unit, open window with traffic or environmental noises). Use of a headset can improve voice quality and eliminate environmental sounds. Wireless headsets are available for practitioners who may need to demonstrate movement-based activities during telehealth sessions.

Telehealth Competencies

Telehealth competencies can be conceptualized as technical, administrative, or clinical (Richmond et al., 2017). Often, these functions overlap. For example, ensuring privacy and security can fall within both the administrative and technological domains.

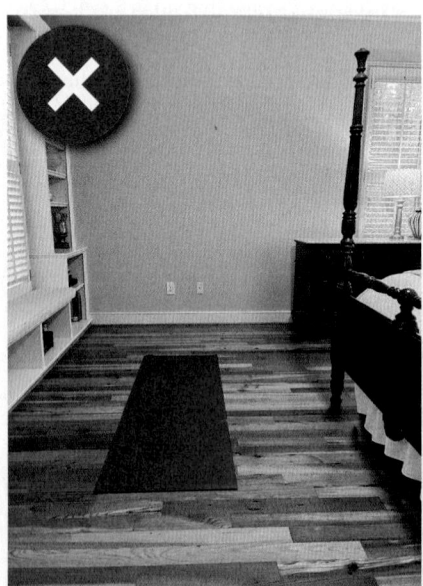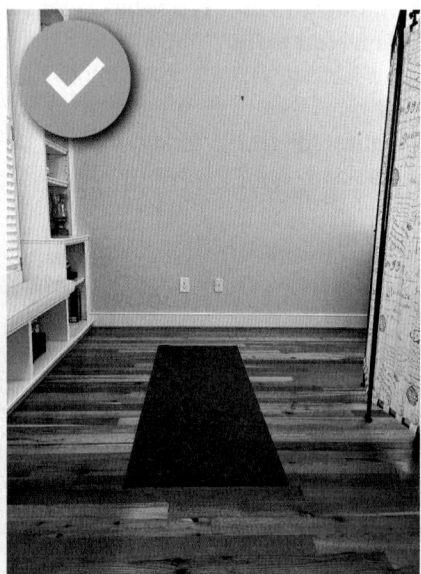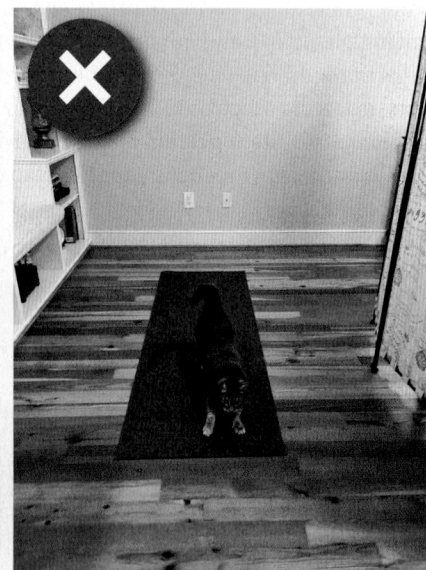

FIGURE 67.2 A screen or room divider can be used to modify the background view if the room where telehealth sessions occur is a multipurpose space. Pets may pose a safety hazard (e.g., tripping/falling) and should be removed from the room during telehealth sessions.

Technical Competencies

In addition to administrative and clinical competencies, OT practitioners should have technical competencies for telehealth. These include having skills to address minor technical issues that may arise during telehealth sessions and the ability to connect with information technology (IT) support personnel to address more complex technical issues. OT practitioners should have knowledge of and employ technical settings (e.g., enabling encryption, using strong passwords) that support compliance with relevant laws and regulations to protect health information. Prior to engaging in telehealth, OT practitioners should practice using the telehealth technology, including role-play with a colleague or friend, to increase skill and confidence prior to implementing telehealth with clients.

OT practitioners can gain telehealth competencies by participating in a combination of professional development activities including, but not limited to, telehealth-related continuing education courses, mentorship from practitioners who have experience with telehealth, role-play, practice with telehealth technologies, reading telehealth-related research, and reviewing telehealth resources created by professional associations, licensure boards, and other organizations. OT students gain knowledge of telehealth through foundational textbooks, classroom assignments, and lived experiences during fieldwork and community engagement.

Technical and Administrative Competencies: Privacy and Security

OT practitioners must implement procedures to safeguard clients' **protected health information** (PHI). According to the HIPAA, PHI includes personal identifiers (e.g., name, address, birth date, phone number, Social Security number) that can link health information to an individual (U.S. Department of Health and Human Services, 2003). Similarly, the Family Educational Rights and Privacy Act (FERPA) requires protection of **personally identifiable information** (PII) in academic settings from preschool through postsecondary education (U.S. Department of Education, 2016). OT practitioners should review organizational policies regarding the sharing of PHI and PII. Specific to telehealth, OT practitioners should enable computer privacy and security features (e.g., password protected access, automatic logout). Videoconferencing platform privacy and security features should also be enabled, including virtual waiting rooms and password entry into telehealth sessions. Strategies to protect PHI and PII in email communications may include the use of encrypted email, strong passwords to protect email access, sending only necessary information in the body of the email, double checking the recipient's email address before sending, attaching files that require a password to open, and making sure the correct file is attached before sending (U.S. Department of Education, 2016). Whether providing services in person or through telehealth, OT practitioners must implement policies and procedures to protect privacy, confidentiality, and security of client information.

Administrative Competencies: OTAs and E-Helpers

OTAs are instrumental in the delivery of OT services. In the United States, each state has its own statutes and regulations on the use of telehealth and OTA supervision requirements (AOTA, 2021a, 2021b). For example, some states permit "face-to-face" supervision to occur through telehealth using videoconferencing, whereas other states require periodic in-person supervision (AOTA, 2021b). OT practitioners should consult the state licensure board in the state(s) in which they practice to determine if OTA supervision may occur through telehealth and state-specific documentation requirements for OTA supervision.

Additionally, there are times it may be deemed necessary to have an **e-helper** (client support person/caregiver) present to facilitate a client's participation and to maintain the client's safety during telehealth sessions. The OT practitioner is responsible for training and supervising such e-helpers.

Clinical Competencies: Telehealth Evaluation

Many assessment publishers have online evaluation platforms that facilitate administration of OT assessments through telehealth, including scoring and producing reports (Pearson, 2021a; Western Psychological Services, 2021b). These publishers provide guidance and tips for telehealth assessment administration (Pearson, 2021b; Western Psychological Services, 2021a). Interview and questionnaire-based assessments generally translate well to a telehealth service delivery model. Some performance-based assessments have also been validated for administration through telehealth. See Commentary on the Evidence for an overview of OT assessments with evidence supporting their delivery through telehealth.

COMMENTARY ON THE EVIDENCE

Jana Cason

Globally, there is a growing body of evidence that demonstrates the efficacy of telehealth for the delivery of OT services. Systematic and scoping reviews have found telehealth to be as effective, and in some cases more effective, than in-person therapy services (Chen et al., 2015; Kairy et al., 2009; Önal et al., 2021). Generally, telehealth results in outcomes comparable to in-person OT services and leads to a high level of satisfaction among clients and practitioners.

Evidence supports administration of some OT assessments through telehealth. OT telehealth assessments have been validated for measuring activities of daily living (ADL) status and hand function in individuals with Parkinson disease using the motor component of the Functional Independence Measure, selected items from the Unified Parkinson Disease Rating Scale, the Nine Hole Peg Test, Jamar dynamometer, and Preston pinch gauge (Hoffmann et al., 2008). Other assessments that have been evaluated for telehealth administration include the Montreal Cognitive Assessment (Abdolahi et al., 2014; Stillerova et al., 2016), Mini-Mental State Exam (Ciemins et al., 2009; McEachern et al., 2014), Functional Reach Test and European Stroke Scale (Palsbo et al., 2007), Timed Up and Go Test (Hwang et al., 2016), Kohlman Evaluation of Living Skills, and the Canadian Occupational Performance Measure (Dreyer et al., 2001).

Additionally, Worboys et al. (2018) examined the validity of a traditional clinical model hand therapy assessment administered in person and through telehealth. An allied health assistant who had earned a level IV certificate in Allied Health Assistance (Queensland Government, n.d.) facilitated objective measurements. In addition, the allied health assistant had completed a 1-hour training led by the occupational therapist to acquire the nuances of managing the videoconferencing connection, facilitating correct use of equipment (i.e., tape measure, dynamometer, pinch gauge, goniometer) during objective measurements, and communicating subjective information to the remote therapist (Worboys et al., 2018). The remote occupational therapist led the assessment and coached the allied health assistant to optimally engage with the client and assist with aspects of the assessment. The researchers found a high level of agreement between in-person and telehealth evaluation for all objective measures, including dynamometer, pinch gauge, goniometer flexion and extension, circumference in millimeters, judgments of scar and general limb function, exercise compliance, pain severity and sensitivity location, ADL, global ratings of change scores, and therapeutic recommendations (Worboys et al., 2018). The validity and reliability of musculoskeletal examinations for shoulder disorders conducted through telehealth have also been established (Steele et al., 2012), as well as the validity and reliability of several smartphone applications for goniometric measurement (Lin et al., 2020; Wellmon et al., 2016).

Pre-admission orthopedic OT home visits were also found to be feasible and accurate using telehealth technologies. Hoffmann and Russell (2008) compared data collected from an in-person therapist and an online therapist obtained during a home evaluation. The online therapist completed the Home Environment Questionnaire through client interview, observed the client completing transfers (chair, bed, shower/bath, and toilet), measured furniture height using a tool within the telehealth platform, and reviewed pictures of different areas of the home. The in-person therapist simultaneously collected data. The mean percentage exact agreement between the in-person and online therapist for items related to the home environment was 98.9% and for transfers 100%, and mean absolute difference in measured heights ranged from 0.1 to 3.3 cm (Hoffmann & Russell, 2008). Similarly, Ninnis et al. (2019) found agreement between traditional methods and technologically based methods of home assessment to be high; however, in-home assessment was reported to be more sensitive to detecting potential fall hazards.

OT practitioners may use a variety of criterion-referenced and norm-referenced assessments during OT evaluations. Criterion-referenced assessments compare an individual's performance to a set criteria or benchmark and are often used to establish baseline performance and to document progress over time. In contrast, norm-referenced assessments compare an individual's performance against a normative sample (usually same age peers) and are often used to determine eligibility for services. Altering the testing protocol of a normed assessment invalidates the score and ability to compare performance with the normative sample. Any variance from testing protocols should be documented (AOTA, 2018b). If administering a normed assessment through telehealth has not been validated by the developers for telehealth administration, the assessment should not be scored. However, skilled clinical observations during the assessment may provide meaningful information as part of the evaluation process.

OT practitioners must adhere to their country's copyright laws when using assessment materials. In general, it is not permitted to photocopy, scan, or duplicate assessment materials, including scoring forms. OT assessments with test protocol booklets or standardized materials may need to be mailed to clients prior to the OT evaluation. If mailing material is not an option, an alternative assessment should be considered. An increasing number of OT assessments are available for telehealth administration from publishers through their secure online evaluation portals.

The following are considerations for OT evaluation through telehealth:

- Ensure that the client has access to telehealth technologies, including hardware with a speaker, microphone, and camera.
- Prepare the client prior to the evaluation with instructions on how to access the telehealth session and any materials that will be needed to complete the evaluation.
- In some situations, it may be appropriate to mail assessment materials to a client with an enclosed postage-paid envelope to return the materials following the evaluation.
- If the evaluation includes viewing alternate angles such as tabletop activities, movement-based activities, transfers, or the home environment, ask if the client has access to a mobile device (smartphone/tablet) that could be used during the evaluation.
- As permitted by your organization, consider using video and digital images to compliment synchronous telehealth evaluation components.
- Where there are safety concerns that cannot be overcome with the use of an e-helper or if components of the evaluation are not conducive to telehealth, an in-person or hybrid service delivery model may be used.

Clinical Competencies: Telehealth Intervention

Benefits of a telehealth service delivery model include facilitating carryover of therapeutic strategies through provision of services in natural contexts, decreased travel, and flexibility in scheduling, such as brief check-ins, scheduling therapy sessions to coincide with targeted activities, and scheduling therapy sessions outside of typical work/office hours. For example, an occupational therapist working with a child and family targeting sleep issues and bedtime routines may schedule an evening therapy session during the time the routine naturally occurs. Using videoconferencing, the therapist observes the child's routine and coaches the caregiver on strategies to resolve the sleep issues and improve bedtime routines.

Telehealth enables caregivers to participate in OT sessions and support groups when time and distance may otherwise prevent participation. In addition, evidence demonstrates that telehealth empowers caregivers through their participation in OT telehealth sessions (Little et al., 2018; Nissen & Serwe, 2018).

Similar to in-person sessions, telehealth sessions should flow with a beginning, middle, and end. It is important to plan the telehealth session in advance and communicate with the client (and caregiver, if applicable) any materials needed for the session. OT practitioners should plan interventions using materials that a client has available (e.g., using water bottles or canned vegetables as weights). Immediately upon initiating the telehealth session, greet the client. If the telehealth session is occurring through videoconferencing,

make eye contact with the client by looking directly into the camera. Confirm your technology is working properly and assist the client to troubleshoot any technical issues.

As you begin the OT telehealth session, discuss any new concerns the client may have and explore how recommended therapeutic strategies or home program activities were implemented since the last session. Next, engage the client in targeted interventions planned for the therapy session (e.g., therapeutic activities, therapeutic exercise, patient education). Finally, wrap up the session by taking a few minutes to commend the client's engagement and summarize the interventions and skills that were targeted during the therapy session. Answer any questions the client may have, provide guidance on integrating the therapeutic strategies into daily routines, and discuss plans for the next session. This may include identifying the focus of the next session and materials needed. Immediately after the session, or within a short timeframe thereafter, send the client/caregiver any information or resources needed to support implementation of recommendations provided during the session and reiterate the plan for the next session, including the schedule and materials needed (e.g., specific household items that will be used during the session, worksheets to be printed). It is helpful to send a reminder within 24 hours of the next scheduled appointment and include session access information and materials, if any, that may be needed for the session. See Box 67.1, for "pearls of wisdom" with important telehealth technology tips. And see Expanding Our Perspectives, for clinical experiences that affirm the ability to engage in therapeutic use of self when providing OT services through telehealth.

BOX 67.1 TELEHEALTH TECHNOLOGY PEARLS OF WISDOM

- Record basic technology information and troubleshooting strategies. These recordings can be shared with clients to help them prepare for telehealth sessions and resolve common technical issues.
- Always turn your computer on at least 15 minutes prior to a telehealth session in order to avoid delays associated with automatic software updates.
- Set software updates to occur at times when you will not be using your devices.
- Assure that you and your clients update videoconferencing software as updates become available. This will enable features to work properly during telehealth sessions.
- Before the telehealth session begins, open videos, websites, or documents that you plan to share during the session.
- Close out of your email and turn off automatic message alert notifications that may pop up while sharing the screen with clients.

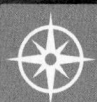

EXPANDING OUR PERSPECTIVES

Therapeutic Use of Self and Telehealth

Jana Cason

There is a misperception that with telehealth one is not able to establish meaningful therapeutic relationships with clients or engage in therapeutic use of self. I'd like to share some experiences as a pediatric occupational therapist that dispel this myth. Because of access barriers, many of my clients received OT services exclusively through telehealth. During the telehealth evaluation, I complete an occupational profile; identify interests, strengths, and challenges; and measure skills through assessments and skilled observation. As I plan telehealth interventions, I consciously incorporate the child's interests to increase motivation and persistence with therapeutic activities.

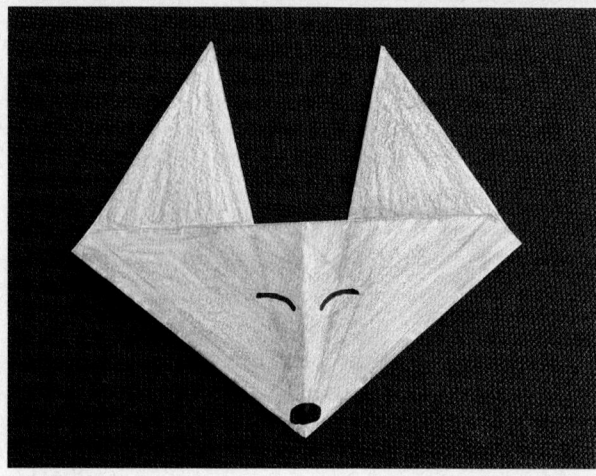

One child that I worked with exclusively through telehealth had an interest in origami, but because of limited fine motor skills, he was unable to fold paper. With the help of his caregiver, foundational skills were targeted and connected to his interests. Specifically aligned with his interest in origami, he first learned to fold a washcloth in half, then a piece of paper, then learned how to make paper snowflakes (requiring multiple paper folds), and eventually he mastered simple origami designs as his fine motor skills improved. The joy on his face as he finished his first origami design, a fox face, left a lasting impression on me. Each week he looked forward to our sessions and greeted me with excitement. A lasting therapeutic relationship was formed, and I still receive updates from his parents on his school successes and extracurricular activities years after he was discharged from OT services.

Another experience reflects humor that can occur during OT telehealth sessions. One day, I was working with a 9-year-old boy diagnosed with a learning disability and fine motor deficits impacting school performance. We were about midway through our telehealth session when suddenly the audio went out, or so I thought. I could see his mouth moving, but there was no sound. As I began to troubleshoot, he burst out laughing, and I realized that he was playing a trick on me and was simply mouthing the words. We both laughed. He tried to trick me on a few more occasions in subsequent sessions, though I didn't fall for it. Nonetheless, the experience reflects the humor and therapeutic relationship we shared.

Working with families through telehealth has helped me develop my coaching skills. Through modeling, verbal cuing, joint problem-solving, and providing opportunities for reflection and feedback, I've supported and empowered caregivers to implement therapeutic strategies into their child's daily routines.

So many clients come to mind as I reflect on my many years of experience with telehealth. These experiences affirm that telehealth supports therapeutic use of self and client-centered therapy.

Telehealth Documentation

Documentation is an important part of the OT process and should reflect the clinical reasoning of the OT practitioner, the nature of the skilled OT services provided, and the relationship of the services to the client's outcomes (AOTA, 2018a). Regardless of service delivery model, OT practitioners should explicitly link interventions and objective data with functional performance and participation.

The client's response to OT services and progress toward treatment goals should also be documented. Treatment goals should be client-centered, occupation-based, and measurable.

When using a telehealth service delivery model, OT practitioners should document that the service was delivered through telehealth. Technical issues impacting the OT session, if any occurred, should also be documented. OT practitioners should follow payer guidance on billing codes, use of modifiers, and location of service codes to appropriately identify services provided through telehealth.

The PACE Framework

The PACE Framework provides a systematic approach to documenting the efficacy and impact of OT services delivered through telehealth (Little et al., 2021a, 2021b). The framework consists of four domains: (a) *Population and health outcomes*, (b) *Access for all clients*, (c) *Costs and cost effectiveness*, and (d) *Experiences of clients and OT practitioners*. Each domain has subdomains, operational definitions, and examples of outcome measures. The PACE Framework facilitates documentation of individual and program-level outcomes of OT services delivered through telehealth and supports evidence-based practice (Little et al., 2021b). See www.paceframework.org, for more information about the PACE Framework and resources to support its use in OT practice.

Telehealth Informed Consent

In the United States, state laws variously dictate the telehealth informed consent process. Some states require written consent, whereas others accept verbal consent documented by the healthcare provider. Practitioners should follow the laws and regulations, including the OT scope of practice and telehealth informed consent requirements, where the client is located as that is deemed the location of service.

Content of a telehealth informed consent may include potential benefits, risks, efforts to protect privacy and security of PHI, and the client's rights and responsibilities. In addition to laws and regulations, OT practitioners should consult their organization's policies and procedures related to the informed consent process and documentation requirements for OT services provided through telehealth.

Conclusion

Telehealth enables OT practitioners to provide services to clients, who are in different physical locations, using information and communication technologies. Benefits of telehealth include improved access, decreased travel and expenses associated with travel, and increased ability to schedule therapy during daily routines when and where they naturally occur. Research validates telehealth as an effective OT service delivery model with high satisfaction among practitioners and clients. Although traditional, in-person therapy will remain central to OT practice, telehealth and hybrid models will be seamlessly integrated as another way in which OT services are provided.

Lippincott® Connect *For additional resources on the subjects discussed in this chapter, visit Lippincott Connect.*

REFERENCES

Abdolahi, A., Bull, M. T., Darwin, K. C., Venkataraman, V., Grana, M. J., Dorsey, E. R., & Biglan, K. M. (2014). A feasibility study of conducting the Montreal Cognitive Assessment remotely in individuals with movement disorders. *Health Informatics Journal, 22*(2), 304–311. https://doi.org/10.1177/1460458214556373

American Occupational Therapy Association. (1993). Core values and attitudes of occupational therapy practice. *American Journal of Occupational Therapy, 47*(12), 1085–1086. https://doi.org/10.5014/ajot.47.12.1085

American Occupational Therapy Association. (2005). Telerehabilitation position paper. *American Journal of Occupational Therapy, 59*(6), 656–660. https://doi.org/10.5014/ajot.59.6.656

American Occupational Therapy Association. (2017). *Advisory opinion for the ethics commission: Telehealth.* https://www.aota.org/-/media/corporate/files/secure/practice/ethics/advisory/telehealth-advisory.pdf

American Occupational Therapy Association. (2018a). Guidelines for documentation of occupational therapy. *American Journal of Occupational Therapy, 72*(suppl. 2), 7212410010. https://doi.org/10.5014/ajot.2018.72S203

American Occupational Therapy Association. (2018b). Telehealth in occupational therapy. *American Journal of Occupational Therapy, 72*(suppl. 2), 7212410059. https://doi.org/10.5014/ajot.2018.72S219

American Occupational Therapy Association. (2020a). AOTA 2020 Occupational Therapy Code of Ethics. *American Journal of Occupational Therapy, 74*(3), 7413410005. https://doi.org/10.5014/ajot.2020.74S3006

American Occupational Therapy Association. (2020b). *Billing telehealth services to Medicare.* https://www.aota.org/advocacy/advocacy-news/2020/billing-telehealth-services-medicare

American Occupational Therapy Association. (2020c). Occupational therapy practice framework: Domain and process (4th ed.). *American Journal of Occupational Therapy, 74*(Suppl. 2). https://doi.org/10.5014/ajot.2020.74S2001

American Occupational Therapy Association. (2021a). *Occupational therapy and telehealth: State statutes, regulations and regulatory board statements.* https://www.aota.org/-/media/Corporate/Files/Advocacy/State/telehealth/Telehealth-State-Statutes-Regulations-Regulatory-Board-Statements.pdf

American Occupational Therapy Association. (2021b). *OTA state statutes and regulations.* https://www.aota.org/-/media/corporate/files/secure/advocacy/licensure/stateregs/supervision/ota-supervision-requirements---10-2022.pdf

California Telehealth Resource Center. (2021). *Program developer toolkit.* https://www.caltrc.org/wp-content/uploads/2021/05/CTRC_ProgramDevToolkit_2021Layout.pdf

Center for Medicare and Medicaid Services. (2021, March). *Telehealth for providers: What you need to know.* https://www.cms.gov/document/telehealth-toolkit-providers.pdf

Chen, J., Jin, W., Zhang, X.-X., Xu, W., Liu, X.-N., & Ren, C.-C. (2015). Telerehabilitation approaches for stroke patients: Systematic review and meta-analysis of randomized controlled trials. *Journal of Stroke and Cerebrovascular Diseases, 24*(12), 2660–2668. https://doi.org/10.1016/j.jstrokecerebrovasdis.2015.09.014

Ciemins, E. L., Holloway, B., Coon, P. J., McClosky-Armstrong, T., & Min, S. J. (2009). Telemedicine and the Mini-Mental State Examination: Assessment from a distance. *Telemedicine Journal and e-Health, 15*(5), 476–478. https://doi.org/10.1089/tmj.2008.0144

Dreyer, N. C., Dreyer, K. A., Shaw, D. K., & Wittman, P. P. (2001). Efficacy of telemedicine in occupational therapy: A pilot study. *Journal of Allied Health, 30*(1), 39–42.

Federal Trade Commission. (n.d.). *The Antitrust Laws.* https://www .ftc.gov/tips-advice/competition-guidance/guide-antitrust-laws/ antitrust-laws

Guilfoyle, C., Wootton, R., Hassall, S., Offer, J., Warren, M., & Smith, D. (2003). Preliminary experience of allied health assessments delivered face to face and by videoconference to a residential facility for elderly people. *Journal of Telemedicine & Telecare, 9*(4), 230–233. https://doi .org/10.1258/135763303322225571

Hoel, V., von Zweck, C., Ledgerd, R., & World Federation of Occupational Therapists. (2021). Was a global pandemic needed to adopt the use of telehealth in occupational therapy? *Work, 68*(1), 13–20. https://doi.org/10.3233/WOR-205268

Hoffmann, T., & Russell, T. (2008). Pre-admission orthopaedic occupational therapy home visits conducted using the internet. *Journal of Telemedicine & Telecare, 14*(2), 83–87. https://doi.org/10.1258/ jtt.2007.070808

Hoffmann, T., Russell, T., Thompson, L., Vincent, A., & Nelson, M. (2008). Using the internet to assess activities of daily living and hand function in people with Parkinson's disease. *NeuroRehabilitation, 23*(3), 253–261. https://doi.org/10.3233/nre-2008-23307

Hwang, R., Mandrusiak, A., Morris, N. R., Peters, R., Korczyk, D., & Russell, T. (2016). Assessing functional exercise capacity using telehealth: Is it valid and reliable in patients with chronic heart failure. *Journal of Telemedicine and Telecare, 23*(2), 225–232. https://doi .org/10.1177/1357633X16634258

Kairy, D., Lehoux, P., Vincent, C., & Visintin, M. (2009). A systematic review of clinical outcomes, clinical process, healthcare utilization and costs associated with telerehabilitation. *Disability & Rehabilitation, 31*(6), 427–447. https://doi.org/10.1080/09638280802062553

Lin, N. C. J., Hayward, K. S., D'Cruz, K., Thompson, E., Li, X., & Lannin, N. A. (2020). Validity and reliability of a smartphone inclinometer app for measuring passive upper limb range of motion in a stroke population. *Disability & Rehabilitation, 42*(22), 3243–3249. https://doi.org/10.1080/09638288.2019.1585972

Little, L. M., Cason, J., Pickett, K. A., & Proffitt, R. (2021a). Keeping PACE with the new normal: A framework for telehealth practice, research, and policy. *OT Practice, 26*(8), 10–15. https://www.aota.org/ publications/ot-practice/ot-practice-issues/2021/pace-framework

Little, L. M., Pickett, K. A., Proffitt, R., & Cason, J. (2021b). Keeping PACE with 21st century healthcare: A framework for telehealth research, practice, and program evaluation in occupational therapy. *International Journal of Telerehabilitation, 13*(1), 1–20. https://doi .org/10.5195/ijt.2021.6379

Little, L. M., Pope, E., Wallisch, A., & Dunn, W. (2018). Occupation-based coaching by means of telehealth for families of young children with autism spectrum disorder. *American Journal of Occupational Therapy, 72*(2), 7202205020. https://doi.org/10.5014/ajot.2018.024786.

Liu, L. (2000). Position statement on telehealth and tele-occupational therapy. *Canadian Journal of Occupational Therapy, 67*(5), 362–364.

McEachern, W., Kirk, A., Morgan, D. G., Crossley, M., & Henry, C. (2014). Reliability of the MMSE administered in-person and by telehealth. *Canadian Journal of Neurological Sciences, 35*(5), 643–646. https:// doi.org/10.1017/S0317167100009458

Miyazaki, M., & Liu, L. (2002). Tele-occupational therapy: Making occupational therapy services accessible. *Occupational Therapy Now, 4*(5), 16–19.

Ninnis, K., Van Den Berg, M., Lannin, N. A., George, S., & Laver, K. (2019). Information and communication technology use within occupational therapy home assessments: A scoping review. *British Journal of Occupational Therapy, 82*(3), 141–152. https://doi .org/10.1177/0308022618786928

Nissen, R. M., & Serwe, K. M. (2018). Occupational therapy telehealth applications for the dementia-caregiver dyad: A scoping review. *Physical & Occupational Therapy in Geriatrics, 36*(4), 366–379. https://doi .org/10.1080/02703181.2018.1536095

Önal, G., Güney, G., Gün, F., & Huri, M. (2021). Telehealth in paediatric occupational therapy: A scoping review. *International Journal of Therapy & Rehabilitation, 28*(7), 1–16. https://doi.org/10.12968/ ijtr.2020.0070

Palsbo, S. E., Dawson, S. J., Savard, L., Goldstein, M., & Heuser, A. (2007). Televideo assessment using Functional Reach Test and European Stroke Scale. *Journal of Rehabilitation Research and Development, 44*(5), 659–664. https://doi.org/10.1682/JRRD.2006.11.0144

Pearson. (2021a). *Q-global.* https://www.pearsonassessments.com/ professional-assessments/digital-solutions/q-global/about.html

Pearson. (2021b). *Staying connected through telepractice: News and how-tos including COVID-19 resources.* https://www.pearsonassessments.com/ professional-assessments/digital-solutions/telepractice/about.html

Queensland Government. (n.d.). *Allied health assistants.* https://www .health.qld.gov.au/ahwac/html/ahassist

Radley, L. G., & Rumery, E. (2021). Ethical telehealth practice. *OT Practice, 26*(7), 34–36. https://www.aota.org/-/media/Corporate/ Files/Publications/CE-Articles/CEA_July_2021.pdf

Richmond, T., Peterson, C., Cason, J., Billings, M., Terrell, E. A., Lee, A. C. W., Towey, M., Parmanto, B., Saptano, A., Cohn, E. R., & Brennan, D. (2017). American Telemedicine Association's principles for delivering telerehabilitation services. *International Journal of Telerehabilitation, 9*(2), 63–68. https://doi.org/10.5195/ijt.2017.6232

Sanford, J., Jones, M., Daviou, P., Grogg, K., & Butterfield, T. (2004). Using telerehabilitation to identify home modification needs. *Assistive Technology, 16*(1), 43–53. https://doi.org/10.1080/10400435.2004 .10132073

Sing-Fai, T., Wai, K. M., Hui-Chan, C. W. Y., Lau, A., Yip, B., & Cheung, W. (2003). Evaluating the efficacy of tele-cognitive rehabilitation for functional performance in three case studies. *Occupational Therapy International, 10*(1), 20–39. https://doi .org/10.1002/oti.175

Steele, L., Lade, H., McKenzie, S., & Russell, T. (2012). Assessment and diagnosis of musculoskeletal shoulder disorders over the internet. *International Journal of Telemedicine & Applications, 2012,* 1–8. https://doi.org/10.1155/2012/945745

Stillerova, T., Liddle, J., Gustafsson, L., Lamont, R., & Silburn, P. (2016). Could everyday technology improve access to assessments? A pilot study on the feasibility of screening cognition in people with Parkinson's disease using the Montreal Cognitive Assessment via internet videoconferencing. *Australian Occupational Therapy Journal, 63*(6), 373–380. https://doi.org/10.1111/1440-1630.12288

U.S. Department of Education. (2016, October 12). *Email and student privacy.* https://studentprivacy.ed.gov/training/email-and-student-privacy

U.S. Department of Health and Human Services. (2003). *Summary of the HIPAA Privacy Rule.* https://www.hhs.gov/sites/default/files/ocr/ privacy/hipaa/understanding/summary/privacysummary.pdf

Wellmon, R. H., Guliek, D. T., Paterson, M. L., & Guliek, C. N. (2016). Validity and reliability of 2 goniometric mobile apps: Device, application, and examiner factors. *Journal of Sport Rehabilitation, 25*(4), 371–379. https://doi.org/10.1123/jsr.2015-0041

Western Psychological Services. (2021a). *Assessment telepractice overview.* https://pages.wpspublish.com/telepractice-101

Western Psychological Services. (2021b). *Online Evaluation System*™. https://platform.wpspublish.com/account/login

Worboys, T., Brassington, M., Ward, E. C., & Cornwell, P. L. (2018). Delivering occupational therapy hand assessment and treatment sessions via telehealth. *Journal of Telemedicine & Telecare, 24*(3), 185–192. https://doi.org/10.1177/1357633X17691861

World Federation of Occupational Therapists. (2021). *Occupational therapy and telehealth.* https://wfot.org/resources/occupational-therapy-and-telehealth

Occupational Therapy Practice Through the Lens of Primary Health Care

Sivuyisiwe Khokela Toto and Karen Ching

LEARNING OBJECTIVES

After reading this chapter, you will be able to:

1. Understand the philosophy of primary health care (PHC), its history, and links to wider healthcare debates in the Global South.
2. Distinguish between comprehensive and selective PHC approaches and their significance in the evolution of PHC since 1978.
3. Understand the practice landscape of PHC.
4. Articulate the role of occupational therapists in the context of PHC.

Introduction

The COVID-19 pandemic has, with devastating effect, illustrated the intrinsic link between health and human development and exposed the inequalities in healthcare provision within and between countries. All sectors and industries have a vested interest in the health system, health policy, and health financing and resources. Health is necessary for all human development contributing to economic growth, creativity, and innovation at national and international levels (Bloom & Canning, 2000; Liu et al., 2003; Sen, 1999). Therefore conceptions of and about health and how to achieve health for all are necessarily sociopolitical, sociohistorical, socioeconomic, and sociocultural. It is against this backdrop that this chapter situates primary health care (PHC) as a philosophy and approach to healthcare provision, grounded in the notion that health is not merely the absence of disease but rather a state of physical, mental, and social well-being. PHC pays specific attention to the social determinants of health in addressing health concerns at the individual, family, community, and population levels. Social determinants of health (SDHs) are "the sociopolitical, economic and historical conditions in which people are born, grow, work, live, and age, and the wider set of forces and systems shaping the conditions of daily life. These forces and systems include economic policies and systems, development agendas, social norms, social policies, and political systems" (World Health Organization [WHO], 2008a).

Although "primary health care" is often used interchangeably with "primary care," they mean very different things in the context of this chapter. Primary care is a term commonly used in the United States and the United Kingdom to denote generalist doctor services rendered to individuals, whereas PHC is a much broader concept that expands beyond individual patient care to include population health outcomes and involves a range of healthcare workers. This chapter specifically refers to the role of occupational therapy (OT) in the context of the broader understanding of the concept of PHC, focusing on contexts of the Global South. The term "Global South" refers to contexts of historical and/or current oppression and marginalization of people across all areas of life in Africa, Latin America, Asia, and other parts of the world; we also acknowledge that the Global South transcends geography to also include locations in the Northern hemisphere that share the same experience of hegemony and subjugation such as the First Nations of Canada (Abrahams et al., 2022).

The History of Primary Health Care

Community-oriented primary care (COPC) is considered to be the original conceptualization of the PHC philosophy and stemmed from the work of two South African doctors who practiced in rural KwaZulu-Natal (KZN) in the 1940s (Kark & Cassel, 1956). As early as 1944, when World War II was drawing to a close, it became clear that healthcare provision needed to move past the medical care of the sick, which had been the dominant model of care, to incorporate preventive and promotive health services by opening meaningful lines of communication about health matters between healthcare workers and communities (Kark & Cassel, 1956). This new approach advocated for a model of care that integrated *primary care* with *population health strategies* to improve the health status of all citizens (Gofin et al., 2015). As originally conceptualized, COPC is an iterative process conducted in collaboration with community members and involves the following six steps (Gervits & Anderson, 2014):

1. Defining a community
2. Characterizing its problems
3. Prioritizing these problems
4. Analyzing the selected health conditions
5. Intervening to address the priority problems
6. Conducting evaluations

The biomedical model of care has dominated healthcare provisioning, wherein services are institutionalized, individualized, and unidirectional. The biomedical model refers to a Western approach to healthcare that emphasizes diagnosis of health issues and assumes all health problems can be reduced to their physiologic symptoms and organic causes. It positions the medical professional as the knower of what needs to be "fixed" while positioning the patient as a passive recipient of treatment.

The treatment plans formulated by healthcare professionals for their patients are informed by research, evidence, and a standardized public health approach where national or international guidelines are implemented (Abrahams et al., 2022; Verboven et al., 2022). However, Pillay and Kathard (2015) note that the biggest beneficiaries of the medical model are White, middle-class, English-speaking people from a dominant culture, even in contexts of the Global South where they may be a minority. This is in part because of the fact that healthcare has been racialized and subsequently commercialized (Abrahams et al., 2022; Coetzee, 2018; Pellegrino, 1999; Ramugondo & Emery-Whittington, 2022). COPC challenges the medical model by shifting the focus of care toward prevention and health promotion and the authority to determine health priorities to a partnership with internal and external health and social care providers as well as local communities (Kinkel et al., 2013). This partnership is built on mutual empowerment where authority, responsibility, and capacity are shared (Kinkel et al., 2013). Multidisciplinary cooperation and nonhierarchical collaboration are the cornerstones of COPC (Lenihan & Iliffe, 2001).

The Declaration of Alma-Ata

The WHO further refined this thinking and approach, and the concept of PHC was eventually endorsed at the 1978 Alma-Ata conference in Kazakhstan, jointly hosted by the WHO and the United Nations Children's Fund (UNICEF). The Declaration of Alma-Ata that emerged from the conference defined PHC as essential healthcare based on scientifically sound and socially acceptable methods and technology made universally accessible at an affordable cost (WHO & UNICEF, 1978). There was deep consensus on PHC as the most effective, equitable, and efficient means to achieving population health and well-being (Kluge et al., 2019). The conference inspired an interpretation of health that went beyond merely the absence of disease to include the social and economic dimensions of health and enshrined health as a basic human right (Rifkin, 2018).

PHC includes promotive, preventive, curative, rehabilitative, and palliative services for common health problems available as close as possible to where people live and work (WHO, 2008b).

At the 1978 conference, the promotion of health was inextricably linked to improving the socioeconomic conditions and the alleviation of poverty (Toole, 1987). This link highlighted the environmental, social, and economic determinants of health status; and in so doing, it was recognized that health cannot be attained by the efforts of the health sector alone, but required an intersectoral approach (WHO & UNICEF, 1978). An intersectoral approach involves a collaboration among government departments, civic society, and industry to address SDH like social development, education, housing, water, and sanitation. The principles of universal access to care, equity and equal access, community participation, appropriate use of resources, and intersectoral collaboration were identified as central to the philosophy of PHC (Du et al., 2019). The PHC places individuals, families, and communities at the center of their own health while drawing on a wide range of stakeholders capable of addressing not only the biomedical aspects but also the broader SDH (Bryant & Richmond, 2016; WHO & UNICEF, 2018). It is considered to be not only an approach to dealing with the problems of ill-health in poor communities but also has the potential to be a major catalyst for self-managed social and economic development (Toole, 1987).

The Theoretical Construct of Primary Health Care and Its Practical Application

The conventional health system is more often shaped by a disproportionate focus on unidirectional (from provider to patient) hospital care and cure (WHO, 2008b). Reorientating health systems to PHC necessitates change in the allocation of roles and responsibilities, resourcing, the structuring of individual organizations, and the health system as a whole. It requires new patterns of interaction within the health system itself and with other agencies, service users, and citizens. In the context of limited consensus on the concept of PHC and how to give effect to it, making the paradigm shift has been fraught with complexity (Bryant & Richmond, 2016). Even though there is widespread acceptance that people should be situated at the heart of health systems, in reality, public engagement in health systems tends to be more perfunctory with less genuine mutuality (Nimegeer et al., 2011). Putting people first has proven to be a major challenge as it requires social and behavioral change operating within complex social and cultural contexts.

Postindustrial culture and thinking are so embedded in the ideas, beliefs, and approaches valued and advocated by medical science that it continues to be extremely challenging to appreciate perspectives of health other than that of medical science (Wilcock, 2006). The Alma-Ata notion of PHC was criticized for being too broad and idealistic. Invariably, a managerial approach dominated the implementation of PHC initiatives, which detracted from the social, political, and economic determinants of health. This resulted in the emergence of *selective PHC* in 1979, which is a top-down approach that targets a limited set of epidemiologically justifiable and technically affordable interventions (Rifkin, 2018; Walraven, 2019). Selective PHC is distinctly vertical in nature and is most often characterized by an approach to healthcare that treats users as passive recipients of medical care. It was meant to rapidly improve access, but only to a limited scope of services.

High-burden diseases such as HIV/AIDS and vulnerable population groups like children and women were targeted with public health interventions dictated by donors and funders. This selective PHC approach was considered to be more feasible, measurable, rapid, and less risky, and it has been favored by global donor organizations (Bryant & Richmond, 2016; Rifkin, 2018; Topp & Abimbola, 2018). Selective PHC is operationalized as a set of standalone vertical health program with a classic public health design, and they do not address the PHC values of social justice, equity, and community participation (Rifkin, 2018; Topp & Abimbola, 2018). Although there has been some success with improving disease-specific outcomes using selective PHC approach, the unintended consequences have included the fragmentation of healthcare with higher costs for reduced value (Heath et al., 2009).

Primary Health Care Today

A strong PHC service is central for realizing the 2030 Agenda for Sustainable Development. In 2015, all United Nations (UN) member states adopted 17 sustainable development goals (SDGs), which are "an urgent call for action by all countries—developed and developing—in a global partnership. They recognize that ending poverty and other deprivations must go hand-in-hand with strategies that improve health and education, reduce inequality, and spur economic growth—all while tackling climate change and working to preserve our oceans and forests" (UN, 2022). PHC was originally conceived as a global strategy to address inequalities in health and universal health coverage (UHC) was identified as a way to protect people from the financial hardship that often comes with accessing healthcare services (WHO, 2008a). SDGs resonate well with the PHC philosophy, in particular SDG 1, which is "end poverty in all its forms everywhere," and SDG 3, which pertains to "ensur[ing] healthy lives and promote well-being for all at all ages" (UN, 2015, p. 18). PHC, as conceptualized at Alma-Ata, remains an important force in thinking about healthcare (WHO, 2008b). It strives to diminish the consequences of socioeconomic injustices by addressing the SDH.

According to the 2021 Global expenditure on health report, costs related to healthcare have more than doubled in the last 20 years, reaching US$8.5 trillion globally in 2019 or 9.8% of global gross domestic product (WHO, 2021). The report further notes that the governments of high-income countries (e.g., Australia, Canada, Finland, Germany, the United Kingdom, the United States) increased their public spending on health since the 2000s, whereas in low-income countries (e.g., Ethiopia, Eswatini, Lesotho, Bangladesh, Zambia, Botswana) that receive external aid, governments have decreased their spending, such that health in low-income countries is financed primarily through high out-of-pocket spending (Maeda et al., 2014; WHO, 2021). Spending on healthcare in today's world is expensive, even for individuals in high-income countries where health spending per capita averaged US$ 4,491 in 2019 (WHO, 2021). Costs related to healthcare can push people into poverty, especially those living with chronic illness or disability in low-income countries.

UHC is a means to ensure that all people have access, without discrimination, to needed promotive, preventive, curative, rehabilitative, and palliative care services and essential, safe, affordable, effective, and quality medicines without experiencing financial hardship. It is a means to attaining equitable access to health services—a core principle of PHC philosophy. Genuine attempts to achieve UHC are fraught with challenges because budget allocation, health workforce recruitment and retention, and design and implementation of health programs depend on the decisions of multiple interest groups, including the private healthcare sector; international agencies such as the World Bank, International Monetary Fund, departments, and agencies specific to each country; and civic society (Maeda et al., 2014). The influence of decisions on UHC by multiple interest groups often involves political compromises, which, at times, may lead to suboptimal outcomes regarding the necessary service delivery reforms needed to ensure health systems are capable of providing accessible basic quality health services (Maeda et al., 2014; Reich et al., 2016; Sanders et al., 2019; Stigler et al., 2016).

In 2018, at the global conference on PHC held in Astana, Kazakhstan, there was a renewed commitment made to PHC and all its values and principles, in particular to justice and solidarity (Rifkin, 2018). As part of the deliberations, PHC was redefined as

> a whole-of-society approach to health that aims equitably to maximize the level and distribution of health and well-being by focusing on people's needs and preferences (both as individuals and communities) as early as possible along the continuum from health promotion and disease prevention to treatment, rehabilitation and palliative care, and as close as feasible to people's everyday environment. (WHO & UNICEF, 2018, p. 2)

Now more than 40 years later, the Alma-Ata vision of "health for all" remains largely unfulfilled, and although people are healthier, wealthier, and living longer than in 1978, there continues to be significant and growing health inequalities in the world. PHC remains underdeveloped and underfunded, with significant workforce challenges (The Lancet, 2018). Approximately half of the population of the world still lacks full coverage of essential health services (WHO, 2019). In low- and middle-income countries (LMICs), an estimated 1 billion people are unable to afford healthcare, with poor people benefiting least from healthcare utilization (Gordon et al., 2020). In 2017, roughly 66% of the world's maternal deaths occurred in sub-Saharan Africa, and only 55.5% of women had their family planning needs met (WHO, 2020). Sub-Saharan Africa accounts for a fifth

of the global disease burden with 93% of deaths because of communicable and noncommunicable disease (NCD; Biney et al., 2020). By 2030, deaths because of NCD are estimated to rise to 52 million globally, with 80% occurring in LMICs (Ndinda et al., 2018). The health systems in LMICs are primarily designed for acute, episodic care and are ill-equipped to meet the needs of people across their life span and the demands of a growing NCD burden (Schwarz et al., 2020).

The entire world is experiencing rapid economic, environmental, technologic, and demographic changes, and these changes have implications for health and well-being. There is evidence to suggest that the majority of a person's health needs can be addressed by a well-functioning PHC service (Lahariya, 2019; WHO, 2019). In countries where these systems are inspired by Alma-Ata such as Japan, France, Brazil, Thailand, and Turkey, there is strong evidence of better health outcomes and reduced inequality at a lower cost (Du et al., 2019; Maeda et al., 2014; Reich et al., 2016; Walraven, 2019). Health systems that embody the principles of PHC are known to respond better and faster to the health challenges of a rapidly changing world (Topp & Abimbola, 2018; WHO, 2008b, 2019).

Unpacking the PHC Continuum

The PHC approach is about ensuring that all people receive a wide and full range of healthcare services to improve their quality of life, health status, and well-being. This means that different populations have different health needs and therefore require different healthcare services. The PHC continuum therefore refers to how the components of a health service are organized to meet and suit the health needs of defined populations. These five components are as follows:

- Health promotion
- Prevention (of disease and illness)
- Treatment (or curative care)
- Rehabilitation
- Palliative and end-of-life care

These components are complementary, integrated, and have a singular goal—the health and wellbeing of all. Each component has a unique focus and adopts tailored strategies to achieve and maintain health and promote well-being. The following sections provide further details on the PHC continuum as well as the role that OT plays in each healthcare component.

Health Promotion

Health promotion is both a form of healthcare service and one of the principles of the PHC approach (Puoane & Hutchings, 2018). In 1986, the WHO and the Canadian government convened an international conference on health promotion that was attended by more than 200 delegates from 38 countries. This conference built on progress made 8 years earlier through the Declaration of Alma-Ata and subsequently adopted a Charter for action to achieve health for all by the year 2000 and beyond (WHO, 1986). This came to be known as the Ottawa Charter for health promotion. It defines health promotion as:

> …the process of enabling people to increase control over, and to improve, their health. To reach a state of complete physical, mental and social well-being, an individual or group must be able to identify and to realize aspirations, to satisfy needs, and to change or cope with the environment. Health is, therefore, seen as a resource for everyday life, not the objective of living. Health is a positive concept emphasizing social and personal resources, as well as physical capacities. Therefore, health promotion is not just the responsibility of the health sector but goes beyond healthy lifestyles to wellbeing. (WHO, 1986, p. 1)

This definition resonates well with the philosophy of the OT profession, including its ideals and values. Unlike other forms of healthcare services championed through PHC, health promotion uses a wider lens to understand health (Puoane & Hutchings, 2018), thus transcending the medical model (Ramugondo & Emery-Whittington, 2022). It accounts for multiple factors and influences beyond organic causes that may impact health, and it uses multiple strategies to achieve health and well-being for the greatest number of people. The WHO (1986) tacitly identifies health promotion as an occupation in itself, thereby strengthening the core assumption of OT that occupation is the natural biologic mechanism for health (Wilcock, 1998) and that health is influenced by the ordinary and extraordinary things that people do in their lives every day (Hocking, 2015; Ramugondo, 2017).

Furthermore, it is useful to think of WHO's definition of health promotion as a collective occupation. Collective occupation has been defined by Ramugondo and Kronenberg (2015) as "occupations that are engaged in by individuals, groups, communities and/or societies in everyday contexts; these may reflect an intention towards social cohesion or dysfunction, and/or advancement of or aversion to a common good" (p. 10). The "common good" being "healthy lives and promotion of well-being for all at all ages" (SDG 3) (UN, 2015). Working toward the "common good" involves a collaborative effort between all healthcare workers, including indigenous and "alternative" healing practitioners (i.e., multidisciplinary collaboration), families, communities, and civic society as well as professions, disciplines, and trades outside of healthcare working together to achieve health for all. OT Story 68.1 illustrates the need for collaboration while highlighting people's different lived realities.

OT STORY 68.1 WAISTBANDS: A HEALTH HAZARD OR A TOOL FOR MONITORING GROWTH AND WARDING OFF EVIL SPIRITS

In 2012, all second-year Audiology, Physiotherapy, Occupational Therapy, and Speech-Language Pathology students at the University of Cape Town were required to conceptualize and implement a health promotion project as part of a shared course. Students were placed in multiprofessional groups of 8 to 10. One such group was placed at an early childhood development center (crèche) in a periurban, low socioeconomic informal settlement in Cape Town. The crèche catered to approximately 60 children between the ages of 2 to 6 years. As part of the students' context-related assessment, they observed that most of the children in the crèche wore strings or bands around their waists. The waistbands naturally accumulated grime because when children play, especially outside, they tend to get dirty. This was what concerned the students; they concluded that the waistbands were unhygienic and therefore a health risk, and they then decided to implement a campaign to remove the waistbands. The students arranged with the preschool teachers to invite the children's parents for a health talk to educate parents about the relationship between hygiene and health. But days after the health talk, the children were still wearing their waistbands.

Evidently, the health talk was unsuccessful. Part of the issue was that the students did not consult the parents and caregivers about what the purpose of the strings was to understand the context better. A PHC nurse, who shared the same culture as the parents, intervened by alerting the students to the significance of waistbands for this community. The nurse explained that waistbands in some African cultures are for monitoring children's growth and for protection against spiritual attacks. Weight is easy to track—if the waistband is loose, it means that the child is losing weight, just as if it is tight, it indicates weight gain. As the children grow, the string is adjusted so that it sits comfortably. The waistband is not only useful for individual growth and weight monitoring but it is also a communal way of monitoring all the children in that community. Thus, the waistbands were, in fact, a contextually situated form of health promotion.

Questions

1. What model of care or health paradigm were the students operating from?
2. What assumptions did the students hold?
3. Reflect on the context-related assessment conducted by the students and what aspects do you think were missing?
4. How could have the students engaged with parents?

This story illustrates how the medical paradigm, as a dominant Western discourse of health (Ramugondo & Emery-Whittington, 2022), has often discredited occupations, activities, and practices of indigenous people as strange, nonsensical, and even pathologic (Ramose, 2022; Said, 1979; Toto, 2021). In fact, the framing of "strange" behavior as pathologic has been associated with the colonial encounter (Ramugondo & Emery-Whittington, 2022; Said, 1979). Western health professions and disciplines established themselves in Africa as the only producers and sources of legitimate knowledge (Okazaki et al., 2008) while concurrently discrediting indigenous ways of knowing (Dastile & Ndlovu-Gatsheni, 2013). Even though PHC as an approach to healthcare is ideologically conversant with indigenous knowledge systems, our training as occupational therapists still reflects attitudes and knowledge inherent in Western medical care.

The Occupational Therapist's Role in Health Promotion

The Ottawa Charter identified three main strategies for health promotion (WHO, 1986), and these can be used by OT students and practitioners in informing their role in PHC settings. These strategies include advocacy, enabling, and mediating.

Advocacy. Socioeconomic and health inequalities between people and communities are driven by powerful social structures based on coloniality, neoliberal policies, racism, sexism, and commercialization of healthcare to the disadvantage of poor communities (van Wees, 2020).

Coloniality refers to hegemonic ways of being, thinking, doing, becoming, and belonging that have outlived colonial administrations, but are imposed by the Western world upon the rest of the world such that there is a dominant, global sociopolitical architecture that defines culture, labor, intersubjective relations, and knowledge production (Maldonado-Torres, 2007). Coloniality takes on many forms. Through an occupational lens, coloniality may have some associations with occupational apartheid, which Kronenberg et al. (2015, p. 22) defines as:

> …the segregation of groups of people through the restriction or denial of access to dignified and meaningful participation in occupations of daily life on the basis of race, colour, disability, national origin, age, gender, sexual preference, religion, political beliefs, status in society, and pervasive social, cultural, and economic consequences jeopardize health and wellbeing as experienced by individuals, communities, and societies.

Coloniality, among its many forms, may express also itself through neoliberal policies. These refer to political and legislative mechanisms of governance that emphasize economic growth through the lowering of corporate tax and privatization of public goods over social justice and redistribution thereby concentrating wealth, resources, and power to the elite while simultaneously stripping the poor of any resources or power (Madlingozi, 2007; Mwipikeni, 2019; Phiri, 2021).

These hegemonic structures are powerful and pervasive, but their elusiveness makes it difficult to articulate them. This further entrenches powerlessness of marginalized others. Thus the role of occupational therapists must involve creating and facilitating opportunities for occupational consciousness. Occupational consciousness has been coined by Ramugondo (2009, p. 221; see also Chapter 11) as an "ongoing awareness of the dynamics of perpetuating hegemonic practices, including personal and collective contributions through the occupations of daily life, and how all this impacts on individual and collective well-being." This construct can be used by occupational therapists to conceptualize interventions that promote social, economic, and occupational justice, as they help communities to reflect on the impact of their actions (and inactions) on their own health (Ramugondo, 2009).

The colonial and apartheid regime in South Africa systematically underdeveloped infrastructure, housing, and recreational spaces in Black communities. Almost 30 years after the abolishment of apartheid in South Africa, its legacy is still alive such that Black children have limited play and recreational spaces, as a result they have no option but to play in busy streets with oncoming traffic. In a 2016 report by the South African Department of Transport, there were 12,944 fatalities, 81.4% were Black individuals, 16.3% were children younger than 10 years, and a 20.8% were children 14 years or younger (South African Department of Transport, 2016). To respond to this dire situation, some communities dig potholes across the road to force motor vehicles to slow down. However, government departments responsible for road maintenance often repair the potholes without asking themselves why they keep getting potholes in the same areas nor engaging the communities themselves.

It is clear that serious health promotion programs and interventions are needed, as well as active collaboration between all affected parties. Thus, the role of an occupational therapist may involve advocating for children's safety and for the creation of safe play and recreational spaces. Occupational therapists working in government departments such as Department of Health, Department of Basic Education, and Department of Social Development inherently have access to governmental networks and resources that could help improve road safety and promote safe and healthy environments. Moreover, occupational therapists in nongovernmental organizations (NGOs) often have access to community networks; thus, their role would involve awareness raising.

Enabling. Health promotion actions that is advocating, enabling, and mediating are often integrated, indivisible, and complementary. According to the Ottawa Charter, health promotion focuses on achieving equity in health and ensuring equal opportunities and resources to enable all people to achieve their fullest health potential (WHO, 1986). In Africa and other Global South contexts, people who need health promotion the most often are subjected to unsuitable and terrible living and working conditions, unemployment, poverty, marginalization, and sociopolitical oppression. Ramugondo and Emery-Whittington (2022) advocate for a decolonizing approach to health promotion where the voices of marginalized and oppressed people inform teaching, research, and practice.

Although the 1948 WHO definition of health can be applied across contexts, it is not all encompassing given that spirituality as an aspect of health is neglected (Ramugondo, 2017). Thus, the health promotion of enabling may involve helping individuals and communities to incorporate their spiritual practices with Western healthcare approaches. For example, in some African contexts, particularly in South Africa, many Black people often are ashamed or do not feel comfortable in sharing with their Western trained health providers that they are also receiving attention from traditional healers. This can have a negative impact on their health, because sometimes the practices/medicines prescribed by traditional healers may counteract Western health interventions. Thus, the role of the OT is to enable people to have open conversations about all their health-seeking behaviors, which may have a bearing on their outcomes.

Mediating. The architecture underlying the PHC approach is based on interrelationships and connectedness between sectors, systems, and processes in government departments, NGOs, and public benefits organizations and institutions. Mediating involves harmonizing indigenous health systems with Western approaches to healthcare. This gives occupational therapists working in the public health sector the ability to connect with and collaborate on programs outside of the ministry of health such as local municipalities; education, housing, social development, community safety, and labor departments; traditional healers; higher education institutions; and so on. In this way, public sector OT practitioners are uniquely positioned to create, assist in creating, facilitate, and explore:

- Engagement and participation in meaningful, health-promoting (collective) occupations for individuals, groups, and communities
- Opportunities and spaces for personal and collective sensemaking with individuals, groups, and communities
- Social, economic, and occupational justice alongside marginalized people and advocate for individuals, groups, and communities

In keeping with the values and principles of the comprehensive PHC and with an occupational perspective that is intrinsic to the practice of OT, occupational therapists in the service of health promotion can be:

- *Enablers* of human development with a profound appreciation for the resilience and ingenuity of the human spirit
- *Facilitators* of social change who work respectfully and thoughtfully with existing forces of change
- *Partners* in the enactment of empathy who reflect a sound grasp of the views and feelings of others
- *Boundary spanners* who are capable of the artistry of establishing rapport with individuals, families, communities, and populations nested within everyday engagements
- *Catalysts* for unlocking the potential of occupations to inform innovative way to manage the risks associate with the social determinants of health

Prevention

PHC invests significantly in the potential of health promotion and prevention to reduce the global burden of disease and creates the opportunity to shift the focus of health systems from solely focusing on the sick to including the healthy. The responsibility is for the health of a defined population in its entirety, for both those who choose to use health services and those who don't (WHO, 2008b). The boundaries between health promotion, prevention of ill-health, and treatment are fluid as achieving their desired impact relies on synergy among all, three especially when mitigating the risks associated with the SDH (Haque et al., 2020; WHO, 2008a). Prevention is fundamentally concerned with improving health status to reduce the likelihood of morbidity and mortality as a consequence of a health condition or injury. This means that prevention overlaps with health promotion as it also addresses SDH. However, the main focus is on building health consciousness. Health consciousness refers to self-awareness about one's and the willingness to engage in behaviors that promote health and well-being (Espinosa & Kadić-Maglajlić, 2018). Prevention strategies may also include improving health literacy—the ability of an individual to obtain and translate knowledge and information in order to maintain and improve health (Liu et al., 2020) and creating agency for behavior change.

Prevention interventions target specific at-risk populations such as children or high-burden diseases such as NCDs. Prevention interventions are typically categorized into primary prevention (the actions taken to prevent the onset of symptoms), secondary prevention (which seeks to halt the progression of clinical illness through early and asymptomatic detection and remediation), and tertiary prevention (which mitigates against disease progression and additional disease complications once clinical disease is apparent) (Haque et al., 2020; Obas et al., 2022; Peckham et al., 2017).

The Occupational Therapist's Role in Prevention

In keeping with the values and principles of the comprehensive PHC and with an occupational perspective that is intrinsic to the practice of OT, occupational therapists in the service of disease prevention can be:

- *Catalysts* for unlocking the potential of occupations to inform innovative ways in managing the risks associate with the SDH
- *Proponents* for the understanding of people as occupational beings in the design of secondary and tertiary prevention interventions for people with a long-term or a complex disabling condition
- *Supporters* of the actions people take to restore and maintain their health and well-being when at risk of developing an impairment
- *Connectors* to ensure people have timely access to resources that can support them to enhance their health and well-being

- *Partners* in the enactment of empathy that reflects a sound grasp of the views and feelings of another
- *Boundary spanners* capable of the artistry of establishing rapport with individuals, families, communities, and populations nested within everyday engagements
- *Facilitators* of maintaining and promoting occupational integrity for people with complex disabling conditions by expanding the focus of therapy beyond "doing" to interventions at the level of the person and identity, supporting people to identify their strengths, values, and purpose that is meaningful and satisfying for them, and then designing and living their lives in congruence (Pentland & McColl, 2008).
- *Guides* in supporting people to build the resilience to live well with a long-term or a complex disabling conditions

The Expanding Our Perspectives box illustrates how primary care services as defined in this chapter might be provided in the United States.

OT Story 68.2 illustrates the need for collaboration while highlighting people's different lived realities.

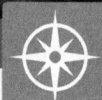

EXPANDING OUR PERSPECTIVES

Primary Care in a Temporary Shelter for Unaccompanied Minors

Claudette Fette

In early 2021, the US border patrol facilities found themselves overcapacity as an unprecedented number of unaccompanied minors entered the United States on its southern border. Most had made treacherous journeys across Mexico from South American countries where their lives were threatened by violence. Some made the journey alone and others began with a parent who died along the way north. Some reported having lived as much as a year in unsafe conditions just on the other side of the border waiting to be allowed to seek asylum in the United States. Several large temporary shelters were created to more effectively process the sheer number of youth.

My experience with the massive unaccompanied minor's shelter near me began with an urgent call for help from a statewide Latina advocate. She reported that the boys' primary occupation in the shelter was waiting in lines to eat, to use the bathroom, to shower, to call home, and for their 30 minutes of recreation every other day. Additionally, she expressed concern that some of the hastily hired staff were bullying the boys to keep them moving through the routines.

From the start, I used a health **promotion** and **prevention** approach. The first thing I did was to initiate the development of a simple trauma 101 training to help staff

recognize trauma responses. I and another faculty member began volunteering in the shelter as **enablers** while we recruited and oriented students. The large convention center space was broken into a grid that organized pods of approximately 50 cots each with one to two staff. The pods were labeled alphabetically, at one point going through the alphabet three times to accommodate as many as 3000. Some boys sat, others lay in their cots, and some with the covers over their head. Their shirts were color-coded, blue if they had a parent as their sponsor, green was for a close family sponsor such as a sibling, brown if the family sponsor was a more distant relative, and a black T-shirt meant they had no sponsor and would be going into foster care.

In the shelter, I acted as a **catalyst**, speaking to everyone who would listen about the boys' need for meaningful occupation in the pods and about the trauma responses I was seeing, and the need for training so that the pod leaders could more effectively support the boys. Our students began volunteering and interacting with the boys. We acted as **facilitators, proponents,** and **boundary spanners**, modeling therapeutic use of self, trauma-sensitive practice, and use of occupation as part of teams partnering our students and staff to bring meaningful activity to the pods. We started by incorporating an idea that a staff member had for a Mother's Day mural for which the boys could create flowers for mothers that they could then choose to attach to panels that we hung near the phones so they could see them. We did activities helping youth identify strengths and goals to use them for the

EXPANDING **OUR PERSPECTIVES** (*continued*)

next year. They worked on a variety of projects and helped those of us with halting Spanish to improve our language skills while we left them with sorting cards to help them in turn build English language skills they would need. As the distinct cultures across the Central American countries soon became apparent, for example the Guatemalan youth were expert weavers and began teaching students their crafts, and we were **partners** and **supporters** of their striving. We were **connectors** with the goal of assuring that the boys experienced no further harm along their journey. We were **guides**, mindful that the deep connections that they needed to forge to help them work through their trauma were to be found at their next stop. We were just working to assure their experience of occupational justice along the way.

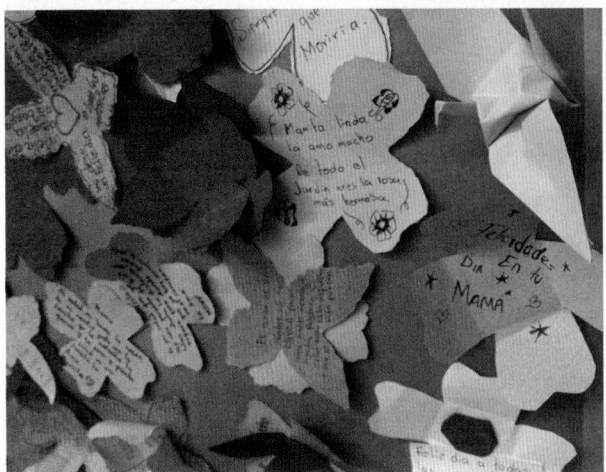

OT STORY 68.2 LIVING WITH A LONG-TERM CONDITION

In South Africa, it is common for people to visit family and friends for extended periods during the summer holidays, and this story is about an elderly woman who came from her hometown in another province to visit her family in Cape Town. During her stay, the family and their neighbors noticed that over time the woman started to "shake" and have odd "facial twitches" more and more. They became increasingly concerned and some where even afraid, thinking the elderly woman had been possessed or a victim of a curse. A neighbor eventually asked the local community rehabilitation worker (CRW) to visit the family as the elderly woman needed assistance with her activities of daily living and was no longer able to walk independently. The CRW in a panic described what she witnessed to her fellow CRWs, and this story about a possessed elderly woman started to do the rounds in the NGO who employed her.

The CRW's supervising occupational therapist also became aware of this story and asked the CRW to describe what she observed on her visit, systematically working through the home visit screening tool, which the CRW had failed to complete as she was convinced the elderly woman was possessed. The occupational therapist then went to visit the family together with the CRW, who was too afraid to enter the home and engage the elderly woman in conversation. The occupational therapist in talking to the elderly woman and doing a basic assessment discovered the woman actually had Parkinson disease. She had run out of her medication as she had visited longer than she originally intended and wasn't able to renew her prescription at the local health facility as she wasn't a local resident.

Consequently, her tremors became more severe, and her family didn't understand when she tried to explain her condition and so did not get the medical help she needed but rather sought the advice of a traditional healer as they too thought she was possessed. The elder woman was desperate to get back home but with her deteriorating mobility and increasing dependence on others to assist her with daily living activities she was not able to travel alone.

Questions

1. Can you identify what form of preventive intervention the elderly woman requires?
2. What is the role of the occupational therapist in this situation, and how can she support the elderly woman in asserting what she needs?
3. In considering that prevention overlaps with health promotion and rehabilitation components of the PHC continuum, can you identify any health promotive or rehabilitative interventions that would need to be considered in this situation?
4. What are key considerations for the occupational therapist in working respectfully and thoughtfully with the culture dimension of this situation?
5. As there are usually an influx of visitors during the summer months, are there any steps the occupational therapist can take to ensure this situation does not arise for other visitors with a similar health status, especially in the households that fall within the geographical area covered by the NGO she works for?

Treatment

Treatment, which is based on the medical model, is perhaps the most dominant form of healthcare across most health professions. In fact, health sciences faculties around the world spend most of their time and resources training students on how to diagnose and treat medical conditions. The curative approach, as it is also known, usually involves a one-on-one service, wherein an individual experiencing occupational dysfunction because of disease, disorder, or disability receives OT services. Therefore, this form of healthcare has been historically based on therapist-centered care, often taking place in clinical settings. However, in recent years, there has been a shift toward patient-centered care, which refers to customized and personalized healthcare services that hone in on individuals' specific health needs and expected health outcomes (NEJM Catalyst, 2017; Reynolds, 2009; Verboven et al., 2022). In this context, occupational therapists usually adopt treatment models or frameworks to inform their treatment approaches. Examples include:

- Canadian Occupational Performance Measure (COPM; Law, 2020)
- Person–Environment–Occupation Performance (PEOP; Baum et al., 2015)
- Model of Human Occupation (MOHO; Kielhofner, 2008)
- Kawa model (Lim & Iwama, 2011)

Increasing Levels of Complexity

One of the challenges in the Global South is the high clinical load with few OT practitioners, especially in rural areas, to address this crisis (Day & Gray, 2016; Rege et al., 2017). Therefore, occupational therapists practicing in resource-limited PHC settings need to explore innovative and creative ways of extending their clinical services to greater numbers of people. Such an approach combines health promotion and disease prevention strategies. A useful strategy might involve investigating and exploring health-promoting collective occupations already embedded in the community's everyday living that could extend treatment beyond the clinic. Another consideration to take into account is that the acute medical conditions that need specialized care are often referred to secondary and tertiary health facilities. Conversely, the need to address SDH and occupational risk factors usually takes place in health facilities closest to the community, that is, at the primary level.

Occupational risk factors refer to occupational experiences that lead to ill-health and diminishing well-being, examples include stress, occupational imbalance, alienation, and deprivation (Townsend & Wilcock, 2004). Occupational imbalance pertains to "a state that occurs because people's engagement in occupation fails to meet their unique physical, social, mental or rest needs and allows insufficient time for their own occupational interests and growth as well as for the occupations each feels obliged to undertake in order to meet family, social, and community commitments" (Townsend & Wilcock, 2004, p. 138). For example, people who work long hours for very low wages sometimes may even hold two jobs to make ends meet; they often have no time to engage in leisurely or restorative occupations. This situation can lead to occupation deprivation; this occurs when an external agency or circumstance (such as overworking, unemployment, or poverty) deprives a person from acquiring, using, or enjoying something (Townsend & Wilcock, 2004, p. 145). Occupational alienation is when a person is estranged from fulfilling occupation. For example, immigrants or refugees may find it difficult to pursue their passions in foreign countries. Intervention, therefore, depends on the presenting challenges faced by those who need OT services. PHC strongly emphasizes a multidisciplinary approach to healthcare services; unfortunately, when this important principle is neglected, the following can happen and often it is service users that suffer the most. OT Story 68.3 illustrates the need for multidisciplinary teamwork and what may go wrong when need for multidisciplinary teamwork in clinical settings is ignored and undermined.

OT STORY 68.3 NEO'S STORY

While working as a junior occupational therapist at a district hospital in the Eastern Cape province of South Africa, I was called into the casualty department to help Neo, a 20-year-old female, calm down. She arrived on a stretcher, highly agitated because of pain in her right ankle and foot. The doctors were unable to examine her, because she was highly agitated; hence, the reason for my call. Through simple breathing exercises, I managed to calm Neo down and asked her to tell me her story and what had brought her to the emergency unit. We soon learned that as she had suddenly lost consciousness, when she couldn't breathe. She was outside packing farming equipment into the toolshed during a heavy thunderstorm. Her right foot got trapped into a ditch as she lost consciousness. Luckily, some of her family members were around the farm when this happened, and they managed to help her and got her to the hospital.

As she told her story, it became clear that she had suffered an asthma attack and a panic attack at the same time. After a brief discussion with the three doctors that were attending to her, I explained to Neo that I needed to assess her foot for injuries, and I assured her that I would be gentle as I palpated her lower limb. On examination, she had full passive range of motion in her ankle and foot. However, she was adamant that she had broken a bone, so I asked the doctors who had called me to order an x-ray, just to make sure (because hairline fractures are not easy to diagnose without an x-ray). The x-ray revealed that she had underdeveloped metatarsal bones, but no history of immobility nor discomfort. The attending doctor decided to admit her overnight for observation. The following day she could walk; however, I noticed that during the gait assessment, she had decreased balance. So I referred her to neurologist at a tertiary hospital as I suspected that she had a cerebellar disorder; however, her attending doctor overrode my referral and insisted that Neo had an orthopedic issue and therefore needs to consult with an orthopedic surgeon.

A few weeks later, Neo was referred by the orthopedic surgeon back to the OT department, but she had a knee and leg cast and crutches on either side. This was confusing to me because there was no indication for it when I last saw her. She explained that the orthopedic surgeon told that

she needs a cast, but did not bother to refer her medical records or perform a clinical examination. The nurses that put her in the cast were merely following "doctor's orders." I explained to Neo that immobilizing her leg would actually worsen things, and upon consultation with a physiotherapist, we advised her to have it removed immediately. Once removed, together with the physiotherapist, we gave her strengthening and balance exercises and referred her to another provincial hospital. We also proceeded to lodge a formal complaint against the orthopedic surgeon, as well as the referring doctor, for medical negligence.

Questions

1. Which other health professions should have been involved in Neo's care, and justify your response?
2. How would you engage with other health professionals when there is disagreement about the diagnosis or which intervention to take?
3. Do you think multidisciplinary teamwork is useful in clinical settings? Why?

The Occupational Therapist's Role in Treatment

Treatment approaches or clinical intervention are dependent on the type of occupational dysfunction a client/patient may present with as well as the client's desired health outcomes. Some interventions in OT may involve the following, but the list is not exhaustive:

- Promoting occupation as both a means and ends (Gray, 1998)
- Involving the family in intervention sessions
- Prescribing assistive devices such as splints or wheelchairs
- Adapting or modify the clients' environment
- Creating home programs
- Linking clients to support groups and NGOs in their locales

In keeping with the values and principles of the comprehensive PHC, and with an occupational perspective that is intrinsic to the practice of OT, occupational therapists in the service of treatment can be:

- *Enablers* of recovery in the event of an impairment
- *Partners* in the enactment of empathy that reflects a sound grasp of the views and feelings of another
- *Boundary spanners* capable of the artistry of establishing rapport with individuals and their families to promote recovery
- *Connectors* to ensure people have timely access to resources that can support them in their recovery

Rehabilitation

When a person experiences difficulty in performing everyday activities like walking, dressing, conducting a conversation, keeping a job, or maintaining relationships as a consequence of a health condition, they require rehabilitative care (Cieza, 2019). The WHO defines rehabilitation as a set of interventions designed to optimize functioning and reduce disability in individuals with health conditions in interaction with their environment; where a health condition is understood to be a disease (acute or chronic), disorder, injury, or trauma and may also include other circumstances such as pregnancy, aging, stress, congenital anomaly, or a genetic predisposition (WHO, 2017). It is characterized by interventions designed to address impairments, activity limitations, and participatory restrictions in the context of personal and environmental factors that impact on functioning (WHO, 2017). Achieving and maintaining the best outcomes from other clinical interventions like surgery often depends on the provision of rehabilitation. Thus, it is not solely for people with disabilities; anyone with a health condition that limits function will need rehabilitation to recover.

As healthcare becomes more accessible, more people are likely to survive injuries and illness, and ultimately live longer. This reality coupled with current shifts in demographic and health profiles of populations has resulted in a rapid increase of people experiencing disability or decline in functioning for prolonged periods of their lives (Cieza et al.,

2020). Globally, at least one in every three people will need rehabilitation at some point in the course of their illness or injury (Cieza et al., 2020). Health systems are under increasing pressure to provide services that target improvement in functioning, in addition to those that reduce mortality, and therefore rehabilitation has become essential to ensuring people live longer and better lives (WHO, 2017). Although the demand for rehabilitation is growing, the capacity for rehabilitation in many parts of the world is unable to meet the existing needs of populations (WHO, 2017).

Community-Based Rehabilitation

Rehabilitation, together with health promotion, prevention, and treatment, plays an integral part in addressing the full scope of health-related needs of a population (WHO, 2017). The inclusion of rehabilitation as a core component of the PHC continuum of care in the Declaration of Alma-Ata has helped to promote a political commitment to improve access to rehabilitation (WHO, 2018). To further these aspirations, in 1979 the WHO developed community-based rehabilitation (CBR), a strategy within general community development for rehabilitation, poverty reduction, equalization of opportunities, and social inclusion of people with disabilities (Ayalew et al., 2020; Blose et al., 2021; Iemmi et al., 2015). The initial conception of CBR focused on access to health and rehabilitation services. It has since evolved to become a multisectorial strategy (Blose et al., 2021; Iemmi et al., 2015).

There was increasing recognition of discrimination, exclusion, and the need to address the social and political aspects of disability (Hartley et al., 2009; Rule et al., 2006). CBR was thus expanded to include socially oriented, rights-based approaches with a focus on empowerment, human rights, equal opportunities, and social inclusion of people with disabilities and their families, particularly in LMICs (Ayalew et al., 2020; Hartley et al., 2009; Rule et al., 2006). It involves targeted interventions at different aspects of life, including health, education, livelihoods, social development, and empowerment (Hartley et al., 2009; MacLachlan et al., 2011; Rule et al., 2006). Fundamental to this approach is that people with disabilities be active partners and through this experience are empowered to take control of their own lives and play a central role in their services (Hartley et al., 2009; Iemmi et al., 2015; Rule et al., 2006). CBR largely shares most of its inherent values with the health promotion principles of empowerment, enablement, social justice, and respect for cultural differences (Fransen, 2005).

The Occupational Therapist's Role in Rehabilitation

In keeping with the values and principles of the comprehensive PHC and with an occupational perspective that is intrinsic to the practice of OT, occupational therapists in the service of rehabilitation can be:

* **Enablers** of clinical recovery in the event of an impairment
* **Facilitators** of personal recovery in the event of an impairment
* **Partners** in the enactment of empathy that reflects a sound grasp of the views and feelings of another
* **Boundary spanners** capable of the artistry of establishing rapport with individuals, families, communities, and populations nested within everyday engagements
* **Connectors** to ensure people with disabilities have timely access to resources that can support them in enhancing and maintaining their health and well-being
* **Guides** in supporting disabled people to unlock their own potential for creating meaningful social change
* **Advocates** of occupational justice in supporting disabled people to realize their occupational potential (see Chapter 10, for more information)

OT Story 68.4 illustrates the occupational therapist's role in rehabilitation.

OT STORY 68.4 CRAFTING A PERSON-CENTERED CARE PATHWAY

In a township in urban South Africa, a CRW was asked to visit a man who used a wheelchair and lived alone, as his neighbors had become increasingly concerned about his well-being. In more recent months, he had increasingly isolated himself and had become quite hostile, which led to many conflicts with the households around him. He no longer welcomed visitors who just came round to chat and check if he needed anything. The neighbors had become increasingly concerned as he was inclined to fling his full bedpan at anyone who attempted to enter his home and was unwilling to accept any of the usual assistance they had provided him over the years. On the first visit, the CRW unfortunately fell victim to a full bedpan and was unable to gain entry to the home or get the man to talk with her outside. What little she was able to observe was that the home was very well kept, everything had a place, and the man had arranged his home in a manner that enabled his independence in his activities of daily living. In speaking to the neighbors, it became apparent that the man was well-respected in his immediate community and was known to be fiercely independent. Although he did accept assistance, it was always with the understanding that it was on his terms. They were, however, concern that his health had deteriorated, and he needed more help to take care of himself but was too stubborn to ask for or accept assistance.

It took multiple subsequent visits to build sufficient trust with the man for the social worker and occupational therapist to eventually be invited into his home. The man had lived on his own for many years and deeply valued this independence and freedom to manage his own life, which was hard earned when he became a paraplegic. He was now almost 70 years old and no longer able to cope as well as he had in the past. He had also developed arthritis, which placed further limits on his ability to manage his daily activities of living as a paraplegic. Consequently, he had become less active and spent more time in bed, and this further exacerbated his functional decline. What he was most afraid of was being placed in an old age home, and as he was poor, he did

not welcome the realities of the state-funded facility. Being a paraplegic, he knew there was a high likelihood he'd be sent to a frail care facility and this terrified him. Even though he was well aware of the resources available to him and how to access the local health and social care services, this fear that he would be forced into a frail care facility stopped him from accessing these services.

Questions

1. How would you have built a rapport with the man to gain his trust?
2. Can you identify key assets in the man's current support network that might be of help to addressing his care needs without compromising his independence to much?
3. In thinking about the principles of CBR, what interventions can the occupational therapist employ to safeguard the man's independence; also consider interventions at a societal level?

Palliative and End-of-Life Care

The Hospice and Palliative Care Association of South Africa (2022) defines palliative care as "the physical, psychological, social, and spiritual [or existential] care provided by a multi-disciplinary team of experts to anyone with a life-threatening illness and their families; [commencing] from a point of diagnosis and extends to bereavement support if needed." It is concerned with ameliorating suffering and pain (including psychological, social, existential, and/or spiritual pain) as well as improving the quality of life of terminally ill and dying people (WHO, 2020). These services also extend to family and loved ones of the dying person (Gwyther, 2019). Palliative care is about upholding and affirming life and about helping everyone involved to see dying, as a normal human phenomenon (Gwyther, 2019; Soogun, 2019). Gwyther (2019) reminds us that palliative care encourages early identification and prevention of further deterioration. For occupational therapists, it is clear that continued participation in valued and meaningful occupations is necessary to maintain the health and well-being of people who need palliative care services. A useful approach for occupational therapists working in palliative care is described by Murray et al. (2005), wherein care is tailored according to the different needs for the different illness trajectories of functional decline, namely, rapid decline, intermittent decline, and gradual decline.

The Occupational Therapist's Role in Palliative Care

Occupational therapists must use their clinical reasoning skills and take a person-centered approach in determining the suitability and appropriateness of valued occupations according to each person's trajectory and health needs. The opportunity to engage in desired occupations, even to participate, is central in maintaining a person's sense of dignity even as they experience progressive decline. At the heart of palliative care is a concern to conserve human dignity even as a person's physical integrity is challenged (Chochinov, 2007; Gwyther, 2019; Haraldsdottir et al., 2020). A life-threatening condition can debilitate a person's sense of dignity and their occupational lives, further diminishing their health status. Therefore, occupational therapists assist terminally ill persons to continue doing things they love. When people do what they love doing, their dignity is conserved. Pentland and McColl (2008) refer to this as occupational integrity, that is, the alignment between a person's occupations, personal values, strengths, and the meaning they attribute to their occupational experiences. This occupational construct can be blended with a practice model. For example, Essential Yeh and McColl (2019) published a practice model on palliative care. They speak about five themes: (a) the importance of valued occupations even at the end of life; (b) an exploration of how occupations change over the trajectory of a terminal illness; (c) the balance between affirming life and preparing for death; (d) valued occupations might be doing, being, becoming, or belonging occupations; and (e) the emphasis of a safe and supportive environment as an essential dimension for effective palliative care.

Although palliative care emphasizes individualized care in institutionalized settings, it stresses the need for a multidisciplinary approach (Haraldsdottir et al., 2020). The role of OT in palliative care services unfolds in context. It includes educating other team members about the role and value of OT, collaborating with, as well as learning about the services of other team members (Talbot-Coulombe & Guay, 2020). In South Africa, palliative care is scarce, especially in rural areas. Rural OT practitioners therefore need to explore community-wide approaches to meet the palliative needs of not just a single individual, but whole communities. A starting point could be exploring with communities the collective occupations associated with, caring for those who are dying.

In keeping with the values and principles of the comprehensive PHC, and with an occupational perspective that is intrinsic to the practice of OT, occupational therapists in the service of palliative and end-of-life care can be:

- *Facilitators* in maintaining and promoting occupational integrity
- *Guides* in supporting people to build the resilience to live well with a life-threatening condition
- *Enablers* in supporting people to prepare for death
- *Connectors* to ensure people have timely access to resources they need to manage their life-threatening condition and die with dignity
- *Partners* in the enactment of empathy that reflects a sound grasp of the views and feelings of another
- *Boundary spanners* capable of the artistry of establishing rapport with individuals and their families nested within everyday engagements

The PHC Practice Landscape

By design, PHC as the first level of contact with the health system should bring promotion, prevention, treatment, rehabilitation, and palliation closer to people in a safe, effective, and socially productive manner at the interface between the population and the health system (WHO and UNICEF, 2018). The intention is to provide comprehensive, accessible, quality, and cost-effective care throughout a person's life span (Kredo et al., 2020). The social dimensions of disease highlight the need for a PHC service design that enables person-centered, comprehensive, and integrated care provision. PHC services need to span a range of risks and illnesses; recognize people as partners in managing

their own health and that of the broader community; and reorientate care around people's needs and expectations. PHC services are thus ideally designed around the health needs of the population in a clearly delineated geographical area, with the intention of making services more socially relevant to produce better health outcomes. It requires an understanding of the human experience and translating that understanding into new service futures (Patrício et al., 2020). The complexity of the health challenges we face necessitates that interventions be:

- Iterative and integrate continues learning
- Cocreated, gathering, and sharing knowledge from a broad range of stakeholders
- Flexible to allow nuancing for local context by automatic adjustment or deliberation

The processes and structure of PHC services are highly dependent on the nature of each society and its healthcare system. First, contact care is most often a missed opportunity as curative, clinical recovery-based interventions dominate, crowding out more promotive, preventive interventions. PHC services are generally organized geographically with a focus on the entire population as opposed to just the sick. Care settings are varied and largely influenced by the accessibility of the health sector's infrastructure footprint and the available workforce. Thus, in countries like the United Kingdom and the United States, you will find general medical practitioners anchor PHC services, whereas in LMICs, nurses together with community health workers (CHWs) form the backbone of the PHC service. In LMICs, people accessing health systems often experience significant frustrations in trying to navigate care continuums as more often than not; they have to undergo many separate assessments; repeat their story multiple time; and are confronted with the inherent delays in the system because of challenges with the transmission of information and environmental factors. PHC services cannot provide for all aspects of health problems, and, in such instances, is responsible for facilitating access to the other levels of care in the health system and/or broader social care services as required by individual users. The design would thus need to have clear mechanisms to enable expedient access to more specialized health services and/or social care services for those who need it. Robust referral systems with clearly defined packages of care for PHC and in-patient care settings are essential for continuity of care.

Community-Based Care Settings

Community-based care settings include the living, learning, working, and social and/or play spaces of a defined population. Health activities would thus take place in people's homes, old age homes, schools/crèches, factories, church/mosque, sports facilities, local parks/playgrounds, and so on. Community-based PHC services are by design ideally embedded in local context involving a comprehensive array of context-sensitive interventions that positively influence environmental and personal factors and recognize people's capacity for self-help. They support the actions people take to maintain health and well-being (health promotion); prevent illness and injury (primary and secondary prevention); treat minor ailments (treatment); enable people to adapt and live well with long-term conditions (tertiary prevention); and recover from periods of acute illness and hospitalization (rehabilitation). The community-based delivery model is population-based with a team being assigned the responsibility for a group of households in a demarked geographical area. The delivery model is anchored by a health facility, most often a clinic, to facilitate seamlessly connecting people to the health system. In LMICs, CHWs with the support ideally of a multidisciplinary team (however, it is more often a nurse) are the primary providers of healthcare in this setting. The community-based care team takes on the role of gatekeeper to the health system, helping people navigate the labyrinth of care continuums.

Community-based services from a health promotion perspective invest in human development, in particular the mobilization of agency at individual, household, and community levels, which dovetails with CBR interventions for people with disabilities. Primary prevention strategies include, for example, supporting breast feeding and investing in early childhood development. Secondary prevention in this setting is about active screening and testing, where appropriate of conditions that drive the burden of disease. The rehabilitation focus is more on personal recovery and to a lesser extent on clinical recovery as interventions center around both activity limitations and participation restrictions. Rehabilitation intervention aimed at addressing function, participation, and social inclusion, and it works hand-in-hand with tertiary prevention strategies, which are intended to prevent relapse and re-admission, shorten hospitalizations, reduce risks, and ultimately interrupt downward social drift. Social drift refers to the gradual downward socioeconomic trajectory that occurs as a consequence of a long-term health condition. Community-based palliative care is becoming increasingly common as people are choosing to die at home surrounded by their friends and family, and in resource-constrained environments, there simply are not enough hospital beds. Palliative care intervention in this setting focuses predominantly on supporting primary caregivers to manage pain and other symptoms at home as well as providing psychosocial support. Interventions in this delivery context have a decidedly promotive, preventive, and rehabilitation orientation, as illustrated in Figure 68.1.

Facility-Based Care Settings

Facility-based services in a PHC context are generalist and ambulatory in nature, serviced by a multidisciplinary team, and ideally organized in a dense network of small service points that are close to users. These teams operate in a seamless manner with the community-based teams and should anchor community-based services. The focus in this setting is on primary prevention strategies like immunization, secondary prevention and treatment particularly as it relates to early diagnosis and a return to previous health status, and tertiary prevention strategies to manage long-term conditions. Rehabilitation interventions have a decidedly clinical recovery orientation that addresses problems in body structure and function and complements tertiary prevention strategies for people with a long-term condition and/or a disability by minimizing the risks of activity limitations and participatory restrictions. The facility-based care settings have the clinical amenities necessary for generalist ambulatory care that allows for more secondary/tertiary prevention, clinical recovery, and treatment type interventions (see Figure 68.2), and in most instances provides basic diagnostic and pharmacy services with access to a doctor.

Occupational Therapy Practice in a Primary Health Care Context

The occupation-focused philosophy and theory of OT offer a distinct perspective that recognizes the inherent links among occupation, health, and well-being, and that engagement in occupations has considerable potential to either enhance or decrease health and well-being (Kim, 2020; Parnell & Wilding, 2010; Wilcock, 2006). An occupational perspective is concerned with what people do daily on their own and with others; how they live and meet their need for subsistence, protection, affection, understanding, participation, idleness, creation, identity, and freedom; organize their habits, routines, and choices; and how engagement is either enabled or restricted by the context in which it is situated (Kim, 2020; Max-Neef, 1991; Njelesani et al., 2014; Wilcock, 2006). It views people as occupational beings and is considered a way of looking at or thinking about human doing (Njelesani et al., 2014; Wilcock, 2006). The occupation theory and reasoning of the profession offer a unique perspective from which to view health and well-being and in finding novel ways to address health issues.

OT views occupational performance as the dynamic interaction between people and their environments, and its practice is concerned with enabling occupational engagement and performance for individuals, families, communities, and

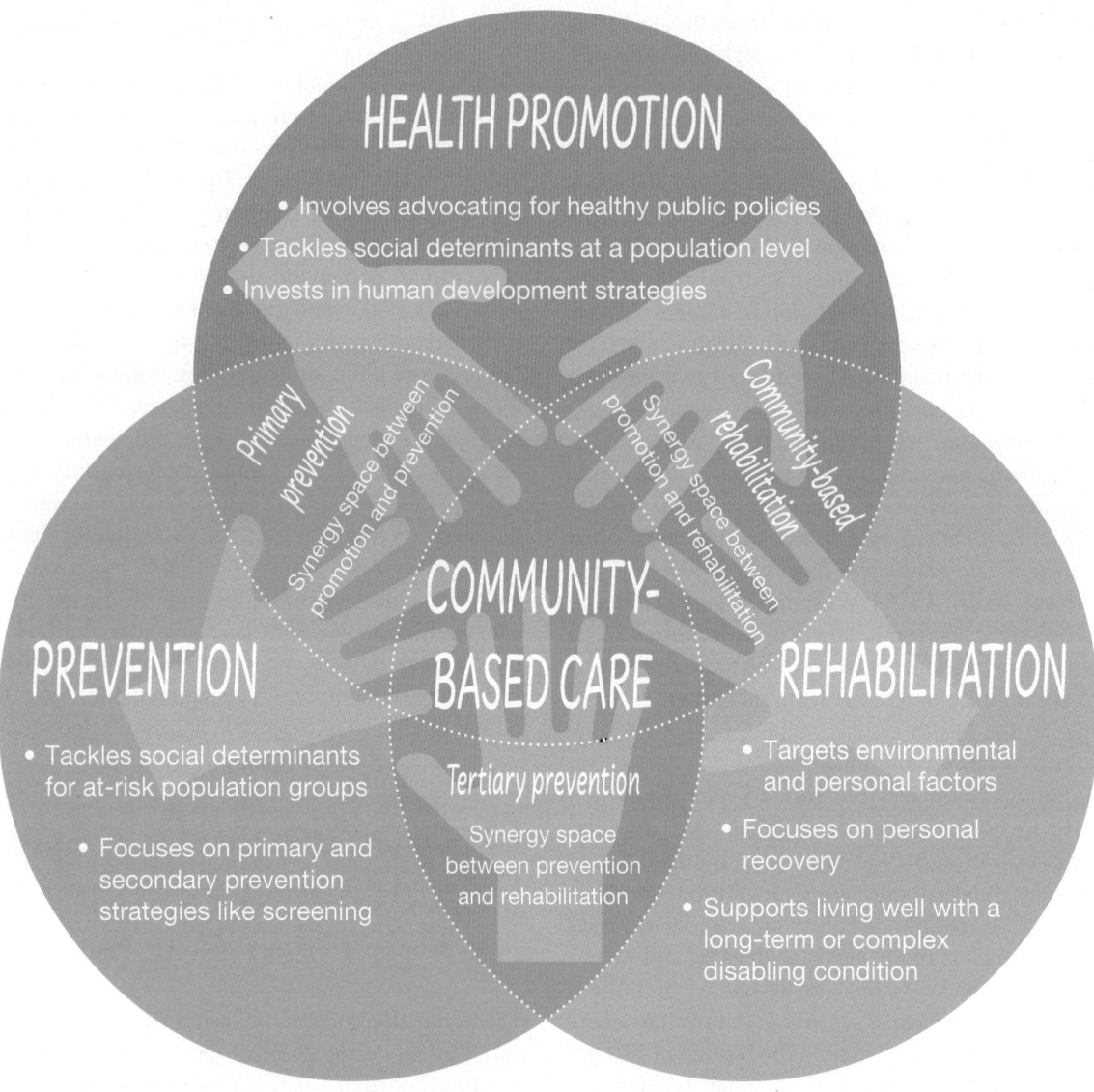

FIGURE 68.1 The service orientation of a community-based care setting.

populations (Fransen, 2005; Parnell & Wilding, 2010). The profession's intrinsic grasp of the relational complexities that exist between the environment and occupation extends far beyond the physical components, and its appreciation for how the environment can either facilitate or restrict choice and engagement in occupations is pivotal in understanding the social constructs of health. The practice of OT takes a problem-based approach to occupations and values the transformational nature of "becoming able" (Fransen, 2005). The very practical approach to dealing with people's occupational engagement challenges and the innovative ways occupational therapists tailor solutions to meet people's needs is particularly valuable in resource-constrained situations. These characteristics of OT practice have deep resonance with the core values and principles of a comprehensive PHC approach.

The OT service design for PHC must consider two important questions: (a) What must the service do? (b) How does the service work in practice?

What Must the Service Do?

The PHC approach asserts the need for people to assume greater responsibility for their own health. It is most often the first point of contact with the health system for the vast majority of people and is rooted in honoring the resilience and ingenuity of the human spirit, creating the space for finding ways of improving health and well-being that is owned and sustained by local communities (Rifkin, 2018; Walraven, 2019). In attempting to understand the likely health needs of a geographically defined population, it is

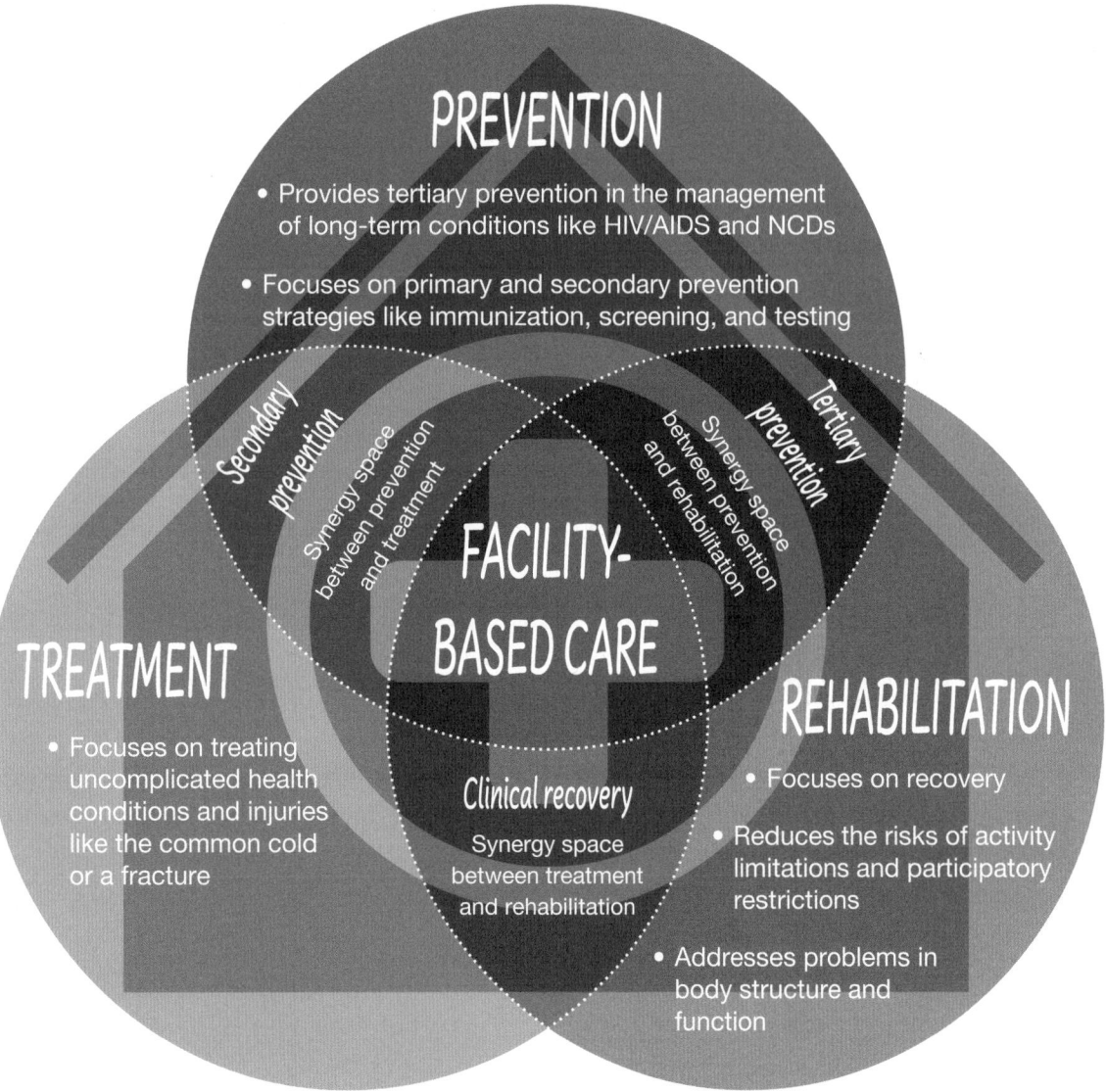

FIGURE 68.2 **The service orientation of a facility-based care setting.**

useful to consider that at any given time the population can be divided into four broad groups:

1. People who are ***mostly healthy***
2. People who access the health system for a ***defined episode of care*** (e.g., pregnancy, broken bone, gunshot and/or stab wound, common cold)
3. Those with ***one or more long-term conditions*** (e.g., diabetes, HIV/AIDS, psychiatric disorder, blindness)
4. Those with ***complex disabling conditions*** (e.g., degenerative neurologic disorders, genetic disorders, complex trauma injuries)

This generic population profile is a useful way to consider what the service must do for each component of the PHC continuum of care, and Figure 68.3 provides guidance on how to go about answering this question. Framing the service in this way facilitates taking a population approach

to understanding health needs across the full spectrum of possible interventions and allows for nuancing interventions based on local context.

How Does the Service Work in Practice?

Once you have a sense of what the service must do, it is now important to consider how the service works in practice. Essentially, this is about defining the OT service delivery model in terms of where best interventions are situated within the local PHC practice landscape, with due consideration for the clinical and social complexities of the care needs. The service delivery model should:

• Place people at the center of their care, with due consideration for their goals, needs, and lifestyle wishes

	Mostly Healthy	Defined Episode of Care	One or More Long-Term Conditions	Complex Disabling Condition
By design	A service that builds the resilience of individuals, families, communities, and populations	A service that returns people to their previous health status	A service that builds capacity for self-management based on active choice, self-empowerment, and hope	A service that builds capacity to attain and sustain the best possible quality of life
PROMOTION	By providing interventions that: • Build people's resilience • Positively influence environmental and personal factors to support the actions people take to maintain health and well-being		By providing interventions that: • Enhance the user's capacity to meaningfully engage in occupations that promote a sense of health and well-being	By providing interventions that: • Enhance the user's capacity to function with fulfillment and a feeling of well-being
PREVENTION	By providing primary interventions that: • Target environmental factors that are negatively impacting on health and well-being in the living, learning, working, and play/social spaces of specific at-risk groups	By providing primary and secondary interventions that: • Enable the early and asymptomatic detection and remediation of ill health • Build people's health consciousness, improve their health literacy, and develop agency for behavior change	By providing secondary and tertiary prevention interventions that: • Lead to symptom reduction and minimize the likelihood of further complications • Support users to develop and sustain self-management techniques	By providing tertiary prevention interventions that: • Halt or retard the progression of the condition(s) • Limit the likelihood of complications
TREATMENT		By providing interventions that: • Restore disruptions to the body structure or its function that were a consequence of illness and/or injury		
REHABILITATION		By providing interventions that: • Enable return to previous levels of function • Facilitate and enable recovery	By providing interventions that: • Focus on function, participation, and social inclusion to promote recovery, prevent unplanned care contacts, and interrupt downward social drift	By providing interventions that: • Focus on function, participation, and social inclusion to promote recovery, prevent unplanned care contacts, and interrupt downward social drift
PALLIATION			By providing interventions that: • Support coping and living well with a life-threatening condition	By providing interventions that: • Provide proactive symptom management to ensure comfort • Support coping with death and dying

FIGURE 68.3 Defining what an occupational therapy service must do in a primary health care (PHC) context.

- Respect the basic values of choice, dignity, diversity, and equality
- Be gender- and culture-sensitive

Reliable systems for clinical support, referral, and record-keeping are essential, and robust working practices for referral, assessment, and reporting are central to the provision of effective health services. The design of these systems must support working seamlessly across care settings, interprofessional collaboration, and strong feedback loops that allow care to evolve with changing user needs throughout their life span. The delivery model should ideally:

1. ***Respect, protect, and contribute to the progressive realization of human rights:*** Occupational therapist have a moral obligation to become actively involved in human rights and the responsibility to meaningful contribute to the realization of these rights. The design of the delivery model should be grounded in the values of mutuality, freedom, and equality, particularly when considering the accessibility and the geographical and population coverage arrangements. Mutuality is an observed principle of life that recognizes the social interdependence of people, valuing respect and solidarity across the boundaries between people, connecting with one another in our common humanity. It is important to note that the lived reality of people in LMICs requires practical, concrete action in response to the basic needs of survival, dignity, and quality of life and necessitates collaborative intervention strategies.

2. ***Proactively engage people around their health and well-being:*** Health services are commonly designed from the perspective of health workers and can be quite difficult for the people needing services to navigate. Delivery models also tend to be reactive and target those who are sick. It is crucial to place people at the center of the design and involve them in the process of determining what delivery model would work best for them. The delivery design must enable person-centered care by supporting a practice that respects the basic values of choice, dignity, diversity, and equality.

3. ***Support users in navigating the local health and social care networks, ensuring they access the right care, at the right time, in the right place, and at the right price:*** The OT delivery model would need to have the flexibility to tailor care to the goals, needs, and lifestyle wishes of not only individuals, but also households, communities, or specific population groups. The delivery model must optimally integrate care and provide continuity within and across care settings, and it should ensure a seamless experience for people as they traverse the health and social care networks.

   Be capable of mobilizing a broader range of resources in support of attaining and sustaining health and well-being: Considering the SDH necessitates collaboration with multiple stakeholders within and outside of the health system, across organizational and sector boundaries. Investing in building social capital is essential to the mobilization of a broader range of resources for health. Social capital refers to resources like information, ideas, leads, trust, and so on, embedded in our relationships with others. Social capital facilitates interpersonal cooperation through the norms of reciprocity, shared values, mutual trust, and a shared understanding that are central to being able to connect people with the right health and social care resources.

Conclusion

Historically, medical professionals have abrogated the right of individuals and communities to make decisions about their own health and well-being, resulting in unequal power dynamics between medical professionals and their patients. Although the biomedical model of care is still useful, it has, unfortunately, led to the commercialization of healthcare, often at the expense of marginalized and poor people. In the Global South, this has also led to disempowerment of entire communities, the destruction of indigenous knowledge systems through disregarding indigenous perspectives on health and well-being. However, PHC philosophy, although Western in its orientation, recognizes the need for people to be actively involved in their own healthcare. Health and well-being must be promoted, ill-health must be prevented, and where prevention fails, treatment and rehabilitation must be acceptable, appropriate, and affordable. And even when both treatment and rehabilitation no longer respond, palliative and end-of-life care must still affirm life. This is the PHC philosophy.

In its original meaning, philosophy was a discipline and study that concerned itself with topics about human flourishing, that is, well-being. Therefore, it makes sense that PHC is sometimes referred to as a philosophy. PHC is concerned with human flourishing, because it is underpinned by an unwavering commitment of health for all and social justice because ill-health is often brought about by social inequalities. PHC is about ensuring access to quality affordable, acceptable, and appropriate healthcare to diverse populations in the most equitable manner without undermining the principle of equal access to all.

Where people live; where people work, play, grow, and age; and all conditions that affect their everyday doing have a significant and direct impact on the status of their health and well-being. PHC is the most ideal way to ensure healthy lives and promote well-being for all people because it guarantees comprehensive healthcare services. The multipronged nature of PHC is useful for addressing SDH and occupational risk factors, especially when they undermine health. A key feature of PHC that makes it the best way to address all health challenges is because it has a strong emphasis on community participation, multidisciplinary teamwork, and intersectoral collaboration.

Lippincott® Connect *For additional resources on the subjects discussed in this chapter, visit Lippincott Connect.*

REFERENCES

Abrahams, K., Mallick, R., Hohlfeld, A., Suliaman, T., & Kathard, H. (2022). Emerging professional practices focusing on reducing inequity in speech-language therapy and audiology: A scoping review protocol. *Systematic Reviews, 11*(1), 1–7. https://doi.org/10.1186/s13643-022-01953-0

Ayalew, A. T., Adane, D. T., Obolla, S. S., Ludago, T. B., Sona, B. D., & Biewer, G. (2020). From Community-Based Rehabilitation (CBR) services to inclusive development. A study on practice, challenges, and future prospects of CBR in Gedeo Zone (Southern Ethiopia). *Frontiers in Education, 5*, 506050. https://doi.org/10.3389/feduc.2020.506050

Baum, C. M., Christiansen, C. H., & Bass, J. D. (2015). The person-environment-occupation-performance (PEOP) model. *Occupational Therapy: Performance, Participation, and Well-Being, 4*, 49–56.

Biney, E., Amoateng, A. Y., & Ewemooje, O. S. (2020). Inequalities in morbidity in South Africa: A family perspective. *SSM - Population Health, 12*, 100653. https://doi.org/10.1016/j.ssmph.2020.100653

Bloom, D. E., & Canning, D. (2000). The health and wealth of nations. *Science, 287*(5456), 1207–1209. https://doi.org/10.1126/science.287.5456.1207

Blose, S., Cobbing, S., & Chetty, V. (2021). Community-based rehabilitation implementation for people with disabilities in South Africa: A protocol for a scoping review. *Systematic Reviews, 10*(1), 279. https://doi.org/10.1186/s13643-021-01839-7

Bryant, J. H., & Richmond, J. B. (2016). Alma-Ata and primary health care: An evolving story. In W. Cockerham (Ed.), *International encyclopedia of public health* (2nd ed., pp. 83–102). Elsevier Science & Technology. https://doi.org/10.1016/B978-012373960-5.00001-0

Chochinov, H. M. (2007). Dignity and the essence of medicine: The A, B, C, and D of dignity conserving care. *BMJ, 335*(7612), 184–187. https://doi.org/10.1136/bmj.39244.650926.47

Cieza, A. (2019). Rehabilitation the health strategy of the 21st century, really? *Archives of Physical Medicine and Rehabilitation, 100*(11), 2212–2214. https://doi.org/10.1016/j.apmr.2019.05.019

Cieza, A., Causey, K., Kamenov, K., Hanson, S. W., Chatterji, S., & Vos, T. (2020). Global estimates of the need for rehabilitation based on the Global Burden of Disease study 2019: A systematic analysis for the Global Burden of Disease Study 2019. *The Lancet, 396*(10267), 2006–2017. https://doi.org/10.1016/S0140-6736(20)32340-0

Coetzee, D. (2018). Introduction to health and health care in South Africa. In D. Coetzee (Ed.), *Primary health care: Fresh perspectives* (2nd ed., pp. 1–12). Pearson.

Dastile, N. P., & Ndlovu-Gatsheni, S. J. (2013). Power, knowledge and being: Decolonial combative discourse as a survival kit for Pan-Africanists in the 21st century. *Alternation, 20*(1), 105–134. https://eref.uni-bayreuth.de/id/eprint/69264

Day, C., & Gray, A. (2016). Health and related indicators. *South African Health Review, 2016*(1), 243–347. https://journals.co.za/doi/pdf/10.10520/EJC189304

Du, S., Cao, Y., Zhou, T., Setiawan, A., Thandar, M., Koy, V., Nurumal, M. S. B., Anh, H., Kunaviktikul, W., & Hu, Y. (2019). The knowledge, ability, and skills of primary health care providers in SEANERN countries: A multi-national cross-sectional study. *BMC Health Services Research, 19*(1), 602. https://doi.org/10.1186/s12913-019-4402-9

Espinosa, A., & Kadić-Maglajlić, S. (2018). The mediating role of health consciousness in the relation between emotional intelligence and health behaviors. *Frontiers in Psychology, 9*, 2161. https://doi.org/10.3389/fpsyg.2018.02161

Essential Yeh, H., & McColl, M. A. (2019). A model for occupation-based palliative care. *Occupational Therapy in Health Care, 33*(1), 108–123. https://doi.org/10.1080/07380577.2018.1544428

Fransen, H. (2005). Challenges for occupational therapy in community-based rehabilitation: Occupation in a community approach to handicap in development. In F. Kronenberg, S. Algado, & N. Pollard (Eds.), *Occupational therapy without borders: Learning from the spirit of survivors* (pp.166-182). Elsevier Churchill Livingstone.

Gervits, M., & Anderson, M. (2014). Community-oriented primary care (COPC) in Barcelona, Spain: An urban COPC experience. *International Journal of Health Services, 44*(2), 383–398. https://doi.org/10.2190/HS.44.2.m

Gofin, J., Gofin, R., & Stimpson, J. P. (2015). Community-oriented primary care (COPC) and the affordable care act: An opportunity to meet the demands of an evolving health care system. *Journal of Primary Care Community Health, 6*(2), 128–133. https://doi.org/10.1177/2150131914555908

Gordon, T., Booysen, F., & Mbonigaba, J. (2020). Socio-economic inequalities in the multiple dimensions of access to healthcare: The case of South Africa. *BMC Public Health, 20*(1), 289. https://doi.org/10.1186/s12889-020-8368-7

Gray, J. M. (1998). Putting occupation into practice: Occupation as ends, occupation as means. *American Journal of Occupational Therapy, 52*, 354–364. https://doi.org/10.5014/ajot.52.5.354

Gwyther, E. (2019). *How is palliative care part of the right to health? The South African evidence* [Doctoral thesis, University of Cape Town]. OpenUCT. http://hdl.handle.net/11427/30368

Haque, M., Islam, T., Rahman, N. A. A., McKimm, J., Abdullah, A., & Dhingra, S. (2020). Strengthening primary health-care services to help prevent and control long-term (chronic) non-communicable diseases in low- and middle-income countries. *Risk Management and Healthcare Policy, 13*, 409–426. https://doi.org/10.2147/RMHP.S239074

Haraldsdottir, E., Donaldson, K., Lloyd, A., Barclay, I., & McCormack, B. (2020). Reaching for the rainbow: Person-centred practice in palliative care. *International Practice Development Journal, 10*(1), 1–14. https://doi.org/10.19043/ipdj.101.005

Hartley, S., Finkenflugel, H., Kuipers, P., & Thomas, M. (2009). Community-based rehabilitation: Opportunity and challenge. *The Lancet, 374*(9704), 1803–1804. https://doi.org/10.1016/S0140-6736(09)62036-5

Heath, I., Rubinstein, A., Stange, K. C., & van Driel, M. L. (2009). Quality in primary health care: A multidimensional approach to complexity. *BMJ, 338*, b1242. https://doi.org/10.1136/bmj.b1242

Hocking, C. (2015). Editorial: Special issue on contextual and evolutionary perspectives of occupation. *Journal of Occupational Science, 22*(1), 1–2. https://doi.org/10.1080/14427591.2015.990083

Hospice and Palliative Care Association of South Africa. (2022). *What is palliative care?* https://hpca.co.za/palliative-care/

Iemmi, V., Gibson, L., Blanchet, K., Kumar, K. S., Rath, S., Hartley, S., Murthy, G. V., Patel, V., Weber, J., & Kuper, H. (2015). Community-based rehabilitation for people with disabilities in low- and middle-income countries: A systematic review. *Campbell Systematic Reviews, 11*, 1–177. https://doi.org/10.4073/csr.2015.15

Kark, S. L., & Cassel, J. (1956). International report: The Pholela health centre. *Health Education Journal, 14*(2), 101–109. https://doi.org/10.1177/001789695601400208

Kielhofner, G. (2008). *A model of human occupation: Theory and application* (4th ed.). Lippincott Williams & Wilkins. http://www.loc.gov/catdir/enhancements/fy0740/2007031774-d.html

Kim, H. (2020). Introduction to an occupational perspective of health. *Global Journal of Intellectual & Developmental Disabilities, 6*(5), 555700. https://doi.org/10.19080/GJIDD.2020.06.555700

Kinkel, H., Marcus, T., Bam, N., Hugo, J., & Memon, S. (2013). Community oriented primary care in Tshwane district, South Africa: Assessing the first phase of implementation. *African Journal of Primary Health Care and Family Medicine, 5*(1), 1–9. https://hdl.handle.net/10520/EJC133127

Kluge, H., Kelley, E., Birtanov, Y., Theodorakis, P. N., Barkley, S., Aidossov, S., & Valderas, J. M. (2019). Implementing the renewed vision for Primary Health Care in the Declaration of Astana: The time is now. *Primary Health Care Research & Development, 20*, e158. https://doi.org/10.1017/S1463423619000719

Kredo, T., Cooper, S., Abrams, A. L., Muller, J., Schmidt, B.-M., Volmink, J., & Atkins, S. (2020). "Building on shaky ground"—challenges to and solutions for primary care guideline implementation in four provinces in South Africa: A qualitative study. *BMJ Open, 10*(5), e031468. https://doi.org/10.1136/bmjopen-2019-031468

Kronenberg, F., Kathard, H., Rudman, D. L., & Ramugondo, E. L., (2015). Can post-apartheid South Africa be enabled to humanise and heal itself? *South African Journal of Occupational Therapy, 45*(1), 20-27. https://dx.doi.org/10.17159/2310-3833/2015/v45no1a4

Lahariya, C. (2019). "More, better, faster & sustained": Strengthen primary health care to advance universal health coverage. *Indian Journal of Medical Research, 149*(4), 433. https://doi.org/10.4103/ijmr.IJMR_753_19

Law, M. (2020). *COPM Canadian occupational performance measure: Revised.* Schulz-Kirchner Verlag GmbH.

Lenihan, P., & Iliffe, S. (2001). Community-oriented primary care: A multidisciplinary community-oriented approach to primary care? *Journal of Community & Applied Social Psychology, 11*(1), 11–18. https://doi.org/10.1002/casp.605

Lim, K. H., & Iwama, M. K. (2011). The Kawa (river) model. In E. A. S. Duncan (Ed.), *Foundations for practice in occupational therapy* (pp. 117-135). Elsevier Health Sciences. http://ebookcentral.proquest.com/lib/uoct/detail.action?docID=1721292

Liu, C., Wang, D., Liu, C., Jiang, J., Wang, X., Chen, H., Ju, X., & Zhang, X. (2020). What is the meaning of health literacy? A systematic review and qualitative synthesis. *Family Medicine and Community Health, 8*(2), e000351. https://doi.org/10.1136/fmch-2020-000351

Liu, Y., Rao, K., & Hsiao, W. C. (2003). Medical expenditure and rural impoverishment in China. *Journal of Health, Population and Nutrition, 21*(3), 216–222. http://www.jstor.org/stable/23499219

MacLachlan, M., Mannan, H., & McAuliffe, E. (2011). Staff skills not staff types for community-based rehabilitation. *The Lancet, 377*(9782), 1988–1989. https://doi.org/10.1016/S0140-6736(10)61925-3

Madlingozi, T. (2007). Post-apartheid social movements and the quest for the elusive "new" South Africa. *Journal of Law and Society, 34*(1), 77–98. https://doi.org/10.1111/j.1467-6478.2007.00383.x

Maeda, A., Araujo, E., Cashin, C., Harris, J., Ikegami, N., & Reich, M. R. (2014). *Universal health coverage for inclusive and sustainable development: A synthesis of 11 country case studies.* World Bank Publications.

Maldonado-Torres, N. (2007). On the coloniality of being: Contributions to the development of a concept. *Cultural Studies (London, England), 21*(2–3), 240–270. https://doi.org/10.1080/09502380601162548

Max-Neef, M. (1991). *Human scale development.* The Apex Press.

Murray, S. A., Kendall, M., Boyd, K., & Sheikh, A. (2005). Illness trajectories and palliative care. *BMJ, 330*(7498), 1007–1011. https://doi.org/10.1136/bmj.330.7498.1007

Mwipikeni, P. (2019). Ubuntu, rights, and neoliberalism in South Africa. *International Journal of African Renaissance Studies – Multi-, Inter- and Transdisciplinarity, 14*(2), 81–102. https://doi.org/10.1080/18186874.2019.1688096

Ndinda, C., Ndhlovu, T. P., Juma, P., Asiki, G., & Kyobutungi, C. (2018). The evolution of non-communicable diseases policies in post-apartheid South Africa. *BMC Public Health, 18*(S1), 956. https://doi.org/10.1186/s12889-018-5832-8

NEJM Catalyst. (2017). What is patient-centered care? *NEJM Catalyst, 3*(1). https://catalyst.nejm.org/doi/full/10.1056/CAT.17.0559

Nimegeer, A., Farmer, J., West, C., & Currie, M. (2011). Addressing the problem of rural community engagement in healthcare service design. *Health & Place, 17*(4), 1004–1006. https://doi.org/10.1016/j.healthplace.2011.04.013

Njelesani, J., Tang, A., Jonsson, H., & Polatajko, H. (2014). Articulating an occupational perspective. *Journal of Occupational Science, 21*(2), 226–235. https://doi.org/10.1080/14427591.2012.717500

Toole, M. (1987). Primary Health Care: More than just health care. In A. Bloom (Ed.), *Primary Health Care.* Australian Council of Overseas Aid.

Obas, K. A., Bytyci-Katanolli, A., Kwiatkowski, M., Ramadani, Q., Fota, N., Jerliu, N., Statovci, S., Gerold, J., Zahorka, M., & Probst-Hensch, N. (2022). Strengthening primary healthcare in Kosovo requires tailoring primary, secondary and tertiary prevention interventions and consideration of mental health. *Frontiers in Public Health, 10*, 794309. https://doi.org/10.3389/fpubh.2022.794309

Okazaki, S., David, E. J. R., & Abelmann, N. (2008). Colonialism and psychology of culture. *Social and Personality Psychology Compass, 2*(1), 90–106. https://doi.org/10.1111/j.1751-9004.2007.00046.x

Parnell, T., & Wilding, C. (2010). Where can an occupation-focussed philosophy take occupational therapy?: VIEWPOINT. *Australian Occupational Therapy Journal, 57*(5), 345–348. https://doi.org/10.1111/j.1440-1630.2010.00860.x

Patrício, L., Sangiorgi, D., Mahr, D., Čaić, M., Kalantari, S., & Sundar, S. (2020). Leveraging service design for healthcare transformation: Toward people-centered, integrated, and technology-enabled healthcare systems. *Journal of Service Management, 31*(5), 889–909. https://doi.org/10.1108/JOSM-11-2019-0332

Peckham, S., Hann, A., Kendall, S., & Gillam, S. (2017). Health promotion and disease prevention in general practice and primary care: A scoping study. *Primary Health Care Research & Development, 18*(06), 529–540. https://doi.org/10.1017/S1463423617000494

Pellegrino, E. D. (1999). The commodification of medical and health care: The moral consequences of a paradigm shift from a professional to a market ethic. *The Journal of Medicine and Philosophy, 24*(3), 243–266. https://doi.org/10.1076/jmep.24.3.243.2523

Pentland, W., & McColl, M. A. (2008). Occupational integrity: Another perspective on "life balance." *Canadian Journal of Occupational Therapy, 75*(3), 135–138. https://doi.org/10.1177/000841740807500304

Phiri, S. (2021). South Africa and xenophobic violence: A critical analysis of the post-colonial state. In S.O. Abidde & E. K. Matambo (Eds.), *Xenophobia, nativism and Pan-Africanism in 21st century Africa* (pp. 137–153). Springer.

Pillay, M., & Kathard, H. (2015). Decolonizing health professionals' education: Audiology & speech therapy in South Africa. *African Journal of Rhetoric, 7*(1), 193–227. https://hdl.handle.net/10520/EJC172807

Puoane, T., & Hutchings, C. (2018). Health Promotion. In D. Coetzee (Ed.), *Primary health care: Fresh perspectives* (2nd ed., pp. 259–286). Pearson.

Ramose, M. B. (2022). Better see than look at ramose: A reply to Cees Maris. *South African Journal of Philosophy, 41*(1), 1–27. https://doi.org/10.1080/02580136.2021.2004799

Ramugondo, E. L. (2009). *Intergenerational shifts and continuities in children's play within a rural Venda family in the early 20th and 21st centuries* [Doctoral thesis]. University of Cape Town. OpenUCT. http://hdl.handle.net/11427/12113

Ramugondo, E. L. (2017). Human occupation and health. In S. A. Dsouza, R. Galvaan, & E. L. Ramugondo (Eds.), *Concepts of occupational therapy: Understanding Southern perspectives* (pp. 32–48). Manipal University Press.

Ramugondo, E.L., & Emery-Whittington, I. (2022). A Decolonising approach to health promotion. In S. Kessi, S. Suffla & M. Seedat (Eds.), *Decolonial enactments in community psychology* (pp. 191-211). Springer.

Ramugondo, E. L., & Kronenberg, F. (2015). Explaining collective occupations from a human relations perspective: Bridging the individual-collective dichotomy. *Journal of Occupational Science, 22*(1), 3–16. https://doi.org/10.1080/14427591.2013.781920

Rege, S., Acharya, V., & Dsouza, S. A. (2017). Practice settings for occupational therapy. In S. A. Dsouza, R. Galvaan, & E. L. Ramugondo (Eds.), *Concepts in occupational therapy: Understanding southern perspectives* (pp. 110–121). Manipal University Press.

Reich, M. R., Harris, J., Ikegami, N., Maeda, A., Cashin, C., Araujo, E. C., Takemi, K., & Evans, T. G. (2016). Moving towards universal health coverage: Lessons from 11 country studies. *The Lancet, 387*(10020), 811–816. https://doi.org/10.1016/S0140-6736(15)60002-2

Reynolds, A. (2009). Patient-centered care. *Radiologic Technology, 81*(2), 133–147. https://pubmed.ncbi.nlm.nih.gov/19901351/

Rifkin, S. B. (2018). Alma Ata after 40 years: Primary Health Care and Health for All—from consensus to complexity. *BMJ Global Health, 3*(suppl. 3), e001188. https://doi.org/10.1136/bmjgh-2018-001188

Rule, S., Lorenzo, T., & Wolmarans, M. (2006). Community-based rehabilitation: New challenges. In B. Watermeyer, L. Swartz, T. Lorenzo, M. Schneider, & M. Priestley (Eds.), *Disability and social change: A South African agenda* (pp. 273-290). HSRC Press.

Said, E. W. (1979). *Orientalism* (1st Vintage books ed.). Vintage Books.

Sanders, D., Nandi, S., Labonté, R., Vance, C., & Van Damme, W. (2019). From primary health care to universal health coverage—One step forward and two steps back. *The Lancet, 394*(10199), 619–621. https://doi.org/10.1016/S0140-6736(19)31831-8

Schwarz, D., Duong, D., Adam, C., Awoonor-Williams, J. K., Back, D., Bang, A., Bang, R., Beebe, M., Bhatt, S., Campbell, J., Conteh, M., Dimitrova, D., Dimovska, D., Dossou, J.-P., Evans, T., Gadir, M., Islam, K., Kasyaba, R., Kumar, P., … Ellner, A. (2020). Primary Care 2030: Creating an enabling ecosystem for disruptive primary care models to achieve universal health coverage in low- and middle-income countries. *Annals of Global Health, 86*(1), 9. https://doi.org/10.5334/aogh.2471

Sen, A. (1999). Health in development. *Bulletin of the World Health Organization, 77*(8), 619–623. https://apps.who.int/iris/handle/10665/267897

Soogun, O. (2019). *An assessment of the current status of integration of palliative care into primary health care centers in Alexandra community* [Master's thesis]. Faculty of Health Sciences, University of Cape Town. OpenUCT. http://hdl.handle.net/11427/31269

South African Department of Transport. (2016). *Cost of crashes in South Africa. Research and development report.* Road Traffic Management Corporation. https://www.rtmc.co.za/images/rtmc/docs/research_dev_rep/September%202016.pdf

Stigler, F. L., Macinko, J., Pettigrew, L. M., Kumar, R., & van Weel, C. (2016). No universal health coverage without primary health care. *The Lancet, 387*(10030), 1811. https://doi.org/10.1016/S0140-6736(16)30315-4

Talbot-Coulombe, C., & Guay, M. (2020). Occupational therapy training on palliative and end-of-life care: Scoping review. *British Journal of Occupational Therapy, 83*(10), 609–619. https://doi.org/10.1177/0308022620926935

The Lancet. (2018). The Astana Declaration: The future of primary health care? *The Lancet, 392*(10156), 1369. https://doi.org/10.1016/S0140-6736(18)32478-4

Topp, S. M., & Abimbola, S. (2018). Call for papers—the Alma Ata Declaration at 40: Reflections on primary healthcare in a new era. *BMJ Global Health, 3*(2), e000791. https://doi.org/10.1136/bmjgh-2018-000791

Toto. (2021). *The nature and enactment of African dance that produces neurogenic tremors* [Master's thesis]. Faculty of Health Sciences, University of Cape Town. OpenUCT. http://hdl.handle.net/11427/36209

Townsend, E., & Wilcock, A. A. (2004). Occupational justice and client-centred practice: A dialogue in progress. *Canadian Journal of Occupational Therapy, 71*(2), 75–88. https://doi.org/10.1177/000841740407100203

United Nations. (2015). *General Assembly Resolution A/RES/70/1. Transforming Our World, the 2030 Agenda for Sustainable Development.* https://sdgs.un.org/sites/default/files/publications/21252030%20Agenda%20for%20Sustainable%20Development%20web.pdf

United Nations. (2022). *Do you know all 17 SDGs?* https://sdgs.un.org/goals

van Wees, S. H. (2020). We need to talk about guilt in global health education. *The Lancet, 395*(10217), 32. https://doi.org/10.1016/S0140-6736(19)32965-4

Verboven, L., Calders, T., Callens, S., Black, J., Maartens, G., Dooley, K. E., Potgieter, S., Warren, R. M., Laukens, K., & Van Rie, A. (2022). A treatment recommender clinical decision support system for personalized medicine: Method development and proof-of-concept for drug resistant tuberculosis. *BMC Medical Informatics and Decision Making, 22*(1), 1–11. https://doi.org/10.1186/s12911-022-01790-0

Walraven, G. (2019). The 2018 Astana Declaration on Primary Health Care, is it useful? *Journal of Global Health, 9*(1), 010313. https://doi.org/10.7189/jogh.09.010313

Wilcock, A. A. (1998). Occupation for health. *British Journal of Occupational Therapy, 61*(8), 340–345. https://doi.org/10.1177/030802269806100801

Wilcock, A. A. (2006). *An occupational perspective of health* (2nd ed.). SLACK Incorporated.

World Health Organization. (1986). *Ottawa charter for health promotion, 1986* (No. WHO/EURO: 1986-4044-43803-61677). Author. Regional Office for Europe.

World Health Organization. (2008a). *Closing the gap in a generation: Health equity through action on the social determinants of health.* Author. Retrieved September 11, 2022, from https://apps.who.int/iris/rest/bitstreams/65985/retrieve

World Health Organization. (2008b). *Primary health care: Now more than ever.* Author. https://apps.who.int/iris/bitstream/handle/10665/43949/9789241563734_eng.pdf?sequence=1&isAllowed=y

World Health Organization. (2017). *Rehabilitation: Key for health in the 21st century.* Author. https://www.who.int/news-room/events/details/2017/02/06/defaukt-calendar/rehabilitation-2030-a-call-for-action

World Health Organization. (2019). *Primary health care fact sheet.* https://www.who.int/news-room/fact-sheets/detail/primary-health-care

World Health Organization. (2020). *World Health Statistics 2020—Monitoring Health for the SDGs.* Author. https://www.who.int/data/gho/publications/world-health-statistics

World Health Organization. (2021). *Global expenditure on health: Public spending on the rise.* Author.

World Health Organization and UNICEF. (1978). *Report of the international conference on primary health care.* World Health Organisation & United Nations Children's Fund. http://whqlibdoc.who.int/publications/9241800011.pdf

World Health Organization and UNICEF. (2018). *A vision for primary health care in the 21st Century: Towards universal health coverage and the Sustainable Development Goals (Technical Series on Primary Health Care).* World Health Organization and the United Nations Children's Fund. https://www.who.in/oc/efault-sourc/rimary-healt/ision.pdf

ADDITIONAL RESOURCES

Ramugondo, E. L., & Emery-Whittington, I. (2022). A Decolonising approach to health promotion. In S. Kessi, S. Suffla & M. Seedat (Eds.), *Decolonial enactments in community psychology* (pp. 191 - 211). Springer.

The Barefoot Guide Collective have a series of practical guides that you may find useful to support your practice in an LMICs PHC context. It is a free resource and you can download the guides from https://www.barefootguide.org/

Providing Occupational Therapy Services for Persons With Childhood Trauma

Erin Connor

LEARNING OBJECTIVES

After reading this chapter, you will be able to:

1. Articulate the prevalence of trauma in childhood and the impact that is has on occupational performance throughout the lifetime.
2. Understand the impact of childhood trauma on the individual, the family, community, and the global society.
3. Prioritize trauma-informed practices across all settings, ages, and populations.
4. Develop trauma-informed interventions that are culturally sensitive and support the decolonization of health and well-being.
5. Reframe the impact of childhood trauma to encourage strength and resilience in our clients and ourselves.

Introduction

Trauma is a scary word. It evokes an intense range of emotions regardless of the audience. In contrast, it is also a word that can be callously thrown around without a lot of consideration of the impact. Think about how many times you have heard someone in your life make a statement like "Ugh that restaurant was terrible, I'm traumatized and never going back there again." Obviously, in this instance, the term is being used as colloquialism, intended to amplify the impact, and convey emotion. However, it suggests that trauma and the effects it has on an individual, family, or community are misunderstood. There are several reasons for this, but I would suggest that the most profound one is our own resistance to looking in a mirror. Let me explain what I mean.

In her TED talk about childhood trauma, Dr. Nadine Burke-Harris states "I used to think that it was so hard to get support because these things don't apply to us . . . now I am beginning to believe that we marginalize the issue because it DOES apply to us" (Burke-Harris, 2015). This is especially true when the qualifier of *childhood* trauma is added. Horrible things and events exist that are very hard for the typical person to wrap their head around, and when they recognize that most of these atrocities are committed against populations that are immensely vulnerable, it becomes almost unbearable. No one wants to think about children being abused, starving, growing up in war-torn countries, witnessing violence, devastation, and death. But it is EXACTLY our refusal or inability to look at this that allows these patterns to continue, to fester, and permeate our daily lives.

My own history with trauma has been more of a teacher to me than any class, program, or assignment I was given in school. One of the bigger challenges of personal trauma work is what is known as fraud or imposter syndrome. Very often, individuals can convince themselves that their experiences were not "that bad," or that other people had it worse than them. Due to the nature of traumatic memories, the cover-up or avoidance of acknowledging these events leads individuals to constantly question whether what they feel is real, which makes it difficult to connect these events to whatever symptoms they are having. This was certainly the case for me. I come from a very loving family, with parents and siblings who were supportive and encouraged me. It is also true that I experienced treatment from someone outside my immediate family that was abusive, and that I was not believed when I asked for help. This resulted in my doubting and questioning any memory, sensation, or thought I had well into my early adulthood.

Once I accepted that this was part of me, it became painfully obvious that trauma was everywhere. Being able to see trauma—in people's faces in their eyes, to feel it in their touch, or in the way they move—becomes like a sixth sense (or ninth sense if you are an occupational therapist). As the mental health field progresses, the occupational therapy (OT) community is beginning to realize the importance of lived experience and empathetic connection in the treatment and support of individuals with mental health challenges. This is never truer than when OT practitioners consider traumatic impact. Considering the immensely high incidence of traumatic experiences that exist in our world, there is significant potential for healing. However, we cannot hope to utilize this powerful treatment method without doing our own work and being willing to acknowledge whatever level of traumatic response is present in our own lives.

I volunteered to write this chapter for the same reason that I teach at a college. It helps me with my meaning making (you will understand that term by the end of this chapter) of doing everything I can to ensure that the warning signs and impact of trauma do not get missed, like they did for me. The things I experienced as a young girl shaped my understanding of the world, and it led me to believe for an exceedingly long time that I was the problem, that I was dramatic, or difficult, that it was my fault. It has taken an immense amount of support, therapy, self-reflection, and honestly, poor decision-making to finally arrive at a place where I understand the cycle that allowed the events of my life to take place. Unless we are in a place where we agree to address our shadows and blind spots, we continue to perpetuate the culture of don't ask, don't tell.

That being said, I want to end this introduction with a trigger warning. It is likely that you will relate to this material in some very personal way. Research suggests that two-thirds of children report at least one traumatic event before the age of 16 (Substance Abuse and Mental Health Services Administration [SAMSHA], 2022). If you consider the events of the past few years including the worldwide pandemic, severe political unrest, and the threat of a third world war, I will argue that number increases to 4 out of 4. The first step is acknowledging it and accepting it, so you can breathe and integrate these experiences into your ego. That process is incredibly challenging and requires a lot of support, self-awareness, and self-care. If you find this material disturbing, please seek out support for yourself. But please do not turn away, the people you serve need you to be the best version of yourself you can be. Sometimes that means doing demanding work and facing uncomfortable truths about yourself and the world. I am asking you to be the safe adult that I needed when I was younger, and maybe the one that you needed as well (Box 69.1).

History and Prevalence

Diagnostic Evolution

Occupational therapy has a strong historical tie to the treatment of trauma. Our profession was started with the mission of supporting soldiers returning from war, treating what was known then as "shell shock." During the reintegration process from combat, medical professionals were noting the extreme difficulty of the soldiers to be able to find purpose and meaning in their lives. OT was able to provide these soldiers with opportunities to be successful, re-engage in their daily lives, and find purpose through hands-on activities.

Shell shock eventually became known as post-traumatic stress disorder (PTSD). This was diagnosed by a psychiatrist if the client had met five criteria listed in the Diagnostic and Statistical Manual (*DSM-5*): direct experiencing, intrusive symptoms, avoidance symptoms, altering of mood or cognitive status, and alterations in arousal and reactivity. The manual also states that the symptoms need to be present for longer than a month and cause a significant disruption to the individual's functioning. It should also be clear that the symptoms are not the result of using a substance (American Psychiatric Association, 2022). These symptoms had to be present for at least 1 month and impact an individual's ability to function. There is an additional categorization for children under the age of 6, that makes some adjustments for the differences in how trauma presents itself in children. The categories of symptoms remain the same but the examples as well as the number of symptoms present in each

BOX 69.1 NARRATIVE PERSPECTIVE: WHILE FOCUSING ON RECOVERY, I FORGOT TO GET A LIFE

I was struggling with starting to write this chapter. I found myself procrastinating, doubting myself, being all talk, and very little action. I'd do a bunch of research, and then not look at it for weeks. I'd read an article or two, and then go down a rabbit hole of memes and videos. One day when I was berating myself for being so far behind and needing to get moving on this work, I came across a document that was sent to me by the publisher entitled "While Focusing on Recovery, I Forgot to Get a Life." I read this chapter by Gloria Dickerson from the previous W&S edition, and I read it all the way through in one sitting. Gloria shares her story of growing up in 1950s Alabama as a young Black girl, living a life riddled with trauma and challenges.

On an instinct, I reached out to the publishers and asked if they would be able to connect me with Gloria. She was gracious enough to offer to talk with me on the phone, and

I am going to share what I learned from her on that phone call. She was exactly how I pictured her from her story. Despite having her own health challenges and having just finished writing her own workbook on Creating Resilience, she made time to listen to my fears, offered me encouragement, and supported a total stranger. Her advice was to just start writing and write like I was telling a story. She told me to write like I talk, that even in our brief email interactions she could tell that I was a good communicator and had clarity that would translate. I could feel the warmth of her statement through the phone. I thanked her, hung up, and wrote this section of my chapter almost immediately. Gloria embodies resilience, strength, and compassion. All things that are required of those of us who are working with trauma, either our own or with our clients. Please read her story, which can be found on Lippincott Connect.

category is lower. It is important for practice to consider that with children, how the symptoms present themselves may change. Children will often show symptoms behaviorally, they may act out, run away, or display tantrum-like behavior. Children may experience frightening dreams that may seem unrelated to trauma and can have limited fear responses initially after the incident(s) (Davis, 1999).

Over the past 10 years or so, professionals have identified that this diagnosis of a singular incident was not thorough enough to encompass the chronic stress that some individuals live with. Bessel Van Der Kolk, and his team at the Justice Resources Institute coined the phrase C-PTSD, or Complex PTSD. This term is used to address children and individuals who live with almost constant traumatic stress, which has a different impact than a singular event (Van der Kolk, 2000). For example, a child who grows up in a household with a parent who is abusive experiences multiple events, including but not limited to the abuse itself, lying and hiding from others, protecting siblings, or the other parent, all of which is further complicated by the fact that the child has to rely on said parent for food, clothing, and shelter. This creates what is known as *cognitive dissonance*, or inconsistent or conflicting thoughts or ideas. In contrast, a child who experiences a singular traumatic event such as a car crash, or the loss of a loved one has potentially fewer complications to manage and typically has a better prognosis than a child with C-PTSD. This has been somewhat of a controversial proposal that is still being debated within the mental health community.

Although diagnosis is outside of the OT scope of practice, the point about the evolution of this diagnosis, and the continued lack of understanding it by the medical and

mental health community, is an important one to consider. There have been additional suggestions regarding diagnostic categorization made to the DSM committee by van der Kolk and his team, including but not limited to Developmental Trauma Disorder and Childhood Trauma Disorder, all of which have been rejected by the DSM committee. Bremness and Polzin (2014) state the following about the importance of having an accurate and comprehensive diagnosis. "Current clinical practice often reveals no diagnosis, inaccurate diagnosis, or inadequate diagnosis ... all of which leads to misguided or complete lack of treatment plans. Further, because there is almost always considerable dysregulation of body (sensory and motor), affect (explosive/irritable or frozen/restricted), cognition (altered perceptions of beliefs, auditory and sensory-perceptual flashbacks and dissociation) and behavior (multiple forms of regression), the diagnoses of bipolar, oppositional defiant disorder/conduct disorder, attention deficit hyperactivity disorder (ADHD) or other anxiety disorders are confusingly made" (Bremness & Polzin, 2014, p. 143).

Adverse Childhood Experiences

The best explanation of trauma comes from studies on **adverse childhood experiences (ACEs)** done by the Centers for Disease Control and Prevention (CDC) and Kaiser Permanente (ACE Response, 2022). The original ACE study was conducted at Kaiser Permanente from 1995 to 1997 with two waves of data collection. Over 17,000 health maintenance organization members from southern California who were receiving physical examinations completed confidential surveys regarding their childhood experiences and current health status and behaviors. The body of evidence has continued to be built and collected over the years, with the original researchers recognizing gaps in the initial research (e.g., poverty, diversity, systemic marginalization, and oppression). According to the CDC, ACEs are potentially traumatic events or circumstances that occur during a child's development (from birth through age 17). These include events such as physical, emotional, or sexual abuse; witnessing violence; or the unexpected death of a family member. Additionally, these can also be experiences that undermine or threaten a child's safety or stability in their home. For instance, having a parent who is mentally ill, is struggling with substance addiction, or has been incarcerated (CDC, 2021).

The results of this study were revolutionary in terms of understanding the impact of trauma, which will be discussed later in this chapter. Of course, adults can be traumatized by circumstances that overwhelm their sense of safety; however, the impact on children is significantly increased due to the fragile state of their development, potential lack of a support system, or that support system being the origins of the traumatic event(s).

Prevalence and What's Missing

According to the SAMSHA (2016), approximately two-thirds of children report a traumatic event before the age of 16. In the United States alone, there are approximately 1,000 children a day who receive treatment in an emergency department for some type of assault. According to the American Occupational Therapy Association (AOTA), a report of child abuse is made every 10 seconds nationally (AOTA, 2015). And the World Health Organization (WHO) says that each year there are approximately 40,000 deaths of children under 18 worldwide, with indication that a sizable portion of these can be attributed to neglect and maltreatment (Kessler et al., 2017).

However, the prevalence of traumatic experiences can be a challenge to accurately assess, both locally and globally. Let us look at some of the potential reasons for this:

1. *Significant underreporting.* Due to the nature of many of these experiences, it is quite common that individuals will not disclose that they have been victimized. For example, based on a study conducted by Viola et al. (2016), the occurrence of child abuse is significantly lower in China. However, if you consider the cultural and political values within the Chinese culture, specifically preferences of dealing with things within the family, lofty expectations of childhood behavior, and elevated levels of obedience, it is possible that is a result of inhibited disclosure.

2. *Lack of knowledge or understanding.* Relatively speaking, the concept of trauma and its impact on individuals is a rather new concept. It negates the strict medical model of identifying the symptom and eliminating it. Understanding trauma requires practitioners to consider the whole person.

3. *Cultural variances.* The term "abuse" is extremely subjective, and it is difficult to maintain a consistent definition throughout the entire world. For example, something like physical punishment (spanking, hitting, etc.) is still utilized in many parts of the world where it is seen as completely appropriate parenting. While in other locations it has become taboo and results in referrals to child protective services, loss of custody, or criminal charges for the parents or guardians.

4. *Inadequate screening and assessment tools.* The most used child trauma assessment is called the Childhood Trauma Questionnaire, which was developed by the National Institute of Mental Health (Pennebaker & Susman, 1988). This assessment is a self-report questionnaire, and although it is effective and widely used, it lends itself to the concerns mentioned above of underreporting or misunderstanding. There are a few other screening tools, but most are focused on diagnosis. As OT practitioners we need to understand the importance of how trauma impacts how we gather data and assess progress of our clients.

5. *Colonization and lack of cooperation.* The WHO states that child maltreatment is the abuse and neglect that occurs to children under 18 years of age. It includes all types of physical and/or emotional ill-treatment, sexual abuse, neglect, negligence, and commercial or other exploitation, which results in actual or potential harm to the child's health, survival, development, or dignity in the context of a relationship of responsibility, trust, or power (Kessler et al., 2017). Having a universal definition is a good start; however, measuring the occurrence of trauma in the world requires us to collaborate and work together. This is a challenging conquest for many reasons, even just considering the disproportionate availability of mental health professionals, treatment, and education regarding trauma, and the limitations that creates.

Regardless of the variations in reportability, it is becoming increasingly clear that traumatic experiences are incredibly common. In the aftermath of the worldwide COVID-19 pandemic that we collectively experienced over the past few years; it will be almost impossible to find an individual who has not been potentially impacted by trauma (Figure 69.1). As an OT practitioner, you will encounter individuals daily that have been through things they do not talk about but that affect every interaction they have and every activity they engage in. It is our responsibility to work as therapists to understand these circumstances and how to treat our individual clients and work toward preventive measures.

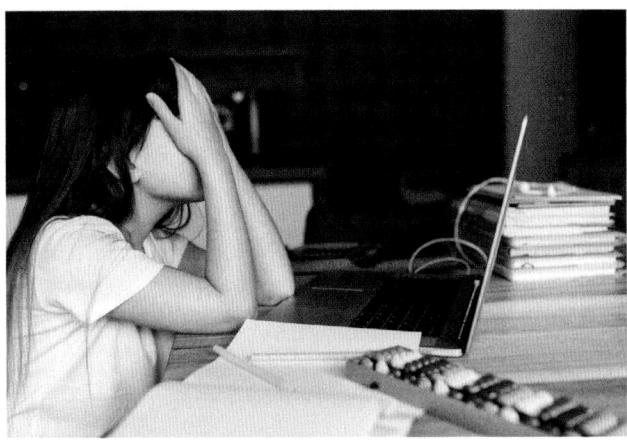

FIGURE 69.1 During the COVID-19 pandemic, online schooling was traumatic for many children and families.

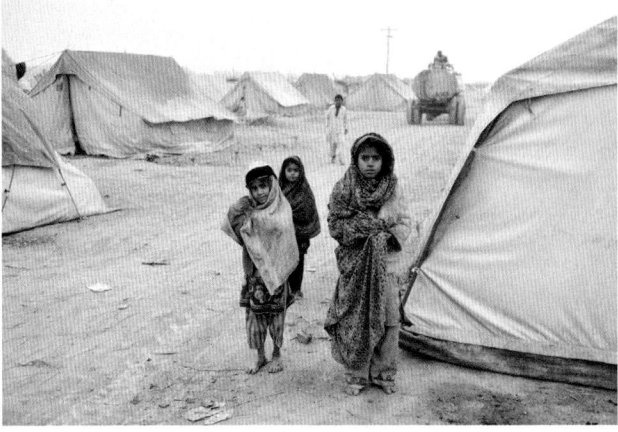

FIGURE 69.2 Pakistani children experience acute trauma due to a flood, and then Type Two trauma because it resulted in dislocation to a refugee camp.

Types of Trauma

When a child experiences one or more instances of trauma, it creates a sense that overwhelms the child's ability to cope, and a situation where the symptoms will continue to interfere with their lives even after the traumatic situation is over. The threat of death or injury or the perceived threat of death or injury creates a sense of feeling traumatized by the event, leading to intrusive symptoms that require intervention and treatment.

While there is some debate over the categories of trauma, as well as the inclusion of different human experiences as traumatic, for the purposes of this chapter, we will be utilizing the categories according to the National Child Traumatic Stress Network (NCTSN, 2022). There are three categories of traumatic events:

- *Type One* is known as acute trauma. This is a one-time incident or event, such as a singular attack, that causes the individual severe stress. This is the most well-known and traditional example of a trauma, which most closely fits the diagnosis of PTSD. Think about a child who is bitten by a dog and then becomes terrified of all dogs. While these singular events are still subject to the compounding factors of severity, response to the incident, and potential consequences or repercussions, they tend to have a better prognosis and a wider range of treatment options.
- *Type Two* is identified as individual identity or complex trauma. This is where a person experiences multiple traumatic events over the course of their lifetime, or a person lives in a chronic state of traumatic stress. For example, growing up in an abusive or neglectful household, living in a refugee camp, or serving in the military during combat time (Figure 69.2). As one would imagine, these individuals experience more complicated feelings and greater impact to the prolonged exposure, and they develop defense mechanisms to endure that experience. Think about

a soldier that develops a "dark" sense of humor to cope with the difficulty of what they have been exposed to while engaging in combat.
- *Type Three* is referred to as collective identity or continuous traumatic stress. This category is newer and is being included to address the traumatic impact of things like racism, sexism, homophobia, and so on. Research is beginning to acknowledge that the defenses that developed for groups of individuals who are "othered," or not of the majority, are the same as those who have grown up in abusive households or spent time in an incarceration center. Collectively, these groups experience the treatment they receive as a generalizable experience. Consider the circumstances around the Black Lives Matter protests where an entire racial group shared the lived experiences of being treated differently by law enforcement due to the color of their skin. Black mothers everywhere shared the experience of training their sons to navigate police interactions safely from an incredibly early age. This is not a universally shared experience, and it begins to create an awareness in a young Black child that there is the potential for danger that is solely connected to an identity they hold.

Please see Box 69.2 for further details on the three types and read OT Story 69.1 about Lana for an example.

Impact on Occupational Engagement

Skill Deficits and Barriers

According to the NCTSN (2022), the most common symptoms of childhood exposure to traumatic events can be broken into four categories: (a) Neurological or cognitive; (b)

BOX 69.2 TYPES OF TRAUMA WITH EXAMPLES

Type One

Acute Trauma/PTSD: Short-term, unexpected event

- **Examples:** one-time rape, car accident, natural disaster

Type Two

Individual Identity/Complex Trauma: Sustained, repeated ordeal stressors

- **Examples:** ongoing abuse, combat, domestic violence, prostitution, captivity, torture, incarceration

Type Three

Collective Identity Trauma/Continuous Traumatic Stress: Ongoing systemic and/or cultural oppression

- **Examples:** discrimination, racism, sexism

Data from Kira, I., & Fawzi, M., & Fawzi, M. (2013). The Dynamics of Cumulative Trauma and Trauma Types in Adults Patients With Psychiatric Disorders Two Cross-Cultural Studies. *Traumatology. 19.* 179–195. https://doi.org/10.1177/1534765612459892

OT STORY 69.1 LANA'S STORY

Lana is a 16-year-old adolescent who lives in an apartment with her maternal grandmother. Lana identifies as nonbinary and uses they/them pronouns. Lana has been having difficulties at school including but not limited to truancy, behavioral outbursts, severe resistance to authority, as well as vaping at school. Lana has been referred to an intensive outpatient program, where you work as an occupational therapist. The goal is to provide stability and skill development to improve her occupational engagement.

Lana grew up in a rural area with their biological mother until the age of 10. Lana's father left their mother before they were born. Lana's mother worked several jobs to make ends meet which meant that Lana spent a lot of time in the care of babysitters. Lana's mother unfortunately passed away in a car accident when Lana was 10. She was on her way to pick Lana up from school. This was a huge loss for Lana, and she has blamed herself since.

It has recently come to light that as a child, at least one of the babysitters mistreated and abused Lana. They report nightmares, intrusive thoughts, and an over-reactive fight or flight response when presented with certain stimuli, such as men with beards, or being closed in a small space. Lana's grandmother has sought help for them through individual therapy, which has led to some discovery of repressed memories. Lana and their therapist have been working on recovering some memories, and the therapist believes that this may be a factor in Lana's school behavior.

The intake assessment for Lana involved them and their grandmother. They were able to get a release signed by the therapist to involve her in Lana's care. It was revealed that Lana has been engaging in self-harm behaviors and has become very overwhelmed with the process of memory recovery. You are completing the safety and group assessment with Lana to determine what level of groups they would benefit from. Please consider the following questions in your approach with Lana.

Questions

1. Which of the three types of trauma do you think that Lana has experienced? Why do you think that?
2. What challenge would you address with Lana first?
3. How would you approach Lana and what things would you consider when developing a therapeutic relationship with them?

Sensory; (c) Social and emotional; and (d) Sense of self or control. Trauma targets an individual's nervous system, and it places demands on the body and mind that are not sustainable or functional. As has been noted, the current top practitioners in the field are advocating for a wider understanding of how these symptoms manifest in complex and collective trauma.

- **Neurological or cognitive symptoms** also have a variety of implications. Arguably, the most exhausting of the trauma symptoms is what is known as *hypervigilance* or an over-reactivity of the body's fight-or-flight system. This system is designed to warn the body and brain of potential danger. Once activated, it puts the body into a kind of survival mode, so that if we need to be prepared to defend ourselves or escape to safety we are equipped to do so. In this state, people will experience heightened sensation, increased blood flow and respiration, muscle tension, and the ability to direct their focus for a singular purpose. When a child is experiencing a traumatic symptom, particularly relevant for those clients who fall in the category of complex trauma or collective identity trauma, this system that is designed only for emergencies is ALWAYS on. This results in anything and everything feeling potentially dangerous. This has implications for musculoskeletal issues, behavioral dysregulation, difficulty storing and integrating memories, high-risk behavior, and substance use or misuse.

- *Sensory issues* can present themselves as a heightened sensitivity to varied sensory experiences, particularly one that reminds them of their traumatic experience. This is commonly referred to as a trigger, meaning that an individual is presented with a stimulus that could be either external (such as a smell or sound) or internal (such as feelings of hunger) that then causes them to feel emotional distress. In an extreme form, a trigger for a traumatic event can cause the individual to re-experience the trauma, meaning they feel as though they are living through the experience all over again. This is commonly known as a "flashback." In these cases, the client will disconnect or dissociate from reality, and their body and mind become immersed in the memory of the traumatic experience. A common situation that can instigate a flashback for veterans or those who have experienced combat is the sound of fireworks. According to these individuals, a firework sounds very similar to a gunshot. This results in the individual reverting to behaviors that they would have been exhibiting during combat, such as dropping to the ground, covering their head, or running for cover.
- *Social and emotional issues* are important when attempting to understand childhood trauma reactions. Children often communicate through behavior and social interactions, so observing them in those states can provide important treatment information. Trauma impacts a child's ability to communicate, to self-regulate, or navigate their social environments. Due to the abovementioned symptoms, children can develop varied unhealthy coping strategies. The difficulty becomes that despite being potentially necessary for their home where the abuse or trauma is happening, they become inappropriate or maladaptive in nontraumatic settings. For example, a child who runs and hides in their room when their parents begin to argue then also utilizes isolation and silence when encountering adversity at school.
- *Sense of self or control* is impacted by trauma in a comparable way. A child who is being abused, neglected, or exposed to a traumatic event may experience a disconnect between their experience and their intuition. They may crave connection and time with a parent but experience that parent being violent and angry. They may have a biological pleasant physical reaction to an inappropriate touch but feel violated and angry at the same time. This creates a cognitive dissonance, or mismatch in their experience that leads them to not trust their instincts, or not feel solid in their identity, self-control, or body autonomy. Without a sense of self, the child can feel disconnected, unable to make a decision, have difficulty tolerating frustration or failure, and become increasingly susceptible to peer pressure or other influences.

Areas of Occupation

Now that we have learned about the ACE studies and additional skill deficits that can be the result of traumatic experiences, let's look at each area of occupation and how it may impact children who have been traumatized (see Table 69.1). It is important to note that all children are different, and any one of these issues does not automatically mean that the child may be experiencing trauma. It is also important to always consider context when assessing the following areas of occupation. This is not an exhaustive list and should be viewed as such. These are guidelines that may encourage the practitioner to ask further questions and consult with colleagues (AOTA, 2020).

Traumatic or Traumatizing

There needs to be a separation between what is considered a traumatic event and a child becoming traumatized. It is entirely possible, and research would suggest common in fact, that an individual can experience a traumatic event but not develop traumatic symptoms. The NCTSN outlines several factors that contribute to how a child experiences a potentially traumatic event (NCTSN, 2022).

- *Severity of the event.* How serious was the event? How badly was the child or someone they loved physically hurt? Did they or someone they love need to go to the hospital? Were the police involved? Were children separated from their caregivers? Were they interviewed by a principal, police officer, or counselor? Did a friend or family member die? See Figure 69.3.
- *Proximity to the event.* Was the child at the place where the event occurred? Did they see the event happen to someone else or were they a victim? Did the child watch the event on television? Did they hear a loved one talk about what happened? See Figure 69.4.
- *Caregivers' reactions.* Did the child's family believe that the child was telling the truth? Did caregivers take the child's reactions seriously? How did caregivers respond to the child's needs, and how did they cope with the event themselves?
- *Prior history of trauma.* Children continually exposed to traumatic events are more likely to develop traumatic stress reactions.
- *Individual person factors.* In OT we identify client factors as values and beliefs, body functions, and body structures. There are many factors that impact an individual's ability to process a traumatic event, including level of cognitive functioning, basic temperament, and the presence of additional diagnoses or disabilities. For example, a child with a strong value of overcoming adversity might be more likely to engage in treatment and have stronger family support.

• *Family and community factors.* The culture, race, and ethnicity of children, their families, and their communities can be a protective factor, meaning that children and families have qualities and or resources that help buffer against the harmful effects of traumatic experiences and their aftermath. One of these protective factors can be the child's cultural identity. Culture often has a positive impact on how children, their families, and their communities respond, recover, and heal from a traumatic experience. However, experiences of racism and discrimination can increase a child's risk for traumatic stress symptoms.

TABLE 69.1	**Areas of Occupation and Possible Skill Deficits**
Area of Occupation	**Targets for Intervention**
Social Participation	• Poor eye contact • Difficulty maintaining friendships • Poor interpersonal boundaries • Preference for isolation • Bullying (victim or offender) • Emotional dysregulation-impairing social skills
Activities of Daily Living	• Poor hygiene • Limited capacity for routine • Difficulty with bladder or bowel control (after potty training) • Hoarding food or odd mealtime behaviors • Irrational fear of showers/bathrooms, bedrooms, etc. (can be associated with where abuse happened)
Education	• Difficulty with executive function • Impulsive/Inattentive • Poor decision-making skills • Poor attendance or work completion • Acting out/ Issues with authority
Work	• Lack of insight or self-management • Difficulty managing emotions • "Over-reactive" to stressful situations • Poor communication skills
Play/Leisure	• Decreased interest in play or healthy leisure • Withdrawal from activities • Acting out abuse scenarios during play
Rest and Sleep	• Difficulty falling or staying asleep • Increased frequency of nightmares or sleep disruptions • Bedwetting or enuresis • Increased fears/ asking to sleep with caregivers

Adapted from American Occupational Therapy Association. (2015). *Childhood trauma.* https://www.aota.org/~/media/Corporate/Files/Practice/Children/Childhood-Trauma-Info-Sheet-2015.pdf

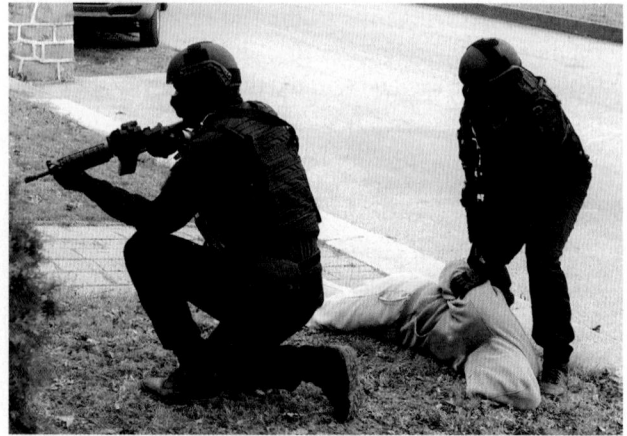

FIGURE 69.3 The involvement of police in tactical gear potentially increased the severity of this event.

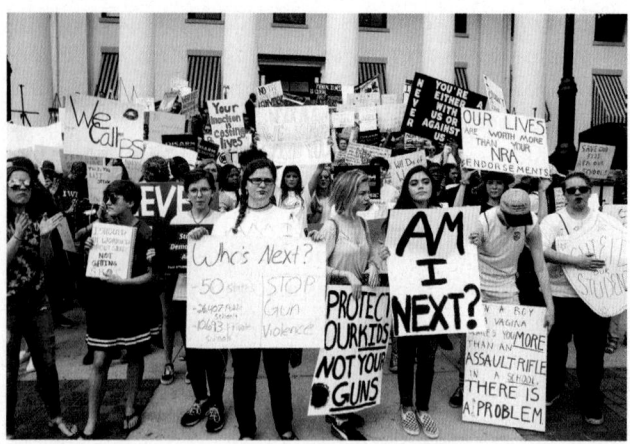

FIGURE 69.4 Even if not present at a school shooting, the event can make other students feel vulnerable.

From a prevention perspective, these factors can be developed and utilized to increase the resiliency, or coping ability, of a child's family or community. Understanding the factors that allow a child to process and integrate a traumatic experience helps to identify important skill development, caregiver training, and even community programming that can help prepare children to manage adversity in their lives more readily (Cloitre et al., 2009).

Considering these factors, as well as simple biological makeup and temperament, it becomes clear that the impact of trauma requires the consideration of several factors and perspectives. Even in the same family, individuals who experience the same traumatic incident can develop drastically different symptoms or defenses. Please see OT Story 69.2 about the Juarez family and Expanding Our Perspectives for further understanding of this concept.

Developmental Perspective

"A developmental approach to understanding disorders of trauma would support the imperative notion that such a diagnosis is complicated, in that there are constant changes with the individual child/youth/adult (genetically and otherwise) that are further complicated by the individual's interaction with his/her environment. Further, a developmental approach would appropriately recognize the interactive effect of such dynamics of familial systems, as well as cultural and societal expectations. In children and youth, the altered trajectory of development from ongoing trauma from caregivers over several developmental periods is simply more profound and evident across a wider spectrum of developmental domains than adults."

— Bremness and Polzin (2014, p. 142)

The above quote is from an article in the *Journal of Canadian Academy of Child and Adolescent Psychiatry.* It is a commentary on the importance of understanding the impact of trauma from a developmental perspective. As mentioned earlier, the impact of traumatic events is more severe in children due to their personality and cognitive structure being so malleable and open to change. Our role as OT practitioners in childhood trauma is around both treatment and prevention. Traumatized children grow up to be traumatized adults. While it is true that the impact of trauma is more severe in children due to still being in development, the same can be said for their adaptability and receptivity to treatment and intervention.

OT STORY 69.2 THE JUAREZ FAMILY

Marco (age 10), Evan (age 8), and Josie (age 7) are siblings growing up in an inner city in the United States whose parents were going through a divorce. The family has a history of DCF (Department of Children and Families) involvement, due to domestic violence in the home. All three children have witnessed their father's abusive treatment of their mother from an incredibly young age. In addition to witnessing violence in their home, the family has experienced food insecurity, unstable housing, and maternal mental illness. Things became worse when the parents decided to separate. The children were supposed to split their time between their mothers' and fathers' houses. The father has been very up and down with them, showering them with gifts one day, and then punishing them severely for minimal mistakes the next day. The mother has been extremely depressed, often not feeding the children, or forgetting to pick them up from school.

The three siblings all attend the public school where you are employed as an OT practitioner. Despite all having the same experience, the three children display extremely different behavior.

Marco started having behavioral issues at age 6. He would become violently angry, throw desks and chairs, threaten other children in school, use violent and inappropriate language, and show a strong resistance to authority.

Evan demonstrated "perfect child" syndrome. He never got a poor grade, never was in trouble at school, and sat silently and alone at lunch and recess reading. His teachers would have described him as a model student. The only time he ever had a recorded incident in school was when a peer was bullying his sister. Upon witnessing the bully corner his sister and grab her arm, Evan became extremely upset. He pushed himself in between his sister and the bully, grabbed them by their shirt and pushed them up against the wall. The recess monitor was able to intervene and separate the two children.

Josie would show up to school at least twice a week with a new injury. Scratches, bite marks, cuts, and bruises on her knees. When asked about these, she would often shrug and claim to "not know where they came from." However, her teachers have observed her scratching at her wrists with a broken pencil in school, which is how she was referred to the behavioral specialist at the school who contacted you for a consultation.

Questions

1. Why do the three siblings present so differently despite having the same experiences?
2. Would you work with all three siblings together or individually? Why?
3. What, if anything, is your role in engaging the parents?
4. What other professionals should you consult with to ensure that these three siblings are being supported?

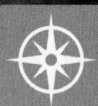

EXPANDING OUR PERSPECTIVES

Nurturing Sensitivity and Developing Strategies to Address Childhood Trauma

Anonymous

I am a clinician practicing OT for the past 20 years. I primarily work with adults with varying physical and mental disabilities in long-term care facilities in an urban setting.

It did not take long for me to realize that long-term care facilities in urban areas tend to be used as "catchment institutions" for many people across different age groups with varying degrees of impairments/disabilities, often unable to cope with the demands of independent living in community settings.

In my clinical work, I often encounter young adults who are recovering from stroke, musculoskeletal injuries, traumatic brain injuries, mental illness, and chronic illnesses such as diabetes and chronic obstructive pulmonary disease. I also need to contend with narrowly defined OT goals dictated by stringent insurance requirements. Thus, OT goals tend to address basic self-care and physical impairments like strength, balance, activity tolerance, and functional mobility.

Many times, even after achieving such goals and providing home health services, some individuals are unable to cope with independent living. After listening to my patients' narratives, it became evident that many of them experienced complex childhood trauma including abusive/unstable family structures, homelessness, unhealthy relationships with adults, and trauma from systemic issues like racism and homophobia.

As a clinician and as someone who has also experienced childhood trauma, it began to dawn on me that addressing these past traumas was a key part of ensuring successful OT outcomes, especially if independent living in the community is a desired outcome. When preparing patients for community transitions, we often consider social support networks without recognizing that, for patients with childhood trauma, such networks are often fractured or imbued with complicated emotions. Working with other team members and advocating to establish safe and stable social networks should therefore be a key priority.

Being an occupational therapist, I realized we are equipped with using the concept of "therapeutic use of self" in assisting patients to identify and develop meaningful positive occupations (including hobbies, interests, and self-care routines) to deal with and possibly replace maladaptive coping patterns. Addressing childhood trauma is a new and challenging area for clinical practice. Nurturing sensitivity and developing strategies to address this issue can be an important variable for meaningful OT outcomes.

Mosey's Development of Adaptive Skills

Anne Cronin Mosey's Development of Adaptive Skills outlines skill levels that a person requires to develop a solid sense of self (Mosey, 1980). If we look at trauma through the lens of Mosey's adaptive skills (see Table 69.2), you can see the detriment that having traumatic experiences can have on a child's ability to grow and develop appropriate skills to interact in the world. While there is an indicated hierarchy of skill areas, particularly when considering the subskills in each of the areas, many of these stages overlap and occur simultaneously. An individual who has not mastered the previous set of subskills will struggle and encounter barriers when attempting a higher-level interaction. Instead of viewing them as steps to conquer, I will suggest that they serve the purpose of identifying deficits and informing treatment plans and interventions.

Integration of Skill Deficits

Through this perspective, the main point of occupational engagement during childhood is to develop an individual's sense of self. Namely, the self-identity stage of Mosey's Development of Adaptive Skills. Imagine a child growing up in a home where they never knew what to expect. The person who they relied on for food, clothing, and shelter was also the person who hurt and abused them. This leaves them with a skill deficit around assessing the safety of another person, a vital skill for dyadic interaction. This could show itself in multiple ways, over attachment to relationships, codependence, severe isolation, narcissistic manipulation, and eventually severe mental health issues or personality disorders. Inability to master dyadic interaction skills has permeating effect in all areas of performance. As an adult, this individual appears unstable, often floating from job to job, hobby to hobby, social circle to social circle. They learned not to count on their family, so they never learned to rely on anyone else. If you cannot accurately assess the safety of one other person, that impacts your group's skills, has implications for your sexual identity, and so on. How would you see that lack of skill development manifest in their later stages of development?

Mosey suggests that we organize our treatment of our clients around the concept of Recapitulation of Ontogenesis. To review a child's skills and abilities, identify the gaps, and create treatment opportunities around recapturing that

| TABLE 69.2 | Trauma Through the Lens of Mosey's Adaptive Skills |||

Mosey Skill Level	Important Subskills	Targets for Intervention	Potential Impact of Trauma
Sensory Integration Skills	Receive, select, and combine sensory skills	• Hyper/hypo sensitivity to stimuli • Reactive or inappropriate responses to stimuli	• Inability to tolerate different environments • Poor emotion regulation • Behavioral dysregulation
Cognitive Skills	Perceive, represent, or organize sensory information	• Initiation or termination • Time management • Decision making	• Difficulty problem-solving • Obsessive thought patterns • Poor memory • Difficulty following directions
Dyadic Skills	Participate in a variety of dyadic relationships	• Emotion regulation • Communication skills	• Resistance to authority • Unstable friendships • Isolative
Group Interaction Skills	Ability to engage in a variety of primary groups	• Divided attention • Sequencing • Heeds/regulates Self	• Social anxiety • Substance misuse • Unstable relationships
Self-Identity Skill	Perception of self Autonomy Permanence Holistic view	• Chooses/ decision making • Communication skills • Self-expression	• Poor self-esteem • Lack of boundaries • Emotional repression
Sexual Identity Skill	Acceptance of sexual nature Ability to engage in healthy sexual relationships	• Initiation or termination • Self-regulation • Safety awareness	• Sexual confusion, • Unhealthy or codependent relationships • Repeating patterns of abuse, neglect

Adapted from Mosey, A. C. (1980). A model for occupational therapy. *Occupational Therapy in Mental Health, 1*(1), 11–32. https://doi.org/10.1300/J004v01n01_02

missed skill or area of development. Consider the above-mentioned person, who finds themselves unable to connect with another individual due to difficulty with assessing a person's safety, or genuineness. This client may benefit from group therapy where they can be supported in interpreting other members' actions. You might engage them in role-play activities to learn methods for asking direct questions and setting boundaries. Improving their communication and conflict management skills would increase their ability to connect with another person in an authentic way. If you understand the goal and the circumstances that created the deficit, then your options for treatment are only limited by your creativity.

Breaking the Cycle

When treating children, it is necessary to include the larger family unit in assessment, treatment, and outcomes measures. Children are reliant on caregivers for survival, and often in the cases of trauma, there are complex family dynamics that are contributing factors to how a child is impacted by stressful events.

The term *generational trauma* is used to describe trauma that is passed down from generation to generation. The idea comes from the science of epigenetics (DeAngelis, 2019), meaning how your DNA is designed and expressed.

It considers the possibility that, for example, exposure to stress hormones in utero can cause changes in a developing fetus' DNA. This would cause traumatic exposure to imprint itself into our biology, allowing it to be transmitted over generations.

A long-time argument in the world of mental health care is the nature or nurture debate. Essentially, can we determine for sure if mental health problems are caused by nature (biology, genetic makeup, chemical imbalances) or nurture (environmental exposure and risk factors). There does not seem to be a simple answer, even in the field of trauma. As OT practitioners it is essential that we understand how a family's story creates a context in which a child will be growing, maturing, and becoming themselves. When the parent or guardian has also experienced trauma, this creates a complicated treatment environment that can be challenging to navigate. OT practitioners are taught to see the client from a holistic point of view. This means that we cannot simply support the child if we are going to then send them back to a toxic or unsupportive home. This perspective is critical when the parent has experienced childhood trauma (Whitney, 2021). Parents who have unresolved traumatic histories are more likely to pass along their own negative beliefs and behavior patterns, and they are also in need of treatment.

The most research on this topic has been within families who had a relative live though the Holocaust. Several studies have found atypically higher occurrences of depression, anxiety, and substance abuse in children who were direct descendants of a Holocaust survivor (Sangalang & Vang, 2017).

This type of research is newer and needs further exploration, however as OT practitioners, we know that context and environment is a very important part of assessing and treating an individual. Families who have a child that has experienced trauma need support, resources, parenting training, community and outreach, psychoeducation, and much more. Without treatment and intervention that supports the whole family, the cycles of violence and abuse can continue to affect all generations to come. Families can heal with the right kind of intervention and holistic approach.

Evidence-Based Treatment and Advocacy

The evidence around treatment for trauma has recommendations at both the individual level and the systemic level. This section of the chapter will look at both of those avenues. Our role as OT practitioners is not drastically different from how we engage our clients with any other diagnosis. We identify the barriers to occupational engagement and work to create new patterns, restore previous functions, or develop adaptations that support our client's function capabilities. Additionally, we have an obligation to advocate and support our clients on a policy and procedural level. There are many opportunities for direct care treatment, as well as implementation of practice and policies that can significantly reduce the occurrence of traumatic instances, and the impact these experiences have on individuals and society. BOTH avenues are extremely important to effectively address the epidemic of childhood trauma and maltreatment.

Stages of Trauma Treatment

In her extensive work with this population, Judy Herman (2015) outlines three stages of trauma treatment:

1. *Safety and stability:* Creating a support system, identifying coping skills, working through automatic thoughts and behaviors
2. *Re-telling of traumatic events:* Processing the event or events, integrating memories.
3. *Re-establishing connections or meaning making:* Identifying a purpose and integrating this experience into your self-concept.

As OT practitioners, our work is within both stage 1 and stage 3 of this process. For stage 1 this work may look like:

- Development of healthy coping skills (writing, exercise, relaxation skills, meditation, creative expression, or creating routines and structure)

- Identifying needs for adaptations (planning social events, managing sensory needs, organizing spaces to optimize performance)
- Creating a support system (caregiver or family education, identifying appropriate resources and support groups, developing a care team).

For stage 3 work, this may look like:

- Identifying new interests (hobbies, volunteer work, career paths) that previously felt unattainable
- Creating new routines and habits (self-care, bedtime routines, integration of healthy habits)
- Developing new skills for new roles (parenting, intimate relationships, work roles)
- Re-establishing previously valued occupations or roles that had become unmanageable due to traumatic symptoms.

It is vitally important that OT practitioners do **not** engage in stage 2 work without additional training or support. This work requires an extreme level of understanding of trauma and how to integrate memories that the typical practitioner does not possess. Trying to process traumatic events with your client without the proper knowledge and safety measures in place can have a detrimental impact and leave them re-traumatized. OT practitioners can, however, engage in therapies like cognitive-behavioral therapy (CBT), exposure therapy, or other cognitive retraining exercises. It is also an option for OT practitioners to get further training in methods like eye movement desensitization and reprocessing (EMDR), a type of therapy that helps an individual change the way that they process memories.

The challenge of this comes when clients choose to disclose information to OT practitioners who then need to help the clients find a safe way to process that information. Listening and supporting clients in a compassionate way is ALWAYS the responsibility of practitioners. The difference here is that OT practitioners are not qualified to do the *processing* of the event that is outside of scope of OT practice. For some clients, processing their trauma will be a lifelong struggle that may never fully be healed, but it can be integrated into identity and functionality that allows them to participate in their occupations in a way that is meaningful and valued.

Trauma-Informed Care

Trauma-informed care is a model of practice that encourages practitioners to consider the high likelihood that a significant number of their clients have experienced a traumatic event and would benefit from an approach that aims to decrease the possibility of re-traumatization (Piller & Achord, 2022). The model has a wide range of applications in multiple different settings, including but not limited to hospitals, schools, community outreach, home care, and educational programs. Imagine trauma-informed care as similar to universal precautions for your emotional safety.

According to the NCTSN (2022) Trauma Informed Care should include the following elements:

1. Routinely screen for trauma exposure and related symptoms.
2. Use evidence-based, culturally responsive assessment and treatment for traumatic stress and associated mental health symptoms.
3. Make resources available to children, families, and providers on trauma exposure, its impact, and treatment.
4. Engage in efforts to strengthen the resilience and protective factors of children and families impacted by and vulnerable to trauma.
5. Address parent and caregiver trauma and its impact on the family system.
6. Emphasize continuity of care and collaboration across child-service systems.
7. Maintain an environment of care for staff that addresses, minimizes, and treats secondary traumatic stress, and that increases staff wellness.

Trauma-informed care requires a collaborative and holistic approach and is strongly aligned with OT core values and domain of concern. Read OT Story 69.3 to see an example of applying a trauma-informed approach in a school system.

Comprehensive and Inclusive Programs

The great news is that there are new and exciting updates in trauma treatment and prevention program development. Below are a few examples of programs and initiatives that have already had a significant impact on how the world views this issue, and what OT practitioners, educators, communities, and families need to know to address it.

- Using a sensory integration lens, Tina Champagne (OTD) and her team at Cutchins Programs for Children and Families in North Hampton, Massachusetts, US, have developed a trauma-informed treatment program that includes a comprehensive online resource. The program includes family support, art therapy, neurofeedback, wrap-around services (support provided to families in the United States to manage all the professionals working on their case, to ensure collaboration and integrative care), restraint, and seclusion reduction, and many more elements. They have created a multidisciplinary, child-centered, and family-inclusive program that addresses all areas of occupation. To find out more about this program you can visit their website at https://cutchins.org/
- The International Trauma Center is a community-based international training program, whose mission is to guide and support the natural resiliency responses of

OT STORY 69.3 THE LEARNING TOGETHER CHARTER SCHOOL

The Learning Together Charter School is an inner-city charter (alternative) public school. The school is open to children in Kindergarten through eighth grade who live in the immediate neighborhood of the school. The school currently has approximately 650 students. The school is diverse, serving a variety of racial and ethnic backgrounds. Approximately 75% of the students live just at the poverty line, and another 50% report being exposed to violence or danger of some kind in or around their homes.

At the beginning of the 2019 school year, the school administration observed a disturbing trend. The school had seven students that were hospitalized for mental health concerns all within the first month of school. Teachers were reporting high levels of behavioral acting out, lack of attention or follow through with assignments, and stated that they felt they were spending so much time teaching basic social skills that they were unable to get to any curriculum. There was a high level of teacher and staff burnout, which led to multiple position turnovers and a high level of instability.

One of the fourth-grade classrooms began using a social–emotional curriculum that taught the children about communication, self-regulation, and being a community. They noticed dramatic results, the children began to show increased self-esteem, positive social behaviors, and community responsibility. The administration was made aware of this progress and consulted with the school occupational therapist to develop an initiative around including this curriculum at the school. The OT practitioner had just finished reading about the ACE studies and attended a conference at Harvard University on the Trauma and Learning Policy Initiative (2022). She suggests looking into a trauma-informed school consultant and developing a training program for staff and faculty. The administration agrees that the school would benefit from a trauma-informed approach and puts the OT practitioner in charge of coordinating this effort for the school.

Questions
1. What policies and procedures may you consider when implementing trauma-informed care?
2. How might you engage the students in this process?
3. What is your role in supporting the implementation of this plan.

multicultural recovery into hope, healing, and renewed strength for individuals and communities suffering from violence and trauma. The organization is comprised of teams of experts who engage in training and program development across some of the most dangerous and impacted areas of the world, such as Burundi, Cambodia, Palestine, and the United States. Their unique focus around developing the resiliency of a community empowers these populations to take ownership of these programs, utilize trauma-informed practice and care in all settings, and drastically improved health and educational outcomes. To find out more about this program you can visit their website at https://internationaltraumacenter.com/.

- The WHO in collaboration with the CDC, UNICEF, and several other worldwide agencies launched the Inspire Program in 2016. This program identifies seven strategies for ending violence against children. They include items such as implementation of guidelines and laws, creating safe environments, parental and caregiver support, and income and economic strengthening. Designed as a how-to guide, this program addresses the individual ground-floor work that needs to be done, while also assessing the systemic issues that allow these atrocities to take place at all. The full program can be downloaded from the WHO webpage at https://www.who.int and is available in over 13 languages.

This is an evolving specialty in the medical, mental health, and educational communities. It is only with increased collaboration, communication, and understanding that we can begin to provide safer, stronger, and more effective programming that adequately addresses the root causes, detrimental impacts, and continuous cycle of childhood trauma and maltreatment.

Conclusion: Trauma-Informed Everything

While of course specific treatment strategies and evidenced-based care are certainly important, the MOST beneficial thing we as OT practitioners can do is what we do best: consider the context. There are many ways that we can go about creating a more trauma-informed world and educating ourselves is the first step. The existence and prevalence of trauma and traumatic responses need to be considered in ALL things. From each interaction you have with a client, to what types of music or art you have in your clinic, what your intake procedures encompass, the hiring and staff support structure, and your own practice in professional development and self-care. A fundamental part of this is that when your client tells you they experienced something traumatic, you BELIEVE THEM. It is not our role or duty to figure out if they are telling us the truth or not. There are plenty of other agencies and avenues for that. The desire to get to the bottom of a story or prod and ask questions is about our own needs, and not what is best for the client. They will spend plenty of time defending and explaining themselves, you need to be a person that they can trust and rely on.

Consider one last example of thinking from a trauma-informed perspective. A child on your case load in a school district is continually missing homework or not completing work in a timely manner. Most of us would assume the child is just not interested or being lazy. Consider the alternative that the child is living with a parent who is mentally ill, and they are responsible for caring for their siblings at home. This leaves them no time to complete homework, or study, resulting in poor school performance. Instead of giving the child a consequence of low grades or holding them back in school, we should be offering support to this family, providing access to childcare services, giving them food assistance, and medical and mental health care for the family. What other things can you think of that would make a difference for this child and their family?

Trauma-informed thought is about changing the way we look at a situation. In Occupational Therapy we ask what matters to you, instead of what is the matter with you. In trauma-informed care, we ask what happened here, instead of what is wrong with you. Trauma-informed care helps us see that there are potentially other explanations for an individual, group, or communities' behavior or performance. It is important to note that this is not an excuse or permission for individuals to engage in any behavior they deem fit. Consequences and structure are paramount features of trauma-informed care. This is simply about assessing context and addressing barriers in a collaborative and supportive way. It is about understanding the holistic view of a client, so we can ensure that they have the tools to be successful and healthy.

As OT practitioners I would suggest to you that we are uniquely qualified to identify, develop, and implement this type of thinking across all settings and populations. Our holistic approach, coupled with our understanding of contextual factors and our presence in many diverse types of treatment facilities provides us with the amazing opportunity to really make an impact on how society functions and supports each other. The theoretical foundations of our profession provide us with the wisdom and knowledge to make a difference. To be the change we wish to see in the world.

Lippincott® Connect *For additional resources on the subjects discussed in this chapter, visit Lippincott Connect.*

REFERENCES

ACE Response. (2022). *What is ACE response?* http://www.aceresponse.org/

American Occupational Therapy Association. (2015). Childhood trauma. https://www.aota.org/~/media/Corporate/Files/Practice/Children/Childhood-Trauma-Info-Sheet-2015.pdf

American Occupational Therapy Association. (2020). Occupational therapy practice framework: Domain and process—Fourth edition. *American Occupational Therapy Association, 74*(Suppl. 2), 7412410010p1–7412410010p87. https://doi.org/10.5014/ajot.2020.74S2001

American Psychiatric Association. (2022). *Diagnostic and statistical manual* (5th ed., revised). Author.

Bremness, A., & Polzin, W. (2014). Commentary: Developmental trauma disorder: A missed opportunity I DSM V. *Journal of the Canadian Academy of Child and Adolescent Psychiatry, 23*(2), 142–145. https://www.ncbi.nlm.nih.gov/pmc/articles/PMC4032083/

Burke-Harris, N. (2015). *How childhood trauma affects health across a lifetime* [Video]. TED Talks. https://www.ted.com/talks/nadine_burke_harris_how_childhood_trauma_affects_health_across_a_lifetime?language=en

Centers for Disease Control and Prevention. (2021). *Adverse childhood experiences (ACEs).* https://www.cdc.gov/violenceprevention/aces/index.html

Cloitre, M., Stolbach, B. C., Herman, J. L., van der Kolk, B., Pynoos, R., Wang, J., & Petkova, E. (2009). A developmental approach to complex PTSD: Childhood and adult cumulative trauma as predictors of symptom complexity. *Journal of Traumatic Stress, 22*(5), 399–408. https://doi.org/10.1002/jts.20444

Davis, J. (1999). Effects of trauma on children: Occupational therapy to support recovery. *Occupational Therapy International, 6*, 126–142. https://doi.org/10.1002/oti.93

DeAngelis, T. (2019, February 1). The legacy of trauma. *Monitor on Psychology, 50*(2). https://www.apa.org/monitor/2019/02/legacy-trauma

Herman, J. L. (2015). *Trauma and recovery: The aftermath of violence, from domestic abuse to political terror.* Basic Books.

Kessler, R. C., Aguilar-Gaxiola, S., Alonso, J., Benjet, C., Bromet, E. J., Cardoso, G., Degenhardt, L., de Girolamo, G., Dinolova, R. V., Ferry, F., Florescu, S., Gureje, O., Haro, J. M., Huang, Y., Karam, E. G., Kawakami, N., Lee, S., Lepine, J. P., Levinson, D., . . . Koenen, K. C. (2017). Trauma and PTSD in the WHO world mental health surveys. *European Journal of Psychotraumatology, 8*(Suppl. 5), 1353383. https://doi.org/10.1080/20008198.2017.1353383

Mosey, A. C. (1980). A model for occupational therapy. *Occupational Therapy in Mental Health, 1*(1), 11–32. https://doi.org/10.1300/J004v01n01_02

National Child Traumatic Stress Network. (2022). https://www.nctsn.org/

Pennebaker, J. W., & Susman, J. R. (1988). Disclosure of traumas and psychosomatic processes. *Social Science and Medicine, 26*, 327–332. https://doi.org/10.1016/0277-9536(88)90397-8

Piller, A., & Achord, A. (2022, July). Defining trauma-informed care in OT. *American Journal of Occupational Therapy, 76*(Suppl. 1), 7610505061p1. https://doi.org/10.5014/ajot.2022.76S1-PO61

Sangalang, C. C., & Vang, C. (2017). Intergenerational trauma in refugee families: A systematic review. *Journal of Immigrant and Minority Health, 19*, 745–754. https://doi.org/10.1007/s10903-016-0499-7

Substance Abuse and Mental Health Services Administration. (2016). *DSM-5 changes: Implications for child serious emotional disturbance.* Substance Abuse and Mental Health Services Administration (US); DSM-5 Child Mental Disorder Classification. https://www.ncbi.nlm.nih.gov/books/NBK519712/

Substance Abuse and Mental Health Services Administration. (2022). *Understanding childhood trauma.* https://www.samhsa.gov/child-trauma/understanding-child-trauma#:~:text=More%20than%20two%20thirds%20of,Community%20or%20school%20violence

Trauma and Learning Policy Initiative. (2022). History and Background. https://traumasensitiveschools.org/

Van der Kolk, B. (2000). Posttraumatic stress disorder and the nature of trauma. *Dialogues in Clinical Neuroscience, 2*(1), 7–22. https://doi.org/10.31887/DCNS.2000.2.1/bvdkolk

Viola, T. W., Salum, G. A., Kluwe-Schiavon, B., Sanvicente-Vieira, B., Levandowski, M. L., & Grassi-Oliveira, R. (2016). The influence of geographical and economic factors in estimates of childhood abuse and neglect using the Childhood Trauma Questionnaire: A worldwide meta-regression analysis. *Child Abuse & Neglect, 51*, 1–11. https://doi.org/10.1016/j.chiabu.2015.11.019

Whitney, R. V. (2021). Understanding the role of adverse childhood experiences (ACEs) on family quality of life: A descriptive case study using the occupational profile. *American Journal Occupational Therapy, 75*(Suppl. 2), 7512515372p1. https://doi.org/10.5014/ajot.2021.75S2-RP372

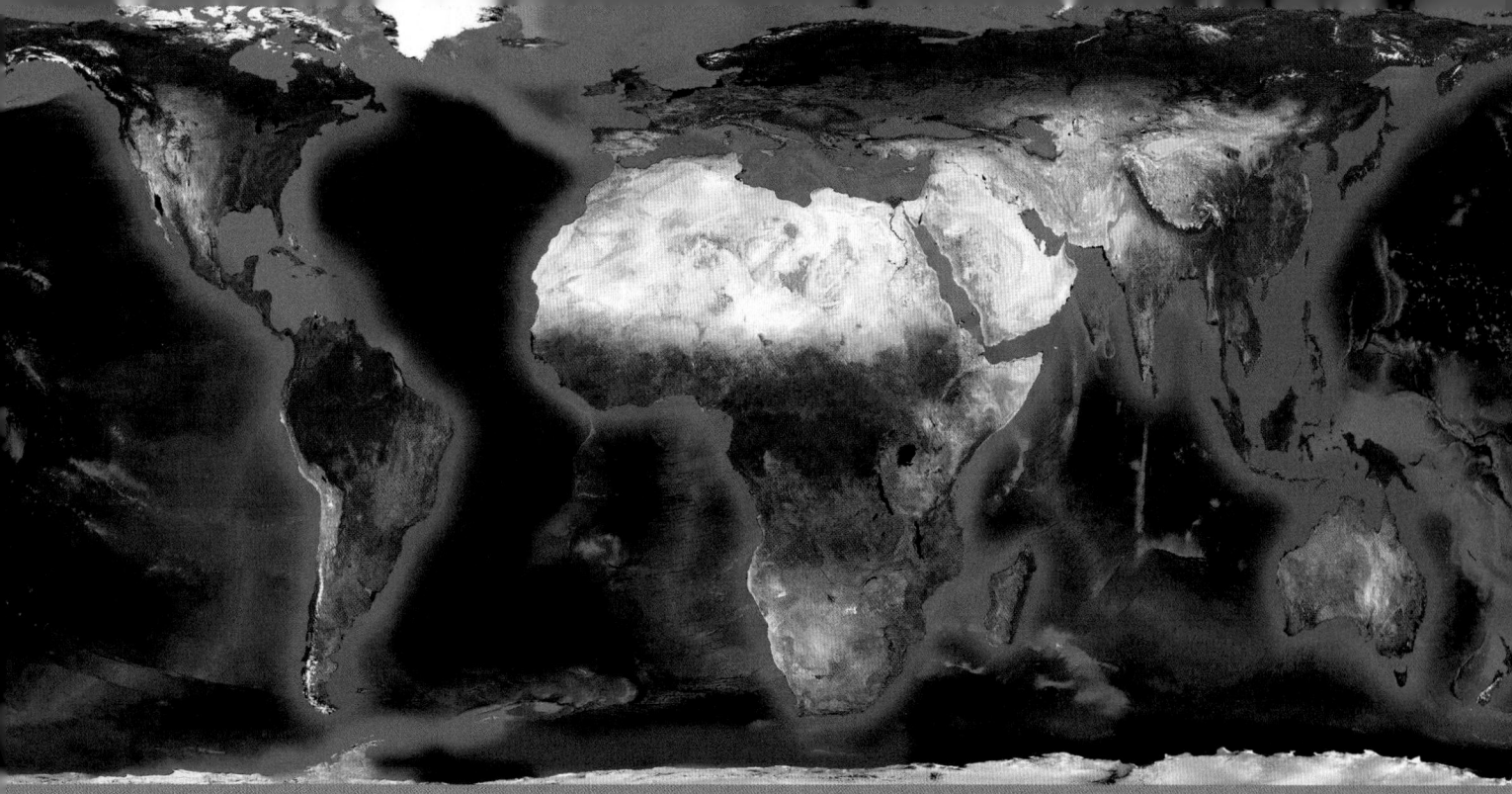

UNIT X

Occupational Therapy Education

Media Related to Occupational Therapy Education

Readings
- *Thinking Fast and Slow:* Daniel Kahneman's book helps us understand how we think and make decisions and how cognitive biases interfere with sound judgment. It includes techniques for better thinking. (2013)
- *I Hate the Ivy League: Riffs and Rants on Elite Education:* Malcolm Gladwell describes how higher education in the United States rewards the elites and proposes ways to do a better job of making college more affordable, fair, and accessible to everyone. (2022)

- *Being Mortal:* Surgeon Atul Gawande writes about how we should reconsider the care people receive at the end of life. (2007)

Movies
- *Dear White People:* A dark comedy that depicts the perspective of Black students at a predominately White Ivy League College in the United States (2014)

Theater
- *The 25th Annual Putnam County Spelling Bee:* A musical comedy about children competing in a spelling bee and share their strategies for winning. (2005)

Fieldwork, Practice Education, and Professional Entry

Emily Zeman Eddy, Amanda Mack, and Mary E. Evenson

LEARNING OBJECTIVES

After reading this chapter, you will be able to:

1. Comprehend how fieldwork or practice education is integral to the educational curriculum and one's own professional development.
2. Identify the requirements, types, and levels of experiential learning, fieldwork, and practice education in the United States and international academic occupational therapy programs.
3. Compare different types of fieldwork experiences and supervision models.
4. Analyze the roles and responsibilities of those stakeholders who are involved in the fieldwork education process.
5. Analyze the process and types of learning criteria that are used to evaluate student fieldwork performance.
6. Explore the dynamic nature of the personal and professional transitions that are inherent in the role shifts from that of being a student to assuming the role of a professional.
7. Explain individual responsibilities for meeting professional credentialing requirements for certification and licensure/registration.
8. Compare the entry-level requirements for both occupational therapists and occupational therapy assistants.

Introduction

This chapter addresses the purpose and goals of fieldwork, or practice education, along with various models associated with that form of education. Roles and responsibilities of students and educators are identified. Shifts in the learning context and expectations related to the transition from student to professional are discussed, including special considerations for students with disabilities. Lastly, factors associated with professional entry into employment are described.

Fieldwork or practice education placements are structured learning experiences that are formally administered by academic programs in partnership with facilities that offer training experiences. Fieldwork or practice education provides students the opportunity to "integrate knowledge, professional reasoning and professional behaviour within practice, and to develop knowledge, skills, and attitudes to the level of competence required" (World Federation of Occupational Therapists [WFOT], 2016). The consensus within the occupational therapy (OT) profession is that the fieldwork or practice education experience plays an integral role in professional development. Through progressively more challenging requirements, designed as a part of each academic program's curriculum, students gain exposure to individuals across the life span with different health needs in different practice contexts (Accreditation Council for Occupational Therapy Education [ACOTE], 2017; WFOT, 2016).

Purpose and Goals of Fieldwork

The purpose of fieldwork education is to provide students with opportunities to apply the knowledge, skills, and attitudes learned in the classroom by putting them into practice in the fieldwork setting (AOTA, 2016; Costa, 2015). Fieldwork experiences provide students with opportunities to carry out professional responsibilities under supervision of professionals who also act as role models (ACOTE, 2017). Working in the context of real-life or simulated practice and through a variety of different delivery systems enables students to develop a multitude of skills. The two main categories of skill development inherent in fieldwork are (a) the core skills and techniques that are relevant to OT service delivery for a given setting and (b) the personal skills that evolve and transform one's level of professional behavior (Missiuna et al., 1992). For example, fieldwork interactions with clients[1] and team members from other disciplines provide significant learning opportunities in the development of one's therapeutic use of self (Taylor et al., 2009) and in gaining awareness of the impact of cultural diversity on service provision (Murden et al., 2008).

---

1 According to the American Occupational Therapy Association (AOTA, 2020d, p. S75), the term *client* refers to *persons* (including those involved in care of a client), *groups* (a collection of individuals having shared characteristics or common or shared purpose, e.g., family members, workers, students, and those with similar interests or occupational challenges), and *populations* (aggregates of people with common attributes such as contexts, characteristics or concerns, including health risks). However, in countries other than the United States, the term *client* often refers to persons who are paying for their care directly. In most countries, *patient* is used to describe persons who are in hospital or rehabilitation. *Service user* and *person* are terms in general use that describe those in need of OT services. For this chapter, we are using *client* without implying the source of payment for services.

Fieldwork is one major venue for enculturation into the field. The interplay between the student as a person, the profession, and the environment supports the development of a professional identity along with a set of basic professional competencies (Alsop & Donald, 1996). This component of education functions as the gateway into the profession because it enables students to establish the fundamental skills of the profession that will support them in transitioning from the role of student into employment as a practitioner. The ultimate goal of fieldwork is to prepare students to be able to enter the workforce as a generalist practitioner. Beyond establishing basic skills in service provision, fieldwork also enables students to engage in advocacy, leadership, and managerial/administrative learning activities that require critical thinking, communication, collaboration, and ethical reasoning.

Types of Fieldwork or Practice Education Experiences

Fieldwork or practice education occurs in many different contexts, using many different education models and methods, and may combine a variety of approaches. Some of the most common types of fieldwork or practice education experiences are described in the following sections with the goal of providing a broad overview of what a student might expect during their experience. In the United States, Level I fieldwork introduces students to the OT process through observational learning within practice contexts, or experiential learning within the academic or practice settings, enriching classroom learning. Level II fieldwork aims to develop students into competent, entry-level, generalist practitioners.

Simulation and Standardized Patient Encounters

Simulation is "a technique, not a technology, to replace or amplify real experiences with guided experiences, often immersive in nature, that evoke or replicate substantial aspects of the real world in a fully interactive fashion" (Gaba, 2004, p. i2). Simulation activities are provided on a continuum from *low to high fidelity* (Maran & Glavin, 2003). *Low-fidelity* simulation activities, through the use of case studies, task trainers, and the like, provide opportunities for learners to practice discrete tasks, parts of a process, or other isolated skills. Practicing one-handed dressing techniques on a mannequin or role-playing how to respond to a given practice scenario are examples of low-fidelity simulation (Herge et al., 2013). *High-fidelity* simulation involves integration of knowledge, skills, and concepts and immersing the participant in a situation that mimics an actual circumstance. This might involve the use of equipment or life-like mannequins that enable students to respond as though they were with a real patient. Alternatively, live actors, known as *simulated* or *standardized patients*, might be hired and trained to play the part of a patient in a standardized way for educational purposes (Giles et al., 2014). Other simulation possibilities involve use of computerized simulation technology to simulate various practice conditions and scenarios. Computerized simulation may be low or high fidelity. Examples of low-fidelity options include videos and simple case studies; high-fidelity experiences may include learning techniques like interactive virtual reality scenarios (Grant et al., 2021). The use of computer-based simulation, including the use of video simulation platforms like Simucase™, has become increasingly utilized by academic programs to meet fieldwork needs (DeIuliis et al., 2021; Mattila et al., 2020).

Though the evidence on the outcomes of the use of simulation as fieldwork and practice education in OT education is still developing, there have been studies that support the use of simulation and have shown similar outcomes for students who complete simulated learning versus traditional fieldwork or practice education experiences (Imms et al., 2018). Students in both nontraditional fieldwork and traditional fieldwork settings have demonstrated improvements in critical thinking skills (Nielsen et al., 2020). The use of computer-based simulation cases for Level I fieldwork has also been shown to improve clinical reasoning and clinical learning, as well as reflection and debriefing skills (Mattila et al., 2021). Students can expect to learn and practice OT skills and reasoning through a variety of fieldwork approaches.

Interprofessional Education, Faculty Practice, and Student-Run Clinics

Innovative health professions educational methods are being explored for promoting interprofessional collaboration and community service (Institute of Medicine, 2015). Core competencies for all health professions have been identified as strategies to promote person-centered care that is accessible, equitable, and cost effective, while considering diverse factors, and taking into account the work life of health providers to prevent burnout and dissatisfaction (Bodenheimer & Sinsky, 2014; Interprofessional Education Collaborative, 2016). Person-centered care places the person's interests, goals, and preferences at the center of interprofessional practice, giving attention to ethical, quality services that respectfully acknowledge shared values and uphold privacy and dignity. Understanding the roles and responsibilities of other providers and colleagues is essential to working

together to assess and address the health needs of individuals and populations. Teamwork and communication skills are foundational to promoting meaningful, effective, and efficient healthcare.

Faculty-led programs and clinics, otherwise known as *faculty practice*, can provide a venue to role-model quality OT practice, teamwork, and interprofessional collaboration, while also providing community-based services to underserved populations (Boshoff et al., 2020; Rogers et al., 2017). Similarly, student-run and faculty-supervised clinics provide opportunities for students to practice OT skills while addressing a specific community need; these clinics may also involve interprofessional learning experiences while increasing exposure to a diverse client population (Copley et al., 2007; Wilbur et al., 2017). These learning experiences may occur on campus or within the community context. Examples include occupational therapists' role in assessing clients' functional capacities in relation to daily habits and routines to facilitate coordination services, such as primary care (Andreae et al., 2021); providing community mental health services for individuals with chronic mental illness and substance abuse or experiencing homelessness (Drummond et al., 2021; Wilbur et al., 2017) or school-based programming with school staff and teachers for refugee students (Copley et al., 2011).

Telehealth

OT is one of many health professions embracing the use of technology as a service delivery tool. With an increasing demand for telehealth services from organizations and clients, the need for telehealth, or telepractice, education and supporting students in developing competencies, is more important than ever. Telehealth is broadly defined by the AOTA as the delivery of consultative, preventive, evaluative, and therapeutic services through information technologies (AOTA, 2018), provided through either synchronous or asynchronous means. For OT educational programs, one telehealth-specific standard exists, standard b.4.15 (ACOTE, 2018, p. 31), that addresses students' requirement to understand the use of information and communication technologies in practice. The accreditation requirement includes not only understanding telehealth technology but also being familiar with and using electronic medical record systems and virtual environments across various platforms (ACOTE, 2018). AOTA's position paper on telehealth outlines guidelines for use in practice, underscoring the importance of clinical reasoning and adhering to the AOTA Code of Ethics (2020); following state regulatory boards' rules and regulations; and making decisions on a case-by-case basis.

Historically, in the United States, telehealth has expanded access to OT clients, while ensuring continuity of care and remote consultation between professionals (AOTA, 2018). Examples include clients being served in rural or underserved areas and children with cancer accessing services safely from home. With the onset of the COVID-19 pandemic, state and federal guidelines for OT and other health professions allowed emergency expansion to telepractice, which included students utilizing technology for virtual service delivery and also virtual supervision during their fieldwork education (Peart et al., 2021). After the emergent phase of COVID-19, when all practitioners were required to shift practice to virtual service delivery, continued payor coverage of telehealth and use of telehealth became part of the therapist's toolkit for client care. Globally, telepractice has not only increased access to care but also has supported continuity of services while offering different delivery systems to clients. Fieldwork student preparation, specifically for the virtual patient-care context, is essential to keep up with the pace of integrative technologies that allow OT practitioners the ability to offer accessible, secure, continuous, and effective care. With these fluctuating changes, students are expected to engage in in-person and telehealth client care to align with the different delivery systems.

Models of Supervision

Traditionally, in the United States, fieldwork or practice education occurred with one student learning from one supervisor. Supervision models have evolved to models outside the one-to-one supervision model. In some settings, a student may be paired with multiple supervisors, or sometimes one or more supervisors may provide oversight for multiple students simultaneously. A variety of other models are used, including peer-mentorship models, inter- and intraprofessional models, and others. Notably, practitioners tend to prefer 1:1 supervision models, though there is an ongoing need for innovative supervision models to help address an ongoing shortage of fieldwork or practice education experiences (Forfa et al., 2022). For a summary of

various fieldwork or practice education models and their benefits and challenges, see Table 70.1.

Fieldwork Education and Capstone Experiences in the United States

Level I Fieldwork Experience

Level I fieldwork offers students practical experiences that are integrated throughout the academic program. For both OT and OT assistant students, the goal of Level I fieldwork is to "introduce students to fieldwork, apply knowledge to practice, and to develop understanding of the needs of clients" (ACOTE, 2018, p. 41).

Through Level I experiences, students are exposed to the values, routines, and customs of OT practice and have the opportunity to examine their reactions to clients, systems of service delivery, related personnel, and potential role(s) within the profession. Because the academic Level I performance expectations, learning objectives, and specific purposes of the Level I fieldwork experience vary in each OT curriculum, the timing, length, requirements, and specific focus of the experience are determined by each academic program on an individual basis (ACOTE, 2018). For example, schedule options may include full or half days throughout an academic term, a 1-week placement, or otherwise prearranged visits or activities. Schedule flexibility is often required as various learning activities involving more than one visit may evolve during a semester or at multiple points across a curriculum in a programmatic approach.

There are many different models of Level I fieldwork experiences. For example, Level I fieldwork may include a project-based practice placement in a community-based setting that is organized as a service learning experience (Hansen et al., 2007). International placements may also

TABLE 70.1	**Educational Requirements Practice Education and Level II Fieldwork**		
	Occupational Therapist in the US (ACOTE, 2018)	Occupational Therapy Assistant in the US (ACOTE, 2018)	WFOT (2016)
Duration	24 weeks full time	16 weeks full time	1,000 hours, some placements—8 weeks
Settings	Minimum of one setting if reflective of more than one practice setting; maximum of four settings	Minimum of one setting if reflective of more than one practice setting; maximum of four settings	Different levels of healthcare: acute care, rehab, disability, community, and wellness
Supervisor qualifications	Occupational therapist with 1 year of experience	Occupational therapist or OT assistant with 1 year of experience	No requirement for on-site supervisor

ACOTE, Accreditation Council for Occupational Therapy Education; WFOT, World Federation of Occupational Therapists.

be used as they provide opportunities to learn cross-culturally and practice many collaborative practice skills (AlHeresh & Cahn, 2020; Brown & Stav, 2020; Saviers et al., 2021). Standardized patients/clients, faculty-led site visits, simulated environments, and/or faculty practice may also be considered Level I experiences according to the academic program's curricular design (ACOTE, 2018).

Level II Fieldwork Experience

The goal of Level II fieldwork for the OT and OT assistant (OTA) student is "to develop competent, entry-level, generalist" practitioners (ACOTE, 2018, p. 42). Accreditation standards state that "Level II fieldwork must be integral to the program's curriculum design and must include an in-depth experience in delivering occupational therapy services to clients, focusing on the application of purposeful and meaningful occupation" (ACOTE, 2018, p. 42). Occupational therapy students at the doctoral and master's degree levels also have a goal to incorporate research, administration, and management of OT services. Although 24 weeks of full-time Level II is required for OT students and 16 weeks for OTA students, it may be completed on a part-time basis as long as it is at least 50% of a full-time position at the placement site (ACOTE, 2018). ACOTE also recommends that students are exposed to "a variety of clients across the lifespan and to a variety of settings," and requires that students participate in Level II fieldwork in a minimum of one setting (with more than one practice area) or up to four settings (OTs) or three settings (OTAs) (ACOTE, 2018, p. 42). For more information about duration of placements, settings, and supervisor qualifications, see Table 70.2.

TABLE 70.2 Fieldwork and Practice Placement Supervision Models

Fieldwork Model and Definition	Benefits/Opportunities	Challenges/Drawbacks
Same-Site Model of Fieldwork *Level I and Level II fieldwork in the same-site employing developmental learning approach* (Diambra et al., 2004; Evenson et al., 2002)	• Gain familiarity with site • Increase comfort, decrease anxiety • Early learning experience builds foundational skills and confidence for Level II Fieldwork	• Decreased exposure to alternative practice settings in the profession • Negative Level I can increase anxiety
Project-Focused/Role-Emerging/Off-Site Supervision Models *Designed to promote OT services in settings where the occupational therapist role has not yet been established; focuses on occupational needs, with emphasis on skills in direct practice and program development; often in community settings; supervision may be fully or partially provided "off-site" or remotely* (Clarke et al., 2015; Dancza et al., 2013; Hanson & Nielsen, 2016; Linnane & Warren, 2017; Schmitz et al., 2018)	• Increased self-confidence, flexibility, perseverance, and problem-solving • Project management skills • Develop skills for consultancy role • Strengthened professional identity • Opportunity to integrate theory into practice and program planning	• Coordination of on-site supervision with occupational therapist supervision • Students experience a wide variety of emotions • Time challenges • Lack of occupational therapist role modeling • Purpose of placement may be obscured if on-site staff have alternative expectations • Additional support needed from academic program
Collaborative/Peer-Assisted Learning Models *Students at a similar level of education work together collaboratively to acquire knowledge and skills; usually with one supervisor* (Flood et al., 2010; Forfa et al., 2022; Hanson & Deluliis, 2015; Hong Meng Tai et al., 2016; Price & Whiteside, 2016)	• Positive interdependence • Face-to-face interaction skills • Cooperative, group problem-solving • Supports both collaborative and autonomous learning • Equips students to be peer educators • More supportive of adult learning principles and development of teamwork skills commonly applied in OT education • Social support for students	• Interpersonal difficulties or incompatibility between students • Individualization of student grading and maintenance of student confidentiality • Requires established structure and practices along with advance orientation for all parties to support optimal outcome • Supervisor workload • Client safety in high-acuity medical settings • Clinician buy-in due to unfamiliarity with the model and expectations of medical hierarchy

TABLE 70.2 **Fieldwork and Practice Placement Supervision Models (*continued*)**

Fieldwork Model and Definition	Benefits/Opportunities	Challenges/Drawbacks
Multiple Mentoring/Shared Supervision Model *Multiple mentors share in the supervision of one or more students.* (Copley & Nelson, 2012; Forfa et al., 2022; Nelson et al., 2010; O'Connor et al., 2012)	• Mentors learn from one another. • Increased access of students to multiple mentors and practice areas • Increased independence and development of a range of skills	• Preplanned structure and organization needed to support student learning • Consistency among mentors in grading or expectations
Intraprofessional OT–OT Assistant Education Model *OT and OT assistant students share practice activities to explore roles and promote understanding.* (Costa et al., 2012; Jung et al., 2008)	• Develops relationship of trust, mutual respect • Facilitates understanding of roles • Enhanced communication skills • Development of competence and confidence in skills and abilities	• Care given to site selection and preceptor preparation • Coordinating schedule between occupational therapist and OT assistant programs • Additional tutorial once per week with resources binder
Interprofessional Experience *Trainees collaborate with two or more professions in provision of client intervention.* (Ford et al., 2013; Precin, 2007; Sheppard et al., 2015)	• Increased respect for the benefits of teamwork • Increased understanding of own role and the role of other professions • Development of skills for collaborative interprofessional communication • Increased quality of client care	• Students may underestimate skills and knowledge until they orient the next cohort • Coordination of placement schedules across disciplines may be challenging • Inconsistency in discipline participation
Hybrid Model *Multiple models are combined to meet learning objectives for fieldwork or practice education placements; may include combining simulation with other models* (Knightbridge, 2014; Reed, 2016; Thew et al., 2018)	• Provides a variety of learning experiences to better meet objectives of experience • May allow for targeted exposure to different settings, populations, or service delivery models, etc. within the same experience • Facilitates meaningful experiences that best meet current educational environment limitations	• Students may have difficulty managing expectations presented by multiple models • Management, scheduling, and coordination of hybrid placements • Difficulty with consistent student evaluation

ACOTE, Accreditation Council for Occupational Therapy Education.

Generally, during a Level II placement, students initially work under direct supervision. They test firsthand the theories and facts learned in academic study and have a chance to refine skills through interaction with clients across the life course, with clients' families, and with team members while working in various service delivery settings and systems. As students' abilities grow, supervision may become less direct as appropriate for the setting and the severity of the client's condition. A developmental model of supervision can be applied as an approach for planning, intervening, and evaluating the students' readiness for learning and participation throughout the trajectory of a fieldwork placement. Within a developmental framework, the learner and supervisor relationship progresses through four different phases: directive, coaching, supportive, and delegation (Barnes & Evenson, 2000). Throughout the placement, the fieldwork educator is responsible to assess the level of student competency for engaging in direct care and retains legal obligations for service provision in the fieldwork experience. In all, supervision of students must meet existing local, state/provincial, and/or federal/national safety and health requirements for relevant policies, laws, and regulations for OT practice.

Doctoral Capstone and Baccalaureate Projects

In the United States, entry-level doctoral degree programs must include a doctoral capstone component that is completed after finishing Level II fieldwork (ACOTE, 2018, pp. 44–46), and threaded throughout the curriculum design. The doctoral capstone consists of two parts: a *capstone project* and a *capstone experience*. Completion of the *capstone project* includes a literature review, needs assessment, goals/objectives, and an evaluation plan, as well as dissemination of the project. The *capstone experience* requires a 14-week, 560-hour full-time immersive experience. This in-depth experience includes one or more of the following areas: clinical practice, research, program and policy development, education, administration, leadership, advocacy, or theory development (ACOTE, 2018). Determination of faculty, student, and site mentor roles and responsibilities, as well as individualized learning objectives, are agreed on and documented in a memorandum of understanding (ACOTE, 2018). For example, some students may participate in faculty-led research, whereas others may be leading a pilot implementation of community-based educational services in a

BOX 70.1 REQUIREMENTS AND QUALIFICATIONS FOR GLOBAL FIELDWORK OR PRACTICE PLACEMENTS

- Language fluency
- Support on local dialects and customs
- Knowledge of healthcare regulations and practices
- Immunization requirements
- Personal safety
- Insurance
- Criminal records/police checks
- Travel advisories

- Conflict areas
- Housing
- Finances
- Contract between academic program and training facility
- Presence of qualified supervisors
- Duration of placement (meets curricular/accreditation standards)

role-emerging setting (DeIuliis & Bednarski, 2020; Evenson & Connor, 2015). Students complete their capstone under the supervision of a mentor with expertise consistent with the student's area of focus, though the mentor does not need to be an occupational therapist (ACOTE, 2018, p. 46).

OTA students receiving a bachelor's degree are required to complete a baccalaureate project. The goal of this project is to "demonstrate application of knowledge gained" and to "provide an in-depth experience in one or more of the following: clinical practice skills, administration, leadership, advocacy, and education" (ACOTE, 2018, p. 44). This project must align with the curriculum designed and include individualized specific objectives. The student(s) must present a report of the project following completion.

Practice Placements: International Perspectives

Educational Standards

Internationally, the WFOT *Minimum Standards for the Education of Occupational Therapists, Revised 2016* require that students complete 1,000 practice placement hours in different healthcare settings. Within these settings, practice education must provide students with the opportunity to implement an OT process "involving human interaction" with clients (individual, family, group, or community to business, institution, agency, or government) delivering interventions that focus on the person, the occupation, and the environment (WFOT, 2016, p. 49). Targeted learning outcomes for graduates of WFOT-approved educational programs are to demonstrate knowledge, skills, and attitudes in the following competencies: the person-occupation-environment and its relationship to health, therapeutic and professional relationships, OT processes, professional reasoning and behavior, the context of professional practice, and the application of evidence to promote best practice (WFOT, 2016, p. 29). The Minimum Standards for Education have aligned with the WHO and United Nations Educational, Scientific and Cultural Organization (UNESCO) with the goal of advancing "human rights

in global society" (WFOT, 2016, p. 3). Position statements on a variety of topics serve as resources for educators, practitioners, and students, including environmental sustainability, human displacement, universal design, vocational rehabilitation, and diversity and culture (WFOT, 2016, p. 19).

Placements

For students who are interested in international placements, the WFOT Website lists "Country Profiles" with contact details for national OT associations. It is recommended that students and academic programs allow at least 18 months for advance planning, working through the resources of the WFOT member country association in order to understand the supervision requirements of the country of interest as well as to assess individual student qualifications (WFOT, n.d.; Box 70.1). As an alternative, non-fieldwork experiences abroad may be more readily accessible with wider choices and greater flexibility for scheduling when organized through volunteer organizations, charitable mission trips, faculty initiatives, or university global center institutes. With any type of intercultural learning experience, it is important to explicitly acknowledge and address differences between healthcare providers and recipients of services, including belief systems, political systems, social structures, health status, educational level, and wealth (Whiteford & McAllister, 2007). Internationally, health educators have identified a number of factors that are influencing fieldwork education.

Roles and Responsibilities of Students and Educators

Students are eligible to begin fieldwork experiences upon completion of the prerequisite academic coursework or concurrent with specific course(s) within the curriculum. Academic fieldwork coordinators or designated faculty are responsible for administrative arrangements to support student participation in fieldwork experiences, commensurate with the goals of the curriculum and accreditation standards as well as with the policies of affiliated practice settings and healthcare systems (Figure 70.1). Clearly defined objectives and guidelines can help to organize student efforts toward

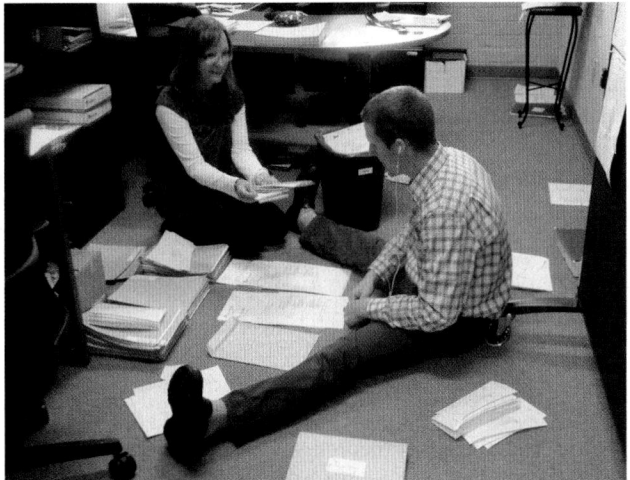

FIGURE 70.1 **A fieldwork coordinator and her assistant sort through required paperwork.**

achieving professional competence. Working toward mastery of the entry-level skills required for high-quality client care is a mutual undertaking between fieldwork educators in academic and professional practice and students. If a fieldwork or practice education takes place using an alternative model, like simulation or other experiential learning approaches, the academic fieldwork coordinator may play a more active role in developing and executing the experience.

Fieldwork or practice educators assume primary responsibility for the process of evaluating student progress and modifying the learning experience within the environment, in consultation with the academic fieldwork coordinator, as appropriate. Professional confidence, which is "an understanding of and a belief in the role, scope of practice, and significance of the profession" (Holland et al., 2012a, p. 222) is also nurtured during the Level II fieldwork experience. See Table 70.3 to gain insight into how each person contributes to and participates in the overall fieldwork process.

Many sites also utilize a site coordinator to help manage logistics of fieldwork and practice education placements. These support people may or may not be occupational therapists and may have limited or extensive contact with each student. Their role is to help support both the students and the fieldwork or practice educators as the need arises.

TABLE 70.3 Roles and Responsibilities in Fieldwork

Roles	Responsibilities
Academic fieldwork coordinator (AFWC)	• Serves as a liaison and collaborator with faculty and fieldwork educators to ensure integration of curricular goals with fieldwork (ACOTE, 2018) • Develops site relationships; selects training sites or learning experiences, and assigns students • Oversees administrative requirements, such as contracts and student health records • Available for consultation to fieldwork educators and students
Site coordinator of fieldwork	• Addresses administrative details of the fieldwork placement on behalf of the facility, serving as the fieldwork sites' formal representative and liaison to the academic institution • Serves as a resource/support to the fieldwork educator
Fieldwork/practice educator	• As a credentialed occupational therapist or OT assistant, meets requisite eligibility for supervisory role as applicable (ACOTE, 2018; Committee on University Fieldwork Education, Association of Canadian Occupational Therapy University Programs, 2011) • Engages in administrative collaboration with site coordinator of fieldwork (if applicable) and AFWC to determine and schedule assignments • Provides day-to-day student supervision • Completes evaluation of student performance as designated • Structures learning and create a positive learning environment
Site educator	• Represents a professional discipline at the site or within the learning experience, not a credentialed occupational therapist or OT assistant • Provides direct day-to-day supervision when a role-emerging model is used or during a Level I fieldwork
Student	• Fulfills all duties identified by the fieldwork educators and academic fieldwork coordinators within the designated time lines • Complies with the professional standards identified by the fieldwork facility, the education program, and the Occupational Therapy Code of Ethics (AOTA, 2020c)

ACOTE, Accreditation Council for Occupational Therapy Education.

Fieldwork Educator Guidelines

In the United States, the role for the people who are responsible for providing student supervision is formally titled *fieldwork educator*, although the terms *clinical educator*, *fieldwork supervisor*, *student supervisor* (AOTA & Commission on Education and Fieldwork Issues Committee, 2000), or *practice educator* (Turpin et al., 2011) are also commonly used. Although the minimum requirement is 1 year of experience to supervise Level II students in the United States, fieldwork educators should be competent practitioners who meet governmental practices acts and regulations and serve as good role models or mentors for future practitioners. This implies that the educator should demonstrate best practices in the OT services they deliver to their clients, as well as model professional behaviors and demonstrate the principles of justice, equity, diversity, and inclusion in their interactions with peers, clients, OT students, and others (Salavant et al., 2021).

Supervising students can be beneficial in keeping up to date with research evidence and professional theoretical frameworks to guide occupation-based interventions. Additionally, serving in the role as a fieldwork educator enables practitioners to hone their teaching skills in fostering the professional development of future colleagues. Beyond training students, supervision is fundamentally viewed as supporting the overall quality of service delivery and development of the workforce (College of Occupational Therapists, 2015).

In the United Kingdom, national initiatives address the provision of training to support the professional development and accreditation of practice placement educators via either a course taught by a program endorsed by the Royal College of Occupational Therapists or an experiential routine and application (The Royal College of Occupational Therapists [RCOT], 2022). In the United States, AOTA has continued offering a Fieldwork Education Certificate Program with the curriculum centered on the Self-Assessment Tool for Fieldwork Educator Competency (AOTA & Commission on Education, 2009) that addresses five areas: professional practice, education, supervision, evaluation, and administration. Regional workshops are instructed by a team of a practice educator and an academic educator. In Canada, the Preceptor Education Certification Program for Health Professionals and Students consists of seven modules to guide learning (Bossers et al., n.d.). In Australia, an online training package is freely available to support the use of the Student Placement Evaluation Form–Revised (Second Edition) (SPEF-R2), including resources addressing the use of the tool, various assessment processes, and approaches for providing feedback (Caine et al., 2021; Turpin et al., 2011). Each of these training programs serves as a tool to assist the fieldwork educators who strive to develop and provide the best opportunity for the implementation of theoretical concepts offered as part of the academic educational program while creating an environment that facilitates learning, inquiry, self-direction, and reflection on practice. However, it remains the responsibility of each fieldwork educator to ensure they are delivering effective, equitable, and inclusive supervision to OT students to facilitate a bias-free learning environment (Johnson et al., 2021). This will often require participation in ongoing continuing education and other learning opportunities to ensure the fieldwork educator is adequately prepared to provide quality mentorship and supervision to students, especially for those students from marginalized groups (see Expanding Our Perspectives).

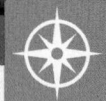

EXPANDING OUR PERSPECTIVES

The Significance of Fieldwork Advocacy

Arameh Anvarizadeh

As an academic fieldwork coordinator (AFWC), my main focus was always on student success. I ensured success by providing safe spaces for students, developing trust and rapport with them, engaging in meaningful conversations about their goals and aspirations, understanding their strengths and areas needing improvement, and fostering learning environments that helped them prepare for fieldwork. Additionally, practicing mock fieldwork interviews, reviewing resumes, role-playing learning and teaching styles with students, emphasizing the importance of practicing with cultural humility, and providing opportunities to analyze what professionalism looks like in fieldwork were just a few concrete examples of how I provided student support. More importantly, genuinely getting to know students was key to placing them at a site where they could thrive and have a meaningful experience.

While establishing my new role and identity as an AFWC, I developed the philosophy that successful fieldwork experiences are not solely the student's responsibility. The relationship between the student, the AFWC, and the fieldwork educator (FWE) is critical. We need to expand on the concept that the student is the only driver of a successful learning experience because it's the duty of all three parties: the student, the educational program, and the site.

Among the positive student fieldwork experiences, there are some fieldwork sites and educational programs with severely unsupportive practices, causing the student's stress

⊕ EXPANDING OUR PERSPECTIVES (*continued*)

and anxiety levels to increase, leading them to question their ability to pass the rotation. During those times, students must have the tools and confidence to communicate their needs in hopes the educational program and the site can create a meaningful, individualized plan to support their experience. And while the strategies for successful outcomes may come in many forms, the core should reflect justice, equity, diversity, and inclusion (JEDI) principles. Below are a couple of examples of my own fieldwork advocacy, which emphasize this reflection and also the significance of teaching the skills to students.

I recall a time when I sent my students to a site that would often sign up to take multiple students at once for both Level I rotations, and always sign up for at least one Level II rotation for each cohort. This eagerness is a dream come true for any AFWC. I was new to the role when I first learned of this site having just taken over for the previous AFWC. The students were already placed and were at the midpoint of their fieldwork. At the time, there was one Level II student at the site. He did not do well; however, since I didn't know the students nor the site dynamic and was a very new AFWC, I was naïve and didn't immediately recognize the problem.

Fast forward, I sent a few Level I students at that site together and then a Level II student. I had taught and mentored this cohort since the start of the program and knew them very well. I was also honing my skills as an AFWC and developing my unique style. As those students began to struggle, they shared deep concerns about the site, particularly the fieldwork educator. I began to see consistent red flags and took several steps to address the situation. However, ultimately, because I implemented support strategies from the beginning, I had empowered my students to be open and direct. From that moment forward, I never sent another fieldwork student to that site because I knew my students, who were all minoritized students, were being targeted to fail.

What advocacy looked like here: Students spoke up. I listened, acted, and developed a clear protocol on steps moving forward interacting with that particular site. Students were safe, no longer traumatized, and began having more positive fieldwork experiences. It came down to being intentional about building a solid student-AFWC relationship.

Another example is when my students were interested in completing a rotation at a competitive fieldwork site. Some of the guidelines were very detailed and included a panel interview with several interested students at once. The students were to provide their resumes with photos attached before the interviews. Although I would role-play interviews with students and review their resumes, a few problematic practices led to an increased bias toward the students. Requesting photos ahead of time is just one highlighted issue. Students of color began to express deep feelings of impostor syndrome and concern about judgment before the interview. They spoke up, and I could affirm they were right. These interview practices were outdated and discriminatory. I had an impactful conversation with the site, resulting in a change to the interview policy.

What advocacy looked like here: Students felt heard, they felt the interview process was more equitable and inclusive, and they felt it reflected less implicit bias. This positive advocacy outcome was again due to being intentional about building an open and robust AFWC-fieldwork site/educator relationship. And like the previous example, it shows the power of student voices igniting the change for more empowering and meaningful learning experiences.

Although I'm no longer an AFWC, the skills I learned and practiced stay close to my heart. Students from across the country often contact me, disclosing fieldwork concerns and seeking support and strategies to advocate for themselves. Since fieldwork is another way to gatekeep, students should always feel empowered to advocate for themselves, without fear of retaliation. If students do not have the tools and confidence to speak up in a time of need, we are doing a disservice to our future generation of leaders.

Taking ownership of one's learning demonstrates courage, emotional maturity, reflective practices, and effective communication skills. If the entire team: the student, the educational program, and the site are all implementing JEDI principles during the fieldwork selection process and throughout the rotation, the outcome will be meaningful for everyone. Fieldwork is more profound than simply placing a student somewhere. Fieldwork advocacy is a way to hold systems accountable to ensure all students have just, equitable, inclusive, diverse, and dynamic learning experiences.

Considerations for Improving Accessibility for Students

Although occupational therapists are skilled in adaptation, education in the practice context presents legal, administrative, and emotional issues that impact supervision, including for students with disabilities (Tee & Cowen, 2012). There is an increasing number of postsecondary education students who have disabilities and may require the use of accommodations to successfully participate in fieldwork or practice education (U.S. Department of Education, National Center for Education Statistics, 2019). Nearly

17% of OT students reported having a disability in a study by Ozelie et al. (2019), with the most commonly reported disabilities being anxiety disorder, depression, migraines, attention-deficit/hyperactivity disorder, and learning disability. These numbers seem to be rising; in 2020, during the COVID-19 pandemic, Chirikov and colleagues reported that across all disciplines in the United States, 35% of undergraduates and 32% of graduate and professional students were classified as having major depressive disorder, with 39% of those in the study screening positive for generalized anxiety disorder (Chirikov et al., 2020). Clearly, there is an increasing need to address the accessibility of fieldwork and practice education experiences for many students.

In the United States, Section 504 of the Rehabilitation Act of 1973 and Titles II and III of the Americans with Disabilities Act of 1990 (ADA) as well as the amendment in 2008 provides for equal access to educational opportunities for students with a physical or mental disability. Students with a documented disability may request "reasonable accommodations" to help them meet the academic and technical standards of their educational program, including the fieldwork component of the program. Accommodations must be provided by the institution as long as the accommodations or aids do not result in fundamental alteration of the program or cause undue burden to the institution. Students may find that the physical or behavioral requirements of the fieldwork setting differ from academic requirements and that difficulties that might have been manageable during the academic program become significant during fieldwork education. For example, the academic class schedule typically allows for breaks during the day and across the week, whereas placements are generally full time, which may require a schedule accommodation for part-time accommodations. There may be challenges for students with complex or multiple disabilities in determining, from the fieldwork site perspective, whether a proposed accommodation is reasonable, and from the academic program perspective, whether an accommodation fundamentally alters program requirements (Katsiyannis et al., 2009).

Before the start of the placement, all students are advised to review with an OT faculty member (usually the AFWC) the technical standards of the academic program to determine institutional expectations and, if applicable, the need to request accommodations before fieldwork placement (Dupler et al., 2012). All students and both academic and fieldwork educators alike benefit from a learning context that supports proactive communication to plan for meeting the fieldwork experience's expectations. With a supportive learning environment, students with disabilities can be encouraged to self-advocate to enhance the planning process.

Students who decide to disclose their disability will find that campus resources, such as student support services and disability or accessibility services, will help them to determine what accommodations might be needed for fieldwork and to complete the paperwork associated with an accommodation request (Meeks & Jain, 2016). Academic fieldwork coordinators are often knowledgeable about specific site requirements and policies and can advise on performance expectations to help students determine what accommodations might be helpful (Taguchi Meyer, 2014). In contrast, a student who chooses not to self-identify disability status to the fieldwork site is not entitled to accommodations as provided by the law and risks the possibility of failing fieldwork if unable to meet the performance expectations without accommodations (Griffiths et al., 2010).

There are both benefits and drawbacks to advance disclosure for students who have a disability. A survey of students and OT practice educators with experience supervising students with disabilities revealed that most educators were able to implement reasonable accommodations for students with disabilities once disclosed, and the majority felt that the placement environment had the facilities to support students with disabilities to demonstrate competency (Nolan et al., 2015). Practice educators did express concerns about being able to give extra time to students with disabilities. The most common concern reported by practitioners occurred when the disability was not disclosed until the clear emergence of a health issue interfered with the student's ability to meet the placement requirements. In these situations, they were uncertain how to maintain safety for their clients while also supporting student performance. The main reason offered by students surveyed for not disclosing was fear of being treated differently or judged as less capable. On the other hand, factors encouraging disclosure were knowing that supports were available; the knowledge that rules are in place to avoid discrimination; and the availability of supportive staff. Ozelie et al. (2019) found similar results in a survey of students with disabilities, finding that the main reasons provided for not disclosing a disability were fear of stigmatization and feeling that it would not be beneficial to the educational experience to disclose. It is hoped that the awareness of the experiences of these educators and students will help to motivate educators to provide all students with a safe and trustworthy learning space, especially those with disabilities, so that if or when they communicate a disability status, supportive actions steps are taken to accommodate them.

Disclosure of disability status is a personal choice, and students are not required to disclose their disability diagnoses to a faculty member or fieldwork educator; they need only to request accommodation based on a recognized disability status (Sharby & Roush, 2009). Students who are aware of their disability have an opportunity to be self-advocates and disclose their status in advance of fieldwork to enable collaboration between themselves, the academic program and fieldwork coordinator, other health professionals, and the prospective fieldwork site(s) (Brown et al., 2006). As educators provide safe and empowering learning spaces in the academic context, a student's decision to disclose can promote an open dialogue in exploring strategies and barriers and types of support available from the university, placement site, family and friends, and personal healthcare providers (Brown et al., 2006; Griffiths et al., 2010). Recommendations in advance of placements are to obtain a job description and to clarify the essential performance requirements. If a student has decided to disclose, it can be useful for the student to visit the fieldwork facility to plan ahead for accommodations and to explore what modifications may be necessary and those which are deemed reasonable by the training facility (Tee & Cowen, 2012). In addition to these preparatory steps, key strategies identified by individuals with disabilities include setting personal goals, learning from prior experiences, identifying coping actions, and maintaining a positive attitude (Brown et al., 2006). Regardless of the degree of advance planning, it is also possible that the student may not realize all accommodation needs until fully immersed in the training setting, and therefore, communication between the student and fieldwork educator should be ongoing throughout the placement (Andrews et al., 2013). Overall, students identified the value of support during placements as an important component contributing to a positive educational experience (Brown et al., 2006; Nolan et al., 2015). Students who seek assistance in building confidence to take initiative in identifying and negotiating strategies and accommodations can plan for positive placement experiences and develop self-advocacy skills that will be needed in the future.

Evaluation of Student Performance

Both formal and informal mechanisms for providing feedback and evaluation of performance, judgment, and attitude are built into the fieldwork experience. These evaluations have two distinct purposes, which are referred to as formative and summative processes. The formative process occurs throughout the fieldwork experience so that students and their fieldwork educators can compare perceptions, assess which learning activities are important and which are less so, review objectives, plan new learning opportunities, and make necessary modifications in behaviors and expectations. The summative process serves to document the level of skills attained. This cumulative review requires documentation of performance at the midpoint of the placement and upon completion of the fieldwork experience.

In the United States, a Level I Fieldwork Competency Evaluation for OT and OTA students assesses performance skills that build a foundation for Level II fieldwork (AOTA, 2017b). The Level I Evaluation addresses skill assessment in the areas of fundamentals of practice, foundations of OT, professional behaviors, screening and evaluation, and

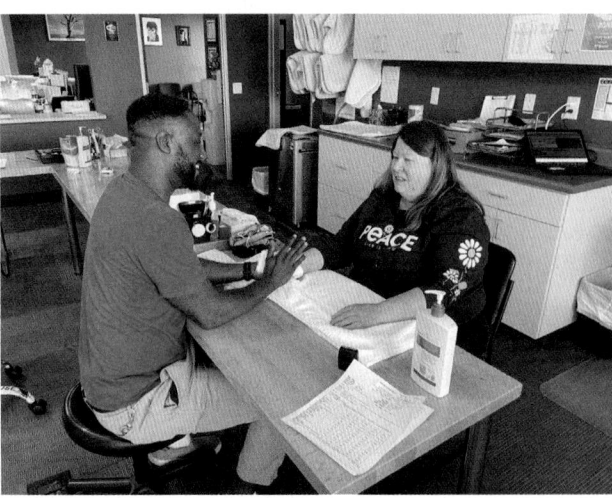

FIGURE 70.2 Loren Battieste provides therapy during his OTA Level II fieldwork at a hand clinic.

intervention. For Level II, the Fieldwork Performance Evaluation for the Occupational Therapy Student (FWPE/OTS) (AOTA, 2020b) and the Fieldwork Performance Evaluation for the Occupational Therapy Assistant Student (FWPE/OTAS; AOTA, 2020a) are companion instruments (AOTA, 2017a, p. 4). Apart from a numeric rating system, the forms provide space and opportunity for supervisors to add or qualify their scoring with written descriptions and comments (Atler, 2003). The intent of the fieldwork evaluation is not to differentiate between students but to measure the achievement of specific entry-level competencies. A profession usually defines its boundaries by setting up criteria for entry. In OT, the fieldwork experience is an essential component of the entry criteria. Successful completion of Level II fieldwork is a requirement for certification as a credentialed occupational therapist or credentialed OTA (see Figure 70.2; National Board for Certification in Occupational Therapy, n.d.). Future employers want assurance that students satisfy the entry-level requirements. The FWPE data may be synthesized to provide the foundation for employment references.

Internationally, there is a trend toward the use of standardized approaches for the evaluation of student fieldwork performance. However, students are advised to verify the tool being used by their individual academic program. The Competency Based Fieldwork Evaluation for Occupational Therapists (CBFE-OT; Bossers et al., 2007), widely used across English Canada and the United Kingdom, is designed for use in any level of fieldwork and within any placement area. This instrument is used in conjunction with a learning contract associated with each competency. In Australia, SPEF-R has been revised and included as part of an online package of resources (Allison & Turpin, 2004; Turpin et al., 2011), and is in another state of revision as the SPEF-R2 (Caine et al., 2021). A unique aspect of the SPEF-R tool is

TABLE 70.4	Fieldwork Evaluation in the United States, Australia, Canada, and the United Kingdom			
	FWPE/OTS (United States)	**FWPE/OTAS (United States)**	**SPEF-R2 (Second Edition) (Australia)**	**CBFE-OT (Canada, United Kingdom)**
Fieldwork evaluations and authors	AOTA (2020b)	AOTA (2020a)	Caine et al. (2021)	Bossers et al. (2007)
Purpose	To measure entry-level competence of the OT student	To measure entry-level competence of the OT assistant student	To assess student performance for professional practice and behavior	To evaluate a student's performance and learning
Content: areas of competency	• Fundamentals of practice • Basic tenets • Evaluation/screening • Intervention • Management of OT services • Communication • Professional behavior	• Fundamentals of practice • Basic tenets • Evaluation/screening • Intervention • Communication • Professional behavior	• Professional behavior • Self-management skills • Coworker communication • Communication skills • Documentation • Information gathering • Service provision • Service evaluation/reflection	• Practice knowledge • Clinical reasoning • Facilitating change with a practice process • Professional interactions • Communication • Professional development • Performance management
Number of items	37	31	38, or Variable; stream selected by practice educator; items vary for • Direct client contact, including case management • Project management/consultancy	Variable; learning objectives are written by each fieldwork site as relevant to the setting.
Rating scale	4 points	4 points	5 points	3 points
Evaluation	Midterm, final	Midterm, final	Midterm (half-way), final	Midterm, final

CBFE-OT, Competency-Based Fieldwork Evaluation for Occupational Therapists; FWPE/OTAS, Fieldwork Performance Evaluation for the Occupational Therapy Assistant Student; FWPE/OTS, Fieldwork Performance Evaluation for the Occupational Therapy Student; SPEF-R2, Student Practice Evaluation Form–Revised (Second Edition).

the option to select domains that relate to the streams of either direct service provision or project management/consultancy. Additionally, a comment bank has been developed to support selection of comments that are consistent with the rating scale (Rodger, Turpin, et al., 2014). It is noteworthy that each of these fieldwork evaluation tools is intended to be used across and within all practice contexts and experiences. Furthermore, similar content and competency areas are evident among these tools, as noted in Table 70.4.

Student Evaluation of the Fieldwork Experience

Students also provide their fieldwork or practice educators and the placement facility with feedback. The AOTA Student Evaluation of Fieldwork Experience Task Force (2016) recommends the Student Evaluation of Fieldwork Experiences (SEFWE) form. This form allows students to provide feedback about orientation, caseload, and OT process;

theory, frames of reference, and models of practice; fieldwork assignments; supervisor interactions; aspects of the environment, such as team relationships; and how the entire learning experience related to the academic curriculum and to one's own professional development. In Canada and Australia, similar forms are used for students to provide feedback to placement sites. Overall, documentation of students' feedback regarding their participation in fieldwork experiences provides valuable program evaluation information to both the training site and the academic program.

Transition from Classroom to Fieldwork

The shift from the academic setting to the fieldwork setting is an obvious, yet often underestimated, life change. As a student, this shift entails making the environmental transition from the classroom to the fieldwork setting while simultaneously

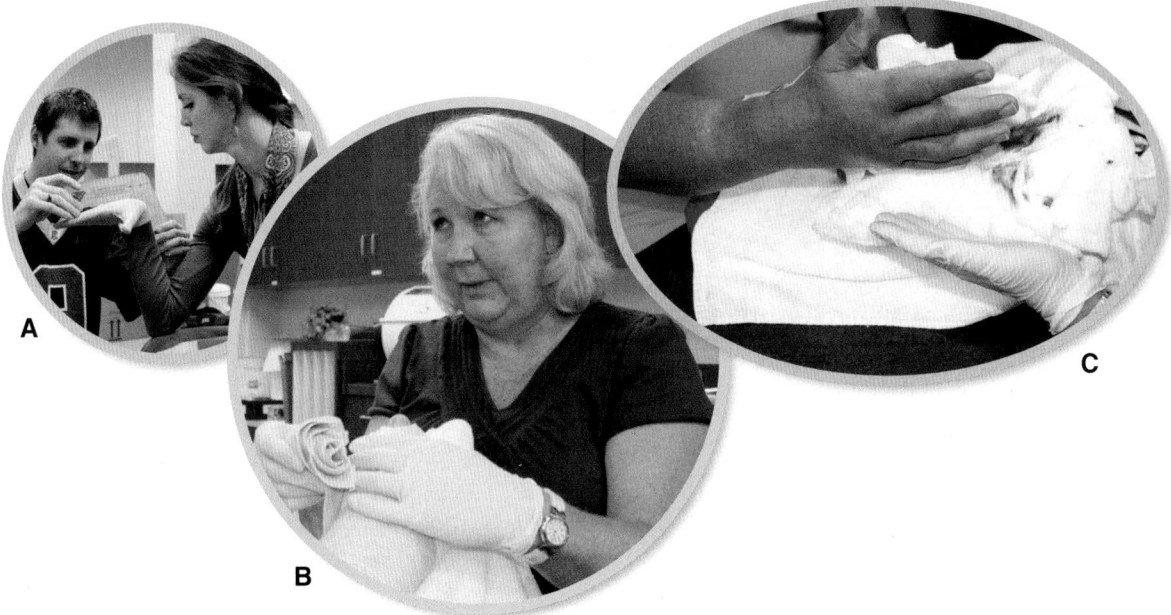

FIGURE 70.3 Moving from classroom to fieldwork: a lot to think about. Practicing techniques in the classroom can be very different than doing them with a client, as shown in these examples related to assessing wrist range of motion. **A:** The students are practicing how to measure wrist motion. **B:** The occupational therapist is unwrapping a man's hand during his first therapy session after hand surgery. This requires her to remove his dressings and manage any postoperative bleeding from his wound. **C:** The occupational therapist is observing how well he can move his wrist. She may eventually measure his wrist mobility using a similar technique as the students did during lab. Note how in the classroom, students can worry less about the client's fear and pain and focus on the technique. In practice, the therapist has to carefully monitor the client's response and postsurgical precautions while observing universal precautions and functional range of motion.

(Photos courtesy of Krisi Probert and Barbara Schell.)

emerging from the role and mindset of student into the role and mindset of OT practitioner (Figure 70.3). As with any transition, leaving academia triggers a process of change from one structure, role, or sense of self to another. The challenge to assimilate into a new environment and to develop a new role can jolt students into disequilibrium, and some students have trouble adjusting to the novel responsibilities and balancing their professional and personal lives. As is true of all life changes, this time of flux can be an opportunity for growth, especially in the context of a supportive supervisory relationship (Opoku et al., 2020).

The nature of the fieldwork context is fundamentally different from that of the academic context. Knowing and acknowledging some of the distinctions between the two may ease the transition and provide support and insight to accept the challenges of fieldwork experiences (Table 70.5). Within the fieldwork context, the learning focus shifts to the application or implementation of therapy techniques in an applied interpersonal context. Techniques that were introduced in a simulated context now must be mastered and applied with attention to the client's emotional needs in real time.

Abstract questions that are appropriate in the academic environment shift to pragmatic questions to reduce the possibility of error in one's thinking. For example, rather than thinking about a client's function in the kitchen from an abstract perspective, the new practitioner has to think about the client's function in the context of a specific kitchen in a certain small apartment and attend to the client's concerns about their roles, activities, family, and home environment. Recognizing that actions have an influence on the client's life, supervisor tolerance for ambiguity or uncertainty by the student declines during fieldwork.

In the academic setting, students are accountable primarily to self and peers, and performance is evaluated on a summative basis through tests, assignments, and grades. Students can choose whether to disclose grades to family or peers, and performance may have little effect on others. In the fieldwork placement, a student's performance is evaluated on a formative basis and may be observed by the entire healthcare team, especially at team meetings. Performance shifts from "safe" competencies, simulations, interprofessional teamwork, and service learning to actions that have

TABLE 70.5 Distinctions Between Academic and Practice Contexts

Characteristic	Academic Context	Practice Context
Purpose	Dissemination of knowledge, development of creative thought, student growth and reflection	Provide high-quality client care
Faculty/supervisor accountability	To student, to university/college, program	To client and significant others, to fieldwork center, to organizational team, to student
Student accountability	To self	To clients and significant others, to supervisor and organizational team, to fieldwork center
Pace	Depends on curriculum; adaptable to student and faculty needs	Depends on clients' needs; less adaptable; shaped by facility procedures
Student/educator ratio	Many students to one faculty member or a few faculty	One student to one supervisor, small group of students to one supervisor, one or two students to two supervisors
Source of feedback	Summative at midterm or end of term; provided by faculty	Provided by clients and significant others, supervisor, and other staff; formative
Degree of faculty/supervisor control of educational experience	Able to plan, controlled	Limited control; various diagnoses and length of client stay, pace of setting, and size of caseload varies across different practice contexts
Primary learning tool	Books, journal articles, lectures, audiovisual aids, case studies, online or in-person simulations, technology, Internet	Situation of practice; clients, families, significant others, and staff; may be face to face or virtual (e.g., videoconferencing, e-mail, telehealth)
Conceptual learning	Abstract, theoretical	Pragmatic, applied in interpersonal context
Learning process	Teacher directed	Client, self, peer, supervisor-directed
Tolerance for ambiguity	High	Low
Lifestyle	Flexible, able to plan time around class schedule	Structured, flexible time limited to evenings and weekends or days off
Contexts	University or college classroom, on-campus center, online learning, simulated contexts	Hospitals, schools, nursing homes, day care centers, day treatment programs, community-based agencies, clients' homes, telehealth

OT STORY 70.1 MANAGING DIFFICULT MOMENTS

Georgie is participating in an outpatient fieldwork placement, finishing up their fifth week. Georgie's skills and confidence are growing, and their supervisor has assigned primary responsibilities for several individuals on their shared caseload. Georgie is treating a woman who sustained a wrist fracture because of a fall (unknown etiology). They are working in a large therapy gym with multiple client sessions ongoing. They have established a friendly and open rapport while working with this client for the last few weeks. However, the client enters the clinic for an intervention session, noticeably distressed. It is apparent she has been crying with red, puffy eyes, and she is acting withdrawn and not making eye contact, while limiting her normal conversation with Georgie to curt answers. Georgie notices that she has a bandage on her arm with an open wound that is showing and appears to have a need for stitches. The client's cell phone rings and vibrates continuously throughout the session. Finally, she apologizes and tells Georgie her partner keeps calling her and she is

afraid to talk to them because they had a fight before coming to the clinic. The client breaks down crying as she explains to Georgie loudly that she does not feel safe to return home. Another client at a table nearby seems to have overheard the conversation, suddenly stating, "I would call the police. Do you want me to do it for you?" Georgie freezes.

Questions

1. What initial strategies do you recommend for Georgie to address both the client and the nearby client who was listening?
2. Did Georgie do anything to violate the client's privacy?
3. After managing the circumstance, Georgie goes home and has a hard time sleeping the next few nights, thinking about the client and doubting their skills at handling future difficult moments during fieldwork. What are some options for Georgie so that they can navigate this placement while balancing personal life, too?

direct and critical consequences for clients, and often ethical dilemmas (see OT Story 70.1). Colleagues, clients, and their families may offer meaningful feedback during fieldwork that fosters skill development and growing understanding of the therapeutic relationship and practice patterns. Although all these opportunities may create uncertainty or tension, they also constitute new ways to learn about self and the profession. The broad and diverse practice activities within fieldwork experiences present challenges to students to redefine their sense of self and evolving professional identity while learning from their supervisor(s). Remaining open to learning can counter negative feelings related to criticism, judgment, failure, and self-doubt that may come from supervisor and/or client feedback during fieldwork. Such personal and professional growth can be supported through the use of mindful, self-care protocols to mitigate stress and burnout. Resources and strategies about mindful awareness and self-care may enable students to access adaptive coping skills to orchestrate their student role with their personal life (Zeman & Harvison, 2017).

Examination of supervisor perceptions of what makes up a quality fieldwork experience includes the need for students to be well prepared for the caseload, to demonstrate professional work behaviors, and to also be open to a variety of diverse experiences and exposure to various conditions (Jensen & Daniel, 2010; Rodger et al., 2011; Ryan et al., 2018). A Delphi study of 49 fieldwork educators revealed adaptability and teamwork as essential professional behaviors as well as being open to constructive criticism (Campbell et al., 2015). Student characteristics desired by fieldwork educators across healthcare professions included willingness to take responsibility for their own time management and learning, while remaining open to implementing constructive criticism and willingness to engage in learning activities (Chipchase et al., 2012; Kemp & Crabtree, 2017), while remaining proactive and professional in technical development

of communication skills (Mason et al., 2020). Other desired characteristics include having theoretical knowledge in and enthusiasm for the profession; knowing how to assess information when there is a gap; being on time, prepared, and dressed appropriately; managing stress effectively; and engaging in creative problem-solving (Chipchase et al., 2012). There is also an immediate need for students, as future practitioners, to demonstrate culturally sensitive care (Ford et al., 2021). Awareness of these attributes and characteristics, in addition to positive coping strategies, can aid students in preparing for and participating in their fieldwork.

Both external and internal factors impact the development of professional confidence in OT students during fieldwork (Holland et al., 2012b). External factors include positive role modeling by an occupational therapist; opportunities for practice; positive grades during fieldwork; a supportive, encouraging supervisor; the support of peers; positive feedback from patients, family members, and supervisors; increased competence; and the overall reputation of the profession within the facility as well as the reputation of the facility for providing quality care. Internal determinants of confidence included students' ownership and personal responsibility for their professional confidence, use of a variety of coping mechanisms to address stress and anxiety, including those that foster resilience, and ability to adapt to language and cultural differences. In an exploratory study of undergraduate OT students, professionalism was a predictor of many variables of fieldwork performance at the half-way point during their fieldwork experience (Brown et al., 2020).

Students experiencing difficulty during fieldwork should communicate directly with their fieldwork supervisor and contact the academic program as a resource as soon as possible. Besides the fieldwork program, students may also want to access the resources and supports within their professional program or academic institution for solutions. See Box 70.2 for a list of behaviors that may put students at

---

BOX 70.2 BEHAVIORS THAT PUT STUDENTS AT RISK

Affective Behaviors

- Making excuses or blaming others
- Being defensive, not receptive to feedback
- Allowing fear/anxiety to interfere with new learning and risk taking
- Making insensitive/unfiltered comments to others, including racist or discriminatory comments
- Difficulty upholding professional demeanor, appearing sleepy/sluggish, disinterested, distracted
- Becoming avoidant/passive or overwhelmed/shut down

Performance and Judgment Behaviors

- Arriving late in the morning to client sessions or to meetings

- Being disorganized or unprepared, such as misplacing schedule, documentation, etc.
- Failing to change behavior/performance after repeated feedback and redirection from supervisor
- Inconsistently maintaining your level of performance, "backsliding," regressing
- Violating facility policies, such as dress code, cell phone usage/texting
- Demonstrating a lack of culturally responsive care
- Lacking ability to "think on your feet"
- Demonstrating poor safety awareness and adherence to precautions
- Breeching confidentiality by posting client or facility-related information to social media or other websites

risk for not succeeding in fieldwork placements. Often, an action plan can be developed with specific strategies to address any identified challenges. The Fieldwork Experience Assessment Tool (FEAT) can be a useful method to help clarify which key components of fieldwork might be posing the greatest challenges, whether related to the student, the fieldwork educator, and/or the learning environment (AOTA & The Fieldwork Research Team, 2001).

Transition from Fieldwork to Employment

For all students, the overarching purpose of the fieldwork experience is to gain mastery of OT professional reasoning and techniques to develop entry-level competence. Effective oral and written communication of ideas and objectives that are relevant to the roles and duties of an occupational therapist or OTA, including professional interaction with clients and staff, is expected of all students. Students are responsible for demonstrating sensitivity to and respect for client confidentiality and site policies and procedures, establishing and sustaining therapeutic relationships, and working collaboratively with others. Another expectation, more internal to the students' development of positive professional identity, includes taking responsibility for maintaining, assessing, and improving self-competence. Students are responsible for articulating their understanding of theoretical information and identifying their abilities to implement evaluation or intervention techniques. Moreover, the ability to benefit from supervision as a resource for self-directed learning is *crucial* to professional development, establishing valuable habits that will support and sustain growth as a new practitioner.

Fieldwork has long been associated with employment, with students gaining important insights into practice demands, their preferences, and directions for the future (Rodger et al., 2007). A recent study confirmed the critical influence of fieldwork on preferred future practice areas. Findings from a study of 152 entry-level OT students indicate the most influential factors for future practice area preference are fieldwork experiences with clinical supervisors, fieldwork experiences with peers, social factors, college course, and future work experiences (Chiang et al., 2013). Thus, the fieldwork experience can be rich and rewarding, and as such, it is likely to have a tremendous bearing on career choices.

Recruitment of students into paid employment positions has been identified as a benefit to organizations offering fieldwork placements (Hanson, 2011; Rodger et al., 2007). However, in order to be eligible for employment, students in the United States and Canadian provinces must first apply for and successfully meet requirements for national certification and state or provincial licensure or registration, as applicable to laws and regulations for healthcare practitioners. In the United Kingdom, individuals must register with the Health and Care Professions Council, upon proof of approved training, and show evidence of indemnity insurance and meeting of continuing professional development criteria (RCOT, n.d.). Initial certification often involves successfully passing a national examination once all degree requirements are completed and verified by the university or college, including utilizing any helpful study guides and online resources for navigating the board exam. New graduates must take responsibility to investigate and adhere to professional credentialing requirements and procedures. Once certification and licensure/registration, as applicable, have been granted, new graduates are ready to search for and accept a job position.

Once they enter the workforces, studies report that new graduates may experience a range of feelings and stages of adjustment in regard to professional confidence and competence. Novice therapists describe professional confidence as a phenomenological experience, rooted in knowing and believing in yourself, your professional skills and knowledge, and your role (Holland et al., 2013). Hodgetts et al. (2007) identify that 6 months to 2 years of practice is often required for practitioners to feel competent. An online survey of new graduate occupational therapists in Australia and Aotearoa/New Zealand found that new graduates felt competent in "managing inwards" such as interpersonal and technical skills for assessment and intervention but less confident in tasks requiring interactions with other professionals and using evidence/resources (Gray et al., 2012).

Tryssenaar and Perkins (2001) describe four stages associated with the first year of practice: "Transition, Euphoria and Angst, Reality of Practice, and Adaptation" (p. 19). Seah et al. (2011) found similar themes in their study of graduate students transitioning to the practitioner role. They noted the excitement of challenging work and the need to normalize the challenges by gaining emotional and practical support from a community of practice, including OT colleagues, other professionals on site, and networking with peers. Opoku et al. (2020) found in a systematic review that as graduate health professionals moved into new roles, four themes prevail describing the transition: systems and structures; personal capacities; professional competence; and mediating processes. Morley and colleagues (2007) found that the transition from academia to novice OT practitioners comes with increasing self-sufficiency and lessening peer contact. A more positive experience was found when supervisors of entry-level therapists clarified job duties, procedures, and provided resources during the entry, such as job guidelines and planned mentorship.

Mentorship is another avenue for entry-level practitioners in onboarding to a new professional role and setting. New practitioners can utilize local resources for mentorship offered by state professional organizations, or the national organization, AOTA. The Special Interest Sections (SIS) within AOTA provide mentorship groups for new practitioners within a multitude of practice areas, including academic education (AOTA, n.d.) and state organizations may do the same.

Viewing the entry to employment as a time of predictable stress and rapid professional development can aid new graduates in seeking jobs that provide support and supervision to ease this transition (Robertson & Griffiths, 2009). For example, the United Kingdom has a 1-year preceptorship, whereby newly qualified National Health Service (NHS) practitioners are paired with senior colleagues who serve as day-to-day role models and resources (Morley et al., 2007). The AOTA has supported a number of fellowships across the country to allow new graduates to spend an extra year developing specific skills and competencies, much like the medical model of residency, including participating in special concentration areas of geriatrics in the Veterans Administration (VA) system, acute care, and behavioral health (AOTA, 2022). Evaluation of this model revealed that new graduates were experiencing increased demands for autonomy and valued access to informal, accessible support from coworkers and the opportunity to observe more experienced practitioners (Morley, 2009). In Australia, an Occupational Therapy Clinical Learning Framework (OTCLF) was developed and refined to support new graduates in their clinical learning and professional development (Fitzgerald et al., 2015). Overall, these studies illustrate the importance of acknowledging that a transition period is normal for new practitioners entering employment.

This recognition is apparent in a survey of what attributes employers seek when hiring therapists employers have fewer or modified expectations for new graduates (Adam et al., 2011; Mulholland & Derdall, 2004). Besides background experience, employers sought job candidates who possess attributes in teamwork, communication, interpersonal skills, and specific practice competencies role. These findings can offer important insights to new graduates who are marketing themselves to prospective employers along with a realistic understanding of expectations for entry-level competencies.

Conclusion

Participating in fieldwork or practice placements, successfully completing this component of an academic program, and entering employment are influential rites of passage in becoming an OT practitioner. Historically and in contemporary practice, fieldwork functions as a critical link between the academic world of theory, the scientific world of research, and the world of practice, now and in the future (Costa, 2015; Santalucia & Johnson, 2015). Quality fieldwork involves an investment of all parties to promote successful experiences (Kirke et al., 2007; Rodger et al., 2011). The depth of the experience depends greatly on the degree to which students and fieldwork educators share the responsibility for teaching and learning. Today's rapidly changing health and human service delivery systems are providing new opportunities for OT practice and fieldwork education. Globally, the profession is giving attention to innovative approaches to improving the quality of fieldwork while taking into consideration each country's health, economic, educational, and social status (McAllister et al., 2010). To be successful in these dynamic and complex situations, student-practitioners must be able to make judgments based on thoughtful inquiry, analysis, and reflection on practice, while working effectively with interprofessional colleagues, groups, and communities. As students navigate fieldwork placements, they have the opportunity to develop competence in professionalism and practitioner skills, in their new vocation, in order to support their clients in improving their participation in daily and social activities and overall quality of life.

Acknowledgments

A special "thank you" to Deb Hanson for her collaboration and efforts on previous versions of this chapter. Additionally, we would like to acknowledge everyone involved in the fieldwork and practice education process: academic faculty and educators, students, and our dedicated fieldwork and practice education educators, along with their interprofessional colleagues.

Lippincott® Connect *For additional resources on the subjects discussed in this chapter, visit Lippincott Connect.*

REFERENCES

Accreditation Council for Occupational Therapy Education. (2017). *ACOTE 2027 mandate and FAQs.* https://acoteonline.org/wp-content/uploads/2019/02/December2017ACOTEActions.pdf

Accreditation Council for Occupational Therapy Education. (2018). 2018 Accreditation Council for Occupational Therapy Education standards and interpretive guide. *The American Journal of Occupational Therapy, 72*(Suppl. 2), 7212410005p1–7212410005p83. https://doi.org/10.5014/ajot.2018.72S217

Adam, K., Gibson, E., Strong, J., & Lyle, A. (2011). Knowledge, skills and professional behaviours needed for occupational therapists and physiotherapists new to work-related practice. *Work, 38,* 309–318. https://doi.org/10.3233/WOR-2011-1134

AlHeresh, R., & Cahn, P. S. (2020). Expanding global rehabilitation services through international academic-community partnerships. *Annals of Global Health, 86*(1), 71. https://doi.org/10.5334/aogh.2876

Allison, H., & Turpin, M. (2004). Development of the student placement evaluation form: A tool for assessing student fieldwork performance.

Australian Occupational Therapy Journal, 51, 125–132. https://doi.org/10.1111/j.1440-1630.2004.00414.x

Alsop, A., & Donald, M. (1996). Taking stock and taking chances: Creating new opportunities for fieldwork education. *British Journal of Occupational Therapy, 59,* 498–502. https://doi.org/10.1177/030802269605901102

American Occupational Therapy Association. (2016). Occupational therapy fieldwork education: Value and purpose. *American Journal of Occupational Therapy, 70,* 7012410060p1–7012410060p2. https://doi.org/10.5014/ajot.2016.706S06

American Occupational Therapy Association. (2017a). Fieldwork performance evaluation validation study. *OT Practice, 22*(14), 4. https://higherlogicdownload.s3-external-1.amazonaws.com/AOTA/d4359e4b-aebd-fe77-eced-236a5f867e30_file.pdf?AWSAccessKeyId=AKIAVRDO7IEREB57R7MT&Expires=1680115673&Signature=CQsse8QvNEcwEp%2BA1SArYLpdHiI%3D

American Occupational Therapy Association. (2017b). *Level I fieldwork competency evaluation for OT and OTA students.* https://www.aota.org/~/media/Corporate/Files/EducationCareers/Educators/Fieldwork/LevelI/Level-I-Fieldwork-Competency-Evaluation-for-ot-and-ota-students.pdf

American Occupational Therapy Association. (2020a). *Fieldwork performance evaluation for the occupational therapy assistant student.* Author.

American Occupational Therapy Association. (2020b). *Fieldwork performance evaluation for the occupational therapy student.* Author.

American Occupational Therapy Association. (2020c). Occupational therapy code of ethics. *American Journal of Occupational Therapy, 74,* 7413410005p1–7413410005p13. https://doi.org/10.5014/ajot.2020.74S3006

American Occupational Therapy Association. (2020d). Occupational therapy practice framework: Domain and process, 4th edition. *American Journal of Occupational Therapy, 74*(Suppl. 2), 7412410010. https://doi.org/10.5014/ajot.2020.74S2001

American Occupational Therapy Association. (2022). *The AOTA fellowship program.* https://www.aota.org/career/career-center/fellowship-program

American Occupational Therapy Association, & Commission on Education. (2009). *The AOTA self-assessment tool for fieldwork educator competency.* Author. https://www.aota.org/education/fieldwork/-/media/c7fc694ef1f44315a3e052bc7e63c853.ashx

American Occupational Therapy Association, & Commission on Education and Fieldwork Issues Committee. (2000). *Guidelines for an occupational therapy fieldwork experience: Level II.* Author.

American Occupational Therapy Association Student Evaluation of Fieldwork Experience Task Force. (2016). *Student evaluation of fieldwork experience.* Author. https://www.aota.org/Education-Careers/Fieldwork/StuSuprvsn.aspx

American Occupational Therapy Association, & The Fieldwork Research Team. (2001). *Fieldwork Experience Assessment Tool (FEAT).* Author. http://www.aota.org/Students/Current/Fieldwork/FEAT.aspx?FT=.pdf

Americans with Disabilities Act Amendments of 2008, Pub. L. No. 110-325, § 122 Stat. 3553 (2008).

Andreae, B., Chang, W., Fisher, T. F., & Bakshi, P. (2021). Primary care: A service-learning environment for occupational therapy students. *Open Journal of Occupational Therapy, 9*(4), 1–13. https://doi.org/10.15453/2168-6408.1792

Andrews, E., Kuemmel, A., Williams, J., Pilarski, C., Dunn, M., & Lund, E. (2013). Providing culturally competent supervision to trainees with disabilities in rehabilitation settings. *Rehabilitation Psychology, 58,* 233–244. https://doi.org/10.1037/a0033338

Atler, K. (2003). *Using the fieldwork performance evaluation forms: The complete guide.* American Occupational Therapy Association.

Barnes, M. A., & Evenson, M. E. (2000). Supervision and mentoring. In S. C. Merrill & P. A. Crist (Eds.), *Meeting the fieldwork challenge: A self-paced clinical course* (pp. 9–12). American Occupational Therapy Association.

Bodenheimer, T., & Sinsky, C. (2014). From triple to quadruple aim: Care of the patient requires care of the provider. *Annals of Family Medicine, 12,* 573–576. https://doi.org/10.1370/afm.1713

Boshoff, K., Murray, C., Worley, A., & Berndt, A. (2020). Interprofessional education placements in allied health: A scoping review. *Scandinavian Journal of Occupational Therapy, 27*(2), 80–97. https://doi.org/10.1080/11038128.2019.1642955

Bossers, A., Bezzina, M. B., Hobson, S., Kinsella, A., MacPhail, A., Schurrs, S., & Jenkins, K. (n.d.). *Preceptor education program (PEP) for health professionals and students.* University of Western Ontario. http://www.preceptor.ca

Bossers, A., Miller, L. T., Polatajko, H. J., & Hartley, M. (2007). *Competency based fieldwork evaluation for occupational therapists.* Delmar Thomson Learning.

Brown, K., James, C., & Mackenzie, L. (2006). The practice placement education experience: An Australian pilot study exploring the perspectives of health professional students with a disability. *British Journal of Occupational Therapy, 69,* 31–37. https://doi.org/10.1177/030802260606900106

Brown, J., & Stav, W. (2020). International fieldwork: A qualitative analysis of the lived experiences of OT students in Ecuador. *American Journal of Occupational Therapy, 72*(Suppl. 1). https://doi.org/10.5014/ajot.2020.74S1-PO4025

Brown, T., Yu, M., Hewitt, H., & Etherington, J. (2020). Professionalism as a predictor of fieldwork performance in undergraduate occupational therapy students: An exploratory study. *Occupational Therapy in Health Care, 34*(2), 131–154. https://doi.org/10.1080/07380577.2020.1737896

Caine, A. M., Copley, J., Turpin, M., Fleming, J., & Herd, C. (2021). Development of the student practice evaluation form-revised (Second Edition) (SPEF-R2): The first action research cycle. *Australian Occupational Therapy Journal, 68*(1), 21–31. https://doi.org/10.1111/1440-1630.12702

Campbell, M., Corpus, K., Wussow, T., Plummer, T., Gibbs, D., & Hix, S. (2015). Fieldwork educators' perspectives: Professional behavior attributes of level II fieldwork students. *The Open Journal of Occupational Therapy, 3,* 7. https://doi.org/10.15453/2168-6408.1146

Chiang, H.-Y., Liu, C.-H., Chen, Y., Wang, S.-H., Lin, W.-S., Su, F.-Y., Su, C.-T., Pan, C.-H., & Wang, C.-A. (2013). A survey of how occupational therapy fieldwork influences future professional preference. *Hong Kong Journal of Occupational Therapy, 23,* 62–68. https://doi.org/10.1016/j.hkjot.2013.09.003

Chipchase, L., Buttrum, P., Dunwoodie, R., Hill, A., Mandrusiak, A., & Moran, M. (2012). Characteristics of student preparedness for clinical learning: Clinical educator perspectives using the Delphi approach. *BMC Medical Education, 12,* 112. https://doi.org/10.1186/1472-6920-12-112

Chirikov, I., Soria, K. M., Horgos, B., & Jones-White, D. (2020). *Undergraduate and graduate students' mental health during the COVID-19 pandemic.* Center for Studies in Higher Education. https://escholarship.org/uc/item/80k5d5hw

Clarke, C., Martin, M., de Visser, R., & Sadlo, G. (2015). Sustaining professional identity in practice following role-emerging placements: Opportunities and challenges for occupational therapists. *British Journal of Occupational Therapy, 78,* 42–50. https://doi.org/10.1177/0308022614561238

College of Occupational Therapists. (2015). *Supervision: Guidance for occupational therapists and their managers*. Royal College of Occupational Therapists Limited. https://www.rcot.co.uk/files/supervision-guidance-occupational-therapists-and-their-managers-2015

Committee on University Fieldwork Education, Association of Canadian Occupational Therapy University Programs. (2011). *Canadian guidelines for fieldwork education in occupational therapy (CGFEOT): Guiding principles, responsibilities and continuous quality improvement process*. http://www.caot.ca/pdfs/Exam/June7.pdf

Copley, J., Allison, H. D., Hill, A. E., Moran, M. C., Tait, J., & Day, T. (2007). Making interprofessional education real: A university clinic model. *Australian Health Review, 31*, 351–357. https://doi.org/10.4276/030802212X13496921049662

Copley, J., & Nelson, A. (2012). Practice educator perspectives of multiple mentoring in diverse clinical settings. *British Journal of Occupational Therapy, 75*, 456–462. https://doi.org/10.4276/0308022 12X13496921049662

Copley, J., Turpin, M., Gordon, S., & McLaren, C. (2011). Development and evaluation of an occupational therapy program for refugee high school students. *Australian Occupational Therapy Journal, 58*, 310–316. https://doi.org/10.1111/j.1440-1630.2011.00933.x

Costa, D. (Ed.). (2015). *The essential guide to occupational therapy fieldwork education: Resources for today's educators and practitioners* (2nd ed.). American Occupational Therapy Association.

Costa, D., Molinsky, R., & Sauerwald, C. (2012). Collaborative intra-professional education with occupational therapy and occupational therapy assistant students. *OT Practice, 17*(21), CE1–CE7. https://higherlogicdownload.s3-external-1.amazonaws.com/AOTA/OTP%20Vol%2017%20Issue%2017.pdf?AWSAccessKeyId=AKIAVRDO7IEREB57R7MT&Expires=1680115746&Signature=DWu4oNQWM0cnMMnaTsBaPEwMmh8%3D

Dancza, K., Warren, A., Copley, J., Rodger, S., Moran, M., McKay, E., & Taylor, A. (2013). Learning experiences on role-emerging placements: An exploration from the students' perspective. *Australian Occupational Therapy Journal, 60*, 427–435. https://doi.org/10.1111/1440-1630.12079

DeIuliis, E. D., & Bednarski, J. (2020). *Entry-level occupational therapy capstone: A framework for the experience and project*. SLACK Incorporated.

DeIuliis, E. D., Mattila, A., & Martin, R. M. (2021). Level I FW in a simulated environment: A blueprint on how to use Simucase™. *Journal of Occupational Therapy Education, 5*(2). https://doi.org/10.26681/jote.2021.050215

Diambra, C., Cole-Zakrzewski, K., & Booher, J. (2004). A comparison of internship stage models: Evidence from intern experiences. *Journal of Experiential Education, 27*, 191–212. https://doi.org/10.1177/105382590402700206

Drummond, R., Koziol, C., Yeats, H., & Tyminski, Q. (2021). Occupational therapy student-run free clinic: Mutual benefits in expanded homeless and health services and clinical skills development. *Journal of Student-Run Clinics, 7*(1). https://studentrunfreeclinics.org/journalsrc.org/index.php/jsrc/article/view/248

Dupler, A. E., Allen, C., Maheady, D. C., Fleming, S. E., & Allen, M. (2012). Leveling the playing field for nursing students with disabilities: Implications of the amendments to the Americans with Disabilities Act. *Journal of Nursing Education, 51*, 140–144. https://doi.org/10.3928/01484834-20120127-05

Evenson, M. E., Barnes, M. A., & Cohn, E. S. (2002). Perceptions of level I and level II fieldwork in the same site. *American Journal of Occupational Therapy, 56*, 103–106. https://doi.org/10.5014/ajot.56.1.103

Evenson, M. E., & Connor, L. T. (2015). Perspectives on the doctoral experiential component. *OT Practice, 20*(8), 17–19. https://higherlogicdownload.s3-external-1.amazonaws.com/AOTA/9cc22e8c-2caa-2207-4209-7eb4473439fe_file.pdf?AWSAccessKeyId=AKIAVRDO7IEREB57R7MT&Expires=1680115805&Signature=wmjJ09MmmMn7rxJA518BZvsZVaY%3D

Fitzgerald, C., Moores, A., Coleman, A., & Fleming, J. (2015). Supporting new graduate professional development: A clinical learning framework. *Australian Occupational Therapy Journal, 62*, 13–20. https://doi.org/10.1111/1440-1630.12165

Flood, B., Haslam, L., & Hocking, C. (2010). Implementing a collaborative model of student supervision in New Zealand: Enhancing therapist and student experiences. *New Zealand Journal of Occupational Therapy, 57*, 22–26.

Ford, A. R., Smith, D. L., & Banister, G. E. (2021). Recruitment and retention of occupational therapy practitioners and students of color: A qualitative study. *American Journal of Occupational Therapy, 75*(1), 7501205150p1–7501205150p8. https://doi.org/10.5014/ajot.2020.039446

Ford, C., Foley, K., Ritchie, C., Sheppard, K., Sawyer, P., & Swanson, M. (2013). Creation of an interprofessional clinical experience for healthcare professions trainees in a nursing home setting. *Medical Teacher, 35*, 544–548. https://doi.org/10.3109/0142159x.2013.787138

Forfa, M., Helfrich, C., & Simon, R. (2022). Perceptions on non-traditional models of fieldwork supervision. *Journal of Occupational Therapy Education, 6*(1). https://doi.org/10.26681/jote.2022.060111

Gaba, D. M. (2004). The future vision of simulation in health care. *Quality and Safety in Health Care, 13*(Suppl. 1), i2–i10. https://doi.org/10.1136/qshc.2004.009878

Giles, A., Carson, N., Breland, H., Coker-Bolt, P., & Bowman, P. (2014). Conference proceedings—use of simulated patients and reflective video analysis to assess occupational therapy students' preparedness for fieldwork. *American Journal of Occupational Therapy, 68*, S57–S66. https://doi.org/10.5014/ajot.2014.685S03

Grant, T., Thomas, Y., Gossman, P., & Berragan, L. (2021). The use of simulation in occupational therapy: A scoping review. *The Australian Occupational Therapy Journal, 68*, 345–356. https://doi.org/10.1111/1440-1630.12726

Gray, M., Clark, M., Penman, M., Smith, J., Bell, J., Thomas, Y., & Trevan-Hawke, J. (2012). New graduate occupational therapists feelings of preparedness for practice in Australia and Aotearoa/New Zealand. *Australian Occupational Therapy Journal, 59*, 445–455. https://doi.org/10.1111/j.1440-1630.2012.01029.x

Griffiths, L., Worth, P., Scullard, Z., & Gilbert, D. (2010). Supporting disabled students in practice: A tripartite approach. *Nurse Education in Practice, 10*, 132–137. https://doi.org/10.1016/j.nepr.2009.05.001

Hansen, A. W., Munoz, J., Crist, P. A., Gupta, J., Ideishi, R. I., Primeau, L. A., & Tupe, D. (2007). Service learning: Meaningful, community-centered professional skill development for occupational therapy students. *Occupational Therapy in Health Care, 21*, 25–48. https://doi.org/10.1300/J003v21n01_03

Hanson, D. J. (2011). The perspectives of fieldwork educators regarding Level II fieldwork students. *Occupational Therapy in Health Care, 25*, 164–177. https://doi.org/10.3109/07380577.2011.561420

Hanson, D. J., & DeIuliis, E. D. (2015). The collaborative model of fieldwork education: A blueprint for group supervision of students. *Occupational Therapy in Health Care, 29*, 223–239. https://doi.org/10.3109/07380577,2015.1011297

Hanson, D., & Nielsen, S. K. (2016). Introduction to role-emerging fieldwork. In D. Costa (Ed.), *The essential guide to fieldwork education* (2nd ed., pp. 341–368.). American Occupational Therapy Association.

Herge, A., Lorch, A., DeAngelis, T., Vause-Earland, T., Mollo, K., & Zapletal, A. (2013). The standardized patient encounter: A dynamic educational approach to enhance students' clinical healthcare skills. *Journal of Allied Health, 42*, 229–235.

Hodgetts, S., Hollis, V., Triska, O., Dennis, S., Madill, H., & Taylor, E. (2007). Occupational therapy students' and graduates' satisfaction with professional education and preparedness for practice. *Canadian Journal of Occupational Therapy, 74*, 148–160. https://doi.org/10.1177/000841740707400303

Holland, K., Middleton, L., & Uys, L. (2012a). Professional confidence: A concept analysis. *Scandinavian Journal of Occupational Therapy, 19*, 214–224. https://doi.org/10.3109/11038128.2011.583939

Holland, K., Middleton, L., & Uys, L. (2012b). The sources of professional confidence in occupational therapy students. *South African Journal of Occupational Therapy, 42*, 19–25. https://sajot.org.za/index.php/sajot/article/view/107

Holland, K., Middleton, L., & Uys, L. (2013). Professional confidence: Conceptions held by novice occupational therapists in South Africa. *Occupational Therapy International, 20*, 105–113. https://doi.org/10.1002/oti.1340

Hong Meng Tai, J., Canny, B. J., Haines, T. P., & Molloy, E. K. (2016). Implementing peer learning in clinical education: A framework to address challenges in the "real world." *Teaching and Learning in Medicine, 29*, 162–172. https://doi.org/10.1080/10401334.2016.1247000

Imms, C., Froude, E., Chu, M. Y., Sheppard, L., Darzins, S., Guinea, S., Gospodarevskaya, E., Carter, R., Symmons, M. A., Penman, M., Nicola-Richmond, K., Hunt, S. G., Gribble, N., Ashby, S., & Mathieu, E. (2018). Simulated versus traditional occupational therapy placements. A randomized controlled trial. *The Australian Journal of Occupational Therapy, 65*(6), 556–564. https://doi.org/10.1111/1440-1630.12513

Institute of Medicine. (2015). *Building health workforce capacity through community-based health professional education: Workshop summary.* National Academies Press. https://www.nap.edu/catalog/18973/building-health-workforce-capacity-through-community-based-health-professional-education

Interprofessional Education Collaborative. (2016). *Core competencies for interprofessional collaborative practice: 2016 update.* Interprofessional Education Collaborative.

Jensen, L. R., & Daniel, C (2010). A descriptive study on Level II fieldwork supervision in hospital settings. *Occupational Therapy in Health Care, 24*, 335–347. https://doi.org/10.3109/07380577.2010.502211

Johnson, R., Browning, K., & DeClerk, L. (2021). Strategies to reduce bias and racism in nursing precepted clinical experiences. *Journal of Nursing Education, 60*(12), 697–702. https://doi.org/10.3928/01484834-20211103-01

Jung, B., Salvatori, P., & Martin, A. (2008). Intraprofessional fieldwork education: Occupational therapy and occupational therapy assistant students learning together. *Canadian Journal of Occupational Therapy, 75*, 42–50. https://doi.org/10.2182/cjot.06.05x

Katsiyannis, A., Zhang, D., Landmark, L., & Reber, A. (2009). Postsecondary education for individuals with disabilities: Legal and practice considerations. *Journal of Disability Policy Studies, 20*, 35–45. https://doi.org/10.1177/1044207308324896

Kemp, E., & Crabtree, J. L. (2017). Matching student abilities to level II fieldwork sites. *American Journal of Occupational Therapy, 71*(4_Suppl. 1), 7111510173p. https://doi.org/10.5014/ajot.2017.71S1-PO1125

Kirke, P., Layton, N., & Sim, J. (2007). Informing fieldwork design: Key elements to quality fieldwork education for undergraduate occupational therapy students. *Australian Occupational Therapy Journal, 54*, S13–S22. https://doi.org/10.1111/j.1440-1630.2007.00696.x

Knightbridge, L. (2014). Experiential learning on an alternative practice education placement: Student reflections on entry-level competency, personal growth, and future practice. *British Journal of Occupational Therapy, 77*(9), 438–446. https://doi.org/10.4276/030802214X14098207540956

Maran, N., & Glavin, R. (2003). Low- to high-fidelity simulation—A continuum of medical education? *Medical Education, 37*, 22–28. https://doi.org/10.1046/j.1365-2923.37.s1.9.x

Mason, J., Hayden, C. L., & Causey-Upton, R. (2020). Fieldwork educators' expectations of level II occupational therapy students' professional and technical skills. *Open Journal of Occupational Therapy, 8*(3), 1–16. https://doi.org/10.15453/2168-6408.1649

Mattila, A., DeIuliis, E. D., Martin, R., & Casile, E. (2021). Investigating student satisfaction and perception in clinical reasoning skills with simulated case-based learning as a level I fieldwork experience. *American Journal of Occupational Therapy, 75*(Suppl. 2). https://doi.org/10.5014/ajot.2021.75S2-RP50

Mattila, A., Martin, R. M., & DeIuliis, E. D. (2020). Simulated fieldwork: A virtual approach to clinical education. *Education Sciences, 10*(10), 272. https://doi.org/10.3390/educsci10100272

McAllister, L., Paterson, M., Higgs, J., & Bithell, C. (2010). *Innovations in allied health fieldwork education: A critical appraisal.* Sense.

Meeks, L. M., & Jain, N. R. (Eds.). (2016). *The guide to assisting students with disabilities: Equal access in health science and professional education.* Springer.

Missiuna, C. A., Polatajko, H. I., & Ernest-Conibear, M. (1992). Skill acquisition during fieldwork placements in occupational therapy. *Canadian Journal of Occupational Therapy, 59*, 28–39. https://doi.org/10.1177/000841749205900105

Morley, M. (2009). Contextual factors that have an impact on the transition experience of newly qualified occupational therapists. *British Journal of Occupational Therapy, 72*, 507–514. https://doi.org/10.4276/030802209X12577616538753

Morley, M., Rugg, S., & Drew, J. (2007). Before preceptorship: New occupational therapists' expectations of practice and experience of supervision. *British Journal of Occupational Therapy, 70*, 243–253. https://doi.org/10.1177/030802260707000604

Mulholland, S., & Derdall, M. (2004). Exploring what employers seek when hiring occupational therapists. *Canadian Journal of Occupational Therapy, 71*, 223–229. https://doi.org/10.1177/000841740407100407

Murden, R., Norman, A., Ross, J., Sturdivant, E., Kedia, M., & Shah, S. (2008). Occupational therapy students' perceptions of their cultural awareness and competency. *Occupational Therapy International, 15*, 191–203. https://doi.org/10.1002/oti.253

National Board for Certification in Occupational Therapy. (n.d.). *Online certification examination handbook.* Author. http://www.nbcot.org/pdf/eligibility_01.pdf

Nelson, A., Copley, J., & Salama, R. (2010). Occupational therapy students' perceptions of the multiple mentoring model of clinical supervision. *Focus on Health Professional Education, 11*, 14–27.

Nielsen, S., Klug, M., & Fox, L. (2020). Impact of nontraditional level I fieldwork on critical thinking. *American Journal of Occupational Therapy, 74*(3), 1–7. https://doi.org/10.5014/ajot.2020.036350

Nolan, C., Gleeson, C., Treanor, D., & Madigan, S. (2015). Higher education students registered with disability services and practice educators: Issues and concerns for professional placements. *International Journal of Inclusive Education, 19*, 487–502. https://doi.org/10.1080/13603116.2014.943306

O'Connor, A., Cahill, M., & McKay, E. (2012). Revisiting 1:1 and 2:1 clinical placement models: Student and clinical educator perspectives. *Australian Occupational Therapy Journal, 59*, 276–283. https://doi.org/10.1111/j.1440-1630.2012.01025.x

Opoku, E., Van Niekerk, L., & Jacobs-Nzuzi Khuabi, L. A. (2020). Exploring the factors that affect new graduates' transition from students to health professionals: A systematic integrative review protocol. *British Medical Journal Open, 10,* e033734. https://doi.org/10.1136/bmjopen-2019-033734

Ozelie, R., Delehoy, M., Jones, S., Sykstus, E., & Weil, V. (2019). Accommodation use by individuals with disabilities in occupational therapy fieldwork. *Journal of Occupational Therapy Education, 3*(4). https://doi.org/10.26681/jote.2019.030407

Peart, A., Wells, N., Yu, M., & Brown, T. (2021). "It became quite a complex dynamic": The experiences of occupational therapy practice educators' move to digital platforms during the COVID-19 pandemic. *Australian Occupational Therapy Journal.* https://onlinelibrary.wiley.com/doi/10.1111/1440-1630.12767

Precin, P. (2007). An aggregate fieldwork model: Interdisciplinary training/intervention component. *Occupational Therapy in Health Care, 21,* 123–131. https://doi.org/10.1080/J003v21n01_09

Price, D., & Whiteside, M. (2016). Implementing the 2:1 student placement model in occupational therapy: Strategies for practice. *Australian Occupational Therapy Journal, 63,* 123–129. https://doi.org/10.1111/1440-1630.12257

Reed, H. (2016). Student responses to the use of simulation in combination with traditional level I fieldwork. *American Journal of Occupational Therapy, 70*(Suppl. 1), 7011505105p1. https://doi.org/10.5014/ajot.2016.70S1-PO1075

Robertson, L., & Griffiths, S. (2009). Graduates' reflections on their preparation for practice. *British Journal of Occupational Therapy, 72,* 125–132. https://doi.org/10.1177/030802260907200307

Rodger, S., Fitzgerald, C., Davila, W., Millar, F., & Allison, H. (2011). What makes a quality occupational therapy practice placement? Students' and practice educators' perspectives. *Australian Occupational Therapy Journal, 58,* 195–202. https://doi.org/10.1111/j.1440-1630.2010.00903.x

Rodger, S., Thomas, Y., Dickson, D., McBryde, C., Broadbridge, J., Hawkins, R., & Edwards, A. (2007). Putting students to work: Valuing fieldwork placements as a mechanism for recruitment and shaping the future occupational therapy workforce. *Australian Occupational Therapy Journal, 54,* S94–S97. https://doi.org/10.1111/j.1440-1630.2007.00691.x

Rodger, S., Turpin, M., Copley, J., Coleman, A., Chien, C., Caine, A., & Brown, T. (2014). Student Practice Evaluation Form–Revised edition online comment bank: Development and reliability analysis. *Australian Occupational Therapy Journal, 61,* 241–248. https://doi.org/10.1111/1440-1630

Rogers, O., Heck, A., Kohnert, L., Paode, P., & Harrell, L. (2017). Occupational therapy's role in an interprofessional student-run free clinic: Challenges and opportunities identified. *Open Journal of Occupational Therapy, 5*(3), 1–15. https://doi.org/10.15453/2168-6408.1387

Ryan, K., Beck, M., Ungaretta, L., Rooney, M., Dalomba, E., & Kahanov, L. (2018). Pennsylvania occupational therapy fieldwork educator practices and preferences in clinical education. *The Open Journal of Occupational Therapy, 6*(1), Article 12. https://doi.org/10.15453/2168-6408.1362

Salavant, S., Kleine, E. A., & Gibbs, V. D. (2021). Be heard – we're listening: Emerging issues and potential solutions from the voices of BIPOC occupational therapy students, practitioners, and educators. *The American Journal of Occupational Therapy, 75*(6), 7506347010. https://doi.org/10.5014/ajot.2021.048306

Santalucia, S., & Johnson, C. (2015). Transformative learning: Facilitating growth and change through fieldwork. In D. Costa (Ed.), *The essential guide to occupational therapy fieldwork education: Resources for educators and practitioners* (2nd ed., pp. 15–24). American Occupational Therapy Association.

Saviers, B., Traywick, L. S., & Meaux, J. (2021). Effect of an international level I fieldwork experience on interprofessional and cultural competencies [conference presentation at AOTA INSPIRE Conference]. *American Journal of Occupational Therapy, 75*(Suppl. 2). https://doi.org/10.5014/ajot.2021.75S2-RP177

Seah, C., Mackenzie, L., & Gamble, J. (2011). Transition of graduates of the master of occupational therapy to practice. *Australian Occupational Therapy Journal, 58,* 103–110. https://doi.org/10.1111/j.1440-1630.2010.00899.x

Sharby, N., & Roush, S. E. (2009). Analytical decision-making model for addressing the needs of allied health students with disabilities. *Journal of Allied Health, 38,* 54–62.

Sheppard, K. D., Ford, C. R., Sawyer, P., Foley, K. T., Harada, C. N., Brown, C. J., & Ritchie, C. S. (2015). The interprofessional clinical experience: Interprofessional education in the nursing home. *Journal of Interprofessional Care, 29,* 170–172. https://doi.org/10.3109/13561820.2014.942776

Taguchi Meyer, J. T. (2014). Ensuring a diverse workforce: Fieldwork success for occupational therapy students with disabilities [Fieldwork issues]. *OT Practice, 19*(20), 18–19. https://higherlogicdownload.s3-external-1.amazonaws.com/AOTA/3dd0d79c-ad17-23a9-db15-6e3d9ad7479a_file.pdf?AWSAccessKeyId=AKIAVRDO7IEREB57R7MT&Expires=1680116063&Signature=w%2BFqUsuLMxqFPn47BNsCroikfBk%3D

Taylor, R. R., Lee, S. W., Kielhofner, G., & Ketkar, M. (2009). Therapeutic use of self: A nationwide survey of practitioners' attitudes and experiences. *American Journal of Occupational Therapy, 63,* 198–207. https://doi.org/10.5014/ajot.63.2.198

Tee, S., & Cowen, M. (2012). Supporting students with disabilities—Promoting understanding amongst mentors in practice. *Nurse Education in Practice, 12,* 6–10. https://doi.org/10.1016/j.nepr.2011.03.020

The Royal College of Occupational Therapists. (2022). *Accreditation of practice placement educators [APPLE].* https://www.inpractice.org/cot/apple/index.php

The Royal College of Occupational Therapists. (n.d.). *Health and care professions council.* https://www.rcot.co.uk/about-occupational-therapy/become-an-occupational-therapist/hcpc

Thew, M., Thomas, Y., & Briggs, M. (2018). The impact of a role emerging placement while a student occupational therapist, on subsequent qualified employability, practice, and career path. *Australian Occupational Therapy Journal, 65*(3), 198–207. https://doi.org/10.1111/1440-1630.12463

Tryssenaar, J., & Perkins, J. (2001). From student to therapist: Exploring the first year of practice. *American Journal of Occupational Therapy, 55,* 19–27. https://doi.org/10.5014/ajot.55.1.19

Turpin, M., Fitzgerald, C., & Rodger, S. (2011). Development of the Student Practice Evaluation Form revised edition package. *Australian Occupational Therapy Journal, 58,* 67–73. https://doi.org/10.1111/j.1440-1630.2010.00890.x

U.S. Department of Education, National Center for Education Statistics. (2019). *Digest of education statistics, 2017 (2018-080).* Chapter 3. https://nces.ed.gov/fastfacts/display.asp?id=60

Whiteford, G. E., & McAllister, L. (2007). Politics and complexity in intercultural fieldwork: The Vietnam experience. *Australian Occupational Therapy Journal, 54,* S74–S83. https://doi.org/10.1111/j.1440-1630.2006.00607.x

Wilbur, K., Zylstra, S. L., & Pitonyak, J. S. (2017). Innovative level I fieldwork opportunities as a method to promote health in diverse populations. *OT Practice, 2*(4), 31–33. https://higherlogic download.s3-external-1.amazonaws.com/AOTA/45e93a68-b3b2-6000-afc9-1927046c5e3b_file.pdf?AWSAccessKeyId=AKIAVRDO7IEREB57R7MT&Expires=1680116245&Signature=11uF7Ae67kOtFkuFIy6DH1iQp0A%3D

World Federation of Occupational Therapists. (2016). *Minimum standards for the education of occupational therapists, revised 2016.* http://www.wfot.org/

World Federation of Occupational Therapists. (n.d.). *FAQ—Education.* https://wfot.org/faqs

World Health Organization. (2010). *Community-based rehabilitation guidelines.* https://www.who.int/publications/i/item/9789241548052

Zeman, E., & Harvison, N. (2017). *Burnout, stress and compassion fatigue in occupational therapy practice and education: A call for mindful, self-care protocols* [Commentary]. National Academy of Medicine. https://nam.edu/Burnout-Stress-and-Compassion-Fatigue-in-Occupational-Therapy-Practice-and-Education-A-Call-for-Mindful-Self-Care-Protocols/

CHAPTER

71

Competence and Professional Development

Winifred Schultz-Krohn

LEARNING OBJECTIVES

After reading this chapter, you will be able to:

1. Discuss the professional expectation of an individual as well as accountability for pursuing continuing competence and professional development.
2. Differentiate the terms *competency* and *continuing competence* and explain the variables influencing each concept.
3. Examine the basic differences in competency expectations for occupational therapists and occupational therapy assistants.
4. Explain how to engage in continuing competence on an ongoing basis through self-assessment, individualized professional development, and clear outcomes while developing the routine of lifelong learning.
5. Identify available resources and the steps in the process of creating a professional development plan, including beneficial learning activities for plan implementation.
6. Assess the role of certification, licensure, and advanced and specialty certifications for practice.
7. Compare and contrast the merits of practice competence and practice excellence.
8. Identify the characteristics of positive mentorship.

Introduction

Occupational therapy practitioners (OTPs) are expected to deliver competent services. The delivery of these services is guided by an ethical foundation as described by the American Occupational Therapy Association's (AOTA) 2020 Code of Ethics (AOTA, 2020a) and the World Federation of Occupational Therapy's (WFOT) Code of Ethics (WFOT, 2016). Included in these documents is a clear recognition that the profession of occupational therapy (OT) and the provision of these services are dynamic, responsive to societal needs, and proactive in promoting participation and inclusion in occupational pursuits. The dynamic nature of OT services requires the practitioner to consider the complexities of clients' occupational needs, various models of service delivery, and reimbursement issues, along with laws and regulations governing services. The cornerstones or foundation of OT identifies the distinct contributions of the profession with occupation being a core value and a clear understanding of the therapeutic use of occupation (AOTA, 2020c). To authentically provide OT, the OTP continuously examines and expands skills in the therapeutic use of self and occupation to meet the clients' needs.

There is an expectation that all OTPs engage in continuing competence and professional development to meet the changing needs of clients and societies (AOTA, 2017). The WFOT supports the development of competency standards within all member countries (WFOT, 2012). In this chapter, the examples are drawn primarily from the United States; however, the concepts are likely to be applicable to other countries and cultures.

This chapter describes the process of moving from initial (entry-level) competencies to advanced skills through continuing competence and professional development. This process is self-directed and requires the practitioner to systematically examine current skills and abilities while anticipating future service demands. The process is applicable to all OTPs regardless of entry-level education.

Continuing Competence

The terms *continuing competence* and *competency* are not interchangeable. The term *competence* refers to the *capacity* to perform a task, function, or role and the performance meets or exceeds a prescribed standard (Institute for Credentialing Excellence [ICE], 2020). The term *continuing competence* reflects the "ongoing process of building ... capacity to perform a task, function, or role" (AOTA, 2021e).

Competency refers to the observed performance of a specified skill or ability measured against an expected performance (criterion) or outcome (AOTA, 2021e). The AOTA's Standards for Continuing Competence identify a need for every OTP to not only maintain the skills needed to competently practice but also develop skills needed for future demands. This process of engaging in continuing competence requires OTPs to enhance practice knowledge, professional reasoning, interpersonal abilities, performance skills, and ethical practice on an ongoing basis (AOTA, 2021e). The OTP seeks to provide service that is more effective by engaging in continuing competence activities and, through this process, moves from an entry-level practitioner to one with more advanced skills (Unsworth, 2001).

Entry-Level Competencies

The Accreditation Council for Occupational Therapy Education's (ACOTE) Standards, adopted in 2018, identify the entry-level expectations for OTPs at the associate, baccalaureate, master's, and doctoral degree levels of educational preparation in the United States (ACOTE, 2021). These entry-level competencies identify the performance expectations at each level of educational preparation. The entry-level competencies are directed toward delivery of OT services as a generalist and specify that an entry-level OTP is one who has less than 1 year of experience (Table 71.1).

TABLE 71.1	Differences in Occupational Therapists and Occupational Therapy Assistant (OTA) Standards of Practice—United States		
Occupational Therapy Process		**Occupational Therapist; Master's or Doctoral Degree**	**Occupational Therapy Assistant; Associate or Baccalaureate degree**
Education, Examination, and Licensure Requirements			
1. Graduated from an OT program accredited by ACOTE		x	x
2. Successfully completed a period of supervised fieldwork		Master's: 24 weeks Doctoral: 24 weeks fieldwork and 14 weeks doctoral capstone experience	16 weeks
3. Passed nationally recognized entry-level examination for occupational therapist		x	x
4. Fulfills state requirements for licensure, certification, or registration		x	x
Professional Standing and Responsibility			
1. Delivers OT services that reflect the philosophical base of OT and are consistent with the established principles and concepts of theory and practice (OTPF-4; AOTA, 2020c)		x	x
2. Knowledgeable about and delivers OT services in accordance with AOTA's standards, policies, and guidelines and state, federal, and other regulatory and payer requirements relevant to practice and service delivery		x	x

| TABLE 71.1 | Differences in Occupational Therapists and Occupational Therapy Assistant (OTA) Standards of Practice—United States (*continued*) |

Occupational Therapy Process	Occupational Therapist; Master's or Doctoral Degree	Occupational Therapy Assistant; Associate or Baccalaureate degree
3. Maintains current licensure, registration, credentialing, or certification as required by law or regulation	x	x
4. Abides by the Occupational Therapy Code of Ethics (AOTA, 2020a)	x	x
5. Abides by the Standards for Continuing Competence (AOTA, 2021e) by establishing, maintaining, and updating professional performance, knowledge, and skills	x	x
6. Responsible for all aspects of OT service delivery and is accountable for the safety and effectiveness of the OT service delivery process	x	
7. Responsible for providing safe and effective OT services under the supervision of and in partnership with the occupational therapist and in accordance with laws or regulations and AOTA documents		x
8. Maintains current knowledge of legislative, political, social, cultural, societal, and reimbursement issues that affect clients and the practice of OT	x	x
9. Knowledgeable about evidence-based research and applies it ethically and appropriately to provide OT services consistent with best practice approaches	x	x—service implementation
10. An occupational therapist uses professional and clinical reasoning to evaluate, analyze, and diagnose occupational challenges and provide occupation-based interventions (ACOTE, 2018; AOTA, 2020c, 2021a).	x	NOTE: An OTA uses occupation-based interventions to address client factors, performance patterns, and performance skills (ACOTE, 2018; AOTA, 2020c 2021a).
11. An OTP obtains the client's consent before and throughout the OT process.	x	x
12. An OTP is an effective advocate for the client's intervention and accommodation needs.	x	x
13. An OTP is an integral member of the interprofessional collaborative team and works to ensure the client-centeredness of the service delivery process.	x	x
14. An OTP provides client-centered services and demonstrates cultural humility, recognizes gaps in cultural knowledge and maintains a constant process of learning, understands differentiations between and within cultures, acknowledges implicit and explicit bias, and recognizes power dynamics in the delivery of services (Agner, 2020; AOTA, 2020d).	x	x
Service Delivery		
1. An OTP provides skilled OT services through a direct service delivery approach when interventions are completed in direct contact with clients and families during in-person meetings, group sessions, and telehealth and mHealth interactions (AOTA, 2020c, 2021a).	x	x
2. An OTP may provide skilled OT services through an indirect service delivery approach. Such services include consultation to entities such as teachers and school systems, participation on multidisciplinary teams and community planning agencies, and advocacy on behalf of their clients (AOTA, 2020c).	x	x

(continued)

TABLE 71.1	Differences in Occupational Therapists and Occupational Therapy Assistant (OTA) Standards of Practice—United States (*continued*)		
Occupational Therapy Process		Occupational Therapist; Master's or Doctoral Degree	Occupational Therapy Assistant; Associate or Baccalaureate degree
Service Delivery			
3. An OTP is responsible for ensuring client safety throughout the OT process and service delivery.		x	x
4. An OTP is responsible for the continual evaluation of the effectiveness of OT processes and service delivery within the practice setting.		x	x
Screening, Evaluation, and Reevaluation			
1. Responsible for all aspects of the screening, evaluation, and reevaluation process		x	
2. Accepts and responds to referrals in compliance with state laws or other regulatory requirements		x	
3. In collaboration with the client, evaluates the client's ability to participate in daily life activities by considering the client's capacities, the activities, and the environments in which these activities occur		x	
4. Initiates and directs the screening, evaluation, and reevaluation process and analyzes, interprets, and synthesizes the data in accordance with federal and state laws, other regulatory and payer requirements, and AOTA official documents and determines what assessments can be delegated to the OTA (AOTA, 2020b)		x	NOTE: An OTA may contribute to the screening, evaluation, and reevaluation process in accordance with federal and state laws, other regulatory and payer requirements, and AOTA official documents.
5. Uses evidence-based, standardized, and/or structured assessment tools and protocols and conducts needs assessments during the screening, evaluation, and reevaluation process (AOTA, 2018a)		x	x
6. Completes, documents, and synthesizes the results of the OT evaluation. An OTP abides by the time frames, formats, and standards established by practice settings, federal and state laws, other regulatory and payer requirements, external accreditation programs, and AOTA official documents.		x	NOTE: An OTA may contribute to the documentation of evaluation results.
7. Communicates screening, evaluation, and reevaluation results within the boundaries of client confidentiality and privacy regulations		x	x
8. Recommends additional consultations or refers clients to appropriate resources when the needs of the client can best be served by the expertise of other		x	
9. Educates current and potential referral sources about the scope of OT services and the process of initiating OT		x	x
Intervention			
1. Has overall responsibility for the development, documentation, and implementation of the OT intervention based on the evaluation, client goals, current best evidence, and clinical reasoning; delegates intervention to the OTA as appropriate with supervision		x	
2. Ensures that the intervention plan is documented within the time frames, formats, and standards established by the practice settings, agencies, external accreditation programs, state and federal laws, and other regulatory and payer requirements		x	Contributes as delegated by occupational therapist
3. Collaborates with the client to develop and implement the intervention plan to facilitate engagement in occupation on the basis of the client's needs and priorities, safety issues, and relative benefits and potential harms of the intervention and service delivery		x	x

TABLE 71.1	Differences in Occupational Therapists and Occupational Therapy Assistant (OTA) Standards of Practice—United States (*continued*)		
Occupational Therapy Process		**Occupational Therapist; Master's or Doctoral Degree**	**Occupational Therapy Assistant; Associate or Baccalaureate degree**
Intervention			
4.	Coordinates the development and implementation of the OT plan of care with the intervention provided by other professionals when appropriate	x	x
5.	Uses professional and clinical reasoning, best available evidence, and therapeutic use of self to select and implement the most appropriate types of interventions. Types of interventions implemented may include occupations and activities, interventions to support occupations, education and training, advocacy, group interventions, and virtual interventions (AOTA, 2020c). All interventions are used to facilitate engagement in occupation.	x	x
6.	Selects, implements, and makes modifications to OT interventions consistent with demonstrated competence levels, client goals, and the requirements of the practice setting, including payment source requirements (AOTA, 2020b)	x	In collaboration with the occupational therapist
7.	Modifies the intervention plan throughout the intervention process and documents changes in the client's needs, goals, and performance	x	NOTE: An OTA contributes to the modification of the intervention plan by exchanging information with and providing documentation to the occupational therapist about the client's responses to and communications throughout the intervention.
8.	Documents the OT services provided within the time frames, formats, and standards established by the practice settings, agencies, external accreditation programs, federal and state laws, other regulatory and payer requirements, and AOTA official documents (AOTA, 2018a)	x	x
Outcomes, Transition, and Discontinuation			
1.	Responsible for determining outcomes of the OT intervention and selecting appropriate outcome measures to identify the client's ability to engage in their desired occupations	x	
2.	Responsible for implementing and interpreting outcome measures and documenting progress toward occupational performance, engagement, and participation	x	Responsible for implementing delegated outcome measures and reporting results to the occupational therapist
3.	Responsible for documenting changes in the client's performance and capacities and for transitioning the client to another type or intensity of service or discontinuing services when the client has achieved identified goals, reached maximum benefit, or does not desire to continue services	x	
4.	Prepares and implements a safe and effective transition or discontinuation plan based on the outcomes of the intervention and the client's needs, goals, performance, and appropriate follow-up resources	x	Contributes to the transition or discontinuation plan by providing information and documentation to the occupational therapist related to the client's progress toward goals, needs, performance, and appropriate follow-up resources

(continued)

TABLE 71.1	Differences in Occupational Therapists and Occupational Therapy Assistant (OTA) Standards of Practice—United States (*continued*)		
Occupational Therapy Process		Occupational Therapist; Master's or Doctoral Degree	Occupational Therapy Assistant; Associate or Baccalaureate degree
Outcomes, Transition, and Discontinuation			
5. Facilitates the transition or discontinuation process in collaboration with the client, family members, significant others, other professionals (e.g., medical, educational, social services), and community resources, when appropriate		x	x
6. Ethically reports outcomes to payers and referring entities as well as to relevant local, regional, and national databases and registries, when appropriate		x	x

ACOTE, Accreditation Council for Occupational Therapy Education; AOTA, American Occupational Therapy Association; OT, occupational therapy; OTP, occupational therapy practitioner.

NOTE: *Occupational therapy practitioner (OTP) includes the occupational therapist and OTA ACOTE, Accreditation Council for Occupational Therapy Education.*

Source: Adapted from American Occupational Therapy Association. (2021f). Occupational therapy scope of practice. *American Journal of Occupational Therapy, 75*(suppl. 3), 7513410030. https://doi.org/10.5014/ajot.2021.75S3005

Although the ACOTE's Standards and Interpretive Guide differentiates entry-level competencies for OTPs by the level of educational preparation (ACOTE, 2021), there are similarities noted. Foundational skills such as knowledge of the biologic, social, and behavioral sciences are expected for all practitioners, as are the basic tenets of the profession. The depth and application of this knowledge differs across the educational levels. These are the entry-level skills to practice as an OT generalist at the designated practitioner level (occupational therapy assistant [OTA] or occupational therapist). The minimum standards of practice for OT delineate the occupational therapist and OTA roles and provide a starting point as the individual enters the field of practice (ACOTE, 2021; AOTA, 2020b). See Chapter 74, for more information on these roles. So how does the OTP advance skills and how would an OTP, at all levels of educational preparation, engage in continuing competence and professional development?

Continuing Professional Development

OT practice is constantly changing in response to new evidence, advancements in technology, health policy modifications, institutional changes, novel diseases and disorders, and emerging areas of practice that create new employment options and practice needs. As a result, advancing practice skills is not a matter of longevity in a specific job or position but a process of engaging in self-directed professional knowledge and skills gap assessments that lead to the acquisition of knowledge and skills through the use of professional development activities, products, and resources

(AOTA, 2017). In addition, practitioners may seek new employment opportunities necessitating new knowledge to meet job expectations, practice setting, or both. Clients, employers, third-party reimbursement resources, licensure boards, accreditation agencies, and society, in general, expect occupational therapists and OTAs to proactively anticipate and meet changes in practice by maintaining and upgrading their skills and abilities to deliver effective OT services.

Meeting these expectations can be challenging for several reasons (Moyers, 2009, p. 241):

- The skills and abilities of all practitioners fade with lack of practice, feedback, or administrative/systems support.
- The rapid expansion of information makes it challenging to systematically focus on learning and upgrading practice knowledge and skills.
- Significant sophistication is required to translate new knowledge into practice that meets the client-centered and culturally appropriate services.
- The pressure from complex healthcare and social systems creates barriers to practice enhancements.
- Rapid shifts in health policy and third-party reimbursement processes modify intervention delivery and outcome expectations.

The AOTA provides a guide with a five-step process to support OTPs as they engage in continuing professional development (CPD; AOTA, 2017).

Step 1: Reflect

First, the practitioner reflects on current service delivery demands with anticipated advancements and/or pressures that impact practice. This first step is not only an externally driven process but also includes intrinsic motivation and personal goals.

Step 2: Assess Practice

The next step in the process is assessing professional development in terms of the AOTA's Standards for Continuing Competence (AOTA, 2021e). These standards identify the components to address during this step and include the practitioner's *knowledge* related to current and anticipated future demands. For example, an OTA and an occupational therapist are practicing in a school system. The school system is considering the use of new technology to enhance student learning. Both levels of OTPs would need to be able to use the technology effectively to support student access. *Professional reasoning skills*, another standard for continuing competence, would need to be assessed as the practitioner considers how new evidence can be incorporated into current practice and what decisions need to be made to upgrade practice skills. *Interpersonal skills* are critical in the process of assessing practice and require the practitioner to consider the relationships and communications with others. For example, a hospital is providing a new oncology service to support clients in their homes. An occupational therapist, who developed relationships within the hospital, could advocate for OT services to be included to support clients. *Performance skills* are the standards that address the OTP's therapeutic use of self, client-centered occupations and activities, consultation, and education as part of service delivery (ACOTE, 2021; AOTA, 2021e). An example is seen with the arena of telehealth and access to service. An OTP, working in early intervention in a rural area, plans to provide services using telehealth (Kronberg et al., 2021). The practitioner would need to acquire the performance skills to competently deliver OT services using this model (Fitzgerald et al., 2015; Moyers & Metzler, 2014). The final standard is that of *ethical practice* and refers to the application of ethical principles and adherence to the OT's Code of Ethics (AOTA, 2020a). In examining one's practice, these standards are used and combined with feedback obtained from performance reviews, self-assessment tools, and consumer ratings.

Step 3: Develop the Continuing Professional Development Plan

Developing the plan is the third step in the process and includes setting measurable goals with strategies to meet these goals. This includes reflecting on learning styles and abilities (Fitzgerald et al., 2015; Haywood et al., 2012). These goals should provide incremental steps to be successfully implemented along with a completion date.

Step 4: Implement the Plan

The fourth step includes selecting opportunities that will best fit the goals. For example, an OTP plans to pursue the AOTA's Professional Certificate in Home Modifications and Fall Prevention to meet a personal goal and better serve clients to safely remain in their home. To meet this goal, the practitioner selects a variety of strategies such as online educational courses, in-person workshops with the opportunity to practice new techniques, and engaging in a mentorship relationship with another practitioner who holds a current AOTA's Professional Certificate in Home Modifications and Fall Prevention.

Step 5: Document Effectiveness of the Continuing Professional Development Plan

The final step considers the completion of the plan in terms of client outcomes, external expectations, and personal satisfaction. The benefits of using a systematic plan can be seen in the trajectory of professional growth (Haywood et al., 2012; Roessger, 2015). If the plan has brought about improved client outcomes, greater job satisfaction in performance, and better service delivery, the plan would be considered a success. Often, a plan reveals a pattern of strengths and weaknesses. As the OTP evaluates the effectiveness of the plan, the practitioner may need to return to the first step of engaging in reflection and consider why the client outcomes improved but personal job satisfaction did not substantially change. This may be the impetus to initiate a new plan.

What Does It Mean to Be Competent?

The term *competent* refers to the knowledge, skills, and ability to practice as an OTP. This does not only refer to entry-level competence but also refer to practitioners as they shift areas of practice. For example, an occupational therapist practicing in an acute care hospital setting accepts a new position in a skilled nursing facility. A majority of the clients in this setting have unique sensory needs because of vision and hearing loss. The occupational therapist has the foundational skills to practice but needs to expand knowledge and practice skills to competently work with clients who have vision and hearing compromises (Wittich et al., 2017). Competency is the *actual performance* of competence; an example of competency would be an OTP fabricating a specific hand orthosis (splint) using the correct materials and accurately fitting the orthosis to the client's hand. The OTP demonstrates competent splinting skills with this action (competency). **Competence** is the result of combining one's knowledge base, current practice skills, and abilities along with client outcomes and comparing your competence with a specific criterion such as using evidence-based practice on a consistent basis. Substantiating competence implies internal self-determination coupled with external validation regarding one's effectiveness in performing certain skills or behaviors. Although practice guidelines are available for specific arenas of services, this poses a problem for emerging practice areas (Knightbridge, 2014). For emerging practice areas, the OTP will have far fewer external benchmarks to use as a comparison between current performance and desired performance skills. This will require a greater degree of reflection on professional behaviors and further development of professional reasoning skills (Unsworth & Baker, 2016).

Ensuring competence and practicing competently is a dynamic and evolving process requiring lifelong learning. Determining the currency of one's competence requires self-evaluation of existing abilities according to criteria such as completing a self-development tool, a periodic peer review, a knowledge examination, a refresher course offered by the employer, or even recalibrating oneself against published standardized procedures for an assessment tool or meeting continuing education (CE) requirements for licensing or certification. Also, one may seek out professional development opportunities to identify and enhance a skill set to ensure implementation of contemporary approaches during practice, particularly using current evidence in practice. Common approaches include pursuing post-professional education or workshops, reading scholarly publications and/or evidence-based practice briefs, securing additional certifications, participating in local special interest practitioner groups, or attending focused in-service or conference presentations. Participation in these activities provides several benefits such as validation of current practice skills, acquisition of advanced knowledge and practice skills, and opportunities for further inquiry in the selected topic.

AOTA and the Choosing Wisely Campaign

As of 2017, AOTA joined the Choosing Wisely Campaign initiated by the American Board of Internal Medicine (ABIM) in 2012 (Gillen et al., 2017). The impetus for this campaign was to foster meaningful conversations between practitioners and clients in the selection and implementation of services. Overuse of medical procedures has substantially increased healthcare spending and generated concern (Morgan et al., 2016). A systematic review of medical literature found overuse of medications, advanced technological treatments and tests, and that clinicians were slow

to discontinue use of these options when evidence identified approaches that were more effective. The AOTA joined this campaign as a member-driven organization to improve communication among OTPs, clients, consumers, and other service providers. The purpose of joining this effort is specifically to improve communication to implement the most effective OT service, not as a guide for reimbursement (Gillen et al., 2017). Services provided should be evidence-based, not duplicate other services, be free from harm, and be truly necessary (Gillen et al., 2019). The Choosing Wisely Campaign surveyed members to identify the top five practices that should be question by OTPs and clients. The member survey identified (a) providing nonpurposeful activities as part of OT services, (b) sensory-based interventions that are not based on systematic assessment results, (c) use of physical agent modalities without purposeful activities, (d) use of pulleys for clients with a hemiplegic shoulder, and (e) cognitive-based interventions that are not directly related to occupational performance (Gillen et al., 2019). As an OTP, providing authentic OT services necessitates use of occupation- and evidence-based practices to foster occupational engagement and performance of clients. An example of authentic OT services can be seen when an OTP works on vocational skills (e.g., interviewing skills, applying for positions using online applications) with a formerly incarcerated client, who now lives in a homeless shelter.

Costs of Ineffective Practice

Competent service delivery is a core professional value and is essential when providing effective healthcare services to clients (AOTA, 2021a). The consequences of providing ineffective OT service harm not only the client/consumer but also the profession. All stakeholders, including the clients, their family, employers, payers, and social service agencies, expect at least minimally effective practice, and for the most part, the use of best practices grounded in evidence that suggests the intervention selected will lead to desired outcomes. This requires the OTP to systematically monitor advances in practice and upgrade skills to provide effective service. Examples can be seen when new evidence reports an effective method of functional retraining for individuals who sustained a stroke, or an investigation identifies better outcomes using an intervention for individuals who have autism compared to current interventions. Professional ethics and accountability requires the practitioner to be aware of such innovations and engage in continuing competence and professional development on an ongoing basis. Not knowing about new evidence or seeking relevant training for practice approaches supported by evidence represents unethical and neglectful practice and may lead to charges of malpractice. Waiting for external funding from employers or others to be educated is not sufficient. An ethical, responsible OTP needs to proactively advocate for and complete continuing competence activities to ensure the provision of best practice in the delivery of OT services. Self-funding is a clear option to enhance one's professional responsibility to prevent neglect or harm, which includes delivering the most effective intervention available.

Evidence-Based Practice

Evidence-based practice has been adopted by the profession of OT for several decades and was a clear directive for OTPs in Dr. Holm's 2000 Eleanor Clarke Slagle address (Holm, 2000). The foundation of evidence-based practice combines clinical expertise, client input with the best current evidence to direct decisions regarding client services (Holm, 2000; Sackett et al., 1996). This requires all OTPs to carefully and consistently examine available evidence with an understanding of current and future client needs. With the expansion of available information, this can appear to be a daunting task, but a systematic approach can offer guidance in examining available evidence. The process may begin with a review and discussion of a specific publication related to the area of practice and expands into a journal club where articles are selected and reviewed periodically (Davis, 2014). The AOTA Website provides evidence-based practice resources to support OTPs (AOTA, 2021d). Further examination of the topic may result in the OTPs generating a critically appraised topic (CAT) that can be shared with other OTPs to advance the professional use of evidence. The AOTA provides a CAT Website with topics

aligned with clients' occupational needs, practice settings, and intervention approaches. These can serve as an avenue to enhance the continuing competence of the OTP and affords an opportunity to share expertise with other practitioners. Refer to Chapter 26, for an in-depth discussion of evidence-based practice.

Professional Development and Resources in the United States

The continuing competency journey begins with becoming familiar with external guides and resources. These resources and guides are often developed by organizations and agencies committed to ensuring a work force well equipped to provide quality OT services. Professional organizations, certification agencies, institutional accreditation programs, and state regulatory groups each play a unique and pivotal role in defining and applying standards related to competence and continuing competence. For OTPs in the United States, the primary ones are AOTA, state professional organizations supporting OT, National Board for Certification in Occupational Therapy (NBCOT), governmental programs, state regulatory agencies, and institutional accreditation bodies. Each of these previous mentioned groups has a unique mission and purpose and, as a result, a healthy tension exists that supports quality service delivery, promotes the profession, honors all the stakeholders, and protects professional domains of concerns. The focus of these groups varies as can be seen in Table 71.2.

TABLE 71.2 **Organizations and Focus Related to Continuing Professional Development in Occupational Therapy**

Name	American Occupational Therapy Association (AOTA; State Professional Associations)	National Board for Certification in Occupational Therapy (NBCOT)	State Regulatory Agencies	Institutional Accreditation Bodies
Website	AOTA, http://www.aota.org (state associations parallel)	NBCOT, http://www.nbcot.org	Check each state's government site.	Example: The Joint Commission
Purpose	Support the profession by setting standards to assure high-quality services; represent the interests and concerns of OT practitioners, students, and educational programs to the public and to policy groups; improve consumer access to healthcare services; and promote the professional development of members	Initial certification of OT practitioners; develop, administer, and continually review a certification process based on current and valid standards that provide reliable indicators of competence for the practice of OT	Oversee implementation of laws or statutes enacted by legislators who are elected public officials; regulations specifically describe how the intent of the laws will be carried out	Quality assurance; indicate service provider's commitment to continually improve services, encourage feedback, and serve the community

(continued)

TABLE 71.2	Organizations and Focus Related to Continuing Professional Development in Occupational Therapy (*continued*)			
Name	American Occupational Therapy Association (AOTA; State Professional Associations)	National Board for Certification in Occupational Therapy (NBCOT)	State Regulatory Agencies	Institutional Accreditation Bodies
Oversight responsibilities	Profession, member-driven	Certificants (initial) and those who voluntarily recertify after initial certification	State government regulators who are appointed public officials of various departments or boards in state government to enact state law	Nonprofit agencies offering accreditation to institutions
Responsible to	Profession, members of the association	Consumers of practice or intervention	Citizens of the state	Consumers of services
OT practitioner input	Occupational therapist and OTA members elect key leaders and representatives who make decisions. Appointed or elected volunteer committees make recommendations to decision-makers.	OTR® and COTA® representatives along with public representatives appointed by the governing board	Government-appointed board members oversee regulations (writing and ensuring implementation). Occupational therapists can be appointed to a board.	Experts invited by agency to set standards and accredit institutions *Standards developed independently but seek input from related professions*
Professional development	Provides standards and guidelines for practice, self-assessment tools, profession-focused continuing education, and advanced board and specialty certification processes	Certification renewal requires acquisition of professional development unit, self-assessment tools, and verification documents.	Requirements for continuing education established by each state	Standards related to continuing competency promote institutional supports.
Value	Supports occupational therapist and OTA members by promoting the profession, educating the public, and advancing the profession	Public, regulatory groups, and employers by providing certification examination, verification of credentials, disciplinary actions, and oversight of ongoing general professional certification	Public health and welfare	Public health and welfare, including third parties who provide service reimbursement

COTA®, certified occupational therapy assistant; OTA, occupational therapy assistant; OTR®, certified (registered) occupational therapist.

The promotion of the profession comes from each of these organizations being well established to oversee and promote valuable change in practice in response to challenges and opportunities. Engaging in continuing competency is complex and multifactorial endeavor. Thus, it benefits practitioners to have several resources to guide and/or support professional development in OT.

The AOTA is committed to ensuring quality service delivery and has several resources that are useful: "AOTA's Standards for Continuing Competence" (AOTA, 2021e) and the "AOTA's Standards of Practice for Occupational Therapy" (AOTA, 2021a). Together, these outline core performance expectations that oversee all practice. The *Standards for Continuing Competence* describes the process as multidimensional including the following standards to support the individual practitioner's roles and responsibilities:

- *Knowledge:* the process of acquiring, assessing, and appraising knowledge to meet multiple roles and responsibilities
- *Professional reasoning:* used to make sound judgments and decisions requiring reflection on one's own practice
- *Interpersonal skills:* developed and maintained for professional relationships and communication

- *Performance skills:* demonstrates the ability to enhance or enable occupational participation and competently provide OT services using a client-centered approach that is inclusive
- *Ethical practice:* responding responsibly to ethical issues and dilemmas in the changing context of roles and responsibilities

In addition, AOTA publishes various practice guidelines and related documents that are specific to practice with specific populations, conditions, and/or contexts. The AOTA's (2003) *Professional Development Tool* provides a process for self-assessing professional development interests and needs and then presents a guide for planning. The AOTA also provides a CE Recording Form (https://www.aota.org/~/media/Corporate/Files/EducationCareers/CE/CE-Recording-Form.pdf) that fosters the application of new knowledge to practice. The recording form is more than a simple log of attendance. This form prompts the OTP to consider the application of the new knowledge to practice with a prompt to return to the form to reflect on the changes in practice upon using this form (Schultz-Krohn et al., 2017). This AOTA CE Recording Form can be used in conjunction with a larger professional development plan as the form includes sections for the OTP to decide on next steps and future pursuits.

An OTP may want to pursue advanced certification such as the AOTA's Advanced Certifications and Professional Credentials. These certifications are focused on continuing competence and quality service delivery in advanced or specialty practice areas that exceed the profession's core expectations. To complete these AOTA programs, the applicant engages in self-assessment, a systematic program to increase skills, as well as successful completion of objective assessment to examine knowledge.

State professional associations, similar to AOTA, provide opportunities for the OTP to engage in continuing competence through education. Additionally, state licensing boards may have additional credentialing programs. The state professional associations are designed to serve specific state interests, particularly desired by the state government agencies or programs. The goal of state professional associations is to represent and advocate for practice opportunities and challenges at the state level, where many states require some form of continuing competence engagement. State associations also closely monitor and even provide suggestions regarding the state regulations on continuing competency. The AOTA provides a list of licensure requirements for occupational therapist and OTA in each state (https://www.aota.org/Advocacy-Policy/State-Policy/Licensure/StateRegs.aspx).

Some form of *government-based state regulation of practice* is present in the United States in all 50 states plus the District of Columbia, Puerto Rico, and Guam for OTPs in some capacity. The major purpose of regulation is to protect consumers in a state or jurisdiction from unqualified or unscrupulous practitioners (AOTA, 2021b, 2021c). State laws and regulations significantly affect the practice of OT. Over 90% of the states have a continuing competency or education requirements for renewal of a license (AOTA, 2020f). These requirements may be in terms of submitting evidence of continuing education units (CEUs) or professional development units (PDUs) (Box 71.1).

The NBCOT (https://www.nbcot.org/Certificants/Certification) administers the initial certification examination for occupational therapists and OTAs, which, when successfully passed, allows the applicant use of the occupational therapist, registered (OTR*) or certified OTA (COTA*) credential. The "NBCOT also serves the public interest by developing, administering, and continually reviewing a

BOX 71.1 WHAT IS A CONTINUING EDUCATION UNIT?

The award of a continuing education units (CEUs) is often dependent on the number of hours of instruction, where 10 hours of formal instruction equals 1 CEU. Courses can be approved for CEUs through the International Association for Continuing Education and Training (IACET), but CEUs can also be obtained by completing post-professional academic coursework offered by an accredited institution. Professional development units (PDUs) can include a wider variety of activities such as engagement in journal clubs, involvement in a mentee/mentor relationship with specific objectives, or by attending post-professional workshops or seminars. The AOTA provides a voluntary, approved continuing education (CE) provider screening and designating process called the AOTA's Approved Provider Program

(APP) that aligns with the professional association's mission. Generally, 1 CEU equals 10 PDUs. The decision to select the CEU or PDU activity is based on several variables, including professional goals, client needs, emerging practice demands, and workplace expectations, along with the costs of engaging in these continuing competence activities. Engaging in self-assessment and then searching for literature in rigorous journals is a frequent method of professional development by OT practitioners (Coffelt & Gabriel, 2017). The use of journal clubs and literature search to support professional development may be accepted for state licensure purposes (AOTA, 2021b, 2021c); however, the types and amount of qualified professional development activities vary among states.

certification process that reflects current standards of competent practice in occupational therapy" (NBCOT, 2021a, 2021b). The professional development requirement for NBCOT recertification asks the OTP to demonstrate continuing competency to the public, be it consumers, employers, agencies, and so on. To retain use of the OTR* or COTA* professional certification designations, one must apply for certification renewal every 3 years and be able to present documentation regarding continuing competency activities. One of the goals regarding recertification is to engage OTPs at all levels of experience in self-reflective assessment of one's current levels of proficiency or efficacy leading to ongoing, role-related engagement in continuing competency activities. Certification renewal requires assembling documentation of continuing competence activities called PDUs. In addition, the NBCOT provides self-assessment tools to self-identify professional developmental needs in the highest frequency practice areas for the OTR and COTA (NBCOT 2021a, 2021b).

OT Story 71.1 provides an illustration of creating and implementing a professional development plan for an occupational therapist.

Factors Motivating Continuing Competence

The process of engaging in continuing competence is dynamic with multiple factors influencing decisions (Moyers, 2009). The new OTP may have specific goals to accomplish within the first few years of practice. The transition from student to OTP requires both time and systematic planning to gain the skills needed to be proficient in the practice area (Fitzgerald et al., 2015; Wallingford et al., 2016). This process requires the OTP to consider the knowledge necessary to provide service within the specific setting, the critical reasoning needed to select the best intervention for clients, and the skills to ethically implement these services (AOTA, 2021a, 2020a). Additionally, interactions with others involved with the client requires a clear understanding of the role of OT. Consider the varied factors presented in OT Story 71.1, in which Sienna, as a new OTP, is seeking guidance and support from coworkers, whereas Luis is interested in expanding the fieldwork program and Sarah is pursuing a Professional Certificate as a means to recognize her expertise and guide her further development as a school-based OTA. Factors motivating continuing competence can be viewed along a continuum from self-determined to primarily external factors. Practitioners often have specific professional interests, and with experience and professional self-reflection, they identify their particular therapy talents. These internal motivations may also be influenced by their desire to provide more expert care for specific groups of clients. In addition to these personal motivations, external requirements from employers,

regulators, and accreditation agencies provide external pressure to gain skills. All of these factors may influence practitioner's choices to engage in continuing competence programs, obtain advanced certification or credentials, seek additional knowledge to support evidence-based practice, or add new skills to meet new or expanding job responsibilities.

Regardless of the motivating factors, engagement in thoughtful, continuous professional development processes is essential for all OTPs (AOTA, 2017; Coffelt & Gabriel, 2017; Schultz-Krohn et al., 2017). A practitioner must also critically evaluate who determines competence when implementing a continuous, goal-directed professional development plan that is not only individually relevant but also ethically reflects external practice demands.

Who Determines Whether Someone Is Competent?

Competent practice is the expectation and responsibility of every OTP (AOTA, 2021a, 2021e; Coffelt & Gabriel, 2017; Fitzgerald et al., 2015). In addition, the profession and public use credentials as indicators that the OTP has met minimal standards to provide safe, quality practice. The most common approaches to determining competency are entry-level education expectations, testing, credentialing, and requiring position-related CE (Coffelt & Gabriel, 2017; Fitzgerald et al., 2015; Moyers, 2009; Wallingford et al., 2016). Graduation from an accredited educational program, meeting licensure requirements from state or government agencies, and/or professional certification is presumed to protect the public from incompetent practitioners. Both entry-level OTPs and those practitioners with several years of experience report consistent expectation when asked about the importance of entry-level competence (Wallingford et al., 2016).

State regulatory authorities and NBCOT protect the public by providing practice credentials to qualified individuals. This is referred to as credentialing. In the United States, initial credentialing is met by graduating from an ACOTE-accredited academic program, completing the required fieldwork experience and then successfully passing the NBCOT examination. State credentialing involves licensure to practice and may require additional documentation from the applicant. Both state regulatory boards and the NBCOT grant credentials to practitioners who meet the required standards, and they also remove credentials from individuals if the practitioner is either not able or unwilling to act according to established standards. This information is of particular interest to current or future employers. On finding significant misconduct or malpractice, practice credentials can be removed, reprimanded, or censored. Most states have licensure portals that readily identify the current state-credentialed practitioners.

Sienna, who uses the pronouns she, her/s, is an entry-level occupational therapist and accepted her first position in a school district. The current OT services consist of a full-time occupational therapist (Luis) and a full-time OTA (Sarah). Luis has been at the school district for 6 years and Sarah, the OTA, has been with the district for 7 years. Sienna is replacing an occupational therapist who recently resigned to pursue another job opportunity. Sienna completed a Fieldwork (FW) Level II 3-month placement at a public school and has reviewed the laws and regulations related to school-based practice.

Both Luis and Sarah are active in the state OT association and participate in a journal club with other school-based OTPs. Additionally, Luis recently contacted a local university with an OT program to provide FW Level I experiences at the school. The FW Level I program would provide an OT student 40 hours of experience as part of the academic program during the semester. Luis established an FW Level II program with that same university and typically provides one FW Level II 3-month experience per school year. Sienna knows that with less than 1 year of experience, she would not be able to supervise an FW Level II OT student but is interested in participating in the FW Level I program. Sienna examines her knowledge base regarding expectations and support she could offer in the FW Level I program. As a newly hired employee of the school district, she had to complete several training modules regarding the federal law, Individuals with Disabilities Education Act (IDEA). She also needed to complete training modules addressing the Family Educational Rights and Privacy Act (FERPA), Every Student Succeeds Act, and the Americans with Disabilities Act (ADA). Sienna asks Luis if she could help with the FW Level I program by providing a brief orientation to the students regarding the laws guiding school-based OT practice. Luis and Sienna collaborate on the development of the program including the orientation of the FW Level I students and the selection of teachers and classrooms where the OT student could complete the FW Level I requirements. Sienna's initial step of self-assessment and consideration of how she could become involved in the FW Level I program represents the basic start of a professional development plan.

Sienna was excited to participate in the FW Level I program with Luis. The collaborative interactions provided the support for Sienna to begin the process of developing a systematic professional development plan. She discussed her short- and long-term goals with Luis and Sarah during the next OT staff meeting. Sienna identified a goal of obtaining her AOTA Fieldwork Educator Certificate by completing the program outlined by AOTA. Sarah suggested reaching out to the journal club hosted by the OT state association, to see if other members were interested in pursuing the Fieldwork Educator Certification program. Sarah, the OTA at the school, was in the journal club and was examining information related to fostering social interaction skills for students with mental health issues such as anxiety and autism. Another occupational therapist in the journal club, Ahmed, was working on the requirements to obtain an AOTA Professional Certificate in Participation, Resilience, and Wellness. Ahmed and Sarah exchanged various articles to address social participation within the school system with a particular interest in fostering resilience for older students in preparation for their transition to the community. Luis previously completed the process to be Board Certified in Pediatrics (BCP) through AOTA and was mentoring Sarah and Ahmed with a focus on supports needed for students transitioning from the public school to the community. This collaborative mentoring supported Sarah and Ahmed to incorporate evidence into practice to meet specific student needs. Sienna was interested in incorporating this information into the FW Level 1 experience because there are fewer school-based occupational therapists working with older students to support transitions to the community.

Following the staff meeting, Sienna developed a plan with clear goals to work toward obtaining her Fieldwork Educators Certificate from AOTA and orienting students in the FW Level I program. She discussed that an additional goal would be to expand the FW Level II program that Luis started by connecting with other universities and potentially adding an OTA FW program at the school within 2 years. She knew that a substantial number of OTPs work in schools and many school systems faced difficulties in recruiting and retaining OTPs. Her professional interests seemed well aligned with supporting OT students to understand the role of the OTP in schools. Sienna used the suggestions provided by Luis and Sarah to identify the steps to take to reach these goals using the journal club, contact with the local OT program, and connecting with her previous professors to ask for guidance.

Sienna engaged in the process of professional development by creating a plan with systematic steps and clear outcomes. She developed a method to meet her goals that included several activities not only attending conferences but also engaging in additional professional development activities. She collaborated with other practitioners and sought their support and guidance as she moved toward her goal.

Questions

1. What improved client outcomes could Sienna identify as a result of her professional development plan?
2. What challenges might Sienna face in implementing her professional development plan?
3. What suggestions would you provide Sienna to diminish the impact of these challenges in completing her professional development plan?
4. What additional skills, supports, and resources would be needed to assist Sienna in completing her professional development plan?

Planning and Engaging in Continuing Professional Development

CPD refers to the process of engaging in "lifelong learning aimed at maintaining practice competence, ensuring client safety and quality outcomes, enhancing or expanding professional practice, and reaching career goals" (AOTA, 2017). This process is self-directed and requires a reflective process to establish goals and a plan to meet the goals. The OTP considers not only current skills but also skills needed to meet future client needs, anticipated roles, and educational activities suited to meet these goals (Dik et al., 2008; Haywood et al., 2012; McMahon et al., 2015). All professional development planning is based on continuous self-reflection and critical analysis regarding one's current practice competence and one's career aspirations coupled with sustained environmental scanning of practice standards and expectations.

Evaluating the quality of professional development opportunities is essential to develop a productive CPD plan (AOTA, 2017). The process is more than just acquiring specific skills or enhancing competence-related knowledge. The OTP seeks to improve critical and ethical reasoning processes and requisite interactional skills. Use of audio or video recording of the OTP's intervention session can be used for both experiential self-learning and during a mentor/mentee session. Consent should always be obtained when recording a session with a client. Numerous approaches and tools are available to implement a CPD plan. Literature reviews including critically appraised papers and CATs, journal clubs, and mentee/mentor relationship in addition to attending CE courses are only a few examples of professional development activities that can be used to reach a CPD goal. *Competence is continually enhancing "best practice" to achieve the highest potential or outcome for the client that is possible according to evidence and applied knowledge in the practice area.*

The outcomes of CPD are only as good as the quality of learning activities and the successful integration of the knowledge and skills into more competent practice (Coffelt & Gabriel, 2017). Selecting activities that best support the achievement of CPD goals is an important part of the CPD process. For example, gaining information about billing and documentation may be achieved through literature review, but learning a new intervention approach often requires guided practice and support from a mentor. Because competence is usually not achieved on the first attempt, repeated practice including systematic reflection on and comparing results to benchmark outcomes is expected. The following questions guide individual reflection on the results of competency-based learning:

- What are my outcomes in relation to predicted ones in using the new skill(s)?
- How can I improve effective, efficient evidence-based practice?
- When does the approach work best or worst?
- What are cues that I can use to move forward?
- When should I withhold using this approach when cues suggest difficulty or failure in achieving desired results?

Regardless of the educational program attended, learning will not be translated into practice without an opportunity to test and refine skills to guide future application (Coffelt & Gabriel, 2017; Doyle et al., 2019). Evidence found in systematic reviews indicates that workshops that mix interactive components with didactic information are better integrated into intervention processes than educational meetings that only have didactic components. Experiential learning activities such as case history reviews and simulated practice adapted to self-study can all be effective. Problem-based learning can be implemented through the use of study groups, conference calls, and networking through electronic systems. Assistance from a more expert practitioner can include mentoring and structured observation of your practice in which newly acquired skills are used (Doyle et al., 2019). The key in self-directed learning is to consider integrating any continuing competency into practice coupled with continuous feedback and reflection regarding practice results. See Expanding Our Perspectives.

EXPANDING OUR PERSPECTIVES

The Strong Advice Is to Keep Moving

María Agostina Ciampa

When I was first asked to write about this box, I started reviewing my professional path since I graduated in 2010, in Buenos Aires, Argentina. It is very common to feel a bit unprepared when we are about to begin delivering our services as occupational therapists. So, I thought it would be a good idea for me to work at a place where I could work within a team of occupational therapists, some with more experience and advanced skills who could supervise my work and I could learn with. I was lucky enough to find a position at a prestigious neurocognitive institute. I stayed there for almost 10 years.

I said I was lucky enough, but let me share with you I don't believe in luck. Instead, I prefer this definition: *"Luck is when preparation meets opportunity"* (attributed to Seneca). I am convinced that in order to promote our competence and professional development, we need to have opportunities, of course, and never take them for granted, but we also need to have resources that enable us to continue our competence and professional development.

One way to promote competence and professional development is to apply evidence-based practice (EBP) in those cases where the evidence is relevant not only to the population but also to the context and to the meaningful occupations implied. As the years go by, I'm more and more convinced that context sensitivity is a truly relevant and sensitive matter. It should be part of a competence, don't you think?

When I began working at this prestigious institution, I was searching for evidence that could support our practice almost every day. I must confess to you that the evidence I used back then to support my daily practice in a Latin-American context was mostly written in the Global North. I can tell that some were easily replicable, but

some others were not. Especially when I started using a person-centered approach and I understood that the people I was working with didn't want to be more independent in feeding but wanted to work, to make friends, and share their lives with a partner. I tried to apply the evidence that I was learning about, but I didn't reach the expected results, so I had to use my OT lens to understand all the variables that were impacting on that occupational injustice.

So the uncovered problem is: What can we do when we find that the available evidence is not enough? The answer is: Get out, and create your own.

I enrolled myself in postgraduate courses, in a PhD program, and here I am, walking this path. Sometimes, pursuing our competence and professional development is not like playing one general hopscotch, it is more about being open to look at our local needs and trying to find suitable answers. Enrolling in courses, entering postgraduate programs, reading and publishing in journals, attending and disserting at national and international congresses, writing books, designing postgraduates programs ourselves, and participating actively in professional associations are different blocks in our own personalized hopscotch. It's up to us where we'd like to throw the small stone, and where to go next. But the strong advice is to keep moving.

Advanced and Professional Certification

Specialization refers to becoming proficient in a particular practice area, diagnostic procedure or evaluation tool, or intervention approach (Moyers, 2009). The growing use of phrases such as advanced practice and *advanced practitioner* raises the issue of what is meant by the term *advanced*. Advanced practitioners possess a higher level of practice expertise resulting from engagement in theory-informed, evidence-based practice. In addition, expertise is developed and improved with proactively planned CPD with sustained focus on reflections, skill enhancement, applied ethics, and strategically planning a career. An example is seen in the area of providing OT services for those with compromised vision and hearing (Wittich et al., 2017) or driving rehabilitation services.

The AOTA provides *board certifications* of advance practice (for occupational therapists only) and *professional certifications* (for both occupational therapists and OTAs). The AOTA defines advanced practice as knowledge and skills regarding both the breadth and depth of a major practice area such as mental health, pediatrics, gerontology, and physical rehabilitation. In contrast, professional certification reflects expertise in a more precise or definitive intervention

skill area such as community mobility. Additional professional certifications are being developed by AOTA to meet the evolution of OT practice. Post-professional credentialing is available from other groups invested in being able to document and attest to specific practitioner competencies (see Table 71.3).

Changing Areas of Practice, Pursuing Emerging Areas, or Reentering the Field

Sometimes during one's career, the opportunity presents itself to take professional work in a new direction such as with changing practice focus, seeking a new emerging practice area, or reentering after a leave of absence from practicing. All these require professional development considerations. Changing practice areas requires careful analysis of specific theories and skills relevant to the new or emerging practice area, with attention to both prospective clients and the practice context. Further work is often necessary when practitioners have opted to leave practice and then return.

For a variety of reasons, an OTP may choose to leave the field for a period of time and then return. In these cases,

TABLE 71.3	Entry-Level (Initial) and Post–Entry-Level (Specialty) Certifications for Practice in the United States		
Credentials[a]		**Granting Organization**	
Entry-Level Credentialing and Certification Renewal			
OTR®	Occupational therapist, registered (professional level)	NBCOT	http://www.nbcot.org/
COTA®	Certified OT assistant (technical level)	NBCOT	http://www.nbcot.org/
AOTA Board Certification (Advanced Practice for Occupational Therapists Only)			
BCG	Board Certification in Gerontology	AOTA	https://www.aota.org/Education-Careers/Advance-Career/Board-Specialty-Certifications-Exam/recertification-requirements.aspx
BCP	Board Certification in Pediatrics	AOTA	https://www.aota.org/Education-Careers/Advance-Career/Board-Specialty-Certifications-Exam/recertification-requirements.aspx
BCPR	Board Certification in Physical Rehabilitation	AOTA	https://www.aota.org/Education-Careers/Advance-Career/Board-Specialty-Certifications-Exam/recertification-requirements.aspx
Other Specialty Certifications (Professional Level Varies)			
ATP	Assistive Technology Practitioner	RESNA	http://resna.org/
CCM	Certified Case Managers	CCMC	http://www.ccmcertification.org/
CDRS	Certified Driver Rehabilitation Specialist	ADED	http://www.driver-ed.org/
CHT	Certified Hand Therapist	HTCC	http://www.htcc.org/
CLVT	Certification in Low Vision Therapy	ACVREP	http://www.acvrep.org/
CPE	Certified Professional Ergonomist	BCPE	http://www.bcpe.org/
CPRP	Certified Psychiatric Rehabilitation Practitioner	PRA	https://www.psychrehabassociation.org/certification/cprp-certification
CVE	Certified Vocational Evaluation Specialist	CRCC	http://www.crccertification.com/
PC or CC	Professional Coach Certification	ICF	(PC) http://www.coachfederation.org/
MPC, CMC, or MMC	Masteries Practitioner Coach, Certified Masteries Coach, or Master Masteries Coach	IAC	(CC) https://certifiedcoach.org/about/
SMS	Seating and Mobility Specialist	RESNA	http://resna.org/certification/

[a]Note that credentialing starts with graduation from Accreditation Council for Occupational Therapy Education (ACOTE)–accredited educational program. ACVREP, Academy for Certification of Vision Rehabilitation & Education Professionals; ADED, Association for Driver Rehabilitation Specialists; AOTA, American Occupational Therapy Association: Board Certification; BCPE, Board of Certification in Professional Ergonomics; CCMC, Commission for Case Manager Certification; CRCC, Commission on Rehabilitation Counselor Certification; HTCC, Hand Therapy Certification Commission; IAC, International Association of Coaching; ICF, International Coach Federation; NBCOT, National Board for Certification in Occupational Therapy; RESNA, Rehabilitation Engineering and Assistive Technology Society of North America.

guidelines have been established to support the practitioner who has left OT practice for over 24 months and decides to return to provide OT services (AOTA, 2020e). These Guidelines for Reentry into the Field of Occupational Therapy identify basic expectations to return to practice as an OTP, but all state licensure and regulatory requirements must be met in addition to workplace requirements.

Reentering occupational therapists and OTAs are defined as individuals who previously practiced in the field of OT, who have not engaged in the practice of OT for a minimum of 24 months, and who wish to return to the profession in the capacity of delivering OT services to clients (AOTA, 2020e). Regardless of the reason for change, practitioners have the ethical accountability to ensure high standards of practice competency and skills. The AOTA's (2020e) "Guidelines for Reentry into the Field of Occupational Therapy" contain procedural recommendations to follow for returning to practice after an extended absence. These strategies can also be used and adapted when entering new areas of unfamiliar practice.

Professional Sustainability: Mapping and Documenting

Sustainability is the capacity to persist. For OTPs, engagement in CPD is sustainability. Responsible, systematic advancement of knowledge and skills enables the OTP to remain productive and effective over time. Professional development stems from a commitment not only to personal competence but also to maintaining ethical practice and upholding the social justice of providing the best practice possible coupled with the economic value associated with this promise and obligation. Sustaining professional competence reflects continuous, dynamic engagement in one's professional development.

Beneficial tools and resources to sustain professional development processes specific to OT are the following:

The AOTA:
Professional Development Tool (AOTA, 2003)
Fieldwork Educators Certificate (AOTA, 2018b)
The NBCOT:
COTA Self-Assessment Tool (NBCOT, 2021a)
OTR Self-Assessment Tool (NBCOT, 2021b)

Creating a Routine for Lifelong Learning

Integrating information from the professional development self-assessment process becomes the basis on which to develop an individualized, professional development plan. Effective development plans answer the following questions:

- Where are the gaps between my current competence and what is expected or possible?
- What new learning will fill these gaps in my practice competence to ensure best practice?
- What evidence can I accumulate to demonstrate my acquired competencies?

Reflection on the first two questions provides a personalized map or plan for professional development. The last one calls for the development of a reflective portfolio to collect ongoing activities and evidence of competence.

A reflective portfolio is a dynamic, flexible, self-directed tool designed to document CPD through thoughtful engagement with artifacts created and accumulated in pursuit to achieve professional goals and desired roles (Schultz-Krohn et al., 2017). The CPD is a cyclical process initiated by reflection. The OTP reflects on current practice skills by identifying important situations within the environment and the ability to respond to those situations. These situations

can be external factors such as changes to reimbursement, changes in practice area, or derived from internal personal goals. The OTP then completes an analysis of practice that may include consumer ratings, peer reviews, or assessing skills through use of the continuing competence document (AOTA, 2017). A CPD plan is then developed including specific goals with the methods to achieve the stated goal. The next phase of the process is the implementation of the CDP plan. The final step is documenting the effectiveness of the plan, which then returns the OTP to the first step of reflection to determine new goals to be addressed. This circular process provides an ongoing and advancing systematic approach to engaging in CPD. The process of engaging in continuing competence is an iterative process whereby the changes in any of the above-mentioned situations can serve as the impetus to revise and upgrade the CPD to meet the new and anticipated demands.

Mentoring

The term **mentoring** connotes a relationship where there is a minimum of two individuals, the mentor and the mentee. This relationship can serve a variety of purposes (Doyle et al., 2019). The interaction between the two or more individuals can be focused on knowledge exchange where the mentor has greater experience and knowledge in a select area and the mentee is seeking to acquire this expertise. But mentorship goes beyond knowledge acquisition and often includes support for the mentee engaging in systematic continuing competence (VanderKaay et al., 2019). A positive mentoring relationship is distinct from a supervisory relationship where the supervisor has the responsibility of evaluating an employee's performance on a periodic basis. In a positive mentoring relationship, it is the mentee who initiates and directs the process in collaboration with the mentor. This relationship assumes mutual trust and respect between the mentee and mentor. The mentee establishes the outcome measures and evaluates if the relationship is supporting the trajectory toward meeting the desired outcome. An example would be an entry-level OTP who seeks advanced skills in the area of dysphagia. The mentee may be focused on a specific client population, such as children diagnosed with cerebral palsy. The mentee may request support and guidance from another OTP with far more experience and skills in working with this population including addressing issues of dysphagia. The mentee creates the intended outcomes of the mentoring relationship and the timeline for accomplishment. As an entry-level OTP, actively seeking out another OTP to serve as a mentor is one method to support and guide a CPD plan. Often a mentor can suggest a progression of activities that fosters reaching the desired outcome or goal, but it is the mentee who determines the desired outcome or goal. A positive mentoring relationship varies in length from a few months to 1–2 years, depending on the goal. The mentoring relationship is often sought after the entry-level OTP completes the self-assessment and determines what skills are needed to best serve clients.

Conclusion

Rapid changes in healthcare, knowledge, and technology require constant reevaluation and modification of the role and functions of every OTP. Our clients, their families, our employers, the profession, and the public expect every occupational therapist and OTA to provide the highest quality services possible. Engaging in CPD is an essential responsibility for every OTP to ensure continuing competence and competency. Professional development results from continuous, reflective self-assessment accounting for client outcomes, job responsibilities, and context as well as future trends in practice (AOTA, 2017; Schultz-Krohn et al., 2017). Professional development is individualized, goal-directed learning that advocates for, responds to, and initiates change in practice delivery and competence and ultimately enhances the profession.

The universal standard is to deliver best practices with encouragement to strive for practice excellence. Self-responsibility for engaging in continuous professional development is primary. Seeking support and guidance to engage in CPD and assistance in selecting the best suited activities to meet CPD goals is beneficial for all OTPs.

Lippincott® Connect *For additional resources on the subjects discussed in this chapter, visit Lippincott Connect.*

REFERENCES

Accreditation Council for Occupational Therapy Education. (2021). *2018 Accreditation Council for Occupational Therapy Education (ACOTE) standards and interpretative guide: August 2021 interpretative guide version.* https://acoteonline.org/

Agner, J. (2020). The Issue Is—Moving from cultural competence to cultural humility in occupational therapy: A paradigm shift. *American Journal of Occupational Therapy, 74,* 7404347010. https://doi.org/10.5014/ajot.2020.038067

American Occupational Therapy Association. (2003). *Professional development tool.* Author. https://www1.aota.org/pdt/index.asp

American Occupational Therapy Association. (2017). Continuing professional development in occupational therapy. *American Journal of Occupational Therapy, 71,* 7112410017p1–7112410017p5. https://doi.org/10.5014/ajot.2017.716S13

American Occupational Therapy Association. (2018a). *Board and specialty certifications.* https://www.aota.org/Education-Careers/Advance-Career/Board-Specialty-Certifications.aspx

American Occupational Therapy Association. (2018b). *Fieldwork educators certificate workshop.* https://www.aota.org/Education-Careers/Fieldwork/Workshop.aspx

American Occupational Therapy Association. (2020a). AOTA 2020 occupational therapy code of ethics. *American Journal of Occupational Therapy, 74*(suppl. 3), 7413410005. https://doi.org/10.5014/ajot.2020.74S3006

American Occupational Therapy Association. (2020b). Guidelines for supervision, roles, and responsibilities during the delivery of occupational therapy services. *American Journal of Occupational Therapy, 74*(suppl. 3), 7413410020. https://doi.org/10.5014/ajot.2020.74S3004

American Occupational Therapy Association. (2020c). Occupational therapy practice framework: Domain and process (4th ed.). *American Journal of Occupational Therapy, 74*(suppl. 2), 7412410010. https://doi.org/10.5014/ajot.2020.74S2001

American Occupational Therapy Association. (2020d). Occupational therapy's commitment to diversity, equity, and inclusion. *American Journal of Occupational Therapy, 74*(suppl. 3), 7413410030. https://doi.org/10.5014/ajot.2020.74S3002

American Occupational Therapy Association. (2020e). Guidelines for reentry into the field of occupational therapy. *American Journal of Occupational Therapy, 74*(suppl. 3), 7413410010. https://doi.org/10.5014/ajot.2020.74S3003

American Occupational Therapy Association. (2020f). *Occupational therapy profession—Continuing competence requirements.* https://www.aota.org//media/Corporate/Files/Advocacy/Licensure/StateRegs/ContComp/Continuing-Competence-Chart-full.pdf

American Occupational Therapy Association. (2021a). Standards of practice for occupational therapy. *American Journal of Occupational Therapy, 75*(suppl. 3), 7513410050. https://doi.org/10.5014/ajot.2021.75S3004

American Occupational Therapy Association. (2021b). *OT licensure requirements.* https://www.aota.org/-/media/Corporate/Files/Secure/Advocacy/Licensure/StateRegs/Qualifications/OT-qualifications-licensure-requirements-by-state.pdf

American Occupational Therapy Association. (2021c). *OTA licensure requirements.* https://www.aota.org/-/media/Corporate/Files/Secure/Advocacy/Licensure/StateRegs/Qualifications/OTA-qualifications-licensure-requirements-by-state.pdf

American Occupational Therapy Association. (2021d). *AOTA's evidence-based practice &research.* https://www.aota.org/Practice/Researchers.aspx

American Occupational Therapy Association. (2021e). AOTA 2021 standards for continuing competence in occupational therapy. *American Journal of Occupational Therapy, 75*(suppl. 3), 7513410040. https://doi.org/10.5014/ajot.2021.75S3009

American Occupational Therapy Association. (2021f). Occupational therapy scope of practice. *American Journal of Occupational Therapy, 75*(suppl. 3), 7513410030. https://doi.org/10.5014/ajot.2021.75S3005

Coffelt, K. J., & Gabriel, L. S. (2017). Continuing competence trends of occupational therapy practitioners. *The Open Journal of Occupational Therapy, 5*(1), 4. https://doi.org/10.15453/2168-6408.1268

Davis, S. (2014). Evidence-based practice and the new practitioner. *OT Practice, 19*(22), 17–18. ISSN: 1084-4902.

Dik, B. J., Sargent, A. M., & Steger, M. F. (2008). Career development strivings: Assessing goals and motivation in career decision-making and planning. *Journal of Career Development, 35,* 23–41. https://doi.org/10.1177/0894845308317934

Doyle, N. W., Lachter, L. G., & Jacobs, K. (2019). Scoping review of mentoring research in occupational therapy literature, 2002–2018. *Australian Occupational Therapy Journal, 66,* 541–551. https://doi.org/10.1111/1440-1630.12579

Fitzgerald, C., Moores, A., Coleman, A., & Fleming, J. (2015). Supporting new graduate professional development: A clinical learning framework. *Australian Occupational Therapy Journal, 62,* 13–20. https://doi.org/10.1111/1440-1630.12165

Gillen, G., Hunter, E. G., Lieberman, D., & Stutzbach, M. (2019). The Association—AOTA's top 5 Choosing Wisely® recommendations. *American Journal of Occupational Therapy, 73,* 7302420010. https://doi.org/10.5014/ajot.2019.732001

Gillen, G., Lieberman, D., Stutzbach, M., & Arbesman, M. (2017). Five interventions/assessments our clients should question: AOTA joins Choosing Wisely. *OT Practice, 22*(15), 19–20. ISSN: 1084-4902.

Haywood, H., Pain, H., Ryan, S., & Adams, J. (2012). Engagement with continuing professional development: Development of a service model. *Journal of Allied Health, 41*, 83–89. ISSN: 0090-7421.

Holm, M. B. (2000). The 2000 Eleanor Clarke Slagle lecture. Our mandate for the new millennium: Evidence-based practice. *American Journal of Occupational Therapy, 54*, 575–585. https://doi.org/10.5014/ajot.54.6.575

Institute for Credentialing Excellence. (2020). *I.C.E. Basic guide to credentialing terminology* (2nd ed.). https://www.credentialing excellence.org/blog/term20-ice-basic-guide-tocredentialing-terminology-(2nd-edition)

Knightbridge, L. (2014). Experiential learning on an alternative practice education placement: Student reflections on entry-level competency, personal growth, and future practice. *British Journal of Occupational Therapy, 77*, 438–446. https://doi.org/10.4276/030802 214X14098207540956

Kronberg, J., Tierney, E., Wallisch, A., & Little, L. M. (2021). Early intervention service delivery via telehealth during COVID-19: A research-practice partnership. *International Journal of Telerehabilitation, 13(1)*, e6363. https://doi.org/10.5195/ijt.2021.6363

McMahon, M., Forde, C., & Dickson, B. (2015). Reshaping teacher education through the professional continuum. *Educational Review, 67*, 158–178. https://doi.org/10.1080/00131911.2013.846298

Morgan, D. J., Dhruva, S. S., Wright, S. M., & Korenstein, D. (2016). 2016 update on medical overuse: A systematic review. *JAMA International Medicine, 176*, 1687–1692. https://doi.org/10.1001/jamainternmed .2016.5381

Moyers, P. (2009). Occupational therapy practitioners: Competence and professional development. In E. B. Crepeau, E. S. Cohn, & B. A. B. Schell (Eds.), *Willard & Spackman's occupational therapy* (11th ed., pp. 240–251). Lippincott Williams & Wilkins.

Moyers, P. A., & Metzler, C. A. (2014). Interprofessional collaborative practice in care coordination. *American Journal of Occupational Therapy, 68*, 500–505. https://doi.org/ajot.2014.685002

National Board for Certification in Occupational Therapy. (2021a). *COTA self-assessment tool manual.* https://www.nbcot.org/Certificants/Certification#Self-Assessments

National Board for Certification in Occupational Therapy. (2021b). *OTR self-assessment tool manual.* https://www.nbcot.org/Certificants/Certification#Self-Assessments

Roessger, K. M. (2015). But does it work? Reflective activities, learning outcomes and instrumental learning in continuing professional development. *Journal of Education and Work, 28*, 83–105. https://doi .org/10.1080/13639080.2013.805186

Sackett, D. L., Rosenberg, W. M., Gray, J. A. M., Haynes, R. B., & Richardson, W. S. (1996). Evidence-based medicine: What it is and what it isn't. *British Medical Journal, 312*, 71–72. https://doi.org/10.1136/bmj.312.7023.71

Schultz-Krohn, W., James, A., & Nonaillada, J. (2017). Continuing professional development—How if fits with practice. *OT Practice, 22*(5), 22–24. ISSN: 1084-4902.

Unsworth, C. A. (2001). The clinical reasoning of novice and expert occupational therapists. *Scandinavian Journal of Occupational Therapy, 8*, 163–173. https://doi.org/10.1080/110381201317166522

Unsworth, C., & Baker, A. (2016). A systematic review of professional reasoning literature in occupational therapy. *British Journal of Occupational Therapy, 79*, 5–16. https://doi.org/10.1177/0308022615599994

VanderKaay, S., Jung, B., Letts, L., & Moll S. E. (2019). Continuing competency in ethical decision making: An interpretive description of occupational therapists' perspectives. *Canadian Journal of Occupational Therapy, 86*, 209–219. https://doi.org/10.1177/0008417419833842

Wallingford, M., Knecht-Sabres, L. J., Lee, M. M., & St. Amand, L. E. (2016). OT practitioners' and OT students' perceptions of entry-level competency for occupational therapy practice. *The Open Journal of Occupational Therapy, 4*(4), 10. https://doi.org/10.15453/2168-6408.1243

Wittich, W., Jarry, J., Barstow, E., & Thomas, A. (2017). Vision and hearing impairment and occupational therapy education: Needs and current practice. *British Journal of Occupational Therapy, 80*, 384–391. ISSN: 0308-0226.

World Federation of Occupational Therapists. (2012). *The World Federation of Occupational Therapists (WFOT) Position Statement on Competency and Maintaining Competency* (CM2012). http://www. wfot.org/ResourceCentre.aspx

World Federation of Occupational Therapists. (2016). *The World Federation of Occupational Therapists (WFOT) Code of Ethic (Revised CM2016).* http://www.wfot.org/ResourceCentre.aspx

Preparation for Work in an Academic Setting

Catana Brown, Tamara Turner, and Glen Gillen

LEARNING OBJECTIVES

After reading this chapter, you will be able to:

1. Describe academic settings for occupational therapists and occupational therapy assistants.
2. Explain the process for developing a college course.
3. Summarize the skills needed for carrying out research in an academic setting.
4. Depict the different types of service involved in being a faculty member.
5. Understand the tenure and promotion process.

Introduction

Recently, the Accreditation Council for Occupational Therapy Education or ACOTE (American Occupational Therapy Association [AOTA], 2018) introduced new standards (effective July 2020) focused on preparing for work in an academic setting. The standards require occupational therapy (OT) programs to provide students with coursework related to instructional design and teaching and learning so that students will be prepared to teach in OT or occupational therapy assistant (OTA) programs.

The information contained in this chapter is appropriate not only toward meeting these standards but for those practicing clinicians who are contemplating a shift to academia.

What to Know About Academia

The following chapter sections will focus on types of educational settings, degrees that are required to obtain a faculty position, the interviewing process, World Federation of Occupational Therapy (WFOT, n.d.) requirements for education programs, and understanding the tenure and promotion process.

Types of Educational Settings for Occupational Therapy Programs in the United States

Accredited OT programs can exist in a variety of educational settings. Specifically, accredited OT educational programs are established in senior colleges, universities, or medical schools for OT programs. For OTA education programs, settings may include community, technical, junior, and senior colleges; universities; medical schools; or military institutions (AOTA, 2018).

In addition, the settings where OT education takes place must be accredited by an institutional accrediting agency recognized by the US Department of Education (USDE). For OT programs in countries other than the United States, the ACOTE determines an equivalent external review process (AOTA, 2018).

Degrees Needed for a Faculty Position in Occupational Therapy in the United States

ACOTE has developed specific degree requirements for faculty hired by these institutions (AOTA, 2018). For institutions granting an entry-level OT degree, all full-time core OT faculty must have a doctoral degree and at least 50% of the faculty must have a post-professional doctorate. For OT programs granting an entry-level OT degree at the masters level, 50% of full-time core faculty must hold a doctoral degree and all must hold a minimum of a master's degree. At baccalaureate-level OTA programs, the majority of full-time core faculty must hold a master's degree, and for OTA programs granting an associate's degree, all full-time core faculty must have a baccalaureate degree.

Interviewing Process for an Academic Position

Interviewing for a faculty position is typically an arduous process requiring multiple steps. This process usually begins with the established search committee reviewing your curriculum vitae and letter of intent. The search committee may consist of current OT faculty members as well as faculty from related departments.

The search committee's first charge is to rank order applicants and decide which candidates will be called in for the interview process. If a candidate is called in for interview, it is prudent that the candidate does their "homework" prior to the interviews. This "homework" should consist of knowing the backgrounds of the faculty and search committee members, gaining knowledge of the mission and vision of the institution and the department, knowing the scholarship agenda of the department as well as individual faculty members, and preparing answers to potential questions that may be asked during the process by the search committee, program director, faculty, students, and so on. During the interview, it is important to discuss the teaching, scholarship, and service expectations.

The interview process itself will most likely consist of a series of interviews with individuals and groups. Potential interviews may include meeting with:

- Search committee members
- Faculty
- Groups of students
- The Program Director
- The Dean or Provost
- A group at a social event such as lunch or dinner

The interview day(s) will also include a professional presentation or "job talk." This is arguably one of the most important parts of the interview process. Your topic may be chosen for you, focus on current and future scholarship, or an area of clinical specialty. Presentations are usually 60 minutes including questions.

If you are asked back for a continued interview, you will want to ask questions that are more specific to the job. Topics to inquire about include:

- Rank, promotion, and salary
- The tenure process
- Length of the appointment
- Research expectations
- Internal funding opportunities
- Teaching credit load
- Institutional review board requirements
- Benefits
- Grading policies
- Committee requirements
- Advising requirements
- etc.

In OT Story 72.1, Ali de la Montaigne describes her process of transitioning from clinician to becoming an OT faculty member.

Concerns Related to Diversity, Equity, and Inclusion in Academia

A survey by the Institute of Education Sciences (2018) indicates that women and people of color are underrepresented as faculty across all disciplines. Women make up 44% of faculty. The numbers of faculty for some racial groups are sparse with only 3% Black, 3% Hispanic, and 1% First Nations/Indigenous faculty. Asians are not

OT STORY 72.1 ALI DE LA MONTAIGNE

During my time as an occupational therapist, I have worked in all areas of adult practice, with the bulk of my experience in acute care. Whenever asked about my favorite part of being an OT practitioner, I without hesitation say patient care. I love being an occupational therapist and helping clients see hope for their future during the darkest time in their life.

In 2018, I had worked in acute care for 5 years. I noticed I was becoming too routine in my day-to-day practice and I was searching for some new tools and inspiration. I decided to attend the AOTA conference with another colleague from the hospital. During the conference, I attended a "meet-up" event with my alma mater where I was introduced to the faculty member who taught the adult practice courses. By the end of the event, I was asked to do a guest lecture on "Occupational Therapy in the ICU," and I gladly accepted. I knew nothing about teaching and even though the last time I presented I was in OT school, I was excited for the challenge.

After the two-day guest lecture and simulation lab, I remember feeling so fulfilled. In many ways, this felt very similar to seeing a breakthrough with a client who had been intubated and sedated for months in the intensive care unit (ICU) and finally was able to brush their teeth at the side of the bed or after advocating for a patient who clearly needed acute rehab and finally got insurance authorization. I had no idea this was just the start of my journey, but as a practitioner eager to learn and explore new opportunities, I was excited at the thought of more opportunities like this one.

A few months later I was asked if I was interested in being hired on as adjunct faculty. This involved assisting with class content and discussion, grading assignments, and co-facilitating the labs. Whenever asked about my interest in academia, my answer was always, "I don't know that I can

give up patient care." For the next year, I continued helping with courses as an adjunct faculty and loved taking on new opportunities to teach a lecture or facilitate a lab activity. The course director increased my responsibilities as my teaching skills and abilities improved. I eventually became the course director and was finally offered a full-time faculty position in the fall of 2020.

As stated best by the department chair of the university where I teach, as an OT educator, you get to work with thousands of clients through your students. What I love about teaching is not just the desire to teach about practice areas that I am passionate about, but also the opportunity to help future practitioners along their path, just like we do as OT practitioners with our clients. I strongly believe that if you work hard and are open to challenging yourself, you will find your path. Two years later I have started the dissertation candidacy in my doctoral program where I am pursuing a doctorate in education with an emphasis in instructional leadership. I also teach the adult practice courses and co-teach the evidence-based practice series in the curriculum. The conference I attended to get a few additional tools to improve my practice introduced me to an entirely different sector of OT practice. Teaching OT students how to be effective evidence-based practitioners is an honor and a privilege.

Questions

1. Have you ever thought about teaching? What about it appeals to you?
2. What strengths do you have that you could bring to an academic setting? What skills would you need to develop?

underrepresented in academia with 12.2%. The specific numbers for women and people of color in OT academia is unknown; however, the AOTA workforce summary (2019) indicates although women are not underrepresented in OT, the OT workforce is identified as 3% Black, 0.3% Indigenous, 5.8% Asian, and 3.6% Hispanic/*Latinx*.

There are many reasons why people of color, especially female people of color, are likely to feel marginalized in academic environments (Lin & Kennette, 2022). People of color are more likely to be hired in nontenure-track positions making career advancement more difficult. Affirmative action can lead to negative stereotypes and psychological pressure to overachieve just to be seen as legitimate. Because of underrepresentation, faculty of color may feel unsupported and isolated. People of color are often expected to take on more service responsibilities, especially on committees related to diversity, which can interfere with research and teaching eventually impacting the tenure process.

Diversity increases understanding and can reduce bias among coworkers. A diverse faculty is more likely to attract a diverse student body, thereby increasing the diversity of the OT workforce. The advantages to having a more diverse faculty require that OT education programs consider ways to mitigate the challenges. Some strategies for increasing recruitment and retention of faculty from underrepresented groups include creating supportive environments, developing mentorship programs, removing barriers to advancement, and ensuring equity in resources (Crooks et al., 2021).

WFOT Requirements for OT Programs

The WFOT is an international organization representing occupational therapists in over 100 countries. WFOT has established educational standards for OT known as the minimum standards for the education of occupational therapists (WFOT, n.d.). The WFOT reviews documents for educational institutions that are submitted through the country's national association. If the country does not have a national organization, then the educational institution can submit the documents directly. Expert reviewers analyze the documents to determine if the curricula meet the minimum standards.

As these are minimum standards, graduation from a WFOT Approved Education Program does not automatically make the graduate eligible for certification and/or licensing in some countries that may have additional standards. You can find a list of approved programs on their website at https://www.wfot.org/programmes/education.

Understanding Promotion and Tenure

Tenure is an academic appointment available at most universities. Tenure offers protection to faculty such that the tenured professor can only be fired for cause or extraordinary circumstances. The modern view of tenure in the United States was established in 1940 by the American Association of University Professors (AAUP, 2006). Tenure was developed to support academic freedom, which means that teachers are entitled to present their views in the classroom and in research without fear of censorship or retaliation. Tenure promotes innovation and prevents teachers and researchers from being controlled by special interest groups or political organizations.

Not all teachers at the university level are tenured or in a tenure-track position (working toward tenure). Adjunct faculty are not eligible for tenure, and many colleges and universities have nontenure-track positions that may have titles such as clinical associate professor, lecturer, or instructor. Faculty in a nontenure-track position often spend a larger percentage of their time focused on one specific area such as teaching or research.

The Process for Obtaining Tenure

There are three components to tenure-track positions: teaching, research/scholarship, and service. The amount of time spent in each component varies depending on the institution and the needs of your department. In a large university dedicated to research, you may spend the majority of your time conducting research. In a teaching-focused university, teaching will be your primary focus. The amount of time spent in the three components of teaching, scholarship, and service is something that you should negotiate with the chair of the department at the outset of your employment.

It typically takes 6 years before a faculty member can apply for tenure. The 6 years are a probationary period and a time for meeting the tenure criteria. Most universities will have guidelines regarding the expectations in terms of teaching, scholarship, and service. This information is available in the faculty handbook. These guidelines will include criteria such as expectations for teaching evaluations, innovations in the classroom, number of publications, grant application, and committee work. In many institutions, you will receive an early review of materials to make sure that you are on track.

As a tenure-track faculty, you will create a dossier so that your work at the university can be reviewed. The dossier is a comprehensive document that includes letters of recommendations and evidence (e.g., copies of publications, ratings on teaching evaluations) that you have met the established criteria for your institution. Typically, the chair of your department or a committee within your department will review your dossier first. If approved, it will go to a tenure and promotion committee, and eventually to the Provost or President of the university. The process will take several months.

Tenure-Track Positions

A faculty member that is on a tenure-track position will traditionally start out as an Assistant Professor. If the faculty member's application for tenure is accepted after the 6-year process, they will be promoted to the position of Associate Professor. In some institutions, if a faculty member is denied tenure, they are terminated from their position at the end of year. Full professors are tenured faculty that have achieved a higher level of academic rank. These faculty have an established body of scholarly work and have taken a leadership role at the university and/or within their profession.

Teaching

In most academic positions, teaching responsibilities take up the largest component of your time. This includes not only the classroom delivery of content, but also the preparing of the course, meeting with students outside of class, and assessing and revising your teaching.

Preparing a Course

Preparation of the course is key to success and significant time must be dedicated to course preparation. The purpose of teaching is not to deliver content, but rather to create optimal learning (Fink, 2013). When preparing to teach, there are four essential steps to follow that will lead to good teaching and optimal learning (Diamond, 2008). The final piece is a syllabus, which summarizes all the information about the course so that students know what to expect.

1. Conduct a needs assessment
2. Develop course objectives
3. Determine specific content
4. Develop learning assessments

Conducting a Needs Assessment

The first step in preparing a course is to conduct a needs assessment. This might sound or feel intimidating at first thought, but really a needs assessment is just finding the answers to the questions you have. These can be broken into three categories: questions about the curriculum, questions about the students, and questions about the learning environment.

- *Curriculum:* You will want to know how the course you are designing fits into the overall curriculum. You need to know what students have already learned, what they will be concurrently learning, and how this course will prepare them for future courses. You will also want to know the depth of their knowledge, that is, was a particular concept introduced only or has it been further developed? You may identify standards that must be met and discover that there are holes you can fill. Finding these answers allows you to design your course to support the curriculum and enhance student learning.
- *Students:* You will want to know about your students. How many students are in class? What is their age range? How long have they known each other? Is attendance mandatory or voluntary? Do students bring computers to class? What are the students' expectations? Knowing more about your students will help you to better tailor your teaching to meet their needs.
- *Learning environment:* You will want to have an idea about your learning environment. Will you be teaching in person, online, or hybrid? Will you be in a classroom with desks or in a lab with room to move around? Will you have rectangular tables or circular tables? Can you request a particular classroom setup? What media resources are available? What supplies are available? Knowing more about the learning environment will help you to plan your content delivery.

The needs assessment is an essential first step in instructional design. As you learn how the course fits into the curriculum, who your students are, and where the teaching and learning will take place, you will be ready to complete the next steps of preparing the course.

Developing Course Objectives

The second step to preparing a course is to develop the course objectives. These should be learner-centered and outcome-driven. Objectives will be written based on what you want your students to know, be able to do, and value. (You might think of course objectives as akin to goals for a client's plan of care.) The objectives you develop will influence your teaching methods, guide your learning assessments, and help you assess your teaching effectiveness.

Bloom (1956) identified three domains of learning: cognitive, psychomotor, and affective. The **cognitive domain** is looking at knowledge. For example, OT practitioners are expected to determine the appropriate adaptive equipment for a client. They will do this based on their knowledge of adaptive equipment and a variety of diagnoses and treatment approaches. When they combine this knowledge, they can apply their learning by selecting the most appropriate adaptive equipment for a particular client. The **psychomotor domain** is looking at motor skill development. For example, OT practitioners are expected to transfer a client from a wheelchair to a toilet. They do so by first learning safe transfer techniques, practicing in lab, adjusting technique after receiving feedback, and finally applying this skill in the field. The **affective domain** refers to values, beliefs, attitudes, and behaviors. For example, OT practitioners use person-first language rather than referring to a client by their diagnosis or their room number. Before being made aware of this concept, a student may not understand why this matters or even be able recognize it in action. Once taught the concept, the student can then practice implementing person-first language and may even find themselves annoyed when someone doesn't implement person-first language. The student's values, beliefs, attitudes, and behavior have changed.

Bloom's Taxonomy of Educational Objectives (Bloom, 1956; Krathwohl et al., 1964; Simpson, 1972) delves deeper into each domain looking at levels of knowledge from basic exposure to content mastery. See Table 72.1, for these levels of learning that progress from low- to high-level learning. When developing course objectives, you should consider

TABLE 72.1 Bloom's Taxonomy

Level of Learning	Cognitive Domain	Psychomotor Domain	Affective Domain
Low	Knowledge	Perception	Receiving (attending)
	Comprehension	Set	Responding (complying)
	Application	Guided response	Valuing (accepting)
↓	Analysis	Mechanism	Organization (integrating)
	Synthesis	Complex overt response	Characterization (internalizing)
High	Evaluation	Adapt	
		Origination	

each domain of learning in addition to the level of learning you expect your students to achieve. For example, if you are first introducing adaptive dressing equipment, you may have a simple objective about the student's knowledge of adaptive dressing equipment. As the student learns more about when adaptive dressing equipment is appropriate, you may have an objective related to the student's comprehension. This deepening of cognitive learning will help your students to attain synthesis and evaluation skills related to adaptive dressing equipment. Table 72.2 provides example objectives from low- to high-level learning across each domain.

Determining Specific Content

Now that you have written your course objectives, you are ready to determine the specific content that you will cover. Reread each course objective and determine what the students need to learn, practice, and/or value to meet that objective. For example, if one course objectives is "By the end of this course, students will identify appropriate discrete theories for the neurological client," you know the students will need to learn common neurologic diagnoses and common discrete theories. You might then determine to spend a class session on degenerative neurologic conditions, one class session on cerebral vascular accidents and acquired brain injuries, and another on facilitation and inhibition strategies.

Once you've determined the specific content, you can also identify reading assignments to prepare for or support the in-class learning. These can come from textbooks, peer-reviewed articles, resource websites, and more.

Note: This is a good time to create a course schedule. A course schedule allows you to see the layout of your course and which topics should be grouped together. One technique is lay this out in a table with a column for each day the course meets and a row for each week of the term. You can then add reading assignments, assignment due dates, and any other helpful information that the students can see at-a-glance.

TABLE 72.2 Sample Objectives

Domain	Level	Objective
Cognitive	Knowledge	Students will identify adaptive dressing equipment options.
	Comprehension	Students will identify suitable adaptive dressing equipment option for orthopedic conditions.
	Application	Students will demonstrate how selected adaptive dressing equipment will be used for an assigned case.
	Analysis	Students will determine suitability of adaptive dressing equipment based on client's performance.
	Synthesis	Students will determine when and how to introduce adaptive dressing equipment in the Plan of Care.
	Evaluation	Students will determine the efficacy of adaptive dressing equipment based on client's occupational performance.
Psychomotor	Perception	Students will use proprioceptive and kinesthetic feedback to position self for a safe transfer.
	Set	Students will recognize their mental, physical, and emotional dispositions prior to completing transfers.
	Guided response	Students will identify unsafe transfers with instructor feedback and guidance.
	Mechanism	Students will be able to replicate safe transfer with basic steps for stand pivot transfers.
	Complex overt response	Students will complete efficient and safe transfers.
	Adapt	Students will demonstrate the ability to modify a transfer technique to ensure a safe patient transfer.
	Origination	Students will develop a new transfer technique based on client's performance skills and environmental demands.
Affective	Receiving (attending)	Students will attend person-first presentation.
	Responding (complying)	Students will recognize when they can use person-centered language.
	Valuing (accepting)	Students will self-correct to appropriately use person-first language.
	Organization (integrating)	Students will educate an interprofessional peer about person-first language.
	Characterization (internalizing)	Students will consistently use person-first language appropriately.

Developing Learning Assessments

Learning assessments are how you will measure whether the course objectives have been met. Learning assessments fall into one of two categories: formative assessments and summative assessments.

- *Formative assessments* are designed to give you an idea of how the students are coming along in their learning. The stakes are usually lower and give the students an opportunity to demonstrate what they know yet will often also learn from the experience. Some examples of formative assessments are quizzes, discussion posts, lab activities, and small group discussions.
- *Summative assessments* are designed to showcase the student's knowledge gained over a period of time. This is often a synthesis of what the student has learned and the stakes are usually higher. Some examples of summative assessments are midterm and final exams, term papers, oral exams, final projects, and practical exams.

A well-written multiple-choice exam will take a long time to write, but will be very quick to grade; on the other hand a well-written short answer or essay exam is rather quick to write, but will take a long time to grade. Weigh the pros and cons of your exam delivery and decide on which question style will best showcase the students' knowledge for that particular learning item.

As you design your learning assessments, you may consider developing a rubric to guide your grading. A rubric will help your students know what you want them to include and will help you to grade fairly across all submissions. As a word of caution, a very detailed rubric can lead to "cookie-cutter" responses from your students. Check with your institution as they may have guidelines or expectations regarding rubric development.

Developing the Syllabus

The course syllabus has many purposes from providing course information and expectations to establishing the course's place in the professional development process (O'Brien et al., 2008). The course syllabus is the culmination of all the preparation you have completed for the course. The syllabus should include:

1. Instructor information
2. Course description and course objectives
3. Required and suggested textbooks
4. Course schedule (content, readings, assignment due dates)
5. Course requirements (assignments and their descriptions)
6. Grading procedures
7. Policies and expectations (attendance, late or missed assignments, professional behaviors, academic honesty, and disability access)

Teaching the Course

Now that you have prepared the course, you need to look at how you'll teach the course. What do the best college teachers do (Bain, 2004)? How can you best help, support, and encourage your students in their development of skills, knowledge, and values?

Teaching theory is called **pedagogy**. Pedagogies guide how you conduct your class, the expectations you have, and how you treat your students (Bain, 2004). Shulman (2005) introduced the term **signature pedagogy** to describe discipline-specific pedagogies. Schaber and Candler (2020) looked at the profession of OT and the disciplinary practices that we bring to the classroom in order to identify the signature pedagogies in OT, which they list as relational learning, affective learning, and highly contextualized, active engagement.

Relational Learning: A Signature Pedagogy in Occupational Therapy

Relational learning relies on the teacher-to-student connection. As we get to know our students and they get to know us, relational learning occurs. We model the relationship between therapist and client. We share stories to highlight our clinical reasoning. As we build relationships with our students, we "guide the student experience by reflection in action, stimulating reflection, and providing feedback on student responses and behaviors" (Schaber & Candler, 2020, p. 50). This relational learning also occurs with student-to-student relationships in small group work (Schaber & Candler, 2020).

Affective Learning: A Signature Pedagogy in Occupational Therapy

Affective learning occurs when a student's core values have changed or deepened. "The goal of the professional program is to transform the occupational therapy student emotionally to fit into a cultural ethos embraced by the profession" (Schaber & Candler, 2020, p. 50). Students form a new identity through affective learning. This learning is akin to transformation learning theory, in which there is personal change through learning. The student embraces the professional ethics and core values of the profession and is in a sense a new person through this learning and growth (Schaber & Candler, 2020).

Highly Contextualized, Active Engagement: A Signature Pedagogy in Occupational Therapy

Highly contextualized, active engagement is "learning through doing." The profession of OT began in the field by doing. We continue to learn through doing, certainly

1. Start with a motivational hook—some kind of attention-getter. This will pull your students in. You can use an interesting fact, a video clip, a story from practice, and so on.
2. Start the class period with an overview of what you'll cover that session.
3. Avoid rushing through the material. Don't mention running out of time, as this distracts from your content.
4. Don't lecture for more than 20 minutes straight without stopping for a learning activity.
5. Use slide shows as a visual aid, rather than a place to put all the information. Keep it simple and let the students take notes.
6. End the class period with a summary of what you covered that session.

not only during fieldwork and service-learning opportunities, but also in the classroom through active learning (Schaber & Candler, 2020).

It is easy to get caught up in the idea of fitting your content into the class period and not being satisfied with how much material you covered. You might even be tempted to exclude learning activities because you "don't have enough time." Keep in mind that learning the material is different from covering the material, and it is better to help your students to learn something well than to hope that they grasped the key concepts from your lecture. When deciding what to include in your class period, think about what the students need to know for entry-level practice. Focusing on what your students need to know will actually give you more time to include active learning, which in turn makes your students more likely to process and retain the information (Plack & Driscoll, 2017).

Active learning strategies should be designed to promote critical thinking, allow time to process the new information, and begin to own that knowledge. There are many evidence-based active learning strategies, including using learning stations, case presentations, think-pair-share, concept mapping, debates, and many more. If you notice your students' engagement declining, it is time to stop the lecture and introduce an application activity, whether preplanned or thought up in the moment. See Box 72.1, for teaching tips.

Evaluating and Revising the Course

How do you evaluate your teaching? Is it about whether you wrote clearly on the white board and gave prompt assignment feedback or is it about what the students have learned...or maybe a combination? There certainly is value in what you do as an instructor, but measuring what the students have learned over your course is of even higher value. Here are four questions from Bain (2004, p. 164) to ask yourself: "(a) Is the material worth learning (and, perhaps appropriate to the curriculum)? (b) Are my students learning what the course is supposedly teaching? (c) Am I helping and encouraging the students to learn (or do they learn despite me)? (d) Have I harmed my students (perhaps fostering short-term learning with intimidation tactics, discouraging rather than stimulating additional interest in the field, fostering strategic or bulimic rather than deep learning, neglecting the needs of a diverse student population, or failing to evaluate students' learning accurately)?"

One method to determine whether your students are learning what you've intended is to review student work and responses to exam questions. Look at themes where more students didn't perform as expected, whether in written work or exams, in class activities and discussions, or practical labs and exams. This allows you to look into their understanding of the material, their ability to think critically, and see how they apply the knowledge gained. You also should reflect on your assessment methods to ask yourself if they showcased the students' abilities, knowledge, and values the way you intended.

Students are often asked to rate the course and the instructor at the end of the term. Additionally, you can provide your own set of questions for the students to evaluate and provide feedback. This can be done at the end of the term, but also in the middle, allowing you to adjust your methods to better meet the students' learning needs. Some teachers pass out index cards halfway through the term and ask students to write down things they like about the class and things they'd like to change. Others create an end-of-course survey asking the students to rate various learning activities and how well they met each objective. One great moment for any teacher is seeing students long after graduation and hearing them say that the way you taught changed the way they practice.

"Excellent teachers develop their abilities through constant self-evaluation, reflection, and the willingness to change" (Bain, 2004, p. 172). For another view on teaching, see Expanding Our Perspectives.

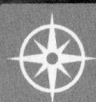

EXPANDING OUR PERSPECTIVES

Becoming an OT Professor: My Learning Experience

Carmen Gloria de las Heras de Pablo

As a devoted OT practitioner for 40 years, I was inspired to share my theoretical and practical knowledge as a clinical educator, university professor, and guest lecturer to teach a range of topics in my specialty: Human Occupation, Occupational Therapy Foundations, and the Model of Human Occupation (MOHO). My skills as an educator have developed mainly through experience and study. One of my challenges in my role as international professor has been to carry out needs assessments to better understand the professional knowledge of my audience, their predominant culture, the characteristics of each group of participants and professors, and the objectives prioritized in each academic curriculum. Based on this information, I have had to quickly adapt to the different ways of presenting educational programs in English and in Spanish according to the format used in different countries and universities. In addition, I learned the administrative procedures of each educational entity. I would say that I never stop learning and that *diversity is what has taught me to be flexible enough to manage these issues at ease in the present.*

Thinking of my learning process to become a better professor, I remember my first experience of teaching courses in which *my essence as a person made me trip.* My essence includes being a very giving person. This drove me to share myself as much as I could, "all" my knowledge with OT professionals and OT students, even in short periods of time. It was hard for me to handle the idea of not doing this.

The first introductory MOHO courses I taught were delivered in South America between the late 1980s and 1990s. These courses lasted 4 days in a row consisting of 9–10 clock hours each (not including breaks). I did well organizing the content in a proper sequence and including clear examples along with group exercises. I communicated the content with great passion, dedication, and conviction, using the existing media of the times, such as projecting transparencies using an overhead projector, writing on a blackboard, and projecting handmade slides. I observed that participants were highly motivated, active, and content. *However, they were also exhausted.* I really think that what kept them alert and sitting in awkward chairs all day long was their motivation. From their feedback and that of other beloved colleagues, I became aware of the immensity of the content I delivered, and the

little time participants had to assimilate it. Although I gave participants manuals as a guidance, these also contained too much content.

What was most evident was that *affective learning did occur.* Participants described a new connection with the profession ("falling in love with the profession again," "what the real OT was," "realizing that the principles of OT could be applied in practice"). These transformational experiences were really impressive as they were charged with strong positive emotions. I realized that the basic level of cognitive and affective objectives was met. The more complex cognitive objectives I set for these courses were well above what could be expected for a short, intensive course.

Since then, I have learned I need to program courses at a pace that allows participants to accomplish the cognitive and affective learning objectives—*time for reflection, critical thinking, and active learning.* I shifted the format into a 300-hour advanced postgraduate course, which consists of three consecutive modules implemented over a 1-year time period. These modules were organized to progressively address the development of integrative therapeutic reasoning skills. Each of the three modules included one course over 4–5 days, an applied project in each participant's OT practice; self-study using shared materials, manuals, and books; and tutoring to support application of the project in practice. Courses are organized interweaving lecture with learning activities during class time such as forums, debates, video analysis, OT stories presentations, group, and individual project presentations.

Convinced that learning through doing/experience is best to internalize the theory and practice of MOHO, these courses follow a cycle of a continuing exercise going "from practice to theory and theory to practice," highlighting the participant's personal occupational experience and progressive self-knowledge, thus, doing my best to foster an affective, relational, highly contextualized, and engaging learning process.

I became a professor through self-learning, being open to students' and colleagues' feedback. Today, I can tell, in all my teaching, I am better able to prioritize a clear summary of current theory and application of the model and follow through with a combination of reflection, discussion, lectures, and learning activities. So different from how I approached it at the beginning!

Once again. I never stop learning...Flexibility, humility, and passion have been my best allies. My essence continues being the same.

Scholarship

In most academic settings, faculty are expected to contribute to the development of new knowledge, otherwise known as **scholarship** or research. This is especially true if you are a faculty member on a tenure-track position, in which case conducting research and publishing that research is a very important consideration in the tenure decision.

Expectations for Scholarship

The expectations for conducting research will vary greatly depending on your position and the type of educational institution where you work. The degree to which you desire to perform research is an important consideration when selecting an academic institution that best fits your personal goals. If you are an adjunct faculty member, then you will have specific expectations for teaching, and scholarship is likely not a part of your contract. There are other situations in which research obligations are minimal, such as clinical faculty who provide clinical services and do some teaching or faculty at a community college. Conversely, faculty on a tenure track will be expected to do more research than nontenure-track faculty. Universities will also vary in terms of their emphasis on teaching versus research, so it is important to know the university culture before accepting a position. If you are on a tenure track at a research university, there are typically guidelines available to give you a sense of what you will need to produce to be considered eligible for tenure. Factors under consideration typically go beyond the number of publications to include the quality of the journal in which articles are published and the number of publications in which the faculty member serves as the first author. Presentations at scientific meetings are also considered scholarship, but do not receive as much weight as publications.

Even though scholarship can be the most important factor in a tenure decision, it is often challenging for new faculty to establish a routine and focus on research. It is impossible to ignore teaching requirements when your course(s) meets regularly for 3 hours every week throughout the semester. Similarly, you will be missed if you don't show up at a committee meeting. However, it is mostly on you to maintain your momentum toward your research undertakings.

Therefore, if your academic position has high expectations for research, it is important that you figure out ways to stay productive in this area. Some useful strategies include:

1. Finding a research mentor and/or collaborator(s)
2. Creating or joining a research or writing group
3. Setting realistic goals
4. Dedicating time every week to your research agenda
5. Setting deadlines with accountability from peers or supervisors

It is easy to abandon the time set aside for research. Students, colleagues, and supervisors as well as your teaching and service obligations will put demands on your time. But in this case, you need to be selfish with your time. Unless you make scholarship a priority, it will not get done. For more information on scholarship, see Chapter 6.

The Process of Scholarship/Research

The process of scholarship is discussed in greater detail in Chapter 6: Scholarship in Occupational Therapy, but scholarship as a component of your job responsibilities in academia is presented in a condensed form here. Generally speaking, the steps of scholarship include identifying a research agenda, obtaining funding, conducting the research, and disseminating the findings.

Creating a Research Agenda

You will be more productive as a researcher if you can establish an area of expertise, instead of following different projects without a focus. With an area of concentration, projects will build on one another, and you don't have to start from scratch in terms of learning the literature, creating contacts, identifying collaborators, and establishing credibility. You might be able to build upon your dissertation or other graduate research or you may pursue areas of interest in which you already have some familiarity clinically. As a faculty member, you may be interested in studying the best methods for student learning, otherwise known as **scholarship of teaching and learning.** See the Commentary on the Evidence box, for an example of scholarship of teaching and learning.

COMMENTARY ON THE EVIDENCE

Occupation is a core concept of our profession. However, how instructors assess student knowledge related to the concept of occupation is not well known. In a study that would fit the classification of scholarship of teaching and learning, Price et al. (2021) used qualitative methods to examine practices that educators use to assess knowledge of occupation. They randomly selected 25 OT and OTA programs in the United States and collected data from 29 educators from those programs. Data collection included interviews, classroom videos, and artifacts such as exams, papers, and lab practicals. The data were sorted into direct versus indirect

(continued)

learning of occupation and whether the activities met the criteria for a robust assessment.

Results indicated that OT programs varied greatly in their methods for assessing learning related to occupation and that many creative methods were used. However, most assessments of knowledge of occupation were indirect and did not meet the criteria for robust assessment. The researchers make recommendations to enhance assessment of student knowledge of occupation such as using backward course design, establishing clear learning objectives that target knowledge of occupation, and identifying clear performance criteria for assessing knowledge.

Obtaining Funding

Much of the research conducted in OT requires some funding. Initially, you will likely be operating from smaller pools of money. If you are lucky, your department may offer you start-up funds to get your research program off the ground. In addition, or instead of start-up funds, most universities will have internal sources of funding that allow you to obtain pilot data for your research. You will have to prepare a small grant proposal for these internal funds. It is useful to find a mentor who has experience with the process to assist you with your first submission. Later on, you can use the pilot data from these studies to apply for federal or foundation grants.

Conducting Research

Carrying out a research project takes a lot of organization and planning. As mentioned previously, it is important to create time for yourself during the work week to do the research. This will include time for recruiting participants, collecting data and, if you are conducting an efficacy study, administering some sort of intervention. You may be working with research assistants, possibly students or people who are hired with your grant funding. The research assistants can be very helpful, but they will require training and oversight. After the data collection is complete, you will need to analyze the data. In some instances, this may require the services of a biostatistician. Some colleges will have statisticians available to assist faculty with their research. In other instances, you may find a colleague with statistical expertise that is willing to assist with the process and in doing so is included in the publication.

Disseminating Findings

The two primary ways in which research findings are disseminated is through scholarly presentations and publications. The process of publication is a lengthy one, so you may first present your research at local or national conferences that are interested in your topic. When selecting a conference, you want to consider your intended audience and how best to reach those individuals. The same is true with publications, but in getting your work published there is also the desire to publish in a reputable journal.

In addition to identifying journals that peer review their submissions, you can also consider the **impact factor** of a journal. All journals are required to publish their impact factor on their website. The impact factor represents the average number of times articles in that journal are referenced in peer-reviewed publications.

The process of publication is a humbling one. You should be prepared for your submission to be rejected outright or for the editor to suggest that you revise the article and resubmit. It is extremely rare for an article to be accepted as is with the first submission. Consequently, the opportunity to revise and resubmit a manuscript is encouraging. However, rejection is commonplace and not a reason to give up. There are many journals that publish OT research, so if your manuscript is rejected, it is worthwhile to seek other journals that are relevant to your topic.

Service

Service in academia refers to contributions made by faculty to the university and society as a whole. Faculty members are expected to serve on committees and potentially be involved in other acts of service. It is not only important to do your share of committee work so that you are seen as a collegial faculty member, but it is also important to be mindful of the amount of time you spend in service. Recognize that service is often given less weight for faculty that are on the tenure track.

Department, School/College, and University Committees and Service Work

The committees in academia are charged with specific duties associated with the running of the school. The different levels of committee work include department, school or college, and university. Your involvement in committee work is likely to start at the department level. There are many committees that are common to departments, but there may be some that are unique to your institution. For example, your OT department will have a curriculum committee that determines the philosophy and structure of the department's curriculum, the courses that will be offered, the sequence in which the courses are offered, the congruence between the curriculum and ACOTE standards, and many other concerns related to the department's courses. Other department committees might include admissions, which oversee the selection of the incoming class, and an academic review committee that determines the status of students that are not meeting academic standards. There will also be a curriculum committee at the school or university level that reviews changes in curricula or courses.

Other school or university level committees include the Institutional Review Board, which makes decisions about research that is being conducted at your school; a Faculty Senate, which forms rules and regulation for the governance of the university; and Student Affairs, which considers nonacademic topics such as campus life, student housing, and health and safety of students. More recently, departments and universities have created diversity, equity, and inclusion (DEI) committees that work to create and sustain practices that reflect core values associated with DEI. This is a very small sample of the numerous committees found in an academic setting.

As a faculty member you usually have some input into which committees you would like to serve on. At the department level, depending on the size of the department, there may be some committees that all faculty serve on. For other committees, you can typically negotiate with your chair as to what committees you would like to be assigned to. The university often has a Committee on Committees (yes, that's a real thing), or something like it that identifies faculty interests and makes assignments to the various university committees. Early on you will likely serve as just a member of committees, but eventually you will be expected to take on leadership roles and serve as the chair of some committees. One of the benefits of school and university committees is that you get to work alongside faculty from a variety of departments, many that might be quite different from your own, especially if you work in a large liberal arts university.

Some universities have expectations for community outreach work or clinical practice as components of university service. For example, one university provides interdisciplinary healthcare services to four homeless shelters in the area. A faculty member from each participating department provides coordination and supervision of students. Other universities have OT clinics, and faculty may spend some of their work time within those clinics.

External Service Work

Many faculty are also involved in service work that happens outside of their university environment. For example, you may serve on a committee or in a leadership role in your local- or national-level OT organization. OT faculty are often involved in organizations associated with their areas of interest in research or teaching. For example, a faculty member might serve on the board of an agency that provides services to people with disabilities or act as a consultant for a newly developing OT department. External service work can complement and enhance your research and teaching and for that reason is often desirable for both the faculty member and the university.

Conclusions

With the rapid growth of OT programs in the United States and worldwide, there is a shortage of faculty. This chapter provides a basic introduction to the role of a faculty member, so that you might consider the prospect of working in an academic setting. There are not only many challenges, but also much reward in academia.

Lippincott® Connect *For additional resources on the subjects discussed in this chapter, visit* Lippincott Connect.

REFERENCES

American Association of University Professors. (2006). *1940 statement of principles of academic freedom and tenure – AAUP.* https://www.aaup.org/report/1940-statement-principles-academic-freedom-and-tenure

American Occupational Therapy Association. (2018, November/December). 2018 Accreditation Council for Occupational Therapy Education (ACOTE˚) Standards and Interpretive Guide (effective July 31, 2020). *American Journal of Occupational Therapy, 72* (suppl. 2), 7212410005p1–7212410005p83. https://doi.org/10.5014/ajot.2018.72S217

American Occupational Therapy Association. (2019). *2019 workforce and salary survey.* AOTA Press.

Bain, K. (2004). *What the best college teachers do.* Harvard University Press.

Bloom, B. S. (Ed.). (1956). *Taxonomy of educational objectives: Book 1 cognitive domain.* David McKay.

Crooks, N., Smith, A., & Lofton, S. (2021). Building bridges and capacity for Black, Indigenous, and scholars of color in the era of COVID-19 and Black Lives Matter. *Nursing Outlook, 69*(5), 892–902. https://doi.org/10.1016/j.outlook.2021.03.022

Diamond, R. M. (2008). *Designing and assessing courses and curricula: A practical guide* (3rd ed.). Jossey-Bass.

Fink, D. (2013). *Creating significant learning experiences: An integrated approach to designing college courses* (2nd ed.). Jossey-Bass.

Institute of Education Sciences. (2018). *Race/ethnicity of college faculty.* National Center for Education Statistics. https://nces.ed.gov/fastfacts/display.asp?id=61

Krathwohl, D. R., Bloom, B. S., & Masia, B. B. (1964). *Taxonomy of educational objectives: Book 2 affective domain.* Longman.

Lin, P. S., & Kennette, L. N. (2022). Creating an inclusive community for BIPOC faculty: Women of color in academia. *SN Social Sciences, 2*(11), 246. https://doi.org/10.1007/s43545-022-00555-w

O'Brien, J. G., Millis, B. J., & Cohen, M. W. (2008). *The course syllabus: A learning-centered approach* (2nd ed.). Jossey-Bass.

Plack, M. M., & Driscoll, M. (2017). *Teaching and learning in physical therapy: From classroom to clinic*. Slack.

Price, P., Hooper, B., Krishnagiri, S., Wood, W., Taff, S. D., & Bilics, A. (2021). Toward robust assessments of student knowledge of occupation. *American Journal of Occupational Therapy, 75*(2), 7502205120. https://doi.org/10.5014/ajot.2021.038224

Schaber, P., & Candler, C. (2020). Signature pedagogies and learning designs in occupational therapy education. In S. Taff, L. C. Grajo, & B. R. Hooper (Eds.), *Perspectives on occupational therapy education: Past, present, and future* (pp. 45–53). Slack.

Shulman, L. S. (2005). Signature pedagogies in the professions. *Daedalus, 134*(3), 52–59. https://doi.org/10.1162/0011526054622015

Simpson, E. J. (1972). *The classification of educational objectives in the psychomotor domain*. Gryphon House.

World Federation of Occupational Therapy. (n.d.). *Education*. https://www.wfot.org/programmes/education

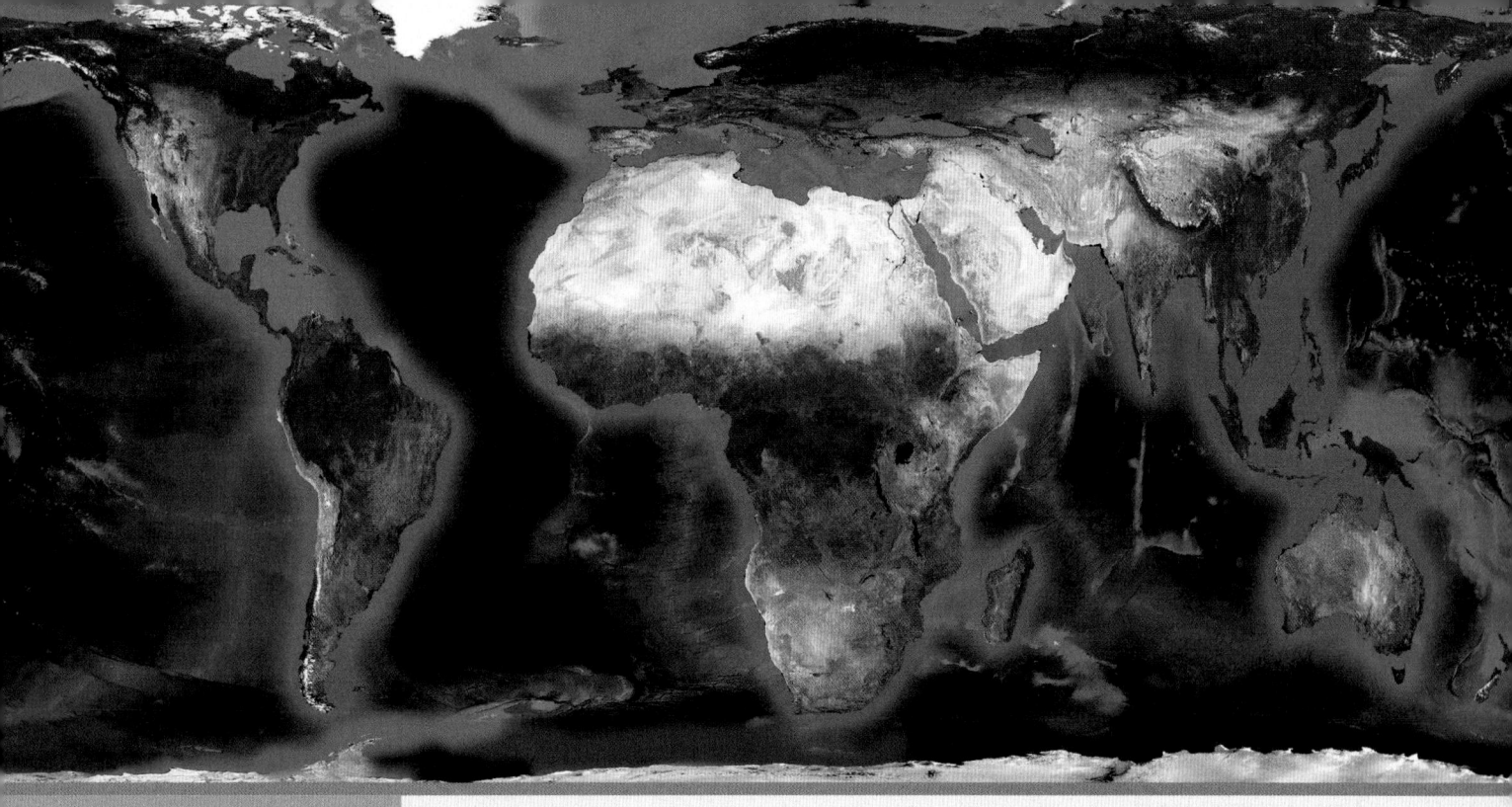

UNIT
XI

Occupational Therapy Management

Media Related to Occupational Therapy Management

Readings

- *Don't Sweat the Small Stuff at Work:* Richard Carlson describes how to stop worrying about the aspects of your work that are beyond your control and interact more effectively and joyfully with colleagues, clients, and managers. (1998)
- *The Coaching Habit: Say Less, Ask More & Change the Way You Lead Forever:* Michael Bungay Stanier's book makes coaching a regular, informal part of your day so managers and their teams can unlock their potential, work less hard, and have more impact. (2016)

Movies

- *Sicko:* Michael Moore looks at healthcare in the United States as provided by profit-oriented health maintenance organizations (HMOs) compared to free, universal care in Canada, the United Kingdom, and France. Moore contrasts US media reports on Canadian care with the experiences of Canadians in hospitals and clinics there.

He interviews patients and doctors in the United Kingdom about cost, quality, and salaries. (2007)

- *Invictus:* The film explains the series of events in South Africa before the 1995 Rugby World Cup and competition. Mandela, the first Black president in South Africa, seeks to end the racial tension in his country through rugby. This movie gives a complete picture of what inspirational leadership is and the heights it can take a team to. (2009)
- *The Desperate Hours: One Hospital's Fight to Save a City on the Pandemic's Front Lines:* Marie Brenner shares a remarkable depiction of New York based on reporting in the New York-Presbyterian Hospital system that captures the resilience, peril, and compassion of the early days of the COVID pandemic. She tells the stories of the those who tried to save lives across the city in secure ICU units, sealed operating rooms, locked executive suites, unknown basement workshops, and makeshift clinics. (2022)

Management of Occupational Therapy Services

Brent Braveman

LEARNING OBJECTIVES

After reading this chapter, you will be able to:

1. Analyze and explain the relationship and differences between administrators, managers, supervisors, and leaders in the oversight of work activities in organizations.
2. Identify and explain examples of the common roles, functions, and responsibilities of managers.
3. Identify and explain the areas of knowledge and skills necessary for a manager to demonstrate competency.

Management Can Mean Many Things

Becoming an occupational therapy (OT) or interdisciplinary manager is just one of the many professional roles that an OT practitioner may assume over their career. Being a "manager" can mean many different things depending on the setting in which you practice, the scope of duties included in your job description, and the related roles and functions assumed by others in that setting. There is a wealth of information to guide management practice, including theory, research and other types of evidence, formal education, continuing education and training, publications, and other scholarly forms. Investigators and practitioners in a variety of disciplines such as organizational development, business psychology, business administration, and human resource management have contributed to this knowledge base over the past decades. Consequently, many resources to guide managers in their jobs are readily available on the Internet, in bookstores, and through educational courses offered at colleges and universities or at continuing education events, such as professional conferences. Resources are also available from the American Occupational Therapy Association (AOTA) and the World Federation of Occupational Therapists (WFOT).

Similar to clinical practice within OT, demonstrating effective practice as an OT manager is dependent on familiarity with the relevant theories and the ability to apply these theories based on the most current evidence. Just as there are multiple clinical practice models that OT practitioners draw on depending on the area of practice and the needs of the client, there are multiple theories and skill sets on which a manager draws to guide effective

	Administration, Management, Supervision, and Leadership Defined
TABLE 73.1	

Function	Definition
Administration	The process of guiding an organization through the authoritative control of others and overseen by the governing body of the organization
Management	The process of guiding a work unit by planning for future work obligations, organizing employees into functional units, directing employees in the process of completing daily work tasks, and controlling work processes and systems to ensure adequate quality of work output
Supervision	The control and direction of the work of one or more employees in a manner that promotes improved performance and a higher quality outcome
Leadership	The process of creating structural change where the values, vision, and ethics of individuals are integrated into the culture of a community as a means of achieving sustainable change

managerial practice. Becoming an effective OT manager is a complicated and time-intensive process. Therefore, this chapter focuses on introducing the reader to the scope of what an OT manager *is* and what an OT manager *does*. Chapter 74 provides a complementary discussion that focuses on supervision and the roles and functions that OT supervisors perform.

In order to truly understand and appreciate the variety of roles and functions that an OT manager can serve, it is critical to recognize that most managers function in ways often described as supervisors and leaders. Table 73.1 provides definitions of administration, management, supervision, and leadership.

An administrator may be defined as a member of a *governing body*, such as a board of directors of an organization; the top officials, such as the president or chief executive officer of an organization; or that official's leadership team. Together, administrators perform the key function of being responsible for the overall welfare and direction of the organization, including oversight of financial affairs, establishing the major policies and procedures that guide operations, and planning for the health and future of the organization. Administrators typically supervise others but usually are only indirectly responsible for the oversight of the day-to-day work of the organization. They frequently delegate authority for much of the day-to-day coordination of organizational functioning to managers.

Managers are responsible for oversight of work units (such as an OT department or a program for head injury

survivors) and of their contributions to the organization's mission. Managers put the policies and directives of administration into action in measurable and visible ways. The specific responsibilities of a manager have been traditionally categorized according to four major functions, which are (a) planning, (b) organizing, (c) directing, and (d) controlling. Staffing is a management function that is sometimes grouped with organizing (e.g., organizing and staffing). These four functions are briefly defined in Table 73.1 and further discussed in the next sections of this chapter.

Supervisors are responsible for direct oversight of employees who perform the work of the organization. Although managers are typically given the ability to decide who becomes part of their work unit through the ability to hire and fire, there are many supervisory roles in organizations that do not perform this or many other functions of the manager. Understanding the important concept of requisite managerial authority can help us to further clarify how an OT manager is different from an organizational administrator or from an OT supervisor. Elliot Jaques (1998) defined minimum requisite managerial authority as the level of control and discretion that a manager must have to be fairly held responsible for the outcomes of work groups (p. 69).

For example, requisite managerial authority includes the authority to hire and fire employees and to determine within reason how rewards are distributed. However, in OT, it is not uncommon for therapists to accept a formally named position within an organization in which they have supervisory responsibilities but do not have requisite managerial authority. An example of such a position would be that of a *senior therapist or senior therapy assistant*—an individual who might have specialized or advanced skills and who might provide clinical supervision to other practitioners but who does not have the full range of managerial responsibilities.

Administrators, managers, and supervisors may often be viewed as *leaders* by virtue of their formally named positions in an organization, although there are typically many informal leaders in organizations as well. One conceptualization of the relationship between management and leadership is that the role of a manager is to maintain stability in the organization, whereas a leader guides change. Effective leadership is a topic that has been the focus of much research, and several leadership theories have been investigated in depth. A brief description of five of the most commonly cited theories of leadership is presented in Table 73.2.

Administrators, managers, and supervisors all perform various tasks related to the four functions of management described in Table 73.3, but the scope of these tasks varies for the different levels of leadership. Table 73.4 provides a comparison of sample functions of administrators, managers, and supervisors organized according to the traditional four functions of management. See OT story 73.1 regarding acclimating as an occupational therapy manager.

| TABLE 73.2 | Common Theories of Leadership |

Theories of Leadership	Primary Focus
Supervisory Theories	
Path–Goal	Leaders increase personal payoffs for subordinates for goal attainment and make the path to these payoffs easier to travel by reducing obstacles, thereby improving performance.
Transactional	Leaders promise rewards and benefits to subordinates for meeting work goals, and leaders and subordinates agree through transactions on what will lead to reward and how to avoid punishment.
Strategic Theories	
Charismatic	Stresses the personal identification of followers with the leader who formulates an inspirational vision and impression that the leader's mission is extraordinary.
Transformational	Leaders achieve change by expressing the value associated with outcomes and by articulating a vision of the future, resulting in commitment, effort, and improved performance on the part of subordinates.
Situational	Leaders should adopt a leadership style that best fits the developmental level of their subordinates' competence and commitment.

OT STORY 73.1 FINDING SOLID GROUND AS AN OCCUPATIONAL THERAPY MANAGER

Ten years after accepting a position as the director of the department of rehabilitation services at a large, internationally renowned cancer research and treatment center, Brent has finally begun to feel that he is standing on solid ground. Thirty-six years earlier in his career, Brent accepted his first management position as the director of OT at a small acute care hospital. In that first job, Brent treated patients half the time and supervised just four OT practitioners. Today, he works full days as a manager and leads a department of over 145 OT and physical therapy practitioners and support staff.

Reflecting on his experiences, Brent realizes that despite the many changes that have occurred in healthcare over 36 years and the differences in size and scope, his current job holds many of the same challenges as his first. In both experiences, he had to (a) manage the expectations, satisfaction, and performance of employees as well as the expectations of patients and those of his boss; (b) navigate complex organizations while promoting the distinct value of OT; (c) promote the development of clinical competencies and the professional development of the therapy practitioners; and (d) develop a variety of skills including human resources, program development and evaluation, continuous quality improvement, financial planning and budgeting, and others.

Questions

As you read this chapter, consider Brent's situation and ask yourself the following questions:

1. What challenges OT managers face no matter how big or small the department they lead?
2. What types of managerial knowledge and skills do all OT managers need to develop?
3. What would be examples of the traditionally identified management functions of planning, organizing, directing, and controlling that most managers perform?
4. What questions can any OT manager ask to guide themselves toward useful management theory and evidence to make their practice as a manager more effective?

| TABLE 73.3 | The Four Traditional Functions of Management |

Function	Definition
Planning	The process of deciding what to do by setting performance goals and identifying the specific objectives and activities that need to be carried out to accomplish these objectives
Organizing	Designing workable units, determining lines of authority and communication, and developing and managing patterns of coordination
Controlling	Providing guidance and leadership so that the work that is performed is congruent with goals
Directing	Establishing performance standards, measuring, evaluating, and correcting performance

TABLE 73.4	Comparisons of Sample Functions of Administrators, Managers, and Supervisors		
Management Function	**Organizational Administration**	**Occupational Therapy Managers**	**Occupational Therapy Supervisors**
Planning	• Establishment of organizational mission and vision • Creation of an organizational culture • Strategic planning • Financial forecasting • Establishing organization policies and procedures	• Interpreting the organizational mission and vision for the staff • Aligning the departmental mission and vision with the organizational mission and vision • Establishing departmental objectives • Creating and implementing the departmental budget • Establishing departmental policies and procedures	• Integration of the mission and vision of the organization and department in the daily work of the department and staff • Oversight of work tasks related to achievement of departmental objectives • Ensuring that work is completed effectively and efficiently
Organizing and staffing	• Oversight of the organizational chart and determination of primary organizational structure • Establishing systems for staff functions such as human resources and marketing[a]	• Recruiting, hiring, orienting, and training staff • Appraising performance, determining rewards, and overseeing disciplinary actions	• Providing management with feedback related to the appropriateness of staffing levels • Provide daily supervision, coaching, and feedback to line staff
Directing	• Development of parameters for staff training, education, and development • Mentoring and coaching middle managers	• Mentoring and coaching supervisors • Implementing staff training, education, and development programs	
Controlling	• Establishing systems to measure organizational performance and achievement of key organizational goals • Setting expectations for performance for management	• Oversight and implementation of departmental continuous quality improvement and quality control systems • Establishing performance expectations and measures for department functions and outputs	• Ensuring compliance with policies and procedures • Measuring and recording quality indicators • Alerting management to systems problems

[a]Staff functions relate to the overall maintenance and management of an organization (e.g., human resources, housekeeping, or marketing). Line functions relate to carrying out the primary work of the organization (e.g., OT, physical therapy, or social work in medically oriented organizations).

The Four Functions of Management

Planning

Planning is the first of four critical functions that managers perform in an organization. Planning is the process of establishing short- and long-term goals, measurable objectives, and action plans that are both congruent with the mission of the organization and consistent with the vision that current organizational leaders have established. An organization's mission is typically established by its founders and remains relatively stable. It is often expressed in the form of a mission statement that sets forth the organization's purpose, products, and services. *Mission statements* succinctly describe (a) why an organization exists or the function the organization performs in society or in a community,

(b) who the organization serves or who its customers are, and (c) an indication of how an organization goes about achieving its purpose.

A *vision statement,* by contrast, expresses an aspirational message about what a department or organization would like to become as it seeks to fulfill its mission. Vision statements are inherently future-oriented and therefore are helpful management tools in long-term planning. Both missions and visions are often communicated in *statements,* but the process itself of developing a mission statement or vision statement can be of tremendous value to an organization.

One example of a mission statement and vision statement are those developed by the University of Texas MD Anderson Cancer Center in Houston, Texas. The mission of the University of Texas MD Anderson Cancer Center is to "eliminate cancer in Texas, the nation, and the world through outstanding programs that integrate patient care, research and prevention, and through education for undergraduate and graduate students, trainees, professionals, employees and the public" (MD Anderson Cancer Center, 2022, para. 1). The vision statement for MD Anderson reads, "We shall be the premier cancer center in the world, based on the excellence of our people, our research-driven patient care and our science. We are Making Cancer History" (MD Anderson Cancer Center, 2022, para. 2).

It is common to distinguish between strategic planning or long-range planning and the shorter term day-to-day planning that most managers complete. Strategic planning is "a deliberative, disciplined effort to produce fundamental decisions and actions that shape and guide what an organization (or other entity) is, what it does, and why" (Bryson et al., 2017, p. 317). Strategic plans are often developed with 3- to 5-year time frames in mind, although hopefully the top leadership of an organization (e.g., administration) is thinking much further into the future. The *goals* included in the strategic plan are a reflection of the scope of the desired outcomes such that they can be broad and encompass the full breadth of organizational activities or they can be more focused on critical segments of an organization. *Objectives* are the measurable steps that are taken to reach each goal. The discreet objectives for each goal are commonly based on a 1-year period that corresponds with an organization's financial cycle, or *fiscal year*. Fiscal years may correspond with a calendar year or may be reflective of some other time cycle such as an academic calendar. It is common for organizations to have fiscal years that begin on July 1st and end on June 30th.

Operating in an environment in which change occurs frequently, such as the healthcare arena, may make long-term planning more difficult than in industries or environments that are more stable. When an organization experiences significant change, the processes of mission review and visioning previously discussed become even more important (Braveman, 2022b). The scholarship on change management has focused on four principal aspects: (a) theoretical models and frameworks that reveal and guide organization members' and researchers' thinking about organization change, (b) approaches and tools for creating and managing change, (c) factors that are important to successful change management, and (d) outcomes and consequences of the process of change management (Errida & Lotfi, 2021; Kuipers et al., 2014). It is strongly recommended that new managers become familiar with theories of change and strategies for promoting successful change. For example, Kurt Lewin (1997) proposed a prominent and relatively simple approach to understanding change still commonly employed today that includes three stages, as shown in Figure 73.1. These three stages are (a) unfreezing or recognizing the need to change, (b) changing, and (c) refreezing or standardizing new procedures or ways of behaving.

Managers can apply this theory by identifying different strategies to use with employees during each of the three

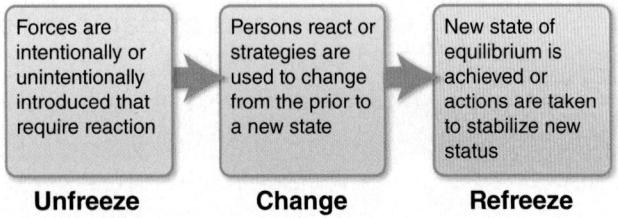

Forces are intentionally or unintentionally introduced that require reaction	Persons react or strategies are used to change from the prior to a new state	New state of equilibrium is achieved or actions are taken to stabilize new status
Unfreeze	**Change**	**Refreeze**

FIGURE 73.1 Lewin's three-stage model of change.

stages to facilitate the change process. Two other theories that are often used to understand change include the following:

- Prochaska and DiClemente's transtheoretical stages of change model, which conceptualizes change in five stages: (a) precontemplation, (b) contemplation, (c) preparation, (d) action, and (5) maintenance (Prochaska, 2020; Del Rio Szupszynski & Ávila, 2021)
- Social cognitive theory, which focuses on change in individuals who can learn by direct experiences, human dialogue and interaction, and observation (Luszczynska & Schwarzer, 2020; University of Twente, 2017)

Although the transtheoretical stages of change model and social cognitive theory have most often been applied to change as it relates to health behaviors, they can also be useful in understanding how humans interpret and respond to change in the workplace.

In addition to establishing goals and objectives, planning includes determining the needs for the human resources, materials, supplies, facilities, and equipment required to meet goals and objectives. Financial planning and budgeting and the writing of policies and procedures that guide the use of materials, supplies, facilities, and equipment are also commonly considered components of planning.

Organizing and Staffing

Typically, an organization's administration will determine the overall structure of the organization, including how line authority will be organized and how employees may be grouped into departments. Organizational structures can vary in complexity. An organizational chart helps to facilitate understanding of an organization's structure. Liebler and McConnell (2017) explain that an organizational chart is a management tool that visually depicts the following aspects of an organization:

- Major functions, usually by department
- Relationships of functions or departments
- Channels of supervision
- Lines of authority and of communication
- Positions by job title within departments or units

When one examines an organizational chart, one must keep in mind that it is a static picture of how the organization is structured at one point in time. It might not reflect recent changes, vacancies, or informal relationships because written charts typically indicate only formal lines of command. Earlier, it was noted that there are many informal leaders in organizations, and these sources of knowledge, power, and influence are not communicated in an organizational chart. The organizational charts of many large organizations support the notion that systems are often quite organic in how they grow and are restructured over time.

Although few large organizations fit the perfect theoretical profile of any formal organizational form or structure, there are a few basic structures commonly found in healthcare and service organizations and systems that are useful for a new manager or practitioner to understand. These structures include the dual-pyramid form of organizing, product line or service line organizations, and hybrid or matrix organizations.

The term *dual pyramid* has been used to describe the common structure found in many medical model settings, such as acute and general hospitals. The pyramid structure is also commonly found in community-based organizations, although the second pyramid representing medical staff might be absent in these cases. A pyramid is typically used to represent an organization of personnel with upper management at the top and line staff at the bottom (Figure 73.2).

In the dual-pyramid form of organizing, the traditional relationship between medical staff and administration results in the structure shown in Figure 73.2, in which two supervisory pyramids are arranged side by side. One pyramid represents the structure of the professional staff that is organized in departments, including administration (with the chief executive officer at the top of the pyramid); health professionals such as occupational therapists, physical therapists, and social workers; and all support services such as engineering, housekeeping, and human resource personnel. A second pyramid mimics that structure but represents the organization of the medical staff with the chief medical officer at the top of the pyramid, department heads as middle management, and staff physicians as line employees (Braveman, 2022b). Although the medical staff, professional staff, and support staff all ultimately report to a board of trustees or board of directors, there are two distinct chains of command that result in the authority and accountability systems being separated. So, for example, physicians, nurses, occupational therapists, and physical therapists all work together as part of an interdisciplinary team. However, the physicians on a particular service (e.g., cardiovascular) report to a department head (also a physician) who reports to the chief medical officer, who in return reports to the chief executive officer. The other members of the team report to a supervisor and/or a department director who in turn may report to a vice president who reports to the same chief executive officer as the chief medical officer.

A second common form of organizational structure is the *product line*, or *service line*, structure. In a product line structure, personnel are organized according to the service or product that they provide rather than according to the specific function that they complete or their departments. A board of directors maintains ultimate authority, and the chief executive officer and chief medical officer often still maintain parallel but distinct responsibilities and authority. An example of the organizational chart for a product line form is provided in Figure 73.3. Additional ways of structuring organizations may combine elements of the dual pyramid and product line structures and may function in a more *matrixed* manner with many interconnections between departments, dual-reporting structures where some employees report to more than one manager, and heavy use of internal consultants.

Each of the methods of organization has advantages and disadvantages, and understanding how structure influences

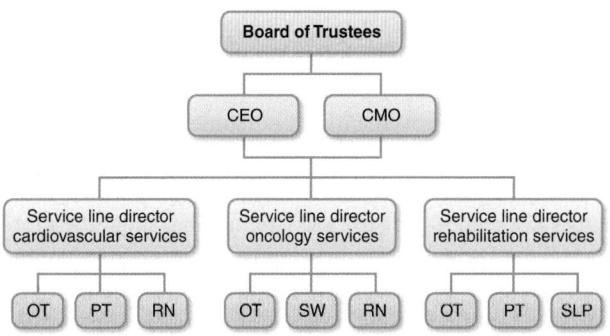

FIGURE 73.3 A sample product line management form of organizing. CEO, chief executive officer; CMO, chief medical officer; OT, occupational therapist; PT, physical therapist; RN, registered nurse; SLP, speech-language pathologist; SW, social worker.

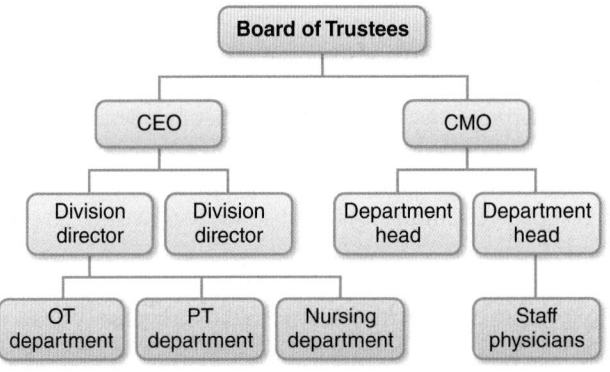

FIGURE 73.2 A sample dual-pyramid form of organizing. CEO, chief executive officer; CMO, chief medical officer; PT, physical therapy.

TABLE 73.5	Advantages and Disadvantages of Common Forms of Organizing	
	Pyramid	**Product Line**
Communication	• Communication within a discipline is facilitated.	• Communication between disciplines becomes harder.
Planning	• Planning for activities such as professional development and clinical supervision is facilitated, but program planning becomes harder.	• Program planning and planning for interdisciplinary activities such as program evaluation is facilitated, but planning functions within disciplines becomes harder.
Budgeting	• Tracking and planning for finances related to single-discipline costs are facilitated, but tracking and planning for interdisciplinary activities (e.g., cost per unit of care) are harder.	• Tracking and planning for finances related to programmatic costs are facilitated (e.g., cost per unit of care), but tracking and planning for discipline-specific activities are harder.
Staffing	• Some needs such as providing coverage for leaves or vacancies may be easier, but the need to communicate with other managers increases. Recruitment activities are facilitated.	• Staffing activities influenced by other disciplines such as scheduling programmatic elements may be facilitated, but coverage for leaves or vacancies becomes more difficult. Recruitment of staff may be more difficult, or you might need to rely on managers from other disciplines for assistance.
Process improvement, program evaluation, and outcomes	• Improving discipline-specific processes is easier as is measuring single-discipline outcomes and indicators of program evaluation, but interdisciplinary programs require extra effort.	• Improving interdisciplinary or program processes is easier, as is measuring program outcomes and indicators of program evaluation, but discipline-specific elements require extra effort.
Professional development	• Development of discipline-specific skills related to assessment and intervention may be facilitated by the ease of access to disciplinary specialists.	• Development of interdisciplinary skills related to the needs of a population or program development or implementation may be facilitated.

the function of an organization can help one to capitalize on the system's benefits and compensate for its limitations. For example, healthcare organizations that have a dual-pyramid structure rely on departments structured by discipline or professional education and training to provide for strong supervision of staff and their clinical performance. Thus, communication within a professional discipline is facilitated, and the discipline-specific daily work of a unit may be completed more efficiently. Because a department manager or supervisor representing each discipline has direct access to staff and to the data related to routine processes and interventions, performance improvement and outcome measurement using these data may also be easier in a dual-pyramid organization. Nonetheless, in this form of organizing, communication across disciplines (e.g., from OT to nursing) might be more complicated, which can pose potential hazards for developing and managing new programs. Problem-solving and process improvement in existing programming can be cumbersome when staff members feel that it is necessary to communicate up through the chains of command. The advantages and disadvantages of the dual pyramid and the product line forms of organizing are summarized in Table 73.5.

Once decisions have been made about how an organization or a department is to be structured, administrators and managers ideally work together to develop plans for staffing and human resources management. Functions related to recruitment and staffing, such as advertising job vacancies or the development of policies and procedures related to employment, may be performed by a human resources department. OT managers are frequently involved in a number of other staffing-related activities. The following is a list of some of these activities:

- *Human resources planning:* Collaborating with administrators and supervisors at all levels of the organization to forecast the short- and long-term personnel needs of the organization based on the organizational mission, leadership vision, and strategic plans
- *Recruitment:* Seeking out and attracting adequate numbers of diverse, qualified personnel to meet ongoing organizational needs, including contingencies, such as resignations and leaves of absence for medical or personal reasons
- *Hiring:* Selecting the appropriate personnel for vacant positions and activities related to the hiring process, such as benefits counseling and overseeing background and reference checks
- *Orientation:* Introducing the new employee to organizational policies, benefits, procedures, values, personnel, and environments

- *Training and development:* Meeting the short- and long-term educational and professional development needs of employees at all levels of the organization
- *Separation:* Terminating the employment of personnel because of resignation or inadequate job performance or that which may come about as the result of a decrease in organizational resources

Maintaining a viable workforce by retaining a diverse, qualified, and competent staff is perhaps one of the most important functions of the manager for an organization. Retention of staff can also be very difficult in professions such as OT and physical therapy where much of the workforce is young and mobile, and the demand for staff far outnumbers the supply. Maintaining staff satisfaction and retention of staff are two areas where the OT manager can benefit from considerable research and evidence (Bolding et al., 2021; Eckhaus, 2021; Mertala et al., 2021). Similar to the topics of leadership and change, an in-depth discussion of theories related to staff retention and satisfaction are beyond the scope of this chapter, and managers would benefit from a thorough review of contemporary literature. A few examples of theories that have evolved regarding employee satisfaction and retention are the following:

- Self-determination theory, which explores the relationship of intrinsic and extrinsic motivators to work motivation (MacDonald & Zitomer, 2021)
- Need theories such as Maslow's hierarchy of needs and McClelland's need theory that focus on identifying physiologic and psychological needs of employees with the rationale that satisfying these needs will lead to employee satisfaction (Acquah et al., 2021)
- Expectancy theory, which holds that people are motivated to behave in ways that produce expected and desired combinations of outcomes (Zeb et al., 2021)

Directing

Directing is the management function that involves giving guidance, instruction, and leadership to subordinates so that work that is performed is goal-oriented and contributes to meeting organizational or departmental requirements. More specifically, a manager could assign and manage the workload, develop and implement policies and procedures to guide others in uniform completion of their work, provide mentoring and coaching for improved future performance, and appraise performance by providing feedback to employees about current performance.

Managing the workload is a complicated and multistep process that involves projecting the amount of work to be done, determining which resources are necessary to complete the work, and managing these resources to make certain that the appropriate person with the right skills and right equipment and space is available when needed. The

workload is typically projected on a yearly basis as part of planning a departmental budget, but it may also be done on a week-to-week, day-to-day, or even hourly basis. Effective workload management requires flexibility, creativity, a commitment to planning, and advanced problem-solving skills.

Writing policies and procedures to guide staff in their daily tasks in a standardized manner, as well as their use of materials, supplies, facilities, and equipment in ways that are compliant with accreditation and other standards, is a specific aspect of directing that is typically the responsibility of a department manager. Policies are statements of values that are congruent with the organizational or departmental mission and justify the boundaries that govern the services provided. They set parameters for making decisions about day-to-day operations. Procedures outline the specific tasks that should be completed or that provide specific direction about how a policy should be implemented. A manager should not only be able to cite a policy or procedure but also be able to give the underlying logic for the policy's existence.

Most organizations follow a prescribed standard format that guides managers in deciding what to include in a department's policy and procedure manual. If a policy and procedure format is not provided, the organization may purchase existing customizable resources on the Internet. It is typical for managers to network with others, both locally and nationally, and most managers will freely share nonproprietary information such as a policy and procedure. The basic components of a policy and procedure protocol are presented in Box 73.1.

Managers also serve as mentors, coaches, and appraisers of overall work performance; resources to develop the skills and knowledge necessary for these functions should be sought out both from within the profession of OT and from outside of it. The AOTA has a number of resources related to supervisory tasks specific to occupational therapy assistants (OTAs) or to OT aides (http://www.aota.org). For more generic information on models of supervision, theories of motivating others, developing effective performance appraisal systems, or providing effective mentoring or coaching, managers should look outside the OT literature. For example, associations such as the American Management Association (http://www.amanet.org) or the National Association for Employee Recognition (http://www.recognition.org/) provide resources about how one may become an effective supervisor. See OT story 73.2 related to developing skills around the concepts of Justice, Equity, Diversity, and Inclusion (JEDI).

Controlling

Controlling is a management function that relates to the processes of establishing specific work performance standards and the measurement, evaluation, and correction of performance. A key responsibility of managers is to promote the delivery of appropriate intervention through the use of quality control (QC) mechanisms and performance

---

BOX 73.1 BASIC COMPONENTS OF A POLICY AND PROCEDURE

Organizations often have policy manuals either in print or stored online. Manuals consist of many policies and related procedure statements, each of which typically includes the component listed below.

- Policy statement(s): brief statements of the guiding principles to be communicated
- Purpose statement(s): brief statements that outline the reasons for inclusion of the policies or procedures
- Applicability: lists the employee groups to which the policy and procedure applies (e.g., all occupational therapy [OT] department staff members)

- Procedures: statements outlining the specific actions to be taken by the identified employee groups and criteria for determining adherence to the policy
- Responsibility: identifying the individuals who are responsible for oversight of the policy and procedure (e.g., all OT team leaders)
- Review period: lists the date of the last review and update of the policy and procedures (typically, policies and procedures are reviewed on an annual basis)

OT STORY 73.2 A MANAGER LEARNS MORE ABOUT JUSTICE, EQUITY, DIVERSITY, AND INCLUSION (JEDI)

Shammi is a manager and the director of a mid-sized department of rehabilitation services. She has assumed that her staff perceive her, the rest of her leadership team, and the department staff in general to be inclusive and respectful of diversity. Her leadership team and staff are made up of leaders from diverse racial and ethnic backgrounds and she is a member of the LGBTQIA+ community. Given this, she was surprised that on a recent organization-wide employee satisfaction survey, her department scored below the organizational mean on the question, "I work in an environment that is free of discrimination and offensive behavior."

Shammi and her leadership team took several steps to learn more about the experiences of her staff. They developed and distributed an anonymous feedback survey asking staff to describe behavior that they encountered that they perceived as discriminatory or offensive. They developed a Justice, Equity, Diversity, and Inclusion (JEDI) Committee that was chaired by a member of the staff. Finally, they included questions about discrimination and offensive behavior in employee rounding meetings, which are short face-to-face meetings between leadership team members and staff to provide an opportunity for feedback.

Shammi learned that many members of the department had encountered discriminatory and offensive language in staff offices and break rooms. Microaggressions or incidents of subtle discriminatory language were not uncommon. Two examples provided were (1) staff hearing, "That is so Gay" and (2) reported being told, "You speak great English for someone from India." In response, Shammi and her leadership team developed several mandatory online learning modules that described the desired culture of the department regarding JEDI, introduced staff to microaggressions and other discriminatory and offensive behavior, and presented strategies for responding when encountering these situations. Shammi was pleased that the staff responded positively to these actions but decided that continued attention was necessary. She hoped to see more positive results on the next employee satisfaction survey.

Questions

1. Has Shammi taken effective steps to respond to her current situation?
2. What additional strategies would you recommend to Shammi to help her further promote JEDI in her department?

---

improvement (PI), which is sometimes also called continuous quality improvement (CQI). The QC and PI are related functions, but each serves a different purpose and relies on different philosophies, strategies, tools, and techniques. The focus of QC is to intervene when the quality or quantity of work output falls below predetermined measures (indicators). The focus of PI is to improve customer satisfaction by constantly striving to meet customer expectations

through enhancing critical processes. A critical process is defined as any process that is performed to produce the work of an organization. Examples of OT critical processes include responding to referrals for service, administering assessments, fabricating adaptive equipment, and making postdischarge referrals. PI projects may be complex and time-intensive because they rely on decision-making based on data and therefore require an organized and structured

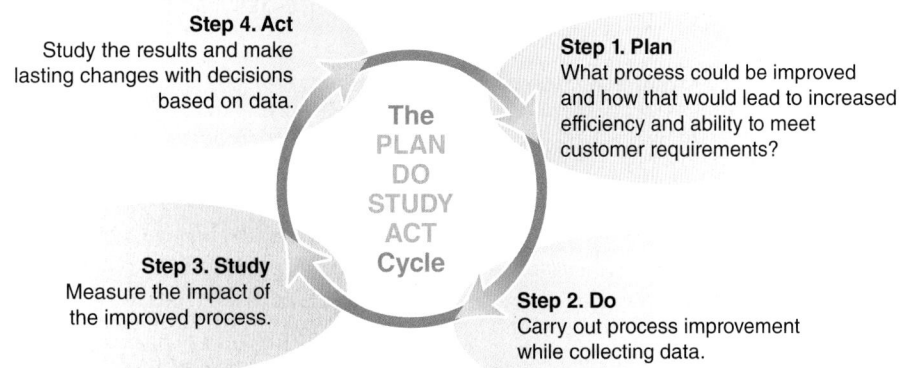

FIGURE 73.4 The Plan, Do, Study, Act (PDSA) cycle.

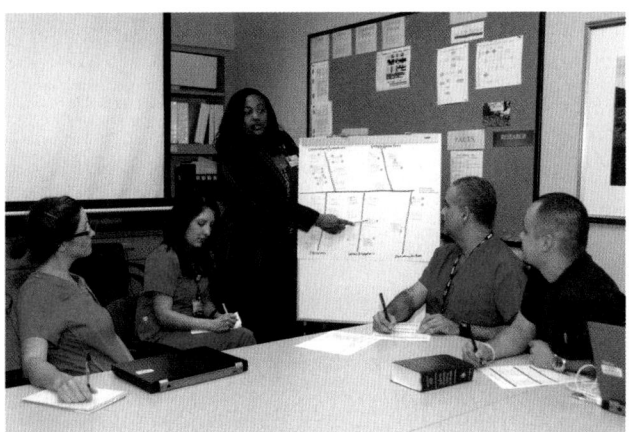

FIGURE 73.5 Staff members complete a cause-and-effect diagram to identify potential root causes of a problem as part of a formal performance improvement project.

approach to gathering and analyzing data. Explaining PI in depth is beyond the scope of this chapter, but Figure 73.4 provides a brief overview of commonly identified steps to choose a critical process and implementing steps that improve its performance. The Plan, Do, Study, Act (PDSA) cycle may be invoked under other names or acronyms, but the steps of the PI process remain constant (Figure 73.5). The most common tools and techniques and their uses are presented in Table 73.6.

Financial Management

An important function of most managers is the planning and controlling of a department budget. Budgets are typically planned for a calendar year or a fiscal year (e.g., many organizations operate on a fiscal year that runs from July 1 to June 30). The process of planning and managing a budget

TABLE 73.6 Common Process Improvement Concepts, Tools, and Techniques

	Use/Importance/Summary
Core Concepts	
The Plan, Do, Study, Act (PDSA) cycle	The overarching framework for guiding and ordering process improvement activities
Critical processes	The important processes that are repeated again and again to complete the organization's or department's work
Operational definitions	A quantifiable description of what to measure and the steps to follow to measure it consistently
Customers and customer requirements	Identifying internal and external customers or individuals who receive the output of your work and their valid requirements
Quality indicators	Quantitative measures of compliance to valid customer requirements
Variation	The spread of process output over time; discriminating between natural "common cause" variation that is inherent in a process and the uncommon "special cause" variation that you want to eliminate from a process or emulate if positive
Strategies	
Ground rules for meetings	Explicit agreements about how a team will work together and behave as team members
Roles for effective meetings	Assigning roles such as the leader, scribe, facilitator, and timekeeper can lead to more effective meetings

(continued)

TABLE 73.6	Common Process Improvement Concepts, Tools, and Techniques (*continued*)
	Use/Importance/Summary
Consensus	A method for reaching agreement whereby all members agree to fully support a decision even if it is not how they would act if they were acting alone
Tools	
Process flowcharts	A visual representation of the steps in a process used to highlight redundancies, rework, or bottlenecks
Control charts	A chart with statistically determined upper and lower control limits used to determine whether a process has changed and to highlight variation
Cause-and-effect diagrams	A tool to assist in determining possible root causes to a problem
Proposed options matrix	A tool for comparing possible options for action against a set of predetermined criteria
Techniques	
Data stratification	Methods for categorizing collection of data; it is important to decide how to stratify data before you collect it
Designing an effective data collection tool	Tools to gather facts on how a process works or its effectiveness that allows for accurate collection of data in the simplest manner
Balancing tasks and people	Attending to both the needs of team members and the work to be completed to maintain team motivation
Icebreakers	Short activities to help team members learn about each other or to become more comfortable interacting with each other
Brainstorming	A method for creatively generating lists of possible causes of problems, solutions, or processes to improve
Multivoting	A decision-making method to narrow a larger number of options to a number that can be reasonably discussed individually

requires that a manager have a comprehensive understanding of the goals and objectives of the larger organization so that he or she can establish priorities for funding that support this mission over time.

OT practitioners who want to become managers or directors of an OT department or to own and operate their own businesses are encouraged to learn financial planning and management and to become well versed in the use of information management technologies, such as spreadsheets or other financial management tools. Braveman (2022a) notes that effective financial planning and management requires a working knowledge of the following:

- Healthcare systems, including city, county, state, and national systems
- Payment and reimbursement structures, such as Medicare, Medicaid, Workers' Compensation, private insurance, and grants or foundation support
- Human resources systems and costs, including salary and benefit administration, training and educational costs and systems, and recruitment and retention structures
- Equipment and materials purchasing and management, including medical supplies such as splinting or assistive and adaptive equipment, office supplies, and other supportive supplies
- Facilities management, maintenance, and improvement protocols, including cleaning and maintenance of physical plant structures

Budgets may also include revenue and expenses, although it is not uncommon for a community-based organization manager to have oversight of only expenses with no control over direct sources of revenue. Typically, the revenues and expenses associated with each department in an organization are given some sort of marker or code in the organization's accounting system that indicates how the subset of revenues and expenses relate to that department. These subsets of revenues and expenses are commonly referred to as *cost centers*. They may represent the budget of a single department or of several related services. Common examples of revenues and expenses are shown in Table 73.7 and are further explained in the following section.

Forecasting revenue requires that the manager be able to accurately predict the volume of work that a department will deliver and how that work will happen. In some settings, almost all OT intervention is provided to consumers on a one-to-one basis, whereas in some settings, intervention is provided in groups, and elsewhere, there can be a combination. There can be great pressure on OT managers to forecast revenue accurately and to increase revenue by increasing productivity demands. This can sometime lead to ethical dilemmas.

Regulations regarding group treatment or treating more than one patient at a time have changed over time, and managers must remain current in their understanding of regulations regarding billing and coding of services. By accurately predicting the total volume of work for a year,

TABLE 73.7	Examples of Revenues and Expenses
Revenues	**Expenses**
Individual 15 minutes: ADL treatment	Variable expense—salary
Individual 15 minutes: cognitive remediation	Variable expense—wages
Individual 15 minutes: community reintegration	Variable expense—office supplies
Individual 15 minutes: neuromuscular facilitation	Variable expense—splinting supplies
Group 15 minutes: home management	Fixed expense—phone
Group 15 minutes: communication skills	Fixed expense—rent
Group 15 minutes: community reintegration	Fixed expense—utilities

ADL, activities of daily living.

managers are able to predict the total gross revenue by multiplying the number of work units (e.g., a 15-minute unit of therapy) by the charge for each unit of service. It is important to note that in the current managed care environment, few payers reimburse at the full rate that is billed, and the net revenue, or the amount of revenue after all discounts to insurers and nonreimbursed charges are accounted for, is typically much less than gross revenue.

Expenses typically include costs associated with personnel, supplies, facilities management, and equipment. As part of the process of forecasting the expense budget, managers determine the number of full-time equivalent (FTE) employees that will be required to handle the projected work volume. Generally, an FTE represents an employee who will be paid 2,080 hours in a year (i.e., 40 hours $\times$ 52 weeks). Setting productivity standards (e.g., the amount of work a practitioner is expected to perform in a given period such as a day or week) and helping staff to meet such standards is a common challenge faced by OT managers. Personnel expenses can include salary expenses for professional staff who are exempt from the labor laws that require an organization to pay extra for overtime effort and wages for support staff who are nonexempt. Occupational therapists are often categorized as exempt, and OTAs and OT aides are often categorized as nonexempt.

Nonpersonnel expenses such as supplies, equipment, food, phone, continuing education, or travel allowances must also be projected. In private businesses, expenses for utilities and rent must also be considered. These expenses are categorized as either fixed or variable expenses. Fixed expenses are costs that are not directly influenced by changes in client volume, such as expenses budgeted for employee continuing education, heating costs, or monthly rent if space is leased. Variable expenses are those that are directly influenced by changes in client volume. For example, you may use more of some types of office supplies, food used for meal preparation activities, or splinting or medical supplies if patient volumes rise and less if they are lower. Although there might not always be a direct correlation, over time, one will be able to estimate how an increase or decrease in volume might affect expenses.

To effectively plan and control a budget, managers must learn many useful concepts and strategies. Some organizations may provide training or orientation for new managers, but, most often, it is assumed that a new manager understands the basic information needed to develop and oversee a budget. People who are assuming their first management position would benefit from additional education or training in financial management and from networking with experienced managers. The AOTA provides networking opportunities such as the professional networking site *CommunOT* and resources for managers through its Administration & Management Special Interest Section (AMSIS). More information on AMSIS, *CommunOT*, and other resources can be found at http://www.aota.org. OT associations in other countries should be consulted for resources relevant to OT management in systems outside the United States.

Technology and Management

The technological advances in medicine, information management, communication, and related areas that have occurred over the last few decades are astounding. Managers must evaluate and integrate a wide range of technology into their departments, ranging from computer software programs to clinical equipment, such as driving simulators or environmental controls. Choosing and successfully integrating a new technology requires that managers synthesize information, including costs of initial purchase, maintenance, space, and training requirements and the rate at which the specific technology is advancing so that an estimate can be made of when the current technology may become outdated.

One major area of technology used by managers is that employed in information management, which includes the use of computers for documentation, billing, and financial management as well as data collection and analysis for outcomes management. Table 73.8 lists common types of data

TABLE 73.8   Common Types of Data, Sources, and Possible Uses

Types of Data	Sources	Uses
Demographics (age, sex, educational level, etc.)	• Admissions records • Public data sets	• Program planning • Program evaluation
Revenue (payer source, rates, discounts)	• Accounting • Budget reports	• Budgeting • Program planning
Expense (accounts payable)	• Financial reports • Purchasing records	• Budgeting • Program planning and evaluation
Payroll (salary, benefits, leave usage)	• Accounting • Budget reports	• Staffing plans • Recruitment and retention
Productivity (visits, staff activity)	• Automated charge systems • Department billing records or productivity tracking sheets	• Staffing plans • Performance appraisal • Recruitment
Personnel (licensure, competencies, professional development, performance)	• Human resources • Departmental personnel files • Professional association data sets	• Accreditation visits • Staffing plan development • Professional development plans
Clinical (diagnosis, intervention, outcomes)	• Medical records • Outcome databases	• Process improvement • Program evaluation
Legal (contracts, leases)	• Legal or grants and contracts department	• Facility planning

and information that must be collected and managed and their possible uses. Becoming skilled at the use of common software programs such as managing a spreadsheet to organize and analyze the large amount of data available to most managers has become a common expectation of most managers.

Marketing

OT managers are often responsible for assessing the needs of the target populations served by their department or organization; determining programmatic strategies for meeting these needs; designing, implementing, and evaluating the interventions to meet identified needs; and promoting the intervention to consumers, payers, physicians, and others. These processes, collectively, are called *marketing*. Traditionally, the following four steps are identified in the marketing process:

- *Organizational assessment*: Examination of the factors within an organization that will influence the development and promotion of a new product or service
- *Environmental assessment*: Examination of the data and other forms of evidence, including the needs of the target population that will guide the development and promotion of a new product or service
- *Market analysis*: Use of the information gained during organizational and environmental assessments to validate perceptions of the wants and needs of the target populations that will receive a new product or service
- *Marketing communications*: Packaging and promoting a product so the target populations and other key

stakeholders in the new product or service have a clear understanding of what the product or service is and how it may be accessed

In larger organizations, other professionals, such as members of a marketing department, often perform portions of the marketing process such as collecting demographic and other data about potential consumers or may be called on to collaborate with a manager to perform these functions. However, OT managers who are also business owners or who work in community-based, nonprofit organizations might need to learn the marketing process in greater depth. These managers benefit from establishing effective networks with other managers and becoming active in professional organizations, such as their state and national OT associations, diversity organizations, and business-oriented groups such as the local chamber of commerce.

Who Should Be a Manager?

Over the last two decades, numerous professions have addressed managerial competencies with increasing urgency and concern, emphasizing the need to determine the initial competence of health professionals, to assess specific job competencies as professionals are hired and begin to work, and to promote the professionals' continuing development of competence (Henry & Braveman, 2022). The assessment of initial competency and facilitation of continuing development of staff competency is a function of the OT manager.

Before assuming a role as an OT manager, one should assess one's own level of preparedness to perform the tasks associated with the role. Although the assessment of competencies for managers has not received the same attention by certifying or regulatory bodies such as accrediting agencies, competency development and assessment have been addressed, and some empirical investigations of managerial competencies have been conducted by a number of professions (Henry & Braveman, 2022).

Some competencies might be considered "universal" for managers. One method of identifying managerial competence is to compare their performance against the "yardstick" of previously described traditional managerial functions (e.g., planning, organizing and staffing, directing, controlling). As a guide for this process, each of the management functions is listed subsequently with sample areas for assessment of competency provided for each. (See Box 73.2 for additional areas, for development of competencies.)

Other managerial competencies will depend on the nature of the manager's job. Not all managers perform the same tasks and functions, so it is important that before accepting a management position, one understands what will be expected of one and have done a thorough assessment of readiness by identifying strengths and areas in which help might be needed.

BOX 73.2 SAMPLE AREAS FOR ASSESSMENT OF COMPETENCY FOR MANAGERS

Planning

- Use of goal setting
- Financial management skills
- Understanding the changing healthcare environment

Organizing and staffing

- Understanding team structure and flexible work design
- Designing and leading effective teams
- Applying coordination techniques

Directing

- Interpersonal competencies
- Communication skills

- Communicating with the boss
- Communicating with peers and others
- Communicating with employees
- Being politically astute
- Managing conflict
- Managing diversity

Role model competencies

- Demonstrating professionalism in conduct and demeanor
- Enhancing technical competence

Controlling

- Empowering employees
- Applying continuous quality improvement efforts

COMMENTARY ON THE EVIDENCE

The State of Evidence Related to Management

Decades of evidence on management theory, effective managerial strategies, and practices have been produced by multiple disciplines and fields such as business, organizational development, organizational psychology, social work, and nursing. The topics that have been investigated are quite diverse; examples include effective leadership strategies, performance appraisal processes, factors affecting recruitment and retention, effective recognition and reward structures, change management, and performance improvement.

A variety of forms of evidence, including the results of empirical studies, program descriptions, and descriptions of managerial interventions, are published widely in a range of professional journals, websites, and books.

Although the body of evidence specifically related to management in healthcare organizations might be more limited, it is growing, and OT managers who wish to use an *evidence-based* approach to management will benefit from research and science conducted by other disciplines such as those mentioned.

Particularly in the last decade, there has been a movement toward discussions of *evidence-based management* as the role of evidence in guiding decision-making has become more prevalent in healthcare and other industries. However, caution has been advised to address the worry that application of evidence can become too rote and prescriptive. For example, Arndt and Bigelow (2009, p. 206) cautioned that managers should use all available information and data when planning and implementing decisions, and evidence from research should play a

(continued)

role in that. At the same time, in a turbulent and uncertain environment, creativity and risk-taking also will be important, and unanticipated outcomes may result from, among other factors, limits on human cognition, unknowable differences in initial conditions in organizations, and adaptive responses to change as it is implemented.

Current trends in management research include efficient and effective use of technology, including the electronic health record, change management, personalization of care, workforce diversity and safety, cost-effectiveness strategies, and managing access to care (Economist Intelligence, 2021; Martin, 2021). For an additional viewpoint, see Expanding Our Perspectives.

Although OT managers can certainly make valuable judgments by generalizing from evidence produced in other disciplines, the profession would benefit from research specifically related to OT. Questions for investigation might include the following:

- How will healthcare reform and other societal influences affect the profession?
- How might OT managers influence the delivery of culturally responsive services as we have become more globally connected?
- What are the most effective strategies for retaining OT practitioners within the profession across the life course to prevent attrition from the discipline?

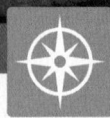

EXPANDING OUR PERSPECTIVES

Facilitating JEDI-based Management Practice

Arameh Anvarizadeh

As an OT practitioner, educator, and leader, one of my core values is providing culturally responsive care no matter the setting. Prioritizing justice, equity, diversity, and inclusion (JEDI) as the gold standard and having my team practice this is the ultimate goal to maximize the quality of life for all people, populations, and communities. Addressing barriers, having difficult conversations, advocating for resources, and working through implicit bias are just a few essential leadership skills every manager should strive for as they build and maintain diverse and influential teams.

One aspect of managing with a JEDI lens is recognizing where health disparities persist and identifying the barrier to provide access in bridging those gaps. I recall managing a fieldwork department at an OT educational program. When I started the position, the fieldwork department was pretty new, only having a few fieldwork contracts and only having placed one very small cohort. My job was to grow the department by solidifying more sites, developing relationships with fieldwork educators, placing students at fieldwork sites, and teaching all fieldwork courses. I also had the task of establishing a fieldwork team to help support the department's needs. Managing hundreds of sites, students, and a team was incredibly demanding yet immensely rewarding to see my students and team thrive.

One of the areas we were committed to growing were nontraditional fieldwork sites that served marginalized communities. These sites needed OT services but did not know they needed them or did not have funding to provide them. As a leader/manager, being innovative takes vision, courage, and skill to assess the marginalized community's needs and then create culturally responsive interventions that address their occupational performance.

One example of fostering access is building a relationship with a women's emergency shelter and transitional housing facility in the heart of Los Angeles, California. This shelter provides a safe, structured living environment that empowers and encourages individuals and families to move from dependence to independence through comprehensive, supportive services. Providing OT services, advocating for funding, and developing daily interventions were strategic ways to decrease barriers and increase access for a marginalized community. By sharing the vision with the team and teaching the students to be creative, culturally humble, and provide best practice, we were able to see positive client outcomes and increased satisfaction in occupational performance. Not only did the students learn how to provide OT in a nontraditional setting, but the women in the emergency shelter were also able to accomplish so many meaningful goals, such as building a garden. Their garden served as a way to identify healthier food options, leading them to cook more nutritious meals. It was also an opportunity for developing their entrepreneurial and money management skills.

As a leader, seeing the vision through is critical, but recognizing there will be pushback while managing several individuals and creating new systems is key. The easy way would be to continue securing sites that already existed and that were traditional. The challenge, which is the part that truly tests your leadership/managerial skills, is finding the need, creating the opportunity, and taking the leap to execute the plan. First, empowering my team by sharing the vision of the significance of serving marginalized communities was essential because it aligned everyone to the ultimate goal. Then, accomplishing tasks such as creating a budget, making an OT curriculum, getting buy-in from the university, identifying an occupational therapist to supervise the students, and developing a long-term plan to remain at the site are examples of a manager leading with a clear vision and purpose. Moreover, especially when working with and advocating for marginalized communities, being equipped to address implicit and unconscious bias, microaggressions, oppressive language, and discrimination are critical issues to navigate and communicate with your team and stakeholders. Creating nontraditional fieldwork sites, such as providing OT at the women's transitional home, is just one example of

a manager's impact on innovating and leading a team to bridge health disparity gaps and uplift marginalized communities through OT services.

Whether managing a rehab unit or a community-based nonprofit organization, every team member should feel seen and heard. By focusing on the team's strengths and emphasizing their value, managers can home in on the power and significance of having a diverse staff. Furthermore, as a manager, having the skills outlined in this chapter is essential for successfully running a facility or program. However, in addition to those skills, it is also vital to always consider a JEDI lens and be an advocate when disparities are present. By managing in this way, you can positively impact healthcare disparities, address the occupational needs of marginalized communities, and be a role model to your team in providing culturally responsive care.

Conclusion

This chapter has provided an overview of the numerous tasks, functions, and responsibilities that an OT manager may perform. Readers are encouraged to appreciate the variety and complexities of a manager's responsibilities and the need for a beginning manager to get appropriate training and education. Managers work closely with the administrators and supervisors in large organizations, but small business owners and entrepreneurs also function independently as managers. Fortunately, many resources are available that are specific to OT managers, and more resources may be found in other fields, including business, psychology, and organizational development, that are useful guides for a manager performing his or her job.

Lippincott® Connect *For additional resources on the subjects discussed in this chapter, visit Lippincott Connect.*

REFERENCES

Acquah, A., Nsiah, T. K., Antie, E. N. A., & Otoo, B. (2021). Literature review on theories of motivation. *EPRA International Journal of Economic and Business Review, 9*(5), 25–29. https://doi.org/10.36713/epra2012

Arndt, M., & Bigelow, B. (2009). Evidence-based management in health care organizations: A cautionary note. *Health Care Management Review, 34,* 206–213. https://doi.org/10.1097/HMR.0b013e3181a94288

Bolding, D. J., McCallister, C., Poisson, K., Pufki, D. M., Ramirez, A., Rickly, C., & Scattini, V. (2021). Incivility in the occupational therapy workplace: A survey of practitioners. *American Journal of Occupational Therapy, 75*(3), 7503205020p1–7503205020p8. https://doi.org/10.5014/ajot.2021.046698

Braveman, B. (Ed.). (2022a). Roles and functions of managers: Planning, organizing, controlling and directing. In *Leading and managing occupational therapy services: An evidence-based approach* (pp. 187-216). F. A. Davis.

Braveman, B. (Ed.). (2022b). Understanding and working within organizations. In *Leading and managing occupational therapy services: An evidence-based approach* (pp. 186–216). F. A. Davis.

Bryson, J. M., Edwards, L. H., & Van Slyke, D. M. (2017). Getting strategic about strategic planning research. *Public Management Review, 20*(3), 317–339. http://www.tandfonline.com/doi/abs/10.1080/14719037.2017.1285111

Del Rio Szupszynski, K.P., de Ávila, A.C. (2021). The Transtheoretical Model of Behavior Change: Prochaska and DiClemente's Model. In Andrade, A.L.M., De Micheli, D., Silva, E.A.d., Lopes, F.M., Pinheiro, B.d.O., Reichert, R.A. (eds.), Psychology of Substance Abuse. Springer, Cham. https://doi.org/10.1007/978-3-030-62106-3_14

Eckhaus, E. (2021). The fourth dimension of happiness and work satisfaction. *Management & Marketing. Challenges for the Knowledge Society, 16*(2), 118–133. https://doi.org/10.2478/mmcks-2021-0008

Economist Intelligence. (2021). *Healthcare in 2022.* https://www.eiu.com/n/campaigns/healthcare-in-2022/

Errida, A., & Lotfi, B. (2021). The determinants of organizational change management success: Literature review and case study. *International Journal of Engineering Business Management, 13,* 18479790211016273. https://doi.org/10.117/18479790211016273

Henry, T., & Braveman, B. (Ed.). (2022). Assessing and promoting clinical and managerial competency. In *Leading and managing occupational therapy services: An evidence-based approach* (pp. 379–410). F. A. Davis.

Jaques, E. (1998). *Requisite organization.* Cason Hall.

Kuipers, B. S., Higgs, M., Kickert, W., Tummers, L., Grandia, J., & Van der Voet, J. (2014). The management of change in public organizations: A literature review. *Public Administration, 92,* 1–20. https://doi.org/10.1111/padm.12040

Lewin, K. (1997). *Resolving social conflict and field theory in social sciences.* American Psychological Association.

Liebler, J. G., & McConnell, C. R. (2017). *Management principles for health professionals* (7th ed.). Jones & Bartlett.

Luszczynska, A., & Schwarzer, R. (2020). Changing behavior using social cognitive theory. In M.S. Hagger, L.D. Cameron, K. Hamilton, N. Hankonen, & T. Lintunen (Eds.), *The handbook of behavior change* (pp. 32–45). Cambridge University Press.

MacDonald, C., & Zitomer, M. R. (2021). Experiences of therapeutic horseback riders in their youth: A self-determination perspective. *European Journal of Adapted Physical Activity, 14*(1), 5. https://doi.org/10.5507/euj.2020.017.

Martin, G. (2021). *Top 10 emerging trends for healthcare 2021: The new normal.* https://trustees.aha.org/top-10-emerging-trends-health-care-2021-new-normal

MD Anderson Cancer Center. (2022). *About MD Anderson.* https://www.mdanderson.org/about-md-anderson.html

Mertala, S. M., Kanste, O., Keskitalo-Leskinen, S., Juntunen, J., & Kaakinen, P. (2021). Job satisfaction among occupational therapy practitioners: A systematic review of quantitative studies. *Occupational Therapy in Health Care, 36*, 1–28. https://doi.org/10.1080/07380577.2021.1964146

Prochaska, J. O. (2020). Transtheoretical Model of Behavior Change. In Gellman, M.D. (eds.), *Encyclopedia of Behavioral Medicine.* Springer. https://doi.org/10.1007/978-3-030-39903-0_70

University of Twente. (2017). *Social cognitive theory.* https://www.utwente.nl/en/bms/communication-theories/sorted-by-cluster/Health%20Communication/Social_cognitive_theory/

Zeb, A., ur Rehman, F., Arsalan, Y., & Usman Khan, M. (2021). Does organizational justice enhance job performance through high-performance human resource practices? *WPOM-Working Papers on Operations Management, 12*(2), 16–40. https://doi.org/10.4995/wpom.15497

CHAPTER 74

Supervision of Occupational Therapy Practice

Patricia A. Gentile

LEARNING OBJECTIVES

After reading this chapter, you will be able to:

1. Explain the roles and functions of supervision.
2. Differentiate types of supervision.
3. Examine supervisory processes and implementation.
4. Compare and contrast approaches to managing performance.
5. Apply American Occupational Therapy Association's (AOTA) guidelines for appropriate supervision of occupational therapy personnel in the United States.

Introduction

Supervision is a distinct professional activity that is an integral part of occupational therapy (OT) service provision. The supervisory process is consciously used in our profession to ensure that our clients receive safe, effective, and evidence-based OT services. Although the ability to supervise skillfully is developed throughout one's practice career, the entry-level practitioner must be knowledgeable about the supervisory process and have a beginning understanding of how to give and receive supervision in a manner that is consistent with the profession's values and expectations. This chapter provides you with an overview of what supervision is and introduces you to basic information you will need to develop positive and effective supervisory relationships. Supervisory best practices and expectations in general are explained, along with supervisory standards specific to practice in the United States.

Supervision Embedded in Practice

The supervision process is an everyday feature of each practitioner's work experience. It is a process that supports effective job performance as well as personal growth. Read OT Story 74.1 about Elena, an OT practitioner, and Pam, an occupational therapy assistant (OTA), which describes their career experiences with supervision.

OT STORY 74.1 ELENA AND PAM: SUPERVISION EMBEDDED IN PRACTICE

Elena has been working as an occupational therapist in a pediatric hospital since graduating from her OT program. She worked with three other therapists and was supervised by Andre, the senior occupational therapist in the setting. In addition to Elena's regular supervisory meetings with Andre, she also sought and received feedback and guidance from Marilyn, another staff occupational therapist, who was experienced in working with children with complex orthopedic injuries. Elena integrated feedback from both Andre and Marilyn to advance her knowledge and develop her professional reasoning skills. After working in the department for a year, Elena began supervising volunteers who provided service in a playtime program for hospitalized children. She was responsible for orienting and training these volunteers. Elena would also make time to observe their interactions with the children and was always available for questions. After 1 year of practice, Elena began to supervise Level I OT and OTA students. She enjoyed sharing her knowledge with these students. At the end of her second year of work, Elena was assigned her first Level II OT student, whom she supervised on a daily basis. As the department's caseload expanded, Pam, an OTA was hired. Elena was assigned as Pam's supervisor and oriented Pam to the hospital and the department's policies and procedures. Elena supervised Pam as they worked together to provide OT services to patients. Initially, Elena closely observed Pam's treatments and/or cotreated with her to establish Pam's level of competency. Although Pam came to the hospital with 5 years of experience with children, her prior work had been in a school setting, so she was not familiar with OT interventions involving acute medical conditions. After working in the department for 9 months, Pam was assigned responsibility for supervising the playtime program volunteers. Pam frequently consulted with the recreational therapist at the hospital about strategies for expanding the play activities and improving volunteer participation.

In this case scenario, supervision played a regular part in Elena's and Pam's daily work experience. Supervision provided feedback, direction, and support to enable them to carry out responsibilities effectively as well as support them in their personal professional development to gain additional competencies. Elena and Pam had a designated formal supervisor, but both of them sought out informal peer supervision from other therapists. The collegial nature of the department and everyone's interest in providing the best possible care allowed this type of supervision to occur naturally. Adding supervisory responsibilities to their jobs expanded both Elena's and Pam's job roles and provided opportunities for personal growth.

As the OT Story illustrates, practitioners are involved in giving as well as receiving supervision. In the United States, supervisory skills are an expected entry-level competency for occupational therapists who are responsible for supervising OTAs (American Occupational Therapy Association [AOTA], 2020b). Entry-level OTAs may be responsible for supervising OT aides and later may move into supervisory roles with other OTAs. All practitioners should know how to effectively provide supervision and benefit from it. Before exploring how to best provide supervision, let us first look at what supervision is and how it fits into the overall management structure of a work setting.

Questions

1. Why is it important to include both observation and joint treatment sessions in the supervisory process?
2. What are two specific ways that adding supervisory responsibilities to your role as an occupational therapist can help to increase your own professional and personal skills?

Formal Supervision

Definition and Focus

Dictionaries trace the roots of the term *supervise* to the Latin roots *super-*, "over," + *videre-*, "to see" (Stevenson, 2010). **Supervision** is a process that involves "overseeing" or "watching" the work of another. The employer gives a supervisor formal authority to watch the work of others and ensure that the work meets the organization's goals and objectives. To effectively oversee the work of others, supervisors need to be familiar with the work of the positions they supervise. Individuals assuming supervisor positions, who do not have advanced knowledge or experience in the supervisee's job description, would be expected to familiarize themselves with the job tasks and responsibilities. This background allows them to provide the support and direction that supervisees need to solve work problems, to learn and grow in their jobs, and to better meet the organization's objectives (Figure 74.1).

It is important to consider where a supervisor fits in the management structure of an organization. Braveman (2016) offers insight into the relationship of the two by defining *supervision* as "the control and direction of the work of one or more employees in a manner that promotes improved performance and a higher quality outcome" (p. 187). Although supervisors may participate in all functions of management (planning, organizing, directing, and controlling), they typically spend the majority of their time focused on the directing and controlling functions by overseeing employee progress and productivity in their daily work (Braveman, 2016, p. 187). (See Chapter 73, for a discussion of management functions.) When considering the supervisor's placement within the management hierarchy, this becomes easier to understand (Figure 74.2). Supervisors are typically positioned immediately above the staff level in an organization and typically do not supervise others who are in management positions. Supervisors are generally considered to

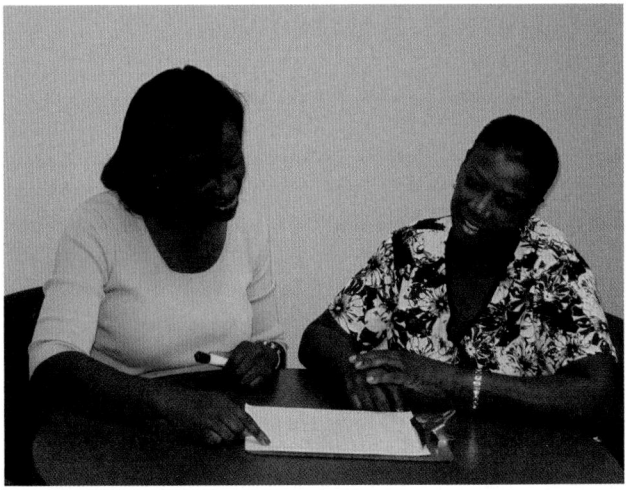

FIGURE 74.1 Discussing weekend coverage plans and how they will be implemented is a common supervisory task in hospital-based OT. OT, occupational therapy.

be the first line of management. Although they have some management responsibilities, they are not considered to be managers.

The emphasis primarily on the directing and controlling functions of management rather than the planning and organizing functions does not diminish the importance of the supervisor's role. Formal supervisors, because of their placement within the organization, serve as a bridge between the staff and higher levels of management. In this position, the supervisor must support, interpret, and implement management decisions as well as relay staff concerns to higher management, which can influence planning and organizing functions. The supervisors' ability in conveying management concerns to staff and staff concerns to management is crucial to the organization's effectiveness and ability to adapt to change.

In addition to organizational success, supervision takes on an added dimension and responsibility when people who are members of a profession (e.g., OT, nursing, psychology) take on responsibilities to supervise other members of their profession in a work setting. Providing professional supervision that is consistent with the profession's values and standards and supports the professional growth and development of the supervisees should be integrated with the supervisor's responsibility to meet the organization's needs. For example, the supervisor must not assign tasks and responsibilities that are outside of the supervisee's professional scope of practice. The supervisor must be cognizant of the profession's standards and guidelines regarding

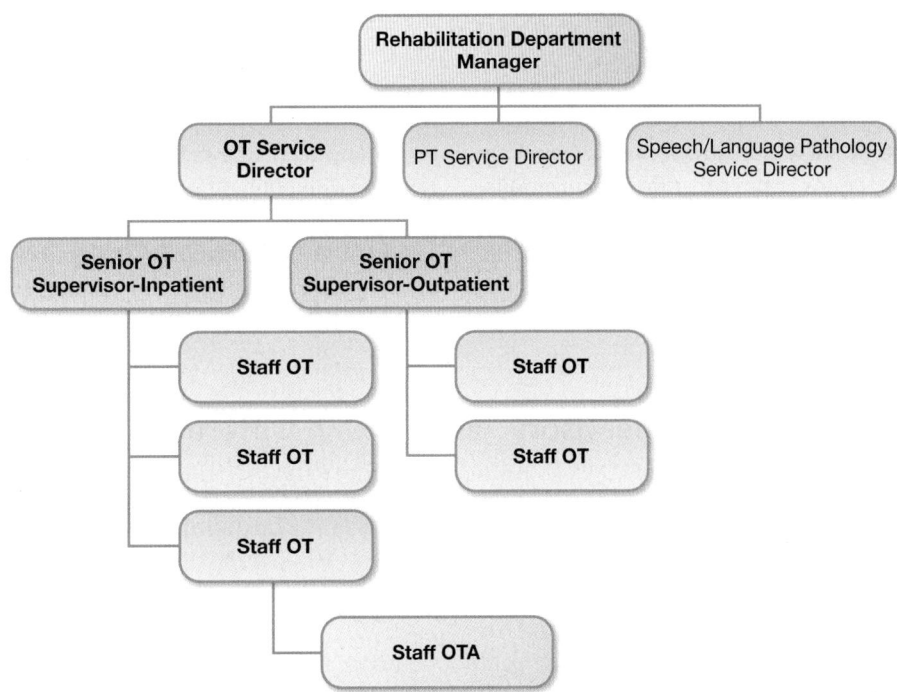

FIGURE 74.2 In this organization, the senior occupational therapists are supervisors and the OT service director is a manager. OT, occupational therapy; OTA, occupational therapy assistant; PT, physical therapist

frequency of supervision and requirements for training and competency. Overall, the supervisor must manage and supervise work in a manner that respects the profession's scope and that supports the supervisee's development of continuing competence.

The supervisor who is providing professional supervision must continually ask two related but different questions, which will guide the supervisor's observations, analysis, decisions, and actions.

1. Is the supervisee successfully accomplishing the work?
2. Is the supervisee demonstrating continued professional growth and development?

Supporting the supervisees' efforts to maintain and develop continuing competence should complement supporting the supervisee's successful accomplishment of work duties. As individuals develop new skills and abilities, clients receive better care and organizations benefit from workers' improved expertise. The supervisor should be concurrently providing feedback on performance and assessing the supervisee's learning and professional development needs.

Functions of Supervision in a Professional Practice Setting

The supervisor's role in a professional practice setting encompasses three broad functions that are carried out under the broader management functions of directing and controlling. These functions are administrative, educational, and supportive functions (Kadushin, 1992). Table 74.1 lists examples of supervisory tasks for each function.

Administrative functions are directed toward managing the day-to-day work performance and process. Checking that all clients were seen and assigning clients to specific supervisees are examples of administrative tasks. Carrying out administrative functions ensures that the organization's day-to-day work is accomplished. The educational function is focused on the worker and is concerned with teaching and training, providing feedback about performance, and remediating and disciplining, if necessary. Educational

functions assist the supervisee to be effective in meeting job demands and also can help to promote the supervisee's own professional growth and development. The supportive function is directed toward relationships—both individual and group relationships within the workplace. This function focuses on developing harmonious relationships that will maintain a positive work environment in which people can be productive and successful.

Informal Supervision: Peer Supervision

Although supervision is typically understood as a formalized process that occurs in a work setting in which a person's work is supervised by a formally designated supervisor, peer supervision can be perceived as a method of mutual accountability and commitment to the profession's obligation to provide the best quality of services to clients.

In a healthcare professional practice environment where all staff members are committed to providing the best quality of service, informal peer supervision may also occur. Peer supervision is oversight that is provided by another professional who has no formal authority to provide supervision. The peer supervisor provides feedback and shares knowledge with the intent of influencing the peer professional's practice in order to improve client outcomes.

Peer supervision is a natural extension of each professional's responsibility to ensure that clients receive the highest quality of care. It may or may not be solicited by the "supervisee" practitioner. In OT Story 74.1, Elena sought input from her peers as a way of continuing to learn and grow as a professional, but not all practitioners seek input from others. When a peer therapist provides peer supervision and feedback that is not requested, the intent is to improve client outcomes by offering information that could help other practitioners improve their services.

In a professional and collegial work environment, peer supervision often occurs spontaneously and is seen as a benefit of working with others. Exchange and feedback

---

TABLE 74.1   Examples of Supervisory Tasks Within Different Supervisory Functions

Administrative Function	Educational Function	Supportive Function
• Plan and assign workload • Make schedules • Set priorities for work activities • Check performance against work standards • Interpret policies and procedures • Delegate work • Provide written and verbal reports to managers	• Orient new staff • Identify training needs • Develop and provide training programs • Identify and provide educational resources • Assess performance and provide feedback • Remediate, discipline	• Hold group meetings to allow for expression of concerns • Meet individually with supervisee on a regular basis to check on progress toward work goals • Provide informal and formal support for performance

among practitioners frequently occur as colleagues explore how to solve clinical problems and seek the best solutions for their clients. Such exchanges can be energizing for both parties. In addition to helping to solve clinical problems, peer supervision can also "assist practitioners in navigating challenging situations with supervisors, resulting in more effective self-advocacy, better problem solving and, ultimately better clinical outcomes and professional development" (Golia & McGovern, 2015).

Mentoring

Being mentored by another professional is often confused with supervision. Mentorship and supervision are different types of relationships. In a mentoring relationship, the mentor's primary concern is the personal and professional growth of the mentee (Braveman, 2016). The goal of the mentor is to "guide, counsel and support professional development in regard to the mentee's career, knowledge and skill" (Waite, 2014). The mentor does not necessarily have any formal authority to oversee the mentee's work. Although the mentor is interested in the work the mentee is doing, the focus is on the mentee and not on work performance per se. Instead, discussions between the mentor and mentee center on career options and decisions, identification of personal and professional growth needs and resources, and feedback about the mentee's behaviors and choices. A mentor relationship may be sought by the mentee who is feeling the need of guidance and direction in professional growth and development. Mentoring relationships have been found to improve staff satisfaction and increase productivity, and many organizations have implemented formal mentoring programs (Newstrom, 2013). Generally, the mentor is a more experienced professional and is seen as a trusted adviser.

Mentor–mentee relationships may also occur spontaneously between two professionals. In these instances, the mentee usually is attracted to the mentor's knowledge, skills, and accomplishments, and the mentor is attracted to the mentee's talent and potential as well as the opportunity to contribute to another professional's development.

True mentoring relationships are acknowledged by both parties and require formal commitment of time and effort. Mentor and mentee discuss and agree on learning needs and goals for the relationship as well as the structure for the mentoring process.

Mentee–mentor relationship can also develop within a supervisory relationship. When this happens, for example, a person who is functioning in the role of a mentor might recognize that a mentee would benefit from staying in one clinical setting for several months to allow for solidification of learning. However, this same person, functioning as a supervisor, recognizes that staffing limitations require that the supervisee must be rotated to a new clinical setting each month. Hence, it is important to be clear about the different responsibilities of each role. Table 74.2 offers a comparison of supervision, mentorship, and peer supervision.

Mentoring should not be confused with role modeling. A role model is an individual whose example, such as their behaviors or successes, are looked up to and imitated by others. Role models are usually watched and admired by practitioners, but the role models do not have a reciprocating active interest in the development of others and might not even be aware that they are serving as role models (Urish, 2004).

The Supervisory Process

The overseeing of work is an *ongoing* process: It occurs repeatedly across time and is embedded in the everyday work experience. A supervisor, both formally and informally,

TABLE 74.2	Comparison of Supervision, Mentorship, and Peer Supervision		
	Supervision	**Mentorship**	**Peer Supervision**
Authority	Provided by the work organization	No formal authority	No formal authority; supported by professional responsibility
Nature of relationship and how it is established	Formal—established by the workplace	Personal, voluntary	Informal, spontaneous, ad hoc
Purpose	To support growth and development that will benefit the organization	To foster personal and professional growth and development that will benefit the mentee	To support growth and development that will ensure best outcomes for clients
How established	Assigned	Sought by the mentee and mutually agreed on	Offered by a peer or may be solicited by a practitioner
Accountability for performance	Organizational	Personal	Professional
Whose needs are met—outcomes expected	Needs of organization—work meets organizational objectives and needs	Needs of mentee—mentee achieves personal and professional growth	Needs of mentee and clients—clients receive best services

observes and checks on the work of supervisees by talking to them about their work as well as observing them on a regular basis. A supervisor who observes the work of supervisees only occasionally and meets with them during an annual performance review is not providing adequate supervision. Supervisors should have a presence in the workplace and have regular contact with their supervisees.

Supervision is an *orderly* process. A good supervisor establishes a process in which the supervisee understands when regular contacts and meetings will occur. The supervisor is clear about performance expectations and consistent in providing feedback. The supervisory process, although orderly and expected, is also *dynamic*. It changes as people grow and work demands shift. Upon initial hiring, the supervisor might observe an employee daily and meet weekly. After several weeks, the employee might practice more independently without daily observation. Any changes in supervisory expectations should always be clearly communicated.

Finally, supervision is an *interactive* process. It is based on an exchange or communication between the supervisor and the supervisee. This exchange is central to the development and maintenance of professional competence. For example, the AOTA (2020b) document "Guidelines for Supervision, Roles, and Responsibilities during the Delivery of Occupational Therapy Services" describes supervision as "a cooperative process in which two or more people participate in a joint effort to establish, maintain, and/or elevate a level of competence and performance" (p. S1).

In this description, the AOTA authors see supervision as a two-way street. Supervision is viewed as a cooperative process in which both parties have professional responsibility. This cooperative approach to supervision stems from the profession's ethical responsibility to demonstrate concern for the safety and well-being of their clients (e.g., see Principle 1: Beneficence; AOTA, 2020a) and the profession's responsibility to abide by standards directed to establishing, maintaining, and updating professional performance, knowledge, and skills (AOTA, 2015, 2020b).

The AOTA's (2020b) "Guidelines for Supervision, Roles, and Responsibilities during the Delivery of Occupational Therapy Services" describe the supervisory process as having two purposes that relate to these responsibilities: (a) to ensure safe and effective delivery of OT services and (b) to foster professional competence and development (p. S1). These objectives reflect the organizational duties of the supervisor as well as professional practice obligations. All practitioners have a common interest in providing the best possible care to their clients, and all practitioners are obligated to demonstrate continuing competence. The supervisory process is the tool that occupational therapists and OTAs use to reach these goals.

Developing a Supervisory Relationship

The supervisory relationship is central to the supervisory process. An effective supervisory relationship is built on trust and integrity. To develop trust and integrity, supervisors need to create and foster respectful, inclusive environments and be approachable and open to the supervisee's questions and concerns; the supervisee, likewise, must be open and willing to share observations, perceptions, and ideas.

Both must value and respect the input of the other. The supervisor must be responsive and follow through with actions that indicate that the supervisee's concerns were considered; the supervisee will feel valued and confident in their personal abilities, and commitment to the organization will increase. The supervisor must be clear about expectations and provide regular objective feedback about performance; the supervisee will understand what is expected and feel more competent in the job. The supervisor must be consistent in their interactions; the supervisee will develop a level of trust in how they will be treated. When the supervisor is approachable and responsive, the supervisory relationship can thrive. Box 74.1 provides some additional examples of supervisory behaviors that build trust and integrity.

BOX 74.1 IMPORTANT BEHAVIORS IN SUPERVISION

Key Positive Supervisory Behaviors

- Praises others
- Accepts criticism and suggestion without judging
- Tells the truth
- Is supportive of supervisee—goes to bat for supervisees
- Gives credit for accomplishments
- Abides by the same rules as expects others to abide by
- Gives clear and frequent feedback
- Is dependable
- Is loyal to organization—makes decisions that are in best interest of organization
- Is respectful of differences

Key Positive Supervisee Behaviors

- Accepts feedback
- Seeks feedback
- Provides information
- Asks for clarification
- Attempts to integrate feedback to improve performance
- Shares ideas and concerns in a direct but not critical manner
- Sensitive to feelings and needs of supervisor

Supervisor's Role in Building the Relationship

Both supervisee and supervisor bring their own values, beliefs, and attitudes about supervision to the relationship. Each brings past experiences with other supervisors and authority figures, which may have been positive or negative.

Supervisors must be able to establish effective supervisory relationships with an increasingly diverse set of supervisees. Supervisors' cultural competence and humility within the supervisory relationship has been found to positively relate to supervisees' satisfaction with supervision (Wilcox et al., 2021). Refer to Chapter 14 to learn more about cultural competence considerations.

It is the supervisor's responsibility to set the tone for the relationship in a job setting and to take actions that will support an ongoing positive relationship. The following four steps will help to ensure that a positive supervisory relationship is initiated and developed:

1. ***Learn about the supervisee.*** Remember that you are responsible for guiding the learning of this new employee. To do this effectively, you need to understand what your new supervisee knows and how the person learns best. Assess whether the person's knowledge and skills match with those that are needed for this job. Interviewing the new employee about past experiences and asking for current strengths and learning needs sends the message that you are interested in building on what the person knows and that you value the person's experiences. You might wish to develop a skills checklist that the employee can fill out to supplement the interview process. Learning about a supervisee's abilities is an ongoing process, but gathering this information formally during orientation to design training and learning experiences is very helpful. Identifying the employee's learning styles and preferences can facilitate the learning process on the new job and avoid wasted time and effort for both parties.

2. ***Be clear about expectations.*** During the initial orientation and training, the supervisor needs to clearly outline the performance expectations for the job. The job requirements and expectations should have been broadly discussed during the job interview and hiring process. Now it is a good time to revisit this discussion and provide more specifics. Reviewing the job description is an objective method for beginning this discussion. Expectations about productivity and quality of work should be made clear to the employee. Be honest and open about consequences for various behaviors—rewards as well as punishments. In addition, organizational cultural expectations such as attitudes and behaviors employees are expected to exhibit in interdisciplinary, peer, and client/family interactions should be addressed. These expectations are often not included in a job description but are central to acceptable performance. Discuss your expectations regarding the supervisee's responsibility to learn and grow.

3. ***Develop and implement a supervisory plan.*** As noted earlier, the supervisory process is a collaborative one. During the orientation, discuss how you view the supervisory process and work together to develop a supervisory plan. Discuss topics such as frequency of supervisory contact (e.g., daily, three times per week, weekly), types of contact (e.g., informal, spontaneous, formal scheduled meeting), methods of contact (e.g., face-to-face, e-mail, phone, text, written), and preferred supervisory methods (e.g., observation, cotreatment, dialogue, documentation review). Be clear about the obligations and expectations you have of the supervisee; for example, explain that you expect the supervisee to initiate contact with you if more frequent feedback or supervision is needed.

4. ***Document supervision that is provided.*** Document when you meet with your supervisee and what was discussed. A supervisory log can be used to keep a record of incidents, observations, and meetings. This log allows you to track and note changes in performance. The log record provides concrete examples that can be used to provide feedback and during performance review meetings. Regulatory laws in some states in the United States require supervisory logs be kept to document the supervisory process that occurs between an occupational therapist and an OTA to maintain current licensure.

For a glimpse at a supervisee's experience, see Expanding Our Perspectives.

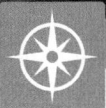

EXPANDING OUR PERSPECTIVES

Surviving Supervision

So Sin Sim, OT PhD Candidate

I would like to share some perspectives both as an international student who survived supervision in a cross-cultural environment and as one who is passionate about supporting the emotions of students during fieldwork placements. Barely 3 months into my OT program in the United Kingdom, I received my posting to my first-year 3-week observation placement. My considerate fieldwork coordinator had paired me up with another student who was local and could drive, which was important for this

(continued)

placement because we were going to be living in the middle of the woods, in a cozy cottage, where there was no transport, and driving daily to the placement site that was accessible only via car. It was a mixed bag of excitement and nervousness.

Having moved to the United Kingdom from Singapore, I was familiar only with high-rise flats, so living in the woods sounded really cool. Although I did not know much about the client group I was attached to, I set off in good spirits and went off with the girl that I have just met briefly.

This was a placement in a day and group home setting for people with severe learning disabilities, and the set up was lovely. There were lots of activities and very nice staff. What really got me stressed was anticipating the behaviors of the clients and knowing what to do. It was the first time I have met people with such severe disabilities and I was just shocked and lost. Meanwhile, I watched my schoolmate confidently helping and interacting with the clients. It was not a great feeling.

The second shock I had was to do with the lovely cottage I was living in. It's quite a laugh when I recall now. Firstly, I got told off by my landlady for wetting her bathroom (we have "wet room" bathrooms in Singapore); secondly, I did not use a coaster and made burn marks on her table (we do not have expensive wooden antique tables at home); thirdly, there was huge sheep dog that lived in the house that liked to lie in front of and scratch at my door. I was so terrified of the dog that I would stay in my room until he moved away. In sum, my feelings included embarrassment, being stressed out, and feeling incompetent.

This walk down memory lane reminds me of the importance of empathy for students and to be sensitive to cultural differences as supervisors and lecturers.

Cultural differences can lead to differences in expectations, learning style, and communication, which can adversely affect how fieldwork might go. The supervisors' openness, school's facilitation, and the students' initiative need to go together to ensure the best learning environment for the student. Here are some quick tips on surviving fieldwork from all three parties' perspectives:

- *Fieldwork supervisor:* Keep close communication with the school to check in on expectations and to understand your student behaviors and motivation. Make time for the student on a regular basis to pick up on areas of support students might need. When in doubt, contact the school.
- *School's facilitation:* The school knows the student and the learning content; therefore, the school is in the best position to advise what kind of support students might need or what learning gaps they might have. The school can also provide some general tips for supervisors on cross-cultural exposure.
- *Student on placement:* Most supervisors want to help you learn but they may not know how. Do not be afraid to approach your school fieldwork team if you are unable to communicate with your supervisor or you think you might not be doing well. It is best to nip the problem early so that there will be time for intervention.

Supervisee's Role in Building the Relationship

Supervision occurs as an ongoing process of involving the exchange of information about the job and feedback about performance. The feedback process is a two-way street, with both the supervisor and supervisee playing important roles. Positive feedback and constructive criticism should be provided on a regular basis by the supervisor, as described in the next section. However, the supervisee also has a responsibility to regularly seek feedback as a way to validate work performance and identify areas for further professional development. In order to be effective, this is a reciprocal process. The supervisor needs to be skilled in delivering feedback, and the supervisee needs to be skilled in seeking and responding to feedback.

How does a supervisee respond effectively to feedback? First and most importantly, the supervisee needs to view the supervisory relationship positively and be open to receiving feedback. Feedback provided by a supervisor

provides honest information about how work is to be done and behaviors and performance are perceived. This information can be used to develop new skills, refine current skills, and monitor personal growth and development. Sometimes, hearing how others see you can be difficult to accept. Avoid responding defensively by explaining your behavior or by discounting the feedback as uninformed. Neither strategy will promote the supervisory relationship nor lead to professional growth. If aspects of the information received are unclear because the feedback may not have been behaviorally specific enough, the supervisee should ask for clarification and/or concrete examples of the performance in question. If the feedback is based on incomplete information, the supervisee should provide more information in a calm and matter-of-fact manner. Exchanges that occur during supervisory sessions can help to clarify performance for both the supervisee as well as the supervisor and contribute to the collaborative supervisory relationship. Some general guidelines for receiving feedback are outlined in Box 74.2.

BOX 74.2 GUIDELINES FOR RECEIVING FEEDBACK

- Listen openly. Assume feedback is being shared with positive intentions.
- Make sure you understand what is being said. Paraphrase what you have heard to check for accuracy.
- Ask for clarification or examples if feedback is unclear.
- Pause and think before you respond. If you want some time to consider feedback, ask for it.
- Acknowledge mistakes.

- Avoid interrupting or becoming defensive. Provide justification only if asked.
- Seek a solution to problems presented. Ask for examples of how you could perform better.
- Thank the person for providing you with the feedback.
- Make appropriate changes.
- Initiate a follow-up discussion to assure that needed changes have occurred as expected.

After feedback has been received, the supervisee needs to reflect on how to respond to it. Consideration should be given as to how this new information can be integrated into your daily work performance and how this new information can influence your professional development.

Perhaps, your supervisor pointed out how your ability to communicate succinctly in team meetings has improved. Based on this feedback, you decide you would like to offer to more frequently attend team meetings when others cannot. Perhaps, your supervisor has observed that your skill in wheelchair assessment and positioning are weaker than required by your role. Based on this feedback, you decide to look for a continuing education opportunity in this skill area. Feedback can sensitize you to behaviors, attitudes, and skills that validate your abilities and can also help to provide direction for new learning and growth.

Performance Evaluation: A Supervisory Responsibility

All supervisory actions are directed toward managing the supervisee's work performance. The purpose of performance management is to encourage the supervisee to meet or exceed the established job performance standards and behave safely and appropriately at work (Newstrom, 2013, p. 265). Supervisors use a variety of methods in managing performance (e.g., incentives, job structure), but providing ongoing evaluation of performance by providing both formal and informal feedback is a central supervisory responsibility and skill.

Providing Feedback

Effective feedback is the supervisor's primary tool in influencing the employee's job performance. The supervisor is responsible for letting employees know if they are meeting job performance standards or not. When positive supervisory relationships have been established, feedback occurs naturally and informally throughout the work week. The supervisor comments on what they have observed and uses the feedback to point out when performance needs to be changed as well as to verify and praise effective performance. Effective feedback needs to be descriptive rather than evaluative.

Evaluative: The splint you fabricated does not fit well.
Descriptive: The splint you fabricated has rough edges that may cause skin breakdown.

Effective feedback also needs to be specific rather than general.

General: Your time management skills are poor.
Specific: Your treatment notes are not filed in the medical record within 24 hours of completion in accordance with the department policy.

It is important to provide feedback that is descriptive and specific. This will keep the focus on the effectiveness of the supervisee's work behaviors and not on personal characteristics or personality. This distinction is critical to the supervisee's being able to "hear" and respond to the feedback. Other suggestions for giving feedback are listed in Box 74.3.

BOX 74.3 GUIDELINES FOR GIVING FEEDBACK

- Provide timely feedback—give feedback as close to when the behavior was observed as is possible.
- Provide balanced feedback—point out what is working as well as what needs to be changed.
- Provide feedback on behaviors that can be changed.
- Use "I" statements.
- Avoid the use of generalizations such as "always," "never," and "all."
- Ask the supervisee if they understood what you said; ask them to restate it in their own words.
- Ask for feedback about your feedback—how did you do?

Remember that the purpose of supervision is to support effective work performance. When supervisors evaluate employees, they are evaluating what employees do—how they behave, how they act, and how effectively they are accomplishing the work. The focus of feedback in supervision—both informal and formal—should be on the task, not the person. The purpose is to relay information about performance to the performer so that actions can be taken to maintain or improve performance.

Performance Evaluation and Appraisal

Newstrom (2013, p. 311) points out four basic reasons for appraising an employee's performance:

1. To encourage good behavior or to correct and discourage below-standard performance
2. To satisfy employees' curiosity to know how they are doing
3. To provide an opportunity for developing employee skills
4. To provide a firm foundation for later judgments that concern an employee's career such as promotions, pay raises, and transfers

A supervisor should be regularly evaluating the supervisee's performance and providing feedback. However, at least once or twice a year, the supervisor should meet with the employer and provide a formal and systematic evaluation of how the person is performing, using a structured performance appraisal format. Most organizations have formal performance appraisal systems and appraisal forms. Appraisal methods and formats may vary and could include written narratives, behaviorally anchored rating scales, management by objectives, or 360-degree feedback. In a formal performance appraisal, the employee's performance is compared to established standards.

As a supervisor, you might be asked to develop job standards for OT personnel. Professional organizations such as the AOTA can help you to identify standards. For example, AOTA's "Standards of Practice" (AOTA, 2021) and the "Guidelines for Supervision, Roles, and Responsibilities during the Delivery of Occupational Therapy Services" (AOTA, 2020b) are important resources for supervisors practicing in the United States. The World Federation of Occupational Therapists (WFOT) (http://www.wfot.org) provides a listing of member OT professional organizations throughout the world, each of which is likely to have resources relevant to practice within that region. Refer to Chapter 5, for more information on professional organizations in OT. Equally important are worksite job descriptions. Standards will vary by workplace, but all standards should include *what* performance or behaviors are expected, *how* performance will be *measured*, and *when* performance is to occur. An example of a standard that includes all of these criteria is "Evaluations are completed and distributed within 24 hours of initial contact with the client." Standards for each job title should be clearly outlined in the employee's job description.

In preparing a formal performance appraisal, the supervisor needs to complete three steps:

1. ***Gather information about the employee's performance.*** Review your supervisory logs, noting key incidents that you recorded. Record additional information that might have been overlooked. Review other employee records, such as attendance, training and educational records, and competency check-off completions. Review the previous year's performance appraisal. Talk to other members of the team, both within and outside of your department, to understand how the employee's performance is viewed by others. Ask the employee to perform a self-appraisal of their work, identifying accomplishments, strengths, and weaknesses. You can ask the employee to give this to you before the performance appraisal or have the employee bring it to the performance appraisal meeting.
2. ***Compare current performance to standards.*** Note areas of strength and areas in which improvement may be needed.
3. ***Reflect on and synthesize information.*** Consider the needs of the department as well as the professional growth needs of the supervisee. Provide feedback about the effectiveness, efficiency, and safety of performance. Note how the employee has contributed to the department's achievements. Document your comments, including both positive feedback and constructive criticism. Avoid allowing an employee's positive or negative qualities in one area to influence your assessment in other areas. Be objective and balanced and focus feedback on task performance. Numerous Websites and management literature offer information on how to perform effective performance evaluations and can alert you to additional factors to be aware of.

When the performance appraisal is completed, it is time to meet with the employee. The purpose of this meeting is to provide an opportunity for the supervisor and supervisee to discuss the employee's job performance and to collaborate on ways to improve it. Unfortunately, performance appraisal meetings are often viewed as anxiety-provoking events that focus on what the employee has done wrong. The common emphasis on the supervisor's rating of the employee tends to detract from a collaborative educational process during which supervisee and supervisor share perspectives and work together to identify barriers to improved performance. The supervisor can use several approaches to correct this problem:

1. ***Demystify the process.*** Orient the employee to the evaluation process ahead of time. If a standard form is used, make sure the employee has seen it and understands any terminology or rating scales that are used. Make

sure the employee is aware of the job expectations and standards. Involve the employee in the appraisal process by using a self-assessment.

2. ***Plan ahead.*** Notify the employee in advance as to when the meeting will occur and allow the employee time to prepare.

3. ***Establish a comfortable climate for the exchange.*** Set a time to meet in private without interruptions. Allow adequate time for discussion. Put the employee at ease in the beginning and explain that you view this time as an opportunity for mutual sharing on how to improve job performance for the benefit of the employee and the organization.

During the performance appraisal interview, be prepared to collaborate with the employee and exchange ideas. Share accomplishments and review what has not been accomplished. If performance ratings are provided, be sure to provide reasons for your ratings that are based on actual job performance. If the employee is surprised by any of your ratings or comments, you probably have not provided enough regular feedback during the year. Take note and work to correct that. The appraisal interview offers another opportunity to realign expectations about job performance and to target goals for the future.

Handling Work Performance Problems

Although there are numerous types of performance problems in professional practice settings, the most common ones are behavior or conduct problems in which a rule is broken, performance that falls below the expected standards, and interpersonal issues that interfere with department morale and effectiveness. Each type of problem is handled differently, but in all situations, the actions that are taken are directed toward helping the employee to improve performance and meet job expectations.

Behavior or Conduct Problems

Behavior or conduct problems are handled by disciplining. Behavior or conduct problems may include absenteeism, chronic late arrival, intoxication, insubordination, sexual harassment, negligence in following procedures, and falsification of records. These are all serious infractions and should not be allowed to persist. Although individual facilities may adopt their own specific procedures for disciplining a variety of infractions, in unionized environments, the disciplinary process is highly prescribed. Regardless of setting, disciplining is generally handled in a progressive manner. In a progressive discipline approach, the employee is counseled repeatedly if performance does not improve, and the penalties for noncompliance with the rules become increasingly harsh (Figure 74.3). In rare cases, conduct

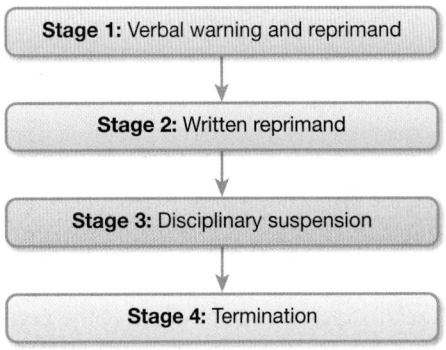

FIGURE 74.3 Using a standard sequence for dealing with performance problems is required in many formal organizations and is considered good practice in most settings.

problems may be grounds for immediate dismissal as delineated in organizational policies.

In the first stage of progressive disciplining, the performance problem is discussed with the employee, clear expectations for acceptable performance are outlined, and consequences of not improving are described. In the second stage, the process is repeated, and this time, a written record of the exchange is documented. Both the supervisor and the employee sign it, and it is placed in the employee's personnel file. If the behavior persists, in the third stage, the employee is suspended for a period of time and is told that once they have returned to work, the behavior must be corrected or the employee will be terminated. The last stage occurs if the employee returns to work and another infraction occurs, at which time the employee is terminated.

A useful analogy for administering any discipline is the "red-hot stove" rule. The analogy likens the process of administering discipline to that of touching a red-hot stove and points out the four essential characteristics of a good disciplinary policy and practice. Discipline should be administered in the following manner:

- ***With advance warning.*** When you see a red-hot stove, you know that if you touch it, you will be burned. Employees should know what will happen if they break a rule or policy.
- ***Immediately.*** When you touch a red-hot stove, you will be burned right away. Administration of discipline should be done as soon after the occurrence of the behavior as possible.
- ***Impartially.*** No matter who touches a red-hot stove, the person will be burned. Supervisors should not play favorites in administering discipline. Everyone should receive the same penalty for the same infraction.
- ***Consistently.*** Every time you touch a red-hot stove, you get burned. Discipline should be administered the same way with each occurrence.

Performance Problems

Problems of substandard performance may occur in professional practice. When dealing with these types of problems, the supervisor needs to adopt an approach of collaborating with the supervisee and enlisting their help in resolving the problem. Typical steps in dealing with this type of problem after the performance problem is identified include the following:

1. Meet with supervisee and point out the performance problem. Review the standard and describe the expected performance.
2. Collaborate with the supervisee to determine reasons for the problem.
3. Work together to develop and implement an action plan with time frames to improve performance.
4. Monitor performance.
5. Repeat the process if needed.
6. Inform employee of consequences if the standard is achieved and if the standard is not achieved.

Interpersonal Work Issues

Interpersonal work issues vary in scope and complexity and are common in all work groups. In a professional practice environment in which teamwork is central to the department's effectiveness and to the achievement of positive client outcomes, problems among workers should not be ignored. Interpersonal issues can arise among practitioners in the OT department or among team members from different disciplines. These types of work problems often stem from miscommunication and/or differences in communication styles or personalities. Lack of clarity about job roles or about expectations can also lead to interpersonal problems.

Just because two people are different or disagree does not mean that they cannot work effectively together. The supervisor's role in resolving these types of performance issues should focus not on personalities, individuals, or differences but on the job tasks and mutual goals that need to be accomplished. The first approach to take when an employee complains to you about another employee is to listen carefully and encourage the person with the complaint to talk directly to the other individual. You should help the person to clarify his or her concerns and frame them in terms of how the other person's actions are affecting the person's ability to get their own job done. This approach often works and begins the process of opening communication.

When this approach does not work, you might need to take further action by talking to each of the parties involved. You might want to do this individually at first and then together, or you might want to approach the problem by talking to the parties at the same time. In either case, you will want to interview both to understand all of the facts and frame the issues or problems in terms of specific behavior and job performance expectations that are being affected. As the supervisor, you also must be clear about your expectations for job performance actions and attitudes and remind both of them about the department's expectations. During this discussion, each party should become more aware of their own behaviors as well as the behaviors of the other and how the interaction of their choices is affecting their work. Your goal in this exchange is for both parties to work out a solution that does not compromise the work of either and allows the work of the department to continue more effectively.

Supervision of Occupational Therapy Personnel

Effective supervision of OT personnel is necessary to ensure safe and effective delivery of services. As was mentioned at the beginning of this chapter, supervision is embedded within the OT process. However, OT practitioners work in a broad range of work environments (medical, educational, and community-based settings). To guide practitioners in developing effective supervisory practices in these different situations, professional organizations may develop supervisory guidelines that can be applied in all settings. These guidelines describe how the profession views the supervisory process, who needs to be supervised, the methods and frequency of supervision, and supervisory responsibilities of different OT personnel.

Occupational Therapists

The AOTA describes occupational therapists as "autonomous practitioners who are able to deliver services independently" (AOTA, 2020b, p. S1). Likewise, the WFOT endorses the autonomy of the profession (World Federation of Occupational Therapists [WFOT], 2007) and describes the minimum qualifications for OT practitioners (WFOT, 2008). In the United States, entry-level occupational therapists are qualified to practice without supervision. The therapist's professional education and training prepares to deliver services independently, which in the United States includes a minimum of 6 months of supervised fieldwork experience and successful completion of the initial certification exam. Entry-level occupational therapists are trained as generalists and are qualified to enter general practice settings as autonomous therapists. Although entry-level therapists do not require supervision, "occupational therapists are encouraged to seek peer supervision interprofessional collaboration, and mentoring to promote their ongoing professional development and to ensure they are using best practice approaches in the delivery of services" (AOTA, 2020b, p. S1).

This statement underscores each therapist's professional responsibility to maintain the competencies that are needed to provide safe and effective services. The therapist who enters a work setting where professional supervision is not provided should carefully compare their current competencies with the demands of the work setting. When this comparison reveals that current knowledge and skills may need further support or development, the therapist should seek supervision or mentoring to ensure competent practice and professional growth. Although this is not required, many entry-level therapists seek first-time jobs in which supervision will be available. These positions allow them more time to solidify clinical skills and develop confidence. Therapists beyond entry level should continue to assess their need for professional supervision if it is not provided in their work setting. Career changes, such as switching practice settings (from school to nursing home) or types of clients treated (autistic children to adults with spinal cord injuries), may challenge the therapist's current competency and trigger the need to seek supervision or mentoring (AOTA, 2015; Youngstrom, 1998).

In many OT practice settings, there may be no formal supervision by another OT practitioner. In these situations, OT practitioners often seek informal peer supervision from OT practitioners in similar settings. They ask for feedback from each other and share case information, often problem-solving together to plan effective interventions. The advent of social networking and Web-based resources has expanded the informal consultation resources available to practitioners. This is a positive and proactive approach that helps to ensure effective professional practice and personal competence. See Chapter 71, for an extended discussion of competence and professional development.

Occupational Therapy Assistants

Although OTAs are used in as many as 36 other countries throughout the world (WFOT, 2020), supervisory guidelines are most fully developed in the United States. This discussion of OTA supervision is based on current practice in the United States. Occupational therapists working with OTAs in other countries will want to contact the professional association in those countries to determine if supervision requirements are different.

In the United States, OTAs who deliver OT services must be supervised by an occupational therapist (AOTA, 2015, 2020b). OTAs are trained and educated in basic OT approaches and techniques, and their role is one of assisting the professional level therapist with the delivery of services.

The occupational therapist is responsible for all aspects of service delivery and works in partnership and collaboration with the OTA to provide appropriate services to clients. The inclusion of OTAs as OT service providers helps to ensure increased access to OT for all clients (AOTA, 2019). Entry-level occupational therapists are expected to be able to supervise OTAs and to be knowledgeable about the collaborative supervisory relationship that the profession values (Accreditation Council for Occupational Therapy Education [ACOTE], 2018). Entry-level OTAs are expected to be knowledgeable of the supervisory partnership and to seek supervision appropriately. In the United States, OTAs, by virtue of their training and education, are often well qualified to take on related work roles (e.g., assistive technologists, activity program directors). When they do assume these roles, they are not providing OT services and consequently do not need to be supervised by an occupational therapist.

Fieldwork Students

Level II fieldwork students at the therapist and assistant level both must be supervised by OT practitioners. In the United States, OT students must be supervised by an occupational therapist who has at least 1 year of experience after being initially certified by the National Board for Certification in Occupational Therapy (ACOTE, 2018). OTA students may be supervised by either an occupational therapist or an OTA, both of whom also must have at least 1 year of experience after initial certification (ACOTE, 2018). If an OTA is providing the Level II supervision for the OTA student, it is understood that the supervising assistant is supervised by an occupational therapist. According to ACOTE, personnel who are qualified to supervise Level I OT or OTA students include all credentialed OT personnel as well as individuals from other disciplines such as nursing, psychology, social work, and teaching (ACOTE, 2018).

To benefit from Level II fieldwork supervision, the OT student needs to seek and respond to feedback that is given. The supervisory relationship that is established during fieldwork is similar to a professional supervisory relationship. Chapter 70 discusses the nature of supervision in the fieldwork setting, and Expanding Our Perspectives discusses fieldwork from the student perspective.

Other Personnel

Other types of personnel who may assist with the provision of OT services or the management of services delivery, such as administrative assistants, OT aides, or volunteers, may be supervised by either occupational therapists or OTAs. Table 74.3 provides an overview of whom various personnel may supervise.

TABLE 74.3 **Patterns of Supervision: Who Can Supervise Whom?**

Type of Supervisor	OTA	OT Aide	Volunteer	OT Fieldwork Student Level I	OT Fieldwork Student Level II	OTA Fieldwork Student Level I	OTA Fieldwork Student Level II	Occupational Therapist
Entry-level occupational therapist	X	X	X	X	X			
Occupational therapist with more than 1 year of experience	X	X	X	X	X	X	X	X
Entry-level OTA		X	X					
OTA with more than 1 year of experience	X	X	X	X		X	X	

OT, Occupational therapy, OTA, occupational therapy assistant.

Types of Supervision: Overseeing Various Aspects of Work

Work is a complex activity. The responsibility for supervising various aspects of work is sometimes assigned to different people. It is not uncommon for an OT practitioner to receive supervision from more than one person for different aspects of their work performance. Discussion of three distinct aspects of work performance and the type of supervision used to oversee that performance will help you to see how supervision in some settings may require a multifaceted approach.

Administrative Supervision

Administrative supervision is focused on monitoring performance and making sure that the supervisee's work performance and professional development meet the objectives and standards of the employing organization. Administrative supervisors focus on the administrative aspects of job performance, such as attendance, schedules, benefit usage, and checking for appropriate completion of assigned job tasks. This type of supervision correlates closely with the administrative function of supervision discussed earlier.

Administrative supervision can be provided by an occupational therapist or an OTA to other occupational therapists and OTAs or to members of other disciplines. Likewise, members of other disciplines can administratively supervise OT practitioners and OTAs. This type of supervision commonly occurs in public school settings in which school principals or special education administrators are the designated supervisors for the OT staff. As the supervisor, the principal or special education administrator would be supervising the administrative aspects of the OT's work. Similarly, in rehabilitation settings, an occupational therapist may function in a management role and, thus, provide administrative supervision to members of other disciplines such as physical therapy or speech-language pathology.

Clinical or Professional Practice Supervision

Supervision that is aimed at providing support, training, and evaluation of a supervisee's professional performance and development is called professional practice supervision or clinical supervision. The term *clinical supervision* was the most commonly used term in the past to describe this type of supervision. However, as more OT practitioners have moved into work settings outside the clinical medical model (e.g., school settings, community centers), the term *clinical supervision* seems less appropriate than the broader term **professional practice supervision.** In professional practice supervision, the supervisor's responsibilities extend beyond the purely administrative aspects of job performance and are additionally aimed at assisting and supporting the supervisee's development of professional discipline-specific skills, such as interviewing skills, appropriate use of selected therapeutic techniques, and professional reasoning.

Professional practice supervision can appropriately be provided only by a member of the supervisee's discipline. Consequently, it would not be appropriate for a physical therapist to provide professional practice supervision or clinical supervision to an occupational therapist. Likewise, an occupational therapist cannot be expected to provide professional practice or clinical supervision for a physical therapist. Professional practice supervision is the type of supervision that is provided by fieldwork educators during Level II fieldwork experiences. (Fieldwork educators also provide administrative supervision to students.) An occupational therapist may provide professional practice supervision to other occupational therapists and OTAs, and an OTA may provide professional practice supervision to other OTAs. This type of supervision correlates closely with the educational and supportive supervisory functions.

Functional Supervision

A third type of supervision that is seen in some OT practice environments is functional supervision (AOTA, 1993, p. 1088). In **functional supervision,** a specific aspect of work or a "function" of professional practice is delegated to a specified individual to provide training and oversight in that aspect of work. The supervisor who is providing only functional supervision generally has advanced knowledge, skill, and competence in the area being supervised. For example, an OT supervisor of a new employee might request that another OT who is experienced in wheelchair assessment and positioning provide functional supervision to the new employee in this area. When providing functional supervision, the supervisor is not responsible for the entire supervisory process but rather supervises the person's performance and development of specific skills or competency in only the selected job function area.

Methods of Supervision

A professional practice supervisor needs to consider what supervisory methods will be most effective in developing and monitoring performance. Supervisees have different learning styles. Worksites have varying caseload demands, administrative requirements for supervision, and time available to provide supervision. Supervisory methods need to be selected to meet the supervisee's needs and the demands of the worksite.

The supervisor is responsible for initially orienting and training the supervisee and then supporting the supervisee's professional growth and development. From the organization's perspective, it is important that information provided while training the supervisee be delivered in a manner to promote safe and effective outcomes and positive client experiences (Laverdure et al., 2017). To achieve this, consideration should be given to the type of teaching methods that will be most effective in learning new information and developing work skills. Varying the methods used and selecting the ones that will mesh with the learner's skill and comfort level can be most effective. Involve the supervisee in the process by asking what learning approaches they prefer. Box 74.4 lists examples of various learning methods.

To monitor and evaluate performance, the supervisor can use direct and indirect approaches.

Direct or Line-of-Sight Supervision

In direct or line-of-sight methods of supervision, the supervisor is present when the employee is performing the job and actually observes performance. When considering

---

BOX 74.4 EXAMPLES OF LEARNING METHODS

- Provide written protocols or instructions.
- Have the learner report back on what they learned from reading.
- Provide articles or books to read or use as reference.
- Demonstrate and have the learner return the demonstration.
- Provide a verbal explanation or lecture that covers the content.
- Provide videotapes with questions about content to answer at end.

- Have the learner participate in small group discussion to problem-solve clinical situations.
- Discuss cases or problems presented, either one on one or in small groups.
- Role-play situations.
- Provide repeated practice opportunities to apply new knowledge and skills.
- Observe others carrying out tasks; ask the learner to describe what they observed.
- Model desired performance and behaviors.

COMMENTARY ON THE EVIDENCE

Supervision in Occupational Therapy

The majority of research in supervision has been conducted by business and management researchers. Within the healthcare professions, nurses, social workers, and counseling psychologists have been the primary contributors to the research on clinical supervision. In OT, direct empirical evidence to support effective supervisory practice is lacking. The research that is available in OT is often

related to management issues and/or is descriptive in focus. For example, OT managers, concerned with employee satisfaction and retention, have shown that factors such as feedback and recognition of accomplishments, realistic workloads, and autonomy and opportunities for professional growth and skill development all influence job satisfaction (Barnes, 1998; Smith, 2000). Relationships with other therapists on the team and the immediate supervisor or manager have also been found to contribute to

(continued)

job satisfaction and reduce burnout (Mason & Hennigan, 2019; Park, 2021). Although these studies did not directly look at supervision, the factors that were identified are all factors that a supervisor can affect, so effective supervision should attend to these factors.

Two studies have provided some insight into current supervisory practices. Johnson et al. (2006) reported that more fieldwork educators who supervise Level I fieldwork students are not occupational therapists (OT practitioners) than in the past. In April 2006, the National Board for Certification in Occupational Therapy reported the results of a 2005 online survey of OT and OTA certification exam candidates that included data on who the practitioner's primary supervisor was and the number of hours of direct supervision received per week (Bent & Conway, 2006). Thirty-eight percent of occupational therapists and 23% of OTAs were supervised by members of other disciplines. Thirty-one percent of occupational therapists and 18% of OTAs received zero hours of direct supervision per week. Descriptive statistics such as these prompt us to ask other questions: How does being supervised by someone who is not an OT practitioner affect practitioners' professional growth and commitment to occupation-based practice? Does frequency of direct supervision affect the quality of services delivered and the rate of professional growth?

Research about supervision readiness and practices with OT fieldwork students is somewhat more prevalent. Researchers have explored the supervisory experiences of fieldwork educators (Karp et al., 2021; Richard, 2008) to identify supervision issues as well as their readiness to provide telesupervision (Calabrese et al., 2021). The effectiveness of different models of supervision including the use of non-OT supervisors for Level I fieldwork experiences (Heine & Bennett, 2003), faculty-driven Level I fieldwork experiences (Ciro & Isaacson, 2016), and aggregate fieldwork models (Precin, 2009) have also been examined.

Both descriptive and empirical studies of supervision in OT are needed. How do supervisory practices vary by setting? What is the most efficient and effective way to establish service competency with an OTA? What supervisory approaches are most effective in supporting professional growth and development with supervisees? These are only a few of the many questions that need to be answered to provide supervisors with the evidence they need to supervise effectively.

supervision methods, this approach is generally the first one that comes to mind. Direct observation provides firsthand information to the supervisor, but is time-consuming, and it is not always practical to use as the only method of supervision.

Indirect Supervision

Indirect methods allow the supervisor to ascertain how the job was performed by gathering this information after performance occurs. Indirect methods include communicating with the supervisee (via phone, e-mail, or written correspondence) after performance, looking at written records (attendance records, documentation), or receiving reports from others (clients, parents, other staff, or team members) about the supervisee's performance. Listening to what others say provides information about the employee's performance and provides feedback about how others perceive the performance. Supervising performance in a clinical setting by reading the supervisee's documentation is a frequently used indirect method in OT practice. Reviewing documentation tells the supervisor what happened when clients were seen and provides insight into the supervisee's clinical reasoning and documentation skills. However, using only the indirect method of supervision without also periodically observing performance would not give the supervisor a well-rounded picture of the employee's performance in areas such as interpersonal skill, technique application, adaptability in spontaneous clinical situations, and problem-solving. Both indirect and direct methods need to be used to develop an accurate and complete picture of employee performance.

Telesupervision

With the advances in and widespread access to technology, increased attention has been given to the use of telesupervision in the health professions, including OT (Brandoff & Lombardi, 2012). **Telesupervision** refers to clinical supervision provided with communication technology and includes the use of videoconferencing, telephone, e-mails, chats, podcasts, or the use of social networks (Brandoff & Lombardi, 2012; Kind et al., 2014). Telesupervision has primarily been used in rural or remote areas or when having to supervise staff working in multiple sites (Dudding & Justice, 2004; Martin et al., 2015). Increased use of telesupervision has been noted in response to the COVID-19 global pandemic (Robinson et al., 2021).

The format of telesupervision varies and depends on the particular setting, available technology, supervisee's needs, and supervisor availability (Miller et al., 2003). For instance, an OT supervisor may lead a chat session with a group of supervisees to review documentation requirements, whereas another OT supervisor may observe a supervisee via videoconference to assess their ability to perform a seating assessment.

Factors that have been identified as contributing to effective use of telesupervision include previous face-to-face contact, access to high-quality technical systems, continuity, careful participant selection, and well-planned supervisory sessions (Martin et al., 2017, 2018). OT supervisors planning to use telesupervision should consider these factors when developing these programs. Supervisors will also need to be aware of and comply with any applicable governmental regulations or institutional policies related to employee and patient privacy when using telesupervision (e.g., the need to obtain consent for videotaping and the use of encrypted transmitted data).

Frequency of Supervision

One of the first decisions a supervisor must make when developing a supervision plan is to determine how frequently to have contact with the supervisee to teach, train, monitor, and evaluate performance. The members of the profession have considered this question in relation to how frequency of supervision should be determined in supervising OTAs (AOTA, 2020b, p. S2). The factors that are outlined next can be considered in all supervisory situations. In determining frequency of supervisory contact, the supervisor should consider the following:

1. *The skills of the supervisor.* Supervisors who are new and just developing their skills might require more frequent contact with the supervisee because they are less efficient in observing and analyzing performance. They might need more time to recognize possible performance issues and to provide supervisory interventions. The supervisor who has had more experience and/or who has previously supervised in a similar setting might be clearer about performance expectations and able to anticipate problems and provide guidance and direction sooner.

2. *The skills of the supervisee.* New employees who come to a job with background and experience in a similar job probably bring the needed skills to the new job. Generally, these employees will require less

initial training and often move very quickly to a point at which they need less frequent supervision. The supervisor, however, must individually evaluate each employee because experience does not always guarantee effective performance. The employee's speed and style of learning will also affect the frequency of supervision needed.

3. *The nature of the work.* Work that is more varied and complex might require more frequent supervisory contact to allow the supervisor to observe performance at different times under various conditions and levels of complexity. The new practitioner working in a rehabilitation hospital whose caseload consists only of patients who had stroke might require less frequent supervision than the new practitioner who is working in an acute care setting seeing clients with orthopedic, neurologic, and acute medical conditions.

4. *The expectations and requirements of the work setting.* In various work settings, standards and expectations may have developed, based on experience in that setting, that require certain levels of supervision. Although an experienced supervisor might think that weekly contact is sufficient, a worksite might require daily contact.

5. *The expectations and requirements of external regulatory or legislative agencies.* Federal or state practice acts and regulations, accrediting agencies, and third-party papers may specify certain methods of oversight and contact that must occur between the occupational therapist and the OTA. When these requirements apply, it is essential that the occupational therapist comply and provide supervision in accordance with.

Frequency of supervision is generally viewed as occurring on a continuum. At the high end of the continuum, the supervisor is continually in sight of the supervisee who is working. At the low end of the continuum, the supervisor contacts the supervisee only as needed. The supervisor needs to be flexible in dealing with the wide variety of practice setting and supervisory demands that exist within the profession and consider these demands carefully when determining supervision frequency.

There are, however, two firm directives regarding need for supervision based on professional documents:

1. Entry-level OT practitioners do not *require* supervision. They are, however, "encouraged to seek peer supervision, interprofessional collaboration, and mentoring to promote their ongoing professional development and to ensure they are using best practice approaches" (AOTA, 2020b, p. S1; WFOT, 2007).

2. OTAs must *always* receive some level of regular supervision from an occupational therapist when they are providing OT services in the United States (AOTA, 2020b).

The Occupational Therapist–OTA Supervisory Relationship

In the United States, where the role of the OTA has been developed over a longer period of time, the supervisory relationship between the OT practitioner and OTA is characterized as a partnership. The discussion that follows describing the OT practitioner–OTA supervisory relationship is based on this partnership perspective.

Both levels of practitioners in the United States are trained and educated within the profession but at different levels. The occupational therapist is educated at the professional knowledge and skill level and receives an entry-level graduate degree. The OTA is currently educated at the technical level and receives an associate of arts or bachelor's degree (ACOTE, 2018). Each level of practitioner has complementary but distinct roles. The occupational therapist is responsible for overall service provision and can carry out all facets of service provision (i.e., evaluation, intervention planning, intervention implementation and review, and outcomes assessment). The OTA's primary role is in the implementation phase of service provision. They may contribute to other aspects of service provision, such as performing selected assessments for which they have demonstrated service competence, or recommending intervention changes, but only under the supervision of the occupational therapist.

The "Guidelines for Supervision, Roles, and Responsibilities during the Delivery of Occupational Therapy Services" (AOTA, 2020b) outline the roles and responsibilities of each level of practitioner during the delivery of services. For the partnership to be successful, each practitioner must have a clear understanding of each other's role and respect and value the contribution that each practitioner makes. When the occupational therapists and OTAs work as a team, they are able to use and build on each other's skills and expand the number and kinds of services that can be provided to clients. When an occupational therapist partners with an OTA, the professional level therapist is often able to see more clients and to use the assistant's personal expertise in specific practice areas or techniques to improve client care. See OT Story 74.2, for dilemmas that can occur when supervising an OTA.

OT STORY 74.2 CHANGING PRACTICE PATTERNS: TAYLOR SUPERVISES AN OCCUPATIONAL THERAPY ASSISTANT

Taylor recently started a new job as an occupational therapist at a large long-term care facility in her community. She works with a team of two other occupational therapists and two OTAs. She is responsible for supervising Diane, one of the OTAs. Diane has been working at this facility for 5 years and considers herself very experienced in dealing with this population. When Taylor started the job, she met with Diane to discuss their supervisory relationship and to determine how they would conduct their partnership. Taylor spent time observing and working with Diane and found Diane to be very helpful in orienting her to the facility and familiarizing her with the patients and the typical OT interventions that were being used.

Taylor has now worked at the facility for more than 6 months and is more familiar with the clients and their individual needs. She is interested in developing intervention plans that are more individualized and that use intervention activities that relate to each patient's own needs and personal lifestyle choices, whether they will return home or remain in the nursing home's long-term care wing. Interventions in the past have been focused primarily on self-care issues, and Taylor, although not wanting to ignore these occupations, would like to emphasize more instrumental activities of daily living and leisure occupations in which patients will want to engage if they return home or that might allow them to increase their sense of self-efficacy and control if they remain in long-term care. She has communicated this goal to Diane, and when they develop intervention plans, individualized goals are developed in these areas. However, as she follows up with Diane and observes interventions and monitors patient progress, Taylor has noted that Diane is not choosing to address these goals and continues to use the routine types of tasks and activities that she was previously using.

Questions

1. How would you define the supervisory issues and problems in this situation?
2. As a supervisor in this scenario, what are Taylor's responsibilities?
3. As a supervisee in this scenario, what are Diane's responsibilities?
4. What do you think might be some of the reasons for Diane's behavior?
5. How would you suggest that Taylor approach Diane and address this problem?
6. What do you think might be some supervisory interventions that Taylor could take that would help to improve this situation?

Service Competency

The purpose of the supervisory process is to ensure that safe and effective services are delivered and that professional competence is fostered. The occupational therapist who is responsible for overall service delivery needs to ensure that any OTAs they are supervising are performing effectively. To ensure that services provided by both levels of practitioners are safe and effective, the occupational therapist establishes service competency with the OTA.

Service competency is the process of teaching, training, and evaluating in which the occupational therapist determines that the OTA performs tasks in the same way that the occupational therapist would and achieves the same outcomes (AOTA, 2020b).

When the occupational therapist and OTA initially start working together, the occupational therapist will establish service competency for overall job performance. In the early stages of the work relationship, the therapist will need to determine what knowledge and skills the OTA has. The establishment of service competency is integrated into the normal supervisory process as the supervisor orients and trains the new employee and begins comparing the employee's performance to the established professional and worksite standards and expectations. The occupational therapist should identify the primary job tasks and skills that are needed for the OTA's job. These tasks will vary by site and service setting. The therapist will observe and train the assistant to determine whether they can perform the identified skills and tasks and whether intervention outcomes are similar to those normally achieved by the occupational therapist. Examples of job tasks or skills for which service competency may be established include reviewing the medical record, being able to record appropriate and pertinent information, and being able to appropriately grade an activity to increase its cognitive difficulty.

The concept of service competency is based on the assumption that the supervising therapist is competent in the skills for which competency is being established. Both levels of practitioners are responsible for being aware of each other's competent behaviors and providing feedback to inform each other of possible problem areas.

It is important that the supervisor establish an acceptable standard of performance or level of agreement for skills and tasks on which service competency is being established. For example, when observing client ability to dress, the OTA will rate the client's level of independence at the same level as the occupational therapist 95% of the time. The comparison of outcomes between practitioners is an approach that helps to ensure that services clients receive are of comparable quality. It supports the validity of delegating to the OTA and ensures consistency of services. The methods the therapist can use while establishing service competency could include observation, cotreatment, return demonstration of techniques or skills, review of documentation, testing for knowledge and its application, and discussion of cases to ascertain clinical reasoning and judgment.

After initial service competency is established, the therapist supervisor will need to periodically recheck service competency to ensure that it is maintained. The occupational therapist may also select new tasks and skills in which to establish service competency with the OTA. For example, the occupational therapist might decide to train the assistant in how to carry out and score a particular structured assessment tool. After service competency has been established, the therapist can delegate the administration of this assessment to the assistant and be assured that the results of the assistant's giving the test will be comparable to the results that would be obtained if the occupational therapist administered the test. Service competency does not mean that the OTA will perform the task in exactly the same manner as the OTA would—only that the outcomes will be similar. Note that in all cases, the occupational therapist is responsible for interpreting the assessment results as part of the overall evaluation process.

Frequency and Type of Occupational Therapy Assistant Supervision

The decisions about frequency of supervision for the OTA will vary with practice setting and should be decided based on the five factors previously discussed: skills of the supervisor, skills of the supervisee, nature of the work, expectations and requirements of the work setting, and expectations and requirements of external regulatory or legislative agencies. The OTA's level of service competency and skill will influence the frequency of supervision needed. If service competency has already been established, the need for supervision might be less frequent. When service competency is being established in a new area or skill, the supervisor will need to change the frequency of supervision until competency is established.

Work factors that can affect frequency of supervision needed by an OTA include increased complexity of client's needs and diagnoses, rapidity of client change, more involved or complex types of interventions, and increased number and diversity of clients in the assistant's caseload. When the client population is complex and/or rapidly changing, frequent reevaluation and adjustment in types of interventions and implementation plans are needed, which require the clinical reasoning and evaluation skills of the OT practitioner. Frequency of supervision needs should be regularly reassessed as workplace demands, client needs, and supervisee skills change.

Because the supervisory process with the OTA is collaborative and both practitioners are responsible for providing safe and effective services, the occupational therapist and OTA should discuss the decision about the frequency of supervision. Supervision frequency and methods should be mutually decided on.

Although frequency of supervision can vary, OTAs who are providing OT services will always need some level of regular supervision. Supervision of the OTA on an irregular, spontaneous, or as-needed basis is not appropriate. It does not demonstrate that the occupational therapist is providing the ongoing oversight required to ensure safe and effective services nor does it validate that high-quality OT services are being provided. Many external regulatory and legislative agencies specify the frequency and type of supervisory contact that must take place between the occupational therapist and OTA. The Centers for Medicare and Medicaid Services (CMS) states that the OTA providing services to Medicare patients under an occupational therapist working in a physician's office must have direct or onsite (in the building but not in the line of sight) supervision on the day of treatment (CMS, 2012). CMS requires that occupational therapists must write a progress report every 10 treatment days or once every 30-day interval and that they perform or actively participate in treatments at this frequency level if the treatments have been delegated to an OTA (Thomas, 2006). This requirement necessitates that the therapists have regular contact with the client and with the OTA who is providing services.

Many state regulatory agencies outline specific supervision requirements in their laws for OTA supervision, and CMS requires that the supervisor provided complies with these regulations. OT practitioners should contact their regulatory boards for information about specific supervisory requirements.

Effective OTA Supervisory Relationships

The occupational therapist–OTA relationship should be collaborative in nature. The OT supervisor has the obligation and responsibility to supervise the OTA, and the OTA has the obligation and responsibility to seek supervision. In writing about their own collaborative relationship, Hanft

and Banks (1999) identified six qualities that support the development of collaborative supervisory relationships:

1. *Sensitivity,* for perceiving and responding to one another's professional and personal needs
2. *Dependability,* for keeping commitments and responding to unexpected situations
3. *Attentiveness,* for actively listening to one another
4. *Respectfulness,* for appreciating one another's distinct knowledge, experiences, and judgment
5. *Collaborativeness,* for working toward a common goal and representing OT services together as a unit
6. *Reflection,* for an ability to use self-observation to review situations objectively from different perspectives (p. 31)

It is essential when establishing a collaborative relationship that the OT practitioner and OTA understand each other's roles, responsibilities, experience, competence, and learning styles (Thomas, 2019).

The occupational therapists need to actively involve the OTA in the supervisory process and need to tailor the experience to meet individual needs of the OTA and the worksite. Box 74.5 presents a summary of the primary steps that should be taken in supervising an OTA.

Supervising Occupational Therapy Aides

Occupational therapy aides are individuals with no formalized education in the provision of OT services who are hired to provide supportive services to OT practitioners. Aides are trained on the job to meet the specific needs of the individual department. Aides do not provide skilled OT services, and the types of activities they can perform with clients are clearly prescribed for therapists in the United States in the "Guidelines for Supervision, Roles, and Responsibilities during the Delivery of Occupational Therapy Services" (AOTA, 2020b). Aides can perform two types of tasks within the department: they can carry out (a) non–client-related tasks such as clerical work, clinic maintenance tasks, and preparation of work

---

BOX 74.5 SUMMARY OF STEPS TO TAKE IN SUPERVISING AN OCCUPATIONAL THERAPY ASSISTANT

1. Orient OTA to worksite.
2. Discuss job and professional expectations.
3. Identify OTA's skill level.
4. Identify OTA's learning needs and methods of learning

5. Establish service competency.
6. Collaborate with OTA to establish methods and frequency of ongoing supervisory plan
7. Document ongoing supervision.

areas and equipment and (b) selected client-related tasks that are routine and supervised by an occupational therapist or an OTA (AOTA, 2020b). For a task to be considered routine, it must meet the following four criteria:

1. The outcome anticipated for the delegated task is predictable.
2. The situation of the client and the environment is stable and will not require that judgments, interpretations, or adaptations be made by the aide.
3. The client has demonstrated some previous performance ability in executing the task.
4. The task routine and process have been clearly established (AOTA, 2020b).

These criteria are based on the understanding that aides do not have the knowledge and skill to evaluate or make changes in an intervention activity but can be helpful in providing oversight or practice of selected activities when change and judgment are not anticipated.

Before a selected task can be delegated to an aide, the practitioner must be assured that the aide can carry out the task safely and effectively. They must instruct and assess their competency in performing the delegated task. The aide also must be aware of all precautions and signs or symptoms that a particular client might demonstrate that would indicate that the aide needs to seek assistance (AOTA, 2020b). Each of these requirements is intended to ensure that the aide's interaction with the client will be safe and effective. Practitioners can appropriately use aides to oversee clients who are practicing certain skills after the process has been set up (e.g., one-handed shoe tying and activity routines). Aides can also provide another pair of hands during physical activities when additional help is needed to engage the client in an activity as when providing assistance to transfer a patient. Aides can be supervised by either an occupational therapist or an OTA. However, when the OTA supervises the aide, the occupational therapist maintains overall responsibility for the process through the occupational therapist's supervision of the OTA.

Frequency of supervision will vary with tasks assigned and the aide's skill. Client-related tasks may require closer supervision because of the importance of patient safety and intervention effectiveness. The supervisory plan and process need to be documented to demonstrate accountability.

Supervising Non–Occupational Therapy Personnel

The same basic guidelines and process for effective supervision should be followed in supervising non-OT personnel. The OT practitioner who assumes a supervisory or management role may supervise personnel from other disciplines who provide direct services to clients (e.g., physical therapists, psychologists, recreational therapists) as well as personnel who provide support services for the department (e.g., administrative assistants, information technology specialists). The type of supervision the OT practitioner will provide to personnel from other disciplines will be administrative. Occupational therapy practitioners cannot provide professional practice supervision or clinical supervision because OT practitioners are not trained in the other individuals' professions. Supervisors will ensure that their supervisees from other disciplines seek and have access to professional practice supervision or mentoring and will consult with members of the supervisee's discipline to assist them in evaluating the supervisee's professional practice performance.

Conclusion

Supervision is a dynamic and person-oriented process—much like OT. The OT supervisor must continually balance the needs of the organization with the needs of supervisees to provide safe and effective services to clients. Awareness of the basic functions of supervision and an understanding of the supervisory process make up the first step in preparing practitioners for the supervisory role.

Acknowledgments

The author thanks Mary Jane Youngstrom for previous contributions to this chapter. Her knowledge, expertise, and perspective remain an inspiration.

Lippincott® Connect *For additional resources on the subjects discussed in this chapter, visit* Lippincott Connect.

REFERENCES

Accreditation Council for Occupational Education. (2018). Accreditation Council for Occupational Therapy Education (ACOTE®) standards. *American Journal of Occupational Therapy, 72*, S1–S83. https://doi.org/10.5014/ajot.2018.72S217

American Occupational Therapy Association. (1993). Occupational therapy roles. *American Journal of Occupational Therapy, 47*(12), 1087–1099. https://doi.org/10.5014/ajot.47.12.1087

American Occupational Therapy Association. (2015). Standards for continuing competence. *American Journal of Occupational Therapy, 69*, 6913410055p1–6913410055p3. https://doi.org/10.5014/ajot.2015.696S16

American Occupational Therapy Association. (2019). Value of occupational therapy assistant education to the profession. *American Journal of Occupational Therapy, 73*(suppl. 2), 7312410007. https://doi.org/10.5014/ajot.2019.73S209

American Occupational Therapy Association. (2020a). AOTA 2020 occupational therapy code of ethics. *American Journal of Occupational Therapy, 74*(suppl. 3), 7413410005. https://doi.org/10.5014/ajot.2020.74S3006

American Occupational Therapy Association. (2020b). Guidelines for supervision, roles, and responsibilities during the delivery of occupational therapy services. *American Journal of Occupational Therapy, 74*(suppl. 3), 7413410020. https://doi.org/10.5014/ajot.2020.74S3004

American Occupational Therapy Association. (2021). Standards of practice for occupational therapy. *American Journal of Occupational Therapy, 75*(suppl. 3), 7513410050. https://doi.org/10.5014/ajot.2021.75S3004

Barnes, D. S. (1998). Job satisfaction and the rehabilitation professional. *Administration & Management Special Interest Section Quarterly, 14*(4), 1–2.

Bent, M. A., & Conway, S. (2006). *Results of a national study profiling the 2005 certification candidate population.* http://www.nbcot.org

Brandoff, R., & Lombardi, R. (2012). Miles apart: Two art therapists' experience of distance supervision. *Art Therapy, 29*(2), 93–96. https://doi.org/10.1080/07421656.2012.683729

Braveman, B. (2016). *Leading and managing occupational therapy services: An evidence-based approach* (2nd ed.). F. A. Davis.

Calabrese, J. A., Coviello, J. M., Grasso, A. Y., Otchet, K. A., Pugh, E. A., Thomas, M., & Trivinia, B. (2021). Use of a webinar to assess fieldwork educator readiness to provide occupational therapy services and supervise students through telehealth. *Journal of Occupational Therapy Education, 5*(2). https://doi.org/10.26681/jote.2021.050212

Centers for Medicare & Medicaid Services. (2012). *Part B billing scenarios for PTs and OTs.* https://www.cms.gov/Medicare/Billing/TherapyServices/Downloads/11_Part_B Billing Scenarios_for_PTs and_OTs.pdf

Ciro, C. A., & Isaacson, M. (2016). Student rating of skill performance opportunities in faculty-directed research. *The Open Journal of Occupational Therapy, 4*(3), Article 3. https://doi.org/10.15453/2168-6408.1184

Dudding, C. C., & Justice, L. M. (2004). An e-supervision model: Videoconferencing as a clinical training tool. *Communication Disorder Quarterly, 25*(3), 145–151. https://www.learntechlib.org/p/98025/

Golia, G. M., & McGovern, A. R., (2015). If you save me, I'll save you: The power of peer supervision in clinical training and professional development. *The British Journal of Social Work, 45*(2), 634–650. https://doi.org/10.1093/bjsw/bct138

Hanft, B., & Banks, B. (1999). Competent supervision: A collaborative process. *OT Practice, 4*(5), 32–34.

Heine, D., & Bennett, N. (2003). Student perceptions of level I fieldwork supervision. *Occupational Therapy in Health Care, 17*(2), 89–97. https://doi.org/10.1080/j003v17n02_06

Johnson, C. R., Koenig, K. P., Piersol, C. V., Santalucia, S. E., & Wachter-Schutz, W. (2006). Level I fieldwork today: A study of contexts and perceptions. *American Journal of Occupational Therapy, 60*(3), 275–287. https://doi.org/10.5014/ajot.60.3.275

Kadushin, A. (1992). *Supervision in social work* (3rd ed.). Columbia University Press.

Karp, P., Lavin, K., & Collins, T. (2021). Exploring preparedness for competency in the role of fieldwork educator. *The American Journal of Occupational Therapy, 75*(suppl.2), 7512505185p1. https://doi.org/10.5014/ajot.2021.75S2-RP185

Kind, T., Patel, P. D., Lie, D. L., & Chretien, K. C. (2014). Twelve tips for using social media as a medical educator. *Medical Teacher, 36*(4), 284–290. https://doi.org/10.3109/0142159x.2013.852167

Laverdure, P., Smith, L. C., DuPrey, J., Lynn, J., & Swope, K. (2017). Beyond the badge: Supporting the orientation and training of new employees across practice settings. *OT Practice, 22*(17), 8–13.

Martin, P., Kumar, S., & Lizarondo, L. (2017). Effective use of technology in clinical supervision. *Internet Interventions, 8,* 35–39. https://doi.org/10.1016/j.invent.2017.03.001

Martin, P., Kumar, S., Lizarondo, L., & VanErp, A. (2015). Enablers of and barriers to high quality clinical supervision among occupational therapists across Queensland in Australia: Findings from a qualitative study. *BMC Health Services Research, 15*(413), 1085–1088. https://doi.org/10.1186/s12913-015-1085-8

Martin, P., Lizarondo, L., & Kumar, S. (2018). A systematic review of the factors that influence the quality and effectiveness of telesupervision for health professionals. *Journal of Telemedicine and Telecare, 24*(4), 271–281. https://doi.org/10.1177%2F1357633X17698868

Mason, V. C., & Hennigan, M. L. (2019). Occupational therapy practitioners' ratings of job satisfaction factors through a lens of social capital. *Occupational Therapy in Health Care, 33*(1), 88–107. https://doi.org/10.1080/07380577.2018.1543912

Miller, T. W., Miller, J. M., Burton, D., Sprang, R., & Adams, J. (2003). Telehealth: A model for clinical supervision in allied health. *The Internet Journal of Allied Health Sciences and Practice, 1*(2), 6. http://nsuworks.nova.edu/ijahsp/vol1/iss2/6/

Newstrom, J. W. (2013). *Supervision: Managing for results* (10th ed.). McGraw-Hill.

Park, E. Y. (2021). Meta-analysis of factors associated with occupational therapist burnout. *Occupational Therapy International, 2021,* 1226841. https://doi.org/10.1155/2021/1226841

Precin, P. (2009). An aggregate fieldwork model: Cooperative learning, research, and clinical project publication components. *Occupational Therapy in Mental Health, 25,* 62–82. https://doi.org/10.1080/01642120802647691

Richard, L. F. (2008). Exploring connections between theory and practice: Stories from fieldwork supervisors. *Occupational Therapy in Mental Health, 24,* 154–175. https://doi.org/10.1080/01642120802055259

Robinson, L., Brown, T., Fossey, E. M., Yu, M-L., Barclay, L., Chu, E., Peart, A., & Callaway, E. (2021). Practice education in lockdown: Lessons learned during the COVID-19 global pandemic. In D. Nestel, G. Reedy, L. McKenna, & S. Gough (Eds.), *Clinical education for the health professions: Theory and practice* (pp. 1–20). Springer.

Smith, V. (2000). Survey of occupational therapy job satisfaction in today's health care environment. *Administration & Management Special Interest Section Quarterly, 16*(4), 1–2.

Stevenson, A. (Ed.). (2010). *The new Oxford American dictionary* (3rd ed.). Oxford University Press.

Thomas, H. (2019). Working with occupational therapy assistants. In K. Jacobs & G. L. McCormack (Eds.), *The occupational therapy manager* (6th ed., pp. 385–392). AOTA Press.

Thomas, J. (2006). Interpreting Medicare's documentation requirements. *OT Practice, 11*(7), 8.

Urish, C. (2004). Ongoing competence through mentoring. *OT Practice, 9*(3), 10.

Waite, A. (2014). Guiding forces: Finding and benefiting from occupational therapy mentors. *OT Practice, 19*(17), 7–10.

Wilcox, M. M., Drinane, J. M., Black, S. W., Cabrera, L., DeBlaere, C., Tao, K. W., Hook, J. N., Davis, D. E., Watkins, C. E., & Owen, J. (2021). Layered cultural processes: The relationship between multicultural orientation and satisfaction with supervision. *Training and Education in Professional Psychology.* Advance online publication. https://doi.org/10.1037/tep0000366

World Federation of Occupational Therapists. (2007). *Professional OT autonomy—Revised 2007.* http://www.wfot/ResourceCentre/positionstatements.aspx

World Federation of Occupational Therapists. (2008). *Occupational therapy entry-level qualifications* (CM2008). http://www.wfot.org/ResourceCentre/positionstatements.aspx

World Federation of Occupational Therapists. (2020). *OT human resources project 2020—Numerical.* http://www.wfot.org/ResourceCentre/humanresourceproject.aspx

Youngstrom, M. J. (1998). Evolving competence in the practitioner role. *American Journal of Occupational Therapy, 52*(9), 716–720. https://doi.org/10.5014/ajot.52.9.716

Consultation as an Occupational Therapy Practitioner

Paula Kramer

LEARNING OBJECTIVES

After reading this chapter, you will be able to:

1. Understand and analyze the knowledge and skills necessary to be successful as a consultant.
2. Articulate the step-by-step process of consulting.
3. Appraise the content areas where occupational therapy (OT) practitioners may choose to engage in a consulting practice.
4. Appreciate how your OT knowledge paired with an understanding of business skills can aid in the consultation process.
5. Articulate the elements of the consulting process, including establishing consulting relationships, developing a proposal and the contract for engagement, and completing the project.
6. Analyze the challenges and ethical considerations associated with the role of consultant.
7. Explore the opportunities for OT consultants.

Introduction

This chapter presents the role of consultant for occupational therapy (OT) practitioners. Within the practice of OT, we have always advised individuals using our services about their conditions, interventions, and involvement in daily occupations. We have consulted with other professionals and the families of those in our care. This chapter focuses on how to use that knowledge and combine it with business skills to enter the less traditional role of consulting with organizations and institutions. Although the role of the consultant is still part of the helping relationship, it is a way that we can reach out and support interventions with organizations reaching out to individuals, groups, and communities. It also bridges staffing gap in some areas such as nursing homes, where OT services may be scarce. It also provides opportunities to showcase an occupation-centered model of care delivery to other disciplines, which is important for our profession.

This chapter is focused on the basic knowledge that the OT practitioner needs to move into the consulting realm. It includes a step-by-step guide to developing a consulting practice and learning to work within larger organizations and systems. Most systems in which we consult are complex, and the chapter discusses working within larger organizations and effecting positive change. The challenges and ethical issues of consulting are also presented. Consulting is discussed as an exciting arena for OT practitioners.

An Overview of Consultation

What Is Consultation?

Consultation comes from the word *conference*, as when two or more individuals meet to discuss or confer (Dictionary.com, 2021). Generally, it begins with a person or organization seeking help from someone who has knowledge or expertise in a specific area. Therefore, the concept of providing help is basic to the consultation process. A person or organization is either seeking for or providing help to another. The need for help or desire to help may be used by clients, families, other professionals, organizations, and communities. Consultation is a collaborative process of giving advice, something we do on a frequent basis with both clients and friends. However, in the professional consultative relationship, there is a combination of helping and business principles. You are generally contracted by a person, organization, or agency to provide a specific service or achieve a particular outcome. That service might be, but is not limited to, designing or developing a program, organizing a particular project, providing input on a current operation, or writing a document that will be used with professionals or clients. Thus, consultation involves a contract defining the consultant's role, the desired outcome, and/or the specific help the consultant will provide to the client or organization to reach that desired outcome. As consultants, we are responsible or accountable for delivering the product as outlined in the contract. This responsibility or accountability, as defined by the contract, is what makes consultation different from just giving advice.

Consultation, in the most general sense, describes any action one might take with a system expressing a need for assistance in moving forward or making changes (Block, 2011). The consultant has no power to make decisions or implement a program within an organization but can be influential in the organization based on their suggestions. A consultant is not a manager, as the manager has direct responsibility for decision-making and implementing programs and making changes in programs within their purview (Braveman, 2016). The consultant generally works with managers or higher administrators rather than with clients or staff members.

The recipients of the consultant's expertise are generally called clients; although in the world of management and marketing, they may be referred to as customers (Anastasi, 2014; Block, 2011). Sometimes, the client is a single individual and at other times an organization. In some cases, it may be several organizations. The client is the person or persons with whom the consultant interacts. The process of consulting is a collaborative relationship. The consultant needs to establish a relationship with the client on a personal level. It is critical that the consultant understands the needs of the client and understands the organization involved. The consultant makes recommendations and suggestions related to the areas that have been outlined by the clients but does not prescribe what should be done. Consultants use their knowledge and expertise to help the client achieve their goals for the organization.

Steinberg (2016) identifies that there are three general types of consultation in healthcare: clinical consultation, systems consultation, and organizational consultation. He views consultation as an "informed partnership" (p. 1) between parties.

Similarities Between Consulting and Traditional OT Practice

Traditionally, in OT practice we evaluate an individual or group, consult with them on setting goals, identify a theoretical approach to reach those goals, proceed with the intervention, and then reevaluate to determine whether the goals have been reached. Through our intervention process, we hope to promote changes in the individual or group through specific interventions and then either adjust the intervention to promote additional change or terminate the treatment. The consultation process is similar to the process we use with individuals or groups, but not the same. The organization or community may come to us with a problem already identified or may ask us to assess the situation to identify areas that should be changed or modified. Establishing a relationship with the client is very similar to establishing a rapport with an individual patient or client. In order to feel comfortable with the consultant, the client needs to know that you have the appropriate knowledge and expertise to understand their organization and to be responsive to concerns of the managers and administrators in the organization. Together with the client, the consultant will set goals and establish a time frame for reaching those goals. As the process continues, the consultant makes suggestions, offers potential changes, and introduces strategies for change, but cannot make change occur directly. It is important to ensure that the recommendations are compatible with and achievable by the organization. Consultants should not tell organizations what to do, but instead should offer suggestions based on knowledge and expertise and be open to discussing alternate ways to approach a particular problem (Anastasi, 2014; Block,

2011). It is important to keep in mind that consultation is generally descriptive, not diagnostic or prescriptive (Steinberg, 2016), and that maintaining a descriptive perspective takes experience and skill. The descriptive perspective requires the consultant to explain different ways to solve a problem, rather than telling someone what should be done.

Most often, OT practitioners consult within the type of organizations where occupational therapists tend to work, such as hospitals, educational institutions, community organizations, nursing homes, and outpatient facilities. Generally, these are same type of institutions where occupational therapists have developed specific expertise related to practice, education, and research. The American Occupational Therapy Association (AOTA, 2007) Centennial Vision developed in 2006 stressed the importance of focusing on trending populations, such as health and wellness, productive aging, and work and industry. Vision 2025 (AOTA, 2019) mentions the importance of serving all peoples, populations, and communities. Further, the Accreditation Council for Occupational Therapy Educational (ACOTE) Standards (2018) identifies the need to teach OT practitioners to work with persons, groups, and populations, rather than just focus on individuals. These are areas that are ripe for consultation. Almost all the individuals, groups that we treat, and systems that occupational therapists treat can benefit from occupation-centered consultation to promote occupational participation.

Your career as an OT practitioner will change over time. You may start in one area of practice and move on to other areas of practice. You may find that opportunities present themselves that help you grow and develop in different ways. Lifelong learning is key to the development of a true professional. You will follow your interests and develop different areas of expertise in areas of practice such as education, administration, and research. Within these areas you may build new programs, modify and improve existing programs, or continue with the status quo. You might help a department or division become more occupation-centered, guiding them in the choice of theories, frames of reference, or approaches. Maybe you will become a student supervisor in a new setting and develop a manual that will help students acclimate easier to your setting and understand what will be expected of them weekly. In OT Story 75.1, the occupational therapist's knowledge and experience is used to develop a new program in a community setting.

As you progress in your career and gain experience, your potential to become a consultant increases. Becoming a subject-matter expert is only the first step in becoming a consultant. You will need to understand the business aspects of consulting and develop the interpersonal skills needed to become a consultant. According to Anastasi (2014), subject-matter expertise for which you are hired and paid is generally "only about 75% of what is required" (p. 19) to deliver successful consulting

OT STORY 75.1 MOVING INTO A NEW ROLE AND DEVELOPING AN OCCUPATION-BASED PROGRAM IN AN ASSISTED LIVING FACILITY

Tisha is an occupational therapist who has worked with older adults for 7 years in various settings including rehabilitation and nursing homes. Although she has never worked as a consultant before, one of her former employers recommended her to an administrator of a local-assisted living facility. The administrator of the facility, Mr. Gomez, was concerned that many of the residents were spending much of their time in their rooms and were not involved in socialization or activities. He was interested in assistance from a consulting occupational therapist to create a program that would get the residents more involved in meaningful occupations, encourage them to interact more with each other, and eventually be able to have the residents run the program with some outside supervision or continued consultation from an occupational therapist. Tisha found herself pondering the following questions:

1. Did she have the skills necessary to be a consultant?
2. Was she capable of taking on this project?

3. Would she be able to translate her direct intervention knowledge into program development?

Do you think there are other questions Tisha should be considering?

Tisha's questions are all valid. Although she had never been a consultant, she had a strong working knowledge of the population involved in this project. Further, her practice had always been occupation-based. Her experience has led her to understand how new programs are developed and implemented. The only question left was her questioning her own capabilities to be a consultant.

To address her concerns, Tisha met with Mr. Gomez to gain a better understanding of what he expected and what the project would entail. We will revisit this example again later in the chapter.

Question

1. What specific questions should Tisha ask Mr. Gomez?

professional services. The remaining skills are those that will help you successfully manage your relationship with your client(s).

Starting Out as a Consultant

The first step in being a successful consultant involves self-exploration to identify your areas of expertise. Be honest about what you have to offer another organization or system (see Box 75.1). Think about whether you have specific educational and experiential background that will be useful to an individual or an organization. Do you have specific credentials that will appeal to an organization? Be aware that advanced doctoral education is common for those who consult in education and in research. In addition, OT consultants must have a firm foundation in the theories and skills that support entry-level practice. An awareness of professional history is also useful in that we can learn from the past about the importance of both content and context. Initially, consulting opportunities often come through our professional networks. Presenting posters or workshops at conferences may offer your first consulting invitations outside of your day-to-day employment. Participation in conferences, state, national, and international organizations like AOTA and World Federation of Occupational Therapists (WFOT) provides great opportunities for learning and gaining expertise, as well as networking. The author's personal experience as a faculty member, department chair, and volunteer at AOTA and ACOTE provided an invaluable knowledge base, extensive experience, and a basis for networking.

Beyond this, most consultants have some years of clinical practice, and many have achieved advanced education and practice in one or more areas of interest. Consulting in community programming and nonprofit development is being done by all levels of practitioners generally with an entrepreneur's ability to explore and learn as you go. Think about ways that you can use this information about yourself to promote your future as a consultant.

Once you have foundational knowledge and skills and have established a professional arena where you are comfortable with your expertise, there are questions for you to consider. Do you already have some consulting experience?

Has your current employer asked you to develop a new program in your own facility, such as adding an outpatient program or replicating a current program in another facility owned by the same organization? Although this may not sound like consulting, it is, and this is a very common beginning for many consultants in OT. This should go without saying, but do not consult in areas that are outside of your expertise.

Make sure that your resume includes the following:

- Targets your area(s) of expertise and includes any internal consulting that you have already done
- Identifies presentations that you have made that demonstrate your area(s) of expertise
- Lists any articles you have published on the topic
- Describe relevant experience such as:
  - Developing an effective fieldwork/internship/residence model
  - Functioning as an internship supervisor or academic fieldwork coordinator
  - Creating an innovative program that assists students or the academic institution

Review your resume and make sure that your expertise comes across loud and clear. Some consultants choose to actively market their services as a consultant and have effectively used social media, especially those who are looking to grow a business. When people need consultants, they tend to contact each other for recommendations so the more you work, the more work you'll have. Remember to acknowledge those who have recommended you and keep in contact with those who may serve as references for you. Consulting and marketing are very personal businesses, and there is nothing more powerful than a personal recommendation (Lowe, 2016; Weiss, 2019).

The strongest points for marketing yourself are what Fazio (2017) describes as *personal selling*. You represent yourself as a professional with skills and expertise, and most of all, you must have integrity. You are committing to do what you state you will do, and you know that you cannot promise anything that you will be unable to deliver. Make sure that you have the skills required for the job!

Let's return to the case of Tisha (see OT Story 75.2).

BOX 75.1 WILL YOU BE A GOOD CONSULTANT?

As you're learning more about what it means to be a consultant, consider these basic questions:

- Do you have a defined area of expertise?
- Do you know your strengths and limitations?
- Do you know your biases?
- Are you a good communicator?

- Are you a good manager of time and tasks?
- Can you negotiate?
- Can you be assertive when necessary?

OT STORY 75.2 INITIAL MEETING WITH MR. GOMEZ

Tisha is meeting with Mr. Gomez. She first asks him to describe the project to see if she feels her expertise matches with the program he is looking to develop. Another thing that she asks about is the timeline for developing this program and if there will be continued OT involvement in the program once it is up and running. She also asks about the budget for starting this program. As she learns more about the proposed program, Tisha finds that her confidence is building, and she feels capable of entering this consultative role.

Questions

1. Are there any other things you would have asked Mr. Gomez?
2. Are there any things that Tisha asked that you would not have asked? Why?

The Consultation Process

The process of consultation can be outlined in five steps, which are listed here and described in detail below.

1. Review the project being proposed and make sure you have the required expertise to complete the project to the client's satisfaction.
2. Understand the environment.
3. Establish the agreement, including a proposal, scope of work, costs and fees, and a legal contract.
4. Begin the actual consulting, including analyzing the project and establishing a plan for taking action that includes goals and deadlines.
5. Oversee the implementation of the project, providing suggestions and direction as necessary.

    Complete the project or extend the work, establishing new or revised goals (Block, 2011; Lowe, 2016).

Review the Project and the Needed Expertise

When you first meet the client and learn of the proposed project, you need to explore exactly what the client is looking for and what will be expected of you as a consultant. You will have to decide if you have the necessary experience to meet their expectations, the time to devote to this project, and the ability to deliver the product or program that they want.

Understand the Environment

Healthcare and educational organizations in general are complex systems. Consulting typically starts with investigation of the immediate environment of the client; however, it rarely ends there. The client's environment may consist of many involved agencies and organizations and, ultimately, may interact with various governmental agencies at local, state, national, and international levels. Sometimes, the client may not be fully aware how all of these interrelated systems assist or constrain the goals of their organization. For this reason, it can also be important, once the consultation has begun, to visit the site where the consultation will take place. This helps the consultant to understand the culture of the organization. Though the pandemic has made this difficult, it is still an important area to consider.

    Some environments will accept change, whereas others may make it very difficult to effectively complete the project as defined. In order to assist your client, it will be your task to adapt to this environment, to come to understand its complexity, and to work effectively within it. Sometimes, the consultant is able to see something within the environment than those working there on a regular basis do not see. The consultant can identify "blind spots" that people have within the organization, Additionally, understanding the environment may be helpful to you as the consultant to identify those who may support the completion of the project and those who may make your work more difficult.

Establish the Agreement

There are many steps involved in establishing a consulting agreement. Keep in mind that agencies may have their own process for establishing an agreement.

Develop a Proposal

Once you have had the initial meeting with the client, you have gained the information that you need to understand their expectations for the project and what will be expected of you. You have determined that you are interested in taking on this project.

    It is then advisable to draft a *proposal* of the work you are recommending to be done. Most clients will require this before you initiate a more formal contract. The proposal isn't a finished document and will likely be altered by you and your client. It generally states what you will do specifically, what will be included in the process, the outcome or deliverables, and the time frame for completion of the project. Sometimes, costs are included at this point. You might request a meeting or a conference call, after your client(s) have read the proposal.

This proposal is not a formal contract and does not have to be signed by both parties (Weiss, 2019). It serves as a point of discussion for what will be included in the *formal contract* or *consultation agreement*. In some cases, the proposal may be referred to as a *letter of intent* (LOI) or a *memorandum of understanding* (MOU). In most cases, there is a good deal of verbal exchange during this process. Often this will become the basis of the formal contract. In other cases, organizations have a specific contract for consultants and will attach the proposal document to the contract with specific monetary amounts for tasks included. This is generally done by mutual agreement between the consultant and the client.

In its simplest form, Anastasi (2014) states that the proposal should include the following:

- A detailed description of the project (the *scope*)
- The effort it is expected to take to achieve the scope
- The price to be charged

If you are taking on a project for your present employer, keep in mind that you are still acting as a consultant to some degree. The scope of work should be documented in some way, along with the proposed timeline and outcome, and if there will be any additional pay or release time to complete this work. Depending on your circumstances, this may be more of a social contract with a present employer designed not so much for enforcement but for clear communication.

Some refer to the culmination of the proposal in a document as a *conceptual agreement* (Weiss, 2019); in other cases a formal contract is required. The proposal should include:

- What are the objectives to be achieved through this project?
- What will and will not be included in the project?
- How will progress be measured? And how will success be measured?
- What is the timeline for completion of the project?
- What are the expected outcomes for the project?
- What is the value of this project to the organization?
- What is the proposed cost of the project?

The most critical expectations of the client are written in this document and/or the contract. Most critical are the *scope* of your engagement as a consultant, the necessary *effort* for you as a consultant, and the expected *time* for this project to take (Anastasi, 2014). These three areas are interdependent, meaning that if any one of these areas changes, the other two areas will probably change as well (Anastasi, 2014).

The clarity and specificity of this document are critically important. If any of the areas are not clearly delineated, then the expectations may be misunderstood. If, during the project, the consultant finds that there is a misunderstanding or a difference of expectations, then the consultant should address this immediately. This may be something as simple as who will cover travel expenses (and what specific expenses will not be covered) or specific materials needed for the project. The detailed proposal should make expectations and assumptions clear (Lowe, 2016).

If you choose, or the organization requires, the use of a formal contract, this final legal agreement provides a clear vision of the plan to complete the project and to ensure that the vision to complete the engagement aligns perfectly with the previous discussions and the earlier proposed plan.

Establish Costs and Fees

Consulting costs are generally composed of your fee (which should be based on the time the project will take) and travel. You should include your fees and costs in your proposal. Your communication from the point that you establish the proposal or contract with the site should be included in your fee. Initially it will be hard to estimate the fee for your time, but this will improve as you gain more experience as a consultant. Some consultants set a flat fee for each section of a project and others estimate at an hourly rate and then set the fee per section of the project, with a total amount for the project overall. As you continue to consult, you will be far better able to anticipate a fairly accurate budget, although there will often be unanticipated surprises. With experience, you'll come to a point where you know well what a project is worth and how much time it will require, particularly if you specialize in an area and consult with different organizations. It is important for you to understand the type of organization you are working with. Smaller organizations often have smaller budgets. Not all organizations have similar monies in their budgets, particularly for consultants. Not-for-profit organizations sometimes have smaller budgets, but not always. Take time to learn about the organization.

Sometimes discussing fees is the first difficult conversation you may have with your client (Lowe, 2016). Once you are established, you will feel more confident with this discussion. After this discussion, your fee is specified in the proposal when you define the deliverables of the project and establish the estimated timeline to completion of the project. How and when you will be paid is included as well. Many consultants prefer to be paid in phases, receiving some payment in advance of the completion of the project.

Consulting fees are quite subjective, and consultants usually do not want to disclose their fee to potential competitors. Only you really know what your time is worth. You can ask around, particularly of those who have hired consultants who do what you are proposing, or you can ask colleagues and mentors, and hopefully you will get a range for hourly or project task fees. Many business consulting books offer resources for fee setting. However, keep in mind that these are usually geared to purely business environments and not healthcare, education, or research environments.

As a consultant, you need to recognize your value. Sometimes those in helping professions have difficulty putting a value on their services. Consulting is not a charity, it is a business. Although you might want to engage in project pro bono to gain experience or to sell yourself to a client, that is fine, but generally you need to value your services. This requires some personal confidence. Sometimes you do need to make a change to your initial estimates, such as if the scope of the project suddenly changes once you are immersed in it or you miss a deadline that may change the timeline for the project. If such situations occur, meet with your client as soon as possible and reach a solution. If you are responsible for the change or underestimated the time involved, then you should absorb the cost of the delay.

Although initially you may not accurately estimate the cost/budget (your fee and project costs), it is often an assumption of the client that the estimated fee is the actual fee, and it prompts a breach in communications if you must come in later with a fee adjustment (which is seldom lower than your initial estimate). Thus, it is better to be specific that the fee/cost quotes may change once the needs assessment and analysis of the project details are complete and assumptions are validated. Do this verbally as well as point it out in your written agreement.

Sometimes clients may have unrealistic expectations of the time and funds required to achieve their desired goals. These are their goals, not yours, but most clients rely on you to help refine them, make the goals measurable, and achievable. This may require a change at the contract level. If there are new versions of the contract that may require approval by one or more people, then you will want to keep a written history of their status and note when they are actually approved. Keeping good records is important for your business.

Legal Contracts

In this author's experience as a consultant in healthcare and educational environments, most organizations have a set or blueprint of a legal contract for consultants, which they always use and which they are reluctant to revise. For this reason, they use their blueprint contract and attach the detailed proposal to the contract. In this way, they are conforming to their business standards yet acknowledging the specifics for the project. In the business world, the contract is a must. Anastasi (2014) cautions the consultant that an explicit and detailed contract is critical because it is the most effective way to manage expectations for all concerned.

One other area where confusion may occur is in the management of actual materials you may produce as part of your work. If you are providing materials as part of the contractual agreement, then you should specify how that material will be used. Identify at the beginning whether these materials are your intellectual property or the property of the organization with which you are consulting. In the author's personal experience, this is usually set out in a formal contract.

Begin the Actual Consultation

The consultation consists of analyzing the project, setting goals, and establishing a plan for taking action that includes deadlines for each phase.

Analyze the Project

The actual work most often begins with a series of interviews with all persons involved who will continue to carry out the work and sustain the project following the consultant's exit. It is best to do these interviews in person and on the site of the consultation so that one begins to understand the culture of the organization. However, during the pandemic, this was not usually possible, resulting in interviews and meetings over the Internet. Although not optimal, this can still be effective if one is a good interviewer and observer.

The person who has hired you for the consultation can give you some guidance about the key people with whom you should meet. You should discuss who the stakeholders are and who the influential people in the organization are. This will vary based on the setting of the consultation. Persons interviewed should include those who will be supportive of the project and can be helpful to you as well as those who may not be supportive of the project and whom you might need to win over. Kavanaugh (2018) states that the main components of communication in business is to convey information and to persuade people; however, another purpose of communication in consulting is to effectively gather information. To do this effectively, you need to be prepared. You must know who you are talking to and what information you want to gather. As an occupational therapist, you should already have good interviewing skills; however, Fazio (2017) provides a good resource for conducting effective interviews, and Kavanaugh (2018) notes that effective communication can be learned and should be learned as it is essential to successful consulting. These interviews will help you understand the environment and the culture of the site, which is why it is most effective to conduct these interviews in person, whenever possible. Beginning with a series of interviews is not common in management consulting. However, in those community-based projects, often involving patients/clients, or educational environments, understanding the situation can lead to a more successful outcome and future sustainability.

Set Goals

Once you have a firm understanding of the project, the environment, and the individuals involved, you need to set goals for each step of the project. This involves planning your approach, deciding what you will do first and who will be involved in each phase of your work. Identify what are the deliverables for each stage of the project. These should be clearly stated as your goals. Your goals should match the items that you have identified in your proposal. Now that you know the participants in the consulting environment, you will be able to find people who can provide the information that you need and can support your project. It is often helpful to check in with your client to ensure that both of you agree on the goals.

Establish a Plan and Deadlines

It is up to you to establish a plan for completing the project and define the deadlines. The plan involves how you will go about meeting the goals you have set. Will you be working independently and then present it to the client? Will you be onsite discussing your suggestions and proposed changes with employees? Will you do some work on your own and have some meetings with key personnel? It is important for the consultant to know who they are accountable to and be prepared to provide that individual(s) with regular updates. All of these depend on the particular project that you are working on.

Deadlines are critical. Sometimes they are clearly stated in the proposal. Other times, you are setting them as you go along. It is important to your credibility as a consultant that you meet your deadlines, whether internally or externally imposed. Often deadlines are externally set (such as in accreditation issues), and at times, they are decided on internally between the consultant and the client. If, for any reason, the tasks cannot be completed on time, the consultant should discuss this with the client to ensure that this will not create additional problems and that the client still wants the consultant to continue working on the project. It is the consultant's responsibility to deliver the completed project in a timely manner. In most of the author's consulting experience, an externally imposed timeline has been critical to the process, and it is generally related to the goals identified in the proposal. If the products are not completed by the deadlines, particularly external deadlines, then the project is not successful.

Complete the Task

It is important to understand the format that the client wants for the final product. Knowing what *done* looks like requires that everyone (consultant and client) understand the mutually agreed criteria that will determine successful conclusion. Make sure that your communications are clear with all parties and that the expectations of all are considered. This relates to meeting deadlines as discussed above. When you as a consultant feel that the task has been completed, it is useful to meet with the client to review the project and come to an agreement on whether the project is completed as expected and if all goals have been met.

Sometimes a review of the final project will result in the identification of new or altered goals, causing an extension of the work. This will usually require an additional agreement and often an extension of the contract. It is up to the consultant to determine if they are capable of working

on these new goals and if they want to extend the contract. Most often this is an expression of support by the client and a positive outcome for the consultant.

Foundational Skills for the Consultant

There is a general business career path called *management consulting*. Most of the consultants in this career are experts in business/management/leadership and/or technology and consult to their specific expertise. Peter Block (2011) and many of the other authors cited in this chapter (Anastasi, 2014; Kavanaugh, 2018, Schein, 2016) have had long careers as management consultants. Block describes his work as being about empowerment, stewardship, chosen accountability, and the reconciliation of community. In his continuing career, he has stated that "[we] must begin to organize consulting from its' original model of providing information and solutions to one that focuses on discovering the strengths, positive examples, and 'gifts' of the client organization" (Block, 2011, pp. 10–11). Differing from earlier approaches to the consulting relationship seen in management consulting, today's consultants must develop a capacity for authentic behavior, deeper relatedness, and partnership in their consulting roles (Block, 2011; Wickham & Wilcock, 2016).

Kavanaugh (2018) also stressed the need for authenticity, innovation, and creativity when relating to clients. OT practitioners are well prepared for this type of consulting relationship, and with the expertise they bring to the table, they should be very effective in helping their clients meet the challenges of the evolving health and wellness industry.

Understanding and Managing Change

All of consulting is about *change*, sometimes chosen by the organization and sometimes externally imposed. Regardless of the area where you choose to consult, you can anticipate that at least some of your client's goals will be about trying to stay afloat or maximize their market share in a competitive marketplace. This, likely, will require much of your existing skills plus those that are specific to understanding and managing the change process (Block, 2011; Heifetz et al., 2009). If you want to help your organization, your community, and your society thrive in the world today, you must anticipate working with the change process.

Levels of organizational change include individuals, groups, and larger systems. At the individual level, most often consultants are involved in training, coaching, and counseling, and they should always be aware of analyzing issues that arise critically and with creativity (Kavanaugh, 2018). Although creativity is not a word frequently used in business, it is becoming more popular in texts (Kavanaugh, 2018) and is an area where OT practitioners excel. Handling resistance and helping individuals cope with change also is relevant. At the group level, agendas may include team building and intergroup relations. At the larger systems level, all the previously mentioned concerns still hold, but contextual issues may take the forefront as changes of larger institutions (local, state, national, and international) may influence practice.

There are several models and frameworks used to help an organization develop lasting change. One of the most common frameworks that is used in many settings as a method of analysis is the Strength, Weaknesses, Opportunities, and Threat (SWOT) format, which is outlined in Box 75.2 (Kavanaugh, 2018). This involves identifying the strengths of the organization, the weaknesses of the organization, the opportunities that may be available to the organization, and threats to the organization that can be both internal and external. Organizational change management (OCM) is a structured approach used in organizations for ensuring that changes are smoothly and successfully implemented and that the lasting benefits of change are achieved (Gilley et al., 2009). Organizational change models, as with most other models, link theory with practice. They help us to understand what happens during the change process, why it happens, the predictability, and/or randomness of the actions and reactions (Burke, 2018). There have been numerous conceptual models for content (what to change) and process (how to change) as well as practice frameworks to explain phases of planned change (Burke, 2018).

As someone who wants to consult, you likely desire to mobilize greater progress on the issues that are important to you, and in doing so, you want to strengthen your practice of communication and leadership so that you can help others strengthen their capacity for change (Block, 2011; Kavanaugh, 2018). To do this, you will work on your skills of training, coaching, and facilitating (see OT Story 75.3). Much of this will relate to your OT skills.

BOX 75.2 SWOT ANALYSIS

A SWOT analysis is a method used to determine the areas that will potentially support or hinder the development of a new program. The boxes show possible examples of each area.

Strengths
- The health of the organization
- The abilities of the staff
- The willingness to embrace new ideas

Weaknesses
- Lack of specifically trained staff for the program
- Budgetary restrictions
- Need for organizational changes to support the program …

Opportunities
- There is little or no competition for the proposed program
- The proposed program will offer new areas of revenue
- The new program will promote the organization's mission in a new way

Threats
- Internal threats might be a lack of support from key personnel
- A lack of willingness to provide the budget necessary for the program
- External threats might be a lack of community support
- The need for external state approval for the new program

OT STORY 75.3 A CAREER PATH LEADING TO EXPERT CONSULTATION IN CLINICAL INTERNSHIP DESIGN

Midral is an occupational therapist with 9 years of practice experience in adult rehabilitation. Seven of those years he also supervised Level I and Level II OT and occupational therapy assistant (OTA) fieldwork students. Two years ago, he completed his OT post-professional doctorate and focused his final project on fieldwork supervision. He is now a clinical faculty member in an OT academic program and serves in the role of the academic fieldwork coordinator (AFWC). He has always been an active member of AOTA and his state association, and he has frequently presented posters on fieldwork supervision and fieldwork programming topics at national and state meetings.

Questions

1. Is Midral ready to market himself to other academic programs and/or facilities offering fieldwork to OT and OTA students?
2. Do you think there may be gaps in his experience? If so, what are these gaps?
3. Are there any specific ways that he might become better prepared to be a consultant?

The Role of Helping and Coaching in Consultation

As OT practitioners, we are skilled at working with people, although maybe not in the role of a consultant. We understand the therapeutic use of self and can put it to good use in the consulting role. These skills can be effectively transferred to the consultation role. Several areas are important to consider when interviewing and working with individuals or groups.

- *Mindfulness:* Jon Kabat-Zinn (2003) offers an operational working definition of *mindfulness* as "the awareness that emerges through paying attention on purpose, in the present moment, and nonjudgmentally to the unfolding of experience moment by moment" (p. 144).
- *Active and effective listening:* Good listening skills are critical to the ongoing process of consultation and work well as a companion to mindfulness (Fazio, 2017). Listening is an art, and it is at the core of both the helping relationship and the consulting relationship (Green & Howe, 2012). Active listening takes simple listening to the next level, making it a true therapeutic skill, and it enhances the consultant–client relationship (Figure 75.1).
- *Flexibility:* The consultant needs to be open-minded and ready to understand the environment, rather than bringing their own agenda. The consultant has the expertise but has to be ready to accept different ideas, structures, and ways of assisting change.
- *Empathy:* Another area that can be helpful is empathy (Norfolk et al., 2007). As you are consulting in an area that you know well, you may have had experiences similar to those of your client(s). Using your understanding of your own experiences can help you to understand your client better.

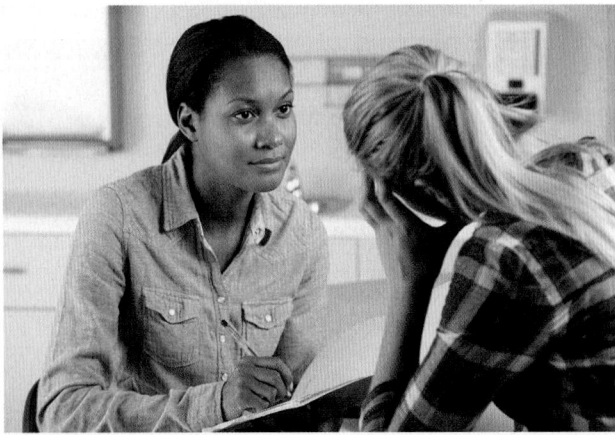

FIGURE 75.1 Active listening is a therapeutic skill that is critical to the act of coaching.

Mindfulness, active listening, empathy, and a genuine desire to help come together in what may be described as the act of coaching. Elements of coaching such as suggesting, empowering, and supporting change can be very useful in the consulting relationship with client(s). Even though consultation is different from patient/client intervention, it is critical to remember foundational therapeutic skills and use them in the consulting process. Layering your newly learned consultation skills on top of your core caring and helping skills will become your personal strength in this new role.

Challenges in Consulting

Controlling Chaos

Although chaos does not always occur in consulting projects, it can occur and can derail a project. The basis for avoiding chaos in consulting is to maintain good communication with your client. This includes phone calls, meetings, and email to keep the lines of communication open (Block, 2011; Lowe, 2016). If you have a large meeting, it is often helpful to debrief afterwards with the person you are responsible to, to make sure that you have both heard the same thing and agree in the approach to move forward.

Chaos and problems in your consulting relationship can also be a direct result of your inability to manage the project. You need be aware of your potential role when chaos occurs. You may inadvertently be the cause of the chaos. If you tend not to respond to deadlines or manage your actions well, then you may not be ready to help larger groups attain their goals (Hattori, 2015; Rasiel & Friga, 2002). This is something to consider carefully as you review your skills and attributes in preparation to consult. Even as an experienced consultant, there are times when an organization is resistant to change, which can result in chaos. Sometimes chaos occurs despite the consultant and/or the client's best efforts.

Managing Expectations, Assumptions, and Difficult Conversations

Management consultants talk about honesty and integrity as foundation skills for the consultant and the need to have difficult conversations early on as well as managing the expectations of your client(s) (Anastasi, 2014; Block, 2011; Lowe, 2016). It is important to remember that you, the consultant, have assumptions, expectations, and perhaps biases. Know what they are and try to work through them to stay focused on the client and their needs. One of the most difficult conversations you may have either early on or midway through the process is to correct a misalignment in expectations for what the finished product will include. Usually this does not occur when you have a well-developed detailed proposal. But sometimes it does happen, often because of extenuating circumstances beyond anyone's control. Anastasi (2014) suggests that "a consultants true worth is measured by the speed at which issues are brought to the customer's attention regardless of who is at fault, or the difficulty of the conversation" (p. 134). Remember that your client is taking risks. It is your task as a consultant to mitigate these risks. Keeping in regular contact with the person to whom you are accountable can assist in this process.

Consulting With Large Group of Participants or a Board: Managing Meetings for Action

It is usually most efficient for the consultant to report to one person who will then share findings with board or organization members and stakeholders rather than hold meetings with large groups. In this author's experience consulting in academic settings as well as in community settings, there is often the need to have larger meetings where everyone involved can hear what is occurring directly from the consultant. They are often led as focus groups with participants given the opportunity to provide feedback.

As a consultant, it is important to know your audience and focus your communication to that particular audience. There are times that you will be expected to present to a Board of Directors, which will be concerned with the costs of projects and the potential benefits. Preparing carefully for the audience and conducting a meeting, whether large or small, is a critical skill that all consultants must master (Robinson et al., 2015). In addition, developing comfort in public speaking and developing presentations contribute greatly to a good meeting.

Ethical Responsibilities of the Consultant: Building Credibility and Trust

Consultants have an obligation to provide services that meet the standards for the profession. The work of OT practitioners uniquely focuses on the capabilities and opportunities for individuals and for groups to engage in occupations (AOTA, 2020; WFOT, 2016). Throughout this chapter, areas have been presented where the consultant's ethical responsibilities may be challenged and/or compromised. Consultants are more likely to work alone as they engage in the consulting process, and, at times, they may not appreciate the complexity involved in working within a given system. The role of consultant is as an expert advisor, and this can create situations fraught with potential ethical problems and dilemmas (Purtillo & Doherty, 2015). As the expert, your clients are relying on your ability to guide them to realistic and achievable expectations while delivering on your commitment to their success. *Guide* is an important word here. Do not promise your clients something that you cannot deliver. As a consultant, you may be an expert, but you seldom have all the answers. The challenges of the consulting relationship and your need to help may test your integrity. It is best to hold fast and admit you don't know something, but let the client know that you will find the answer. Building credibility and trust is never ending; each interaction must be the best that you can offer (Robinson et al., 2015). It is critical that all practitioners, consultants, and private practitioners understand ethical principles and related standards so that they are prepared to resolve ethical dilemmas that may occur (see Chapter 27, for an in-depth discussion of ethics as they may apply to the OT practitioner).

Keeping Boundaries as a Consultant

As a consultant, you often have access to the higher levels of administrators. They are the ones to whom you are generally responsible and often report to. Although it is important to establish positive relationships with all levels of staff, you are not there to become their friends. You are there to complete a specified job and make suggestions that will improve the organization. The consultant does not dictate changes but recommends ways to help the organization move forward. You are not teaching them to become occupational therapists but showing them effective ways to use OT and occupation-based interventions. And the organization is not required to take all of your suggestions. So be aware that your role is to provide ideas, not enforce the recommended changes.

The Consultant as Social Entrepreneur

In recent years, the term *social entrepreneur* has become a popular way to define those entrepreneurs who have the public good as their agenda. Scofield (2011) refers to this as "righting the unrightable wrong and finding your mission possible" (p. 1). He goes on to say that it's likely that many of these social entrepreneurs will come from the healthcare sector where they have been exposed to frequent inequities in the distribution of opportunity for health-promoting environments. Block (2011) has identified both healthcare and education as two sectors of society where the call for change and reform has been blatant for years. OT practitioners fit this description, and many are being prepared for this entrepreneurial work in their basic education as they develop the skills and knowledge

for program design and development, particularly those who are engaged in OT doctoral education (Fazio, 2017). It makes sense that as these students enter the practice environment, they will gravitate toward social entrepreneurship and/or engage in the consulting role to bring about positive change wherever they choose to work. Further, with the additional emphasis on health and wellness and populations and communities in Vision 2025 (AOTA, 2019), OT practitioners are in a perfect position to become consultants in healthcare, education, and community services.

EXPANDING OUR PERSPECTIVES

Consultation Work

So Sin Sim

Consultation work is a place where some occupational therapists find themselves land, especially with a general shortage of OT services and increasing emerging practice areas. Consultation work allows clients, who otherwise cannot access OT services, to receive intervention that is directed at increasing their meaningful engagement in occupations and supporting people's valued roles. The impact factor of consultation work is far-reaching and occupational therapists who are well-trained in program development, occupational science, and health and well-being make very good consultants for places typically short of occupational therapists such as residential facilities, group homes, workplace organizations, schools, and other community settings or even the setting up of services in less developed countries.

I have been involved in both formal and informal consultation work. One of the memorable ones would be being a part of a team that flew into East Timor from 2002 to assist in the recovery of the community following the 1999 East Timorese crisis. I worked alongside with psychiatrists, psychologist, and social workers to educate and equip them on posttraumatic stress disorder and useful interventions for rebuilding the community. It was challenging because there were no infrastructure and the people we were training were community volunteers and leaders who want to help their villagers and loved ones. The trainees were essentially nurse, OT, social worker, and psychologists all in one. The usual discussion surrounding professional boundaries and regulations seemed to become so unimportant in war-torn areas where people struggle with even basic needs. The science of occupations and clinical reasoning were not important to articulate, but I relied on my intuition and years of experience of training as an occupational therapist to adapt and be creative about my contribution to the project in recovering the community.

Another work that I have done is with community mental health facilities where my role was to set up programs for the staff of the day program. The work surrounds assessing the needs of clients and providing activity scheduling with therapeutic intent. I find consultation work satisfying because I know that I am working through the hands of other people and the impact factor is greater than if I worked individually. Besides education, consultancy allows me to share my years of experience with mental health clients, which eventually benefits clients.

Sometimes, our consultancy work could be informal when we exercise our influence in boards and committees or workgroups. I have had the privilege to work in dementia workgroups contributing to the building of dementia-friendly environment and programs for a facility, groups looking into workplace mental health promotion program and systems to better the well-being of students in schools. Typically, I worked alongside the multidisciplinary team whose function was less related to professional boundaries as compared to focusing on the project outcome. The challenge that comes alongside this type of work is when you are less experienced, you might find yourself feeling a loss of professional identity and even a lack of recognition, which can be disconcerting and disillusionment, and could contribute to burnout. What helped me personally was to keep connected to the profession through continuing education, teaching into OT programs, and being involved in association and special interest groups to keep reminding myself of who I am, why I am doing, what I am doing, and am I making a unique contribution through my years of being an occupational therapist.

Overall, I think that consultancy work is immensely satisfying and a very creative process where you get to decide what is your contribution as an occupational therapist to better the lives of clients and their families. It is a good career progression when you have years of experience on the ground and looking to do something different from a specific season.

Conclusion

Consultation is a growing area of practice for OT practitioners. This chapter outlines the knowledge needed from the business, management, and leadership world and how this knowledge when combined with our therapeutic skills and understanding of the helping relationship can provide a unique consulting relationship. It provides a step-by-step guide to implement a consulting project. Keep in mind that the first step is to become proficient in a specific content area. Content areas where OT consultants are often sought are practice, education, community programs, administration/supervision and research, or a combination of any of these. Once you have developed a strong background and a clear content area of expertise, you are in a perfect position to influence healthcare, communities, education and others with our distinctive perspective.

Acknowledgment

The author thanks Linda Fazio for her immense contribution to the previous edition of this chapter.

Lippincott® Connect *For additional resources on the subjects discussed in this chapter, visit Lippincott Connect.*

REFERENCES

Accreditation Council for Occupational Therapy Education. (2018). Standards and interpretive Guide. *American Journal of Occupational Therapy, 72*(suppl. 2), 721241000583p1–721241005p83. https://doi.org/10.5014/ajot.2018.72S217

American Occupational Therapy Association. (2007). AOTA's centennial vision and executive summary. *American Journal of Occupational Therapy, 61*(6), 613–614. https://doi.org/10.5014/ajot.61.6.613

American Occupational Therapy Association. (2019). AOTA board expands vision 2025. *American Journal of Occupational Therapy, 73*(3), 7303420010p1. https://doi.org/10.5014/ajot.2019.733002

American Occupational Therapy Association. (2020). AOTA code of ethics. *American Journal of Occupational Therapy, 74* (Suppl. 3), 7413410005p1–7413410005p13. https://doi.org/10.5014/ajot.2020.74S3006

Anastasi, S. (2014). *The seven principles of professional services: A field guide for walking the consulting tightrope.* PS Principles.

Block, P. (2011). *Flawless consulting: A guide to getting your expertise used* (3rd ed.). Jossey-Bass.

Braveman, B. (2016). *Leading & managing occupational therapy services: An evidence-based approach* (2nd ed.). F. A. Davis.

Burke, W. (2018). *Organization change: Theory and practice* (5th ed.). Sage.

Dictionary.com. (2021). *Consultation.* https://www.dictionary.com

Fazio, L. S. (2017). *Developing occupation-centered programs with the community* (3rd ed.). Slack.

Gilley, A., McMillen, H., & Gilley, J. (2009). Organizational change and characteristics of leadership effectiveness. *Journal of Leadership and Organizational Studies, 16*(1), 38–47. https://doi.org/10.1177/1548051809334191

Green, C. H., & Howe, A. P. (2012). *The trusted advisor fieldbook: A comprehensive toolkit for leading with trust.* Wiley.

Hattori, S. (2015). *The McKinsey edge: Success principles from the world's most powerful consulting firm.* McGraw-Hill.

Heifetz, R., Linsky, R., A., & Grashow, A. (2009). *The practice of adaptive leadership: Tools and tactics for changing your organization and the world.* Harvard Business Press.

Kabat-Zinn, J. (2003). Mindfulness-based interventions in context: Past, present, and future. *Clinical Psychology: Science and Practice, 10*(2), 144–156. https://doi.org/10.1093/clipsy.bpg016

Kavanaugh, J. (2018). *Consulting essentials: The art and science of people, facts, and frameworks.* Lioncrest.

Lowe, R. (2016). *How to manage a consulting project.* The Writing King.

Norfolk, T., Birdi, K., & Walsh, D. (2007). The role of empathy in establishing rapport in the consultation: A new model. *Medical Education, 41*(7), 690–697. https://doi.org/10.1111/j.1365-2923.2007.02789.x.

Purtillo, R., & Doherty, R. (2015). *Ethical dimensions in the health professions* (6th ed.). Elsevier Saunders.

Rasiel, E., & Friga, P. (2002). *The McKinsey mind: Understanding and implementing the problem-solving tools and management techniques of the world's top strategic consulting firm.* McGraw-Hill.

Robinson, D. G., Robinson, J. C., Phillips, J. J., Phillips, P. P., & Handshaw, D. (2015). *Performance consulting: A strategic process to improve, measure, and sustain organizational results.* Barrett-Koehler.

Schein, E. (2016). *Humble consulting: How to provide real help faster.* Berrett-Koehler.

Scofield, R. (2011). *The social entrepreneur's handbook: How to start, build, and run a business that improves the world.* McGraw-Hill.

Steinberg, D. (2016). *Complexity in healthcare and the language of consultation: Exploring the other side of medicine.* Taylor & Francis Group.

Weiss, A. (2019). *Getting started in consulting* (4th ed.). Wiley.

Wickham, L. & Wilcock, J. (2016). *Management consulting* (5th ed.). Pearson.

World Federation of Occupational Therapists. (2016). *World Federation of Occupational Therapists code of ethics.* http://www.wfot.org/ResourceCentre/tabid/132/did/780/Default.aspx

Payment for Healthcare Services

Helene Lohman, Angela Patterson, and Angela M. Lampe

LEARNING OBJECTIVES

After reading this chapter, you will be able to:

1. Describe the impact of policy related to payment of occupational therapy (OT) services in the United States.
2. Explain the key types of payments received in OT practice.
3. Describe payment terminology for Medicare reimbursement.
4. Distinguish between skilled and unskilled services.
5. Discuss emerging payment systems in the United States.
6. Explain the status of the uninsured and underinsured in the United States and what practitioners can do to advocate for reimbursement of OT services.
7. Discuss how practitioners can be advocates for clients related to payment issues impacting practice.
8. Explain examples of global healthcare payment models.

Payment for Services in Healthcare

Payment for services in healthcare is complex, particularly in the United States, and complicated by multiple stakeholders (clients, providers, payers, and sometimes employers). Furthermore, there are many options for payment for healthcare services ranging from private pay to employer and government-funded programs. In this chapter, we largely discuss payment for services in the United States but also offer a global perspective on healthcare payment models given the diversity and world mobility of the clients we serve.

With over 19% of the American gross domestic product (GDP), approximately $4.1 trillion dollars, spent on healthcare (Centers for Medicare & Medicaid Services [CMS], 2021a), payment for healthcare is of high importance to many stakeholders, including occupational therapy (OT) practitioners. Payment structures and systems change frequently. All practitioners must understand that the clients we serve come from diverse backgrounds and have different perspectives on payment for healthcare services. Practitioners must also be knowledgeable about payment sources, have a professional responsibility to understand how payment systems influence practice nationally and internationally, and advocate for payment of needed services for the diverse clients they serve. Some practitioners may depend on the facility's billing department or the therapy manager to keep them abreast of payment policies and procedures, but regardless they should stay informed (Sieck et al., 2017). Other practitioners, for example, private practice practitioners who handle their own billing, may be intimately aware of the regulations affecting payment.

As you read this chapter, open your mind to learn not only about payment for therapy services in the United States but also gain more of a global perspective about the diversity of practice in other healthcare systems. The chapter begins with a historical perspective about policy and payment in the United States followed by an overview of private and governmental payments. The second part of the chapter overviews payment trends in the United States as well as considers the uninsured, underinsured, pro-bono intervention and advocacy. The final section generally explores global healthcare models followed by a specific focus on Canada, the United Kingdom, Australia, and Korea as exemplars of different systems throughout the world.

Before we dive into this chapter about payment for healthcare services, let us first start with a personal story intended to expand our perspective of healthcare services. The Expanding Our Perspectives story below was written by Said Naif who shares a perspective about healthcare services in his home country of Morocco.

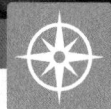 **EXPANDING OUR PERSPECTIVES**

Payment for Healthcare in Morocco

Said Naif

Growing up in the city of Kenitra, Morocco, was full of mixed blessings. Amazingly, my siblings and I were born in alternating gender birth order to parents who were quite young by U.S. standards. We were boy (Ahmed, died at 3 months), girl (Khadija), boy (myself), girl (Samira), boy (Nabil), girl (Siham), and boy (Mouhcine). Although technically the second son and third child, I was considered the eldest boy and the expectations on me to help the family financially started young, mainly due to the nature of the Moroccan public healthcare system.

When I was seven, I vividly remember walking home from school with my big sister, where we found our mother crying over our baby brother. She sobbed that "something is wrong with Nabil, his legs won't move anymore" as the previously robust 7-month-old infant cried in obvious pain.

Our regional hospital did not have the expertise to diagnose or treat the sudden onset of flaccidity in my brother's legs. The only option left was traveling to the pediatric hospital in the capital Rabat. It was a day's journey and cost more than my father's daily income to get there, even though my mother carried my brother on her back the final miles, walking from bus depot to hospital to save the taxi fare.

The medical payment system in Morocco is either public or private. Private care is better than the public care, but we could not afford it on my father's sole income. Every cent was desperately needed, not only to feed and house the family but also to pay for medicine and transportation to hospitals.

It is hard to understand from a Western perspective, but public healthcare in Morocco means that after waiting in seriously overcrowded waiting rooms, sometimes for days, a doctor may briefly see you and if you are very lucky, you receive a hospital stay. You bring your own food, bed linens, and have to send someone to the pharmacy outside the hospital grounds to pay cash for any prescribed medicine. At the hospital a family member as a caregiver must stay with the child at all times even when they need to get food and medicine or use the bathroom due to nursing staff being overburdened and often unavailable. Even in 2022, you can see people passing food through windows of the hospital to loved ones.

While my mother was pursuing healthcare for Nabil in the following months, my father ended up hospitalized for a stomach ulcer operation. I remember visiting him, despairing that he would ever come home. At this point, there was nothing left but for my mother to part with her life savings of gold jewelry and for me to start selling fruit on the streets after school by the age of 10, while my big sister Khadija helped take care of the family and home.

Eventually, doctors explained that my brother "must have polio or some type of infection" that affected his lower extremities. They told us he would never stand or walk. However, by the time he turned ten, with the help of orthotics, Nabil managed to stand and walk. He currently ambulates short distances using just one forearm crutch. The years of my mother's dogged advocacy pursuing various technically "free" therapies and treatments had long-term costs for our family.

An Historical Look at How Policy Has Influenced Payment in the United States

Legislation, the economy, technology, and many other factors have all influenced payment for the profession of OT. The success of any profession depends on how well it responds to and adapts to such changes. Since the inception of OT in 1917, numerous forces have shaped its trajectory. The major events that have influenced OT payment and practice beginning with the growth of private insurance in the 1940s up to the Patient Protection and Affordable Care Act (PPACA) in 2010 are summarized in a table on Lippincott Connect.

Types of Payment in the United States

This section briefly describes varied methods of payment for OT services in the United States. The status of how Americans are insured is presented in Figure 76.1, which will guide this discussion. Figure 76.2 presents United States spending figures of where the nation's healthcare dollars originate.

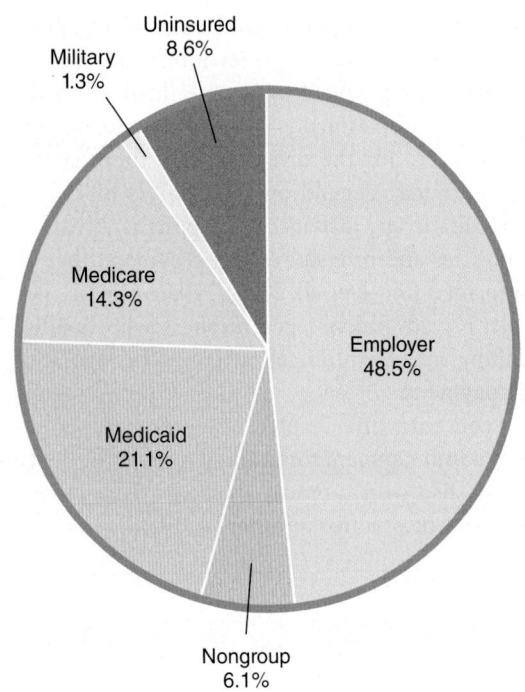

FIGURE 76.1 Health insurance coverage of the U.S. population.

(Data from Kaiser Family Foundation. [2019]. *Health insurance coverage of the total population.* https://www.kff.org/other/state-indicator/total-population/?currentTimeframe=0&sortModel=%7B%22colId%22:%22Location%22,%22sort%22:%22asc%22%7D)

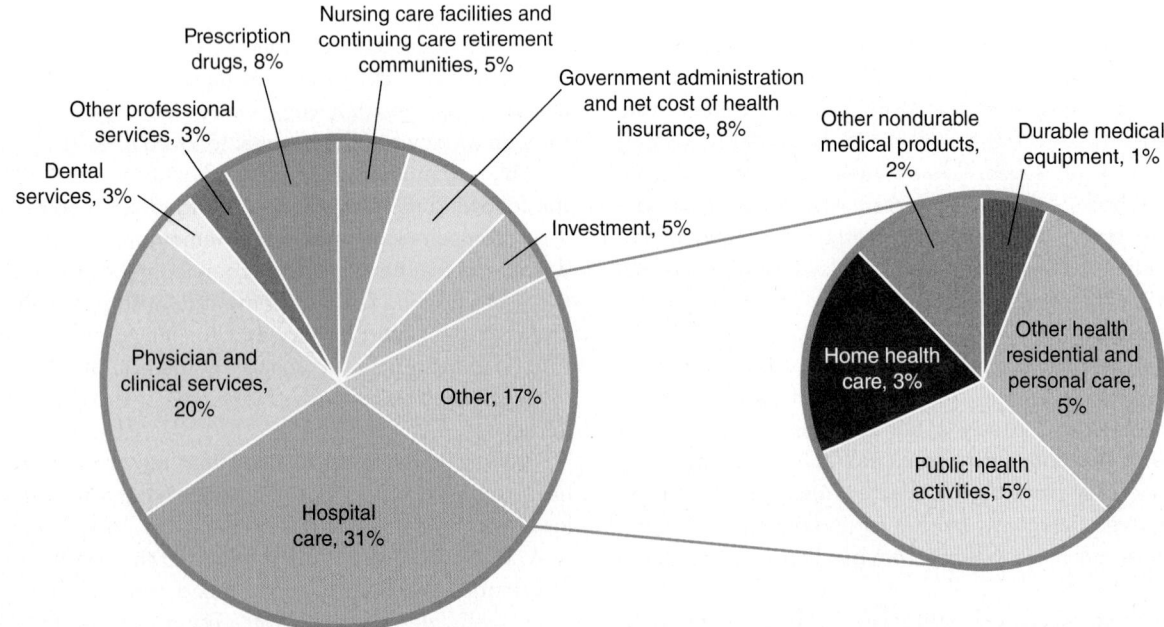

FIGURE 76.2 The nation's health dollar, 2020.

(Data from Centers for Medicare & Medicaid Services. [2020]. *The nation's health dollar ($4.1 trillion), calendar year 2020, where it came from.* https://www.cms.gov/files/document/nations-health-dollar-where-it-came-where-it-went.pdf)

Private Employer-Based Insurance

Nearly half of healthcare insurance in the United States is employer-based or purchased privately. Health insurers, such as United Healthcare and Blue Cross/Blue Shield offer a range of for-profit and not-for-profit options for consumers. Most health insurance plans include varying levels of inpatient coverage; however, not all plans include outpatient coverage, and those that do can vary greatly. See Box 76.1 for a list of common abbreviations used in the insurance industry.

The original employer-based insurance was based on a fee-for-service model in which the insured paid 20% of the costs. In 1974, federal regulation, the Employee Retirement Income Security Act encouraged larger employers to develop self-funded plans. With self-funded plans, the employer takes fiscal responsibility for some or all the healthcare services (benefits) of their workers (Kaiser Family Foundation [KFF], 2021a). Self-funded health plans currently cover 64% of workers in the United States (KFF, 2021b). Forty-six percent of employer-based insurance is a type of managed care plan called preferred provider organization (PPO) (KFF, 2021b). These PPOs involve a group of providers that the insured can access. The second most common plan type is a high-deductible health plan (HDHP) with a health savings account (HSA) (28% in 2021) (KFF, 2021a). As the name implies, the insured pays a high deductible (typically a dollar amount paid by the insured before insurance benefits apply)

BOX 76.1 FREQUENTLY USED ABBREVIATIONS

CDHP	Consumer-directed health plan
CHAMPVA	Civilian Health and Medical Program of the Department of Veterans Affairs
CHIP	Children's Health Insurance Program
CMS	Centers for Medicare & Medicaid Services
COBRA	Consolidated Omnibus Budget Reconciliation Act of 1985
CPT	Current Procedural Terminology
DME	Durable medical equipment
DRG	Diagnostic-related group
EPSDT	Early and Periodic Screening, Diagnosis, and Treatment
HSA	Health savings account
HCPCS	Healthcare Common Procedure Coding System
HDHP	High-deductible health plan
HHA	Home health agency
HMO	Health maintenance organization
IDEA	Individuals with Disabilities Education Act
IRF	Inpatient rehabilitation facility
IRF-PAI	Inpatient Rehabilitation Facility-Patient Assessment Instrument
LCD	Local coverage determination
MAC	Medicare administrative contractor
MCO	Managed care organization
MDS	Minimum Data Set
OASIS	Outcome and Assessment Information Set
POS	Point of service
PPACA	Patient Protection and Affordable Care Act
PPO	Preferred provider organization
PPS	Prospective payment system
PT	Physical therapy
SLP	Speech language pathology
SNF	Skilled nursing facility
TRICARE	Military insurance plan
VA	Department of Veteran's Affairs
VD-HCBS	Veteran-Directed Home and Community Based Services
VHA	Veterans' Health Administration

for coverage and contributes to medical costs through a tax-free savings account. With most employer-based plans, the employee pays a percentage of the charge or coinsurance (typically a percentage of total charges to be paid by the insured) and a deductible out-of-pocket amount per year. More information about managed care and HDHP/health savings accounts (HSAs) is discussed later in this chapter.

Managed Care

Managed care, and specifically PPOs, has dominated the employer-based healthcare market for several years (KFF, 2021a). The many definitions of managed care emphasize controlling and reducing healthcare costs. Managed care "integrates the functions of financing, insurance, delivery, and payment within one organization" (Shi & Singh, 2004, p. 326). Most managed care organizations (MCOs) include primary and preventive care services (Shi & Singh, 2004). Health maintenance organizations (HMOs), PPOs, and point of service (POS) plans are examples of managed care options.

To receive payment, OT practitioners need to understand how specific managed care plans work and recognize managed care plans often include strategies to reduce cost. For example, some plans require preauthorization or precertification before beginning intervention and may demand authorization for the number of treatments and treatment continuation. As new systems evolve, such as value-based care, it is possible managed care will have a decreased role in the private healthcare marketplace

Government Payment in the United States

Although the United States does not have universal healthcare like the other major industrial countries (e.g., Canada, United Kingdom), government funding accounts for a large percentage of the U.S. healthcare dollar. The following sections outline key government payers including Medicare, Medicaid, the Children's Health Insurance

Program (CHIP), Individuals with Disabilities Education Act (IDEA), which are combined federal/state programs, and Workers' Compensation, which is a state-administered program, funded by employers, designed for employees who get sick or injured on the job.

Medicare

Medicare is a federal health insurance system overseen by the CMS (2022a). CMS is the largest purchaser of healthcare and the biggest government health insurance program in the United States (CMS, n.d.-a). Medicare covers people who are 65 or older, people under 65 with certain disabilities, and people of any age with end-stage renal disease (ESRD) (CMS, 2022a). Medicare is financed primarily by general revenues, payroll taxes, taxation income taken from social security benefits, and Part A premiums (Cubanski & Neuman, 2021). In the Medicare system, patients are called "beneficiaries."

Medicare consists of four main parts:

- A (inpatient or hospital insurance)
- B (outpatient or medical insurance)
- C (Medicare Advantage)
- D (prescription coverage) (CMS, 2022a)

Medicare Parts A, B, and C are related to reimbursement for OT practice and are briefly discussed with information that is current at the time of this writing.

Medicare Part A All Medicare beneficiaries are covered under Part A, which incorporates inpatient hospitalization and critical access hospitals, skilled nursing facilities (SNFs) (excluding custodial or long-term care), home health agencies (HHAs), inpatient rehabilitation facilities (IRFs), and hospice care. Medicare beneficiaries pay deductibles and may purchase coinsurance plans to supplement coverage in these practice settings. The payment method for Part A is a prospective payment system (PPS) related to the different practice settings. (Refer to Table 76.1 for an overview of Medicare Part A payment in different settings.)

TABLE 76.1 An Overview of Medicare Part A Payment in Different Settings

Facility Type	Basis of Payment
Inpatient prospective payment system (IPPS hospital) acute hospital	Diagnostic-related group (DRG)
Inpatient rehabilitation facility	Case mix group based on patient assessment instrument
Critical access hospitals	Rehabilitation services are paid at cost
Inpatient psychological hospitals	DRG
Part A skilled nursing facility	A per-diem rate part of the patient driven payment model (PDPM) which includes occupational therapy (OT), physical therapy (PT), speech language pathology (SLP), nursing, and non-therapy ancillary based on coding for clinical categories in the Minimum Data Set (MDS).
Home health	Thirty-day payment period based on 432 case mix groups considering twelve different subgroups for broad categories as entered into the Outcome and Assessment Information Set (OASIS) as part of the PDGM. A plan of care is established and services including OT if appropriate must be listed along with goals, duration of care, and treatment course.

Payment Coverage for Medicare: Skilled Care When working in any setting with beneficiaries covered by Medicare, it is imperative that OT practitioners critically consider whether their services are truly skilled. Skilled OT services mean the expertise of OT practitioners is necessary to treat the patient properly and safely based on the complexity of the patient's condition. Thus, if the same service could be provided by an aide or caregiver, then the service would be considered unskilled and consequently not payable by Medicare. An example of an unskilled service provided by an OT practitioner would be general fitness training or supervised daily repetitive exercises. Providing skilled therapy must be appropriate for the nature and severity of the illness or injury and medical needs (CMS, 2018a). For example, therapy would be considered unskilled if upper extremity dressing was addressed for a patient who sustained a total hip replacement. Other factors are whether the intervention is "reasonable and necessary" for the patient's condition to obtain functional improvement, or to prevent deterioration. Thus, therapy does not necessarily always depend on improving the patient's functional status but rather on skilled needs.

The court case *Jimmo v. Sebelius* brought about changes in the interpretation of the Medicare law to allow skilled therapy coverage to prevent or slow down functional loss and help maintain a level of function even when no improvement is expected (CMS, 2013). Therapy timeframes for intervention must be reasonable for the intervention and not excessive. Seeing a patient for several months after an acute condition is considered excessive unless there is strong justification to continue skilled intervention. Acceptable standards of practice must guide OT intervention. For example, delivering acupuncture for pain relief would not be considered acceptable practice. In certain cases, OT practitioners may develop maintenance programs based on the skilled needs of the patient to help maintain function, deter, or slow down functional regression. For example, the skilled expertise of the OT practitioner may be necessary to supervise a patient to safely perform exercises with the correct positioning for a person with a Colles fracture. Boxes 76.2 and 76.3 provide more details about the important concept of skilled services.

Medicare Part A Coverage in Acute Care Hospitals

Acute care hospitals receive payment for all services under a prospective, predetermined, payment rate based on diagnostic-related groups (DRGs). A DRG is a statistical system of classifying possible diagnoses of patients into groups for the purpose of inpatient hospital stay payment. All services (e.g., treatments provided, such as OT) and treatment supplies (e.g., medication and equipment) are included in the DRG rate. Research found higher utilization (spending) of OT services lowered hospital readmission rates for persons with heart failure, pneumonia, and myocardial infarction (Rogers et al., 2017).

Medicare Part A Coverage in Skilled Nursing Facilities: The Patient-Driven Payment Model (PDPM)

On October 1, 2019, the CMS instituted the most major change in payment in 20 years in SNFs called the PDPM. This model focuses on patient considerations addressing value of care rather than the volume of care provided, decreases administrative responsibilities like scheduled regular assessments throughout a beneficiaries' care, and improves payments for patients with certain characteristics (CMS, n.d.-b). Along with this new focus was a switch to a per-diem, or daily rate for payment, with five case-mix adjusted components based

---

BOX 76.2 UNSKILLED THERAPY SERVICES AND REASONS FOR NONPAYMENT WITH MEDICARE

- Services not reasonable and necessary for treatment
- Services inappropriate to the setting or condition
- Services performed by an unqualified person (e.g., by certified nursing assistant [CNA])
- Services that do not require the skills of a therapist or carried out by an unskilled person (e.g., caregiver doing repetitive range of motion program)
- Services that are for fitness, diversion, motivation, or for a transitory condition (e.g., endurance training with an older adult)
- Services not under a therapy plan of care that supports the diagnosis being treated

- Services not considered to be acceptable by standards of practice
- Services that are too long for the condition and do not benefit the patient
- Services with unclear vague documentation about the skilled need for therapy
- Documentation does not include objective evaluations (therapy provided, and patient response)

Adapted from Centers for Medicare & Medicaid Services. (2022e). *Medicare benefit policy manual. Chapter 15 — covered medical and other health services.* https://www.cms.gov/Regulations-and-Guidance/Guidance/Manuals/downloads/bp102c15.pdf

BOX 76.3 GUIDELINES FOR DETERMINING OCCUPATIONAL THERAPY COVERAGE

- Treatment must be provided under a plan of care certified by a physician or non-physician practitioner (NPP). Physician order recommended, not required, and plan of care created before beginning of treatment (CMS, 2022e).
- Treatment must be completed by a qualified occupational therapist or occupational therapy assistant (OTA) under the supervision of a qualified occupational therapist. The occupational therapist provides correct level of supervision for the OTA based on state and local law with a minimum of general supervision (CMS, 2022e).
- Treatment must be of reasonable duration, and necessary intervention must be at the level of complexity requiring the "skilled" intervention of an occupational therapist. Treatment must be appropriate for the patient's condition.

- Medicare typically does not cover long-term supportive care.
- Documentation should be legible, signed, and include a national provider number (CMS, 2022e).
- Documentation follows Medicare guidelines for type of documentation (e.g., progress notes provide justification of the medial necessity of treatment/continued treatment and must be completed by the occupational therapist every 10 days).
- Occupational therapist must follow Medicare policies and should refer to CMS Benefit Policy Manual 100-02 Chapter 15, Section 220-230 for specific payment and documentation requirements.

on data and patient characteristics. *Case mix* refers to "the type or mix of patients treated by a hospital or unit" (PALLIPEDIA, 2022).

The PDPM considers the needs, characteristics, and goals of patients as addressed by the components of the five case-mix adjusted components (CMS, n.d.-b). Besides OT, the other four case-mix adjusted components are PT, SLP, nursing, and non-therapy ancillary (NTA). NTA refers to charges such as for medications and medical supplies. Payment is taken from the established per diem rate for OT and for any of the other four case-mix components. Classification for OT and PT is based on a clinical category (e.g., major joint replacement or spinal surgery) as well as a functional score. Together the scores from OT and PT assign residents to one of 16 case-mix groups for payment (CMS, n.d.-b). The patient's functional score is determined from ten items in Section GG, a tool that assesses functional self-care abilities and mobility. Section GG is utilized in SNFs and across the post-acute healthcare arena in long-term care hospitals, IRFs, and home health Part A to encourage better coordination of care and consistency of data collection.

In SNFs, Section GG is located in the MDS 3.0, a standardized assessment and care management tool that continues to be provided as an integral part of the regulatory structure in SNFs (CMS, 2022b). Besides Section GG the MDS addresses many other areas of relevance to therapy intervention such as cognitive patterns, hearing, speech, vision, mood, and behavior (CMS, 2022c). The PDPM also regulates other aspects of therapy such as group and concurrent therapy (working with two residents on different activities). OT practitioners working in SNFs need to be efficient, have good interdisciplinary communication skills, and keep up with regulatory changes (see OT Story 76.1 for an example).

Medicare Part A Coverage in Inpatient Rehabilitation Facilities Patients are admitted to IRFs, which can be a freestanding facility or a specialized unit in an acute care hospital, when they require complex nursing, medical care, and rehabilitation from an interprofessional team (CMS, 2018b). Payment in IRFs at the time of this writing is through a PPS and includes an evaluation tool called the Inpatient Rehabilitation Facility-Patient Assessment Instrument (IRF-PAI), which also monitors quality of care (CMS, 2022d). Medicare beneficiaries receiving services in an IRF are classified in several ways based on clinical, demographic, and anticipated needs of resources (CMS, 2022d).

There are specific regulations for IRFs that guide patient care and are required for reimbursement. Regulations necessitate 60% of patients in IRFs have one of 13 diagnoses (American Hospital Association, 2022) including but not limited to stroke, spinal cord injury, brain injury, amputation, major multiple trauma, and burns. Patients with knee or hip replacement must be 85 years or older to be admitted to an IRF (CMS, n.d.-c). Additionally, therapy provided in an IRF setting must equate to a minimum of 3 hours of skilled services 5 days per week. Patients are expected to be medically stable enough to participate and make gains from that intense of therapy (CMS, 2018b). If patients cannot participate in or tolerate the minimum hours of therapy, or if they are not making gains in therapy, the patient will be discharged. As mentioned, self-care and mobility data in Section GG is also collected in IRFs, which allows consistency of documentation in all post-acute systems.

Medicare Part A Coverage in Home Health Agencies and the Patient-Driven Groupings Model (PDGM) HHAs provide a variety of services in the patient's home including skilled nursing care, PT, OT, SLP, medical social

OT STORY 76.1 FIELDWORK STUDENT IN SKILLED NURSING FACILITY (SNF)

Kelly is an OT student on Level II fieldwork at an SNF. She has been treating an 82-year-old Medicare beneficiary, Carol, under the supervision of her fieldwork educator, Ben. Carol has been a patient at the SNF for 10 days due to a stroke. Carol has made good progress during OT sessions but continues to require minimal assistance with bathing and toileting. Carol uses a raised toilet seat for toileting and an extended tub bench for bathing. Carol is reaching the end of her allotted days in the SNF. The interprofessional team meets to discuss Carol's progress and discharge planning. Kelly reports that Carol is having difficulty with toileting and bathing and will require durable medical equipment (DME) upon discharge. The physical therapist reports similar findings with mobility and transfers and recommends that Carol stay at the SNF for one additional week and discharge with a hemi walker. The speech-language pathologist states Carol has met all SLP goals, and she will be discharged from SLP. Carol's family agrees Carol should stay one more week and wants the recommended DME for discharge, only if covered by insurance. Kelly informs Ben that she has one week to order the DME and mentions she is positive that insurance will cover the DME for toileting and bathing. Ben corrects the student's misperception and responds that Carol's insurance coverage is Medicare and that Medicare does not

cover bathroom DME. Ben advises Kelly that she needs to inform the family that Medicare does not cover the raised toilet seat and extended tub bench. Ben educates Kelly that Medicare will reimburse the cost of the hemi walker because it is utilized for safe mobility and PT obtained a prescription for the device. The next day, Kelly discusses with Carol and her family the DME Medicare will cover. Carol states, "Well I guess I will not be able to go home." Kelly states she is happy to work with Carol and her family to find an alternative to purchasing the bathroom DME out of pocket. Carol suggested local senior centers and community organizations that offered free or reduced price DME. By discharge, Carol's family was able to obtain DME and Carol discharged to home.

Questions

1. Where might Kelly the OT student have found out more information about Medicare coverage for DME equipment?
2. What DME equipment does Medicare cover?
3. Since Medicare does not cover bathroom DME what are some possible community resources that can be researched in your community?

work, and aide services. Medicare beneficiaries utilizing HHAs for either Part A or Part B must meet eligibility criteria for coverage including being *homebound,* or confined to the home. The regulations for qualifying for homebound status specify reasons such as the need for supportive devices, special transportation, and/or requiring assistance from others in order to leave the home. Another consideration for homebound status is that the person has an inability to leave the home, or it would require much effort to leave. In most cases, beneficiaries should only leave home for unique or infrequent events, such as to receive healthcare treatment (CMS, 2021b). Other eligibility requirements for HHAs include the patient's need for skilled services (nursing and/or therapy), having a plan of care created by the physician, and a visit with a physician or allowed non-physician practitioner (NPP) in an established timeframe. This plan of care should include measurable treatment goals, duration, and course of therapy based on the therapist's assessment of function (CMS, 2021b).

A recent, major change in home health regulations was a provision allowing OT practitioners to open home health cases when they are listed on the plan of care along with PT or SLP without skilled nursing services. Within OT's scope of practice, OT practitioners can then perform the initial and comprehensive assessment as part of the plan of care.

However, the original eligibility criteria of requiring skilled PT, SLP, and/or nursing services on an intermittent basis and/or continual skilled OT intervention remains in place (CMS, 2021b).

HHAs use a screening tool called the OASIS which is completed by nursing and used to evaluate the beneficiary's status and monitor outcomes for quality of care. OT practitioners consult with nursing regarding the primary diagnosis for which home healthcare is needed and the patient's functional status. HHAs are paid prospectively an established amount calculated every 30 days based on a classification system that identifies patient characteristics and other factors (CMS, 2019a). Scoring certain items on the OASIS determines functional levels and the therapist's evaluation is a strong contribution to the functional levels. Established by the physician-assigned diagnosis the patient is placed in one of 12 clinical subgroups (CMS, 2021c). Two of the clinical subgroups (musculoskeletal rehabilitation and neuro/stroke rehabilitation) specify therapy and others mention nursing. However, regardless of the grouping assignment, intervention should be a multidisciplinary benefit and cover all needs in the plan of care (CMS, 2019b).

Therapy is paid out of the consolidated billing regulations (CMS, 2021b) and payment is bundled to cover all vital services specified in the person's plan of care (CMS, 2019b).

To receive payment, Medicare stipulates occupational therapists, not OT assistants, must perform the ordered service visit, assessments, and documentation of evaluation and therapy (CMS, 2021b). This reimbursement rate made to HHAs under the PPS consists of all services provided (e.g., therapy) and medical supplies. DME is not included in HHAs PPS.

Medicare Part B   Many Medicare beneficiaries elect to purchase optional Medicare Part B coverage, which includes coverage for outpatient OT, PT, and SLP; and some DME (CMS, 2022a). In several Medicare settings, people can also be reimbursed under Medicare Part B guidelines for a less intensive level for therapy (e.g., hospital outpatient departments, HHAs, SNF, outpatient rehabilitation facilities, and private practice) (Medicare Payment Advisory Commission [MedPAC], 2021). Medicare Part B beneficiaries pay a set fee per month, and 20% of costs after a yearly deductible to cover utilized services.

All Medicare patients receiving outpatient services have an individualized written treatment plan developed by the therapist, physician or by a NPP who consults with the therapist (MedPAC, 2021). Plans of care for OT are certified initially by the physician/NPP and should include diagnoses, long-term goals, and details about the "type, amount, duration and frequency of therapy services" (CMS, 2022e, p. 167). Recertifications signed off by the physician/NPP are completed every 90 days and/or for significant modifications in the plan of care. With Medicare, a certified plan of care is necessary for payment and not necessarily a physician order. However, a physician/NPP order is helpful as it provides confirmation of the need for therapy and demonstrates that the patient is under physician/NPP care (CMS, 2022e).

Durable Medical Equipment   To qualify for reimbursement under Medicare Part B, DME must be prescribed by a physician to be used for a medical reason by the beneficiary in the home environment (Medicare.gov, n.d.). Examples of covered DME include commodes, walkers, wheelchairs, hospital beds, and patient lifts. Items like bathtub grab bars and raised toilet seats are not reimbursed under Medicare Part B coverage.

Current Procedural Terminology and Medicare Physician Fee Schedule   Currently, payment for Medicare Part B is completed using the Medicare Physician Fee Schedule (MPFS) established by the American Medical Association (AMA), which lists the fees used by physicians and other providers for healthcare services and products. All healthcare services are categorized and documented using the Healthcare Common Procedure Coding System (HCPCS) or Current Procedural Terminology (CPT) codes (MedPAC, 2021). Choosing the right code for evaluation involves critically assessing the beneficiary's occupational profile and history, occupational performance, and the degree of clinical decision-making involved with intervention (AOTA, 2016). (Refer to Table 76.2 for an explanation of payment terminology for Medicare Part B.)

Therapy Thresholds   Every patient receiving Medicare Part B services has an annual threshold amount for therapy services. This therapy threshold replaced the longstanding therapy cap that was allocated annually by Congress until it was repealed in 2018 as a result of advocacy efforts by many organizations, including American Occupational Therapy Association (OATA). There is one amount for OT (e.g., $2,150 in 2022) and a shared threshold amount for PT and SLP. With Medicare Part B, therapy providers certify therapy services are necessary when treatment exceeds the threshold amount, which requires application for extension of services with the addition of a modifier (KX) to the outpatient claim. The modifier attests services billed and provided are medically necessary. A CMS "targeted" medical review by Medicare contractors occurs when OT service charges reach a second larger amount or "threshold" ($3000 in 2022) (CMS, 2021d; MedPAC, 2021). Providing thorough documentation supporting OT services is always important for payment and essential for CMS review.

Medicare Part C   Medicare Advantage, or Medicare Part C, is the private part of Medicare that beneficiaries can elect to use instead of the traditional program. Medicare Part C plans are typically overseen by managed care commercial payers, such as HMOs or PPOs, and may provide expanded services (e.g., vision, dental, hearing). Each Medicare Part C plan administers Medicare Part A and Part B benefits, including therapy. However, each Part C plan is different with its own requirements for patient out-of-pocket expenses and authorization for therapy services (CMS, 2022a).

Keeping Up With Medicare-Related Payment Changes   Medicare regulations related to therapy are continuously updated, and OT practitioners must keep current with the changes. The CMS website is a good source for current information on Medicare. Practitioners should access the CMS Internet-only manuals and specifically the Benefit Policy Manual 100-02 Chapter 15, Section 220-230 (CMS, 2022e). The AOTA Website is another good source of information OT practitioners can utilize to stay abreast of healthcare changes impacting payment.

OT practitioners must also be aware of regional Medicare Administrative Contractors (MACs) who oversee regional Medicare coverage and payment (CMS, 2022f). Each regional MAC may have its own interpretation for therapy coverage (AOTA, 2021a). Personnel in MACs can be valuable resources for answering payment questions. OT practitioners should pay close attention to policies related to payment established by the MACs, called local coverage determinations (LCDs; AOTA, 2021a).

TABLE 76.2 **Payment Terminology for Medicare Part B**

Type	Definition	Application
MPFS: Medicare Physician Fee Schedule	Fee schedule for physicians and other health professionals used for Medicare billing in outpatient settings. A separate unit of payment is for each individual outpatient service as identified by the Healthcare Common Procedure Coding System codes (MedPAC, 2021, p. 2)	Used by therapists and other qualified healthcare providers to bill Medicare Part B
CPT codes: Level I Healthcare Common Procedure Coding System/Current Procedural Terminology	"Identifies medical services and procedures" (CMS, 2021e, para. 1)	Typically, therapists apply timed and untimed codes. Timed codes are based on an *8-min rule* for 15 minute units of service. Many insurance carriers besides Medicare may utilize this system (AOTA, 2021b) and untimed or service codes are billed once daily (CMS, 2019).
HCPCS codes: Level II Healthcare Common Procedure Coding System	"Identifies products, supplies, and services not included in the CPT codes such as durable medical equipment, prosthetics, and orthotics and supplies" (CMS, 2021e)	Used for payment of "durable medical equipment, prosthetics, orthotics, and supplies not listed as a CPT code" (CMS, 2021e)
RVU: Relative Value Unit	Payment rate for CPT codes "based on a relative weight . . . which account for the relative costliness of the inputs used to provide the service: the clinician's work, practice expense and professional liability insurance" (MedPAC, 2021, p. 2)	Therapists should bill appropriately for services provided.
CCI: Correct Coding Initiative	"National correct coding methodologies and to control improper coding leading to inappropriate payment in Part B claims" (CMS, 2022h, para. 3)	Used to review claims for improper coding (CMS, 2022h, para.2) particularly bundling of pairs of CPT codes. There are specific requirements for billing certain codes together (Robinson, 2007).
MPPR: Multiple Procedure Payment Reduction	Method of avoiding duplication of services when "more than one unit or procedure is provided to the same patient on the same day" (CMS, 2022i, p. 33)	Therapists should be aware that full payment is made for the unit or procedure with the highest practice expense (PE) payment. Beyond that, 50% of the PE is paid daily for second and additional codes for the same Medicare beneficiary and same provider (CMS, 2019b).
ICD-11 codes: *International Statistical Classifications of Diseases* codes	"The ICD is the foundation for the identification of health trends and statistics globally, and the international standard for reporting diseases and health conditions. It is the diagnostic classification standard for all clinical and research purposes" (World Health Organization, 2022). These codes are found on billing claims forms.	Therapists select the most appropriate codes to explain the primary medical condition and primary and secondary therapy diagnoses.

Medicaid

Medicaid, or Title XIX of the Social Security Act, enacted in 1965, historically has helped cover persons of low-income status including older adults, children, parents of dependent children, parents of other nonelderly adults, pregnant women, and people with disabilities who meet the eligibility requirements (Congressional Research Service, 2021). Medicaid is the largest government program for low-income Americans covering one in five people and financing about a fifth of all healthcare spending in the United States (Rudowitz et al., 2019). Nearly 43% of Medicaid recipients are children and one in four Medicaid enrollees are older adults and people with disabilities (Rudowitz et al., 2019). Relevant to therapy provision is that Medicaid finances 48%

of children with special needs and six out of ten nursing home residents (Rudowitz et al., 2019). Yet, older adults and persons with disabilities covered through Medicaid account for two-thirds of Medicaid spending because of extensive use of acute and long-term care services (Rudowitz et al., 2021). Medicaid pays for approximately 50% of long-term care services in home/community and nursing homes (Rudowitz et al., 2019).

Medicaid administered federally by the CMS is jointly financed by federal and state governments and regulated differently in each state (Rudowitz et al., 2021). Medicaid is a *means-tested* program as people qualify if their assets and income levels are below standards set by the program (Shi & Singh, 2004). States can choose to expand their baseline

Medicaid coverage and income eligibility requirements beyond the federal minimal requirements. Resulting from the PPACA and a subsequent Supreme Court ruling, many states have elected to expand Medicaid coverage to nonelderly adults with incomes up to 138% of the federal poverty level. Medicaid programs vary as each state provides different services and different systems for delivery. Quite often, programs are administered with a managed care approach and managed care accounts for nearly half of Medicaid payments (Rudowitz et al., 2021). Each state has a plan that documents how the program is administered, eligibility requirements, as well as required and optional health services. OT is one of the optional services; therefore, in some states, OT might not be a covered benefit (KFF, 2018).

Medicaid and Other Programs Covering Children Beyond Medicaid coverage for children with disabilities is provided by another program called the Children's Health Insurance Program (CHIP). CHIP provides reasonable health coverage for children in families that are low-income but earn too much to meet Medicaid qualifications (HealthCare.gov, n.d.). The CHIP is financed through federal and state governments; however, states administer their own programs (Medicaid.gov, n.d.).

The Early and Periodic Screening, Diagnosis, and Treatment (EPSDT) benefit covers a large amount of screening and diagnostic services for children up to the age of 21 years, such as medical, vision, hearing, and dental screenings (KFF, 2017). With Medicaid, OT services are covered for children, including EPSDT benefits.

In school systems or with early intervention programs, Medicaid is required to pay for educationally related services that are medically necessary (AOTA, 2022a). Besides funding from Medicaid, school-based services are financed partially by the IDEA with federal/state cost sharing and money from taxpayers in local school districts (Car Autism Roadmap, 2020). Thus, funding will vary for special educational programing throughout the United States.

When Payment Gets Denied

Therapy documentation is reviewed by third-party payers for payment for people with private and public insurance and services can be denied. Within the Medicare system, MACs and other private contractors are responsible for reviewing therapy records. MACs establish guidelines and LCDs describe criteria for coverage. Medicare denials can be for many reasons. A common reason is for technical errors, such as incomplete billing codes, not having legible documentation, or a missing physician signature on a Medicare plan of care. Other reasons for denial are for not following the Medicare regulations, such as the therapy service provided is not reasonable or necessary or a skilled level of therapy is not provided (refer to Boxes 76.2 and 76.3). Beyond Medicare, knowledge about how OT services are covered in any insurance plan can prevent denials. Appealing a denial for therapy that is perceived as justifiable is one way to advocate for clients.

The Patient Protection and Affordable Care Act

The PPACA was signed into law in 2010. Factors behind the development of PPACA were the large numbers of uninsured and underinsured people, the rising contribution of healthcare to the gross national product, and the inefficiencies in the healthcare market (ObamaCare Facts, 2020). The PPACA was a primary piece of legislation reforming the U.S. healthcare system and was intended to address many problems. The PPACA has many important provisions impacting payment for OT including, for example, expanded coverage of preventive health services, enhanced support for Medicaid and CHIP programs, linking payment to outcomes for Medicare, and creating healthier communities through prevention of chronic disease and access to preventive services (PPACA, 2010).

The PPACA impacts the quality, accessibility, and affordability of healthcare by extending insurance to over 31 million uninsured Americans through expanded Medicaid coverage in some states and providing benefits (U.S. Department of Health and Human Services, 2021). Insurance "exchanges" or marketplaces were created for the purchase and comparison of private health insurance by individuals, families, and small businesses.

Other provisions impacting payment for OT services under the PPACA include the following:

- Requiring insurers to cover mental health, substance abuse, rehabilitation, habilitative, and chronic disease management services
- Improving coverage through eliminating lifetime and annual limits and extending dependent coverage
- Prohibiting insurance companies to deny coverage or raise rates for preexisting conditions, guaranteeing renewability of coverage, and prohibiting discrimination in healthcare (PPACA, 2010)

Veteran's Administration

The Department of Veterans Affairs (VA) is the single largest employer of OT practitioners in the United States (U.S. Department of Veterans Affairs, 2020). Veterans receiving free or reduced healthcare must have actively served in the military and be enrolled in the VA's comprehensive Medical Benefits Package managed by the Veterans Health Administration (VHA; Benefits.gov, n.d.). OT practitioners are employed by the VA in all practice settings. They also treat uniformed military and veterans in private healthcare facilities. Interventions and DME are covered under various forms of VA insurance plans such as TRICARE for Life, TRICARE, CHAMPVA for Life, or Veteran-Directed Home and Community Based Services (VD-HCBS) (Paying for Senior Care, 2022). Active uniformed service members and National Guard/Reserve members and their families are covered under TRICARE as well as others with a military connection (TRICARE, 2022). The National Defense Authorization Act signed into law for fiscal year 2018 designated OTAs as providers under TRICARE (AOTA, 2017) and provision of services provided by the OTA under TRICARE follows Medicare guidelines (AOTA, 2020a).

Workers' Compensation

Workers' Compensation programs are state programs that address multiple needs of people who became ill or injured while working for private companies or state and local governments. The U.S. Department of Labor's Office of Workers' Compensation Programs covers federal workers. OT practitioners provide services with the primary goal of returning the ill or injured person to work. Programs financially support medical and rehabilitation services, partial payment of lost wages, and short- and long-term disability. Programs also reimburse partial as well as permanent disability. Payment for permanent disability may be provided if the condition is expected to last greater than 1 year, or result in death (Social Security Administration, 2021). Programs may include services such as vocational rehabilitation, medical rehabilitation, job placement, and social services. Many of the state programs are instituted with a managed care approach. Each state has a governing body that determines the administration and funding; therefore, Workers' Compensation programs vary from state to state for non-federal workers.

Consolidated Omnibus Budget Reconciliation Act of 1985

The Consolidated Omnibus Budget Reconciliation Act of 1985 (COBRA) gives workers and their families who lose health benefits the right to temporary group health benefits. Several circumstances may result in the loss of health benefits. Qualification for COBRA includes voluntary or involuntary loss of employment, reduction in hours worked, transition between jobs, death, divorce, and other life events

(U.S. Department of Labor, n.d.). OT practitioners may provide services to persons covered by COBRA insurance.

Trends in Payment Systems in the United States

Several trends to reduce the cost of care have emerged in the healthcare marketplace: consumer-driven healthcare, value-based care, telehealth, and a movement toward healthcare in outpatient and community settings.

Consumer-Driven Healthcare

Consumer-driven healthcare is an economically driven approach involving lowering healthcare expenditures while simultaneously providing consumer control over health plans. Thus, decision-making about healthcare moves to the consumer instead of to the insurer, and consumers with these plans should become engaged in researching healthcare options and costs (Vanetine & Masters, 2017). An example of consumer-driven healthcare is an HDHP often accompanied by an HSA. The HDHPs and HSAs, also known as consumer-directed health plans (CDHPs), allow people to save and apply pre-tax dollars to health-related payments. Pre-tax dollars can be used to pay for deductibles, coinsurance, copayments, and health insurance premiums, which are traditionally paid for with after-tax dollars. The consumer can choose areas for healthcare intervention that are not always covered by traditional insurance. Consumer-driven plans are growing and are predicted to continue to grow, with recent data indicating 45.6% of persons younger than 65 years old with private health insurance are enrolled in an HDHP, 20.6% are enrolled in a CDHP, and 25% are enrolled in an HDHP without an HSA (Terlizzi et al., 2019). Because these plans provide an incentive not to spend healthcare dollars, practitioners need to educate consumers about the value of therapy services.

Value-Based Care

The shift from paying for quantity of care (volume-based) to paying for the value of care (value-based) will likely continue and is embraced by many payers, including Medicare. Increasing cost of healthcare coupled with subpar outcomes, the aging population, and healthcare reform all support a continued focus on expanding value-based care payment models (Bristol & Joshi, 2014). Value-based payment models are a component of CMS's quality strategy to reform the delivery and payment of healthcare and support CMS's goal of providing better care for individuals and populations at a lower cost (CMS, 2022g).

OT practitioners should be knowledgeable about the aim of value-based payment models and utilize patient-centered and evidenced-based care to reduce cost and improve the quality and safety of patient care regardless of practice setting. Such knowledge is supportive of AOTA's Vision 2025 which calls for members of the profession to "maximize health, well-being, and quality of life for all people, populations, and communities through effective solutions that facilitate participation in everyday living" (AOTA, 2022b, para.3).

Telehealth

OT practitioners utilize telehealth technologies for the provision of OT evaluation, intervention, supervision, and education. Historically reimbursement for telehealth was not widespread among the various types of reimbursement mentioned in this chapter (Cason, 2014). Reimbursement coverage for telehealth expanded in 2020 because of the public health emergency with the COVID-19 pandemic. With schools, clinics, and the ability to enter a client's home shut down, OT services via telehealth grew in multiple areas of practice across the United States. At the time of this book publication, AOTA is advocating for permanent telehealth coverage inclusive of Medicare beneficiaries (AOTA, 2022c). Private insurance reimbursement for telehealth varies among companies and client populations and should be verified by the provider before telehealth service delivery. OT practitioners should refer to state regulatory boards for determining Medicaid coverage for telehealth. The VHA covers telehealth including OT (Cason, 2014).

Movement Toward Outpatient and Community Care

Reflecting on considerations about the high cost of healthcare, consumer demands, the growth of value-based care, and advances in technology, there continues to be a movement toward delivering healthcare services in community settings (Gerhardt & Arora, 2020). Because of advances in technology some procedures, such as for joint replacement, are now available in outpatient settings (Webb, 2021). With Medicare, outpatient therapy services (Part B) are now being provided in the home, which differs from the traditional home health Part A regulations. With Medicaid, federal funds have expanded home care services for older adults and people with disabilities (Simmons-Duffin, 2021). Remote monitoring of patients will become more of a norm (Gerhardt & Arora, 2020). Medicare is piloting providing acute hospital care at home (Donlan, 2021). With this concept, patients will be cared for in their home at an inpatient hospital level. OT practitioners should be aware of these trends so that they can strategically plan to work in these developing practice settings. Along with awareness of these trends is knowledge about payment sources for therapy in the outpatient and community arena.

The Uninsured, Underinsured, and Pro Bono Therapy Intervention

Health insurance is essential; however, a portion of Americans are either uninsured or underinsured. Without insurance, severe health consequences can happen, especially if a preventable condition could have been treated (Garfield et al., 2019). Public concern about the large number of Americans lacking insurance (44 million in 2013) was behind much of the discussion leading to the PPACA. Due to the PPACA, gains have been made resulting in fewer uninsured people (27.5 million in 2021). The uninsured are lower income, more likely to be people of color, have one employed worker in a family, or are undocumented immigrants. Approximately 64% of uninsured citizens claim the high cost of insurance premiums prohibited purchase of health insurance (Tolbert et al., 2022), and they must consider the costs of paying for healthcare against other life necessities (Garfield et al., 2019). As discussed with the PPACA, there was a lack of Medicaid expansion in some states. This lack of expansion left certain citizens caught between not qualifying for Medicaid and unable to afford insurance in the marketplaces. This is because the original intent of the PPACA was to expand Medicaid coverage in all states. Not understanding the insurance system is another reason for people being uninsured (Tolbert et al., 2020).

Even with insurance, approximately 44 million U.S. citizens are underinsured. Underinsured adults may have insurance, but coverage is limited, often because their deductibles are too high in relation to their income. Underinsurance can lead to increased medical debt and not seeking out healthcare services (The Commonwealth Fund, 2019, 2020a), including OT.

The uninsured or underinsured individual can elect to privately pay for OT services, but often, they must pay the full cost of service versus the negotiated rates of insured individuals (Garfield et al., 2019). As alternatives, the OT practitioner can look for community-based grants or provide pro bono services to increase access to OT services. Providing pro bono services is supported by the OT profession as stated in the Occupational Therapy Code of Ethics: practitioners should "provide information and resources to address barriers to access for persons in need of occupational therapy services" (AOTA, 2020b, p. 7).

Advocacy for Payment

Every time OT practitioners experience problems with payment for services, they should critically consider how best to obtain and advocate for reimbursement. Advocacy for payment can occur in many ways. For example, effective communication with case managers or other key people in an insurance system may be all it takes to obtain payment. Providing evidence of the efficacy and value of the intervention is often helpful. Following through with the processes in place, such as an appeals system, can result in payment for services. Specific appeal requirements exist with different payment resources. Accessing resources beyond the traditional system to get funds through charitable and/or community organizations may be an option. Beyond advocating for the client in a clinical situation, practitioners can advocate for improved payment in the healthcare system when patient-centered care and quality is compromised.

Global Healthcare Payment Models

U.S. healthcare includes multiple payment systems. Globally there are four additional models of healthcare that are the foundation for payment of healthcare services. These models are the Beveridge model, the Bismarck model, the National Health Insurance model, and the "Out of Pocket" model (Table 76.3) (Princeton Public Health Review, 2017; Washington State, n.d.). Although categorized separately, most countries blend multiple models of healthcare together. Understanding the differences among the models assists in identifying the payment systems that exist within a particular country. U.S. OT students and practitioners who intend to go abroad to do fieldwork or work in another country should be familiar with the healthcare payment model of that particular country.

Table 76.3 can be generalized to healthcare services within a country. To understand the specifics of how OT services are paid, OT practitioners or students completing international fieldwork experiences should access government resources, national OT organizations, or speak to knowledgeable practitioners from the country. The following discussion elaborates on the healthcare systems in Canada, the United Kingdom, Australia, and Korea.

Canada

The Canadian Association of Occupational Therapists (CAOT) provides information for payment of OT services in Canada (CAOT, 2016). Government funding is the primary source of payment for therapy services in Canada. Provincial health insurance plans fund OT in hospitals, community health centers, rehabilitation centers, home care programs, and schools. Additional funding models are accessible as well. Extended health insurance plans from employers may include OT services as a benefit. If a person has a work-related injury, a worker's compensation referral to OT will cover the payment. Auto insurance plans may cover OT services when someone is injured in a car crash. Those on long-term disability may also get OT services covered. A veteran of the Canadian armed forces may receive coverage from the Department of Veteran Affairs (CAOT, 2016).

United Kingdom

OT services can be accessed for free in the United Kingdom through the National Health Service (NHS), or a local council. For short-term conditions such as following a surgery, OT is accessed through the NHS. In cases that are long-term such as permanent physical disability, OT is accessed through a local council or a Health and Social Care Partnership. Qualification for OT services is determined through a health and social care assessment. OT equipment and home modifications may also be paid for if the assessment deems them necessary. OT practitioners also practice in the private healthcare sector in the United Kingdom. Access to private OT services does not require a referral from a general practitioner (NHS Inform, 2020). Private OT services are paid for out of pocket or by private health insurance. Private health insurance may be paid for by an employer or directly by the consumer. However, only an estimated 10.5% of the UK population obtain private insurance (The Commonwealth Fund, 2020b).

Australia

The Australian Medicare Benefits Schedule outlines coverage for OT, which is covered for five sessions and must be referred by a medical practitioner (Australian Government, n.d.). Australians who have a permanent and significant disability can receive funding for OT through the National Disability Insurance Scheme (NDIS). Participants in NDIS receive a plan that includes their goals and their eligible funding. They can utilize the funding to purchase OT services (NDIS, 2021). Private health insurance in Australia provides coverage for costs of services that Medicare does not cover and allows private patient treatment in hospitals. Purchasing private health insurance may allow people to avoid paying a Medicare levy surcharge that is assessed on people who do not have private hospital coverage or earn income over a certain level (Australian Government, 2021).

TABLE 76.3 **Global Healthcare Models**

	Bismarck Model	Beveridge Model	National Health Insurance Model	"Out of Pocket" Model
Description	Social health insurance model	National health service	National health insurance	Market-driven healthcare
Sample Countries	Austria Belgium France Germany Japan Switzerland The Netherlands	Australia Cuba Denmark Finland Greece Iceland Ireland Italy Italy New Zealand Norway Portugal South Korea Spain Sweden United Kingdom	Canada Taiwan	*Market-based plans:* Argentina Chile South Africa The Bahamas Uruguay *Minimal health plan structures:* Rural areas of Cambodia China India Nigeria Sudan
General Structure	• De-centralized • Employers and employees support "sickness funds" created by compulsory payroll deductions. • Private insurance plans cover everyone regardless of preexisting conditions	• Government acts as the single payer through the establishment of a central national health service that delivers the care	• Publicly run insurance program that every citizen pays into • Uses private sector providers • The universal insurance does not deny claims	• Wealthier able to purchase commercially offered insurance • If no insurance available or can't afford, patients must pay for procedures out of pocket
Eligibility	All legal citizens	All legal citizens	All legal citizens	N/A
Benefits	• Set by a federal committee in collaboration with the regional "sickness funds" • Use evidence in decision making	• Access to a standardized set of benefits available across the country • Evidence-based decision-making in benefit selection	• Medically necessary defined federally, but local decisions vary on benefit package • Evidence-based decision-making	• Varies
Costs	• For example, some copays in Germany for nursing homes, pharmaceuticals, and medical aids • Government tightly controls prices while insurers do not make a profit, even if more than one health plan option	• Free at point of service; no out of pocket costs • Government controls prices	• Government processes all claims; aims to reduce the amount of duplication of services • Financial barriers to treatment are generally low • Patients usually can choose their healthcare providers	• No cost controls in place

TABLE 76.3 **Global Healthcare Models (*continued*)**

	Bismarck Model	Beveridge Model	National Health Insurance Model	"Out of Pocket" Model
Administration	De-centralized regional administration with national role	Central/national government administration	For example, in Canada it is administered by provinces and territories	N/A
Delivery System	• Health providers are generally private institutions • Social health insurance funds are considered public	• The government owns majority of hospitals and clinics • Most doctors are government employees	• Hospitals and providers remain private	• Majority are private entities • Some countries have some public investment in hospitals
Health Plans	Some have a single insurer (France, Korea); other countries may have multiple, competing insurers (Germany, Czech Republic) or multiple, noncompeting insurers (Japan).	Government run; eliminates competition in the market	In some countries, can purchase private insurance for additional needs or in substitution	More availability of health plans emerging; if can afford
Funding	Payroll deductions	Income taxes	Income taxes	Predominately self-pay

Adapted from Washington State. (n.d.). *High level overview of major international models.* https://www.hca.wa.gov/assets/program/major-final-frameworks-international-models.pdf

Korea

The National Health Insurance (NHI) system in Korea provides healthcare insurance to all citizens. Fee-for-service is the payment model for the majority of inpatient and outpatient care (Health Insurance Review & Assessment Service [HIRA], 2017). The insurance fee system has 44 rates for rehabilitation with OT only able to act on three classifications and five codes. The three code areas are OT (simple, complex, special), ADL training, and rehabilitation dysphagia therapy. Much advocacy is necessary to expand payment for OT's scope of practice (Song & Cha, 2015). NHI provides long-term care insurance. To qualify for long-term care insurance, a person receives an approval score based on their physical and mental health. OT practitioners participate in determining the disability grade score based on level of independence and completion of activities of daily living (Long Term Care Insurance, 2010).

Medical Tourism

Medical tourism is a term to describe the process of traveling outside of one's country of residence to receive medical care. There are many reasons for medical tourism including

to receive medical care that may be cheaper in another country, that is timely, and that may be or perceived to be of a higher quality. Other reasons are to receive medical care from a provider who shares the traveler's language and culture, or for care that is not available or approved in one's country of residence (AMA, n.d.; Centers for Disease Control and Prevention [CDC], 2021). Individuals opting to complete medical tourism trips recognize that they self-pay for procedures although costs can be lower in other countries (CDC, 2021; Global Protective Solutions, n.d.). Medical tourism trips most commonly include travel to receive dental care, surgery, cosmetic surgery, fertility treatments, organ and tissue transplantation, and cancer treatment (CDC, 2021). Although medical tourists may receive safe and effective care, both the AMA (n.d.) and the CDC (2021) advise there are risks to medical tourism. These risks largely revolve around safety and quality of medical care such as infections, substandard surgical care, antibiotic resistance, communication, and continuity of care challenges. Some insurance options exist for complications that can occur (CDC, 2021). Individuals opting to travel outside of their country are advised to thoroughly research the providers who will be providing the care, get a pre-travel consultation form, maintain their health and medical records, and arrange for follow-up care (CDC, 2021).

Conclusion

Dealing with payment issues is a regular part of OT practice. OT practitioners may work with a variety of payment systems. On the surface, knowledge about payment systems might seem overwhelming because the financial system for healthcare and social services in the United States is very complex. Yet, it is every practitioner's professional duty to learn about these systems to provide needed OT services and to advocate for payment or changes with policies/systems when considered necessary (AOTA, 2020c). Payment systems change, and these changes often occur because of new or amended legislation. Keeping current with policy and legislation that affect payment for one's area of practice is essential for successful practice.

Lippincott® Connect *For additional resources on the subjects discussed in this chapter, visit Lippincott Connect.*

REFERENCES

American Hospital Association. (2022). *Fact sheet: Inpatient rehabilitation facilities (IRFs).* https://www.aha.org/factsheet/2018-03-19-fact-sheet-inpatient-rehabilitation-facilities-irfs

American Medical Association. (n.d.). *Medical tourism: Code of medical ethics opinion 1.2.13.* https://www.ama-assn.org/delivering-care/ethics/medical-tourism

American Occupational Therapy Association. (2016). *New occupational therapy evaluation coding overview.* https://www.aota.org/~/media/Corporate/Files/Advocacy/Federal/Evaluation-Codes-Overview-2016.pdf

American Occupational Therapy Association. (2017, December 12). *Bill to designate OTAs as Tricare providers signed into law.* https://www.aota.org/advocacy/advocacy-news/legislative-issues-update/bill-to-designate-otas-as-tricare-providers-signed-into-law

American Occupational Therapy Association. (2020a, April 24). *OTAs added as authorized TRICARE providers.* https://www.aota.org/advocacy/advocacy-news/2020/otas-added-authorized-tricare-providers

American Occupational Therapy Association. (2020b). AOTA 2020 occupational therapy code of ethics. *The American Journal of Occupational Therapy, 74*(suppl. 3), 7413410005p1–7413410005p13. https://doi.org/10.5014/ajot.2020.74S3006

American Occupational Therapy Association. (2020c). Occupational therapy practice framework: Domain and process (4th ed.). *The American Journal of Occupational Therapy, 74*(suppl. 2), 7412410010. https://doi. org/10.5014/ajot.2020.74S2001

American Occupational Therapy Association. (2021a, June 10). *Medicare.* https://www.aota.org/advocacy/advocacy-news/medicare

American Occupational Therapy Association. (2021b). *Coding and billing resources.* https://www.aota.org/practice/practice-essentials/coding#TimedCodes-8MinRule

American Occupational Therapy Association. (2022a). *Medicaid and occupational therapy.*

American Occupational Therapy Association. (2022b). *About AOTA.* https://www.aota.org/about/mission-vision

American Occupational Therapy Association. (2022c, March 10). *Congress extends occupational therapy telehealth waivers for 151 days beyond expiration of PHE.* https://www.aota.org/advocacy/advocacy-news/2022/omnibus-telehealth-extension

Australian Government. (n.d.). *Medicare benefits schedule – item 10958.* http://www9.health.gov.au/mbs/fullDisplay.cfm?type=item&q=10958&qt=item

Australian Government. (2021, August 18). *About private health insurance.* https://www.health.gov.au/health-topics/private-health-insurance/about-private-health-insurance

Benefits.gov. (n.d.). *Basic medical benefits package for veterans.* https://www.benefits.gov/benefits/benefit-details/303

Bristol, S., & Joshi, M. S. (2014). Transforming the healthcare system for improved quality. In M. S. Joshi, E. R. Ransom, D. B. Nash, & S. B. Ranson (Eds.), *The healthcare quality book: Vision, strategy, and tools* (3rd ed., pp. 541–559). Health Administration Press.

Canadian Association of Occupational Therapists. (2016). *How are occupational therapy services paid for?* https://caot.in1touch.org/site/aboutot/howotservicesfunded?nav=sidebar

Car Autism Roadmap. (2020, May 26). *Who pays for special education services?* https://www.carautismroadmap.org/who-pays-for-special-education-services/

Cason, J. (2014). Telehealth: A rapidly developing service delivery model for occupational therapy. *International Journal of Telerehabilitation, 6,* 29–35. https://doi.org/10.5195/ijt.2014.6148

Centers for Disease Control and Prevention. (2021). *Medical tourism: Travel to another country for medical care.* https://wwwnc.cdc.gov/travel/page/medical-tourism

Centers for Medicare & Medicaid Services. (n.d.-a). *CMS roadmaps overview.* https://www.cms.gov/medicare/quality-initiatives-patient-assessment-instruments/qualityinitiativesgeninfo/downloads/roadmapoverview_oea_1-16.pdf

Centers for Medicare & Medicaid Services. (n.d.-b). *SNF PPS: Patient Driven Payment Model* [PowerPoint slides]. Medicare Learning Network® Event. https://www.cms.gov/Medicare/Medicare-Fee-for-Service-Payment/SNFPPS/Downloads/MLN_CalL_PDPM_Presentation_508.pdf

Centers for Medicare & Medicaid Services. (n.d.-c). *Fact sheet #1 inpatient rehabilitation facility classification requirements.* https://www.cms.gov/Medicare/Medicare-Fee-for-Service-Payment/InpatientRehabFacPPS/downloads/fs1classreq.pdf.

Centers for Medicare & Medicaid Services. (2013). *Jimmo v. Sebelius settlement agreement fact sheet.* https://www.cms.gov/medicare/mdicare-fee-for-service-payment/snfpps/downloads/jimmo-factsheet.pdf.

Centers for Medicare & Medicaid Services. (2018a, March). *Home health prospective payment system.* https://www.cms.gov/Outreach-and-Education/Medicare-Learning-Network-MLN/MLNProducts/Downloads/Home-Health-PPS-Fact-Sheet-ICN006816.pdf

Centers for Medicare & Medicaid Services. (2018b, December 20). *Inpatient rehabilitation facility (IRF) medical review changes.* https://www.cms.gov/Outreach-and-Education/Medicare-Learning-Network-MLN/MLNMattersArticles/Downloads/SE17036.pdf

Centers for Medicare & Medicaid Services. (2019a, November 25). *MLN matters: Overview of the patient driven group model.* https://www.cms.gov/files/document/se19027.pdf.

Centers for Medicare & Medicaid Services. (2019b). *Medicare claims processing manual: Chapter 12 - Physicians/nonphysician practitioners.* https://www.cms.gov/files/document/medicare-claims-processing-manual-chapter-12

Center for Medicare & Medicaid Services. (2021a, December 15). *NHE fact sheet.* https://www.cms.gov/Research-Statistics-Data-and-Systems/Statistics-Trends-and-Reports/NationalHealthExpendData/NHE-Fact-Sheet

Center for Medicare & Medicaid Services. (2021b). *Medicare benefit policy manual: Chapter 7 - home health services.* https://www.cms.gov/Regulations-and-Guidance/Guidance/Manuals/Downloads/bp102c07.pdf.

Center for Medicare & Medicaid Services. (2021c, December 1). *Home health patient-driven groupings model.* https://www.cms.gov/Medicare/Medicare-Fee-for-Service-Payment/HomeHealthPPS/HH-PDGM

Centers for Medicare & Medicaid Services. (2021d, December 1). *Therapy services.* https://www.cms.gov/Medicare/Billing/Therapy Services

Centers for Medicare & Medicaid Services. (2021e). *HCPCS - general information: What's new.* https://www.cms.gov/Medicare/Coding/MedHCPCSGenInfo

Centers for Medicare & Medicaid Services. (2022a). *Medicare & you 2022.* https://www.medicare.gov/pubs/pdf/10050-Medicare-and-You.pdf

Centers for Medicare & Medicaid Services. (2022b, February 26). *Minimum Data Set (MDS) 3.0 for nursing homes and swing bed providers.* https://www.cms.gov/Medicare/Quality-Initiatives-Patient-Assessment-Instruments/NursingHomeQualityInits/NHQIMDS30

Centers for Medicare & Medicaid Services. (2022c, March 22). *Minimum Data Set (MDS) 3.0 Resident Assessment Instrument (RAI) manual.* https://www.cms.gov/Medicare/Quality-Initiatives-Patient-Assessment-Instruments/NursingHomeQualityInits/MDS30RAIManual

Centers for Medicare & Medicaid Services. (2022d, February). *Medicare payment systems.* https://www.cms.gov/Outreach-and-Education/Medicare-Learning-Network-MLN/MLNProducts/html/medicare-payment-systems.html#Intro.

Centers for Medicare & Medicaid Services. (2022e). *Medicare benefit policy manual. Chapter 15 — covered medical and other health services.* https://www.cms.gov/Regulations-and-Guidance/Guidance/Manuals/downloads/bp102c15.pdf

Centers for Medicare & Medicaid Services. (2022f). *What's a MAC?* https://www.cms.gov/Medicare/Medicare-Contracting/Medicare-Administrative-Contractors/What-is-a-MAC.html

Centers for Medicare & Medicaid. (2022g). *What are the value-based programs?* https://www.cms.gov/Medicare/Quality-Initiatives-Patient-Assessment-Instruments/Value-Based-Programs/Value-Based-Programs

Centers for Medicare & Medicaid Services. (2022h). *National correct coding initiative edits.* https://www.cms.gov/Medicare/Coding/NCCI-Coding-Edits

Centers for Medicare & Medicaid Services. (2022i). *Medicare claims processing manual: Chapter 5 - part B outpatient rehabilitation and CORF/OPT services.* https://www.cms.gov/Regulations-and-Guidance/Guidance/Manuals/Downloads/clm104c05.pdf

Congressional Research Service. (2021, February 22). *Medicaid: An overview.* https://crsreports.congress.gov/product/pdf/R/R43357

Cubanski, J., & Neuman, T. (2021). *FAQs on medicare financing and trust fund solvency.* Kaiser Family Foundation (KFF). https://www.kff.org/medicare/issue-brief/faqs-on-medicare-financing-and-trust-fund-solvency/

Donlan, A. (2021, April 19). *CMS Hospital-at-Home program closing in on 200 participants.* Home Health Care News. https://homehealthcarenews.com/2021/04/cms-hospital-at-home-program-closing-in-on-200-participants/

Garfield, R., Orgera, K., & Damico, A. (2019, January 25). *The uninsured and the ACA: A primer – key facts about health insurance and the uninsured amidst changes to the Affordable Care Act.* Kaiser Family Foundation (KFF). https://www.kff.org/uninsured/report/the-uninsured-and-the-aca-a-primer-key-facts-about-health-insurance-and-the-uninsured-amidst-changes-to-the-affordable-care-act/

Gerhardt, W., & Arora, A. (2020, February 21). *Hospital revenue trends: Outpatient, home, virtual, and other care settings are becoming more common.* Deloitte. https://www2.deloitte.com/us/en/insights/industry/health-care/outpatient-virtual-health-care-trends.html

Global Protective Solutions. (n.d.). Category archives: Medical tourism. https://www.globalprotectivesolutions.com/category/medical-tourism/

HealthCare.gov. (n.d.). *The Children's' Health Insurance Program (CHIP).* https://www.healthcare.gov/medicaid-chip/childrens-health-insurance-program/

Health Insurance Review & Assessment Service. (2017). *Health security system.* http://www.hira.or.kr/dummy.do?pgmid=HIRAJ010000006002

Kaiser Family Foundation. (2017, February 15). *Key issues in children's health coverage.* http://www.kff.org/medicaid/issue-brief/key-issues-in-childrens-health-coverage/

Kaiser Family Foundation. (2018). *Medicaid benefits: Occupational therapy services.* https://www.kff.org/medicaid/state-indicator/occupational-therapy-services/?currentTimeframe=0&sortModel=%7B%22colId%22:%22Location%22,%22sort%22:%22asc%22%7D

Kaiser Family Foundation. (2019). *Health insurance coverage of the total population.* https://www.kff.org/other/state-indicator/total-population/?currentTimeframe=0&sortModel=%7B%22colId%22:%22Location%22,%22sort%22:%22asc%22%7D

Kaiser Family Foundation. (2021a, November 10). *2021 employer benefits survey.* https://www.kff.org/health-costs/report/2021-employer-health-benefits-survey

Kaiser Family Foundation. (2021b). *Employer health benefits: 2021 summary of findings.* https://files.kff.org/attachment/Summary-of-Findings-Employer-Health-Benefits-2021.pdf

Long Term Care Insurance. (2010). *What is judgment rating?* https://www.longtermcare.or.kr/npbs/e/e/100/htmlView?pgmId=npee301m03s&desc=JudgmentRating

Medicaid.gov. (n.d.). *CHIP state program information.* https://www.medicaid.gov/chip/state-program-information/index.html

Medicare.gov. (n.d.). *Durable medical equipment (DME) coverage.* https://www.medicare.gov/coverage/durable-medical-equipment-coverage.html

Medicare Payment Advisory Commission. (2021, November). *Outpatient therapy services payment system.* https://www.medpac.gov/wp-content/uploads/2021/11/medpac_payment_basics_21_opt_final_sec.pdf

NDIS. (2021, September 14). *What is NDIS?* https://www.ndis.gov.au/understanding/what-ndis

NHS Inform. (2020, February 14). *Occupational therapy.* https://www.nhsinform.scot/tests-and-treatments/counselling-and-therapies/occupational-therapy#how-to-access-it

ObamaCare Facts. (2020, August 14). *ObamaCare: Everything you need to know about the ACA.* https://obamacarefacts.com/obamacare-everything-you-need-to-know-about-the-aca/

PALLIPEDIA. (2022, August 8). *Case-mix.* https://pallipedia.org/case-mix/

Patient Protection and Affordable Care Act, 42 U.S.C. § 18001. (2010, March 23). https://www.gpo.gov/fdsys/pkg/PLAW-111publ148/pdf/PLAW-111publ148.pdf

Paying for Senior Care. (2022, September 20). *Veterans assistance for durable medical equipment: TRICARE, CHAMPA & VD-HCBS.* https://www.payingforseniorcare.com/durable-medical-equipment/help-for-veterans.html

Princeton Public Health Review. (2017, December 2). *Health care reform: Learning from other major health care systems.* https://pphr.princeton.edu/2017/12/02/unhealthy-health-care-a-cursory-overview-of-major-health-care-systems/

Robinson, M. (2007). Medicare 101: Understanding the basics. *OT Practice, 12*(2), CE1–CE7.

Rogers, A. T., Bai, G., Lavin, R. A., & Anderson, G. F. (2017). Higher hospital spending on occupational therapy is associated with lower readmission rates. *Medical Care Research and Review, 74*(6), 668–686. https://doi.org/10.1177/1077558716666981

Rudowitz, R., Garfield, R., & Hinton, E. (2019, March 6). *10 things to know about Medicaid: Setting the facts straight.* Kaiser Family

Foundation (KFF). https://www.kff.org/medicaid/issue-brief/10-things-to-know-about-medicaid-setting-the-facts-straight/

Rudowitz, R., Williams, E., Hinton, E., & Garfield, R. (2021, May 7). *Medicaid financing: The basics.* Kaiser Family Foundation (KFF). https://www.kff.org/medicaid/issue-brief/medicaid-financing-the-basics/

Shi, L., & Singh, D. A. (2004). *Delivering health care in America: A systems approach* (3rd ed.). Jones & Bartlett Learning.

Sieck, R., Lohman, H., Stupica, K., Minthorne-Brown, L., & Stoffer, K. (2017). Awareness of Medicare regulation changes: Occupational therapists' perceptions and implications for practice. *Physical & Occupational Therapy in Geriatrics, 35,* 67–80.

Simmons-Duffin, S. (2021, October 21). *New federal funds spur expansion of home care services for the elderly and the disabled.* Shots – Health News from NPR. https://www.npr.org/sections/health-shots/2021/10/21/1048082143/new-federal-funds-spur-expansion-of-home-care-services-for-the-elderly-and-disab

Social Security Administration. (2021, April). *Disability benefits* (Publication No. 05-10029). https://www.ssa.gov/pubs/EN-05-10029.pdf

Song, Y. J., & Cha, Y. J. (2015). Occupational therapy medical insurance review of issues and improvement of the system in Korea. *Korean Journal of Occupational Therapy, 23*(1), 123–125. https://doi.org/10.14519/jksot.2015.23.1.10

Terlizzi, E. P., Cohen R. A., & Martinez, M. E. (2019, February). *Health insurance coverage: Early release of estimates from the National Health Interview Survey, January–September 2018.* National Center for Health Statistics. https://www.cdc.gov/nchs/data/nhis/earlyrelease/insur201902.pdf

The Commonwealth Fund. (2019, February 7). *Underinsured rate rose from 2014-2018, with greatest growth among people in employer health plans.* https://www.commonwealthfund.org/press-release/2019/underinsured-rate-rose-2014-2018-greatest-growth-among-people-employer-health.

The Commonwealth Fund. (2020a, August 19). *U.S. health insurance coverage in 2020: A looming crisis in affordability: Findings from the Commonwealth Fund biennial health insurance survey, 2020.* https://www.commonwealthfund.org/publications/issue-briefs/2020/aug/looming-crisis-health-coverage-2020-biennial.

The Commonwealth Fund. (2020b, December). *International profiles of health care systems.* https://www.commonwealthfund.org/sites/default/files/2020-12/International_Profiles_of_Health_Care_Systems_Dec2020.pdf

Tolbert, J., Orgera, K., & Damico, A. (2020, November 6). *Key facts about the uninsured population.* Kaiser Family Foundation (KFF). https://www.kff.org/uninsured/issue-brief/key-facts-about-the-uninsured-population/

Tolbert, J., Drake, P., & Damico, A. (2022). Key facts about the uninsured population. Kaiser Family Foundation (KFF). https://www.kff.org/uninsured/issue-brief/key-facts-about-the-uninsured-population/

TRICARE. (2022, March 2). *Eligibility.* https://tricare.mil/Plans/Eligibility

U.S. Department of Health and Human Services. (2021, June 5). *New HHS Data show more Americans than ever have health coverage through the Affordable Care Act.* https://www.hhs.gov/about/news/2021/06/05/new-hhs-data-show-more-americans-than-ever-have-health-coverage-through-affordable-care-act.html

U.S. Department of Labor. (n.d.). *Continuation of health coverage COBRA.* https://www.dol.gov/general/topic/health-plans/cobra

U.S. Department of Veterans Affairs. (2020, March 12). *Rehabilitation and prosthetic services: Occupational therapy.* https://www.rehab.va.gov/pmrs/Occupational_Therapy.asp

Vanetine, S. T., & Masters, G. M. (2017, January 30). *Healthcare forecast 2017: Top trends driving board strategic priorities.* NRC Health. https://nrchealth.com/resource/healthcare-forecast-2017-top-trends-driving-board-strategic-priorities/

Washington State. (n.d.). *High level overview of major international models.* https://www.hca.wa.gov/assets/program/major-final-frameworks-international-models.pdf

Webb, J. (2021, April 1). *Same-day joint replacement surgery possible.* Mayo Clinic Health System. https://www.mayoclinichealthsystem.org/hometown-health/speaking-of-health/same-day-joint-replacement-surgery-possible

World Health Organization. (2022). *International statistical classification of diseases and related health problems (ICD).* https://www.who.int/standards/classifications/classification-of-diseases.

Appendix I: Table of Interventions: Listed Alphabetically by Title

Cheryl Lynne Trautman Boop

Appendix I summarizes many of the interventions mentioned in the 14th edition. For each intervention, the following information is included: the intervention name, the publisher and/or contact information if applicable, the ages for which it is intended, and the stated purpose.

Appendix II: Table of Assessments: Listed Alphabetically by Title

Cheryl Lynne Trautman Boop

Appendix II summarizes many of the assessments mentioned in the 14th edition. For each assessment, the following information is included: the assessment name and author, the publisher and/or contact information, the ages for which it is intended, the stated purpose, and the areas assessed.

Appendix III: First-Person Narratives

Following an introductory chapter on the importance of narratives (Chapter A), Appendix III includes nine first-person narratives of people with various occupational challenges (Chapters B–J).

- A: Narrative as a Key to Understanding, *Ellen S. Cohn, Elizabeth Blesedell Crepeau*
- B: Who's Driving the Bus? *Laura, Craig, and Will Horowitz*
- C: Homelessness and Resilience: Paul Cabell's Story, *Paul Carrington Cabell III, Sharon A. Gutman, Emily Raphael-Greenfield*
- D: While Focusing on Recovery, I Forgot to Get a Life, *Gloria F. Dickerson (updated for the 14th edition)*
- E: Mom's Come to Stay, *Jean Wilkins Westmacott*
- F: Journey to Ladakh, *Beth Long*
- G: Experiences With Disability: Stories From Ecuador, *Kate Barret*
- H: An Excerpt From *The Book of Sorrows, Book of Dreams, Mary Feldhaus-Weber, Sally A. Schreiber-Cohn*
- I: He's Not Broken—He's Alex, *Alexander, Laurie S., Lon McIntosh*
- J: The Privilege of Giving Care, *Donald M. Murray*

GLOSSARY

The following definitions are drawn from the chapters in this book and are intended as a resource for understanding. The Glossary also includes definitions from the American Occupational Therapy Association (AOTA) "Occupational Therapy Practice Framework, 4th Edition"; these definitions are indicated by the abbreviation OTPF-IV. Likewise, there are definitions from the World Health Organization (WHO); the WHO International Classification of Functioning, Disability and Health (ICF); and the Centers for Disease Control and Prevention (CDC). Readers should cite the original citations when referring to these constructs.

Ableism The oppression that disabled people experience.

Accessible design Also referred to as *barrier-free design*, adds accessibility to otherwise inaccessible buildings, products, and services to enable persons with disabilities to function independently.

Actigraphy The use of recordings of body motion to display activity patterns across many consecutive days and nights.

Active assistive range of motion (AAROM) Arc of motion through which the joint passes when moved by muscles acting on the joint in conjunction with external assistance.

Active range of motion (AROM) Arc of motion through which a client can move a joint (without assistance) using the adjacent muscles.

Activities of daily living (ADL) Activities that are oriented toward taking care of one's own body such as bathing/showering, bowel and bladder management, dressing, feeding, functional mobility, personal device care, personal hygiene and grooming, sexual activity, and toilet hygiene.

Activity "The execution of a task or action by an individual." (WHO)

Activity analysis An examination of an activity to distinguish its component parts with the goal of designing an evaluation or an intervention.

Activity limitations "Difficulties an individual may have in executing activities." (WHO)

Acute care Short-term medical treatment, usually in a hospital, for individuals having an acute illness or injury, recovering from surgery, or requiring medical stabilization due to safety concerns.

Adaptation A change in response approach generated when encountering a challenge. It also refers to therapeutic intervention in which task demands are changed to be consistent with the individual's ability level; may involve modification by reducing demands, use of assistive devices, or changes in the physical or social environment.

Adaptation gestalt Relative balance of sensorimotor, cognitive, and psychosocial functioning that the individual creates internally in order to carry out an adaptive response.

Adaptive capacity Apparent capability of the individual to perceive the need for change and draw from a repertoire of adaptive responses that will enable him or her to experience mastery over the environment.

Adaptive occupation Occupations such as cooking, exercise, and helping others used by forced migrants as coping strategies or a way of filling the abundance of unstructured time when living in refugee camps and asylum centers.

Adaptive repertoire An individual's ability to make adaptive transitions by applying past occupational experiences to new or evolving circumstances.

Adaptive response (adaptiveness) A successful environmental interaction in which the individual meets the demands of the task demand; requires adequate sensory integration.

Adenotonsillar hypertrophy Adenoid and tonsillar enlargement that may cause airway obstruction.

Administration The process of guiding an organization to meet its objectives by using the authoritative control of others.

Administrative supervision Aspect of supervision directed toward managing the day-to-day work performance and process; includes tasks such as scheduling, monitoring performance, and delegating.

Advanced practice (practitioner) Practice or practitioners who possess a higher level of expertise in professional practice.

Adverse childhood experiences (ACEs) Potentially traumatic events or circumstances that occur during a child's development (from birth through age 17), including events such as physical, emotional, or sexual abuse; witnessing violence; or the unexpected death of a family member.

Affective domain The domain of learning that includes attitudes, values, and interests of learners, which allows internalization of new ideas.

Ageism Stereotypic and often negative bias against older adults; a form of discrimination based on age.

Aging in place The ability to remain in one's current home while growing older. Also, designing dwelling units such that residents, if they so choose, can occupy their home from childhood to old age unless illness or impairment comes into play.

Agnosia Inability to recognize incoming sensory information in spite of intact sensory capacities.

Airborne infection isolation room (AIIR) Single-occupancy patient room for patients with an airborne infectious disease. Also referred to as a negative pressure room.

Americans with Disabilities Act (ADA) US federal law that prevents discrimination against persons with disabilities.

Anthropometry Field of science that studies and defines the physical measures of a person's size (e.g., overall height and weight, length of leg, elbow, height in sitting and standing, size of head) and functional capacities (e.g., range of motion, strength, and aerobic capacity).

Any mental illness (AMI) Term that encompasses all recognized mental illnesses.

Apnea A cessation of breathing.

Apnea/hypopnea index (AHI) An index of obstructive sleep apnea severity.

Apraxia Inability to perform motor activities, although sensory motor function is intact and the individual understands the requirements of the task.

Areas of occupation Various kinds of life activities in which people engage, organized into categories, such as self-care, productivity, and leisure, or the nine categories used by the AOTA.

Arena Describes the places in which activities occur, such as a library, school, or hospital.

Assessment Specific method, instrument, tool, or strategy that is used as part of the evaluation process.

Assistive technology(ies) Devices, adaptive equipment, or products that are designed to enable persons with disabilities to engage in daily occupations within their home, school, workplace, and communities.

Assumptions In science, refers to ideas that really cannot be definitively proven true or false, for example, the idea that people have an inherent drive for mastery of their environment.

Asylee A person granted asylum and therefore allowed to legally stay in a country other than their country of origin (also used interchangeably with "refugee," see definition later).

Asylum center A residential facility, also referred to as a transit/reception center, that offers temporary accommodation, food, and other basic services to asylum seekers and refugees.

Asylum seeker A person who claims refugee status, has applied for legal protection in another country, and whose application is yet to be processed (Migration Data Portal, 2022). Many countries have their own system in place to verify and review individuals' claims for asylum.

Asynchronous telehealth Electronically shared data (e.g., video, digital images, data from wearable devices/sensors, text messaging, e-mail, and other forms of communication) between the practitioner and client that does not include real-time interaction.

At-homeness The taken-for-granted situation of feeling completely comfortable and intimately familiar with the world in which one lives their everyday life.

Atonia Muscle paralysis.

Atopic dermatitis An inflammatory, chronically relapsing, noncontagious, and pruritic skin disorder.

Attention The cognitive ability to focus on a task, issue, or object.

Autism spectrum disorder (ASD) A spectrum of disorders characterized by a confluence of challenges in verbal and nonverbal communication and restricted and repetitive behaviors.

Autonomy The ability to act freely and independently on one's own decisions. It is often called the principle of self-determination.

Avoiding (sensory pattern) A sensory pattern characterized by low thresholds and an active self-regulation approach; avoiders want less input.

Axiology The theory of values; asks the question "what are right actions?"

Background question A type of question used to obtain general knowledge to understand the nature of a problem.

Behavioral theory Theory that focuses on how observable, tangible behaviors are learned in response to some environmental stimulation.

Beliefs Something that is accepted, considered to be true, or held as an opinion. (OTPF-IV)

Beneficence Actions done on or for the benefit of others.

Benign prostatic hypertrophy Benign enlargement of the prostate.

Biofeedback The process of becoming aware of various physiologic functions using instruments that provide information on the activity of those same systems, with a goal of being able to manipulate them at will.

Biomechanical approach Therapeutic intervention focused on improving body movement and strength; typically identified with remediation or improvements in strength, range of motion, or endurance.

Bipolar disorder A mental illness characterized by severe mood swings, episodes of depression, and at least one episode of mania.

Birth cohorts Groups of people who were born about the same time and for which the sum effects of the times and the people around them affect the trajectory of their lives.

Body functions Physiologic processes of the body. (ICF)

Body structures Anatomic parts of the body such as bones and organs. (ICF)

Broad theory Overarching model that helps to explain a large set of findings or observations.

Bruxism Grinding of the teeth (during sleep); typically includes clenching of the jaw.

Business Associate Agreement (BAA) An agreement required by the Health Insurance Portability and Accountability Act of 1996 (HIPAA) between a healthcare practitioner and a third-party vendor (e.g., video-conference platform providers, billing services, etc.) that requires the third-party vendor to adhere to the same confidentiality, privacy, and security requirements as the practitioner in order to protect clients' protected health information.

Cataplexy An abnormal sudden paralysis of some or all skeletal muscles brought on by strong emotions such as those that accompany laughter and anger.

Centers for independent living A nonresidential, private, nonprofit agency providing an array of independent living services that are consumer controlled, community based, cross disability, and designed and operated within a local community by individuals with disabilities. Core services include information and referral, independent living skills training, individual and systems advocacy, and peer counseling.

Certified Community Behavioral Health Clinics (CCBHCs) Clinics that are required to provide coordinated integrated care that is person centered and recovery oriented and to integrate physical and behavioral healthcare.

Chaining A stepwise process for teaching a multistep task.

Chaining strategy Integrating a new activity within an existing routine to increase the likelihood of it becoming a habit.

Classical test theory (CTT) Also called classical reliability theory; centers around the notion that each observation or test score has a single true score and yields a single reliability coefficient and that the observed or test score has two components: the true score and the measurement error score.

Clinical importance The practical application of research results; it considers whether the magnitude and scope of the results are sufficient to suggest that using the intervention will produce changes that will improve the outcomes for actual patients in the outcomes tested in the study.

Clinical reasoning Process used by practitioners to plan, direct, perform, and reflect on client care. See *Professional reasoning* for a term that is considered to be broader.

Cognition The mental processes involved in perceiving, understanding, organizing, assimilating, and processing information.

Cognitive behavioral therapy (CBT) A psychotherapeutic approach that combines cognitive and behavioral therapy techniques, aiming to solve problems concerning dysfunctional emotions, behaviors, and cognitions through a goal-oriented, systematic procedure.

Cognitive control The ability to actively guide performance of a task including choosing strategies, coordinating, and regulating responses.

Cognitive domain The domain of learning that includes recall or recognition of knowledge and the development of intellectual abilities and skills.

Cognitive functional capacity evaluation A clinical evaluation to determine an individual's cognitive capacity to perform work activities related to job demands.

Cognitive impairments Cognitive deficits such as memory loss, attention deficits, lack of awareness, and decreased executive function that affect an individual's ability to perform ADL, IADL, education, work, play, leisure, social participation, and role competence.

Cognitive interventions Interventions focused on information processing such as thinking, paying attention learning, remembering, and solving problems that improve engagement and participation in everyday activities.

Cognitive rehabilitation Therapy to increase a person's sense of competence, self-efficacy, and self-esteem, in adapting to the demands of everyday living and adopting to the new "self" postinjury.

Cognitive work hardening Uses graded work tasks to simulate a person's actual work tasks and/or the cognitive demands of the person's job to develop the cognitive skills required for job performance.

Collectivist societies Those that put more value on the family structure or community than the individual. Interdependence is valued, and decisions are made by the group or family who consider what is good for the entire group before focusing on the individual.

Communicable diseases An infectious disease acquired through transmission from an infected individual or contact with a contaminated surface.

Communities of practice Informal or formal groups of people that have a common interest and come together for the process of sharing knowledge.

Community development Strategies that aim to create supportive environments and strengthen the capacity of communities to respond to health problems. (WHO)

Community integration Attaining the personal, social, and vocational competency to successfully participate in the community.

Community participation Active participation of individuals who both benefit and contribute to the community through their actions, ideas, knowledge, or skills.

Community program Occupational therapy programs that address the needs of groups of people, where the *community* is the client.

Community(ies) Specific group of people, often living in a defined geographical area, who share a common culture, values, and norms, are arranged in a social structure according to relationships that the community has developed over a period of time. (WHO)

Compensation (in occupational therapy) Bypassing or minimizing the effects of impairment by teaching the person to use methods that capitalize on their strengths and reduce demands on areas of weakness.

Compensatory strategies Strategies provided by the therapist and taught directly or integrated within metacognitive strategy approaches that promote strategy generation and use guided learning methods.

Competence The result of combining one's knowledge base, current practice skills, and abilities along with client outcomes and comparing your competence with a specific criterion such as using evidence-based practice on a consistent basis.

Competency The observed performance of a specified skill or ability measured against an expected performance (criterion) or outcome.

Conditioning A behavior modification process that increases or decreases the likelihood of a behavior being performed.

Confusional arousals Parasomnia sleep disorder that causes the affected person to act in a nonresponsive and confused manner.

Constraint-induced movement therapy (CI or CI therapy) A form of rehabilitation therapy that constrains the less involved upper limb, engages the more affected limb in intense repetitive practice, and provides behavioral strategies for generalization. The goal is to improve everyday function in the more involved limb after central nervous system damage.

Construct validity Establishes whether the assessment measures a construct and the theoretical components underlying the construct. A construct is an abstract idea that cannot be observed directly.

Constructivist theory Theory that explains the process where people seek, find, and integrate information for themselves.

Consultant Person in a position to have some influence over an individual, a group, or an organization but has no direct power to make changes or implement a program.

Consultation A collaborative process completed with clients, families, other professionals, organizations, or communities to identify and solve problems with participation in occupations; describes any action one might take with a system expressing a need for assistance in moving forward or making changes.

Consumer-driven healthcare An economically driven approach involving lowering healthcare expenditures while simultaneously providing consumer control over health plans. A high-deductible health plan accompanied by a health savings account is an example of a consumer-driven healthcare approach.

Content validity The extent to which an empirical measurement reflects a specific domain of content.

Context Factors that transact with the performance of occupations including personal, physical, cultural, social, spiritual, temporal, and virtual environments.

Continuing competence An ongoing process of building capacity to perform a task, function, or role for the future.

Continuing professional development The process of engaging in lifelong learning aimed at maintaining practice competence, ensuring client safety and quality outcomes, enhancing or expanding professional practice, and reaching career goals.

Continuous positive airway pressure (CPAP) A treatment for obstructive sleep apnea in which a continuous stream of air under pressure is delivered through a mask worn over the nose, or nose and mouth, to keep the sleeper's airway open.

Continuum of care Term used to summarize the range of healthcare, educational, residential, employment, and social settings, which may be necessary to meet a client's needs over time.

Controlling (in management) Function that relates to the processes of establishing specific work performance standards and the measurement, evaluation, and correction of performance.

Convergent validity Level of agreement between two tests that are being used to measure the same construct.

Co-occupation An occupation that implicitly involves two or more individuals.

Coping Conscious, volitional efforts to regulate emotion, cognition, behavior, physiology, and the environment in response to stressful events or circumstances.

Credentialing Process of obtaining or demonstrating accepted forms of proof of professional knowledge and skills.

Criterion validity Implies that the outcome of one assessment can be used as a substitute test for the established gold standard criterion test. Criterion validity can be tested as concurrent validity or predictive validity.

Cryotherapy The use of therapeutic low temperatures such as ice packs to relieve symptoms.

Cultural dexterity Refers to skills that facilitate effective collaboration and communication among people across multiple dimensions of diversity.

Cultural humility Refers to an attitude and process in which OT providers try to address issues of power differences between professionals and service users and to value and respect service users by continuously engaging in self-reflection, lifelong learning, and reflective practice.

Cultural intelligence Using metacognition (having knowledge of your own attitudes, values, and skills, as well as those of your clients) to interact effectively with clients and ensure effective encounters.

Cultural responsiveness An approach that communicates a state of being open to the process of building mutuality with a client and to accepting that the cultural-specific knowledge one has about a group may or may not apply to the client they are currently treating.

Cultural safety The acknowledgment that healthcare providers have an unconscious assumption of power over marginalized groups and that clients experience trust and safety when treated with respect and are included in the decision-making process.

Culture The interconnection of significant meanings we use to understand the phenomena or events of everyday life.

Delayed sleep phase syndrome A daily sleep/wake rhythm in which the onset of sleep and the time of awakening are later than desired.

Descriptive research Types of research, such as qualitative studies and case series, whose purpose is to provide information about a population, for example, the prevalence of a disorder or specific characteristics of a disorder.

Diagnostic-related group (DRG) Classification system in the United States for Medicare Part A payments based on groups of diagnoses and procedures.

Dialectical behavioral therapy (DBT) Psychotherapy protocol based on cognitive behavioral principles with a focus on building a life worth living.

Direct action Methods such as protesting, chaining themselves to buses, and getting arrested to push for rights and services.

Directing (in management) Function that involves giving guidance, instruction, and leadership to subordinates so that work that is performed is goal oriented and contributes to meeting organizational or departmental requirements.

Disability Disability is an umbrella term, covering impairments, activity limitations, and participation restrictions. An impairment is a problem in body function or structure, an activity limitation is a difficulty encountered by an individual in executing a task or action, whereas a participation restriction is a problem experienced by an individual in involvement in life situations. Disability is thus not just a health problem. It is a complex phenomenon, reflecting the interaction between features of a person's body and features of the society in which they live. (WHO)

Discrimination Denial of equal treatment to people because of their membership in some group that occurs at many levels including individual, institutional or organizational, or structural.

Diversity Refers to the inclusion of a wide variety of human differences with some sort of organization or institution.

Downward occupational drift Situation experienced by forced migrants with professional background experience as the credentials earned in their home country are not recognized in their country of resettlement and asylum.

Durable medical equipment (DME) In the United States refers to hardware, tools, and devices used by individuals to manage disease or disability or that provides therapeutic benefits.

Early intervention (early intervening) services Multidisciplinary academic and support services provided to children in the United States who have developmental delays or special needs, generally from birth until the child turns 3, or 5, depending on individual state laws/regulations. State law also determines context for service delivery, provided either in a child's home or in an early intervention program facility.

Ecologic models Four models of practice that emphasize the importance of considering the environment in OT practice: the Ecology of Human Performance (EHP) model, the Person Environment Occupational Performance (PEOP) model, the Person Environment Occupation (PEO) model, and the Canadian Model of Occupational Performance (CMOP).

Effectiveness evidence Evidence obtained from effectiveness studies.

E-helper A client support person/caregiver who is present with the client during the telehealth session to facilitate the client's participation and safety.

Electroencephalogram (EEG) A recording of brain waves obtained by attaching flat metal disks (electrodes) to the scalp.

Electromyogram Technology that measures motor activity through electrodes placed on the skin over muscles.

Electronic health record Computerized medical record created in an organization that delivers care.

Electrooculogram Technology that measures eye movements through electrodes placed on the skin around the eyes.

Embodied process Used to reflect a view that the mind and body are not separate but rather one entity. As a facet of professional reasoning in relation to occupational therapy, refers to the wholistic nature of therapeutic actions as experienced by the therapist and the client.

Emotion An evaluative mental state that occurs in the present moment and consists of neurobiological arousal, perceptual-cognitive processes, subjective experience, and affective expression.

Emotion dysregulation Actions or behaviors related to emotional experience that interfere with goal-directed pursuits, interpersonal relationships, or healthy adaptation.

Emotional regulation skills Actions or behaviors a client uses to identify, manage, and express feelings while engaging in activities or interacting with others.

Empathy Awareness of and insight into the feelings, emotions, and behavior of another person and their meaning and significance; not the same as sympathy, which is usually nonobjective and noncritical.

Entry-level competence Denotes successful completion of academic program requirements, classroom, and fieldwork, resulting in eligibility to apply for professional credentials required for employment.

Environment(s) Particular physical, social, cultural, economic, and political features within a person's everyday life that affect the motivation, organization, and performance.

Environmental embodiment The various ways, both sensorially and movement wise, that the lived body engages and coordinates with the world at hand, especially its environmental aspects.

Environmental modifications Internal and external physical adaptations to environments that are necessary to maximize independence and to ensure health and safety.

Environmental supports Supports to help organize a person's environment, including signs, reminders, and checklists. Social supports such as home aides, formal or informal caretakers, and societal attitudes are also included.

Epistemology The theory of knowledge; asks the question "what is knowledge?"

Epworth Sleepiness Scale A self-report scale intended to measure daytime sleepiness.

Equality Concept of the recognition of others as equals; that everyone is entitled to the same rights, resources, and opportunities as any other human being.

Equity Concept that recognizes that individuals and groups of people have different circumstances and needs.

Ergonomics The scientific discipline concerned with the understanding of interactions among humans and other elements of a system, and the profession that applies theory, principles, data, and methods to design in order to optimize human well-being and overall system performance.

Essential functions Component of the US ADA law that describes the basic job duties that all employees must be able to perform with or without reasonable accommodation.

Ethical dilemma Problem for which there are competing possible responses and that requires a morally defensible course of action.

Ethics Branch of philosophy that involves systemic study and reflection providing language, methods, and guidelines to study and reflect on morality.

Ethnicity A social grouping of people who share cultural or national similarities. The most common characteristics of an ethnic group include kinship, family rituals, food preferences, special clothing, and particular celebrations.

Ethnocentrism Tendency of people to put their own group (*ethnos*) at the center; to see things through the narrow lens of their own culture and use the standards of that culture to judge others.

Evaluation The evaluation process is focused on finding out what the client wants and needs to do; determining what the client can do and has done; and identifying supports and barriers to health, well-being, and participation. Evaluation occurs during the initial and all subsequent interactions with a client. The type and focus of the evaluation differ depending on the practice setting; however, all evaluations should assess the complex and multifaceted needs of each client. (OTPF-IV)

Evidence Knowledge gained through systematic appraisal of experience and of scientific studies.

Evidence-based practice (EBP) Healthcare practice that is composed of three equal core components: (1) the current best evidence, (2) the treatment environment, and (3) each client's values and circumstances.

E-visit Defined by the Center for Medicare and Medicaid Services as non–face-to-face patient-initiated communications through an online patient portal.

Executive functions The mental processes that enable us to plan, focus attention, remember instructions, and juggle multiple tasks successfully; composed of a set of interrelated core skills including working memory, inhibition and flexibility, and initiation. These skills are involved in every activity a person does across their lifespan.

Exploratory research Research such as cross-sectional studies and cohort studies that examines a specific phenomenon and its relationship to other factors.

External validity Refers to whether generalizations should be made to the general population.

Extinction (in behavioral theory) The process of reducing the frequency of a behavior by withholding reinforcement.

Face validity Indicates that a measure's items are viewed as plausible.

Factor analysis Statistical process used to identify one or more underlying dimensions of a construct.

Fading Systematic reduction of support (scaffold) to clients so that task demands increase; used when clients improve their skills.

Family Groups of people who identify as family; who share emotional, biologic, or cultural ties; and who participate in shared family occupations.

Family occupation Every meaningful activity and shared experience of family members during daily activities and special events that occur over time with input from family members who may participate in different ways.

Family routines Observable and repetitive patterns involving family members that occur with predictable regularity in family life.

Family-related occupations Refers to occupations that are central to an individual's role within their family, whereas family occupation relates to common occupation shared within the family group.

Fidelity Being faithful to one's promises or commitments; implementing interventions in a way that conforms to the basic principles of the treatment approach.

Fieldwork (practice placements) Structured learning experiences that are formally administered by academic programs in partnership with facilities that offer supervised training experiences.

Fieldwork educator Person responsible for providing student supervision; interchangeable terms include clinical educator, fieldwork supervisor, student supervisor, or practice educator.

Food desert A geographic area where inhabitants "lack access to affordable fruits, vegetables, whole grains, low-fat milk, and other foods that make up the full range of a healthy diet."

Forced displacement/forced migration When people are dislocated from their homes and communities due to persecution, conflict, generalized violence, or human rights violations.

Foreground questions A type of question used to obtain current knowledge related to best practice treatment of specific clients.

Form (of an occupation) In occupational science, the knowledge people share about how something is usually done.

Formative process Evaluation or feedback designed to support continued learning and development.

Framing (of play/leisure) Cues that separate play or leisure from "real life"; generally, the cues tell others how a player or leisure participant wishes to be viewed by others.

Free appropriate public education (FAPE) In the United States, special education and related services provided at public expense that meet the standards of the state education agency (SEA).

Function (of an occupation) In occupational science, refers to the purpose or effect of an occupation.

Functional capacity evaluation A clinical evaluation to determine an individual's capacity to perform work activities related to their participation in employment.

Functional cognition The integration of cognitive skills with motor skills and/or the demands of the activity and environment during the performance of everyday activities.

Functional supervision Supervision over a specific aspect of work or job function.

Generalizability (in research) The applicability of a study result to the population.

Generalizability theory A measurement theory that recognizes multiple different sources of error and attempts to quantify the sources from those various errors.

Global North/South Terms used by development organizations and development scholars to categorize high-income countries in one group, the Global North, and low- and lower middle-income countries in a second group, the Global South. These categories are sometimes criticized for not being geographically consistent and for obscuring differences between countries within the same category.

Grading Systematically increasing the demands of an activity or occupation to stimulate improved function or reducing the demands to respond to client difficulties in performance.

Group An aggregate of people who share a common purpose that can only be achieved through collaboration.

Group home Small, residential facility located within a community, designed to serve children or adults with chronic disabilities. These homes usually have six or fewer occupants and are staffed 24 hours a day by trained caregivers.

Group process The interrelationships and interactions among members, leaders, and within the group as a whole.

Habits Specific, automatic behaviors that are performed repeatedly, relatively automatically, and with little variation.

Habituation The process whereby people organize their actions into patterns and routines.

Habitus A person's overarching character and disposition.

Health "The complete state of physical, mental, and social well-being and not just the absence of disease or infirmity." (WHO)

Health disparity A particular type of health difference that is closely linked with social, economic, and/or environmental disadvantage. Health disparities adversely affect groups of people who have systematically experienced greater obstacles to health based on their racial or ethnic group; religion; SES; gender; age; mental health; cognitive, sensory, or physical disability; sexual orientation or gender identity; geographic location; or other characteristics historically linked to discrimination or exclusion.

Health literacy The degree to which individuals have the capacity to obtain, process, and understand basic health information and services needed to make appropriate health decisions.

Health management "Activities related to developing, managing, and maintaining health and wellness routines, including self-management, with the goal of improving or maintaining health to support participation in other occupations." (OTPF-IV)

Health promotion The process of enabling people to increase control over, and to improve, their health. To reach a state of complete physical, mental, and social well-being, an individual or group must be able to identify and to realize aspirations, to satisfy needs, and to change or cope with the environment. (WHO)

Health savings account (HSA) In the United States, savings account used for medical bills that is not subject to income tax.

Healthcare interpreter Trained interpreters who facilitate communication between the client and the healthcare professional when their primary languages differ.

Healthcare translators People who adapt health education materials into clients' primary languages.

Healthcare-associated infections (HAIs) Infections acquired during a stay at a healthcare facility that was not present at the time of admission. Sometimes called healthcare-acquired infections or nosocomial infections.

High-deductible health plan (HDHP) In the United States, a health insurance plan with lower premiums and higher deductibles than a traditional health plan.

Home healthcare Provision of health-related services to patients in a home setting rather than in a medical facility.

Homeostatic sleep drive The drive to sleep that accumulates during prolonged wakefulness and lessens during sleep. Sleep homeostasis is one of the primary modulators of sleep in humans.

Hospice Palliative care designed to provide medical, emotional, social, and spiritual support to individuals in the final phase of a terminal illness, focusing on comfort and quality of life rather than curative interventions. Aggressive methods of pain control may be used. It is generally provided as home care but can be delivered in freestanding facilities, nursing homes, or within hospitals.

Hybrid telehealth Primarily refers to a combination of in-person and telehealth services; however, it may also refer to a combination of both synchronous and asynchronous telehealth.

Hyperalgesia An increased sensitivity to pain.

Hypnagogic hallucinations Vivid, sometimes frightening images in transition to sleep.

Hypnogram A graph that summarizes the pattern of sleep stages across a night, for instance, as recorded in the sleep laboratory.

Hypothesis testing Statistical process used to determine the likelihood that assumptions (hypotheses) are true or supported by data.

Impact factor A measure of the number of citations of publications from a particular journal.

Impairment A problem with part of a person's anatomy or their physiologic or psychological functioning due to a significant deviation from normal or loss. (ICF)

Implementation (of evidence-based research) An iterative process that addresses a specific setting with the aim to promote the uptake of research and other evidence into practice.

Inclusion State of being able to participate in life activities—often used in relation to removing social and physical obstacles to participation.

Individualistic societies Societies that value self-expression, personal choice, autonomy, individual responsibility, and independence.

Individualized Education Programs (IEPs) In the United States, written plan for the delivery of educationally related services to children ages 3 to 21 years with disabilities, as mandated by the IDEA law.

Individualized Family Service Plans (IFSPs) In the United States, written plan for the delivery of services to children with disabilities ages birth through 2 years; prepares children with disabilities to enter the educational system at age 3 years.

Individuals with Disabilities Education Act (IDEA) US federal law that mandates that educational services must be provided to a child with a disability from birth to age 21 years.

Infection control Procedures that limit exposure to bacteria, viruses, and other transmissible infectious microorganisms and prevent infection spread within healthcare settings.

Inferential statistics Statistics that are used to infer the degree to which a study result from a sample can confidently be applied to the population.

Inpatient rehabilitation Intensive interdisciplinary services (at least 3 hours a day, 5 to 7 days a week of at least two different types of therapy) performed on a discrete, licensed unit either within a hospital or in a free-standing hospital. Specific admission criteria must be met in order for individuals to be eligible for inpatient rehabilitation in the United States.

Insomnia Trouble falling asleep, staying asleep, or waking up too early.

Institutional review board (IRB) A panel of diverse individuals, including organization staff and at least one community member, who are responsible for reviewing all research proposals and grants to ensure that adequate protections for research participants are in place.

Instrumental activities of daily living (IADL) Activities to support daily life within the home and community that often require more complex interactions than self-care used in ADL. IADL include 11 activity categories: care of others, care of pets, child rearing, communication management, community mobility, financial management, home establishment and management, meal preparation and cleanup, religious observance, safety and emergency maintenance, and shopping.

Intentional relationship model A person- and practitioner-centered and an evidence-based conceptual model of practice that is applied across OT with all people in diverse settings and fields. This model has been developed for OT practitioners and students to discover, validate, and improve their natural interpersonal skills and styles they use (or will use) in practice.

Interdisciplinary team Individuals representing different professional disciplines that work together to identify goals and plan intervention collaboratively.

Internal validity Refers to whether or not the assessment measures what it is supposed to measure, that is, a specific trait, behavior, construct, or performance. Also the degree to which the results of a study are accurate and not accounted for by confounding variables.

International Code of Sleep Disorders (ICSD-2) Published by the American Academy of Sleep Medicine. This system classifies sleep disorders into eight major categories.

Interpersonal characteristics Facets of an individual that play a fundamental role in the therapeutic relationship; they include enduring characteristics (that come from an individual's personality and reflect their natural style) and situational characteristics (that are emotional and behavioral reactions to immediate events).

Interpersonal event A naturally occurring communication, reaction, process, task, or general circumstance that occurs during therapy and that has the potential to fortify or weaken the therapeutic relationship, depending on how it is handled.

Interpersonal reasoning A six-step process in which practitioners intentionally evaluate and make decisions of the best ways to relate with people under different circumstances, taking into consideration their historic narrative, interpersonal characteristics, occupational needs, and contextual realities.

Interrater reliability With a statistical approach, it is used to detect differences in scoring between two or more raters who measure the same clients on the same attributes.

Intersectionality Idea that originated in Black feminism explaining that all systems of oppression (e.g., ableism, racism, sexism, heterosexism, cissexism, classism) are intertwined.

Intervention The intervention process consists of services provided by occupational therapy practitioners in collaboration with clients to facilitate engagement in occupation related to health, well-being, and achievement of established goals consistent with the various service delivery models. Practitioners use the information about clients gathered during the evaluation and theoretical principles to select and provide occupation-based interventions to assist clients in achieving physical, mental, and social well-being; identifying and realizing aspirations; satisfying needs; and changing or coping with contextual factors. (OTPF-IV)

Interviewing A vital skill of occupation-based practice for gathering information from a client about their occupational history and concerns.

Intrarater reliability A statistical approach used to detect differences in scoring obtained by the same rater when measuring the same client on the same attributes.

Intrinsic motivation The desire to engage in an activity for its own sake.

Job accommodations Accommodations made to a workplace to address physical, social, and attitudinal factors to enable individuals with occupational performance challenges to enter or return to work and successfully perform their jobs. Also called *workplace accommodations*.

Job analysis A form of activity analysis that is specific to work tasks and includes the process of gathering and analyzing data related to job task requirements or demands, the environment, and human capacities needed to complete job functions.

Justice Fair and equal treatment; it deals with the proper distribution of benefits, burdens, and resources.

Kawa model Model of OT practice comprising four basic constructs that interact to form a river—Water, River walls, Rocks, Driftwood—plus Spaces and Ambient Environment.

Knowledge translation The synthesis, exchange, and application of knowledge by relevant stakeholders to accelerate the benefits of global and local innovation in strengthening health systems and improving people's health. (WHO)

Leadership The process of creating structural change where the values, vision, and ethics of individuals are integrated into the culture of a community as a means of achieving sustainable change.

Learned nonuse A learning phenomenon whereby movement is suppressed initially due to adverse reactions and failure of any activity attempted with the affected limb, which then results in the suppression of behavior.

Least restrictive environment (LRE) In the United States, environment in school that provides maximum interaction with nondisabled peers and is consistent with the needs of the child/student.

Leisure A transaction in which one becomes totally engaged and that is characterized by relative internal control, a high level of motivation, and disengagement from unnecessary constraints of reality; it is often framed in such a way as to clearly indicate it as leisure.

Letter of intent (LOI) In consulting refers to a summary of the work that can be done and that the consultant recommends.

Level I fieldwork In the United States, experiences designed to enrich didactic course work through directed observation and participation in selected aspects of the occupational therapy process.

Level II fieldwork In the United States, an in-depth experience in delivering OT services to clients, focusing on the application of purposeful and meaningful occupation, as integral to the academic program's curriculum design.

Life balance A satisfying pattern of daily activity that is healthful, meaningful, and sustainable to an individual within the context of his or her current life circumstances.

Life course A term (and a field of study) used to describe the patterns of people's lives in context. It considers the determinants and consequences of social relationships, historic events, and government policy for how people live their lives.

Life imbalance A state in which one's activity configurations limit or compromise participation in valued relationships; are incongruent for establishing or maintaining physiologic health and a satisfactory identity; or are mundane, uninteresting, or unchallenging.

Lifeworld The tacit, taken-for-granted context, tenor, and pace of daily life to which people normally give no reflective attention; a major focus of phenomenological investigation.

Lived body A phenomenological concept referring to the ways in which our existence as bodily beings contributes to the constitution of human experience and to the human lifeworld; the phenomenologist argues that the lived body is the primary means of being in, experiencing, and encountering the world.

Local independence An indication of whether the items of an assessment independently contribute to the measurement of a particular trait. That is, some items are redundant or not adding anything new to the measuring of a particular trait.

Lures Use of play, leisure, or other incentives as motivation to participate in therapeutic activities or as rewards for participation in them.

Maladaptive occupations Occupations such as engaging in exploitative occupations including illicit jobs in the informal economy or sex work used by force migrants for survival.

Managed care In the United States, comprehensive healthcare system that provides a variety of health services and facilities with a focus on controlling costs.

Management The process of guiding a work unit by planning for future work obligations, organizing employees into functional units, directing employees in the process of completing daily work tasks, and controlling work processes and systems to ensure adequate quality of work output.

Meaning (of an occupation) In occupational science, the significance of an occupation at a personal level as well as how it is viewed by different groups in society.

Measurement Process of assigning numbers to represent quantities of a trait, attribute, or characteristic or to classify objects.

Mechanisms of action An understanding of how specific intervention strategies lead to particular outcomes including how change proceeds and the particular

conditions under which an intervention achieves the desired results; also called *mechanism of change*.

Medicaid A governmental insurance program in the United States for people with low incomes who meet eligibility requirements.

Medical tourism The process of traveling outside of one's country of residence to receive medical care.

Medicare A US national social insurance program that guarantees access to health insurance for Americans ages 65 years and older and younger people with disabilities as well as people with end-stage renal disease.

Melatonin A hormone secreted by the pineal gland in the brain. It helps regulate other hormones and maintains the body's circadian rhythm.

Memorandum of understanding (MOU) Memorandum summarizing agreements between parties; see also Letter of intent.

Memory Ability to register, retain, and recall past experience, knowledge, and sensation.

Mental health Individuals having the sense that they are able to cope with the normal stresses of life, work, or complete school tasks productively, and participate socially in school, home, work, or community contexts. (WHO)

Mental illness Mental, behavioral, or emotional disorder (excluding developmental and substance use disorders).

Mentoring An at-will relationship between the mentor and mentee that is reciprocal and collaborative in nature to support reaching mentee identified goals.

Meta-analysis A form of systematic review that includes statistical techniques to combine the results of multiple studies into a single effect size.

Metacognition Knowledge or awareness of one's thinking and strengths or weaknesses as well as control or moment-to-moment self-monitoring including ability to recognize potential obstacles, adjust and use strategies effectively, and self-assess performance in comparison to goals or outcomes.

Metacognitive strategy approaches A broad group of interventions that use structured metacognitive processes within the context of occupational performance and focus on cognitive strategies rather than discrete cognitive skills.

Methodology A general approach to practice.

Methods The actual processes and procedures used when working within a given methodology.

Micro-perspective Analyzing activities in terms of how the presence, absence, or impairment of body functions support or limit engagement.

Minimal clinically important difference (MCID) The smallest change in an outcome that will lead to some perceived clinically beneficial improvement.

Mission The core purpose of an organization, often includes why an organization exists, who the organization serves, and how an organization goes about achieving its purpose.

Mission statement A written summary of the core purpose of an organization, often includes why an organization exists, who the organization serves, and how an organization goes about achieving its purpose.

Mode shift A conscious change in the practitioner's mode of relating to a client depending on the person's needs.

Model of Human Occupation (MOHO) Broad model for the practice of occupational therapy that is occupation-focused, theory-driven, and evidence-based; the theory guides thinking about clients and the therapy process.

Modes Six therapeutic modes that describe the specific ways of relating to clients: advocating, collaborating, empathizing, encouraging, instructing, and problem solving.

Moral distress A problem that occurs when practitioners know the right thing to do but cannot achieve it because of external barriers or uncertainty about the outcome.

Moral reasoning The process of reflecting on ethical issues; includes reasoning about norms and values, ideas of right and wrong, and how practitioners make decisions in professional work.

Morality Social conventions about right and wrong human conduct and sets the stage for ethical behavior.

Motor control The ability to regulate or direct the mechanisms essential to movement.

Motor development A process during which a person acquires skills and movement patterns.

Motor learning A set of processes associated with practice or experience leading to relatively permanent changes in the capability for skilled movement.

Motor planning Ability to carry out a skilled, nonhabitual motor activity; process that bridges ideation and motor execution to enable an adaptive response.

Multidisciplinary team A group of individuals from different professional disciplines that serve the client; each individual is responsible for identifying and carrying out one's own discipline-related assessment, intervention plan and implementation, and communicating with each other.

Multidrug-resistant organism (MDRO) Bacteria resistant to being controlled with or killed by antibiotics.

Multilingual learner (MLL) People who are developing proficiency in multiple languages.

Narcolepsy A rare sleep disorder marked by excessive sleepiness or sudden sleep attacks.

National Board for Certification in Occupational Therapy (NBCOT) The credentialing body for occupational therapists and occupational therapy assistants practicing in the United States; organization that develops and administers the initial certification examinations for occupational therapists and occupational therapy assistants.

Naturally occurring retirement community (NORC) Buildings or neighborhoods populated almost exclusively by individuals older than age 65 because young people have moved out. NORCs support positive aging.

Negative predictive value A statistic indicating the likelihood that people with a negative test result would not have a condition.

Neurodiversity Term coined by Judy Singer to reflect an idea that autism and other neurodivergent ways of being should be considered forms of diversity, rather than pathologies that require elimination.

New poor People who have fallen into poverty because of sudden or unexpected circumstances such as serious illness, divorce, or sudden job layoffs related to changes in the structure of the economy, including technology, which continues to replace human workers.

Night terrors Episodes of fear, flailing, and screaming while asleep; also known as sleep terrors, night terrors often are paired with sleepwalking.

Nocturia The need to get up in the night to urinate, thus interrupting sleep.

Nonrapid eye movement sleep (NREM) The stages of sleep that do not include rapid eye movement patterns. According to current guidelines for sleep stage classification, NREM consists of three different stages: N1, N2, and N3.

Nonstandardized assessments Assessments that do not follow a standard approach or protocol. For instance, they may not involve a consistent set of questions, directions, or conditions for administration, testing, or scoring.

Objective Not influenced by personal feelings, interpretations, or prejudice; based on facts; unbiased.

Obstructive sleep apnea (OSA) Apnea caused by partial or complete blockage of airway passages during sleep.

Occupation Everyday personalized activities that people do as individuals, in families, and with communities to occupy time and bring meaning and purpose to life. Occupations can involve the execution of multiple activities for completion and can result in various outcomes. Occupations include things people need to, want to, and are expected to do, such as activities of daily living, instrumental activities of daily living, health management, rest and sleep, education, work, play, leisure, and social participation.

Occupation as end Occupations that constitute the end product of therapy, that is, the occupations to be learned or relearned.

Occupation as means Occupations that act as the therapeutic change agent to remediate impaired abilities or capacities.

Occupational adaptation Normative internal process that is activated by the individual when approaching and adapting to challenges in life; constructing a positive occupational identity and achieving occupational competence over time in the context of one's environment.

Occupational alienation Experienced by people such as forced migrants who are engaged in occupations that are far removed from personal motivation, skills, aptitude, and meaning.

Occupational analysis A broad, overarching analysis of occupation that includes, but is not limited to, gathering information from the person about their occupational history and concerns (e.g., via interview) as well as implementing (a) observation-based performance analyses, (b) observation-based task analyses, and (c) decontextualized activity analyses.

Occupational apartheid Separation between those who have meaningful, useful occupations and those who are deprived of, isolated from, or otherwise constrained in their daily life occupations.

Occupational balance The perception that one's patterns of everyday occupations are satisfactory and include a range of meaningful occupations.

Occupational competence The degree to which one is able to sustain a pattern of occupational participation that reflects one's occupational identity.

Occupational consciousness An ongoing awareness about the dynamics of hegemony, recognizing that dominant practices are sustained through what people do every day, with implications for both personal and collective health.

Occupational deprivation Lack of access to engagement in an array of occupations that have meaning to the individual, family, or community, which can result in ill health.

Occupational disruption When the ability of forced migrants to participate in meaningful occupations of choice is precluded by factors outside their control.

Occupational dysadaptation Performance problems arising from a mismatch between environmental demands and the person's motivation or capacity for response.

Occupational engagement A person's doing, thinking, and feeling under certain environmental conditions in the midst of or as a planned consequence of therapy.

Occupational environment One of the three primary elements in the theory of occupational adaptation. In contrast with other environments, the occupational environment calls for an occupational response from the individual in the context of work, play/leisure, or self-maintenance. The contexts are shaped by unique physical, social, and cultural influences.

Occupational experience Individuals' verbal or nonverbal report of what they experience during occupational performance—their perspective on their doing.

Occupational expressions The unique ways a person performs an occupation at a given moment including the form (i.e., step-by-step process) and style (e.g., cadence, intensity, rhythm, flair, bodily comportment, etc.) of that occupation.

Occupational form The preexisting structure that elicits, guides, or structures performance of daily life activities.

Occupational identity Composite sense of who one is and wishes to become as an occupational being generated from one's history of occupational participation.

Occupational imbalance Situation that occurs when forced migrants are faced with precarious living conditions, resource constraints, and institutional restrictions, and survival occupations such as gathering food and fuel and caring for dependents take precedence over occupations undertaken for self-enhancement and personal fulfillment.

Occupational justice The perspective that holds that people have the right to express their occupations to experience dignity, inclusion, health, and well-being in a context of associated living where their occupational expressions do not oppress the occupational expressions of others.

Occupational knowledge The experiential, observational, and investigatory information acquired by occupational therapy practitioners to understand the form, function, and meaning of engaging in occupations for individuals and society.

Occupational orchestration The capacity of individuals to enact their occupations on a daily basis to meet their own needs and the expectations of the many environments in which they are required to function. This may include attention to habits and routines and the interface of these with the needs and expectations of others.

Occupational participation Engagement in work, play, or activities of daily living that are part of one's sociocultural context and that are desired and/or necessary to one's well-being.

Occupational patterns Habits, routines, roles, and rituals used in the process of engaging in occupations or activities.

Occupational performance Human actions in response to an occupational form. The observable aspects of a person's doing—engaging in activities and performing daily life tasks and enacting occupational performance skills.

Occupational profile The occupational profile is a summary of a client's (person's, group's, or population's) occupational history and experiences, patterns of daily living, interests, values, needs, and relevant contexts. Developing the occupational profile provides the occupational therapy practitioner with an understanding of the client's perspective and background. (OTPF-IV)

Occupational readiness A term that characterizes interventions that are designed to affect the individual's sensorimotor, cognitive, and/or psychosocial deficits.

Occupational risk factors Occupational experiences that lead to ill health and diminishing well-being; examples include stress, occupational imbalance, alienation, and deprivation.

Occupational roles Normative models for behavior shaped by culture and society (e.g., student, friend, worker, and parent). The personally experienced situation of the individual.

Occupational science The study of the things people do; interdisciplinary academic discipline in the social and behavioral sciences dedicated to the study of the form, the function, and the meaning of human occupations.

Occupational skill acquisition Increased proficiency in performance and skill related to a meaningful occupation.

Occupational therapy–directed health promotion The client-centered use of occupations, adaptations to context, or alteration of context to maximize individuals', groups', families', communities', and populations' pursuit of health and quality of life.

Occupational transition Major change in the occupational repertoire of a person in which one or several occupations change, disappear, and/or are replaced by others.

Occupational wholeness (OW) Emerging model of OT practice developed to explain what people experience as life balance and/or occupational balance from their own perspective. It refers to a sense of wholeness through doing.

Ontology An element of philosophy that is concerned with the question "what is most real?"

Organizational health literacy The degree to which organizations equitably enable individuals to find, understand, and use information and services to inform health-related decisions and actions for themselves and others. (CDC)

Organizing (in management) Refers to the overall structure of the organization, including how the line of authority will be organized and how employees may be grouped into departments and relative expectations of employees and groups.

Orientation Awareness of self in relation to time, place, and identification of others.

Orthosis (splint) An orthopedic appliance or apparatus used to support, align, prevent, or correct deformities or to improve function of movable parts of the body.

Outcome(s) Measurable result(s) or consequence(s) of an intervention or other factors.

Outpatient rehabilitation Rehabilitation performed in an outpatient facility that is attached to an acute care hospital, rehabilitation hospital, or freestanding facility.

Oxygen saturation A measure of how much oxygen the blood is carrying.

***p* value** The probability that a study effect, or a larger effect, would be found if in actuality there were no true effect or the effect was due to chance.

Palliative approach (palliation) Providing clients with relief from the symptoms, pain, and stress of a serious illness regardless of the diagnosis with a goal of improving quality of life for both the clients and their family.

Parasomnias Nonsleep behaviors that intrude during sleep, such as sleepwalking and sleep eating.

Partial hospital, partial hospitalization programs (PHPs) In the United States, programs that are intended to divert the person from hospitalization or serve as an intermediary step toward community living after an acute inpatient course of treatment. Also, an outpatient program specifically designed for the diagnosis or active treatment of a serious mental disorder when there is a reasonable expectation for improvement or when it is necessary to maintain an individual's functional level and prevent relapse or full hospitalization.

Participation "Involvement in a life situation." (WHO)

Participation restriction "Problems an individual may experience in involvement in life situations." (WHO)

Passive range of motion (PROM) Arc of motion through which the joint passes when moved by an outside force.

Pedagogy The method and practice of teaching.

Peer review When work is reviewed by experts in the field who provide feedback and contribute to the decision of whether or not the work meets specified criteria for dissemination.

Performance analysis The evaluation of the quality or effectiveness of the motor, process, and/or social interaction skills based on the observation of a person as he or she is engaged in the performance of a desired or needed daily life task and with the goal of evaluating the person's quality of occupational performance.

Performance capacity Ability to do things provided by the status of underlying objective, physical and mental components, and corresponding subjective experience.

Performance skills A component of occupational performance—small observable goal-directed links in a chain of ongoing actions that people perform one by one as they "construct" overall daily life task performances.

Periodic limb movement disorder (PLMD) A sleep disorder characterized by leg movements or jerks that typically occur every 20 to 40 seconds during sleep, causing sleep to be disrupted and leaving the person with excessive daytime sleepiness.

Personal causation A person's thoughts and feelings about their abilities and effectiveness as they engage in everyday occupations.

Personal factors Broad term used to encompass several aspects of the human condition such as body structures and body functions.

Personal health literacy The degree to which individuals have the ability to find, understand, and use information and services to inform health-related decisions and actions for themselves and others. (CDC)

Personal protective equipment (PPE) Equipment that provides a barrier against transmission of infectious organisms. May include wearing a gown, gloves, face mask, face shield, or goggles.

Personally Identifiable Information (PII) A term defined by the Family Educational Rights and Privacy Act (FERPA) related to protected information in educational records including students' names, addresses, social security numbers, and other identifiable information.

Phenomenology (phenomenological) A philosophical tradition that focuses on describing and interpreting human experience. It is also used to indicate experience of occupation.

Physical environment Natural and built nonhuman surroundings and the objects in them. The natural environment includes geographic terrain, plants, and animals as well as the sensory qualities of the natural surroundings. The built environment includes buildings, furniture, tools, and devices. (OTPF-IV)

Physiologic Pertaining to the functioning of an organ as governed by the interactions between its physical and chemical conditions.

Place Any environmental locus that gathers individual or group meanings, intentions, and actions spatially; a fusion of human and natural order and any significant spatial center of a person or group's lived experience.

Plain language Using words and terms an audience perceives as familiar, understands the first time, and feels comfortable with.

Planning (in management) The process of establishing short- and long-term goals, measurable objectives, and action plans that are both congruent with the mission of the organization and consistent with the vision that current organizational leaders have established.

Play A transaction characterized by relative intrinsic motivation, relative internal control, and suspension of reality and that is framed in such a way as to separate it from "real life."

Polysomnography (PSG) The recording of a person's sleep using several physiologic signals such as the brain waves (electroencephalography), eye movements (electrooculography), and muscle activity (electromyography) as well as breathing, the amount of oxygen in the bloodstream, heart rate, etc.; used to evaluate patients in a sleep laboratory for potential sleep disorders.

Population health Health outcomes of a group of individuals, including the distribution of such outcomes within the group; an approach to health that aims to improve the health of an entire human population.

Populations Groups of people within a community who share common characteristics, for example, refugees in a new country, veterans, and people with chronic mental and/or physical disabilities.

Positive aging Maintaining positive quality of life as normal age-related physical and cognitive changes occur.

Positive predictive value Indicates the likelihood that a person with a positive test result would actually have the condition for which the test is used.

Postdoctoral research Research position (postdoc) that provides the individual with additional research experience and training in preparation for a career in academia/research. Postdocs work under a research mentor and contribute to the research mentor's body of work as well as developing their own research focus.

Postural control Controlling or regulating the body's position in space to maintain stability and orientation.

Practice guidelines Documents developed by organizations that synthesize and interpret the research and the expertise of clinicians to serve as a basis for making clinical recommendations for specific populations.

Precision The accuracy or confidence in the results of a measure or assessment.

Prejudice Preconceived ideas and attitudes—usually negative about a particular group of people, often without full examination of the facts.

Preparatory interventions Interventions to support occupations such as physical agent modalities, orthoses, and self-regulation. (OTPF-IV)

Prevention Measures not only taken to prevent disease but also to arrest its progress and reduce its consequences once established. This also refers to injury prevention and prevention of secondary impairments.

Primary healthcare (PCH) A philosophy and approach to healthcare provision, grounded in the notion that health is not merely the absence of disease but rather a state of physical, mental, and social well-being.

Prion Type of protein that triggers healthy proteins in the brain to fold abnormally (e.g., Creutzfeldt–Jakob disease). Prions possess no genetic material and cannot reproduce.

Process skills Refers to how effectively a person organizes objects, time, and space, including sustaining performance, applying knowledge, organizing timing, organizing space and objects, and adapting performance.

Professional practice supervision Supervision of others in the same profession undertaken with an understanding of the profession's values, standards, and ethics aimed at providing support, training, and evaluation of the supervisee's professional performance.

Professional reasoning A complex and dynamic process that is connected directly to therapy action that practitioners use to develop and provide occupational therapy services with individuals, groups, or populations.

Professionalism Concepts that encompass how one presents oneself as a professional and the individual's responsibilities and obligations as a professional and to one's profession.

Propositions Formal statements about causes and effects or the nature of relationships among features of the world.

Prospective payment system (PPS) A method of reimbursement commonly associated in the United States with Medicare. Payment is made based on a predetermined, fixed amount; derived from the classification system of that service (e.g., diagnosis-related groups for inpatient hospital services).

Protected Health Information (PHI) A term defined by HIPAA with personal identifiers that can link health information to an individual.

Protozoa Single-celled, eukaryotic microorganisms where cells have both a nucleus and organelles. Eukaryotes are cells with a nucleus and other membrane-bound organelles enclosed within a nuclear envelope.

Psychomotor domain The domain of learning that includes motor activity and the cognition and affect to complete that motor activity.

Punishment An aversive stimulus that causes a behavior to decrease in frequency.

Quality of life (QOL) A person's overall well-being, including "perceptions of their position in life in the context of the culture and value system where they live and in relation to their goals, expectations, standards, and concerns." (WHO)

Racism The assessment of individual worth on the basis of real or imputed group characteristics, most notably skin color.

Range of motion (ROM) Arc of motion through which a joint moves.

Rapid eye movement (REM) sleep The stage of sleep characterized by a period of intense brain activity often associated with dreams; named for the rapid eye movements that occur during this time. It is also called paradoxical or dreaming sleep.

Reading level Grade level at which one reads; academic level and reading level are often not equivalent.

Reasonable accommodation Component of the US ADA law requiring employers to offer any change or adjustment to a job or work environment that permits a qualified applicant or employee with a disability to participate in the job application process, to perform the essential functions of a job, or to enjoy benefits and privileges of employment equal to those enjoyed by employees without disabilities.

Reasonable and necessary Terms used by payers to determine if services should be covered; based on payer criteria about the likelihood of client change and importance of that change.

Recovery (in mental health) A process experienced by people with mental illness whereby they come to a life that is defined less by illness and pathology and more by a personal sense of purpose, agency, and control and active participation in valued and meaningful activities; a process of change through which individuals improve their health and wellness, live a self-directed life, and strive to reach their full potential.

Reevaluation A systematic evaluation conducted to determine change from initial evaluation; typically performed to determine need for changes in course of intervention.

Reflection Mindfulness and other forms of self-assessment that can be used to improve practice. Developing reflective capacity is a critical element in professional development and competence.

Reflective portfolio A dynamic, flexible, self-directed tool designed to document continuing professional development through thoughtful engagement with artifacts created and accumulated in pursuit to achieve professional goals and desired roles.

Refugee A person who is recognized under the 1951 UN Convention relating to the Status of Refugees, its 1967 Protocol, the 1969 Organization of African Unity (OAU) Convention Governing the Specific Aspects of Refugee Problems in Africa as being "outside their country of origin for reasons of feared persecution, conflict, generalized violence, or other circumstances that have seriously disturbed public order and, as a result, require[in] international protection." (United Nations General Assembly)

Refugee camp A temporary settlement established to provide safe accommodation for persons displaced from their homes and communities. Basic services such as food and household essentials, water, shelter, primary healthcare, and, occasionally, educational opportunities are provided by the UNHCR and NGOs. In protracted refugee situations, people live in camps for years or decades.

Registration (sensory pattern) A sensory pattern characterized by high thresholds and a passive self-regulation approach; bystanders do not know what they are missing.

Rehabilitative approach A therapeutic approach aimed at making people as independent as possible in spite of any residual impairment; includes the concepts of adaptation, compensation, and environmental modifications. This approach places an emphasis on the client's strengths as opposed to their limitations. The ultimate goal is to maximize independence despite the presence of persistent impairments.

Reinforcement A stimulus that causes a behavior to be strengthened and performed again; can be positive or negative.

Relative mastery A person's phenomenological evaluation of the quality of their occupational response. This evaluation has four aspects: efficiency (use of time, energy, resources), effectiveness (the extent to which the desired goal was achieved), satisfaction to self, and satisfaction to society.

Relevance The degree to which a research study answers the clinical question and how well its methods fit within the constraints and resources of the practitioner's context of practice.

Reliability Consistency and repeatability of the outcome of administration of a test across time, parallel forms of the test, and raters. It also refers to the consistency of the internal structure of the test.

Religion A set of shared beliefs and attendant practices used to relate to the sacred.

REM sleep behavior disorder (RBD) A sleep disorder in which one appears to physically act out vivid, often unpleasant dreams with abnormal vocal sounds and movements during REM sleep.

Remediation An intervention approach designed to change client variables to establish a skill or ability that has not yet developed or to restore a skill or ability that has been impaired.

Remote patient monitoring The use of telehealth technologies to collect physiologic health data, either synchronously or asynchronously, within a medical model.

Requisite managerial authority The level of control and discretion that a manager must have to be fairly held responsible for the outcomes of work groups.

Resettlement A formal process overseen by the United Nations High Commissioner for Refugees for transferring refugees from the country where they first sought protection in (typically a country adjacent to their country of origin) to another country that has agreed to admit them and ultimately grant them permanent residence.

Response The reaction to the stimulus.

Rest Period of relaxing or ceasing to engage in strenuous or stressful activity.

Restless leg syndrome (RLS) A disorder in which there is an urge to move the legs to stop unpleasant sensations.

Rhythmic movement disorders in children Neurologic disorder characterized by involuntary (however, may sometimes be voluntary), repetitive movements of large muscle groups immediately before and during sleep.

Rituals Symbolic actions with spiritual, cultural, or social meaning. Rituals contribute to a client's identity and reinforce the client's values and beliefs. (OTPF-IV)

Role(s) A set of socially agreed-on behavioral expectations, rights, and responsibilities for a specific position or status in a group or in society. These may be further conceptualized and defined by individuals enacting the role(s).

Routines A type of higher order habit that involves sequencing and combining processes, procedures, steps, or occupations and provides a structure for daily life.

Sanism Discrimination against people who are thought to be mentally ill or "insane."

Schizophrenia One of several brain diseases whose symptoms may include loss of personality (flat affect), agitation, catatonia, confusion, psychosis, unusual behavior, and withdrawal. The illness usually begins in early adulthood.

Scholarship The development of new knowledge; research.

Scholarship of teaching and learning Studying the best methods for student learning.

Screening Obtaining and reviewing data that are relevant to a potential client to determine the need for further evaluation and intervention.

Secondary insomnia When insomnia is a result of another medical condition, a side effect of a drug, or another similar cause, it is called secondary insomnia.

Seeking (sensory pattern) A sensory pattern characterized by high thresholds and an active self-regulation approach; seekers want more input.

Self-awareness Includes lack of knowledge about one's own cognitive–perceptual limitations and/or functional limitations as well as deficiencies in metacognitive skills.

Self-regulation The individual's ability to alter behavior to match environmental demand; in relationship to sensory integration and processing, this involves intake, integration, and processing of sensation and using it as a foundation for appropriate environmental interaction.

Sensitivity (sensory pattern) A sensory pattern characterized by low thresholds and a passive self-regulation approach; sensors are particular about their input.

Sensitivity (statistics) The predictor test's ability to obtain a positive test when the condition really exists (a true positive).

Sensory integration Model for practice developed by Jean Ayres that incorporated sensory input, integration of sensory inputs, and behavioral outputs into a cohesive set of ideas.

Sensory processing The way a person makes meaning of the sensory input they experience.

Serious mental illness (SMI) A diagnosable mental disorder found in persons aged 18 years and older that is so long lasting and severe that it seriously interferes with a person's ability to take part in major life activities; includes diagnoses such as schizophrenia, bipolar disorder, and major depression when these illnesses have a significant impact on the person's ability to function.

Service (in academia) Contributions made by faculty to the university and society as a whole.

Setting Describes those aspects of the context or arena to which the person attends.

Shaping A strategy to develop closer and closer approximations of behavior.

Shared decision-making The process of information exchange that occurs between the practitioner and the service recipient to facilitate a collaborative agreement regarding the intervention plan.

Shift work A general term to describe a job that requires an individual to work other than the standard working hours of midmorning to late afternoon, Monday through Friday. For instance, shift work may involve working from midnight until 7:00 A.M.

Signature pedagogy The type of teaching that organizes the fundamental ways in which future practitioners are educated for their new professions.

Skilled nursing facility (SNF) In the United States, a hospital unit, nursing home, or distinct part of a nursing home that provides skilled nursing care, medical treatments, and rehabilitation services.

Skilled services In the United States, services that require the expertise of OT practitioners and are necessary to treat the patient properly and safely based on the complexity of the patient's condition.

Sleep debt An individual's accumulated sleep loss from insufficient sleep, regardless of cause.

Sleep diary Self-report system for tracking sleep time and restorative experience.

Sleep hygiene Habits, environmental factors, and practices that may influence the length and quality of one's sleep.

Sleep inertia Period after awakening before full alertness.

Sleep latency Period awake in bed before falling asleep.

Sleep-disordered breathing (SDB) Describes a group of disorders characterized by abnormalities of respiratory pattern (pauses in breathing) or the quantity of ventilation during sleep.

Sleep-wake homeostasis Regulated balance between sleep and waking.

Slow wave sleep (SWS) Often referred to as deep sleep, consists of stages 3 and 4 of NREM sleep.

Smart house (smart house technology) Dwelling design using computer technologies to incorporate robotics, networked appliances, and other digital devices connecting residents with their home and wider community; the house is "smart" in the sense that it can respond, through digital directives, to the residents' everyday needs in terms of lighting, thermal comfort, security, and so forth.

SOAP note Acronym for a type of progress note written in a standard format of Subjective, Objective, Assessment, and Plan so that specific information is easy to find.

Social capital The networks of relationships among people who live and work, enabling a society to function. This is an important precondition for forced migrants for occupational outlets that promote community participation and social integration.

Social class Ranking of people into a hierarchy within a culture, arising from interdependent economic relationships such as "middle class," "upper class," or "lower class"; the more neutral term *social position* is now preferred.

Social cognitive theory Theory that explains learning as occurring in a social context.

Social determinants of health (SDOH) Five broad categories—economic stability, education access and quality, healthcare access and quality, neighborhood and built environment, and social and community context—that are the fundamental social causes of health. The conditions in the places where people grow, live, work, age, learn, and play affect a wide range of health and quality-of-life outcomes. They are the non-medical factors that impact health.

Social inequality Refers to uneven access to and distribution of resources across domains such as education, employment, and health that, in turn, leads to disparities across gender, race, and ethnicity.

Social interaction skills Small, observable actions related to communicating and interacting with others in the context of engaging in a task that involves social interaction with others.

Social media The use of online and electronic tools to create, share, and exchange content and ideas in communities and networks.

Social participation Involvement in a subset of activities that involve social interactions with others and that support social interdependence; organized patterns of behavior that are characteristic and expected of an individual or a given position within a social system and encompasses the individual's engagement with family, peers and friends, and community members.

Social position Indicates social differences between groups.

Socioeconomic status (SES) Status- or prestige-based measure of place in the social hierarchy; measurement of SES includes occupational attainment, education, and income.

Spatial neglect A condition in which, after damage to one hemisphere of the brain (usually right) is sustained, a deficit in attention to and awareness of the opposite side (usually left) of space is observed.

Special education Educational services in the United States that are designed to help a child with a disability learn in a way that is consistent with that child's unique needs.

Specificity The predictor test's ability to obtain a negative result when the condition is really absent (a true negative).

Spirituality A deep experience of meaning brought about by engaging in occupations that involve the enacting of personal values and beliefs, reflection, and intention within a supportive contextual environment.

Standard precautions Previously known as Universal Precautions. Refers to basic infection prevention practices across all healthcare settings, regardless of suspected or confirmed infection status. Standard precautions are considered the primary method of reducing healthcare-associated infections.

Standardized assessments Measurement instrument that has been developed in a rigorous, scientific manner for a defined construct and population with a prescribed process of administration and scoring and with demonstrated psychometric properties.

Stereotyping Attributing certain characteristics to an entire group of people; these can be thoughts about people related to age, race, gender, sexuality, occupation, ethnicity, and physical and mental abilities.

Stimulus Verbal, sensory, or environmental input that prompts a behavior.

Strategic planning The process of ensuring that an organization's current purpose, aspirations, goals, activities, and strategies connect to plans and support its mission.

Substrates of occupation In occupational science, the physical and cognitive attributes of human anatomy, physiology, and consciousness that underpin our capacity to engage in occupation.

Successful aging Moving through late life in a way that enables participation in valued activities and sustains life satisfaction.

Summative process Evaluation or feedback desired to summarize current skills or related current skills to set criteria.

Sundowning Increased confusion or disorientation that occurs at the end of the day; typically seen in people with Alzheimer disease or other dementias.

Supervision The process of overseeing or guiding individuals or an organization through the authoritative control of others authorized by the governing body of the organization.

Supported education An emerging best practice to help individuals with major mental disorders succeed in higher education. Participants receive the education and training they need to achieve their learning and recovery goals and become gainfully employed in the job or career of their choice.

Supported employment Integrated employment, including customized employment or employment in an integrated work setting, in which individuals with significant disabilities receive the supports they need to be successful in a competitive employment position.

Suprachiasmatic nucleus (SCN) Also referred to as circadian clock, circadian pacemaker, or internal biologic clock. The internal circadian pacemaker is a small group of nerve cells located in the hypothalamus that controls the circadian cycles and influences many physiologic and behavioral rhythms occurring over a 24-hour period, including the sleep/wake cycle.

Synchronous telehealth Telehealth that occurs in real time with the practitioner and client engaged in interactive, simultaneous communication.

Systematic review A literature review pertinent to a specific question that aims at identifying, appraising, and synthesizing all the research evidence relevant to that question.

Tacit Implicit or based on information or experiences that we cannot easily put into language.

Task analysis Analysis based on observation of a person performing a task, an evaluation strategy focused on identifying underlying impairments of body functions and/or environmental factors that are speculated to be the reasons for a person's challenges with occupational performance.

Task-oriented approaches A person centered approach that uses functional tasks with everyday objects in familiar environments to improve motor function.

Task-specific strategies Tasks that are taught within targeted tasks and environments and combined with errorless learning and adaptive methods.

Task-specific training Rote repetition of specific tasks or routines within natural contexts to develop habits or functional behavioral routines.

Teach-back technique Having clients return demonstration, repeat in their own words, or explain a concept using a different example to help clients understand the information.

Telehealth The use of technology to deliver OT services when the practitioner and client are in different physical locations at the time of service delivery.

Telehealth hardware Physical devices such as computers (desktop/laptop), electronic tablets, telephones/smartphones, wearables (e.g., smart watches/sensors), and peripheral devices (e.g., headsets, external microphones, document cameras).

Telehealth software Operating information for hardware that enables telehealth; software provides access to client/patient portals, videoconferencing platforms, and applications (apps).

Telesupervision Clinical supervision provided with communication technology and includes the use of videoconferencing, telephone, e-mails, chats, podcasts, or the use of social networks.

Therapeutic mode Six specific ways of relating to a client: advocating, collaborating, empathizing, encouraging, instructing, problem solving.

Therapeutic relationship The alliance created by the OT practitioner and the service user.

Therapeutic use of self Planned use of practitioner's personality, insights, perceptions, and judgments as part of the therapeutic process.

Third-party payer Private company or government agency that provides payment for medical expenses.

Transactional perspective of occupations Offered as an alternative to individualism that presumes the person is separate from life situations; a transactional way of thinking sees interrelated elements where occupations form relationships between the person and life situations. This idea is compatible with contextualism.

Transdisciplinary team Individuals representing different professional disciplines whose role-related functions become interchangeable.

Transitional work Process performed at the client's actual job location and uses the client's job duties to assist in a safe gradual return to work process.

Translational science Theory-driven research focused on developing practical applications that resolve peoples' real-world needs; the process of turning knowledge from basic science into useful applications.

Transmission-based precautions Precautions put in place when standard precautions are inadequate to prevent the transmission of certain infectious diseases. Includes contact, droplet, airborne, and enhanced barrier precautions.

Transtheoretical Model (TTM) Theory of intentional change that was built on multiple theories of psychotherapy to identify an individual's readiness to change and uses stages of change and processes to facilitate one's progress toward goals.

Trauma-informed care A model of practice that encourages practitioners to consider the high likelihood that a significant number of their clients have experienced a traumatic event and would benefit from an approach that aims to decrease the possibility of retraumatization.

Traumatic brain injury (TBI) A complex condition characterized by varying degrees of cognitive, physical, psychological, behavioral, and emotional impairment.

Trustworthiness (in evidence-based practice) The degree to which a research study's conclusions are defensible with respect to the study methods.

Unidimensionality The determination of whether an assessment measures a single trait.

United Nations High Commissioner for Refugees (UNHCR) The United Nations agency in charge of aiding and protecting displaced and stateless people.

Universal design (UD) Design of environments and products to be usable by all people to the greatest extent possible without the need for special arrangements or adaptations; intended to simplify life for everyone by making products, communications, and the built environment more usable by as many people as possible at little or no extra cost.

Universal housing Dwellings, housing, and neighborhoods that address the needs of all users, whatever their age or ability.

Universal performance skills Skills categorized as motor skills, process skills, and social interaction skills, which are considered universal because they can be observed in virtually any daily life task performance and, in the case of social interaction skills, virtually any daily life task performance involving social interaction.

Unskilled services In the United States, services that can be provided by aide or caregiver and do not require the expertise of an OT practitioner.

Validity The degree to which a measurement tool measures what it is supposed to measure (accuracy).

Value-based care As a component of a larger strategy to reform healthcare delivery and payment, the Centers for Medicare & Medicaid in the United States rewards providers for quality versus quantity of care, adherence to best practices, and the patient's experience of care.

Values Acquired beliefs and commitments, derived from culture, about what is good, right, and important to do. (OTPF-IV)

Vector Organism that carries and transmits disease and infectious agents.

Veracity Telling the truth.

Vision statement (in management) An aspirational statement about what a department or organization would like to become as it seeks to fulfill its mission.

Visual perceptual (perception) Cognitive process of obtaining and interpreting visual information from the environment; involves the reception, organization, and assimilation of visual information.

Volition The process by which people are motivated toward and choose occupations.

Wake after sleep onset (WASO) The time spent awake from sleep onset to final awakening.

Well-being "An individual or group must be able to identify and to realize aspirations, to satisfy needs, and to change or cope with the environment." (WHO)

Wellness A conscious, deliberate process that requires a person to become aware of and make choices for a more satisfying lifestyle. The individual's perception of and responsibility for psychological and physical well-being as these contribute to overall satisfaction with one's life situation. It is also the outcome of health promotion.

Work Labor or exertion related to the development, production, delivery, or management of objects or services; benefits may be financial or nonfinancial (e.g., social connectedness, contributions to society, adding structure and routine to daily life). (OTPF-IV)

Work conditioning Intervention that emphasizes physical conditioning and addresses issues of strength, endurance, flexibility, motor control, and cardiopulmonary function to restore the performance of a worker recovering from an injury or illness.

Work hardening A multidisciplinary, highly structured, goal-oriented, individualized treatment program designed to maximize the individual's ability to return to work.

Working memory Involves holding information in mind and mentally working with it (i.e., working with information no longer perceptually present).

Working poor People who maintain full-time jobs but remain in relative poverty according to government-established poverty standards; may have negative net worth and lack the ability to escape their situations.

Workplace accommodations Accommodations made to a workplace to address physical, social, and attitudinal factors to enable individuals with occupational performance challenges to enter or return to work and successfully perform their jobs. Also called *job accommodations*.

INDEX

Page numbers followed by f denote figures, those followed by t denote tables, and those followed by b denote boxes.

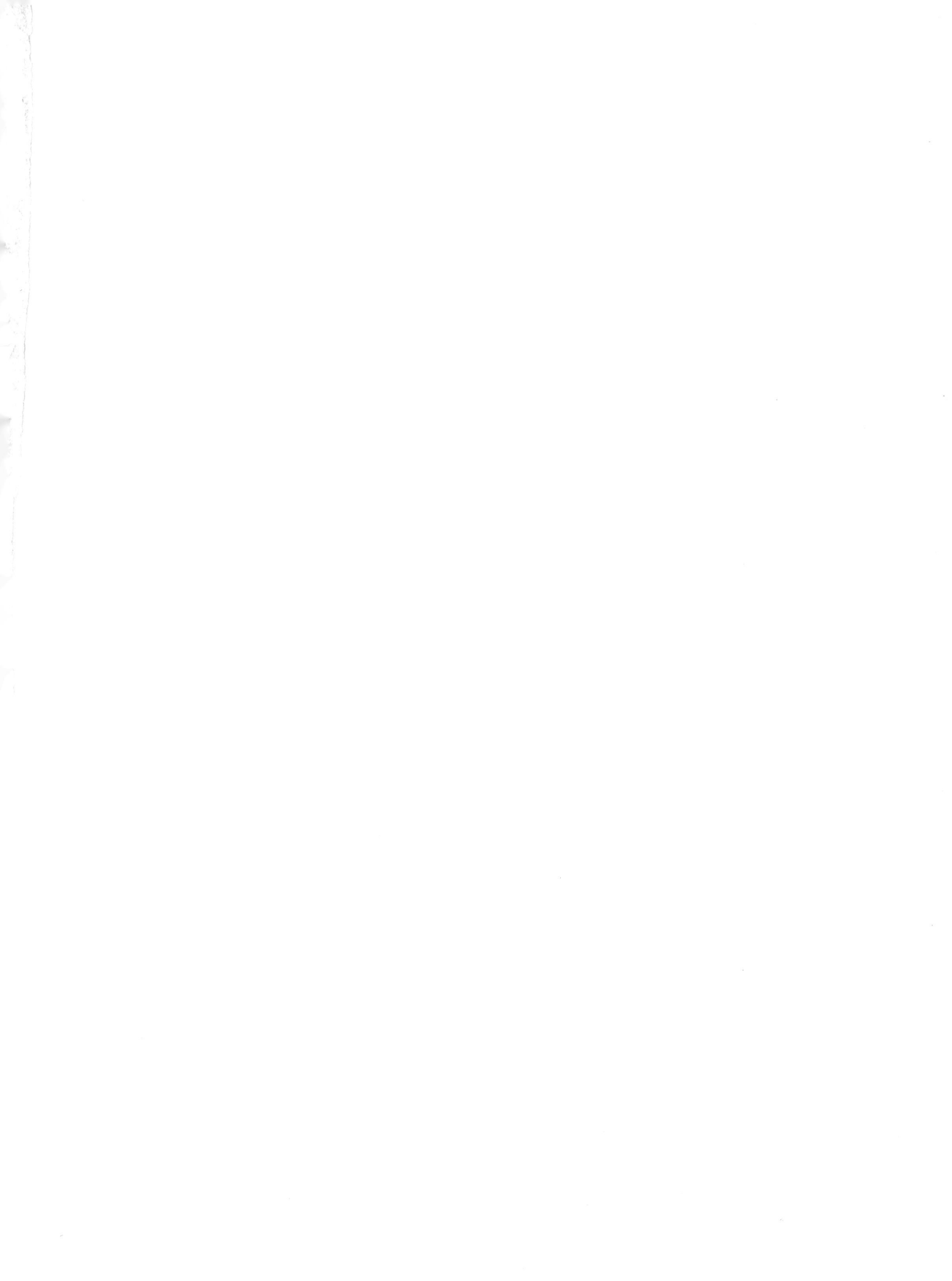